VOLUME TWO

GRADWOHL'S
CLINICAL LABORATORY
METHODS AND
DIAGNOSIS

ALEX C. SONNENWIRTH, Ph.D.

Professor of Microbiology and Immunology, and Pathology, Washington University School of Medicine; Director, Division of Microbiology, Department of Pathology and Laboratory Medicine, The Jewish Hospital of St. Louis, St. Louis, Missouri· Fellow, American Academy of Microbiology; Fellow, American Association for the Advancement of Science; Fellow, American Public Health Association; Fellow, New York Academy of Sciences; Member: Academy of Clinical Laboratory Physicians and Scientists, American Society for Microbiology, American Venereal Disease Association, Association of Clinical Scientists, Association for Practitioners in Infection Control, Conference of Public Health Laboratory Directors, Infectious Diseases Society of America, Society for Applied Bacteriology (Great Britain), Society for General Microbiology (Great Britain); Associate, American Society of Clinical Pathologists; Affiliate, Royal Society of Medicine (Great Britain)

LEONARD JARETT, M.D.

Professor of Pathology and Medicine and Head, Division of Laboratory Medicine, Washington University School of Medicine; Director of Laboratories, Barnes Hospital, St. Louis, Missouri; Fellow, College of American Pathologists; Fellow, American Society for Clinical Pathologists; Member: American Society for Clinical Investigation, Academy of Clinical Laboratory Physicians and Scientists, American Association of Pathology, Endocrine Society, American Society of Biological Chemists, American Diabetes Association, American Association of Cell Biologists, American Association of Clinical Chemists

VOLUME TWO

GRADWOHL'S CLINICAL LABORATORY METHODS AND DIAGNOSIS

EDITED BY

ALEX C. SONNENWIRTH, Ph.D.

Professor of Microbiology and Immunology, and Pathology,
Washington University School of Medicine; Director, Division of Microbiology,
Department of Pathology and Laboratory Medicine, The Jewish Hospital of St. Louis,
St. Louis, Missouri

LEONARD JARETT, M.D.

Professor of Pathology and Medicine and Head, Division of
Laboratory Medicine, Washington University School of Medicine;
Director of Laboratories, Barnes Hospital,
St. Louis, Missouri

EIGHTH EDITION
with 748 illustrations, including 50 in color

The C. V. Mosby Company

ST. LOUIS • TORONTO • LONDON   1980

The C. V. Mosby Company
11830 Westline Industrial Drive, St. Louis, Missouri 63141

Library of Congress Cataloging in Publication Data

Gradwohl, Rutherford Birchard Hayes, 1877-1959.
  Gradwohl's Clinical laboratory methods and diagnosis.

  Includes bibliographical references and index.
  1. Diagnosis, Laboratory.   I.   Sonnenwirth,
Alex C., 1923-   II.   Jarett, Leonard.
III.   Title.   IV.   Title: Clinical laboratory methods
and diagnosis.
[DNLM: 1. Diagnosis, Laboratory. QY4.3 G733c]
RB37.G675   1980   616.07′5   79-26398
ISBN 0-8016-4741-X

TS/CB/B   9 8 7 6 5 4 3 2 1   01/C/030

CONTRIBUTORS

Philip O. Alderson, M.D.
RADIONUCLIDES

Associate Director of Division of Nuclear Medicine and Associate Professor of Radiology and Environmental Health Sciences, Johns Hopkins Medical Institutions, Baltimore, Maryland

David N. Bailey, M.D.
TOXICOLOGY

Assistant Professor of Pathology and Director, Toxicology Laboratory, University of California Medical Center, San Diego, California

John D. Bauer, M.D.
HEMATOLOGY

Assistant Professor of Pathology, Washington University School of Medicine; Chairman, Department of Pathology, DePaul Community Health Center; Director of Laboratories, Faith Hospital, St. Louis, Missouri

Dov L. Boros, Ph.D.
PHAGOCYTOSIS

Associate Professor of Immunology, Department of Immunology and Microbiology, Wayne State University School of Medicine, Detroit, Michigan

C. Lynne Burek, Ph.D.
DETECTION OF AUTOANTIBODIES

Department of Immunology and Microbiology, Wayne State University School of Medicine, Detroit, Michigan

Jan Cejka, Ph.D.
IMMUNOGLOBULINS

Department of Immunochemistry, Children's Hospital of Michigan; Associate Professor, Department of Pediatrics, Wayne State University School of Medicine, Detroit, Michigan

Flossie Cohen, M.D.
CELL-MEDIATED IMMUNOLOGIC RESPONSES

Professor of Pediatrics, Wayne State University School of Medicine; Director of Clinical Immunology, Children's Hospital of Michigan, Detroit, Michigan

Thomas P. Conway, Ph.D.
IMMUNOGLOBULINS

Division of Immunology, Department of Clinical Pathology, William Beaumont Hospital, Royal Oak, Michigan; Department of Immunology and Microbiology, Wayne State University School of Medicine, Detroit, Michigan

Cecilia A. Cronin, M.T.(A.S.C.P.), S.B.B.
COMPATIBILITY TESTING, ANTIBODY DETECTION

Missouri/Illinois Regional Red Cross, St. Louis, Missouri

Hugo L. David, M.D., Ph.D.
MYCOBACTERIA

Chef de Laboratoire, Service de la Tuberculose et des Mycobacteries, Institut Pasteur, Paris, France

Gustave L. Davis, M.D.
MICROSCOPY

Associate Professor of Pathology, Washington University School of Medicine; Department of Pathology and Laboratory Medicine, The Jewish Hospital of St. Louis, St. Louis, Missouri

James E. Davis, Ph.D.
SAFETY, INSTRUMENTATION, SOLUTIONS, AND BUFFERS, ENZYMOLOGY

Assistant Professor of Pathology and Medicine, Washington University School of Medicine; Assistant Director, Clinical Chemistry Laboratory, Barnes Hospital, St. Louis, Missouri

David N. Dietzler, Ph.D.
CARBOHYDRATES, AMINO ACIDS

Associate Professor of Pathology and of Clinical Chemistry in Medicine, Washington University School of Medicine; Associate Director, Clinical Chemistry, Barnes Hospital, St. Louis, Missouri

William R. Dito, M.D.
AMNIOTIC FLUID AND MATERNAL SERUM

Associate Adjunct Professor of Pathology, University of California, San Diego; Head, Laboratory Medicine, Department of Pathology, Green Hospital of Scripps Clinic, Scripps Clinic and Research Foundation, La Jolla, California

Irene Dorner, B.A.M.T.(A.S.C.P.), S.B.B.
ABO BLOOD GROUPS, RH SYSTEM, HEMOLYTIC
DISEASE OF NEWBORN

Clinical Instructor, Department of Medical Technology, School of Nursing and Allied Health Professions, St. Louis University; Instructor, Gradwohl School of Laboratory Techniques; Chief Technologist, Barnes Hospital Blood Bank, St. Louis, Missouri

V. R. Dowell, Jr., Ph.D.
ANAEROBES (ch. 83-85)

Chief of Enterobacteriology Division, Bureau of Laboratories, Center for Disease Control, Atlanta, Georgia

Emanuel Epstein, Ph.D.
ADRENAL MEDULLA AND CORTEX, OVARY, TESTIS

Senior Clinical Chemist, Department of Clinical Pathology, William Beaumont Hospital, Royal Oak, Michigan

Carolyn S. Feldkamp, Ph.D.
ADRENAL MEDULLA AND CORTEX, OVARY, TESTIS

Director, Ligand Assay Laboratory, Department of Pathology, Henry Ford Hospital, Detroit, Michigan

Sydney M. Finegold, M.D.
GRAM-NEGATIVE ANAEROBIC RODS, *BACTEROIDACEAE*

Professor of Medicine, University of California at Los Angeles School of Medicine; Chief, Infectious Disease Section, Wadsworth Veterans Administration Medical Center, Los Angeles, California

Martin Fleisher, Ph.D.
BLOOD GAS ANALYSIS AND ACID-BASE BALANCE

Associate Attending Biochemist, Department of Biochemistry, Memorial Sloan-Kettering Cancer Center, New York, New York

Robert S. Galen, M.D., M.P.H.
STATISTICS

Assistant Professor of Pathology, Columbia University College of Physicians and Surgeons, New York, New York; Associate Director of Laboratories, Overlook Hospital, Summit, New Jersey

Henry Gewurz, M.D.
COMPLEMENT

Chairman and Thomas J. Coogan Professor, Department of Immunology, Rush Medical College, Chicago, Illinois

Millicent C. Goldschmidt, Ph.D.
INSTRUMENTATION, AUTOMATION, AND MINIATURIZATION

Dental Branch: Dental Science Institute, The University of Texas Health Science Center at Houston, Houston, Texas

Dieter H. M. Gröschel, M.D.
STERILIZATION, DISINFECTION, AND ANTISEPTICS

Professor of Pathology and Director of Microbiology, Department of Pathology, University of Virginia School of Medicine, Charlottesville, Virginia

Charles T. Hall, Ph.D.
QUALITY CONTROL IN MICROBIOLOGY LABORATORY
SAFETY IN MICROBIOLOGY LABORATORY

U.S. Department of Health, Education and Welfare, Public Health Service, Center for Disease Control, Bureau of Laboratories, Laboratory Training and Consultation Division, Venereal Disease Training Branch, Atlanta, Georgia

John E. Hammond, Ph.D.
MEASUREMENT OF PROTEINS

Assistant Professor of Pathology, Medicine, and Biochemistry, School of Medicine, University of North Carolina; Associate Director, Clinical Chemistry Laboratory, North Carolina Memorial Hospital, Chapel Hill, North Carolina

W. A. L. Heaton, M.D.
ERYTHROCYTE TRANSFUSION PRODUCTS

Assistant Professor of Pathology, Eastern Virginia School of Medicine; Director, Tidewater Regional Red Cross Blood Services, Norfolk, Virginia; Assistant Professor of Pathology, Eastern Carolina School of Medicine, Greenville, North Carolina

Michael H. Ivey, Ph.D.
MEDICAL PARASITOLOGY

Professor and Chairman, Department of Laboratory Practice, School of Health, University of Oklahoma; Professor of Preventive Medicine and Public Health, University of Oklahoma School of Medicine, Oklahoma City, Oklahoma

Laurence S. Jacobs, M.D.
COMPETITIVE BINDING ASSAY, RADIOIMMUNOASSAY
OF PEPTIDE HORMONES

Associate Professor of Medicine; Associate Chief, Endocrine-Metabolism Unit; Director, Clinical Research Center, School of Medicine and Dentistry, University of Rochester; Senior Associate Physician, Strong Memorial Hospital, Rochester, New York

Bernard M. Jaffe, M.D.
GASTROINTESTINAL HORMONES

Professor and Chairman, Department of Surgery, SUNY Downstate Medical Center, Brooklyn, New York

Leonard Jarett, M.D.
COMPUTERS IN LABORATORY MEDICINE

Professor of Pathology and Medicine and Head, Division of Laboratory Medicine, Washington University School of Medicine; Director of Laboratories, Barnes Hospital, St. Louis, Missouri

Peter I. Jatlow, M.D.
ANALYTICAL TOXICOLOGY

Professor of Laboratory Medicine, Yale University School of Medicine, New Haven, Connecticut

J. Heinrich Joist, M.D., Ph.D.
HEMOSTASIS AND THROMBOSIS, PLATELET
FUNCTION, COAGULATION

Associate Professor of Medicine and Pathology and Co-Director, Division of Hematology-Oncology, St. Louis University School of Medicine, St. Louis, Missouri

J. Mehsen Joseph, Ph.D.
VIRAL AND RICKETTSIAL DIAGNOSTIC PROCEDURES

Director, Laboratories Administration, and Chief, Division of Virology, Maryland State Department of Health; Assistant Professor of Microbiology, University of Maryland, Baltimore, Maryland

George E. Kenny, Ph.D.
MYCOPLASMA

Professor and Chairman, Department of Pathobiology SC-38, School of Public Health and Community Medicine, University of Washington, Seattle, Washington

Karel Kithier, M.D., Ph.D.
TUMOR-ASSOCIATED ANTIGENS

Associate Professor, Department of Pathology, Wayne State University School of Medicine, Detroit, Michigan

George S. Kobayashi, Ph.D.
MEDICAL MYCOLOGY

Professor, Departments of Medicine and Microbiology and Immunology, Washington University School of Medicine; Associate Director, Diagnostic Microbiology Laboratory, Barnes Hospital, St. Louis, Missouri

George P. Kubica, Ph.D.
MYCOBACTERIA

Microbiologist Consultant, Laboratory Training and Consultation Division, Bureau of Laboratories, Center for Disease Control, Atlanta, Georgia

Daniel J. Ladd, M.D.
HEPATITIS TESTING, QUALITY CONTROL IN BLOOD BANKING

Lecturer, Texas A & M University School of Medicine, College Station, Texas; Chief, Hematology and Blood Bank Laboratories, Scott and White Clinic, Temple, Texas

Jack H. Ladenson, Ph.D.
NONANALYTICAL SOURCES OF VARIATION, QUALITY CONTROL, MINERAL HOMEOSTASIS

Associate Professor of Pathology and Assistant Professor of Medicine, Washington University School of Medicine; Co-Director of Clinical Chemistry, Barnes Hospital, St. Louis, Missouri

Robert A. Levine, M.D.
DIGOXIN

Assistant Clinical Professor of Laboratory Medicine, Yale University School of Medicine, New Haven, Connecticut

John W. Lewis III, Ph.D.
INSTRUMENTATION, COMPUTERS

Assistant Professor of Pathology and Electrical Engineering, Washington University School of Medicine; Director of Laboratory Computing, Barnes Hospital, St. Louis, Missouri

John M. Matsen, M.D.
ANTIMICROBIAL SUSCEPTIBILITY TESTS

Professor of Pathology and Pediatrics, Director, Clinical Microbiology Laboratories, Associate Dean for Academic Affairs, University of Utah, College of Medicine, Salt Lake City, Utah

John C. Mauck, Ph.D.
CLINICAL ENZYMOLOGY

Kodak Research Laboratories, Bioscience Division, Rochester, New York

Michael D. D. McNeely, M.D., F.R.C.P.(C)
GASTROINTESTINAL, LIVER, AND RENAL FUNCTION

Island Medical Laboratories, Vancouver Island, British Columbia, Canada

William V. Miller, M.D.
BLOOD DONORS, TISSUE ANTIGENS AND ANTIBODIES, BLOOD TRANSFUSION

Director, American Red Cross Blood Services, Missouri/Illinois Region; Associate Professor of Pathology and Medicine (Visiting Staff), Washington University School of Medicine, St. Louis, Missouri

Erwin Neter, M.D.
BACTERIAL HEMAGGLUTINATION TESTS

Professor of Microbiology and Pediatrics, State University of New York at Buffalo; Consultant Bacteriologist, Roswell Park Memorial Institute, Buffalo, New York

Hipolito V. Niño, Ph.D.
VITAMINS AND TRACE ELEMENTS

Beckman Instruments, Diagnostic Operations, Fullerton, California

Margarita Palutke, M.D.
TRANSPLANTATION IMMUNOLOGY

Associate Professor of Pathology and Head of Hematopathology and Histocompatibility Section, Wayne State University School of Medicine; Associate Director, Clinical Laboratory, Wayne State University Health Care Institute, Detroit, Michigan

Demosthenes Pappagianis, Ph.D., M.D.
MEDICAL MYCOLOGY

Professor and Chairman, Department of Medical Microbiology, School of Medicine, University of California, Davis, California

Miroslav D. Poulik, M.D.
IMMUNOGLOBULINS

Chief, Division of Immunology, William Beaumont Hospital, Royal Oak, Michigan; Adjunct Professor of Immunology and Bacteriology, Wayne State University School of Medicine, Detroit, Michigan

Edward R. Powsner, M.D.
ADRENAL MEDULLA AND CORTEX, OVARY,
AND TESTIS

Director of Clinical Laboratories and Professor, Department of Pathology, Michigan State University, East Lansing, Michigan

Ananda S. Prasad, M.D., Ph.D.
VITAMINS AND TRACE ELEMENTS

Professor of Medicine and Director, Division of Hematology, Wayne State University School of Medicine; Chief of Hematology, Harper-Grace Hospitals, Detroit, Michigan; Veterans Administration Hospital, Allen Park, Michigan

Noel R. Rose, M.D., Ph.D.
IMMUNOLOGIC WORK-UP

Professor and Chairman, Department of Immunology and Microbiology, Wayne State University School of Medicine, Detroit, Michigan

John Savory, Ph.D.
MEASUREMENT OF PROTEINS

Professor of Pathology and Biochemistry and Director of Clinical Chemistry and Toxicology Laboratories, University of Virginia Medical Center, Charlottesville, Virginia

Gustav Schonfeld, M.D.
LIPIDS AND LIPOPROTEINS

Professor of Medicine and Preventive Medicine and Director, Lipid Research Center, Washington University School of Medicine; Assistant Physician, Barnes Hospital, St. Louis, Missouri

Morton K. Schwartz, Ph.D.
BLOOD GAS ANALYSIS

Chairman, Department of Biochemistry, and Vice-president for Laboratory Affairs, Memorial Sloan-Kettering Cancer Center, New York, New York

Laurence A. Sherman, M.D.
BLOOD BANKING, FIBRINOLYSIS, THROMBOSIS, HYPERCOAGULABILITY

Professor of Pathology and Medicine, Washington University School of Medicine; Director, Barnes Hospital Blood Bank, St. Louis, Missouri

Barry A. Siegel, M.D.
RADIONUCLIDES

Professor of Radiology and Director, Division of Nuclear Medicine, Edward Mallinckrodt Institute of Radiology, Washington University School of Medicine, St. Louis, Missouri

Carl Hugh Smith, M.D.
CARBOHYDRATES, AMINO ACIDS

Associate Professor of Pathology and Pediatrics, Washington University School of Medicine; Co-Director, Clinical Chemistry, St. Louis Children's Hospital, St. Louis, Missouri

Alex C. Sonnenwirth, Ph.D.
BACTERIOLOGY, SEROLOGY (ch. 68, 70-72, 75-77, 79, 80, 82-85, 105-107)

Professor of Microbiology and Immunology, and Pathology, Washington University School of Medicine; Director, Division of Microbiology, Department of Pathology and Laboratory Medicine, The Jewish Hospital of St. Louis, St. Louis, Missouri

Lisbeth A. Suyehira, M.T.(A.S.C.P.)
COMPLEMENT

Supervisor, Clinical Immunology, Rush Presbyterian-St. Luke's Medical Center, Chicago, Illinois

Stuart W. Weidman, Ph.D.
LIPIDS AND LIPOPROTEINS

Assistant Professor of Preventive Medicine and Biological Chemistry and Director, Core Laboratory, Lipid Research Center, Washington University School of Medicine, St. Louis, Missouri

Alice Schauer Weissfeld, Ph.D.
NOSOCOMIAL INFECTIONS AND HOSPITAL EPIDEMIOLOGY

Associate in Microbiology, Department of Pathology and Laboratory Medicine, The Jewish Hospital of St. Louis; Instructor, Department of Pathology, Washington University School of Medicine, St. Louis, Missouri

Bennie Zak, Ph.D.
ADRENAL MEDULLA AND CORTEX, OVARY, AND TESTIS

Professor, Department of Pathology, Wayne State University School of Medicine, Detroit, Michigan

TO

**Rosaline Sonnenwirth, Betty Sonnenwirth Ozar and
Stuart Ozar, Maurice Sonnenwirth**

Arlene, Stacy, Douglas, and Jenifer Jarett

who have provided us with the beauty of life

and to

Paul E. Lacy

who has been more than a mentor—a friend

PREFACE

Because of major changes that have occurred in the field of laboratory medicine during the last decade, *Gradwohl's Clinical Laboratory Methods and Diagnosis* has undergone major revisions in its eighth edition. The use of the laboratory grew at an annual rate of 15% during much of this time period, although the rate of increase has slowed during the past 2 years. The complexity of the laboratory in both technology and the biologic processes involved has grown in a logarithmic fashion. This is because newer knowledge of disease is at a molecular level and will most likely be applied to a patient through laboratory procedures. The variety of instrumentation utilized spans the entire range used in the biologic and physical sciences, as well as the latest technology of automation, including computerization. This text still remains as a reference source, laboratory manual, and textbook. However, more detail to each area has been included and the medical overtones emphasized, as well as the potential sources of errors. Older material and procedures have been eliminated or mentioned for historical purposes only. The histology sections have been completely eliminated since they are more appropriate to a surgical pathology text. Electrocardiography was omitted because it is not part of laboratory medicine. General concepts have been stressed and not technics specific to each instrument. It was felt that the instrument manufacturers would' provide the unique methodology for their equipment; thus only manual or generally applicable methods are detailed. The International System of Units (SI, Systeme International) has been used where appropriate throughout the text. Throughout the book authors were chosen on the basis of their expertise in the area about which they have written. Thus no common approach is taken to all chapters, but individual authoritative approaches.

PART I, **GENERAL CONSIDERATIONS,** was designed to cover general principles applicable to many individual sections of the book. Although the safety chapter (Chapter 1) by James E. Davis was written for clinical chemistry, it is applicable to every section of the laboratory (except the clinical microbiology laboratory, which is discussed separately in Chapter 69). This safety aspect of the laboratory cannot be overemphasized in the present age. Gustave L. Davis provides an easily understandable chapter on the use of the light and electron microscopes. James E. Davis and John W. Lewis III have written a detailed chapter on the principles of instrumentation that covers such items as electronics as well as chromatography. Galen has taken a novel approach to statistics by emphasizing the definition of the normal range and the calculation of the predictive value of a laboratory test procedure. The use of competitive binding assays (Jacobs) and radionuclides (Siegel and Alderson) in all areas of the laboratory makes Chapters 5 and 6 essential and informative to all laboratorians. Lewis and Jarett have provided a needed chapter on the role of the computer system in the laboratory, computer terminology, selection of a computer system, and the cost justification of a laboratory computer system. Finally, this part contains a chapter on the fundamental chemistry of preparing solutions and buffers (J. E. Davis).

PART II, **CLINICAL CHEMISTRY,** is all new and markedly expanded. Ladenson has written a classic chapter on the nonanalytical sources of variation in clinical chemistry results. This subject has never been covered in this detail and is essential knowledge for the student, the technologist, the Ph.D., and the physician. This is followed by a chapter detailing the quality control efforts that must be followed to assure quality data. Individual chapters have been devoted to carbohydrates, amino acids (Dietzler and Smith), proteins (Savory and Hammond), and lipids and lipoproteins (Weidman and Schonfeld). Enzymology is treated separately (Mauck and J. E. Davis), and only the well-established "tried and true" methods needed for the practice of modern medicine are discussed. The recognition of the importance of mineral homeostasis (Ladenson) and blood gases and acid-base balance (Fleisher and Schwartz) in disease led to treatment of these subjects in special chapters. The same is true for the emerging field of analysis of vitamins and trace elements (Niño and Prasad). Jatlow and Bailey have detailed toxicologic examinations and covered the more important areas of therapeutic drug monitoring. All areas of hormone analysis have been detailed as well as their pathophysiologic implications (Jacobs). Approaches are described for analysis of amniotic fluid and maternal serum (Dito), which should be standard for assessment of pregnancies at risk. McNeely has provided a beautifully combined medical-technical approach to analysis of the urine and liver and kidney and gastrointestinal function testing. The importance of adrenal function testing and the depth of complexity of steroid hormone metabolism has necessitated individual chapters to be dedicated to the ovary, testis, adrenal medulla, and adrenal cortex. This new addition has been ably handled by Powsner, Epstein, Feldkamp, and Zak. Jaffe, an expert in gastrointestinal hormones, has provided a comprehensive discussion of this new and growing area of medical interest. The reader of this entire part should understand the medical applications and interpretations of clinical chemistry as well as the technics to perform the test.

PART III, **HEMATOLOGY,** by Bauer, was completely revised in the previous edition. It has now been updated and expanded. Heavy emphasis has been placed on quality control and collection and handling of specimens. This is particularly necessary with the advent of automated instruments for cell counts and differentials. Such instruments are discussed and the pros and cons of each reviewed. The coverage of the pathology of the cellular elements of the blood has been expanded by inclusion of the latest scanning and electron microscopic studies, which, coupled with biochemical effects, help explain the individual cellular abnormalities. Not only are the genetics of the hemoglobinopathies discussed, but the role of the fast hemoglobins, particularly A_{1c}, in the monitoring of therapy of diabetes mellitus is examined and the biochemistry of the formation of the glycosylated hemoglobins detailed. The classic and newer staining technics are detailed along with the necessary visual aids. This part of the text is readable by the student or the expert, which indicates the efforts by the author.

A separation of this part, PART IV, **HEMOSTASIS AND THROMBOSIS,** from Hematology has been necessitated by the marked increase in our knowledge of these processes. Joist and Sherman were chosen to write this critical part because of their clinical and laboratory expertise, including their research accomplishments, in this area. Joist has written a simple description of the hemostasis process and the formation of the thrombus. This is followed by a chapter that details the morphologic, numerical, sizing, and biochemical evaluation of platelets and their functional states. Chapter 42, on blood coagulation, details the current knowledge of each coagulation factor and the tests measuring their presence, quantity, and activity. As throughout the book, emphasis has been placed on quality con-

trol and proper collection and handling of the specimens as well as on the other conditions that alter test results. Sherman continues this exciting part by taking the same approach to the testing of fibrinolysis. Knowledge of this area is essential for all laboratory personnel from the student to the laboratory director. This laboratory information then has been integrated into a clinically oriented chapter on the laboratory approach to the bleeding patient. Finally, a chapter is presented that explores the pathophysiology and testing for the hypercoagulable state and thrombosis formation. In all these chapters not only are the procedures for the classic tests described but also the new procedures for the clotting factors and inhibitors.

PART V, **IMMUNOHEMATOLOGY AND TISSUE TYPING,** has been completely rewritten and expanded. No other area of the laboratory has experienced such increasing complexity with potentially fatal or serious consequences. This has come about for a variety of reasons, including governmental regulations, component therapy, tissue typing, phoresis, antibody problems, and hepatitis. The organizers of this part, Sherman and Miller, were chosen not only for their expertise in the field but because they are responsible for a major teaching hospital blood bank and a regional Red Cross blood center, respectively. They have called on Cronin, Dorner, Heaton, and Ladd for assistance in specialized areas. Their insight into the problems has helped bring a state of the art approach to this part, but with a medical basis. All the classic sections are covered, but with the latest immunologic data and technical approaches. Chapter 55, Tissue Antigens and Antibodies, focuses on the use of tissue typing in specific platelet and white cell therapy. The biochemical data relating to blood group substances are detailed, including the rarer antigens. Blood collection and storage are discussed, and emphasis is placed on the quality control standards that must be carried out in a modern blood bank. All aspects of hepatitis biochemistry and testing are discussed.

PART VI, **IMMUNOLOGY,** represents a completely new addition to this edition and was mandated by the great strides made in understanding the body's immune mechanism, discerning those disorders that result from an abnormal or inadequate immune mechanism, and, in general, broadening of the concept of the immunologic response from its role in protection against infection to a cause of several immunologic diseases (i.e., allergic, immune complex, or autoimmune diseases, or those due to malignant change or failure). In Chapter 60, Immunologic Work-up, Rose discusses the major cell types that comprise the immunologic organ (e.g., B- and T-lymphocytes, macrophages, polymorphonuclear leukocytes) and the role of various antibodies and of complement and outlines the general immunologic examination. Cejka, Conway, and Poulik provide a detailed and highly useful chapter, Assessment of Immunoglobulins, that includes technics for radial immunodiffusion, nephelometry, immunoelectrophoretic methods, quantitation of IgE, and estimation of catabolism of proteins. Chapter 62, Complement (Suyehira and Gewurz), provides detailed assays of the complement system and function and discussions of complement as a diagnostic aid, including details of an autoimmune disease laboratory profile.

Cohen has written a detailed chapter, Cell-mediated Immunologic Responses, that includes in vivo skin tests, quantitation of T- and B-lymphocytes, lymphocyte transformation, lymphokine production, and assays of cytotoxicity. In Phagocytosis, Boros discusses in detail the events of the process, disorders in its functions, and various technics for measurement of chemotaxis, degranulation, neutrophil activities, and the nitro-blue tetrazolium test. Burek and Rose provide a most useful chapter, Detection of Autoantibodies, that includes tests for antinuclear, DNA, Sm, and ENA antibodies, rheumatoid factor, and various organ-specific antibodies. In Transplantation Immunology, Palutke focuses in great detail on the HLA system, including the biochemistry and molecular biology of HLA antigens, and the clinical applications and laboratory technics of histocompatibility testing (tissue transplantation, disease association studies, population genetics, and paternity testing), while Kithier, in Tumor-associated Antigens, details procedures for α-fetoprotein, carcinoembryogenic antigen, and paraproteins. This entire part should be highly useful for the laboratory worker, the student, or the expert.

PART VII, **BACTERIOLOGY,** has been completely restructured and revised to allow for a comprehensive treatment of the subject, removal of outdated material, and addition of new, useful, and needed procedures and information. Considerable effort was expended throughout the discussion to update and revise the nomenclature and classification of bacteria to conform, as far as possible, to the decisions of the International Committee on Systematic Bacteriology (International Association of Microbiological Societies) promulgated in the last decade, the changes effected in the eighth edition of *Bergey's Manual of Determinative Bacteriology* (1974), and the changes in nomenclature and taxonomy of Enterobacteriaceae put in effect by the U.S. Center for Disease Control Enteric Section in October 1977. Additions to the text include many new methods and procedures (each accompanied by critical evaluation, description of rationale, and interpretation) and numerous new tables to allow rapid scanning of essential characteristics and reactions useful in identification, as well as several new chapters.

The chapter General Considerations (Sonnenwirth) now includes the classification of bacteria according to the eighth edition of *Bergey's Manual* (1974), characteristics of bacteria, an updated discussion of wall-defective microbial variants, the scope of clinical bacteriology, and a detailed section on the normal flora. Hall furnished the chapter Safety in the Clinical Microbiology Laboratory, by far the most comprehensive and up-to-date chapter in a textbook of this type; it includes laboratory design, preventive medical services, personnel training, and safety regulations. In Bacteriologic Methods (Sonnenwirth) the discussion on anaerobic culture equipment and system is new and greatly enlarged, as is immunofluorescence (IF), which now includes an exhaustive list on the status of IF tests and the direct fluorescent antibody (FA) test for *Legionella pneumophila.*

New or improved methods added in the chapters Stains and Staining Procedures and Media, Tests, and Reagents (Sonnenwirth) are, among others, the Kopeloff-Berman modification of Gram stain (for anaerobes), flagellar stains, modification of the Dieterle spirochete stain (for *Legionella pneumophila*), media for *Campylobacter, Legionella pneumophila, Vibrio cholerae, Vibrio parahaemolyticus,* rapid fermentation test for *Neisseria gonorrhoeae,* detailed descriptions of media and reagents for anaerobes as used by the Center for Disease Control (Dowell et al.) and by the Wadsworth group (Finegold et al.), counterimmunoelectrophoresis, and miniaturized identification systems.

Chapter 73, Quality Control in the Microbiology Laboratory, is new to this volume, and Hall furnishes considerable details on a subject that is now part of the statutes of the federal and state regulatory agencies and is of growing concern to the laboratory. Goldschmidt's very large chapter, Instrumentation, Automation, and Miniaturization, reflects the increasing role of instrumented and noninstrumented procedures applicable to the more rapid detection, identification, and susceptibility testing of microorganisms. This subject has not been covered in such detail in any text, and the chapter represents a veritable storehouse of up-to-date information and informed opinion. It covers mechanized equipment (e.g., blenders, automated plate streakers, replicators, colony counters, pipettors, staining machines), detectors of growth or inhibition (Autobac, AMS, MS-2), chromatographic procedures, liquid and gas liquid chromatography, electrophoresis, impedance, enzyme-ion-sensitive electrodes, bioluminescence, chemiluminescence, calorimetry, radiometry, immunologic technics, counterimmunoelectrophoresis, ELISA, RIA, coagglutination, miniaturized systems for identification and susceptibility testing, immunologic test kits, and computer usage. The chapter is backed by over 350 references; it is truly an essential source for the student, the technologist, the clinical microbiologist, and the physician.

In the completely rewritten voluminous chapter Collection and Culture of Specimens and

Guides for Bacterial Identification (Sonnenwirth), additions and changes include emphasis on prevention of specimen contamination by normal flora, importance of anaerobic collection and transport systems, regulations for shipping of specimens or cultures, tabulation of clinical specimens and media for primary culture, venting of blood culture bottles, investigation of septicemia associated with possible contamination of intravenous fluids, counterimmunoelectrophoresis and lactic acid determinations in meningitis, *Limulus* assay, Jones-Kendrick medium for diagnosis of pertussis, scoring and evaluation of quality of expectorated sputum before culture, isolation of *Legionella pneumophila,* paddle, dip-slide, and coated tube kits for urine culture, anaerobic cultures, detailed discussion of the bacteriology of the female and male genital tract, new information on media and procedures for *Neisseria gonorrhoeae, Corynebacterium* (Hemophilus) *vaginalis, Haemophilus ducreyi,* donovanosis, nongonococcal urethritis, fecal leukocytes and microscopic examination of stool, role and isolation of newer diarrheal agents, i.e., *Yersinia enterocolitica, Vibrio parahaemolyticus, Campylobacter fetus* ssp. *jejuni,* enteropathogenic versus enterotoxigenic or invasive *Escherichia coli,* and discussion of data flow (requisitions, presumptive and final reports, a "panic list," and emergency reports to physician). The "Guide to the Presumptive Recognition of Common Groups of Bacteria" included here has been completely revised, and it now incorporates a number of newly described (or renamed) genera and species. Following, in part, the work of the late Elizabeth King and the concepts of Cowan and Steel, the guide is based on a few key characteristics (such as cell morphology, staining characteristics, oxygen requirements, oxidase and catalase reactions, and nature of attack on carbohydrates, i.e., fermentative, oxidative, or neither) that allow preliminary and presumptive placement of an unknown isolate into a larger group (genus or family); it also indicates additional selected characteristics and reactions most likely to be useful for identification of the unknown. The guide has now been critically evaluated in the laboratory for over a decade and should prove practical and useful in aiding the laboratory worker to make a rational choice, after referring to the appropriate and indicated chapter, for proceeding with a choice of tests that will lead to the identification of the isolate within a reasonable span of time and without undue expenditure of a large number of often irrelevant media and tests.

The chapters Gram-positive and Gram-negative Cocci (Sonnenwirth) and Gram-positive Bacilli (Sonnenwirth) now contain new information on dwarf forms of *Staphylococcus aureus,* β-lactamase detection, group B hemolytic streptococci, detailed procedures for identification of "viridans" streptococci, CAMP test, antibiotic-resistant pneumococci, *Aerococcus, Branhamella,* rapid identification of *Neisseria gonorrhoeae* and *N. meningitidis,* newer *Corynebacterium* species, identification of lactobacilli, *Streptomyces, Rothia, Bacterionema, Nocardia caviae, Rhodochrous,* and identification of *Bacillus* species.

Kubica and David, both renowned experts in their field, contributed a totally rewritten chapter, The Mycobacteria, that represents the latest knowledge on and technics applicable to these organisms; the illustrations accompanying their text are superb and most helpful.

Chapter 79, Gram-negative Bacilli, Vibrios, and Spirilla (Sonnenwirth), is a book-size chapter that includes over 500 up-to-date references and is divided into sections on fermenters, nonfermenters, and miscellaneous fastidious or unclassified rods. New or greatly expanded material in this chapter includes Weaver's (CDC) keys for presumptive identification of aerobic gram-negative rods, the nomenclatural changes in *Bergey's Manual* (eighth edition), Ewing's system, and those effected by the Center for Disease Control in 1977; enterotoxic and invasive *E. coli,* in vitro tests for *E. coli* virulence properties, *Klebsiella oxytoca, Enterobacter agglomerans, E. sakazakii, E. gergoviae, Providencia rettgeri, Morganella morganii,* new biotypes of *Yersinia enterocolitica,* new technics for *Vibrio cholerae,* halophilic vibrios (*V. parahaemolyticus, V. alginolyticus, Vibrio* lac$^+$ species), *Chromobacterium,* and *Kingella.* For the nonfermenters, several identification schemas and technics are presented (CDC, Gilardi, and Pickett); the genus *Pseudomonas* is presented in detail including the fluorescein-producing group, the *pseudomallei* group with *P. cepacia,* and other nonfluorescent pseudomonads. Newly added are *Achromobacter xylosoxidans, Eikenella, Campylobacter, Agrobacterium,* and transformation assay for *Acinetobacter* and *Moraxella.* Among the fastidious rods, additions include *Brucella canis,* a new identification system for *Haemophilus* species with the porphyrin test, *Haemophilus vaginalis,* the DF-2 organism, and *Legionella pneumophila.*

Chapter 80, The Spirochetes (Sonnenwirth), now includes updated information on indigenous treponemes, the two major leptospiral complexes (*biflexa* and *interrogans*), and laboratory technics for their isolation and identification. Kenny furnished a new, succinct, and critical chapter on *Mycoplasma;* in addition to descriptions of *Mycoplasma* and *Ureaplasma* and the pathogenesis of mycoplasma infections, a variety of modern media and technics for isolation and identification are included.

A fundamental change in this edition concerns the creation of 5 new chapters for detailed treatment of the anaerobic bacteria: in the previous edition the anaerobes were segregated within the major chapters (e.g., Gram-positive Bacilli) that also included facultative anaerobes and (obligate) aerobes. The proliferation of information and the growth of technics in anaerobic bacteriology clearly required the separate treatment of anaerobes.

In Anaerobic Bacteria—An Introduction, Sonnenwirth and Dowell survey the evolution of anaerobic technics, specimen selection, collection and transport, various anaerobic culture systems, anaerobic antimicrobial susceptibility tests, anaerobic infections, give details of two major methodologies (Wadsworth group and CDC procedures), and list changes in the nomenclature of anaerobes. They also provide detailed, essential, and up-to-date information and directions in Chapter 83, Anaerobic Cocci, including the newly described genera *Acidaminococcus* and *Megasphaera.*

In Anaerobic Sporeforming Rods Sonnenwirth and Dowell furnish the most complete and up-to-date information on clostridia, with new additions on infant botulism, examination for *C. botulinum* and *C. perfringens* toxin(s), histotoxic infections, and *Clostridium difficile* and its role in pseudomembranous colitis (with description of selective media and isolation procedures). In Gram-positive, Anaerobic, Non-sporeforming Bacilli they describe the genera *Actinomyces, Arachnia, Propionibacterium, Bifidobacterium, Lactobacillus,* and *Eubacterium,* while Finegold, the renowned expert in anaerobic infections, discusses in Gram-negative Anaerobic Rods—Bacteroidaceae this highly important group of (mostly) indigenous organisms, with emphasis on the organisms occurring in humans and producing disease and their role in pathophysiologic states; the chapter includes newly characterized forms, and critical evaluations of all presently used technics for isolation and identification.

Chapter 87, Antimicrobial Susceptibility Testing: Laboratory Testing in Support of Antimicrobial Therapy, by Matsen, is a truly comprehensive, totally new contribution. It furnishes guidelines and details for organism-antimicrobial testing, quality assurance, disk diffusion, agar overlay, agar dilution, macrobroth and microbroth dilution, automated broth dilution, anaerobic susceptibilities, susceptibility tests for fastidious organisms, β-lactamase test methods, synergy testing, assays of antimicrobial agents, and serum bactericidal testing.

In the new chapter Nosocomial Infections and Hospital Epidemiology, Weissfeld details infection control procedures and furnishes modern, up-to-date guidelines and procedures for environmental testing, while Gröschel, in Sterilization, Disinfection, and Antisepsis, provides definitions and current technics for these highly important procedures, as well as some test methods to assay or control their effectiveness.

The gain in knowledge of the biochemical, biophysical, and biologic properties of viruses and the accompanying advances in the laboratory diagnosis of viral diseases are reflected in the extensive revision of PART VIII, **VIRAL AND RICKETTSIAL DIAGNOSTIC PROCEDURES,** by Joseph.

In the chapter Viruses: Classification and General Considerations, viruses are classified on the basis of their chemical composition and architecture of the virion, with the nomenclature employed completely revised. Discussion of non-A non-B hepatitis, EB virus, Norwalk agent, rhabdoviruses, and TORCH complex, among others, have been added, and the material on influenza, adenoviruses, and hepatitis viruses has been brought up to date.

Chapter 91, Tissue Culture and Chick Embryo Technics (Joseph), includes preparation and propagation of several tissue lines and technics for detection and eradication of mycoplasma contamination in tissue cell culture.

In Chapter 92, Routine Procedures for Isolation and Identification of Viruses (Joseph), the discussion on the viral spectrum of tissue cell cultures includes several continuous heteroploid and also diploid cell lines; the detailed, tabular directions on clinical materials to be submitted for diagnosis of viral and related diseases have been revised again; identification of echoviruses by the intersecting serum schema, typing of adenoviruses and enteroviruses by hemagglutination-inhibition tests, and the plaque technic are all included. Totally new material includes detection of viruses by cocultivation, rapid diagnosis by immunofluorescence, diagnosis by electron microscopy (negative staining, immune electron microscopy, microscopy of fecal extracts in gastroenteritis, vesicular fluids, leukocytes), detection of hepatitis B (Australia, HBsAg) surface antigen (agar gel diffusion, counterelectrophoresis, complement fixation, radioimmunoassay, hemagglutination-inhibition), double immunodiffusion for influenza viruses, and differentiation of wild-type and vaccine strains of poliovirus.

Chapter 93, Serologic Diagnosis of Viral Infections (Joseph), incorporates the neutralization test, CF test, various hemagglutination-inhibition technics, the rubella and rubeola hemagglutination-inhibition technics, and the indirect fluorescent antibody (IFA) test for titration of rubella antibodies; detection and titration of Epstein-Barr virus antibody (and other viral antibodies) by indirect fluorescent antibody test have been added. Detailed instructions for the fluorescent antibody (FA) technic for diagnosis of rabies are included in Chapter 94, Cytologic and Cytochemical Technics for Study of Viral Infections (Joseph).

PART IX, **MEDICAL PARASITOLOGY,** again extensively revised by Ivey, treats both protozoa and helminths in complete detail, with methods of transmission, host-parasite relationships, morphology, and laboratory diagnosis presented for each parasite. New illustrations have been added to several chapters. In Chapter 97, Phylum

Protozoa, much new material has been added, e.g., enlarged discussion of leishmaniasis, detailed directions for diagnosis of amebiasis, including a large variety of immunodiagnostic methods, new data on primary amebic meningo-encephalitis, *Babesia*, *Sarcocystis*, and *Pneumocystis carinii.*

Of invaluable aid will be the comprehensive chapter Laboratory Procedures in Parasitology. Among the considerable number of technical procedures included are the trichrome staining technic, a method for permanent mounting of helminth eggs, the Cleveland-Collier medium for *Entamoeba histolytica*, Stoll procedure for egg count, the Tobie and Weinman media for cultivation of trypanosomes, examination of spinal fluid for detection of *Toxoplasma* and soil amebae (*Naegleria*), and directions for examination of duodenal, bile, liver, splenic, and proctoscopic aspirates and for various biopsy materials, lung lesions, and skin scrapings. New material includes chlorazol black E staining, concentration of microfilariae by membrane filtration, and an up-to-date listing of commercially available parasite antigens (with sources given).

Two valuable, concise aids incorporated are a "specimen-parasite summary," which lists the frequency of use of a particular specimen in detection of specified parasites, and the "examination procedure summary," which indicates for each parasite the proper specimen and examination technic to be used—features not usually found in textbooks of laboratory medicine.

PART X, **MEDICAL MYCOLOGY,** has again been revised by Kobayashi and Pappagianis, both of whom have made significant contributions in their field. It is an up-to-date, advanced guide to laboratory technics and a concise description of mycotic diseases. Emphasis has been placed on methods for study of medically important fungi by inclusion of numerous tables and an extraordinarily large number of photomicrographs and other illustrations to facilitate the handling and examination of clinical specimens suspected of containing fungus organisms and their identification on culture. Because of the apparent increase in the incidence of opportunistic fungal infections caused by ubiquitous saprobic fungi, the importance of working knowledge of these organisms is discussed, along with suggested methods for maintenance of stock culture collections.

Chapter 104, The Mycoses, has been organized according to the tissue levels representing the primary focus of infection, i.e., superficial, cutaneous, subcutaneous, and systemic infections. An exception is the material on yeast-like fungi of the genera *Candida* and *Cryptococcus*, since these organisms are handled in the laboratory in a manner different from that used for the filamentous fungi. A comprehensive, detailed tabular listing that indicates for each suspected mycotic disease the specimens needed and the recommended and preferred isolation technics and media should be helpful. Available immunologic technics, i.e., skin tests and serologic procedures, including immunofluorescent methods wherever applicable, are discussed for each mycotic disease.

PART XI, **SEROLOGY OF INFECTIOUS DISEASES,** has been completely revised by Sonnenwirth, and it now focuses on the serology of infectious diseases. Chapter 105, General Considerations, discusses antigen-antibody reactions, equipment, safety devices, micro-technics, and standardization of erythrocyte suspensions. In Chapter 106, Serologic Tests in Infectious Diseases—I. Tests for Syphilis (Sonnenwirth), the newer treponemal hemagglutination tests have been added, with the technic of the microhemagglutination (MHA-TP) test described in detail. Chapter 107, Serologic Tests in Infectious Diseases—II (Sonnenwirth), now includes a large number of new procedures, i.e., the indirect fluorescent test (IFA) for *Legionella* (Legionnaires' disease) antibodies, the latex test for *Cryptococcus neoformans* antigen, immunodiffusion for histoplasma antibodies, the streptococcal multienzyme test, the direct immunofluorescent test for *Treponema pallidum*, as well as the macroscopic and microscopic agglutination, and the hemagglutination test for leptospira antibodies. Chapter 108, Bacterial Hemagglutination Tests, not available in other textbooks of this nature, was again updated and revised by Neter, who was instrumental in conceiving and developing many of these tests.

It is only through the serious effort and the excellent cooperation of all the contributors that the preparation of this text was possible. We wish to express to them our sincere thanks and indebtedness.

Alex C. Sonnenwirth
Leonard Jarett

CONTENTS

COLOR ILLUSTRATIONS

IMMUNOLOGY

60

IMMUNOLOGIC WORK-UP*

Noel R. Rose

The emergence of immunology as a distinct medical speciality has made possible both technical and theoretical advances in the diagnosis of immunologic disorders. From a theoretical point of view, our understanding of the immunologic response has broadened from its role in protection against infection to a cause of several important diseases. Immunologic diseases may be due to interactions with extrinsic antigens (e.g., allergic and immune complex diseases) or intrinsic antigens (autoimmune diseases). Failure of the immunologic response or malignant change may also produce disease. Both protective immunity and disease production are in a sense coincidental by-products of an even more fundamental biologic function of immunity as the basic physiologic process that permits distinction of foreign molecules from constituents of self.

While all cells have some capability for recognition, in vertebrates this function resides in a special organ, the immunologic apparatus. Like other organs the immunologic apparatus is specialized to perform its function in a highly proficient fashion and, like other organs, depends on interactions among several different types of cells. It is subject both to internal controls and to external regulation. Unlike most other organs of the body, however, the immunologic apparatus is not a localized structure but is diffused throughout the body, an arrangement that is particularly favorable for its job of searching for foreign molecules. Fig. 60-1 diagrams our current understanding of the major cell types that comprise the immunologic organ and describes something of their interactions in producing an immunologic response. Although greatly simplified, the diagram will provide a framework for carrying out an orderly clinical examination of the immunologic organ.

The most important cells specialized for immunologic functions are the lymphocytes. The lymphocyte is endowed with a surface receptor or recognition site that allows it to pick out a particular 3-dimensional molecular configuration known as an antigenic determinant. A single lymphocyte seems to be responsive to only 1 (or 2) antigenic determinants, and only a very small number of lymphocytes are programmed to react with any particular determinant. The encounter of the quiescent lymphocyte with its corresponding antigenic determinant perturbs the cell membrane. This event in turn triggers metabolic activation of the lymphocyte. It is evidenced by an increase in the level of DNA synthesis in the nucleus. The lymphocyte enlarges and eventually divides, giving rise to offspring with the same specific recognition site as the parent cell. This process continues until a whole colony or clone of lymphocytes with the same recognition site is produced.

As Fig. 60-1 shows, there are 2 major types of lymphocytes in the immunologic apparatus. The B-lymphocyte derives directly from the bone marrow in adult mammals, but in birds its maturation depends on a unique lymphoid organ, the bursa of Fabricius. When it encounters an antigen for which it has a receptor the B-lymphocyte undergoes proliferation and morphologic change, giving rise eventually to cells with characteristic marginal chromatin in the nucleus and highly basophilic cytoplasm recognized as plasma cells. The plasma cell secretes large amounts of the specialized proteins detectable in the blood serum and other body fluids as immunoglobulins. Five classes of immunoglobulins, IgG, IgM, IgA, IgD, and IgE, are known in humans. Although they serve somewhat different biologic functions, all share the ability to combine with the antigenic determinant that originally stimulated their synthesis, the property that has given rise to the term "antibodies."

A few antigens, particularly large molecules with repeating subunits, are able to trigger proliferation of the B-lymphocyte. Other antigens require cooperation of a T-lymphocyte with the B-lymphocyte for initiating antibody production. After arising in the bone marrow the T-lymphocyte matures under the influence of the thymus gland, probably through the agency of one or more simple peptide hormones produced in the thymus. Like the B-lymphocytes, T-lymphocytes are programmed with the ability to recognize a particular antigenic determinant. Proliferative

*Modified from Rose, N. R.: Medical Opinion **5**:31-35, 1976; **6**:41-47, 1977.

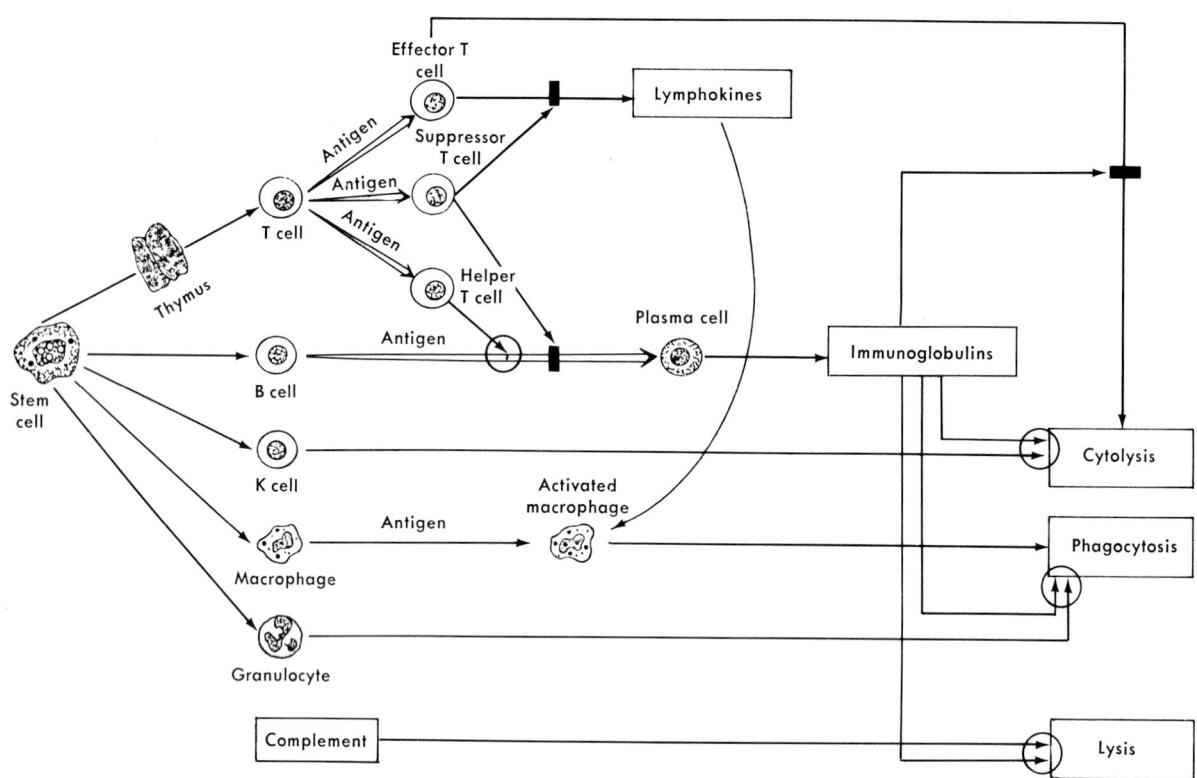

Fig. 60-1. Cellular and humoral interactions in the immune response.

differentiation of the T-lymphocyte may proceed along 3 alternate pathways. After encountering their counterpart antigenic determinant some lymphocytes mature into helper or amplifier T cells with the ability to cooperate with B-lymphocytes in promoting antibody synthesis. Other T cells impede or suppress synthesis of immunoglobulin molecules by B cells. Finally, some T cells are directly involved in cell-mediated (in contrast to antibody-mediated) immunity. These effector T cells produce the typical delayed hypersensitivity skin reaction. When they encounter their corresponding antigenic determinant on cell surfaces the effector T-lymphocytes are capable of inflicting injury referred to as cell-mediated lymphocytotoxicity (CML).

After interacting with their specific antigen the T-lymphocytes in cell-mediated immunity secrete certain soluble agents that affect surrounding cells. These factors released from activated lymphocytes are called lymphokines. They can act on neighboring lymphocytes, causing them to proliferate. Another cell that is highly susceptible to lymphokine is the macrophage, a key component of the immunologic response.

The macrophage, like the lymphocyte, is produced mainly in the bone marrow. It is found in the bloodstream as the relatively quiescent monocyte and in the tissues as the histiocyte. The particular specialty of the macrophage is phago-

cytosis. This function of the macrophage is immunologically nonspecific in the sense that it is governed by the physicochemical properties of the respective surfaces rather than their antigenic determinants. After phagocytosis the hydrolytic enzymes in the cytoplasm of the macrophage are activated so they can break down ingested particles. Some particles, including most bacterial cells, are rather readily digested by the activated macrophage, while others are resistant to hydrolytic breakdown. After ingestion some microorganisms survive and finally kill the macrophage. The tubercle bacillus is a bacterium capable of this. The activated macrophage is richer in the cytoplasmic hydrolytic enzymes that arise from its lysosomes. Such activated macrophages are more adept at engulfing and destroying invading microorganisms than the docile monocyte or histiocyte. Some of the lymphokines produced by the T-lymphocyte are important because of their ability to activate the macrophage before its encounter with invading microorganisms.

Certain classes of antibody, called cytophilic antibodies, are thought to attach firmly to the surface of the macrophage. It has been suggested that these cytophilic antibodies may confer the ability to recognize particular antigens on the macrophage, so they are termed "macrophage arming factors."

There are other types of cells in the immunologic apparatus. One heterogeneous group of cells looks very much like lymphocytes but lacks the characteristic surface markers of mature T-lymphocytes or the B-lymphocytes. Therefore these cells are sometimes called the "null cells." Together with antibody some cells seem to be able to kill certain cellular invaders. Cells active in antibody-dependent cell-mediated cytotoxicity are designated "killer" or K cells.

Another important component of the immunologic system is the polymorphonuclear leukocyte. As the most plentiful member of the circulating white cell population, it is capable of responding rapidly to tissue injury. The neutrophils leave the bloodstream and accumulate at the site of damage, where they go about their specialized duties of phagocytosis. As with the macrophage, phagocytosis by the polymorphonuclear leukocyte is a physical phenomenon depending on the relative surface properties of the phagocyte and the particle. Antibody deposited on the surface of the particle, referred to as opsonizing antibody, increases phagocytosis.

After the combination of antibody with an antigenic determinant at the surface of a particle, other serum proteins are activated that also favor phagocytosis. These serum factors are collectively called "complement." Complement is another important component of the immunologic system. It represents a group of circulating plasma proteins with complex stimulatory and inhibitory interactions. Some of the major complement components have enzymatic functions. After they are activated by splitting from their natural inhibitors these enzymes are capable of weakening or dissolving (i.e., lysing) the walls of certain kinds of cells. Complement can be activated in a variety of ways, such as by the aggregation of immunoglobulin molecules following combination with antigen. In lysis it is the initial interaction of antigen with immunoglobulin that provides specificity. Once activated, complement is nonspecific with respect to antigen.

Having seen the complicated interdigitations of the components of the immunologic apparatus it can be understood that disorders are fairly common. Because of recent technical advances it is often possible to carry out a detailed analysis of the immunologic organ in the human and determine where a lesion occurs. Symptomatic treatment of some immunologic diseases (e.g., by providing antibody in the form of γ-globulin injections) is now quite feasible.

GENERAL EXAMINATION

Like other clinical examinations the immunologic work-up begins with a careful history and physical examination followed by appropriately selected laboratory tests. Because we live in an environment heavily populated with microorganisms, one of the first indications of a defect in immunologic function is repeated infection. Not only the frequency of infection but the nature of infectious agents is significant. The immunologic

Table 60-1. Antibody-mediated immune-deficiency syndrome

Recurrent severe infections: pneumonitis, meningitis, otitis, septicemia, pyoderma, eczema
Organisms: *Staphylococcus, Pneumococcus, Streptococcus, Meningococcus, Pseudomonas, Haemophilus influenzae*

Table 60-2. Cell-mediated immune-deficiency syndrome

Severe infections: rubeola, varicella, cytomegalic inclusion disease, candidiasis, histoplasmosis, generalized tuberculosis, toxoplasmosis
Smallpox vaccination may lead to progressive vaccinia
Severe generalized BCG infection

mechanisms for handling gram-positive cocci, such as staphylococci and streptococci, are quite different from those responsible for protection against intracellular parasites such as tubercle bacilli or *Toxoplasma* (Tables 60-1 and 60-2).

Contact with cytotoxic drugs or environmental toxicants that may affect 1 or more components of the immunologic system should receive special attention during an immunologic history.

As part of the physical examination attention should be given to the skin and mucous membranes, which are important portals of entry for microorganisms. Some lymphoid tissues can be estimated during the physical examination, especially the tonsils and adenoids in younger individuals and the lymph nodes and spleen if they are palpable in adults.

Important additional tests that are part of a general immunologic examination are x-ray studies to permit assessment of the thymus gland and adenoids and sometimes angiography of lymph nodes. Examinations of the blood, including quantitative and qualitative measurement of lymphocytes, monocytes, and polymorphonuclears, are essential. Histologic examination of bone marrow, tissue biopsies, or various fluids sometimes provides evidence of an immunologic disorder.

NONSPECIFIC DEFENSE MECHANISMS

Because they are not immediately dependent on the ability of lymphocytes to recognize an antigen and undergo a proliferative response, the nonspecific defense mechanisms are the first defense against microbial invasion. There are several means by which the phagocytic capabilities of polymorphonuclear leukocytes and macrophages can be determined (see Chapter 64).

Another important component of nonspecific immunity is the complement system. Several practical tests for determining the intactness of this system are now available (see Chapter 62).

B CELL FUNCTIONS

Disorders of the B-lymphocytes can give rise to hypofunction or hyperfunction. Hypofunction is associated with hypogammaglobulinemia or agammaglobulinemia of either the acquired or congenital form. Hyperfunction often signifies chronic antigenic stimulation, sometimes leading to amyloid deposition. Malignancy of the B cell is recognized as multiple myeloma or plasmacytoma as well as B cell lymphomas and leukemias. Therefore careful evaluation of the B-lymphocyte system is an important portion of the immunologic work-up (see Chapters 61 and 64).

The recognition of abnormal antibodies is an important step in the diagnosis of immunologic disease. High levels of IgE antibodies accompany many allergic diseases such as hay fever and extrinsic asthma. A radioimmunoassay for IgE antibodies (RAST) can be used in conjunction with skin tests in an effort to identify the causative antigen. In the case of immune complex diseases deposits of immunoglobulin can be detected, sometimes with complement, at the site of the lesions, such as the renal glomeruli. A number of tests for autoantibodies can be performed with the appropriate tissues or blood cells (see Chapter 65).

T CELL FUNCTION

Both hypofunction and hyperfunction of the T cell system must be considered. Reduced T cell functions may reflect congenital or acquired illness. Important forms of acquired T cell defect are seen in Hodgkin's disease and sarcoidosis but are more often encountered in patients receiving chemotherapy with cytotoxic drugs. Methods to measure T cell functions are given in Chapter 63.

T cells are important effectors of tumor immunity and transplantation. These applications of immunology are discussed in Chapters 66 and 67.

NULL CELLS OR K CELLS

At this time quantitation of null cells is performed by subtraction; that is, the percentage of circulating T cells and B cells is added and subtracted from 100%. A test for killer or K cell function can be performed by using as a standard target the chicken erythrocyte labeled with chromium. Antibody to the chicken erythrocytes plus human peripheral lymphocyte suspensions are mixed with the labeled red blood cells and the amount of chromium release determined.

SUMMARY

The immunologic apparatus, like other organs of the body, is complex. Its proper function depends on the integrity of each component and on a delicately balanced system of checks and balances. The organ is subject to abnormal increase or decrease in function due to congenital or acquired illness and may undergo malignant change. It is now possible to dissect these disorders with a fair degree of precision. The major cell type involved can be defined and a reasonable idea of the basis of the defect made evident. The stage is now set for the next major step forward in clinical immunology, the introduction of specific cellular and molecular factors to correct the precise defect.

61

ASSESSMENT OF IMMUNOGLOBULINS

Jan Cejka
Thomas P. Conway
Miroslav D. Poulik

Introduction of a quantitative immunoprecipitation technic by Heidelberger and Kendall[1] paved the way for application of the immunologic method for quantitative work in this field. The development of immunodiffusion technics by Oudin[2] and double-diffusion technic by Ouchterlony[3] gave impetus for the development of fast, inexpensive, and highly practical methods for quantitation and identification of antigens present in biologic fluids, particularly in serum. There are well over 100 known proteins in serum. Antisera have been produced to practically all of them, and at least 30% are available commercially. In spite of the fact that the first precipitin reaction was noticed in 1897 by Kraus,[4] quantitation of serum proteins by immunologic methods was not begun in earnest until the 1950s and 1960s. This chapter discusses mainly immunoprecipitation technics used currently in a routine immunologic laboratory. Quantitation of IgE immunoglobulins and IgE antibodies (reaginic antibodies) by a radioimmunoassay technic is described as well as methods for the assessment of the catabolism of immunoglobulins. Although immunoglobulins are emphasized the methods described can be used for any antigen present in any biologic fluid.

Quantitation of immunoglobulins by radial immunodiffusion or other methods constitutes at least 50-70% of all serum protein quantitations. Application of the immunoelectrophoretic method is primarily in the field of immunodeficiencies and plasma cell dyscrasias, diseases characterized by changes in quantities of immunoglobulins (e.g., myeloma, Waldenström's disease, and lymphoma). Thus it seems appropriate to discuss, at least in general terms, some properties of the immunoglobulins.

The immunoglobulins are a group of structurally related proteins produced by lymphocytes and plasma cells. The total immunoglobulin spectrum is composed of subpopulations of molecules, each endowed with unique antigenic specificity (idiotype) as well as shared genetic (allotype) and structural (class) specificities. As with other serum proteins the steady state serum concentration of the immunoglobulins is proportional to their synthetic and catabolic rate as well as their concentration in extravascular compartments. Unique to the immunoglobulins is their rapid catabolism following the formation of antigen-antibody complexes (immune elimination). Immunoglobulinopathies may be characterized by increased synthesis (e.g., myeloma), decreased synthesis (e.g., agammaglobulinemia, ataxia telangiectasia), increased catabolism (e.g., intestinal or kidney malfunction), or by variations of these.

An IgG immunoglobulin molecule is composed of 2 pairs of dissimilar polypeptide chains. A major difference between them is the molecular weight of each pair of chains. One pair is of low molecular weight (light chains), and the other is of heavy molecular weight (heavy chains). The light chains are bonded to the heavy chains by covalent bonds (—S—S; disulfide bond) and so are the heavy chains (with the help of noncovalent bonds). This overall structure also holds true for IgA, D, and E immunoglobulins, the major differences among them being the size of the heavy chains and their amino acid sequences. In polymeric immunoglobulins (e.g., IgM and a large percentage of IgA) the monomers have the same overall structure as the monomeric IgG molecules. In the case of IgM 5 monomers make a whole molecule with an additional chain, the so-called J chain. The polymeric serum IgA also contains a J chain. The dimeric secretory IgA molecules contain a J chain and an extra chain, the secretory component (SC). The primary amino acid sequences of these chains as well as their secondary and tertiary structures are responsible for a number of antigenic determinants on the chains as well as the whole molecule. Antibodies produced against the whole γ-globulin molecules or separated chains can distinguish such determinants after proper absorption of the

Table 61-1. Human serum immunoglobulins*

Class	Subclass	Mol. wt.	Concentration (mg/ml)	$T^{1}/_{2}$ (d)
γG	1,2,3,4	145,000	12	18-23
γA	1,2	160,000	2.5	5-6
γM	1,2	900,000	0.93	5
γD		160,000	0.023	2.8
γE		200,000	0.0001	2.4

*Adapted from Waldman, T. A., Blaese, R. M., and Strober, W.: In Rothschild, M. A., and Waldman, T. A., editors: Plasma protein metabolism, New York, 1970, Academic Press.

antisera. This is extremely fortunate because with the aid of such antibodies it is possible to subdivide the heavy chains into γ, α, μ, δ, and ϵ, or in other words into IgG, IgA, IgM, IgD, and IgE classes of immunolgobulins. The light chains carry their own specific determinants called κ and λ. Consequently one can detect in the mixture (e.g., human serum) all these immunoglobulin classes by a specific antiserum against the specific heavy-chain determinant(s) without complicated physicochemical methods. With specific antilight chain antisera it is possible to subclassify them into IgG-κ or -λ, IgA-κ or -λ, and so on. Production of specific antisera went hand in hand with the development of the technics described below. Antisera are also available that distinguish the immunoglobulins on a genetic basis (allotypes, so-called Gm groups) as well as with regard to unique antigenic determinants (idiotypes). Developments of this field grew rapidly since 1961 when the basic structure was discovered[5] and culminated in 1970 when Edelman's group determined the amino acid sequence of 1 myeloma γ-globulin.[6] The interested reader may wish to become familiar with the general structure and functions of the immunoglobulins in order to understand why certain methods are used for a particular purpose. Numerous reviews of the subject have been written; that of Gally[7] is perhaps the most up-to-date. An abbreviated table of immunoglobulin classes is included here as a guide (Table 61-1).

RADIAL IMMUNODIFFUSION

Immunochemical technics are virtually the only methods presently used for accurate quantitation of immunoglobulins as well as other proteins of clinical importance. These technics are sensitive enough for most routine quantitative protein studies and simple enough to be introduced in any clinical laboratory provided specific antisera and suitable standards are available. In addition these methods do not require isolation of the protein under study. Several immunoprecipitation methods have been developed that allow quantitation of plasma and other body fluid proteins, such as single radial immunodiffusion,[8,9] electroimmunoassay,[10] manual or automated immunonephelometric analysis,[11] quantitative immunoelectrophoresis,[12] and numerous modifications thereof. Because it is simple to per-

form, requires no expensive apparatus, and is available commercially in kit form, radial immunodiffusion is currently the most frequently used immunoprecipitin method. The single radial immunodiffusion method was first developed for the quantitation of plasma proteins by Mancini et al.[8] and later by Fahey and McKelvey[9]; through the years the method has been established as a reliable routine clinical procedure for the quantitation of serum immunoglobulins IgG, IgA, IgM, and IgD.

Principle. In the radial immunodiffusion technic an antigen in solution (isolated protein dissolved in an appropriate buffer, solution containing a mixture of proteins, serum, or other biologic fluid) is applied to a cylindrical well cut in an agar gel in which an antiserum specific for the protein studied is evenly distributed. The antigen diffuses radially through the agar gel and forms a circular precipitin ring as a result of the antigen-antibody reaction. At any time the diameter of the ring depends on the time of diffusion, temperature, molecular size of the antigen, its concentration, and the amount of the antibody incorporated in the gel. Since the area enclosed by the precipitin ring is directly proportional to the concentration of the antigen, the measurement of the diameter of the ring formed by the protein quantitated and comparison with the diameter of the precipitin rings produced by standard solutions of known protein concentration provide a simple means for the determination of concentration of the protein under study.

There are 2 basic approaches to the radial immunodiffusion method: (1) the Mancini technic[8] in which the reading of the ring diameters is made after the equilibrium between the antigen and antibody has been reached (i.e., after the end point of immunodiffusion has occurred), and (2) an alternative approach described by Fahey and McKelvey[9] in which the reading of the diameters is made during the early stages of diffusion when the rings are still enlarging. Both methods have their advantages and disadvantages. The Mancini method is more accurate in that the diameters at equivalence are independent of temperature and variations in diffusion rates; they can be read at any time after the equilibrium has been reached. The rather long time needed for complete diffusion (48-72 hours or even more for high-molecular-weight proteins) is a disadvantage of this method, especially if rapid reporting of the results is required. The Fahey technic offers results within a short time (12-24 hours) at the expense of some degree of accuracy and sensitivity.

Equipment. Antiserum specific for the protein studied and a solution of known concentration of this protein (or a standard serum with predetermined concentration of the protein being quantitated) must be available for the radial immunodiffusion method to give meaningful and accurate results. Once the specificity of the antiserum and the concentration of the standard solution have been established, an appropriate amount of antiserum to be incorporated in the gel must be determined. An amount of antiserum is chosen that provides easily readable precipitin rings in the range of concentrations occurring in the serum or other solution studied. Decreasing the concentration of antiserum in the gel will increase the diameter of the ring at a given antigen concentration; since diluting the antiserum makes the precipitate less distinct, the limiting factor is the density and visibility of the precipitin ring. Increasing the antiserum concentration will have the opposite effect; too high an antiserum concentration will limit the use of the immunodiffusion plate at low antigen concentrations.

Immunodiffusion plates are prepared using simple glass plates, Petri dishes, or commercially available plastic disposable plates (Hyland Laboratories, Costa Mesa, Calif.; Miles Laboratories, Elkhart, Ind.) and specific antiserum and purified agar (or agarose), which can be purchased from most manufacturers of immunochemicals. The preselected amount of antiserum is mixed with warm (55 C) agar solution in phosphate-buffered saline and poured onto the plate so that the agar layer is approximately 1 mm thick. After the agar solidifies holes are punched into the agar with a circular gel cutter and the gel plugs removed with a wooden applicator or by suction. Special templates providing different patterns and wells of various diameters are commercially available.

Radial immunodiffusion plates for the quantitation of different plasma proteins including immunoglobulins are now commercially available from a number of manufacturers (Behring Diagnostics, Somerville, N.J.; Hyland Laboratories, Costa Mesa, Calif.; ICL Scientific, Fountain Valley, Calif.; Kallestad Laboratories, Chaska, Minn.; Meloy Laboratories, Springfied, Va.; Miles Laboratories, Elkhart, Ind.; Oxford Laboratories, Foster City, Calif.; Pfizer Diagnostics, New York; and others). Some manufacturers supply immunodiffusion plates with different amounts of antiserum (regular-level and low-level plates) to cover normal as well as subnormal concentrations of immunoglobulins in sera or other fluids with low immunoglobulin concentrations (spinal fluids, urine, pediatric samples). The immunodiffusion kits include directions regarding the storage and handling of the plates, application of standards and samples, method of plotting the calibration curve, and analysis of results.

Standards. Great progress has been made in the past 5 years in the standardization of immunoglobulin quantitation. With the object of improving the uniformity of immunoglobulin quantitations in different laboratories an international reference preparation has been established by the WHO International Center for Immunoglobulins.[13] It has been recommended[14] that the concentration of the individual immunoglobulins be estimated against this reference preparation and expressed in International Units (IU) per milliliter rather than in familiar mass per volume units (mg/100 ml). Because of difficulty in general acceptance of the new, unfamiliar unitage another WHO committee authorized the use of conversion factors[15] to relate the 2 systems of measurement: 80.4 μg IgG, 14.2 μg IgA, or 8.47 μg IgM are equivalent to 1.0 IU. It is now generally agreed that immunoglobulins should always be measured against the International Reference Preparation (lot no. 67/95, available from the NCI Immunoglobulin Reference Center, Springfield, Va.) or against a secondary standard carefully calibrated against this preparation.

Standard serum solutions of known immunoglobulin concentration, necessary for the construction of standard curves, are provided with each kit or are available from the manufacturer. These secondary standards are calibrated against the WHO International Reference Preparation and the concentrations of the individual immunoglobulins expressed in IU/ml and mg/dl. Because of the differences in purified immunoglobulin preparations and in isolation technics used by different manufacturers, somewhat different conversion factors relating International Units to mass per volume units are used by the individual reagent suppliers. These and other problems of immunoglobulin standardization have recently been reviewed by Reimer and Maddison.[16]

Procedure. The filling of wells with reference sera as well as specimens should be performed according to manufacturer's instructions. The greatest precision is obtained if samples (standards and specimens) are applied in duplicate. Either a specified volume is pipetted into the well using disposable micropipets or microliter syringes (e.g., Drummond Microdispenser, Hamilton Microliter Syringe) or the wells are filled to flatness with disposable capillary tubes; in the latter case overfilling or underfilling of wells should be avoided. Care should also be taken not to distort the well with the micropipet or to spill the antigen outside the well. After the wells have been filled the plates are stored in a horizontal position in an immunodiffusion chamber. The samples are allowed to diffuse for a specified time depending on the method used: plates designed for early readings (Fahey method) require 12-24 hours, the end-point plates (Mancini method) 24-72 hours. A developed radial immunodiffusion plate is shown in Fig. 61-1.

The diameters of the precipitin rings are measured to the nearest 0.1 mm using a simple measuring device (Behring Diagnostics), magnifying eyepieces (Hyland, Kallestad, Miles) or special precision viewers (ICL Scientific, Kallestad). Since the precipitin rings continue to enlarge when the Fahey method is used, all readings on a single plate should be done within approximately 15 minutes. The specimens in which precipitin rings are too large and would fall off the standard curve should be diluted and rerun; if

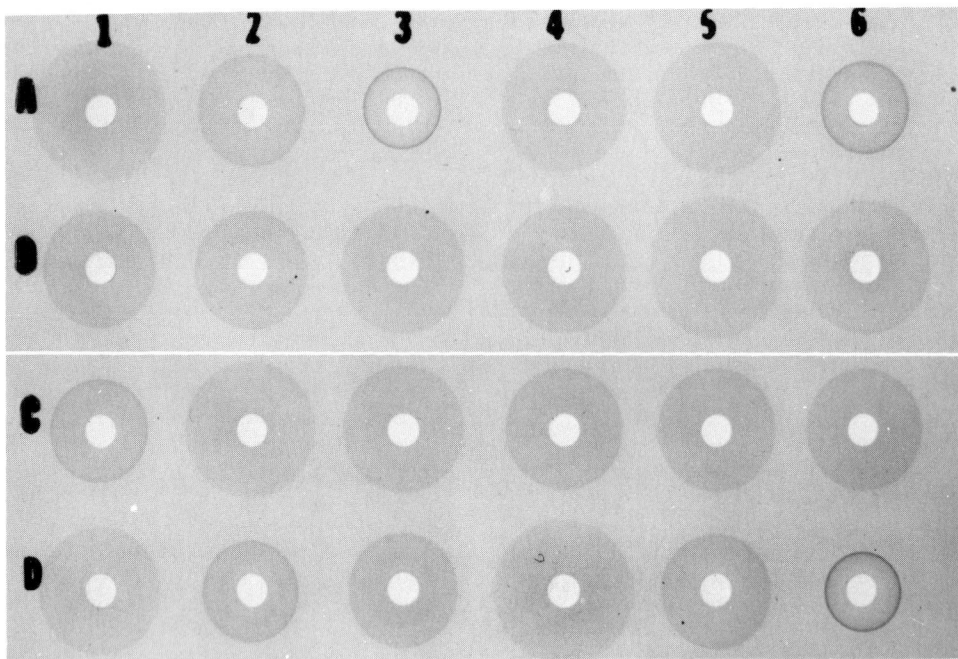

Fig. 61-1. Developed immunodiffusion plate for quantitation of IgG. Standard solutions of decreasing IgG concentrations applied in wells A1, A2, and A3. (Courtesy Meloy Laboratories, Springfield, Va.)

the ring diameter is too small the specimen should be rerun on a low-level plate containing less antiserum.

The calibration curve can be plotted in several ways. The most commonly used plots are d^2 vs. c and log c vs. d, where d is diameter of the precipitin ring and c is concentration of the antigen quantitated. The log c vs. d plot is used with the Fahey method and is constructed by plotting the concentrations of standards (c) on the ordinate (logarithmic scale) and ring diameters (d) on the abscissa using a semilogarithmic paper (Fig. 61-2). A straight line (log $c = d$) is obtained only when early readings are taken; the linearity is progressively lost with increasing time of diffusion, and the curve is completely nonlinear when all circles reach their end points. Commercial plates designed for early readings should never be used for equivalence readings, since such plates work at antigen excess and may not contain a sufficient amount of antibody to react with all of the antigen. With the Mancini method a standard curve is constructed by plotting the diameter squared (d^2) of the precipitin rings produced by the standard protein concentrations vs. the respective concentrations (c) on linear graph paper. The plot becomes progressively linear as time elapses until all the antigen has reacted with the antiserum and no further extension of the precipitin rings occurs; all circles fall on a straight line corresponding to the relationship $c = d^2$ (Fig. 61-3). The diameters at equivalence are independent of temperature or variations in diffusion rates; they can be read at any time after

reaching their end points. The end-point method is slightly more accurate than the early-readout method of Fahey; this is, however, at the expense of prolonged diffusion time (e.g., approximately 24 hours for IgG, 48-72 hours for IgM or other high-molecular-weight proteins). Some commercially available end-point plates allow early readout; this approach does not provide a straight line but results in a curvilinear c vs. d^2 relationship. With both the Fahey and the Mancini methods the extrapolation of the standard curve to lower or higher concentrations is not recommended. The test must be repeated at a lower sample concentration or with a low-level plate if the reading of the test sample falls outside the extreme portions of the standard curve.

Sensitivity. The sensitivity of the radial immunodiffusion method is approximately 1 mg protein per deciliter; the limit of sensitivity depends basically on the ability to see and measure the antigen-antibody precipitates. Commercially available plates are designed for easy and direct reading of the precipitin rings in the selected concentration range. However, in plates intended to measure very low concentrations the visibility of rings can be facilitated by several technics. Staining with amido black after washing the plate in saline or staining with 1% tauric acid have been used. Also 0.1M 3,4-dihydroxyphenylalanine has been recommended for developing faint precipitin rings.

Several methods can be used to increase the sensitivity of radial immunodiffusion. The decrease in the antibody concentration in the gel

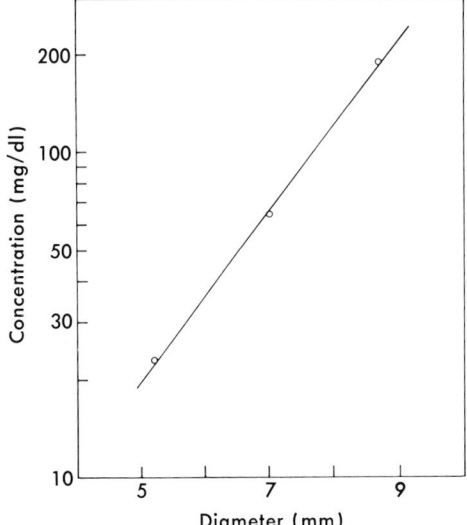

Fig. 61-2. Plot of log *c* vs. *d* according to Fahey method. Numbers correspond to 3 standard solutions of known concentrations.

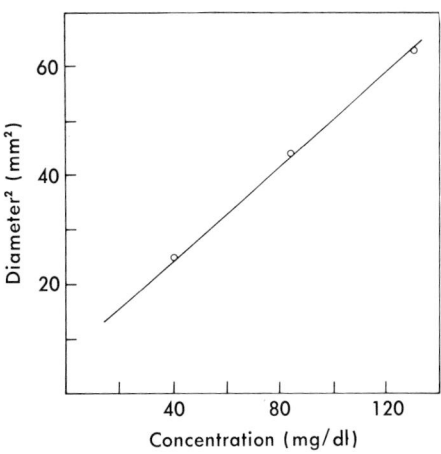

Fig. 61-3. Plot of *d²* vs. *c* according to Mancini (end-point) method.

will result in an increase in the precipitin ring diameter; for better readability of faint rings any of the above-mentioned methods can be used. Also increase in the volume of antigen solution can further lower the minimum concentration of antigen that can be measured. The concentration of the sample (e.g., by ultrafiltration or lyophilization) has also been used, especially with samples containing low immunoglobulin concentrations (spinal fluids, saliva); however, denaturation and subsequent change in antigenic properties of the protein quantitated might lead to erroneous results unless properly tested. An effective method for increasing the sensitivity of quantitation by radial immunodiffusion has been developed by Rowe.[17] In this method a radioactive iodine–labeled second antibody directed against the antibody originally incorporated in the gel is used to make the precipitate visible. After washing and staining the plate the radioactivity attached to the precipitin rings is visualized by exposure of the gel plate to photographic film (e.g., Kodak NS 54 T x-ray film). The method has been used for the quantitation of IgE,[18] β_2-micro-globulin,[19] and other proteins. The sensitivity can be increased 100 times as compared with conventional radial immunodiffusion. A peroxidase-labeled second antiserum can also be used for the same purpose.[20]

Sources of error. Erroneous findings might result from inappropriate handling of the plates. Distorted precipitin rings can occur as a result of a cut in the well or of an uneven layer of the agar gel. Spilling of antigen outside the well, unequal volumes delivered into the wells, or different incubation periods for standards and samples would also create an error. An excess of antigen might lead to a false conclusion of an absence of

antigen due to the formation of a large and actually invisible precipitin ring. Also aggregated or dissociated antigens will give false concentration values. Aggregated proteins (e.g., polymeric IgA, higher IgM polymers) will produce smaller rings and subsequently low readings, whereas fragmented proteins (e.g., 7S IgM) will diffuse faster and lead to erroneously high values. Some serum samples (e.g., sera from IgA-deficient patients) contain antibodies against certain animal proteins; such samples might produce false precipitin rings due to the reaction of the patient's antibodies with an animal protein incorporated in the gel.

Analysis of sera containing monoclonal proteins usually gives spuriously high values for the particular monoclonal immunoglobulin. Since the M protein usually belongs to only 1 subclass of immunoglobulin and contains only a limited number of antigenic determinants as compared with a normal immunoglobulin molecule to which the antiserum has been raised, an apparent antibody deficiency thus formed leads to high false values. Serum protein electrophoresis has been recommended[21] as the most satisfactory technic for the quantitation of M proteins.

Normal values. Immunoglobulin concentration in serum depends primarily on the age of the individual and to a lesser extent on sex, race, and geographic location. Thus each laboratory dealing with pediatric samples should use proper age-related immunoglobulin levels, and, if possible, determine its own normal ranges of immunoglobulin concentrations reflecting the geographic location and race differences. Table 61-2 shows normal concentration of immunoglobulins G, A, and M in healthy children 0.5 month to 16 years of age as used by Meloy Laboratories; simi-

Table 61-2. Serum immunoglobulin concentrations of normal children of different ages

Age	IgG mg/dl*	IgG IU/ml†	IgA mg/dl*	IgA IU/ml*	IgM mg/dl*	IgM IU/ml†
½-3 mo	299-821	36.5-100.2	3-60	2.1-40.2	15-149	18.9-193.9
3-6 mo	142-952	17.3-116.2	4-82	3.0-54.8	18-109	23.7-141.7
6-12 mo	418-1102	51.0-134.4	14-86	9.1-57.6	43-207	56.1-268.9
1-2 y	356-1162	43.4-141.7	13-108	8.8-71.7	37-239	47.5-310.2
2-3 y	492-1224	60.0-149.3	23-124	15.4-82.8	49-190	63.7-246.2
3-6 y	564-1332	68.8-162.5	35-190	23.2-126.7	51-199	66.5-257.9
6-9 y	658-1480	80.3-180.5	29-384	19.6-256.1	50-211	65.1-274.3
9-12 y	625-1541	76.2-188.0	60-270	40.3-180.0	64-258	82.9-335.1
12-16 y	680-1493	83.0-182.1	81-232	53.9-154.4	45-237	57.9-308.4

*Concentrations in mg/dl calculated from IU/ml using conversion factors of 82 for IgG, 15 for IgA, and 7.7 for IgM.
†From Cejka, J., Mood, D. W., and Chung, S. K.: Clin. Chem. **20**:656, 1974.

Table 61-3. Serum immunoglobulin concentrations of normal adults

Protein	White males (n = 681)	White females (n = 660)	Black males (n = 116)	Black females (n = 212)
IgG				
mg/dl	616-1543	629-1604	724-2092	765-2163
IU/ml	75-188	77-196	88-255	93-264
IgA				
mg/dl	71-417	61-371	79-483	83-425
IU/ml	48-279	41-249	53-324	56-285
IgM				
mg/dl	57-343	77-376	63-339	84-374
IU/ml	75-449	101-492	83-444	110-490
IgD				
mg/dl	0.5-19.7	0.5-19.5	0.6-25.0	0.8-23.1

lar tables have been published by other manufacturers (Behring Diagnostics, Kallestad Laboratories). A nationwide survey of normal ranges of 12 serum proteins including immunoglobulins has recently been performed by Meloy Laboratories. Cumulative data on immunoglobulin ranges for the normal adult population in the United States taken from this large-group study is given in Table 61-3.

NEPHELOMETRIC METHODS

The increase in volume of quantitative determination of serum proteins and γ-globulins in particular demanded new technics to handle such a volume and also to alleviate possible errors by technologists performing these tests. Concomitantly with such demand a new principle was applied, namely, nephelometric determination of the antigen-antibody complexes. In dilute solutions antigens and antibodies will form complexes that scatter light that can be measured by nephelometry. In 1959 Schultze and Schwick[22] showed that immune precipitates can be measured by turbidimetry. This lead was not immediately followed, and it was not until 1967 that Ritchie[23] showed that low-level proteins can be analyzed by turbidimetry and 1968 that Alper and Propp[24] used modified fluorometry for the same purpose. A fully automated immunoassay was introduced by Ritchie et al.[25] The method

used only microgram quantities of antigen and microliters of antibodies and so became economically feasible.

The nephelometric methods are based on law of mass action that the antigen-antibody reaction follows. Under appropriate conditions the amount of the complexes formed is a function of both antigen and antibody. Since the amount of antibody supplied is constant the number of complexes varies in direct proportion to the antigen concentration and thus the amount of scattered light. If the amount of scattered light of an unknown sample is compared with the amounts of light scattered by dilutions of a reference serum of known antigen concentration, the antigen concentration present in the unknown sample can be determined.

At the present time several instruments are commercially available: the fully automated A.I.P. (Automated Immuno Precipitin, Technicon Company, Tarrytown, N.Y.), the Laser Nephelometer PDQ (Hyland Laboratories, Costa Mesa, Calif.), Behring Laser Nephelometer (Behring Diagnostics, Somerville, N.J.), Digital Nephelometer (Kallestad, Chaska, Minn.), and Rate Nephelometer Immunochemistry System (Beckman, Fullerton, Calif.). Poulik has used the A.I.P. method for several years. The details of the method can be found in the various manuals supplied by the company as well as in a book by Rose

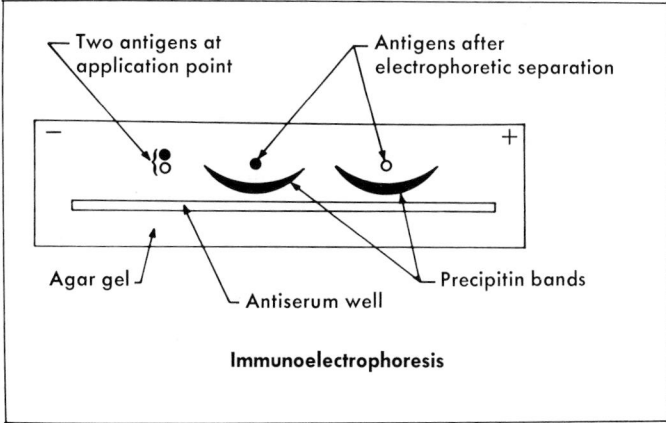

Fig. 61-4. Principle of immunoelectrophoresis (IEP). For details see text. (From Seminar on Basic Immunology, 24th Annual Meeting of the American Association of Blood Banks, Chicago, September 1971.)

and Friedman.[26] Various modifications of the method exist, and a major contribution in this field was the introduction by Hellsing[27] of polyethylene glycol (PEG) to enhance the antigen-antibody reaction. The sensitivity can be increased about 3-fold and the speed of the reaction about 12-fold when this polymer is used with the reagents. Our experience with this technic, after a period of difficulties, is more than satisfactory. The complete automation, which is so far lacking in the other instruments, is the greatest asset. It is the opinion of Poulik that these methods will be replaced in the not too distant future by enzymoimmunoassays. Since only a few (about 50) A.I.P. instruments are in operation in the United States, the method is not discussed in detail here. Laser nephelometry is new in this field, and data obtained in the field are not available as yet. Nevertheless the method is promising, and institutions gaining volume in immunoquantitation should consider this method.

IMMUNOELECTROPHORETIC METHODS

Double-diffusion methods, especially if used for qualitative rather than quantitative purposes, have certain limitations: (1) a single line may be formed by several antigen-antibody complexes that happen to have the proper optimal ratios, (2) the antigen-antibody ratio may be so unbalanced that until it becomes stabilized it may give several precipitin lines, changing with time, and (3) if complex mixtures are investigated (e.g., serum) enumeration of the actual number may not be possible.

In most instances the composition of the reactants is insufficiently known. The same holds true for the antibody as well as the antigen. Consequently it becomes clear that if the complexity of at least 1 of the mixtures could be demonstrated the interpretation of the double-diffusion results could be facilitated. Electrophoresis was exploited for this purpose in the form of immunoelectrophoresis. As the term describes, electro-

phoretic separation of 1 of the mixtures, usually antigen(s), is subjected to radial immunodiffusion.

The principle of immunoelectrophoresis is extremely simple. The antigen sample (e.g., serum, urine, CSF, isolated fraction) is subjected to electrophoretic migration in a supporting medium (e.g., agar, cellulose acetate, filter paper, starch gel, polyacrylamide gel). After completion of this step the separated components are allowed to diffuse from the supporting medium into agar gel (or cellulose acetate, or polyacrylamide gel). Parallel to the axis of the migration of the antigen a trough is dissected and filled with the appropriate antiserum and allowed to diffuse perpendicularly through the agar layer (or other medium). Where the reactants meet in optimal proportions a precipitation line is formed that reveals the presence of a specific antigen. The results can be viewed by the naked eye or made permanent by appropriate staining of the precipitin arcs and eventually photographed. The principle of the method is depicted in Fig. 61-4. Since 1952 a number of immunoelectrophoretic technics have been developed (Table 61-4).

The prototype of the electrophoresis technic[28] was developed by Poulik in 1952. This was of the transfer type (paper-agar). The agar-agar type of electrophoresis[29, 30] was performed by Grabar and Williams in 1953. This method became the most practical and best known through introduction of a micromethod by Scheidegger.[31] However, if more complex mixtures are to be investigated the starch gel–agar method[32] developed by Poulik in 1959 is most advantageous. A still more convenient method, which combines identification of the components and their quantitation in 1 procedure, in the form of electroimmunodiffusion[33] was introduced by Laurell in 1966. Each of these methods has advantages and disadvantages and is progressively more complex technically. In a routine clinical immunodiagnostic laboratory the agar-agar technic is usually

Table 61-4. Types of immunoelectrophoresis

Immunoelectrophoresis
  Electrophoresis and immunodiffusion performed in
  same medium.
    Agar-agar
    Cellulose acetate–cellulose acetate
    Acrylamide-acrylamide
Transfer immunoelectrophoresis
  Electrophoresis and immunodiffusion performed in
  different media.
    Filter paper-agar
    Cellulose acetate-agar
    Starch gel-agar
    Acrylamide-agar
    Sephadex-agar
Crossed immunoelectrophoresis
  Essentially 2-dimensional transfer immunoelectrophoresis. First-dimension electrophoresis performed in agar gel. Agar gel is then transferred into
  agar gel containing antibody. Electrophoresis continued at right angle to first electrophoresis.
Immunoelectro-osmophoresis (IEOP)
  Antibodies move by endosmotic flow to encounter
  antigen(s) migrating "electrophoretically" in opposite direction.

most useful and sufficient for the information
desired. The type of immunoelectrophoresis
used in Poulik's laboratory since 1954 with a
great degree of reproducibility is described in
detail. The following questions can be answered
by this method. What is the minimum number of
antigens present in the mixture? How are the
antigens related immunologically? What is the
concentration of at least some of them? Semiquantitative answers can be obtained by an experienced operator.

Immunoelectrophoresis (IEP)

Apparatus
1. IEP chamber (Brinkmann-Sartorius, LKB, Gra-
   far, or any other suitable chamber; all 3 used in
   Poulik's laboratory)
2. LKB and Gelman cutters (gel punch)
3. Gelman frames, frame holders, diffusion chamber
4. Staining trays

Materials
1. Buffer. Sodium acetate and sodium barbital
   buffer, pH 8.2, ionic strength 0.15

Sodium acetate, fused anhydrous	7.8 g
Sodium barbital, purified	11.8 g
Distilled water, final vol	1 L

   Adjust pH to 8.2 with 1N HCl
2. Agar, 1% solution in buffer, ionic strength 0.05

Ionagar no. 2	4 g
Sodium azide	200 mg
Buffer	132 ml
Distilled water	266 ml

   Bring to boiling 3 times with constant swirling.
   Cool; filter through glass wool; pour 20 ml into
   each tube (sufficient to prepare 8 slides); store in
   refrigerator before use.
   NOTE: sodium azide may be hazardous in certain
   concentrations and in contact with lead (above
   5%).

Procedure
1. Boil 1 tube agar. Slides are prepard by pipetting
   2.5 ml hot agar onto clean labeled slides. Slides
   are cleaned in 95% ethanol and labeled with
   Diamond marking pen in upper right corner. Agar
   is allowed to cool and set.
2. Cut desired pattern with gel punch and remove
   antigen holes only. Do not remove center trough.
   Use larger holes for CSF and urine IgM, IgD, and
   IgE γ-globulins.
3. Samples are applied with fine capillary tubes
   (B6864-12, Scientific Products, Detroit).
4. Electrophoresis can then be performed after
   slides have been placed in carriage and positioned
   in IEP chamber.
5. Paper wicks (22.5 × 6.0 cm) connect slides to
   buffer in buffer chamber.
6. Labeled right upper corner of slides should be
   directed to anode (positive pole, red lead).
7. Buffer polarity should be reversed with each new
   run (not more than 4 times) to compensate for
   changes in pH.
8. Run for 90 min at 75 mA (about 120-130 V total).
9. After 90 min disconnect current and remove wicks
   and agar in trough. Fill trough with appropriate
   antiserum.
10. Let antiserum diffuse for 18-24 h in moisture
    chamber. During this time precipitin lines will
    develop.
11. Precipitin arcs are visible when viewed under
    oblique light with dark background.
12. Place slides in saline wash (0.9% NaCl) with 0.5%
    sodium azide for 24 h to remove any unreacted
    antibody and antigen.
13. Agar with precipitin lines is then dried to surface
    of slide by applying moistened Whatman no. 1
    filter paper strips to agar surface (several hours or
    overnight).
14. When completely dry, carefully remove paper and
    rinse slides in tap water to remove lint.
15. Slides are now ready to be stained.

Staining reagents
1. Amido black dye

Amido black	6 g
Distilled water	405 ml
Methanol	405 ml
Acetic acid (glacial)	90 ml

   Dissolve amido black in distilled water. Add
   methanol and acetic acid. Strain through glass
   wool.
2. Destaining solution

Methanol	405 ml
Distilled water	405 ml
Acetic acid (glacial)	90 ml

   Stain with amido black for 5 min. Transfer into
   destaining solution for 10 min. Repeat destaining 2
   more times. Place slides with agar side up and let dry
   in air.

Applications and pitfalls. The greatest value
of IEP in a routine diagnostic immunology laboratory is in the field of immunodeficiencies and
plasma cell dyscrasias. An immunoelectrophoretic profile in these conditions may provide immediate leads to further tests as well as diagnosis.
Examples are shown in Fig. 61-5. Patterns *a*, *e*,
and *g* are those of normal sera. As can be seen the
precipitin line patterns of even normal sera are
very complicated, and only an experienced
worker will be able to identify all the antigens

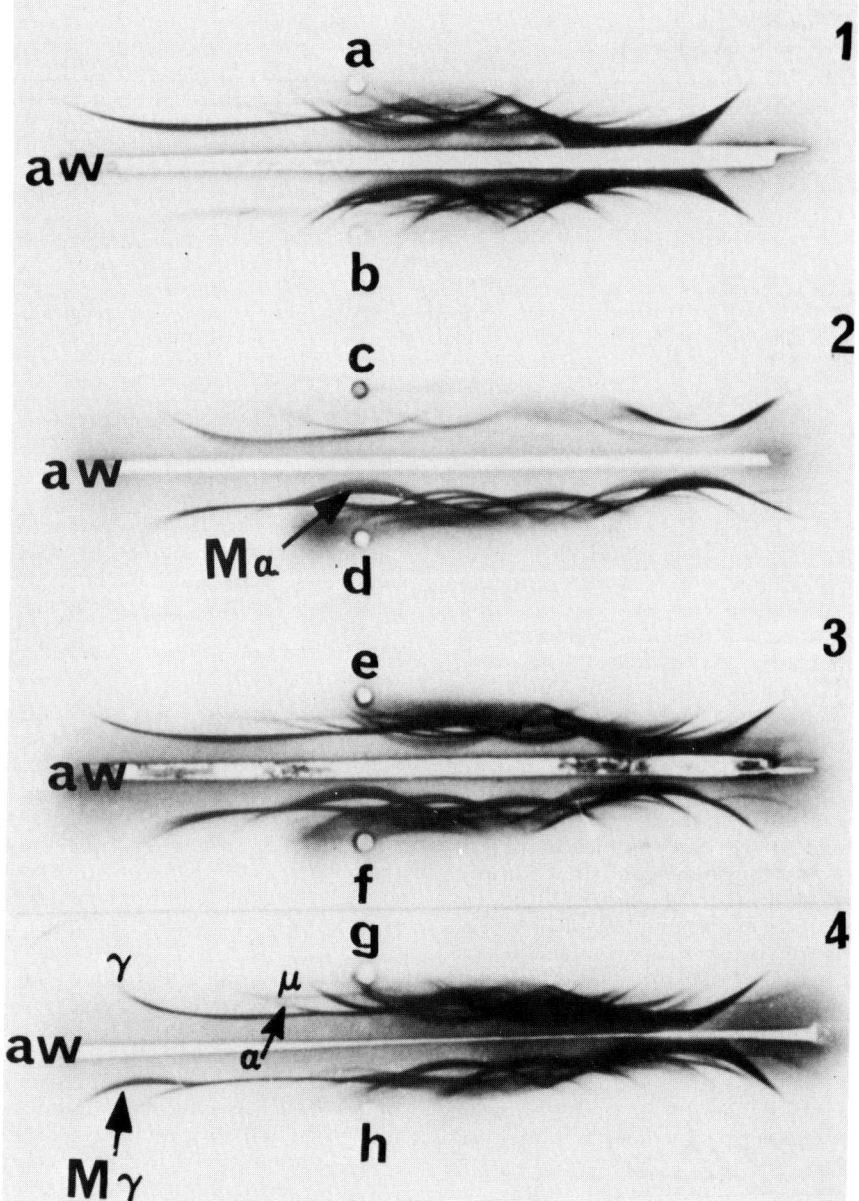

Fig. 61-5. Immunoelectrophoretic patterns of normal and abnormal sera. On 4 slides (1-4) are shown patterns as follows: *a, e, g,* normal sera; *b,* agammaglobulinemia serum; *c,* concentrated normal urine; *d, f, h,* myeloma sera. All patterns were developed with antiserum produced against whole human serum in rabbit. γ, IgG; *M*γ, IgG myeloma; α, IgA; *M*α, IgA myeloma; μ, IgM; *aw,* rabbit anti–whole human serum.

present with certainty. It is a general misconception that routine immunoelectrophoretic patterns of sera are of great diagnostic help. This statement must be qualified, since in some specific conditions the IEP method provides invaluable clues. But in many instances the number of precipitin lines afforded by the α_1- and α_2-globulins as well as β-globulins are very difficult to interpret without the help of additional procedure(s). However, the cathodic portion of the pattern usually affords distinct precipitin lines belonging to the 3 major immunoglobulin classes (IgG, A,

and M) and C3 component of complement. On a well-executed IEP these not only can be identified but can be assessed on a semiquantitative basis as shown in Fig. 61-5. Such precipitin lines are clearly visible in pattern *g* and can be compared with those of patterns *a* and *e*. In agammaglobulinemia shown in pattern *b* most of these proteins are absent, and only a very faint precipitin band(s) belonging to IgA immunoglobulin is seen. There are cases where all 3 immunoglobulin precipitin lines may be missing, but selective deficiency on any of the 3 is possible

Table 61-5. Immunoelectrophoresis precipitin arc position and appearance with varying antigen and antibody concentrations*

Experimental condition	Position of arc	Appearance of arc
Excess antibody concentration	Progressively farther from trough with increasing antibody concentration	Progressively diffuse with increasing antibody concentration
Excess antigen concentration	Progressively nearer to trough with increasing antigen concentration	Dense, elongated arc; sharp edge on sample well side; trough side diffuse; with gross antigen excess precipitate dissolves (prozones) except at tips
Low antibody concentration	Nearer to trough	Elongated arc; sharp edge on sample well side; trough side diffuse
Low antigen concentration	Farther from trough	Indistinct
Weak antibody	Nearer to trough	Diffuse
Weak antigen	Farther from trough	Diffuse

*Adapted from Immunoglobulin abnormality detection by electrophoresis, Bedford, Mass., 1974, Millipore Corp.

(e.g., in ataxia telaniectasia where 40% of patients lack IgA immunoglobulin or in some normal people who totally lack IgA immunoglobulin).

In Poulik's laboratory the electrophoresis conditions are so chosen that endosmotic flow will carry most of the immunoglobulins left to the application well (cathodal end of the slide), and thus they are usually unobstructed by other precipitin lines except by those of C3 of complement and possibly by hemopexin.

Myeloma γ-globulins (M components) are not difficult to detect by IEP. Their electrophoretic mobility may vary considerably as shown in Fig. 61-5, where patterns *d* and *f* show IgA and pattern *h* IgG myeloma immunoglobulins. The methods of identification of M components are discussed in greater detail in another chapter. Immunoelectrophoresis is of great practical help in identification of heavy- and light-chain disease states, antigen-antibody complexes, and so on. This method is practically indispensable for identification of Bence Jones proteins, urine γ-globulin fragments, β_2-microglobulin, and other proteins in urine. However, certain difficulties may be encountered when the amount of these antigens is too high (e.g., Bence Jones proteins, β_2-microglobulin). Due to excess of the antigen the prospective precipitin line may not be found (after 16-18 hours of development), since under these conditions it may be dissolved by the antigen excess. Position of the precipitin arcs depends on the antigen or antibody concentration(s). Useful guidance for understanding these relationships is given in Table 61-5.

It is impossible to give an adequate exposition of all possibilities that IEP offers. Excellent discussion of the technics can be found in a book compiled by Nerenberg.[34] The diagnostic possibilities are described in minuscule detail in a monograph by Arquembourg.[35] The art of diagnosing M components as well as other serum proteins is expertly presented by Ritzman and Daniels[36] and by Kyle.[37] Extremely helpful discussions of immunoglobulin abnormalities for beginners in the field are offered by the Millipore Corp.[38] and by Behring Diagnostics.[39]

Electroimmunodiffusion (Laurell rocket technic)

As pointed out above, IEP methods can provide only semiquantitative estimation of antigens tested. A clever application of electrophoretic methods in combination with immunoprecipitation was devised by Laurell[33] for quantitation of antigens. The principle of the simplest of such methods is as follows. Antigen(s) is migrated by electric current (electrophoresis) into an agar **containing a specific antiserum.** As the antigen migrates it reacts with the constant amount of the antibody in the gel, and where the optimal proportion between antigen and antibody exists, precipitation will occur. The final result is a precipitin line shaped like a rocket; consequently this method is also known as rocket immunoelectrophoresis. The advantage of this technic is that the height of the rocket (i.e., the area under it) is directly proportional to the concentration of the antigen. Consequently this method is admirably suitable for quantitation of antigens present in low concentrations (e.g., factor VIII [AHG-associated antigen], components of complement [C4, C5, etc.], α_1-fetoproteins, and a number of others). The details of the method as used in this laboratory for factor VIII–associated protein are given below.

Factor VIII–associated protein (rocket immunoelectrophoresis method)

Reagents
1. 0.2M Barbital buffer, pH 8.6 (4.12 g sodium barbital + 0.8 g barbital/L)
2. 0.9% Saline
3. Amido black stain (see IEP procedure)
4. 7% Acetic acid (see IEP destaining solution)
5. Plastic film (Cronar clear base, 0.004 in. thick, Dupont Graphic Arts film)

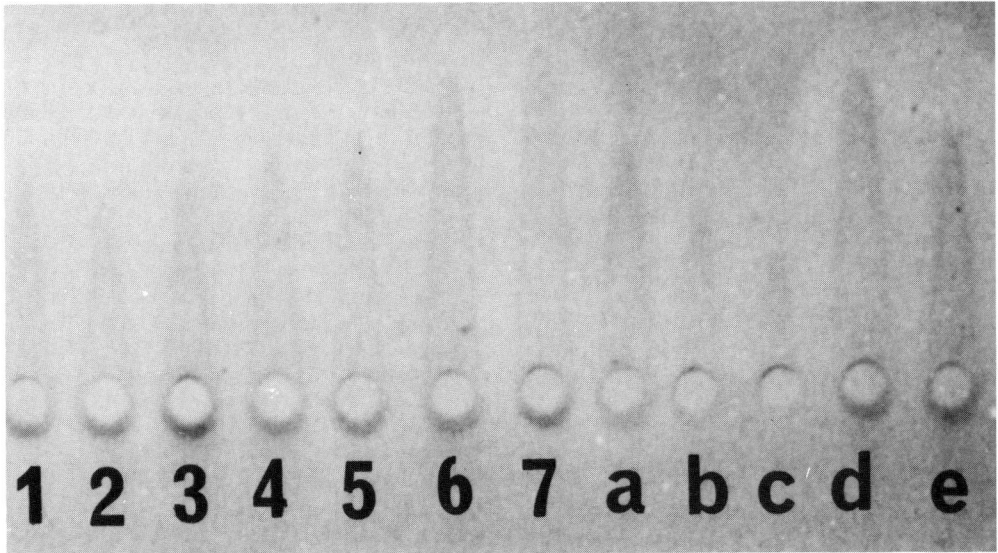

Fig. 61-6. Laurell rocket immunoelectrophoresis (factor VIII-associated protein). *1-7,* Patient plasma; *a,* "Verify" undiluted; *b,* "Verify" diluted 1:2; *c,* "Verify" diluted 1:4; *d,* normal plasma pool (mixture of 20 female and 20 male plasma); *e,* plasma pool.

6. Agarose (SeaKem, MCI, Biomedical, Rockland, Me.)
7. Antiserum (Behring Diagnostics, AHG-associated protein antisera, lot no. 2661) (NOTE: It is important that batch of potent antisera is obtained.)
8. Control. "Verify" normal citrate (General Diagnostics, Morris Plains, N.J.) and prepare according to manufacturer's instructions

Sample preparation. Patient samples should be citrated plasma received **same day.**

Reference curve is made from "Verify" freshly reconstituted with distilled water; use undiluted and with 0.2M barbital buffer, pH 8.6, diluted 1:2 and 1:4. All preparations should be free of floating particles.

Procedure

1. Prepare 20 ml 1% agarose in 0.02M barbital, pH 8.6.
2. Bring to boil with stirring to dissolve agarose (use automatic stirrer). Allow to cool to 56 C.
3. Add antiserum to achieve 0.4% concentration (80 μl Behring anti-AHG, lot no. 2661, added to 20 ml agarose).
4. Mix well and pour onto clean plastic film placed on level stand to ensure uniform thickness of agarose gel.
5. Allow to solidify. Keep in moisture chamber until used (not more than 2 h).
6. Cut 3 mm wells.
7. Use 10 λ Oxford pipet to put exactly 10 μl each standard sample or patient sera (undiluted) into wells (wells should **not** be filled to top).
8. Place slide in Brinkmann electrophoresis chamber with 400 ml 0.02M barbital buffer, pH 8.6, in each buffer chamber.
9. Place filter paper wicks on gel about 5 cm apart and cover chamber.
10. Electrophorese for 16 h at 1 V/cm across gel (actually, ends of wicks).
11. After electrophoresis place film in saline for 24 h.
12. Dry film by compression between filter papers (Schleicher and Schull, 903 grade). Stain with amido black and destain with 7% acetic acid.
13. Measure peak heights in mm and plot curve on logarithmic paper using "Verify" as 100%, 50%, 25%.
14. Determine patient values from above and report as % "Verify" (100%).

Results. A typical result is shown in Fig. 61-6. If immunoglobulins are quantitated by this method the whole serum must first be carbamylated by a procedure described by Weeke.[40] Electroimmunodiffusion technics can also be performed by a transfer technic; this method is then known as crossed immunoelectrophoresis or 2-dimensional immunoelectrophoresis. In principle this method is a combination of single agar gel electrophoresis and electroimmunodiffusion devised by Laurell[41] and developed into a quantitative technic by Clarke and Freeman.[42] This technic is a technically demanding procedure used in specialized laboratories. Genetic polymorphism of proteins present in small quantities (e.g., complement, α_1-fetoprotein) can be evaluated quantitatively by this method. Variations of this technic are tandem immunoelectrodiffusion developed by Kröll[43] and intermediate gel technic introduced by Svendsen and Axelsen.[44] The former method is suitable to demonstrate antigenic identity of antigens and the latter to identify unknown immunoprecipitates. The interested reader should consult references 12 and 45.

Immunoelectro-osmophoresis (IEOP)

This technic is also known as counterimmunoelectrophoresis or crossover electrophoresis. In principle it takes advantage of the endosmotic flow generated during electrophoresis in agar media. The less purified the agar the greater the endosmotic flow. Consequently agarose obtained during purification of agar is the least "endosmotic" supporting medium. The endosmotic flow makes γ-globulins (antibodies) move toward the cathode. If at the same time an antigen (preferably of high mobility or at least of greater mobility than γ-globulin) is moving into the concentrated antibody front, antigen-antibody reaction will ensue and a precipitin line will be formed. Such conditions are easily arranged by proper choice of the application wells. The advantage of this method is the rapidity by which the formation of the precipitin lines can be achieved (within 30-90 minutes). The method was in great demand during the preradioimmunoassay era of hepatitis-associated (Australia) antigen (HAA). In the early stages of screening for HAA of all donor blood for transfusion, this was the method of choice.

An excellent description of the procedure can be found in a manual by Rose and Bigazzi.[46] The method was shown to be more sensitive than the Ouchterlony test by Hanson et al.[47] and by Prince and Burke.[48] A rash of modifications of this technic was made rapidly by a number of manufacturers, but the method was eventually replaced by a more sensitive radioimmunoassay technic. This technic is still valuable for the detection of various microbial antigens, soluble type-specific pneumococcal antigens,[49] group-specific meningococcal antigens,[50] and candidal antigens.[51,52] This method is also suitable for detection of anti-DNA antibodies as well as other specific antibodies. All electrophoretic and immunoelectrophoretic technics are discussed in great detail in a book by Williams and Chase.[53]

QUANTITATION OF IgE IMMUNOGLOBULIN AND IgE (REAGINIC) ANTIBODIES

Immunoglobulin E has molecular weight of 188,000, is heat sensitive, and does not fix complement.[54] IgE participates in the immediate anaphylatic reaction by binding to the cell membrane of basophils and mast cells, which can then be stimulated by antigen to release vasoactive amines.[55-57] In healthy individuals IgE exhibits a skewed distribution of serum concentrations with a mean of 25 U/ml (1 U ≃ 2 ng IgE).[58] Elevated IgE levels (greater than 150 U/ml) are frequently encountered in atopic disease (asthma, hay fever, and similar diseases) and appear to correlate with the degree of allergic hypersensitivity. IgE levels in hypersensitive individuals do not always exceed the normal range but depend on the number and type of allergens as well as the duration of exposure. Measurement of IgE concentration is useful in the diagnosis and treatment of patients with atopic allergy or parasitic infections and in the detection of children who by heredity are predisposed to allergic disease.[59-61] The role IgE plays in body defense is not clear, although markedly elevated levels of IgE are encountered in parasitic infections.[62] Quantitation methods of IgE immunoglobulin(s) and IgE (reaginic) antibodies are only briefly de-

scribed below. The full details can be obtained from the manufacturer of the kits (Pharmacia Fine Chemicals, Piscataway, N.J.).

Serum IgE concentrations can be measured with the commercially marketed radioimmunosorbent test (RIST, Pharmacia Fine Chemicals). In RIST an immunosorbent prepared by covalently linking rabbit anti-IgE to Sephadex is incubated with a mixture of ^{125}I-IgE and IgE (standard or unknown concentration). The presence of unlabeled IgE reduces the amount of ^{125}I-IgE bound to the immunosorbent, and the percent decrease is proportional to the amount of unlabeled IgE. The Phadebas RIST kit contains reagents for 50 IgE determinations with a sensitivity of 10 U/ml and a coefficient of variation of 5% (high values) to 20% (low values). The kit has a shelf life of 4 months and contains lyophilized Sephadex-IgE, IgE standard (800 U), and ^{125}I-IgE (3.7 μCi, 150 ng). By using the buffer supplied with the tests the lyophilized reagents are reconstituted, the IgE standard is diluted over a 1-400 U/ml concentration range, the serum unknowns are diluted 1:10, and the following reagents are added in duplicate to plastic centrifuge tubes:

1. 100 μl each standard
2. 100 μl buffer (zero inhibition)
3. 100 μl unknown
4. 100 μl ^{125}I-IgE (total counts)

With the exception of the ^{125}I-IgE tubes, 100 μl ^{125}I-IgE and 1.0 ml Sephadex–anti-IgE suspension is added to the tubes. The tubes are incubated overnight at 25 C with shaking and centrifuged at 2000 × g for 2 minutes. The supernatant is removed and 2 ml saline added to resuspend the immunosorbent. The tubes are centrifuged once more at 2000 × g for 2 minutes, the supernatant is removed, and the tubes are counted for 2-5 minutes (greater than 5000 counts above background). The background is subtracted, and the count rate (e.g., cpm) is expressed as % mean count rate of zero inhibition (reagent 2) (i.e., cpm standard 1 per mean count rate zero × 100). The standard % count rate is plotted vs. log IgE concentration, and the unknown serum concentrations are estimated from their % count rate and the standard curve. Due to serum factors that interfere with the radioimmunosorbent test, more correct serum concentrations are obtained if the % count rate of sera diluted 1:10 is multiplied by a correction factor of 0.96. If the serum is diluted 1:100 no correction factor is necessary.

An estimate of the quantity of reaginic **antibodies** in a patient's serum that are specific for an allergen can be made using the radioallergosorbent test (RAST, Pharmacia Fine Chemicals). The RAST kit contains rabbit ^{125}I–antihuman IgE (800 ng, 3.5 μCi), the allergen of interest covalently attached to paper disks, and 4 reference sera (approximately 1, 2, 10, and 50 U antibirch pollen antisera) with reference birch pollen paper disks. In the test the patient's serum is incubated with the allergen disk for 3 hours. The disk is then washed and incubated with the radiolabeled anti-IgE for 18 hours. Following a saline wash the disks are counted. A similar procedure is followed using the reference sera and reference disks. The counts per tube of the patient's sera are then compared with the counts per tube of the reference sera and ranked on a scale of 0-4. Variation in the quality of allergen preparations as well as the presence of interfering serum substances (e.g., blocking antibodies) prevent absolute quantitation of allergen-specific IgE at this time. For information on specific allergen paper disks consult the Pharmacia allergen list. Positive RAST scores (2-4) correlate well with in vivo and in vitro estimates of sensitivity (e.g., skin test, provocation test, leukocyte histamine release).[63-65] In addition the risk and inconvenience of in vivo testing are avoided with RAST.

CATABOLISM OF PROTEINS

Although a detailed method is given to measure rabbit immunoglobulins, the principles are the same for estimation of catabolic rate of albumin, transferrin, or any other protein.

Purification of IgG

The following combination of ammonium sulfate precipitation and DEAE chromatography has been found to yield pure IgG fractions from human, goat, bovine, and rabbit serum. Human immunoglobulin and albumin can be obtained from commercial sources.

To 10 ml rabbit serum at 25 C slowly add 4.9 ml saturated ammonium sulfate (767 g/L) with stirring. Centrifuge the mixture at $1000 \times g$ for 20 minutes and resuspend the precipitate in 10 ml distilled water. Dialyze the protein solution against two 1 L vol 0.02M phosphate, pH 7.2, at 4 C. Equilibrate 30 ml DEAE cellulose with 0.02M phosphate, pH 7.2, and apply the protein solution to the column. Under these conditions about 60% of the IgG is not absorbed and passes directly through the column. An estimate of the protein concentration can be obtained by measuring the absorbance at 280 nm ($\epsilon^{1\%} = 13.5$). These proteins can be obtained in pure form from several suppliers.

Radiolabeling of protein

A number of isotopes are commercially available for labeling proteins; however, the most widely used and the ones providing the highest specific activity (dpm/mol isotope) are ^{131}I ($T_{1/2} = 8.1$ days, β^- at 0.608 and 0.355 meV, γ at 0.364 and 0.638 meV) and ^{125}I ($T_{1/2} = 60$ days, γ at 0.035 meV). Although either isotope can be used, if there is to be considerable time between radiolabeling and analysis of the results the longer lived ^{125}I is preferred. There are a number of methods for covalent attachment of iodine to proteins, including iodine monochloride method[66] (problem of strong oxidizing conditions and hazardous gas

production); lactoperoxidase and H_2O_2 method[67] (problem of separating protein from enzyme); chloramine T method[68] (below); and the recent modification of the chloramine T procedure developed by Bolton and Hunter.[69] The basis for these methods is the production by an oxidizing agent of an iodine-free radical or cation, which then covalently bonds (oxidizes) to 1 of the electron-rich side chains of the protein (principally tyrosine, although phenylalanine, histidine, and tryptophan may also react).

Since conjugation of a large number of iodine atoms to a protein will produce functional and structural changes, the concentration of reagents should provide for the attachment of less than 1 mole iodine per mole protein. The specific activity of most commercial radioiodine preparations is from 5-25 Ci/mg ($\sim 10^{18}$ dpm/mol). Thus for a protein with molecular mass of 150,000 daltons, 4-20 mCi/mg protein would be sufficient. In the chloramine T method the following solutions are sequentially added to a 5 ml test tube at 4 C (ice bath) with stirring[70]:

1. 1 ml IgG (1-6 mg/ml) in 0.05M phosphate, pH 7.0
2. 100 μl ^{125}I (4-20 mCi/ml) in 0.05M phosphate, pH 7.0
3. 100 μl Chloramine T (2 mg/ml) in H_2O at 4 C

After 10 minutes the reaction is stopped by adding 100 μl sodium metabisulfite (2 mg/ml) in H_2O at 4 C.

The protein-bound radioactivity is then separated from free radioiodine by dialysis against phosphate buffer or by chromatography on Sephadex G-10 (a disposable 10 ml glass pipet plugged with glass wool is usually adequate). The percent protein-bound radioactivity should be greater than 90% and can be checked by precipitation in trichloroacetic acid (10 μl iodinated protein in 0.5 ml 0.1% BSA and 0.5 ml 12% trichloroacetic acid are mixed and centrifuged at $1000 \times g$ for 10 minutes; supernatant and precipitate are separated and counted). If the iodinated protein is to be injected into humans, special precautions are necessary. The isolated protein (or commercially acquired protein) should be rechromatographed on Sephadex G-200 equilibrated with pyrogen-free saline under sterile conditions. The resulting protein solution should then be checked for pyrogen and bacterial contamination.

Animal injection of protein

During the experiment animals are housed in metabolic cages and allowed free access to food and water containing 0.2% Lugol's solution (5 g I_2 and 10 g KI per 100 ml H_2O) 24 hours prior to injection. The amount of radioactivity injected depends on the size of the animal, the concentration of protein in the serum, and the $T_{1/2}$ of the protein. As an approximation, for a 4 kg rabbit (4% body weight = serum volume) and a protein with $T_{1/2}$ 6 days, 2×10^6 cpm iodinated protein is injected to have 2000 cpm/ml serum at the end of the tenth day.

The iodinated protein is dialyzed against phosphate-buffered saline and carefully injected into the venous system of a preweighed rabbit. The animal is first bled 10 minutes after injection and then at regular intervals until the serum cpm is less than 5% of the 10-minute value. The volume of blood removed should be small (<1% blood volume), or a correction factor for blood dilution must be introduced in calculating the % dose in serum. In addition to the blood samples the urine is collected every 24 hours. To avoid correcting for radioactive decay the serum and urine radioactivities in all samples should be counted within the same time interval at the end of the experiment. The cpm/ml serum and cpm/ml urine are used to calculate the % dose in serum and % dose excreted. Between 60-90% of the total dose should be recovered in the urine. The amount of protein-bound radioactivity in the serum can be measured by precipitation in 6% trichloroacetic acid. The serum value should be >90% after the first 24 hours, and the urine value should be <5% for proteins with molecular mass greater than 50,000 daltons.

Calculation of catabolic rate

After injection the radioiodinated protein rapidly equilibrates with the intravascular fluids (usually complete within 15 minutes), slowly equilibrates with the extravascular fluids (complete within 2-5 days), and is removed from the plasma by the normal catabolic process. In addition during the first 24 hours nonprotein-bound iodine and denatured protein are rapidly removed from the circulation. A number of mathematical models have been developed to describe the process of equilibration and catabolism (for a survey of methods see Donato et al.[71]). Discussion here is confined to the 2-compartment plasma curve method originally developed by Matthews.[72] The validity of this method is based on a number of assumptions: (1) that injection of the radiolabeled protein does not perturb the steady state synthesis and catabolism of the native protein, (2) that it is catabolized in a manner similar to that of the native protein, (3) that there is no reutilization of the radiolabel, (4) that the intravascular protein equilibrates with a single "generalized" extravascular compartment, and (5) that protein catabolism occurs only in the intravascular compartment. Thus at any given time following injection the concentration of protein in the plasma is proportional to the catabolic rate (k_1), the rate of intra- and extravascular equilibration (k_2), and the concentration of protein in the extravascular compartments. The intra- and extravascular protein concentrations are usually expressed as % dose. Thus the plasma % dose = $C_1 e^{-k_1 t} + C_2 e^{-k_2 t}$, where C_1 and C_2 refer to the % dose that would be in plasma and % dose that would be in the extravascular compartment, respectively, if the protein fully equilibrated with

Table 61-6. Calculation of catabolic rate of rabbit IgG in rabbit

	cp/ml Serum	Serum % dose*	$(C_1 e^{-k_1 t})$†	$(C_2 e^{-k_2 t})$‡§
10 min	38,460	100	35.0	65.0
12 h	25,630	66.6	33.1	33.5
24 h	18,750	48.7	31.4	17.3
72 h	10,200	26.5	25.3	1.2
120 h	7,800	20.3	20.3	—
168 h	6,300	16.3	16.3	—
240 h	4,500	11.8	11.8	—

*Following injection of 4.5 10⁶ cpm ¹²⁵I–rabbit IgG into 3 kg rabbit, 10 min value indicates serum vol 117 ml (3.9% body weight).
†k_1 = 0.0045 Corresponds to T½ 153 h or 6.37 d, C_1 = 35%.
‡k_2 = 0.055 Corresponds to T½ 12.6 h, C_2 = 65%.
§Calculated fractional catabolic rate for these data is 26.8%.

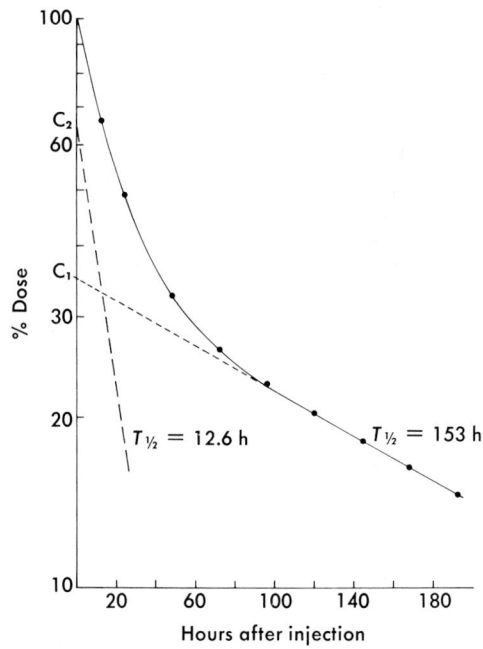

Fig. 61-7. Serum radioactivity following injection of ¹²⁵I–rabbit γG into 3.2 kg rabbit. (From Conway, T. P. Unpublished observations.)

these compartments at the time of injection $(t = 0)$. Obviously 100% = $C_1 + C_2$.

Total dose is calculated from protein solution cpm/ml and the volume injected. The volume may be calculated by weighing the syringe prior to and after injection.

Serum volume is calculated from the ratio of the 10-minute cpm/ml and the total dose.

Serum % dose is calculated by multiplying the cpm/ml serum at a given time by the serum volume and dividing by the total dose (Table 61-6).

A semilog plot of serum % dose vs. time should yield a curve similar to that in Fig. 61-7. As can be seen, after 80 hours the curve becomes linear; that is, the decrease in serum % dose is a function of catabolism only. Thus % dose = $C_1 e^{-k_1 t}$, or $\log_e$ % dose = $\log_e C_1 - k_1 t$. Least-squares analysis of $\log_e$ % dose vs. t will yield a zero time intercept, $\log_e C_1$, and slope k_1 (C_1 = 35% and k_1 = 0.0045/h for the data in Table 61-6 and Fig. 61-7). Sometimes the catabolic rate constant k_1 is expressed as a half-life ($t_{1/2} = 0.693/k_1$), which is the time required to reduce the serum % dose to half its initial value.

Since % dose = $C_1 e^{-k_1 t} + C_2 e^{-k_2 t}$, subtracting $C_1 e^{-k_2 t}$ from % dose yields $C_2 e^{-k_2 t}$ (e.g., in Table 61-6 at 24 hours % dose = 48.7%, C_1 = 35%, and $e^{-k_1 t} = e^{-0.0045(24)} = e^{-0.108} = 0.897$; thus $C_2 e^{-k_2 t} = 48.7\% - 35\% (0.897) = 17.3\%$). A semilog plot of $C_2 e^{-k_2 t}$ vs. time should yield a straight line (Fig. 61-7) with intercept $\log_e C_2$ and slope k_2. For the data in Table 61-6 C_2 = 65% and k_2 = 0.055/h.

Fractional catabolic rate (FCR), or the fraction of intravascular protein catabolized per day, can be calculated from the equation $FCR = (C_1/k_1 + C_2/k_2)^{-1}$, which takes into account the outflux (catabolism) and influx (transport of extravascular protein) into the serum. FCR may also be calculated from the urine data, where FCR is the % dose excreted in the urine over 24 hours divided by the mean serum % dose over the same period. The daily urine FCR values are usually averaged over 3-10 days and reported as the average fractional catabolic rate.

ACKNOWLEDGMENTS

We are indebted to Mrs. Colleen Collier for her unrelenting effort to expedite this manuscript. Supported in part by the National Institutes of Health grant AI-11335, Children's Leukemia Foundation of Michigan, and William Beaumont Hospital Research Institute, Royal Oak, Mich.

REFERENCES

1. Heidelberger, M., and Kendall, F. E.: J. Exp. Med. **55**:555, 1932.
2. Oudin, J.: Compt. Rendu **222**:115, 1946.
3. Ouchterlony, O. In Progress in allergy, vol. 5, 1958, and vol. 6, 1968, Basel, S. Karger.
4. Kraus, R.: Wien. Klin. Wochenschr. **10**:736, 1897.
5. Edelman, G. M., and Poulik, M. D.: J. Exp. Med. **113**:861, 1961.
6. Edelman, G. M.: Biochemistry **9**:3197, 1970.
7. Gally, J. In Sela, M., editor: The antigens, vol. 1, New York, 1973, Academic Press.
8. Mancini, G., Carbonara, A. O., and Heremans, J. F.: Immunochemistry **2**:235, 1965.
9. Fahey, J. L., and McKelvey, E. M.: J. Immunol. **94**:84, 1965.
10. Laurell, C.-B.: Scand. J. Clin. Lab. Invest. **29**(suppl. 124):21, 1972.
11. Ritchie, R. F. In Peeters, H., editor: Protides of biological fluids, 21st Colloquium, Brugge, 1973, New York, 1974, Pergamon Press.
12. Axelsen, N. H., Kröll, J., and Weeke, B.: Scand. J. Immunol. **2**(suppl.):1, 1973.
13. Rowe, D. S., Anderson, S. G., and Grab, B.: Bull. WHO **42**:535, 1970.
14. WHO Expert Committee on Biological Standardization, 23rd report: WHO Tech. Rep. Ser. **463**:20, 1971.
15. Humphrey, J. H., and Batty, I.: Clin. Exp. Immunol. **17**:708, 1974.
16. Reimer, C. B., and Maddison, S. E.: Clin. Chem. **22**:577, 1976.
17. Rowe, D. S.: Bull. WHO **40**:613, 1969.
18. Rowe, D. S., and Wood, C. B. S.: Int. Arch. Allergy Appl. Immunol. **39**:1, 1970.
19. Cejka, J., Cohen, F., and Kithier, K.: Clin. Chim. Acta **47**:59, 1973.
20. Avrameas, S., and Ternynck, T.: Immunochemistry **8**:1175, 1971.
21. Daniels, J. C., Vyvial, T. M., Levin, W. C., et al. Clin. Chem. **21**:243, 1975.
22. Schultze, H. E., and Schwick, G.: Clin. Chim. Acta **4**:15, 1959.
23. Ritchie, R. F.: J. Lab. Clin. Med. **70**:512, 1967.
24. Alper, C. A., and Propp, R. P.: J. Clin. Invest. **47**:2181, 1968.
25. Ritchie, R. F., Alper, C. A., and Graves, J. A.: Arthritis Rheum. **12**:693, 1970.
26. Rose, N. R., and Friedman, H.: Manual of clinical immunology, Washington, D.C., 1976, American Society for Microbiology, p. 8.
27. Hellsing, K. In A.I.P.: New methods, techniques and evaluations, Colloquium on A.I.P., Brussels, 1972, Tarrytown, N.Y., Technicon Corp.
28. Poulik, M. D.: Can. J. Med. Sci. **30**:417, 1952.
29. Grabar, P., and Williams, C. A., Jr.: Biochem. Biophys. Acta **10**:193, 1953.
30. Williams, C. A., Jr., and Grabar, P.: J. Immunol. **74**:397, 1955.
31. Scheidegger, J. J.: Int. Arch. Allergy Appl. Immunol. **7**:103, 1955.
32. Poulik, M. D.: J. Immunol. **82**:502, 1959.
33. Laurell, C.-B.: Anal. Biochem. **15**:45, 1966.
34. Nerenberg, S. T.: Electrophoresis, Philadelphia, 1966, F. A. Davis Co., p. 184.
35. Arquembourg, P. C.: Immunoelectrophoresis, Basel, 1975, S. Karger.
36. Ritzman, S. E., and Daniels, J. C.: Serum protein abnormalities: diagnostic and clinical aspects, Boston, 1975, Little, Brown & Co., p. 351.
37. Kyle, R. A. In Rose, N. R., and Friedman, H.: Manual of clinical immunology, Washington, D.C., 1976, American Society for Microbiology, p. 734.
38. Immunoglobulin abnormality detection by immunoelectrophoresis, brochure AR710, Bedford, Mass., 1974, Millipore Corp.
39. Laboratory notes, no. 3, Somerville, N.J., 1973, Behring Diagnostics.
40. Weeke, B.: Scand. J. Lab. Invest. **22**:107, 1968.
41. Laurell, C.-B.: Anal. Biochem. **10**:358, 1965.
42. Clarke, M.H.G., and Freeman, T.: Clin. Sci. **35**:403, 1968.
43. Kröll, J.: Scand. J. Clin. Lab. Invest. **24**:55, 1969.
44. Svedsen, P. J., and Axelsen, N. H.: J. Immunol. Methods **1**:169, 1972.
45. Axelsen, N. H., editor: Scand. J. Immunol. (suppl. 1), 1975.
46. Rose, N. R., and Bigazzi, P. E.: Methods in immunodiagnosis, New York, 1973, John Wiley & Sons, p. 19.
47. Hansson, B. G., Kindmark, C. O., and Johnsson, T.: Vox Sang. **19**:225, 1970.
48. Prince, A. M., and Burke, K.: Science **169**:593, 1970.
49. Dorf, G. J., Coonrod, J. D., and Rytel, M. W.: Arch. Int. Med. **132**:699, 1973.
50. Edwards, E. A.: J. Immunol. **106**:314, 1971.
51. Remington, J. S., Gaines, J. D., and Gilmer, M. A.: Lancet **1**:413, 1972.

52. Dee, T. H., and Rytel, M. W.: J. Lab. Clin. Med. **85:**161, 1975.
53. Williams, A. C., Jr., and Chase, M. E., editors: Methods in immunology and immunochemistry, vol. 3, New York, 1971, Academic Press.
54. Bennich, H., and Johansson, S. G. O., editors: Advances in immunology, vol. 13, New York, 1971, Academic Press.
55. Ishizaka, K., Ishizaka, T., and Hornbrook, M. M.: J. Immunol. **97:**75, 1966.
56. Ishizaka, K., and Ishizaka, T.: J. Immunol. **101:**68, 1968.
57. Ishizaka, K., and Ishizaka, T.: Clin. Allergy **1:**9, 1971.
58. Nye, L., Merrett, T. G., Landon, J., et al.: Clin. Allergy **1:**13, 1975.
59. Berg, T., and Johansson, S. G. O.: Int. Arch. Allergy **36:**219, 1969.
60. Hamburger, R. A., Lenoin, M., Groshong, T. E., et al.: J. Allergy Clin. Immunol. **53:**94, 1974.
61. Berg, T., and Johansson, S. G. O.: Int. Arch. Allergy Appl. Immunol. **41:**452, 1971.
62. Johansson, S. G. O., Melbin, T., and Vahlquist, B.: Lancet **1:**1118, 1968.
63. Foucard, T.: Int. Arch. Allergy Appl. Immunol. **42:**711, 1972.
64. Berg, T., Bennich, H., and Johansson, S. G. O.: Int. Arch. Allergy Appl. Immunol. **40:**770, 1974.
65. Lichtenstein, L. M., Ishizaka, K., Norman, P. S., et al.: J. Clin. Invest. **52:**472, 1973.
66. McFarlane, A. S.: Biochem. J. **62:**135, 1956.
67. Marchalonis, J. J.: Biochem. J. **113:**299, 1969.
68. Greenwood, F. C., Hunter, W. M., and Glover, J. S.: Biochem. J. **89:**114, 1963.
69. Bolton, A. E., and Hunter, W. M.: Biochem. J. **133:**529, 1973.
70. McConahey, P. J., and Dixon, F. J.: Int. Arch. Allergy Appl. Immunol. **29:**185, 1966.
71. Donato, L., Matthews, C. M. E., Nosslin, B., et al.: J. Nucl. Biol. Med. **10:**3, 1966.
72. Matthews, C. M. E.: Phys. Med. Biol. **2:**36, 1957.

62

COMPLEMENT

Lisbeth A. Suyehira
Henry Gewurz

Complement consists of a group of proteins acting in sequence that mediates reactions of host defense and inflammation. Most of the current knowledge of the complement system is derived from studies involving its ability to lyse sheep erythrocytes coated with antibody.[1-3]

PRIMARY COMPLEMENT PATHWAY

The 11 complement proteins involved in mediating such antibody-initiated hemolysis are the primary (or classic) complement pathway components or subcomponents. They are designated numerically in order of their reaction sequence with 2 exceptions. After its discovery C1 was found to be a macromolecular complex consisting of C1q, C1r, and C1s (C1 esterase) linked by calcium, and the fourth component discovered was later found to be the second to react in the hemolytic sequence but retains its original designation as C4. The reaction sequence is shown in Fig. 62-1. The activated components are designated by an overlying bar and cleavage products by lower case letters.

The primary complement pathway consists of recognition (C1q, C1r, C1s), activation (C4, C2, C3), and attack (C5, C6, C7, C8, C9) mechanisms with respect to its role in antibody-mediated cytolysis.[1] C1 is activated when C1q binds to the Fc portion of antibody (e.g., hemolysin bound to the sheep erythrocyte). Human IgG1, IgG2, IgG3, and IgM, altered either by aggregation or by complexing to antigen, are capable of activating the primary complement pathway by binding C1q.

C$\overline{1}$, via its esterolytic activity, cleaves C4 into 2 fragments, the larger of which (C4b) can bind to the cell surface. C$\overline{1}$ also cleaves C2 into 2 fragments, the larger of which (C2a) can bind to C4b to form a C3 convertase (C4b2a), which is capable of activating C3. C4a and C2b are released into the "fluid phase" as hemolytically inactive fragments whose biologic properties are unknown.

C3 activation involves cleavage by C3 convertase into C3a and C3b; C3b can bind to the cell surface and form the C4b2a3b enzyme, which is capable of cleaving C5 into C5a and C5b. The latter initiates the assembly of the membrane "attack" mechanism by a nonenzymatic absorptive process. C5b may attach to the same cell containing previously activated components or to different cells to initiate "bystander" lysis on binding of later acting components. Each C567 complex on the cell surface binds 1 C8 molecule, which in turn binds up to 6 C9 molecules to produce membrane damage and cytolysis.

ALTERNATIVE COMPLEMENT PATHWAY

An alternative method of complement activation, originally described as the properdin pathway, is capable of initiating the reaction sequence at C3 independent of C1, C4, and C2.[4,5] It involves at least 4 additional proteins, termed initiating factor (IF), factor D, factor B (C3 proactivator), and properdin, in addition to C3 and C3b. This pathway is illustrated in Fig. 63-1.

The alternative pathway may be activated by certain immunoglobulin molecules including classes not generally involved in C1 activation (IgG4, IgA, and IgE) as well as by mechanisms that seem to operate independently of antibody and can initiate all of the known functions attributed to the C3–C9 components.

CONSEQUENCES AND INHIBITORS OF COMPLEMENT ACTIVATION

Activation of the complement system by either pathway results in reactions in addition to cytolysis that contribute to the inflammatory process. C3a and C5a have anaphylatoxic and neutrophil chemotactic activity. Cell-bound C4b and C3b each mediate attachment to B-lymphocytes and (along with C5b) opsonization for phagocytosis. C567 also has neutrophil chemotactic activity, and the C5–9 complex mediates bacterial growth inhibition and cytolysis.

Activation of the complement system is modulated by the lability or short half-life of certain components and intermediates as well as by several protein inhibitors. The first discovered and the most important diagnostically is the C1 esterase inhibitor (C$\overline{1}$-INH), which among its

Revised from Lab. Med. 8(8):29-34, 1977.

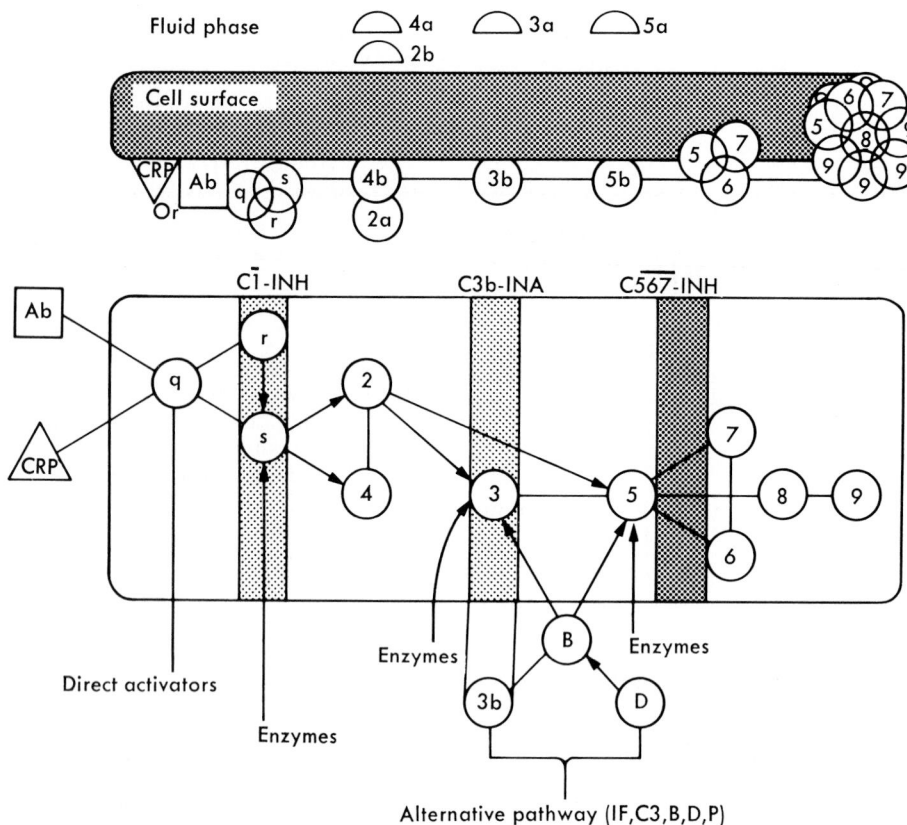

Fig. 62-1. Diagram of primary complement pathway *(enclosed in rectangle)* showing alternative (properdin) pathway and additional modes of complement activation. Enzymatic cleavages are represented by *arrows,* and inhibitory activities are shown by *shading.* Interactions of complement components at cell surface *(stipple)* and cleavage products released into fluid phase are shown at top.

functions inhibits the activation of C4 and C2 by C$\bar{1}$s.

An inborn deficiency or functional abnormality of this protein has been associated with hereditary angioneurotic edema (HAE). The C3b inactivator (C3b-INA) cleaves (and thus inactivates) C3b in the fluid phase and on the cell surface into C3d and C3c. Its deficiency has now been reported in 2 patients with repeated infections; both had severely decreased C3 levels associated with hypercatabolism of C3 and C3b deposition on bystander cells.

Another molecule termed B_1 H, which modulates the function of C3b, and an inactivator of the C3a and C5a anaphylatoxins (the anaphylatoxin inhibitor) have been defined and inhibitors of C5, C6, C7, and C$\overline{567}$ have been described, but deficiencies or clinical associations of these factors have not yet been reported.

LABORATORY ASSAYS OF COMPLEMENT SYSTEM

In sample collection, if serum is used, blood should be clotted for 15-30 minutes at room temperature and 30-60 minutes at 4 C and stored refrigerated until assayed the same day or at −70 C if prolonged storage is necessary.

Total hemolytic complement

Standard assays for complement activity measure the ability of the primary complement pathway to lyse sheep erythrocytes sensitized with optimal amounts of antierythrocyte antibodies (ShEA). Since each of the 11 proteins of the pathway are required for hemolysis, it remains the functional assay of greatest value.

Qualitative screen[6]

Measurement of hemolytic complement activity in plates containing agarose and sensitized sheep cells is valuable to screen rapidly (1 hour) a large number of specimens for inborn or acquired deficiencies. Serum diffuses radially from wells placed in the agarose to produce a ring of lysis approximately proportional to the amount of complement present. Lysis is scored as **normal, low,** or **absent** based on comparison with the activity of normal serum.

Laboratories with access to fresh sheep erythrocytes can inexpensively prepare a large number of plates that should be stable at 4 C for up to 4 weeks. Alternatively test kits for similar assays are available commercially. Each laboratory should establish the normal range for its individual technic before routine clinical use. Those

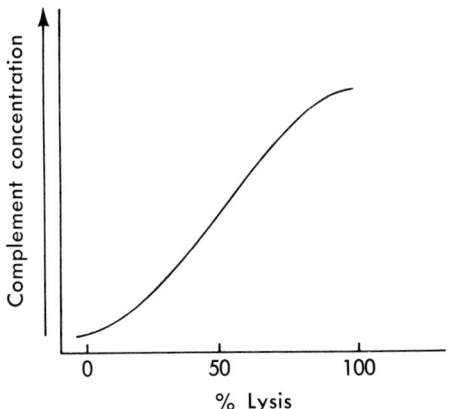

Fig. 62-2. Schema of relationship between complement concentration and percent lysis.

samples giving low or no lysis can be redrawn or retested using a more sensitive and quantitative assay as well as measuring C3, C4, and other complement components by single radial immunodiffusion. Rabbit erythrocytes can be used to prepare plates to screen similarly for the hemolytic capacity of the alternative pathway.

Quantitative assay

The quantitative CH_{50} hemolytic complement assay remains the definitive method for confirming decreased complement levels because of its greater sensitivity and the existence of occasional patients with decreased lysis on the screen plate with a normal CH_{50} level.

The relationship between complement activity present in and the proportion of cells lysed by a given dilution of serum is illustrated in Fig. 62-2. The curve is steepest in the central area of 50% lysis where the degree of lysis is most sensitive to small changes in the amount of complement present. Therefore determination of the amount (serum dilution) of complement necessary to lyse 50% of the cells present provides the most precise estimation of complement activity; this is termed the 50% hemolytic unit of complement or the CH_{50}.

It is important to remember that CH_{50} units are dependent on the cell concentration and fragility, quantity, and quality of antibody used for sensitization, ionic strength, Mg^{++} and Ca^{++} concentration and pH of the assay system, reaction volume, and time and temperature of incubation.

The method most commonly used is that of Mayer.[7] The CH_{50} assay, although quantitative, is insensitive to depletions of up to 50-80% of normal levels of individual components and fails to detect depletions of most of the alternative pathway factors. Thus in certain situations it is valuable to perform specific component assays.

COMPLEMENT PROTEINS

With the isolation and characterization of the complement proteins, immunochemical technics

such as single radial immunodiffusion (RID), in which monospecific antisera to individual components are used, have become the most widely applicable means of assaying complement levels. Application of single RID to component analysis has allowed quantitation by absolute weight rather than arbitrary relative units and offered a markedly increased ease of performance, a high degree of reproducibility, less rigid requirements for serum collection and storage, and easy adaptability into existing laboratory routine.

The advent of commercially available RID plates and antisera has placed the area of component analysis within the reach of any clinical laboratory. C3 and C4 are the components most routinely assayed, although antisera to C1q, C1s, C5, C6, C9, properdin, and factor B are also available. Methods for preparing plates and reference standards are detailed elsewhere.[6]

There are several disadvantages to the RID method of component analysis. Intervals of 24-48 hours are required for the reactions to reach completion. This prolonged incubation time may favor the appearance of falsely elevated serum values when cleaved complement components are present. This also increases the potential for interaction between the agarose and test serum, favoring the possibility that such cleavage products might be formed. It can be minimized by use of EDTA plasma. When routine complement assays are performed infrequently, the time it takes for laboratory results to reach the physician is further increased.

Alternatives to analysis by RID include electroimmunodiffusion by the Laurell technic, an automated, continuous-flow, immunoprecipitation nephelometric method, and most recently an immunoprecipitation method involving laser nephelometry. These newer methodologies offer a sensitivity and turn-around time unequaled by conventional RID assays but involve an additional monetary investment and increased technician time.

Each laboratory must determine the assay system(s) most suitable to its individual application and workload.

OTHER ASSAYS OF COMPLEMENT FUNCTION
C1̄-INH

Antiserum is available to C1-INH, and the inhibitor can be assayed by RID or nephelometric technics. Certain patients, however, may possess normal levels antigenically but decreased levels by functional assay. The definitive titration involves measuring the inhibitory effect of C1̄-INH on C1̄s using the synthetic substrate acetyl-L-tyrosine ethyl ester (ALTEe).

Hemolytic component titrations

Complement components can be assayed hemolytically, either individually or in groups, using sensitized sheep erythrocytes and an excess of other components. The serum in question is tested for the ability to provide the missing component(s) and induce lysis of the reagent erythrocytes. Because of the more complicated nature of these assays and the reagents involved, they mainly are used clinically to detect inborn deficiencies of complement components that cannot be measured by routine laboratory methods and to evaluate presence of complement function as well as protein.

Yeast phagocytosis

An abnormality of C5 manifested by a normal level of C5 protein and hemolytic activity but a decreased ability to opsonize yeast particles for phagocytosis is characteristic of a severe form of Leiner's disease.

In vivo C3 conversion

C3 fragments produced by in vivo conversion can be assayed by methods measuring either changed electrophoretic mobility of C3 or specific antisera to the fragments. These include immunoelectrophoresis, counterimmunoelectrophoresis, and RID with monospecific antisera.

Immunofluorescence

Tissue deposition of complement components can be detected using direct immunofluorescent technics with monospecific antiserum to complement components.

Circulating immune complexes

Because of their frequent association with perturbations of C levels, often it is of value to assay for immune complexes in association with a complete evaluation of the C system. Circulating immune complexes have been described in a variety of diseases including systemic lupus erythematosus (SLE), rheumatoid arthritis (RA), hepatitis, glomerulonephritis, monoclonal gammopathies, and cryoglobulinemia.

COMPLEMENT AS A DIAGNOSTIC AID

Complement levels fluctuate in a variety of disease processes. The most frequently occurring alterations of complement are increased levels, since most components respond as acute-phase reactants. However, the main clinical application of complement assays is the detection of individuals with decreased levels to determine the presence, extent, and possible consequences of an ongoing immune process and when found to serve as an index of therapeutic response. Because of the variation of complement levels during the course of a given disease in a given patient, results must be interpreted in conjunction with other clinical and laboratory parameters as aids to suggesting and confirming diagnoses.

Fig. 62-3 illustrates the autoimmune disease profile instituted by our laboratory in 1972. Samples are routinely screened for acute-phase changes by measurement of the C-reactive protein (CRP) level and Westergren erythrocyte sedimentation rate (ESR). Protein analysis by agarose serum protein electrophoresis (SPE) helps detect polyclonal and monoclonal dysgammaglobulinemic states, acute inflammatory reactions, patterns associated with liver disorders, and so on. The use of rat polysubstrate (stomach, kidney, liver) makes possible the detection of antinuclear antibodies (ANA) as well as antibodies to mitochondria, smooth muscle, and

---

☐ Autoimmune disease profile (acute phase reactants, autoantibodies, protein analysis, complement
☐ Complement profile (all complement assays)   screens, C4, C3)
☐ Autoimmune—complement profile

Acute phase reactants

ESR (Westergren) _____

CRP _____   N = <5 μg/ml

Protein analysis

SPE _____

Autoantibodies

RF FII (latex) _____   N = <1:40 | If indicated:
                                          RF sheep cell _____   N = <1:20

Immunofluorescent analysis: ANA dil: 1:100 _____

ANA (1:20) _____   1:500 _____

Anti-smooth muscle _____   Anti-DNA RIA _____   N = <10%

Anti-mitochondrial _____   Anti-DNA HA _____   N = <1:10

Anti-parietal cell _____   Anti-ENA HA _____   N = <1:100

Other _____

Complement   Hemolytic C (quant) _____   N = 20-40 U/ml

                                         C1q _____   N = 100-210 μg/ml

                                         C5 _____   N = 70-170 μg/ml

Hemolytic C (screen) _____   Properdin _____   N = 10-20 μg/ml

Alternate pathway C (screen) _____ C3PA _____   N = 175-275 μg/ml

C4 _____   N = 200-800 μg/ml   Other _____

C3 _____   N = 800-1800 μg/ml

Fig. 62-3. Autoimmune (collagen) disease profile with basic profile tests *(left)* and follow-up tests *(right)*.

parietal cells by indirect immunofluorescent technics. Sera with demonstrable ANA are screened for anti–double stranded DNA or ENA antibodies, which if present are quantified. Rheumatoid factors are screened by agglutination of IgG-coated latex particles and when present quantified using both these particles and the Waaler-Rose sheep cell agglutination test (SCAT).

Serum samples are screened for classic and alternative hemolytic complement activity, C4, and C3. Samples giving decreased results are tested for C1q, C5, properdin, and factor B proteins and CH_{50} activity. A simplified guide for interpretation of results obtained using this screening procedure is illustrated in Table 62-1.

Complement decreases usually occur because of increased utilization in vivo, decreased synthesis in vivo, or increased conversion in vitro. The first category includes patients with immune-mediated diseases. Immune or inflammatory reactions that consume complement efficiently in vitro result in decreased in vivo complement levels only when utilization is sufficiently intense to overcome the increased synthesis of complement also associated with inflammation; thus patients with both increased utilization and increased synthesis may have normal complement levels.

Complement-consuming processes that result in decreased levels regularly are seen in SLE, acute poststreptococcal glomerulonephritis (AGN), and membranoproliferative glomerulonephritis (MPGN). A characteristic alteration of the component level may be seen in a given disease. Thus active SLE usually causes depressions in C1q, C4, and C3, while in AGN and MPGN often only C3 (of these components) is decreased. Component changes also may reflect superimposed immunopathogenic processes; for example, C1q and C4 often are decreased in association with cryglobulinemia.

Localized rather than systemic complement activation often results in normal or elevated complement levels. Patients with rheumatoid arthritis (RA) usually show normal to increased serum complement levels, while levels of C in the synovial fluid characteristically are low, indicating local activation; however, decreased serum levels (C1q, C4, C3, and total complement) are seen in about 10% of patients with RA who generally have a severe form of the disease.

The second category (decreased synthesis) includes a surprisingly large number of complement deficiencies that have been defined and are briefly summarized in Table 62-2. For example, our laboratory has detected 8 families in which the propositus has lacked complement activity on a genetic basis, involving deficiencies of C1r, C2 (4 patients), C3, C6, and C7 (2 patients), respectively. These individuals frequently exhibit unexplained or unusual responses to infections or an autoimmune "collagen" disease such as SLE. Decreased synthesis of a complement component also occurs on an acquired and transitory basis in certain diseases such as AGN and MPGN associated with complement-consuming processes.

Patients in both categories frequently exhibit a distinctive complement "profile" where total hemolytic complement activity is **greatly** de-

Table 62-1. General guide to evaluation of C4 and C3 protein levels in presence of decreased hemolytic complement activity

	Normal C4	Decreased C4
Normal C3	Alterations in vitro (e.g., improper specimen handling)	Immune complex disease
		Hypergammaglobulinemic states
	Coagulation-associated complement consumption	Cryoglobulinemia
		Hereditary angioedema
	Inborn errors (other than C4 or C3)	Inborn C4 deficiency
Decreased C3	Acute glomerulonephritis	Active SLE
		Serum sickness
	Membranoproliferative glomerulonephritis	Chronic active hepatitis
	Immune complex disease	Subacute bacterial endocarditis
	Active SLE	Immune complex disease
	Inborn C3 deficiency	

Table 62-2. Summary of complement deficiencies in man and their association with repeated infection and/or collagen disease

Deficient component	No. of patients	Disease/symtoms
C1r	4	SLE (1), renal disease (1), repeated infections (1)
C1s	2	SLE (2)
C4	3	SLE (3)
C2	23	LE (7), vasculitis (3), MPGN (1), dermatomyositis (1)
C3	4	Repeated infections (3), fever/rash/arthralgias (1)
C5	3	SLE (1), gonococcal disease
C6	5	Relapsing meningococcal meningitis (4), gonococcal disease (1)
C7	5	Raynaud's disease (1), chronic renal disease (1), gonococcal disease (2), SLE (1)
C8	3	SLE (1), gonococcal disease (1)

pressed or absent, while the protein level of only a single component is depleted. This diagnosis must be established with care, since complement-consuming processes occur with increased frequency in patients with inborn deficiencies.

Complement depressions that occur in vitro (the third category) also tend to be associated with characteristic alterations of the complement profile where the total hemolytic complement activity is usually depressed with normal protein levels of the components tested. These changes may occur from simple "aging" or improper handling of specimens, as in exposure to heat, but also may occur in properly handled specimens when complement-consuming activity (HAE, cryoglobulinemia, certain immune complex diseases) or a recently recognized coagulation-associated complement-consuming process is present.

REFERENCES

1. Muller-Eberhard, J. J.: The molecular basis of the biologic activities of complement. In The Harvey lectures, 1970-71. New York, 1972, Academic Press, pp. 75-104.
2. Ruddy, S., Gigli, I., and Austen, K. F.: The complement system of man, N. Engl. J. Med. **287:**489-494, 545-549, 592-596, 642-646, 1972.
3. Muller-Eberhard, H. J.: Complement, Ann. Rev. Biochem. **44:**697-724, 1975.
4. Gotze, O., and Muller-Eberhard, H. J.: The alternative pathway of complement activation. In Dixon, F. J., and Kunkel, H. G., editors: Advances in immunology, New York, 1976, Academic Press, pp. 1-35.
5. Gewurz, H., and Lint, T. F.: Alternative modes and pathways of complement activation. In Day, N. K., and Good, R. A., editors: Biological amplification systems in immunity, New York, 1977, Plenum Press, pp. 17-45.
6. Gewurz, H., and Suyehira, L. A.: Complement. In Rose, N. R., and Friedman, H., editors: Manual of clinical immunology, Washington, D.C., 1976, American Society for Microbiology, pp. 36-47.
7. Mayer, M. M.: Complement and complement fixation. In Kabat, E. A., editor: Experimental immunochemistry, ed. 2, Springfield, Ill., 1971, Charles C Thomas, Publisher, pp. 133-240.

63

CELL-MEDIATED IMMUNOLOGIC RESPONSES

Flossie Cohen

It is well established that the immune response against foreign stimuli may be humoral or cellular. Evidence for these 2 components of the immune response has been derived from observations in humans with various immunodeficiency diseases and from observations in lower animals subject to ablation studies. Humoral immunity to a specific stimulus can be passively transferred to a nonsensitized subject by serum obtained from a sensitized donor, whereas cell-mediated immunity is not transferred by the serum of sensitized individuals but by the living lymphocytes washed free of surrounding serum.[1] Both humoral and cellular immunity are mediated by lymphocytes, a heterogenous population of cells that may be broadly divided into 2 categories, B-lymphocytes and T-lymphocytes, characterized by different surface markers and functions.

B-lymphocytes (bursa derived) arise from precursor stem cells following their passage through the bursa of Fabricius in the chicken or an equivalent (not yet identified) organ in humans. They mediate humoral immunity and differentiate into plasma cells that secrete specific antibody molecules in response to specific stimuli.

T-lymphocytes (thymus dependent) are also derived from precursor stem cells following their passage through the thymus gland. They mediate cellular immunity either directly or by pharmacologically active lymphokines secreted in response to specific stimuli.

In this chapter measurements of various in vivo and in vitro cell-mediated immunologic responses applicable in clinical medicine are described.

ABSOLUTE NUMBER OF CIRCULATING LYMPHOCYTES

Lymphopenia is a frequent finding in several of the immunodeficiency diseases. An absolute lymphocyte count of 1000-1500/mm³ or greater is normal for both adults and children. Counts below 1000/mm³ are distinctly lymphopenic for any age.

IN VIVO SKIN TESTS

Cutaneous delayed hypersensitivity response is now recognized as an in vivo measure of cell-mediated immunity that constitutes the primary mode of defense against a variety of bacterial, viral, fungal, and protozoan infections as well as heterologous protein, tumor-specific, transplantation, autologous, and other antigens. In general protein rather than polysaccharide antigens induce a delayed hypersensitivity response. The antigen injected intradermally stimulates circulating sensitized T-lymphocytes to undergo blastlike transformation and proliferation. The transformed cells liberate a variety of mediators that attract other cells, primarily monocytes and macrophages but also polymorphonuclear leukocytes (PMNL), eosinophils, and basophils. A positive response is manifested by a complex of factors: lymphocyte-macrophage interaction, nonspecific inflammatory reaction, clotting factors, and the condition of the blood vessels. A positive response is interpreted to indicate intact cellular immunity and successful primary immunization of the individual by the specific antigen. Interpretation of a negative response, on the other hand, may be quite troublesome, since in many instances it may be the result of a lack of previous exposure to the antigen rather than to an impaired cell-mediated immunity, often the case in young pediatric patients.

Cutaneous delayed hypersensitivity testing with microbial antigens

Method. Skin testing is performed as follows. The volar surface of the forearm is cleansed with alcohol, and 0.1 ml antigen contained in a 1 ml tuberculin syringe is injected intradermally through a 26- or 27-gauge hypodermic needle. The bevel of the needle should be directed upward so that the antigen raises a wheal in the skin.

Induration of 5 mm diameter with or without erythema is considered a positive response. However, induration of less than 5 mm, while not a standard positive reaction, is not a totally negative reaction, and the dimension of such a minimal response should be recorded. The injection site should be observed several times during the first 48 hours. An immediate hypersensitivity response in the form of a wheal and flare may appear 15-30 minutes after the antigen is injected intradermally. Induration and erythema 8-10 hours after injection usually indicates an Arthus response resulting from the combination of circulating IgG antibody and the antigen in the vessel wall. This activates the complement system, causing the release of chemotactic factors that attract polymorphonuclear leukocytes, which in turn release enzymes causing tissue damage and the resulting erythema and induration. This antibody response may at times persist and may be misinterpreted for a delayed-type hypersensitivity (DTH) or cell-mediated response at 48 hours. In such situations a biopsy may be necessary to differentiate between the 2 reactions. The Arthus phenomenon typically consists of a PMNL response, whereas DTH has perivascular infiltrates of mononuclear cells, lymphocytes and monocytes, in the deeper part of the dermis.

The following are some of the common microbial antigens used to measure delayed hypersensitivity response:

1. *Candida albicans* extract 1:100 (Dermatophytin "0," Hollister-Stier Laboratories, Spokane, Wash.)
2. Streptokinase/streptodornase (SK/SD), 100 units SK, 25 units SD, in 0.1 ml (Varidase, Lederle Laboratories, Pearl River, N.Y.)
3. Histoplasmin 1:100 (Parke, Davis & Co., Detroit)
4. Mumps skin test antigen (Eli Lilly & Co., Indianapolis)
5. Coccidiodin 1:100 (Cutter Laboratories, Berkeley, Calif.)
6. Intermediate-strength purified protein derivative of tuberculin (0.0002 mg PPD) (Parke, Davis & Co., Detroit)

Contact sensitization with DNCB

1-Chloro-2,4-dinitrobenzene (DNCB) is a chemical used in the photographic industry (Eastman Kodak Co., Rochester, N.Y.). It is a hapten and combines with the lysine groups of epidermal proteins to sensitize the individual. Retesting with a challenge dose 14-21 days after the initial application produces DTH. This test is a useful measure of cellular immunity, since 85-95% of adults and children can be sensitized with it, eliminating any conjecture regarding previous exposure to a particular microbial antigen when there is failure to respond.

Method. Following the suggestion of Catalona et al.[2] 2000 μg DNCB in 0.1 ml acetone "sensitizing" dose is applied within a stainless steel ring 2 cm in diameter held on the volar aspect of the arm previously cleansed with acetone. This is dried rapidly with a hair dryer. At the same time a weaker "challenge" dose of 50 μg DNCB is similarly applied within a ring 2 cm in diameter

held on the precleaned volar surface of the forearm. The smaller "challenge" detects the presence or absence of previous sensitization to DNCB. The sites are covered lightly with adhesive bandages and should not be washed for 24 hours. Varying degrees of erythema and vesiculation are seen at the site of the sensitizing dose within the first 24-48 hours. Seven to 14 days after the initial application a spontaneous flare consisting of erythema and induration may be seen. This is interpreted as evidence of successful sensitization and a subsequent delayed skin hypersensitivity response effected by sensitized lymphocytes and residual antigen at the site. If this reaction is seen at both the sensitizing and the challenge site the reaction is graded as 4+. If the reaction is only at the sensitizing site the reaction is graded as 3+. In the absence of spontaneous "flare" at either site a "rechallenge" dose of 50 μg is applied; this should elicit a positive DTH response at 48 hours, and the response is graded as 2+. An equivocal response should be biopsied, and if microscopic evidence for a DTH response is found (lymphocytes, histocytes, and other cells characteristic of chronic inflammation) the response is graded as 1+.

PHA skin test (purified phytohemagglutinin)

Even though the cellular response elicited by PHA skin test (Burroughs Wellcome, Research Triangle Park, N.C.) resembles a delayed hypersensitivity reaction, it has not often been accepted as a standard measure of cellular immunity. However, several investigators[3-7] have used it to measure the individual's ability to call forth inflammatory cells in response to local stimulation of lymphocytes by the mitogen, which suggests some relationship to cellular immunity.

PHA is a potent nonspecific stimulant of the majority of lymphocytes in a given population and might be expected to elicit a more rapid response under normal conditions than the microbial antigens and a positive response when only a few immunocompetent cells are inadequate to manifest a cutaneous response to specific antigens. The response increases in intensity from infancy to adulthood.

The test is performed like the other DTH tests for microbial antigens, with 0.1 ml containing 2 μg PHA injected intradermally into the volar aspect of the forearm. The test is read at the end of 24-48 hours and, as in the other DTH responses, the extent of induration and erythema are measured. The response is generally greatest at 24 hours and disappears by 72 hours. Erythematous reactions less than 11 mm in adults and less than 4 mm in infants have been considered abnormal.[7] If 2 μg PHA fails to stimulate a response, 5 or 10 μg may be tried.

While the in vivo skin response generally parallels the in vitro response of the lymphocytes stimulated with PHA, discord results from the effect of the factors mediated by stimulated lymphocytes being greater in the in vivo environment than in the in vitro environment. Thus a positive skin test and negative in vitro blastogenesis may indicate adequate mediator release in vivo despite lack of blastogenesis in vitro. Similarly a negative skin test and a positive in vitro blastogenesis may in part be presumed to result from lack of certain mediators in vivo (e.g., lack of migration inhibition factor [MIF] in some patients with chronic mucocutaneous candidiasis but with normal in vitro blastogenesis of their lymphocytes).

SEPARATION OF LEUKOCYTES

To estimate the number and to evaluate the function of T- and B-lymphocytes it is advantageous to separate the lymphocytes from the other blood cells. In general, however, the more complex the procedure to obtain a "pure" population of lymphocytes the greater the loss of lymphocytes and their minor subpopulations and the greater the variance between the in vitro and in vivo immunologic responses of these cells.

A variety of methods have been used to separate lymphocytes: cotton wool filtration,[8-10] magnetic technics utilizing the phagocytic ability of polymorphonuclear leukocytes and monocytes for iron fillings,[11] technics utilizing the adhesive properties of PMNL and monocytes to glass wool[12] or glass beads,[13,14] and gravitational technics.[15,16]

The most popular methods, gravitational technics, are based on the interaction of the size and density of various blood cells, the viscosity, density, and osmolarity of the suspending medium, and the speed, duration, and temperature of centrifugation. In general the heavier cells

sediment first, and of the remaining cells with equal density the larger cells sediment before the smaller ones. Thus erythrocytes, which are smaller than white blood cells, are also more dense and therefore gravitate to the bottom first. Their sedimentation is further enhanced by the use of various erythrocyte clumping agents (e.g., polysaccharide molecules such as dextran, methylcellulose, and Ficoll). The effectiveness of these clumping agents may be further enhanced by electrolytes.

Based on these general principles the procedure described by Boyum[17] with minor changes is presented. The distinguishing characteristic of this procedure is that the clumping mixture does not dilute or mix with the blood.

Reagents
1. Ficoll (Pharmacia Fine Chemicals, Piscataway, N.J.). Add 36.4 g Ficoll to 480 ml distilled water. It dissolves and has relatively low viscosity.
2. Isopaque (Hypaque sodium 50% brand diatrizoate sodium injection, USP; Winthrop Laboratories, Division of Sterling Drug, New York, 30 ml/vial). Add 120 ml Isopaque to 480 ml Ficoll solution. Resulting 600 ml Ficoll-Hypaque has specific gravity 1.076-1.078. Filter 0.45 μm with grid (Falcon Plastics 7102 filter) and store in refrigerator. Dispense 4 ml aliquots into 15 ml conical centrifuge tubes as needed.

Procedure
1. Draw 10 ml blood and place in plastic screw-capped tube containing 100 U heparin (0.1 ml) without preservative (ICN Nutritional Biochem, Cleveland; 100 U/ml in pyrogen-free water, Millipore filtered) at 20 C.
2. Spin tube for 10 min at 800 rpm (International PR-J centrifuge). Remove plasma with platelets and save in plastic tube.

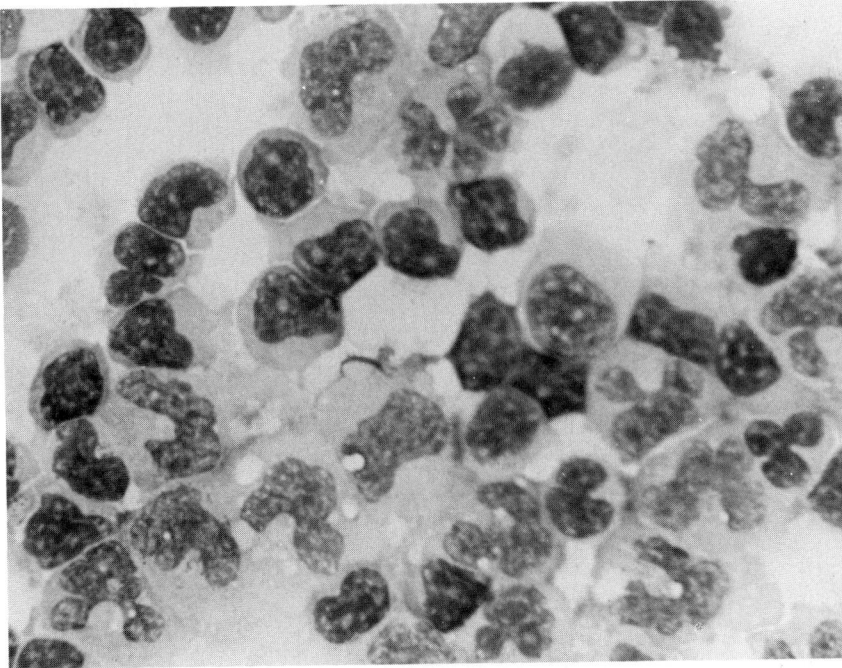

Fig. 63-1. WBC separated on Ficoll-Hypaque.

3. Remove buffy cell layer and some red cells, approximately 3 ml from 10 ml blood, and put into 15 ml conical centrifuge tube.

4. Add plasma from step 2 into original tube with remainder of red cells and spin to recover platelet-free plasma.

5. To tube from step 3 add MEM (minimum essential media [Eagle's] without glutamine for suspension cultures; GIBCO, Grand Island, N.Y.) with heparin (10 U/ml) to make total of 7 ml.

6. Layer this 7 ml on top of 4 ml Ficoll-Hypaque and spin at 1600 rpm for 40 min at 20 C.

7. Remove cell layer at interface of suspending liquid and Ficoll-Hypaque with Pasteur pipet and place in round-bottomed plastic tube, 13 × 100, containing 4 ml MEM-heparin. Spin at 2000 rpm for 10 min, decant supernatant, and repeat process twice at 1600 rpm. Finally add 1-2 ml MEM with heparin and glutamine (L-glutamine, mol. wt. 146, [Sigma Chemical Co., St. Louis]; 2.93 g/100 ml pyrogen-free water, filter sterilized and frozen in 2 ml amounts, 2 ml added to 100 ml MEM) and do cell count.

Lymphocytes are ready for use for variety of tests. Check viability of cells with trypan blue dye exclusion test. To 0.5 ml cells (1-2 × 10^5/ml) in 12 × 75 tube add 0.1 ml 0.4% trypan blue in BSS, mix, let stand 5 min, load hemocytometer chamber, and count. Stained cells are dead. Prepare smear in cytocentrifuge if possible, stain with Wright's stain, and examine. Normally there are 20-35% monocytes, a few basophils, occasional PMNL, and approximately 90% of all lymphocytes (Fig. 63-1).

QUANTITATION OF T- AND B-LYMPHOCYTES

T-lymphocytes

T- and B-lymphocytes can be identified and quantitated in humans by methods that demonstrate their characteristic surface markers.

T-lymphocytes have surface receptors for sheep red blood cells (SRBC) and spontaneously bind them to the surface and form "E" rosettes. The nature of the receptor is not known. It can be inhibited by various agents such as antithymocyte serum and anti–T cell serum. The number of T cells in the circulating blood, determined by their E-binding ability as reported from various laboratories, varies widely (20-80%). This variation is undoubtedly the result of technical differences such as differences in the proportion of SRBC to lymphocytes, age of SRBC, temperature and duration of incubation, dispersion of the cell button, enumeration and interpretation of the preparation, and other factors. The procedure described is based on the method of Jondal et al.,[18] with minor variations adopted in my laboratory.

Method

1. Wash lymphocytes obtained after Ficoll-Hypaque separation of whole blood twice in Hank's balanced salt solution (HBSS). Count lymphocytes and adjust to 2 × 10^6/ml.

2. Wash SRBC (not older than 2 wk) 3 times in HBSS. For first 2 washes spin at 1600 rpm for 10 min, and on third wash spin at 2000 rpm for 10 min to pack cells. Remove supernatant and add enough HBSS to make 5% suspension. Count cell suspension and add additional HBSS so that suspension contains 160 × 10^6 SRBC/ml.

3. Place 0.25 ml lymphocyte suspension containing 0.5 × 10^6 lymphocytes and 0.25 ml SRBC suspension containing 40 × 10^6 SRBC into duplicate tubes (17 × 100 Falcon plastic tubes); SRBC:lymphocytes, 80:1.

4. Place tubes in 37 C water bath for 15 min. Spin at 1000 rpm for 5 min and place in ice bath in refrigerator for 18 h.

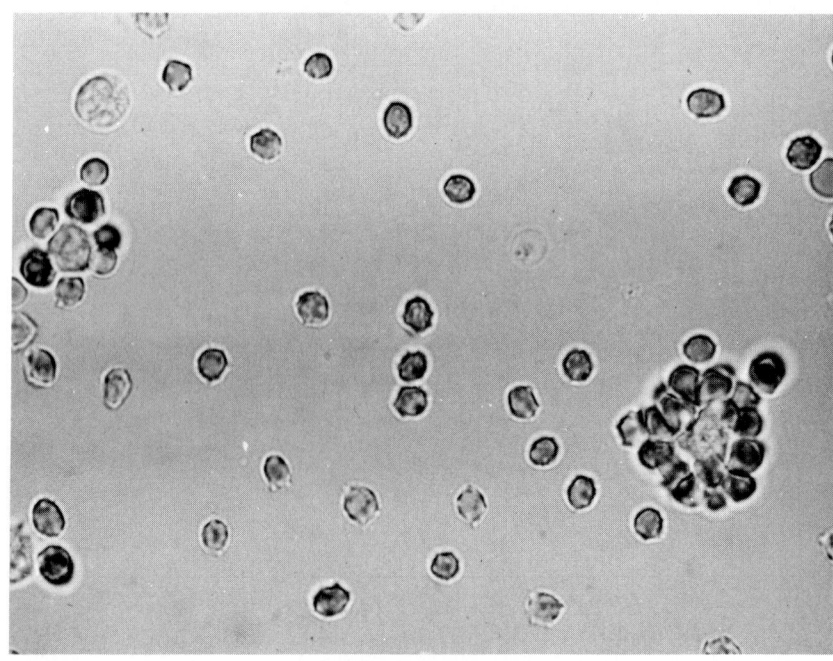

Fig. 63-2. SRBC-binding lymphocytes ("E" rosettes).

5. Aspirate clear supernatant with Pasteur pipet and gently aspirate cell button and place it on 1 of 2 glass slides, cover with 24 × 40 coverslip, seal with nail polish, and examine immediately in microscope fitted with bright-field and phase illumination. Lymphocytes are counted according to number of SRBC attached to them: 0,1,2,3, and >3. Lymphocytes binding 3 or more SRBC are considered to be T-lymphocytes. Normal range is 50-80% with mean of 65 ± 8 (Fig. 63-2).

T-lymphocytes may also be enumerated by their surface antigens using the immunofluorescence technic. Heterologous anti–T cell antiserum is produced against lymphocytes from individuals with congenital agammaglobulinemia (lacking B cells), T cell lymphoblastoid lines, and normal thymocytes. The antiserum is absorbed with B cell lymphoblastoid cell lines or with lymphocytes from patients with chronic lymphocytic leukemia (i.e., with predominantly B-lymphocytes).

Separated lymphocytes are sensitized with the absorbed anti–T cell antiserum and then exposed to species-specific fluorescent anti–Ig serum. (For details of the procedure see identification of B-lymphocytes by immunofluorescence.)

B-Lymphocytes

B-lymphocytes have surface receptors for complement (modified C3). The method to identify this receptor is based on the procedure described by Bianco, Patrick, and Nussenzweig[19] with minor differences.

Method. Preparation of lymphocytes and SRBC is same as that described for quantitation of T-lymphocytes.

SRBC are coated with antibody and complement to prepare "immune SRBC."

1. Add 4 ml 5% SRBC suspension to 4 ml 1:2000 hemolysin (rabbit anti-SRBC hemolysin, Flow Laboratories, Rockville, Md.) and incubate at 37 C for 30 min.
2. Wash cells 3 times with HBSS and resuspend them in 4 ml HBSS.
3. To this add 4 ml 1:40 dilution fresh-frozen pooled AB serum (as source of complement) and incubate at 37 C for 30 min; minimal hemolysis occurs.
4. Wash cells 3 times in HBSS and resuspend to make 0.5% solution.
5. Count cells and adjust to $80 × 10^6$/ml.
6. Set up test in duplicate. Place 0.25 ml lymphocyte suspension and 0.25 ml SRBC suspension in 17 × 100 plastic tubes·and incubate in 37 C water bath for 15 min.
7. Spin tubes at 1000 rpm for 5 min; remove supernatant with Pasteur pipet.
8. Vortex tubes at no. 6 speed (deluxe mixer S8220, Scientific Products, Detroit) for 20 s.
9. Remove cells with pipet, place them on glass slide, cover with 24 × 40 coverslip, seal with nail polish, and examine under microscope with bright-field and phase illumination. Erythrocyte antibody and complement (EAC)–binding lymphocytes are counted similarly as outlined for E-binding lymphocytes. Care should be taken to exclude monocytes, since they also have receptors for complement and may form EAC rosettes.

They may be identified morphologically by phase microscopy. They are considerably larger than lymphocytes and can also be distinguished by their ability to phagocytose latex particles. Normally there are 15-30% EAC-binding lymphocytes, mean 25 ± 5%.

Surface membrane immunoglobulins (SmIg) on B-lymphocytes can be detected by the immunofluorescence technic. The principal requisites for this technic are maximum sensitivity and specificity.

Lymphocytes should be alive.

Wet preparations improve the specificity, since the cells in suspension can be washed more efficiently to remove immunofluorescent material in the suspending media than fixed smears; this leaves only specific antibody attached to reaction sites on the cell membrane.

The heterologous antiserum should be specific; this often requires extensive absorptions with appropriate reagents. It is generally produced in rabbits or goats following immunization with purified myeloma proteins. The antiserum is then fractionated on DEAE cellulose or by other methods such as ammonium sulfate fractionation to obtain the IgG fraction, which is conjugated to the fluorochromes, at optimum F:P (fluorochrome:protein) ratio.[20] Fractionation prior to labeling conserves on the fluorochrome, since albumin has a much greater affinity for the dye than globulins. Specificity of the antiserum is achieved by appropriate absorptions; reaction with the specific antigen followed by elution of the antiserum provides the purest reagent. Commercially labeled antisera with heavy- and light-chain specificity are available and are adequate for clinical use.

Appropriate controls are necessary. A known positive and known negative control are helpful if available. Blocking of the reaction sites with unlabeled antiserum prior to their exposure to labeled antiserum so that no immunofluorescence is seen establishes the specificity of the reagent.

The direct or indirect method may be used. In the direct method the specific antiserum is labeled, and in a first-step reaction the antigenic sites are identified. In the indirect method the cells are reacted with unlabeled antisera and a species-specific labeled antiserum is used to demonstrate the reaction sites. The advantage of this method is that it requires only 1 labeled species-specific antiserum for a large number of specific antisera. Also the layering process increases the final number of antigenic sites with the labeled material, thus increasing the intensity of fluorescence.

The microscope should have a dual light source to view the specimen alternately in tungsten and ultraviolet light. A BG 12 pass filter and an OG 1 barrier filter are best for fluorescein isothiocyanate–labeled material. Double staining is useful to demonstrate the simultaneous presence of immunoglobulins of more than 1 heavy-chain class on a single lymphocyte.

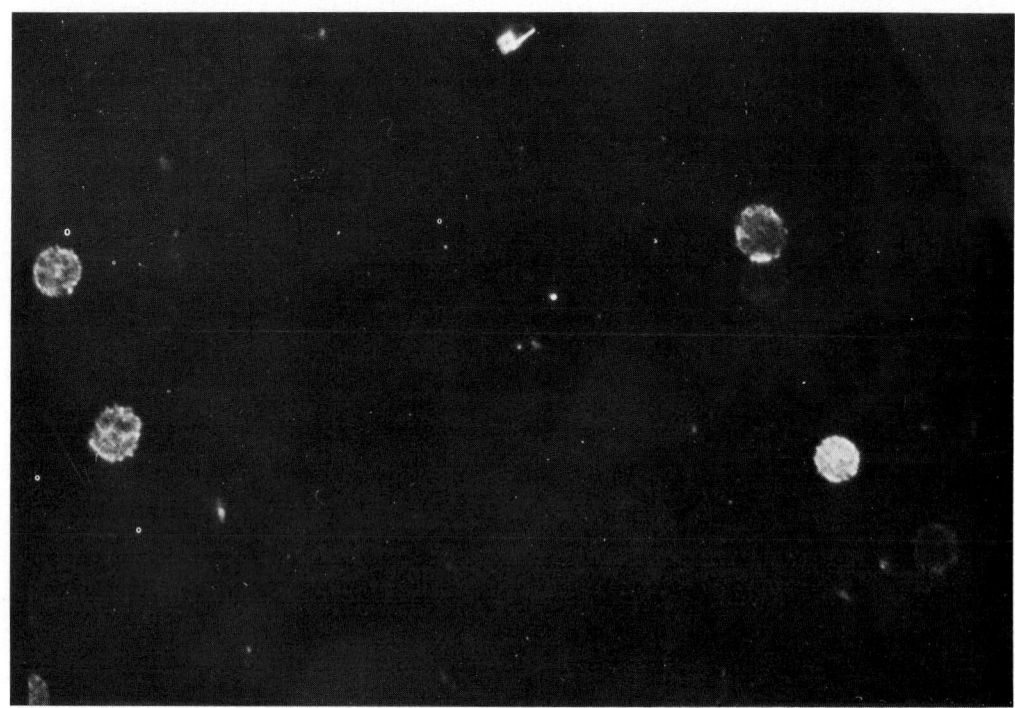

Fig. 63-3. Lymphocytes reacted with fluorescein-labeled anti-IgM showing peripheral, stippled, and patchy fluorescence.

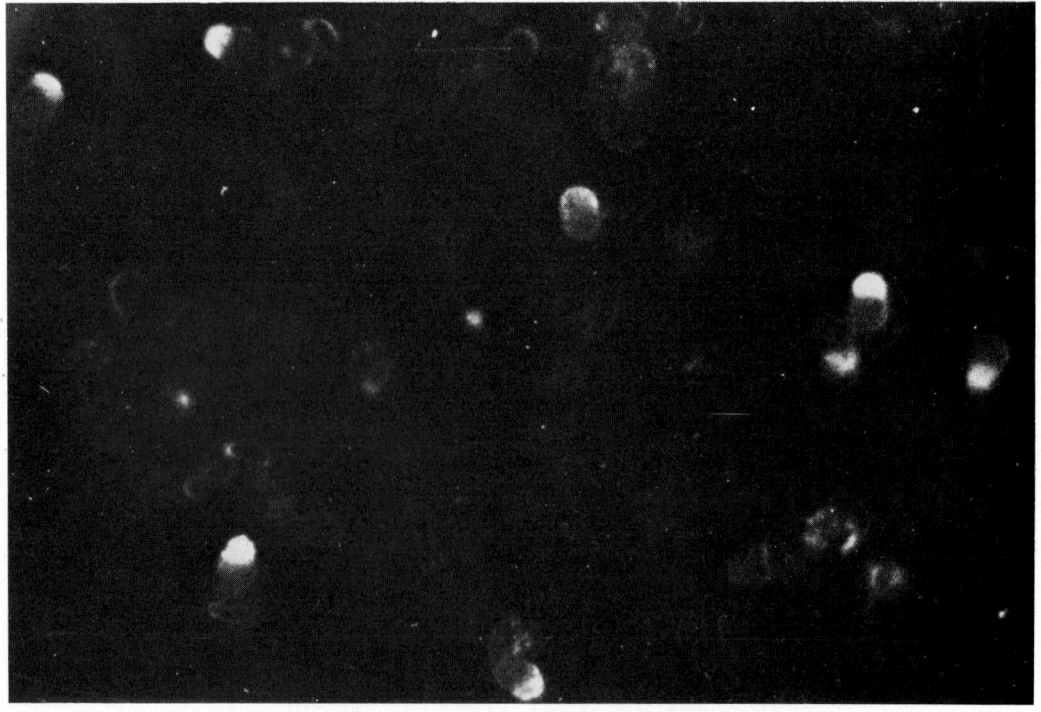

Fig. 63-4. Lymphocytes reacted with fluorescein-labeled anti-IgG showing "capping."

Direct method

1. Wash lymphocytes obtained from Ficoll-Hypaque separation 3 times with phosphate-buffered saline (PBS) with 5% bovine serum albumin (BSA) and 0.02% sodium azide.
2. Suspend lymphocytes in 5% BSA-PBS + Na azide so that there are 5×10^5 lymphocytes/0.1 ml.
3. Incubate 0.1 ml cells plus 0.1 ml fluorescent antiserum for 30 min in ice bath.
4. Wash 3 times with 5% BSA-PBS + Na azide.
5. After last wash decant supernatant.
6. Place cell suspension on glass slide, cover with coverslip, seal with nail polish, and examine under fluorescence microscope. Count only small mononuclear cells (cells less than 8 μm); exclude monocytes. Fluorescence is generally peripheral but may be stippled over entire cell, smooth, or patchy (Fig. 63-3). Due to fluidity of cell membrane, antigens on cell surface combined with fluorescent antiserum may move to 1 end of cell and cause cell to look "capped" (Fig. 63-4). Capping is active process and is inhibited at reaction temperature of 0 C and by Na azide. Sum of cells that react with individual labeled heavy-chain specific antiserum is generally greater than number of cells that stain with single labeled polyvalent antiserum. This may be indicative of more than 1 type of heavy chain on individual cell. Range of means of different laboratories for adults has been given as follows: total Ig 16-28%, IgG 4.0-12.7%, IgA 1.0-4.3%, IgM 6.7-13.0%, IgD 5.2-8.2%.[21]

Indirect method. Lymphocytes are first sensitized with unlabeled specific antiserum by incubating at 37 C for 30 min. Cells are then washed 3 times with 5% BSA-PBS + Na azide and are treated with labeled species-specific antiserum following outline for direct method.

B cells may also be identified by the presence of surface Fc receptors that may bind Fc portion of aggregated γ-globulin. This can be prepared by heating conjugated γ-globulin at 63 C for 15 minutes prior to use.[22]

The normal percentage of lymphocytes with B cell surface markers is approximately 15-30%. Individuals with X-linked hypogammaglobulinemia lack cells with B cell markers, whereas individuals with late-onset acquired hypogammaglobulinemia have normal numbers of B cells, and individuals with primary T cell defects have elevated numbers of B cells.

With appropriate stimulation (e.g., pokeweed mitogen), B-lymphocytes with SmIg convert to plasma cells with cytoplasmic fluorescence prior to the secretion of Ig into the surrounding media (Fig. 63-5). With the fluorescent antibody technic it is possible to identify various blockage points in B cell maturation that result in various types of hypogammaglobulinemia. Thus some patients with hypogammaglobulinemia have no B-lymphocytes with SmIg. (The prototype is X-linked hypogammaglobulinemia.) Other patients with hypogammaglobulinemia have B-lymphocytes with SmIg but do not respond to pokeweed mitogen (PWM) stimulation in vitro and do not have cells with cytoplasmic fluorescence. Finally, some patients with hypogammaglobulinemia have cells with SmIg and cytoplasmic Ig that are unable to secrete Ig into the surrounding media.

LYMPHOCYTE TRANSFORMATION

Lymphocyte transformation (blastogenesis) was first described by Nowell in 1960.[23] Using phytohemagglutinin (PHA, an extract of the red kidney bean *Phaseolus vulgaris*) to separate blood fractions by agglutination of red cells and white cells, Nowell observed that PHA also

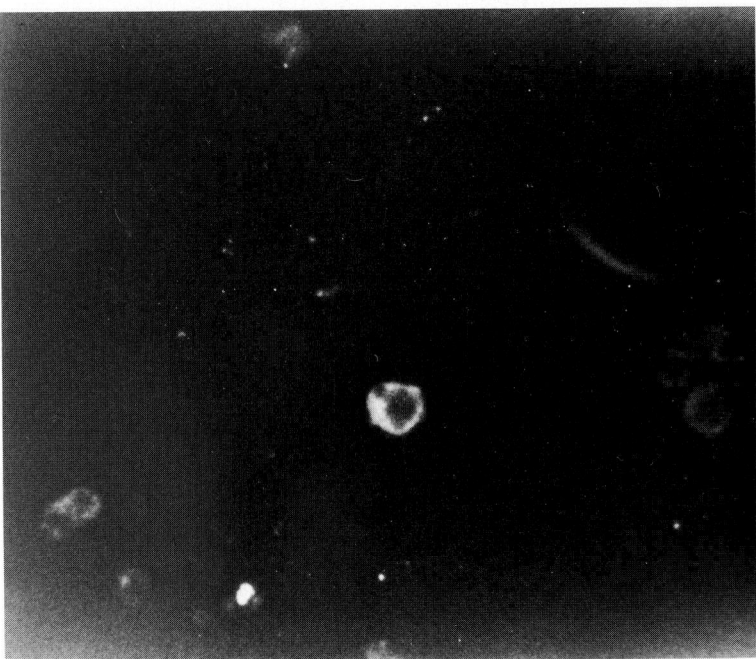

Fig. 63-5. Lymphocytes reacted with fluorescein-labeled anti-IgA showing cytoplasmic fluorescence.

stimulated lymphocytes to undergo blastlike transformation and cell division. This observation was rapidly applied to the study of chromosomes in humans and used to measure the potential of lymphocytes to proliferate, a property essential for cell-mediated immunity. Soon after, other plant lectins, PWM,[24] and concanavalin A (Con A) from the jack bean[25,26] were found capable of stimulating lymphocytes in vitro. In the mouse PHA and Con A primarily stimulate T-lymphocytes, and PWM stimulates both T- and B-lymphocytes.[27,28] A similar selectivity in humans has not been conclusively demonstrated. Nevertheless in vitro lymphocyte transformation is an important measure of cell-mediated immunity and a valuable diagnostic test for the identification of various hereditary and acquired T cell defects.

The precise nature of the surface receptors, the mechanism of interaction between the receptors and the mitogens and antigens, and the subsequent intracellular events are little known. It is probable that different underlying mechanisms produce blastogenesis when nonspecific mitogens and specific antigens are used for in vitro stimulation of lymphocytes. The stimulation of lymphocytes with mitogens and antigens increases cyclic AMP and adenylcylase,[29] lipid turnover,[30,31] pinocytosis,[32] phosphorylation of nucleoprotein,[33] acetylation of histones,[34] RNA and protein synthesis,[35,36] glycogen storage,[37] and DNA synthesis.[38,39] Also 1 of the soluble mediators liberated by the stimulated lymphocytes "recruits" additional cells that amplify the response.

The extent of blastlike transformation can be determined by morphology. The transformed blastlike cell (the pyroninophilic cell) is characterized by large size, dark blue cytoplasm with a perinuclear clear zone, and a large nucleus with nucleoli (Fig. 63-6). Quantitation of the response by morphology is not very precise, especially for the lymphocyte falling between the large, clearly blastlike cells and the very small nonresponsive cells. Furthermore the larger cells tend to stick together, causing underestimation of the degree of blastogenesis. The quantitative uptake of tritiated thymidine into synthesizing DNA is a far more accurate measure of the degree of blastogenesis.

The nonspecific and nonimmunologic stimulation by lectins causes 65-90% of the lymphocytes to undergo blastogenesis and cell division after 2-3 days in culture. The specific stimulation by antigen causes 1% or less of the lymphocytes, those previously sensitized, to undergo blastogenesis and cell division after 5-6 days in culture. The longer culture period allows for several cell divisions, so that the number of responding cells increases and yields a more measurable final response. Antigenic stimulation of lymphocytes in vitro correlates with the in vivo DTH response.

Several facets of the culture system may influence the response of lymphocytes stimulated in vitro by mitogens or antigens.

1. The degree of response varies in proportion to the number of responding cells in the test. With mitogens this factor is not crucial, since the majority of the lymphocytes in a given population are capable of responding; but with antigens few cells respond in a given population, and the larger the number of lymphocytes in the test the better the chance of eliciting a measurable response.

2. The degree of response varies with the types and number of cells associated with the lymphocytes. Although a few PMNL are necessary for an optimum response, an excessive number of PMNL, especially in lymphopenic individuals, is inhibitory. Thus while whole blood may be used to measure lymphocyte response to in vitro stimulation with mitogens

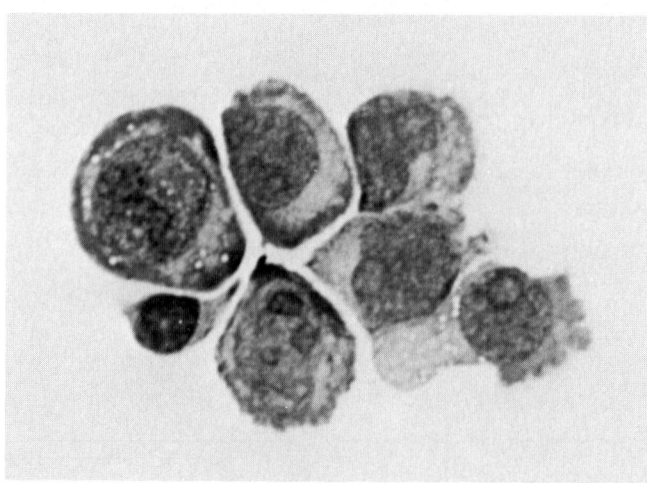

Fig. 63-6. Lymphocytes stimulated with PHA for 3 d showing different sizes of blastlike cells and 1 small unstimulated cell.

and antigens in normal individuals, separated cells composed largely of lymphocytes and containing few monocytes and PMNL are desirable when lymphopenia exists as in certain immunodeficiency states.

3. Lymphocyte response to antigens is weak to absent when macrophages are lacking. Contact between lymphocyte and macrophage is necessary for lymphocyte proliferation to occur. Macrophages seem necessary for the presentation of either the undegraded or the "processed" antigen to the sensitized lymphocytes in order to initiate the proliferative response.

4. The concentration of plasma in the culture media is critical; too low a concentration ($< 10\%$) or too high a concentration ($> 40\%$) is unsuitable for optimum response of in vitro stimulation of lymphocytes by mitogens or antigens.

5. Autologous plasma is generally suitable; however, it may contain inhibitory factors leading to poor response. The presence of inhibitory factors may be verified by substituting pooled serum.

6. Sterility in the test system is essential; most laboratories use 50 U penicillin and 50 U streptomycin per milliliter for this purpose. Using care and a laminar flow hood I have not found this necessary and have had no problems maintaining sterility. This has advantages, since the antibiotics may themselves stimulate the lymphocytes of sensitive individuals.

7. Cultures generally require a moist atmosphere and a pH of 7.2. This is maintained by an atmosphere containing 5% CO_2. This is less crucial if tightly capped vials or tubes are used, but it is essential when microtiter plates are used.

Method

Mitogen stimulation

1. Place 2×10^5 lymphocytes in 1 ml MEM with 20% autologous plasma into 13×100 siliconized glass screw-capped tubes.
2. Add mitogens to each tube. Use different doses, contained in maximum of 0.1 ml, to ensure individual responses. Optimum doses in my laboratory are:

   PHA (purified phytohemagglutin [Burroughs Wellcome, Research Triangle Park, N.C.]), 5 μg and 2.5 μg

   PWM (GIBCO, Grand Island, N.Y.), 1:20 and 1:40

   Con A (Calbiochem, LaJolla, Calif.), 100 μg and 50 μg
3. Set up each mitogen and each dilution in duplicate or triplicate. Include 1 set cell suspension in only MEM and plasma as control. Gently agitate all tubes to obtain uniform suspension.
4. Screw cap tightly and incubate at 37 C for 72 h or place with loosened caps in 5% CO_2 incubator.
5. After 72 h add 50 μl 1:50 dilution (in water) tritiated thymidine (New England Nuclear, Boston), 6.7 Ci/mmol, to each tube (1 μCi/tube).
6. Incubate for additional 2 h at 37 C.
7. Wash with 3 ml 0.85% saline, spin at 2200 rpm (International PR-J centrifuge) for 10 min at 20 C. Pour off supernatant and either freeze pellet at -20 C until further processing or continue as follows.

8. Wash 2 more times with 3 ml 10% trichloroacetic acid (TCA); then spin at 2200 rpm for 10 min. Prior to each spin let tubes stand for 10 min at room temperature after adding TCA.
9. Wash once with 3 ml 80% ethanol, allowing tubes to stand for 10 min prior to spinning.
10. Pour off alcohol, add 0.4 ml NCS solubilizer (Amersham/Searle, Arlington Heights, Ill.) to pellet. Let tubes stand overnight in dark at room temperature. To hasten solubilizing incubate tubes at 37 C for 1-2 h.
11. Rinse tubes twice with 5 ml scintillation fluid (1000 ml toluene, 4 g PPO, and 0.1 g POPOP) and pour into scintillation vial.
12. Count vials in liquid scintillation counter (cpm), correct for quenching and determine percent efficiency from counting efficiency chart, and calculate disintegrations per minute (dpm).

Antigen stimulation. Procedure is basically same as that used for mitogens with following exceptions.

1. Cultures are kept for longer than 3 d (5-7 d) to ensure adequate clonal proliferation of sensitized cells.
2. It is advantageous to increase number of cells per test from 2×10^5 to 5×10^5 per test if possible. This increases initial number of sensitized cells present in population.
3. Antigen is dialysed free of preservatives and similar substances and is added in 0.1 ml aliquots into each tube.

   a. *Candida albicans*, 1:300 (Berry Laboratories, Pompano Beach, Fla.). Dialyse 2 ml against 100 ml HBSS overnight at 4 C. Use at 1:4 dilution.

   b. SK/SD: Varidase SK, 100,000 U; SD, 25,000 U (Lederle Laboratories, Pearl River, N.Y.). Dialyse 2 ml against 100 ml HBSS overnight. Use at 1:25 dilution.

LYMPHOKINE PRODUCTION

Lymphocytes activated by specific antigen or nonspecific mitogens secrete biologically active effector substances (lymphokines) into the surrounding media. Several chemically and functionally distinct lymphokines exist. Some amplify the specific immune response by "recruiting" uncommitted lymphocytes. Others are chemotactic for macrophages, PMNL, eosinophils, and basophils; still others inhibit the migration of these cells and collectively mediate DTH or cell-mediated response.

The macrophage inhibitory factor (MIF) and leukocyte inhibitory factor (LIF) are the most commonly tested lymphokines and seem to be in vitro correlates of DTH or cell-mediated immunity. The first in vitro model for the study of delayed-type hypersensitivity (DTH) was described by Rich and Lewis in 1932[40]; they observed that explants of spleens and lymph nodes from tuberculin-sensitive animals grew poorly in the presence of tuberculin and well in its absence. As a consequence of these observations George and Vaughn in 1962[41] described a simple test using capillary tubes to measure cell migration as an in vitro model for measuring DTH. They showed that peritoneal exudate cells (70% macrophages) migrate from capillary tubes in a tissue culture system. In the presence of purified protein derivative (PPD) the peritoneal exudate cells from animals previously sensitized to PPD failed to migrate from the capillary tubes. This in vitro model was further elaborated by other investigators,[42-46] who identified the soluble factor (MIF) that was capable of inhibiting the spontaneous migration of normal macrophages. Subsequently Søborg and Bendixen[47] showed that the migration of human leukocytes from buffy coat was also inhibited by a soluble substance obtained from lymphocyte activation, making the in vitro assay for MIF much simpler to perform.

Recent studies[48,49] have suggested that MIF and LIF are distinct by virtue of molecular weight and by the cells they inhibit. MIF has a molecular weight of 69,000 daltons and inhibits the migration of guinea pig macrophages and human monocytes. LIF has a molecular weight of 23,000 daltons and inhibits the migration of PMNL but not monocytes and guinea pig macrophages. While the inhibition of cell migration is an accepted in vitro correlate of DTH, predominantly a T-lymphocyte function,[50] MIF and LIF are generated by both T- and B-lymphocytes.

The assay for MIF and LIF may be done in 1 or 2 steps. In the 2-step or indirect method supernatants containing MIF and LIF are collected from culture of lymphocytes with specific antigen or mitogen and reacted with macrophages from nonimmune guinea pig peritoneal exudate cells obtained 4-5 days after intraperitoneal injection of 25-30 ml mineral oil. In the 1-step direct method the migration of human leukocytes incubated together with antigen is determined. Presumably the antigen activates the lymphocytes in the cell mixture to produce MIF and LIF, which in turn inhibits the migration of the monocytes and PMNL. The 1-step procedure is considerably easier to perform and is a good in vitro screening test for DTH. It should, however, be noted that while the lack of migration inhibition may be due to a lack of MIF and LIF, it may also be due to other factors such as a defect of the migratory cells, toxicity of the antigen, improper pH, certain serum factors, and the presence of antigen-antibody complexes.

LIF and MIF assay, in vitro response of lymphocytes stimulated with specific antigens, and in vivo delayed hypersensitivity skin test are all responses arising from the interaction of antigen and sensitized cells and are collectively useful for the assessment of cell-mediated immunity. In vitro stimulation of lymphocytes is perhaps the most sensitive of the 3 tests, followed by LIF and MIF and finally by the in vivo delayed hypersensitivity skin test, which is the most complex of the 3 and involves several sequential cellular and vascular responses.

Method. This method is based on descriptions of Søborg and Bendixen[47] and Rosenberg and David,[51] with modifications adopted in my laboratory.

1. Draw 20 ml blood and place in sterile plastic test tubes containing sterile heparin (without preservative 10 U/ml). Sediment for 1 h at room temperature.

2. To harvest maximum number WBC aspirate plasma with WBC and platelets (buffy count), as RBC settle. This can be done repeatedly during hour of sedimentation as long as tip of Pasteur pipet remains 4-5 mm above level of RBC. All WBC-containing plasma is pooled into another sterile plastic tube.

3. At end of 1 h centrifuge original tubes at 600 rpm (Sorvall GLC-1) for 5 min and aspirate remaining plasma containing WBC and platelets up to 3-4 mm above RBC interface and add to WBC tube.

4. Centrifuge tube with plasma, WBC, and platelets at 1000 rpm for 10 min. Aspirate supernatant plasma containing majority of platelets and save in another container.

5. Resuspend WBC pellet in HBSS containing 1% heparin (without preservative) and wash 3 times. Spin at 2000 rpm for 10 min for each wash.

6. Resuspend washed WBC pellet in tissue culture medium 199 (TC 199) containing 10% horse serum (inactivated at 56 C for 30 min) and adjust cell suspension so that there are 10×10^6 PMNL/ml. Usually 3-4 ml cell suspension is obtained.

7. Divide cell suspension into several plastic tubes (16×100 mm) in aliquots of 1 ml (this amount generally fills about 6 capillary tubes). Spin cell suspensions at 2000 rpm for 10 min, discard supernatant, and resuspend in 1 ml TC 199 with 10% horse serum with various antigens, leaving 1 tube as control with only TC 199 and 10% horse serum.

8. Incubate all tubes at 37 C for 3 h. This increases activity of cells and seems to give more reproducible results.

9. Resuspend cells by gently aspirating them up and down tip of Pasteur pipet.

10. Draw cell suspension for each tube into siliconized sterile capillary pipets ($1.5-2.0 \times 100$ mm) (Kimble Products, Vineland, N.J.) two-thirds of way and seal 1 end with Crito-Seal (Clay Adams, Parsippany, N.J.).

11. Place capillary tubes in individual test tubes with cotton in bottom, unsealed end up, and centrifuge at 600 rpm for 10 min.

12. Wipe outside of capillary tube with alcohol and cut it 1 mm below cell-fluid interface, making sure WBC are up to very edge of cut surface.

13. Place capillary tube on sterile and siliconized coverslip placed in bottom of sterile migrating chamber (Sykes Moore, Bellco Glass, Vineland, N.J.). Dot of silicone grease holds sealed end of capillary tube in place.

14. Cover chambers tightly with another coverslip and screw on ring.

15. Fill chamber with 1 ml TC 199 with 10% horse serum with or without antigen. Avoid air bubbles.

16. Incubate chambers placed flat in a moisture chamber for 18 h at 37 C.

17. Use $4\times$ objective and right-angle projection prism attached to microscope. Area of migration is projected onto wall and drawn on sheet of paper (Fig. 63-7, **A** and **B**).

18. Area of migration is measured with compensating polar planimeter (Kueffel and Esser, Chicago). Average of 3-4 identically treated cultures is computed; there should not be variation greater than ±10%. Migration index = Average migration of

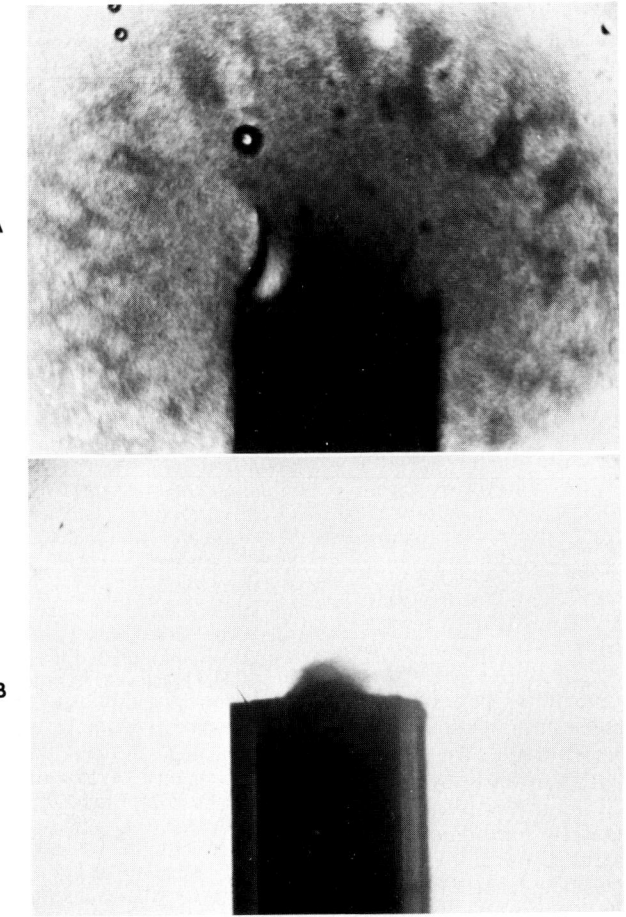

Fig. 63-7. Migration of WBC (LIF) from *Candida*-sensitive individual. **A,** Untreated (normal migration). **B,** Reacted with *Candida* antigen (migration inhibited).

antigen containing culture/Average migration of normal culture. This can be expressed as percent migration; migration index × 100. Positive skin test usually shows 80% or less migration in presence of antigen.[52]

NOTE: Optimum concentration of various antigens must be determined individually. For instance, in my laboratory *Candida* antigen is used as follows: *Candida albicans,* 1:100 (Hollister Stier), is first dialysed against HBSS overnight and is used in concentration of 1:200 (diluted in TC 199 with 10% horse serum) for initial incubation with WBC and in concentration of 1:1000 in TC 199 with horse serum to fill chamber.

CYTOTOXICITY

Cytotoxicity is a complex process by which target cells are killed. The underlying mechanism may be immunologically specific or immunologically "nonspecific." Immunologically specific mechanisms may be accomplished be specific antibody or specifically sensitized lymphocytes. Antibody-mediated cytotoxicity is complement dependent, and although cell-mediated cytotoxicity may occur in the absence of antibody, small amounts of antibody (not enough to bind complement) enhance some forms of cytotoxicity by lymphocytes.

The in vitro assay of immunologically specific lymphocyte-mediated cytotoxicity correlates with the in vivo efferent phases of cell-mediated immunologic reactions involved in tumor rejection, allograft rejection, contact allergy, and certain autoimmune diseases. Cell-mediated cytotoxicity is primarily mediated by living, metabolically active T-lymphocytes capable of establishing contact with the target cells. Approximately 1-2% of a lymphocyte population is cytotoxic,[53] and the approximate ratio of killing lymphocytes to target cells is 1:1. Cytotoxicity occurs prior to DNA synthesis[54] and is independent of blastic transformation. It may be passively transferred by the lymphocytes and not by the serum of sensitized donors to normal recipients.[55]

Specific lymphocyte-mediated cytotoxicity is assayed following in vivo or in vitro sensitization of the lymphocytes. After in vivo sensitization various methods that involve the cytotoxic effect of lymphocytes on specific tissue culture monolayers have been used.[56-58] The degree of cytotoxicity is measured by the amount of isotope (^{51}Cr) released from dead target cells or by counting the unaffected (living) cells. Thus after organ transplantation the recipient's lymphocytes can be tested in vitro for cytotoxicity against the donor's fibroblasts containing the membrane-bound HLA antigens. The in vitro assay correlates with the ability to reject a graft. This form of cytotoxicity is very specific and can be inhibited by specific alloantibodies directed against tranplantation antigens on the surface of the target cells.[59,60] In the same way the ability of the individual lymphocytes to destroy tumor cells can be assayed in vitro.

In the absence of specific in vivo sensitization, lymphocyte cytotoxicity can be measured after first sensititizing the lymphocytes in the mixed leukocyte culture (MLC) with allogeneic cells and then assaying their ability to destory target cells containing the same antigen.[61]

Immunologically nonspecific lymphocyte-mediated cytotoxicity, representing a measurable potential of lymphocytes to become cytotoxic, may be assessed by the effect of normal lymphocytes on target cells in the presence or absence of complement. In these situations B-lymphocytes in addition to T-lymphocytes are sometimes capable of manifesting cytotoxicity.

While lymphocytes sensitized by membrane-bound antigens are specifically cytotoxic to target cells bearing the same membrane antigens, lymphocytes activated by soluble antigens and mitogens are nonspecifically cytotoxic for a variety of target cells. Lymphocytes activated by PHA undergo blastlike transformation and also become highly cytotoxic for a variety of cells. However, lymphocytes activated by Con A undergo blastlike transformation but do not become cytotoxic. By adding Con A to PHA in varying amounts the cytotoxic reaction can be competitively inhibited, whereas transformation remains unaffected.[62]

This form of cytotoxicity may be measured by the amount of ^{51}Cr released from chicken red blood cells (ChRBC) following exposure to PHA-activated lymphocytes or by the amount of ^{51}Cr released from ChRBC coated with rabbit anti-ChRBC antibody and exposed to normal lymphocytes.[63]

"Nonspecific" cytotoxicity is mediated not only by lymphocytes but by macrophages and PMNL, either after they have phagocytised the target cell or perhaps by toxic factors that they secrete. This necessitates care in assigning various cytotoxic effects solely to lymphocytes and has led some investigators[63] to use exhaustive methods for the separation of lymphocytes from other blood cells in order to discriminate the cytotoxic effect of lymphocytes from that of other cells.

Specific lymphocyte-mediated cytotoxicity following in vitro sensitization

This assay system is based on the observation that lymphocytes sensitized by allogeneic cells in the 1-way mixed leukocyte culture (MLC) are rendered specifically cytotoxic to lymphocytes autologous to the sensitizing cells.[61] The sensitivity of the assay is greatly increased by using PHA-stimulated target cells,[64] probably because they are capable of taking up larger amounts of ^{51}Cr than normal lymphocytes. It appears that while differences in the serologically defined antigens (HLA in humans and H-2 in mice) between the responder and stimulator may not be necessary in the MLC,[65] they are essential for effective cell-mediated lymphocytotoxicity (CML).[66,67]

Method. Lymphocytes to be used as responding cells and as stimulating and target cells are obtained from heparinized peripheral blood by separation on Ficoll-Hypaque. Approximately 20-30 ml blood is drawn from donor for both stimulation cells for MLC and target cells for CML.

1. Mix stimulating cells for MLC with mitomycin-C (25 μg/ml) and incubate for 20 min at 37 C. By this process cells can no longer divide but still retain their antigeneic composition and are capable of stimulating other cells.

2. Incubate target cells (1×10^6/ml) in TC 199 with 20% human pooled plasma (TC 199–20) in Falcon plastic bottles (Falcon 3040) for 3 d; then add PHA (1:100 dilution PHA-M) (Difco Laboratories, Detroit). On sixth day centrifuge ($200 \times g$) for 10 min and suspend in 0.3 ml medium (approximately 8×10^6 cells). Label with 250 μCi Na ^{51}Cr O$_4$ (New England Nuclear, Boston). Incubate mixture 1 h with frequent shaking at 37 C. Wash twice with TC 199–20 in refrigerated centrifuge and resuspend at 1×10^5 cells/ml.

3. Put 1.5×10^6 responding and 1.5×10^6 stimulating cells in 2 ml TC 199 supplemented with 20% pooled human serum (TC 199–20) in 16×100 mm glass tubes and incubate at 37 C in 95% air and 5% CO$_2$ for 5 d.

4. On fifth day put 0.2 ml aliquots MLC mixture into Linbro microculture plates with 2 μCi tritiated thymidine (Schwarz-Mann, Orangeburg, N.Y.) (specific activity 1.19 U) and incubate for 12 h.

5. Precipitate cells on glass fiber filters using method of Hartzman et al.[68] and count in scintillation counter. All tests are done in duplicate.

6. Remainder of responding cells from MLC are used as effector cells for CML.

7. For CML assay place 0.1 ml containing 1×10^6 effector cells (based on viable cells, determined by trypan blue exclusion) and 0.1 ml containing 1 $\times$ 10^4 target cells in round-bottom Linbro microculture plates.

8. Incubate 4 h at 37 C in 95% air and 5% CO$_2$.

9. Centrifuge microculture plates at $100 \times g$ for 10 min; remove aliquot and count.

10. Actual test release of ^{51}Cr reflects degree of killing of target cells by effector cells and is derived from formula E-S/T-$S \times 100$, where E is experimental release of ^{51}Cr, S is spontaneous release (target cells incubated alone), and T is total release from same number of target cells after freezing and thawing. Thus E-S reflects degree of killing of effector cells and T-S is maximum amount of chromium available to demonstrate cell destruction.

11. Release of greater than 10% ^{51}Cr is considered significant. Majority of normal individuals effect release generally greater than 20%.

12. Various controls are necessary; for instance, responder cells are stimulated with mitomycin-treated autologous cells in MLC and then reacted against heterologous target cells in CML. Likewise responder cells stimulated by allogeneic cells in MLC are reacted against autologous cells in CML ("autokilling"). Control cells should be used to determine whether lack of CML is inherent characteristic of target cell that precludes killing.

SUMMARY

The various in vitro methods used to measure cell-mediated immunologic responses have a direct application in clinical medicine. In addition to the basic information provided by the tests, they can be varied in design according to individual clinical findings to provide more specific information regarding the underlying mechanism and progress of various disease states. This type of analysis of various disease states has also led to new methods of treatment wherein defective components of the afferent and efferent arcs of the immune system can be reconstituted and overreactive components can be blunted.

REFERENCES

1. Landsteiner, K., and Chase, M. W.: Proc. Soc. Exp. Biol. Med. **9**:688, 1942.
2. Catalona, W. J., Taylor, P. T., Rabson, A. S., and Chretien, P. B.: N. Engl. J. Med. **286**:399, 1972.
3. Shrek, R., and Stefani, S.: Fed. Proc. **22**:428, 1963.
4. Burgio, G. R., Riggoni, G., and Marni, E.: Lancet **2**:411, 1968.
5. Bonforte, R. J., Topilsky, M., Siltzbach, L. E., and Glade, P. R.: J. Pediatr. **81**:775, 1972.
6. Lawlor, G. J., and Stiehm, E. R.: Clin. Res. **20**:667, 1972.
7. Blaese, R. M., Weiden, P., Oppenheim, J. J., and Waldmann, T. A.: J. Lab. Clin. Med. **81**:538, 1973.
8. Fichtelius, K. E.: Ups. J. Med. Sci. **56**:27, 1951.
9. Walker, R. I., Herion, J. C., and Palmer, J. G.: Am. J. Physiol. **201**:1137, 1961.
10. Lamvik, J. O.: Acta Haematol. (Basel) **35**:294, 1966.
11. Levine, S.: Science **123**:185, 1956.
12. Johnson, F. M., and Garvin, J. E.: Proc. Soc. Exp. Biol. **102**:33, 1959.
13. Garvin, J. E.: J. Exp. Med. **114**:51, 1961.
14. Rabinowitz, Y.: Blood **23**:811, 1964.
15. Spriggs, A. I., and Alexander, R. F.: Nature **188**:863, 1960.
16. Coulson, A. S., and Chalmers, D. G.: Lancet **1**:468, 1964.
17. Boyum, A.: Scand. J. Clin. Lab. Invest. **21**(suppl. 97):77, 1968.
18. Jondal, M., Holm, G., and Wigzell, H.: J. Exp. Med. **136**:207, 1972.
19. Bianco, C., Patrick, R., and Nussenzweig, V.: J. Exp. Med. **132**:702, 1970.
20. Goldman, M., and Carver, R. K.: Exp. Cell Res. **23**:265, 1961.
21. WHO/IARC Spec. Tech. Report: Scan. J. Immunol. **3**:521, 1974.
22. Dickler, H. B., and Kunkel, H. G.: J. Exp. Med. **136**:191, 1972.
23. Nowell, P. C.: Cancer Res. **20**:462, 1960.
24. Farnes, P., Barker, B. E., Brownhill, L. E., and Fanger, H.: Lancet **2**:1100, 1964.
25. Douglas, S. D., Kamin, R., and Fudenberg, H. H.: J. Immunol. **103**:1185, 1969.
26. Powell, A. E., and Leon, M. A.: Exp. Cell Res. **62**:315, 1970.
27. Janossy, G., and Greaves, M. F.: Clin. Exp. Immunol. **9**:483, 1971.
28. Janossy, G., and Greaves, M. F.: Clin. Exp. Immunol. **10**:525, 1972
29. Smith, J. W., Steiner, A. L. and Parker, C. W.: Fed. Proc. **29**:369, 1970.
30. Fisher, D. B., and Mueller, G. C.: Proc. Natl. Acad. Sci. **60**:1396, 1968.
31. Kay, J. E.: Nature **219**:172, 1968.
32. Hirschhorn, R., Brittinger, G., Hirschhorn, K., and Weissman, G.: J. Cell Biol. **37**:412, 1968.
33. Kleinsmith, L. J., Allfrey, V. G., and Mirsky, A. E.: Science **154**:780, 1966.
34. Pogo, B. G. T., Allfrey, V. G., and Mirsky, A. E.: Proc. Natl. Acad. Sci. **55**:805, 1966.
35. Cooper, H. L. and Rubin, A. D.: Blood **25**:1014, 1965.
36. Epstein, L. B., and Stohlman, F., Jr.: Blood **24**:69, 1964.
37. Rozensza, L. A., and Fischer, D.: Acta Haematol. (Basel) **42**:138, 1969.
38. Bender, M. A., and Prescott, D. M.: Exp. Cell Res. **27**:221, 1962.
39. Mackinney, A. A., Jr., Stohlman, F., Jr., and Brecher, G.: Blood **19**:349, 1962.
40. Rich, A. R., and Lewis, M. R.: Johns Hopkins Med. J. **50**:115, 1932.
41. George, M., and Vaughan, J. H.: Proc. Soc. Exp. Biol. **111**:514, 1962.
42. David, J. R., Lawrence, H. S. and Thomas, L.: J. Immunol. **92**:279, 1964.
43. David, J. R., Al-Askari, S., Lawrence, H. S., and Thomas, L.: J. Immunol **93**:264, 1964.
44. Bloom, R. B., and Bennet, B.: Science **153**:80, 1966.
45. David, J.: Proc. Natl. Acad. Sci. **56**:72, 1966.
46. Dumonde, D. C.: Br. Med. Bull. **23**:1, 1967.
47. Soborg, M., and Bendixen, G.: Acta Med. Scand. **181**:247, 1967.
48. Rocklin, R. E., Remold, H. G., and David, J. R.: Cell Immunol. **5**:436, 1972.
49. Rocklin, R. E.: J. Immunol **112**:1461, 1974.
50. Yoshida, T., Sonozaki, H., and Cohen S.: J. Exp. Med **138**:784, 1973.
51. Rosenberg, S. A., and David, J. R. In Bloom, B. R., and Glade, P. R., editors: In vitro methods in cell-mediated immunity, New York and London, 1971, Academic Press, p. 297.
52. Rocklin, R. E., Rosen, F. S., and David, J. R.: N. Engl. J. Med. **181**:1340, 1970.
53. Wilson, D. B.: J. Exp. Med. **122**:167, 1965.
54. Mauel, J., Rudolf, B., Chapuis, B., and Brunner, K. T.: Immunology **18**:517, 1970.
55. Medawar, P. B. In Lawrence, H. S., editor: Cellular and humoral aspects of the hypersensitivity states, New York, 1959, Hoeber, p. 504.
56. Perlmann, P., and Holm, G.: Adv. Immunol. **11**:117, 1969.
57. Hellstrom, I., and Hellstrom, K. E. In Bloom, B. R., and Glade, P. R., editors: In vitro methods in cell-mediated immunity, New York, 1971, Academic Press, p. 409.
58. Takasuji, M., and Klein, E. In Bloom, B. R., and Glade, P. R., editors: In vitro methods in cell-mediated immunity, New York, 1971, Academic Press, p. 415.
59. Moller, E.: J. Exp. Med. **122**:11, 1965.
60. Brunner, K. T., Mauel, J., Cerottini, J. C., and Chapuis, B.: Immunology **14**:181, 1968.

61. Solliday, S., and Bach, F. H.: Science **170**:988, 1970.

62. Perlmann, P., Nilsson, H., and Leon, M. A.: Science **168**:1112, 1970.

63. Perlmann, P., and Perlmann, H. In Bloom, B. R., and Glade, P. R., editors: In vitro methods in cell-mediated immunity, New York, 1971, Academic Press, p. 361.

64. Lightbody, J. J., Bernaco, D., Miggiano, V. C., and Ceppellini, R.: G. Batteriol. Virol. Immunol. **64**:273, 1971.

65. Yunis, E. J., and Amos, D. B.: Proc. Natl. Acad. Sci. **68**:3031, 10971.

66. Alter, B. A., Schendel, D. J., Bach, M. L., et al.: J. Exp. Med. **137**:1303, 1973.

67. Eijsvoogel, V. P., duBois, R., Melief, C. J. M., et al.: Transplant Proc. **5**:415, 1973.

68. Hartzman, R. J., Segall, M., Bach, M. L., and Bach, F. H.: Transplant Proc. **2**:268, 1971.

64

PHAGOCYTOSIS

Dov L. Boros

EVENTS IN PHAGOCYTOSIS

Phagocytosis[1,2] is the process of ingestion of particulate substances carried out by cells of mesenchymal origin. In primitive single-cell organisms such as the ameba, ingestion is carried out for nutritional purposes. In the higher organisms phagocytosis serves a protective function by the ingestion and degradation of foreign invaders and the elimination of altered, effete, or dead cells of the body. Essentially 2 major types of phagocytic cells exist in higher organisms: (1) neutrophilic polymorphonuclear leukocytes (neutrophils) and (2) mononuclear phagocytes (monocytes and macrophages). Both cell types originate in the bone marrow and arise from common pluripotential stem cells. The natural habitat of the neutrophils and monocytes is the bloodstream, while various forms of macrophages are found in the tissues. Neutrophils are end cells with a limited life span, whereas tissue macrophages are longer lived and have the capacity to divide and transform into further cell forms.

The phagocytic process can be divided into 4 stages: (1) chemotaxis, (2) attachment, (3) engulfment, and (4) killing and digestion. Each stage is briefly discussed below.

Chemotaxis

During an inflammatory process the phagocytic cells often must migrate toward the target particle to be ingested. This unidirectional migration of phagocytic cells is called chemotaxis. Products of various microorganisms as well as mediators released from activated complement components and lymphocytes possess chemotactic properties that may exert a differential chemotaxis on neutrophils or mononuclears. Bacteria and viruses may release chemotactic products directly or may cleave complement components resulting in strong chemotaxis. Chemotactic factors of complement such as C3a and C5a may be produced following the attachment of specific antibody to the microorganisms and the fixation of C1 (classic pathway) or directly by the activation of C3 component (alternate pathway). Both

neutrophils and mononuclears are influenced by these chemotactic stimuli. Since the former move faster, they are the first cells to appear at the site of an inflammation. Antigen-antibody complex formation and plasma factors such as kallikrein and plasminogen activator released during clotting, as well as tissue breakdown products from collagen and fibrin, can all cause the release of various chemotactic agents. Furthermore, factors released by 1 cell may be chemotactic for another cell type. Examples are the basic peptides released by neutrophils, which attract monocytes, and the lymphocyte-secreted lymphokines, which exert chemotaxis on neutrophils and monocytes alike. The energy necessary for the locomotion of cells during chemotaxis is obtained from the glycolytic pathway. Movement of the phagocytes is carried out by means of subcellular contractile elements composed of myosin-containing microfilaments, which act in a manner similar to the contraction of skeletal muscle.

Attachment

Phagocytes at the site of inflammation or microbial invasion must recognize the target. The mechanism by which recognition functions is still not elucidated, but it seems that cell attachment and subsequent engulfment depend on the surface properties of the target. Negative or positive charges as well as hydrophobic or hydrophilic properties of the target particles are probably important during attachment and engulfment. Both processes are greatly facilitated by the coating of fresh serum on the surface of the particles, a process called opsonization. Encapsulated microorganisms such as pneumococci can be engulfed largely only after successful opsonization. Encapsulated, nonopsonized bacteria, when trapped between phagocytes or on rough surfaces found in the tissues, are also engulfed. This is the phenomenon of surface phagocytosis. Opsonins in part are specific immunoglobulins of the G and M class that may act in collaboration with complement in the recognition and ingestion of the particles. For complete opsonization both the intact Fc and Fab regions of the immunoglobulins are necessary. The Fab portion attaches to the particle, whereas the Fc portion is bound to a specific receptor on the surface of the phagocytes, thus serving as a guiding mechanism. Macrophages possess receptors for the Fc portion as well as the C3 component of the complement. Thus the particle onto which a specific antibody is attached at the Fab region is specifically recognized first as "foreign," then is guided onto the surface of the macrophage, and is finally engulfed by the cell. Some of the heat-labile complement components can also serve as opsonizing agents alone. A split product of C3 deposited on the surface of microorganisms is known to facilitate ingestion.

Engulfment

Following attachment of the particle to the surface of the phagocytic cells pseudopodia are sent out from the ectoplasm, which surround the particle and finally fuse around it. The process of ingestion is energy-dependent requiring the presence of divalent cations and the action of the contractile microfilaments present in the pseudopodia. The particle, which is now interiorized, lies within a vesicle, the so-called phagosome, and migrates toward the interior of the cell. Next granules (lysosomes), which contain hydrolytic enzymes and bactericidal substances, converge on the phagosome; the membranes of the phagosome and the lysosome fuse, and the content of the lysosomes is discharged into the phagosome. The empty granules disappear from the cytoplasm; the cells display degranulation. This process also requires the active participation of microtubules and microfilaments. One distinguishes primary and secondary lysosomal granules in the phagocytic cells. In the neutrophils the primary, large, dense, so-called azurophil granules contain acid hydrolases, myeloperoxidase, and lysozyme, whereas the smaller secondary granules contain alkaline phosphatase and lactoferrin. These 2 types of granules do not discharge their contents simultaneously. In the macrophages the lysosomes contain acid phosphatase, ribonuclease, deoxyribonuclease, lipase, cathepsin D, β-glucuronidase, β-galactosidase, and other enzymes capable of degrading proteins, carbohydrates, lipids, and nucleic acids. Occasionally lysosomal enzymes are liberated from the cells and reach the surrounding tissues, causing damage of various degrees.

Killing and digestion

When the ingested particles are animate, as in the case of various microorganisms, they are killed and then degraded. Many bacteria lose their capacity to multiply following ingestion and can be considered killed. Some organisms, however, such as *Mycobacteria, Brucella, Salmonella,* and *Listeria,* can survive in the intracellular environment and even show multiplication. There are differences between the microbicidal agents utilized by the neutrophils and the mononuclears. An effective bactericidal measure utilized by neutrophils is the lowered intracellular pH. Lactic acid, generated during glycolysis,

may bring the pH down to 4, which alone can kill various organisms or can assist in their degradation by acid hydrolases. Low pH also promotes the generation of hydrogen peroxide (H_2O_2) a powerful bactericidal agent produced within phagocytes during the metabolic events of phagocytosis. As a first step in the production of peroxide, oxygen (O_2) is reduced by an oxidase enzyme into superoxide (O_2^-) and then reduction of superoxide (a highly reactive radical) generates H_2O_2. Superoxide may also react with the H_2O_2 already generated to form very reactive hydroxyl (OH) radicals, which can attack unsaturated fatty acids of the phagosomal membrane and generate bactericidal aldehydes. Superoxides, H_2O_2, and hydroxyl radicals exert their bactericidal effect within the phagosomes. Since superoxide anions and H_2O_2 are toxic, their escape and accumulation in the extracellular medium can be lethal to the neutrophils. To prevent this, various detoxifying mechanisms exist in the cytoplasm.

The most powerful microbicidal system present in the neutrophils consists of a combination of H_2O_2-halide-myeloperoxidase. Chlorides and iodide can covalently bind onto proteins of the ingested particles. Thus it is plausible that halide ions present in the cell participate in the killing. Although the myeloperoxidase enzyme helps the breakdown of H_2O_2, at the same time the capacity of the breakdown product to attack bacterial substrates, perhaps by the formation of reactive aldehydes, is enhanced. While the exact mechanism of microbial killing is still not clear, neutrophils with impaired generation of H_2O_2 display defective bactericidal activity and predispose the patient to recurrent infections.

Other microbicidal functions that are oxygen independent are carried out by lysozyme, lactoferrin, and cationic proteins. Lysozyme is found in large quantities in neutrophils. The enzyme degrades the cell wall of certain bacteria causing direct lysis. It can also act in conjunction with complement and antibody or cation chelators, and following the initial damage by the latter causes lysis of the bacteria. Lactoferrin is an iron-binding protein that may exert its bactericidal effect by chelating the iron required for the microbes. Crude cationic proteins, phagocytins isolated from neutrophils after separation and purification procedures, yield at least 6 basic proteins, each with a specific activity for certain bacteria. The proteins are active in acid pH and exert damage on the bacterial membrane.

Of interest, much less is known about the microbicidal mechanisms utilized by macrophages. These cells do not possess lactoferrin or cationic proteins. Furthermore H_2O_2 production has been observed largely in alveolar but not in peritoneal macrophages, while myeloperoxidase activity is weak compared with that of the neutrophils. Macrophages, however, possess a wide variety of lysosomal enzymes that can degrade effectively most of the ingested materials.

It has been shown that macrophages and also

polymorphonuclear leukocytes can be activated by soluble mediators secreted by lymphocytes. These soluble mediators, termed lymphokines, are nonantibody products secreted by the thymus-derived normal T-lymphocytes stimulated with plant mitogens or are produced by sensitized cells following a stimulus with the specific antigen. Lymphokines have various effects on these cells. Among these effects are mobilization and recruitment of fresh cells from the bone marrow, enhanced chemotaxis and inhibition of migration, increased membrane activity, increased respiration during phagocytosis, increased glucose oxidation, and increased phagocytic and bacteriostatic action.

DISORDERS OF PHAGOCYTIC FUNCTION

Recently it has been realized that some recurrent microbial diseases are associated with defects in phagocytosis and microbial killing by host phagocytes. Impaired phagocytosis may be due to defective humoral factors such as low levels of specific opsonins and disorders of the complement system or to defects in the functions of polymorphonuclear and mononuclear phagocytes. Impaired phagocytic function can occur at any of the steps of phagocytosis. Many of the defects are the result of inborn errors, while some are acquired or iatrogenically induced.

Abnormal chemotaxis[3]

Abnormality in the generation of chemotactic stimuli may occur in the serum or plasma due to a deficiency in the complement or the kinin-fibrinolytic system. Conversely substances may occur in the circulation that inactivate chemotactic factors directed to neutrophils and mononuclears. Finally, a cellular defect may cause the lack of response to normal chemotactic stimuli.

The complement system is one of the most important sources for the generation of chemotactic factors. Genetic deficiencies in humans involving the C2, C3, and C5 components have been described, the most serious being the C3 and C5 deficiencies. The C3 component occupies a key position in the function of both the classic and the alternate pathways of the complement cascade. A deficiency in this important component may occur congenitally or through abnormally fast catabolism, reduced rate of synthesis, or depletion by disease states. Deficiency in another chemotactic plasma system, the kininogen-kinin sequence, also results in diminished chemotactic activity of the serum. This is due to a deficiency in prekallikrein and the diminished rate of Hageman factor activation. Various as yet ill-defined factors have been demonstrated recently in the serum of patients suffering from chronic infections, liver cirrhosis, nephritis, and Hodgkin's disease. These factors can inactivate the chemotactic factors derived from complement and cause diminished chemotaxis in neutrophils and mononuclears. Defects in leukotaxis due to impaired reaction of neutrophils to chemotactic factors have also been described in Chediak-

Higashi syndrome. Another primary defect in the chemotactic migration of neutrophils has been observed in the so-called lazy leukocyte. These cells seem to have normal phagocytic and bactericidal activity but a defective response to chemotactic stimuli. Persons with this syndrome fail to mount an inflammatory response when tested by the Rebuck skin window technic. Acquired defects in cellular chemotaxis are known to occur also in patients with diabetes, recurrent pyogenic infections, mucocutaneous candidiasis, rheumatoid arthritis, and malignant tumors.

Disorders of attachment[4]

Since specific antibodies and complement components are necessary for attachment, defects in either of these humoral factors can cause impaired attachment of the particle to phagocytes. The state of congenital or acquired hypogammaglobulinemia or agammaglobulinemia is known to cause increased susceptibility to recurrent pyogenic infections. Lack of opsonization is especially important in infections caused by encapsulated organisms such as pneumococci and *Haemophilus* because deficient phagocytosis predisposes for septic conditions. It has been shown in vitro that blood leukocyte function from hypogammaglobulinemic persons can be restored to normal by the addition of normal serum or purified immunoglobulin. Opsonization is primarily a function of bound C3b component of the complement. Thus inadequate levels of serum C3 may be the most important factor in the lack of successful opsonization. The C3b fragment binds to bacteria, animal cell membranes, and immune complexes and, aided by an exposed site, can also bind to specific receptors on the surface of the phagocytes. This attachment then induces phagocytosis of the adhering particle. Complement-dependent opsonization may be important in the early phase of bacterial invasion before the production of specific antibodies. Impairment in the classic complement pathway may not render a person vulnerable to infections, since the alternate pathway using the properdin system can also generate opsonizing factors following the attack on the C3 component of complement. Deficiencies in C3 level are acquired in hepatic cirrhosis and nephritis.

Disorders of engulfment and degranulation[4]

Engulfment or ingestion of particles requires the same specific and nonspecific serum factors necessary for attachment. Thus nonopsonized particles are ingested only with difficulty. Deficiencies in both the C3 and C5 components of complement are known to cause decreased ingestion. Hypertonicity of the medium, exposure of the phagocytic cells to immune complexes, the influence of drugs that affect the energy-dependent metabolic pathways of phagocytes, cortisone treatment, which stabilizes the membranes of lysosomal granules, or colchicine, which interferes with microtubule function, all cause impairment of particle ingestion and degranulation. Certain ingested microorganisms may survive the intracellular environment by somehow arresting the fusion of lysosomal granules with the phagosomes. *Toxoplasma* and *mycobacteria* seem to escape intracellular killing by this mechanism. Patients with Chediak-Higashi syndrome show increased susceptibility to pyogenic infection, and giant lysosomal granules appear in the cytoplasm of neutrophils and monocytes. The granules are incapable of migration toward the phagosome and do not fuse with the latter. Consequently the ingested bacteria are not exposed to the hydrolytic enzymes of the granules and escape killing and digestion. The type of lysosomal granules that empty their contents into the phagosomes is also of importance. In the neutrophils the bactericidal effect depends on whether the azurophil granules, which contain the myeloperoxidase, or the lactoferrin containing granules will undergo degranulation.

Defective killing and digestion[5]

Defective killing of ingested bacteria is displayed by phagocytic cells of children with chronic granulomatous disease of childhood. Chronic granulomatous disease (CGD) is a sex-linked inherited defect characterized by marked susceptibility to pyogenic bacteria, lymphadenopathy, appearance of disseminated granulomas with many lipid-containing macrophages, chronic pneumonias, dermatitis, and often early death. The organisms most commonly cultured from patients are *Staphylococcus*, *Klebsiella*, *Serratia*, and *Escherichia*. CGD granulocytes during the ingestion do not develop large phagosomes, but otherwise the uptake of particles, degranulation, distribution pattern of lysosomal enzymes, glucose consumption, and lactate production are normal. Metabolic studies, however, establish that CGD leukocytes do not show the respiratory burst; there is no glucose oxidation to CO_2 through the hexose monophosphate shunt (HMPS) and consequently no accumulation of H_2O_2.

Following ingestion of particles by normal polymorphonuclears there is a noticeable increase in anaerobic glycolysis. Glucose is consumed and lactate is produced. This process yields ATP, which is needed for phagocytosis.

Concurrently there is a respiratory burst evidenced by increased oxygen consumption and oxidation of glucose via the HMPS. During phagocytosis as much as 10% glucose may be oxidized to CO_2 via the shunt (oxidation at glucose-1-C). In addition to energy formation the glycolytic pathway provides reduced nicotinamide adenine dinucleotide (NADH) from nicotinamide adenine dinucleotide (NAD+). Through the catalytic effect of NADH oxidase, NADH and oxygen form H_2O_2. Hydrogen peroxide stimulates the HMPS by oxidizing glutathione, which in turn is reduced by nicotinamide dinucleotide phosphate (NADPH). Oxidized nicotinamide dinucleotide phosphate (NADP+)

is generated by the flow of glucose through the HMPS pathway, which is catalyzed by glucose-6-phosphate dehydrogenase and 6-phosphogluconate dehydrogenase enzymes. Since the most powerful bactericidal system consists of H_2O_2-halide-myeloperoxidase, failure to produce H_2O_2 by CGD leukocytes can account for the defect in the bactericidal mechanism of these cells. Using radioactive iodine, iodination of the bacterial cell walls can be demonstrated in normal but not in CGD leukocytes. Of interest, children with CGD are not prone to pneumococcal or streptococcal infections. These microorganisms apparently are killed in a normal fashion within the CGD leukocytes, presumably because they generate their own H_2O_2 and contribute to their own death. In elegant in vitro experiments the bactericidal capability of CGD leukocytes could be restored following the ingestion of latex particles coated with glucose oxidase, which could initiate HMPS activity.

Additional types of bactericidal defects manifested by impaired oxidative killing are also known. Rare individuals with a total deficiency of myeloperoxidase (MPO) activity in the leukocytes have been identified. Some of these patients have chronic *Candida* infections; the leukocytes are incapable of killing the ingested yeast cells. Compared with patients with CGD, MPO-deficient individuals have a much better clinical prognosis and seem to be freer from recurrent infections. There is a delay in the killing of ingested, catalase-negative and -positive bacteria (probably due to impaired iodination of the organisms), but no absolute defect in killing is observed. Granulocytes with MPO deficiency show normal or even exaggerated oxygen consumption and HMP shunt activity. This in turn ensures an adequate supply of H_2O_2. It seems that the peroxide generated in MPO leukocytes is utilized by an alternative adaptive mechanism with the participation of ascorbic acid, which substitutes for the lack of this important enzyme.

Severe infections can also occur in individuals whose leukocytes are deficient in glucose-6-phosphate dehydrogenase enzyme. While phagocytosis is normal, the lack of HMPS activity, deficient NADH and NADPH content, and the generation of only low levels of H_2O_2 predispose to deficient intracellular killing. Microorganisms such as staphylococci, *Escherichia*, and *Serratia* are not killed within cells, while *Streptococcus* is normally killed, similar to CGD.

Individuals with Chediak-Higashi syndrome contract recurrent severe pyogenic infections and display giant cytoplasmic lysosomal granules in the leukocytes. As mentioned above, the leukocytes are defective in their chemotactic response and show defective intracellular killing of ingested bacteria. While the respiratory burst and H_2O_2 formation are normal during phagocytosis, there is inadequate fusion of the lysosomal granules with the membranes of the phagosomes. This indicates that intracellular killing probably relies on 2 separate steps. The organisms are attacked by lysomal enzymes and subsequently are killed by the myeloperoxidase-halide-peroxide system.

MEASUREMENT OF CHEMOTAXIS[6]

Principle. This test measures in vitro the migratory response of polymorphonuclear neutrophils to a chemotactic stimulus generated across a permeable membrane.

Reagents
1. Methylcellulose, 2%, in normal saline
2. Hank's balanced salt solution without bicarbonate
3. Casein solution (dissolve 5 mg/ml casein in Hank's balanced salt solution and adjust final pH to 5.2)
4. Pooled normal human serum, type AB, as source of complement (stored at -40 C)
5. Mixture of equal proportions of casein solution and human serum
6. Wright's stain
7. Xylene
8. Permanent mounting fluid

Procedure
1. Draw 10 ml peripheral venous blood into heparinized Vacutainer tube.
2. Add to blood 0.75 ml 2% solution of methylcellulose.
3. Gently invert mixture and allow red blood cells and mononuclear leukocytes to settle.
4. After 30-45 min at room temperature remove supernatant plasma layer and make total white cell count.
5. Dilute plasma with Hank's solution to final count of between 7000-10,000 cells/mm³ (75-85% polymorphonuclear content).
6. Deposit cells in center of 25 mm Millipore filter (3 μm pore size), 4-5 drops per slide, and spin in cytocentrifuge at 500 rpm for 5 min.
7. Rapidly remove filter and place in Sykes-Moore tissue culture chamber (Bellco Glass Co., Vineland, N.J.).
8. Construct chamber as follows: 25 mm round coverslip, gasket, Millipore filter with cells, gasket, 25 mm round coverslip; chamber is closed with screw top.
9. Fill chamber through ports in slanted position to prevent air bubbles. Fill upper compartment with Hank's solution (pH 6.8) and lower compartment with casein-serum mixture.
10. Incubate chamber for 3 h at 37 C; then remove filter (do not let it dry!), fix in methanol, and stain with Wright's stain.
11. Treat stained filter with xylene to render it transparent, place filter on microscope slide, fix with permanent mounting fluid, and cover with coverslip.
12. Count cells using 10× ocular and 25× objective of microscope. Count only those cells present at **bottom** of filter (completely penetrated filter). Focus **beyond** cells and count only those cells that appear first in focus as membrane is reached.

Calculation. Count 10 fields at random on each side of filter. Calculate chemotactic index:

$$\text{Chemotactic index} = \frac{\text{No. cells (attractant side)}}{\text{No. cells (starting side)}} \times 100$$

NOTE: Since relative variation of 12% was found on repeated measurements done in single subject, it is advised that test be set up in triplicate for each sample. This reduces error to 7%.

ASSAY FOR DEGRANULATION[7]

Principle. This test measures in vitro the activity of the enzyme, β-glucuronidase, which is liberated from the granules of the polymorphonuclear neutrophils during active phagocytosis.

Reagents
1. 6% Dextran in saline.
2. Ice cold 0.87% ammonium chloride in tris buffer.
3. Phosphate-buffered saline prepared from 0.15M Na_2HPO_4, 0.15M NaCl, 0.6M $CaCl_2$, and 1 mM $MgCl_2$, pH 7.3.
4. Hank's balanced salt solution.
5. Pooled normal human serum, type AB.
6. Zymosan particles, 3-5 μm (Nutritional Biochemicals Corp., Chagrin Falls, Ohio). Particles are suspended in 0.15M NaCl, boiled, washed twice, and resuspended to concentration of 5 mg/ml in Hank's solution supplemented with 10% vol/vol normal human serum. Particles are now opsonized.
7. Acetate buffer. Mix 0.05M sodium acetate and 0.05M acetic acid; pH of mixture, 5.0.
8. Phenolphthalein-glucuronic acid (Sigma Chemical Co., St. Louis).
9. Glycine buffer, 0.2M in 0.2M NaCl, pH 10.4. Prepare glycin buffer by dissolving 16.3 g glycine, 12.65 g NaCl, and 10.9 ml concentrated NaOH solution in 1000 ml distilled water; pH should be 10.4.
10. β-Glucuronidase, bovine liver (Worthington Biochemical Corp., Freehold, N.J.)
11. Triton X 100 detergent (Rohm and Haas, Philadelphia).

Procedure
Preparation of cell suspension and phagocytosis
1. Draw 10-20 ml venous blood into heparinized tube.
2. Sediment erythrocytes at room temperature with dextran saline; add 0.5 vol to each vol blood.
3. After 45-60 min remove supernatant plasma, transfer into conical centrifuge tube, and add to each vol 0.5 vol ice cold ammonium chloride in tris buffer.
4. Invert tube rapidly and centrifuge suspension at $500 \times g$ for 10 min.
5. Resuspend cells in ice-cold phosphate-buffered saline and wash cells twice. Resuspend cells finally in Hank's solution to concentration of 4×10^6 cells per 0.8 ml.
6. Transfer 0.8 ml cell suspension into capped plastic test tubes and incubate for 5 min in shaker water bath at 37 C.
7. Add 1×10^8 opsonized zymosan particles (counted in hemocytometer) in 0.2 ml vol and continue to incubate mixture. Conduct test in duplicates.
8. Set up control tubes containing cells without zymosan and cells with opsonized zymosan particles.
9. Remove duplicate tubes at 15, 30, and 60 min of incubation, cool mixture on ice, and spin cells at $500 \times g$ for 10 min. Supernatants now contain enzyme liberated during phagocytosis.

Assay for enzyme activity[8]
PRINCIPLE. Determine by colorimetry the amount of phenolphthalein liberated from substrate: phenolphthalein-glucuronic acid, following its breakdown by β-glucuronidase.

PROCEDURE
1. Pipet supernatants in 0.1 ml vol into tubes; add 0.9 ml acetate buffer containing 0.01M dissolved phenolphthalein-glucuronic acid. Include blank tube, substituting 0.1 ml buffer for supernatant to be assayed.
2. Incubate mixture for 18 h at 37 C. At end of incubation period stop reaction by addition of ice-cold glycine buffer.
3. Read developed color at 440 nm in colorimeter.

Calculation. Data can be expressed as percent release of enzyme compared with enzyme content of total cell button of 4×10^6 cells lysed with 1 mg/ml Triton X 100 detergent. Absorbance readings are converted into micromoles phenolphthalein cleaved by employing standard curve using β-glucuronidase enzyme and phenolphthalein-glucuronic acid as substrate.

MEASUREMENT OF PHAGOCYTOSIS BY NEUTROPHILS[9]

Principle. This test measures in vitro the ingestion of microorganisms by polymorphonuclear neutrophils using standard microbiologic technics.

Reagents
1. Preservative-free heparin 1000 U/ml.
2. Dextran solution, 6%, in normal saline.
3. Ice-cold 0.87% ammonium chloride. Dissolve NH_4Cl in distilled water and mix 9 vol solution with 1 vol tris buffer. (Tris buffer is prepared by dissolving 20.59 g tris buffer in 1000 ml distilled water; adjust pH with HCl to 7.6.) Final pH NH_4Cl-tris buffer mixture, 7.2.
4. Wright's stain.
5. Gelatin–Hank's solution. Dissolve 100 mg gelatin (Difco Laboratories, Detroit) in 5 ml Hank's balanced salt solution with gentle heating and add Hank's solution to make 100 ml.
6. Pooled normal human serum, type AB, as source of opsonizing agent. Store serum in small aliquots at −40 C.
7. Add 10% vol/vol serum to gelatin–Hank's solution.
8. Trypan blue stain in saline (Grand Island Biological Co., Grand Island, N.Y.).
9. Various gram-positive (e.g., *Staphylococcus epidermidis, Staphylococcus aureus*) and gram-negative (e.g., *Pseudomonas aeruginosa, Salmonella typhimurium*) microorganisms.
10. Normal 0.85% saline.
11. Tryptic soy broth and agar (Difco Laboratories).
12. Methanol.

Procedure
1. Draw 10 ml peripheral venous blood into heparinized Vacutainer tube.
2. Add 5 ml dextran-saline solution to 10 ml blood, mix gently, and allow erythrocytes to sediment at room temperature for 45-60 min.
3. Remove supernatant plasma layer and prepare slide for differential count (Wright's stain). Transfer remainder of plasma into conical centrifuge tube and add ice-cold ammonium chloride to lyse erythrocytes.
4. Centrifuge tube at $500 \times g$ for 10 min. Suspend cell pellet in heparinized saline (0.5 U/ml saline) and wash twice with same.
5. Finally, suspend cell pellet in gelatin–Hank's solution and adjust cell concentration to $1-2 \times 10^7$ cells/ml.

6. Check for viability of cells by adding 1 vol trypan blue stain to 1 vol cells and count at least 200 cells. Blue cells showing uptake of dye are dead.
7. Grow selected test microorganism on tryptic soy broth in 100 ml flasks for 18 h at 37 C. Centrifuge culture on day of cell preparation at $1500 \times g$ for 10 min, wash twice with cold normal saline, and resuspend bacteria in gelatin–Hank's solution to concentration of $1-2 \times 10^7$ organisms/ml. Verify concentration of bacteria by turbidity measurement in colorimeter at 650 nm.
8. Mix 2 ml cell suspension with 2 ml bacterial suspension (optimal cell to bacteria ratio is 1:1). Add 0.4 ml normal human serum and incubate mixture in plastic capped test tubes in shaker water bath at 37 C.
9. Remove 0.5 ml suspension at 0, 30, 60, and 120 min of incubation and add to 1.5 ml ice-cold gelatin–Hank's solution.
10. Sediment polymorphonuclears by centrifuging at $110 \times g$ for 4 min. This speed does not sediment bacteria.
11. Prepare from supernatant fluid serial 10-fold dilutions in saline so that viable microbial count is between 100-1000 bacteria/ml. (Convenient colony count is between 30-300.)
12. Pipet 0.1 ml vol from higher dilutions onto dried surface of tryptic soy agar plates and spread with Drigalski glass rod bent at right angle.

Calculation. Based on colony count, number of bacteria/ml is calculated from mean values of duplicate plates, considering original volume (0.1 ml), dilution factor, and number of microorganisms present at 0 time in reaction mixture.

Remarks. Percentage of cells containing ingested bacteria is determined as follows:
1. Remove 0.5 ml from the bacteria and cell suspension after 15 minutes of incubation and dilute with ice-cold gelatin–Hank's solution.
2. Spin at $110 \times g$ for 4 minutes and wash cells 3 times in same.
3. Prepare a slide from the cell pellet, fix with methanol, and stain with Giemsa stain.
4. Count at least 200 cells to assay the percentage of cells containing ingested bacteria.

MEASUREMENT OF NEUTROPHIL BACTERICIDAL ACTIVITY[9]

Principle. This test measures in vitro the intracellular killing of microorganisms ingested by the polymorphonuclear neutrophils.

Reagents
1. Preservative-free heparin 1000 U/ml.
2. Dextran solution, 6%, in normal saline.
3. Ice-cold 0.87% ammonium chloride in tris buffer, pH 7.2.
4. Wright's stain.
5. Gelatin–Hank's solution, Hank's solution.
6. Pooled normal human serum, type AB. Inactivate serum before use by heating at 56 C for 30 min.
7. Gelatin–Hank's solution with 10% vol/vol human serum.
8. Trypan blue stain in saline.
9. Various gram-positive (e.g., *Staphylococcus epidermidis, Staphylococcus* aureus) and gram-

negative (e.g., *Pseudomonas aeruginosa, Salmonella typhimurium*) microorganisms.

10. Bovine serum albumin, 0.01%, dissolved in distilled water.
11. Normal saline, 0.85%.
12. Tryptic soy broth and agar.

Procedure

1-8. Separation of neutrophils and phagocytosis of microorganisms, identical to procedure for measurement of phagocytosis.
9. Incubate bacteria-cell suspension for 15 min; then remove aliquot of 0.5 ml, add 1.5 ml ice-cold gelatin–Hank's solution, and sediment cells by centrifugation at $110 \times g$ for 4 min.
10. Wash sedimented cells twice in gelatin–Hank's solution; then resuspend in 3 ml Hank's solution containing 10% normal human serum.
11. Incubate cell suspension at 37 C; remove at 0, 30, 60, 90, and 120 min 0.5 ml samples, add equal vol ice-cold Hank's solution, and centrifuge at $110 \times g$ for 4 min.
12. Remove supernatant fluid and lyse neutrophils with 1 ml ice-cold bovine albumin solution and pipettation. Check for complete lysis of cells under microscope.
13. Prepare serial 10-fold dilutions in saline as described previously and plate bacteria on tryptic soy agar.
14. Count colonies of bacteria and calculate number that survived intracellular killing.

Calculation. Killing index K_t can be calculated by:

$$K_t = \log N_0 - \log N_t$$

where N_0 is number of viable intracellular bacteria at start (0 time) and N_t is number of viable intracellular bacteria at time t.

Remarks. The index is valuable for comparative purposes, to establish the differential rate of killing of various organisms by the normal cells as well as the differences in the microbicidal function of healthy and diseased cells.

NITROBLUE TETRAZOLIUM (NBT) REDUCTION TEST[10,11]

Principle. This test measures the diminished bactericidal capacity of polymorphonuclear neutrophils. Defective cells fail to reduce the NBT dye during phagocytosis.

Semiquantitative

Reagents

1. Nitroblue tetrazolium dye (NBT) (Sigma Chemical Co., St. Louis), 0.2% in normal saline
2. Phosphate buffered saline (PBS), 0.15M Na_2HPO_4, 0.15M NaCl, pH 7.2
3. NBT solution, equal vol NBT and PBS
4. Latex particles, 0.8 μm size (Difco Laboratories, Detroit)
5. Pooled human γ-globulin, 1%
6. Wright's stain

Procedure

1. Draw 0.5-1.0 ml peripheral venous blood into heparinized tube.
2. Mix gently and transfer about 0.1 ml blood onto concave microslide (Clay Adams, Parsippany, N.J.). Use only previously acid-cleaned and siliconized slides.
3. Add 0.1 ml buffered NBT solution; keep slide in

humid atmosphere (place on wet gauze in Petri dish) and incubate at 37 C for 15 min.
4. Add bare latex particles or particles coated with human γ-globulin (opsonized). Add vol 0.05 ml from suspension containing 2×10^8 particles/ml.
5. Incubate slide for 15 min at 37 C.
6. After 15 min mix suspension gently with small capillary pipet and prepare cell smear on coverslip. Take care not to damage leukocytes.
7. Air dry coverslip and stain with Wright's stain.
8. Count cells under oil-immersion objective. Between 200-500 cells should be counted to obtain reliable percentage of NBT-positive cells.
9. Establish by differential count total number of neutrophils.

Remarks. A cell is considered NBT positive if it contains large bluish black deposits or stippled granules in the cytoplasm. A positive cell should also have at least 5 phagocytized latex particles in the cytoplasm. Formazan, the reduced form of NBT, when viewed under the microscope has a refractile border that becomes visible when focusing up and down with the micrometer. This helps to differentiate it from other cytoplasmic structures.

About 8-10% of the "resting" nonphagocytizing cells from healthy persons show NBT reduction. During the course of a natural infection (i.e., bacterial meningitis) spontaneous reduction of NBT by neutrophils can be as high as 50%.

NOTE: The test is not applicable during the first 2 months of life due to the elevated metabolic activity of neutrophils.

Quantitative. The quantitative version of this test relies on the extraction of reduced NBT dye and its measurement in a spectrophotometer. The test requires more blood and more extensive facilities (exhaust hood, spectrophotometer) and is more time consuming.

Reagents

1. Heparin
2. Human fibrinogen (Fibro-AHF, Merck, Sharp Dohme, Rahway, N.J.)
3. Ice-cold 0.87% ammonium chloride in tris buffer
4. Krebs-Henseleit bicarbonate buffer, pH 7.4, containing 200 mg glucose/100 ml
5. NBT, 0.1% solution in normal saline
6. Potassium cyanide, 0.01M
7. Latex particles
8. HCl, 0.5N
9. Pyridine

Procedure

1. Draw 25 ml peripheral venous blood into 30 ml plastic syringe containing 0.5 ml 1:1000 heparin.
2. Sediment erythrocytes with 5 ml human fibrinogen.
3. After 60-120 min remove supernatant and lyse erythrocytes with 0.87% ice-cold ammonium chloride.
4. Centrifuge at $120 \times g$ for 5 min at room temperature.
5. Remove supernatant and wash cells twice in Krebs-Henseleit buffer.
6. Suspend cells in same buffer to final concentration of 25,000 cells/mm³.
7. Set up duplicate siliconized 15 ml conical centrifuge tubes and add 0.4 ml buffer (to tubes that also

will receive latex particles add only 0.35 ml), 0.1 ml potassium cyanide, 0.4 ml NBT-saline solution, and 0.05 ml latex particles. No latex particles are added to tubes where "resting" nonphagocytizing cells will be tested.

8. Preincubate tubes in water bath at 37 C for 15 min and then add 0.1 ml final cell suspension to each tube. Incubate tubes for additional 15 min.
9. After incubation add 10 ml HC1 to each tube, centrifuge at $1000 \times g$ in cold for 15 min, and remove supernatant.
10. Extract purple cell button with 2 ml pyridine for 10 min in boiling water bath under exhaust hood.
11. Centrifuge tubes at $500 \times g$, remove supernatant, and repeat extraction of cell button with pyridine.
12. Combine purple fluids and determine absorbance at 515 nm using pyridine as blank.

Remarks. The absorbance of a cell extract and NBT dye incubated for 10 seconds is also determined and the values are subtracted from the others as a reagent blank.

Values obtained from phagocytizing and resting cells are compared and the difference is calculated: Δ absorbance per 15 min per 2×10^6 phagocytes.

Phagocytizing normal cells show values about 5 times higher compared with resting cells. Phagocytizing cells from patients with chronic granulomatous disease (CGD) of childhood have values lower than resting normal cells.

Example:
0.088 "resting" normal cells
0.313 phagocytizing normal cells
0.040 phagocytizing CGD cells

REFERENCES

1. Stossel, T. P.: N. Engl. J. Med. **290:**717, 774, 833, 1974.
2. Elsbach, P.: Phagocytosis: the inflammatory process, vol. 1, New York, 1974, Academic Press.
3. Ward, P. A.: Am. J. Pathol. **77:**520, 1973.
4. Quie, P. G., and Davis, A. T. In Stiehm, E. R., and Fulginiti, V. A., editors: Immunologic disorders in infants and children, Philadelphia, 1973, W. B. Saunders Co.
5. Baehner, R. L.: The phagocytic cell in host resistance, New York, 1975, Raven Press.
6. Baum, J., Mowat, A. G., and Kirk, J. A.: J. Lab. Clin. Med. **77:**501, 1971.
7. Zurier, B. R., Hoffstein, S., and Weissmann, G.: Proc. Natl. Acad. Sci. **70:**844, 1973.
8. Brittinger, G., Hirschhorn, R., Douglas, S. D., and Weissmann, G.: J. Cell Biol. **37:**394, 1968.
9. van Furth, R., and van Zwet, T. L. In Weir, D. M., editor: Handbook of experimental immunology, Oxford, 1973, Scientific Publications.
10. Park, B. H., Fikrig, S. M., and Smithwick, E. M.: Lancet **2:**532, 1968.
11. Baehner, R. L., and Nathan, D. G.: N. Engl. J. Med. **278:**971, 1968.

DETECTION OF AUTOANTIBODIES

C. Lynne Burek
Noel R. Rose

The concept that antibodies do not develop to one's own tissue was first propounded by Erhlich. He coined the term "horror autotoxicus" for the principle that if self-reactive antibodies were produced, the end result might be disease or death. Subsequent investigators have shown that man does develop autoantibodies, although the pathologic significance of these antibodies in many cases is uncertain. There seem to be a number of autoantibodies in normal persons as well as in individuals with various disease processes. In the normal population, autoantibodies appear to be related to age and sex, the highest incidence being in older females and the lowest in younger males.

The term "autoimmune disease" is reserved primarily for those conditions in which the immunologic processes contribute to the pathogenesis of the disease. Criteria for designation of an autoimmune disease were proposed by Witebsky et al. in 1957.[1] They included demonstration of antibodies or cell-mediated immunity operating under physiologic conditions. The responsible antigen should be defined, isolated, and used to induce an immunologic response in experimental animals. Pathologic changes similar to those seen in human disease should appear in the corresponding tissue of the immunized animal.

Autoantibodies are sometimes found when the involvement of the immune system is secondary to an initial infection or other tissue injury. Even in these cases, demonstration of autoantibodies may be valuable in diagnosis. Human disease associated with autoantibody production may range from strictly organ-specific conditions to disorders of a more generalized character. There is often a tendency for more than one autoimmune disorder to occur in the same individual. The overlap is often within the same category of disease, as seen in a patient with multiple endocrine disorders (such as thyroiditis and adrenalitis) or multiple "connective tissue" diseases (such as a patient with Sjögren's keratoconjunctivitis sicca and lupus). In addition there is a significantly higher incidence of autoantibodies to unrelated organ-specific antigens in patients with one autoimmune disease. For example, one-fourth of the patients with thyroiditis have antibodies to gastric parietal cells, while almost half of patients with pernicious anemia have antibodies to a thyroid antigen,[2,3] Twenty-five percent of patients with Addison's disease and 20% of patients with diabetes mellitus have antibodies to thyroid antigen,[3,4] suggesting that an autoimmune factor is also involved in those diseases. The aggregation of autoimmune responses to immunologically distinct organ-specific antigens cannot be explained at this moment except as a genetic predisposition comparable to atopy in the immediate hypersensitivity reactions.

The method of demonstrating autoantibodies is based on the position and properties of the antigen and the desired level of sensitivity. Agglutination tests use stable cell suspensions, especially erythrocytes, either alone or coated with appropriate soluble antigens. Soluble antigens can also be used in precipitation or latex fixation tests. One of the most widely used tests for detection of antibodies directed against tissue antigens is indirect immunofluorescence (IIF). This procedure involves the application of patient serum to a section of appropriate human or animal tissue as substrate, removal of excess globulin by washing, and subsequent addition of antiserum to human globulin, which was prepared by immunization of an experimental animal and which has been conjugated with a fluorescent tag. The site of antibody fixation can be visualized with appropriate fluorescence microscopy. Sometimes demonstration of localized complement is useful as an indicator of antigen-antibody reactions as is a decrease in levels of circulating complement components.

INDIRECT IMMUNOFLUORESCENT TEST FOR ANTINUCLEAR ANTIBODY

Testing for antibody in patient's serum to components of cell nuclei using IIF is one of the

The investigative work of the authors was supported in part by Contract HD-5-2841 from the National Institute of Child Health and Human Development (NICHHD).

most common laboratory procedures for diagnosis of autoimmune disease. Therefore this technic will be described in detail.

Sera from patients with diseases such as systemic lupus erythematosus (SLE), scleroderma, rheumatoid arthritis, and other connective tissue disorders may contain antibodies to nuclear constituents. They are not tissue or species specific, so that sections of any nucleated animal tissue may be used as substrate. The sections are incubated with the individual test serum. Excess globulin is removed by washing, and a fluorescent antiglobulin reagent is applied to the tissue. When viewed by fluorescence microscopy, the deposition of the antibody in the nucleus can be visualized. The most important variables involved in producing a standardized technic are (1) type of substrate, including source, storage, and preparation, (2) duration of staining and washing, and (3) specificity and sensitivity of the conjugate. An essential part of each test is the incorporation of known positive and negative reactive sera as controls.

Materials and methods

The most appropriate and readily available substrate tissue for IIF antinuclear antibody tests is liver of young mice or rats. The animal is exsanguinated and the liver immediately removed, divided into cubes about 5 mm thick, and quickly frozen using dry ice or liquid nitrogen. Tissue blocks can be used for 1 month to 6 weeks if they are stored at -70 C and well sealed to prevent drying. Tissue blocks are mounted in a water-soluble embedding medium usually used for frozen tissue specimens. Sections should be cut at 4 μm with a cryostat, placed on a clean slide, and air dried. Unless special antigens are being investigated, air drying the tissue is suitable for fixation. Other fixative procedures may lower the antigenicity.

Rabbit or goat antisera, prepared by immunization with human globulin or with individual classes of immunoglobulins (H-chains) conjugated to fluorescein isothiocyanate (FITC), are used to locate the site of the reaction of tissue substrate and antibody from the patient's serum. The details of preparing the conjugate have been described by Nairn.[5]

Each conjugated antiserum should be characterized as to its sensitivity and specificity. Sensitivity is dependent on the degree of fluorescein labeling and the potency of the antiserum. The number of fluorescein groups per protein molecule is called the F/P ratio. Most conjugates for IIF have a F/P ratio between 1.0 and 4.5. An F/P ratio that is too great may result in nonspecific staining; if it is too low, staining intensity is low. If the specific antibody content is known (as a titer or mg Ab/ml), the conjugate can be diluted to a satisfactory concentration. Specificity of the antiglobulin can be established by immunoelectrophoresis.

For most clinical laboratory determinations,

commercially available antiglobulin conjugates will be adequate. Different lots, even from the same company, vary considerably. Some suppliers of commercial antisera do not provide the required information about antibody content and F/P ratio. Therefore one must test each conjugated antiserum to determine the appropriate dilution that gives maximum fluorescent staining without significant nonspecific staining. To do this, a checkerboard titration is set up, consisting of multiple dilutions of a known positive patient's serum and multiple dilutions of the FITC-conjugated antiserum.

Commercially available conjugates come in lyophilized form and can be stored for long periods of time. Once reconstituted, they will remain potent for about 2 weeks if stored at 4 C. It is best to divide the conjugate into small samples and store them at -20 C until needed. In this manner, potency will be retained for several months.

Plasma is unsuitable for testing because it causes considerable nonspecific staining of tissue substrate; therefore, only serum should be tested. Since concentrated serum will also cause nonspecific staining and result in unclear results, initial serum dilution of 1:10 is often carried out. Screening of patient sera is conducted routinely at 1 or 2 dilutions (such as 1:10 and 1:20) with subsequent serial dilutions on the positive reactive sera until an end-point titer is reached. Until standard sera are generally available, each laboratory will have to establish its own set of standards with regard to quantitation.

Known positive sera of each recognized pattern, as well as a negative serum, should be included in each run of the test. As a check for conjugate specificity, some sections should be covered with diluent instead of serum, with subsequent application of the conjugate. Another control is a diluent-treated tissue section with no conjugate application. This is necessary because some tissues show autofluorescence under the fluorescence microscope. An untreated tissue section should also be available for reference.

Phosphate buffered saline (PBS), pH 7.2, is used for diluting sera and washing excess globulin and conjugate from substrate tissue. It is made by adding 1 L distilled water to 1.48 g Na_2HPO_4, 0.43 g KH_2PO_4, and 6.80 g NaCl.

Mounting fluid consists of 1 part PBS plus 9 parts glycerol.

FITC conjugate combined with an optional counterstain of Rhodamine B-BSA (Rh B-BSA) will in many cases reduce nonspecific staining and provide good contrast to the FITC conjugate. Twenty μl reconstituted Rh B-BSA is added per milliliter of the appropriate dilution of FITC-conjugated antiserum.

Incubations of the serum or conjugate and substrate tissue are carried out in a humid chamber to prevent drying. This may consist of a level airtight chamber with damp paper toweling in the bottom.

Fluorescence microscopy requires a light source with high emission of light capable of exciting fluorescein and with appropriate primary and secondary filters. The best contrast is achieved with a dark-field condenser. One commonly used light source is the HB–200 W (Osram, West Germany) mercury vapor arc lamp. A primary filter used is a 3 mm BG12 or an FITC interference filter. The secondary filter in this system is usually K530. Different combinations may be used depending on the microscope equipment. Another system utilized is a Halogen Quartz 100 W light source with a 495 nm interference filter and a K530 secondary filter.

Other basic materials used in the immuno-fluorescence test are microscope slides, approximately 1 mm thick; no. 1 coverslips, and nail lacquer.

Procedure
1. Cover individual tissue sections with dilutions of patient serum or control solutions, place in a humid chamber, and incubate for 30 min at room temperature.
2. Drain slides, rinse by dipping in PBS, and then wash in PBS for 30 min with gentle agitation.
3. Drain and dry briefly so that no fluid is seen on the tissue.
4. Cover the tissue sections with an appropriate dilution of FITC-conjugated antiglobulin and incubate in the humid chamber for an additional 30 min.
5. Rinse the slides and wash as before.
6. Add coverslips, using the buffered glycerol as mounting fluid, and seal with nail lacquer.

7. Store the slides at 4 C if they are not to be examined immediately.

Results. Positive and negative controls should be examined first. A positive reaction is bright green. A negative reaction (Fig. 65-1, *A*) can be identified by the lack of stain within the nuclei even though the cytoplasm may take up a small amount of stain nonspecifically. Reference sera from an external source are vital for any laboratory initiating the test.

Different patient sera may produce different patterns of nuclear staining. The most frequent patterns are homogeneous, speckled, peripheral, and nucleolar; the pattern depends on the constituent(s) of the nucleus to which the antibody is directed.

Homogeneous pattern. In the homogeneous pattern the entire nucleus is stained with the same intensity except that in some cases a small round dark spot that represents the nucleolus appears. Antibodies producing the homogeneous pattern are directed against nuclear histone (Fig. 65-1, *B* and *C*).

Peripheral pattern. In the peripheral pattern the staining appears as a bright fluorescent rim surrounding the dark, unstained center of the nucleus. Antibodies of this pattern are directed against DNA.

Speckled pattern. Speckled staining may have a variable appearance ranging from small bright dots to fluorescent threads and variably sized clumps in irregular arrangement. There is some

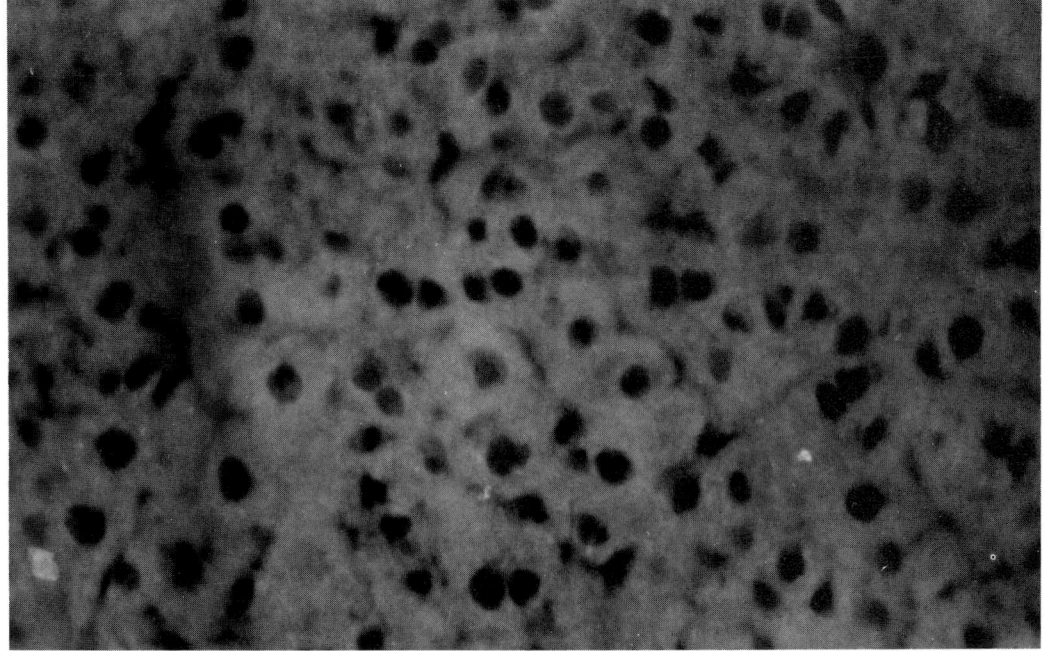

Fig. 65-1. IIF test for antinuclear antibodies. Cryostat sections of mouse liver, 4 μm thick, air dried, and unfixed, were treated with normal human or patient serum containing antinuclear antibodies with subsequent application of goat antihuman gamma globulin conjugated to FITC (FITC conjugate). **A,** Negative reaction due to normal human serum. Nuclei are dark; cytoplasm shows a small amount of nonspecific staining (×450).

Continued.

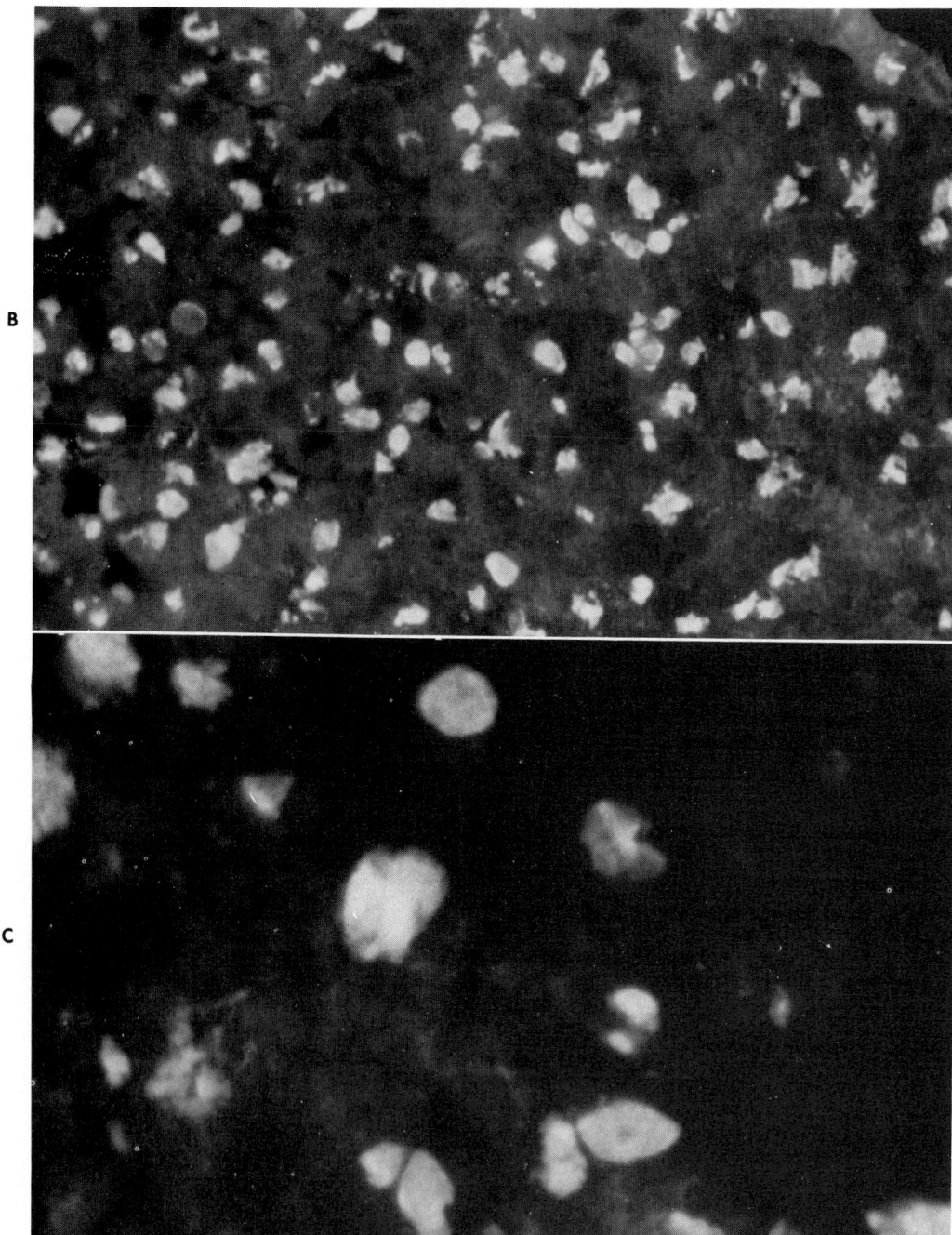

Fig. 65-1, cont'd. B, Positive homogeneous reaction. The entire nucleus appears brightly fluorescent (×450). **C,** Higher magnification of a positive homogeneous reaction (×1125).

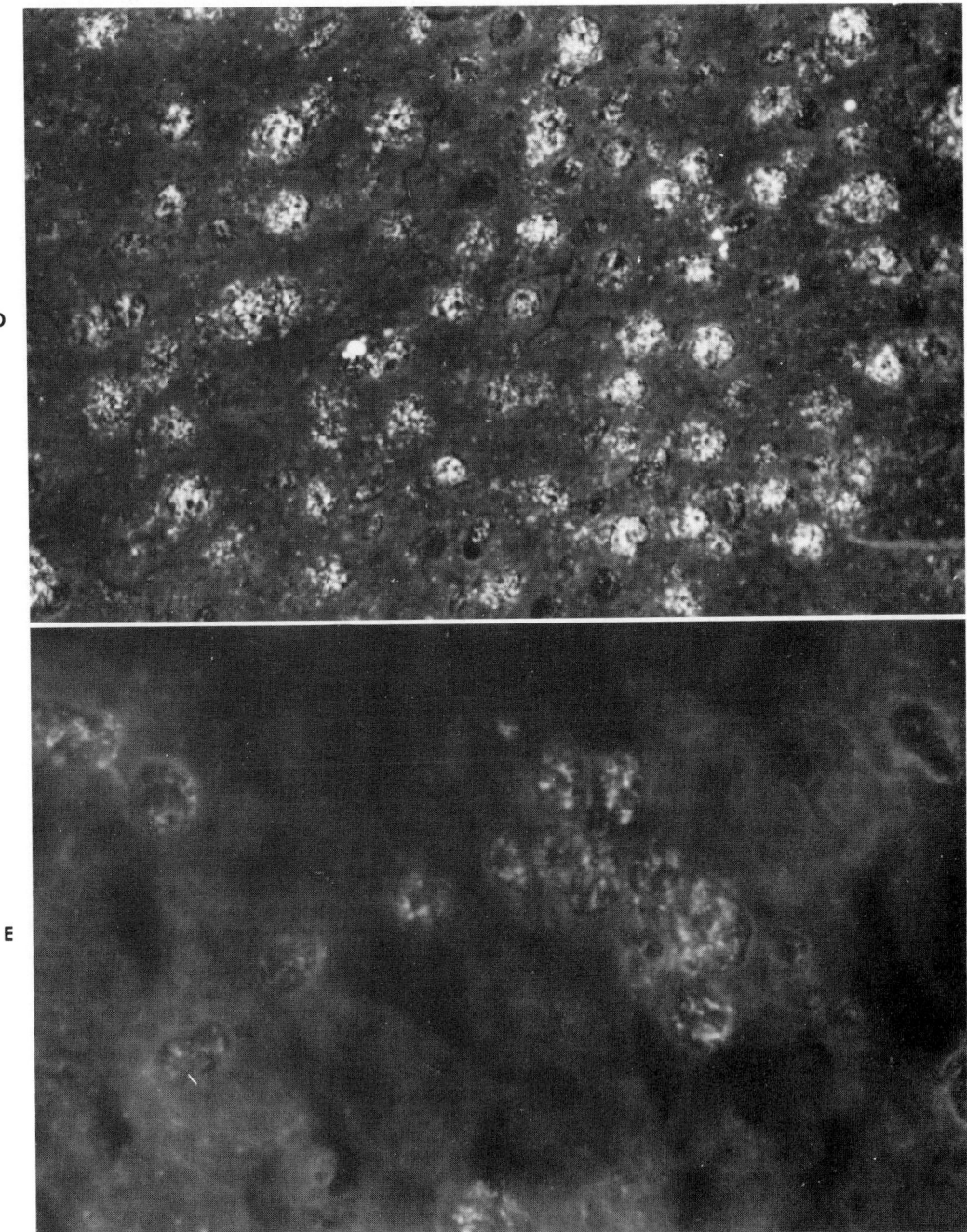

Fig. 65-1, cont'd. D, Positive speckled reaction. Fluorescence appears as scattered areas within the nucleus. This reaction is often difficult to distinguish with low magnification unless very strong (×450). **E,** Higher magnification of a positive speckled reaction. Discrete fluorescent flecks or dots are seen within the nucleus. The appearance caused by other positive serum may vary (×1125).

Continued.

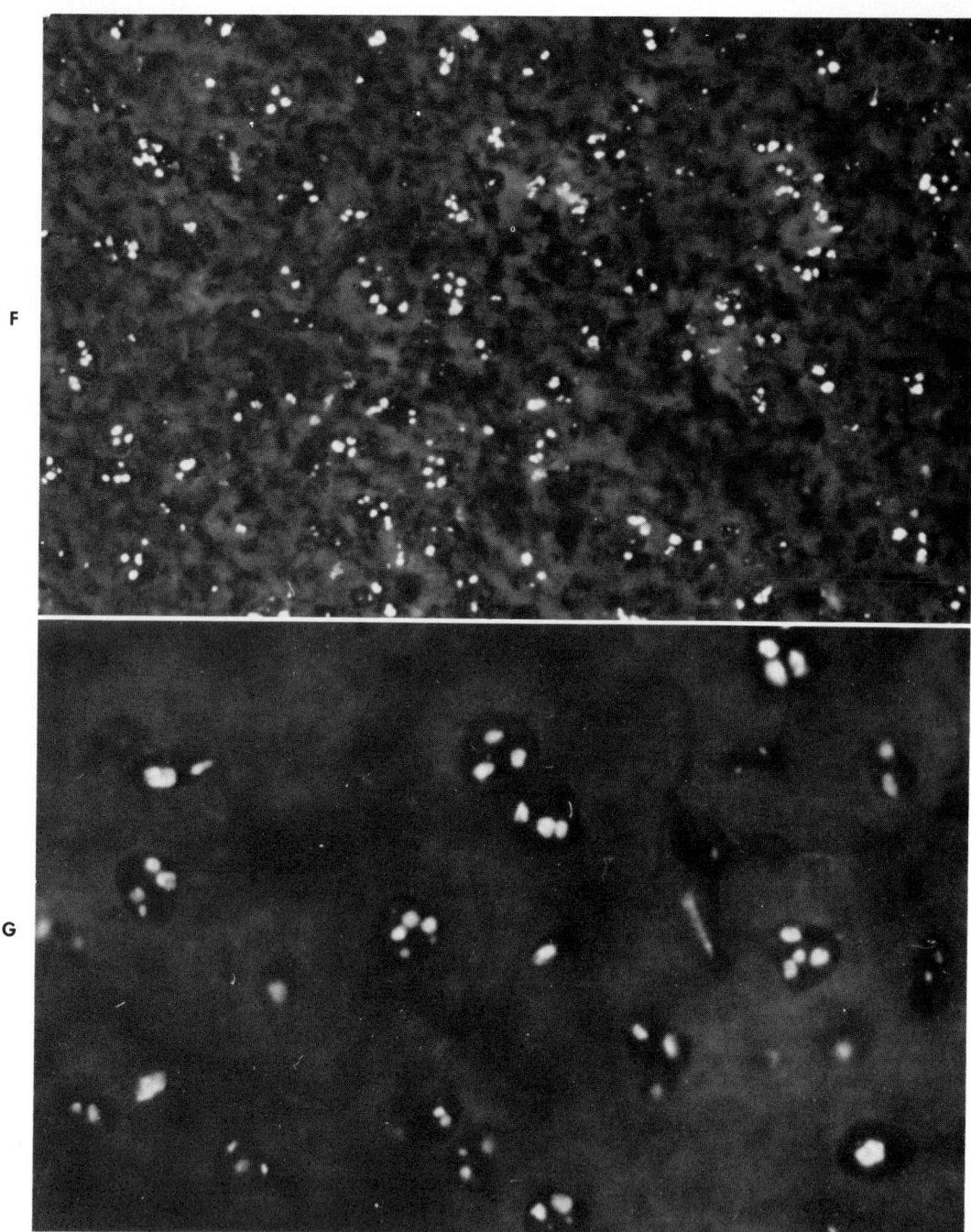

Fig. 65-1, cont'd. **F,** Positive nucleolar reaction. Round discrete fluorescent objects can be seen in the otherwise unstained nucleus (×450). **G,** Higher magnification of a positive nucleolar reaction (×1125).

speculation about the possibility of many subgroups or individual distinctive patterns often included in this category. Burnham et al.[6] describe several different patterns considered under the speckled category. The antibodies associated with speckled staining are those directed against nuclear proteins and are soluble in saline or phosphate buffer (Sm or ENA antigens, see following) (Fig. 65-1, *D* and *E*).

Nucleolar pattern. The nucleolar pattern appears as one or more bright, round structures, variable in size, within the unstained nuclei. The antigen contains RNA and possibly associated protein (Fig. 65-1, *F* and *G*).

• • •

The reciprocal of the highest dilution still giving a definitely positive result (when compared to the normal serum control) should be considered the titer.

Comments. IIF testing for antinuclear antibody (ANA) is primarily of use as a screening procedure. It is a sensitive test but is not diagnostically specific due to the many disorders in which ANA activity is found. There are 3 general considerations in interpretation of the results of ANA testing: whether the test is positive, the pattern of the reaction, and the titer of the serum. The best established correlation between the presence of ANA in the serum and the presence of a disease state is found in patients with previously defined SLE. Over 90% of patients with SLE have positive ANA tests with a predominance of homogeneous and peripheral patterns.[6-8] Speckled patterns are seen in SLE patient serum as well but to a lesser degree and often associated with a variant of SLE known as mixed connective tissue disease.[6,7,9] It is possible that some sera may contain a low titer of antibody causing a speckled pattern that is masked by a higher titered homogeneous reaction. This supposition cannot be verified with the IIF test. Reports state that a correlation exists between the presence of anti-DNA antibodies (peripheral pattern) and lupus nephritis in patients with active disease.[10,11] The prognosis of these subjects is poorer than that of other SLE patients. The clinical course of SLE is reflected by a changing titer of ANA. Those patients treated effectively or those in remission have diminished levels of ANA.

Sera from patients with rheumatoid arthritis (RA) and scleroderma also show a high incidence of ANA, although less frequent and with lower titer than in SLE. Titer and pattern are not as well correlated with severity of disease as in SLE. Many laboratories report a higher incidence of speckled or nucleolar patterns in scleroderma patients. The sera of RA patients show speckled and homogeneous patterns with a lower incidence of peripheral patterns.

Other connective tissue disorders or conditions associated with autoimmune phenomenon exhibit a low incidence of ANA, generally of a low titer (40 or less). The diseases include chronic thyroiditis, chronic active hepatitis, Sjögren's syndrome, discoid lupus erythematosus, pernicious anemia, idiopathic leukopenia, chronic interstitial pneumonia, myasthenia gravis, and Felty's syndrome.[6,7,9]

The occurrence of a low ANA titer is often associated with a variety of nonimmune disorders. Even sera from a normal population of blood group donors show a low incidence of ANA, so interpretation of the test in diagnosis of disease must also be based on other clinical findings and not solely on the results of this test.

IIF as a screening technic for ANA is important in the identification and localization of antibodies directed against nuclear antigens. It is clear that antibodies to the different components result in different IIF patterns, much like a peripheral pattern resulting from DNA-directed antibodies. However, the IIF screening technic has serious limitations. The tissue substrate (mouse liver) is composed of many antigens. There is no separation of the nuclear components, and the reaction can often be unclear, especially if antibodies are directed to more than one nuclear constituent.

Quantitation is another problem. Positive serum can be titered in a semiquantitative fashion, but the examination of the final reaction is often subjective. The intensity of fluorescence judged by different individuals can vary considerably. Each laboratory has also established different criteria on which to base end-point titers, which may not correspond to another laboratory. No standardization exists. Other substrates used are cultured fibroblasts, cultured tumor cells, or imprints of tumor cells, spleen cells, and liver cells, to name a few.[6,12] Each substrate may vary in nuclear components.

It is understandable that correlations linking pattern and disease (other than those with SLE) are difficult to establish using IIF patterns as criteria. For example, it has been reported that speckled patterns can be achieved by having antibodies produced against different nuclear antigens (Sm and ENA).[13,14]

Procedures using isolated products from cell nuclei have been initiated and have a 2-fold purpose—identifying antibody specificity and improving quantitation.

SPECIFIC NUCLEAR ANTIGENS

The specific nuclear components most often used in tests are native DNA (double-stranded), denatured DNA (single-stranded), soluble deoxyribonucleic protein, Sm antigen, and extractable nuclear antigens (ENA).

The DNA-binding assay quantitatively determines antibodies in serum to DNA. This assay has been adapted from the ammonium sulfate globulin precipitation technic of Farr[15] and has been reported to be highly specific and sensitive.[16,17] The principle of the assay depends on the differential solubility of antigen over that of antigen bound to antibody when the immune reaction is precipitated by adding saturated ammonium sulfate to a final concentration of 37% saturation. Serum antibody is proportional to the amount of antibody precipitated. The use of radiolabeled DNA allows rapid and accurate quantitation of the final precipitate.

It is known that SLE patients have DNA antibodies and that the serum titers correlate with disease activity, especially when complicated with lupus nephritis.[18,19] The pathogenic action of DNA antibodies is attributed to immune complex formation. When combined with circulatory DNA, they accumulate in and cause damage to the kidney. Separate demonstrations of DNA and antibodies to DNA in patient serum provide only indirect evidence of this event. However, a method has been proposed to measure DNA–anti-DNA complexes directly in the serum. This procedure measures increased detectable anti-DNA antibodies in serum (by DNA binding) after DNase digestion of the serum sample.[11] If the antibody titer increases after DNase digestion, it indicates that more sites were available for the test DNA because the others had been destroyed by enzyme digestion.

Two antigens have been extracted from soluble fractions of cell nuclei. The antigen known as the Sm antigen was described first and was found to participate in precipitation reactions with a high percentage of SLE sera.[13] It had a relatively acidic nature and was associated with nuclear protein but not histone. Antibodies to the Sm antigen could also be detected by complement fixation.

The other antigen, known as ENA, consists of both RNA and protein and, in some cases, has been called nuclear ribonucleoprotein (RNP). Certain similarities and differences exist between ENA and the Sm antigen.[20] Both antigens were insoluble in ammonium sulfate solutions greater than 35% saturation. Both antigens were soluble in 0-20% ethanol, partly soluble in 20-50% ethanol, and insoluble in solutions greater than 50% ethanol. Both were soluble in 0.15M NaCl but insoluble in water. Repeatedly freezing and thawing the antigens did not alter the precipitating ability, and they were stable at pH values ranging from 5 to 10. Differences were noted in temperature stability and enzymatic digestion. Sm antigen was more stable at higher temperatures for longer periods of time, still maintaining its activity after exposure to 56 C for 60 min, while ENA was unstable. Both antigens were resistant to DNase. Sm antigen was resistant to RNase and partially sensitive to trypsin digestion. ENA activity was destroyed by both RNase and trypsin. It has been reported that serum containing precipitins with either or both of these antibodies cause speckled staining in immunofluorescence ANA testing.[20,21]

Passive tanned cell hemagglutination for specific antigens

The passive tanned cell hemagglutination procedure is a technic that adapts well for the identification of specific nuclear antigens. Red blood cells are treated with tannic acid and coated with antigen in a manner similar to that for the detection of thyroglobulin antibodies.

Materials and methods

Sheep red blood cells (SRBC) stored in Alsever's solution are used from 1-3 weeks after collection. A commercial source may be used.

Two PBSs, pH 7.2 and 6.4, are required in this test. These are prepared from stock solutions of A, 0.15M NaH_2PO_4; B, 0.15M Na_2HPO_4; and C, 0.15M NaCl. The appropriate pH can be obtained by adding different volumes of the stock phosphate buffers and then adding an equal volume of 0.15M NaCl.

Reagents
1. PBS, pH 7.2
   a. Add stock solutions A and B at a ratio of 2:5.
   b. Check with a pH meter.
   c. Add B to the correct pH.
   d. Add an equal volume of 0.15M saline.
2. PBS, pH 6.4
   a. Add stock solutions A and B at a ratio of 5:2.
   b. Check with a pH meter.
   c. Add A to desired pH.
   d. Add an equal volume of 0.15M saline.

Procedure
1. Wash SRBC 3 times with 0.15M PBS, pH 7.2.
2. Prepare a 2.5% suspension using same buffer.
3. Add an equal volume of SRBC suspension to a 1:10,000 dilution of tannic acid in PBS, pH 7.2 (50 mg tannic acid/50 ml PBS). This provides a final dilution of 1:20,000 tannic acid. Incubate mixture for 10 min at 37 C or 30 min at room temperature.
4. Wash cells twice with PBS, pH 7.2, and then once with PBS, pH 6.4. If cells lyse after washing with PBS, pH 6.4, then they are too old and should be discarded.
5. Reconstitute SRBC to a 2.5% suspension with PBS, pH 6.4.
6. Add an equal volume of antigen in PBS, pH 6.4.
7. Incubate for 10 min at room temperature. Wash twice with PBS, pH 6.4, and then once with PBS, pH 7.2.
8. Reconstitute SRBC to a final concentration of 1.25-1.5% with PBS, pH 7.2, with 2% human serum that has been heat inactivated at 56 C for 30 min and adsorbed with antigen-coated SRBC. A separate suspension of SRBC that has been tanned only is similarly prepared as a control for nonspecific reaction to the tannic acid–treated red cells.

Comments. Several nuclear antigens can be used for coating: double-stranded DNA, single-stranded DNA, ENA, and Sm antigen. A solution of double-stranded DNA is prepared from a commerical preparation (no. D-1501 deoxyribonucleic acid from calf thymus, type 1, sodium salt, highly polymerized, Sigma Chemical Co., St. Louis) by dissolving 1 mg in 1.0 ml distilled water and adding 9 ml PBS, pH 6.4. Single-stranded DNA solution is prepared in the same way, then heated in a boiling water bath for 10 minutes and placed quickly in an ice bath. It is kept cold until the test is performed. ENA is made from calf thymus according to the method of Sharp et al.[14] The antigen is prepared for coating cells by adding 5 mg ENA/10 ml PBS, pH 6.4. Sm antigen–coated cells are obtained by RNase treatment of ENA-coated cells.

Test
1. Add equal volumes of 2.5% suspension of ENA-coated red cells (previously washed and ready for use) to an RNase solution consisting of 1.3 mg RNase/ml 0.1M PBS buffer, pH 7.2.
2. Let the mixture incubate 1 h at room temperature.
3. Wash 3 times with 0.15M PBS, pH 7.2.
4. Resuspend with the normal diluent for a working suspension of 1.25-1.5%. Testing for Sm antigen is necessary only if the reaction to ENA is positive, as the ENA contains both antigenic constituents.

Comment. The hemagglutination procedure is

the same as that for thyroid antibodies and is described in some detail later. One important step for these antigens is that of siliconizing the microtiter plates. Because of the charge of DNA and ENA, false-positive results will be produced if this step is not carried out. A solution of silicon, such as Siliclad (Clay Adams, Div. of Becton, Dickinson Co., Parsippany, N.J.), can be made and used according to instructions with the product. Another pitfall to avoid lies in the fact that many human sera have a small quantity of anti-DNA antibodies. Any human serum to be used in the diluent should undergo prior adsorption with tanned and DNA-coated cells.

RHEUMATOID FACTOR

The majority of patients with RA have demonstrable rheumatoid factor. In addition, a certain number of patients with lupus, Sjögren's syndrome, and chronic active hepatitis, as well as a few individuals with other connective tissue syndromes and some with chronic infection, have these factors. In general, patients with variants of RA such as juvenile RA, ankylosing spondylitis, psoriatic arthritis, arthritis associated with ulcerative colitis and regional enteritis, and the form of RA agammaglobulinemia are negative for rheumatoid factor.

The outstanding characteristic of the rheumatoid factors is their ability to react with the Fc portion of aggregated IgG. The antigen is usually attached to SRBC as a subagglutinating dose of rabbit antibody or to latex particles in the form of purified human γ-globulin.

Agglutination of sensitized sheep erythrocytes (Waaler-Rose test)

Waaler in 1939 noted that serum from patients with RA was capable of agglutinating SRBC sensitized by a rabbit anti–sheep erythrocyte serum.[22] This observation was applied to the diagnosis of RA and is the basis of the Waaler-Rose test.[23]

Materials and methods

Serum from the patient should be heat inactivated at 56 C for 30 minutes. Some human serum may contain antibodies to sheep cells, so absorption of the sample should be carried out by the following method:

1. Add 4 vol serum to 1 vol washed, packed sheep cells.
2. Incubate at room temperature for 40 min with occasional gentle shaking.
3. Centrifuge the preparation and draw off the clear serum.

As controls, include a known positive serum and a known negative serum in each test run.

SRBC are used as substrate in the test. The SRBC are washed in 0.15M NaCl, and a 2% cell suspension is made from packed cells with the same saline. A preliminary titration of the rabbit anti-SRBC serum (amboceptor) will determine a subagglutinating dose suitable for the sensitization of SRBC.

Sheep cells are sensitized by combining 3 ml 2% SRBC suspension with 3 ml appropriate dilution of anti-SRBC serum in a 16 × 100 mm test tube. In another tube combine 3 ml 2% SRBC suspension with 3 ml saline for the control SRBC preparation. Incubate both tubes in a 37 C water bath for 15 minutes.

Other materials needed include a 37 C water bath, 16 × 100 mm test tubes, 12 × 75 mm test tubes, and pipets.

Test
1. For each test serum, set up 2 rows of 12 tubes.
2. Label first row a_1 through a_{12} and second row b_1 through b_{12}.
3. Place saline into tubes according to following plan: 0.9 ml in tube a_1, 0.4 ml into tubes a_2 to a_{11}, and 0.2 ml in tubes a_{12} and b_{12} (which are control tubes for sensitized and unsensitized SRBC, respectively).
4. Dilute according to following: a 0.1 ml sample of test serum is placed into tube a_1 and mixed thoroughly (1:10 dilution). Then 0.8 ml is removed from a_1, 0.2 ml is put into tube b_1 and 0.4 ml into tube a_2. Remainder is discarded. Remove 0.6 ml from a_2 after mixing well. Place 0.2 ml into tube b_2 and 0.4 ml into tube a_3 and mix well. Repeat last dilution step through a_{11}, placing 0.2 ml into tube b_{11} and discarding remainder.
5. Add 0.2 ml sensitized SRBC to all tubes in row a and 0.2 ml unsensitized SRBC to all tubes in row b.
6. Shake test tube racks well and incubate overnight at 4 C.
7. Let tubes come to room temperature, and after 30 min read for SRBC agglutination by gently shaking tubes.

Comments. The degree of agglutination is graded +1 to +4. The test is valid only if there is no agglutination in the tubes containing unsensitized SRBC. The titer is expressed as the reciprocal of the highest dilution of patient serum containing agglutination.

Latex agglutination test

A second passive agglutination method for detection of rheumatoid factor involves the use of inert particles coated with a γ-globulin fraction (FII) of human serum.[24] This test was first performed as a tube test. Later a more rapid slide test was developed.

Tube test
Materials and methods

A 0.1% stock latex particle suspension, 0.81 μm in diameter, is made with distilled water. This suspension may be stored in the refrigerator for several months. **Do not freeze.**

A glycine-saline buffer, pH 8.2, is prepared by combining 975 ml 0.1M glycine and 2.5 ml 1N NaOH and adding distilled water up to 1000 ml. Adjust the pH to 8.2, and add 10 g NaCl.

A stock solution of 1% FII of pooled human plasma is made with the glycine-saline buffer.

Patient serum and normal human serum are heat inactivated at 56 C for 30 minutes. Reference standards should be included, consisting of sera with a high titer (e.g., 5120) and one with a low titer (e.g., 160), with each test run.

Other materials to be used in the test are 12 × 75 mm test tubes and pipets.

Procedure
1. Coat latex particles by adding 0.2 ml latex suspension to 20 ml 1% FII.
2. Incubate at room temperature for 10 min.
3. Dilute each test serum initially by mixing 0.1 ml serum with 0.9 ml buffer.
4. Prepare serial dilutions for each test serum.
5. Place 10 tubes in a rack and label them 1 through 10.
6. Add 0.2 ml buffer to all tubes.
7. Place 0.2 ml initial serum dilution into tube 1 and mix thoroughly.
8. Transfer 0.2 ml from tube 1 to tube 2 and mix well; repeat this procedure through 9 tubes and discard remaining 0.2 ml sample. Serum dilutions range from 1:20 to 1:10,240.
9. To each tube add 0.2 ml FII-coated latex particle suspension.
10. Shake tubes well and incubate at 56 C for 90 min; centrifuge at 2000 rpm for 3 min.
11. Allow tubes to cool to room temperature and then incubate overnight at 4 C.
12. A separate tube should be prepared containing only buffer and latex suspension as an additional control.

Result. Read the tubes for agglutination using an oblique light against a dark background. Record the degree of agglutination for each dilution (0-+4). The reciprocal of the highest dilution giving positive agglutination is the titer. An agglutination reaction is considered positive if it occurs at a dilution greater than 1:20. After overnight refrigeration the agglutination becomes greater, and a reaction is considered positive only at a dilution greater than 1:160.

Slide test
Materials and methods

Latex-globulin reagent and glycine-saline buffer diluent, pH 8.2, are available commercially (Hyland Diagnostics Div., Costa Mesa, Calif.). As an alternative, reagents can be prepared as in the tube test method. Patient's serum and normal serum, inactivated at 56 C for 30 minutes, are recommended to improve the specificity and sensitivity of the test.[25] Other materials required for the test are microscope slides, small test tube, capillary pipets, and applicator sticks.

Procedure
1. Dilute test sera 1:20 by adding 1 drop serum to 20 drops diluent.
2. Place 1 drop diluted serum on a microscope slide and add 1 drop latex-globulin reagent.
3. Mix well with an applicator stick and spread over an area approximately 1.5 cm in diameter.
4. Tilt slide side to side and observe for clumping.

Results. A negative reaction appears as a smooth suspension with no visible flocculation.

A weakly reactive reaction will show a visible flocculation but with small aggregates or partial clumping. A strong reaction will cause visible flocculation with large aggregates and complete clumping so that the background is clear. Visible flocculation will usually occur within a few seconds.

The initial dilution of serum can be used as a screening test. Further serial dilution can be made to establish the titer of rheumatoid factor in the serum. With this technic, most adult patients with RA will show a positive reaction, with serum dilutions ranging from 1:160 to 1:2,560.

DETECTION OF ORGAN-SPECIFIC ANTIBODIES IN HUMAN SERA BY IIF

Organ-specific autoantibodies in human sera occur in many conditions, not all of them related to disease. However, most autoantibodies are developed in connection with disease processes. Among the most frequently found antibodies are those to the thyroid gland in patients with chronic thyroiditis or other thyroid diseases. They can be a valuable diagnostic tool, as over 90% of thyroiditis patients have autoantibodies directed against either the epithelial cell microsome, the thyroglobulin, or both. A negative test can virtually exclude thyroiditis. A positive test, however, does not eliminate the diagnosis of such conditions as adenocarcinoma or hyperthyroidism since 20% of these patients have antibodies to thyroid antigen, although titers are generally lower than in those patients with thyroiditis.

The most generally used test to detect tissue autoantibodies is IIF. The procedure for the detection of thyroid autoantibodies will be given in detail.

Materials and methods

The substrate consists of frozen human or monkey thyroid tissue cut into 4 μm sections with a cryostat. For the detection of antibodies directed against the epithelial cells (microsomal membrane components) the tissue should be air dried and unfixed. To detect autoantibodies against thyroglobulin, fixation of the tissue sections with absolute methanol for 10 minutes at 56 C is necessary. This prevents thyroglobulin from leaking out of the follicle during washing.

Patient serum is diluted serially starting as 1:10 with PBS, pH 7.2 (1.48 g Na_2HPO_4, 0.43 g KH_2PO_4, and 6.80 g NaCl, add distilled water up to 1 L).

Controls should include known reactive sera, one with a low titer (e.g., 20) and one with a high titer (e.g., 320), and a negative serum. Several tissue sections should be covered with PBS with and without later addition of conjugated antiglobulin antiserum as a control for nonspecific staining by the conjugate and as a reference specimen for tissue autofluorescence. If any of the control specimens are irregular in staining, then the test run should be repeated.

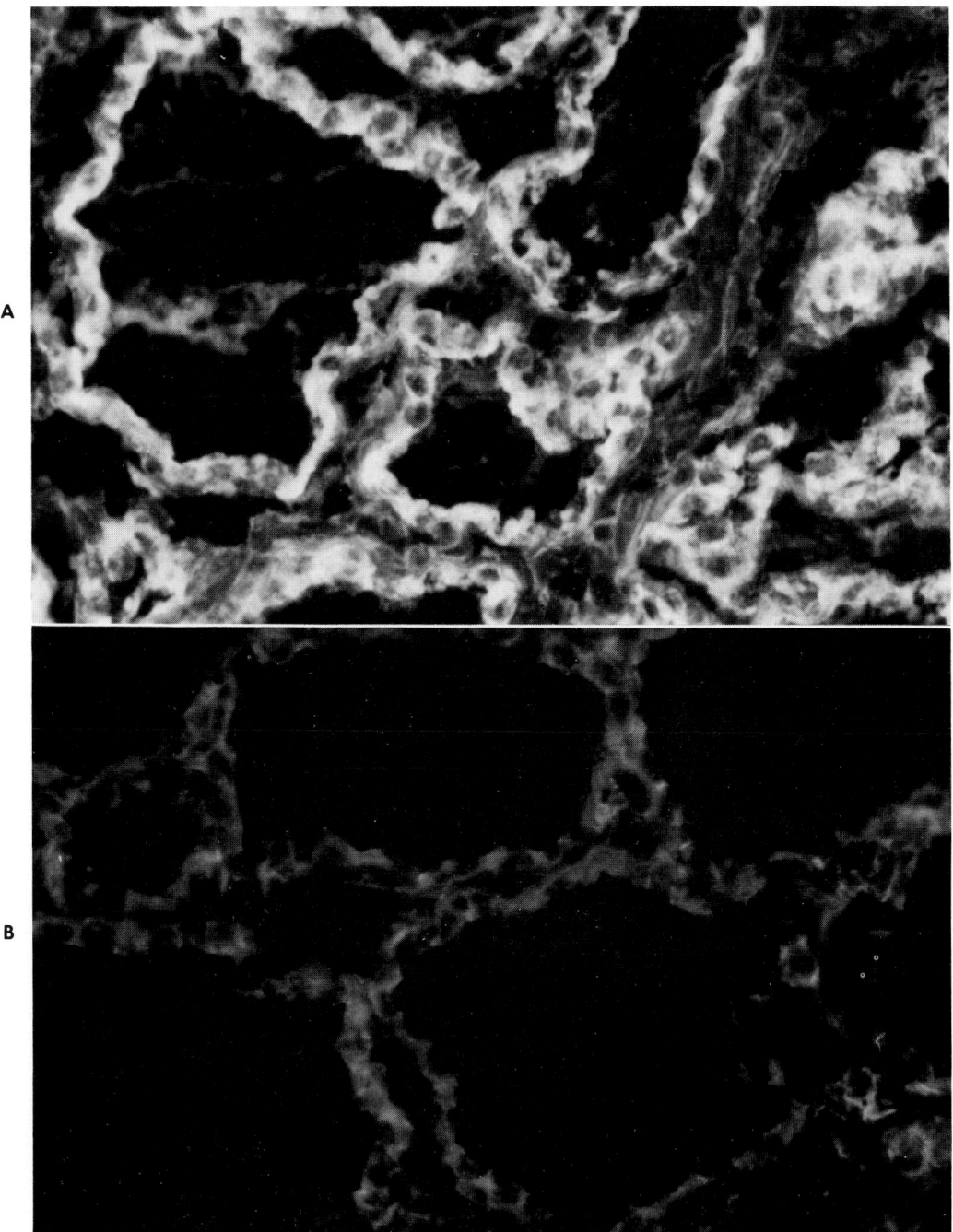

Fig. 65-2. IIF test for thyroid antibodies. Cryostat sections of monkey thyroid, 4 μm thick, air dried, and unfixed, were incubated with normal human or patient serum. After excess serum was washed away, goat antihuman gamma globulin conjugated to FITC was applied. **A,** Positive thyroid microsomal reaction. The cytoplasm of the epithelial cells lining the follicle is brightly fluorescent, while the nuclei are dark (×450). **B,** Negative reaction after incubation with normal human serum (×450).

Goat or rabbit antiserum prepared against human immunoglobulins and conjugated to FITC should be diluted with PBS, pH 7.2, as previously discussed in the section pertaining to the detection of antinuclear antibodies. Indeed, the same conjugate can be used for both tests.

Rh B-BSA is used as an optional counterstain to decrease nonspecific staining and improve contrast. To each milliliter diluted conjugate add 0.2 ml reconstituted stain.

Buffered glycerol as mounting fluid and the equipment for fluorescence microscopy was discussed in the antinuclear antibody section.

Procedure

1. Cover individual tissue sections with dilutions of patient or control sera.
2. Incubate the sections for 30 min at room temperature in a humid chamber.
3. Rinse and wash the slides with PBS for 30 min with gentle agitation.
4. Allow the slides to drain briefly and wipe off excess buffer around the tissue with absorbent paper.
5. Cover the sections with an appropriate dilution of the FITC-conjugated antiserum and incubate for 30 min at room temperature in a humid chamber.
6. Rinse and wash as previously described.
7. Coverslip the slides using buffered glycerol as mounting fluid and seal the coverslips with nail lacquer to prevent drying.
8. Store the slides in the refrigerator until they are examined.

Results. At least 2 distinct autoantibodies can be detected by IIF. They are directed against the thyroid gland epithelial cells or the colloid constituents. A positive test of patient sera on unfixed slides appears as bright fluorescence of the follicular epithelial cells (Fig. 65-2, *A*). The autoantibody responsible for this reaction has been shown to be directed against the microsomal components of the epithelial cell. A slide with control serum should appear dark with perhaps some interstitial connective tissue faintly staining (Fig. 65-2, *B*).

Autoantibodies reacting to colloid can be seen only by using the methanol-fixed slides. The appearance of a negative-reacting serum is presented in Fig. 65-3, *A*. The colloid appears dark. Positive sera can appear in any of 3 patterns.[26] They are as follows: (1) "three-dimensional" floccular pattern (Fig. 65-3, *B*) (usually seen in patients with precipitin-positive sera), (2) crazed pattern with dull staining of colloid spaces and bright fluorescence at the edges and cracks, Fig. 65-3, *C* (tanned cell hemagglutination positive sera), and (3) a uniformly bright-staining colloid pattern (negative by precipitin, tanned cell hemagglutination, and complement fixative tests). The last pattern is attributed to a second colloid antigen (CA_2) not detected by other tests.

Comment. Immunofluorescence as a technic for detection of autoantibodies is advantageous because the reaction site can be visualized

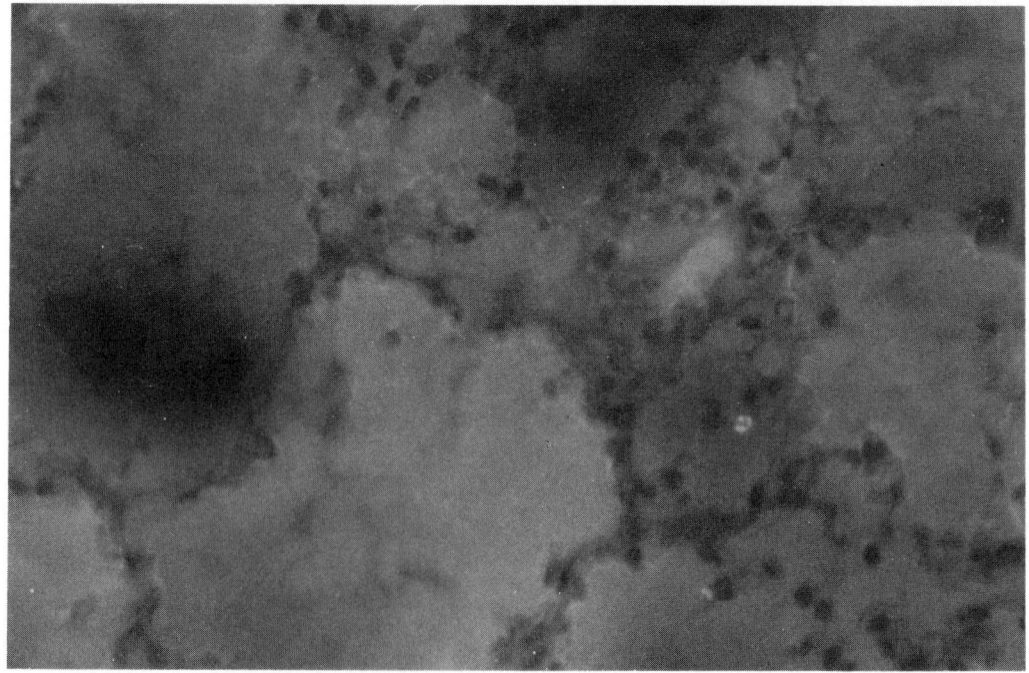

A

Fig. 65-3. IIF test for thyroid antibodies. Cryostat sections of monkey thyroid, 4 μm thick, air dried, and then fixed in methanol at 56 C for 10 min, were incubated with normal human or patient serum. After excess antibody was washed away, the sections were incubated with goat antihuman gamma globulin conjugated to FITC. **A,** Negative reaction after incubation with normal human serum. The follicle contains colloid and appears dark. Epithelial cells are not evident, although occasional dark nuclei can be seen (×450).

and the particular cell antigen can be determined. In addition, a single tissue can sometimes be used for several reactions. For example, thyroid tissue as substrate will react with antinuclear antibody, antithyroid microsomal antibody, and antithyroglobulin antibody. In some laboratories a "composite block" made up of several different tissues is processed at one time to provide a screening test.

Immunofluorescence, although sensitive for demonstration of antibody to microsomal antigens and the second colloid antigen, may not be

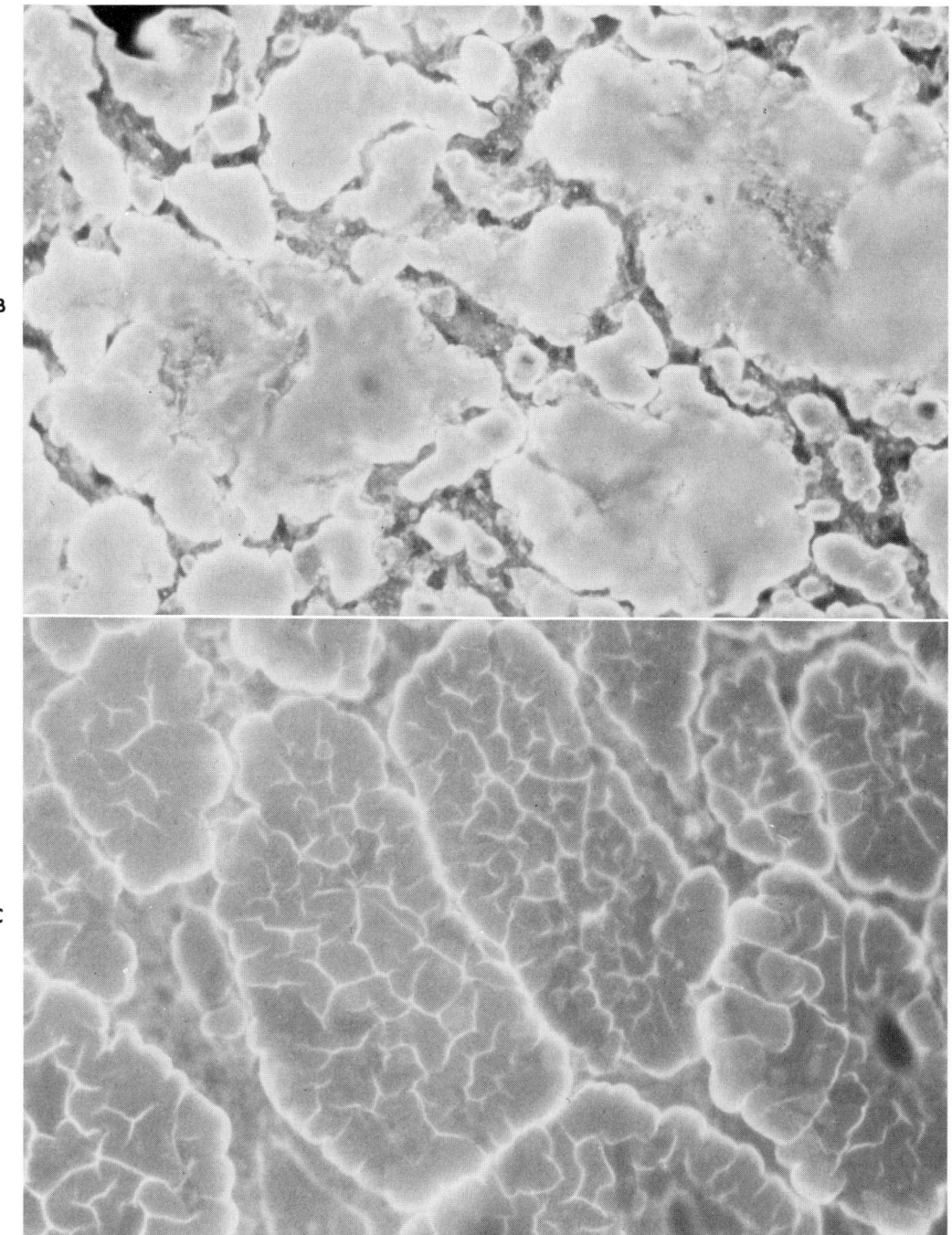

Fig. 65-3, cont'd. B, Positive colloid reaction in a "floccular" pattern. The colloid is brightly fluorescent in a three-dimensional pattern (×450). **C,** Positive colloid reaction in a "crazed" pattern. The edges and cracks of the colloid are brightly fluorescent, while the area between the cracks is dull (×450).

sufficiently sensitive for antibody to thyroglobu-lin. For a complete characterization of the patient's serum, a combination of tests should be performed.

SPECIALIZED TESTS FOR THE DETECTION OF THYROID AUTOANTIBODIES

Several methods are used to detect autoanti-bodies to the thyroid. Precipitation in fluid or gelatinized medium is a simple but relatively in-sensitive method. A microscopic slide agglutina-tion test employing latex particles as a carrier for thyroglobulin is a somewhat more sensitive test than precipitation but seems to lack specificity. The tanned cell hemagglutination and more re-cently the chromic chloride hemagglutination test using modified human O erythrocytes coated with thyroglobulin added to dilutions of anti-serum have a high degree of sensitivity without loss of specificity. A complement fixation test us-ing an optimal dilution of thyrotoxic thyroid ex-tract will detect microsomal antigens, although it is not as sensitive as the immunofluorescence method.

Tanned cell hemagglutination test for thyroglobulin antibodies

In the tanned cell hemagglutination test, human group O erythrocytes are modified by the action of a dilute solution of tannic acid. The tanned erythrocytes are then coated with an op-timal dilution of thyroglobulin, washed, and re-suspended in a dilute normal rabbit serum. The tanned, coated erythrocytes are added to serial dilutions of antiserum and read by patterns of erythrocyte settling after incubation for 3 hours at room temperature.

Materials and methods

Ten ml human group O erythrocytes are col-lected in 1.0 ml 3.8% sodium citrate. The cells should age at least 3 days and can be used up to 2 weeks. Fresh cells will not provide consistent results.

PBS, pH 7.2 ± 0.05, is prepared by dissolving 13.2 g NaCl, 2.96 g Na_2HPO_4, and 0.86 g HK_2PO_4 in 2 L distilled water. Check the pH and adjust if necessary. The buffer is used **cold**.

A tannic acid stock solution is prepared by dis-solving 0.1 g tannic acid in 20.0 ml distilled water. This stock solution is stable for 1 week. Tannic acid from different sources will vary in its effect. Therefore, for use in the test, preliminary testing using various dilutions of the stock tannic acid solution is necessary in treating the eryth-rocytes to obtain the optimal results for antigen coating. The dilution should be at least 1:40 of the stock solution (0.5 ml stock solution up to 20.0 ml PBS), resulting in a final dilution of 1:8000 tannic acid. The proper final dilution may extend as far as 1:60,000 or even 1:80,000. The dilution should be made fresh daily from the stock solu-tion with PBS used as the diluent.

Normal rabbit serum (NRS) dilution is pre-pared from heat-inactivated serum (30 minutes at 56 C) and diluted 1:100 in PBS.

An extract of human thyroid gland can be used in lieu of purified thyroglobulin. An extract is obtained using human thyroid glands from autop-sy or from surgery that have been kept frozen at -70 C until use. The glands are cut into slices 3-4 mm thick and homogenized in approximately an equal volume of 0.9% NaCl in an Omni Mixer (Sorvall) at one-half maximum speed for 2 minutes. The homogenate is extracted overnight at 4 C. Either the clear supernatant of the extract is used or the supernatant is further purified to obtain thyroglobulin by ammonium sulfate pre-cipitation, Sephadex G200 (Pharmacia Fine Chemicals, Piscataway, N.J.) column chro-matography, and DEAE cellulose chromatogra-phy.[27] Protein concentration of the purified thyro-globulin should be adjusted to about 5-10 mg/ml in PBS and stored lyophilized or frozen in small aliquots. Preliminary titrations to determine op-timal antigen dilution for coating of tanned cells must be performed with each new preparation before using. The optimal dilution is usually be-tween 1:25 and 1:200. The crude thyroid extract should be titrated in a similar manner.

For a 1:100 dilution of antigen, add 0.2 ml thy-roglobulin (5.0 mg/ml) to 5 ml PBS in a 50 ml test tube. Place in boiling water for **exactly** 2 minutes. The timing is critical. After boiling, cool the tube under running cold water and add 15.0 ml **cold** PBS.

Patient serum is inactivated for 30 minutes at 56 C and cooled to room temperature. Prepare dilution using the NRS diluent.

As a control, each serum is tested against tannic acid–treated but **uncoated** erythrocytes. Include 2 known reactive sera, 1 weak positive (titer 100-200) and 1 strong positive (titer 10,000-20,000) and 1 nonreactive serum.

Other materials include 12×75 mm and 16×100 mm test tubes, 15 ml graduated centrifuge tubes, and pipets.

Procedure

1. Prepare erythrocytes for tanning and coating with antigen. Wash erythrocytes 3 times with PBS, cen-trifuge at $800 \times g$ for 5 min, and transfer to a 15 ml graduated centrifuge tube to pack and prepare a 4% suspension.
2. Combine 5.0 ml 4% erythrocytes and 5.0 ml tannic acid dilution.
3. Mix by inversion and allow to stand at 4 C for 30 min.
4. In a centrifuge with a horizontal head, wash cells 3 times with PBS for 4 min at low speed. After each wash, check erythrocytes for any graininess. If present, graininess should disappear after the cells are well shaken. IMPORTANT: Prevent eryth-rocytes from having any contact with protein (such as NRS diluent) until they are coated with thyroid antigen.
5. After third washing of tanned erythrocytes, dis-card the supernatant and add PBS up to 10 ml. Suspension is now 2%.
6. Mix by inversion and combine 5.0 ml tanned cells

and 5.0 ml predetermined dilution of thyroglobulin. Mark volume of suspension. Allow preparation to stand at **room temperature** for 30 min.
7. Wash 3 times with NRS diluent and, after final
wash, bring to marked volume with NRS diluent.
Final concentration of erythrocytes is now 1%.
8. Prepare a tube of **uncoated** erythrocytes by combining equal volume tanned erythrocytes with
NRS diluent rather than thyroid antigen.
9. Set up 2 rows of ten 12 × 75 mm test tubes for each
test serum.
10. Add 0.1 NRS diluent to each tube.
11. Prepare a preliminary dilution of 1:5 patient
serum and add 0.1 ml preliminary dilution to first
tube.
12. Mix well and transfer 0.1 ml from first tube into
second; repeat this step until end of row where
remaining 0.1 ml is discarded.
13. Prepare a parallel row of tubes.
14. Add 0.1 ml of tanned and coated erythrocytes to
first row and 0.1 ml of tanned only control erythrocytes to second row.
15. Two extra tubes containing 0.1 ml NRS diluent
and 0.1 ml individual erythrocyte suspension
should be set up as controls for nonspecific agglutination of red cells themselves.
16. Shake well and incubate at room temperature for
3 h.
17. Take first reading at end of this incubation by observing sedimentation pattern at bottom of tube.
18. Transfer racks to refrigerator (4 C) for overnight
incubation and read them again next morning.
19. Resuspend cells by agitation and allow cells to
settle at room temperature for 3 h and reread.
Usually titer does not change.

Reading

++++ Solid compact button on bottom
+++   Solid grainy button with irregular edges
++   Mat covering most of bottom with folded
      edges
+   Mat covering most of bottom without
      folded edges
−   Doughnut with dark red ring outside, light
      red button inside

The titer is the reciprocal of the highest dilution of
patient serum that gives a positive reaction.

Microhemagglutination method

This technic has an advantage over macrohemagglutination because it requires less reagents
and can be performed in much less time. One
disadvantage for high-titered serum is that some
carry-over of the antibody by microdiluters gives
a falsely high titer. This can be overcome by pre-
diluting the serum before dilution by the
microtiter equipment. Some specialized equipment is required.

Materials and methods

Microtiter plates with conical bottoms or U
plates are available through the Dynatech Laboratories, Alexandria, Va. Other equipment obtainable from the same company includes
0.025 ml diluters, standardized prior to use in the
test, and 0.025 ml dropper pipets. Additional
materials are the same as those used for macrohemagglutination test.
Preparation of thyroglobulin-coated erythro-

cytes and control erythrocytes is the same as for
use in the macrohemagglutination test. The final
concentration of red cell suspension, however, is
2%.
Patient serum is inactivated at 56 C for 30
minutes and cooled to room temperature. Prepare an initial 1:5 dilution of patient serum in a
test tube using NRS diluent.

Procedure

1. Place 0.025 ml NRS diluent in each well. Using
0.025 ml diluter, place a loopful of patient serum
into well 1. The diluter is twirled 15 times, carefully removed, and placed into the next well
where it is again twirled 15 times. The process is
repeated throughout all 12 wells.
2. A duplicate row is set up in a similar manner. Add
0.025 ml tanned and thyroglobulin-coated erythrocyte suspension to each well of the first row. A
similar quantity of tanned only cells is added to
each well of the duplicate row of serum dilutions.
3. An additional 2 wells containing only NRS diluent
are set up. One receives 0.025 ml tanned and
coated cells, the other tanned-only cells.
4. The plate is tapped gently to mix.
5. Cover and incubate at room temperature until the
red cells settle (about 1 h) then overnight at 4 C.
6. Read the patterns of sedimentation as for the
macrohemagglutination test.

Comments. The action of tannic acid on red
cells, allowing them to bind antigens, is still unclear. It is noted, however, that tanning the red
cells will change the membrane, producing in
some cases agglutination of the tanned only red
cells by patient and normal sera. This phenomenon usually occurs in the lower dilution range of
serum.
The serum dilutions to which only tanned
erythrocytes have been added are important controls to evaluation of this aspect. If agglutination
occurs, the patient serum should be absorbed
with the group O erythrocytes that have been
tanned.

Chromic chloride coupling for passive hemagglutination test of thyroglobulin

The trivalent metallic cation chromium (Cr^{+++})
will bind protein nonspecifically to red cells.
Because of this property, chromic chloride
($CrCl_3$) solutions have been employed in the
coating of antigens to group O erythrocytes and
subsequently used for passive hemagglutination
test.[28]

Materials and methods

Ten ml human group O erythrocytes is collected in 1.0 ml 3.8% sodium citrate. The cells
can be used fresh to about 10 days.
All solutions should be made in double distilled water. Saline solution (0.85%) consists of
8.5 g NaCl per liter water.
Chromic chloride ($CrCl_3 \cdot 6H_2O$, Fisher Scientific Co., Pittsburgh) stock solution is prepared by
adding 0.125 g $CrCl_3$ to 10 ml saline. This solution is green and will be stable for about 10 days.

A wash solution of $CrCl_3$ is made by adding 0.1 ml stock solution to 100 ml saline. The coating solution of $CrCl_3$ (0.1%) should be made fresh each time from the stock solution and consists of 0.8 ml stock $CrCl_3$ solution and 9.2 ml saline.

NRS is inactivated at 56 C for 30 minutes and diluted 1:100 in saline for use as diluent in the test. A 1:200 dilution of NRS in saline is used for coating control cells. Human thyroid extract or human thyroglobulin is prepared as for the tanned cell hemagglutination test. The remaining materials are the same as those used in the tanned cell macrohemagglutination and microhemagglutination tests.

Procedure

1. Wash erythrocytes 3 times with $CrCl_3$ wash solution and centrifuge at $450 \times g$ for 5 min. After last wash, remove supernatant carefully. Pipet 0.2 ml packed erythrocytes into a 12 ml graduated centrifuge tube. Another tube should be prepared for control cells.
2. To coat cells, add to 0.2 ml packed red cells in the graduated centrifuge tube in the following order: 0.2 ml 0.1% $CrCl_3$ solution and 0.2 ml thyroglobulin (5 mg/ml) or 1:200 dilution of NRS for control cells.
3. Mix with an applicator stick and incubate 4 min at room temperature. Add 10 ml saline to stop reaction and centrifuge as before.
4. Wash twice more in NRS saline diluent.
5. After last wash, resuspend cells up to 10 ml with NRS saline diluent to make a 2% suspension.

Comments. Both macrohemagglutination and microhemagglutination tests are set up in the same manner as for the tanned cell hemagglutination, using the same kind of controls and reading the erythrocyte sedimentation patterns in the same way.

The preparation of erythrocytes using the chromic chloride method of coating antigens on red cells is considerably faster than that used in the tanned cell method. It appears to be about 10-fold more sensitive than the tanned cell test.[29] The nonspecific agglutination of the control nonantigen-coated cell found with tanned only cells is considerably diminished using the chromic chloride–treated red cells.

Hemagglutinating antibodies to thyroglobulin have been found in most patients with Hashimoto's thyroiditis (75-80%). At least one-fourth of them have titers of 1000 or more. Autoantibodies to thyroglobulin are regularly found in patients with other forms of thyroiditis but with a lower incidence and a lower titer.[30] About 60% of patients with Graves' disease and those with primary myxedema have hemagglutinating autoantibodies, but less than 10% have titers of 1000 or more.[30,31] The frequency of thyroglobulin antibodies in normal subjects is greater in women than in men, and the incidence increases with age. As many as 35% of women and 15% of men in the 50- to 70-year age group have detectable antibody, although usually lower titer.[32]

Patients with forms of thyroiditis may have either thyroglobulin or microsomal antibodies or both, so a complete analysis of the patient's status should include testing for both antibodies.

Complement fixation test for thyroid antibodies

The complement fixation test uses an optimal dilution of a thyrotoxic thyroid extract. Serial dilution of antiserum is combined with the thyroid extract and $3CH_{50}$ of complement and incubated at 4 C for 2 hours. The titer is expressed as the reciprocal of the highest dilution of antiserum permitting 50% lysis of sensitized sheep cells. This is for the determination of autoantibodies to thyroid microsomes.

Materials and methods

A stock solution of triethanolamine-buffered saline (TEA) is made by combining 70.6 ml triethanolamine (Eastman Kodak Co., Rochester, N.Y.), 150 g NaCl, 4.8 ml $MgCl_2 \cdot 2H_2O$ (2.08M), and 1.6 ml $CaCl_2 \cdot 2H_2O$ (1.88M) in a 2 L volumetric flask and diluting with approximately 1400 ml distilled water. The pH is adjusted to 7.3-7.4 with 1N HCl (approximately 402.5 ml) and brought up to 2000 ml with distilled water. This 10-fold concentrated stock solution should be stored at 4 C until needed. A working solution is prepared on the day of the test by diluting the stock solution 1:10 with **cold** distilled water. Use cold.

Patient serum is inactivated at 56 C for 30 minutes. For controls, include a known reactive serum with a titer in the range of 32-128 and a known nonreactive serum.

As a complement source, lyophilized pooled guinea pig serum is used. Dilute with **cold** TEA to give $3CH_{50}/0.1$ ml. Keep iced and use after 20 minutes but within 2 hours.

Other materials needed for the test are a 37 C water bath, an ice bath, 12×75 mm test tubes, and 1 ml pipets.

Procedure

1. Prepare a crude suspension of toxic human thyroids as an antigen. Centrifuge lightly. Determine optimal dilution by previous titration with positive antiserum.
2. Sheep erythrocytes are washed 3 times with buffer and adjusted to 5×10^8 cells/ml. Sensitize sheep cells by adding an equal volume of 1:2000 dilution of rabbit antisheep erythrocyte serum (rabbit amboceptor). Incubate at 37 C for 5 min.
3. Prepare a 2-fold dilution of each serum, 1:4 through 1:256. From these dilutions 0.05 ml is pipetted for test itself.
4. In an ice bath, set up test as in Table 65-1.
5. Incubate test tubes for 2 h at 4 C and then for 30 min in a 37 C water bath.
6. Add 0.2 ml of sensitized sheep erythrocytes to each tube and mix well. Tubes are incubated again for 30 min at 37 C.
7. Shake tubes at 10 min intervals during incubation.
8. Transfer immediately to an ice bath.
9. Add 1.5 ml PBS to all tubes, centrifuge, and read absorbency of supernatant at 541 nm in a spectrophotometer.

Text continued on p. 1277.

Table 65-1. Complement fixation test setup

	Serum dilution (ml)	$3CH_{50}$ (ml)	Antigen dilution (ml)	Cold TEA (ml)	Distilled water (ml)
Test					
Patient serum (1:4-1:256)	0.05	0.1	0.1	0.05	—
Controls					
Known reactive serum (1:4-1:256)	0.05	0.1	0.1	0.05	—
Patient serum (1:4-1:256)	0.05	0.1	—	0.15	—
Known reactive serum (1:4-1:256)	0.05	0.1	—	0.15	—
Antigen dilution	—	0.1	0.1	0.1	—
$3CH_{50}$	—	0.1	—	0.2	—
Sensitized sheep erythrocytes	—	—	—	0.3	—
100% lysis	—	—	—	—	0.3

Table 65-2. Antibody detection

Antibodies directed against	Substrate tissue usually used	Fluorescence pattern	Associated diseases or conditions
Adrenal (Fig. 65-4)	Monkey or human adrenal	Glomerular, reticular, and fascicular or reticular and fascicular	Adrenal insufficiency
Gastric parietal cell (Fig. 65-5)	Rat stomach	Parietal cells of the mucosa	Pernicious anemia and atropic gastritis
Kidney—glomerular basement membrane (GBM)	Human kidney biopsies*	Linear pattern, irregular deposits on epithelial side of GBM, and granular pattern	Goodpasture's syndrome, glomerulonephritis, and serum sickness
Liver cytoplasm	Rat liver	Cell cytoplasm	Primary biliary cirrhosis "lupoid" hepatitis
Mitochondria (Fig. 65-6)	Rat kidney	Cytoplasm of duct epithelium	Primary biliary cirrhosis
Muscle			
Cardiac	Rat heart muscle	Striations	Myasthenia gravis
Smooth (Fig. 65-7)	Rat stomach	Muscularis mucosa and muscularis	Chronic active hepatitis
Striated	Rat skeletal muscle	Striations	Myasthenia gravis
Nuclear components (Fig. 65-1)	Young mouse liver	Homogeneous, speckled, peripheral, and nucleolar patterns	Systemic lupus erythematosus, scleroderma, and other connective tissue diseases
Salivary gland	Monkey parotid	Duct epithelium	Sjögren's syndrome
Skin	Monkey esophagus	Intracellular substance of stratified squamous epithelium and basement membrane of stratified squamous and columnar epithelium	Pemphigus vulgaris and bullous pemphigoid
Thyroid (Figs. 65-2 and 65-3)	Monkey thyroid† or human thyroid	Epithelium of follicular cells (microsomes) and colloid	Chronic thyroiditis, Graves' disease, and primary myxedema
Islet	Human or monkey pancreas	Cytoplasm of islet cells	Insulin-dependent diabetes

*Tested with antihuman globulin conjugates.
†Methanol fixation of substrate at 56 C for 10 min to detect colloid antibodies.

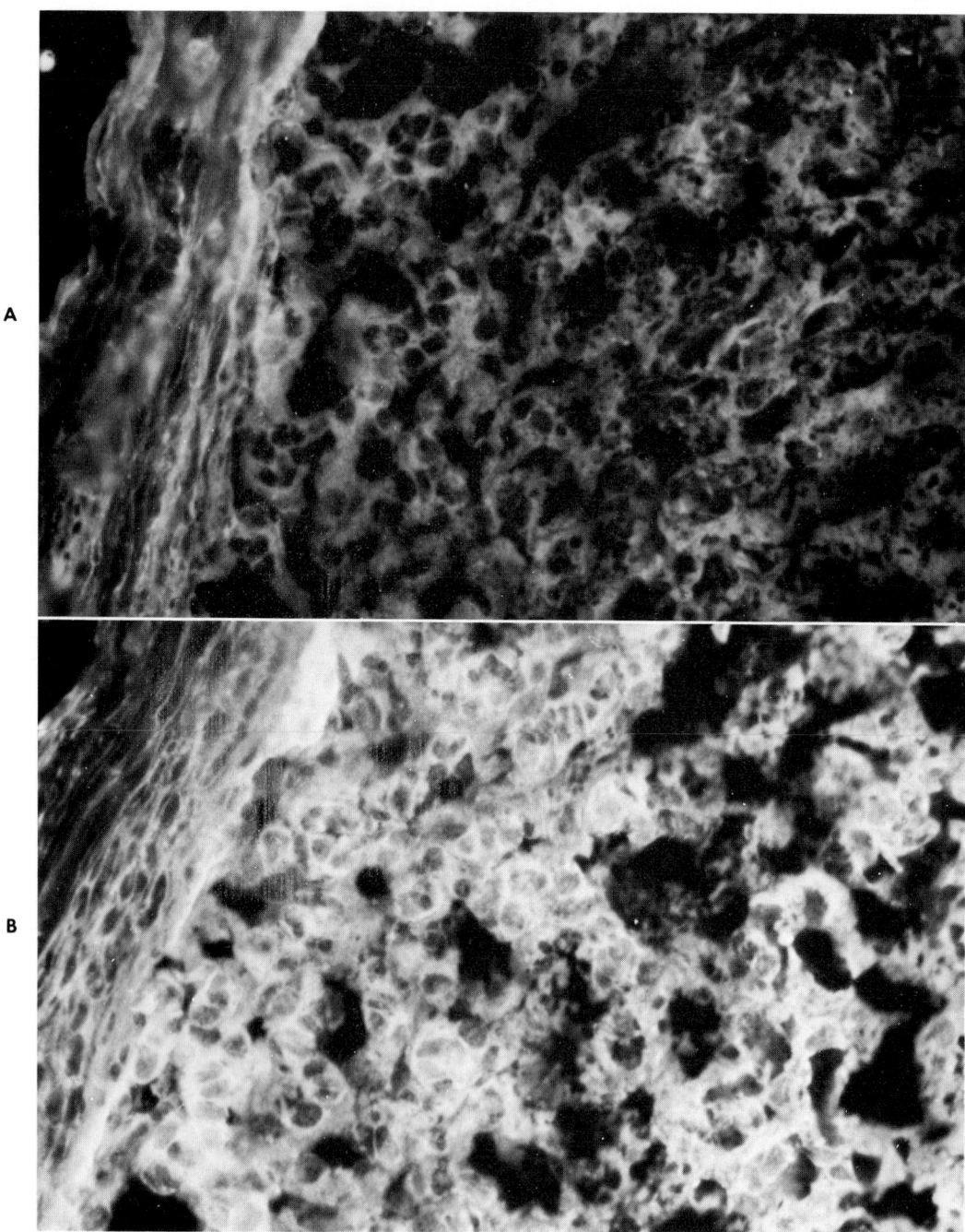

Fig. 65-4. IIF test for adrenal antibodies. Cryostat sections of monkey adrenal, 4 μm thick, air dried, and unfixed, were incubated with normal human or patient serum. After the excess serum was removed, goat antihuman gamma globulin conjugated to FITC was applied. **A,** Negative reaction after incubation with normal human serum. The adrenal capsule, glomerular zone, and part of the fascicular zone are present. There is a small quantity of nonspecific staining (×450). **B,** Positive reaction. Both the glomerular and fascicular zones are brightly fluorescent (×450).

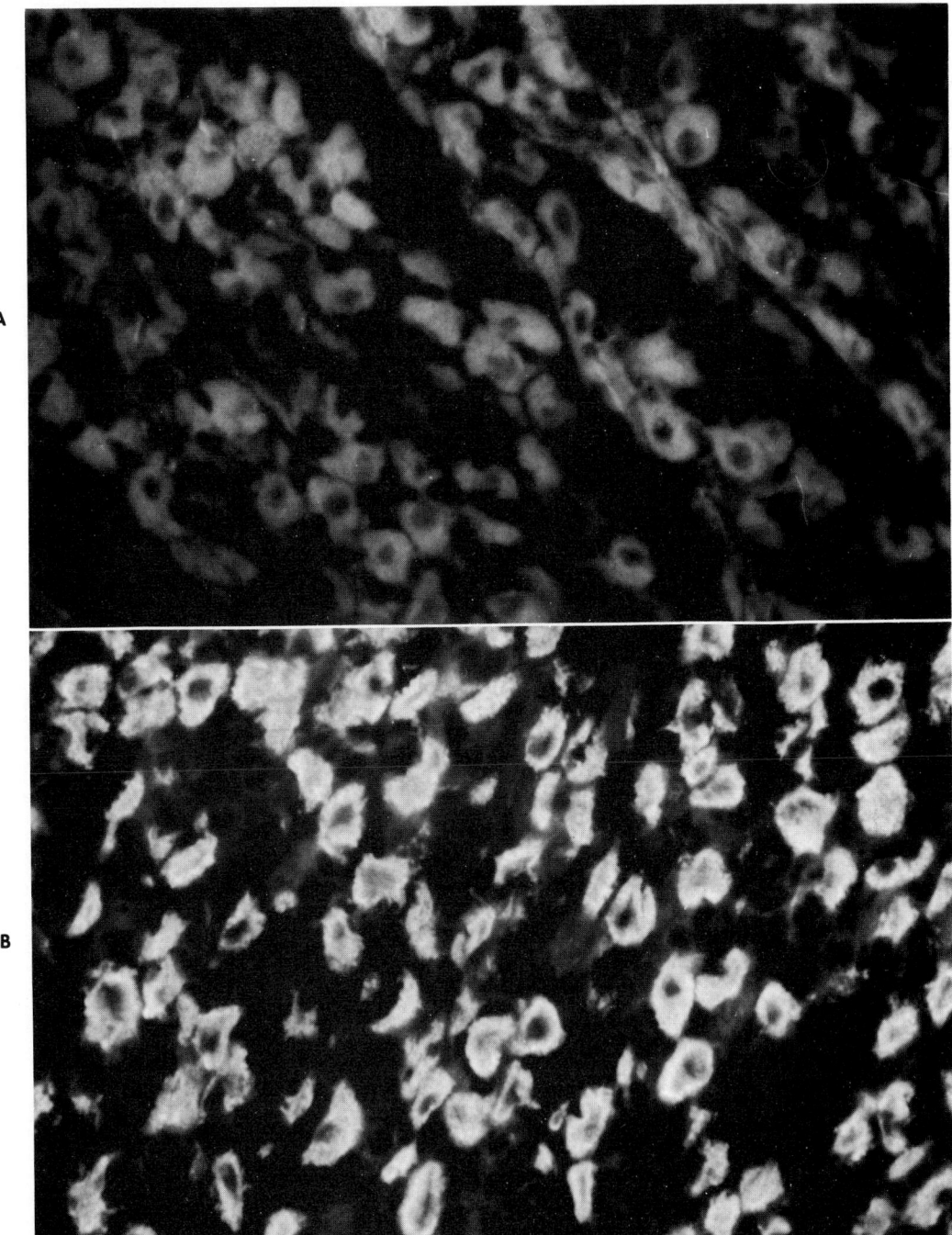

Fig. 65-5. IIF test for parietal cell antibodies. Cryostat sections were prepared from the stomach mucosa of a rat that had fasted. Sections, 4 μm thick, air dried, and unfixed, were incubated with normal human or patient serum. After removal of excess serum, the sections were treated with goat antihuman gamma globulin conjugated to FITC. **A,** Negative reaction due to normal human serum. Parietal cells show a small amount of nonspecific staining ($\times$450). **B,** Positive reaction. Parietal cells are brightly fluorescent ($\times$450).

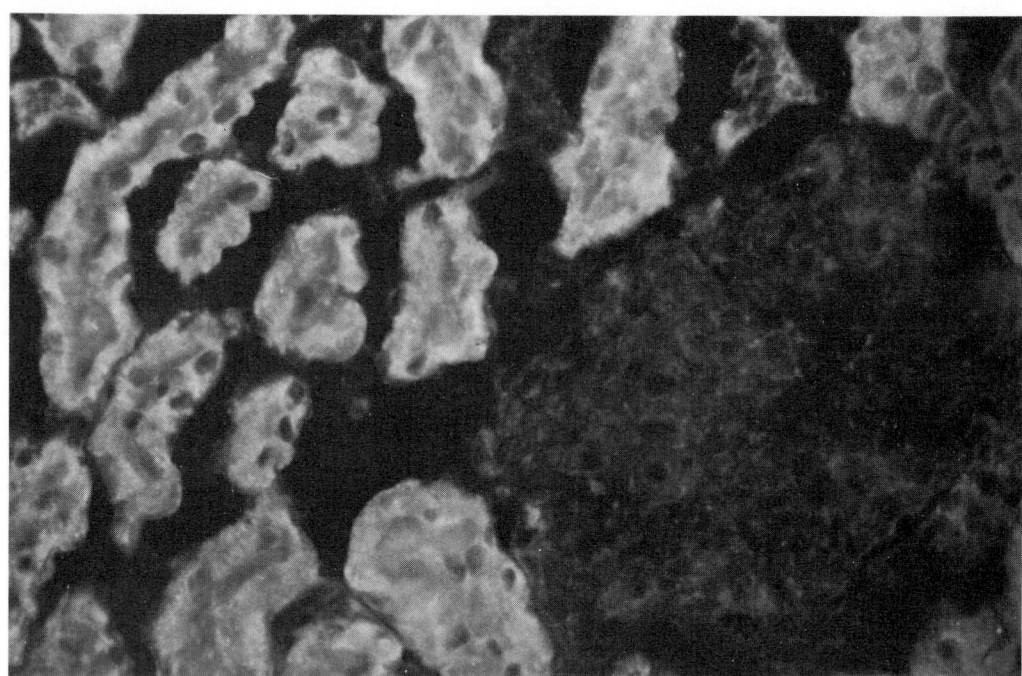

Fig. 65-6. Positive IIF test for mitochondrial antibodies. A cryostat section of rat kidney, 4 μm thick, air dried, and unfixed, was incubated with patient serum (normal human control not shown), washed to remove excess globulin, and then incubated with goat antihuman gamma globulin conjugated to FITC. In a positive result, the cytoplasm of the tubular epithelium is brightly fluorescent. The glomerulus at the right is unstained (×450).

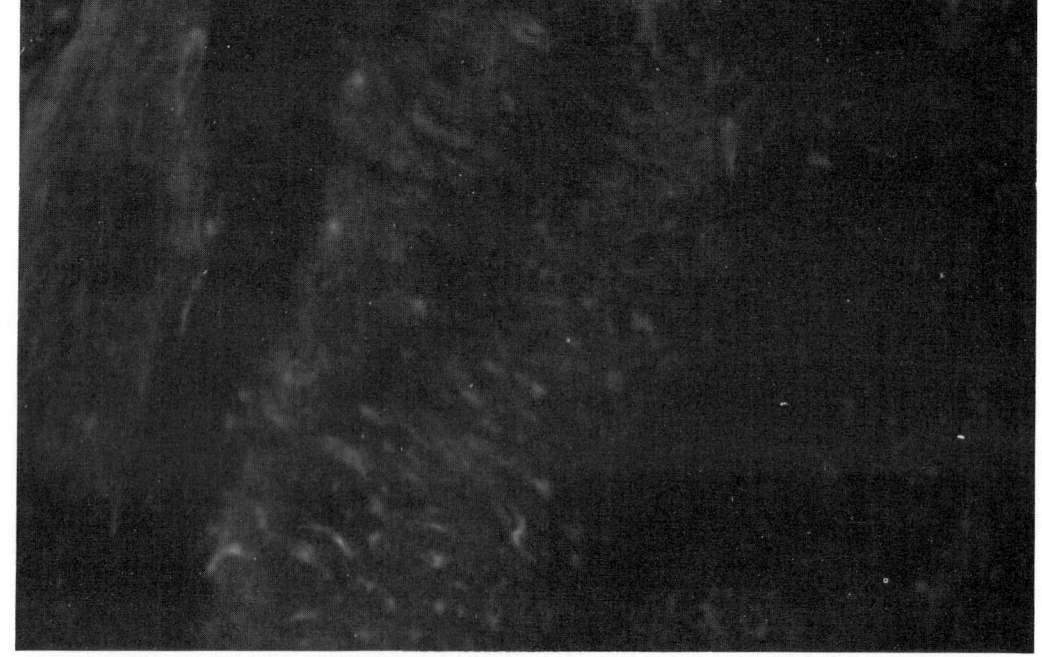

Fig. 65-7. IIF test for smooth muscle antibodies. Cryostat sections of rat stomach muscle tissue, 4 μm thick, air dried, and unfixed, were incubated with normal human or patient serum. Excess serum was removed, and the section was treated with goat antihuman gamma globulin conjugated to FITC. **A,** Negative reaction due to normal human serum. The muscle fibers can barely be seen (×450). **B,** Positive reaction. The muscle fibers, both cross-sectional and longitudinal, are brightly fluorescent (×450).

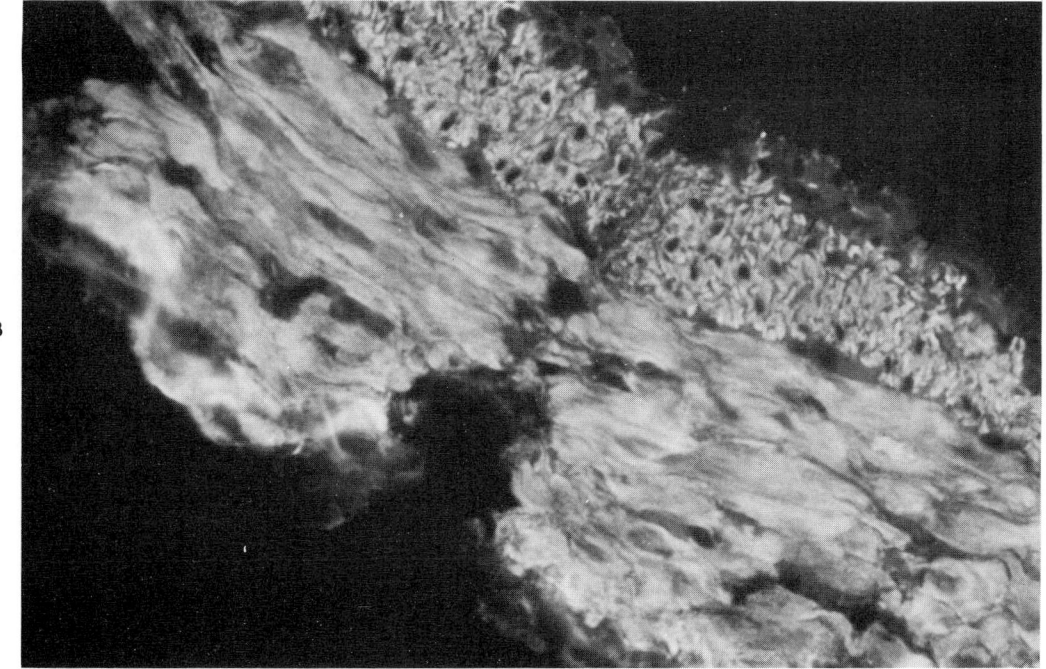

B

Fig. 65-7, cont'd. For legend see opposite page.

Comments. The titer of the patient's serum is expressed as the reciprocal of the highest dilution permitting 50% lysis of the sensitized SRBC. About 65% of serum from thyroiditis patients will give a positive complement fixation test.[33] Immunofluorescent testing for antimicrosomal antibodies is a more sensitive test. Patients with Graves' disease also often will have antibodies to thyroid microsomes. High titers are not unusual. Complement fixation titers of 32 are frequent. Subjects with other diseases of the thyroid such as myxedema (40%), nontoxic nodular goiter (40%), and thyroid carcinoma (20%) demonstrate antimicrosomal antibodies in their serum, although the titer will generally be low.[30,31] Among the normal population, as many as 15% of women over the age of 60 years will have antimicrosomal activity in their serum. The incidence for normal younger women is lower, and the incidence for normal men is even lower. Demonstration of antithyroid antibodies, especially in low titers, is not indicative of disease without other clinical evidence.

The detection of antibodies to other tissues of the body by IIF follows the same procedure as for detection of thyroid autoantibodies, only substituting a more appropriate substrate tissue. Table 65-2 presents a summary of the various antibodies detected with the different substrates, patterns seen, and diseases or conditions usually associated with them. Tissue substrate is cut 4 μm thick using a cryostat, air dried, and unfixed unless otherwise noted.

REFERENCES

1. Witebsky, E., Rose, N. R., Terplan, K., et al.: J.A.M.A. **164**:1439, 1957.
2. Doniach, D., Roitt, I. M., and Taylor, K. B.: Br. Med. J. **1**:1374, 1963.
3. Irvine, W. J., Davies, S. H., Teitelbaum, S., et al.: Ann. N.Y. Acad. Sci. **124**:657, 1965.
4. Whittingham, S., Mathews, J. D., Mackay, I. R., et al.: Lancet **1**:763, 1971.
5. Nairn, R. C.: Fluorescent protein staining, ed. 3, Baltimore, 1969, The Williams & Wilkins Co.
6. Burnham, T. K., and Bank, P. W.: J. Invest. Dermatol. **62**:526, 1974.
7. Lange, A.: Arch. Immunol. Ther. Exp. **20**:209, 1972.
8. Bartholomew, B. A.: Am. J. Clin. Pathol. **61**:495, 1974.
9. Husain, M., Neff, J., Daily, E., et al.: Am. J. Clin. Pathol. **61**:59, 1974.
10. Tan, E. M., Shur, P. H., Carr, R. I., et al.: J. Clin. Invest. **45**:1732, 1966.
11. Carr, R. I., Harbeck, R. J., Hoffman, A. A., et al.: J. Rheumatol. **2**:184, 1975.
12. Hahon, N., Eckert, H. L., and Stewart, L.: J. Clin. Microbiol. **2**:42, 1975.
13. Tan, E. M., and Kunkel, H. G.: J. Immunol. **96**:464, 1966.
14. Sharp, G. C., Irvin, W. S., Tan, E. M., et al.: Am. J. Med. **52**:148, 1972.
15. Farr, R. S.: J. Infect. Dis. **103**:239, 1958.
16. Wold, R. T., Young, F. E., Tan, E. M., et al.: Science **161**:806, 1968.
17. Pincus, T., Schur, P. H., Rose, J. A., et al.: N. Engl. J. Med. **281**:701, 1969.
18. Sharp, G. C., Irvin, W. S., LaRoque, R. L., et al.: J. Clin. Invest. **50**:350, 1971.

19. Reichlin, M., and Mattioli, M.: N. Engl. J. Med. **286**:908, 1972.
20. Northway, J. D., and Tan, E. M.: Clin. Immunol. Immunopathol. **1**:140, 1972.
21. Mattioli, M., and Reichlin, M.: J. Immunol. **107**:1281, 1971.
22. Waaler, E.: A factor in human serum activating the specific agglutination of sheep blood corpuscles, Presented at the Third International Congress for Microbiology, New York, 1939, Abstract Commun.
23. Rose, H. M., Ragan, C., Pearce, E., et al.: Proc. Soc. Exp. Biol. Med. **68**:1, 1948.
24. Singer, J. M., and Plotz, C. M.: Am. J. Med. **21**:888, 1956.
25. Watson, R. G.: Am. J. Clin. Pathol. **43**:152, 1965.
26. Balfour, B. M., Doniach, D., Roitt, I. M., et al.: Br. J. Exp. Pathol. **42**:307, 1961.
27. Rose, N. R., and Stylos, W. A.: Clin. Exp. Immunol. **5**:129, 1969.
28. Gold, E. R., and Fudenberg, H. H.: J. Immunol. **99**:859, 1967.
29. Poston, R. N.: J. Immunol. Methods **5**:91, 1974.
30. Witebsky, E., and Rose, N. R.: N.Y. State J. Med. **63**:56, 1963.
31. Anderson, J. W., McConahey, W. M., Alarcon-Segovia, D., et al.: J. Clin. Endocr. **27**:937, 1967.
32. Doniach, D., and Roitt, I. M.: Autoimmune thyroid disease. In Miescher, P. A., and Müller-Eberhard, H. J.: Textbook on immunopathology, vol. 2, New York, 1968, Grune & Stratton.
33. Belyavin, G., and Trotter, W. R.: Lancet **1**:648, 1959.

TRANSPLANTATION IMMUNOLOGY

Margarita Palutke

HISTORY

It has been clear for many years that there exists in man and animals an antigenic system that is the major barrier to successful tissue transplantation. In man and all animals studied so far a complex of genes responsible for the expression of these antigens in all nucleated cells has been identified. Because of the availability of inbred lines in animals—such as the mouse—it was much easier to demonstrate the relevance of this histocompatibility system to transplantation in animals than it was in man. However, its relevance in man became obvious shortly after the transplantation of human kidneys began. The longest survivals of kidney grafts were in siblings, the intermediate survivals in parent-to-child combinations, and the worst in unrelated individuals.[1] On the basis of these data, Simonsen[2] suggested that there must be a major histocompatibility locus in man, similar to that in the mouse, controlling transplantation antigens responsible for allograft rejection.

Similar conclusions were reached by Ceppellini et al.[3] using experimental skin grafts in human volunteers. Their findings suggested a segregation of antigens controlled by a major locus in siblings.

In 1966 van Rood et al.[4] demonstrated a correlation between the long survival of such grafts and matching of leukocyte antigens in siblings. Although leukocyte typing could be used to predict skin graft survival in siblings, it could not be used for this purpose for grafts between parent and child or between unrelated individuals. This fact has, in large part, held true for kidney transplant survival despite the great strides made in the detection of new histocompatibility antigens.

Histocompatibility antigens were described first in rodents,[4a] then in man and many other animals. Amos,[5] in 1953, was the first to recognize leukocyte alloantigens on mouse leukocytes. Antibodies to these leukocytes were formed in response to allogeneic leukemic cell inoculation in mice. In the same year, Dausset[6] reported leukoagglutinins found in man after blood transfusions, and in 1958 Payne and Rolfs[7] and van Rood et al.[8] independently demonstrated similar antibodies following pregnancy. Dausset[9] is credited with the first characterization of a human leukocyte antigen, Mac, in 1958. The first description of a leukocyte group system, 4a and 4b (FOUR), was made by van Rood[10] in 1962. Payne et al.,[11] in 1964, described a second allelic set of antigens called LA. Although Dausset et al.[12] thought that the 2 sets of antigens were genetically related, Bodmer et al.[13] considered them products of different genetic regions. Ceppellini et al.[14] were able to demonstrate that both concepts were correct because both LA and FOUR antigens are controlled by separate but closely linked loci on the same chromosome. Kissmeyer-Nielsen et al.[15] in 1969 confirmed this concept by finding recombinants between the 2 segregant series. Ward et al.,[16] in the same year, presented similar data to further support the concept of more than 1 genetic region.

Progress in the recognition of new specificities was greatly accelerated when, in 1964, Terasaki and McClelland[17] miniaturized the lymphocytotoxicity technic and Walford et al.[18] found that rabbit serum was the best complement source for this technic. With this stable, reproducible test system that required only minute amounts of valuable antisera and testing cells, it became possible to screen large numbers of cells and sera. Selection of the best antisera was facilitated by the use of computers.[10] New specificities belonging to the 2 antigenic series were rapidly discovered by many groups of investigators in various countries. Several international workshops involving exchange of sera, cells, and information have facilitated and accelerated the definition of antigenic specificities and the understanding of the histocompatibility complex called the HL-A (human leukocyte, locus A) system. Beginning with the international workshop in 1967, a nomenclature committee composed of geneticists and immunologists with special expertise in histocompatibility testing met after each workshop. Antigenic specificities shown to be distinct were numbered and

Table 66-1. Antigens of the 4 genetic loci of the HLA complex[21a]

Locus A Previously first (LA)		Locus B Previously second (FOUR)		Locus C Previously third (AJ)		Locus D Previously LD, MLD-1		Locus DR B cell antigens	
New terminology	Old terminology*	New terminology	Old terminology	New terminology	Old terminology	New terminology	Old terminology	New terminology	Old terminology
HLA-A1	HL-A1	HLA-B5	HL-A5	HLA-Cw1	T1, AJ	HLA-Dw1	LD101	DRw1	WIA1, Te6
HLA-A2	HL-A2	HLA-B7	HL-A7	HLA-Cw2	T2, sa532	HLA-Dw2	LD102	DRw2	WIA2, Te4
HLA-A3	HL-A3	HLA-B8	HL-A8	HLA-Cw3	T3, UPS	HLA-Dw3	LD103	DRw3	WIA3, Te5
HLA-A9	HL-A9	HLA-B12	HL-A12	HLA-Cw4	T4, RH315	HLA-Dw4	LD104	DRw4	WIA4, Te1.1
HLA-A10	HL-A10	HLA-B13	HL-A13	HLA-Cw5	T5	HLA-Dw5	LD105	DRw5	WIA5, Te5.2
HLA-A11	HL-A11	HLA-B14	W14	HLA-Cw6	T7	HLA-Dw6	LD106	DRw6	WIA6, Te10
HLA-A25	W25	HLA-B15	W15			HLA-Dw7	LD107	DRw7	WIA7, Te3
HLA-A26	W26	HLA-B17	W17			HLA-Dw8	LD108		
HLA-A28	W28	HLA-B18	W18			HLA-Dw9	TB9		
HLA-A29	W29	HLA-B27	W27			HLA-Dw10	LD16		
		HLA-B40	W10			HLA-Dw11	LD17		
HLA-Aw19	Li	HLA-Bw4	4a						
HLA-Aw23	W23	HLA-Bw6	4b						
HLA-Aw24	W24	HLA-Bw16	W16						
HLA-Aw30	W30	HLA-Bw21	W21						
HLA-Aw31	W31	HLA-Bw22	W22						
HLA-Aw32	W32	HLA-Bw35	W5						
HLA-Aw33	W19,6 Inc. Fe55, 10.4, Bar 3	HLA-Bw37	TY						
	Malay 1	HLA-Bw38	W16.1, W16, W4, Da31						
HLA-Aw34	Malay 2, HL-A 10.3, Fe26	HLA-Bw39	W16.2, W16, W6, 382						
HLA-Aw36	Mo*, LT	HLA-Bw41	Sabell, LK, Da34						
HLA-Aw43	BK	HLA-Bw42	MWA						
		HLA-Bw44	B12 not TT*						
		HLA-Bw45	TT*						
		HLA-Bw46	HS, SIN2						
		HLA-Bw47	407*						
		HLA-Bw48	KSO						
		HLA-Bw49	Bw21.1						
		HLA-Bw50	Bw21.2						
		HLA-Bw51	B5.1						
		HLA-Bw52	B5.2						
		HLA-Bw53	HR						
		HLA-Bw54	Bw22J						

* For a more extensive list of old terminology, see Table 4 of WHO-IUIS Terminology Committee report.[22]

designated HL-A. Until then they retained a workshop (W) or local designation.

In addition to the 2 antigenic series LA and FOUR (also called first and second series, respectively), a third was suspected by 1970. Shortly thereafter, sera-defining specificities of the third group of antigens, or AJ series, were reported.[19,20] Furthermore, other specificities controlled by yet another locus were discovered through the mixed-lymphocyte culture (MLC) reaction and called lymphocyte-defined (LD) antigens in contrast to the first 3, which were called serologically defined (SD) antigens.[21] The HL-A region became known as the "major histocompatibility complex" (MHC). The appreciation of the complexity of this system has increased with the discovery that genes controlling the levels of several complement components and genes controlling certain immune responses (Ir genes) are probably located in the same region.

In 1975, under the auspices of the World Health Organization and the International Union of Immunological Societies (WHO-IUIS), the WHO-IUIS Terminology Committee adopted a new nomenclature for the 4 best-recognized genetic loci and their respective antigens and alleles in the system (or region) (Table 66-1).[22] The entire complex is now called HLA (without a hyphen). Loci, alleles, haplotypes, and genotypes are italicized or underlined (1 or *Al*) and antigens and specificities are printed in roman type (A1). The loci are designated by a letter following *HLA* and separated by a hyphen (*HLA-A, HLA-B, HLA-C, HLA-D).* The individual alleles of each locus and their respective antigenic specificities receive a number following the locus (or antigenic series) letter (e.g., HLA-A1). Specificities that are still only provisionally identified carry an additional letter w between the locus letter and allele or antigen number (e.g., HLA-B15). Newly recognized loci will receive the next available letter in alphabetical order.

The 1977 workshop was primarily devoted to the characterization of another set of antigens, found primarily on B lymphocytes. These antigens, although identified by serologic methods, appeared to be either identical or closely related to the D locus antigens, which were identified by the MLC method. Thus the locus controlling the expression of these antigens has been called *Dr* (D related).

In addition to the HLA antigens, ABO antigens[23] and possibly organ-specific antigens are considered transplantation antigens. ABO antigens are found on various types of cells, and the ABO barrier in organ transplantation is observed in the same manner as it is in transfusion of red blood cells.

For a more detailed description of the historical aspects of histocompatibility testing, a review by Ceppellini[24] is recommended. In addition, the proceedings of the international workshops in 1964,[24a] 1965,[24b] 1967,[24c] 1970,[24d] 1972,[24e] 1975,[24f] and 1977[24g] provide detailed descriptions of the evolution of the field, as well as the methodologies used in defining the various components of the HLA complex.

THE HLA SYSTEM
Genetics

The genes of this system are located on chromosome 6. Evidence for this has been obtained through somatic cell hybridization and family studies demonstrating that the IPO-B marker and PGM_3, known to be on chromosome 6, and HLA antigens segregate with the same chromosome.[25,26]

Our current understanding of the HLA complex in man has been obtained through the classic tools of formal genetics, including family and population analysis, mendelian segregation, and studies of linkage and crossing-over. The best-defined loci of importance to histocompatibility testing and tissue transplantation are those controlling the SD determinants (HLA-A, B, and C) found on nucleated cells and platelets and those determinants that are identified primarily by MLC (HLA-D).

Genes controlling several complement components (C2, C4, Bf, and C8) and genes controlling Chido (Ch) and Rodgers (Rg) blood groups probably should be assigned to the HLA region on the basis of genetic studies.[22,27] There is also evidence that the genes controlling certain immune responses are in the same region.[22,27]

Although the antigens are designated in alphabetical order (A, B, C, D), the sequence of the gene loci on chromosome 6 is not in that order. Closest to the centromere is D, followed by B, C, and A (Fig. 66-1).[27]

The first described HLA antigens were identified serologically and were found to belong to 2 segregant series—the first, or LA, series and the second, or FOUR, series (now designated A and B), each determined by a single genetic locus. The classic inheritance pattern can most easily be demonstrated using these 2 loci. Although both loci are highly polymorphic, with about 20 presently known alleles for each series, an individual can have no more than 2 antigens in each series, 1 inherited from each parent. The 2 antigens inherited from 1 parent (1 in series A and 1 in series B) comprise the haplotype. The 2 haplotypes determine the phenotype of an individual. The genotype of this individual can be determined when the antigens of the direct

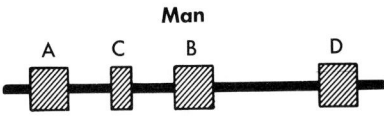

Fig. 66-1. Schema of HLA region or system in humans on chromosome 6 showing 4 genetic loci. D is closest to centromere.

Table 66-2. Examples of possible HLA types in a family

	Locus A antigens	Locus B antigens	Genotype
Father	1,2	8,12	1,8/2,12
Mother	3,w23	7,w16	3,7/w23,w16
Offspring A	1,3	7,8	1,8/3,7
Offspring B	1,w23	8,w16	1,8/w23,w16
Offspring C	2,3	7,12	2,12/3,7
Offspring D	2,w23	12,w16	2,12/w23,w16

family members (parents, sibling, offspring) are known (Table 66-2). The phenotype, genotype, and gene frequencies for the first 2 loci have been studied in great detail at the population level and have been found to conform to the Hardy-Weinberg expectation. Heterozygotes will transmit to their offspring, with equal probability, one or the other antigen, since at meiosis the 2 allelic antigens segregate in different gametes. Occasionally, a new haplotype combination is formed as the result of crossing over at meiosis. This type of recombination between the first 2 loci is estimated to occur with a frequency of 0.8%.[28] Cross-overs between D and B and between C and B also occur, but the frequencies are not definitely established. Considering the number of antigens in the HLA complex, it is obvious why matching of unrelated individuals becomes such a difficult task. The A and B loci alone, with approximately 20 antigens in each locus, provide 400 possible haplotypes, 80,200 genotypes, and 36,481 phenotypes. In contrast to this overwhelming number of possibilities in unrelated individuals, siblings can have only 4 different genotypes, constituting a 25% possibility of an identical match.

One important factor, however, makes matching of unrelated individuals not so completely hopeless a task as these numbers might indicate. The frequencies of the different genes vary greatly in different populations and races[29-30a] (Table 66-3). In addition, because of linkage disequilibrium, certain haplotypes and phenotypes occur much more frequently than would be expected if random assortment of HLA genes took place. Striking examples are the haplotype *HLA-A1, B8* and the phenotypes HLA-A1, A3; B7, B8 and HLA-A1, A2; B8, B12, which are quite common in whites and occur with much greater frequency than would be predicted from the gene frequencies. HLA-A1, which is common in whites, is rarely found in Orientals; and HLA-B17 is common in blacks but rare in whites and Orientals.

Locus C (AJ) antigens, like A and B antigens, fit the Hardy-Weinberg law for true allelism. Proximity of this locus to locus B is suggested by the high linkage disequilibrium value with locus B antigens. In individuals who have shown crossover of A and B alleles, the C alleles have traveled with the B alleles.[19]

Locus D antigens have been detected primarily by the MLC method. In 1964, Bain and

Lowenstein[31] showed that lymphocytes from monozygotic twins did not stimulate or respond in MLC. This remarkable discovery was quickly applied by transplantation immunologists who found that differences in HL-A antigens in man correlated with MLC activation.[32] The HL-A antigens recognized at that time were only those of locus A and B. Since HL-A–identical siblings were found nonstimulatory in MLC, these antigens were initially thought responsible for the MLC reactivity. However, in 1968 Amos and Bach[33] found an HL-A–identical sibling pair that stimulated in MLC culture; this finding suggested that antigens controlled by another locus (called LD by Bach) differing from the SD HL-A antigens were responsible for the stimulation. HLA-identical siblings that stimulated in culture were shown to differ in the MLC (D) locus due to a recombination event in 1 of the parents.[34-36] These studies also suggested that the D locus was peripheral to the second locus, B (Fig. 66-1).

Although in HLA A–, B–, and C–identical siblings instances of MLC reactivity are rare, this is not true for HLA A–, B–, and C–identical unrelated pairs of individuals. Only approximately 10% of the latter combinations are identical for locus D.[37] Of unselected, and therefore HLA nonidentical, individuals such nonstimulatory pairs are extremely low, suggesting considerable polymorphism of the MLC or D locus. However, in view of the 10% identical individuals as determined by identical SD antigens and nonstimulatory MLC, there must be a linkage disequilibrium among A, B, C, and D specificities. This linkage disequilibrium is found mainly with locus B antigens.[37]

Typing for locus D antigens is still done primarily by using the MLC test. Three major approaches have facilitated the identification of locus D alleles. One is the use of reference typing cells from a D-homozygous individual. This type of individual is frequently the offspring of parents who are first cousins and share an HLA haplotype. If cells from another individual are not stimulated by such homozygous cells, one may conclude that the individual carries the gene for that antigen.[40] Another technic is the use of established cell lines as MLC typing cells.[41] The third approach, called primed LD (lymphocyte defined) typing (PLT), introduced by Bach and co-workers,[42,43] involves the use of lymphocytes previously sensitized in a "primary" MLC. These sensitized cells are harvested after 10 days and are designated as PLT cells that, when placed into subsequent MLC with various unknown D locus cells, will undergo a more rapid secondary proliferative response (24 hours). The degree of restimulation is said to correlate with the degree of D antigen incompatibility. At present, MLC typing is performed in only a few centers. Eleven D locus antigens have tentatively been identified. A more detailed recent description of various typing methods, including the use of sperm as stimulator cells for

Table 66-3. HLA-antigen frequencies (%) determined at Seventh International Histocompatibility Workshop (1977)

Antigen	European whites	North American whites	American blacks	African blacks	Japanese	American Indians
HLA-A1	15.8	16.1	8.1	3.9	1.2	2.5
HLA-A2	27.0	28.0	16.3	9.4	25.3	45.3
HLA-A3	12.6	14.1	7.0	6.4	0.7	0.6
HLA-Aw23 }A9	2.4	1.9	10.6	10.8	37.2	23.2
HLA-Aw24 }A9	8.8	7.3	5.1	2.4	37.2	23.2
HLA-A25 }A10	2.0	2.6	0.4	3.5	12.7	0.6
HLA-A26 }A10	3.9	3.4	2.3	4.5	12.7	0.6
HLA-A11	5.1	5.1	2.8	—	6.7	—
HLA-A28	4.4	4.2	5.8	8.9	—	2.8
HLA-A29	5.8	3.6	2.3	6.4	0.2	0.6
HLA-Aw30	3.9	2.9	13.0	22.1	0.5	1.1
HLA-Aw31	2.3	4.5	2.8	4.2	8.7	19.9
HLA-Aw32	2.9	3.7	1.9	1.5	0.5	1.1
HLA-Aw33	0.7	1.2	5.1	1.0	2.0	0.6
HLA-Aw43	—	—	—	4.0	—	—
HLA-B5	5.9	5.9	4.9	3.0	20.9	14.0
HLA-B7	10.4	10.5	12.6	7.3	7.1	0.6
HLA-B8	9.2	10.4	5.5	7.1	0.2	1.7
HLA-B12	16.6	13.8	14.0	12.7	6.5	1.7
HLA-B13	3.2	2.6	0.4	1.5	0.8	—
HLA-B14	2.4	5.1	4.6	3.6	0.5	—
HLA-B18	6.2	3.1	3.6	2.0	—	0.6
HLA-B27	4.6	5.6	0.8	—	0.3	6.2
HLA-B15	4.8	5.9	4.7	3.0	9.3	13.7
HLA-Bw38 }Bw16	2.0	2.5	0.4	1.5	1.8	14.5
HLA-Bw39 }Bw16	3.5	1.4	0.4	1.5	4.7	14.5
HLA-B17	5.7	4.9	11.2	16.1	0.6	—
HLA-Bw21	2.2	3.8	4.4	1.5	1.5	—
HLA-Bw22	3.6	2.3	3.9	—	6.5	0.6
HLA-Bw35	9.9	8.6	12.5	7.2	9.4	22.1
HLA-B37	1.1	1.7	1.2	—	0.8	—
HLA-B40	8.1	9.2	3.9	2.0	21.8	16.6
HLA-Bw41	—	—	—	1.5	—	—
HLA-Bw42	—	—	—	12.3	—	—
HLA-Cw1	4.8	3.7	1.9	—	11.1	10.1
HLA-Cw2	5.4	6.0	9.2	11.4	1.4	4.6
HLA-Cw3	9.4	11.4	8.8	5.5	26.3	16.6
HLA-Cw4	12.6	10.2	12.9	14.2	4.3	23.4
HLA-Cw5	8.4	5.2	1.4	1.0	1.2	1.1
HLA-Cw6	12.6	11.3	—	17.7	2.1	—
HLA-Dw1	7.9	6.8				
HLA-Dw2	9.5	11.7				
HLA-Dw3	9.5	9.0				
HLA-Dw4	5.1	5.2				
HLA-Dw5	9.0	6.1				
HLA-Dw6	11.5	8.9				
HLA-Dw7	5.8	9.8				
HLA-Dw8	2.5	1.6				

locus D antigens, is provided by Bradley and Festenstein.[39a]

There are many unanswered questions about the roles of the various antigens in tissue transplantation and their relationship to each other. One test that until recently appeared to define some of the roles is cell-mediated lympholysis (CML). On the basis of previous experiments demonstrating that mouse[44] and human lymphocytes[45] stimulated in MLC display cytotoxicity toward isogeneic lymphoblastoid cell lines, Lightbody et al.[46] devised a test system, CML, in which the roles of the various HLA antigens could be studied.

This test utilizes 2 lymphocyte culture systems—MLC, which has stimulator and responder cells (see Methods) and a separate lymphocyte culture in which lymphocytes are stimulated to undergo blastogenesis by phytohemagglutinin (PHA). The responder cells in the MLC become the effector cells in the CML. The target cells in the CML test are blasts obtained by PHA stimulation. To study the immunologic and genetic relationships of individuals, various combinations of stimulator, effector, and target cells are used. A positive test is lysis of the target cells (PHA blasts) by the effector cells. If the PHA blasts are HLA identical to the responder or effector cells, there is no appreciable lysis. If they are HLA identical to the stimulator cells, the lysis is marked. Incompatibility between stimulator and responder cells in MLC results in activation of the responder cell and is essential for lympholysis to occur. This lympholysis is produced by the activated MLC responder cell now acting as the CML effector cell when added to the PHA blasts. The production of CML effector cells was thought to be a result of locus D disparity. However, the antigens on the target cells essential for lysis to occur were thought to be those controlled by loci A and B, and possibly C. Eijsvoogel[40] has summarized the results of CML studies of families, demonstrating crossing over and recombinations.

This proposed relationship of the various HLA antigens in the CML test has been challenged and a separate CML locus has been suggested. Long et al.[47] presented evidence that significant locus D disparity may not be necessary for the generation of cytotoxic cells, since the latter were produced when responder and stimulator cells differed by A and B loci alone. Other investigators have found that, in addition, disparity at the first 3 loci may not be necessary for CML to occur.[48] The proposed separate CML locus is thought to be closely linked to locus B. In addition, there is recent evidence that H-Y incompatibility may generate cytotoxic cells leading to graft rejection in humans.[48a,48b]

Immune-response genes and B cell antigens

In the mouse and other animal species a linkage of specific immune-response (Ir) genes to the histocompatibility system has been clearly demonstrated (Fig. 66-2).[49,49a] A similar association is suspected in man because of the association of certain disease states and HLA types (see Clinical Applications).[50,51] In man the Ir region has not been assigned to a specific locus in the histocompatibility system as it has been in the mouse, but it is suspected to be in the area of the D locus.

In the mouse, certain genes of the Ir region (locus Ia) control a series of lymphocyte antigens (Ia) found primarily, but not exclusively, on B-lymphocytes.[52] The relationship of these antigens to genes regulating the MLC response is not clear, although B cell antigens are thought to be MLC activators. In man similar antigens on B cells have been detected. Walford et al.,[53,54] while studying the HLA types of lymphocytes of

patients with chronic lymphocytic leukemia (CLL), detected unexpected reactivities of well-defined HLA typing sera to the CLL cells. Further studies by several groups of investigators[55-57] using CLL cells and lymphoblastoid lines (both of which are now known to be predominantly B-lymphocytes) and isolated peripheral blood B-lymphocyte and T-lymphocyte preparations from normal individuals clearly show a new alloantigenic system on human B-lymphocytes not present on T-lymphocytes. This new antigenic system has been termed the "Merrit system" by Walford et al.,[58] and "B cell antigenic system" by others. B cell antigens have been compared to the Ia antigens of the mouse.[59] These antigens in the mouse have also been detected on macrophages, epidermal cells, and spermatocytes.[60] In humans they have also been demonstrated on blood monocytes.[60a]

The DR antigens seem to follow an inheritance pattern of the type described for HLA haplotypes, and, because of a strong linkage disequilibrium with HLA antigens, a linkage of the genes controlling B cell antigens to those of the HLA system is strongly suspected.[61] Walford et al.,[58] using CLL cell panels, have reported 13 possible factors of the Merrit alloantigenic system, and Billing et al.[62] have mentioned 5 B cell groups. At the Seventh International Histocompatibility Workshop 7 B cell antigens were identified and given the DRw (D related) designation. Another antigen (WIA8) was not granted DRw status as yet.[62a]

B cell (DR) typing is performed with the complement-dependent lymphocytotoxicity assay used for HLA-A, B, and C antigen typing. The preparation of relatively pure B-lymphocyte suspensions and prolonged incubation times required in this test[63] make it more laborious and time consuming than routine HLA typing. Van Rood et al.[64] have used a similar method to detect MLC (HLA-D) determinants. Whether the MLC HLA-D antigens discovered by this method are identical to some or all of the B cell antigens remains to be demonstrated. A review of the DRw antigens by Bodmer[65a] and a critical examination of the relationship of D and DR antigens by Balner[65b] are recommended.

Antibodies to B cells have been found in sera of pregnant women and patients with renal transplants. In the latter the possibility that they represent enhancing, beneficial antibodies, which protect the graft against rejection, has been suggested.[66]

Biochemistry and molecular biology of HLA antigens

Considerable work has been done with antigens controlled by genes of loci A, B, and C in humans and similar H-2 antigens in the mouse.[67,68] The A, B, and C antigens are thought to be globular glycoproteins that float in the lipid bilayer of the cell membrane in the form of dimers linked to β-2-microglobulin by a noncova-

Mouse

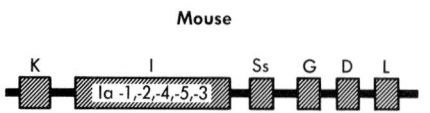

Fig. 66-2. Schema of H-2 region in mouse. Loci H-2K and H-2D correspond to loci A and B. I region genes control MLC reactions and expression of Ia (immune-associated) antigens and certain complement components.

lent bond.[69] HLA-A, -B, and -C antigens are thus composed of 43,000 and 12,000 molecular weight polypeptides linked noncovalently. The smaller polypeptide is the β-2 microglobulin.[69a] The carbohydrate portion has a molecular weight of 3000. The HLA specificity apears to be due to the polypeptide portion of the molecule.

By employing the technic of aggregating and thus removing antigens on the lymphocyte surface into fluorescent "caps" by using specific anti-HLA antisera coupled to either rhodamine or fluorescein dyes, it was shown that the HLA genes of loci A, B, and C control distinctive biochemical molecules that do not interact with each other. This conclusion was based on the fact that the antigens from the different loci did not "co-cap,"[19,70] i.e., antisera to a locus A antigen did not remove the locus B or C antigen and vice versa. With a similar technic the linkage of β-2-microglobulin to all HLA antigens tested was confirmed by demonstrating that antisera to β-2-microglobulin would remove all HLA antigens present on the cell surface, as well as the β-2-microglobulin. The reason for the close association of β-2-microglobulins and HLA antigens remains unclear. Bodmer[71] and Gally and Edelman[72] have proposed the possibility of an evolutionary homology between the genetic regions controlling the HLA antigens and immunoglobulins. Although the β-2-microglobulin gene currently is thought to be on chromosome 15[73] and not on chromosome 6 (the location of the HLA complex), this relationship may still be possible.

Investigation of the biochemical properties of B cell antigens has begun.[74] A 2-chain structure with molecular mass of 28,000 and 33,000 daltons is suggested.[69a] The B cell antigens appear to be distinct from the Fc receptors, which are of a slightly higher molecular mass and have been found separately on certain cell lines. Unlike the HLA antigens A, B, and C, the B cell antigens have not been found in association with β-2-microglobulins.

Relatively little is known about the dynamic aspects of the HLA and B cell antigens in man. They are thought to undergo continuous turnover in living cells. Wernet et al.[75] have found that, whereas B cell antigens are shed spontaneously in vitro, the HLA-A, B, and C antigens shed only after precoating with specific antibody. The shed HLA complexes contain β-2-microglobulin, but the B cell antigens do not.

CLINICAL APPLICATIONS OF HISTOCOMPATIBILITY TESTING

The uses of histocompatibility testing fall into 4 major categories: (1) matching of donor and re-

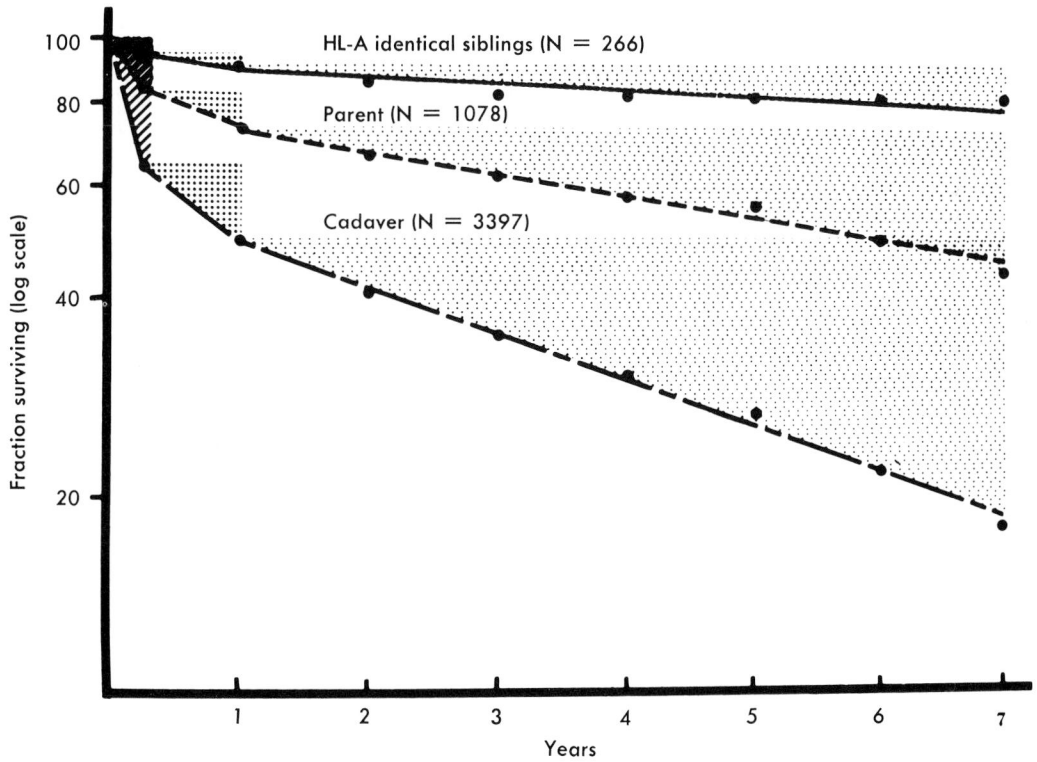

Fig. 66-3. Actuarial survival rates for HL-A–identical siblings, parent, and cadaver-donor transplants. Risk period 1: *slant lines*. Risk period 2: *large dots*. Risk period 3: *small dots*. (From Terasaki, P. I., Opelz, G., and Mickey, M. R.: Transplant. Proc. 6:33, 1974. By permission of author and publisher.)

cipient pairs for tissue transplantation, (2) disease association studies, (3) population genetics, and (4) paternity testing.

Tissue transplantation

The greatest clinical value of histocompatibility testing at present is the matching of donor and recipient pairs for tissue grafting. The tissues of major significance in transplantation currently are kidney, bone marrow, platelets, and possibly granulocytes. Other organ transplants—such as heart, liver, pancreas, lung, and bowel—have been attempted, but with much less success. Recently a correlation between HLA matching and the success or failure of corneal transplants has also been mentioned.[75a]

Kidneys are by far the most commonly transplanted organs. There is little doubt that HLA-identical–ABO-compatible siblings have the best results (Fig. 66-3). Among 215 such sibling transplants, a 90 ± 2% 1-year transplant survival was seen.[76] There still exists, however, a major controversy regarding the relative importance of HLA matching in cadaver-donor renal transplants. The assumption previously had been that the better the match, the better the outcome of the graft. In view of the numerous known and unknown HLA antigens and large number of phenotypes and the difficulty of typing for locus D antigens, it becomes obvious that to find perfectly matched unrelated donor-recipient pairs is a difficult task. The recipient pool must be extensive to allow good matching for the antigens of just the first 3 loci (HLA-A, B, and C). For this purpose many European countries and regions in the United States have established common donor pools. Recent studies, however, seem to indicate that HLA matching for the SD antigens may make little difference in the outcome of renal grafts. The 1-year survival of 402 cadaver transplants unmatched for 3 or 4 antigens (loci A and B) was 49 ± 3%, whereas 21 patients with 4 antigen matches had a 1-year survival of 50 ± 15%.[77]

Similarly, the European Dialysis and Transplant Registry reported a 51% survival for 4 antigen mismatches in 254 patients and 52% survival for 131 patients with 4 antigen matches.[78] Conversely, however, the French-English series showed that 289 patients with 3 and 4 mismatched antigens had a 44 ± 3% 1-year survival and 51 patients with 4 antigen matches had a 70% survival.[79] Nevertheless, considering the overall data from Europe and the United States, it is apparent that HLA matching for the major SD antigens does not ensure better survival in cadaver transplants and suggests that many other factors may be involved.

The fact that sibling donor-recipient combinations that are identical for the serologically recognizable antigens have such good results does not mean that the SD antigens are of primary importance in graft survival. As a rule, such siblings are also identical for the D locus antigens as

shown by nonreactivity in MLC. Jeannet[80] and Hamburger et al.[81] have demonstrated that in parent-child and sibling transplants, even when mismatched for some SD antigens, a low MLC reactivity correlated well with good graft survival. Because of the long period of time necessary for MLC, the use of this procedure for selection of cadaver donors is presently not feasible. Cochrum et al.[82] did a retrospective study on a small group of unrelated donor-recipient pairs and found that even when the pair was incompatible for the SD antigens, low MLC results correlated with better survival than high MLC results in otherwise HLA-identical pairs. Matching for B locus antigens has been considered of greater importance than for A locus antigens by some workers,[83] perhaps because of a greater possibility of finding locus D matching antigens.

Other factors that may be of importance in graft survival may relate to the type of immune response a recipient is able to mount. Opelz et al.[76] found that patients who had received repeated blood transfusions but did not form cytotoxic antibodies had good graft survival. Another interesting finding is that patients who had received no blood transfusions had a poor survival rate.[84] It is notable that transfusions in some people seem to enhance tolerance of the graft, and in others they seem to induce the production of harmful cytotoxic antibodies. The enhancing antibodies may be B cell antibodies.[66] A defect in the formation of cytotoxic T-lymphocytes against donor cells in vitro has correlated with good graft survival in HLA-nonidentical patients.[85]

Bone marrow transplants have been performed primarily in patients with aplastic anemia or acute leukemia after failure of chemotherapy, as well as in rare cases of genetically determined immunologic deficiency disorders in children. Occasionally, patients with carcinoma and lymphoma have also received bone marrow transplants after therapy. A detailed review of the results of a large series of bone marrow transplants in Seattle is available.[86] Unlike kidney transplants, where the majority of donors are unrelated, the donors for bone marrow transplants have generally been identical twins or siblings, matched both for antigens of the SD A, B, and C loci, as well as for the D locus as determined by nonreactivity in MLC. In 2 known cases, donor bone marrow mismatched for A and B antigens but matched for D antigens has been successfully transplanted.[87,88] Both of these cases involved related donors.

A bone marrow transplant is more complicated than other organ or tissue grafts because there exist not 1, but 2 immunologic barriers against a successful outcome. In kidney transplants the host attempts to destroy the graft—the host-versus-graft (HVG) reaction. In bone marrow transplants this problem is encountered, but, in addition, the bone marrow graft itself contains immunocompetent cells capable of mounting a destructive, potentially lethal immunologic reaction against the recipient—the graft-versus-host (GVH) reaction. An exception to this double jeopardy is seen in cases of severely immunologically deficient patients such as those with combined immune deficiency. In these cases the HVG reaction may be completely absent.

For more information on the biology of bone marrow transplantation the reader is referred to the March 1978 Transplantation Proceedings.[88a]

HLA matching of platelets and, to a lesser degree, granulocytes is used in some cases. Platelet and granulocyte transfusions on a short-term basis have usually not involved HLA matching. However, when recipients become immunized against HLA antigens, HLA-matched products, especially platelets, may prove to be lifesaving.[89] In patients with aplastic anemia who need long-term blood component therapy, HLA-identical donors, preferably siblings, are used. If these are unavailable, HLA-identical unrelated donors are generally utilized.[90,91]

At the present time, the necessity for HLA matching for the large number of granulocyte transfusions given to patients with malignant tumors rendered leukopenic by chemotherapy and radiotherapy is uncertain. The great effort required to establish a large enough pool of HLA-matched donors who would undergo leukophoresis is therefore probably not justified.[92,93] That HLA matching of blood components may play a role in granulocyte survival in some cases has been shown in patients with aplastic anemia who, after receiving HLA-incompatible platelet transfusions, developed prolonged granulocytopenia.[94]

Disease association studies

The search for disease association with specific HLA markers has been, and continues to be, active. A similar search for disease associations was undertaken when specific red cell antigens were discovered in man. Although the results of the latter search were not particularly fruitful, some of the associations—such as blood group O with duodenal ulcer and blood group A with gastric carcinoma—have been of interest.

In the case of the HLA system, animal data provided a great impetus to the search for disease association in man. In mice a genetic linkage between the H-2 region and resistance to virus-induced leukemia was suggested in 1964.[95] Subsequently, the discovery of the specific Ir genes and their linkage to the major histocompatibility system, primarily in mice and guinea pigs,[50] stimulated an even greater interest in the search for association between HLA and disease. The clinical significance for man is that if HLA antigens were useful in the early diagnosis of certain diseases, the patient at risk might either be followed more closely or given preventive treatment.

The publications on this subject are numerous and confusing due to conflicting reports from various laboratories. Many studies have been marred by improper sampling, poor or in-sufficient typing sera, and improper statistical analysis. Other discrepancies have remained unexplained. Several recent reviews with detailed bibliographies of this vast and complex field are available.[96,96a] Three reviews—1 by Dausset, Degos, and Koss, another by Vladutiu and Rose, and 1 by McDevitt and Bodmer—are also recommended.[51,97,98]

Some of the diseases for which there is some consensus of opinion will briefly be mentioned here.[96a] The best and most consistent example of HLA-disease association has been the association of HLA-B27 (previously W27) with ankylosing spondylitis and Reiter's disease. The detection of B27 is now a clinically useful tool in the diagnosis of these diseases. B17 has been found in many patients with psoriasis. B8 (formerly HL-A8) has been associated with celiac disease, chronic hepatitis, myasthenia gravis, and dermatitis herpetiformis. Multiple sclerosis has been associated with A3 and B7 in higher than expected frequency. A decreased frequency of A2, A12, B15, and B17 has also been noted in multiple sclerosis. The possible association of leukemias and lymphomas with HLA types, which stimulated so much interest because of the intriguing association in mice, is so far unclear. Hodgkin's disease has been associated with A1, A11, B5, and Bw35.

The association of HLA types and diabetes is more complex. Several different HLA types herald a predisposition to the juvenile-onset type of diabetes.[98a]

Associations with locus D and B cell types are obviously still incomplete because of the recent advances in the identification of these antigens. Dw4 has, so far, been reported with increased frequency in rheumatoid arthritis,[99] and Dw2 in multiple sclerosis.[100] A large portion of the Seventh International Histocompatibility Workshop was devoted to this subject.[96a]

Despite the recognition that certain HLA types—especially those of series B—are frequently associated with certain diseases, many with an autoimmune etiology, a causative nature of this relationship has not been established. It is likely that the observed relationships are not due to the HLA antigens, but rather to the influence of closely HLA-linked "disease-predisposing" or "protecting" genes also in linkage disequilibrium with the HLA genes. These genes may be the same as, or related to, the Ir genes, which have been studied extensively in mice.[51] In mice with autoimmune thyroiditis an association has been established between an H-2 antigen, the antithyroglobulin-antibody response, and the severity of the disease.[101] In humans a similar association was demonstrated between an HLA type, high-titer antiragweed reaginic antibodies, and the classic symptoms of ragweed hay fever and asthma.[102] In the future, identification of the Ir rather than HLA type of an individual may prove valuable in determining the disease predisposition of that individual.[51]

Population genetics

Population genetics, which has contributed data on gene frequency, is of great interest to tissue typers, anthropologists, and others, but this subject is beyond the scope of this chapter. It formed a large part of the Fifth Histocompatibility Testing Workshop.[24e] Use of the HLA system has assisted in tracing the migration of various populations.

Paternity testing

HLA antigens are one of a large battery of cellular and body fluid antigens used in paternity exclusion.

HISTOCOMPATIBILITY TESTING: SEROLOGIC TISSUE-TYPING TECHNICS

Since histocompatibility testing is a relatively new laboratory science, it may be expected that there is no single acceptable method for most of the tests presently used in clinical laboratories. In this chapter I present only the most commonly used procedures such as microlymphocytotoxicity, MLC, cytotoxic antibody screening, crossmatching, and cell freezing. Reference is made to other methods and procedures.[104]

Although HLA antigens are found on all nucleated cells and platelets, tissue typing has been

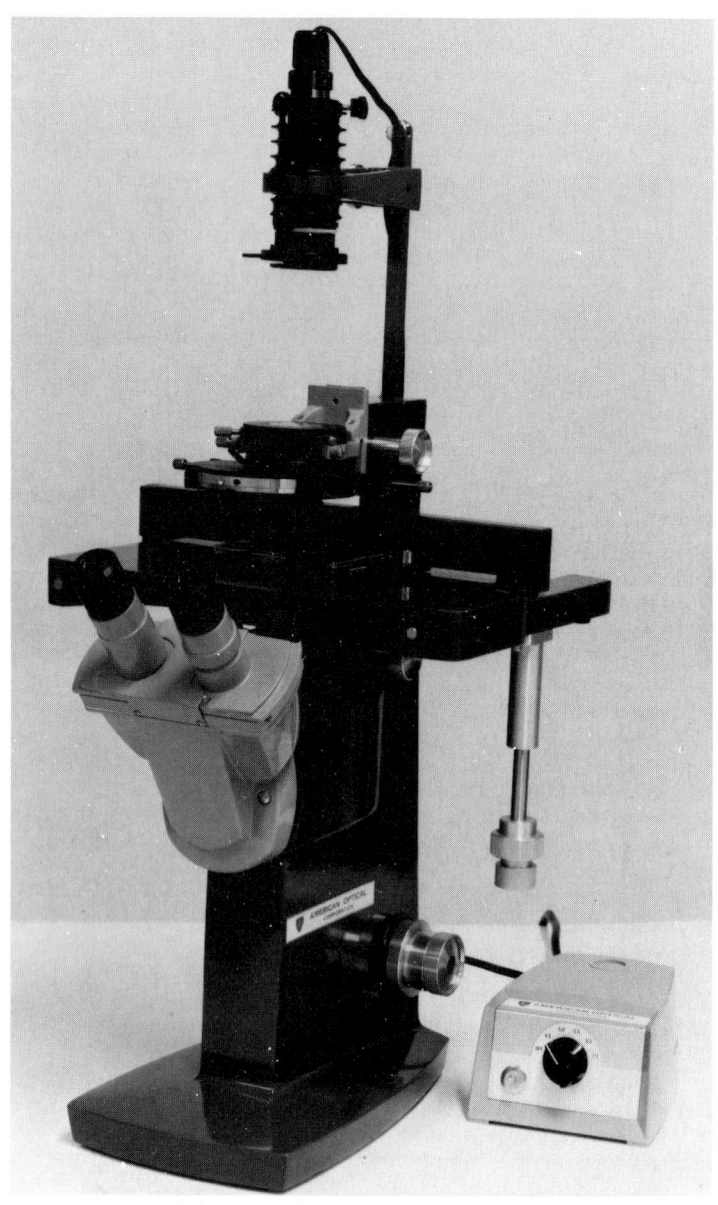

Fig. 66-4. Inverted phase microscope with tissue-typing tray in place. (American Optical, Buffalo.)

performed primarily on leukocytes and, less frequently, platelets because of the easy availability of these cells in the peripheral blood. The early studies of HLA antigens utilized the leukoagglutinin technic. This technic suffered from difficulty in standardization. In 1964, Walford[18] and co-workers introduced the use of a cytotoxic antibody technic to tissue typing, and in the same year Terasaki and McClelland[17] devised the microdroplet technic for the lymphocytotoxicity method of typing. This innovation provided further impetus to the field of tissue typing by conserving valuable antisera and reducing the number of cells required for testing, thus permitting a large battery of antisera to be tested. The test was sensitive and relatively easy to standardize. Presently the leukoagglutinin technic is of value in differentiating neutrophil-specific agglutinins from HLA antibodies. Leukoagglutinin determinations and lymphocytotoxicity cross matches are performed in some centers before granulocyte transfusions are given. The *Manual of tissue typing techniques* provides several methods for leukoagglutinin determination.[104]

A third method for HLA typing is platelet complement fixation. The test is based on the classic principles of complement fixation in which complement is fixed to antigen-antibody complexes.

Free complement in the test system indicates that no antigen-antibody reaction has occurred. The free complement is then measured in a standardized test system using the hemolysis of red cells as the indicator. A microtechnic of this method, agreed upon by several international centers, is presently used.[105] This method has been applied previously only to platelets, but may now also be used for lymphocyte complement fixation. A recent brief review of the method by Colombani and Colombani is available.[106]

The complement fixation method is used much less frequently than the lymphocytotoxicity method. One drawback of its clinical use is that test suspensions of lymphocytes and platelets are not fully reactive in the test immediately after their preparation but should be stored for 2-4 days. An advantage is that the cell suspensions retain their antigenic reactivity for 1-2 months in a +4 C refrigerator and thus avoid lengthy freezing procedures. This method also lends itself to the study of quantitation as well as identification of HLA antigen.

Several variations of the microlymphocytotoxicity technic introduced by Terasaki and McClelland are presently in use at various centers.[104] The basic principle of the test is that

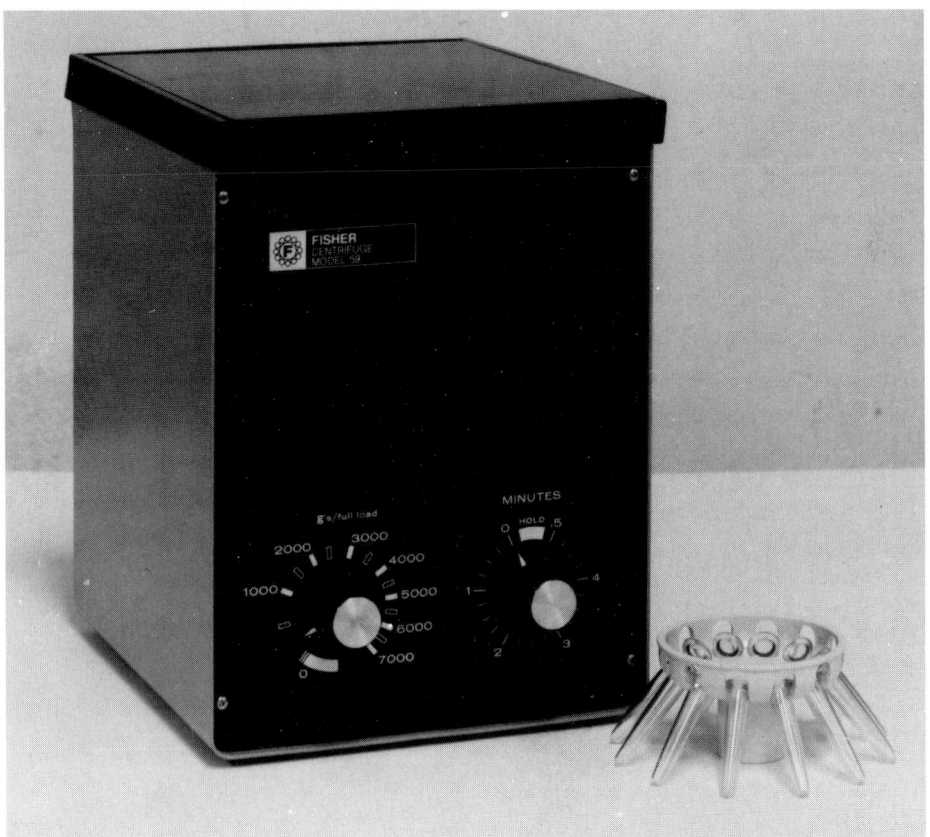

Fig. 66-5. Fisher centrifuge model 59 and Fisher centrifuge tubes. (Fisher Scientific Co., Pittsburgh.)

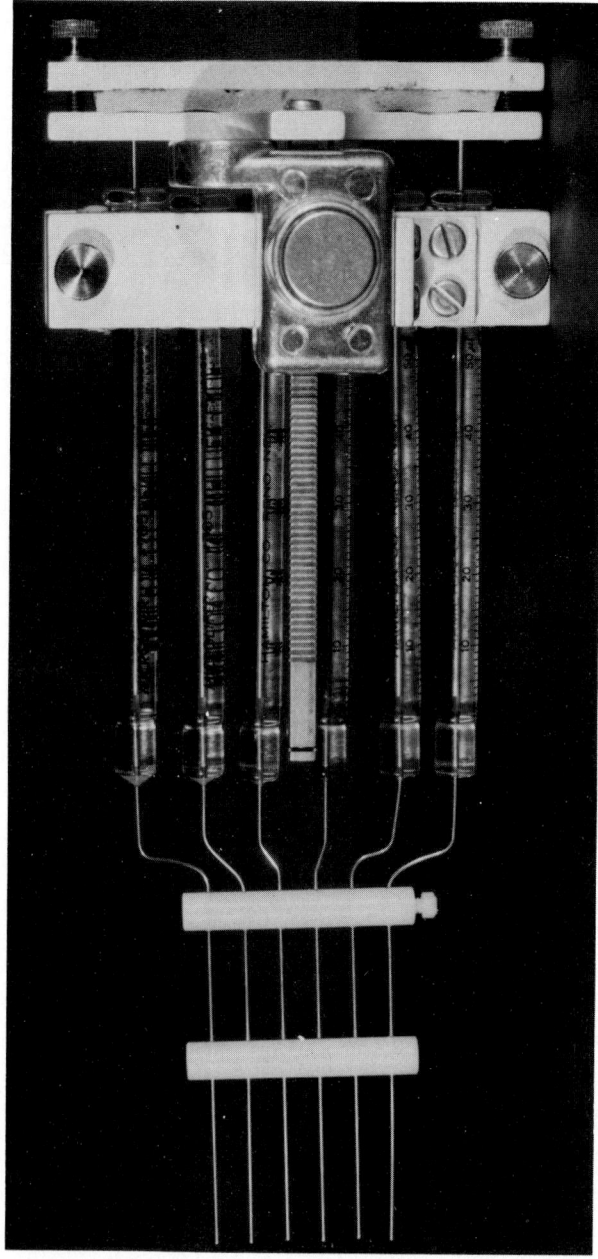

Fig. 66-6. Terasaki multiple repeating dispenser. Each syringe has 50 μl capacity and dispenses 1 μl with each delivery. (Hamilton Co., Reno, Nev.)

lymphocyte suspensions—prepared from blood, lymph node, or spleen—are incubated with antisera containing known cytotoxic antibodies to HLA specificities on the lymphocyte cell membrane. After further incubation with rabbit complement the degree of cell death is measured. Variations in the technic deal with times of incubation, washing of cells before the addition of complement, and the methods used for measurement of cell death.

The following method used in our laboratory (Wayne State University School of Medicine) is based on the National Institutes of Health's (NIH) recommended method of Terasaki's technic.[104]

Microlymphocytotoxicity technic

Equipment and supplies
1. Inverted phase microscope (American Optical [Fig. 66-4] or Carl Zeiss, New York)
2. Light microscope
3. Fisher centrifuge model 59 (Fisher Scientific Co.) (Fig. 66-5)
4. International clinical centrifuge with 6-place

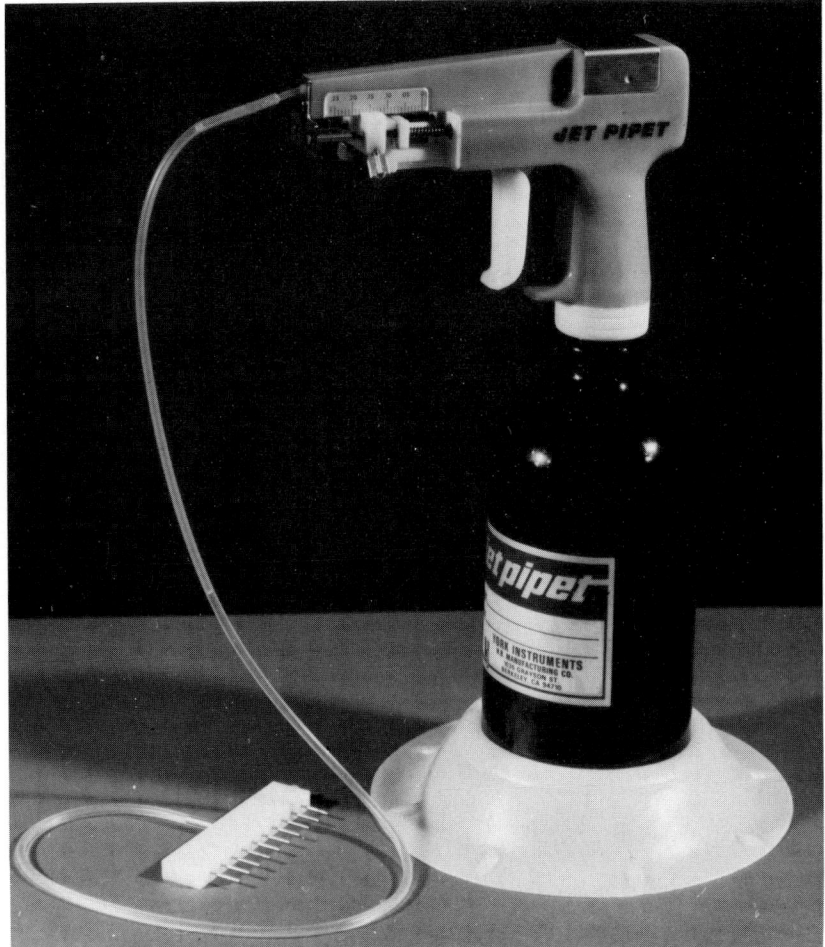

Fig. 66-7. Jet pipet is convenient for dispensing mineral oil, eosin Y, and formalin. (York Instruments, H. B. Manufacturing Co., Berkeley, Calif.)

swinging head (International Equipment Co., Needham Heights, Mass.)

5. Terasaki multiple-needle repeating dispensers—50 μl (Hamilton Co., Reno, Nev.) (Fig. 66-6)
6. Terasaki single needle repeating dispenser—50 μl (Hamilton Co.)
7. Jet pipet (York Instruments, H. B. Manufacturing Co.) (Fig. 66-7)
8. Hemacytometer counting chamber, AO improved double Neubauer ruling
9. Microtest plates (disposable), "Terasaki trays" (Fig. 66-8) (Falcon Plastics, Division of Bioquest, Oxnard, Calif., or CoStar, Cooke Laboratory Products, Alexandria, Va.)
10. Fisher centrifuge tubes (Fig. 66-5)
11. Micro cover slides (50 × 75 mm)
12. Leukopak (Fenwal Laboratories, Division of Travenol Laboratories, Morton Grove, Ill.)
13. Plastic syringe with 20-gauge needle

Reagents
1. Tissue typing sera (see below)
2. Rabbit complement (see below)
3. Lymphocyte suspension (see Preparations of Lymphocytes for Tissue Typing)
4. Hanks balanced salt solution (HBSS) (Grand Island Biological Co., Grand Island, N. Y.)

5. Hypaque, sodium 50% (wt/vol) (Winthrop Laboratories, Division of Sterling Drug, New York)
6. Ficoll (mol. wt. 400,000) (Pharmacia Laboratories, Fine Chemical Division, Piscataway, N. J.)
7. Eosin Y
8. Formaldehyde solution—37% reagent grade
9. Normal saline
10. Mineral oil, white, light
11. Anti-AB blood grouping serum
12. Anti-H blood grouping system

Preparation of antisera trays
1. Add 5 μl mineral oil (to prevent evaporation of typing sera) to each well of microtest trays using Hamilton microtiter dispenser.
2. Add 1 μl tissue-typing sera to each well under oil.
3. Include known positive (anti-human thymus serum) and negative control (known negative serum previously screened for cytotoxic antibodies) on each plate.
4. Cover with lid.
5. Store at −70 C.

Preparation of lymphocyte suspension for tissue typing. Lymphocytes are obtained easily and in large numbers from a lymph node or spleen when these are available (cadaver donors). This tissue is gently forced through stainless steel wire cloth, 80 mesh (Cambridge

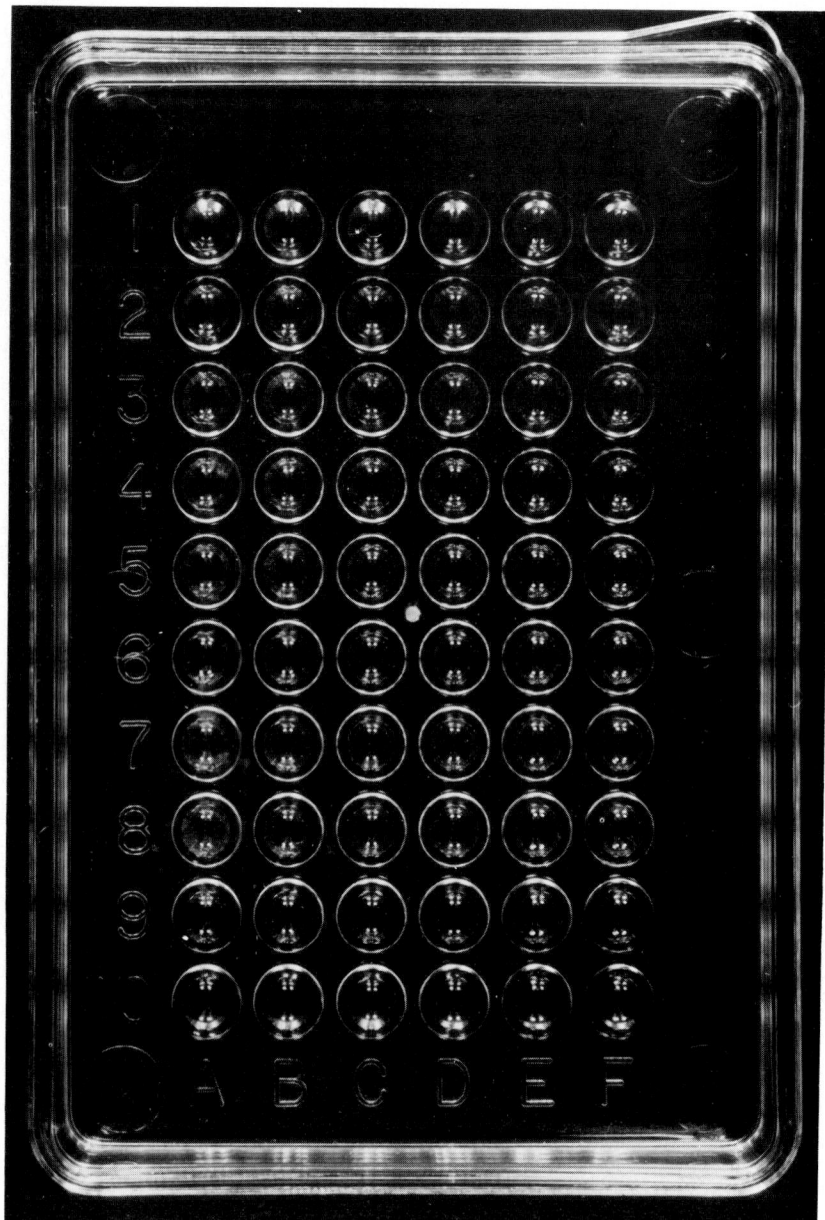

Fig. 66-8. Terasaki tissue-typing tray. (Falcon Plastics, Div. of Bioquest, Oxnard, Calif.)

Wire Cloth Co., Cambridge, Md.), or gently teased into HBSS with forceps and a scalpel. In the case of a lymph node the injection of Hanks solution directly into the lymph node with syringe and needle and collection of lymphocyte-rich Hanks solution escaping from the node frequently yield a good, pure lymphocyte suspension.

The cell preparation from a lymph node generally consists primarily of lymphocytes, but when spleen is used, there frequently are enough contaminating red cells and granulocytes to necessitate further separation, as is always the case when using blood. To ensure accurate reading of the lymphocytotoxicity reaction, a pure lymphocyte suspension is essential; granulocytes may simulate dead lymphocytes, red cells may be

mistaken for lymphocytes, and large numbers of platelets may interfere with the lymphocytic antigen-antibody reaction because of the presence of the same antigens on their surface.

Ficoll-Hypaque separation of lymphocytes

Preparation of Ficoll-Hypaque gradient[107]

1. Prepare solution of 33.9% Hypaque by mixing 20.34 ml 50% Hypaque with 9.66 ml distilled water or 30 ml 50% Hypaque with 14.25 ml distilled water.
2. Prepare a 9% Ficoll solution by dissolving 9 g Ficoll in 100 ml distilled water.
3. Mix 10 parts 33.9% Hypaque with 24 parts 9% Ficoll. The specific gravity must be 1.076-1.078. If it is too high, adjust with distilled water.

4. Solutions may be prepared and stored separately at 4 C. After they are combined, mixture should be used within 2 wk.

Separation of mononuclear cells using Ficoll-Hypaque gradient

1. Pipet 3 ml Ficoll-Hypaque gradient solution into 15 ml plastic (polypropylene) conical centrifuge tube.
2. Carefully layer 5 ml whole blood over gradient solution.
3. Spin at 2000 × g for 30 min at room temperature.
4. Remove lymphocyte layer from interface (Fig. 66-9) into a Fisher tube.
5. Add HBSS and mix.
6. Centrifuge for 2 min; discard supernatant.
7. Resuspend in HBSS (see tissue-typing reagents).
8. Check and adjust cell concentration to 2.0 × 10⁶/ml.

Problems encountered

CONTAMINATION BY GRANULOCYTES AND MONOCYTES. Occasionally, blood from cadaver donors—especially those with head injuries—contains a large number of granulocytes. In these the above separation has on occasion been incomplete and left too many granulocytes. These may be removed by filtration through a nylon column.

1. Remove nylon fiber from Leukopak, shred finely, place in a 5 ml syringe with attached 20-gauge needle, and pack to about the 3-4 ml mark (Fig. 66-10).
2. Pour warm (37 C) HBSS solution through column.
3. Add cell suspension.
4. Collect eluate in Fisher test tubes.
5. Centrifuge all Fisher tubes at 3500 × g for 2 min.
6. Remove supernatant.
7. Resuspend and combine cell buttons in HBSS.
   NOTE: Neutrophils, monocytes, cellular debris, and many B-lymphocytes are retained in the column.

CONTAMINATING RED CELLS. Contaminating red cells may be removed by adding anti-AB or anti-H serum to the cell preparation. The agglutinated red cells are gently spun down for 3 s at 1000 × g in a Fisher centrifuge. The lymphocyte-rich supernatant is removed, centrifuged, and washed to remove the anti-AB or H serum.

EXCESSIVE PLATELETS. Excessive platelets may be removed by differential centrifugation at 600 × g for 1 min. The supernatant containing the platelets is discarded, and the remaining cell button is resuspended in HBSS and plasma. This procedure may be repeated several times.

Alternate methods for removal of contaminating cells are provided by Terasaki and Park.[108]

Procedure

1. Thaw covered trays immediately prior to use.
2. To each well add 1 μl well-mixed lymphocyte suspension (approximately 2000 cells/μl) using multiple Hamilton microtiter dispenser. Mix well by agitating tray but do not touch typing serum with dispensing needle.
3. Incubate for 30 min at room temperature.
4. Add 5 μl rabbit complement to each well using multiple Hamilton microtiter dispenser. Mix gently.
5. Incubate for 60 min at room temperature.
6. Add 3 μl 5% aqueous eosin Y solution to each well using Jet pipet.
7. After 3 min, add 5 μl formaldehyde to each well using Jet pipet.
8. Gently place 50 × 75 mm microscope slide over wells to flatten droplets of fluid in wells.

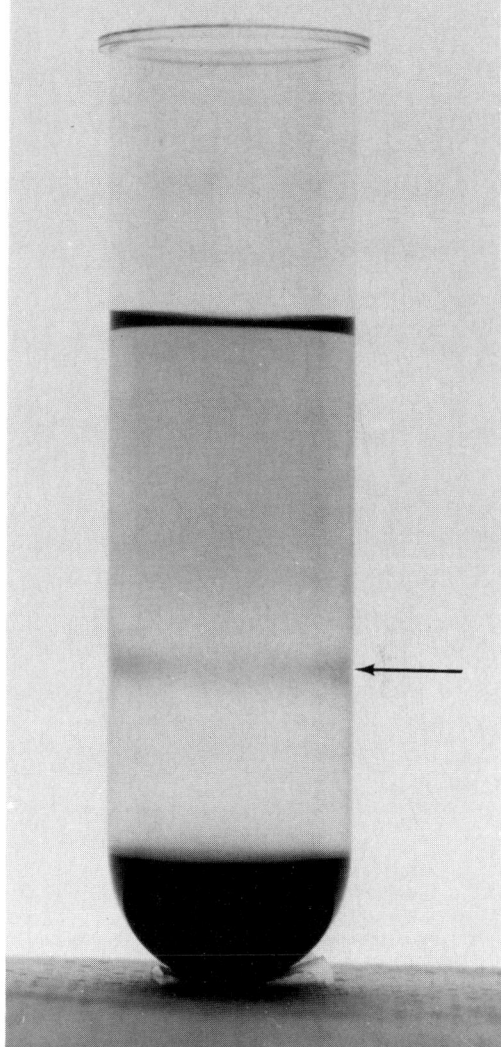

Fig. 66-9. Ficoll-Hypaque density gradient with mononuclear cells at the interface *(arrow).*

9. Seal slide with heated petrolatum if tray is to be saved for future re-reading.

Reading of test. The reactions are read with an inverted phase contrast microscope (Fig. 66-4) using the 10× objective. The stage of the microscope is equipped to hold the typing tray in place.

Living lymphocytes are colorless and refractile; dead ones are larger and dark red when eosin is used (Figs. 66-11 and 66-12), or blue if trypan blue is used. The negative and positive controls are read first. Since some cell preparations contain occasional dead cells from the onset, the percentage of dead cells in the negative control well is used as the baseline for the other positive reactions. The reactions are graded as follows (Figs. 66-11 and 66-12):

1   Negative. Percentage of dead cells is same as control.

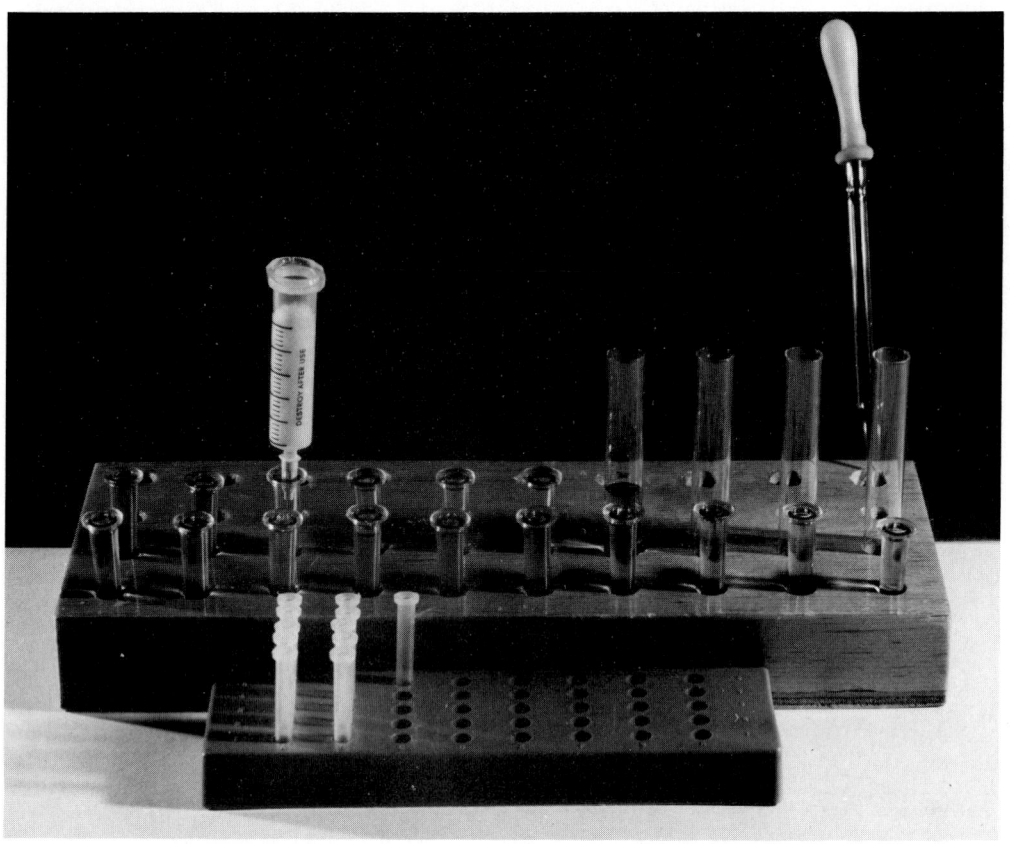

Fig. 66-10. Convenient test-tube holders for variety of test tubes used in tissue typing. One syringe contains nylon fiber used for separation of granulocytes and monocytes. Syringe rests in Fisher test tube. Small test tubes in front are Beckman tubes, convenient for freezing and storing lymphocytes.

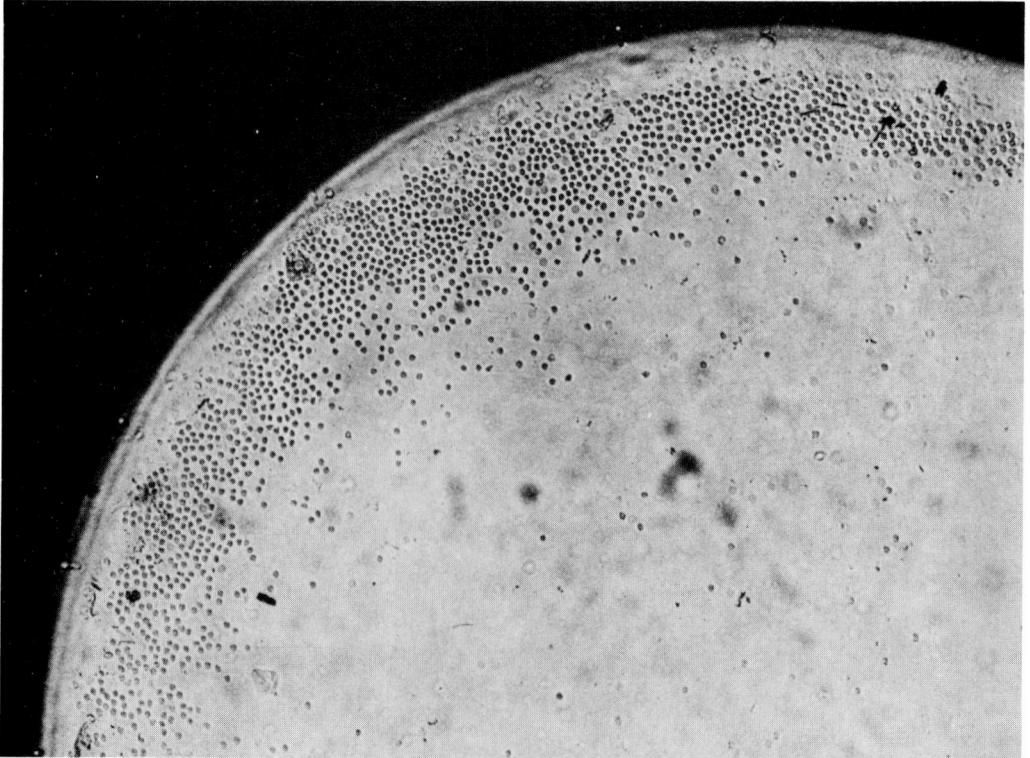

Fig. 66-11. Photograph of edge of well from tissue-typing tray as viewed through 10× objective. More than 90% of cells are dead. (×200.)

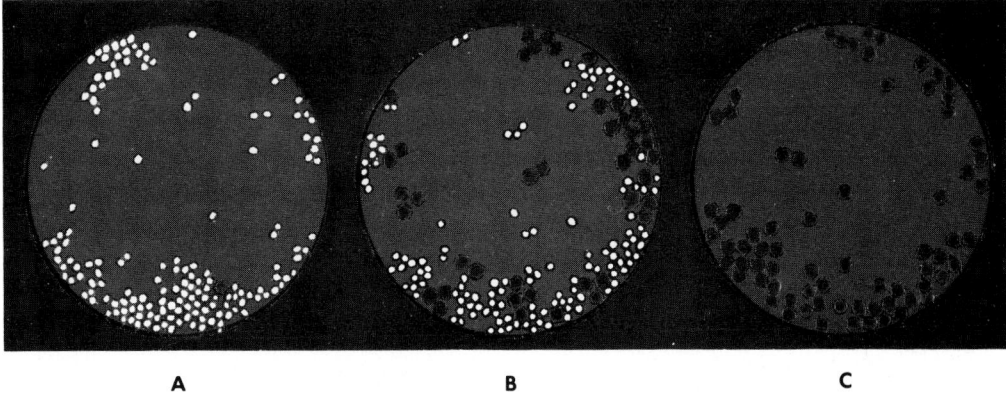

Fig. 66-12. Drawing of 3 wells from tissue-typing tray demonstrating dye exclusion method (eosin Y) in measuring cell death. **A,** Negative (graded as 1). **B,** Doubtful positive (graded as 4). **C,** Strong positive (graded as 8).

2   Doubtful negative. There is an increase in dead cells over negative control (less than 20%).
4   Doubtful positive. Approximately 20-40% of cells are dead.
6   Positive. Between 40 and 80% of cells are dead.
8   Strong positive. More than 80% of cells are dead.
0   Cannot be read due to a variety of reasons (frequently technical problems).

Tissue-typing sera

Antisera are obtained from humans after prior sensitization. This sensitization occurs primarily through multiple pregnancies, multiple blood transfusions, and organ transplants. A few antisera are produced in volunteers willing to be sensitized to specific HLA antigens. It is hoped that animal sera specific for human antigens will be available in the future. Only a few antigens are presently available commercially.

The best sources of antisera at present are multiparous women willing to undergo plasmapheresis. Since patients receiving multiple blood transfusions are being stimulated by a far greater number of HLA antigens, the probability of obtaining antisera with only one or limited numbers of antibody specificities is far less than from multiparous women who are exposed to a limited number of antigens from their fetuses. Patients with organ transplants may yield good antisera, but their availability is limited because of the health status of such patients.

Large laboratories associated with active blood banks, especially regional blood centers, are presently the best equipped for obtaining good tissue-typing sera. Protocols for large-scale screening and preparation of monospecific typing sera are presented by Rodey et al.[109] and Shaw.[110] Since fewer than 20% of the donors will have cytotoxic antibodies, and of these, fewer than half are monospecific or duospecific, the necessity for large-scale screening programs becomes apparent.

Smaller laboratories screen on a smaller scale. They also utilize mother's serum against baby's cells as an effective preliminary screen. The occasionally monospecific antisera detected in the monthly antibody screen obtained from patients awaiting transplants (after several blood transfusions), and those awaiting repeat transplants, are used. A barter system between laboratories is also an effective way to obtain necessary antisera.

The Transplantation and Immunology Branch of the National Institute of Allergy and Infectious Diseases, National Institutes of Health, since 1965 has been the largest distributor of tissue-typing sera, which have been contributed by the various tissue-typing centers. Preloaded tissue-typing trays have been available (at no cost) to qualified laboratories for typing donors and recipients of solid organ and bone marrow transplants. Bulk sera for the purpose of other clinical typings (disease association, granulocytes, and platelet transfusions) and research have also been available free of charge. The individual laboratories use the bulk sera as well as their own antisera in assembling their own tissue-typing trays.

Complement

Rabbit serum has been found to be the most effective source of complement in the cytotoxicity reactions used in human histocompatibility testing, despite the fact that this complement has relatively low reactivity in the hemolytic test system. In 1964, Walford et al.,[18] testing 17 different animal sera (rabbit, hamster, gerbil, rat, mouse, guinea pig, human, rhesus monkey, cat, dog, sheep, goat, chicken, pigeon, frog, alligator, and goldfish), found that only rabbit serum proved entirely satisfactory. The reason for this effectiveness in the lymphocytotoxicity test is not clear. Walford et al. suggested, and Ferrone et al.[111] later demonstrated, that rabbit serum has naturally occurring heteroantibody to human cells that seems to enhance the binding of complement to the HLA antibody.

Rabbit complement may currently be obtained from a variety of sources. A laboratory with animal quarters may keep its own rabbit colony. A pool of at least 6 rabbits should be used. Pooled frozen rabbit serum may be obtained commercially from several companies. Lyophilized rabbit complement is likewise available but is more expensive than the other products.

As with all complement, certain precautions are essential in selecting and using rabbit complement. It should be kept frozen, preferably at -70 C, and repeated freezing and thawing should be avoided through storage in conveniently sized aliquots.

Each batch of rabbit serum should be tested for degree of complement activity in the cytotoxicity reaction and for its heterophile antibody activity. The latter should not be so high as to kill human lymphocytes in the absence of human antibody. By using an adequately large pool of rabbits and diluting high-titered heterophile rabbit serum, the latter problem can be avoided.

Complement titration

Cell and serum combinations with known strongly positive, weakly positive, and negative reactions are selected. When possible, the same cells and sera are used in each titration so that the rabbit complement is the only variable factor in the test system. The data obtained with each successive lot can be compared to previous titrations. Complement for titration should be aliquoted, stored, and thawed in the same manner as that used for daily testing. Various dilutions of complement are run against dilutions of sera (Table 66-4). Serum and complement dilutions should be carried out as far as necessary to demonstrate the decrease in activity. The number of dilutions to be made is dependent upon the titers of the complement and serum used.

The negative serum control, which consists of cells, negative serum (serum found to be negative for cytotoxic antibodies in multiple antibody

screens), and complement, is a check for excessive amounts of anti-human activity in the complement. The serum control, which consists of all serum and cell combinations without complement, is performed to verify that the antibody being tested is a complement-dependent one. The positive control is a 1:1000 dilution of anti-human-thymocyte globulin (ATG).

Procedure
1. Prepare serum dilutions:
   a. Positive 1:1, 1:2, 1:4, 1:8, etc.
   b. Negative—use undiluted.
2. Place 1 μl sera, controls, and cells on tray. Incubate for 30 min at room temperature.
3. Prepare complement dilutions 1:1, 1:2, 1:4, 1:8, 1:12, 1:16, 1:20, 1:24, etc.
4. Add 5 μl complement to trays. Incubate 1 h.
5. Add eosin Y and formaldehyde. Read.

Problems in antibody identification
Cross-reactivity

A major problem encountered in the identification of many of the antigens of the A and B series is cross-reactivity between certain antigens. This cross-reactivity is restricted to antigens within a particular series, i.e., antigens of series A cross-react with other antigens of series A only. The reason for this cross-reactivity is not clear. Although in some instances polyspecific antisera may have been the reason, in many other examples another explanation is required. One theory proposes that HLA specificities can be divided into short (private or subtypic) and long or broad (public or supertypic types).[24,112,113] There is laboratory evidence that long and short specificities may represent different parts of the same molecule on the cell membrane. Thus antisera directed against the long specificity would also react against the short specificity. The short specificity may have been formed as a result of gene mutation or recombination. Examples of very broad specificities are van Rood's 4a and 4b,

Table 66-4. Example of complement titration

Serum dilutions	No complement	Undiluted	Complement dilutions						
			1:2	1:4	1:8	1:12	1:16	1:20	1:24
Strongly positive serum									
Undiluted	1	8	8	8	8	8	6	1	1
1:2	1	8	8	8	8	8	6	1	1
1:4	1	8	8	8	8	8	6	1	1
1:8	1	8	8	8	8	8	4	1	1
1:16	1	4	4	4	4	4	4	1	1
1:20	1	2	2	2	1	1	1	1	1
Weakly positive serum									
Undiluted	1	8	8	8	8	8	4	1	1
1:2	1	6	6	6	6	6	2	1	1
1:4	1	1	1	1	1	1	1	1	1
1:8	1	1	1	1	1	1	1	1	1
Negative serum									
Undiluted	1	1	1	1	1	1	1	1	1
Positive control ATG									
1:1000	1	8	8	8	8	8	8	S	8

later called w4 and w6. Most of the antigens of series B can be grouped with either w4 or w6. Examples of less public specificities are HLA-A2 (long) and A28 (short).

The following is a list of groups of antigens that appear to be related.[30]

A series

HLA-A1, A11, and Aw36 (Mo*). Aw36 is a new specificity recognized in black populations. A separate antiserum is not yet available.

HLA-A9, Aw23 and Aw24. Aw23 and Aw24 are subgroups of A9. The former is more common in blacks, the latter in whites.

HLA-A10 has subdivisions A25, A26, and Aw34. Aw34 is also found primarily in blacks. Other related antigens are A11, Aw32, Aw33, and Aw43.

HLA-Aw19 is a complex that has been subdivided into A29, Aw30, Aw31, Aw32, and Aw33. Cross-reactions frequently occur with the latter 4 antigens.

B series

HLA-B5 cross-reacts with Bw35 and to some extent with Bw18.

HLA-B7 cross-reacts with Bw22, B27, and Bw42.

HLA-B12 has 2 subdivisions, Bw44 and Bw45.

HLA-Bw16 has 2 subdivisions, Bw38, and Bw39.

HLA-Bw21 may have 2 subdivisions, tentatively called Bw21.1 and Bw21.2.

HLA-Bw40 cross-reacts with B13, B7, and B27.

Cross match
Microlymphocytotoxicity cross-match test

In the cross match, recipient's serum is reacted with donor's lymphocytes. The test is performed using the microlymphocytotoxicity technic described for tissue typing. A positive reaction is considered to be any significant cell death in excess of the negative control. This may be as low as 10-20%. As a rule several serum samples from the potential recipient are used. Since a recipient may remain on a waiting list for an organ transplant for many months, during which time he may receive blood transfusions, monthly serum samples are tested for HLA antibodies (see Antibody Screens). Samples of the patient's sera showing a large percentage of antibodies against a cell panel, or sera with defined antibodies to various HLA specificities, as well as the most recent serum sample (preferably within 48 hours from transplant) should be used for the cross match. The sera should be used in several dilutions (1:2, 1:4) and undiluted.

A positive cross match indicates the presence of donor-specific, preformed complement-dependent antibodies. Since the presence of such antibodies has been associated with hyperacute or accelerated allograft rejections, a positive cross match is considered a definite contraindication to transplantation.[114]

To improve the sensitivity of the cross-match test, a number of modifications have been introduced.[66] These have included prolonging the incubation time, enzyme treatment of donor cells, the use of antilymphocyte serum as a potentiating agent, and the use of radioactive target labeling for the measurement of cytotoxicity. In case the donor's lymphocytes might not express all the antigens adequately, other cells such as kidney cells and cultured lymphoblasts have been used. In many centers the antiglobulin microcytotoxicity test[115] is used in conjunction with the standard lymphocyte microcytotoxicity cross match on a routine basis. This involves the addition of carefully determined dilutions of anti-human IgG (heavy-chain specific) prior to the addition of the rabbit complement. The timing, the quality, and proper dilution of the IgG are critical in the proper performance and interpretation of this test. Some workers have found this test too cumbersome and difficult to standardize for use in a busy clinical laboratory.[116]

In light of recent discoveries in renal transplant patients, B-lymphocyte–specific antibodies appear to have no deleterious effect on immediate survival of the graft and may even be enhancing (i.e., favorable to graft survival) antibodies. Ettinger et al.[66] suggest that the increased sensitivity of some of the modifications of the standard cross-match test may be due to less easily detected anti–B cell antibodies. In addition, they raise the possibility that B cell antibodies may be responsible for weak false-positive reactions (10-20% cell death) even with the standard cytotoxicity test. Support for the latter assumption may be found in the fact that Terasaki et al. have reported no hyperacute rejection in approximately 30% of kidneys transplanted across a positive standard cross match.[117] These data were obtained retrospectively, before crossmatching prior to transplantation became common practice. To exclude such false-positive reactions, cross matching against T- and B-lymphocytes separately may have to be performed.

Another false-positive reaction to consider in the routine cross-match test is one in which recipient's serum will kill recipient's own cells. Cross et al.[118] reported a series of patients with such positive reactions and suggest the inclusion of an autocontrol in the standard cross match. The reason for this phenomenon is not known.

Other cross matches

In addition to the previously mentioned modifications of the complement-dependent cytotoxicity cross match, 2 test systems have been employed by several groups of investigators in an effort to produce a more effective cross match and also to detect presensitized cytotoxic T cells. These repeated efforts at developing a better cross match are the result of the fact that within the last few years accelerated acute rejections at 1 month after transplant have, for as yet poorly understood reasons, become a greater problem.[119] The immediate hyperacute rejections, on the other hand, have become rare due to the strict observance of not transplanting organs in the presence of a positive standard complement-dependent cross match. The antibody-dependent, lymphocyte-mediated cytotoxicity test is a highly sensitive assay for antibodies; some of these are not detected by the simple complement-dependent lymphocytotoxicity cross match.[120-122] Direct cell-mediated lympholysis may detect presensitization not detected by the serologic cross matches, since it measures cell-mediated (T cell) cytotoxicity.[123] Both tests are complicated to perform, and definite proof of clinical correlation with test results is still lacking.[123]

Antibody screens

Candidates for organ transplants may have cytotoxic antibodies against HLA specificities. These may have been formed as a result of pregnancy, blood transfusions, previous transplants, or infections.[124] Even if no antibodies have been detected in an initial antibody screen, patients may form antibodies during the sometimes long waiting period, especially when blood transfusions are required. Monthly antibody screens utilizing a large panel of HLA-typed lymphocytes representing all known serologic specificities are performed by many institutions.

The number of cells on the panel varies from institution to institution and with the availability of well-typed lymphocytes. The common specificities are usually well represented with 60 cells. There are several sources of these cells, including those typed in the laboratory for clinical purposes, volunteers ("walking cell panels"), and frozen typed lymphocytes.

The number of positive reactions and the detection of specific HLA antibodies in these patients help the tissue typer to select specific serum samples of the patient to be included in the final cross match against donor cells. Although the last serum drawn from a patient may show a negative cross match, a previous sample, carefully selected, may produce a positive cross match because the antibody level in the patient may have diminished by the time of the final cross match.

It is not clear at present whether the antibody screen is of clinical value in predicting the transplant survival of the patient.

Although some investigators find that patients with HLA antibodies have a poorer prognosis even when the cross match is negative,[76] others

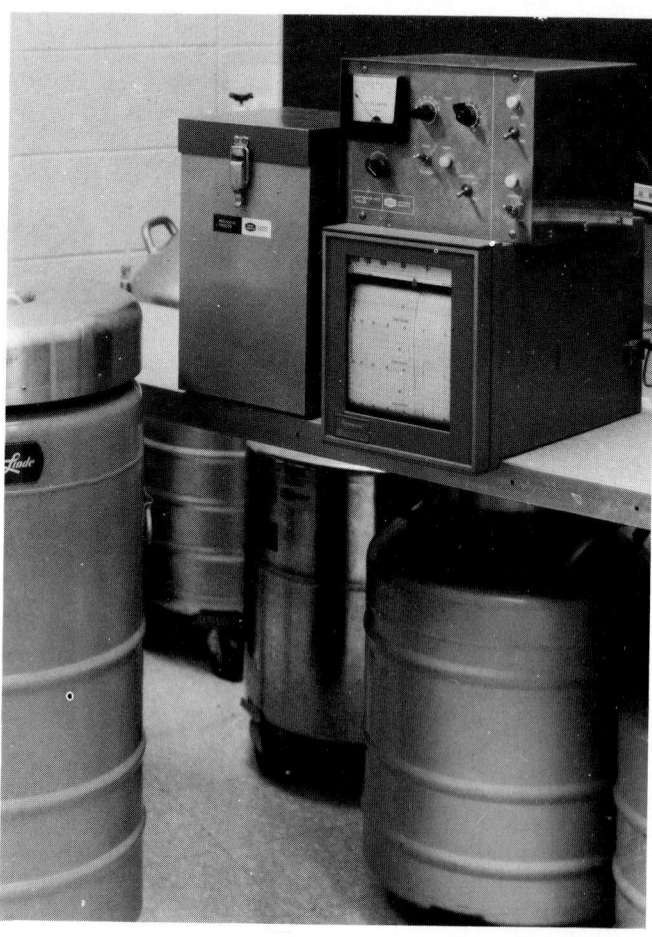

Fig. 66-13. Equipment used for freezing lymphocytes (left to right on table): freezing chamber, recorder, and controller above recorder. Various storage tanks are on floor.

have failed to find this correlation.[125] For the last few years great care was taken to prevent presensitization of patients on dialysis awaiting renal transplants. Blood transfusions were carefully avoided; when absolutely necessary, frozen red cells with few leukocytes were given. Despite these precautions the survival rate of cadaver renal transplant has not improved. The reasons for this are not clear. That blood transfusions may have a beneficial rather than deleterious effect by producing enhancing or B cell antibodies is presently being considered.[66]

Antibody screen procedure. The following procedure has proven to be convenient in our laboratory. Depending on the size and activity of a laboratory, different schedules may prove more efficient.

1. Aliquot each serum sample to be screened and store at −20 C until 29 sera are accumulated. This number is convenient when a 60-well typing tray is used.
2. Worksheets showing name, bleeding date, and location of sera and controls on tray are prepared.
3. When ready to prepare trays, thaw 29 sera, a negative control, and a positive control serum.
4. All sera are centrifuged to remove any cryoprecipitate.
5. 1:2 dilutions in HBSS of each serum are prepared.
6. Undiluted and diluted sera and negative and positive controls are arranged in accordance with worksheet and 1 μl of each is placed in each well of a 60-well tray. Use a multiple repeating dispenser to make 60 trays.
7. When all plates have been loaded, they are stored at −70 C until used.
8. As typed cells become available, they are added to trays.
9. Usual microlymphocytotoxicity procedure is followed.
10. When 60 different cells (all HLA typed) have been used, percentage of positive reactions is calculated and HLA specificity of positive sera is identified, when possible.

Freezing and thawing lymphocytes

Typed lymphocytes are essential for screening of potential typing sera (e.g., serum of previously pregnant women) as well as the patient's antibody screens. Typed lymphocytes can be preserved for years at very low temperatures in order to assure constant availability of such cells.

Equipment (Fig. 66-13)
1. Linde biological freezing controller (Union Carbide, Linde Division, Indianapolis)
2. Linde BF-4 freezing chamber
3. Honeywell electronic strip chart recorder (Honeywell Instruments, Industrial Division, Ft. Washington, Pa.)
4. Linde liquid nitrogen refrigerator
   NOTE: A more compact automatic freezing system has recently become available from Cryo-Med, Division of Weld Metal, Mt. Clemens, Mich.

Supplies and reagents
1. Liquid nitrogen, local supplier
2. Dimethylsulfoxide (DMSO), ACS certified (Fisher Scientific Co., Pittsburgh, Pa.)
3. Hanks balanced salt solution (HBSS) (Grand Island Biological Co., Grand Island, N.Y.)

4. RPMI (Roswell Park Memorial Institute) Media, no. 1640 (Grand Island Biological Co.)
5. Fetal calf serum (Grand Island Biological Co.)
6. Freezing vials, small polypropylene tubes with tightly fitting caps
7. Freezing medium: 16% fetal calf serum and 15% DMSO in RPMI medium

Freezing procedure
1. Prepare cells in same manner as for tissue typing.
2. Concentrate cell suspension by centrifuging and removing half the supernatant, then resuspending cells. Slowly add, dropwise, freezing medium to original volume, mixing continuously.
   NOTE: DMSO must be handled with utmost caution due to its harmful effect on skin and the respiratory tract.
3. Immediately transfer cell suspension to freezing vials, cap tightly, and place in freezing chamber, reserving 1 of these tubes as control for freezing procedure.
4. Insert differential temperature sensor into control vial.
5. Adjust controls to obtain cooling rate of 1 C/min. Observe recorder for sharp temperature rise, which represents latent heat of fusion. Open override switch to admit extra liquid nitrogen to bring temperature back down quickly. After standardization of equipment, temperature at which latent heat of fusion occurs is predictable, and override should begin just prior to expected temperature rise to avoid deleterious effects of heat.
6. When −30 C is attained, freezing rate may be increased to 3½ C/min until final temperature of −125 C is reached.
7. Quickly transfer samples to vapor phase of a liquid nitrogen storage refrigerator (approx. −180 C).

Thawing procedure
1. Remove desired samples from storage refrigerator and thaw by immersing in warm water (approximately 40 C).
2. Centrifuge, remove supernatant, and resuspend in HBSS with 5% fetal calf serum to desired concentration of cells.

This thawing technic works well in our laboratory. Some laboratories find further precautions necessary. For additional methods of freezing and thawing lymphocytes consult the NIH *Manual of tissue typing techniques.*[104]

Mixed-lymphocyte culture test (MLC)

Principle. Lymphocytes from 2 unrelated individuals, when mixed in culture, were found to stimulate each other to undergo blastogenesis and mitosis.[126] By inhibiting the DNA synthesis of 1 of the 2 sets of lymphocytes by using mitomycin C, the reactivity of each of the lymphocyte populations may be measured independently. The mitomycin-inhibited cells are the stimulating cells; the uninhibited lymphocytes, the responder cells. The presence of monocytes in the culture is essential for the reaction to occur.

Lymphocytes from related donors have shown fairly predictable reactions. Serologically HLA-identical siblings—with few exceptions (1%)—do not stimulate each other. Those that differ by 2 haplotypes stimulate strongly, and those that share only 1 haplotype show stimulation of intermediate intensity. It appears that B-lymphocytes

Table 66-5. Example of MLC of a family*

	A_m	B_m	C_m	D_m	X_m	HLA phenotypes
Patient A	153	1402	1635	85	6266	A1, 2; B7, w35
	(9)	(11)	(0.6)		(41)	
Mother B	1140	238	2058	1684	8070	A2, 2; B5, w35
	(5)		(9)	(7)	(34)	
Sibling C	1112	1487	101	1536	3395	A1, 2; B7, 15
	(11)	(15)		(15)	(34)	
Sibling D	134	1708	2113	113	6165	A1, 2; B7, w35
	(1.2)	(15)	(19)		(55)	
Unrelated X	5972	6028	4832	6165	188	A2, 11; B7, 8
	(32)	(32)	(26)	(33)		

*Results are listed in cpm of tritiated thymidine uptake and as SI in parentheses.

at least in large part carry antigens responsible for MLC activation[127,128] but that primarily T-lymphocytes respond to the activation with mitosis and blastogenesis. Only a small proportion of the circulating T-lymphocytes will respond. As previously discussed, antigens responsible for MLC activation (locus D) are different from the SD HLA antigens of loci A, B, and C. Although attempts at identifying the D locus antigens by serologic technics have been made, the MLC reaction is still the primary tool for determining identity or nonidentity for locus D antigens. Because of the long time period (more than 5 days) involved in the performance of the test, its primary clinical use has been for related-donor transplants.

The test is usually run in several combinations, i.e., the recipient (A) and donor (B) and an unrelated control (X) are used both as responder (A, B, X), and as stimulator (A_m, B_m, X_m) cells. The m refers to mitomycin inhibition. The more potential donors there are, the more combinations are performed (Table 66-5).

The reactivity may be expressed in counts per minute (cpm) of tritiated thymidine uptake or as a stimulation index (SI). This is a ratio of the mean radioactivity incorporated in the MLC, e.g., AB_x, over the mean radioactivity incorporated by the autocontrol, e.g., AA_x.

Equipment and supplies
1. Hood, Labconco (Fisher Scientific Co.) (Fig. 66-14)
2. MASH filtering apparatus (Microbiological Associates) (Fig. 66-15)
3. Glass fiber filter paper, 934 AH, Reeve-Angel (Fisher Scientific Co.)
4. Packard scintillation counter (Packard Instrument Co., Downers Grove, Ill.)
5. Scintillation vials, polyethylene, 7 ml (Rochester Scientific Co., Rochester, N.Y.)
6. Centrifuge (International Equipment Co., Needham Heights, Mass.)
7. Incubator, CO_2
8. Media sterilization equipment (Millipore Corp., Bedford, Mass.)
9. Sterile, disposable filter units, 0.45 μm filter with grid, 150 ml capacity (Falcon Plastics no. 7102, Oxnard, Calif.)
10. Microscope
11. Hamilton gastight repeating syringes, 1.0 and 5.0 ml (Hamilton Co.) (Fig. 66-16)
12. Hamilton disposable tips, 1.0 ml (Hamilton Co.)
13. Tissue culture trays and lids (Fig. 66-17) (Falcon Plastics)
14. Tubes, sterile disposable; 50.0 ml centrifuge, 15.0 ml centrifuge, and 10 × 75 mm with caps (Falcon Plastics)
15. Bellco glass tissue culture tubes—16 × 100 mm and plastic caps (Bellco Glass Co., Vineland, N.J.)
16. Media storage and dispensing apparatus (Bellco Glass Co.)

Reagents
1. POPOP-1, 4-bis-[2-(4-methyl-5-phenyloxazolyl)]-benzene (Packard Instrument Co., Downer's Grove, Ill.)
2. PPO (2,5-diphenyloxazole) scintillation grade (Packard Instrument Co.)
3. Toluene, ACS
4. Acid citrate dextrose (ACD) (Grand Island Biological Co., Grand Island, N.Y.)
5. RPMI (Roswell Park Memorial Institute) media no. 1640, with L-glutamine (Grand Island Biological Co.)
6. HEPES (N-2-hydroxyethylpiperazine-N-2-ethanesulfonic acid)
7. Human AB serum
8. $NaHCO_3$
9. Heparin, sodium (preservative free)
10. Ficoll (mol. wt. 400,000) (Pharmacia Laboratories, Piscataway, N.J.)
11. Hypaque, sodium, 50% (wt/vol) (Winthrop Laboratories, Division of Sterling Drug, New York)
12. Mitomycin C (Nutritional Biochemicals Corp., Cleveland, Ohio)
13. Trypticase soy broth
14. Thymidine methyl tritiated (sterile aqueous solution, specific activity 1-13 Ci/mmol) (ICN Pharmaceuticals, Irvine, Calif.)

Working solutions
Mitomycin C
1. Add 4.0 ml sterile RPMI-1640 to bottle of mitomycin C (2.0 mg).
2. Working concentration is 0.5 mg/ml.
3. Store at 4 C protected from light.

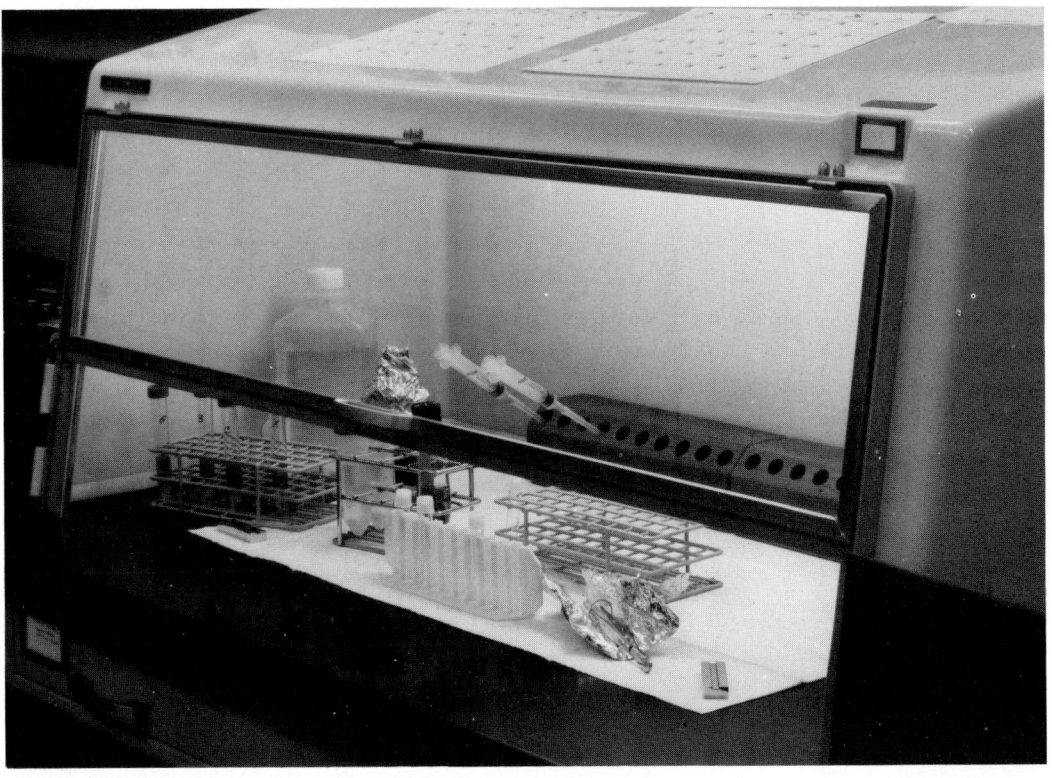

Fig. 66-14. Culture hood containing various equipment used for MLC. (Fisher Scientific Co., Pittsburgh.)

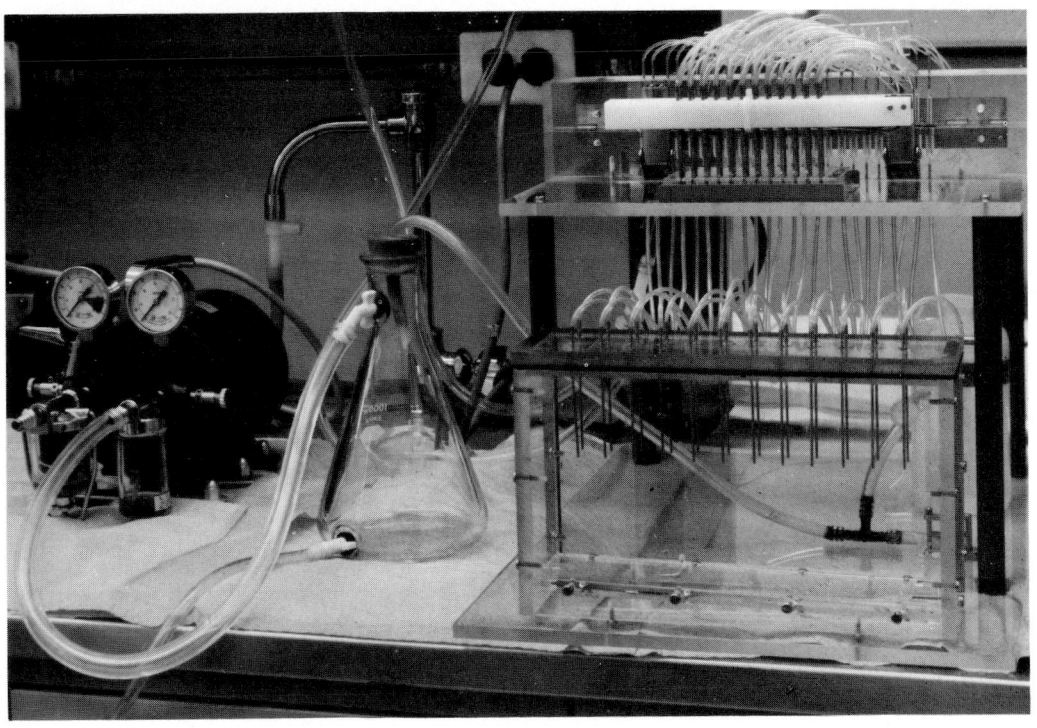

Fig. 66-15. MASH filtering apparatus. (Microbiological Associates, Bethesda, Md.)

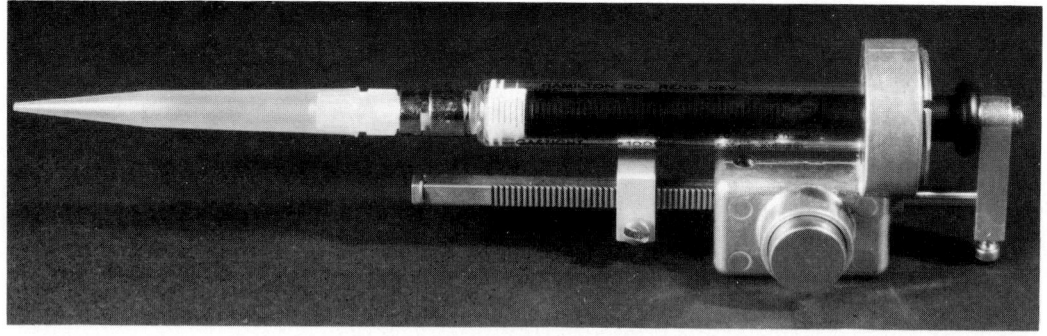

Fig. 66-16. Hamilton gastight repeating syringe. (Hamilton Co., Reno, Nev.)

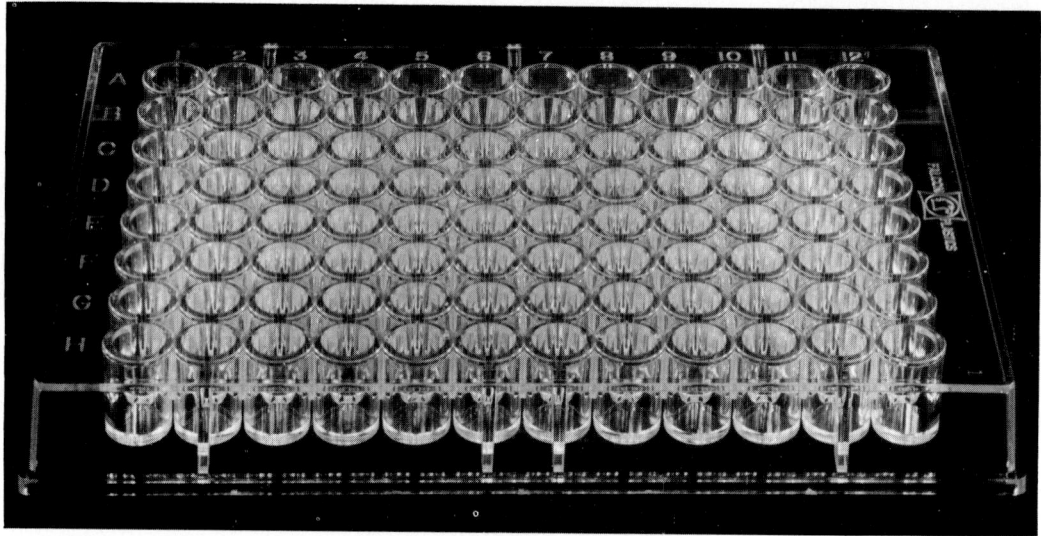

Fig. 66-17. Tissue culture tray for lymphocyte cultures. (Falcon Plastics, Oxnard, Calif.)

Tritiated thymidine
1. To 1.0 ml (1 mCi) of tritiated thymidine, add 49 ml sterile RPMI—1640.
2. Working solution is 20 μCi/ml.
3. Store in refrigerator.

Liquid scintillation fluid
1. Dissolve 0.037 g POPOP and 22.74 g PPO in 3.79 L (1 gal) of scintillation grade toluene.
2. May be stored at room temperature.

RPMI-1640
1. Dissolve preweighed package (10.4 g) in 600 ml triple-distilled water.
2. Rinse inside of package to remove all powder.
3. Add 2.0 g $NaHCO_3$.
4. Add 5.96 g HEPES.
5. Dilute to final volume of 1000 ml with water.
6. Sterilize immediately by membrane filtration.
7. Store at 4 C for no longer than 1 mo.

Preparation of cell suspensions and cultures
1. To a 50 ml sterile centrifuge tube, add heparin or ACD. Heparin is used in a concentration of 20 U (or 0.02 ml)/ml blood. ACD is used in a concentration of 0.15 ml/ml blood; e.g., if 30 ml of blood is needed, use 0.6 ml heparin or 4.5 ml ACD.
2. Collect volume of blood needed from patient, dis-

pense aseptically into centrifuge tube, and mix well.

NOTE: Volume of blood necessary is dependent on WBC count, percent of lymphocytes, and number of specimens to be tested.

3. Prepare mononuclear cell suspension using Ficoll-Hypaque gradient (see Preparation of Lymphocyte Suspension).
4. Wash cells 3 times with 5.0 ml sterile normal saline.
5. Suspend cells in 5.0 ml complete medium (CM) consisting of 90% RPMI (containing glutamine) and 10% human AB serum. Remove small aliquot for WBC count.
6. Adjust responding cell concentration to 1.0 × 10^6/ml. Total volume needed depends upon number of specimens to be tested. Calculate volume of cell suspension needed as 0.1 ml/well. Cultures with cells from 2 people plus control (A, B, and X) will provide 9 combinations with 3 wells each or 27 total wells. Cells from each person require a total of 9 wells, therefore, 1.0 ml each of A, B, and X. If enough cells are available, set up 4 and 5 d cultures (2.0 ml from each individual tested).

7. Mix cell suspension well and divide into 2 groups.
   a. Remove amount of cell suspension needed for responding cells, place in sterile 16 × 100 mm Bellco tube, and label. Add CM to attain proper cell concentration.
   b. Label remaining cell suspension as stimulating cells (e.g., A_m, B_m, etc.). Add CM to bring the volume to 5.0 ml.
8. Add mitomycin C to stimulating cells; 0.25 ml/5.0 ml cell suspension.
9. Incubate stimulating cells at 37 C for 20 min.
10. Centrifuge at 150 × g for 10 min.
11. Wash twice with 5.0 ml sterile normal saline.
12. Resuspend cells in 3.0 ml CM, mix well, remove small aliquot for WBC count.
13. Perform WBC counts.
14. Calculate amount needed for stimulating cells. Stimulating cell concentrations are 3.0×10^6/ml CM. There are 3 people (A, B, and X); 2.0 ml total volume of suspension (containing 6.0×10^6 total number of cells) for each is required.
15. Remove enough cells for proper concentrations. Add enough CM to bring to proper volume. These cells should be prepared in 16 × 100 mm Bellco tubes. Label all tubes.
16. Combinations of cells may be prepared in 16 × 100 mm Bellco tubes at this time, or each person's cells may be put directly onto culture tray (0.1 ml stimulating and 0.1 ml responding cells per well).
17. Triplication of each combination is recommended.
18. Cells are added to wells according to prepared chart. Example:

AA_m	BA_m	XA_m
AB_m	BB_m	XB_m
AX_m	BX_m	XX_m

Hamilton gas tight syringe with repeating dispenser and disposable tips facilitate dispensing of cells.
19. Cover tray with plastic lid.
20. Incubate at 37 C for 4 or 5 d in 5% CO_2.

Incorporation of tritiated thymidine and harvesting
1. After incubation period (morning of day 4 or 5), remove cover from tray.
2. Add 1 μCi tritiated thymidine to each well. Replace sterile cover on tray.
3. Incubate at 37 C for 18 h in 5% CO_2.
4. Harvest cells onto glass fiber filter paper using MASH apparatus. Wash out wells with normal saline 10-15 times.
5. When filtering is finished, wash out MASH apparatus with distilled water.
6. Dry filter paper strips at 150 C for 1 h or allow to dry at room temperature overnight.
7. Place disks into properly labeled scintillation vials; add 4.0 ml scintillation fluid to each vial.
8. Count each vial for 10 min in a Packard liquid scintillation spectrometer.
9. Calculate mean values from triplicates of each combination.
10. Calculate SI.

Example:

$$SI = \frac{cpm \ AB_m}{cpm \ AA_m} = \frac{8500}{102} = 83$$

Problems encountered
1. There may be considerable variation in the degree of MLC reactivity of the same individual on different days. Some of this may be due to technical variation or a change in number of responsive lymphocytes in circulation from day to day.
2. Uremic patients on occasion may have a poor response even to several unrelated controls.
3. Patients with severe immune deficiency diseases may have either too few lymphocytes or nonreactive lymphocytes. In this case, response of donor's lymphocytes must be used as measure of compatibility.
4. SI may be greatly influenced by small variations in background reactivity. Use of selected pools of stimulating cells of unrelated donors to determine true relative response of test reactions has been suggested by Osoba and Falk.[129]
5. In typing for D antigens, MLC results obtained using homozygous stimulating and heterozygous responding cells are rarely negative.[130] "Typing response" representing a weak-to-moderate MLC response is often observed, and a variety of correction factors have been introduced by various investigators to facilitate interpretation of the MLC results.
6. Contamination of culture by microorganisms may give false low or high response. Various solutions used should be checked for sterility on a regular basis.

REFERENCES
1. Barnes, B. A.: Transplantation 3:812, 1965.
2. Simonsen, M.: Lancet 1:415, 1965.
3. Ceppellini, R., Curtoni, E. S., Mattiuz, P. L., et al.: Ann. N.Y. Acad. Sci. 129:421, 1966.
4. van Rood, J. J., van Leeuwen, A., Schippers, A., et al.: Ann. N.Y. Acad. Sci. 129:467, 1966.
4a. Gorer, P. A.: J. Genetics 32:17, 1936.
5. Amos, D. B.: Br. J. Exp. Pathol. 34:464, 1953.
6. Dausset, J.: Presse Med. 61:1533, 1953.
7. Payne, R., and Rolfs, M. R.: J. Clin. Invest. 37:1756, 1958.
8. van Rood, J. J., Eernisse, J. G., and van Leeuwen, A.: Nature 181:1735, 1958.
9. Dausset, J.: Acta Haematol. 20:156, 1958.
10. van Rood, J. J.: Leukocyte grouping, thesis, Leiden, 1962.
11. Payne, R., Tripp, M., Weigle, J., et al.: Cold Springs Harbor Symp. Quant. Biol. 29:285, 1964.
12. Dausset, J., Ivanyi, P., and Ivanyi, D. In Amos, D. B., and van Rood, J. J., editors: Histocompatibility testing, Washington, D.C., 1965, National Academy of Science—National Research Council.
13. Bodmer, W., Bodmer, J., Adler, S., et al.: Ann. N.Y. Acad. Sci. 129:473, 1966.
14. Ceppellini, R., Curtoni, E. S., Mattiuz, P. L., et al. In Curtoni, E. S., Mattiuz, P. L., and Tosi, R. M., editors: Histocompatibility testing, Baltimore, 1967, The Williams & Wilkins Co.
15. Kissmeyer-Nielsen, F., Svejgaard, A., Ahrons, S., et al.: Nature 224:75, 1969.
16. Ward, F. E., Southworth, J. G., and Amos, D. B.: Transplant. Proc. 1:352, 1969.
17. Terasaki, P. I., and McClelland, J. D.: Nature 204:998, 1964.
18. Walford, R. L., Gallagher, R., and Sjaarda, J. R.: Science 144:868, 1964.
19. Mayr, W. R., Bernoco, D., DeMarchi, M., et al.: Transplant. Proc. 5:1581, 1973.

20. Solheim, B. G., Bratlie, A., Sandberg, L., et al.: Tissue Antigens 3:439, 1973.
21. Bach, F. H.: Transplant. Proc. 5:23, 1973.
21a. Bodmer, W. F.: Br. Med. Bull. 34:217, 1978.
22. WHO-IUIS Nomenclature Committee: Transplant. Proc. 8:109, 1976.
23. Dausset, J., and Rapaport, F. T.: Ann. N.Y. Acad. Sci. 129:408, 1966.
24. Ceppellini, R. In Amos, D. B., editor: Progress in immunology, New York, 1971, Academic Press.
24a. Russell, P. S., Winn, H. J., and Amos, D. B., editors: Histocompatibility testing 1964, Copenhagen, 1964, Munksgaard.
24b. Amos, D. B., and van Rood, J. J., editors: Histocompatibility testing 1965, Copenhagen, 1965, Munksgaard.
24c. Curtoni, E. S., Mattiuz, P. L., and Tosi, R. M., editors: Histocompatibility testing 1967, Copenhagen, 1967, Munksgaard.
24d. Terasaki, P. I., editor: Histocompatibility testing 1970, Copenhagen, 1970, Munksgaard.
24e. Dausset, J., and Colombani, J., editors: Histocompatibility testing 1972, Copenhagen, 1972, Munksgaard.
24f. Kissmeyer-Nielsen, F., editor: Histocompatibility testing 1975, Copenhagen, 1975, Munksgaard.
24g. Bodmer, W. F., Batchelor, J. R., Bodmer, J. G., et al., editors: Histocompatibility testing 1977, Copenhagen, 1978, Munksgaard.
25. van Someren, H., Westerveld, A., Hagemeijer, A., et al.: Proc. Natl. Acad. Sci. U.S.A. 71:962, 1974.
26. Lamm, L. U., Kissmeyer-Nielsen, F., Svejgaard, A., et al.: Tissue Antigens 2:205, 1972.
27. Carpenter, C. B.: N. Engl. J. Med. 294:1005, 1976.
28. Svejgaard, A., Bratlie, A., Hedin, P. J., et al.: Tissue Antigens 1:81, 1971.
29. Bodmer, J., Curtoni, E. S., van Leeuwen, A., et al. In Kissmeyer-Nielsen, F., editor: Histocompatibility testing, Copenhagen, 1975, Munksgaard.
30. Duquesnoy, R. J., and Fuller, T. C., editors: Proceedings of the first HLA workshop of the Americas, Bethesda, Md., 1975, National Institutes of Health.
30a. Pickbourne, P., Piazza, A., and Bodmer, W. F. In Bodmer, W. F., Batchelor, J. R., Bodmer, J. G., et al., editors: Histocompatibility testing 1977, Copenhagen, 1978, Munksgaard.
31. Bain, B., and Lowenstein, L.: Science 145:1315, 1964.
32. Bach, F. M., and Amos, D. B.: Science 156:1506, 1967.
33. Amos, D. B., and Bach, F. H.: J. Exp. Med. 128:623, 1968.
34. Plate, J. M., Ward, F. E., and Amos, D. B. In Terasaki, P., editor: Histocompatibility testing, Baltimore, 1970, The Williams & Wilkins Co.
35. Yunis, E. J., Plate, J. M., Ward, F. E., et al.: Transplant. Proc. 3:118, 1971.
36. Eijsvoogel, V. P., van Rood, J. J., du Toit, E. D., et al.: Eur. J. Immunol. 2:413, 1972.
37. Albert, E. D., Mempel, W., and Grosse-Wilde, H.: Transplant. Proc. 5:1551, 1973.
38. Trinchieri, G., DeMarchi, M., Mayr, W., et al.: Transplant. Proc. 5:1631, 1973.
39. van Leeuwen, A., Schuit, H. R. E., and van Rood, J. J.: Transplant. Proc. 5:1539, 1973.
39a. Bradley, B. A., and Festenstein, H.: Br. Med. Bull. 34:223-232, 1978.
40. Eijsvoogel, V. P.: Semin. Hematol. 11:305, 1974.
41. Svedmyr, E. A., Leibold, W., and Gatti, R. A.: Tissue Antigens 5:186, 1975.
42. Bach, F. H., Bach, M. L., Alter, B. J., et al. In Duquesnoy, R. J., and Fuller, T. C., editors: Proceedings of the first HLA workshop of the Americas, Bethesda, Md., 1975, National Institutes of Health.
43. Sheehy, M. J., Sondel, P. M., Bach, M. L., et al. In Ray, J. G., Hare, D. B., Pedersen, P. D., et al., editors: NIAID manual of tissue typing techniques, Bethesda, Md., 1976-1977, National Institutes of Health.
44. Häyry, P., and Defendi, V.: Science 168:133, 1970.
45. Solliday, S., and Bach, F. H.: Science 170:1406, 1970.
46. Lightbody, J., Bernoco, D., Miggiano, V. C., et al.: G. Batteriol. Virol. Immunol. 64:243, 1971.
47. Long, M. A., Mandwerger, B., and Yunis, E. J. In Kissmeyer-Nielsen, F., editor: Histocompatibility testing, Copenhagen, 1975, Munksgaard.
48. Kristensen, T., and Grunnet, N. In Kissmeyer-Nielsen, F., editor: Histocompatibility testing, Copenhagen, 1975, Munksgaard.
48a. Goulmy, E., Termijtelen, A., Bradley, B. A., et al.: Nature 266:544, 1977.
48b. Goulmy, E., Bradley, B. A., Lansbergen, Q., et al.: Transplantation 25:315, 1978.
49. Klein, J.: Biology of the mouse—histocompatibility 2 complex, New York, 1975, Springer Verlag.
49a. Klein, J. In Dixon, F. J., and Kunkel, H. G., editors: Advances in immunology, New York, 1978, Academic Press.
50. McDevitt, H. L. In Landy, M., editor: Genetic control of the immune responsiveness: relationship to disease susceptibility, Perspectives in Immunology Series, New York, 1973, Academic Press.
51. McDevitt, H. O., and Bodmer, W. F.: Lancet 1:1269, 1974.
52. Sachs, D. H., and Cone, J. L.: J. Exp. Med. 138:1289, 1973.
53. Walford, R. L., Smith, G. S., and Waters, H.: Transplant. Rev. 7:78, 1971.
54. Walford, R. L., Waters, H., Smith, G. S., et al.: Tissue Antigens 3:222, 1973.
55. Terasaki, P. I., Opelz, G., Park, M. S., et al. In Kissmeyer-Nielsen, F., editor: Histocompatibility testing, Copenhagen, 1975, Munksgaard.
56. Mann, D. L., Abelson, L., Harris, S., et al.: J. Exp. Med. 142:84, 1975.
57. Winchester, R. J., Fu, S. M., Wernet, P., et al.: J. Exp. Med. 141:924, 1975.
58. Walford, R. L., Gossett, T., Troup, G. M., et al.: J. Immunol. 116:1704, 1976.
59. Arbeit, R. D., Sachs, D. H., Amos, D. B., et al.: J. Immunol. 115:1173, 1975.
60. Hämmerling, G. J., Mauve, G., Goldberg, E., et al.: Immunogenetics 1:428, 1975.
60a. Jones, E. A., Goodfellow, P. N., Bodmer, J. G., et al.: Nature (London) 256:650, 1975.
61. Mann, D. L., Abelson, L., Henkart, P., et al.: Proc. Natl. Acad. Sci. U.S.A. 72:5103, 1975.
62. Billing, R. J., Honig, R., Terasaki, P. I., et al.: Lancet 1:1365, 1976.
62a. Bodmer, J. G. In Bodmer, W. F., Batchelor, J. R., Bodmer, J. G., et al., editors: Histocompatibility testing 1977, Copenhagen, 1978, Munksgaard.
63. Severson, C. D., Blaschke, J. W., and Thompson, J. S. In Ray, J. G., Hare, D. B., Pedersen, P. D., et al., editors: NIAID manual of tissue typing techniques, Bethesda, Md., 1976-1977, National Institutes of Health.

64. van Rood, J. J., van Leeuwen, A., Keunig, J. J., et al.: Tissue Antigens **5**:73, 1975.
65. van Rood, J. J., van Leeuwen, A., Parlevliet, J., et al. In Kissmeyer-Nielsen, F., editor: Histocompatibility testing, Copenhagen, 1975, Munksgaard.
65a. Bodmer, J. G.: Br. Med. Bull. **34**:233, 1978.
65b. Balner, H.: Transplant. Proc. **11**:657, 1979.
66. Ettinger, R. B., Terasaki, P. I., Opelz, G., et al.: Lancet **2**:56, 1976.
67. Snary, D., Goodfellow, P., Hayman, M. J., et al.: Nature **247**:457, 1974.
68. Nathenson, S. G., Shimada, A., Yamane, K., et al.: Fed. Proc. **29**:2026, 1970.
69. Nakamuro, K., Tanigaki, N., and Pressman, D.: Proc. Natl. Acad. Sci. U.S.A. **70**:2863, 1973.
69a. Bamstable, C. J., Jones, E. A., and Crumpton, M. J.: Br. Med. J. **34**:241, 1978.
70. Bernoco, D., Cullen, S., Scudeller, G., et al. In Dausset, J., and Colombani, J., editors: Histocompatibility testing, Baltimore, 1972, The Williams & Wilkins Co.
71. Bodmer, W. F.: Nature **237**:139, 1972.
72. Gally, J. A., and Edelman, G. M.: Ann. Rev. Genet. **6**:1, 1972.
73. Goodfellow, P. N., Jones, E. A., van Heyningen, V., et al.: Nature **254**:267, 1975.
74. Wernet, P., and Kunkel, H. G. In Kissmeyer-Nielsen, F., editor: Histocompatibility testing, Copenhagen, 1975, Munksgaard.
75. Wernet, P., Jersied, C., Cunningham-Rundless, C., et al. In Kissmeyer-Nielsen, F., editor: Histocompatibility testing, Copenhagen, 1975, Munksgaard.
75a. Morris, P. J., Batchelor, J. R., and Festenstein, H.: Br. Med. Bull. **34**:259, 1978.
76. Opelz, G., Mickey, M. R., and Terasaki, P. I.: Transplantation **17**:371, 1974.
77. Terasaki, P. I., Opelz, G., and Mickey, M. R.: Transplant. Proc. **6**:33, 1974.
78. Gurland, H. J., Brunner, F. P., v Dehn, H., et al.: Proc. Eur. Dial. Transplant. Assoc. **10**:17, 1973.
79. Dausset, J., Hors, J., Busson, M., et al.: N. Engl. J. Med. **290**:979, 1974.
80. Jeannet, M.: Helv. Med. Acta **35**:168, 1970.
81. Hamburger, J., Crosnier, J., Descamps, B., et al.: Transplant. Proc. **3**:260, 1971.
82. Cochrum, K. C., Perkins, H. A., Payne, R. O., et al.: Transplant. Proc. **5**:391, 1973.
83. van Hooff, J. P., Schippers, H. M. A., van der Steen, G. J., et al.: Lancet **2**:1385, 1972.
84. Opelz, G., Sengar, D. P. S., Mickey, M. R., et al.: Transplant. Proc. **5**:253, 1973.
85. Thomas, J., Thomas, F., and Lee, M. M.: Transplant. Proc. **9**:85, 1977.
86. Thomas, E. D., Storb, R., Clift, R. A., et al.: N. Engl. J. Med. **292**:832, 895, 1975.
87. Dupont, B., Andersen, V., Ernst, P., et al.: Transplant. Proc. **5**:905, 1973.
88. Gatti, R. A., Meuwissen, H. J., Terasaki, P. I., et al.: Tissue Antigens **1**:239, 1971.
88a. Gale, R. P., and Opelz, G., editors: Immunobiology of bone marrow transplantation, vol. 2, New York, 1978, Grune & Stratton.
89. van Rood, J. J.: Semin. Hematol. **11**:253, 1974.
90. Yankee, R. A., Grumet, F. C., and Rogentine, G. N.: N. Engl. J. Med. **281**:1208, 1969.
91. Yankee, R. A., Graff, K. S., Dowling, R., et al.: N. Engl. J. Med. **288**:760, 1973.
92. Higby, D. J., Yates, J. W., Henderson, E. S., et al.: N. Engl. J. Med. **292**:761, 1975.
93. Graw, R. G., Herzig, G., Perry, S., et al.: N. Engl. J. Med. **287**:367, 1972.
94. Herzig, R. H., Poplack, D. G., and Yankee, R. A.: N. Engl. J. Med. **290**:1220, 1974.
95. Lilly, F., Boyse, E. A., and Old, L. J.: Lancet **2**:1207, 1964.
96. Moller, G., editor: Transplant. Rev. **22**:3, 1975.
96a. Batchelor, J. R., and Morris, P. J. In Bodmer, W. F., Batchelor, J. R., Bodmer, J. G., et al., editors: Histocompatibility testing 1977, Copenhagen, 1978, Munksgaard.
97. Dausset, J., Degos, L., and Koss, J.: Clin. Immunol. Immunopathol. **3**:127, 1974.
98. Vladutiu, A. O., and Rose, N. R.: Immunogenetics **1**:305, 1974.
98a. Cudworth, A. G., and Festenstein, H.: Br. Med. Bull. **34**:285, 1978.
99. Stastny, P. In Kissmeyer-Nielsen, F., editor: Histocompatibility testing, Copenhagen, 1975, Munksgaard.
100. Bertrams, J., Grosse-Wilde, H., Netzel, B., et al. In Kissmeyer-Nielsen, F., editor: Histocompatibility testing, Copenhagen, 1975, Munksgaard.
101. Vladutiu, A. O., and Rose, N. R.: Science **174**:1137, 1971.
102. Levine, B. B., Stember, R. H., and Fotino, M.: Science **178**:1201, 1972.
103. Dausset, J., and Colombani, J., editors: Histocompatibility testing, Baltimore, 1972, The Williams & Wilkins Co.
104. Ray, J. G., Hare, D. B., Pedersen, P. D., et al., editors: NIAID manual of tissue typing techniques, Bethesda, Md., 1976-1977, National Institutes of Health.
105. Colombani, J. In Ray, J. G., Hare, D. B., Pedersen, P. D., et al., editors: NIAID manual of tissue typing techniques, Bethesda, Md., 1976-1977, National Institutes of Health.
106. Colombani, J., and Colombani, M.: Semin. Hematol. **11**:273, 1974.
107. Boyum, A.: Scand. J. Clin. Lab. Invest. **21** (suppl.):97, 1968.
108. Terasaki, P. I., and Park, M. S. In Ray, J. G., Hare, D. B., Pedersen, P. D., et al., editors: NIAID manual of tissue typing techniques, Bethesda, Md., 1976-1977, National Institutes of Health.
109. Rodey, G. E., Anderson, J., and Aster, R. H. In Ray, J. G., Hare, D. B., Pedersen, P. D., et al., editors: NIAID manual of tissue typing techniques, Bethesda, Md., 1976-1977, National Institutes of Health.
110. Shaw, J. F. In Ray, J. G., Hare, D. B., Pedersen, P. D., et al., editors: NIAID manual of tissue typing techniques, Bethesda, Md., 1976-1977, National Institutes of Health.
111. Ferrone, S., Cooper, N. R., Pellegrino, M. A., et al.: J. Immunol. **107**:939, 1971.
112. Ceppellini, R., and van Rood, J. J.: Semin. Hematol. **11**:233, 1974.
113. Thorsby, E.: Transplant. Rev. **18**:51, 1974.
114. Kissmeyer-Nielsen, F., Olsen, S., Petersen, V. P., et al.: Lancet **2**:662, 1966.
115. Johnson, A. H.: In Ray, J. G., Hare, D. B., Pedersen, P. D., et al., editors: NIAID manual of tissue typing techniques, Bethesda, Md., 1976-1977, National Institutes of Health.
116. Ross, J., Dickerson, T., and Perkins, H. A.: Tissue Antigens **6**:129, 1975.
117. Terasaki, P. I., Kreisler, M., and Mickey, M. R.: Postgrad. Med. J. **47**:89, 1971.

118. Cross, D. F., Greiner, R., and Whittier, F. C.: Transplantation **21**:307, 1976.
119. Ting, A., and Terasaki, P. I.: Lancet **1**:304, 1975.
120. Lightbody, J. J., and Rosenberg, J. C.: J. Immunol. **112**:890, 1974.
121. Lightbody, J. J., and Rosenberg, J. C.: In Ray, J. G., Hare, D. B., Pedersen, P. D., et al., editors: NIAID manual of tissue typing techniques, Bethesda, Md., 1976-1977, National Institutes of Health.
122. Garovoy, M. R., Zschaeck, D., Strom, T. B., et al.: Lancet **1**:573, 1973.
123. Dickweiss, E., and Nielsen, L. S.: Tissue Antigens **6**:137, 1975.
124. Rapaport, F. T., and Chase, R. M.: Science **145**:407, 1964.
125. Callender, C. O., Simmons, R. L., Yunis, E. J., et al.: Surgery **76**:573, 1974.
126. Bain, B., Vas, M. R., and Lowenstein, L.: Blood **23**:108, 1964.
127. Opelz, G., Kiuchi, M., and Takasugi, M.: J. Immunol. Genet. **2**:1, 1975.
128. Lohrmann, H. P., Novikovs, L., and Graw, R. G.: Nature **250**:144, 1974.
129. Osoba, D., and Falk, J.: Cell. Immunol. **10**:117, 1974.
130. Thorsby, E., and Piazza, A.: In Kissmeyer-Nielsen, F., editor: Histocompatibility testing, Copenhagen, 1975, Munksgaard.

67

TUMOR-ASSOCIATED ANTIGENS

Karel Kithier

Among the features of the metabolism of a cancer cell is the synthesis of molecules not expressed in healthy cells or an enhancement of normally minute synthesis of such components. Tumor-associated antigens belong to this group of neoantigens.

In the literature many antigens are reported to be associated with cancer or even to be tumor specific. Such antigens have been detected by a variety of technics; among these, immunologic and immunochemical methods play the most important role. At the present time unfortunately a majority of these antigens have not been well characterized physiochemically, and the knowledge of their physiologic and pathologic importance is fragmentary at best. Out of the broad spectrum of various tumor antigens only α-fetoprotein (AFP) and carcinoembryonic antigen (CEA) have gained major attention in laboratory medicine, and both of them have already crossed the borderline between research and clinical applications. These 2 proteins are sometimes called oncofetal antigens because of their occurrence in fetuses as well as in malignant growths. Monoclonal immunoglobulins (paraproteins, M components, etc.), which are also associated with certain malignant tumors, will be discussed here. These components have been studied extensively and have contributed a great deal to the present knowledge of immunoglobulin structure and metabolism. They are routinely detected and evaluated in clinical laboratories.

Literature dealing with these subjects is voluminous, and it is impossible to list here even the most important studies. The reader is advised to consult some of the review articles. The reviews on AFP by Abelev[1] and by Masseyeff[2] are recommended. CEA has recently been discussed by Terry et al.[3] The book by Snapper and Kahn[4] will provide the interested reader with a number of references on the problems of paraproteins and their detection.

α-FETOPROTEIN

α-Fetoprotein (AFP) belongs to the group of plasma proteins sometimes called feto-specific proteins,[5] which are present in high concentrations in fetal sera but absent or not detectable in healthy adults. One of the most interesting features of these feto-specific proteins is that although almost absent from the sera of healthy adults, they are found in some pathologic sera, especially in neoplastic diseases. A number of feto-specific proteins were described in mammals; however, it is AFP that is the most important protein of this group from the clinical viewpoint.

Properties of AFP

AFP was discovered in 2 independent laboratories[6,7] as a normal constituent of human fetal sera. This protein is distinct from fetuin.[8] AFP was isolated in several laboratories by a variety of procedures. Most of them employed gel chromatography, electrophoresis, and immunochemical technics, although some authors also used the classic procedures of salt fractionation. The major problem in purification is the removal of albumin and sometimes α$_1$-antitrypsin. As a source of AFP, human fetal serum, cord serum of newborns, or serum of patients with hepatocellular carcinoma was used.

AFP is a globulin with electrophoretic mobility of fast α$_1$-globulins. The molecular mass of AFP was found to be between 64,600 and 75,500 daltons. The isoelectric point has been reported to be 4.8. AFP contains about 4.3% carbohydrates and 0.9% sialic acid. The molecule appears to be composed of a single polypeptide chain. The amino acid composition of AFP isolated from fetal sera did not show any considerable difference when compared with AFP isolated from sera of patients with hepatomas.[9]

AFP concentration in plasma of human fetuses depends on fetal age. The highest concentration (up to 3 mg/ml) is reached between weeks 12 and 15 of intrauterine development[10]; after this period the concentration decreases gradually until term. At birth, AFP is still detectable by immunodiffusion in most cord sera; however, after the end of the first month of life it is not found in sera by these technics. AFP is not entirely absent from adult body fluids; low serum concentrations (less than 25 ng/ml) were demonstrated by radioimmunoassay in sera of healthy adults.[11,12] The synthesis of human AFP during the fetal period takes place mainly in the liver; however, some other organs also show a certain rate of synthesis (e.g., yolk sac and digestive tract). The biologic role of human AFP has not yet been found. In addition to fetal sera, AFP was also detected in amniotic fluids and maternal sera.

Detection of AFP

Until recently immunodiffusion and electro-immunodiffusion technics (Chapter 61) have been used most frequently for the detection and quantitation of AFP. These technics, although highly specific, are not the most sensitive ones. The introduction of radioimmunoassay (RIA) for AFP enabled its estimation in nanograms per milliliter. Other highly sensitive technics include enzyme-linked immunoassay,[13] hemagglu-tination,[14] and latex fixation.[15]

AFP in disease

AFP was detected by immunodiffusion technics in sera and other body fluids of patients with hepatocellular carcinomas.[16,17] Patients with teratomas were also frequently found to have elevated concentrations of serum AFP.[18,19] Occasionally AFP was observed in other malignant growths and in non-neoplastic disorders. Not all patients with hepatocellular carcinoma showed increased levels of AFP. Using immunodiffusion tests, investigators found elevated levels of AFP in about 40-80% of these patients, and the highest frequency was recorded in countries where this malignant tumor was endemic (e.g., some parts of Africa and Asia). The highest incidence of abnormal AFP serum concentration was found by RIA; however, it was not seen in all patients with hepatocellular carcinoma. For a presently unknown reason, some hepatocellular carcinomas do not produce an appreciable quantity of AFP. Such tumors represent a group of false-negative cases (i.e., patients with hepatocellular carcinoma and normal AFP concentration), which makes the test less specific in terms of diagnosis. The production of AFP in hepatocellular carcinoma does not seem to be related to the microscopic appearance of the tumor. No clear-cut correlation could be established between the degree of tumor differentiation and AFP serum concentration; high and low concentrations were observed in patients with highly, as well as with poorly, differentiated tumors.[20] On the other hand, the total mass of the tumor producing AFP affects its serum concentration. It has been shown[21] that the reduction of the tumor size by partial hepatectomy was accompanied by a drop of AFP serum concentration. Hence, the importance of a serial quantitation of AFP to monitor the progress of the disease after the surgery is obvious. Variations of AFP serum concentration may also reflect the patient's response to chemotherapy. The ages of patients also seem to play a role in the production of AFP. Young patients, especially children, tend to have elevated concentrations more frequently than adults.[2]

Although the AFP test is not entirely specific for the diagnosis of hepatocellular carcinoma, it may be of major value in the diagnostic consideration. Indeed, in several reported cases, the AFP test was the only clue to the definite diagnosis, which was later confirmed by liver biopsy. The importance of this test for the screening of the population, especially in high-risk areas, still awaits evaluation. A large-scale survey has recently been conducted in Shanghai. Out of 66,376 persons, 151 had elevated AFP; of these 151 persons 131 were diagnosed as having primary liver cancer. In some of these patients increased levels of AFP appeared at an early stage of the disease.[22]

Increased AFP serum concentration is also seen in patients with teratomas and with tumors described as "teratoblastoma" or "embryonal carcinoma."[18,19,23] It is believed that AFP synthesis in these tumors is related to the presence of poorly differentiated structures. It has been recently proposed, however, that the synthesis of AFP may depend on the presence of a vitelline component (entodermal sinus tumor) rather than on the presence of a teratoid component or embryonal carcinoma cells.[24] Regardless of this consideration, it is important that the quantitation of AFP in sera of these patients represents a valuable tool in monitoring therapeutic response and detecting recurrence of the disease.[23,25] It is also important in differential diagnosis to note that patients with pure seminomas do not have significantly increased AFP serum concentration.

Occasionally, patients with other malignant tumors, mainly of digestive tract, are found to have increased AFP serum concentrations. The incidence of these false-positive cases is low, especially when immunodiffusion tests are used to detect AFP or when the cut-off level is 500 ng/ml.[26,27]

In nonmalignant diseases of adults, the AFP level may be elevated in patients suffering from liver disorders, i.e., cirrhosis or infectious hepatitis.[26,27] In most cases such an elevation is well below the threshold of the sensitivity of immunodiffusion tests and can be detected only by radioimmunoassay. In pediatric patients, especially infants, the elevation of AFP associated with liver disorders may be high enough to be detected by the Ouchterlony test.[19] The increased AFP concentration in patients with nonmalignant liver diseases is usually transient and may indicate regeneration of the liver parenchyma and improvement of the patient's status.[26]

An interesting finding of increased AFP serum levels in ataxia teleangiectasia has been reported recently.[27] Further studies are still needed to evaluate the possible diagnostic and prognostic significance of AFP testing in nonmalignant diseases.

In addition to its role in oncology, AFP appears to be gaining an importance in obstetrics and neonatology. Quantitation of AFP in amniotic fluids has recently been found to be a promising tool for the diagnosis and management of some pathologic pregnancies. Brock and Sutcliffe[28] reported on the association of high AFP concentrations in amniotic fluids and the presence of neural tube malformations. Grossly elevated levels were observed between weeks 25 and 30 of gestation in pregnancies with anencephalic fetuses or fetuses with spina bifida. This finding was corroborated by other authors, and at the present time there seems to be general agreement that the estimation of AFP concentration in amniotic fluid could be a valuable indicator for the presence of these defects. Whether similar diagnostic information could be derived from the quantitation of AFP in maternal sera is not yet clear. On the other hand, some other pathologic conditions occurring during pregnancy may also lead to increased AFP concentration, e.g., atresia of the fetal digestive canal at different levels. Fetal distress and death in utero may have the same result. Physiologically the concentration of AFP increases in twin pregnancy. The significance of these findings has not yet been evaluated.

In summary, although AFP cannot be seen as a specific tumor marker, as it was once hoped, its detection and quantitation is a valuable tool for the diagnosis of some malignancies, for monitoring patient response to therapy, and for the detection of a remaining or recurrent tumor.

CARCINOEMBRYONIC ANTIGEN

Studies by Gold and Freedman[29] on soluble proteins of tumor tissues demonstrated a special protein in extracts of colon carcinoma. This component appeared to be absent from a healthy, tumor-free colon; however, it was detectable in fetal gut, liver, and pancreas in the first 2 trimesters of fetal development. Because of its occurrence in neoplastic and fetal tissues, the protein has been named carcinoembryonic antigen (CEA). Immunodiffusion technics, which originally demonstrated CEA in tissue extracts, failed to detect it in blood of cancer patients. After the isolation of CEA, radioimmunoassay (RIA) was adapted for its detection and quantitation.[30] This procedure was sensitive enough to demonstrate the presence of CEA in sera of patients with gastrointestinal malignancies, mainly colon carcinomas. Other laboratories tried to eliminate certain drawbacks of the original procedure, and several modifications were developed. The presence of CEA in blood and tissues, originally believed to be specific for entodermally derived tumors of the digestive tract, was also detected in other malignancies and even in certain nonmalignant diseases.

Isolation of and properties of CEA

The first procedure for CEA isolation developed by Krupey et al.[31] used metastatic tissues of colon carcinoma as sources of the antigen. The procedure included tissue hemogenization and extraction with perchloric acid. Subsequent steps employed gel filtration and preparative electro-phoresis. A number of modifications of the original procedure were later developed in other laboratories, some of them circumventing perchloric acid fractionation.

CEA was found to be a glycoprotein soluble in 1M perchloric acid with a molecular mass approximately between 200,000 and 300,000 daltons. The CEA molecule contains about 50% carbohydrate. The amino acid composition indicates a rather high content of carboxyl and hydroxyl amino acids and a low content of basic amino acids.[3] Electrophoretic mobility of CEA in an alkaline pH corresponds to the mobility of serum β-globulins. On polyacrylamide gel electrophoresis and immunoelectrophoresis, CEA often migrates as a broad band or line, respectively, indicating its microheterogeneity. CEA preparations isolated from various donors or from carcinomas located at different levels of the digestive tract may exhibit variations in some physiochemical properties; however, no antigenic differences were observed in such preparations. Immunochemical cross-reactivity of CEA with antisera to various substances has been observed in some laboratories. On the other hand, some antigens were extracted from a variety of tissues (either cancerous or healthy) or from various body fluids that reacted in immunodiffusion experiments with antisera to CEA.[32-34] Some of these components may be different entities or molecules antigenically related to the original CEA described by Gold and Freedman. Some of these results may be due to the use of antisera that were not strictly specific to CEA. To obtain a specific antiserum to CEA often requires an extensive absorption of the antiserum with material derived from various sources, e.g., blood and tissues.[34,35] After the absorption a careful control of the antiserum specificity must be performed, and the antiserum should be compared with another that is known to detect the antigen originally described by Gold and Freedman; this was not always done in studies on CEA.

Detection of CEA

CEA concentrations in most sera are low (nanograms per milliliter); therefore immunodiffusion technics are not suitable for its detection and quantitation. RIA becomes the method of choice for the quantitative study of CEA. In the original procedure[30] CEA is extracted from the serum along with other mucoproteins by perchloric acid. The supernatant containing CEA is dialyzed and lyophilized, and the lyophilized material is used for the RIA procedure. The separation of free from bound CEA is achieved by ammonium sulfate precipitation. Several modifications of RIA for CEA quantitation are presently in use.[3] Hansen's procedure[36] includes perchloric acid extraction; however, patient plasma instead of serum is used, and lyophilization is eliminated. Zirconium gel serves to separate free and bound CEA. This method is often used in clinical laboratories, and the reagents are available commercially. The sensitivity is less than 1 ng CEA per 1.0 ml plasma; the test requires 1.0 ml plasma and can be completed in 2 days. The CEA concentration up to 20 ng/ml is determined by an indirect assay; if the CEA concentration is found to be higher than 20 ng/ml, the quantitation is repeated in a different arrangement (direct assay) in which perchloric acid extraction is not applied. The indirect assay must always be performed first. The exact description of the procedure is supplied with the kit.

Normal values. The cut-off value of normal serum CEA concentration was set up by Thompson et al.[30] at 2.5 ng/ml; so-called positive cases are those showing CEA concentrations in excess of this value. A certain percentage of an apparently healthy population may show slightly elevated concentrations of CEA; for example, Concannon et al.[37] found 16% of 201 healthy volunteers with a CEA level above 2.5 ng/ml. A history of heavy smoking seems to be associated with the elevated CEA concentration; in nonsmokers CEA concentrations above 2.5 ng/ml were seen in 3% of healthy subjects studied by Hansen et al.[38] The cut-off value of 2.5 ng/ml is not generally applicable to all technics of RIA presently used.[34]

Clinical findings

Elevated serum levels of CEA were originally believed to be associated specifically with gastrointestinal malignancies, particularly with colon carcinoma. Thus Thompson et al.[30] found increased serum concentrations of CEA in 35 of 36 patients with colon carcinoma; patients with tumors of non-digestive-tract origin did not show abnormal CEA concentrations. Later, however, increased CEA levels were reported in patients with malignancies of non-gastrointestinal-tract origin (e.g., carcinomas of lung, breast, and urinary system) and also in patients with nonmalignant diseases (for a review see ref. 39). The nature of the CEA molecules circulating in these patients and their relationship to the original CEA of Gold is not clearly understood. These reports resulted from studies done by different technics, using different antisera and antigens from various sources. On the other hand, workers in laboratories employing antisera and antigen supplied by Gold's laboratory also observed elevated serum levels in patients with non-digestive-tract malignancies.[40]

In the group of gastrointestinal malignancies, colorectal carcinomas show the highest incidence of elevated CEA concentrations. The incidence appears higher in patients with cancer localized in the distal parts of the digestive tract as compared with those having the primary tumor in the proximal parts. In colon carcinoma itself, elevated CEA levels are seen more frequently in patients with the tumor localized in the sigmoid colon than in patients in whom the tumor was localized in the cecum. In rectal carcinomas the incidence of increased CEA concentrations is lower than in sigmoid colon cancer;

however, if the CEA serum level is abnormal, a metastatic disease is already present.[41] In colon carcinoma the CEA test positivity appears to be a function of the tumor stage according to Dukes' classification: the lowest incidence of positive results is seen in patients with tumors of stage A; an increasing percentage of positive cases is observed in stages B-D. Thus the diagnostic value of the test depends on the stage of the tumor. A negative result (less than cut-off value) in preoperative CEA determination may indicate a localized tumor; a strongly positive result suggests the presence of metastasis.

Several investigators have found that a serial determination of CEA concentration is of prognostic value in patients with colon carcinoma after surgery.[30,36,42] The return to a normal CEA level after surgery indicates complete removal of the tumor. When the CEA level fails to decrease after such a treatment, the metastatic disease or an incomplete tumor resection should be considered. On the other hand, some patients with a recurrent or remote disease after resection of the colon lesion may not show elevation of CEA values above normal levels.[42]

Increased CEA levels were also found by Ona et al.[43] in a high percentage of patients with pancreatic cancer. Most of these patients had a highly advanced stage of the disease, and resectable tumors usually showed lower values of serum CEA. Patients with carcinoma of the upper part of the digestive tract (esophageal and gastric carcinoma) also show increased CEA levels. The incidence of elevated CEA is believed to be lower than in cases of colon carcinoma.

Abnormal CEA levels were also reported in a variety of tumors derived from tissues outside the digestive system. Carcinomas of lung, breast, female genital system,[44] and urinary tract belong to this group. Also, patients with neuroblastomas and with sarcomas were observed to have abnormal CEA levels. In a group of 115 patients with lung carcinoma[45] 72-100% showed elevated CEA serum concentrations. The incidence appeared to depend on the histologic type of tumors. A decrease in CEA concentration was recorded after successful surgery. Serum levels seen in lung carcinoma were generally lower than those found in colon carcinoma patients, and only 28 of 115 patients had CEA concentrations higher than 15 ng/ml. Most of the patients in this group had advanced disease. Hall et al.[46] studied CEA in the urine of patients with urothelial carcinoma. The urine concentration of CEA was elevated in 20 of 30 male patients; no consistent correlation was seen between the urinary and serum CEA concentrations. Khoo[44] reported abnormal CEA levels in female genital carcinomas; 65% of the patients studied (114 of 175) had values above 5 ng/ml. In noncancerous gynecologic conditions the results of CEA tests were negative.

Reported nonmalignant diseases that may be associated with increased CEA serum concentration represent a variety of disorders. Among these are alcoholic liver cirrhosis and pancreatitis[47] as well as inflammatory bowel diseases.[48] These conditions usually cause a rather low increase in CEA concentration when compared with the malignant diseases.[49] Practically no information is available on CEA levels in pediatric patients. Recently, concentrations higher than 10 ng/ml were found in the plasma of children with a variety of nonmalignant diseases; chronic renal failure was frequently observed to be associated with an abnormal plasma CEA concentration.[50]

It is generally felt that the CEA test in the present situation is unsuitable for screening. On the other hand, its use in the monitoring of therapy and detection of recurrent disease in some malignancies appears to be of practical value. A major problem faced by investigators is the lack of knowledge about the physicochemical and antigenic properties of CEA. Although much investigative work has been done in recent years, the understanding of the CEA molecule and so-called CEA-like antigens and their possible interference in the CEA tests is still far from satisfactory. Part of the problem will be largely overcome once an international CEA standard becomes available.

PARAPROTEINS

Paraproteins are the products of a single clone of immunoglobulin-forming cells. Any given clone forms immunoglobulin molecules of practically identical physicochemical and antigenic properties. In a malignancy such as multiple myeloma, neoplastic cells appear to be of a single clonal origin, and their product is an electrophoretically homogeneous immunoglobulin, a paraprotein. These proteins are called by different terms, and so far no united nomenclature has prevailed. Thus terms such as paraproteins, myeloma proteins, M components, monoclonal immunoglobulins, and homogeneous immunoglobulins are found in the literature. A finding of a paraprotein in serum or urine was considered for a long time to be a specific feature of lymphoreticular malignancies, e.g., multiple myeloma or Waldenström's macroglobulinemia. Clinical and laboratory studies during the past 20 years demonstrated, however, that benign disorders of the immune system associated with paraproteinemia occur more frequently than do the lymphoreticular malignancies.[51]

Detection of paraproteins

Paraproteins can be detected by a variety of electrophoretic technics. Filter paper electrophoresis and more commonly cellulose acetate electrophoresis are routinely used in clinical laboratories. Although these electrophoretic media have many practical advantages, the better resolving power appears to be achieved by the use of agarose gel. A convenient and fast micromodification of cellulose acetate electrophoresis shows any grossly distorted plasma protein patterns; however, it may fail to discern minor abnormalities and demonstrate faint additional bands. In the studies of plasma protein dyscrasias a number of authors prefer agar or agarose gel electrophoresis. Johansson's[52] or Wieme's[53] modification of agar gel electrophoresis is a powerful tool in the study of immunoglobulin abnormalities.

The presence of paraproteins in the body fluids, e.g., serum and urine, is demonstrated as a narrow band on zone electrophoresis or as a tall spike on the scan of the electrophoretic strip. The appearance of the spike, i.e., its height and shape, depends on the concentration of the monoclonal component. In multiple myeloma patients, paraproteins (especially IgG) frequently reach excessive concentrations, and the quantity of the remaining normal immunoglobulins (i.e., those formed by the remaining normal cell population) is declining and may become very low. Sometimes almost all of the immunoglobulins present in the patient's serum are of a monoclonal nature and appear on the zone electrophoresis as a dense band on an almost empty background. Such a band may be found anywhere in the region extending from the γ- to the α-globulins. In other diseases that are sometimes associated with the nonexcessive production of homogeneous immunoglobulins or in cases of so-called benign monoclonal gammopathy or idiopathic paraproteinemia, the changes in the concentration of residual normal immunoglobulins is minimal, and the homogeneous band, which may be delicate, is superimposed on the normal heterogeneous immunoglobulin background. Such faint bands may escape detection, especially when only a scan of the cellulose acetate microelectrophoresis is evaluated. For this reason the electrophoretic strip should always be visually inspected. The possibility of missing paraproteins in low concentrations is minimized if agar or agarose gel electrophoresis is used and supplemented with immunoelectrophoresis (IEP). Immunoelectrophoretic examination is complementary to zone electrophoresis. Paraprotein, which is detected as a homogeneous band on cellulose acetate or agar gel electrophoresis, is classified and typed by immunoelectrophoresis with the use of specific antisera. In addition, immunoelectrophoresis may reveal paraproteins that escaped detection on zone electrophoresis, especially if such proteins are located in the α- or β-globulin region, and their respective bands are overlapped with other α- or β-globulins. To demonstrate the presence of a paraprotein, at least the class of its heavy chain and the type of its light chain should be determined.

A general outline and the principles of IEP are discussed in Chapter 61. In this discussion only typical patterns of the main classes of paraproteinemias will be discussed. IEP patterns encountered in paraproteinemias can be highly variable and cannot be covered here in detail.

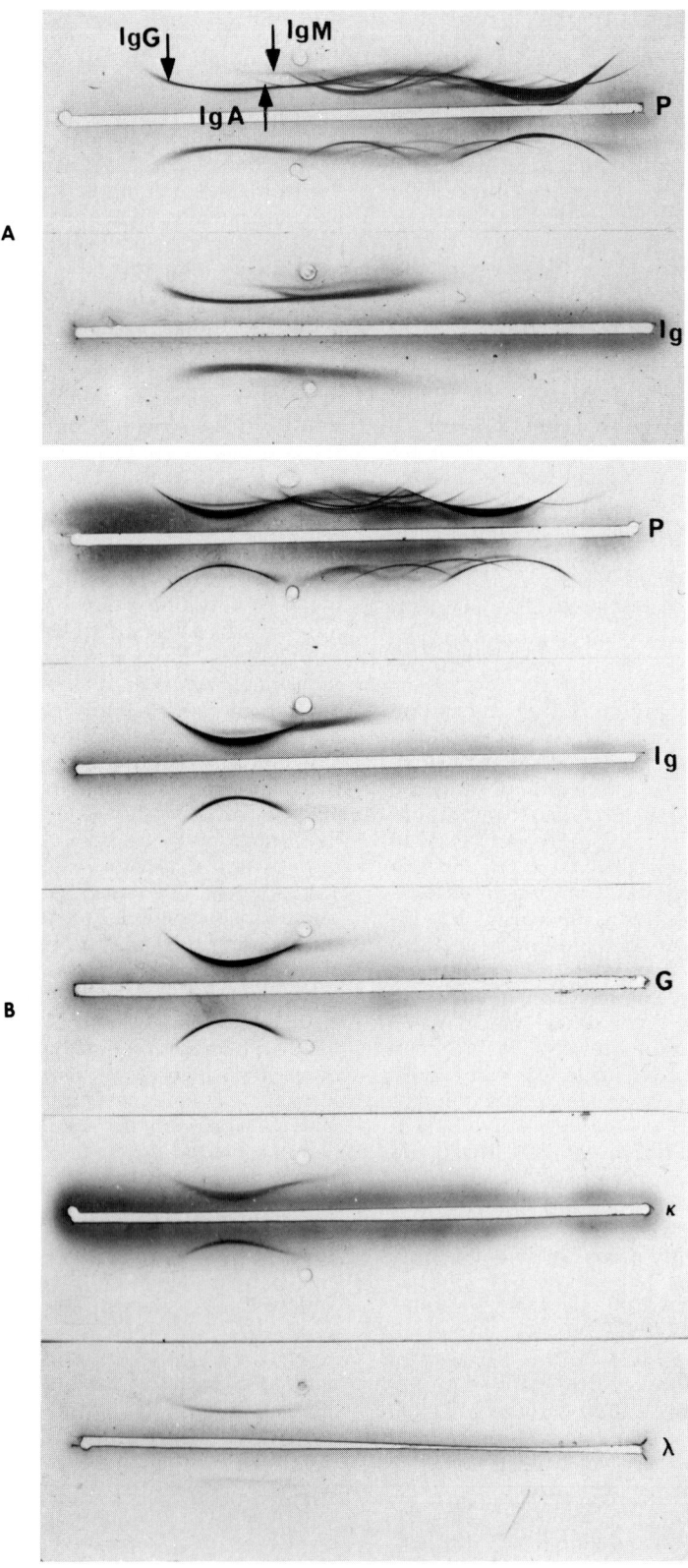

Fig. 67-1. For legend see opposite page.

The reader is advised to consult recent books[54-56] and special publications[57,58] that discuss this matter extensively. In principle, the position of the precipitin line on IEP depends on the molecular size of the studied protein and on the ratio between the concentrations of this protein and reacting antibodies. When a constant volume of the same antiserum is applied, the position of the line between the antigen and antibody wells is influenced mostly by the concentration changes of the antigen. The precipitin line develops closer to the antibody well at higher concentrations of the antigen and closer to the antigen well if its concentration is low. For instance, a highly increased concentration of serum IgG (e.g., in polyclonal hyperimmunoglobulinemia) causes a

shift of the precipitin line toward the antibody well; the shape of the line, however, will not be substantially changed. On the other hand, the immunoelectrophoretic pattern observed in patients with IgG paraproteinemia shows a different feature: the monoclonal IgG due to its homogeneous electrophoretic mobility is limited to a narrow part of the electrophoretic strip. In this particular location the IgG concentration is higher (as compared to the IgG in the remaining zone of γ-globulins) and causes the precipitin line to develop close to the antibody trough. This line or arc fuses with the precipitin line of the remaining, normal IgG. Thus the whole line developed with the specific antiserum to IgG shows a distortion, bending, or so-called parapro-

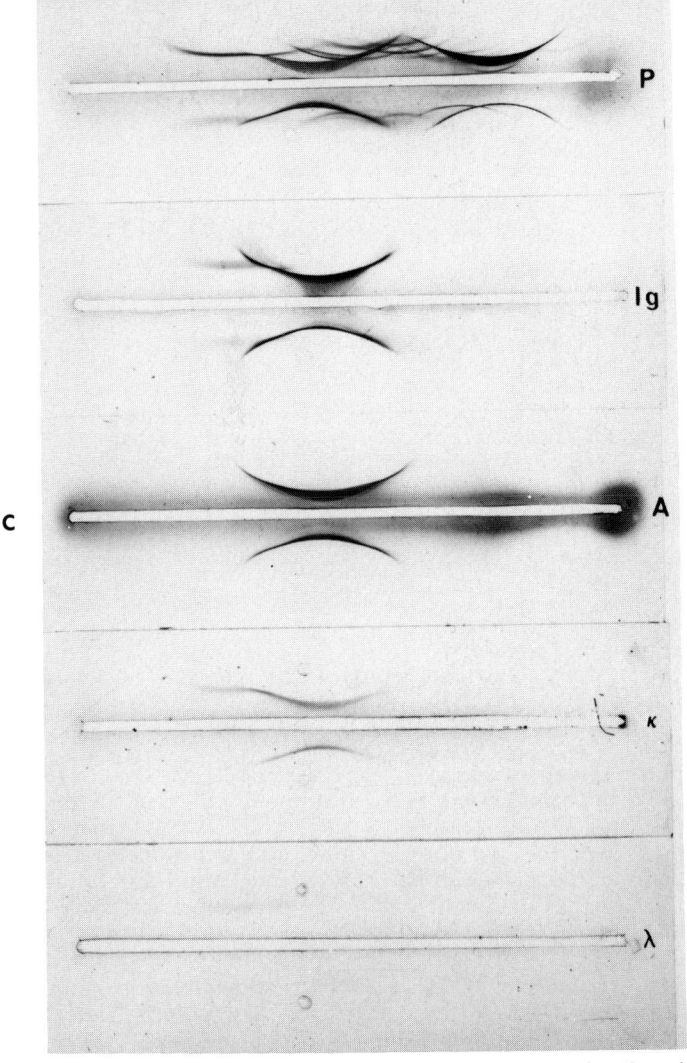

Continued.

Fig. 67-1. Immunoelectrophoresis of **A,** normal human serum; **B,** serum with IgG paraprotein; **C,** serum with IgA paraprotein; and **D,** serum with IgM paraprotein. Upper well = undiluted serum. Lower well = serum diluted 1:4. Antisera: *P* = antiserum to human plasma proteins; *Ig* = antiserum to immunoglobulins G, A, and M; *A* = antiserum to heavy chain of IgA; *G* = antiserum to heavy chain of IgG; *M* = antiserum to heavy chain of IgM; κ, λ = antisera to light chains (bound). Agar gel = 1% Ionagar no. 2, 0.05M barbital buffer, pH 8.4. Anode to right, voltage = 5 V/cm.

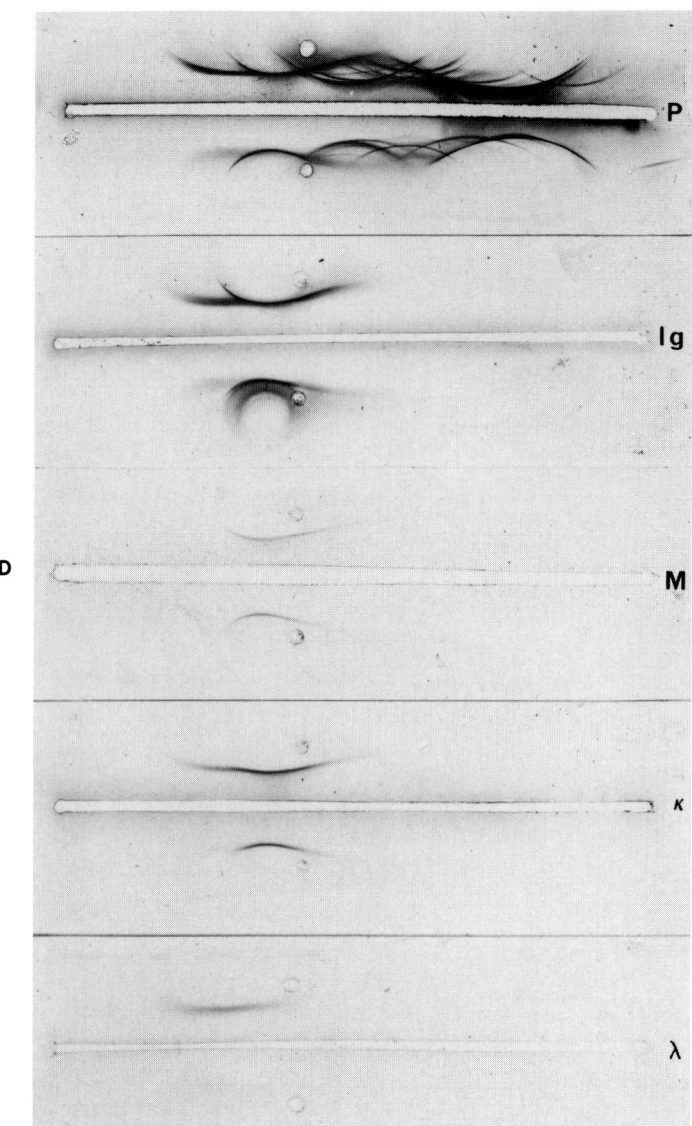

Fig. 67-1, cont'd. For legend see p. 1313.

teinemic bow deformation. Sometimes, due to an excessive concentration of the paraprotein, no precipitin arc is found in its location (prozone phenomenon), and the line of the remaining normal IgG is interrupted and bent toward the antibody trough. In such a case the dilution of the studied sera will facilitate the development of the paraprotein precipitin arc.

For the identification of paraproteins specific antisera are used, which are directed to the 3 main classes of heavy chains (IgG, IgA, and IgM) and to κ- and λ-types of light chains (Fig. 67-1). The deformation of the precipitin line is developed only with the antiserum to the class of the heavy chain carried by the present paraprotein. When its class is determined, the next step is to establish the type of light chain. The shape

of the precipitin line developed with the antiserum to the type of the light chain of the paraprotein has a shape similar to that of the precipitin line developed by the class-specific antiserum; only 1 antiserum (either κ or λ) reacts with the monoclonal component.

Paraproteins of IgG class

Monoclonal immunoglobulins of the IgG class usually pose no problem in determination of the class and type. The deformation of the IgG precipitin line is a striking finding. More than half of all paraproteins detected are of the IgG class. On zone electrophoresis and IEP, monoclonal IgG is found anywhere between the slow γ- and α_2-globulin regions; most frequently, however, it is located in the slow or intermediate γ-globulin region. The concentration may be quite high, and dilution of the serum is frequently required for the IEP studies.

Paraproteins of IgA class

Monoclonal IgA is encountered in 13-36% of all monoclonal gammopathies. The monoclonal component of this class migrates in the region between γ- and α-globulins, most frequently in the β_2-position. The distortion of the precipitin line is less markedly pronounced than in cases of IgG paraprotein. However, a minor deformation when compared with the precipitin line of IgA in normal serum can usually be noticed. When this deformation is present at high concentration, it is usually not difficult to detect IgA paraprotein and to determine the type of light chain. However, IgA paraprotein in a low serum concentration relative to the normal IgG level may pose a problem, particularly for the determination of the light chain type. This is the case when the paraprotein occurring in low concentration has a slow electrophoretic mobility and is found in the region of normal IgG. The attempt to isolate IgA by gel filtration may not help because of the similarity of the molecular weights of IgA and IgG. In such cases special technics, e.g., immunoselection[59] or immunofixation,[60] may facilitate the determination of the light chain type. IgA paraprotein sometimes forms complexes with other plasma proteins and may simulate the presence of 2 M components.

Paraproteins of IgM class

Monoclonal IgM occurs typically in Waldenström's macroglobulinemia. The incidence of monoclonal IgM varies widely; it has been reported between 7-30% of all paraproteinemias. On electrophoresis it is usually located between the β_1-zone and the mid γ-zone. Sometimes the detection of IgM paraprotein is difficult because some of these paraproteins do not penetrate the agar gel and remain in the starting well. The use of buffers with higher ionic strength may alleviate this problem. The presence of IgM polymers with sedimentation constants higher than 20 S or complex formation of the paraprotein with other plasma proteins is occasionally observed. In order to dissociate these polymers or complexes, incubation of the serum with substances containing sulfhydryl groups (e.g., cysteine or penicillamine) is recommended.[58] Low concentrations of monoclonal IgM in sera containing a normal amount of IgG may be a problem in determining the type of light chains: the antiserum to light chain is used up by IgG molecules present at high concentration and diffusing faster than IgM. Separation of monoclonal IgM (most conveniently by gel filtration on Sephadex-200; IgM appears in the void-volume fraction) will circumvent this problem. Special technics of immunofixation[60] or immunoselection[59] can be tried before the time-consuming gel filtration procedure is applied.

Bence Jones protein

Homogeneous free light chains, or Bence Jones protein, are found in the sera and urines of some patients either alone (light-chain disease) or in association with paraproteins. Analysis of the urine for the presence of Bence Jones protein should always be performed when lymphoreticular cancer is suspected. The occurrence of Bence Jones protein in serum and urine may be associated with the decreased concentration of serum immunoglobulins. Very low levels of serum immunoglobulins call for the study of urine for the possible presence of Bence Jones protein.

The heat-precipitability test widely used in the past has presently been replaced by more sensitive and reliable means, e.g., zone electrophoresis and immunochemical methods. Electrophoresis of concentrated urine shows a band anywhere between a γ- and an α_1-zone. On IEP the protein should react with the antiserum to light chains of one type only. It should not react with any class-specific antiserum. When Bence Jones protein is present together with the paraprotein in the serum, the paraprotein reacts with a class-specific antiserum as well as with the antiserum to the corresponding light chains. Bence Jones protein reacts with the latter antiserum only. Antisera to light chains (sometimes called antisera to "bound-light chains" or to "exposed determinants") reacts with the light chains linked with the heavy chains of the intact immunoglobulin molecule as well as with the free light chains. To prove that the detected component corresponds to a free light chain, specific antisera to free light chains should be employed. Such antisera are directed to the "hidden determinants" of the light chains, which are exposed only when the light chains are not bound to the heavy chains. These antisera should not react with the light chain of the intact molecule of the immunoglobulins. It is convenient to use them in a double immunodiffusion test (Ouchterlony test), but sometimes the IEP employing such antisera is necessary to exclude excessive excretion of free heterogeneous light chains. Occasionally, however, special studies of the Bence Jones protein, e.g., gel filtration to determine its molecular weight, are necessary for the proper evaluation of the nature of the protein detected.

Rare forms of paraproteinemias

The occurrence of 2 or 3 paraproteins of different classes is sometimes observed. Biclonal paraproteins may also be of the same class but of a different subclass or light chain type. Some rare conditions that may also be encountered include paraproteinemias of D and E classes. The concentration of these paraproteins may be too low to find any spike on the zone electrophoresis. Class-specific antisera should determine their nature. Other rare pathologic conditions involve the occurrence of free heavy chains or parts thereof in the serum (heavy-chain disease). In this situation the protein detected reacts with the class-specific antisera only, and no reaction takes place with the antisera to light chains. Such a finding calls for special studies, e.g., molecular weight determination or isolation of the component. Sometimes the nature of a detected paraprotein may be quite difficult to establish without detailed studies. In such cases the assistance of specialized immunochemical laboratories (or of the National Cancer Institute, Immunoglobulin Reference Center, Springfield, Virginia 22151) may be obtained.

REFERENCES

1. Abelev, G. I.: Adv. Cancer Res. **14**:295, 1971.
2. Masseyeff, R.: Pathol. Biol. (Paris) **20**:703, 1972.
3. Terry, W. D., Henkart, P. A., Coligan, J. E., et al.: Transplant. Rev. **20**:100, 1974.
4. Snapper, I., and Kahn, A.: Myelomatosis. Fundamentals and clinical features, Basel, 1971, S. Karger.
5. Bull. WHO **43**:309, 1970.
6. Bergstrand, C. G., and Czar, B.: Scand. J. Clin. Lab. Invest. **8**:174, 1956.
7. Halbrecht, I., and Klibanski, C.: Nature **178**:794, 1956.
8. Kithier, K., and Poulik, M. D.: Biochim. Biophys. Acta **278**:505, 1972.
9. Nishi, S.: Cancer Res. **30**:2507, 1970.
10. Gitlin, D., and Boesman, M.: J. Clin. Invest. **45**:1826, 1966.
11. Ruoslahti, E., and Seppälä, M.: Int. J. Cancer **8**:374, 1971.
12. Purves, L. R., Branch, W. R., Geddes, E. W., et al.: Cancer **31**:578, 1973.
13. Belanger, L., Hamel, D., Dufour, D., et al.: Clin. Chem. **22**:198, 1976.
14. Lehmann, F. G., and Lehmann, D.: Z. Klin. Chem. Klin. Biochem. **11**:339, 1973.
15. Cahill, J., Cohen, H., and Starkovsky, N.: Am. J. Obstet. Gynecol. **119**:1095, 1974.
16. Tatarinov, J. S.: Vopr. Med. Khim. **10**:90, 1964.
17. Kithier, K., Houstek, J., Masopust, J., et al.: Nature **212**:414, 1966.
18. Abelev, G. I., Assecritova, I. V., Karevsky, N. A., et al.: Int. J. Cancer **2**:551, 1967.
19. Masopust, J., Kithier, K., Radl, J., et al.: Int. J. Cancer **3**:364, 1968.
20. Kithier, K., Belamaric, J., Al-Sarraf, M., et al. In Masseyeff, R., editor: Alpha fetoprotein, Paris, 1974, INSERM, pp. 275-286.
21. Alpert, E., Starzl, T. E., Schur, P. H., et al.: Gastroenterology **61**:144, 1971.
22. Chin. Med. J., no. 8, p. 98, Aug. 1973.
23. Mawas, C., Buffe, D., Lemerle, J., et al.: Arch. Fr. Pediatr. **26**:779, 1969.
24. Teilum, G., Albrechtsen, R., and Norgaard-Pedersen, B.: Acta Pathol. Microbiol. Scand. [A] **83**:80, 1975.
25. Kithier, K., Lusher, J., Brough, J., et al.: J. Pediatr. **81**:71, 1972.
26. Ruoslahti, E., Pihko, H., and Seppälä, M.: Transplant. Rev. **20**:38, 1974.
27. Waldmann, T. A., and McIntire, K. R.: Cancer **34**:1510, 1974.
28. Brock, D. J. H., and Sutcliffe, R. G.: Lancet **2**:197, 1972.
29. Gold, P., and Freedman, S. O.: J. Exp. Med. **122**:467, 1965.
30. Thompson, D. M. P., Krupey, J., Freedman, S. O., et al.: Proc. Natl. Acad. Sci. U.S.A. **64**:161, 1969.
31. Krupey, J., Gold, P., and Freedman, S. O.: Nature **215**:67, 1967.
32. Martin, F., and Martin, M. S.: Int. J. Cancer **6**:352, 1970.
33. Von Kleist, S., Chavanel, G., and Burtin, P.: Proc. Natl. Acad. Sci. U.S.A. **69**:2492, 1972.
34. Kupchik, H. Z., Zamcheck, N., and Saravis, C. A.: J. Natl. Cancer Inst. **51**:1741, 1973.
35. Kithier, K., Al-Sarraf, M., and Cejka, J. In Anderson, N. G., Coggin, J. H. Jr., Cole, E., et al.: editors: Embryonic and fetal antigens in cancer, vol. 2, Oak Ridge, Tenn., 1972, Oak Ridge National Laboratory.
36. Lo Gerfo, P., Krupey, J., and Hansen, H. J.: N. Engl. J. Med. **285**:138, 1971.
37. Concannon, J. P., Dalbow, M. H., and Frich, J. C.: Radiology **108**:191, 1973.
38. Hansen, H. J., Snyder, J. J., Miller, E., et al.: Hum. Pathol. **5**:139, 1974.
39. Chu, T. M., Holyoke, E. D., and Murphy, G. P.: N.Y. State J. Med. **74**:1388, 1974.
40. Mach, J. P., Pusztaszeri, G., Dysli, M., et al.: Schweiz. Med. Wochenschr. **103**:365, 1973.
41. Shuster, J., Livingstone, A., Banjo, C., et al.: Am. J. Clin. Pathol. **62**:243, 1974.
42. Dhar, P., Moore, T., Zamcheck, N., et al.: J.A.M.A. **221**:21, 1972.
43. Ona, F. V., Zamcheck, N., Dhar, P., et al.: Cancer **31**:324, 1973.
44. Khoo, S. K.: Med. J. Aust. **1**:1025, 1974.
45. Vincent, R. G., and Chu, T. M.: J. Thorac. Cardiovasc. Surg. **66**:320, 1973.
46. Hall, R. R., Laurence, D. J. R., Darcy, D., et al.: Br. Med. J. **3**:609, 1972.
47. Delwiche, R., Zamcheck, N., and Marcon, N.: Cancer **31**:328, 1973.
48. Moore, T. L., Kantrowitz, P. A., and Zamcheck, N.: J.A.M.A. **222**:944, 1972.
49. Neville, A. M., and Laurence, D. J. R.: Int. J. Cancer **14**:1, 1974.
50. Kithier, K., and Cejka, J. In Peeters, H., editor: Protides of the biological fluids, vol. 24, Oxford, 1977, Pergamon Press.
51. Radl, J. In Peeters, H., editor: Protides of the biological fluids, vol. 23, Oxford, 1976, Pergamon Press.
52. Johansson, B. G.: Scand. J. Clin. Lab. Invest. **29**(suppl. 124):7, 1972.
53. Wieme, R. J.: Clin. Chim. Acta **4**:317, 1959.
54. Waldenström, J.: Diagnosis and treatment of multiple myeloma, New York, 1970, Grune & Stratton.
55. Ritzmann, S. E., and Daniels, J. C., editors: Serum protein abnormalities, Boston, 1975, Little, Brown & Co.
56. Kawai, T.: Clinical aspects of the plasma proteins, Philadelphia, 1973, J. B. Lippincott Co.
57. Palmer, D. F., and Woods, R.: Qualitation and quantitation of immunoglobulins, 1972, U.S. Dept. of Health, Education and Welfare Publication no. (HSM) 72-8102.
58. Penn, G. M., and Davis, T.: Identification of myeloma proteins, Chicago, 1975, American Society of Clinical Pathologists.
59. Radl, J.: Immunology **19**:137, 1970.
60. Cejka, J., and Kithier, K.: Immunochemistry **13**(7):629-631, 1976.

BACTERIOLOGY

68

GENERAL CONSIDERATIONS

Alex C. Sonnenwirth

CLASSIFICATION AND NOMENCLATURE

The taxonomic position of microorganisms has been the subject of continuous debate for many years. Bacteria, algae, and fungi were assigned many years ago to the plant kingdom and the protozoa to the animal kingdom. Although many biologists still adhere to this practice, it has become increasingly clear that these microorganisms cannot be assigned unequivocally to either of the 2 kingdoms, since their characteristics cut across the accepted definition of animals and plants. For example, many bacteria are motile (a characteristic of animals) but at the same time possess cell walls (a hallmark of plants). During their growth plants and animals develop highly differentiated tissue forms, consisting of specialized cells, whereas among microorganisms this does not occur; even among the multicellular forms, the cells are essentially alike. The establishment of a third kingdom, the *Protista* (Haeckel, 1866), was proposed to accommodate these microorganisms characterized by relatively simple organization. Although not yet universally accepted, the concept of grouping bacteria, algae, fungi, and protozoa as protists has gained widespread support. Some protists are plantlike or animal-like, and many share certain characteristics common to both animals and plants; however, all are distinguishable from higher animals and plants by virtue of their simple organization.

The protists can be divided into 2 groups on the basis of their cellular structure—the higher protists (most algae, the fungi, and the protozoa) have **eucaryotic** cells, and the lower protists (the blue-green algae and all bacteria) have **procaryotic** cells. The eucaryotic cells are like those of plants and animals; i.e., they possess a nuclear membrane, a mitotic apparatus, more than one chromosome, and mitochondria. The procaryotic cells are smaller, have no nuclear membrane and no mitotic apparatus, and have but a single chromosome (or, in different terms, the nuclear material is not organized into individual chromosomes). One group of infectious agents, the viruses, cannot be discussed in this framework, since their structure (the complete viral particle, the virion) is not comparable to that of a cell, and their mode of multiplication (replication) is fundamentally different from that of cellular organisms in its total dependence on the synthetic system (enzymes and precursors) of the host cell.

It is beyond the scope of this introduction to discuss the difficulties inherent in creating a universally acceptable and applicable system for the classification of bacteria. It should suffice to point out that the classification of higher animals and plants is based on a phylogenetic, natural system in which the organisms are grouped according to the degree of their genetic relatedness and evolutionary relationships, whereas until very recently little or no evidence of such relationships was available for bacteria beyond their procaryotic cell nature. Thus systems of bacterial classification had to be constructed as more or less arbitrary descriptive keys based on a mixture of known structural and physiologic characteristics of bacteria.[1,2]

More recently the chemical study of deoxyribonucleic acid (DNA, the carrier of the genetic code) has shown a promising way of determining the genetic relatedness of bacteria. The DNA molecule is a duplex structure; it consists of 2 strands wound around each other helically. The strands carry sequences of the 4 nucleotide bases: adenine, guanine, thymine, and cytosine. Adenine is always opposite thymine, and guanine is opposite cytosine. The study of DNA base composition, expressed as the mean molar guanine + cytosine content (mole% G + C) has opened up a new approach to establishment of intrageneric and intergeneric relationships.[3] When the base composition of DNA in vertebrates was determined, it was found to be much the same in all vertebrates (approximately 60 mole% adenine + thymine and 40 mole% guanine + cytosine). However, among bacteria the overall base composition of DNA bases varies about 30-80 mole% G + C. Base composition determination of various bacteria has confirmed previously accepted close relationships, whereas others have been shown to be far removed from the species, genus, or even family in which they were previously placed.

A more precise measurement was devised by

determining the ability of DNA strands from 2 different bacteria to form molecular hybrids (hybridization) and thus to ascertain the degree of similarity of the base sequence of the 2 DNAs (homology).[4] By study of the binding DNA fragments to homologous and heterologous DNA immobilized in a gel structure, it is possible to measure quantitatively the genetic relatedness of various strains of bacteria. Since the genetic information is inscribed in the base sequence, the degree and completeness of homology, as measured by hybridization, indicate the degree of genetic relatedness. The determination of DNA base composition and of homology by hybridization has yielded much needed information for the classification of bacteria.[5]

For a more detailed discussion of modern views of microbial taxonomy, classification, and genetics the reader is referred to *The Microbial World* by Stanier et al.[3] and *Microbiology* by Davis et al.[6]

The present systems of bacterial classification were constructed on the basis of a large number of structural and physiologic characteristics of bacteria, e.g., morphology (size, shape, staining properties, presence or lack of flagella, capsule), physiologic and biochemical patterns (growth requirements, fermentation products, utilization of various substrates), presence of specific antigens, and ecology (relation between the organism and its environment, including habitat, and ability to cause disease or to survive in a particular host). Each organism is identified, named, and grouped by determining the combination of the above characteristics it possesses.

The most widely used system of classification and nomenclature in the United States is *Bergey's Manual of Determinative Bacteriology,* the first edition of which appeared in 1923. The system in *Bergey's Manual* has some phylogenetic implications that cannot be verified at the present time[1]; it represents the closest approach to the construction of a natural system on the basis of a mixture of characteristics. Through each succeeding edition of Bergey's, major changes occurred in the basic classification, and the eighth edition (1974) contains substantial revisions of nomenclature and classification. The nomenclature and differentiation of bacteria in this text conforms, wherever possible, to the system used in the eighth edition of *Bergey's Manual.*

In the formal bacterial nomenclature, following the rules of biologic classification, each distinct kind of bacterium is called a **species.** The name of the species is always a latin binomial. The first word, the name of the genus, is always capitalized; the second, the species name, is not capitalized. A **genus** (pl., genera) contains a group of related species (or sometimes only a single species). A group of related genera is placed into a **family** (ending, -*aceae*), related families form an **order** (-*ales*), and related orders are placed into a **class.**

In the eighth edition of *Bergey's Manual,*[5] the newly proposed kingdom *PROCARYOTAE* is divided into the **Cyanobacteria** (division I, blue-green algae, not further discussed in *Bergey's Manual*) and the **Bacteria** (division II, "procaryotic organisms that are not blue-green algae"). Recognizing that provision of a formal, meaningful, and complete hierarchy is not possible at this time, the editors of the eighth edition of *Bergey's Manual* present the material on Bacteria in 19 parts, each of which bears a vernacular name (or sometimes that of a taxon) and is distinguishable by relatively few readily determined criteria. In several parts (1, 5, 11, 13, 14, and 18) all accepted genera are grouped in families; in others "genera of uncertain affiliation" follow the family's description, while in still others genera are simply described in sequence without family or order grouping. It is recognized that further work is required in all phases of bacterial taxonomy and that further revisions will occur in nomenclature and classification.

In line with the evidence indicating that the **rickettsia** (family *Ricketsiaceae*) are bacteria (inhibition by antibacterial agents inactive against viruses, multiplication by binary fission, possession of various enzyme systems related to their metabolic activities, and presence of both ribonucleic acid [RNA] and deoxyribonucleic acid [DNA]), and not a separate group between viruses and bacteria, they are now included among the Bacteria (part 18), together with *Bartonellaceae, Anaplasmataceae,* and *Chlamydiaceae* (**chlamydia** or **bedsonia**). The chlamydia, formerly referred to as **large viruses,** and including the agents of psittacosis, lymphogranuloma venereum, trachoma, and inclusion conjunctivitis, are now also known to be bacteria (based on presence of both RNA and DNA, in contrast to viruses, which have either DNA or RNA but not both; possession of some biosynthetic capabilities; and susceptibility to various antibacterial agents).

A detailed key for determining the generic position of unknown organisms is included in the eighth edition of *Bergey's Manual*[5] and is most useful.

Despite their clearly bacterial nature, the rickettsia and chlamydia are dealt with in the section on viral and rickettsial diagnostic procedures, since the technics for their isolation and identification are similar to those used for viruses and unlike those applied to bacteria.

BACTERIA

Bacteria are small, unicellular microorganisms (0.2-10 μm, average size), most containing no chlorophyll. They possess nuclear material without a nuclear membrane; the cell wall in most cases is rigid. Bacteria reproduce generally by binary fission, resulting usually in the production of 2 daughter cells of equal size. Commonly the cell is enclosed by a rigid wall; some bacteria have a capsule surrounding the cell wall. Some are motile, most by means of **flagella.***

The spherical bacteria, **cocci,** may form pairs, chains, or irregular clusters. **Helical or spiral** forms include the spirochetes (flexible, with a number of coils), spirilla (rigid, one or more portions of a turn), and vibrios (rigid, short, curved rods, with only part of a spiral turn). **Bacilli** are rod-shaped organisms, some of which are capable of forming spores. Filamentous organisms, some growing with branching and forming a mycelium, also occur (actinomycetes).

Most bacteria can be placed in one of 2 groups by their reaction to the **Gram stain** (**gram positive** and **gram negative**), a valuable aid in their identification.

With respect to **oxygen** requirements, **obligate aerobes** grow well only in its presence; **facultative anaerobes** grow either in the absence or presence of oxygen; **microaerophiles** grow only in minimal concentrations; and **strict anaerobes** only in the total absence of oxygen.

Capnophiles require, at least for initiation of growth, increased carbon dioxide tension (3-10%). **Psychrophiles** tolerate very low temperatures and will grow even at 4 C. **Mesophiles** will grow at temperatures of 30-44 C; those inhabiting mammalians grow best at 35-38 C. **Thermophiles** have an optimum temperature of 45-55 C.

Bacteria produce enzymes that enable them to carry out a large variety of chemical activities (fermentation, hydrolysis, etc.); their demonstration is another useful aid in differentiation. Some bacteria, the **saprophytes,** live on dead organic substances; the **parasites** obtain their nourishment from a living host. Certain bacteria are designated as **commensals (amphibionts, symbionts)** implying a normally harmless association with their host. Microorganisms able to cause disease are termed **pathogens;** some do so only under certain conditions (facultative pathogens), whereas a few cause disease almost always (obligate pathogens). The distinction between commensals and pathogens is not absolute; many commensals are potential pathogens, and some pathogens may behave as commensals.

A combination of the various briefly mentioned morphologic, physiologic, and biochemical (as well as antigenic) characteristics forms the basis for the systematic classification of bacteria in *Bergey's Manual of Determinative Bacteriol-*

ogy. In its eighth edition[5] the bacteria are arranged in 19 parts. The details of this system are not reproduced here, but a brief outline of the **medically important parts** only is given for orientation.

Part 5, the **Spirochetes** (order *Spirochaetales,* family *Spirochaetaceae),* includes among its 5 genera the flexuous, helical *Treponema* (some of which are responsible for syphilis, yaws, and pinta), *Borrelia* (relapsing fever), and *Leptospira* (leptospirosis, one type of infectious jaundice).

Part 6, **Spiral** and **Curved Bacteria,** includes the family *Spirillaceae,* with the genera *Spirillum* and *Campylobacter.*

Part 7, **Gram-Negative Aerobic Rods** and **Cocci,** includes, among others, the family *Pseudomonadaceae* (genera *Pseudomonas, Xanthomonas,* and 2 others) and the genera of uncertain affiliation: *Alcaligenes, Acetobacter, Brucella, Bordetella,* and *Francisella.*

Part 8, **Gram-Negative Facultatively Anaerobic Rods,** includes the family *Enterobacteriaceae* with 12 genera (*Escherichia, Edwardsiella, Citrobacter, Salmonella, Shigella, Klebsiella, Enterobacter, Hafnia, Serratia, Proteus, Yersinia,* and *Erwinia*) and the family *Vibrionaceae* (with the medically important genera *Vibrio, Aeromonas,* and *Plesiomonas*) as well as the genera of uncertain affiliation: *Chromobacterium, Flavobacterium, Haemophilus, Pasteurella, Actinobacillus, Cardiobacterium, Streptobacillus,* and *Calymmatobacterium.*

Part 9, **Gram-Negative Anaerobic Bacteria,** includes the family *Bacteroidaceae* with the genera *Bacteroides, Fusobacterium,* and *Leptotrichia* and the genera of uncertain affiliation: *Desulfovibrio, Butyrivibrio, Succinivibrio, Succinimonas, Lachnospira,* and *Selenomonas.*

Part 10, **Gram-Negative Cocci** and **Coccobacilli,** is composed of the family *Neisseriaceae* (genera *Neisseria, Branhamella, Moraxella,* and *Acinetobacter*).

Part 11, **Gram-Negative Anaerobic Cocci,** includes the family *Veillonellaceae* (genera *Veillonella, Acidaminococcus,* and *Megasphaera*).

Part 14, **Gram-Positive Cocci,** includes the aerobic or facultatively anaerobic family *Micrococcaceae* (genera *Micrococcus* and *Staphylococcus*), *Streptococcaceae* (genera *Streptococcus, Leuconostoc, Pediococcus, Aerococcus,* and *Gemella*), and the anaerobic family *Peptococcaceae* (genera *Peptococcus* and *Peptostreptococcus*).

Part 15, **Endospore-Forming Rods** and **Cocci,** consists of the family *Bacillaceae,* which includes the important genera *Bacillus* (aerobic sporeforming rods) and *Clostridium* (anaerobic sporeforming rods).

Part 16, **Gram-Positive, Asporogeneous** (Non-Sporeforming), **Rod-Shaped Bacteria,** includes the family *Lactobacillaceae* and the genera of uncertain affiliation *Listeria* and *Erysipelothrix.*

Part 17, **Actinomycetes** and **Related Or-**

---

*Flagellar types[7]: (1) **polar**—attached to 1 or both poles of the organism: **monotrichous**—1 flagellum at 1 or both poles; **multitrichous**—more than 1 flagellum at 1 or both poles, flagella usually with more than 2 curves; **lophotrichous**—same as multitrichous but flagella usually with 1 or 2 curves; (2) **peritrichous**—flagella attached at various points of the cell wall, both from sides and poles (some may be individually arranged, others may be in tufts); also **amphitrichous**—used by some authors to denote an organism with 1 flagellum at each pole.

ganisms, includes, among others, the genera *Corynebacterium, Kurthia*, the families *Propionibacteriaceae* (genera *Propionibacterium* and *Eubacterium*), *Actinomycetaceae* (*Actinomyces, Arachnia, Bifidobacterium*, and *Rothia*), *Mycobacteriaceae, Nocardiaceae*, and *Streptomycetaceae*.

Part 18, the **Rickettsias,** consists of the order *Rickettsiales* which includes among others the families *Rickettsiaceae* (*Rickettsia, Coxiella*) and *Bartonellaceae* and the order *Chlamydiales*.

Part 19 consists of the **Mycoplasmas,** organisms that possess no cell walls and are the smallest free-living (cultivable) cells known.

Parts 1 (Phototrophic Bacteria), 2 (Gliding Bacteria), 3 (Sheathed Bacteria), 4 (Budding or Appendaged Bacteria), 12 (Gram-Negative, Chemolitotrophic Bacteria), and 13 (Methane-Producing Bacteria) are not discussed further in this volume.

The bacteria included in the above outline are discussed in detail in Chapters 77-83, together with the methods and technics appropriate for their detection, cultivation, and identification. For chlamydia and rickettsia see Chapters 90-95.

Wall-defective microbial variants

L-forms, spheroplasts, protoplasts, and transitional phase variants are cell-wall-deficient bacterial variants.[8]

The first such variants recognized were the **L-forms** (L-phase variants) named after the Lister Institute (London), where they were isolated by Klieneberger in 1935. They occur under certain conditions, i.e., the presence of toxic agents such as penicillin, and high salt concentrations in the medium. On transfer they can be grown (in a hypertonic medium of sucrose or salts, without penicillin); the resulting colonies are small and nondescript, with the organisms being pleomorphic and poorly stained. Some of them, when grown in the absence of, e.g., penicillin, revert to the parent bacterial form (**unstable variants**), a characteristic that distinguishes them from *Mycoplasma* (Chapter 82), which they otherwise resemble; some, however, continue to grow as L-forms (**stable variants**).

Protoplasts are another bacterial variant, artificially obtained from bacteria by eliminating the cell wall through exposure to lysozyme in a hypertonic medium such as 20% sucrose, with consequent release of the cell content. They usually do not multiply in artificial media. **Spheroplasts** are derived from gram-negative organisms by treatment with lysozyme or penicillin; these retain some portions of the wall. Some can be grown on artificial media.

Transitional phase variants have a tendency to revert to bacterial phase; unlike L-forms they do not grow as colonies on special agar.

The role of these bacterial forms in human disease is not yet clearly established. L-forms (and protoplasts) have been considered in relation to the persistence of bacteria in various infections, e.g., carditis, joint disease, urinary tract disease, and Whipple's disease. Since these forms cannot be detected or cultured with ordinary bacteriologic technics, special media and procedures must be employed for their culture. Among others, L-forms (or protoplasts) of streptococci (from the acute stage of rheumatic fever), staphylococci, listeriae, corynebacteria, *Candida* sp., *Proteus* sp., and *Haemophilus influenzae* have been isolated from patients receiving penicillin or other antibiotic therapy.

The concept of an L-phase of bacteria (naturally occurring) has been much debated; some workers believe that L-forms are products of laboratory manipulation of bacteria, while others maintain that L-forms do occur naturally and that they may be implicated in recurrent or persistent infections.

Although the role, if any, of L-forms in human or animal disease continues to be debated, it is most likely that protoplasts, spheroplasts, and transitional phase variants are laboratory products produced by exposure of the bacteria to various enzymes, e.g., lysozyme.

For the technics used and the occurrence of L-forms of various bacteria (naturally occurring or artificially induced), the reader is referred to the review of Eaton,[9] *Biology of the Mycoplasma*,[10] *Pleuropneumonia-like Organisms (PPLO) Mycoplasmataceae*,[11] *Microbial Protoplasts, Spheroplasts and L-forms*,[12] Clasener's review[13] on the pathogenicity of the L-phase of bacteria, *Pathogenic Mycoplasmas*,[14] Madoff and Pachas' chapter[15] on the clinical significance of mycoplasma and bacterial L-forms, and Chapter 82 in this volume.

CLINICAL BACTERIOLOGY

It is customary to state that the concern of clinical bacteriology is the search for pathogens; this is true, with the important qualification that not every bacterium isolated from the human body is a pathogen. Large areas of the human body such as the skin, the upper respiratory tract, the mouth, and the lower intestinal tract are inhabited by bacteria (also yeasts and, in some cases, protozoa), acquired practically from the time of birth, that constitute what is called the **normal flora (indigenous biota)** of man. When a specimen from a patient suspected of having an infectious disease is examined, distinction must be made between specimens that are obtained from **sites with a normal flora** and from **sites** that are **normally sterile** (for a more detailed discussion, see Normal Flora, below).

If the specimen is from a nonsterile site, it is important to determine whether there is a change in the **kind** or **distribution** of the normal flora and to search for any abnormal pathogenic organisms.

On the other hand, **any** organism, even if part of the indigenous flora, recovered from a body site or fluid that is normally sterile should be regarded as a potential pathogen, since many indigenous (and saprophytic) organisms can cause severe and often fatal disease.

The finding of a particular organism is not always indicative of it presumed causative role. For instance, meningococci or pneumococci, usually classified as pathogens, may be present in the upper respiratory tract of man without overt disease (the **healthy carrier**), and typhoid organisms may be present in the **recovered carrier**; the carrier state is not an uncommon phenomenon. Laboratory findings should always be correlated with clinical data (for further details see Normal Flora and Interactions of Some Microorganisms with Man, below).

Since the introduction of chemotherapeutic agents and antibiotics, an increasing number of resistant strains have appeared. Predictions of susceptibility have become unreliable, and it is now necessary to test the susceptibility (sensitivity) of a number of organisms. As a result, **antibiotic susceptibility testing** has become a major responsibility of the clinical bacteriology laboratory. Speed coupled with accuracy, reproducibility, and adequate controls is essential in order to furnish the physician with useful information for rational antibiotic treatment.

Although speed is essential in diagnosis, accurate methods should be used to ensure the validity of findings; close collaboration between the physician and the laboratory in terms of proper specimen collection and furnishing necessary information about the specimen and the patient is vital.

Normal flora (indigenous biota)

Under **normal** conditions certain sites of the human body are sterile, i.e., the central nervous system (spinal fluid), circulatory system (blood), the peritoneal and pulmonary cavity, urinary bladder, posterior urethra, kidneys, prostate, uterus, larynx, trachea, bronchi, alveoli, accessory nasal sinuses, and middle and inner ear.

On the other hand, various species of bacteria inhabit surfaces of the human body. Such **nonsterile** sites range from those sparsely populated (e.g., stomach contaminated by ingestion of food) to others very heavily and invariably populated with a multitude of organisms (e.g., colon). Knowledge and familiarity with the normal inhabitants of these sites are imperative in order to avoid the trap of uncritical attribution of pathologic significance to organisms that usually are present on and are normal inhabitants of the site in question. A brief discussion of the bacterial population of the various nonsterile body sites follows.

Skin. Although considered as a single site, the skin's bacterial flora varies in different anatomical regions. For example, the flora of the facial area reflects that of the oropharynx, whereas the perineal flora is influenced to a considerable extent by the bacteria of the lower intestinal tract. Vigorous scrubbing with soap and water (or other disinfectants) will rid the skin temporarily of most of its surface bacteria; however, organisms sequestered in the hair follicles and sweat glands soon reestablished the surface organisms. The majority of the resident flora consists of gram-positive aerobic cocci (*S. epidermidis*, micrococci) and anaerobic corynebacteria (*Propionibacterium*), with aerobic corynebacteria, *S. aureus*, nonhemolytic streptococci less prevalent; gram-negative bacteria (*Enterobacteriaceae, Pseudomonas*) are found sporadically.

Mouth (including teeth, gingiva, tongue, and saliva). Commonly found are *S. epidermidis*, micrococci, and anaerobic cocci (*Peptostreptococcus* and *Peptococcus*), with nonhemolytic (α and γ) streptococci, including *S. salivarius* and *S. mitis*, present in large numbers in all surfaces of the mouth. *S. mutans* and *S. sanguis* are found mainly on the teeth; moderate numbers of enterococci are also present. Spirochetes (*Treponema macrodentium* and *T. denticola*) and *Bacteroidaceae* (e.g., *Fusobacterium, Bacteroides melaninogenicus*) are found mainly in periodontal pockets or gingival crevices. Various gram-positive anaerobic rods and filaments (*Actinomyces, Propionibacterium, Leptotrichia*) and the facultative rods *Nocardia, Lactobacillus, Rothia*, and *Corynebacterium*, as well as *Candida albicans* and other yeasts, are also present.

Throat, nasopharynx, oropharynx, and tonsils. *S. aureus* is frequently present in the pharynx and on the tonsils, while viridans streptococci are ubiquitous in the throat. *Neisseria* and *S. pneumoniae* (pneumococci) are often present in the healthy throat; *N. meningitidis* occurs infrequently in the healthy nasopharynx. *S. aureus, H. influenzae*, and various enteric bacilli may be isolated from the throat without any evidence that these cause acute pharyngitis in the healthy host. All the other organisms mentioned under **Mouth** are also present with greater or lesser frequency in the throat. The nose is colonized chiefly by staphylococci, and corynebacteria (commonly referred to as diphtheroids); about 20-30% of individuals carry *S. aureus*.

Trachea and lower respiratory tract. The trachea occasionally may contain a few bacteria, but usually it is sterile, as is the normal lower respiratory tract (bronchi, bronchioles, and alveoli).

The gastrointestinal tract. The *esophagus* generally contains only the bacteria swallowed with the saliva and food. Due to the high acidity of the gastric juice, few organisms (predominantly lactobacilli) can be cultured from the normal stomach. The microflora of the **upper small intestine** consists of a sparse population of gram-positive organisms, mostly lactobacilli and enterococci (in concentrations of 10^5-10^7/ml intestinal fluid, depending on the amount of food ingested). In the **lower small intestine** (distal and terminal ileum), the microbial flora changes, with anaerobes and coliform bacteria appearing; the microbial biota of the lower ileum is qualitatively but not quantitatively similar to that of feces. Past the ileocecal valve, the numbers and types of microorganisms change strikingly. The normal colon flora (inferred from the composition of the normal fecal flora) consists of about 10^{11} bacteria/g feces, and about 95-98% of these are obligate anaerobes. The anaerobes outnumber *E. coli* and other facultative enteric bacilli by 1000-10,000:1. When cultured **anaerobically,** (not done in the clinical laboratory), feces yield predominantly the non-spore-forming anaerobes, i.e., bacteroides and bifidobacteria (anaerobic lactobacilli) and smaller numbers of spore-forming clostridia, gram-positive and gram-negative anaerobic cocci, *Eubacterium* (non-sporeforming gram-positive rods), and vibrios. **Aerobic** cultures yield predominantly *E. coli* and smaller numbers of other coliform bacilli (enterobacteria), enterococci, other streptococci, and *Candida* species.

Vagina. During the childbearing years, lactobacilli, *S. epidermidis,* and corynebacteria predominate in the vagina, with a variety of anaerobes (*Bacteroides,* anaerobic cocci) also present in about 70% of women. Others with smaller numbers and lower incidence, are enterococci, α and γ (viridans) streptococci, β-hemolytic streptococci, nonpathogenic neisseriae, enteric bacilli, *Acinetobacter* species, *Hemophilus (Corynebacterium) vaginalis,* and *Mycoplasma* species. In the postmenopausal years the flora seems to remain about the same, with a somewhat greater incidence of gram-negative facultative bacilli (other than *E. coli)* noted in postmenopausal women.[16]

Urethra. The urethra generally contains small numbers of enterococci, staphylococci, corynebacteria, enteric bacilli, *Haemophilus vaginalis, Acinetobacter,* and various species of *Candida,* all usually contaminants from the mucous membranes of the external genitalia.

External genitalia. The surface of the genitalia yields α and γ (viridans) streptococci, *S. epidermidis,* enterococci, various anaerobic cocci, *Bacteroides, Fusobacterium,* corynebacteria, yeasts, and enteric bacilli.

Ear. The external ear canal's microbial biota is similar to that of the skin. The middle ear and inner ear are usually sterile.

Eye. On the conjunctiva *Staphylococcus epidermidis* and *Propionibacterium acnes* are predominant, with small numbers of nonhemolytic streptococci, anaerobic streptococci, *S. aureus,* corynebacteria, lactobacilli, and enteric bacilli occurring less frequently.

• • •

For further details on the distribution of normal flora, see *Microorganisms Indigenous to Man* (Rosebury),[17] *Human Intestinal Flora* (Drasar and Hill),[18] *The Normal Microbial Flora of Man* (Skinner and Carr),[19] the chapter on "Indigenous and Pathogenic Microorganisms of Man" (Isenberg and Painter),[20] and the chapter on "Bacteria Indigenous to Man" (Sonnenwirth).[21]

As stated before, the presence of normal flora organisms in various specimens may be misleading (e.g., the finding of viridans streptococci or of *S. aureus* in a throat swab from a patient with acute pharyngitis is irrelevant, since neither of these normal flora organisms causes pharyngitis), and therefore a general knowledge of the normal biota is essential.

Conversely, members of the normal flora are also important because of their potential association with disease: the incidence of **endogenous infections** (due to members of normal flora, i.e., **indigenous** organisms) has increased considerably. Indigenous organisms (as well as many saprophytes) are responsible for many **opportunistic infections** in **compromised hosts**[22] (patients with impaired antimicrobial defense mechanisms due to, e.g., radiation therapy, immunosuppression, lymphoproliferative disorders, splenectomy, diabetes, extensive surgery) and in nosocomial (hospital-acquired) infections.[20-22]

Practically all members of the normal biota, generally harmless in their habitats, can cause illness when they reach tissues outside their usual location (e.g., *E. coli* from colon appearing in kidneys or bloodstream). Thus a clear-cut division of organisms into "pathogens" and "nonpathogens" has become increasingly difficult.

Importance of properly collected specimens

From the foregoing discussion of the normal flora, it should be clear that the results of bacteriologic culture will be greatly influenced by the proper selection and collection of the specimen.

The specimen must be collected from the suspected lesion and not from an adjacent area; every effort must be made, if at all possible, to avoid contamination of the specimen with the normal flora, and the specimen must be delivered to the laboratory as soon as possible, preferably in transport media, to preserve the viability of the organism(s) and, in the case of mixed cultures (more than one organism), to preserve their orginal ratio in the sample.

Further details on specimen collection are described in Chapter 75.

Interaction of some microorganisms with man

Despite the difficulty of distinguishing between "pathogens" and "nonpathogens," it is possible to distinguish certain organisms in terms of their harmful activities based on their occurrence in and interaction with man. Although the categories are somewhat arbitrary, they are based on Rosebury's well-regarded work.[18]

Obligate pathogens. Obligate pathogens are definitely **not** members of the normal flora. **Infection** of man with, e.g., *Brucella* species, *Yersinia pestis, Francisella tularensis, Pseudomonas pseudomallei,* or various rickettsiae (also encephalitis viruses and rabies virus), almost always results in **disease.** These microorganisms are both virulent (pathogenic) and communicable.

Facultative pathogens. Facultative pathogens include a multitude of organisms, some of which are present in small numbers and irregularly in the normal host without any overt signs of disease: *Hemophilus influenzae*, pyogenic streptococci (β-hemolytic), and *Streptococcus pneumoniae;* they seem to coexist with the host in an uneasy equilibrium. *Neisseria meningitidis* may be present in the "healthy carrier," while *Salmonella* and *Shigella* may be found in the "recovered carrier."

Others, generally (and rightfully) considered pathogens and not generally thought of as occurring in the normal flora, e.g., *Mycobacterium tuberculosis*, *Treponema pallidum*, *Neisseria gonorrhoeae*, *Corynebacterium diphtheriae*, usually but not always cause overt **disease** following **infection.** Some may give rise to **latent** or **inapparent infection** (persistent, but not sufficiently active to be recognized, e.g., latent stages of syphilis and tuberculosis) or to **subclinical infection.** The facultative pathogens are also communicable.

Potential pathogens. Potential pathogens, called also **symbionts** or **commensals,** include members of the indigenous flora (biota) proper; *Bacteroides, Fusobacterium,* anaerobic cocci, lactobacilli, veillonellae, leptotrichia, *Escherichia* and certain species of spirochetes, vibrios, *Enterobacteriaceae* (e.g., the variably occurring *Klebsiella, Proteus, Enterobacter*), clostridia, *Actinomyces,* corynebacteria, neisseriae, streptococci, and staphylococci. These are permanently established in and highly adapted to man; under **normal** conditions they are nonvirulent (nonpathogenic), while under **abnormal** conditions they may be potential (opportunistic) pathogens.

Transient saprophytes. Some organisms, e.g., *Bacillus subtilis, Sarcina,* and aerobic actinomycetes, are not adapted to man and usually are transients. However, infections due to these organisms can occur.

EQUIPMENT[23,24]

The bacteriologic laboratory requires a variety of mechanical equipment. The size of the laboratory and the range of services offered often determine the amount and complexity of the equipment; however there are certain **basic** requirements that must be provided. A brief description of **essential** equipment follows; **automated** or **mechanized equipment** is discussed in Chapter 74.

Incubators providing constant temperature are necessary for growing bacteria. They vary in size from small portables to large walk-in incubator rooms. Maintenance of uniform temperatures is achieved in some types by employing a fan or blower to move the air (mechanical convection) and in others by surrounding the chamber with a water jacket that contains heated water. The water-jacketed type is preferred in work requiring extreme accuracy in maintenance of constant temperature; however, it is considerably more expensive than other types. Gas, oil, or electricity is used to heat incubators, depending on the available facilities. Safety features include recording thermometers and, in large electrically heated incubators, alarms that sound if the set temperature is exceeded or drops too low and a thermostatically controlled safety switch to cut off electricity if the temperature rises above a predetermined amount.

Incubators in the clinical laboratory should be set at 35 C. For many years 37 ± 2 C was considered the optimum temperature for growing medically important bacteria; however, they grow equally well at 35 C, and a rise of 2 C from 35 C would be tolerable, whereas such a rise from 37 C may be highly deleterious to some pathogenic organisms. In CO_2 incubators CO_2 concentrations should be maintained at 5-10% CO_2. Certain organisms require different incubation temperatures, such as leptospira (30 C) and fungi (22 C). For the latter, well-equipped laboratories use so-called room-temperature incubators, which are equipped both with heating and cooling elements (essentially a refrigerator with added heating element and thermostatic regulator).

All incubators should have external thermometers; in large ones especially it is advisable to place a small thermometer in a beaker of water on a shelf. Temperatures should be checked **daily** or a **recording thermometer** should be employed. Keep a container of fresh, clean water in the incubator at all times to prevent the air from becoming dry. The size of the water container and the amount of water needed depends on the size of the incubator (humidity of 40-80% is required).

Refrigerators are necessary for storage of perishables such as media, reagents, antisera, and antibiotic disks. For small laboratories household refrigerators are satisfactory, whereas in large laboratories commercial refrigerators or walk-in cold rooms are provided. If a choice can be made, 2 small refrigerators are preferable to a large one with double capacity, since mechanical breakdown will represent less interruption and possible loss of stored materials. Refrigerator temperature should be kept at 5 ± 2 C; check thermometer inside refrigerator daily. For storage in the frozen state (sera, certain antibiotic disks, etc.) the freezer unit of household refrigerators can be used. Depending on the amount of material to be kept frozen, it may be necessary to purchase a **freezer.** Temperatures of -15 to -20 C are adequate for most purposes; however, for certain specialized purposes (storage of viruses and bacteria) a temperature of -70 to -80 C is needed. This can be accomplished by using a dry ice chest or specially constructed mechanical (deep) freezer.

A compound binocular **microscope** is an integral part of the bacteriology laboratory. Low-power (10×, 16 mm), high dry (45×, 4 mm), and oil immersion (95× or 97×, 1.8 mm) achromatic objectives, a pair of 8× or 10× oculars, a mechanical stage, an achromatic condenser, a substage rack with centering screws, and a good light source are required. A dark-field condenser and a funnel stop for the oil immersion objective are needed for dark-field work (Chapter 80). A dissecting or stereoscopic microscope is very useful for identification of parasites and the study of colony characterics. Phase contrast and fluorescence microscopy are increasingly used (especially the latter). Attachments are available that allowed conversion of a light microscope into either type (special condenser and phase objectives for phase microscopy; filter systems, regular darkfield condenser, and ultraviolet light source for fluorescence microscopy). If fluorescence microscopy is to be used, it is recommended that a complete fluorescence microscope unit, including light source (Chapter 70), be purchased. Provision must be made for a darkroom or cubicle for setting up the fluorescence equipment.

For a more detailed description of the microscope see Chapter 2.

The **centrifuge** is an important item of equipment in the bacteriology laboratory; it allows the speedy separation of bacteria from the liquid in which they are suspended. Two main types are used: the horizontal (swinging) head and the angle head centrifuge. The horizontal centrifuge is equipped with a head that holds cups attached in such a manner that they can swing out and rotate in a horizontal plane during centrifugation. The centrifuge tubes are placed in cups. The head of the angle type contains a number of holes into which the tubes are placed and held at an angle of 30-50°. During rotation of the head, the tubes thus are held in a fixed position. Greater speeds can be obtained with the angle head, but the horizontal head allows better sedimentations. For the average laboratory a small tabletop centrifuge accomodating 10-12 tubes of 15 ml capacity and a floor model taking tubes or bottles of 50 ml (or greater) are needed. The larger units have changeable heads and cups and allow for versatility. An important accessory is the aerosol-free sealed cup that is used for the centrifugation of materials containing highly infectious particles. When centrifuging, always balance units (cups containing tubes) to prevent breaking of tube and damage to centrifuge. Tubes should be placed exactly opposite each other, should be the same weight (e.g., do not balance a heavy-walled tube with a thin-walled one), and should contain the same amount of liquid.

Continuous-flow centrifuges (Sharples type) are also available. In these the fluid is continuously fed into a rotating tube, where the bacteria sediment rapidly on the sides of the tube. The centrifuged liquid flows out of the tube, is collected, and is carried away from the machine. Such centrifuges are used for very large amounts of material in industry and in research laboratories but are not utilized in the routine laboratory.

The acceleration of a particle effected by a centrifuge (i.e., the increase in the force of gravity due to centrifugation) is usually expressed as the relative centrifugal force (RCF) or g.

$$RCF(g) = 1.118 \times 10^{-5} \times R \times N^2$$

where R is the rotating radius, i.e., the distance in **cm** from the center of the centrifuge to the end of the centrifuge tube, and N is the speed of rotation (revolutions per minute [rpm]). Thus, by stating the radius and the speed of a centrifuge, the efficiency of centrifugation can be stated in accurate terms.

Water baths are constant temperature devices, electrically operated and controlled by thermostats that hold the temperature within preset limits. Always install an accurate immersed thermometer in the water bath. A **water still** or a **demineralizer** containing ion exchange resins is needed for furnishing distilled or demineralized water to be used for the preparation of various reagents and media. The **autoclave** is discussed under sterilization (Chapter 70, and in more detail in Chapter 89).

For a discussion of **anaerobic equipment** refer to Chapters 70, 82, and 86.

Manual or **automatic pipettors and dispensers** are instruments designed to dispense an exact, preset amount of liquid, thus circumventing hazards or mouth pipetting, speeding repetitive transfers, and increasing accuracy. A large variety of manual pipettors and dispensers (tip-ejector, fixed-volume pipets; standard, fixed-volume pipets; tip-ejector, multivolume pipets; refilling, syringe type pipet filler; adjustable-volume, syringe type; controlled-volume rubber bulb), as well as automatic pipettors, dispensers, and dilutors (basically syringe-type cylinders or pumps filled repetitively by an electric compressor), are commercially available.

Inoculating wires and **loops** are made of platinum, platinum-iridium, stainless steel, pure nickel, and nichrome. Heavy-gauge platinum, although expensive, is recommended for anaerobic work and for precalibrated loops. Nichrome should not be used; it may cause false-positive oxidase reactions and is not suitable for anaerobic work. Loops should be inspected periodically and maintained at approximately 3 mm diameter.[24]

A **biological safety cabinet** is used when handling specimens or cultures that are suspected or known to contain hazardous organisms (e.g., *M. tuberculosis* and various fungi). Safety cabinets with high-efficiency (HEPA) filter exhaust or recirculation or with an incinerating exhaust are preferred.[24] For further discussion see Chapters 69 and 78.

For further details the reader is referred to *Diagnostic Procedures and Reagents*,[23] *Quality Assurance Practices for Health Laboratories*,[24] and *Medical Microbiology*.[25]

Automation in the bacteriology laboratory. See Chapter 74 for a detailed discussion of mechanization and automation as well as miniaturization in the clinical microbiology laboratory.

• • •

In conformity with the *Système International* (SI) the following abbreviations are used in this text: s, second; min, minute; d, day; mo, month; y, year.

REFERENCES

1. Stanier, R. Y., Doudoroff, M., and Adelberg, E. A.: The microbial world, ed. 2, Englewood Cliffs, N. J., 1963, Prentice-Hall.
2. Stanier, R. Y., Adelberg, E. A., and Ingraham, J. L.: The microbial world, ed. 4, Englewood Cliffs, N.J., 1976, Prentice-Hall.
3. Marmur, J., and Doty, P.: J. Mol. Biol. **5:**109, 1962.
4. McCarthy, B. J., and Bolton, T. E.: Proc. Natl. Acad. Sci. U.S.A. **50:**156, 1963.
5. Buchanan, R. E., and Gibbons, N. E., editors: Bergey's manual of determinative bacteriology, ed. 8, Baltimore, 1974, The Williams & Wilkins Co.
6. Davis, B. D., Dulbecco, R., Eisen, H. N., et al.: Microbiology, ed. 3, New York, 1980, Harper & Row, Publishers.
7. Leifson, E.: J. Bacteriol. **62:**377, 1951.
8. McGee, Z. A., Whittler, R. G., Gooder, H., et al.: J. Infect. Dis. **123:**433, 1971.
9. Eaton, M. D.: Annu. Rev. Microbiol. **19:**379, 1965.
10. Hayflick, L., editor: Biology of the mycoplasma, Ann. N.Y. Acad. Sci. **143:**1, 1967.
11. Klieneberger-Nobel, E.: Pleuropneumonia-like organisms (PPLO). Mycoplasmataceae, New York, 1962, Academic Press.
12. Guze, L. B., editor: Microbial protoplasts, spheroplasts and L-forms, Baltimore, 1968, The Williams & Wilkins Co.

13. Clasener, H.: Annu. Rev. Microbiol. **26:**55, 1972.
14. Pirie, N. W., chairman: Pathogenic mycoplasmas, Amsterdam, 1972, Elsevier.
15. Madoff, S., and Pachas, W. N. In Lorian, V., editor: Significance of medical microbiology in the care of patients, Baltimore, 1977, The Williams & Wilkins Co.
16. Tashjan, J. H., Coulam, C. B., and Washington, J. A.: Mayo Clin. Proc. **51:**557, 1976.
17. Rosebury, T.: Microorganisms indigenous to man, New York, 1962, McGraw-Hill Book Co.
18. Drasar, B. S., and Hill, M. J.: Human intestinal flora, New York, 1974, Academic Press.
19. Skiner, F. A., and Carr, J. G., editors: The normal microbial flora of man, New York, 1974, Academic Press.
20. Isenberg, H. D., and Painter, B. G. Ch. 5, In Manual of clinical microbiology, ed. 3, Washing-ton, D. C., 1974, American Society for Microbiology.
21. Sonnenwirth, A. In Davis, B. D., Dulbecco, R., Eisen, H. H., et al.: Microbiology, ed. 3, New York, 1980, Harper & Row, Publishers, chap. 42.
22. Graevenitz, A. U.: The role of opportunistic bacteria in human disease, Annu. Rev. Microbiol. **31:**447, 1977.
23. Bodily, H. L., Updyke, E. L., and Mason O., editors: Diagnostic procedures and reagents, ed. 5, New York, 1970, American Public Health Association.
24. Inhorn, S. L., editor: Quality assurance practices for health laboratories, Washington, D.C., 1977, American Public Health Association.
25. Cruikshank, R., Inguid, J. P., Marmion, B. P., et al.: Medical microbiology, vol. 2, ed. 12, London, 1975, Churchill Livingstone.

69

SAFETY IN THE CLINICAL MICROBIOLOGY LABORATORY

Charles T. Hall

In the clinical microbiology laboratory relatively small numbers of potentially pathogenic bacteria in patients' specimens are routinely cultured on a variety of recovery media and harvested in populations billions of times more numerous but no less infectious than those encountered in the primary specimens. It is in this environment that the microbiologist performs the routine tasks of isolation and identification, and therefore both laboratory administrator and employee must recognize that some risk is involved for persons working in a clinical microbiology laboratory.

The purpose of a safety program is to reduce this risk to minimal levels so that laboratory-incurred infections become extraordinary rather than inevitable occurrences. In the development of a safety program the subjects of legal liability and responsibility often becomes a controversial issue. Safety programs are sometimes implemented by laboratory administrators in order to avoid liability rather than by both management and staff in an effort to combat a common danger. As a result of this defensive approach to safety, quite often any infected employee is immediately assumed to have incurred the infection outside the laboratory. This approach to laboratory safety is self-defeating. It causes laboratory workers to question whether the administration is interested in their well-being, and even more damaging to the program, it precludes any follow-up or review of laboratory procedures for the purpose of discovering inadequacies in the system or deficiencies in equipment that were responsible for the infection. An acceptable level of safety can be achieved only through the mutual efforts of everyone involved.

ROLE OF LABORATORY MANAGEMENT IN SAFETY PROGRAMS

Once the decision has been made to establish a clinical laboratory, management has tacitly assumed 3 major responsibilities:

1. To protect the laboratory staff against unnecessary and unwarranted exposure to infectious agents
2. To safeguard the integrity of the clinical specimen against degradation or cross-contamination, which might jeopardize the validity of laboratory findings
3. To contain infectious agents within the confines of the laboratory

Safeguarding the integrity of the clinical specimen and assuring the validity of the laboratory findings are discussed in Chapter 73. The quality control efforts of a laboratory are essentially, then, a safety program for the patient's specimen. The protection of the laboratory staff and confinement of recovered infectious agents within the laboratory are discussed in this chapter.

In assuming the responsibility for establishing a laboratory, management must make some profound decisions. What types of specimens will be accepted for analysis? What types of agents might be present in these specimens? What is the probability that they will be present? What technic would be appropriate for processing the specimens without subjecting the staff to undue hazard? What qualifications must the staff possess? What equipment must be obtained? What procedures must be physically separated to protect personnel and the specimen? How do these requirements influence laboratory design and safety? The answers to these questions serve as the basis for establishing laboratory policies. It is only after these policy decisions have been made that a rational approach to safety can be contemplated.

Phillips and Jemski[1] suggested a number of measures that management can implement to control laboratory hazards. These suggestions are directed toward the laboratory worker, who must be the focal point for any safety program. Among the suggestions are the following:

1. Establish written safety regulations and see that they are read and understood by all.
2. Keep safety needs in mind when new employees are selected.
3. Train all employees until it is certain that they understand both the rules and the reasons for making them.

4. Inasmuch as possible, design safety into technic and procedures as they are developed.
5. Establish responsibility for safety. Each supervisor should be responsible for the safety of his people, but each employee should have a personal responsibility. Safety should be a part of every job.
6. Establish a reporting system for infections, accidents, and injuries requiring loss of work time, and insist on prompt reporting.
7. Investigate each illness and each accident to determine what should be done to prevent recurrence.
8. Encourage workers at all levels to suggest means of eliminating laboratory hazards.

LABORATORY DESIGN AND SAFETY

Once it has been decided what kinds of specimens will be processed in the laboratory, then the pathogenic agents that may be present in the samples, their relative pathogenicity, and their modes of transmission can be determined. On the basis of this information an intelligent decision can be made about the levels of security that are required to protect the laboratory staff as well as the surrounding community. The handling of some bacterial and viral agents will require that certain activities be physically isolated in order to protect the staff. Conversely, certain activities will be separated from the mainstream of laboratory activities to protect the integrity of the recovery system (e.g., media preparation and the tissue culture laboratory).

The modern microbiology laboratory is usually divided into several zones described below depending on the level of security required to protect the staff and the integrity of the specimens being studied.

Zone I (clean area). In this area, the routine administrative duties and logistical activities are performed. Personnel offices, libraries, lunchrooms, storerooms, and maintenance shops are housed in this part of the laboratory. Although situated in zone I, the media and reagent preparation areas should be open only to authorized and necessary traffic.

Zone II (moderately hazardous areas). These areas are usually restricted to work with biologic agents of low pathogenicity or to activities involving hazards that can be adequately controlled by implementing conventional isolation and recovery technic and by using safety equipment. These areas should always be considered as potentially contaminated, and despite the routine nature of the work, traffic between this area and zone I should be carefully controlled.

Zone III (hazardous areas). In these areas, highly pathogenic or transmissible agents are investigated. In addition to the diagnostic and research activities, these areas would include the animal crematory or the contaminated waste incinerator areas. In smaller laboratories the hazardous area might contain only the tuberculosis and mycology laboratory, which require the use of biological safety cabinets.

All work with biologic agents should be expressly prohibited in the clean areas. The laboratory should be designed so that no infected materials need to be taken into or through a clean area. Appropriate regulations should assure that persons who work in the moderately hazardous and hazardous areas remove contaminated outer garments before entering the clean area. The storage and consumption of food and beverages in the contaminated areas of the laboratory should be forbidden, and this rule should be strictly enforced.

Entry into moderately hazardous and hazardous areas of the laboratory should be restricted to a few portals through which accessibility can be controlled. Dressing rooms, lockers for personal items, and wash-up or shower facilities should be conveniently located so that the staff members can use them immediately before they enter and after they leave the contaminated areas. All outer garments worn in the laboratory should be discarded in this pass-through area.

Laboratory spaces should be ventilated so that the air will flow from the area of least probable contamination to the most contaminated areas. Chatigny[2] discussed the control of the air supply into the laboratory and the requirements for filtration of air exhaust.

PREVENTIVE MEDICAL SERVICES

A meaningful laboratory safety program should include a systematic procedure for determining whether illness in an employee is caused by a laboratory-acquired infection. The health and well-being of all laboratory workers should be continuously monitored. New employees should be required to give a comprehensive **medical history** and have a **physical examination** (including a Pap smear for females). The examination should include a skin test for tuberculosis, a full-plate chest x-ray film, appropriate serologic tests, selected biochemical tests, a complete blood count, urinalysis, and an electrocardiogram as indicated; appropriate immunizations should be given at this time. At the initial physical examination and at periodic physical examinations thereafter, sera should be collected from each employee and stored in a deep freeze as reference serum samples. These sera and other recorded physical data provide a basis for comparison in the event that a job-related disease occurs, and they can be useful in determining when a particular condition (e.g., tuberculin skin test conversion) occurred.

The appropriate immunization for personnel in the average clinical laboratory is not as easily defined as is that for personnel in a research facility where specific agents are under investigation. In research situations involving identified disease entities, immunization should be provided when warranted and available. However, extensive immunization programs generally are not required in most clinical laboratories. Usually the diphtheria and tetanus toxoids (as contained in standard DTP preparations) and poliomyelitis vaccine should suffice.[3] Ultimately, however, the **immunization requirements** must be established as a matter of laboratory policy.

For a number of years the clinical microbiology laboratory was involved only rarely, if ever, in processing sputum specimens for *Mycobacterium tuberculosis*. Generally these specimens were referred to state public health facilities for testing. However, because of recent advances in technology, increasing numbers of clinical laboratories offer this service, and personnel involved in processing these specimens should be under special surveillance.

Personnel actively engaged in processing sputa should have periodic **tuberculin tests** so that any infection with virulent *M. tuberculosis* can be detected early enough for isoniazid treatment to be given and development of clinical disease prevented. Bacille Calmette-Guérin (BCG) vaccine is an attenuated, live bacterial vaccine prepared from a bovine tubercle bacillus. The organism was originally isolated in 1902 by Nocard, and after more than 200 passages by Calmette and Guérin on a potato medium to which ox bile had been added, it was declared in 1920 to be incapable of producing fatal tuberculosis in cattle, monkeys, guinea pigs, and rabbits. The safety of the vaccine has been attested to by extensive and prolonged use, but unfortunately BCG vaccine does not necessarily prevent infection with virulent tubercle bacilli. It is generally agreed, however, that it prevents disastrous complications of primary infection with virulent tubercle bacilli. Nevertheless, BCG vaccine is not recommended for laboratory personnel, including those working directly with mycobacteria. Since adequately applied modern methods for detection, isolation, treatment, and chemoprophylaxis are highly successful in controlling tuberculosis, BCG should be reserved for situations in which these methods cannot be applied. BCG should be used for a person or small group of persons who are uninfected but live in unavoidable contact with one or more uncontrolled infectious persons who cannot or will not obtain or accept supervised treatment.

Pregnant employees should not be allowed to work in a virus laboratory. Whether pregnancy alters an individual's susceptibility to viral infection has not yet been determined; however, an increase in the abortion rate has been attributed to several viral agents.

The circumstances of each individual case should be thoroughly investigated before vaccines are administered to pregnant employees. The use of live, attenuated viral vaccines such as those for rubella, measles, and mumps is contraindicated for pregnant employees. Pregnant women in high-risk areas or subject to increased chance of exposure to yellow fever or poliomyelitis may require immunization after the relative risks have been considered.

One hazard to laboratory personnel that has gained widespread attention in recent years is **viral hepatitis.** As commonly used, the term "viral hepatitis" applies to 2 diseases that are clinically quite similar but virologically, immunologically, and epidemiologically distinct.

Table 69-1. Guidelines for ISG prophylaxis against hepatitis A*

Person's weight (lb.)	ISG dose (ml)
50	0.5
50-100	1.0
100	2.0

*From Lab Safety at the Center for Disease Control, DHEW Publication No. CDC-75-8118, Atlanta, Center for Disease Control, pp. 11-29.

These diseases are hepatitis A (formerly infectious hepatitis) and hepatitis B (formerly serum hepatitis). Immune serum globulin (ISG) provides highly effective protection against the clinical manifestations of hepatitis A but is ineffective for hepatitis B. Therefore accurate diagnosis of the kind of viral hepatitis, insofar as is possible with methods presently available, is crucial to the effective use of ISG. Distinguishing individual cases of hepatitis A and hepatitis B on the basis of clinical manifestations is extremely difficult, but differentiation of these diseases often is possible by careful evaluation of epidemiologic evidence and blood tests for hepatitis B. The usual incubation period of hepatitis A is 15-50 days (average = 25-30). Stools from patients with hepatitis A have been shown to be infected for as long as 2-3 weeks before and 2 weeks after the onset of jaundice. Blood is infective at least 2 weeks before but less than 1 week after the appearance of jaundice, so parenteral transmission of hepatitis A is also possible. Routine prophylactic administration of ISG to hospital and laboratory personnel is not indicated, but sound hygienic practices should be emphasized. Intensive continuing education programs pointing out the risks of exposure to hepatitis and the recommended precautions are very important for hospital and laboratory personnel who have close contact with patients or infective materials. For a person accidentally inoculated with blood or serum from a hepatitis patient (e.g., by needle puncture), ISG prophylaxis should be used only if the inoculum is suspected of containing hepatitis A. Then ISG should be given in the dose specified in Table 69-1. Provision should be made in the laboratory to obtain immune serum globulin for treatment of personnel within 48 hours after the possible risk of exposure to hepatitis A has been assessed. ISG should be given as soon as possible after known exposure. Its prophylactic value is greatest when given early in the incubation period and decreases with time after exposure. The use of ISG more than 6 weeks after exposure or after onset of clinical illness is not indicated.

PERSONNEL INDOCTRINATION AND TRAINING

In too many laboratories new personnel are assigned to routine tasks without any indoctrination that will enable them to identify potential hazards associated with assigned duties or any instruction in approved procedures for their prevention and control. This is particularly true for support personnel (secretaries, janitors, maintenance men, etc.) who are assigned service responsibilities. These personnel should be instructed in their specific job assignments and made aware of the laboratory hazards in proximity to their working areas. Under routine conditions these personnel should be restricted to "clean areas" in the laboratory, and their entry into potentially contaminated areas of the laboratory should be authorized only by the laboratory technical supervisor. The personnel should be instructed in how to conduct their activities in an area of potential hazard. In many laboratories specimens are opened and entered in the work log by secretarial and clerical staff. Specimens should be received and processed only by personnel specifically trained to handle infectious materials.

Especially important is the decontamination of all equipment needing repair or maintenance. It should be laboratory policy that no potentially contaminated equipment be removed from the laboratory to outside service areas and no maintenance personnel be admitted to perform on-site service until the equipment bears a tag denoting the completion of decontamination procedures. The tag should bear the date the equipment was disinfected, the method of decontamination used, and the name of the person who performed the procedure.

Even technically trained personnel assigned to microbiology, biochemistry, or radiology units should be required to attend a safety indoctrination program based on specific job assignments. It is not good policy to assume that even technically trained personnel are knowledgeable in safe laboratory practices. The indoctrination program should identify potential hazards related to the job assignment and instruct the employee in the approved procedures for preventing and controlling them. In the microbiology laboratory new employees should be provided with pertinent information on the possible etiologic agents they may encounter and on the approved methods of inactivation or decontamination. In the event of a laboratory accident, the employees should know the procedure for reporting it and the importance of placing themselves under a physician's care.

TRANSMISSION OF INFECTION IN LABORATORY

Laboratory-associated infections are an enigma to the laboratory worker. In a study of 3921 laboratory infections reported by Pike[4] in 1976, only 703 (18%) of the infections were attributable to known accidents or identifiable breaches of aseptic technic. The figure compares favorably with the findings of Sulkin and Pike[5] in which only 16% of infections in their study population could be traced to specific documented incidents. Of

Table 69-2. Probable or proved sources of 3921 laboratory-associated infections*

Source	No.
Accident	703
Animal or ectoparasite	659
Clinical specimen	287
Discarded glassware	46
Human autopsy	75
Intentional infection	19
Aerosol	522
Worked with agent	827
Other	16
Unknown or not indicated	767
TOTAL	3921

*From Pike, R. M.: Health Lab. Sci. **13**:105, 1976.

the remaining 3218 laboratory-associated infections in Pike's study, a probable source of infection could be assigned to approximately three-fourths of these cases. Unfortunately in many instances the association of disease with the laboratory could only be implied by the fact that the infected person had worked with the organism. These findings would indicate that approximately 80% of laboratory workers who are infected while performing routine laboratory functions do not know when or how they acquired the infection.

Reitman[6] stated that as a result of all manipulations required during a routine day in the microbiologic laboratory, aerosols are produced that contaminate the environment. In Table 69-3, several routine laboratory activities are listed in the sequence in which they might be performed on any given day in a laboratory. Included in this list are several miniaccidents, which might, and often do, occur during these routine manipulations. As indicated in Table 69-3, even the common, routine laboratory functions produce retrievable bacterial aerosols in the immediate working area. Accidents (e.g., the breaking of a tube during centrifugation or spilling of a culture) also are potential sources of infection to the laboratory staff.

In the average clinical laboratory, the laboratory worker may by chance be exposed to the potential infectious agent several times each day. Fortunately most organisms encountered in the clinical laboratory exhibit low invasiveness for man even through the specimen under scrutiny was obtained from an infected individual. When reasonable precautions are taken and classic aseptic technics are used, most bacteria do not constitute a great danger to the laboratory staff. Four factors determine whether the chance encounter between man and microbe will result in infection:

1. Virulence of the organism
2. Dosage or numbers of organisms encountered
3. Route of introduction
4. Resistance of the host to the agent

Table 69-3. Infection hazards of various laboratory procedures as revealed by air-sampling technics[*]

Infection hazard	Average no. of organisms recovered from air (1 ft³/min)
Streaking agar plate with inoculum from agar colony	0.1
Shaking loopful of culture in test tube	0.5
Inserting hot loop into broth culture in	
Test tube	0.1
250 ml flask	8.7
Inserting cold loop into broth culture in	
250 ml flask	0.8
Pipetting 30 ml culture (1×10^9 cells/ml) into 50 ml centrifuge tube	1.2
Drop of culture falling 30 cm onto	
Stainless steel	49.0
Painted wood	43.0
Dry hand towel	28.0
Hand towel wet with 5% phenol	4.0
Pan of 5% phenol	0.1
Breaking tube during centrifugation	
Cracked but retained in cup (10 ft³ air sample)	4.0
Shattered and culture spilled into chamber (10 ft³ air sample)	1183.0
Removing 1 cotton plug after centrifuging (2 ft³ air sample)	2.3
Removing 30 ml supernatant	
Decanting 1 tube into flask	17.6
Siphoning 30 ml supernatant from each of 10 tubes	3.0
Adding 30 ml saline to 1 tube packed centrifuged cells and resuspending by mixing through alternate sucking and blowing with pipet	4.5
Bursting film in inoculating loop	0.2
Placing inoculum for plate count in Petri dish with pipet and blowing out last drop	3.8

[*]Adapted from Reitman and Phillips[7,8] and Reitman and Wedum.[9]

Table 69-4. Types of laboratory accidents causing 703 laboratory-associated infections[*]

Type of accident	Percent
Spill/splatter	27
Syringe/needle	25
Broken glass/sharp object	16
Animal-related	14
Pipet	13
Other	5

[*]Adapted from Pike.[4]

fire extinguishers, the type of extinguisher and the type of fire for which it is intended, and the location of emergency showers. On completion of the indoctrination, it is the responsibility of management to discipline personnel who either blatantly ignore the regulations or inadvertently jeopardize co-workers by not performing routine tasks as quickly as possible. A meaningful program is one that is monitored and enforced.

From the compilation of laboratory accidents resulting in infections (Table 69-4), Pike deduced that the greatest single source of laboratory infections was the spill or splatter type of accident: the dropping of a flask or a culture tube and the breaking of a container of dried material and contamination of the worker or work area by infected tissues.

The second most common accident involved the syringe and needle. Such accidents included not only the penetration of the skin by the needle but also contamination when the needle separated from the syringe. Injuries were inflicted by broken glass and sharp objects during autopsies on both animals and humans. Infections were also transmitted by animal bites and the bites of insect vectors. Not surprising was the finding that aspiration of infectious material through the pipet was responsible for 13% of the documented laboratory-incurred infections. Had Pike's study been limited exclusively to the clinical microbiology laboratory, accidents occurring during autopsies and through animal bites would probably have been less frequent. Nevertheless, the general categories of laboratory accidents are applicable to average clinical laboratory circumstances.

Spills and splatter

Little can be done to prevent the inadvertent spilling or dropping of viable cultures in the laboratory. In research laboratories where highly infectious agents are studied, the pathogenic agent is physically separated from personnel by erecting maximun containment facilities. In these circumstances the microbial agent is placed in a sealed chamber, and the investigator either manipulates the culture mechanically through a glass partition or enters the chamber in a sealed suit, the internal suit environment of which is supplied from the "clean" area. For the Marburg virus or the Lassa fever virus, such precautions

Essentially a safety program developed in the microbiology laboratory provides for the control of one or more of these factors.

SAFETY REGULATIONS IN MICROBIOLOGY LABORATORY

The task of developing laboratory safety regulations must not be taken lightly. The rules imposed on laboratory workers must be both realistic and recognizably beneficial. The imposition of idealistic regulations that impair or disrupt the routine performance of duties encourages employees to selectively ignore regulations that they feel are irrational. However, once regulations have been developed and approved, management is responsible for providing written copies of the regulations to every individual and for training employees until they understand the rules. Every employee should be aware of the nearest fire exit and should know the location of are advisable and, in fact, imperative. In the average clinical laboratory such precautions are unnecessary, and class I (negative pressure) or class II (laminar flow) biological safety cabinets provide sufficient containment capabilities to satisfy safety requirements for working with the organisms encountered. A chemical fume hood is not acceptable for use with infectious agents.

Nevertheless, the dangers presented by the spilling or dropping of a routine culture should not be underestimated, nor should the response be too casual. Work areas where spills occur should be decontaminated immediately. The area of the spill should be flooded with a strong (0.5-1.0%) hypochlorite solution. Household bleach contains a 5% solution sodium hypochlorite, and therefore rubber gloves should be used when a 1:5 or 1:10 dilution is applied. In small-scale spills the hypochlorite solution can be applied from a spray bottle. At the end of each working day in which potentially infectious material has been handled, the workbench surface should be washed thoroughly with the strong solution. For cleaning corrodible surfaces, 2% buffered glutaraldehyde may prove preferable to hypochlorite.

Dropping a flask culture is particularly hazardous because of the initial aerosol generated. The room should be evacuated for at least 10 minutes to allow the larger aerosol particles to settle and for ventilation and air exchange to dilute the aerosolized particles. Those personnel in close proximity to the accident should be restricted in their movements outside the contaminated area until soiled clothing has been removed and placed in a disinfecting solution.

Centrifuge

Centrifuge accidents are generally of 2 types: the breaking of a tube producing a potentially infectious aerosol or lacerations or breaks from being struck by rotor blades. The breakage of tubes in the centrifuge can constitute a significant hazard to laboratory personnel. Reitman and Phillips[8] reported that when the shattered tube or bottle collapsed down into the trunnion cups, few aerosolized bacteria were released into the laboratory environment. However, loss of the culture into the centrifuge chamber releases large numbers of bacteria into the laboratory air. Some alternatives for circumventing this problem are available. In some laboratories the large centrifuges are placed together in one room, thus removing the danger of an infectious aerosol from the work area and also allowing more efficient and economical utilization of equipment. Before the centrifuge is used, all tubes should be inspected for cracks. The interior of the trunnion cups should be checked for materials that might crack the tubes. The bottoms of the trunnion cups should be checked for the presence of rubber cushions, which should be clean and free of bits of glass or abrasive materials. Trunnion cups with screw caps are prefer-

able for spinning down infectious materials, and this type of cup must be used for centrifuging specimens possibly containing mycobacteria.

If a tube is broken in an open trunnion, the centrifuge should be turned off, personnel removed from the room, and the area left unattended for at least 10 minutes until the aerosol has settled and ventilation and air exchange have reduced the inhalation hazard. Appropriate supervisory personnel should be informed of the accident immediately so that suitable decontamination procedures can be expedited. The interior of the centrifuge chamber should be washed in 2% glutaraldehyde and removable parts left to soak in the solution. After an hour the interior walls and parts should be washed with distilled water.

Laboratory workers sometimes reach into the centrifuge chamber to hurry deceleration of the rotor. When one considers that this rotor is spinning in excess of 1000 rpm and that, even at maximum power, an airplane propeller may approach only 2500 rpm, it is obvious that this practice constitutes a wanton disrespect for safety.

Syringe and needle

Whenever a needle and syringe are used to collect or transfer infectious material, a laboratory accident can occur. The separation of the needle from the syringe can result in leakage of the material and, quite often, in production of an aerosol. A needle-locking hypodermic syringe should be used any time that infectious material is involved.

Little can be done to prevent needle stab wounds in the laboratory other than to stress that needles must be handled very carefully. Disposable needles should not be tossed loosely into discard pans containing glassware that must be retrieved; they should be separated from the syringe and stabbed into a cork before they are sterilized. Reusable needles should be separated from the syringe with forceps and placed carefully into a Petri dish or beaker for sterilization. In the event of a puncture wound by a contaminated needle, the area around the wound should be squeezed until blood is forced to flow freely. This initial reduction in inoculum may aid the body in warding off an infection. An appropriate disinfectant should be applied to the wound.

Pipet

Most laboratory infections associated with the pipet are due to aspiration of liquid rather than inhalation of aerosol. The practice of mouth pipetting should no longer be tolerated in the laboratory. A variety of other pipetting devices are available commercially (Fig. 69-1). Although early models of these devices were cumbersome, slow, and difficult to manipulate, a number of recently marketed pipetting devices do not have these disadvantages. In addition, for some uses, e.g., mixing serum dilutions in serologic titra-

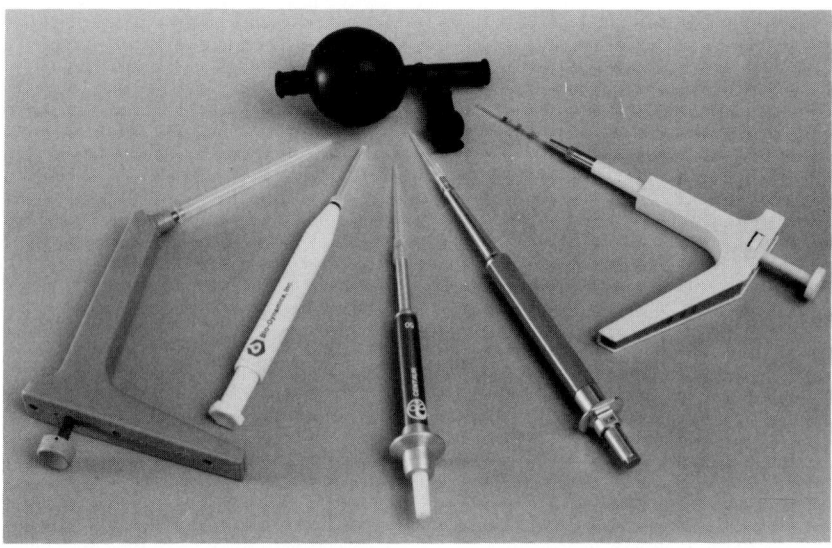

Fig. 69-1. Pipetting devices that have proven to be accurate, rapid, and easy to manipulate under routine laboratory conditions. At top: Spectroline Pipette Filler (Spectronics Corp., Westbury, N.Y.). Left to right: Selectopette (Clay-Adams, Division of Becton, Dickinson & Co., Parsippany, N.J.), Biodynamics Automatic Pipette (Bio-Dynamics, Indianapolis, Ind.), Centaur Pipette (Centaur Chemical Co., Stamford, Conn.), MLA Precision Pipette (Medical Laboratory Automation, Mt. Vernon, N.Y.), and Micro-Selectopette (Clay-Adams, Division of Becton, Dickinson & Co., Parsippany, N.J.).

tions, these devices are superior to the old practice of mouth pipetting.

In selecting a pipetting device with disposable glass or plastic tips, an important consideration is the manner in which the contaminated tip must be removed from the device. Some devices have been designed to automatically eject the used tip into a disinfecting solution so that the tip does not have to be pulled free by hand. Regardless of the pipetting device selected, in transferring, mixing, and dispensing infectious materials the workers must be careful not to create aerosols by the too vigorous and forceful ejection of the material from the device.

Eye protection

Good safety practices dictate that suitable protective eye and face equipment be used when there is a reasonable probability of injury from flying objects, glare, liquids, injurious radiation, or a combination of these factors. For more hazardous operations a face shield should be used.

Contact lenses do not provide eye protection. The capillary space between the contact lens and the cornea may trap material present on the surface of the eye. Chemicals trapped in this space cannot be washed off the surface of the cornea. Contact lenses must not be worn by persons exposed to hazardous chamicals unless goggles or plastic face masks or both are also worn. It is the responsibility of supervisors to identify employees who wear contact lenses.

Supplies of caustic chemicals, i.e., ammonia solution, liquid phenol, strong bases, acids, etc.,

should not be stored higher than counter-top level to minimize the possibility of facial and upper-body burns in the event that they are spilled or their containers are broken. It is also good practice to use the smallest container compatible with the need.

Plastic eye-wash bottles currently available from many laboratory supply firms do not meet the standards of the Occupational Safety and Health Administration (OSHA) or the Joint Commission for Accreditation of Hospitals (JCAH) for emergency eye-wash facilities. Two major problems are associated with these bottles: the quantity of the water supply and the distinct possibility that the water supply in these wash bottles may be contaminated with bacteria. Growth of various gram-negative bacteria, including *Pseudomonas* species, in distilled water has been well documented in many instances. These organisms can be present in concentrations up to 10^7 bacteria/ml without producing visible turbidity. The use of such colonized water on corneal and conjunctival tissues that are already traumatized significantly increases the risk of superimposing a bacterial infection.

Both the OSHA safety and health standards and the JCAH accreditation standards state that facilities for quick drenching or flushing the eyes and body with large quantities of water should be provided within or near the work area in which injurious corrosive, caustic, or toxic materials are used. An adequate quantity of water is defined as a sufficient amount to flush the eyes or body for 15 continuous minutes. Most eye-wash bottles contain less than a 1-minute supply of water.

General laboratory practices

Because of the nature of the laboratory environment, certain practices cannot be condoned. Storing edibles in laboratory refrigerators or freezers and consuming food in the work area are dangerous practices. A dining area should be available to the laboratory staff in the "clean" area of the laboratory. Outer garments worn when laboratory procedures are performed should not be worn into the clean area, and the use of washroom facilities before a clean area is entered should be encouraged.

Long hair in the laboratory can be dangerous, particularly around open flames, and invariably it must be brushed aside by hands that have handled infectious material. While working in the laboratory, persons with long hair should wear it in such a manner as not to constitute a hazard.

Considerable confusion exists about using refrigerators to store flammable solvents. A flammable solvent is defined as a liquid substance having a flash point below 140 F and having a vapor pressure not exceeding 40 psi at 100 F. Therefore in many cases it is better to store them on well-ventilated open shelves. A refrigerator provides a cold, relatively safe place to keep some kinds of solvents provided the internal wiring of the refrigerator has been modified to make it safe for storing flammable solvents and provided the flash point of the solvent is above the temperature of the refrigerator. Ethyl ether, for example, has a flash point of −40 F and should not be kept even in modified refrigerators. There are other disadvantages to refrigerator storage. Cold solvents pick up atmospheric moisture much faster when opened than do those kept at ambient temperature. It is recommended that only the smallest volumes of flammable solvents compatible with the immediate needs of the laboratory be stored in the laboratory. All volumes of flammable solvents greater than 2 L should be stored in cabinets that meet the specifications of the National Fire Protection Association (NFPA). When the cumulative amount of flammable solvents in one laboratory room exceeds 7.5 L, the solvents should be removed to an appropriate storage cabinet.

Wedum[10] has prepared the following excellent list of laboratory regulations applicable to most laboratory situations in which infectious agents are involved.

1. Never pipet infectious or toxic fluids by mouth.
2. Plug pipets with cotton.
3. Do not blow infectious material out of pipets.
4. Do not mix infectious material by bubbling expiratory air through liquid by pipet.
5. Use alcohol-soaked pledget around stopper and needle when removing syringe and needle from rubber-stoppered bottle.
6. Use only needle-locking hypodermic syringes.
7. Expel excessive fluid and bubbles from syringe vertically into cotton pledget soaked with disinfectant or into small bottle of cotton.
8. Before and after injecting an animal, swab site of injection with disinfectant.
9. Sterilize discarded pipets and syringes in pan in which they were first placed after use.
10. Before centrifuging, inspect tubes for cracks. Inspect inside of trunnion cup for rough walls caused by erosion or adhering matter. Carefully remove all bits of glass from rubber cushion. Germicidal solution added between tube and trunnion cup not only disinfects both surfaces, but also provides cushion against shocks that otherwise might break tube.
11. Use centrifuge trunnion cups with screw caps or equivalent.
12. Avoid decanting centrifuge tubes. If you must decant, subsequently wipe off outer rim with disinfectant. Avoid filling tube to point that rim becomes wet with culture.
13. Wrap lyophilized culture vial with disinfectant-wetted cotton before breaking it open.
14. Make sure that discarded infectious material is easily identified as such or is sterilized immediately.
15. Sterilize all contaminated discard material.
16. Periodically clean deep freeze and dry ice chests in which cultures are stored to remove any broken ampules or tubes. Use rubber gloves and respiratory protection during this cleaning.
17. Use rubber gloves when handling diagnostic serum specimens posing risk of infectious hepatitis.
18. Develop habit of keeping your hands away from your mouth, nose, eyes, and face. This may prevent self-inoculation.
19. Avoid smoking, eating, and drinking in laboratory.
20. Make special precautionary arrangements for oral, intranasal, and intratracheal inoculation of infectious materials.
21. Use operating room gowns that fasten at back when available.
22. When there is danger of hand contamination because of procedure or agent used, wear gloves or use forceps.
23. Wear only clean laboratory clothing in dining room, library, etc.
24. Shake broth cultures in manner that avoids wetting plug or cap.

Postaccident surveillance

While the major objective of a safety program is to prevent accidents, the action taken after an accident is also of critical importance. The supervisor is the key to a postaccident follow-up. Of immediate concern should be the comfort and well-being of any injured personnel. The supervisor should be trained in first-aid technics or have immediate access to trained medical personnel. An immediate course of action should be initiated to treat burns from fire or from corrosive substances. All personnel should be able to locate eye-wash bottles, emergency showers, and fire extinguishers without hesitation. Personnel exposed to infectious agents must be removed from the probable contaminated area until aerosols have settled or dissipated. Their contaminated clothing and footwear should be collected and disinfected and the personnel exposed should be restricted to a limited area until the severity of the accident is assessed. The supervisor should direct the clean-up operation and disinfection of the affected area. The director of the laboratory should be notified of the accident as soon as possible after it occurs.

Once the immediate emergency has been resolved, the supervisor should determine precisely when, where, and how the accident occurred. Notes should be recorded immediately, before small but critical facts are overlooked and forgotten. In instances involving biologic agents, the supervisor must determine the type of material involved in the accident and, if at all possible, the probable agent or agents to which the personnel were exposed. Susceptibility patterns should be determined by searching the routine workup on the organism involved in the accident or if need be by performing susceptibility testing for future reference. On subsequent days all personnel exposed to the potentially infectious agent should be placed under discreet surveillance to determine whether any illnesses can be associated with the accident. Unexcused absences or requests for sick leave should be noted by the supervisor and the laboratory director should be given periodic reports of any illness or injury that might be attributable to the accident. All information concerning the accident and pertinent recommendations should be forwarded to those individuals charged with the administration of the laboratory safety program.

BIOSAFETY AND CONTROL OF DISCARD MATERIALS

Although the primary mission of the laboratory is to aid the physician in diagnosing pathologic disorders, responsibility to the community for the containment of disease entities within the laboratory cannot be overlooked.

The handling of discarded materials poses a threat to laboratory staff members, particularly cleaning service personnel, and to the surrounding community. Inevitably, service personnel without technical training will handle dirty and contaminated glassware and materials and will retrieve and clean reusable items. Laboratory management is responsible for developing a system to protect these personnel and to assure that hazardous materials are disinfected or sterilized before the retrievable items are cleaned or the discarded ones are removed from the premises. The practice of dumping discarded laboratory material into sanitary landfills without sterilizing it is not recommended or justifiable. The retrievable equipment and disposable materials should be separated at the bench immediately after they are used. This can be achieved readily by placing appropriate pans of different sizes, colors, or labels at the bench for glassware, pipets, and disposable items. This routine sorting of used materials by the technical staff keeps service personnel from being needlessly exposed to possible infection. The pans must be inspected for pinholes or leaks before being distributed to the laboratory. This can be achieved by inverting the pans and totally immersing them upside down in a deep sink filled with water. Pans that leak a stream of air bubbles should be discarded or repaired.

Lids of all bottles, test tubes, and vials should be loosened before they are placed in the discard pan to allow steam to reach all surfaces during autoclaving. Reusable needles and syringes should be placed in a container used exclusively for their retrieval to reduce the risk of stab wounds during sorting operations. Syringe plungers and the barrels should be carefully separated so that steam can come in contact with all surfaces, and both should be totally immersed in water as soon as possible after use to prevent material from drying on surfaces. Approximately 2.5 cm water should be added to all discard pans containing bottles or tubes before they are taken from the laboratory to be autoclaved. This additional liquid in the pan provides sufficient moisture during the late stages of the autoclave cycle to assure that residual solid material does not bake on the surface of the glassware and impede cleaning of the glassware. The discard containers should be tagged with an indicator tape that changes color and verifies that the pan and its contents have been sterilized.

A recent innovation in the handling of disposable contaminated materials has been the use of the autoclavable plastic bag. However, the autoclavable bag is not without its limitations. In quality control studies of these bags, it was found that in some of them, especially the tightly closed bags, the steam failed to penetrate the plastic cover and as a result bacterial spores survived. To be effectively sterilized all contents of the bag must be exposed to the steam. An additional hazard of plastic bags is that infectious materials may leak through breaks or tears caused by slides, applicator sticks, and plastic implements. If plastic bags are used, sterilization procedures must be strictly monitored.

Incineration of infected animals is recommended. It is advisable, however, to autoclave small animals infected with highly virulent organisms for an extended time (about 1 hour) before they are placed in a plastic bag and then transported to the incinerator.

When there is no reasonable evidence to indicate that clinical specimens or other materials may contain an infectious agent, the materials can be discarded into the municipal sewer system without sterilization. Materials that may be discarded directly into the sanitary sewer include (1) uninoculated liquid media, tissue cultures, and nutrient fluids; and (2) serum, plasma, or blood (provided that the specimens are not believed to contain any agent that might not otherwise enter the sanitary sewer system).

SAFETY COMMITTEE

Successful safety programs do not just happen, nor are they invoked by administrative edict. While the responsibility for enforcement and regulation of the safety program rests ultimately with the laboratory director, the program must be developed by individuals specifically charged with this responsibility, i.e., the safety committee. The safety committee should be representative of the various scientific disciplines and services within the laboratory, including the clerical staff and central services (i.e., reagent and media preparation, janitorial services, glassware cleaning, and animal caretakers). In many laboratory situations potentially infectious materials are received, opened, and logged into the laboratory by members of the clerical staff who have little understanding of the hazards of the operation. It is ironic that the disposal of infectious cultures and contaminated glassware is often delegated to service personnel with no technical training. It is imperative therefore that these groups have a voice in the development of laboratory safety policies. The presiding officer of the safety committee should serve in the official role as safety officer and be directly responsible to the director of the laboratory.

The safety committee has 4 major functions:

1. Prevention of accidents and establishment of health safeguards
2. Investigation of every reported laboratory accident to establish cause
3. Monitoring and surveillance of personnel with excessive sick leave absenteeism
4. Recommendation of remedial actions

It is the responsibility of the safety committee to develop regulations that are applicable to the specific needs of the laboratory. However, such regulations require periodic review and reassessment, and new regulations should be developed when needed. By immediate investigation of laboratory accidents, the safety committee can assess the effectiveness of current regulations. The abuse of a particular safety regulation, as evidenced by recurring accident reports, may indicate a need for more strict enforcement or a renewed training program. As the result of a particular accident, a new laboratory hazard requiring the development of corrective measures may be revealed. Through regularly scheduled training sessions, employees must be made aware of the problem, acquainted with the newly established laboratory policy, and observed to see that they adhere to the new regulation.

Reacting to documented accidents or to probable exposures to infectious agents that are reported from within the laboratory is not difficult. The challenge is to anticipate a hazardous condition before it becomes recorded history. The employee must be encouraged to report probable sources of danger.

The most difficult problem facing the safety committee is the detection of possible laboratory-associated infections in members of the staff. Problems related to this responsibility are discussed above.

Absenteeism is a serious drain on laboratory resources, both economically and physically. However, chronic and recurring absenteeism among staff members engaged in a particular activity or discipline may serve as an indication of a laboratory safety problem. The safety committee should constantly review records of injury and sick leave, and if there are recurring infections among staff members, the appropriate supervisor should be notified of the suspicious nature of this evidence. The committee should scrutinize activities and procedures within the affected group or discipline closely and make sure that conformance to the established protocol is followed. When a hazard is detected, corrective action must be initiated. Periodically thereafter, the adequacy of the committee action must be substantiated by an obvious alleviation of the problem.

In summary, laboratory safety must be a mutual endeavor of both management and staff working together through a committee that represents the interests and needs of the laboratory personnel. It is only through the efforts of a group which is directly involved and specifically charged with this responsibility that a meaningful safety program can be achieved.

REFERENCES

1. Phillips, G. B., and Jemski, J. V.: Lab. Anim. Sci. **13**(1):13, 1963.
2. Chatigny, M. A.: Adv. Appl. Microbiol. **3**:1, 1961.
3. Lab safety at the Center for Disease Control, DHEW Publication no. CDC-75-8118, Atlanta, 1974, Office of Biosafety, Center for Disease Control, pt. II, pp. 23, 26, 38, 40.
4. Pike, R. M.: Health Lab. Sci. **13**:105, 1976.
5. Sulkin, S. E., and Pike, R. M.: Am. J. Public Health **41**:780, 1951.
6. Reitman, M.: Am. J. Med. Technol. **22**:12, 1956.
7. Reitman, M., and Phillips, G. B.: Am. J. Med. Technol. **21**:338, 1955.
8. Reitman, M., and Phillips, G. B.: Am. J. Med. Technol. **22**:14, 1956.
9. Reitman, M., and Wedum, A. G.: Public Health Rep. **71**(7):659, 1956.
10. Wedum, A. G.: Bacteriol. Rev. **25**:210, 1961.

70

BACTERIOLOGIC METHODS

Alex C. Sonnenwirth

CLEANING OF GLASSWARE

All glassware used in bacteriologic work must be cleaned adequately before use. The presence of free alkali (occasionally given off by certain types of new glassware), grease, and coagulated protein as well as any trace of detergents will interfere with the successful cultivation of bacteria.

All contaminated glassware and contents (specimens, used culture media, etc.) must be sterilized in the autoclave before cleaning. After sterilization discard any medium or other foreign matter from the glassware, then proceed with cleaning and washing. Mechanical glassware washing machines are available in several varieties and are extremely useful. Pipet washing is best done in an automatic pipet washer, utilizing the siphon principle.

Procedure

1. Remove all dirt, grease, or coagulated proteins from glassware by using stiff brushes. It is often necessary to soak glassware containing coagulated proteins in a protein-digesting detergent for 18-24 h before washing.
2. Wash all glassware with water and soap or good detergent cleaner (Alconox or similar product). For machine washing, use detergent recommended by manufacturer. If glassware remains dirty, boiling it in detergent or soap solution may be necessary. If this is done, do not permit water to dry on glassware.
3. After washing, rinse glassware several times with running hot and cold water to remove all traces of detergent or soap. Detergent or soap must be completely removed before heat sterilization (autoclave or dry heat oven); otherwise glassware may become coated with white precipitate that is difficult, if not impossible, to remove.
4. Wash with distilled water, employing 3 rinses.
5. Allow glassware to drain and dry it in a low-temperature (80-90 C) dry heat oven in an inverted position.

Although the use of **dichromate–sulfuric acid cleaning solution** has been advocated for many years, to use it at all times is unnecessary. It is most often used for pipets and other glassware employed in biochemical and serologic procedures. Some workers prefer to soak new glassware in 1% hydrochloric acid for 2-3 hours to remove alkali from the glass. If this procedure is used, the glassware should be first washed with detergent, rinsed well, and then placed in the 1% HCl solution. Afterward, rinse several times in hot and cold tap water, followed by 3 rinses of distilled water.

If mechanical glassware washing machine is used, it is imperative to follow directions of the manufacturer regarding washing and rinsing procedures. New slides should be washed in detergent, then rinsed as other glassware. Afterward immerse in 95% alcohol and dry with an old linen cloth. The cloth must be free of lint. Used slides are best discarded; however, if they are to be reused, clean with an abrasive soap before washing with a detergent. Precleaned slides are available commercially.

PLASTIC LABORATORY PRODUCTS

Within the last decade a large variety of useful plastic laboratory products became available. Some of these are intended for single use (disposables) and are generally sold presterilized in sealed, sterile packages; others withstand repeated autoclaving and can be reused. There is little doubt about the convenience and labor-saving aspects of disposable labware (Petri dishes, pipets, small test tubes, evacuated specimen collection tubes), and their availability has been of great help, especially to smaller laboratories faced with a shortage of trained help. Cost and availability of storage space still present problems. Disposable, presterilized Petri dishes have been universally accepted due to their greatly reduced cost versus autoclaving and washing of individual glass dishes. Many other products such as disposable reagent bottles, culture tubes, supports, beakers, etc., are used, depending on the facilities and needs of the individual laboratory.

Disposable plastic products are usually sterilized by ethylene oxide, dry heat, tyndallization, or ionizing radiation in a linear accelerator, depending on their heat stability. Disposables manufactured of **polyethylenes** (polymers of ethylene), **polystyrene,** and **cellulose nitrate** cannot be autoclaved or subjected to intense heat.

The major factor to be considered in the use of disposable, **presterilized** products is the adequacy of the manufacturer's sterility control procedures, since not too many laboratories are equipped or prepared to run periodic sterility checks on these products. The reputable manufacturer will test each product lot and will package the sterilized product in moisture-resistant paper or polyester film. Products for parenteral use (syringes, needles, tubing) should also have been tested for acute and chronic toxicity, pyrogenicity, skin reactivity, and tissue sensitivity. Prepackaged and presterilized products remain sterile for at least 1 year (or longer), **provided that the package remains intact.** Should the seal or package be broken, the product can no longer be regarded sterile. It is recommended that lot numbers of presterilized products used be recorded to allow for checking in case of problems.

Reusable plastic products are usually made of **polypropylene** (polymers of propylene) and **polycarbonate;** nylon and polytetrafluoroethylene (Teflon) are also used. These withstand autoclaving and include items such as centrifuge tubes (both high-speed and screw-capped types), cylinders, pipets, tubing, etc. Many available and widely used products are reusable but **not** autoclavable: bottles, beakers, carboys, wash bottles, flasks, etc. These are used when sterility is not required (mostly polyethylene ware, unbreakable and lightweight).

Various physical properties and the chemical resistance of the above-listed materials must also be considered before use.

Opaque: polyethylene, nylon, Teflon
Translucent: polypropylenes
Clear: polystyrene, polycarbonate, cellulose nitrate

The effect of laboratory reagents (acids, alkalies, organic solvents) on these materials varies widely and should be carefully ascertained before use. Polyethylene tubes and bottles can be used for freezer storage to −50 C and polycarbonates to −100 C; however, polypropylenes are not recommended for freezer applications. The laboratory worker using plastic ware should be familiar with the limitation(s) of the product and should use it according to the manufactuuer's instructions.

STERILIZATION

In this section a brief outline of sterilization methods is given, together with some details on the use of the autoclave as well as various filters.

For a considerably more detailed treatment of sterilization methods and their quality control, as well as disinfection and antisepsis, see Chapter 89.

Sterilization is defined as a process that completely destroys all types of microbial life, including bacteria and spores (and viruses). It differs from **disinfection,** a procedure that may remove a large number of susceptible organisms, thereby reducing the capacity to cause infection, but usually will not destroy resistant organisms such as bacterial and fungal spores, tubercle bacilli, enteroviruses, and hepatitis viruses.

For bacteriologic work involving the isolation, progagation, and maintenance of pure cultures, sterile containers, glassware, instruments, and culture media are absolutely essential. Adequate knowledge of proper sterilization procedures is therefore indispensable for those working in the bacteriology laboratory.

There are 2 major groups of methods whereby sterilization can be achieved—chemical and physical methods.

Chemical methods

Although a variety of chemicals is widely used as "sterilizing" agents, in reality they are either disinfectants or antiseptics.[1] Chemicals used to disinfect inanimate objects (instruments, floors, furniture) are known as "disinfectants" ("germicides"), whereas those used for disinfection of living tissue (e.g., body surfaces) are termed "antiseptics." The majority of chemical disinfectants are toxic and therefore cannot be used on living tissue. Since most of them kill only vegetative cells and have no effect on spores, they cannot be considered sterilizing agents. Of the large variety of chemical disinfectants such as iodine, chlorine compounds, alcohols, aldehydes, phenols, quaternary ammonium compounds, mercurials, and gaseous disinfectants (ethylene oxide and β-propiolactone), only a very few are sporicidal: (1) glutaraldehyde, related to formaldehyde; (2) a combination of 70% isopropyl alcohol and 8% formaldehyde, called Bard-Parker germicide; (3) ethylene oxide; and (4) β-propiolactone.

Some of the agents listed are widely used in the laboratory, mainly for disinfection of workbenches and other surfaces as well as for the temporary storage of contaminated materials such as glassware and swabs. Among these are the quaternary ammonium compounds ("quats")—the main shortcoming of which is their ineffectiveness against tubercle bacilli—the phenolic compounds, and the iodophores (iodine complexed with nonionic detergents). The phenolics and the iodophores are effective against tubercle bacilli when used in the proper concentration. Other agents are utilized as preservatives, e.g., sodium ethylmercurithiosalicylate (Merthiolate) in 1:10,000 dilution is used to preserve various sera. Finally, thymol, a crystalline phenol, can be used for the sterilization of certain thermolabile culture ingredients (see sterilization of media).

Among the gaseous compounds, ethylene oxide is widely used in various commercial processes for sterilization of many materials, and it is also used in hospitals for sterilizing such items as may be damaged by heat (rubber and plastic materials, mattresses, etc.). Some attempts were made to utilize ethylene oxide in the laboratory as a sterilizing agent; however, its usefulness is limited and it is not used in the laboratory.

For further details on disinfection and antiseptics see Chapter 89.

Physical methods

Physical methods of sterilization include radiation, filtration, and heat.

Radiation

Ultraviolet light is bactericidal beginning at the wavelength of 333 nm and increasing in bactericidal effectiveness at lower wavelengths. Low-pressure mercury vapor lamps produce intense ultraviolet light (250-260 nm). Such "germicidal" lamps have been found effective in reducing the number of airborne bacteria in surgical operating rooms, infectious animal quarters, and laboratories in which highly infectious material is handled. It is recommended that areas of the laboratory in which tuberculosis work is carried out should be equipped with such ultraviolet lamps.

Ionizing radiation (x-rays, beams of high-speed electrons such as cathode rays, β-rays of radioactive substances, and various other high-energy particles produced by accelerators) is lethal to all cells—including bacteria and spores—when used in sufficient dosage. Industry has made considerable use of this killing effect by applying it to the sterilization of disposable items that cannot withstand heat. However, ionizing radiation is too cumbersome and expensive for use in the clinical laboratory.

Filtration

This method is used for sterilization of various solutions that cannot tolerate the high temperatures employed in heat sterilization, such as media containing labile carbohydrates or other culture ingredients, antibiotic solutions, and sera. Sterilization is attained by passing the fluid through filters that have pore sizes of 1.0 μm or less and thus retain bacteria. Many types of filters have been devised: various infusorial earths (Berkefeld), unglazed porcelain (Chamberland), compressed asbestos (Seitz), sintered (fritted) glass, and celluose membranes. The asbestos Seitz filter, still used, has the disadvantage of being adsorptive. Instructions for its use are described under sterilization of media. Modifications of the unglazed porcelain filter (Selas) and the sintered glass filters are very effective and absorb little; however, they are expensive and require considerable care.

The earlier type (gradocol) **membrane filters** were prepared from an ether-alcohol solution of collodion (nitrocellulose) and were used mostly for the determination of particle size of viruses and macromolecules. The newer membrane filters are thin porous structures composed of cellulose acetate or mixed esters of cellulose. The pores of these filters are uniform in size; the filters are nonadsorptive and have a much higher flow rate than the conventional filters. A major advantage of the membrane filters is that the bacteria retained on the filter can be subsequently grown by placing the filter in contact with culture media to grow visible colonies on the filter surface. These can then be examined, stained, and counted. Thus they can be used both **for sterilization** and for the **isolation and counting** of bacteria (see below).

The membranes composed of cellulose esters are widely used and are commonly referred to as Millipore filters, since they were first developed by the Millipore Corp. (Bedford, Mass.). Other manufacturers* in the United States and abroad are now also producing similar membrane filters. The Millipore filters are presently available in pore sizes ranging from 14 μm to 10 nm (0.01 μm). The most frequently used types for sterilization are the HA (0.45 μm) and GS (0.22 μm) filters. The 0.22 μm pore size filter will effectively remove all bacteria (but not viruses) from the liquid being filtered.

It should be remembered that fluids do not pass easily through filters by gravity. Therefore it is necessary to apply pressure. Negative pressure (suction) is used most often to draw the solution into a sterile container. In certain instances positive pressure is used to force the material through the filter.

Heat

Sterilization by heat can be accomplished by using either dry heat or moist heat. Dry heat generally requires longer periods of time and higher temperatures for sterilization than moist heat. It is therefore not used for materials that would be charred or otherwise destroyed by high temperatures.

Dry heat

Dry heat can be applied in several forms. **Flaming** is used for sterilizing the mouths of flasks and culture tubes, slides, coverslips, or various instruments, whereas **burning** is used for sterilizing spatulas and inoculating loops by keeping them in the flame of a gas burner until they turn red hot.

The **dry heat oven,** which may be heated by electricity or gas, is used mostly for glassware, metal instruments, and other materials that are heat stable and are required to be dry for use and for storage. Various powders, oils, and petrolatum are also sterilized in the dry heat oven, since they are not penetrated by moisture. Modern ovens usually have a fan or blower to assure the circulation of air and uniform heating. In such ovens sterilization for 1 hour at 160 C is usually recommended. However, for heavy loads in ovens without blower or fan or for oils and powders, 2 hours at 160 C are recommended. It

---

*Gelman Instrument Co., Ann Arbor, Mich.; Oxoid, Ltd., Southwark Bridge Rd., London SE1, England; Schleicher & Schuell, Keene, N.H.

should be remembered that the temperature of the air in the oven must first reach 160 C, as shown by the thermometer, before timing of the 1- or 2-hour period begins. Do not pack oven too tightly with material. Close door tightly before sterilization. After cutting off the heat, be sure not to open the oven until the contents have cooled (at least 1 hour); otherwise the glassware may crack.

Moist heat

The superior effectiveness of moist heat as a sterilizing agent is probably due to the participation of water in the coagulation and denaturation of proteins, the mechanism most likely involved in the killing of microorganisms by moist heat.

Boiling at 100 C, usually for 15-30 minutes, is employed for materials such as metal and glass syringes, instruments used in minor surgery, and rubber goods that cannot withstand higher temperatures. It does **not** ensure total sterility, since some spores may survive as much as 2 hours of boiling.

Complete sterilization is attained by applying moist heat at temperatures above 100 C, by using saturated steam under pressure in the **autoclave** for specified periods of time and temperature (autoclaving). Steam at a pressure of 15 lb/sq in. (psi) above atmospheric pressure has a temperature of 121 C. Even the most resistant spores are killed by steam at 121 C, 15 psi, in 15 minutes, whereas in the dry heat oven, killing of the same spores requires 1 hour at 160 C.

Most media, contaminated glassware, and instruments for major surgery are sterilized in the autoclave, usually at 15 psi, 121 C for 15 minutes (exposure to steam at 132 C, 27 psi will produce sterility in 2 minutes; used only in emergencies).

It is extremely important when using an autoclave that all air be displaced from the autoclave chamber by the flowing steam, since the presence of air results in a lower temperature at a given pressure; air will also settle in the bottom part of the autoclave, forming an unheated layer there. Thus it is imperative in manually operated autoclaves that all the air be allowed to escape before the outlet valve is closed.

A variety of autoclave types are available. The nonjacketed autoclave, containing its own water supply for producing steam, has been replaced by the steam-jacketed type. Some of these are manually operated; others have automatic gravity discharge controls for air and water (steam condensate). Unless the autoclave has an automatic process control system that handles the entire sterilization cycle, it requires the attention of an operator throughout the cycle.

Sterilization in autoclave

General procedure
1. Follow operating instructions of manufacturer.
2. Heat jacket by introducing steam into it at beginning of workday and keep it at 121 C (15 psi) throughout day.

3. Load chamber, close door, and let steam enter chamber. In 10-15 min, all air should be displaced. Check thermometer in **exhaust line** at bottom of sterilizer; steam should register 121 C.
4. Start timing at this point. At end of 15 min (if normal procedure is followed), cut off steam supply to chamber. Cooling begins and pressure goes down.
5. If liquids are sterilized, let cooling proceed for about 15-30 min. When pressure falls to 0 psi, door should be opened. Remove materials after they have cooled in air for about 5 min. If chamber pressure is reduced too rapidly (by opening discharge valve), liquids in chamber will boil over.
6. When contaminated materials (used media) are sterilized, place tubes and plates into deep trays or metal buckets so that melted agar does not clog pipelines.
7. Do not use cork and rubber plugs for glassware sterilized in autoclave. Tubes that are to be closed with rubber stoppers must be sterilized with cotton plugs in autoclave. Sterilize rubber stoppers separately (wrapped in paper or in large test tubes) and exchange them for cotton plugs under sterile precautions after autoclaving.
8. **Disposable plastic Petri dishes** should be autoclaved in trays or buckets, since they melt.

For control measures for the autoclave (e.g., recording thermometer, spore strips, and indicators,[2,*]), see Chapter 73.

Sterilization of glassware

All glassware must be cleaned and sterilized before use. Metal closures, plastic plugs, or nonabsorbent cotton plugs are used for closing tubes. All glassware to be sterilized in the dry heat oven must be completely dry.

Procedure
Metal closures for culture tubes. Metal closures for culture tubes are available; they are economical and are easily manipulated. The Morton closure is made of stainless steel; others, of aluminum.

Screw-capped tubes and flasks. Screw-capped tubes and flasks in various sizes with cap liners that withstand autoclaving are useful for storage of media. Good protection against evaporation is afforded by screw-capped tubes.
1. When empty screw-capped tubes or flasks are sterilized, screw caps on partially to allow air to escape. Sterilize in dry heat oven at 160 C for 2 h.
2. Wrap glass **Petri dishes** in paper or put in metal cans before sterilization.
3. Place loose plug of nonabsorbent cotton in pipets and droppers and wrap in paper before sterilization.
4. Secure paper wrapping at delivery end by folding over, and at mouth end by twirling; use of **metal cans** is also recommended.
5. Keep cans containing sterile pipets in horizontal position at all times. Place some glass wool in bottom of pipet cans to prevent breakage of pipet tips.

---

*Available commercially as Kilit sporestrips or Kilit ampule from BBL, Division of BioQuest, Cockeysville, Md.; Spordex bacterial spore strips from Amercian Sterilizer Co., Erie, Pa.; and Oxoid sporestrips from Oxoid, Ltd., Southwark Bridge Rd., London SE1, England (K.C. Biologicals, Lenexa, Kan. in U.S.).

6. Sterilize clean, dry pipets in dry heat oven at 160 C for 2 h.

Nonabsorbent cotton plugs

1. Separate approximately quadrangular piece of nonabsorbent cotton from roll. Fold 2 sides of this piece inward to about ¼ its width. Firmly roll cotton along longitudinal axis and insert plug by gentle rotation.
2. Protect inner end of cotton plugs for flasks with 1 or 2 layers of gauze or cheesecloth. Cut quadrangular piece of gauze. Put inner end of cotton plug in its middle, then lift corners and insert whole into flask in such a way that neck of flask is not in contact with cotton.
3. Covering plug and neck of bottles with paper and fastening this cover with string around neck is helpful.
4. Sterilize **empty**, plugged test tubes and flasks by dry heat at 160 C for 2 h. Let temperature of oven fall to 100 C before taking out glassware to prevent cracking of nonresistant glass.

Sterilization of media

Heat, filtration, or chemical substances are employed for sterilization of media.

Steam under pressure. Most media are sterilized in the autoclave at temperatures in excess of 100 C. Do not pack the autoclave too tightly, or sterilization will not take place. Cover the plugs of the flasks with wrapping paper tied with a string around the necks of the flasks. Sterilize test tubes standing in racks, with the exception of media containing eggs or serum or other coagulable substances. These must be slanted during sterilization.

Different **media** require differing pressures for various lengths of time. It is essential not to oversterilize because the media suffer by prolonged or too intensive heating. The length of time necessary for sterilization also varies with the amount of media in the flasks. It is essential that baskets not be packed too tightly with tubes. Screw caps of bottles should be applied loosely.

It is important that the autoclave not be exhausted, but that the steam pressure be allowed to drop slowly. The best method is to shut off the steam immediately after sterilization and to allow the autoclave to cool. The media are taken out when the temperature has dropped to 30 C or lower and the steam pressure in the chamber is equal to that outside. Tighten screw caps firmly.

Flowing steam. Flowing steam is produced by leaving the door of the autoclave ajar. Carefully watching the thermometer is necessary to be certain that the inside of the autoclave reaches the proper temperature. The temperature may vary in different parts of the inner chamber, depending upon the location of the steam inlets. Media sterilized by flowing steam must be exposed to the steam for 30 minutes on 3 successive days; between these periods the media are kept at room temperature to allow spores that are **not** killed by the flowing steam to germinate. The vegetative bacteria are readily killed by the steam. This technic of fractional sterilization is known as **tyndallization.** The procedure is not

employed often; its use is restricted to media such as milk or others that may be damaged by autoclave sterilization.

Inspissation. Inspissation is the coagulation of media containing proteins (mostly serum or eggs). To obtain a smooth surface of the tubed media, great care must be exerted. Some laboratories use special inspissators; others perform this task in the autoclave. In the latter case slant the tubes on a tray or rack and cover with newspaper. Then close the exhaust and the air outlet valve. Lock the door and let steam in slowly, to 15 psi. After 10 minutes slightly open the air outlet so that the pressure remains constant between 14.75 and 15.25 psi. Sterilize for 20 minutes more; then shut off the steam and let the autoclave cool before opening the door.

Filtration. Certain media cannot be subjected to the very high temperatures used in autoclaving or treating with flowing steam. Various carbohydrate solutions, serum, ascitic fluid, urea, and some others must be sterilized without using heat. For such materials, filtration is employed.

Seitz filter. Seitz filter makes use of asbestos pads for removal of bacteria from liquids during filtration process. Asbestos filters are disk shaped and vary in size and in grades of porosity. For bacterial work specify E. K. grade of porosity when ordering the disks.

1. To use Seitz filter, assemble apparatus by fitting asbestos disk into special metal container.
2. Below asbestos disk place metal screen that comes with apparatus.
3. Place screen and disks in metal container and then tighten by means of set screws.
4. Cover metal container with asbestos in place with tinfoil, then fit tightly into opening of 1-hole rubber stopper that is placed in a Pyrex filtering flask.
5. Plug arm of filtering flask with nonabsorbent cotton and sterilize whole apparatus in autoclave at 15 psi for 30 min.
6. Attach apparatus as assembled to vacuum pump.
7. When filtration begins, if there is foaming around asbestos disk simply tighten screws that hold it in metal shield.
8. After use either burn or autoclave and then discard disks.

Membrane filter. As described above there are now several manufacturers of membrane filters. For the use of each type of filter, it is essential that the manufacturer's instructions are followed. Millipore and other membrane filters are preferable to the Seitz filter because they are less adsorptive (Fig. 70-1). The Swinny filter* is of considerable help in sterilizing small amounts of solutions. The filter holder attaches to any syringe having Luer fittings. The filter is placed into the filter holder, and the unit is autoclaved. The material to be filtered is drawn into the syringe, and the sterile filter holder unit is attached. A sterile hypodermic needle is attached to outlet of the unit. By applying pressure to the syringe plunger, the material is forced through the filter into a sterile container (Fig.

---

*Swinny filter holder, stainless steel, for small volumes; microsyringe filter holder, for volumes of 10-50 ml; Swinnex disposable filter unit, presterilized, available from Millipore Corp.

70-2). For sterilizing larger volumes, the Millipore Sterifil system or stainless pressure filter holder should be used; with proper precautions the Teflon-treated Millipore Pyrex filter holder or the Hydrosol stainless filter holder can also be used.

NOTE: Membrane filters from various manufacturers have been found to contain detergents, representing 2-3% of the filters' dry weight, necessary for efficiency of filtration and to allow autoclaving of the filters. Cahn[3]

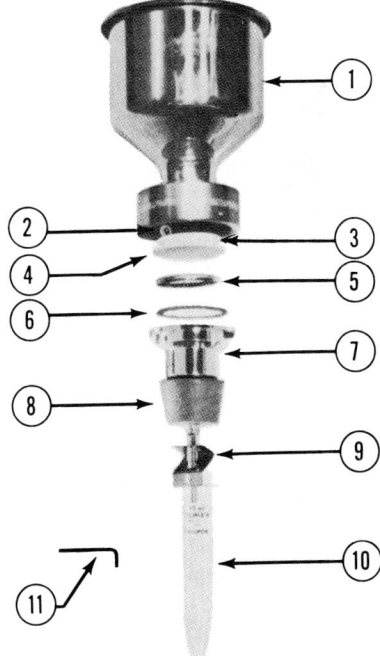

Fig. 70-1. Exploded view of stainless steel holder (Hydrosol) for membrane filtration. *1,* Stainless steel funnel and aluminum locking ring assembly; *2,* nylon lockwheels; *3,* prefilter; *4,* Millipore filter; *5,* stainless steel support screen assembly; *6,* Teflon flat gasket; *7,* stainless steel base with support screen, gasket, and stopper; *8,* neoprene stopper; *9,* centrifuge tube holder, stainless steel; *10,* centrifuge tube; *11,* Allen wrench. (Courtesy Millipore Corp., Bedford, Mass.)

demonstrated a toxic effect of eluates from unwashed filters containing detergents; tissue cells cultured in media filtered through washed (detergent-free) filters have higher plating efficiencies and a higher percentage of differentiation than do cells cultured in media filtered through unwashed (detergent-containing) filters. Accordingly, it is suggested that for critical studies involving tissue cells, membrane filters should be washed prior to use or detergent-free filters should be employed (furnished upon request by Millipore or Gelman).

Chemical sterilization of solutions

1. Use thymol, a crystalline phenol, for sterilization of certain thermolabile materials if filtration facilities are not available.
2. Add thymol to concentrated solutions of material to be sterilized.
3. Use 1 g thymol for 20% solution of carbohydrate in 100 ml water.
4. Let solution stand at room temperature for 24 h.
5. Make dilutions for use, thus nullifying bactericidal effect of thymol.

Disposition of contaminated material

Procedure

1. To prevent accidental infection of laboratory workers and drying of proteinaceous materials in or on glassware, all contaminated glassware (such as pipets, syringes, and slides) should be placed, immediately after use, into discard containers filled with reliable disinfectant (e.g., Amphyl, Lysol). For pipets, plastic cylinders are recommended. Enough disinfectant should be placed in these cylinders so that pipets can be completely immersed.
2. For other contaminated glassware such as slides, syringes, disposable Pasteur pipets or for needles, use stainless steel pans with tops; these will withstand repeated autoclaving.
3. When working with specimens suspected of containing acid-fast bacilli or when handling mycobacterial cultures, immerse all glassware used (pipets, slides, syringes) in 5% phenol.
4. Place all specimens, contaminated swabs, wooden spatulas, Petri dishes containing cultures, etc., into deep trays or pails and sterilize in autoclave. All contaminated glassware and containers into which they were placed must be sterilized by

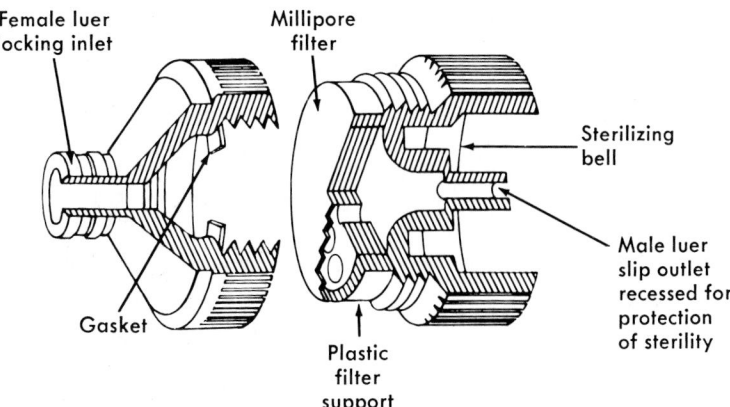

Fig. 70-2. Schematic cutaway view of Swinny filter unit (Swinnex-25). (Courtesy Millipore Corp., Bedford, Mass.)

autoclaving at 15 psi for 30 min. Afterward glassware can be cleaned and washed.

Preparing sterile capillary tubes

Material

1. Pieces of glass tubing about 45 cm long of 7 mm caliber

Procedure

1. Cut a number of these tubes into 45 cm lengths.
2. Stopper them at each end with piece of cotton.
3. Wrap them in separate bundles in paper or in metal cans and sterilize in dry heat oven at 170 C for 2 h.
4. When sterile capillary tube is required, open package, remove 1 tube, heat it over Bunsen burner (Figs. 70-3 to 70-5), and draw it out to desired length and thickness.

5. By turning tube in flame, uniform degree of heat is obtained.
6. When at least 7.5 cm are well heated, under rotation, take tube out of flame, rapidly pull in straight manner, and cut.
7. These tubes can then be made into capillaries for drawing up blood, or they can be used as sterile droppers.
8. **Disposable, predrawn capillary pipets** are available from several manufacturers. Sterilize in cans or wrap in paper.

CULTURE METHODS
General technics

Materials collected for diagnostic purposes are plated on media in Petri dishes or slants in tubes

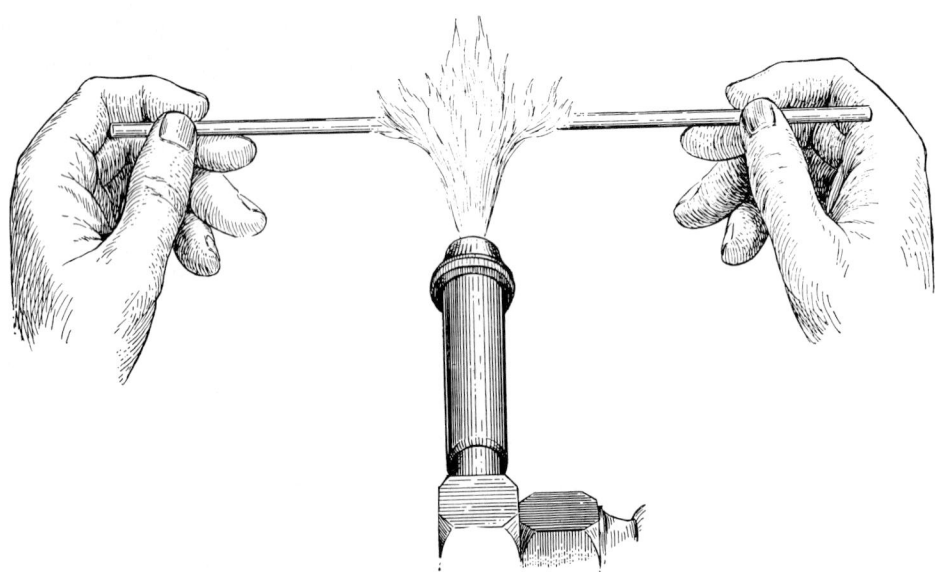

Fig. 70-3. Heating glass tubing before drawing a capillary.

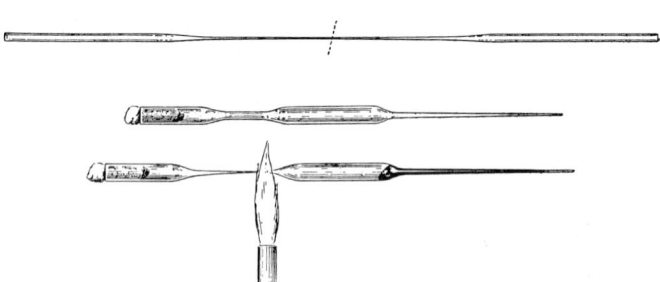

Fig. 70-4. Cutting capillary, *top;* sealing capillaries, *bottom.*

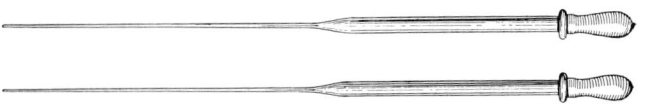

Fig. 70-5. Completed capillaries.

and into tubed liquid media. In some cases an enrichment fluid is inoculated first; then after sufficient incubation, plates are streaked from this fluid. In other cases a carrying medium or a preservative (such as buffered glycerol saline for bacillary incitants of diarrhea) is used, chiefly for transportation of the specimens. Best results are attained when a proper scientific selection of methods is combined with reliable, sterile technic and rapid work.

Preserving fluids or carrying media must be inoculated with a proper amount of material. Too much material impairs the efficacy of the preservative, whereas too little may cause false-negative results. The technic of the use of preservatives for transportation of material is described in detail in the section dealing with diagnostic methods (Chapter 75).

Enrichment fluids must be handled in a manner similar to that used for perserving fluids. In addition to the proper amount of inoculum, temperature and length of incubation are of paramount importance to prevent the overgrowth of "contaminating" microorganisms.

Plating media must be prepared and kept under conditions prescribed for the respective medium. Plating is the only reliable technic for isolation of bacteria in pure culture. It is usually done by streaking the material on the surface of media in Petri dishes.

Streak plates

Only proper streaking can ensure isolated colonies. It is a waste of time and material to smear a specimen over a plate or a section thereof and expect to make a bacteriologic diagnosis. The art of streaking a plate is not inborn in bacteriologists but has to be learned by hard daily practice.

If the streaks "did not come out" so that no isolated colonies were obtained, a fresh specimen must be requested. An honest laboratory worker will avoid issuing a negative report when distinctly isolated colonies have not been seen on the plates.

Replating may help in an emergency but should not be practiced.

Method I. "Streak" method
1. Have on hand Petri dish containing culture medium on which organism to be isolated grows characteristically.
2. Pick up loopful of material to be plated and streak out over upper part of culture medium across from one side to the other. Be careful to touch surface of medium, but do not dig into agar.
3. Flame platinum wire. Allow to cool.
4. Streak out at right angles to the original line of inoculation, making streaks about 1.25 cm distant from each other.
5. Flame platinum wire. Allow to cool.
6. Turn plate and streak at right angles to parallel lines just made, so that result is a series of lines forming small squares over surface of medium.
7. Flame platinum wire.
8. Throughout procedure use precautions to eliminate contamination with air bacteria.

9. Turn plate **upside down** and place in incubator for 24 h or longer at 35-37 C until good growth has been obtained.
10. By fishing out typical colony under microscope and inoculating on a slant or another Petri dish of same medium as that used in the isolation process, pure culture is obtained.
11. Amount of material taken in original loopful must be gauged by possible number of bacteria in specimen. There should be few enough bacteria so that distinct colonies appear at ends of streaks.
12. If there is growth of bacteria in centers of squares formed by streaking process, these, obviously, are contaminants.
13. If medium is very moist, the water of condensation will carry bacteria over surface of plate and render it unfit for isolation purposes. Care should be taken, therefore, to eliminate as much of water as possible.

Method II. "Clock streak"
1. Pick up a loopful of material to be plated and streak out over the upper $^1/_5$ of plate.
2. Flame loop and cool it by stabbing it once or twice into the medium in some place that was not streaked.
3. Turn plate about 70°.
4. Take some material from streaked area by drawing loop through it in a straight line and streak out over next $^1/_5$ of plate. Return loop to streaked portion, draw line through it, and streak material out.
5. Flame loop and cool it by stabbing it once or twice into the medium in some place that was not streaked.
6. Turn plate about 70°.
7. Take some material from part last streaked and streak out as before.
8. Repeat this procedure once more (Fig. 70-6).
9. Proceed in manner described in **Method I.**

Method III. "Z" method
1. Prepare Petri dish of desired culture medium and allow it to solidify.
2. Pick up loopful of material to be plated and streak over surface of agar in such a way that letter Z is formed and covers surface of plate. Flame loop and allow to cool.
3. Streak out from initial line of inoculation; flame loop and allow to cool; streak out from another point on line; flame loop; continue this process until many steaks have been made, flaming loop between each streak. Flame loop and allow to cool.
4. Place plate upside down in incubator at 37 C for 24 h or longer and proceed in the manner described under **Method I.**

Method IV. "Compass" method
1. Prepare Petri dish of desired medium and allow it to solidify.
2. Along radius of circle (Petri dish) place 3 small loopfuls of material to be isolated.
3. Prepare piece of capillary glass by heating glass tubing in flame, pulling it out to a capillary, and then, while still hot, bending it to a 45° angle. (These capillaries may be prepared, wrapped, and sterilized, ready for use.)
4. Using capillary as compass, describe circle over surface of medium in such way that 3 loopfuls of material are spread in thin layer over entire surface.
5. Burn capillary in flame.
6. Turn plate upside down in incubator at 37 C for 24

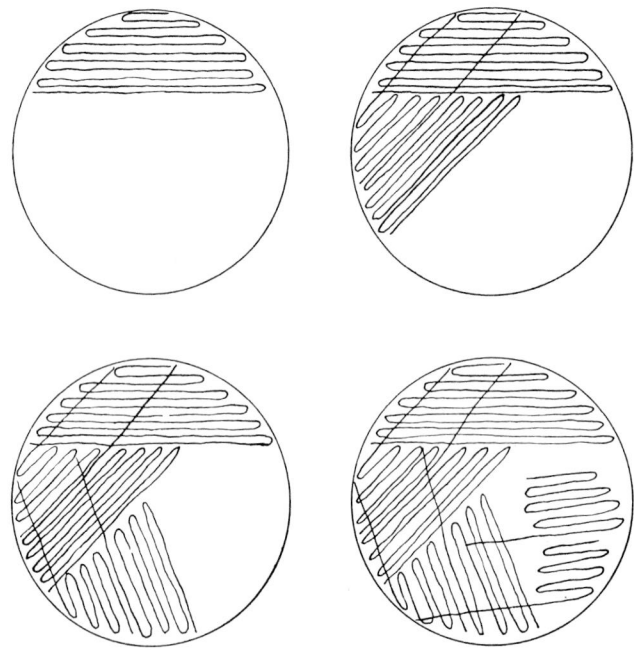

Fig. 70-6. Steps used in performing "clock" streak. (Courtesy Dr. Oscar Felsenfeld.)

h or longer, then proceed in manner described in
Method I.

Method V. Spreading with glass rod
1. Prepare glass rods by bending them at 90° angle. Short end of rod should be about ⅓ diameter of plates used, longer arm about 12.5 cm long.
2. Wrap each rod in paper and sterilize in dry heat sterilizer.
3. Place drop of material to be examined on plate of culture medium.
4. Rub it in with sterile glass rod.
5. Without taking fresh material, rub same glass rod over surface of a second plate.
6. Proceed as in **Method I.**

Some precautions in plating

The surface of the plate must be dry but not dried out.

To avoid contamination, do not keep the plates open too long. Lay the lid on the laboratory table upside down. Hold the bottom of the Petri dish (the part that contains the medium) in a vertical position, with the medium turned toward the worker, to prevent settling of organisms from the air.

When plates are examined or inoculated, it is imperative that the worker does not speak. Contaminated fishings are sometimes due to the selection of colonies that are too near the others. Contamination during the "fishing" process is often due to conversation while the covers are removed. Cultures are exposed during this time, and precautions must be taken not to contaminate them.

Do not cut the medium with the inoculating loop. If this should occur on soft media, interrupt the streak and take fresh material from another part of the surface of the plate for continuance of the streak. Bending the wire at the point where the loop is formed to make a slight angle assists in avoiding this difficulty.

Always keep Petri dishes upside down, except when streaking them or during inspection or fishing.

Inoculation of liquid media

Procedure
1. Using all sterile precautions (i.e., flaming mouths of containers from which specimen is taken and of tube containing liquid medium and holding plugs between fingers), pick up loopful of material to be planted, using a sterile platinum or Nichrome wire.
2. Make emulsion of material on side of tube just above liquid.
3. Replace cotton plug, flame wire, and mix emulsion with liquid by rotating.

Inoculation of butts

Procedure
1. Using all sterile precautions (i.e., flaming mouth of tube from which material is taken and of tube containing medium and holding plugs between fingers) pick up some of material, using sterile platinum or Nichrome wire.
2. Introduce this material with one stab into medium, stabbing down to bottom of test tube. Replace cotton plug and flame wire.

Inoculation of slants and butts

Procedure
1. This method is often used in examination of enteric organisms.
2. With usual precautions, first stab needle to bottom of medium, then streak material remaining on needle over surface of slant.
3. When inoculating butts, take special care that entire wire is well flamed (sterilized) and that contaminants from holder are not added to medium. This often occurs when using fluid media if loop is shaken to force more material into the liquid.
4. Success in growing pure cultures depends greatly on proper plugging of containers. If medium is allowed to flow down neck of tubes during tubing

process, particles of cotton often adhere to glass. This greatly increases chances of contamination.

"Fishing" or "picking" colonies

Procedure
1. For most purposes, it is usually possible to select macroscopically the colony to be transferred from plate to differentiating medium. Use daylight coming in through window and not direct sunshine. Using wax pencil, draw circle on bottom of Petri dish around colony to be fished.
2. Flame platinum or Nichrome wire.
3. Raise bottom of Petri dish to eye level, holding it in a vertical position.
4. Cool needle in air.
5. Pick up colony, taking care not to touch another colony in so doing. If using selective media that retard the growth of contaminants but do not kill them, pick up only center of the colony.
6. Replace Petri dish in its cover.
7. Holding needle between index finger and thumb and using same hand, pull plug of tube containing differentiating medium held in other hand. To accomplish this, use little finger of hand, bending it against palm, with top of cotton plug between finger and palm of hand.
8. Flame neck of tube.
9. Inoculate medium in tube.
10. Again flame neck of tube and replace plug.
11. Flame needle.
12. If hands of worker are unsteady, it is best to rest elbows on table while picking colonies. It is also possible to lean hand holding plate against hand holding needle by touching proximal parts of both antithenars.
13. When fishing with aid of microscope is indicated, following procedure is recommended:
    a. Focus colony on Petri dish with lid open, using 16 mm objective of microscope. Leave Abbé condenser in microscope. Keep edge of colony in sharp focus.
    b. Flame platinum or Nichrome loop.
    c. Steady arm on table.
    d. Holding platinum loop between first and second fingers to make it easy to manipulate and guiding it with thumb, place hand on stage of the microscope with little finger resting on stage. Place wire over area of colony. Look into microscope at colony and introduce wire until it appears in the field of vision.
    e. Remember that an invert image is presented and that a loop introduced from right side appears on left side of microscopic field.
    f. Pick up colony that has been selected.
    g. Withdraw wire, taking care that it does not touch any spot on medium.

Pour plate methods

The approximate number of viable organisms in a liquid (blood, milk, water, broth culture) can be determined by the use of pour plates. The findings are reported as the plate or colony count/ml of material that was examined. Pour plates, using an agar medium with added blood, are also very useful for determining the nature of hemolysis produced by deep colonies of streptococci.

Generally, to prepare a pour plate, serial dilutions of the specimen are made. In this manner

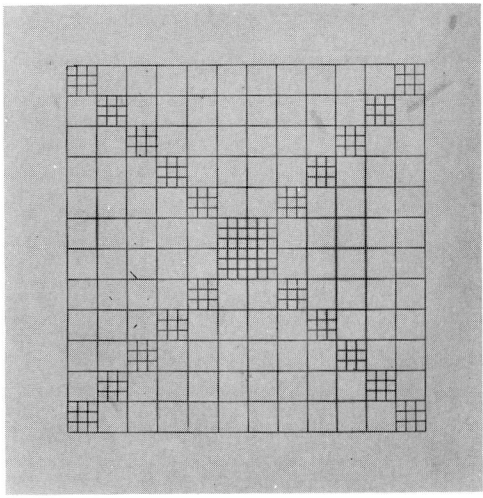

Fig. 70-7. Wolffhuegel counting plate used in Quebec colony counter. (Courtesy American Optical Co., Buffalo, N.Y., and Aloe Scientific Division, Brunswick Corp., St. Louis, Mo.)

isolated colonies may be obtained. A prescribed volume of the dilutions is pipetted into sterile Petri plates, and melted and cooled medium is poured into the plates. Thorough mixing is obtained by rotating the plates. After the agar solidifies, the plates are incubated. After incubation, the number of colonies growing throughout the medium is determined, or, as in the case of streptococci, their hemolytic activity is noted (α or β).

The greatest accuracy in counting the number of organisms in a pour plate is accomplished when using plates on which between 30 and 300 colonies developed. This allows differentiation or "fishing" of colonies. Counting can be done on a counting plate, ruled off in square centimeters. Count the number of colonies per square in 5 or 10 squares, calculate the average, and multiply the average by 62.5 (the average, 90 mm inside diameter Petri dish has an area of 62.5 cm²) to obtain the estimated number of colonies per plate. A guide plate used in the Quebec colony counter is shown in Fig. 70-7.

Membrane filtration culture technics
General principle

Bacteria larger than the pore size of the membrane filter used for filtration are retained on the filter surface. Membrane filters and their use for sterilizing filtration were discussed earlier. The membrane filter is aseptically transferred to an appropriate growth medium by rolling it onto the surface of the medium (to prevent entrapping bubbles). Conventional solid media may be used, or the membrane filter is placed on a pad saturated with liquid medium (usually doublestrength broth) in a Petri dish. The medium diffuses into the membrane filter; after appropriate incubation colonies grow on the surface of the filter, where they can be examined and counted (Fig. 70-8). For detection only, the membrane filter can be placed into a tube or flask of liquid (as in sterility testing). Colonies can be picked for further selective growth or staining. Various micromethods can be used for examination of colonies directly on the filter membrane (oxidase test for *Pseudomonas,* plate bile-solubility test for pneumococci).

Membrane filter cultures offer a number of intrinsic advantages: (1) many organisms grow somewhat more rapidly on membrane filters than on conventional plates, (2) antibiotics and other bacterial inhibitors can be removed by washing the filter after the sample has been filtered, and (3) organisms in low concentrations in large volumes can be easily detected.

Applications

The membrane filter culture technic has been used in a number of areas, but it has not gained general acceptance in the clinical laboratory, despite numerous publications describing its successful application to the isolation of a large variety of medically important microorganisms.

A few procedures are described below; for details, the interested reader is referred to the original publications and the instruction manuals of the manufacturers.*

Generally, 47 mm filter holders with 0.45 μm pore size membrane filters (grid type) are used for clinical applications.

Blood culture. The original approach[4,5] depended upon lysis or digestion of the blood to prepare it for filtration. Winn et al.[6] successfully diagnosed bacteremia by removing the formed elements of the blood and filtering only the plasma (and extracellular bacteria). Their method also allows quantitative distinction of extracellular bacteremia from intraleukocytic and erythrocyte-associated infection. The procedure proved effective in a clinical trial.[7]

Isolation of Mycobacterium tuberculosis. Haley and Arch[8] describe technics for the culture of *M. tuberculosis* from spinal fluid, sputum, urine, and other body fluids. Rose[9] described cultivation of *M. tuberculosis* from sputum, using N-acetyl-cysteine for digestion before filtration.

Examination of water and wastewater. The membrane filter method for the determination of coliform bacteria was adopted as a standard technic in 1960. For details consult edition 14 of *Standard Methods for the Examination of Water and Wastewater* (1975).[10]

MEDIA—GENERAL FACTS AND METHODS

Culture media are divided into **collecting, preserving (transport), plating, and diagnostic**

Manual ADM-40, Millipore Corp., Bedford, Mass; *Procedures, Techniques and Apparatus for Bacteriological Analysis,* Gelman Instrument Co., Ann Arbor, Mich.

media. **With the exception of a few very selective media, all media must be sterile.** Heat sterilization, however, may harm certain ingredients. It is of paramount importance, therefore, to adhere rigorously to the directions concerning sterilization. The glassware in which the media are stored or used must be chemically clean and sterile. No traces of the cleaning solution must remain on the glassware. The tubing of media and the pouring of plates must be carried out in a dust-free room. Speaking and walking in the laboratory are to be avoided during these operations. Routine dry sweeping in laboratory rooms causes extensive contamination.

Each tube or plate must be correctly labeled immediately after sterilization to indicate its content.

Media should not be reheated or resterilized more often than allowed in the formula.

In addition to proper composition and sterilization, the **pH of the medium** and the final reaction are very important. This is checked by the use of indicators or preferably with a pH meter.

Every bacteriologist, clinical pathologist, and laboratory technologist should realize that proper media are the most essential tools in bacteriologic work. Proper preparation and proper keeping of the media are of such importance that this cannot be emphasized too strongly.

Culture media are divided into **fluid, semifluid, semisolid, and solid media** according to their consistency. Isolated colonies can be obtained only on solid media. The other media serve as collecting, preserving, and enrichment fluids, for the study of pure cultures, or for the cultivation of anaerobes (thioglycollate media and others). Solid media, except for certain coagulated media, are frequently used in plates. They may be poured into Petri dishes so that the material to be examined can be spread on the surface. Or the material to be examined may be mixed with the melted medium and this mixture poured into plates and allowed to solidify. In this way colonies may be isolated and selected for further study.

Agar is used as the solidifying agent. When 0.05-0.2% agar is added to the medium, the medium will be semifluid. Such a solution supports the growth of neisseriae, clostridia, etc. **Semisolid tubes** contain 0.3-0.5% agar. For a **solid plate,** 1.5-1.7% agar is required.

Media containing agar become liquid when heated to about 96 C and solidify again when the temperature falls to about 45 C. Tubes are placed in a boiling water bath to liquefy the medium. Sometimes it is necessary to melt the agar in a flask over a Bunsen flame, protecting the flask with a wire-and-asbestos net, e.g., for dissolving dehydrated media when preparing them for use. In such cases it is necessary to shake the flask frequently to prevent the ingredients from sticking to the bottom. If the agar burns, the culture medium must be discarded.

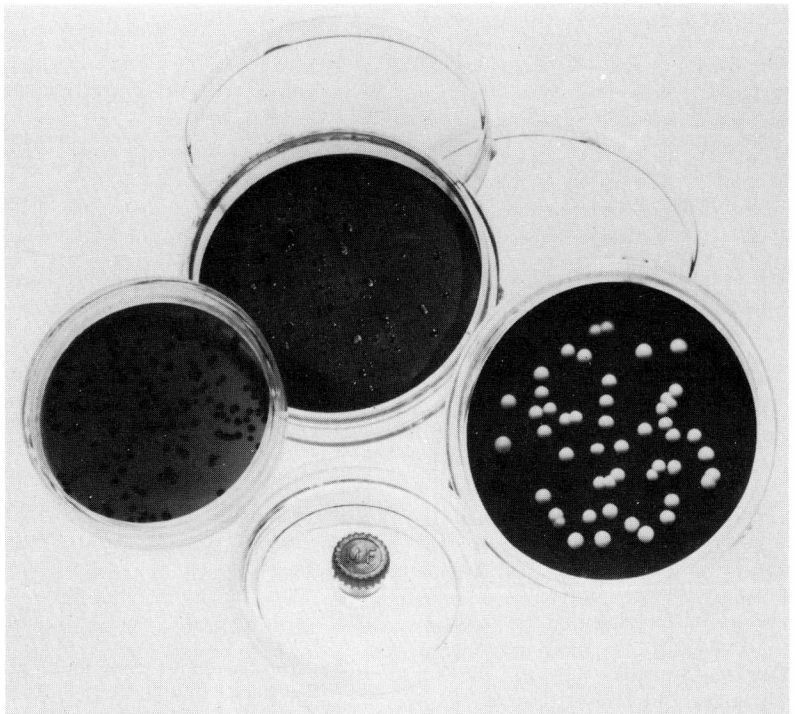

Fig. 70-8. Membrane filters used for filtration of various fluids and cultured on surface of medium in Petri dishes, showing identifiable colonies that developed from bacteria retained on filter surface. (Courtesy Millipore Corp., Bedford, Mass.)

Gelatin is the most reliable measure of bacterial proteolysis ("gelatin liquefaction").

Distilled water should be used for the preparation of culture media.

All chemicals must be chemically pure.

Most media contain **peptone** in one form or another. Peptone (Difco) and polypeptone (BBL) satisfy most requirements. Pancreatic digest of casein (Difco) has been used widely as an all-purpose peptone. Tryptone (Difco) and trypticase (BBL) are recommended for indole production; proteose-peptone (Difco) and thiotone (BBL), for hydrogen sulfide production. Phytone (BBL) is a papaic digest of plant material. Most media require 0.5-2% peptone.

Meat is essential for many media. Meat extract is used routinely, but for more fastidious bacteria, infusions of heart, liver, brain, etc., are indicated. Some authors suggest "hormone" and tryptic digest broths that have growth-supporting properties. These hormone media require special care, and for this reason the ready-made commercial products are used in most laboratories. Meat extracts, however, often give false-positive fermentation reactions and are therefore bypassed whenever possible in such media.

Yeast extract, Casamino acids (Difco), and supplements are required for a number of media. Yeast extract, 0.3-1%, strongly supports the growth of many microorganisms and may be substituted for a part or all of the meat extract when so indicated in the formula.

Fermentable substances—carbohydrates, alcohols, glucosides, and urea—are often destroyed by heat. They are therefore frequently added to the previously sterilized "base" after filtration of the concentrated solutions through a membrane or Seitz filter.

Hemolysis must never be evaluated on plates containing fermentable substances, notably dextrose or sodium azide, since these materials cause false readings.

Negative indole tests will sometimes be observed when media containing carbohydrates are used for this reaction.

Some laboratories prepare media from their basic ingredients; most purchase commercially prepared dehydrated media. The choice is usually dictated by the extent of available facilities. Dehydrated media are convenient, simple to prepare, and reliable. Excellent desiccated media are available commercially. **Many laboratories purchase media ready made, sterilized, plated or tubed.***

Approximately 500 media in dehydrated form are available commercially in the United States; peptones, additives, yeast extracts, meat extracts, and various supplements are also widely available. There is little doubt about the great convenience and economy afforded by the use of dehydrated media. They are, on the whole, manufactured under rigid control measures and are reliable. However, unsatisfactory media can be obtained from excellent dehydrated media if certain precautions are not observed[11]:

1. Stocks of dehydrated media should be periodically checked and rotated. Moisture, oxidation, and heat are all deleterious to desiccated media, and

---

*BBL, Division of BioQuest, Cockeysville, Md.; Gibco, Grand Island, N.Y.; Scott Labs, Fiskeville, R.I.; Pfizer Labs, New York, and many others.

contents of bottles previously opened should be carefully inspected for "caking" and discoloration. Dehydrated material should be kept for 1 y at most (sealed) and less if in opened bottles.
2. Dry material should be weighed accurately.
3. Measure water to be used for reconstitution accurately; do not use tap water.
4. Avoid overheating or heating for prolonged periods beyond manufacturer's instructions.
5. Use clean glassware free of detergents.

Details for preparing media from basic ingredients are listed in Chapter 72; see also quality control, Chapter 73.

Selection of media

The quality of results in the bacteriology laboratory depends to a considerable extent on the proper selection of media. It is possible, by judicious application of basic criteria, to limit the media to a manageable number. General purpose media are used for the initial isolation and specific-purpose media for selection and identification of bacteria.

Among the medically important bacteria, some can grow on relatively simple media, whereas the more fastidious ones require complex media. Since their nutritional requirements vary widely, it must be emphasized that there is no single medium that would allow the growth of all cultivable bacteria. Therefore, usually more than one medium is employed for initial isolation; depending on the specimen and the bacteria searched for, a variety of special purpose media is employed.

Media for **primary** culture, **selective, differential,** and **enrichment** media, and media for special purposes are discussed in Chapter 72; specific recommendations for use of specific media are also made throughout the following chapters dealing with various groups of bacteria.

Sterilization of media

Sterility of the medium to be used for bacteriologic procedures is essential.

Preparation of solutions

PRECAUTIONS. Peptones, agar, and gelatin often adhere to walls or to bottom of flask and burn when flask is heated. This spoils the medium; it may also cause sticking of cotton plug. To avoid adhesion of these materials to glass surfaces, observe following precautions.

Pour small amount of water in flask before adding ingredients. If, for example, medium is to be made by dissolving ingredients in 1000 ml water, first pour about 500 ml water into the flask; then add ingredients. Finally, pour rest of water into flask to wash inside of neck of flask. This washes into contents of flask any powder adhering to neck.

Capacity of flask should be double the amount of the medium to be made. Erlenmeyer flasks with wide necks and without pour-outs are preferred.

Pouring plates

Procedure
1. Pour plates under sterile conditions. Repeatedly flame necks of flasks or tubes between pouring plates. Hold plug of flask in such a position that it does not become contaminated.
2. Media should not be warmer than 60 C when poured. This will reduce the formation of water of condensation.
3. It is best to leave plates on laboratory table until media have solidified, then store the plates upside down in refrigerator.
4. Mark each plate to indicate its contents.
5. Never use dried-out plates or plates showing growth of contaminants.
6. If surface of plate is moist, put plate, with partly removed lid, in a dust-free incubator until surface is dry. Do not open incubator during this procedure except to take out drying plates.
7. Some very selective media, such as those used for stool work, may be dried on laboratory table with partly removed lids.
8. Proper amounts of medium/100 mm plate, if not directed otherwise, are 17-20 ml.

Tubing media
Procedure
Media sterilized after they have been tubed
1. Attach piece of rubber tubing to short-stemmed 10-15 cm glass funnel (Fig. 70-9). Size of funnel varies according to amount of medium.
2. Insert dropper into other end of rubber tubing so that pointed end of dropper is free.
3. Place this tubing apparatus in ring stand high enough that space remains to operate outlet. Put Moore or Cenco clamp on rubber tubing to allow interruption of flow and close clamp.
4. Fill funnel with medium. To fill tubes, place dropper well into tubes so that medium will flow into tubes without soiling upper parts that come in contact with plug.
5. Plug tubes and sterilize them.
Media tubed under sterile conditions
1. Safest procedure is to use sterile pipets and distribute medium into sterile test tubes. It is best to have an assistant to flame necks of tubes and insert plugs.
2. Another method is to prepare a tubing apparatus using a 500 ml (or larger) bottle, Pyrex glass, with

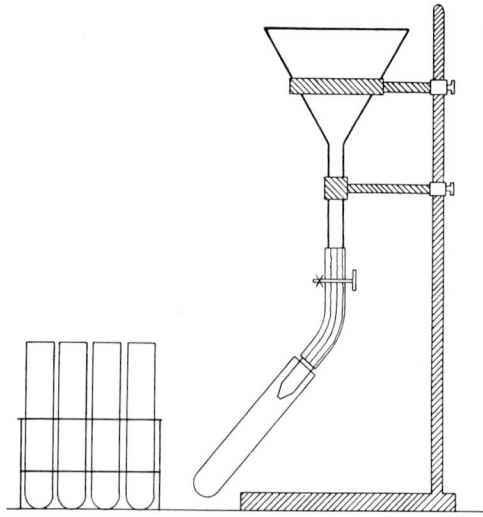

Fig. 70-9. Apparatus for tubing culture media. (Courtesy Dr. Oscar Felsenfeld.)

a tube at bottom. Adjust rubber tubing and dropper as they were adjusted to funnel, as described above. Wrap entire apparatus in paper and sterilize.

3. Protect outlet of apparatus against contamination during operation by covering it with sterile test tube between fillings.
4. All media tubed after sterilization must be checked for sterility by incubation at 35-37 C for 24-72 h, according to the medium.

Storage of media

Most media are stored in the refrigerator to avoid dehydration and deterioration of certain labile components. Dried-out media cannot be used because a certain water content is essential for growth of most organisms. Bulk storage of plating media in screw-capped bottles or flasks reduces evaporation considerably and also protects against contamination. Poured plates stored preferably in metal containers with tight-fitting closures or protected with foil or Mylar plastic bags will keep for several weeks under refrigeration. Without such protection, refrigerated media in glass or plastic plates should be kept no longer than 1-2 wk. Tubed media are usually closed with rolled cotton plugs, metal closures, plastic caps, paraffined corks, or preferably with tightly fitting screw caps. Refrigeration is necessary for most tubed media; some media, when kept in tightly closed (screw-capped) tubes, may be stored at room temperature. Tubed media with cotton plugs, loosely fitting metal closures, or plastic caps, even when refrigerated, should not be stored for more than 2 wk.

Prepared media in sealed plates are available from several commercial sources.* Such sealed plates are eminently suitable for small laboratories or physicians' offices, since they may be stored in the refrigerator for relatively long periods. Prepared, sterilized, and ready-to-use media in bottles, in tubes, or as slants are also available from the sources listed.

Preparation of eggs

Procedure

Whole eggs
1. Scrub fresh eggs with soap; then wash with water and put into 70% alcohol for 30 min or longer.
2. Prepare large, strong-walled bottle containing numerous glass beads; plug with nonabsorbent cotton and sterilize in dry heat oven.
3. Take eggs out of alcohol and wrap them in sterile towel. When they are dry, open them with sterile knife, nicking both ends, and collect contents under sterile conditions in sterile bottle. Shake bottle until eggs are homogeneous.
4. Take care not to touch ends of eggs after taking them out of alcohol.

Egg yolks
1. Clean and sterilize eggshells as for collection of whole eggs, previously described.
2. It is best for operator to wear sterile rubber gloves. If he does not, then he must scrub his hands clean before handling eggs.
3. Open eggs by breaking shell in middle and parting halves. Separate yolks and whites. Pour yolks into sterile bottle and save egg whites for other purposes.

---

*BBL, Division of Bioquest, Cockeysville, Md.; Hyland Laboratories, Los Angeles, Calif.; Gibco Laboratories, Grand Island, N.Y.; and others.

Media

Formulas for various media are listed in Chapter 72.

ANAEROBIC CULTURE EQUIPMENT AND SYSTEMS

General principles

Until recently the importance of obligate anaerobes in infections has been frequently overlooked. Anaerobic culture was neglected partly because many pathogens that cause illness grow well in air and partly because of alleged technical difficulties and the lack of adequate information about methods allowing the cultivation of anaerobes with comparative ease. Stokes (1958)[12] found anaerobes in up to 32% of clinical specimens from tissues and fluids normally sterile, all of which must be therefore considered as potential pathogens.

To many clinicians the term "anaerobic infections" used to indicate gas gangrene or tetanus. However, many other anaerobes—among them bacteroides, streptococci, veillonellae, corynebacteria, micrococci, actinomycetes—occur much more frequently in infections, many of them severe and often fatal. In the absence of anaerobic cultures, such specimens would be reported "sterile" or, in the case of mixed aerobic-anaerobic infections, only the organisms growing in air would be recognized. With the availability of antibiotics, it is imperative to isolate and to identify anaerobes so that successful therapy may be instituted.

Definition

Organisms that require a low (reduced) oxidation-reduction potential, attainable by removal or exclusion of atmospheric oxygen, alone or concomitantly with reducing agents included in the medium, are defined as obligate anaerobes.[13]

As a matter of convention, any organism is considered an anaerobe if, when plated on (1) blood agar, incubated in air plus 5-10% CO_2, and (2) anaerobically, it appears on the anaerobic but not on the aerobic plate.

Growth in liquid anaerobic medium and no growth on air-incubated plates does not necessarily mean the presence of an anaerobe. Growth in the lower part of a liquid anaerobic tube is only presumptive evidence; growth in the upper layer, up to the surface, usually means the presence of an aerobic or facultative organism.

Anaerobic methods

Until the end of the 1960s, anaerobic methods in most clinical laboratories fell into 2 categories: (1) minimal, i.e., cultivation of specimen in liquid anaerobic medium only, with no further attempt to produce anaerobic plate cultures, and (2) cultivation in liquid anaerobic medium, with consequent plating on anaerobic plates for purification and isolation. Following Stokes's report[12] (see above) a number of major developments occurred in anaerobic methodology: antibiotic-containing media selective for anaerobes were developed[14] and the GasPak (BBL, Cockeysville, Md.), a self-contained combustion jar system with its own gas-generating package,[15] anaerobic chambers,[16] and the VPI (roll-tube) method[17] were introduced. All of these improvements were eventually introduced in the clinical laboratory.

Currently, research laboratories studying the normal flora or attempting to define the role of certain anaerobes in specific disease entities and some clinical laboratories use the roll-tube (Hungate or VPI) method or the anaerobic chamber (glovebox); for most clinical laboratories, the anaerobic jar methods, widely used, are sufficient. For a survey of the evolution and present status of anaerobic culture technics, see Sonnenwirth[18, 19]; see also Chapter 82.

Although there are advantages and disadvantages to each system, recent studies have shown that all of the systems are suitable for isolation of the **commonly** encountered anaerobes responsible for human infections if certain principles of anaerobic bacteriology are followed[20, 21]:

1. Specimens must be properly collected and handled to exclude atmospheric oxygen.
2. Fresh or prereduced media must be used.
3. The anaerobic system must be properly used by providing an active catalyst in the system to allow effective removal of residual oxygen.

Roll-tube method (VPI)

The method was developed by Hungate[22] for the isolation of anaerobes from the rumen and was simplified by Moore.[17] It involves preparation of media, inoculation, incubation, and transfer in an oxygen-free atmosphere. The medium is melted, then inoculated, and the tube is rolled as the agar cools. The organisms grow in a thin layer of agar around the sides of the tube. The technic is used to grow the most fastidious anaerobes; however, it requires specialized equipment and is demanding.

The prereduced anaerobically sterilized (PRAS) media used in this technic are sterilized under oxygen-free gas in rubber stoppered tubes. The tubes of media should remain reduced up to and during the time they are inoculated. Oxygen-sensitive indicators, e.g., resazurin, included in the PRAS media are used to monitor the oxidation-reduction potential of the media. Oxygen is excluded from the tubes when cultures are inoculated or transferred by inserting a sterile cannula and passing a gentle stream of oxygen-free CO_2 into the neck of the tube until the stopper is replaced. This maintains anaerobic conditions in the tube and **allows each tube to serve as an anaerobic culture system** that can be incubated in an ordinary incubator and inspected at any time without exposure to atmospheric oxygen. PRAS media can be prepared in the laboratory if time and available personnel permit or may be ob-

tained commercially.[23,*] Detailed methodology, description of media, equipment, and identification methods are described by the staff of the Virginia Polytechnic Institute (VPI) Anaerobe Laboratory in Anaerobe Laboratory Manual (1977).[24]

Anaerobic plate cultures

There are several methods for the surface cultivation of anaerobic bacteria in an environment from which atmospheric oxygen has been excluded. The choice among these must by necessity rest with the individual laboratory, depending on available space, equipment, manpower, and financial considerations; however, the availability of relatively inexpensive equipment and materials places the recommended technics, e.g., the **replacement** or **combustion** methods (see below), within the reach of even the smallest laboratory.

Replacement method

In this method the oxygen-containing atmosphere is replaced with an inert gas such as nitrogen, illuminating gas, or helium.

Both plates and tubed media can be used in various airtight containers that allow removal of a large part of the oxygen-containing atmosphere by means of a vacuum pump or water aspirator. All apparatus described in this and the following section can also be used for creating **a partial CO_2 atmosphere.**

The replacement method is not wholly without disadvantages. A certain amount of oxygen is left behind in the jars (repeated "flushing" with gas may somewhat alleviate this problem) that may interfere with the growth of some anaerobes. The illuminating gas used by some laboratories is not of uniform quality and in some localities has been found to inhibit the growth of anaerobes.

> **Accessory equipment**
> 1. Source of vacuum, bottled gas with appropriate regulators and gauges **that are different for various gases**
> 2. Two- and 3-way stopcock arrangements for vacuum and gas connections
> 3. Manometer
>
> **Brewer jar.** Although it can be used as an evacuation-replacement jar, the Brewer jar is mainly useful in the combustion method (Fig. 70-10). The use of jars **without** catalyst is **not** recommended.

Combustion method

It is generally agreed that oxygen removal can be accomplished most efficiently by using Laidlaw's principle[24] of combustion. With the use of jars expressly designed for this purpose, hydrogen or illuminating gas is admitted into an evacuated (as completely as possible if a water pump is used, or to 600 mm Hg negative pressure if a vacuum pump is used) jar. The lid of the jar

---

*Scott Laboratories, Fiskeville, R.I.; Gibco Labs, Grand Island, N.Y.

contains a catalyst (palladium or platinum) with the aid of which the **oxygen** present combines with **hydrogen** to form water or, in the case of illuminating gas, water and CO_2, thus removing the free oxygen from the jar.

Gases used. Earlier, there had been considerable controversy regarding the various gases used in the combustion method. Many workers

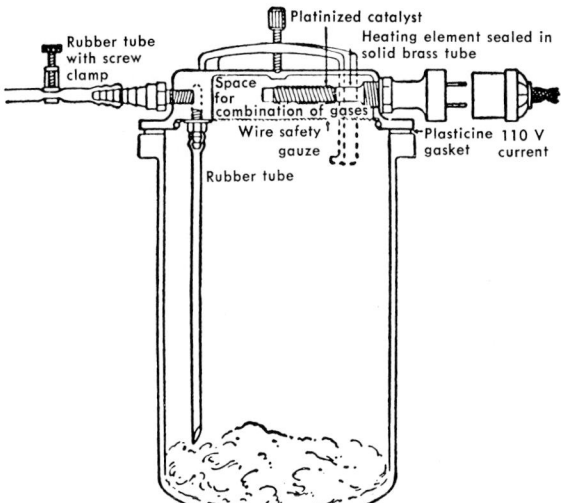

Fig. 70-10. Diagram of Brewer anaerobic jar. (Courtesy BBL, Division of BioQuest, Cockeysville, Md.)

preferred to use pure hydrogen; others used natural or coal gas (the latter 2 are not satisfactory in all areas).

Recently a gas mixture consisting of 80% or 85% nitrogen, 5% or 10% CO_2, and 10% hydrogen has gained considerable popularity; it is less explosive than pure hydrogen. Its use eliminates an extra step—the need for addition of CO_2; the advisability of adding 5-10% CO_2 to anaerobic jars is universally accepted. A disposable hydrogen and CO_2 generator (GasPak) is now available and is widely used (BBL, Division of BioQuest, Cockeysville, Md.). It is somewhat expensive but is easy to use and should prove useful for the laboratory with limited facilities.

Brewer jar.[26] As mentioned before, the Brewer jar is a multipurpose container. The platinized catalyst in the head is activated by heat (electricity) and is shielded from the jar by a heavy, fine mesh screen to minimize explosion hazards. The most efficient results are obtained if it is employed as an evacuation-replacement jar with catalyst using hydrogen or hydrogen mixture.

Evacuation-replacement technic using catalyst (combustion)[23]

Fig. 70-11 illustrates the evacuation-replacement technic in which a Brewer jar is used. If a manometer is not available, a balloon can be connected to the system to serve as a pressure indica-

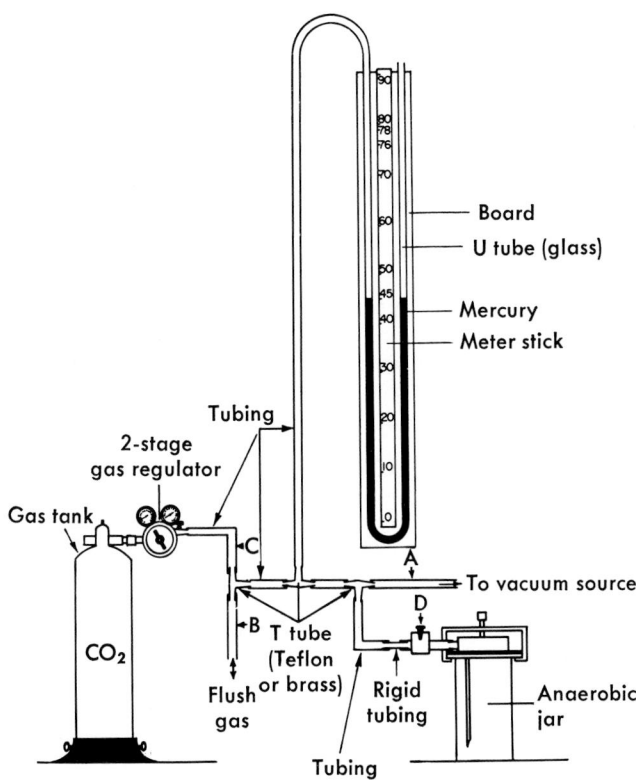

Fig. 70-11. Evacuation replacement technic using a Brewer jar.

tor during the evacuation and replacement procedure. The procedure is performed as follows:

1. Place material to be incubated inside jar.
2. In a 15 × 25 mm test tube, place indicator (methylene blue–NaHCO$_3$–glucose mixture). If anaerobic conditions are achieved, methylene blue indicator solution will be colorless after overnight incubation; otherwise, solution will be blue. Place tube in jar. Disposable methylene blue (GasPak) anaerobic indicator strips (BBL) are also suitable.
3. Seal lid to jar with Plasticine or use stopcock lubricant such as "Cello Seal" (BBL) and fasten lid with clamp.
4. Connect outlet on jar lid to vacuum-gas-manometer assembly.
5. Evacuate to 30 cm Hg.
6. Clamp off tubing to vacuum pump and turn off vacuum pump motor.
7. Slowly fill jar with gas mixture (80% N$_2$, 10% CO$_2$, 10% H$_2$) (Matheson Co., East Rutherford, N.J., and branches). A full tank of gas has approximately 1500 pounds pressure; therefore, tanks must be securely fastened to a post or wall bracket and reducing valve used that has been adjusted to 4-5 pounds pressure.
8. Remove clamp on tubing to vacuum pump.
9. Repeat steps 5-8.
10. Repeat steps 5-7.
11. Tighten clamp on jar outlet tubing.
12. Disconnect jar from vacuum gas assembly.
13. Remove clamp on tubing to vacuum pump.
14. Connect electrical element and heat for 10 min.
15. Disconnect electrical element and place jar in incubator.

The evacuation-replacement technic is used with other types of containers (Torbal, vented GasPak jar, vacuum dessicator, and so on) exactly as described for the Brewer jar, except step 14 is omitted.

If 3-gas mixture is not available, use jar by attaching to separate hydrogen cylinder and CO$_2$ cylinder. By using a 2-way stopcock, separate filling with CO$_2$ and H$_2$ can be done.

For a somewhat different arrangement and detailed instructions for exchanging atmosphere in anaerobic jars (using helium or nitrogen as flush gas), see Fig. 86-1 and Table 86-2.

Some workers recommend[27] that the evacuation and replacement procedure be performed 3 times when hydrogen is used; the final charge is then allowed to react in the presence of the heated catalyst (i.e., the jar head is **not** connected to electric current until the final charge of hydrogen is admitted).

McIntosh-Fildes jar, modified.* A modification of the McIntosh-Fildes jar that is of all metal construction, a distinct advantage, was described by Stokes.[28] A rubber gasket for the lid eliminates the need for Plasticene or grease. The catalyst, made of pellets of alumina coated with palladium and contained in a Monel metal gauze envelope,

---

*Baird & Tatlock, Hatton Garden, London ECl, England (Baird-Tatlock jar); Torsion Balance Co., Clifton, N.J. (Torbal jar).

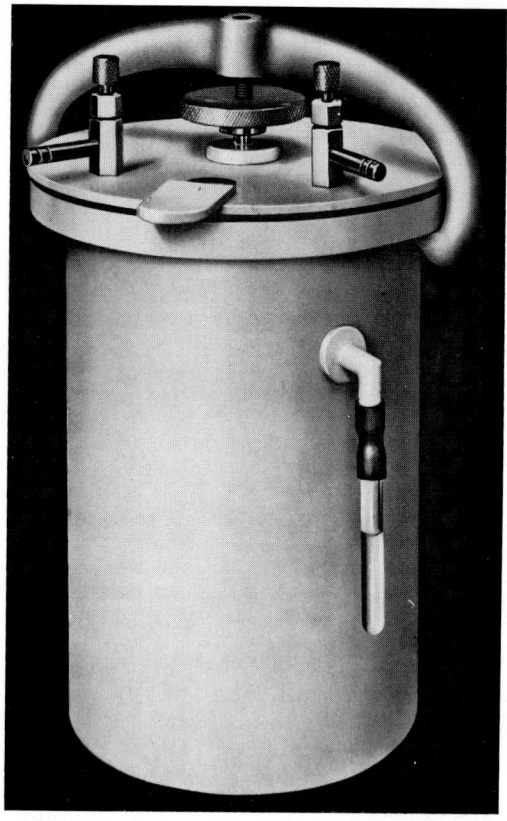

Fig. 70-12. Modified McIntosh-Fildes (Torbal) anaerobic jar. (Courtesy Torsion Balance Co., Clifton, N.J.)

is active at room temperature and dispenses with the need for electricity, thus reducing the danger of explosion. The lid has 2 needle valves, one for attachment to vacuum and manometer and one for attachment to gas sources (Fig. 70-12).

Remove air until there is a negative pressure in the jar of 60-70 cm Hg. Close the vacuum valve and open the valve to the gas source and admit a small amount, 2-5%, CO$_2$. Then add hydrogen, passing through a wash bottle, to atmospheric pressure (at about 2 ω). Adjust the flow of gas so that about 1 bubble/s is seen, keep it flowing for about 2 minutes, then close the valve, and incubate the jar. The jar can be set up in about 3 minutes. (Instructions available from manufacturer.)

This modified jar is convenient to use and easy to maintain; because of the room temperature ("cold") catalyst, its use results in considerable saving of time, as compared to the electrically heated catalyst-equipped jars.

Modernization of Brewer jars. Brewer and other anaerobic jars using electrically heated catalysts can be converted into cold-catalyst types by the simple expedient of removing the original catalyst and attaching the cold-catalyst sachet (available from manufacturers of Baird-Tatlock and Torbal jars).[29] This can be done by employing one of the screws holding the large disk of wire gauze or by fixing it under the short gas nozzle protruding from the underside of the lid. The cold catalyst does not require heating; thus the jar can be filled in 1-2 minutes with hydrogen (after evacuation) and then incubated, since the catalyst continues to operate at incubator temperature.

Precautions with combustion technic. Jars should be inspected for cracks before use. The metal screen of the Brewer jar lid must be intact as well as the metal gauze sachet of the McIntosh-Fildes jar. A safety shield should be placed on the glass jar when the procedure is followed.

Gas containers as well as connecting rubber tubings should be periodically checked for leakage. No smoking is permitted when gas is flowing.

Indicators for efficiency of anaerobiosis

For all types of jars and methods, except individual plating systems, **it is essential to use an indicator tube that shows the presence of oxygen.** The most commonly used system utilizes the change of methylene blue from the colored (oxidized) state to the leuko form (reduced state).

Methylene blue indicator. Among a number of available methods, the following formula has been used with success:

Methylene blue, 1:1000, in distilled water	0.2 ml
0.2M Na_3PO_4	0.1 ml
0.2M Na_2HPO_4	1 ml
Glucose, 4%, in distilled water	1 ml

When mixed in these proportions, pH is 9. Mix solutions immediately before use and boil until colorless. Place in jar immediately and begin procedures. If anaerobiosis is satisfactory, color will not reappear. Occasionally some color will reappear briefly and then disappear as anaerobiosis develops. If at the end of the incubation period the indicator tube shows color, no satisfactory anaerobiosis was achieved.

Lucas semisolid indicator (Torsion Balance Co., Clifton, N.J.). The McIntosh-Fildes modified jar, being constructed of metal, requires an external indicator.

Indicator is prepared by adding 2 drops phenol red and 12 drops 9% thioglycollic acid to 5 ml 2% borax solution in a boiling tube. Methylene blue solution, 10 ml, and melted watery agar, 10 ml, are then added. Blue mixture is boiled until it becomes colorless. With a warmed Pasteur pipet, mixture is transferred into warm ampules that are sealed immediately. When needed, ampule is opened, and tube is attached to side arm of jar with piece of rubber tubing. Indicator should just set when cool; this may require adjustment of proportion of watery agar. If too firm, color of indicator changes too slowly. When oxygen is present, indicator becomes blue to depth of about 5 mm. Indicator is inspected before jar is opened; if trace of blue shows, anaerobiosis in jar was not adequate and culture should be repeated.[28]

In my laboratory it was found that commercially available Stuart transport medium, with added methylene blue (0.1 ml 1:1000 methylene blue solution added to 10 ml melted Stuart transport medium) is a satisfactory and easily prepared substitute.*

GasPak system (Brewer cold-catalyst jar). A self-contained hydrogen–carbon dioxide anaerobic system was developed by Brewer and Allgeier (available from BBL, Division of Bio-Quest, Cockeysville, Md., as GasPak Anaerobic Jar, GasPak Generator Envelope, BBL anaerobic indicator, and catalyst replacement charge).[30] The system eliminates the need for gas cylinders, vacuum pumps, valves, and gauges. It makes use of the standard Pyrex glass anaerobic jar with a new anaerobic lid that is fitted with a snap-in rubber gasket, a double stainless steel gauze flash arrestor, and a catalyst holder that contains alumina pellets coated with 0.5% palladium. **This catalyst is active at room temperature and does not require heating.** The system uses a disposable hydrogen–carbon dioxide generator and a disposable methylene blue anaerobic indicator (Fig. 70-13). For further details see GasPak technic.

The hydrogen–carbon dioxide generator[30] (GasPak [BBL]) contains a hydrogen-producing sodium borohydride tablet and a citric acid plus sodium bicarbonate tablet that produces carbon dioxide. It is activated by cutting off the corner and adding 10 ml water with a pipet. The lid is clamped in place, and the jar is placed in the incubator.

The **disposable methylene blue indicator** gradually changes from blue to colorless as the oxygen in the jar is utilized. This occurs within several hours.

GasPak disposable methylene blue indicator. A modified methylene blue indicator, described by Brewer et al.,[31] is contained in a Teflon sachet attached to a polyethylene-coated card. The sachet contains 1 ml indicator solution, composed of equal parts of 0.02% methylene blue, 4% dextrose, and 60% tris(hydroxymethyl) aminomethane (Tris); it may be sterilized, prior to attachment to the card, by ethylene oxide gas (1.5 hour at 20 psi). The indicator, in a convenient unit form, ready for use, is available commercially (Anaerobic indicator, BBL, Division of Bio-Quest, Cockeysville, Md.) and can be used in the Brewer jar with an electrically heated catalyst or in the GasPak jar.

Changing catalysts

It is important to keep the lids of anaerobe jars clean and dry when not in use to prevent inactivation of catalyst. The **catalyst** (palladium-coated alumina pellets) used with the GasPak system is

---

*OR indicator agar, dehydrated or in prepared vials, is available from Difco Laboratories, Detroit, Mich. It contains sodium thioglycollate (1.7 g), sodium glycerol phosphate (10 g), calcium chloride (0.1 g), methylene blue (0.006 g), and agar (15.0 g); all amounts are given/L.

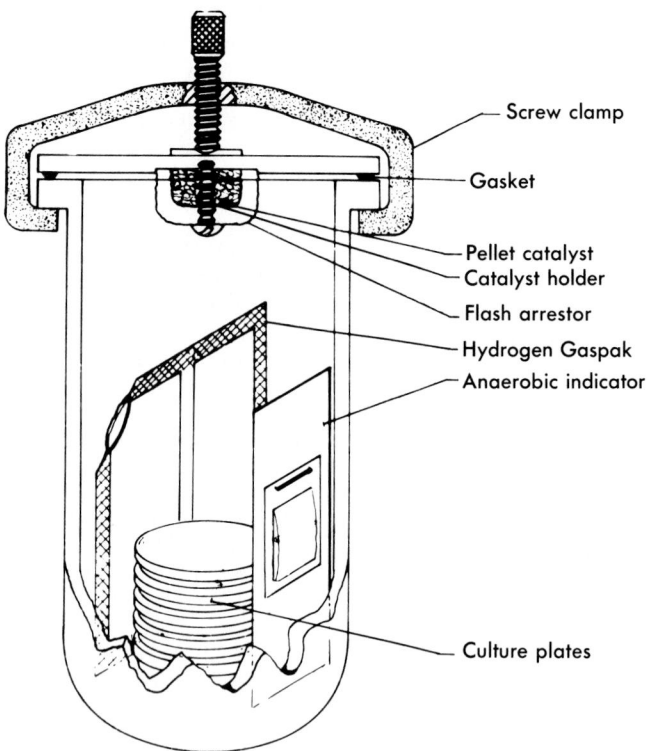

- Screw clamp
- Gasket
- Pellet catalyst
- Catalyst holder
- Flash arrestor
- Hydrogen Gaspak
- Anaerobic indicator
- Culture plates

Fig. 70-13. Schematic cutaway view of Brewer cold-catalyst anaerobic jar using GasPak hydrogen and CO₂ generator. (Courtesy BBL, Division of BioQuest, Cockeysville, Md.)

known to be **inactivated** ("poisoned") by hydrogen sulfide, chlorine, and sulfur dioxide gases. Therefore, the pellets must be replaced at frequent intervals (**preferably each time the jar is used**) with new or "rejuvenated" pellets. The activity of used catalyst can be restored ("rejuvenated") by heating the pellets in a dry heat oven at 160-170 C for 2 hours. After rejuvenation, store the pellets in a clean, dry container away from contaminating gases until they are used.

GasPak technic[23]

Three types of GasPak anaerobic systems are now available: (1) GasPak anaerobic system (polycarbonate jar) (A larger version of this jar that will accommodate twelve 150 mm Petri dishes is now available from BBL. Because of the larger volume, 3 GasPak hydrogen plus carbon dioxide generator envelopes are required to provide anaerobic conditions in the jar. An adaptor is also available from BBL that permits evacuation and replacement of this system as described in "evacuation-replacement" technic.); (2) Gas-Pak anaerobic system, vented (polycarbonate jar); and (3) GasPak disposable anaerobic system. Each of these is a self-contained anaerobic system in which hydrogen and carbon dioxide are supplied from the disposable GasPak hydrogen plus carbon dioxide generator envelope. The evacuation-replacement technic can also be used with the **vented** system.

The polycarbonate GasPak systems (vented or unvented) are used as follows:

1. Remove used catalyst from lid of the jar and replace with equal quantity of new or rejuvenated pellets.
2. Place material to be incubated and methylene blue indicator in jar.
3. Cut corner off GasPak hydrogen plus carbon dioxide generator envelope, spread foil to form opening, and place in jar in upright position.
4. Pipet 10 ml water through opening into envelope. Do not insert pipet.
5. Quickly place GasPak lid on jar. Apply clamp and secure it until "hand-tight."
6. Place jar in incubator.

The disposable GasPak anaerobic system is assembled and used as follows:

1. Assemble carrier and mount hydrogen plus carbon dioxide generator and indicator in proper slot of carrier as directed (cut off one corner of envelope and spread foil to form opening).
2. Place material to be incubated into carrier and pipet 10 ml water into open corner of envelope. Do not insert pipet.
3. Immediately place carrier in flexible plastic container so that GasPak envelope faces a side seam of bag, fold over plastic bag, and press it flat on top of carrier to express as much air as possible.
4. Next fold top edge of bag over sponge strip and fold again.
5. Then take plastic clamp and, beginning at one end, place clamp over folded edge and slide until en-

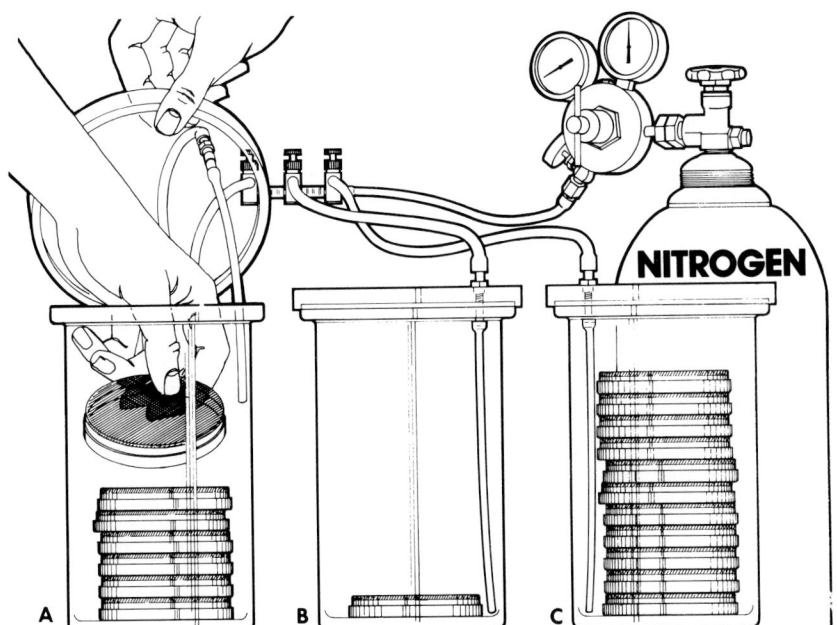

Fig. 70-14. Holding-jar procedure using GasPak jars. **A,** Uninoculated plates. **B,** Plates with growing colonies. **C,** Inoculated plates to be incubated.

tire top edge is clamped. Final clamped edge must be smooth to prevent leakage.

6. Place system in incubator.

NOTE: Catalyst in carrier of disposable GasPak system is not replaceable, and number of times system can be used will depend on degree of exposure to hydrogen sulfide and other gases that inactivate the catalyst. After catalyst is expended, it is still possible to use bag (if there are no leaks) by adding packet of catalyst pellets (palladium-coated alumina) as described above for the evacuation-replacement technic.

Holding jar procedure

Two special problems are associated with the anaerobic jar system: (1) when plates are inoculated, they are often put into a jar that is left open until more cultures arrive to fill the jar before it is sealed, and thus the plates are exposed to oxygen; (2) sometimes properly and promptly sealed jars will be opened to add new plates, again resulting in repeated exposure to oxygen.

By using Martin's **holding-flush jar arrangement**,[32] these problems can be easily solved. Inoculated plates are placed into a storage jar (GasPak, vented) covered with an unclamped vented lid through which oxygen-free CO_2 is passing continuously until enough plates accumulate to fill the jar, sealing it and setting up anaerobiosis. The same can be done with media held before inoculation and with plates for subculture. The most economical way to obtain oxygen-free CO_2 is to use a tube filled with copper shavings heated in a thermostatically controlled small electric oven (Sargent-Welch furnace S-36517, tube S-36518); the CO_2 passes through the hot copper, oxidizing it as the O_2 is removed from the CO_2. The copper can be

reduced periodically by passing gas containing 3% hydrogen through the heated copper for a few minutes.[23]

Allen et al.[33] have modified Martin's procedure as follows:

Agar media are placed in cellophane bags and stored in refrigerator for up to 6 wk. Plates are held in anaerobic glovebox or a GasPak jar for 18-24 h **prior** to inoculation. As needed, reduced media are placed in holding jar or other container and continuously flushed with gentle stream of nitrogen (N_2). Plates of reduced media are surface inoculated in ambient air and immediately placed in holding container and flushed with N_2. After jar is filled, plates are then incubated in conventional anaerobic system at 35 C. During examination and subculture of colonies, 3 jars are used to prevent undue exposure of uninoculated media, colonies, and inoculated plates of media to O_2 (Fig. 70-14).

Anaerobic glovebox technic[23]

An anaerobic glovebox is a self-contained anaerobic system. With the glovebox, most bacteriologic technics involved in the isolation and identification of anaerobic bacteria can be performed under anaerobic conditions without exposing the microorganisms to air. The first practical, inexpensive glovebox for cultivation of anaerobes was described by Aranki et al.[16] Since then the equipment has been improved considerably and it is now available in various sizes commercially (Coy Manufacturing Co., Ann Arbor, Mich. 48104—flexible glovebox; Forma Scientific Corp., Marietta, Ohio—rigid box), Fig. 70-15.

The **flexible glovebox** consists of a chamber of pressed clear vinyl with a floor, fitted with one or 2 pair of gloves, a metal lock entry, and unheated

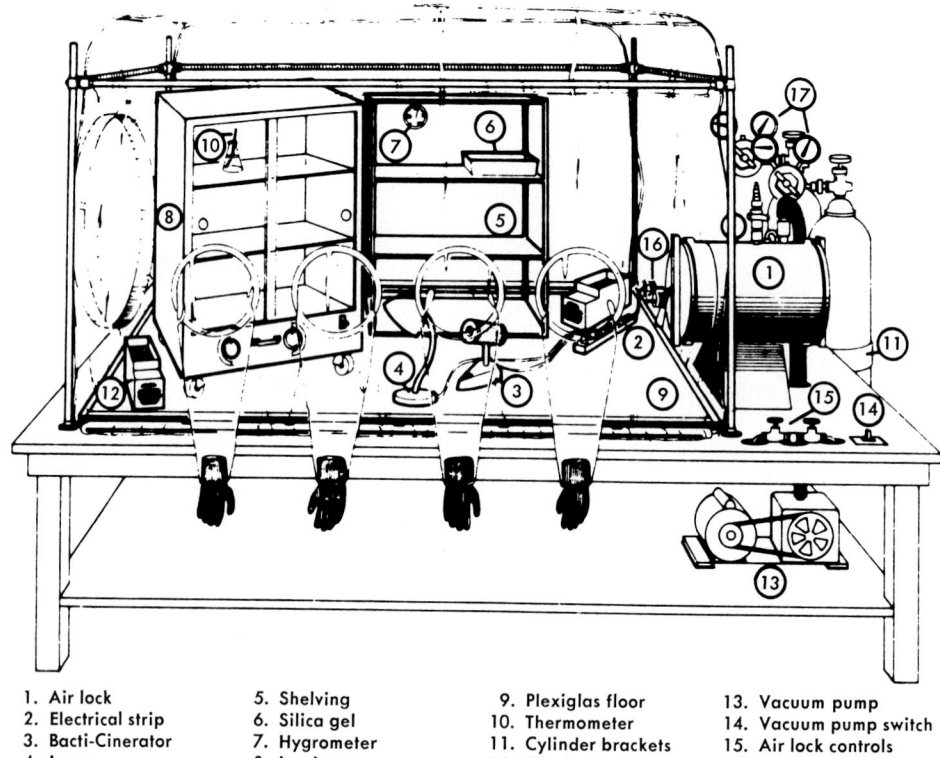

Fig. 70-15. Anaerobic glovebox.

1. Air lock
2. Electrical strip
3. Bacti-Cinerator
4. Lamp
5. Shelving
6. Silica gel
7. Hygrometer
8. Incubator
9. Plexiglas floor
10. Thermometer
11. Cylinder brackets
12. Catalyst tray
13. Vacuum pump
14. Vacuum pump switch
15. Air lock controls
16. Access nipple
17. Gas regulators

catalyst boxes to be used with palladium-coated alumina catalyst pellets (Deoxo); it also includes an incubator, an electrical heater for sterilization of bacteriologic loops or wires, and a vacuum pump. After the glovebox is assembled and sealed, the chamber is partially evacuated and filled 10 times with technical grade nitrogen and 10 times with a gas mixture of 5% CO_2 (bone dry), 10% H_2, and 85% N_2. Approximately 0.45 kg of catalyst pellets in each of the catalyst diffusion boxes aids in the removal of residual oxygen.

The relative humidity of the chamber is regulated with a drying agent (Tel-Tale silica gel, desiccant, grade H type IV, Davison Commercial Chemical Corp., Baltimore, Md. 21223) reusable by heating in a dry-heat oven at 160 C to remove moisture. Anaerobic conditions are maintained in the glovebox by replacing the catalyst pellets with new or "rejuvenated" catalyst at frequent intervals (at least once per week).

The oxygen concentration can be monitored, if desired, with an oxygen analyzer. Use of an oxygen analyzer is not absolutely necessary if the catalyst is changed frequently and oxygen-sensitive indicators are used to monitor anaerobic conditions.

When material is passed into the chamber, the lock is evacuated and replaced twice with nitrogen and once with the gas mixture (5% CO_2, 10% H_2, 85% N_2) before the inner door is opened. The

same procedure in reverse is used when removing materials from the chamber. Media prepared in the usual manner are passed into the chamber and **reduced** 48 hours before they are used. PRAS media can also be used in the glovebox if desired. Cultures are incubated within the chamber and can be inspected and subcultured at any time without exposure to air.

The use of an anaerobic glovebox has several advantages:

1. Either conventional media (prereduced in the chamber) or prereduced anaerobically sterilized media (PRAS) can be used.
2. Clinical specimens are not exposed to aerobic conditions during culture procedures.
3. The need for boiling liquid media just before use is eliminated.
4. Conventional plating technics can be used.
5. Cultures can be incubated under anaerobic conditions, inspected, and subcultured at any time without exposing the bacteria to air.
6. Using the system is economical. The only major operating cost is for gases that are used when materials are passed into and out of the chamber.

Liquid media

General. The addition of various reducing agents, sodium thioglycollate (0.3-0.5%), cysteine, cooked meat, and 0.1-0.3% agar to liquid media will reduce the oxygen potential sufficiently to permit anaerobic growth in the depth of the tubed column.

Thioglycollate broth, enriched with vitamin K (0.1 μg/ml) and hemin (5 μg/ml), and chopped meat–glucose medium are widely used as "backup" media; i.e., they are examined only when there is no growth on anaerobic plates.

Addition of blood (5%), serum (10%), ascitic fluid (10-25%), or Fildes enrichment (5%) to thioglycollate broth improves growth of anaerobes significantly. **Selectivity** can be obtained by adding 100 μg/ml kanamycin **or** neomycin (both are autoclavable), which prevent the growth of many aerobic organisms. **Do not use selective medium without using nonselective medium in parallel.**

If specimen is liquid, inoculate thioglycollate tubes with Pasteur pipets (or long capillary pipets, available commercially), taking care that no air is introduced.

Petrolatum-sealed tubes
1. Use tubes of any suitable medium, e.g., fluid thioglycollate, chopped meat, or similar medium. Heat in boiling water bath for 10 min to expel oxygen.
2. Cool and inoculate medium.
3. Pour over medium a layer of sterile liquid petrolatum, using sterile precautions. The layer should be about 1.5 cm high.
4. Replace plug and incubate.

PRECAUTIONS. Thioglycollate medium should not be refrigerated, since it absorbs more oxygen at lower temperatures. Store in the dark at room temperature.

Other anaerobic methods
Deep agar column

The deep agar tube method was originally developed by Veillon and Zuber[34] and has been used extensively by French workers at the Pasteur Institute.[35] Details of the technic have been described, in English, by Fredette[36] and Quinto.[37] It involves the use of beef and liver medium (VF medium), acidified with HCl and digested with pepsin, employed in deep agar columns, serially inoculated with a long capillary pipet. When colonies appear, the wall of the tubes is scraped with a file, cracked with a red-hot tip of a small glass rod, and broken apart; the desired colony is then removed with a capillary pipet and subcultured. Differential tests (proteolysis, nitrate reduction, indole, and H_2S production) are determined, using VF broth or agar columns with the appropriate substrate added. The broth tubes are evacuated and sealed. Antibiotic sensitivities are performed with disks suspended in deep agar tubes or in Petri pour plates. No specialized equipment is required for this technic. However, it has a number of disadvantages: small numbers of organisms may not be detected, single colonies are difficult to pick, and opaque media cannot be used. The method is chiefly used in France and French Canada but not in the United States or Great Britain. The required media are not available commercially and the method is time consuming.

Phosphorus jar

The phosphorus jar is a reasonably effective method for obtaining anaerobiosis. At one time it was widely used, since the materials needed are inexpensive, and with reasonable care to prevent accidental burns of the operator, there is no danger involved. **Its use is not recommended, except in emergencies or if no other equipment is available.**

Materials
1. Stocks of white (yellow) phosphorus (keep in water, in tightly stoppered widemouthed bottle)
2. Pair of long forceps or tongs
3. Lubriseal or Plasticene
4. Pyrex cylinder (jar) and lid

The Varney jar, produced expressly for the phosphorus method, is no longer available commercially. On the other hand, any glass (Pyrex) museum jar can be modified by the workshop so that it can be conveniently used for this method. The lid and the jar should have ground glass surfaces. A metal framework (rack) for Petri dishes is easily fabricated. To hold the phosphorus a metal can is needed, with a lid and a wire gauze cylinder.

CAUTION. **Never handle phosphorus without using tongs or forceps.** At the time the container is opened, remove the phosphorus with the tongs and return to container with water.

Procedure
1. Keep phosphorus in water in glass jar inside metal jar so that in the event inner jar should be broken, metal can would still contain both phosphorus and water.
2. Streak cultures on blood agar or other media, wrap in paper towel, and place in inverted position in metal framework.
3. Cover bottom of small metal can with Drierite before it is placed in jar. (Drierite particles on ground surfaces can prevent good seal, as can cotton fibers; always use paper towel or other lint-free material to wipe surfaces.)
4. Grease ground glass surface of both lid and jar with Lubriseal.
5. Place metal can in jar. Then remove phosphorus from water in which it is stored, place immediately in can, and place small lid in position quickly.
6. Close jar quickly and clamp shut. White smoke settling as a yellow precipitate indicates that phosphorus has burned. Remainder of phosphorus should burn when jar is opened. This is proof that anaerobic conditions have been attained.

Alkaline pyrogallol method—Spray

This method utilizes the oxygen-absorptive capacity of the reaction between alkali and pyrogallic acid. Spray[38] devised a special dish for use with pyrogallic acid and sodium hydroxide. The dishes are expensive and subject to considerable breakage. Use only if no other equipment is available.

Fill one-half of bottom of dish with 4 ml 20% solution pyrogallic acid. Fill other half with 10 ml 2.5N NaOH solution. Do not mix chemicals before closing cover. Place lid, with culture medium down, over dish. Seal with modeling clay or paraffin. Tilt dish gently so that the 2 solutions mix. Do not splash solution onto medium. Incubate.

CULTIVATION IN AIR WITH INCREASED CARBON DIOXIDE CONTENT

Many organisms grow better if incubated in air plus 5-10% CO_2. Certain organisms such as *Brucella abortus, Vibrio fetus,* and *Haemophilus vaginalis* are CO_2 dependent for initiation of growth; others such as *Neisseria gonorrhoeae* and *N. meningitidis* as well as certain streptococci grow faster initially under increased CO_2 tension.

There are several methods for producing such an atmosphere.

Procedures
"Candle jar" method
1. Place inoculated plates in a container that can be tightly covered; e.g., desiccator jar, Pyrex preparation jar, Petri dish container, coffee can, or any other available container. Place lighted, smokeless candle in container and close lid. Flame consumes oxygen, and enough CO_2 is produced for culture needs of bacteria.
2. Brewer jar can be used as CO_2 jar by evacuating 10% of air and replacing it with CO_2 from a cylinder. If used in such manner, rubber tubing attached to bottom of lid should be removed.
3. Place plates in a tin can that can be tightly covered. If V = volume of container in **L**, add $0.25 \times V$ g marble chips to $2.5 \times V$ ml 25% hydrochloric acid in the can. This will give an approximately 5% CO_2 atmosphere.
4. Place in one half of bottom of Spray dish 0.5 g sodium bicarbonate with enough distilled water to dissolve it. In other half place 3% sulfuric acid. Place lid containing inoculated culture medium over Spray dish, medium side down, and seal with modeling clay. Shake dish from side to side to mix the contents in bottom of dish, taking care not to splash liquid on medium.
Method of Ellner-Elbogen-Frankel[39]
1. Although this technic was originally designed for use in cultures for acid-fast bacilli, it can now also be used for blood cultures, and so on. It is applicable wherever **closed** container (blood culture bottle, TB medium bottle), usually employing screw cap with self-sealing rubber liner is used. Tank of 5% CO_2 in air, filled with needle valve, serves as source of gas mixture. Meter gas through flowmeter (no. 8021, Gelman Instrument Co., Ann Arbor, Mich.) at 0.5 L/min and filter through membrane filter (Gelman GA Metricel filter mounted in syringe filter holder no. 4320). Attach sterile, 20-gauge Yale, 1 in. disposable needle to discharge end of filter holder. Loosen cap of container, insert needle through rubber liner, and let the gas flow for 10 s. Withdraw needle and tighten cap. Change filter attachment after 200 bottles have been filled, since mold spores present in gas may contaminate cultures. This method is prac-

tical, fast, and, with reasonable care, safe and efficient.
2. Carbon dioxide incubators are commercially available and are used in large laboratories. They require gas cylinders and have to be refilled with CO_2 after each opening of the incubator. Laboratories doing large volume of TB work prefer use of CO_2 incubators.

NOTE. None of the methods described above, including the candle jar method, results in anaerobiosis; this is a commonly held misconception. **Anaerobic conditions** can be obtained only by the use of methods described under anaerobic methods and **not** by the methods used for increased Pco_2.

EGG CULTURE METHODS

Egg culture methods have been used not only for the propagation and isolation of viruses, but also for diagnosis of certain bacterial diseases. The special value of this living medium has been demonstrated for culturing organisms such as *H. influenzae, Bordetella pertussis, B. abortus, Pasteurella tularensis,* meningococci, pneumococci, and certain fungi.

Because of the speed of growth of bacteria in this medium, the method was an important factor in the early diagnosis of various bacterial diseases. The egg as a culture medium has been applied particularly to the culture of spinal fluids in meningitis. The routine methods employed in many hospital bacteriologic laboratories have in the past frequently failed to yield the etiologic agent of this disease. In many cases of meningitic infections, growth of bacteria can be demonstrated by egg inoculation when simultaneous agar cultures fail to permit their detection.

However, with the advent of many newer and sensitive culture media (as well as the introduction of immunofluorescence methods), little use is made today of egg cultures in the isolation of bacteria.

Those interested in this technic should refer to Chapter 91, where there is an extensive description of the various methods employed in chick embryo work, together with detailed drawings.

EXPERIMENTAL ANIMALS FOR CLINICAL DIAGNOSTIC PURPOSES

The use of experimental animals is sometimes necessary to verify certain bacteriologic procedures. The animals of choice are white mice, white rats, guinea pigs, and rabbits. It is necessary to procure healthy animals. For this purpose, one must be sure to buy animal stock from reliable animal dealers.

The animals must be kept in cages that can be readily cleaned. Cages of all experimental animals must be kept clean and must be disinfected at intervals.

Care and feeding of animals

Mice. Mice may be fed on white bread and oats. Drinking water may be supplied through the special drinking apparatus that was introduced by Ehrlich and modified by Dunker.

Guinea pigs. Guinea pigs must be kept in dry roomy cages, preferably with the bottoms covered with straw. They should be protected against sudden changes in temperature conditions. Artificially prepared foods can be obtained for mice, guinea pigs, and rabbits. A moderate amount of green vegetables, cabbage, etc., should also be given. When guinea pigs are being fed on cabbage or vegetables in summer, it is well to give them very little water, but when they are given dry food, they should be freely supplied with water.

Rabbits. Rabbits should be kept in roomy cages. Their food requirements are about the same as for guinea pigs.

Injection of animals

Materials
1. Clean, sterile 2 ml syringes
2. 23-gauge 1 in. needles

Procedure
White mice
1. Seize mouse at nape of neck.
2. Lay mouse on its back, holding tail or hind legs stretched out and immovable.
3. Make subcutaneous injection by lifting skin, after disinfection with iodine, and inserting needle through skin.
4. Take care in working around abdomen not to penetrate the abdominal wall.

Guinea pigs
1. Secure in same position as white mice.
2. For intra-abdominal or intraperitoneal injections, lift abdominal wall with fingers so that no part of intestine comes along with it.
3. Make injection in such a manner as to avoid puncture of the intestines.

Rabbits
1. For intra-abdominal or intraperitoneal injections, use same procedure as for guinea pigs.
2. For intravenous work, select marginal vein in ear.

METHOD I
1. Place rabbit on table.
2. Assistant holds him securely while one or the other ear is selected for injection.
3. With fine pair of scissors, clip off hair along marginal vein.
4. Few brisk rubs with small amount of xylol on cotton sponge will dilate vein. Disinfect skin with bichloride of mercury or small dab of iodine.
5. Thrust needle into the marginal vein.
6. Make injection.

METHOD II. A very ingenious method for holding a rabbit so as to facilitate the injection of solutions into the marginal ear veins is the use of the Beohm device. This permits one to see that the needle is securely in the vein and that the blood is being pushed back through the venous system and not going out into the tissues. It consists of a light unit attached to a rabbit box; a spotlight bed lamp also works very well. This can be clamped to the edge of the table so that the rabbit's ear can be held out over the lens.

After the inoculation
1. Sterilize all instruments.
2. Mark animal.
   a. Mice: Place 1 or 2 drops aniline dye on fur.
   b. Guinea pigs and rabbits: Thrust very fine staple holding numbered tag through ear; numbered tags can be bought from any supply house.
3. Make records and observe animals.

The date of inoculation, number of tag, material, etc., should be entered in a notebook. The animal should be observed at frequent intervals. Notes should be made regarding any signs of sickness. When animals die, they must be autopsied. Mice are autopsied by being placed on a board and tacked down with a tack through each extended extremity. Use sterilized instruments. Make the median incision with a pair of fine scissors and observe the visceral conditions. Bacteriologic cultures sometimes must be made from autopsies of animals. These must be taken under strict aseptic conditions. The same method may be applied in autopsies on rabbits and guinea pigs.

Laboratory animals may be used in the diagnosis of rat-bite fever (*Spirillum minor*), leptospirosis, relapsing fever (some species of *Borrelia*), tuberculosis, anthrax, and for determination of the toxigenicity or pathogenicity of certain organisms (such as *Corynebacterium diphtheriae* and clostridia). For details of these procedures, reference should be made to the section on the specific organism.

MAINTENANCE AND PRESERVATION OF BACTERIAL CULTURES; STOCK CULTURES

Teaching institutions and type-collecting agencies* maintain many cultures at great expense and effort. In clinical laboratories it is necessary to preserve cultures for teaching purposes, for use in testing newly prepared batches of reagents, or to allow work at length with cultures isolated from clinical material that may present difficulties in identification. The main concern in maintenance of cultures is to preserve their typical biologic characteristics; this is not always easy, since bacteria have great capacity to undergo variation.

Standard organisms for control purposes can be obtained from the American Type Culture Collection (ATCC). Isenberg and Berkman[40] list a large number of strains they recommended for maintenance in the clinical laboratory; a limited number of strains from their list and a few others are recommended as the minimum needed for stock cultures: *Actinomyces israelii* (ATCC no. 12102), *Alcaligenes faecalis* (8750), *Arizona arizonae* (13314), *B. abortus* (9539), *Clostridium haemolyticum* (9650)—for control of anaerobic procedures, *Escherichia coli* (11775), *Herellea anitratus* (9955), *Klebsiella-Aerobacter* (13048), *Listeria monocytogenes* (13932), *Mycobacterium kansasii* (12478), *Nocardia asteroides* (3308), Providence sp. (9886), *Sarcina lutea* (9341)—widely used for control of antibiotic sensitivity testing, *Salmonella schottmuelleri* (*S. paratyphi* B, 10719), *S. typhi* (9992V), *Shigella boydii* (9207), and *Serratia marcescens* (13880). For

*American Type Culture Collection, 12301 Parklawn Drive, Rockville, Md. 20852; National Collection of Type Cultures, Central Public Health Laboratory, Colindale Ave., London NW9, England.

those interested, a strain of *Yersinia enterocolitica*, indole positive (ATCC no. 23715; NCTC no. 10598, which I deposited) may be valuable. The characteristics of these strains are stable, since most are maintained by the ATCC in the lyophilized state. The organisms can be maintained in cystine trypticase agar (CTA) medium (BBL) at room temperature for 6 months; some will survive better on nutrient agar or tryptose agar slants at room temperature. Mycobacteria can be maintained on Lowenstein-Jensen medium slants, in screw-capped tubes for 6 months at room or refrigerator temperature.

See also Chapter 73, "Quality control."

Lyophilization

Probably the most useful and successful of all methods is freeze-drying, in which dense growth of the organism to be preserved—usually suspended in serum, milk, or 3% lactose—is placed in small vials. These are quick frozen in a mixture of dry ice and 95% alcohol and then are evacuated while frozen, until completely desiccated; finally the vials are sealed hermetically while evacuated. Freeze-drying apparatus is available commercially. It should be noted that some fastidious organisms do not tolerate lyophilization well.

Oil seal

Morton and Pulaski[41] worked out a method of preservation under paraffin oil that they claim has many advantages; it reduces contamination, especially with molds. No preliminary treatment of the cultures is necessary. All the organisms tested lived longer under oil than in the control tubes. Changes in cultural and biochemical characteristics have not been observed. The cultures are available at all times for transplantation without interfering with the preservation of the stock culture. The method is applicable to single colonies or mass cultures. It is advantageous in working with unstable variants, for which occasional transferring to fresh media or growth in mass culture results in a change in the developmental stage of the strain. No seals such as rubber caps, waxes, cements, etc., are needed. No special apparatus is needed, such as a centrifuge, desiccator, or vacuum pump. The method of choice recommended by these workers is as follows:

Organisms are grown on appropriate solid media, such as infusion agar, blood agar, etc., slanted to avoid giving too long a slant. After good growth has taken place, the slant is covered with sterile heavy paraffin oil, or mineral oil, to a height of 1 cm above the top of the slanted surface.

Attention must be called to the following points. The oil should be well above the uppermost level of the medium. The medium is this way cannot dry out and separate from the wall of the tube and float to the surface of the oil, in which event the organisms are usually found dead. The quality of the oil is very important, as any rancidity or toxic substance is harmful to the organisms. It is preferable to sterilize the oil by auto-claving at 15 psi for 1 h and then heating in a drying oven at 110 C for 1 h to drive off any entrapped moisture. Precaution is necessary in flaming the loop after it has been withdrawn from the oil, since plunging directly into the flame results in spattering. This may be prevented by warming the loop very gently before heating to redness, or by plunging into a beaker of boiling water, then flaming to redness in the usual manner. *Mycobacterium* and *Salmonella* do not preserve well under oil seal.

Freezer storage

Rosebury and Frances[42] have successfully employed storage in a dry ice chest. Dense growth in appropriate liquid culture media is placed into 1 ml constricted-neck ampules; these are flame sealed and immediately placed in the dry ice chest.

Temporary storage in commercially available media

Many organisms can be maintained for varying lengths of time by simply inoculating appropriate media and keeping the cultures at recommened temperatures. Screw-capped tubes are preferable to cotton-plugged tubes, since dehydration is greatly retarded. Most coliform organisms can be maintained in cooked meat medium or nutrient agar slants at room temperature for about 1 year or on trypticase agar base for 6-12 months at room temperature or in the refrigerator. *Brucella, Neisseria, Pasteurella, Listeria,* pneumococci, and streptococci can be maintained in BBL CTA at room temperature for 3-6 months. *Salmonella* and *Shigella* organisms should be maintained in Difco cooked meat medium or in nutrient broth at room temperature (will survive for 1 year or more). Molds are best maintained on BBL mycophil agar under oil (6 months, room or refrigerator) or Difco Sabouraud maltose agar. Castellani[43,44] recommends inoculating tubes containing 6, 8, or 10 ml sterile distilled water, plugged with cotton wool, with large inocula of pathogenic fungi, especially dermatophytes, for preservation at room temperature for 12 months.

Castellani's procedure was evaluated by McGinnis et al.[45] who found it simple, inexpensive, and reliable with filamentous fungi, yeasts, and aerobic actinomycetes.

Glycerol broth at −50 C.[46] A large variety of nutritionally fastidious organisms and anaerobes have been maintained in glycerol broth at −50 C for at least 2 years without loss of viability. The medium used is trypticase soy broth with 15% glycerol (sterilized by autoclaving or by filtration, final pH 7.0-7.5). Glycerol broth in 3 ml volume is placed in Pyrex tubes (22 × 160 mm); about one dozen growing colonies (or 0.5 ml of liquid suspension) are added to glycerol broth.

Place tubes immediately in a deep freezer at −50 C. When needed, thaw the frozen tube at room temperature and inoculate directly onto broth or solid medium.

Table 70-1. McFarland nephelometer standards

Tube	Sulfuric acid, 1% aqueous solution (ml)	Barium chloride, 1% aqueous solution (ml)	Corresponding density of bacteria (approx. million/ml)	International Units (IU) of opacity[50]
1	9.9	0.1	300	3
2	9.8	0.2	600	7
3	9.7	0.3	900	10
4	9.6	0.4	1200	12
5	9.5	0.5	1500	15
6	9.4	0.6	1800	—
7	9.3	0.7	2100	20
8	9.2	0.8	2400	—
9	9.1	0.9	2700	—
10	9.0	1.0	3000	30

STANDARDIZATION OF BACTERIAL SUSPENSIONS—McFARLAND NEPHELOMETER STANDARDS*

1. Make set of nephelometric tubes by mixing 1% sulfuric acid, cp, with 1% barium chloride, cp, according to Table 70-1.
2. Tubes must be of uniform size and of resistant glass.
3. Plug tubes with rubber stoppers and carefully seal with paraffin. Set tubes up in rack.
4. For estimation, compare bacterial suspensions with standards.
5. This set serves to determine approximately number of bacteria present in saline suspension. To estimate bacterial density in broth cultures, make set by dissolving sulfuric acid and barium chloride in sterile broth.
6. Some more modern procedures use photelometers. Standardize curve by using McFarland standards (Table 70-1). Select filter according to photelometer and color of the fluid in which organisms are suspended.

FLUORESCENCE MICROSCOPY METHODS

Certain substances, said to be **fluorescent,** absorb light energy of one wavelength ("activation" or "excitation" light) and emit light of another wavelength, usually within 10^{-7} to 10^{-9} seconds. (When the absorbed light is emitted over a longer period, the substance is said to be **phosphorescent.**) Fluorescence is essentially an electronic phenomenon and involves light of wavelengths of 200-800 nm (mμ), e.g., ultraviolet light, 200-400 nm, and visible light, 400-800.

A number of organic and inorganic substances are fluorescent, i.e., can be excited by a shorter wavelength light and will as a result emit light of a longer wavelength (e.g., if excited by ultraviolet light, will emit light in the visible spectrum). Among the organic substances that show fluorescence are those that are aromatic or contain conjugated double bonds (have alternating single and double bonds between atoms); these are said to have "native" fluorescence. Many nonfluorescent substances can be converted by

*Available commercially as McFarland barium sulfate standards, Difco Laboratories, Detroit, Mich.

chemical reactions into fluorescent ones. The fluorescent properties of various compounds (such as certain proteins, aromatic amino acids, porphyrins, purines, vitamins, hormones, and a large number of drugs) are of considerable importance in medicine; however, it is not possible to describe all their applications here. Only those applications of fluorescence of interest in the diagnostic microbiology laboratory will be discussed.

The interested reader is referred to the review of Williams and Bridges,[47] to Udenfriend's *Fluorescence Assay in Biology and Medicine,*[48] and to Nairn's *Fluorescent Protein Tracing.*[49]

Direct fluorescence—nonimmunologic
Autofluorescence

Most biologic tissues are autofluorescent, i.e., possess natural fluorescence that is a mixture of the blue, blue-green, and green emissions of the various molecules making up the tissue. Fluorescence microscopy without stains has been used to study, among others, the autofluorescence of porphyrins and vitamin A in the skin. Characteristic red fluorescence has been shown in the skin of patients with various types of porphyria.[51]

Fluorescent dyes

A number of synthetic and natural dyes show substantial fluorescence. Some have a selective affinity for various bacteria, tissue cells, and their components and therefore can be used for identification purposes. Among these, auramine O, acridine orange, rhodamine B, and trypaflavine are widely used. Acridine orange has been used for staining fungi to visualize some internal structures poorly stained by other reagents and also for staining skin scrapings containing superficial fungi. Acridine orange–stained slides examined with ultraviolet light are used as a screening procedure for suspected skin tumors and for studying the growth of viruses in their host cells; ribonucleic acid (RNA) shows red to orange fluorescence, whereas deoxyribonucleic acid (DNA) fluoresces yellow-green.

Normal cells have less RNA and DNA, whereas tumor cells show increased amounts and hence fluorescence; the same applies to viruses in host cells where DNA or RNA can be visualized during the replication of viruses.[51]

Auramine and rhodamine are used for staining mycobacteria (especially *M. tuberculosis* and groups I, II, and III of the atypical mycobacteria). The stain is retained by the acid-fast organisms; upon excitation of the stain by light of a suitable wavelength the organisms fluoresce, which can be detected by dark-field or bright-field microscopy. Background light is absorbed by a filter system that allows only the transmission of the light caused by fluorescence. There has been a renewed interest in the use of fluorescence microscopy for acid-fast organisms.[52] The modifications introduced by Silver et al.[53] have made the procedure more effective and easier to perform than the Ziehl-Neelsen procedure. When auramine and rhodamine are used, ultraviolet light is not absolutely necessary, since they can be excited by light of up to 496 nm.

Direct fluorescent tracing of proteins, consisting of injection of labeled serum proteins into animals and their detection in tissues or body fluids, is also used. According to Nairn,[49] fluorescent protein tracers can be detected by fluorescence microscopy in animal tissues at a concentration of 1 μg protein/ml body fluid. The method has been used for studying the distribution and metabolism of proteins, the determination of sites of enzyme and antibiotic action, and the mechanism of pinocytosis.

Immunofluorescence—fluorescent antibody (FA) methods

Fluorescent antibody methods are, in effect, an outgrowth of the vexing problem facing workers who tried to determine the distribution of soluble antigens in the animal body. Haurowitz and Breinl[54] injected into rabbits horse serum coupled with diazotized arsanilic acid and then sacrificed the animals and assayed their organs for arsenic content. Heidelberger et al.[55] introduced the chemical labeling of antigens by the use of color. They coupled a salt of benzidine into egg albumin by means of a diazo linkage and thus obtained a red azoprotein that could be measured by spectrophotometric methods. Radioactive isotopes for labeling antigens were introduced by Libby and Madison,[56] who injected such labeled antigens into mice and then determined the radioactivity in various organs.

The chemical methods of labeling antigens described were not completely satisfactory, since they altered the antigenic character of the labeled protein.

Marrack[57] found that antibody proteins could be conjugated with single chemical compounds without altering their specificity and thus preserving their capacity to react with their corresponding antigens. He obtained red antityphoid and antichlorea antibodies using a dye, and when he mixed the antibodies with the organisms, the bacteria were seen to be specifically reddened by the colored antibody. Coons[58] conceived the idea of labeling antibodies with fluorescent compounds. With his collaborators[59,60] he showed that pneumococcal antibody labeled with fluorescein isocyanate could detect pneumococci and pneumococcal polysaccharide in the tissues of mice injected with pneumococci.

All presently used methods employing fluorescent antibodies are either the direct or indirect products of Coons's investigations. The major applications of the technic for the next decade were essentially studies of the fate of antigenic material (proteins, antigens, virus, toxins) and of antibody formation in the animal body. These studies were extensively reviewed by Coons.[61-64] Both antibodies and antigens have been labeled with fluorescent dyes. The reviews of Beutner[65] and of Borek[66] should be consulted for details.

Since 1956 there has been rapid development in the use of fluorescent antibody technics for the diagnosis of various infections (by visualizing and identifying bacterial, viral, parasitic, and mycotic antigens), for the visualization of animal tissue antigens and the localization of antibody in tissues (in a modified form), and for the detection and characterization of serum antibody (used diagnostically, among others, as the fluorescent treponemal antibody test, the antinuclear and antithyroid FA procedures).

The reviews of Beutner,[65] Coons,[67] the excellent monograph[68] on FA technics in diagnostic bacteriology, the technical manual of Cherry et al.[69] and of Jones et al.[50] are recommended for anyone wishing to use FA methods for diagnostic purposes. Important source books for FA work, dealing with the principles of fluorescent protein tracing, together with details of making conjugates and their application in direct fluorescence and immunofluorescence, are Nairn's *Fluorescent Protein Tracing*[49] and Goldman's *Fluorescent Antibody Methods*.[70]

It should be emphasized that FA technics require special equipment and well-trained workers familiar with principles of immunology and serology. There are numerous pitfalls in FA procedures, and a thorough understanding of the principles involved and meticulous care in technics are mandatory.

The FA method is a new way of detecting conventional antigen-antibody reactions. It is a specific staining procedure in which specimens containing the antigen (bacteria, viruses, fungi, protozoa) are treated with appropriate fluorescein-labeled (conjugated) antibody and are then examined under the fluorescence microscope. The light causes the antigen-antibody complex to become fluorescent and to emit a brilliant green-yellow (direct FA staining; other methods are described below).

The only labeling substance of practical use until 1958 was fluorescein isocyanate, chosen by

Coons[60] because of the brilliant yellow-green fluorescence of its protein conjugates. The conjugation procedures with this substance were cumbersome and complicated. A much simpler conjugation method using fluorescein isothiocyanate (FITC), introduced by Riggs et al. in 1958,[71] represented a major advance and contributed greatly to the intensification of FA work. Dyes that fluoresce in the red portion of the spectrum are also used for labeling proteins (rhodamine B isothiocyanate, lissamine rhodamine B, and others). Rhodamine-conjugated normal globulins are used for staining tissue or cellular debris present in the specimen to be examined. Immune globulin conjugated with rhodamine can be used in polyvalent globulins, in which the components have been labeled separately with dyes of contrasting colors and then mixed. Such a mixture may make it possible to identify different antigens or organisms in the same preparation at the same time. (The fluorescein isothiocyanate label will fluoresce green while the rhodamine label will fluoresce red.)

The specimens used can be either tissues (both frozen and paraffin embedded) or smears containing bacteria, fungi, parasites, and viruses from cultures or clinical material.

In contrast to conventional bacteriologic and serologic technics, requiring from 1 to several days for definitive diagnosis, FA technics are rapid; in some instances, results can be obtained from clinical specimens in 1-4 hours. The procedure in some respects is more sensitive than cultural methods. Nonviable organisms can be detected with FA, but instances in which FA technics failed to detect organisms grown later in cultures also occur.

In 1960-1961 Cherry et al.[69] strongly emphasized that FA technics are **not** to be considered as a replacement for bacteriologic procedures but as an adjunct to conventional methods. At the time of writing, this warning is still valid for many FA procedures. Cherry and Moody in their extensive review,[68] Eveland,[72] and Nahmias et al.[73] emphasize that of the many FA procedures (applied to approximately 30 genera or species of bacteria), only a limited number have been standardized and evaluated to the point where they are recommended as routine procedures in the diagnostic laboratory (and as **possible** replacements for the standard cultural technics). They also repeatedly point out the need for well-trained personnel, adequate equipment, and carefully controlled reagents and procedures in the performance of FA tests.

Fluorescent antibody tests in diagnostic microbiology

Cherry and Moody[68] noted that among the applications of the FA technic to diagnostic bacteriology, only the following have been evaluated fully and are in routine use: (1) the identification of group A streptococci in nasopharyngeal exudates,[74-79] (2) the serogrouping of the enteropathogenic E. coli in fecal smears,[80-87] (3) the identification of N. gonorrhoeae in exudates from the genital tract,[88-93] and (4) the use of the indirect FA test for detection of syphilitic antibody in human serum (as a confirmatory test for reactive nonspecific tests, such as the VDRL test). They listed a number of other procedures that are less well evaluated or standardized, such as the FA technic for detection of S. typhi[94] and Shigella sp., the identification of the whooping cough organism (B. pertussis),[95] the screening of sediments from spinal fluids for agents of bacterial meningitis, and the rapid presumptive diagnosis of the diphtheria organism.[97]

Nahmias et al.[73] and Biegeleisen et al.[97] have obtained good results with FA methods in the screening of spinal fluid sediments from cases of meningitis. N. meningitidis, Streptococcus (Diplococcus) pneumoniae, and H. influenzae were correctly diagnosed by the use of conjugate pools (pool of 3 groups for the meningococcus, pool of 31 types for the pneumococcus, and pool of 6 types for the influenza bacillus). These workers, along with Cherry and Moody,[68] state that in their opinion the FA technic will prove to be a valuable adjunct in the rapid and specific diagnosis of certain bacterial infections. However, they caution against discarding the use of the Gram stain and of cultural procedures.

In their 1978 monograph, Jones et al.[50] tabulated the bacteria, diseases, and summaries of the status of the FA tests that may be applied for their detection (Table 70-2).

Diseases other than bacterial for which FA procedures were available were listed by Casey[143] as follows:

Fungal diseases (see Part X, Medical Mycology). Histoplasmosis, coccidioidomycosis, sporotrichosis, North American blastomycosis, and paracoccidioidomycosis.

Parasitic diseases (see Part IX, Medical Parasitology). Toxoplasmosis, malaria, trichinosis, and schistosomiasis.

Viral and rickettsial diseases (see Part VIII, Viral and Rickettsial Diagnostic Procedures). Rabies (widely used for early specific identification of agent), rubella, smallpox, and herpes simplex.

FA methods

Only an outline of the methods used in FA technics for the diagnosis of various microorganisms can be presented here. The reader is referred for details to Cherry and Moody,[68] Cherry et al.,[69] and especially Jones et al.[50]

Optical equipment. Standard diagnostic microscopes equipped with glass (as opposed to quartz) optics are suitable for FA work. Dark-field condensers are used by most workers with various combinations of oculars and objectives. High-pressure mercury arcs enclosed in quartz envelopes provide the bright light source needed to produce visible fluorescence with the minute amounts of fluorescein involved in FA reactions. Small arcs are available that emit a major percentage of their energy in the ultraviolet and blue portion of the spectrum. The Osram HBO-200 high-pressure mer-

Table 70-2. Status of immunofluorescence (IF) tests*

Organism	Disease	Status	Reference
Direct IF tests			
1. Group A streptococci	Acute pharyngitis and scarlet fever	Most highly evaluated and most extensively used of all IF tests for bacteria; sensitive and specific for detecting Group A streptococci from throat cultures	68
2. Group B streptococci	Acute rheumatic fever Neonatal sepsis and meningitis and bovine mastitis	Polyvalent reagent containing both type and group antibody gave 99.1% agreement between IF and culture-precipitin tests on 833 clinical isolates and 97% agreement on 99 vaginal swabs; 8 false + reactions occurred in 982 clinical specimens; IF detected 9 nonhemolytic Group B's not detected by culture	98
3. Escherichia a. E. coli (EEC)	Infant diarrhea	Highly effective for rapid screening of saline suspensions of feces; eliminates culture of negatives	68, 99
4. Salmonella typhi	Typhoid fever	Vi conjugate equals culture for detection of chronic carriers; make smears directly from saline susp. of feces; less effective than culture for use on acute cases; use OVi conjugate on smears of acute specimens prepared directly from saline susp. and from enrichments	68, 100, 101
5. Salmonellae (most serotypes)	Gastroenteritis, enteric fever, meningitis	Use a polyvalent conjugate covering O groups A-S to screen smears from tetrathionate or selenite enrichments of feces, foods, and environmental samples; very sensitive but gives 1-20% IF positives on culture negative specimens; culture all IF positives	102-107
6. Shigella a. S. sonnei	Shigellosis	Sensitive and specific for screening saline suspensions of fecal smears; well-evaluated	108, 109
b. S. flexneri		Appears promising for screening of fecal smears but needs further evaluation	110, 111
7. Bordetella a. B. pertussis b. B. parapertussis	Whooping cough	A rapid, sensitive, specific, and simple test for an organism for which culture is difficult; stain pernasal-pharyngeal smears with specific conjugates	68, 112, 113
8. Haemophilus a. H. influenzae type b and/or types a-f	Bacterial meningitis	These reagents when applied to CSF's are comparable in sensitivity to culture and Gram stain, but are rapid, have immunologic specificity, and will detect bacteria in partially treated patients; superior for use on CSF's containing small numbers of organisms	68, 97, 114
9. Streptococcus a. S. pneumoniae	Bacterial meningitis	Complex polyvalent conjugates needed for good coverage of capsular types (1-31); quite specific	68, 97, 114
10. Neisseria a. N. meningitidis (groups A-C)	Bacterial meningitis	Polyvalent conjugate stains groups A and C well and group B less well; also stains N. gonorrhoeae; may be used on smears from petechiae	68, 97, 114
11. Legionella pneumophila (Legionnaires' bacterium)	Lobar pneumonia	Excellent for specific detection of organisms in formalin-fixed, paraffin-embedded lung tissues, lung tissue imprints, lung exudates, and cultures, including colonies from plates	115
12. Listeria monocytogenes	Listeriosis	Excellent for specific detection of organisms in formalin-fixed, paraffin-embedded tissues, tissue imprints, body fluids, and cultures, including colonies from plates	68

Continued.

Organism	Disease	Description	References
13. *Brucella* a. *B. suis* b. *B. abortus* c. *B. melitensis*	Brucellosis	Sensitive, rapid and specific for smooth strains of these species in culture and tissues; indirect FA tests for serum antibody offer no advantage over agglutination	68, 116, 117
14. *Yersinia pestis*	Plague	Excellent for rapid diagnosis when used on blood, stored animal tissues, and stomach contents of vectors; organisms stain well in tissue impression smears or in frozen or freeze-dried sections, but not in routinely prepared formalin-fixed, paraffin-embedded sections; conjugate is specific if carefully prepared or sorbed	68
15. *Francisella tularensis*	Tularemia	Rapid, sensitive, and specific for detection of organisms in culture, impression smears, and frozen or freeze-dried sections of infected tissue specimens; does not cross stain *F. novicida* or *Brucella*; may stain *E. insidiosa* and some *Pseudomonas*	68, 118
16. *Bacillus anthracis*	Anthrax	Rapid and sensitive for detection of anthrax organisms in culture, in tissue imprints, or in formalin-fixed, paraffin-embedded tissues of man or other infected animals; cross stains some strains of *B. megaterium* and *B. subtilis*	68
17. *Mycobacterium tuberculosis*	Tuberculosis	Rapid and sensitive for detection of *M. tuberculosis* in direct sputum smears or digests; 98% of 96 culturally positive sputa were + by IF; 0 of 6 other mycobacterial species were +; conjugates specific for *M. kansasii, M. phlei, M. marium,* and the V subgroups of Runyon's Group III have been prepared and tested	119, 120
18. *Campylobacter fetus* var. *venerealis*	Vibriosis	Reliable, simple, rapid means of diagnosing bovine vibriosis in the cow; use filtered cervical-vaginal mucus; does not differentiate *C. fetus* var. *venerealis* from *C. fetus* var. *intestinalis*	121
19. *Erysipelothrix insidiosa*	Infections in many animal species	Rapid, sensitive, and specific for detection of bacteria in cultures, blood, tissue imprints, and in histologically processed tissue sections; labeled antibody to major shared antigens is used; sensitivity compared to culture may be inadequate for routine diagnostic use on swine tissues	122, 123
20. *Actinomyces* a. *A. israelii* b. *A. naeslundii* c. *A. eriksonii*	Actinomycosis	Rapid, sensitive, and specific for species determination, and for serotyping of *A. israelii* and *A. eriksonii* in pure or mixed cultures; also useful with Gram-staining for detecting organisms in human tonsils and other tissues or exudates	124, 125
21. *Clostridium* a. *C. botulinum*	Botulism	Conjugates are available for differentiating toxin types A, B, and F from toxin types C and D, and from type E in cultures and in foods	126, 127
b. *C. chauvoei*	Blackleg in cattle and other animals	Sensitive, rapid, and specific staining of bacteria in culture and in tissue imprints and sections, with a single "O" conjugate	128
c. *C. septicum*	Braxy of sheep, maligant edema, gas gangrene	Same as above with a conjugate containing antibodies to the 2 "O" group antigens	128
d. *C. novyi*	Gas gangrene, necrotic hepatitis	Same as above with a single "O" conjugate	129
e. *C. tetani*	Tetanus	Same as above with a single "O" conjugate	129

*From Jones, G. L., Herbert, G. A., and Cherry, W. B.: Fluorescent antibody techniques and bacterial applications, Atlanta, 1978, U.S. Dept. H.E.W., Center for Disease Control.

Table 70-2. Status of immunofluorescence (IF) tests—cont'd

Organism	Disease	Status	Reference
Direct IF tests—cont'd			
22. *Leptospira* a. Multiple serotypes	Leptospirosis	Excellent for rapid and sensitive screening of formalin-preserved or fresh tissue scrapings or imprints, and for cultures and urine sediments for the presence of pathogenic leptospires; use a single group—specific conjugate	130
23. *Neisseria gonorrhoeae*	Gonorrhea	Usefulness limited to staining of organisms in pure culture, in conjunctivae, skin lesions, and joint fluids and to screening mixed cultures for rapid presumptive information; not recommended for **diagnosis** or for **test of cure;** use only conjugates tested for specificity by the CDC	131
24. *Chlamydia trachomatis*	Trachoma	IF is most sensitive method for detecting intracellular inclusions of the trachoma-inclusion conjunctivitis group of agents; it is highly specific	132, 133
25. *Mycoplasma* sp.	Respiratory diseases, genital infections and arthritis	Sensitive, rapid, and specific for detecting colonies by flooding plates with conjugate and observing by incident illumination	134
26. *Pseudomonas* a. *P. pseudomallei* b. *P. mallei*	Melioidosis Glanders	Rapid and sensitive for detecting bacteria in culture, exudates, and tissue imprints of infected animals; conjugate for *P. pseudomallei* will also detect *P. mallei*; may cross react with other *Pseudomonas* species	135, 136
27. *Treponema pallidum*	Syphilis	Rapid procedure for detecting *T. pallidum* in early syphilitic lesions; still experimental, but specificity appears adequate to differentiate saprophytic organisms from *T. pallidum*	137
28. *Bacteroides fragilis*	Bacteremia	Potentially valuable for detecting *Bacteroides fragilis* subspecies in blood, other clinical specimens, and in culture; commercial sera and conjugates available for both indirect and direct FA tests	138, 139
Indirect IF tests			
Treponema pallidum	Syphilis	FTA-ABS test should be used for verification and not for routine tests; most sensitive of treponemal tests with specificity equal to the TPI; not useful for evaluating therapeutic response; recent data show that FTA-ABS tests for IgM antibody to *T. pallidum* in congenital infections may not be disease specific	140-142

cury vapor lamp is one that is widely used. Johnson et al.[144] state that an iodine-quartz lamp, less expensive than the mercury vapor lamp, is satisfactory when used with a combination of 2 Wratten primary filters (32 and 28A) and a yellow secondary filter.

Filters are employed between the lamp and object with only fluorescence-exciting wavelengths being passed (such as the Schott BG-12 filter used with the heat-absorbing filters, Schott BG-14, or BG-22), and between object and observer (barrier filter in the eyepiece, such as Schott OG-1) to remove ultraviolet light and to transmit visible wavelengths of light characteristic of the specimen's fluorescence. In this manner the excitation light that would mask the fluorescent images is removed before it reaches the eye of the observer. Different filter combinations are used, depending on the material examined.

Transmitted-light fluorescence. Fluorescence excitation with transmitted light is the classic method. Light from the source must be critically centered to a 45° mirror and directed upward into a dark-field condenser beneath the specimen. When the dark-field condenser is properly aligned, the specimen is illuminated from below in the form of a hollow cone. This means that none of the exciting light can enter the objective. The dark background of the microscopic field provides an increased contrast for viewing weak fluorescence.

Incident-light fluorescence. With incident light, the exciting radiation is directed at the specimen from above, through an incident-light illuminator with dichroic beam splitting mirrors. The light travels downward through the microscope objective; thus the full aperture of the objective is used for excitation. Incident light gives a high fluorescence intensity because, unlike the situation with transmitted-light excitation, no light can be lost through scattering or primary absorption in the specimen.

Because the intensity of the exciting radiation depends on the numerical aperture (N.A.) of the objective used, microscope objectives with the largest possible aperture should be used for incident-light excitation. Thus oil immersion objectives are desirable for all magnifications, including 10X, since the N.A. is increased by immersion.

Materials and solutions[50]

1. Phosphate buffered saline (PBS), pH 7.6, 0.01M
   a. Concentrated stock solution (pH will not be 7.6)

Na_2HPO_4 (anhydrous; reagent grade)	12.36 g
$NaH_2PO_4 \cdot H_2O$ (reagent grade)	1.80 g
NaCl (reagent grade)	85.00 g
Distilled water to make final volume	1000 ml

   Dibasic salt dissolves much more readily in water at 37 C than at 25 C.
   b. Working solution (pH 7.6; 0.01M buffer; 0.85% NaCl):

Concentrated stock solution	100 ml
Distilled water to make final volume	1000 ml

2. Buffered glycerol mounting fluid (approx. pH 9.0):

Glycerol, reagent grade	90 ml
0.2 M Na_2HPO_4	10 ml

3. Polyvinyl alcohol semipermanent mounting medium
   a. Elvanol, 10% or 15%

Elvanol 51-05	10 or 15 g
0.85% NaCl to pH 7.4 with 0.01 M Na_2HPO_4-KH_2PO_4	70 ml

Glycerol	30 ml
1% Merthiolate	1 ml

   Add Elvanol to buffered saline, heat to approx. 75 C or until Elvanol dissolves; cool to room temperature. Add glycerol, mix, check pH, and adjust to pH 7.4. Add Merthiolate, mix, and store in air-tight bottle.
   b. Gelvatol, 5%

Gelvatol 3-60	5 g

   Prepare as for Elvanol, with the same reagents.
4. Formalinized saline
   a. 0.5% Formalinized, 0.85% NaCl

Formaldehyde (36-38%)	5.0 ml
NaCl	8.5 g

   Dissolve NaCl in distilled water and bring to 1 L vol. Autoclave 15 min at 121 C and cool to room temperature. Add formaldehyde.
   b. 0.6% Formalinized, 0.85% NaCl (for *Salmonella*)

Formaldehyde (36-38%)	6.0 ml
NaCl	8.5 g

   Prepare as for the 0.5% above.
   c. 0.5% Formalinized, 0.5% NaCl (for *E. coli*)

Formaldehyde (36-38%)	5.0 ml
NaCl	5.0 g

   Prepare as for the 0.5% above.
5. Kirkpatrick's fixative

Absolute ethanol	60 ml
Chloroform	30 ml
Formalin (37%)	10 ml

   Mix thoroughly. Use as fixing solution for smears.
6. Sorensen's phosphate buffer, pH 7.4, M/15
   a. Stock solutions
   (1) Na_2HPO_4 9.46 g
      Dissolve and bring to 1 L with distilled water.
   (2) KH_2PO_4 9.07 g
      Dissolve and bring to 1 L with distilled water.
   b. Working buffer, pH 7.4

Solution 1	800 ml
Solution 2	200 ml

7. Buffered cotton swabs. Boil cotton swabs in Sorensen's phosphate buffer M/15 at pH 7.4 for 5 min to neutralize acids from the wood and cotton of the swabs. Shake off excess solution, place in suitable container, autoclave, and dry before use.
8. Deparaffin of tissue for FA staining
   a. Cut very thin sections (4 μm or less) from paraffin block.
   b. Heat for approximately 15 min at 58-60 C to fix sections to slides.
   c. Dip slides through series
   (1) 2 dishes xylol
   (2) 2 dishes absolute ethanol
   (3) 2 dishes 95% ethanol
   (4) 2 dishes water
   d. Allow slides to air dry.

Reagents. FA reagents are immune globulins (antibodies) labeled ("tagged") with fluorescein; these may be specific for a given microbial species such as tagged antistreptococcal sera, or they may be labeled antiglobulins (Coombs serum) for globulins of various species such as man, guinea pig, etc. Purified globulins rather than whole antisera are used for labeling, since the labeling agent attaches itself to nonantibody as well as antibody globulin; this would be wasteful. In addition, the use of whole antisera increases the chance for nonspecific staining.

Many labeling compounds, antisera, and finished conjugates are now available from commercial sources.

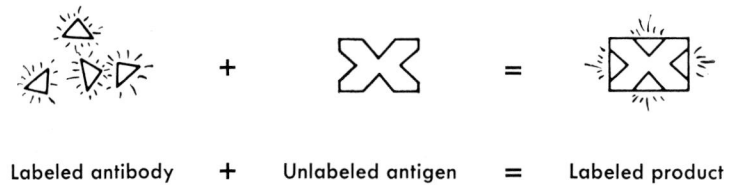

Labeled antibody   **+**   Unlabeled antigen   **=**   Labeled product

Fig. 70-16. Schematic representation of direct staining with fluorescent antibody. (From Cherry, W. B., Goldman, M., Carski, T., et al.: Fluorescent antibody techniques in the diagnosis of communicable diseases, PHS pub. no. 729, Atlanta, 1960, Communicable Disease Center.)

For details about the preparation and characterization of FA antibody reagents, see Hebert et al.[145]

Direct staining[50, 67, 68]

The basic reaction is shown schematically in Fig. 70-16. **Labeled antibody** is applied to smears of antigen fixed on slides. After a suitable interval, previously determined by experimentation, the excess antibody is washed off, and the mounted (coverslipped) preparation is examined with a fluorescence microscope. This is the simplest form of FA test and is employed to identify unknown antigen by using known labeled antibody as the staining agent. The labeled antibody will be adsorbed onto the homologous antigen; the combined antibody-antigen particles will appear as fluorescent bodies.

Fluorescent antibody procedure for rapid identification of group A streptococci[50]

Reagent. *Streptococcus* group A FITC-labeled immune globulin is prepared from rabbit *Streptococcus* Group A antiserum. This grouping serum is fractionated by the ammonium sulfate method, and the resultant globulin mixture is conjugated with FITC to yield a fluorescein to protein ratio (F/P) of 25 μg FITC/mg protein.

The appropriate **dilution for routine use** of Group A antistreptococcus conjugate must be determined for each new lot of reagent. The dilution of conjugate selected is based upon (1) the brilliance of the fluorescence reaction with Group A streptococci and (2) the extent of fluorescent cross-reactions with Groups C and G streptococci and with *Staphylococcus aureus*.

Significant **cross-reactions** that sometimes remain for certain strains of Groups C and G streptococci and *S. aureus* after absorption of conjugates with Group C streptococci usually can be inhibited with a mixture of equal parts of appropriately diluted conjugate and selected normal rabbit serum or Group C antistreptococcus serum.

A satisfactory working dilution of the test reagent is one that stains all of the Group A strains at a 3+ to 4+ fluorescence intensity and the other strains not more than 1+ to 2+.

The reagents may be stored at 2-10 C and used until the supply is exhausted or no longer satisfactory. The reagents should be tested periodically with known Group A, C, and G streptococci and *S. aureus* to ascertain their reactivity.

Conjugates with inhibiting sera added are available commercially. These conjugates are normally already diluted to titer (or recommended for reconstitution to titer from the lyophilized state), but the dilution should be confirmed. The conjugates should also be checked

for cross-reactions and rechecked periodically with known cultures as outlined above.

Preparing and fixing of smear

1. Place throat swabs in 1 ml broth (Todd-Hewitt, trypticase soy, or heart infusion) and incubate for 2-5 h at 37 C.
2. Remove swab from broth and place in sterile tube.
3. Centrifuge broth for 5 min at approximately 2,000 rpm.
   NOTE. If Kirkpatrick's fixative (see below) is used, broth culture will adhere to slides and centrifugation in step 3 is not necessary, unless needed to concentrate cells.
4. Pour off broth into disinfectant solution and wipe lip of tube with disinfectant-soaked cotton; resuspend cells in 1 ml sterile phosphate buffered saline (PBS), pH 7.6, and recentrifuge.
5. Pour off buffered saline into disinfectant solution. Wipe lip of tube with disinfectant-soaked cotton while tube is in inverted position to remove all visible diluent.
6. Place tube in rack for 2-3 min and let residual buffered saline collect in bottom of tube. (Usually no additional diluent will be needed.)
7. Mix cells thoroughly in diluent.
8. With Pasteur capillary pipet, transfer sediment to area within circles on FA slide. Try to transfer most of sediment to smears.
9. Let smears dry in air. If atmosphere is humid, smears may be dried in 37 C incubator.
10. Cover each smear with 95% ethanol. Keep wet for 1 min, then let ethanol evaporate. After smears are thoroughly dry, stain them or freeze and store and if **absolutely no thawing** occurs, stain later.

Alternate procedure for preparing smears. The most satisfactory procedure for screening large numbers of throat swabs is to inoculate a blood agar plate culture and 18-24 h later stain smears prepared from β-hemolytic colonies with *Streptococcus* Group A conjugate.

1. Inoculate throat swab onto a **sheep** blood agar plate, streaking for isolated colonies. For primary isolation, sheep rather than rabbit blood should be used to prepare plates because sheep blood contains a factor that inhibits the growth of *H. haemolyticus*. Blood agar medium for primary isolation should contain no added glucose.
2. Incubate plates 18-24 h at 35 C under anaerobic conditions or, at a minimum, make some cuts into the agar to assure growth away from oxygen for poor surface-hemolyzing Group A streptococci.
3. Pick β-hemolytic colonies to small amount of sterile buffered saline, pH 7.6, in small test tube. Adjust density to that through which printed letters can be easily read; prepare smears.
4. For better definition of cells (chaining) or for plates that contain few β-hemolytic colonies, pick

colonies to 1 ml of broth, incubate 2-5 h, adjust density, and prepare smears.

5. Fix the smears either with 95% ethanol or Kirkpatrick's fixative.

NOTE. After desirable sensitivity and specificity of a particular vial of Group A antistreptococcus conjugate has been established with Groups A, C, and G streptococci and with *Staphylococcus aureus* control cultures only a known positive *Streptococcus* Group A control slide is needed with each day's run.

Staining. Apply procedure to thoroughly dried, fixed smears. Include a known positive control slide in each test run.

1. Cover smears with Group A antistreptococcus conjugate.
2. Spread conjugate over entire smear with applicator stick held in horizontal position.
3. Incubate 30 min at room temperature in moist chamber. Half of 15 cm Petri dish fitted with moist filter paper is suitable chamber.
4. Drain excess conjugate onto disinfectant-soaked paper towel.
5. Dip slides momentarily into buffered saline, pH 7.6, in a staining dish.
6. Transfer to second vessel of buffered saline and let stand for 10 min.
7. Dip momentarily into distilled water and air dry (do not blot).
8. Add drop of buffered glycerol mounting fluid, pH 9.0, and cover slip. Keep bubbles from forming in mounting fluid. Apply drop of nail polish (or similar adhesive) to each corner of 1 cover slip. If necessary, refrigerate but do **not** freeze.
9. Stained and mounted smears stored in refrigerator may be examined anytime within 24-48 h without significant loss of brilliance of fluorescence. If smears are to be used later for reference purposes, they may be stored for longer periods. If they are stored longer than 48 h, however, there may be a gradual loss in staining intensity. Slides to be stored in refrigerator overnight or longer should be sealed completely with nail polish.

Interpretation of results. *Streptococcus* Group A strains exhibit 3+ to 4+ cell-wall fluorescence with sharply defined, nonstaining cell centers. Heterologous streptococci (non–Group A) and staphylococci usually do not exhibit more than 1+ cell-wall fluorescence with indistinguishable cell centers.

Test limitations. The testing of smears made directly from throat swabs is not entirely satisfactory and is therefore not recommended. Optimal results are obtained by testing cells from 2- to 24-hour broth cultures or suspensions of growth of β-hemolytic streptococci from blood agar plates.

As a confirmatory diagnostic procedure for the detection of Group A streptococci, the direct FA test is comparable in accuracy and reliability to the Lancefield capillary precipitin test (≥95% agreement).

Direct fluorescent antibody procedure for Legionella pneumophila (Legionnaires' disease bacterium)[50, 115]

This organism causes a severe pneumonia, particularly in compromised patients. The direct FA test is used for detection of the organism in lung tissue or exudates therefrom.

Reagents. The specific reagent may consist of a single high-titered conjugate that has been evaluated for adequate detection of all known strains of the Legionnaires' bacterium. A conjugate prepared from hyperimmune rabbit antiserum for the Knoxville strain has this characteristic. At its diagnostic use dilution of 1:80, it will stain the following strains to an intensity of 3-4+: Philadelphia numbers 1, 2, 3, and 4; Flint 1 and 2; Knoxville; Pontiac, Burlington; Albuquerque; Berkeley; and Birmingham. The Bellingham strain is stained only 3+, but this is adequate for its detection in clinical specimens. Conjugates to other Legionnaires' strains may require much lower-use dilutions for adequate detection of the first 12 strains, and they may be inadequate for demonstrating the Bellingham strain. Eventually, a single pooled or polyvalent conjugate that will stain all known strains satisfactorily may become available. The control reagent may be a normal rabbit conjugate.

Preparation of specimen material

Tissue scrapings of formalin-fixed tissue

1. Select one or more areas of the lung or other tissue for testing. With lung tissue, choose dense areas of grey or reddish consolidation.
2. Transfer each tissue block to sterile Petri dish.
3. With sharp scalpel, cut through these areas to produce new tissue faces for scraping.
4. Grasp tissue with forceps and holding scalpel at right angle to the tissue face, scrape it to produce fine puree of tissue particles. (Lung tissue of victims of Legionnaires' disease is usually quite friable.) If tissue is rubbery or spongy, positive test is unlikely.
5. Using scalpel blade, smear particles of tissue and tissue juices onto two 1.5 cm circles on a microscope slide.
6. Let smears air dry. Gently heat fix.

Fresh or fresh-frozen tissue (autopsy or biopsy): Tissue should be processed in a safety cabinet.

1. Using sterile instruments, cut fresh face of tissue and with forceps press and squeeze tissue against clean slide, making at least 2 smears. If tissue is so moist that smears may be too thick, blot on sterile gauze or culture media before imprints are made. If tissue is to be cultured, do not touch tissue to slide first because the slide may not be sterile.
2. Air dry and heat fix.
3. Fix smears for 5 min by covering them with a solution of 10% neutral formalin in a Coplin jar. During fixation each patient's material should be processed in a separate jar to prevent carry-over.
4. Drain off formalin and gently and briefly dip each slide into distilled water to remove remainder of formalin.
5. Air dry.

Tissue sections

Legionnaires' bacteria maintain their serologic integrity through histopathologic processing and can easily be demonstrated in tissue sections if they are reasonably numerous. They are not as easily demonstrated in sections, however, as in scrapings of formalin-fixed lung or in imprints of fresh lung tissue. This is because many of the bacteria are intracellular, lie at many different levels in the section, and are shrunken by the histologic processing. Counterstains, such as rhodamine-labeled rabbit serum or rhodamine-labeled bovine serum albumin, make the organisms much more visible in tissue sections. Evans blue and other counterstains will also probably be helpful, but they have not been sufficiently studied.

1. Tissue sections should be cut as thin as possible (4 μm or less) from paraffin blocks.
2. Fix the sections by heating for approximately 15 min at 58-60 C.
3. Deparaffin by 2 passages through xylol followed by 2 passages each through absolute ethanol, 95% ethanol, and water.
4. Air dry.

Exudates from the lung (process in safety cabinet). Sputum, transtracheal aspirates, bronchial washings, or other specimens from the lower respiratory tract are satisfactory materials for study. Legionnaires' disease patients frequently do not produce much sputum, and what is produced may or may not be purulent. The secretions are, however, usually extremely viscid and tenacious. Counterstains are needed; see above.

1. Select viscous portion of specimen and prepare 2 smears of moderate thickness on one or more microscope slides.
2. Air dry and heat fix.
3. Fix in formalin as for fresh tissue, as described above.
4. Drain off formalin and dip slides briefly into distilled water.
5. Air dry.

Pleural fluids (process in safety cabinet)

Pleural fluids should be cultured for attempted isolation of the Legionnaires' organism. Since these fluids are obtained aseptically, overgrowth of the Legionnaires' organisms by contaminants is not a problem. Two of the available isolates were obtained in this way.

Prepare thin smears, air dry, heat fix, and process as described for lung exudates above.

NOTE. Pleural fluids tend to form a fibrin clot on the slide and, unless handled carefully, the entire film may be dislodged during processing.

Culture smears (process in safety cabinet)

1. Make suspensions of cultures of known or suspected Legionnaires' bacteria in 1% buffered formalin to give a light turbidity.
2. Prepare smears on double ring or on multiwell slides.
3. Air dry and heat fix.

Controls. The most important controls consist either of (1) preimmune conjugate from the same animals that furnished the specific reagent or (2) conjugates prepared from the serum of unimmunized animals of the same species as those immunized. These control reagents should have approximately the same protein content and F/P ratio as the specific conjugate.

As controls, the conjugates should be used at either the same dilution as that of the specific conjugate or, preferably, at twice that concentration, as a margin of safety.

Each specimen preparation showing specific staining must be tested with the control reagent to ensure that the observed reaction is serologically specific. Other essential controls are culture suspensions and positive and negative preparations of tissue scrapings, tissue imprints, sections, and smears of lower respiratory tract secretions, depending upon the types of diagnostic material being submitted for examination.

Positive and negative smears should be carried through the specimen staining procedure each time a group of specimens is processed. Negative smears may be made from suspensions of any heterologous bacteria not related serologically to the Legionnaires' bacterium.

FA staining procedure

1. Stain all preparations by covering smear nearest labeled end of slide with 1-2 drops (0.05 ml) of the preimmune or other control conjugate.
2. Cover other smear with 1-2 drops of use dilution of Legionnaires' conjugate.
3. Place slides in covered chamber to prevent evaporation during staining.
4. Stain for 20 min or other suitable period as previously determined.
5. Remove excess conjugate by holding slide level, but perpendicular, and tapping it against towel. Quickly and gently rinse smears with stream of phosphate-buffered saline (PBS) from wash bottle while holding slides horizontally with long edge tipped downward. Prevent specific conjugate from coming into contact, even momentarily, with control smear.
6. Immerse slide in PBS for 5 min.
7. Dip slide in distilled water.
8. Air dry.
9. Add small drop of buffered glycerol (pH 9.0) and a Corning 1 or 1½ coverslip to the smears.

Examination of stained slides. Examine first under the 10X objective of the fluorescence microscope. In strongly positive preparations the bacteria will be visible as uniformly sized dots. Select areas of the smear where organisms may be present and switch to the oil immersion objective. The bacteria will be visible as single short rods or small intracellular or extracellular clumps of organisms showing strong peripheral staining with darker centers.

Interpretation of results. In clinical specimens, except sputum, the following criteria are used to evaluate the test results:

Result	Report
>50 strongly fluorescing bacteria/field (oil-immersion objective)	FA + (many)
2-50 strongly fluorescing bacteria/field	FA + (moderate numbers)
1 strongly fluorescing bacteria/field	FA + (few)
<25 strongly fluorescing bacteria/*smear*	Report numbers only
O strongly fluorescing bacteria/smear	FA −

In sputum, organisms are never numerous. Thus, the observation, per smear, of 5 or more brightly stained small rods—morphologically typical of the Legionnaires' bacterium—is considered a positive result.

Test limitations. Direct FA staining of scrapings or of sections of formalin-fixed lung, of fresh lung imprints, or of cultures or pleural fluids is rather straightforward. Organisms in culture are usually longer rods than those seen in tissues. In older cultures long filaments, swollen rods, and other bizarre forms may be seen.

Interpretation of the results of staining lower respiratory tract specimens is more difficult. Tissue and white blood cells may be highly autofluorescent. Bacteria such as staphylococci, diplococci, and streptococci may fluoresce because of natural antibodies in the serum of the immunized rabbit. Familiarity with the morphology and staining characteristics of the Legionnaires' organism is imperative if false-positive diagnoses are to be avoided. One strain of *Pseudomonas fluorescens* has recently been found that is brightly and specifically stained by the working dilution of a Legionnaires' conjugate. The fluorescent *Pseudomonas* rods may, however, appear wider than the Legionnaires' rods. Relatively few Legionnaires' bacteria are seen in lower respiratory tract specimens, so a smear should not be called negative until after at least a 5-minute search.

The use of counterstains for sputum and tissue examination has proven very helpful. Because of the size of the particles of tissue obtained by scraping formalin-fixed lung, many particles are lost from the slide during processing. The free bacteria and tissue cells will, however, remain on the slide to give a very good test substrate.

Because of its rapidity and sensitivity, the direct FA test is now the method of choice for diagnosis of Legionnaires' disease. Results can be obtained on autopsy or biopsy tissue more quickly by the direct FA test than by pathologic examination. The most important advantage emerging, however, is the rapid detection of the organisms in appropriately selected lower respiratory tract specimens. This permits appropriate antibiotic therapy to be selected much earlier in the course of the disease, at a time when it may be lifesaving.

The direct FA test has a dimension of serologic specificity that the Dieterle silver stain and other stains used to demonstrate the organisms in tissue do not have.

Performance characteristics

1. Diagnostic dilution of FA conjugate should stain all known strains of Legionnaires' bacteria at least to a 3+ intensity.
2. Corresponding control conjugate at its use dilution should not stain any of stock strains to more than 1+ intensity.

Fluorescent antibody procedure for enteropathogenic E. coli

The serogrouping of enteropathogenic *E. coli* in fecal smears has been proved to be an excellent and rapid screening procedure, yielding a higher percentage of positive findings than the conventional culture technic. The great value of the test is in its use for screening negative specimens that require no culture. FA-positive specimens (direct smear) are cultured, and isolates are serogrouped by immunofluorescence.[50, 68] The excess of positive FA over positive cultural results seems to represent increased sensitivity of the FA procedure, since enteropathogenic *E. coli* can be isolated by repeatedly culturing specimens originally culture negative and also since few heterologous staining reactions are encountered when *E. coli* conjugates are tested against a variety of Enterobacteriaceae. For details of the procedure see Jones et al.[50]

Fluorescent antibody procedures for identification of N. gonorrhoeae

The FA technic for the identification of gonococci, using the delayed (enrichment) technic, decreased the time necessary to identify the gonococcus from 4-8 days necessary for cultural technics (especially when purification measures were needed) to approximately 20 hours. It also was shown to be two thirds more efficient than the conventional culture in detecting gonorrhea in women. When the **highly selective Thayer-Martin medium** (see media), which allows the growth of gonococci and meningococci but not of saprophytic neisseriae or other contaminating organisms, and the delayed FA procedure were compared (in the female), they were found to be of equal efficiency if multiple sites were examined[146]; however, if only one site is examined, the culture is more productive. In addition, it was found that the FA procedure detected dead bacterial forms; for this reason, the FA procedure is said by Lucas et al.[146] to be suitable for the primary diagnosis of gonorrheal specimens, but it should not be used as a test of cure (after penicillin or other antibiotic therapy). For details of the procedure see references 89-93 and 50. Neither the direct nor the delayed FA technic is recommended for primary diagnosis of gonorrhea or for test of cure.

Indirect staining

In this method, shown in Fig. 70-17, **unlabeled antibody** is used in the first stage of the reaction. To determine whether the unlabeled antibody and the antigen have combined, a **labeled antiglobulin** specific for the unlabeled antibody is added. Excess antibody is washed off and the preparation is examined with the fluorescence microscope.

Fluorescence indicates a reaction between the antigen and the unlabeled specific antibody employed in the first stage. The method can be used for detection of **unknown antibodies** (Chapter 75) (using known antigen and unknown, unlabeled antibody followed by labeled antiglobulin) or for identification of an **unknown antigen** (using known, unlabeled antibody, followed by labeled antiglobulin).

An example of indirect FA staining is the fluorescent treponemal antibody (FTA-ABS) test described in Chapter 106. In this test the unlabeled serum of the patient suspected of having antibody against *Treponema pallidum* is added to treponemes fixed on a slide. After suitable reaction time the excess serum is washed off and labeled antihuman globulin (Coombs serum) is added. Fluorescence of the treponemes indicates a reaction between antibody in the patient's serum and the treponemes.

Inhibition staining

The inhibition staining reaction, shown in Fig. 70-18, is based on the blocking of specific antigen-antibody reactions by reacting the antigen

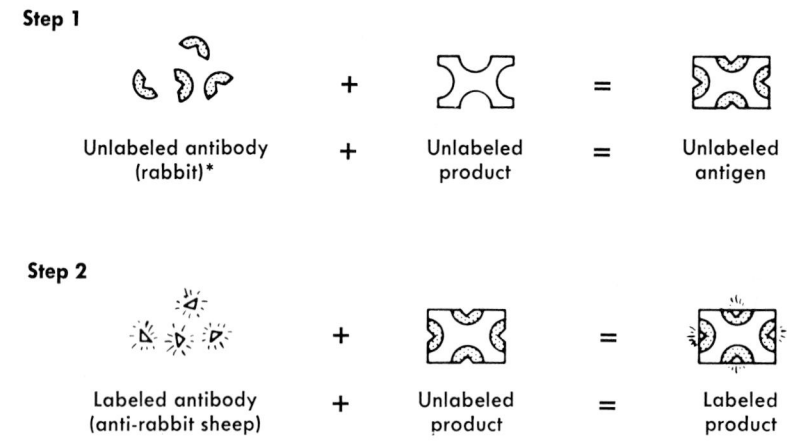

Step 1

Unlabeled antibody (rabbit)* + Unlabeled product = Unlabeled antigen

Step 2

Labeled antibody (anti-rabbit sheep) + Unlabeled product = Labeled product

*Antibody from other species may be used in conjunction with homologous antiglobulin

Fig. 70-17. Schematic representation of indirect fluorescent antibody staining reaction. (From Cherry, W. B., Goldman, M., Carski, T., et al.: Fluorescent antibody techniques in the diagnosis of communicable diseases, PHS pub. no. 729, Atlanta, 1960, Communicable Disease Center.)

Step 1

Unlabeled antibody + Antigen = Unlabeled product

Step 2

Labeled antibody + Unlabeled product = Unlabeled product (inhibition of staining by unlabeled antibody)

Fig. 70-18. Schematic representation of fluorescent antibody inhibition staining reaction. (From Cherry, W. B., Goldman, M., Carski, T., et al.: Fluorescent antibody techniques in the diagnosis of communicable diseases, PHS pub. no. 729, Atlanta, 1960, Communicable Disease Center.)

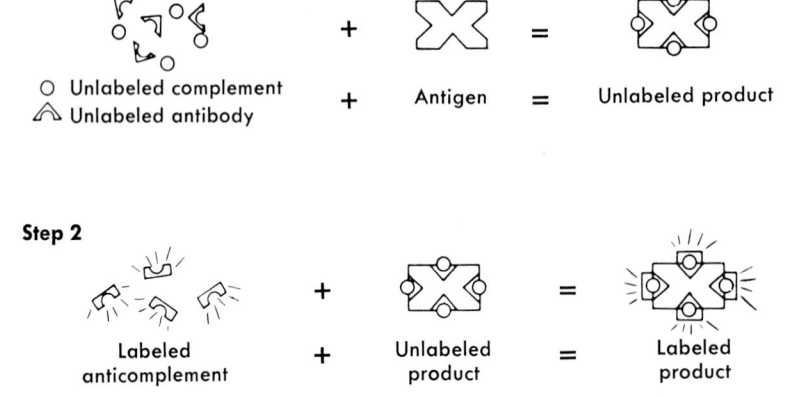

Step 1

○ Unlabeled complement
△ Unlabeled antibody + Antigen = Unlabeled product

Step 2

Labeled anticomplement + Unlabeled product = Labeled product

Fig. 70-19. Schematic representation of complement staining with fluorescent antibody. (From Cherry, W. B., Goldman, M., Carski, T., et al.: Fluorescent antibody techniques in the diagnosis of communicable diseases, PHS pub. no. 729, Atlanta, 1960, Communicable Disease Center.)

with unlabeled specific antibody. In this manner
the antigen becomes saturated with antibody,
and upon the addition of labeled specific antibody, no reaction will occur due to inhibition of
staining by the unlabeled antibody. The inhibition technic, as mentioned earlier, is also employed as a test for specificity of the direct technic.

Complement staining

Complement staining is similar to the indirect procedure. However, the labeled antiglobulin used in the second step of the reaction
is not directed against the species supplying the
antiserum (used in the first step) but against the
species supplying the complement. Fig. 70-19
illustrates the principles involved. The technic
can be used for identification of an unknown
antigen or an unknown antibody.

Preparation of labeled globulins
(fluorescent conjugates)

Only an outline of the methods used can be
presented here. Usually antiserum is first fractionated by conventional ammonium sulfate precipitation (half-saturation) to obtain a globulin
preparation. The precipitated globulin, left overnight at 0-5 C, is separated by centrifugation, dissolved in distilled water, and reprecipitated 2
more times. It is then dialyzed against 0.85%
NaCl at 0-5 C until free of sulfate.

The globulin labeling procedure generally
consists of the following steps:

1. Determine protein content of globulin solution by
   the Biuret test.
2. Adjust protein content before conjugation. Some
   workers use a 1% protein concentration; others
   use 2-3% concentration for conjugation.
3. Adjust pH of globulin solution to 8.8 with 0.5M
   carbonate-bicarbonate buffer.
4. Add fluorescein isothiocyanate powder (0.05
   mg/mg protein) to constantly stirring refrigerated
   globulin solution. Conjugate for 18 h at 0-4 C.
5. Dialyze conjugate against phosphate buffered
   saline (pH 7.6) or process through chilled dextran
   column (Sephadex G-25) to remove unbound dye
   from conjugate.
6. Conjugate may be absorbed with animal tissue
   powders or processed through diethylaminoethyl
   (DEAE) cellulose column to reduce nonspecific
   staining.
7. Store conjugate frozen in small aliquots or lyophilize.

For further details refer to Hebert,[145] Nairn,[49]
Cherry et al.,[69] Goldman,[70] Marshall et al.,[147] and
McKinney et al.[148]

REFERENCES

1. Spaulding, E. H.: J. Hosp. Research **3**:1, 1965.
2. Brewer, J. H., and McLaughlin, C. B.: J. Pharm.
   Sci. **50**:171, 1961.
3. Cahn, R. D.: Science **155**:195, 1967.
4. Tidwell, W. L., and Gee, L. L.: Proc. Soc. Exp.
   Biol. Med. **88**:561, 1955.
5. Randriambololona, R., and Dodin, A.: Ann. Inst.
   Pasteur Lille **99**:278, 1960.
6. Winn, W. R., White, M. L., Carter, W. T., et al.:
   J.A.M.A. **197**:111, 1966.
7. Sullivan, N., Sutter, V. L., and Finegold, S. M.: J.
   Clin. Microbiol. **1**:30, 1975; **1**:37, 1975.
8. Haley, L. D., and Arch, R.: Am. J. Clin. Pathol.
   27:117, 1957.
9. Rose, R.: Detection of M. tuberculosis using MF,
   Millipore Corp., 1967 (personal communication).
10. Standard methods for the examination of water
    and wastewater, ed. 14, New York, 1975, Ameri-
    can Public Health Association, American Water-
    Works Association, Water Pollution Control
    Federation.
11. Vera, H. D.: Guide lines for control of routine
    microbiology, presented at American Society for
    Microbiology meeting, May 1, 1967, New York,
    N.Y.
12. Stokes, E. J.: Lancet **1**:668, 1958.
13. McClung, L. S., and Lindberg, R. B. In Society of
    American Bacteriologists. Committee on Bac-
    teriological Technic: Manual of microbiological
    methods, New York, 1957, McGraw-Hill Book Co.
14. Finegold, S. M., Miller, A. B., and Posnick, D. J.:
    Ernaehrungsforschung **10**:517, 1965.
15. Brewer, J. H., and Allgeier, D. L.: Appl. Environ.
    Microbiol. **14**:985, 1966.
16. Aranki, A., Syed, S. A., Kenny, E. B., et al.: Appl.
    Environ. Microbiol. **17**:568, 1969.
17. Moore, W. E. C.: Int. J. Syst. Bacteriol. **16**:173,
    1966.
18. Sonnenwirth, A. C.: Am. J. Clin. Nutr. **25**:1295,
    1972.
19. Sonnenwirth, A. C.: Metronidazole proceedings,
    Montreal, May 1976, p. 236, Excerpta Medica,
    1977.
20. Rosenblatt, J. E., Fallon, A. M., and Finegold, S.
    M.: Appl. Microbiol. **25**:77, 1973.
21. Killgore, G. E., Starr, S. E., Del Bene, V. E., et al.:
    Am. J. Clin. Pathol. **59**:552, 1973.
22. Hungate, R. E.: Bacteriol. Rev. **14**:1, 1950.
23. Dowell, V. R., Jr., and Hawkins, T. M.: Laboratory
    methods in anaerobic bacteriology, Atlanta, 1977,
    CDC Laboratory Manual, U.S. Department of
    Health, Education, and Welfare, Public Health
    Service, Center for Disease Control.
24. Holdeman, L. V., and Moore, W. E. C., editors:
    Anaerobe laboratory manual, ed. 4, Blacksburg,
    Va., 1977, Virginia Polytechnic Institute and State
    University Anaerobe Laboratory.
25. Laidlaw, P. P.: Br. Med. J. **1**:497, 1915.
26. Brewer, H.: J. Lab. Clin. Med. **24**:1190, 1939.
27. Holdeman, L. V.: Public Health Lab. **22**:164,
    1964.
28. Stokes, E. J.: Clinical bacteriology, ed. 2, London,
    1960, Edward Arnold Ltd.
29. Khairat, O.: J. Bacteriol. **87**:963, 1964.
30. Brewer, J. H., and Allgeier, D. L.: Appl. Micro-
    biol. **14**:985, 1966.
31. Brewer, J. H., Allgeier, D. L., and McLaughlin, C.
    B.: Appl. Microbiol. **14**:135, 1966.
32. Martin, J. W.: Appl. Microbiol. **22**:1168, 1971.
33. Allen, S. D., Lombard, G. L., Armfield, A. Y., et
    al.: Abstr. Ann. Meeting Am. Soc. Microbiol.,
    1977, Abstr. C 142, p. 59.
34. Veillon, A., and Zuber, A.: Soc. Biol. **49**:253, 1897.
35. Prévot, A. R.: Manuel de classification et de déter-
    mination des bactéries anaérobies, Paris, 1957,
    Masson et Cie.
36. Fredette, V.: Manual of methods for the selective

isolation, rapid identification and antibiogrammetry of the anaerobic bacteria, Montreal, 1960, University of Montreal.

37. Quinto, G.: Am. J. Med. Technol. **30:**304, 1964.
38. Spray, R. S.: J. Lab. Clin. Med. **16:**203, 1930.
39. Ellner, P. D., Elbogen, S., and Frankel, H.: Am. Rev. Respir. Dis. **95:**107, 1967.
40. Isenberg, H. D., and Berkman, J. I.: Recent practices in diagnostic bacteriology. In Stefanini, M., editor: Progress in clinical pathology, New York, 1966, Grune & Stratton.
41. Morton, H. E., and Pulaski, E. J.: J. Bacteriol. **35:**163, 1938.
42. Rosebury, T., and Frances, S.: Oral Surg. **3:**1557, 1950.
43. Castellani, A.: Ann. N.Y. Acad. Sci. **93:**159, 1962.
44. Castellani, A.: J. Trop. Med. Hyg. **70:**181, 1967.
45. McGinnis, M. R., Padhye, A. A., and Ajello, L.: Appl. Microbiol. **28:**218, 1974.
46. Park, C. H.: Am. J. Clin. Pathol. **66:**927, 1976.
47. Williams, R. T., and Bridges, J. W.: J. Clin. Pathol. **17:**371, 1964.
48. Udenfriend, S.: Fluorescence assay in biology and medicine, New York, 1962 (3rd printing, 1964, with literature appendix 1962-1964), Academic Press.
49. Nairn, R. C., editor: Fluorescent protein tracing, ed. 4, Edinburgh, 1976, Churchill Livingstone.
50. Jones, G. L., Hebert, G. A., and Cherry, W. B.: Fluorescent antibody techniques and bacterial applications, Atlanta, 1978, U.S. Department of Health, Eduction, and Welfare, Center for Disease Control.
51. Mescon, H., and Grots, I. A.: J. Invest. Dermatol. **41:**181, 1963.
52. Truant, J. P., Brett, W. A., and Thomas, W., Jr.: Henry Ford Hosp. Bull. **10:**287, 1962.
53. Silver, H., Sonnenwirth, A. C., and Alex, N.: J. Clin. Pathol. **19:**583, 1966.
54. Haurowitz, F., and Breinl, F.: Z. Physiol. Chem. **205:**259, 1932.
55. Heidelberger, M., Kendall, F. E., and Soo Hoo, C. M.: J. Exp. Med. **58:**137, 1933.
56. Libby, R. L., and Madison, C. R.: J. Immunol. **55:**15, 1947.
57. Marrack, J.: Nature **133:**292, 1934.
58. Coons, A. H.: J. Immunol. **87:**499, 1961.
59. Coons, A. H., Creech, H. J., and Jones, R. N.: Proc. Soc. Exp. Biol. Med. **47:**200, 1941.
60. Coons, A. H., Creech, H. J., Jones, R. N., et al.: J. Immunol. **45:**159, 1942.
61. Coons, A. H.: Ann. Rev. Microbiol. **8:**333, 1954.
62. Coons, A. H.: Int. Rev. Cytol. **5:**1, 1956.
63. Coons, A. H.: Ann. N.Y. Acad. Sci. **69:**658, 1958.
64. Coons, A. H.: Schweiz. Z. Path. Bakt. **22:**693, 1959.
65. Beutner, E. H.: Bacteriol. Rev. **25:**49, 1961.
66. Borek, H.: Bull. W.H.O. **24:**249, 1961.
67. Coons, A. H.: Schweiz. Z. Path. Bakt. **22:**700, 1959.
68. Cherry, Q. B., and Moody, M. D.: Bacteriol. Rev. **29:**222, 1965.
69. Cherry, W. B., Goldman, M., Carski, T. R., et al.: Fluorescent antibody techniques in the diagnosis of communicable diseases, PHS pub. no. 729, Atlanta, 1960, United States Department of Health, Education and Welfare, Communicable Disease Center.
70. Goldman, M.: Fluorescent antibody methods, New York, 1968, Academic Press.
71. Riggs, J. L., Seiwald, R. J., Burckhalter, J. H., et al.: Am. J. Pathol. **34:**1081, 1958.

72. Eveland, W. C.: Public Health Lab. **24:**41, 1966.
73. Nahmias, A. J., Brahen, L., and Luce, C.: Antimicrobial agents and chemotherapy—1965, Ann Arbor, Mich., 1966, American Society for Microbiology.
74. Moody, M. D., Ellis, E. C., and Updyke, E. L.: J. Bacteriol. **75:**553, 1958.
75. Warfield, M. A., Page, R. H., Zuelzer, W. W., et al.: Am. J. Dis. Child. **101:**160, 1961.
76. Peeples, W. J., Spielman, D. W., and Moody, M. D.: Public Health Rep. **76:**651, 1961.
77. Redys, J. J., Parzick, A. B., and Borman, E. K.: Public Health Rep. **78:**222, 1963.
78. Moody, M. D., Siegel, A. C., Pittman, B., et al.: Am. J. Public Health **53:**1083, 1963.
79. Smith, T. B.: J. Bacteriol. **89:**198, 1965.
80. Whitaker, J., Page, R. H., Stulberg, C. S., et al.: Am. J. Dis. Child. **95:**1, 1958.
81. Thomason, B. M., Cherry, W. B., and Ewing, W. H.: Bacteriol. Proc., p. 90, 1959.
82. Nelson, J. D., and Whitaker, J. A.: J. Pediatr. **57:**684, 1960.
83. Cohen, F., Page, R. H., and Stulberg, C. S.: Am. J. Dis. Child. **102:**82, 1961.
84. Thomason, B. M., Cherry, W. B., Davis, B. R., et al.: Bull. W.H.O. **25:**137, 1961.
85. Thomason, B. M., Cherry, W. B., and Pomales-Lebron, A.: Bull. W.H.O. **25:**153, 1961.
86. Cherry, W. B., Thomason, B. M., Pomales-Lebron, A., et al.: Bull. W.H.O. **25:**159, 1961.
87. Martin, A. J., and O'Brien, M.: J. Bacteriol. **89:**570, 1965.
88. Deacon, W. E., Peacock, W. L., Freeman, E. M., et al.: Proc. Soc. Exp. Biol. Med. **101:**322, 1959.
89. Deacon, W. E., Peacock, W. L., Freeman, E. M., et al.: Public Health Rep. **75:**125, 1960.
90. Deacon, W. E.: Bull. W.H.O. **24:**349, 1961.
91. Thayer, J. D., Garson, W., and Deacon, W. E.: Conococcus—procedures for isolation and identification, Atlanta, 1960, Public Health Service, Communicable Disease Center.
92. Kellogg, D. S., and Deacon, W. E.: Proc. Soc. Exp. Biol. Med. **115:**963, 1964.
93. Peacock, W. L., and Thayer, J. D.: Public Health Rep. **79:**1119, 1964.
94. Thomason, B. M., McWhorter, A., and Sanders, E.: Bacteriol. Proc., p. 56, 1964.
95. Kendrick, P. L., Eldering, G., and Eveland, W. C.: Am. J. Dis. Child. **101:**149, 1961.
96. Moody, M. D., and Jones, W. L.: J. Bacteriol. **86:**285, 1963.
97. Biegeleisen, J. Z., Mitchell, M. S., Marens, B. B., et al.: J. Lab. Clin. Med. **65:**976, 1965.
98. Romero, R., and Wilkinson, H. W.: Appl. Microbiol. **28:**199, 1974.
99. Thomason, B. M., and Cherry, W. B.: Am. J. Med. Technol. **37:**258, 1971.
100. Thomason, B. M., and McWhorter, A. C.: Bull. W.H.O. **33:**681, 1965.
101. Bissett, M. L., Powers, C., and Wood, R. M.: Appl. Microbiol. **17:**507, 1969.
102. Thomason, B. M., and Wells, J. G.: Appl. Microbiol. **22:**876, 1971.
103. Thomason, B. M., and Hebert, G. A.: Appl. Microbiol. **27:**862, 1974.
104. Dimissie, A.: Acta Pathol. Microbiol. Scand. **67:**393, 1966.
105. Stulberg, C. S., Caldwell, W. J., Kennedy, D. W., et al.: J. Epidemiol. **83:**518, 1966.
106. Mohr, H. K., Trenk, H. L., and Yeterian, M.: Appl. Microbiol. **27:**324, 1974.

107. Insalata, N. F., Dunlap. W. G., and Mahnke, C. W.: Appl. Microbiol. **25:**202, 1973.
108. Taylor, C. E. D., Heimer, G. V., Lea, D. J., et al.: J. Clin. Pathol. **17:**225, 1964.
109. Taylor, C. E. D., and Heimer, G. V.: Br. Med. J. **2:**165, 1964.
110. Thomason, B. M., Cowart, G. S., and Cherry, W. B.: Appl. Microbiol. **13:**605, 1965.
111. Thomason, B. M., Nahmias, A. J., and Mathews, A. D.: Appl. Microbiol. **15:**912, 1967.
112. Whitaker, J. A., Donaldson, P., and Nelson, J. D.: N. Engl. J. Med. **263:**850, 1960.
113. Pittman, B.: *Bordetella.* In Lennette, E. H., Spaulding, E. H., and Truant, J. P., editors: Manual of clinical microbiology, ed. 2, Washington, D. C., 1974, American Society for Microbiology.
114. Fox, H. A., Hagen, P. A., Turner, D. J., et al.: Pediatrics **43:**44, 1969.
115. Cherry, W. B., Pittman, B., Harris, P. P., et al.: J. Clin. Microbiol. **8:**329, 1978.
116. Biegeleisen, J. Z., Jr., Bradshaw, B. B., and Moody, M. D.: J. Immunol. **88:**109, 1962.
117. Henderson, R. J., Hill, D. M., Vickers, A. A., et al.: J. Clin. Pathol. **29:**35, 1976.
118. Pittman, B., Shaw, E. B., Jr., and Cherry, W. B.: J. Clin. Microbiol. **5:**621, 1977.
119. Jones, W. D., Beam, R. E., and Kubica, G. P.: Am. Rev. Respir. Dis. **95:**516, 1966.
120. Jones, W. D., Jr., and Kubica, G. P.: Zentralbl. Bakteriol. **175:**582, 1968.
121. Shires, G. M. H., and Kramer, T. T.: J. Am. Vet. Med. Assoc. **164:**398, 1974.
122. Marshall, J. D., Eveland, W. C., and Smith, C. W.: Am. J. Vet. Res. **20:**1077, 1959.
123. Harrington, R., Jr., and Wood, R. L.: Am. J. Vet. Res. **35:**461, 1974.
124. Blank, C. H., and Georg, L. K.: J. Lab. Clin. Med. **71:**283, 1968.
125. Brock, D. W., and Georg, L. K.: J. Bacteriol. **97:**581, 1969.
126. Walker, P. D., and Batty, I.: J. Appl. Bacteriol. **27:**140, 1964.
127. Midura, T. F., Inouye, Y., and Bodily, H. L.: Public Health Rep. **82:**275, 1967.
128. Batty, I., and Walker, P. D.: Bull. Off. Int. Epiz. **59:**1499, 1963.
129. Batty, I., and Walker, P. D.: J. Pathol. **88:**327, 1964.
130. Maestrone, G.: Can. J. Comp. Med. Vet. Sci. **27:**108, 1963.
131. U. S. Department of Health, Education, and Welfare: Criteria and techniques for the diagnosis of gonorrhea, PHS, Atlanta, 1973, Communicable Disease Center.
132. Tarizzo, M. L., editor: Field methods for the control of trachoma, Geneva, 1973, World Health Organization.
133. Hanna, L., Schachter, J., and Jawetz, E.: Chlamydiae (Psittacosis-lymphogranuloma venereumtrachoma group). In Lennette, E. H., Spaulding, E. H., and Truant, J. P., editors: Manual of clinical microbiology, ed. 2, Washington, D.C., 1974, American Society for Microbiology.
134. Del Giudice, R. A., Robillard, M. F., and Carski, T. R.: J. Bacteriol. **93:**1205, 1967.
135. Moody, M. D., Goldman, M., and Thomason, B. M.: J. Bacteriol. **72:**357, 1956.
136. Thomason, B. M., Moody, M. D., and Goldman, M.: J. Bacteriol. **72:**362, 1956.
137. Wallace, A. L., and Norins, L. C.: Progress Clin. Pathol. **11:**198, 1969.
138. Stauffer, L. R., Hill, F. O., Holland, J. W., et al.: J. Clin. Microbiol. **2:**337, 1975.
139. Abshire, R. L., Lombard, G. L., and Dowell, V. R., Jr.: J. Clin. Microbiol. **6:**425, 1977.
140. U.S. Department of Health, Education, and Welfare: Manual of tests for symphilis, PHS pub. no. 411 (rev.), Washington, D.C., 1969, U.S. Government Printing Office.
141. U.S. Department of Health, Education, and Welfare: The laboratory aspects of syphilis, PHS, Atlanta, 1971, Communicable Disease Center.
142. Reimer, C. B., Black, C. M., Phillips, D. J., et al.: Ann. N.Y. Acad. Sci. 1975.
143. Casey, H. L.: Importance of control mechanisms in diagnostic bacteriology, presented at American Society of Microbiology Meeting, New York, May 1, 1967.
144. Johnson, G. D., Beutner, E. H., and Holborow, E. J.: J. Clin. Pathol. **20:**720, 1967.
145. Hebert, G. A., Pittman, B., McKinney, R. M., et al.: The preparation and physiocochemical characterization of fluorescent antibody reagents, Atlanta, 1972, Center for Disease Control.
146. Lucas, J. B., Price, E. V., Thayer, J. D., et al.: N. Engl. J. Med. **276:**1454, 1967.
147. Marshall, J. D., Eveland, W. C., and Smith, C. W.: Proc. Soc. Exp. Biol. Med. **98:**898, 1958.
148. McKinney, R. M. Spillane, J. T., and Pearce, G. W.: Anal. Biochem. **7:**74, 1964.

71

STAINS AND STAINING PROCEDURES

Alex C. Sonnenwirth

GENERAL PRINCIPLES

Biologic stains are dyes that are adapted for special purposes. Clark[1] lists the uses of biologic stains in the following procedures: animal histology, including general tissue, connective tissue, neurologic, blood, bone, fat, and glycogen stains; plant anatomy, histochemistry, cytology, and cytogenetics; and, in microbiology, for staining microorganisms in smears, for differentiation by Gram stain and acid-fast staining, for various cell components (e.g., capsule, spores, lipid, cell wall flagella, and granules), and for staining rickettsiae and chlamydiae and protozoa, as well as for staining microorganisms in sections.

The microbiologic use of stains includes the staining of bacteria, yeasts, fungi, and protozoa. The stains are also employed as constituents of culture media, either as indicators or because of their selective inhibitory activity of certain bacterial species or genera. Bacteriologic stains are used for the study of bacterial cytology, for staining bacteria in dried smears or in tissue.

Biologic stains sold in the United States are certified by the Biological Stain Commission when submitted by the manufacturer on a voluntary basis. The purpose is to ensure that the stains sold are of the best quality possible and that their performance will be uniform and reproducible. Certified batches of stains are now designated with the initials "C.C." or the words "Cert." or "Certified for use" placed after the name of the dye; they are sold in containers bearing a special certification label furnished by the commission that states the purpose for which the dye is certified. The use of certified stains is strongly recommended for diagnostic work.

Bacterial dyes are synthetic coal-tar dyes, derived from substances found in coal tar. The term aniline dye is being abandoned, since many dyes now in use are not derived from aniline, in contrast to some of the earliest synthetic dyes, which actually were produced from aniline. The coal-tar dyes are classified as "acid" or "basic"

dyes. These terms are misleading, since they do not refer to the dye in question as being a free acid or free base. The true dyes are the **salts** of the free color acids and bases. According to the definition of Conn et al.,[3] an acid dye is the salt of a color acid and a basic dye is the salt of a color base; e.g., acid dyes are anionic and basic dyes are cationic. The actual reaction of a dye in solution depends on the proportion of the dye ion and the cation or anion with which it is combined in the dye salt. Nuclei of cells are best stained by basic dyes, whereas the cytoplasm is stained better by acid dyes. Since the nuclear material of bacterial cells seems to be distributed throughout their bodies, basic dyes are generally used to stain them.

The reader is warned about the existence of various synonyms for biologic stains, which occasionally leads to some confusion. A list of stains with their synonyms can be found in *Conn's Biological Stains*[2] and in *Staining Procedures Used by the Biological Stain Commission,*[1] the most useful references in this area. They contain detailed information regarding the chemical nature and formulas of dyes and their use in various procedures and list their color index (C.I.) number. For detailed information on staining technics see Clark's *Staining Procedures Used By the Biological Stain Commission,*[1] *Manual of Microbiological Methods,*[3] and *Manual of Clinical Microbiology.*[4]

Preparation of smears

Smears from pure cultures of bacteria are usually prepared by making an aqueous suspension of the organisms, drying a drop of this on a slide or coverslip, and fixing by gentle heat. Because of their extremely tiny size and their stiff walls, bacteria do not undergo the shrinkage and distortion such a method of fixation would cause with higher forms of life. A small amount of the material is removed and suspended in a drop of distilled water on a slide. This must be done carefully to avoid making too thick a preparation. It should be of a faint turbidity, and solid masses of bacteria should be avoided. A drop of a broth culture is sometimes used to make smears, but solids from the culture material may interfere with the stain, and for this reason this method is not always satisfactory. If a smear shows no areas where the bacteria are separated from each other, more water should be added to dilute the smear.

Several smears may be made on the same slide. A slide with frosted edges is used. It is divided into the necessary number of fields by lines drawn with a wax pencil. A corresponding number of lines are drawn with a graphite pencil on the frosted part of the slide. The code numbers of the smears made on the slide are written on the frosted surface with the same pencil. Eight to 12 smears may be stained on the same slide.

Several methods of fixing are in use. The preferred method is to dry the smear and then pass it rapidly through a Bunsen flame 2 or 3 times or to allow the smear to dry on a flat, moderately hot plate of nonrusting metal on a boiling water bath. Overheating (burning) may be prevented by careful checking of the temperature of the slide, by just touching the back of the slide to the back of the hand each time the slide has been passed through the flame. Staining without fixation after drying in air is not recommended. Special staining methods may call for special fixing methods, in which case the method will be given.

It is preferable to use new slides for all bacteriologic stains, and it is imperative to do so for acid-fast and flagella stains. It is essential that, after staining, the back surfaces of the slides be wiped clean with a piece of cloth or a paper towel.

Staining formulas

Most of the staining technics that follow are intended for use in study of pure cultures; various common staining formulas used in routine laboratory diagnosis of disease are also given. The literature contains many inaccuracies in staining methods. Few can be accepted in the light of present knowledge without some degree of interpretation to make them more explicit. In some cases the author's intentions are evident, whereas in others they must be inferred. Blind adherence to a staining technic is no guarantee of satisfactory results. **Always check a technic on known organisms for controls,** checking the solutions and water to make sure they are free from bacteria and spores.

STAINING TECHNIC*
Preparation and fixation of bacteriologic smears

1. Slides should be fat-free and free from lint or any other foreign substance.
2. Place a loopful of distilled water in center of slide.
3. Flame platinum wire.
4. Remove plug from culture tube (or lift cover of Petri dish or other container), flame mouth of container, and hold stopper between third and fourth fingers.

*Some staining methods not included in this section may be found throughout the text. Consult the index for other stains.

5. With cooled loop (which has been cooled inside tube or other container) pick up a portion of material to be smeared.
6. Replace plug after flaming mouth of container.
7. Holding slide in 1 hand, gently emulsify material on platinum loop in water or saline on the slide.
8. Flame loop.
9. Material on the slide should dry immediately.
10. Fix smear by passing it 3 times through flame, holding it in upper portion of flame 1 s at a time.
11. Allow to cool before staining.
12. If fixation by alcohol instead of dry heat is desired, slide is placed in a Coplin jar of methyl alcohol for 5 min or in ethyl alcohol for 20 min. Other fixatives, such as bichloride of mercury and acetic acid, may be used, time varying according to fixative.

CAUTION: Avoid spattering droplets on slide or bench top when working with pathologic material; dangerous aerosols are formed that may be inhaled or deposited on worker's hands or clothing. Regardless of heating and staining, some organisms may remain viable. Handle slides and blotting paper as contaminated material.

Used slides are placed in benzalkonium chloride (Roccal) or some other disinfectant solution. Boil them in tap water for 1-2 h and then clean in same manner as slides for hematologic work. When possible, do not use a slide more than once.

Stains, staining solutions, and staining technic
Points to be considered in making staining solutions

1. Stains used should preferably be those bearing the certification label of the Biological Stain Commission.
2. All dyes should be weighed accurately on an analytical balance.
3. The dyes should be ground in a mortar with the diluent, adding a small amount of the diluent at a time until all has been added.
4. All staining solutions should be filtered before use, but not before they have been allowed to stand for at least 24 hours.
5. No solutions should be used after precipitation has occurred. When precipitation occurs, discard the solutions from the bottom of the bottle after the rest of the stain has been used or filter and use the filtrate.
6. Diluted solutions should be made in small quantities. The stock solutions keep for a much longer period of time than the diluted solutions.
7. All solutions should show on their labels the concentration of the dye present and the date of preparation. Use stain-fast labels.
8. Keep all staining solutions out of direct sunlight.
9. Keep all staining solutions in glass-stoppered bottles.

Bacteriologic stains*

Formula numbers are given at the left of each formula: (S-1), (S-2), etc. Stock solutions to be

*This is not intended to be a complete catalog of staining solutions. Other staining solutions are found throughout the text. Consult the index for special stains.

diluted before use are indicated by an additional letter: (S-1,a), etc.

(S-1) Hucker crystal violet*

a.	Crystal violet (certified)	2 g
	Alcohol, 95%	20 ml
b.	Ammonium oxalate	0.8 g
	Distilled water	80 ml

1. Dissolve crystal violet in alcohol (solution a).
2. Dissolve ammonium oxalate in distilled water (solution b).
3. Mix solutions a and b; filter through filter paper after 24 h.

(S-2) Carbol gentian violet made from stock saturated alcoholic solution

Saturated alcoholic solution of gentian violet	10 ml
Carbolic acid solution, 1%	100 ml

1. Add 10 ml saturated alcoholic solution of gentian violet (S-2,a) to 50 ml carbolic acid solution in a 100 ml graduated cylinder.
2. Dilute to 100 ml with 1% carbolic acid solution.
3. Filter after 24 h.

(S-2,a) Saturated alcoholic solution of gentian violet, stock

Gentian violet	5 g
Alcohol, 95%	100 ml

1. Grind gentian violet in a mortar, adding alcohol slowly until all dye is in solution.
2. Place in a glass-stoppered bottle and filter through filter paper after 24 h.

(S-3) Carbol gentian violet made from crystals

Gentian violet	1 g
Carbolic acid crystals	2 g
Absolute alcohol	10 ml
Distilled water	100 ml

1. Rub up gentian violet and alcohol in a mortar.
2. Add carbolic acid crystals and mix.
3. Add two-thirds of water, a small amount at a time, stirring constantly.
4. Pour mixture into a graduated cylinder and rinse mortar with distilled water, adding it to mixture in graduate. Dilute to 100 ml.
5. Filter through filter paper after 24 h.

(S-4) Kopeloff modification, crystal violet†

Solution I

Crystal violet	10 g
Distilled water	1000 ml

Solution II

NaHCO₃	50 g
Distilled water	1000 ml

Solution I is used for flooding slide; about 5 drops solution II is added to solution I on slide.

(S-5) Kopeloff-Bermann gentian violet

a.	Aqueous gentian violet, 1% or crystal violet or methyl violet 6B	150 ml
b.	Aqueous sodium bicarbonate, 5%	50 ml

1. Prepare solution a and solution b, separately, in distilled water.
2. Just before use, mix solution a and solution b; or mix 15 ml solution a with 5 ml solution b just before use.

(S-6) Gram's iodine*

Iodine crystals	1 g

Potassium iodide	2 g
Distilled water	300 ml

1. Mix iodine crystals and potassium iodide in a mortar.
2. Add distilled water in small amounts.
3. Store in amber glass bottle.

(S-7) Gram's iodine made from stock Lugol solution

1. Add 10 ml Lugol solution to about 100 ml distilled water in a graduated cylinder.
2. Dilute to 150 ml with distilled water and mix.
3. Filter after 24 h.

(S-7,a) Lugol stock solution

Iodine, resublimed	5 g
Potassium iodide	10 g
Distilled water	100 ml

This solution is 15 times the strength of Gram's iodine solution and may be used as a stock from which Gram's iodine is made.

1. Rub up iodine, resublimed, and potassium iodide in a mortar until they are thoroughly mixed.
2. Add distilled water, a small amount at a time, and grind it into the mixture until all the water has been added.
3. Allow to stand in a glass-stoppered bottle and filter after 24 h.

(S-8) Kopeloff modification, iodine*

1. NaOH

NaOH	4 g
Distilled water	25 ml

2. Add

Iodine	20 g
Potassium iodide	1 g

3. Let dissolve. Add gradually, mixing well, 975 ml distilled water.

(S-9) Kopeloff-Bermann iodine

Sodium hydroxide	4 g
Iodine, resublimed	10 g
Distilled water	500 ml

1. Weigh sodium hydroxide into a 500 ml glass-stoppered flask.
2. Add 50 ml distilled water. Shake until disolved.
3. Add iodine. Shake until dissolved.
4. Dilute to 500 ml with distilled water.
5. Let stand in a dark place for 24 h, and then filter through filter paper into a brown glass-stoppered bottle.

(S-10) Safranin, 0.25% solution†

Stock solution

Safranin O (certified)	25 g
Ethyl alcohol, 95%	100 ml

1. Rub up safranin with alcohol in a mortar.
2. Pour into a flask. This is stock solution.

Working solution

Stock solution	10 ml
Distilled water	90 ml

(S-11) Safranin, 1% aqueous solution

Safranin	1 g
Distilled water	100 ml

1. Dissolve safranin in distilled water by grinding it in a mortar and adding water, a small amount at a time, until all dye has been dissolved.
2. Filter after 24 h.

(S-12) Safranin-Kopeloff modification

Safranin	20 g

1. Add slowly just enough ethyl alcohol, 95%, to dissolve safranin. Then add distilled water, 1000 ml.

---

*Recommended for Gram stain (general).
†Recommended by Virginia Polytechnic Institute (VPI) workers for use in Kopeloff's modification of the Gram stain for staining anaerobic bacteria.[5]

*Recommended by VPI workers for use in Kopeloff's modification of Gram stain anaerobes.[5]
†Recommended for Gram stain (general).

(S-13) Meyrick-Harrison neutral red fuchsin

Neutral red in distilled water,	
1% solution	150 ml
Carbolfuchsin	10 ml

1. Add carbolfuchsin to neutral red solution.

(S-14) Neisser Bismarck brown

Bismarck brown Y	0.2 g
Distilled water	100 ml

1. Dissolve Bismarck brown Y in boiling distilled water.
2. Filter through filter paper while still hot.

(S-15) Ziehl-Neelsen carbolfuchsin

a. Alcoholic basic fuchsin (saturated solution)*

Basic fuchsin	3 g
Ethyl alcohol, 95%	100 ml

b. Phenol, 5%

Phenol	5 g
Distilled water	100 ml

1. Dissolve basic fuchsin in alcohol (solution a).
2. Melt phenol crystals with gentle heat and add distilled water (solution b).
3. To prepare *carbolfuchsin,* mix 10 ml solution a and 90 ml solution b.

(S-16) Kinyoun carbolfuchsin, cold stain*

Basic fuchsin	4 g
Ethyl alcohol, 95%	20 ml
Distilled water	100 ml
Phenol crystals	8 g

1. Dissolve basic fuchsin in alcohol.
2. Add distilled water slowly while stirring.
3. Melt phenol crystals with gentle heat and add to fuchsin solution.

Used in Kinyoun cold staining procedure.

(S-17) Muller-Chermock carbolfuchsin-Tergitol stain*

Carbolfuchin (Ziehl-Neelsen)	25 ml
Tergitol†	1 drop

1. Mix carbolfuchsin (S-15) with 1 drop Tergitol.

Used in Muller-Chermock cold staining procedure.

(S-17,a) Cooper carbolfuchsin

Carbolfuchsin (S-15)	100 ml
Sodium chloride, 10% solution	3 ml

1. Mix carbolfuchsin and sodium chloride, 10% solution. Keep in the refrigerator.

(S-18) Carbolfuchsin made from crystals

Basic fuchsin	1 g
Phenol crystals	5 g
Absolute alcohol	10 ml
Distilled water	100 ml

1. Dissolve 5 g phenol in 100 ml distilled water. Pour 50 ml of solution into a 100 ml graduate cylinder.
2. Dissolve 1 g basic fuchsin in 10 ml absolute alcohol by grinding in a mortar.
3. Pour the basic fuchsin solution into the graduate (containing 50 ml phenol).
4. The mixture should be diluted with the phenol solution to 100 ml. Wash the mortar and pestle with aliquots of phenol solution; add aliquots to graduate to 100 mark.
5. Filter after 24 h.

(S-19) Methylene blue (Ziehl-Neelsen counterstain)*

Methylene blue chloride	0.3 g
Distilled water	100 ml

The chloride salt is water soluble, eliminating the need for alkalinized alcoholic solutions of the dye.

(S-19,a) Brilliant green counterstain*

Sodium hydroxide	0.01 g
Brilliant green	1 g
Distilled water	100 ml

1. Dissolve sodium hydroxide in distilled water.
2. Dissolve brilliant green in the mixture, grinding the dye with small amounts of the alkaline solution at a time.
3. If staining is too intense at this concentration, dilute 1:20 with distilled water.

(S-19,b) Picric acid counterstain*

Picric acid	0.75 g
Distilled water	100 ml

1. Dissolve picric acid in the distilled water.

NOTE: This stain is recommended for **color-blind workers.** Although it does not give good color contrast with acid-fast bacilli, it has the advantage of not selectively staining cellular material.

(S-19,c) Cooper brilliant green

a. Brilliant green | 1 g
Distilled water | 100 ml
b. Sodium hydroxide | 0.1 g
Distilled water | 10 ml

1. Dissolve brilliant green in distilled water.
2. To 100 ml brilliant greeen solution (solution a) add 1 ml 1% solution of sodium hydroxide (solution b).

(S-19,d) Loeffler methylene blue counterstain

1. Prepare methylene blue stain (S-20).
2. Dilute 1:20 with distilled water before use.

(S-20) Methylene blue stain made from stock solution

Distilled water	100 ml
Potassium hydroxide, 10% solution	0.1
Saturated alcoholic solution of methylene blue (S-20,a)	30 ml

1. Add 0.1 ml 10% potassium hydroxide to 100 ml distilled water.
2. Add 30 ml saturated alcoholic solution of methylene blue (S-20,a).
3. Filter through filter paper after 24 h.

When a certified stain is used, the addition of potassium hydroxide is optional.

(S-20,a) Saturated alcoholic solution of methylene blue, stock

Methylene blue	1.5 g
Alcohol, 95%	100 ml

1. Rub up methylene blue with alcohol in mortar, adding the alcohol, a small amount at a time, and grinding in the mixture.
2. Store in glass-stoppered bottle.
3. Filter after 24 h.

(S-21) Methylene blue stain made from crystals—Loeffler

Distilled water	100 ml
Potassium hydroxide, 10% solution	0.1 ml
Methylene blue, certified	0.3 g
Alcohol, 95%	30 ml

1. Rub up methylene blue with alcohol in a mortar.
2. Transfer to a flask.
3. Add potassium hydroxide to distilled water and wash the mortar with the mixture.
4. Pour the washings into the flask, using all the mixture.
5. Filter through filter paper after 24 h.

(S-22) Manson methylene blue

Methylene blue	2 g

---

*Prepare all reagents for acid-fast stains with freshly distilled water.

†Terigitol Anionic 7 (sodium heptadecyl sulfate), Union Carbide, New York, N.Y.

*Prepare all reagents for acid-fast stains with freshly distilled water.

| Borax (sodium tetraborate crystals) | 5 g |
| Distilled water | 100 ml |

1. Dissolve the borax in the distilled water.
2. Grind the methylene blue in the borax solution, a small amount at a time, and pour into a bottle.
3. Filter after 1 wk.

(S-23) Gabbett methylene blue

| Methylene blue | 2 g |
| Sulfuric acid, 25% | 100 ml |

1. Place methylene blue in a bottle; pour sulfuric acid over it.
2. Filter after 24 h.

(S-24) Leifson stain
Formula 1

Potassium alum in distilled water 5% solution	10 ml
Tannic acid in distilled water, 2% solution	10 ml
Basic fuchsin in 9% alcohol, 1% solution	10 ml

1. Mix in order.

Formula 2 (using commercially prepared stain)
1. Dissolve 1.5 g BBL flagella stain in a mixture of 35 ml 95% alcohol and 65 ml distilled water.
2. Allow to stand for 10 min, shaking several times. The stain remains stable for several weeks if kept in a tightly stoppered bottle.

(S-25) Leifson stain, flagellar, modified[6,7]*
Solution A

Distilled water	100 ml
Sodium chloride	0.75 g
Tannic acid	1.5 g

Solution B

Basic fuchsin (certified for flagella staining)*	0.6 g
or	
Pararosanilin acetate*	0.45 g
and	
Pararosanilin hydrochloride*	0.15 g
Ethyl alcohol, 95%	50 ml

Shake and let stand overnight to dissolve.
1. Combine solutions A and B; mix thoroughly.
2. pH should be 5.0 ± 0.2. If too low, adjust slowly and carefully with 1N NaOH.
3. The stain can be used immediately; however, it improves after storage for 2-4 d.
4. Store aliquots of the stain frozen in screw-cap tubes; tighten caps. It is stable when frozen for several months.
5. After thawing, mix well, since the alcohol and water separate during freezing. The thawed stain should be stored refrigerated (4 C); it is stable at this temperature about 1 mo.

(S-26) Flagella stain—Leifson, Clark modification[8]
Solution A

| Basic fuchsin (certified for flagella staining) | 1.2 g |
| Ethyl alcohol, 95% | 100 ml |

1. Mix and leave at room temperature.

Solution B

Tannic acid	1.5 g
Sodium chloride	0.75 g
Distilled water	100 ml

1. Mix equal volumes of solutions A and B, and adjust, if needed, with 1N NaOH to pH 5.0.
2. Store frozen in 50 ml aliquots Storage times are the same as for S-25.

(S-27) Silver plating stain for flagella[9]
Mordant—solution 1

Aluminum potassium sulfate, saturated aqueous solution	25 ml
Tannic acid, 10% solution	50 ml
Ferric chloride, 5% solution	5 ml

The mixture is black and should be stored in the dark at 5 C.

Stain—solution 2

| Ammonium hydroxide, conc. | 2-4 ml |
| Silver nitrate, 5% solution | 90 ml |

1. Prepare solution 2 by slowly adding the concentrated ammonium hydroxide to the 5% silver nitrate solution until the brown precipitate redissolves. Add more silver nitrate solution dropwise until a faint cloudiness persists (will take 2-20 ml). Store solution 2 at 5 C in the dark.

(S-28) Gray stain, flagellar
Mordant—Solution A

Saturated solution of potassium alum, aqueous	5 ml
Tannic acid, aqueous, 20% solution	2 ml
Saturated solution of mercuric chloride, aqueous	2 ml

1. Mix ingredients in order listed.
2. Solution may be kept indefinitely.

Solution B

| Methyl alcohol | 10 ml |
| Basic fuchsin in distilled water, 1% solution | 10 ml |

1. Mix ingredients.
2. Solution may be kept indefinitely.

(S-29) Dieterle spirochete stain,[10] Van Orden and Greer modification[11]
Reagents

| a. Uranyl nitrate | 50 g |
| Ethyl alcohol, 70% | 1000 ml |

   1. Store in refrigerator.

| b. Gum mastic* | 100 g |
| Alcohol, absolute | 1000 ml |

   1. Allow 2 days to dissolve; then filter and store in stoppered bottle in refrigerator.

| c. Silver nitrate | 10 g |
| Distilled water | 1000 ml |

   1. Store in refrigerator. If solution becomes dark, discard.

   d. Developer. Mix in order:

Hydroquinone	15 g
Sodium sulfite	2.5 g
Distilled water	600 ml
Acetone	100 ml
Formalin (37-40%)	100 ml
Pyridine	100 ml
Gum mastic, 10% (see b)	100 ml

Solution becomes milky yellow as gum mastic solution is added and medium brown on standing in a well-lighted area. Developer should be made up when the procedure is begun, as aging of the developer is required for proper development—about 6 h. Developer may be used for 2-3 d or until the color becomes dark brown.

(S-30) Hiss capsular stain
1. Mix 5 ml saturated alcoholic solution of gentian violet in 95 ml distilled water.

---

*Special stain for flagella (**basic fuchsin**, certified, for flagella staining, C. I. 42500), Eastman Organic Chemicals, Division of Eastman Kodak Co., Rochester, N.Y., may be substituted for the 2 dyes. Also available from Matheson, Coleman and Bell, and National Aniline Division, Allied Chemical Corp., Morristown, N.J.

*O. G. Innes Corp., 10 E. 40th Street, New York, New York 10016.

(S-31) MacNeal
Eosin Y, certified	1 g
Methylene blue, certified	1 g
Azure A	0.6 g
Methylene violet, Bernthsen	0.2 g
Methyl alcohol, neutral, acetone-free	1000 ml

1. Mix ingredients.
2. Heat to 50 C for 30 min.
3. Keep at 37 C for 2 d, shaking several times a day.
4. Filter through filter paper.

It is preferable to purchase the stain in dry form or in solution.

(S-32) Lawson mordant
1. Prepare 5% solution of phosphomolybdic acid in distilled water.

(S-33) Lawson stain
Wright stain	10 ml
Glycerin	5 ml

1. Add glycerin to Wright stain just before use.

(S-34) Ljubinsky, granule stain
Crystal violet	0.25 g
Glacial acetic acid	5 ml
Distilled water	95 ml

1. Add glaceal acetic acid to distilled water.
2. Dissolve crystal violet in acetic acid solution.

(S-35) Neisser stain
Methylene blue	0.1 g
Absolute alcohol	2 ml
Glacial acetic acid	5 ml
Distilled water	95 ml

1. Dissolve the methylene blue in the absolute alcohol in a mortar.
2. Mix the acetic acid with the distilled water.
3. Add the acetic acid mixture to the solution of methylene blue, a small amount at a time.
4. Filter after 24 h.

(S-36) Albert stain—Laybourn modification
Solution A
Toluidine blue	0.15 g
Malachite green	0.2 g
Glacial acetic acid	1 ml
Ethyl alcohol, 95%	2 ml
Distilled water	100 ml

1. Add 1 ml glacial acetic acid to 100 ml distilled water.
2. Dissolve 0.15 g toluidine blue and 0.2 g malachite green in 2 ml 95% ethyl alcohol by grinding in a mortar.
3. Add the acetic acid solution and mix.

Solution B
Potassium iodide	3 g
Iodine	2 g
Distilled water	300 ml

1. Dissolve potassium iodide in 5 ml distilled water.
2. To potassium iodide solution add the iodine and dissolve by shaking.
3. Add the remainder of the distilled water. Shake vigorously.

(S-37) India ink
Pelikan Drawing Ink, 17 Black (India ink),* is recommended.

1. As a preservative, add 0.3% tricresol.
2. India ink can become contaminated with microorganisms. It is important to examine every new bottle purchased to rule out contamination; if it is present, bottle should not be used.

(S-38) Nigrosin solution—Dorner
Nigrosin	10 g
Distilled water	100 ml

1. Boil 30 min in an Erlenmeyer flask.
2. Add as preservative 0.5 ml formalin (40%).
3. Filter twice through double filter paper and store in serologic test tubes, about 5 ml to the tube. Stopper tubes with aluminum-foiled corks.

(S-39) Dienes stain
Methylene blue	2.5 g
Azure II	1.25 g
Maltose	10 g
Sodium carbonate	0.25 g
Distilled water	100 ml

1. Dissolve and filter before use.

(S-40) Wayson stain[12]
Solution 1
Basic fuchsin	0.3 g
Absolute alcohol	8 ml

Solution 2
Methylene blue	0.75 g
Absolute alcohol	12 ml

1. Mix solutions 1 and 2. Add phenol, 5%, in distilled water, to make 200 ml. Mix, boil, and let stand for 48 h.
2. Filter the stain, and store in a dark bottle.
3. Storage of the preparation for 1-2 y enhances its staining ability. For use of stain see *Yersinia pestis* (Chapter 79).

Decolorizing agents

Distilled water. Distilled water is a decolorizing agent. If water is allowed to remain on slides after they have been stained, it will remove part of the stain. After staining and washing preparations, always stand them on end to dry if they cannot be blotted.

Absolute alcohol. Absolute alcohol is sometimes used as a decolorizing agent. For the **Gram stain,** 95% alcohol is recommended.

Acetone-alcohol for Kopeloff modification of Gram stain. Mix acetone, 300 ml, with 95% ethyl alcohol, 700 ml.[5]

Acid-alcohol (for Ziehl-Neelsen stain). Add 3 ml conc. hydrochloric acid, cp, to 97 ml 95% ethyl alcohol.

Acid alcohol decolorizer for fluorochrome stain. Add 0.5 ml conc. hydrochloric acid to 100 ml 70% ethyl alcohol.

•   •   •

Various acids and alkalies act as decolorizing agent. Where a special decolorizing solution must be used, it will be described with that staining technic.

STAINING METHODS*†
Simple stains for morphology

The following stains serve for study of the general morphology of the microorganisms. The slides are fixed over the flame before staining.

Methylene blue
1. Use methylene blue prepared according to directions under methylene blue (S-20 or S-21).

*For each staining technic use the staining formula indicated to the **left** of each stain—(S-1), (S-2), etc.
†For a detailed listing of modifications and special procedures see Society of American Bacteriologists: Manual of microbiological methods, New York, 1957, McGraw-Hill Book Co.; and Clark, G., editor: Staining procedures used by the Biological Stain Commission, ed. 3, Baltimore, 1973, The Williams & Wilkins Co.

2. For staining microorganisms in blood films use Manson methylene blue (S-22).
3. Flood the slide with methylene blue and stain for 1½-3 min.
4. Wash with distilled water.
5. Dry by draining, and examine.
Dilute carbolfuchsin
1. Flood slides with diluted carbolfuchsin (S-18, diluted 1:10 with distilled water) for ½-1 min.
2. Wash with distilled water.

Negative demonstration of bacteria

1. India ink (S-37) diluted with equal parts of distilled water or nigrosin (S-38) is used.
2. Mix a loopful of the bacterial suspension on the slide with the same amount of India ink or nigrosin solution. Make a very thin smear. Examine after drying.

Gram stain

The Gram stain is one of the most widely used and important stains in bacteriology. Originally devised by Hans Christian Gram (Denmark, 1884), it permits the differentiation of 2 groups of organisms, 1 group called **gram-positive,** the other **gram-negative.** With the Gram-staining method the gram-positive organisms stain purple, whereas gram-negative organisms stain red. The Gram reaction is correlated with certain basic chemical and physiologic properties of bacteria, and their identification is greatly facilitated by its use.

According to Salton,[13] the color differentiation is due to the formation of a crystal violet–iodine complex "trapped" in the organism, probably by a barrier consisting of the dehydrated and mordanted cell wall. In gram-positive cells the barrier becomes impenetrable after treatment with mordant and iodine; in gram-negative cells the barrier is more penetrable and the solvent extracts the iodine–crystal violet complex. The molecular basis of the reaction is not known; however, in addition to aiding in recognition and identification of organisms, the gram-staining properties seem to denote some very fundamental biologic differences between the "gram-positives" and "gram-negatives" (differential susceptibility to various antibiotics, to lysozyme, etc.). Because of the danger of overstaining or overdecolorizing, it is recommended that at least once a day known gram-negative and gram-positive organisms be stained at the same time as the cultures that are being examined. The following methods of gram-staining technic are commonly used: Hucker modification, original Gram stain, Gram stain, Kopeloff modification, Kopeloff-Bermann modification, and Gram stain for the color-blind.

Hucker modification (recommended method)
1. Fix the slide in the flame and allow to cool.
2. Stain with Hucker crystal violet (S-1) 60 s.
3. Wash with tap water.
4. Stain with Gram's iodine (S-6) 1 min.
5. Wash with tap water.
6. Decolorize with 95% alcohol until no further violet comes away (20-30 s).

7. Wash thoroughly with distilled water.
8. Counterstain with 0.25% safranin (S-10) 20 s.
9. Wash with tap water.
10. Dry in air and examine.
Original Gram stain
1. Fix the slide in the flame and allow to cool.
2. Stain with carbol gentian violet (S-3 or S-2) 60 s.
3. Wash with water.
4. Stain with Gram's iodine (S-6 or S-7) 30 s.
5. Wash with water.
6. Decolorize in 95% alcohol until no further violet comes away.
7. Wash thoroughly with water.
8. Counterstain with 1% aqueous safranin (S-11) 2 min.
9. Wash with water.
10. Dry in the air and examine.
Gram-positive organisms stain purple. Gram-negative organisms stain red.
Gram stain, Kopeloff modification. This is recommended by the VPI Anaerobe Laboratory group for staining of anaerobes.[5]
1. Stain with Kopeloff modifications of crystal violet (S-4) and iodine (S-8).
2. Decolorize with acetone-alcohol (see decolorizing agents).
3. Counterstain with safranin (S-12).
Kopeloff-Bermann modification
1. Fix the slide in the flame and allow to cool.
2. Stain with Kopeloff-Bermann gentian violet (S-5) 5 min.
3. Pour off stain.
4. Flood slide 2 or 3 times with Kopeloff-Bermann iodine solution (S-9).
5. Decolorize with 100% acetone until no further violet comes away.
6. Dry in the air.
7. Counterstain with freshly prepared 1:1000 watery basic fuchsin or Meyrick-Harrison neutral red fuchsin (S-13) 20-30 s.
8. Wash with water.
9. Dry in the air and examine.
10. No water should be used in this procedure before the application of fuchsin.
Gram stain for the color-blind
1. Stain with any accepted modification.
2. Instead of safranin, pyronin, or fuchsin, counterstain with Bismarck brown (S-14) 30-60 s.
Gram-positive organisms are purple. Gram-negative organisms are yellowish brown.

Acid-fast stain*

Acid-fast organisms stain with some difficulty, but once stained, they resist decolorization with mineral acids or acid alcohol. Staining may be facilitated in several ways: (1) application of heat, (2) increased concentration of phenol and dye in the stain solution, (3) prolonged contact of stain with smear, and (4) addition to stain of wetting agents such as Tergitol (Union Carbide). When using the fuchsin stains here described, the acid-fast bacilli stain red. Because basic fuchsin varies in quality and purity, each new lot should be tested for staining ability *before* all of a previously good lot is exhausted.

Various counterstains may be used in the Ziehl-Neelsen procedure outlined later; al-

---

*Contributed by G. P. Kubica and H. L. David (see Chapter 78).

though methylene blue is listed in the directions, brilliant green (S-19,a), picric acid (S-19,b), and others have been employed. It is important that any counterstain used not stain the background debris so intensely that it obscures acid-fast bacilli. Picric acid is especially helpful for color-blind workers or as counter stain for exceptionally thick smears (when other stains might obscure fuchsin-stained mycobacteria).

To minimize cross contamination of slides (1) fix smears properly, (2) stain slides individually or on a rack where they may be kept separated (i.e., do not batch stain in vats of dye), and (3) wipe oil immersion objective with lens paper after examining each slide.

To prevent contamination of slides or stains with extraneous, environmental acid-fast bacilli (1) prepare all reagents with freshly distilled water, (2) check tap water and distilled water reservoirs and delivery tips for such organisms, (3) do not use reagent solutions that are too old, and (4) use both positive and negative control smears as a check on reagents and staining procedures.

Recommended procedures

Ziehl-Neelsen stain[14]

1. Cut pieces of filter paper 2 × 4 (or 5) cm, i.e., just slightly smaller than microscope slide but large enough to cover fixed smear. Place filter paper over smear. This holds stain on slide, prevents drying, and minimizes deposition of any precipitated crystals onto smear area.
2. Cover fixed smear with Ziehl-Neelsen carbolfuchsin (S-15) and steam gently with Bunsen burner or on electric staining rack.
   a. When using Bunsen burner, heat gently until stain begins to steam (do not boil) and allow to stand 5 min without further heating. If necessary, replenish stain, but do not reheat.
   b. If using electric staining rack, allow slides to stand 15 min after stain is added and switch is first turned on. If rack has been preheated, 7-10 min may be sufficient time.
3. Remove filter paper strips using forceps.
4. Rinse slides with tap water.
5. Decolorize with acid-alcohol (see decolorizing agents) until no more stain washes from the smear (ca. 2 min).
6. Counterstain with methylene blue (S-19) for 30-60 s.
7. Wash with water, drain, and air dry. Do not blot.

Kinyoun cold stain[15]

1. Cover smear with Kinyoun stain (S-16).
2. Stain 5 min. Heat is not needed.
3. Rinse slides with distilled water.
4. Decolorize with acid-alcohol (see decolorizing agents) for 3 min.
5. Rinse with distilled water.
6. Repeat decolorization until no red color appears in the wash.
7. Rinse with distilled water.
8. Counterstain with methylene blue for 1 or up to 4 min.
9. Rinse with distilled water.
10. Air dry. Do not blot.

· · ·

Alternate methods for acid-fast staining

Cooper modification

1. Fix slide in flame.
2. Stain with Cooper carbolfuchsin (S-17,a) 3-5 min, gently heating slide so that steam develops.
3. Wash with distilled water.
4. Decolorize with 5% nitric acid in 95% alcohol.
5. Wash with distilled water.
6. Counterstain with Cooper brilliant green (S-19,c) 30 s or longer.
7. Wash with distilled water.
8. Dry and examine.

Gabbett modification

1. Fix slide, stain with carbolfuchsin (S-15), and wash with distilled water.
2. Decolorize and counterstain at same time with Gabbett methylene blue solution (S-23) 20-30 s.
3. Wash with distilled water.
4. Dry in the air and examine.

Muller-Chermock carbolfuchsin-Tergitol cold stain method

1. Cover smear with carbolfuchsin containing 1 drop Tergitol no. 7 (Union Carbide) to each 25 ml stain (S-17). Allow to stain for 2 min without heat.
2. Wash with tap water.
3. Decolorize with acid-alcohol until smear is colorless.
4. Wash with water.
5. Counterstain with methylene blue (S-19,d) for approximately 5-15 s, depending on thickness of smear.
6. Wash with water and dry.

Exposure of smears to carbolfuchsin for 15-60 min at temperatures ranging from 37-80 C also has been reported.

Fluorochrome stains for acid-fast bacilli*

Like the fuchsin stains, fluorochrome dyes also stain acid-fast bacilli; the only difference is that the primary stain will fluoresce when properly excited, so that the bacilli, rather than being red, will fluoresce. The tissue debris and other background material is washed free of fluorescing dye with acid alcohol. Residual fluorescence of background debris may be minimized by a counterstain such as potassium permanganate or may be changed to a contrasting background by using acridine orange.

A number of microscope-light-filter arrangements are available for examination of fluorochrome-stained smears. The equipment here described has worked well for us. A Leitz SM microscope equipped with an HBO 200 mercury vapor lamp, KG-1 heat-absorbing filter, BG-38 red-absorbing filter, BG-12 (3 mm) exciter filter, OB-1 barrier filter, and bright-field, dry condenser (or dark-field condenser) provides ultraviolet excitation for stained smears. In recent years a more convenient setup for fluorescence microscopy has been employed that uses a high-intensity tungsten filament lamp (blue light): a 6V-15W tungsten filament lamp operated at 8 V to provide necessary light intensity, bright-field, dry condenser, combinations of BG-12 (4 mm) exciter filter with GG-50 barrier (ocular) filter or BG-12 (3 mm) with GG-53 barrier filter are satis-

*Contributed by G. P. Kubica and H. L. David.

factory. With 10× oculars, smears may be scanned at 100-250× (10× or 25× planachromat objectives), and bacillary morphology may be confirmed at 450-630× total magnification (45× or 63× objectives).

With the preceding combinations, bacilli fluoresce with a yellow glow against either a dark (permanganate) or orange (acridine orange) background. With the low-power objectives, smears may be scanned much more rapidly than with carbolfuchsin stains, thereby providing considerable time savings for the microscopist.

Although a number of fluorochrome procedures are available, the following have worked well in our hands.

Auramine O fluorochrome stain
Stain
a. Alcoholic auramine solution
Auramine O	0.1 g
Ethyl alcohol, 95%	10 ml
b. Phenol
Phenol crystals	3 g
Distilled water	87 ml
1. Dissolve auramine O in alcohol (solution a).
2. Melt phenol crystals and carefully add distilled water (solution b)
3. Mix all of solution a with all of solution b.

Potassium permanganate (counterstain for fluorochrome stain for AFB)
1. Dissolve 0.5 g potassium permanganate in 100 ml distilled water.
2. Store in brown bottle.

Acridine orange (counterstain for fluorochrome stain for AFB)
Dibasic sodium phosphate, anhydrous (Na_2HPO_4)	0.01 g
Distilled water	100 ml
Acridine orange	0.01 g
1. Dissolve sodium phosphate in distilled water.
2. Add and dissolve acridine orange.
3. Store in tightly stoppered or closed brown bottle.

Procedure
1. Flood smear with auramine O stain (S-5). Do not use filter paper strips as in Ziehl-Neelsen stain.
2. Allow stain to remain on smears at room temperature for 15 min. Do not heat.
3. Rinse with distilled water.
4. Decolorize with acid-alcohol (S-6) for 2 min.
5. Rinse with distilled water.
6. Flood smear with permanganate solution (S-7)[16] or with acridine orange counterstain (S-8)[17] for 2 but no more than 4 min.
7. Rinse with distilled water.
8. Drain; air dry. Do not blot.

Read smears as soon as possible (within a few hours) after staining because fluorescence will fade with time. Smears that cannot be read the same day may be held overnight in the refrigerator, but this procedure is not encouraged. Many rapidly growing mycobacteria fluoresce poorly, even though they stain well with carbolfuchsin.

• • •

Richards-Miller fluorescence microscopy (modified)[18]
1. Decontaminate and concentrate clinical specimen.
2. Prepare smears and fix in usual manner.
3. Stain smears for 4-5 min in 0.1% aqueous solution of fluorescent dye auramine O, to which 3% liquid phenol has been added.
4. Rinse with water.
5. Decolorize for 4-5 min is 70% ethyl alcohol containing 0.5% hydrochloric acid and 0.5% sodium chloride.
6. Rinse in water again.
7. Allow to dry in air.
8. Read with Leitz fluorescent antibody (FA) equipment using OG-1 and BG-12 filters. Scan with high dry magnification and verify with oil-immersion objective.

With this method acid-fast bacilli fluoresce with a characteristic golden glow against a dark background. This typical appearance, in addition to the clear morphology of the bacilli, permits relatively easy differentiation from unclear artifacts that exhibit fluorescence with a characteristic yellow glow.

Silver-Sonnenwirth-Alex modification of fluorescence microscopy[19]
Stain
Auramine-O (C. I. 14100D)	1.5 g
Rhodamine B	0.75 g
Glycerol	75 ml
Phenol crystals liquefied at 50 C	10 ml
Distilled water	50 ml
1. Keep stock solution at room temperature and filter before use through W. and R. Balston Whatman no. 2 filter paper.
2. Dry slides in air at 37 C and fix afterward using a Bunsen burner.
3. Stain for 30 min at 37 C on a staining rack.

Decolorization and counterstaining
1. Decolorize for 10 min with the following solution:
HCl	0.5 ml
Ethyl alcohol, 70%	99.5 ml
NaCl	0.5 g
2. Counterstain for **2 min** with the following solution:
Potassium permanganate	0.5 g
Distilled water	100 ml

The slides are examined with a microscope equipped with dark-field or bright-field condenser, using an HB-200 high-pressure mercury burner, 2 heat-absorbing filters—the KG-1 (2 mm) and BG-38 (4 mm), the BG-12 excitation filter, and the OG-1 barrier filter, which filters out the blue light of the background when placed in the ocular. *Mycobacterium tuberculosis* and groups I, II, and III of atypical mycobacteria fluoresce a reddish, golden yellow against a black background. Artifacts are hazy yellow or gray-green and lack the reddish tinge. (Tissue appears dark, pale green.)

Tissue that has been deparaffinized by washing in 3 changes of xylene for 1.5 min and hydrated by dipping in (1) absolute alcohol, (2) 95% alcohol, (3) 10% alcohol, and (4) water can be stained with the stain listed previously. Staining should be done in stain preheated to 60 C. Slides should be immersed in preheated stain for 10 min, and slide rack should be kept at 60 C in incubator. After staining, proceed as follows:
1. Wash for 2 min.
2. Decolorize with 0.5% HCl in ethyl alcohol (2-3 min).
3. Rinse in tap water for 2 min.
4. Counterstain with potassium permanganate solution listed above (0.5%) for 1 min.
5. Wash for 2 min.
6. Dry by blotting.
7. Dehydrate for 15 s in absolute alcohol.
8. Dip for clearing into xylol.
9. Coverslip: D.P.X. mounting medium is best; Per-

mount is adequate. Fluormount is unsatisfactory, since it imparts excessive fluorescence to the entire slide.

Staining flagella[6,7,19]
General method of applying flagella stains

For staining flagella very young and vigorous cultures must be procured. In general, 12- to 24-hour growths on surface of agar are satisfactory. If stock cultures are used, make daily transplants for several days before studying, to restore vigor.

Use agar slants with plenty of water of condensation. Transfer a loopful of this water of condensation from a 24-hour culture to a second slant; then 24 hours later pour off 1 or 2 drops of condensation water aseptically into a tube of sterile distilled water of the same temperature as the culture. Incubate at optimum temperature of the organism for 48-72 hours. Johnston and Mack recommend a similar method. Others find that bacteria have a tendency to shed their flagella if left in water for as long a period as 48-72 hours. One worker obtained excellent results when bacteria were in the water only 7 hours.

The coverslip or slide must be scrupulously clean. Place in hot cleaning solution, clean in strong sodium or potassium hydroxide, rinse in weak hydrochloric acid, and then rinse in distilled water. Keep in alcohol until ready for use. Burn off alcohol from coverslips just before use, holding them in the flame with forceps. Plimmer and Paine recommend baking slides on a wire gauze mat over a Bunsen burner just before using.

Greatly dilute the growth in distilled water, place tiny drops or streaks on the coverslip; discard those showing signs of grease. Preparations should be thin enough to dry immediately. Fixation of films by heat, although recommended by some authors, may destroy the flagella. Plimmer and Paine recommend scrupulously clean slides instead of coverslips, heated before use and cooled to body temperature. Using a 3 mm loop, place a drop of culture fluid on 1 end of the slide and tilt to allow the suspension to run down the slide. Slide should be warm enough to allow rapid drying. Gray's method is to place a large loopful of the culture suspension on 1 end of a slide and spread gently with a strip of unsized paper (e.g., typing paper).

Poor results are caused by greasy coverslips or slides, old cultures, unsatisfactory medium, too slow drying of the smear, too thick suspensions of bacteria, insufficient or excessive mordanting, understaining, or overstaining. Most poor results come from improper handling of the culture or from greasy slides or coverslips. The personal equation also enters the picture. Best results seem to have been obtained with the Leifson and Gray methods, although success has been reported when other methods were used.

Leifson
1. Prepare 3 slides.
2. With a wax pencil make a heavy, continuous line along the edges of the slides, leaving about 2 cm on one end free for handling. Place a large loopful of bacterial suspension on one end and tilt the slides so that the suspension runs down.
3. Dry in the air.
4. Add to each slide 0.8-1 ml Leifson stain (S-24). Stain first slide 8 min, second slide 10 min, and third slide 12-15 min.
5. Wash with tap water.
6. Drain and examine when dry.
7. If counterstain is necessary, stain with 1:1000 methylene blue in a 1:2000 aqueous solution of borax for 10 min.

Leifson (modified)[6,7]
1. Prepare a fresh slant culture, 16-20 h old, at temperature below optimum growth temperature (usually room temperature).
2. Add 2-3 ml distilled water by running down the glass side of slant.
3. Let stand at room temperature for 1 h.
4. With a Pasteur pipet transfer 5 or 6 drops liquid from the butt area into 10% formalin (40% formaldehyde). Make a slightly turbid suspension.
5. Pipet 1 drop formalinized suspension onto clean, dry slide on incline so that drop slowly runs down slide. The slide must be **thoroughly** clean.
6. Dry in air.
7. Stain with Leifson stain, alternate (S-35). If kept frozen, restore homogeneity of stain by shaking. With a pipet add 1 ml stain to the slide. Leave at room temperature for 10 min.
8. Rinse with tap water under faucet. Do not pour stain off before rinsing.
9. Counterstain if needed with 1% solution of methylene blue in water.
10. Dry in air and examine.
11. Bacterial bodies are blue; flagella, red.

Leifson-Hugh modification*
1. Inoculate organism to be stained into flagella broth (pH 7).

   Flagella broth
Tryptone	10 g
Sodium chloride	2.5 g
Dibasic potassium phosphate	1.0 g
Distilled water	1000 ml

   Place 6 ml quantities in 16 × 125 ml test tubes. Autoclave at 121 C for 15 min. Incubate overnight.
2. Add 0.25 ml formaldehyde (37-40%) to 5 ml flagella broth culture in a 15 ml centrifuge tube. Mix **gently**, allow to stand at room temperature for 15 min.
3. Fill tube with distilled water, mix well, and centrifuge at 2000 rpm for 30 min.
4. Using Pasteur pipet, **carefully** remove supernatant; do not disturb pellet. Resuspend pellet gently in 1 ml water. Repeat step 3.
5. Remove supernatant, resuspend pellet in 1 ml distilled water.
6. Slowly add distilled water until suspension is slightly opalescent. Do **not** invert tube.
7. Preparation of slides: Soak slides in a mixture of 3% conc. HCl in 95% ethyl alcohol solution. Dry with clean linen towel. Heat slides in **blue** portion of Bunsen burner flame.
8. Immediately after heating, draw a line about one-third distance from frosted end of slide with a wax pencil. Slide should be sufficiently hot to melt wax.
9. After slides have cooled, rest them "wax side" up

---

*From Analytab Products, Inc., Plainview, N.Y., 1977.

on a slight incline with frosted end high. This may be easily accomplished by elevating frosted end with a pencil.

10. With an inoculating loop, apply 1 loopful to upper portion of slide a few millimeters down from wax line. Allow to air dry. Do not heat fix.
11. Place slides on a staining rack. Apply 1 ml stain (S-25) to marked area of each side.
12. Staining time is generally in the range of 5-15 min. Allow stain to remain approximately 1 min after a precipitate is observed in staining solution.
13. Without removing slide from rack, gently wash stain off, making sure that stain has been completely removed before slide is lifted from rack.
14. Wipe back of slide and let air dry or blot before examining.
15. Examine slides in area where suspension was applied. The optimally stained area is generally found approximately one-third the distance from the bottom.

Silver-plating stain for flagella[9]
1. Grow organisms in a semisolid motility medium or trypticase soy agar (TSA) slants at 25 C (room temperature) for 18-24 h.
2. Use slides precleaned by manufacturer; before use, wipe with lens paper.
3. Place 4 loopfuls of sterile distilled water on each slide.
4. Collect organisms with an inoculating needle from the original stab line in the motility medium and with a loop from the liquid formed at the base of the TSA slant (use 1 loopful). Mix the organisms into the water on the slide.
5. Cover each smear with solution 1 (mordant) silver-plating stain (S-27) for 4 min.
6. Rinse gently with distilled water. Cover with solution 2 (stain) (S-27). Apply heat until steam forms; allow stain to remain on slide for 4 min.
7. Rinse slide gently with distilled water while holding slide horizontally. Air dry.

Gray
1. Prepare film as directed in general method and dry.
2. Apply Gray mordant (S-28) 5-10 min.
3. Wash with distilled water.
4. Stain with carbolfuchsin (S-15) 5-10 min.
5. Wash with tap water.
6. Drain and examine when dry.

Stain for *Legionella pneumophila* (Legionnaires' bacterium) in tissue.[11] The modified **Dieterle's silver stain** for spirochetes[10] stains the Legionnaires' organism in tissue.

Tissue handling
1. Fix tissue in formalin, embed in paraffin, cut at 4-6 μm, and affix to glass slides either with egg albumin or by the use of gelatin in the flotation water bath.
2. Use glass or plastic staining racks for staining 10-25 slides at a time.
3. Use a **known** positive control in **each** staining rack.*

Staining procedure
1. Preheat the 5% alcoholic uranyl nitrate solution (A, S-29) and the 1% silver nitrate solution (C, S-29) in a 55-58 C oven for at least 30 min. (Do not exceed temperature of 60 C as silver will precipitate.)

---

*Control tissue is available from Center for Disease Control, Control Tissue Repository, Pathology Division, Bldg. 1-2330, Atlanta, Ga. 30333.

2. Deparaffinize and hydrate sections to distilled water.
3. Place sections in preheated 5% alcoholic uranyl nitrate in 55-58 C oven for 30 min to 1 h.
4. Distilled water—1 dip.
5. 95% Alcohol—1 dip.
6. 10% Alcoholic gum mastic (B, S-29)—3 min.
7. 95% Alcohol—1 quick dip.
8. Dip in distilled water for 1 min, then allow slides to drain for 15-20 min until almost dry (may be left overnight).
9. Place sections in preheated 1% silver nitrate solution in 55-58 C oven, in the dark, for 4 h.
10. Distilled water—2 dips.
11. Developer (D, S-29)—dip until sections are pale yellow to light tan.
12. Distilled water—2 dips.
13. 95% Alcohol—2 dips.
14. Acetone—2 dips.
15. Xylol I—2 dips.
16. Xylol II—2 dips.
17. Coverslip with Permount or Protex.

Results
Spirochetes, bacteria—dark brown to black
Background—pale yellow to tan
Other structures that stain—melanin granules, chromatin, formalin pigment, and some foreign material in macrophages

Capsule stains

The capsules of bacteria are often detectable as unstained halos surrounding the bodies of the organisms. In many cases, however, special staining methods are necessary to ascertain the presence or absence of the capsules. The following methods give good results.

Hiss
1. Mix material to be stained with an equal amount of serum. Make thin smear.
2. Allow to dry in air.
3. Fix either in the flame or in 1:10 diluted commercial formalin.
4. Cover with Hiss stain (S-30) or 1% aqueous solution of crystal violet, and heat to steaming for a few seconds.
5. Wash off the stain with a 20% watery solution of copper sulfate.
6. Dry in air and examine.
Bacterial bodies, cells, and background stain purple. Capsules are colorless or pale lavender.

MacNeal
1. Make thin smear.
2. Allow to dry in air.
3. Cover with MacNeal tetrachrome stain (S-31) 3-5 min.
4. Wash carefully with distilled water.
5. Dry in air and examine.
Capsules are colorless or pale.

Lawson
1. Prepare direct smear from the culture without using a diluent.
2. Dry in air.
3. Cover film with mordant (S-32) 30 s.
4. Wash the slide with methyl alcohol.
5. Cover with 20 drops stain (S-33) 2 min.
6. Add 30 drops distilled water, mix stain on slide with water, and allow to act 10-20 min.
7. Rinse with distilled water.
8. Drain slide and examine when dry.
9. Capsules are colorless or pale.

Granule stains

Granule stains serve for the study of bacterial morphology.

Smears must be dried and fixed over the flame before the granule stain is applied.

Ljubinsky
1. Stain with Ljubinsky stain (S-34) 2 min.
2. Wash with distilled water.
3. Stain with Bismarck brown (S-14) 30 s.
4. Wash with distilled water.
5. Dry and examine. Granules are deep purple; bodies are brownish.

Methylene blue
1. Apply methylene blue (S-20 or S-22) 1-2 min.
2. Wash with distilled water.
3. Dry in air and examine.
4. Granules are deep blue; bodies are lighter blue.

Gohar
1. Stain with methylene blue (S-20) 5 min.
2. Quickly decolorize with 1:1000 sulfuric acid.
3. Rapidly wash with distilled water.
4. Stain with Gram's iodine (S-6 or S-7) 10 s.
5. Wash with distilled water.
6. Counterstain with 1% eosin in distilled water 30 s.
7. Wash with distilled water.
8. Dry in air and examine.
9. Granules are dark; bodies are yellowish.

Neisser
1. Stain with Neisser solution (S-35) 30-60 s.
2. Wash with distilled water.
3. Stain with Bismarck brown (S-14) 10 s.
4. Wash with distilled water.
5. Dry in air and examine.

Albert
1. Stain with Albert stain (S-36), solution A, 5 min.
2. Drain; do no wash.
3. Apply (S-36), solution B, 1 min.
4. Wash briefly with tap water.
5. Dry and examine.
6. Metachromatic granules stain black, bars of diphtheria cells, dark green to black, and body of cells, light green.

Staining spores

If a special method is not used but the Gram or a simple bacterial stain is applied, spores appear as unstained holes in the bacterial body. To visualize spores more clearly, special methods must be applied.

Dorner
1. Make a heavy suspension of organism in 3-4 drops distilled water.
2. Add 3-4 drops Ziehl-Neelsen carbolfuchsin (S-15).
3. Boil for 10-15 min.
4. Mix loopful of preparation on slide with loopful of nigrosin, Dorner solution (S-38).
5. Make thin smear.
6. Spores are red, vegetative cell, unstained, and background, gray.

Wirtz-Conklin
1. Make thin smears and fix in flame.
2. Cover with 5% aqueous malachite green and steam 3-6 min.
3. Wash with distilled water.
4. Stain **either** with 0.5% aqueous safranin or 5% aqueous merbromin (Mercurochrome) 30-60 s.
5. Wash with distilled water.
6. Dry and examine.

7. Spores are green; bodies of bacteria are pink.

Abbott
1. Make thin smears and fix in flame.
2. Cover with methylene blue (S-20 or S-22) and heat, bringing the stain to boiling several times but not continuously for 1 min.
3. Wash in distilled water.
4. Cover with a mixture of 1 part saturated alcoholic eosin Y solution and 9 parts distilled water 5-10 s.
5. Rinse with distilled water.
6. Blot.
7. Mount in balsam and examine.
8. Spores are blue; bodies of bacteria, pink.

Staining mycoplasma colonies

The Dienes stain (S-39) is used to distinguish mycoplasma colonies from artifacts.

1. Place a small amount of the stain next to a suspected colony (with loop or cotton swab).
2. The stain will diffuse and the colony will become blue if it is mycoplasma. Live bacteria decolorize the stain in a few minutes.

See also Chapter 81.

Staining yersiniae

For discussion of staining yersiniae see Wayson stain (S-40) and *Yersinia* (Chapter 79).

Staining rickettsiae and inclusion bodies

For discussion of staining rickettsiae and inclusion bodies see Chapter 95.

Staining fungi

For discussion of staining fungi see Chapter 103.

REFERENCES

1. Clark, G., editor: Staining procedures used by the Biological Stain Commission, ed. 3, Baltimore, 1973, The Williams & Wilkins Co.
2. Lillie, R. D., editor: Conn's biological stains, ed. 9, Baltimore, 1977, The Williams & Wilkins Co.
3. Society of American Bacteriologists: Manual of microbiological methods, New York, 1957, McGraw-Hill Book Co.
4. Lennette, E. H., Spaulding, E. H., and Truant, J. P.: Manual of clinical microbiology, ed. 2, Washington, D.C., 1974, American Society for Microbiology.
5. Holdeman, L. V., and Moore, W. E. C., editors: Anaerobe laboratory manual, ed. 3, Blacksburg, Va., 1975, Anaerobe laboratory, Virginia Polytechnic Institute and State University.
6. Leifson, E., and Hugh, R.: J. Bacteriol. **65**:263, 1953.
7. Leifson, E.: Atlas of bacterial flagellation, New York, 1960, Academic Press.
8. Clark, W. A.: J. Clin. Microbiol. **3**:632, 1976.
9. West, M., Burdash, N. M., and Freimuth, F.: J. Clin. Microbiol. **6**:414, 1977.
10. Dieterle, R. R.: Arch. Neurol. and Psychiat. **18**:73, 1927.
11. Van Orden, A., and Greer, P.: Modification of the Dieterle spirochete stain, Atlanta, 1977, Histopathology Laboratory, Pathology Division, Bureau of Laboratories, Center for Disease Control.
12. Goldenberg, M. I.: Health Lab. Sci. **5**:38, 1968.
13. Salton, M. R. J.: The bacterial cell wall, Amsterdam, 1964, Elsevier Publishing Co.

14. Vestal, A. L.: Procedures for the isolation and identification of mycobacteria, Atlanta, 1975, Center for Disease Control.

15. Kinyoun, J. J.: Am. J. Public Health **5:**867, 1915.

16. Truant, J. P., Brett, W. A., and Thomas, W. Jr.: Bull. Henry Ford Hosp. **10:**287, 1962.

17. Smithwick, R. W., and David, H. L.: Tubercle **52:**226, 1971.

18. Koch, M. L., and Cote, R. A.: Am. Rev. Respir. Dis. **91:**283, 1965.

19. Silver, H., Sonnenwirth, A. C., and Alex, N.: J. Clin. Pathol. **19:**583, 1966.

20. Leifson, E.: J. Bacteriol. **62:**37, 1951.

72

MEDIA, TESTS, AND REAGENTS*

Alex C. Sonnenwirth

For **mechanized, automated,** and **miniaturized** methods, including kits, see Chapter 74.

MEDIA

General facts concerning media preparation, including methods for their sterilization, are discussed in Chapter 70.

Quality control procedures essential for media use (laboratory prepared or purchased commercially) are described in Chapter 73.

Indicators added to culture media

Andrade indicator. For carbohydrate fermentation tests, media containing Andrade indicator are recommended.[1]
1. Dissolve 0.5 g acid fuchsin in 100 ml distilled water; then add 16 ml 1 N sodium hydroxide.
2. It may be necessary to add 1 or 2 drops NaOH after several hours if fuchsin is not sufficiently decolorized. Amount of alkali to be used with any particular batch of fuchsin is usually specified by manufacturer on fuchsin bottle label.
3. Use 10 ml indicator for each liter of medium.
4. Indicator is colorless; acid production in media containing this indicator is shown by change to reddish pink color.

Other indicators such as bromthymol blue, bromcresol purple, or phenol red may also be used.

Bromthymol blue
1. Dissolve 0.4 g bromthymol blue in 12.8 ml 0.05N sodium hydroxide by grinding in mortar.
2. Dilute to 100 ml with distilled water.
3. Use 2-4 ml for each 1000 ml culture medium.
4. pH range is 6.1 (yellow) to 7.7 (blue).

Bromcresol purple
1. Dissolve 0.4 g bromcresol purple in 13.8 ml 0.05N sodium hydroxide by grinding in mortar.
2. Dilute to 100 ml with distilled water.
3. Use 2-4 ml for each 1000 ml culture medium.
4. pH range is 5.4 (yellow) to 7.0 (purple).

Phenol red
1. Dissolve 0.4 g phenol red in 23.5 ml 0.05N sodium hydroxide by grinding in mortar.
2. Dilute to 100 ml with distilled water.
3. Use 2-4 ml for each 1000 ml culture medium.
4. pH range is 6.9 (yellow) to 8.5 (red).

pH meter

The pH of desiccated media should be checked after solution in water, using a **glass electrode pH meter.** Determine the pH of the final medium **after** it has cooled to room temperature.

Macerate agar media and place in beaker or cup used with the meter. Surface electrodes are useful in testing plated media.

A flat-bottom electrode, O-I model 2000,*[2] has been used successfully to measure pH of media in dishes without penetrating the agar surface. The pH value of all media must be within the range specified by the manufacturer of the dehydrated base used to prepare the media or ±0.2 pH units of the value specified in the formulation used.

• • •

Formulas of culture media

This section is not intended to be a complete catalogue of media. There are literally hundreds of media in use, and it is impossible to list more that those considered essential for the methods described. **Many additional media and their composition are found throughout the text. Consult the index for media not listed in this section.†**

• • •

Media for mycobacteria, anaerobes, and for fungi are listed separately at the end of this section.

• • •

*The portions of this chapter contributed by George Kubica, Hugo David, V. R. Dowell, Jr., and Sydney M. Finegold have been indicated by the name of the contributor in parentheses. All other portions of the chapter were contributed by Alex C. Sonnenwirth.

*Corporate Technology, Owens-Illinois, Inc., Toledo, Ohio.
†**Dehydrated media:** BBL, Div. of BioQuest, Cockeysville, Md.; Difco Laboratories, Detroit, Mich.; Oxoid Ltd., Wade Road, Basingstoke, Hampshire, England (in United States, K. C. Biologicals, Inc., Lenexa, Kan.).
Ready-to-use media: BBL; Difco; Scott Laboratories, Fiskeville, R. I.; Gibco Diagnostics, Madison, Wis.; and many other regional and local companies.

Alkaline peptone water. See *Vibrio cholerae* media, below.

Aronson medium. See *Vibrio cholerae* media, below.

Acetate agar[1]

Sodium acetate	2 g
Sodium chloride	5 g
Magnesium sulfate	0.20 g
Monoammonium phosphate	1 g
Dipotassium phosphate	1 g
Bromthymol blue	0.08 g
Agar	20 g
Distilled water	1 L
Final pH 6.7 ± 0.2	

1. Dissolve and dispense into tubes for 2.5 cm butts and 3.8 cm slants.
2. Autoclave at 121 C for 15 min.
3. Inoculate and incubate in the same manner as Simmons citrate agar.

Actinomyces media (isolation, maintenance, fermentation, etc.). See Chapter 77.

Alkaline seawater—Venkatraman-Ramakrishnan[4]

1.
Sodium chloride	27 g
Potassium chloride	1 g
Magnesium chloride	3 g
Distilled water	100 ml

Dissolve ingredients in distilled water in order given.

2.
Boric acid	12.405 g
Potassium chloride	14.912 g
Hot distilled water	800 ml

Dissolve ingredients in hot distilled water. Dilute solution 2 to 1000 ml with distilled water.

3.
Sodium hydroxide, 8%, aqueous solution	135.5 ml

4. For use, mix in a graduate:
Sea salt solution (1)	20 ml
Boric buffer (2)	250 ml
Sodium hydroxide solution (3)	135.5 ml

5. Add distilled water to make 1000 ml.
6. Distribute in 10 ml quantities in screw-capped bottles of 30 ml capacity.
7. Sterilize in autoclave 20 min at 15 psi.

Anthrax differential and selective media. See *Bacillus*, Chapter 77.

Aronson medium. See *Vibrio* media.

Azide blood agar base

Tryptose	10 g
Beef extract	3 g
Sodium chloride	5 g
Sodium azide	0.2 g
Agar	15 g

1. Dissolve, with heat, in 1000 ml distilled water.
2. Sterilize at 15 psi for 15 min.

Commercial product. Azide blood agar base, dehydrated, is available from several manufacturers.

Bile agar[5]

Bile, 10%

Ox bile, dehydrated*	10 g
Serum, sterile (filtered), or blood	50 ml
Nutrient agar	1000 ml

1. Melt nutrient agar. Add bile. Mix until dissolved.
2. Autoclave at 10 psi for 20 min. Cool to about 55 C and add serum or blood aseptically.
3. Mix and pour in plates.

Bile, 40%. Use 40 g dehydrated ox bile.

---

*Dehydrated ox bile, available as Oxgall from Difco Laboratories, Detroit, Mich., in 10% solution equals fresh bile.

Bile broth

Ox bile, dehydrated*	10 g
Glycerol	80 ml
Peptone	20 g
Distilled water	1000 ml

1. Mix dry peptone and dehydrated dry ox bile thoroughly and add distilled water slowly to 500 ml.
2. Add glycerol and make up to 1000 ml.
3. Autoclave 15 ml vol in flask or bottle at 15 psi for 15 min.

The medium is used by some workers as an enrichment medium in the isolation of *Salmonella typhi* and other salmonellae.

Bile esculin agar

Beef extract	3.0 g
Peptone	5.0 g
Agar	15.0 g
Oxgall	40.0 g
Ferric citrate	0.5 g
Water	1 L

1. Dissolve first 3 ingredients in 400 ml water. Dissolve Oxgall in 400 ml water. Dissolve ferric citrate in 100 ml water.
2. Combine solutions and mix well. Heat to 100 C for 10 min.
3. Autoclave at 121 C for 15 min. Cool to 50 C.
4. Aseptically add 100 ml water containing 1 g esculin previously heated gently to obtain solution and filter-sterilized.
5. Dispense in sterile screw-capped tubes. Tighten caps and cool in slanted position.

Dehydrated medium of this formula is available; prepare according to directions.

Bismuth sulfite agar—Hajna-Perry

Agar base

Agar	30 g
Beef extract	5 g
Peptone	10 g
Sodium chloride	5 g

1. Suspend in 1000 ml distilled water and dissolve in autoclave.
2. Adjust reaction to pH 7.4-7.6.
3. Sterilize in autoclave 30 min at 15 psi and store in refrigerator.

Hajna-Perry reagent

1. Dissolve 80 g anhydrous sodium sulfite, Baker, in 400 ml boiling distilled water.
2. Add 40 ml distilled water to 24 g bismuth citrate, cp, mix to paste, and add at once 10 ml pure ammonia (sp. gr. 0.897) and then drop by drop add more ammonia until mixture is only fluorescent. Dilute to 200 ml with distilled water.
3. Mix sodium sulfite and the bismuth solutions (1) and (2).
4. Add 42 g anhydrous dibasic sodium phosphate, Baker, to above mixture and mix well until nearly dissolved.
5. Dissolve 3.2 g crystalline ferrous sulfate, cp, in 40 ml distilled water.
6. Add 2 drops concentrated hydrochloric acid, and add this solution to above mixture. Cover mixture with beaker and boil carefully until color turns slate gray. Store in dark, tightly stoppered bottle.

Brilliant green, "certified for media," 1%, aqueous solution

For use:

1. To 1000 ml melted, partly cooled base, add 10 g

---

*Dehydrated ox bile, available as Oxgall from Difco Laboratories, Detroit, Mich., in 10% solution equals fresh bile.

glucose, 70 ml Hajna-Perry reagent, and 3-4 ml brilliant green solution.

Bismuth sulfite agar—Wilson-Blair, modified

Peptone	10 g
Beef extract	5 g
Dextrose	5 g
Disodium phosphate	4 g
Ferrous sulfate	0.3 g
Bismuth sulfite indicator	8 g
Agar	20 g
Brilliant green	0.025 g

Dissolve in 1000 ml distilled water.
The medium is available in dehydrated form from several manufacturers.

Blood agar base. This medium is identical with meat infusion agar to be described, except that a peptone such as tryptose, tryptone, or trypticase, more favorable for growth of fastidious organisms, is substituted for simple peptone.

BBL or Difco blood agar base, available in dehydrated form, are excellent for this purpose. Prepare according to manufacturer's instructions.

Blood agar, method 1. Blood agar is a mixture of sterile blood in sterile blood agar base. As it cannot be sterilized after it is made, utmost care is necessary in preparing it.

For blood agar, sheep or rabbit blood is preferable to human blood, as it does not inhibit growth of pathogenic bacteria to same extent as human blood. Blood must be taken in sterile manner and must be kept sterile throughout entire procedure. Agar to be used should be blood agar base previously made and sterilized. It should be liquefied and kept at a temperature of 47-50 C to prevent hemolysis of blood cells that are to be added.

Medium may be made either in sterile Petri dishes or in sterile test tubes.

Procuring rabbit blood

MATERIALS AND REAGENTS. Assemble the following:
1. Rabbit and rabbit board
2. Necessary equipment for ether anesthesia
3. 5 ml Luer syringe with a 21-gauge, 1½ inch needle previously sterilized in dry heat sterilizer at 170 C for 2 h.
4. A bottle, 100 ml, widemouthed, to which have been added sterile glass beads (for defibrination, preferred) or 10 drops 20% solution neutral potassium or sodium oxalate; bottle and contents sterilized in dry heat sterilizer at 170 C for 2 h (sodium oxalate, if used, remains as a fine white powder in bottom of bottle)
5. Tincture of iodine
6. Sterile sponges
7. Alcohol to remove iodine
8. Bunsen burner

PROCEDURE
1. Place animal on animal board.
2. Shave skin over heart area.
3. Give animal light anesthetic.
4. Locate heart by palpation.
5. Place generous quantity of iodine on skin over area of heart to sterilze surface.
6. Plunge needle attached to syringe into heart and withdraw 5 ml blood.
7. Flame mouth of bottle.
8. Eject contents of syringe into bottle, flaming needle before ejecting blood. Replace cork.
9. Shake bottle thoroughly to defibrinate (shake 5 min) or to oxalate blood.
10. Remove iodine from animal's chest with alcohol, and release from board.

Defibrinated sheep blood is used in many laboratories for preparation of blood agar plates. Human blood (usually from discarded blood bank bottles) should not be used. See discussion under streptococci.

Sheep blood and rabbit blood are available commercially.

Preparing agar
1. Liquefy sterile blood agar base in tubes and keep at temperature of 47-50 C.
2. If blood agar is to be made in slants, there should be 5 ml agar in each tube; if it is to be made in 75 mm Petri dishes, use tubes containing 10 ml agar; if using 100 mm Petri dishes, use tubes containing 15 ml agar base.

To make blood agar in Petri dishes
1. Place 0.5 ml oxalated blood in center of sterile Petri dish, using sterile pipet to measure blood. If 100 mm Petri dishes are employed, use 0.75 ml blood. Care should be taken to exclude all possibility of air contamination during this procedure.
2. Add to Petri dish enough liquefied agar (temperature 47-50 C) to fill plate.
3. Mix thoroughly by rotating plate. Be sure that even mixture is obtained. Bubbles are undesirable because they obscure colony study.
4. Allow to solidify.

To make blood agar in test tubes
1. Keep blood agar base in 5 ml quantities in test tubes.
2. Liquefy and keep at temperature of 47-50 C in water bath.
3. Using sterile precautions, add 0.25 ml oxalated blood to each test tube by means of sterilized graduated 1 ml pipet.
4. Replace cotton plug and rotate tube vigorously between palms of hands.
5. Slant immediately and allow to solidify.
6. Place in incubator at 37 C for 3 days for sterility test.

Blood agar, alternate formula
1. Melt blood agar base, and when cooled to 45 C, add to each 100 ml of medium 5 ml sterile defibrinated human, rabbit, or horse blood.
2. If base is kept in tubes each containing 15 ml agar, melt agar by placing tubes in water bath and add to each tube, when cooled to 45 C, 0.75 ml blood, using sterile syringe.
3. Pour into sterile Petri dishes.
4. Before solidification, flame surface of plates with Bunsen buner to free plate of air bubbles.

Bordet-Gengou agar

Potatoes, peeled and sliced	125 g
Glycerol	10 ml
Sodium chloride	5.60 g
Agar	22.5 g
Distilled water	1.0 L

1. Mix potatoes and glycerol with 500 ml distilled water. Boil, and when soft, dilute to volume with distilled water.
2. Strain through gauze.
3. Allow to settle.
4. Use clear supernatant fluid. Restore to voulme.
5. Add other ingredients.
6. Dissolve by boiling.
7. Distribute in flasks and sterilize in autoclave 15 min at 15 psi; cool to 45 C.
8. Add 50 ml fresh human, rabbit, horse, or sheep blood to each 250 ml base.
9. Pour into plates.

Base may be purchased as **Difco** or **BBL Bordet-**

Gengou agar base. Addition of 125 U of penicillin per 250 ml of base just before pouring is recommended.

Brain-heart infusion broth and agar

Calf brain infusion	200 ml
Beef heart infusion	250 ml
Proteose-peptone	10 g
Dextrose	2 g
Sodium chloride	5 g
Disodium phosphate	2.5 g

1. Mix ingredients.
2. Add distilled water to 1000 ml. For preparation of infusions see Infusion broth.

Commercial dehydrated medium

1. To dehydrate, dissolve indicated amount to dehydrated product in 1000 ml distilled water.
2. To make **brain-heart infusion agar** add 15 g agar.

Brilliant green agar—Christensen-Kauffmann

Meat or yeast extract	3-5 g
Peptone	10 g
Sodium chloride	5 g
Lactose	10 g
Sucrose	10 g
Phenol red	0.08 g
Brilliant green	0.0125 g
Agar	20 g

1. Dissolve in 1000 ml distilled water.
2. Sterilize in autoclave. Final reaction should be about pH 7.2.

BBL and Difco duplicate this formula. Prepare according to manufacturer's instructions.

Bromcresol purple iron milk. See Iron milk.

Broth, pH 9.6. See Glucose phenolphthalein broth.

Brucella medium

1. Petri plates with media for *Brucella* can be prepared as follows:

Brucella agar (Difco)	43 g
Distilled water	1000 ml
or	
Trypticase soy broth (BBL)	30 g
Agar	15 g
Distilled water	1000 ml
or	
Trypticase soy agar	40 g
Distilled water	1000 ml

2. Autoclave at 15 psi for 15 min.

If above media are not available, use Liver infusion agar.

For *Brucella* blood culture see Castañeda medium.

Brucella selective medium

Brucella agar (Difco)	1000 ml
Ethyl (or crystal) violet	1.4 mg
Actidione*	100 mg
Polymyxin B	6000 units
Bacitracin	25,000 units

1. Add ethyl violet to agar, when melted, before autoclaving.
2. Prepare antibiotics in stock solutions and sterilize by passage through Seitz filter. Keep under refrigeration no longer than 1 wk.
3. Add antibiotics to medium after autoclaving, when agar has cooled to about 50 C.

Brucella broth for Campylobacter. See *Campylobacter* media.

Campylobacter media[6-9]

1. Selective medium for *Campylobacter fetus* ssp *jejuni*.[6]
   a. Blood agar base no. 2 (Oxoid*) is prepared ac-

cording to manufacturer's instructions. Sterilize at 121 C for 15 min, cool to 50 C.
   b. Add the following:

Vancomycin	10 μg/ml
Polymyxin B	2.5 IU/ml
Trimethoprim	5 μg/ml
Lysed horse blood	70 ml/L

Oxoid makes available vials of 3 antimicrobics sufficient to supplement 500 ml agar base. Lysed horse blood is/ prepared by freezing and thawing defibrinated horse blood 4 times.

2. Brucella broth media for *Campylobacter* differentiation.
   a. Brucella broth (BB) is base medium used for detecting H_2S with lead acetate paper, growth in 1% glycine, growth in 3.5% NaCl, and growth at 25 C and 42 C. It is prepared as follows:

Brucella broth	29 g
Agar (Difco)	1.6 g
Distilled water	1 L
Adjust to pH 7.0	

   b. Dissolve ingredients, dispense 10 ml into 16 × 150 mm screw-top tubes, and sterilize at 121 C 15 min. For *Campylobacter* differentiation, use as:
   (1) *Glycine medium.* Add 1% glycine to BB before sterilization.
   (2) *NaCl medium.* Add 3.5% NaCl to BB before sterilization.
   (3) *H_2S detection by lead acetate.* Add either 0.05% L-cystine or 0.02% L-cysteine hydrochloride to BB before sterilization.
   c. Suspend lead acetate paper above medium after it has been inoculated.

Carbohydrate fermentation broth base.[10] This medium is recommended for fermentation reactions, especially with *Enterobacteriaceae*.

Peptone	10 g
Meat extract	3 g
Sodium chloride	5 g
Andrade indicator	10 ml
Distilled water	1000 ml

1. Adjust reaction to pH 7.1-7.2.
2. Tube with inverted insert tubes and sterilize at 121 C for 15 min.
3. Add carbohydrates to aliquots of base as follows: glucose, lactose, sucrose, mannitol, 1% (1 g/100 ml), dulcitol, salicin, and others, 0.5% (0.5 g/100 ml).
4. The following can be added to base before sterilization: glucose (dextrose), mannitol, dulcitol, salicin, adonitol, inositol. Others such as lactose, sucrose, xylose, and arabinose should be sterilized by filtration (10% water solution) through Seitz or Millipore filter or should be autoclaved at 15 psi for 10 min and then added to sterile base medium.

A variety of fermentation media are available commercially (phenol red broth, phenol red agar, purple broth, purple agar). For *Enterobacteriaceae*, medium just described is to be preferred.

NOTE: Acid formation in media containing Andrade indicator (see indicators) is shown by change from colorless to reddish pink.

Carbohydrate fermentation medium for clostridia. See media for anaerobes.

---

*The Upjohn Co., Kalamazoo, Mich.

*In the United States, Oxoid media are available from K.C. Biologicals, Inc., P.O. Box 54411, Lenexa, Kan. 06215.

Carbohydrate fermentation medium for Listeria[11]

Beef extract	1 g
Proteose-peptone no. 3 (Difco)	10 g
Sodium chloride	5 g
Bromcresol purple	0.1 g
Distilled water	1000 ml

1. Dissolve with aid of heat.
2. Autoclave at 15 psi for 20 min.
3. Divide medium into aliquots and add glucose, raffinose, salicin, rhamnose, and dulcitol or others, as required (see *Listeria*) in 0.5% concentration.

Carbohydrate medium for Neisseria gonorrhoeae.[12]
Cystine trypticase agar (CTA [BBL]) is used as base. Composition of medium is as follows (per 1000 ml water):

Cystine	0.5 g
Trypticase	20 g
Agar	2.5 g
Sodium chloride	5 g
Sodium sulfite	0.5 g
Phenol red	0.017 g

1. Using commercial medium, add 4.3 g CTA medium, dehydrated, to 150 ml distilled water.
2. Shake to suspend and heat to dissolve.
3. Cool and adjust to pH 7.4-7.6 with 1N NaOH.
4. Dispense 50 ml to each of 2 Erlenmeyer flasks (250 ml).
5. Autoclave at 15 psi for 15 min. Cool flasks.
6. Prepare 20% solutions of glucose and maltose in distilled water; autoclave separately.
7. To flask 1 add 2.5 ml sterile 20% glucose solution.
8. To flask 2 add 2.5 ml sterile 20% maltose solution.
9. After thorough mixing of flasks, dispense media in 2 ml amounts into sterile 10 × 100 ml tubes.
10. Replace cotton stoppers of tubes with corks dipped in hot paraffin. Screw-capped tubes can also be used.

For small laboratories it may be practical to purchase ready-made CTA medium in tubes already containing carbohydrates. These are furnished in screw-capped tubes (BBL) and can be kept for considerable time without loss of water.

For rapid (4 h) fermentation test for Neisseria gonorrhoeae, see *Neisseria*, Chapter 76.

Carbohydrate fermentation medium for differentiation of Staphylococcus and Micrococcus

Tryptone (Difco)	1.0 g
Yeast extract (Difco)	0.1 g
Bromcresol purple	0.004 g
Glucose **or** mannitol	1.0 g
Agar	0.22 g
Distilled water	100 ml

1. Tube in 16 × 120 mm tubes to depth of 7-8 cm.
2. Before use, steam 10 min, cool rapidly.
3. Inoculate heavily by stabbing to bottom.
4. Incubate under anaerobic conditions.

Carbohydrate fermentation slants, 10%[13]

Lactose 10% slant

Trypticase	10 g
Sodium chloride	5 g
Phenol red	0.018 g
Agar	15 g
Lactose	100 g

Phenol red broth base, dehydrated (Difco or BBL), can be used (contains trypicase, sodium chloride, and phenol red in above quantities).

1. Melt 15 g agar in 1000 ml distilled water by heating.
2. Cool to 50-60 C. Add:

Lactose	100 g
Phenol red broth base	15 g

3. Mix well. Tube in 6-8 ml amounts. Autoclave at **10 psi** for 10 min. Remove from autoclave and place tubes in slanting position.

Glucose 10% slant. Prepare exactly as lactose 10% slant, except:
1. Substitute glucose for lactose.
2. Adjust pH to 7.7 before autoclaving.

Casein medium. See *Nocardia*, Chapter 77.

Castañeda medium

1. | | |
   |---|---|
   | Trypticase soy agar (BBL) | 40 g |
   | Agar | 10 g |
   | *or* | |
   | Brucella agar | 43 g |
   | Agar | 10 g |

(Brucella broth, 28 g, and an additional 15 g agar can be substituted for Brucella agar.)
   a. Add to either:
Sodium citrate	5 g
Distilled water	1000 ml
   b. Dissolve ingredients in water by heating.
   c. Adjust to pH 7.4.
   d. Place 15 ml melted medium into Castañeda bottle or similar screw-capped bottle.
   e. Autoclave at 15 psi for 15 min. Allow to solidify, laying bottles on flat side to obtain slants.

2. | | |
   |---|---|
   | Trypticase soy broth, dehydrated (BBL) | 30 g |
   | *or* | |
   | Brucella broth, dehydrated | 28 g |

   a. Add to either:
Sodium citrate	20 g
Distilled water	1000 ml
   b. Sterilize in autoclave 15 min at 15 psi.
   c. When surface of agar 1 is hard, add 10-15 ml of mixture 2.

Cetrimide agar

Heart infusion agar	100 ml
Cetyltrimethyl ammonium bromide* (cetrimide), pH 7.2	0.5 g

1. Autoclave at 121 C for 15 min.
2. Cool tubed medium to solidify in slanted position. Final concentration of cetrimide is 0.5%.

Cetrimide agar, alternate medium

Heart infusion agar	100 ml
Hexadecyltrimethyl ammonium bromide*	0.09 g

Autoclave as above. Some workers prefer to add hexadecyl bromide after autoclaving. If preferred, proceed as follows:
1. Prepare 6% solution of hexadecyltrimethyl ammonium bromide (3 g in 50 ml distilled water).
2. Sterilized by Seitz or membrane filtration.
3. Add 15 ml sterile solution to 1000 ml melted and cooled heart infusion agar (final concentration, 0.09%).

Medium is inoculated lightly from agar slant culture and is observed daily (1-7 d) for presence of growth.

Chapman-Stone medium

Yeast extract	2-2.5 g
Trypticase *or* tryptone	10 g
Gelatin	30 g
D-Mannitol	10 g
Sodium chloride	55 g
Ammonium sulfate	75 g
Dipotassium phosphate	5 g
Agar	15 g
Distilled water	1000 g

Final reaction should be pH 7±.

---

*Distillation Products Industries, Division of Eastman Kodak Co., Rochester, N.Y.

Commercial medium

1. Suspend 20.2 g BBL or Difco dehydrated material in 100 ml distilled water.
2. Allow to stand 5 min.
3. Mix to obtain uniform suspension.
4. Heat and boil 1 or 2 min or until solution is complete.
5. Pour into plates while hot, being careful to avoid formation of bubbles. After solidification, medium should be white and opaque.
6. If medium cannot be used on day of preparation, it should be dispensed and sterilized by autoclaving at 121 C (15 psi) for 15 min.

Chocolate agar, selective for N. gonorrhoeae and N. meningitidis. See Thayer-Martin medium, recommended for 2 species.

Chocolate agar I, with IsoVitaleX enrichment (BBL), nonselective. This medium incorporates a chemically defined supplement, instead of yeast extract, and is recommended for isolation and cultivation of fastidious organisms.

1. Prepare double-strength base by suspending 7.2 g **GC agar base** (BBL or Difco) in 100 ml distilled water, using 500 ml flask. Mix well. Heat with agitation and boil 1 min until completely dissolved.
2. Prepare **double-strength hemoglobin solution** by mixing 2 g hemoglobin in 100 ml distilled water. Start by mixing 2 g hemoglobin with about 3 ml water until smooth paste is achieved. Add water with constant stirring until suspension is homogeneous.
3. Sterilize GC agar base and hemoglobin solution, separately, in autoclave at 15 psi (121 C) for 15 min.
4. Cool solutions to 50 C.
5. Reconstitute **IsoVitaleX enrichment** (BBL), 2 ml vial, aseptically with 2 ml sterile rehydrating fluid (BBL). Shake to dissolve completely.
6. Add aseptically hemoglobin and IsoVitaleX solution to sterile cooled GC agar base.

Chocolate agar II, nonselective. This medium is made from dehydrated GC agar base (BBL or Difco), the composition per liter of which is as follows:

Proteose-peptone no. 3 (Difco) *or*	
Polypeptone (BBL)	15 g
Cornstarch	1 g
Dipotassium phosphate	4 g
Monopotassium phosphate	1 g
Sodium chloride	5 g
Agar	10 g

1. a. Prepare a double-strength **GC medium base** by suspending 7.2 g in 100 ml cold distilled water and steaming or boiling to dissolve medium completely.
   b. For occasional cultures disperse in 10 ml amounts in tubes; for storage, place 250 ml medium in 500 ml flask.
   c. Stopper with cotton, cap with wrapping paper, and sterilize at 15 psi for 15 min.
2. a. Prepare double-strength **hemoglobin solution** by placing 2 g hemoglobin in dry flask and adding 100 ml cold distilled water while flask is being agitated vigorously.
   b. Shake hemoglobin suspension intermittently 10-15 min to break up all aggregates and to effect complete solution.
   c. It is advisable to filter hemoglobin solution through double layer of cheesecloth.
   d. Sterilize 15 min at 15 psi.
3. a. Allow sterile solutions to cool to 56 C in water bath.

b. Add 1% Bacto supplement A* (2 ml/100 ml double-strength GC medium base) to GC base, **not** to hemoglobin solution.
c. Mix and add equal volume of sterile double-strength hemoglobin solution.
d. Pour 15-20 ml into Petri dishes (sterile).

Plates should not be used if stored longer than 1 wk (in refrigerator) and should always be warmed to room temperature before use.

Christensen citrate agar[10]

Sodium citrate	3 g
Glucose	0.2 g
Yeast extract	0.5 g
Cysteine monohydrochloride	0.1 g
Ferric ammonium citrate	0.4 g
Monopotassium phosphate	1 g
Sodium chloride	5 g
Sodium thiosulfate	0.08 g
Phenol red	0.012 g
Agar	15 g

1. Dissolve ingredients in 100 ml distilled water.
2. Tube and sterilize at 15 psi for 15 min.
3. Slant in such a manner that approximately 1 inch butt and 1.5 inch slants result.

Christensen urea agar. See Urea agar—Christensen.

Citrate agar—Simmons. See Simmons citrate agar (for routine citrate test).

CLED agar.[14] Cystine lactose electrolyte deficient (CLED) agar is recommended for use in enumerating and presumptively identifying bacterial flora of urine. It supports growth of urinary pathogens and contaminants but prevents undue swarming of *Proteus* species due to its lack of electrolytes.

Gelysate peptone	4.000 g
Trypticase peptone	4.000 g
Beef extract	3.000 g
Lactose	10.000 g
L-Cystine	0.128 g
Bromthymol blue	0.020 g
Agar	15.000 g
Distilled water	1000 ml

Final pH is 7.3 ± 0.2.

1. Suspend 36 g powder in 1 L purified water.
2. Heat with agitation until solution occurs.
3. Sterilize at 121 C (15 lb pressure) for 15 min.
4. Cool to 50 C and dispense aseptically.

Columbia agar base—Ellner et al.[15]

Polypeptone (BBL) *or* Pantone (Difco)	10 g
Biosate (BBL) *or* Bitone (Difco)	10 g
Myosate (BBL) *or* tryptic digest of beef heart (Difco)	3 g
Sodium chloride	5 g
Cornstarch	1 g
Agar	15 g
Distilled water	1000 ml

1. Suspend materials in water. Heat with frequent agitation and boil 1 min.
2. Dispense and autoclave at 121 C for 15 min. Final pH is 7.3 at 25 C.

The basal dehydrated medium is available from BBL and Difco. It was designed for use as a general solid culture medium as well as a basal medium that can be employed for preparing other media.

Blood agar. Cool sterile base to 45 C and add 5% sterile defibrinated sheep blood.

Selective medium for gram-positive cocci. To blood agar add 10 mg colistin and 15 mg nalidixic acid (in 5 ml solution)/L at same time blood is added. Final concen-

---

*Bacto supplement A (Difco) is a yeast concentrate with 1:6000 crystal violet.

tration will be 10 μg colistin and 15 μg nalidixic acid/ml medium.

Chocolate agar
1. To base at 45 C add 10% sterile defibrinated sheep blood and heat to 85 C.
2. Cool to 45 C and add supplement B (Difco).
3. To prepare **Thayer-Martin medium,** add vancomycin, colistin, and nystatin (as described under Thayer-Martin [selective] medium [see below]).

Tinsdale medium. Add 1 ml Tinsdale enrichment (Difco) and 2 ml KL virulence enrichment (Difco) to 10 ml base (45 C).

Lactose–egg yolk–milk agar

Columbia agar base	42.5 g
Lactose	12 g
Agar	1 g
Neutral red, 1%, aqueous	3.25 ml
Distilled water	1000 ml

1. Heat to boiling.
2. Adjust pH to 7.0.
3. Autoclave at 121 C for 15 min.
4. Cool to 55 C and aseptically add 150 ml sterile milk and 36 ml sterile 50% egg-yolk saline.
5. A **selective medium for clostridia** may be prepared by adding sterile solution of 20 ml, containing 180 mg neomycin sulfate and 240 mg sodium azide.

Cooked meat medium. See Chopped meat medium (anaerobes).

Corynebacterium diphtheriae virulence test medium. See Elek, King, et al. medium.

CYE agar[16]

Yeast extract	10.0 g
Activated charcoal (Norit A)	1.5 g
L-Cysteine HCl · H$_2$O	0.4 g
Ferric pyrophosphate soluble*	0.25 g
Agar	17.0 g
Distilled water	1.0 L

1. Add all other ingredients of CYE agar **except** L-cysteine HCl and soluble ferric pyrophosphate to 980 ml distilled water; dissolve by boiling.
2. Autoclave at 121 C for 15 min and then cool to 50 C in water bath.
3. Prepare fresh solutions of L-cysteine HCl (0.40 g in 10 ml distilled water) and soluble ferric pyrophosphate* (0.25 g in 10 ml distilled water). Membrane filter-sterilize each solution separately. Add L-cysteine HCl to basal medium first.
4. Adjust complete medium to pH 6.90 at 50 C by adding 4.0-4.5 ml 1.0N NaOH. pH of this medium is critical.
5. Pour 20 ml quantities of media into sterile Petri dishes (15 × 100 mm). Swirl medium between pouring plates to keep charcoal particles suspended.

The pH of the solid medium must be 6.9 ± 0.05 to be confirmed either with a surface electrode (if available) or by emulsifying agar from 1 plate in distilled water and measuring with a combination electrode. pH is critical. If lots of ingredients used yield a medium of different pH, adjust pH of the complete liquid medium by adding 1N HCl or 1N NaOH.

Store medium in the dark, in sealed plastic containers, in a refrigerator. (Media have been used successfully for growing LDB after being stored for up to 2 months under these conditions.)

*For source of ferric pyrophosphate, and for precautions about its use, see **FG agar.**

The medium is used for isolation and propagation of Legionnaires' disease bacterium (LDB) (*Legionella pneumophila*).

Cystine glucose blood agar—Francis

Meat infusion agar	100 ml
Cystine	0.1 g
Dextrose	1 g

1. Dissolve cystine and dextrose in meat infusion agar, using flowing steam for 1 h.
2. Cool to 45 C and add 7-8 ml defibrinated rabbit blood.
3. Keep in water bath at 60 C for 2 h.
4. Pour in plates or dispense under sterile conditions into sterile test tubes.
5. Place in incubator for 24 h to test sterility.

Difco-cystine heart agar, 102 g dissolved in 1000 ml distilled water, duplicates above formula.

Cystine trypticase medium (CTA)

Cystine	0.5 g
Trypticase	20 g
Agar	3.5 g
Sodium chloride	5 g
Sodium sulfite	0.5 g
Phenol red	0.017 g

1. Dissolve in 1000 ml distilled water.
2. Final reaction will be pH 7.3±.

Commercial dehydrated medium

Suspend 29.5 g BBL powder in 1 L distilled water. Add carbohydrate (0.5 or 1%, as preferred) if desired. Addition of more than 0.5% carbohydrate may necessitate adjustment of pH, but with most carbohydrates there will be relatively little change in reaction.

1. Mix thoroughly.
2. Heat gently with frequent agitation.
3. Boil about 1 min or until solution is complete.
4. Tube and sterilize at 115-118 C, never over 12 psi, for 15 min.
5. Cool in upright position and store at room temperature. **Do not refrigerate.**

Decarboxylase media.[10] Decarboxylase base (Moeller) as well as decarboxylase medium base (Falkow) is now available in dehydrated form. The Moeller base is recommended (BBL, Difco).[17]

Moeller method[18]

Orthana special peptone*	5 g
Beef extract	5 g
Bromcresol purple, 1.6%	0.625 ml
Cresol red, 0.2%	2.5 ml
Glucose	0.5 g
Pyridoxal	5 mg

1. Dissolve ingredients in 1000 ml distilled water.
2. **Adjust pH to 6.0.**
3. Divide basal medium into 4 equal portions. Portion 1 is tubed without any addition, to serve as control. Portion 2 receives 1% L-lysine dihydrochloride; portion 3, 1% L-arginine monohydrochloride; and portion 4, 1% L-ornithine dihydrochloride. Dispense 3-4 ml media in small screw-capped tubes and autoclave at 15 psi for 10 min.
NOTE: Adjust portion 4 to pH 6.0.[10]
4. After inoculation add to each tube a 4-5 mm layer of sterile mineral oil. Always inoculate control tube.
5. Positive decarboxylation is indicated by change from yellow to violet or reddish violet.

*A/S Orthana Kemish Fabrik, Copenhagen, Denmark.

Falkow modification[19]

Peptone, Bacto	5 g
Yeast extract, Bacto	3 g
Dextrose	1 g
Bromcresol purple	0.02 g
Distilled water	1000 ml

1. Suspend 9 g dehydrated product in 1000 ml distilled water and dissolve by heat.
2. Add 5 g L-lysine, ornithine, and arginine/L medium to separate aliquots of medium. Dispense in 5 ml amounts into screw-capped tubes and autoclave 15 min at 15 psi.

NOTE: pH of aliquot containing ornithine should be adjusted to 6.7-6.8 prior to sterilization.[10]

When growth occurs, these media first become yellow due to acid formation from glucose; later, if decarboxylation occurs, the medium becomes alkaline (purple). Control tube (inoculated) should remain acid (yellow).

Demain medium. See Phenylketonuria (PKU) test materials.

Deoxycholate agar—Leifson

Peptone	10 g
Sodium chloride	5 g
Lactose	10 g
Agar	17-20 g

1. Soak in 1000 ml distilled water for 15 min.
2. Dissolve by heating.
3. While still hot, add quickly and in following order:

Anhydrous dipotassium phosphate	2 g
Ferric ammonium citrate "green scales"	2 g
Sodium deoxycholate	1 g

4. Adjust reaction to pH 7.4.
5. Add 3 ml 1% aqueous solution of neutral red.
6. Heat in steam 15 min.
7. Pour plates in 17-20 ml quantities.
8. Allow to solidify, with covers partially removed, about 1 h.
9. Store in refrigerator.

BBL deoxycholate agar, 46 g dissolved in 1000 ml distilled water, duplicates formula.

Deoxycholate-citrate (DEC) agar—Panja-Ghosh[20]

Beef extract (Lemco or other)	5 g
Peptone (Difco)	5 g
Sodium taurocholate	8.5 g
Agar	25 g

1. Dissolve in 1000 ml distilled water.
2. Steam 1 h.
3. Adjust reaction to pH 7.0.
4. Sterilize in autoclave 20 min at 15 psi.
5. For use, melt and add in order named:

Sodium citrate, crystals	8 g
Sodium thiosulfate, crystals	8.5 g
Disodium phosphate, crystals	7.5 g
Lactose	12.5 g
Ferric citrate "green scales"	3 g

6. Adjust reaction, if necessary, to pH 7.4.
7. Add 15 ml 0.25% solution neutral red and 5 ml 2N sodium hydroxide.
8. Boil 2 min.
9. Pour in plates.

Deoxycholate-citrate (DCA) agar—Leifson

1. Infuse 1000 g ground lean pork meat in 3000 ml distilled water at room temperature 3 h.
2. Add 10 ml 1N hydrochloric acid and boil 1 min.
3. Squeeze through gauze a small amount at a time, then filter through filter paper.
4. Add to filtrate 10 ml 1N sodium hydroxide.
5. Boil 1 min and dilute to 3000 ml with distilled water.

6. Add 30 g peptone (Thio or Wilson B).
7. Adjust reaction to pH 7.5.
8. Boil 5 min and filter through filter paper.
9. Add 60 g agar.
10. Add 15 ml 1N sodium hydroxide.
11. Allow to soak at room temperature 15 min.
12. Boil in steam 20 min.
13. Place in Erlenmeyer flasks in 1000 ml quantities (or smaller amounts).
14. Add the following to each 1000 ml:

Lactose	10 g
Crystalline sodium citrate	20.6 g
Sodium deoxycholate (optional 10 ml 0.35% aqueous lead chloride solution)	5 g

15. Adjust reaction to pH 7.4.
16. **Either** store in refrigerator immediately **or** add at once 2 g ferric ammonium citrate "green scales" and 3 ml 1% aqueous solution of neutral red.
17. Pour in plates, 15-17 ml in each. Allow to dry with partially removed covers for 1½ h. Store in refrigerator.

Small dewdrop-like crystals of sodium deoxycholate appear on surface of medium during storage. Their presence does not influence quality of medium. "Drops" disappear when plate is incubated.

DCA medium is available in dehydrated form.

DNase test medium[21]

Deoxyribonucleic acid	2 g
Trypticase	15 g
Phytone	5 g
Sodium chloride	5 g
Agar	15 g

1. Suspend ingredients in 1000 ml distilled water. Mix thoroughly.
2. Add (for staphylococci only):

Mannitol	10 g
Bromthymol blue	0.025 g

3. Heat, and boil 1 min. Sterilize at 121 C for 15 min.

Double sugar iron agar—Kligler

1. To each 100 ml melted nutrient agar, pH 7.4, add the following:

Lactose	1 g
Ferric ammonium citrate	0.05 g
Sodium thiosulfate	0.05 g
Dextrose	0.5 ml
Phenol red, 0.5% watery solution	0.5 ml

2. Tube and sterilize 20 min at 15 psi in autoclave.
3. Slant with long butts and short slants.

This medium may be purchased from commercial laboratories.

Egg-yolk medium[22] **(Nagler, modified; lecithinase medium)**

1. Use fresh hen's egg. Scrub well and sterilize with dilute mercuric chloride or by immersion of egg for 1 h in 95% alcohol. Discard egg white by aspiration; obtain yolk by aspiration and transfer to sterile tube. Add equal amount of sterile saline. Mix; test for sterility by inoculating 1 ml into thioglycollate tube. If sterile, egg yolk can be kept 2 wk at 4-10 C.
2. Prepare one of the following base media:

   a.

Proteose-peptone no. 2	40 g
Dextrose	2 g
Na_2HPO_4	5 g
KH_2PO_4	1 g
NaCl	2 g
$MgSO_4$	0.1 g
Agar	25 g
Distilled water	1000 ml

   Final pH should be 7.6; autoclave at 15 psi for 15 min.

or

b. Beef extract (Oxoid) — 10 g
   Bacteriologic peptone (Oxoid) — 10 g
   NaCl — 10 g
   Ionagar no. 2 (Oxoid) — 10 g
   Distilled water — 1000 ml
   Final pH 7.5 Autoclave at 121 C for 15 min.

or

c. Infusion broth (heart, meat) — 1000 ml
   Agar — 20 ml

or

d. Blood agar base (dehydrated), according to manufacturer's instructions.

Bases c and d are to be autoclaved at 15 psi (121 C) for 15 min.

3. Add aseptically:
   Egg-yolk solution, sterile — 10 ml
   Base medium: Either a, b, c, or d (sterile), melted and cooled — 90 ml
   Mix and pour plates.

NOTE: **Egg yolk,** sterile, concentrated emulsion, is available from Oxoid, Ltd. (K. C. Biological, Inc., Lenexa, Kan.); it saves time and is convenient. Base a or b is recommended.

The medium is used for demonstration of lecithinase activity of certain organisms (*Bacillus* species, certain staphylococci, and especially *Clostridium perfringens* and *C. bifermentans*). See **Nagler reaction.** See also Media for anaerobes.

Elek, King, et al. medium[23-25]

Proteose-peptone — 20 g
Agar — 15 g
Sodium chloride — 2.5 g

1. Dissolve in 1000 ml distilled water.
2. Adjust reaction to pH 7.8.
3. Place in 10 ml quantities in test tubes and sterilize at 15 psi for 15 min.
4. Before use, melt and add to each tube 2 ml fresh, **nonhemolyzed** rabbit or horse serum.

The difficulties encountered with various batches of animal sera in this test are obviated by use of **KL virulence agar and KL virulence enrichment** (Difco). The medium and enrichment are based on the modification of Hermann et al.[25]

1. Suspend 37.5 g Bacto-KL virulence agar in 1000 ml distilled water.
2. Heat to boiling and sterilize at 15 psi for 15 min.
3. Cool medium to 55 C and add 2 ml Bacto-KL virulence enrichment and 0.5 ml Bacto-Chapman tellurite solution to as many sterile 100 mm Petri dishes as desired.
4. Add 10 ml cooled agar to each plate and rotate 20 times to obtain even mixture.

Elek toxigenicity medium, CDC modification. See *Corynebacterium*, Chapter 77.

EMB (eosin-methylene blue) agar

Peptone — 10 g
Lactose — 5 g
Sucrose — 5 g
Dipotassium phosphate — 2 g
Agar — 13.5 g
Eosin Y — 0.4 g
Methylene blue — 0.065 g
Distilled water — 1000 ml

Methylene blue can be added as 0.5 ml 2% aqueous solution; eosin Y as 2 ml 2% aqueous solution.

Commercially prepared dehydrated EMB media can be used.

Endo agar

Peptone — 10 g
Lactose — 10 g

Dipotassium phosphate — 3.5 g
Agar — 15 g
Basic fuchsin — 0.5
Sodium sulfite — 2.5 g

1. Mix ingredients in 1000 ml cold distilled water and heat to boiling to dissolve completely.
2. Autoclave 15 min at 121 C (15 psi).

The medium is available in dehydrated form from several manufacturers.

Esculin medium (broth)

Peptone (Bacto or equivalent) — 5 g
Dipotassium phosphate — 1 g
Esculin — 3 g
Ferric citrate — 0.5 g
Andrade indicator — 10 ml
Distilled water — 1000 ml

1. Heat gently to dissolve ingredients and dispense in 3 ml amounts in 3 × 100 mm tubes with inverted insert tubes.
2. Sterilize at 121 C for 10 min. **Hydrolysis of esculin** is indicated by formation of black precipitate.

Esculin medium (slant)

Esculin — 1.0 g
Ferric citrate — 0.5 g
Heart infusion agar — 40.0 g
Distilled water — 1000.0 ml

1. Adjust pH to 7.0.
2. Tube 5 ml amounts in 15 × 125 mm tubes.
3. Autoclave at 121 C for 15 min and slant.

FG agar[16,26]

Casein (acid hydrolysis) — 17.5 g
Beef extractives — 3.0 g
L-Cysteine HCl · H_2O — 0.4 g
Ferric pyrophosphate soluble* — 0.25 g
Starch — 1.5 g
Agar — 17.0 g
Distilled water — 1.0 L

PRECAUTION: Soluble ferric pyrophosphate must be kept dry and stored in the dark; it is no longer usable if its color changes from green to yellow or brown. A freshly mixed solution of the compound is required each time it is needed in preparing media. Do not heat over 60 C to dissolve. Mixture can be readily dissolved by placing in 50 C water bath.

1. pH of solid media must be 6.9 ± 0.05 to be confirmed either with a surface electrode (if available) or by emulsifying agar from 1 plate in distilled water and measuring with combination electrode. pH is critical. If lots of ingredients used yield a medium of different pH, adjust pH of complete liquid medium by adding 1N HCl or 1N NaOH.
2. Store media in dark in sealed plastic containers in refrigerator. (Media have been used successfully for growing LDB after being stored up to 2 mo under these conditions.)

The FG agar is used for isolation and propagation of legionnaires' disease bacterium (LDB) (*Legionella pneumophila*).

Fermentation media. See Carbohydrate fermentation media.

Fermentation, rapid, for Neisseria gonorrhoeae. See *N. gonorrhoeae*, Chapter 76.

Fildes enrichment[27,28]

Physiologic saline — 150 ml
HCl — 6 ml

*Available on request from Dr. Morris Suggs, Director, Biological Products Division, Center for Disease Control, Atlanta, Georgia 30333.

Sheep blood, defibrinated   50 ml
Granulated pepsin   10 g

1. Mix ingredients.
2. After shaking, place in 56 C water bath 14-16 h.
3. After heating, add 12 ml NaOH, 20%; pH should
   be 7.6.
4. Adjust, if necessary.
5. Add to heart infusion broth or agar in 5% concentration.

Fildes enrichment, prepared (Difco), can be used for
above. Enrichment cannot be heated and must be
added aseptically to media that have been sterilized
and cooled to 50-55 C.

Fletcher medium. See *Leptospira*, Chapter 80.

GC medium. See Thayer-Martin medium.

Gelatin. See Nutrient gelatin, Iron gelatin, and Thioglycollate gelatin.

Gluconate broth[5]

Yeast extract   1 g
Peptone   1.5 g
K_2HPO_4 1 g
Potassium gluconate   40 g
Distilled water   1000 ml

1. Heat until dissolved; adjust to pH 7.
2. Filter; sterilize 20 min at 115 C. Dispense in 1 ml
   aliquots in tubes.
3. Sodium gluconate, 37.25 g, can be substituted for
   potassium gluconate.
4. Prepared gluconate tablets* can be used in place
   of above broth.

Glucose phenolphthalein broth, pH 9.6[5]

1. Prepare glycine buffer:
   Glycine   0.6 g
   NaCl   0.35 g
   Freshly boiled distilled water   60 ml
   0.1N Sodium hydroxide   40 ml
   Dissolve sodium chloride and glycine in water;
   then add sodium hydroxide.
2. Prepare glucose broth:
   Glucose, 20% aqueous solution   50 ml
   Nutrient broth   950 ml
3. Prepare glucose phenolphthalein broth:
   Glucose broth   900 ml
   Glycine buffer   100 ml
   Phenolphthalein, 0.2% solution   5 ml
4. Mix and refrigerate overnight in stoppered flask.
   Sterilize by filtration. Check pH (9.6). Distribute
   into 5 ml screw-capped tubes; check sterility by
   overnight incubation. Discard any tubes not
   showing definite pink color.

**The medium is used for determining growth at pH
9.6.** Strains growing at pH 9.6 will show heavy growth
and will decolorize indicator.

Glycerol fuchsin broth—Stern
Solution 1:
   Meat extract   10 g
   Peptone   20 g
   Tap water   1000 ml
   Adjust pH to 8.0.
Solution 2:
   Basic fuchsin, 10%, saturated alcoholic solution
Solution 3:
   Sodium sulfite, anhydrous, 10%, fresh aqueous
   solution
Mixture:
   Solution 1   100 ml
   Solution 2   0.2 ml
   Solution 3   1.66 ml
   Glycerol   1 ml

---

*Key Scientific Products Los Angeles, Calif.

1. Tube and autoclave at 15 psi for 12 min.
2. Inoculate from agar slant; incubate at 37 C.
3. Observe daily 8 d, noting development of deep
   red color as compared to uninoculated control
   tube incubated with cultures under examination.

GN broth—Hajna[29]

Tryptose   20 g
Dextrose   1 g
d-Mannitol   2 g
Sodium citrate   5 g
Sodium deoxycholate   0.5 g
Dipotassium phosphate   4 g
Monopotassium phosphate   1.5 g
Sodium chloride   5 g

1. Dissolve in 1000 ml distilled water.
2. Distribute in tubes and sterilize in autoclave at 10
   psi (116 C) for 15 min.
3. Final reaction will be pH 7.0.

Difco GN broth or BBL GN broth, dehydrated, duplicate above formula.

Taylor and Harris[30,31] found that GN broth is more
effective in the recovery of shigellae than are other
enrichment media.

Inoculate medium **lightly** with stool specimen. Incubate at 35-37 C for 6-18 h. Transfer to selective and
differential media. It is important to realize that an
overwhelming inoculum (such as more than 1 g feces to
10 ml broth) will totally obviate enhancement features
of medium.

Guthrie inhibition assay medium. See Phenylketonuria (PKU) test materials.

Heart infusion broth and agar. See Infusion broth.

Heart infusion broth with tryptose (Difco). Dissolve
15 g desiccated powder in 1000 ml distilled water.

Heart infusion agar. Add 15 g agar to above.

Hektoen enteric agar

Proteose peptone   12.0 g
Bile salts   9.0 g
Yeast extract   3.0 g
Lactose   12.0 g
Salicin   2.0 g
Sucrose   12.0 g
Sodium chloride   5.0 g
Sodium thiosulfate   5.0 g
Ferric ammonium citrate   1.5 g
Agar   14.0 g
Acid fuchsin   0.1 g
Bromthymol blue   0.065 g
Distilled water   1000 ml

Hippurate broth

Sodium hippurate   1 g
Infusion broth   100 ml

1. Add sodium hippurate to infusion broth.
2. Preferably, sterilize medium by passing it through
   Seitz filter and then tubing 3 ml amounts with
   sterile precautions into small tubes. If no filter is
   available, medium should be **tubed in 3 ml
   amounts** and sterilized at 121 C for 15 min.

Hiss serum water. See Chapter 77.

Indole medium. See Peptone water.

Infusion broth from meat, heart, liver, or brain

1. a. Chop meat, heart, liver, or brain and mix 500 g
      of it for "single-strength" or 1000 g for "double-
      strength" infusion with 1000 ml distilled water
      in enamel or stainless steel pot.
   b. Let stand at 4-6 C overnight in refrigerator.
   c. Skim off fat with metal or enamel spoon.
   d. Heat to 45 C in water bath and keep at this
      temperature 1 h.
   e. Boil without stirring 30 min.
   f. Filter through glass wool.
   g. Dilute to 1000 ml with distilled water.

2. a. Add 10 g tryptose or trypticase (double strength add 20 g) and 5 g sodium chloride (double strength add 10 g).
   b. Adjust reaction to pH 7.4-7.6. Heat to boiling point, allow to cool, and adjust reaction, if necessary.
   c. Distribute in test tubes or flasks.
   d. Sterilize in autoclave 20 min at 15 psi.

IsoVitaleX enrichment. See Thayer-Martin medium.

Jones-Kendrick charcoal agar.[32] This is a blood-free medium for the transport and growth of *B. pertussis*. It is superior to any "transport" media commonly used previously, since it not only maintains viability, but also supports growth of *B. pertussis* while in transit. In addition, these cultures can be incubated for growth without subculture to another medium.

Soluble starch (BBL)	10 g
Yeast extract (Difco)	3.5 g
Heart infusion broth (Difco)	25 g
Bacto agar (Difco)	20 g
Distilled water	1.0 L

1. Dissolve ingredients over open flame. Add 4.0 g charcoal (Norit FQP).
2. Mix well and autoclave at 15 lbs/15 min.
3. Add 30 units penicillin/100 ml autoclaved cooled agar.
4. Dispense 10 ml agar into widemouth bottle, approximately 7 cm by 3 cm (adjust volume according to size of bottle used), and slant to give as broad streak surface as possible, without slant extending into neck of bottle.
5. Make sure caps are securely attached before placing in refrigerator at about 5 C.

Shelf-life of this medium under these conditions is 2-3 mo.

KCN broth[33]

1.
Peptone, Orthana special*	10 g
Sodium chloride	5 g
Monobasic potassium phosphate	0.225 g
Dibasic sodium phosphate	5.64 g

   a. Dissolve in 1000 ml distilled water.
   b. Adjust to pH 7.6.
   c. Sterilize at 15 psi for 15 min.
   d. Refrigerate until chilled.
2. a. Prepare KCN solution by adding 0.5 g KCN to 100 ml cold sterile distilled water.
   b. Add 15 ml KCN solution to chilled KCN broth base.
   c. Tube medium in 1 ml amounts in sterile tubes. Use corks heated in paraffin and stopper immediately. Medium can be stored 2 wk in refrigerator.[10]

NOTE: Extreme care should be exercised in handling potassium cyanide.

Difco KCN broth base (substituting proteose-peptone no. 3 [Difco]) in dehydrated form can be employed. Use 13.8 g dehydrated product in 1000 ml distilled water. Prepare as previously described.

Positive results are indicated by growth in presence of KCN.

KCNS-tryptose broth. See *Listeria*, Chapter 77.

KL virulence agar and KL virulence enrichment. See Elek, King, et al. medium.

Lactobacillus selective agar. See *Lactobacillus*, Chapter 77.

Lecithinase or lecithovitellin medium. See Egg-yolk medium.

Legionella pneumophila (Legionnaires' disease bacterium) isolation media. See descriptions of **choc-olate agar I with IsoVitaleX enrichment, Mueller-Hinton agar with IsoVitaleX and hemoglobin (MH-IH), CYE medium,** and **FG agar.**

Legionnaires' disease bacterium (LDB) media. See *Legionella pneumophila* media.

Levinthal medium[34]

Levinthal stock
1. Bring to boiling brain-heart infusion broth (Difco), prepared according to manufacturer's directions.
2. Add defibrinated horse blood, 10 ml to each 100 ml medium.
3. Filter through Whatman filter paper no. 12.
4. Sterilize filtrate by passing it through Seitz filter.

Levinthal broth
1. Mix together 1 part sterile Levinthal stock and 3 parts sterile neopeptone broth (made as follows).
2. *Neopeptone broth*[35] is prepared by using beef infusion broth, single strength, with 4 g/L sodium phosphate (Na_2HPO_4) and 10 g/L neopeptone (Difco) added. Boil mixture 1 min; filter through filter paper while hot. Make up to 1000 ml and adjust pH to 8.0 with 2N NaOH; boil until mixture becomes clear, but no longer. Sterilize by autoclaving at 15 psi for 15 min.

Levinthal agar
1. Mix together 1 part sterile Levinthal stock and 1 part sterile melted agar (made as follows).
2. Agar used is made by adding 45 g proteose no. 3 agar (Difco) to 15 g Bacto agar/L distilled water.

"Liquoid" broth[36, 37]
1. a. Mix together 1 g Liquoid (sodium polyanethol sulfonate)* and 20 ml physiologic saline (0.85%).
   b. Sterilize in autoclave at 121 C for 15 min.
2. a. Mix together 10 ml "Liquoid" solution (1), sterile, and 1000 ml nutrient broth.
   b. Check pH. Adjust, if necessary, to 7.6.
   c. Distribute in 40 ml quantities in 2 oz screw-capped bottles.
   d. Sterilize as above. Screw on caps tightly.

Loeffler blood serum medium

Preparation of blood serum
1. Obtain beef blood in sterilized, colorless, wide-mouthed quart bottle.
2. Allow coagulation to take place without agitation of container or contents.
3. Place in refrigerator until coagulation is complete.
4. Loosen clot from sides of bottle by means of sterile stirring rod.
5. Place in refrigerator until serum separates from clot.
6. Remove serum from clot either with transfer pipet or by pouring into glass container.
7. Centrifuge serum in 50 ml centrifuge tubes at high speed 15 min under sterile precautions.
8. Decant clear straw-colored supernatant serum, placing it in glass container.

Preparation of medium
1. Dissolve 1 g dextrose in 100 ml infusion broth.
2. Add 300 ml fresh blood serum (cow, sheep, horse, or pig).
3. Distribute into sterile test tubes.
4. Slant in autoclave.
5. Inspissate and sterilize as described in Chapter 70.

Difco-Loeffler blood serum, 80 g, dissolved in 1000 ml distilled water, and BBL-Loeffler medium, 83 g, dissolved in 1000 ml distilled water, may be used instead of above medium.

---

*See Decarboxylase media.

*Hoffmann-La Roche, Inc., Nutley, N.J.

Lysine iron agar—Edwards-Fife[38]

Peptone (Bacto) or Gelysate (BBL)	5 g
Yeast extract	3 g
Dextrose	1 g
L-Lysine	10 g
Ferric ammonium citrate	0.5 g
Sodium thiosulfate	0.04 g
Bromcresol purple	0.02 g
Agar	15 g

1. Suspend ingredients in 1000 ml distilled water.
2. Mix thoroughly, heat, and boil 1 min.
3. Dispense in tubes (preferably with screw caps).
4. Sterilize 12 min at 121 C by autoclaving.
5. Cool in slanted position to form slants with deep butts.

Medium is available in dehydrated form (BBL and Difco).

Lysozyme broth. See *Nocardia*, Chapter 77.

MRS medium. See *Lactobacillus*, Chapter 77.

MacConkey medium

Peptone	20 g
Sodium chloride	5 g
Sodium glycocholate	5 g
or	
Taurocholate	5 g
or	
Bacto-bile salts no. 3	1.5 g
Agar	13.5 g
Lactose	10 g
Aqueous neutral red, 1%	3-4 ml

1. Suspend peptone in 1000 ml distilled water.
2. Add sodium chloride, sodium glycocholate, and agar. Soak 15 min; then dissolve by heating.
3. Adjust reaction to pH 7.4.
4. Add lactose to warm agar.
5. Sterilize in autoclave at 15 psi for 20 min.
6. Add, with sterile precautions, 3-4 ml 1% aqueous neutral red "certified." Boil neutral red solution in tube 5 min before adding to medium.
7. When partly cooled, pour in Petri dishes, about 18-20 ml/dish. Allow to stand with slightly removed tops 1 hr in dust-free place at room temperature.
8. Store in refrigerator.

There are numerous modifications of MacConkey medium. Several commercial preparations are excellent: they contain 0.001 g crystal violet/1000 ml medium. This combination inhibits gram-positive microorganisms.

Malonate broth. See Sodium malonate broth.

Mannitol salt agar

Mannitol	10 g
Beef extract	1 g
Proteose-peptone no. 3 *or* polypeptone	10 g
Sodium chloride	75 g
Agar	15 g
Phenol red	0.025 g

1. Dissolve ingredients in 1000 ml distilled water. Boil 1-2 min.
2. Dispense and sterilize in autoclave 15 min at 15 psi. Final pH will be 7.4.

Commercial dehydrated medium can be substituted for formula.

McBride medium, modified[11]

Phenylethanol agar (Difco or BBL)	35.5 g
Glycine, anhydride	10 g
Lithium chloride	0.5 g

1. Dissolve in 1000 ml distilled water by heating.
2. Sterilize at 15 psi for 20 min.

Meat extract broth

Peptone	10 g
Sodium chloride	5 g
Beef extract	3 g
Distilled water	1000 ml

1. Weigh beef extract on piece of wax paper.
2. Heat some of water to 60 C in beaker. Drop paper with beef extract into beaker.
3. Dissolve salt and peptone in some water.
4. Mix beef extract solution and salt-peptone solution.
5. Add rest of water. Filter through filter paper.
6. Adjust reaction to pH 7.2-7.4.
7. Distribute into test tubes or flasks.
8. Sterilize in autoclave 20 min at 15 psi.

BBL extract broth, 18 g, desiccated powder dissolved in 1000 ml distilled water, may be used instead of formula.

Meat infusion agar

Infusion broth, double-strength	500 ml
Agar	15-20 g

1. Dissolve agar in 500 ml distilled water by autoclaving or by careful heating. Mix agar solution and infusion.
2. Readjust reaction to pH 7.0.
3. Distribute into tubes or flasks.
4. Sterilize in autoclave at 15 psi for 20 min.

Membrane filter media. Numerous media for membrane filter procedure are available in dehydrated form (Difco, BBL). Most of these are modifications of existing enrichment, differential, and selective media, often in double strength. For formulas see manufacturer's product descriptions, where they are described with prefix m- or M-, to denote their use in membrane filter procedures.

Methyl red (MR) test medium

Polypeptone (BBL) *or* buffered peptone (Difco)	7 g
Glucose	5 g
Dipotassium phosphate	5 g

1. Dissolve ingredients in 1000 ml distilled water by gentle heating.
2. Sterilize at 121 C for 15 min.

BBL and Difco dehydrated products, **MR-VP medium,** are recommended. Medium is also used for Voges-Proskauer (VP) test.

Milk media

Bromcresol purple milk

Skim milk, dehydrated	100 g
Bromcresol purple	0.02 g
Distilled water	1000 ml

1. Mix and heat, not over 50 C, until uniform suspension is obtained.
2. Autoclave at 10 psi (113-115 C) for 20 min.

Methylene blue milk

Skim milk, dehydrated	100 g
Methylene blue, 1%, aqueous	100 ml
Distilled water	900 ml

1. Mix and heat gently.
2. Sterilize by autoclaving at 10 psi for 10 min.
   or
1. Skim milk, fresh — 1000 ml
   Autoclave at 115 C, 10 psi, 15 min.
2. Methylene blue — 1.5 g
   Dissolve in distilled water — 30 ml
   Sterilize by filtration.
3. Add 20 ml methylene blue solution, aseptically, to skim milk.

Skimmed milk. Use fresh, clean, skimmed cow's milk.

1. Dispense in tubes and sterilize either by tyndallization (flowing steam for 30 min on 3 successive days) or in autoclave at 10 lb pressure for 10 min.
2. Commercial dehydrated skimmed milk can also be used.

Dissolve 10% dehydrated skimmed milk in distilled water. Sterilize as described under 1.

Litmus milk

Skimmed milk powder	100 g
Litmus	5 g
Distilled water	1000 ml

Autoclave at 10 lb for 10 min.

Monsur solution. See *Vibrio cholerae* media, below.

Monsur agar. See *Vibrio cholerae* media, below.

Motility medium for clostridia. See Thioglycollate medium, motility.

Motility medium for Listeria[39]

Tryptose (Difco)	10 g
Sodium chloride	5 g
Agar	5 g
Glucose	1 g

1. Dissolve in 1000 ml distilled water, with aid of heat.
2. Sterilize at 121 C for 20 min.

Motility test medium. This medium is recommended by Ewing[1] for motility test with members of family *Enterobacteriaceae*.

Beef extract	3 g
Peptone	10 g
Sodium chloride	5 g
Agar	4 g

1. Dissolve in 1000 ml distilled water.
2. Adjust pH to 7.4.
3. Distribute about 8 ml/tube.
4. Sterilize at 15 psi for 15 min.

Mueller-Hinton medium[40]

Beef infusion	300 g
Casamino acids, technical (Difco)	17.5 g
or peptone	
Starch	1.5 g
Agar	17 g

Casamino acids, technical (Difco) is acid hydrolyzed casein, prepared according to the method of Mueller.[41]

1. Suspend materials in 1000 ml cold distilled water. Heat to boiling to dissolve completely.
2. Distribute in tubes or flasks, and sterilize 10 min at 10 psi (116 C). Final reaction should be pH 7.4.

Mueller-Hinton medium with IsoVitaleX and hemoglobin (MH-IH)

Component A	
Mueller-Hinton agar	38 g
Distilled water	490 ml
Component B	
Hemoglobin powder	10 g
Distilled water	490 ml
Component C	
IsoVitaleX	20 ml

1. Prepare components A and B separately.
2. Autoclave at 121 C for 15 min; Cool to 50 C, mix together, and hold at 50 C in water bath.
3. Prepare component C by adding 10 ml sterile distilled water to each of two 10 ml vials of IsoVitaleX. Add contents of both vials to A-B mixture.
4. Check pH of medium and adjust as needed to final cold pH of 6.9.
5. Pour 20 ml quantities into plastic dishes (15 × 100 mm).

Mycoplasma media. See Chapter 81.

Nalidixic acid medium for Listeria. See *Listeria*, Chapter 77.

Nagler medium. See Egg-yolk medium.

Naylor medium[42]

| Lab-Lemco beef extract* | 3 g |

*Lab-Lemco agar, complete, or ingredients can be obtained from Oxoid Southwark Bridge Rd., Ltd., London SE1, or from Colab Laboratories, Chicago Heights, Ill.

| Peptone (Oxoid L 37) | 5 g |
| Agar (Oxoid) | 15 g |

1. Dissolve in 1000 ml distilled water by gentle heating.
2. Adjust pH to 7.4.
3. Sterilize at 121 C for 15 min.
4. Pour plates from sterile medium and dry at 37 C for 15 min.

Medium is useful for preventing swarming of *Proteus* species.

Nitrate medium. This medium is recommended by Ewing[1] for nitrate reduction test.

Tryptone	5 g
Neopeptone	5 g
Agar	2.5 g

1. Suspend ingredients in 1000 ml distilled water.
2. Boil and adjust pH to 7.3-7.4 (when cooled).
3. Add the following:

| KNO_3 (nitrite-free) | 1 g |
| Glucose | 0.1 g |

4. Sterilize at 121 C for 15 min.

The Center for Disease Control (CDC laboratory methods in special medical bacteriology, 1976) lists the following media for testing of reduction of nitrates and nitrites.

Routine nitrate formula

Bacto peptone (Difco)	20 g
Potassium nitrate, cp	2 g
Distilled water	1000 ml

1. Adjust to pH 7.0.
2. Tube in 15 × 125 mm tubes with gas inserts, 4.0 ml per tube.
3. Autoclave 15 min at 121 C.

Special nitrate formula

Heart infusion broth (Difco)	25 g
Potassium nitrate, cp	2 g
Distilled water	1000 ml

1. Adjust to pH 7.0.
2. Tube in 15 × 125 mm tubes with gas inserts, 4.0 ml per tube.
3. Autoclave 15 min at 121 C.

Test reagents and procedures are the same as with the routine formula given above. (See nitrate reduction under Tests and Reagents.)

Nitrite formula

Heart infusion broth (Difco)	25 g
Potassium nitrite, cp	1 g
Distilled water	1000 ml

1. Adjust to pH 7.0.
2. Tube in 15 × 125 mm tubes with gas inserts, 4.0 ml per tube.
3. Autoclave 15 min at 121 C.

Examine 48 h nitrite broth cultures for nitrogen gas in insert tubes and add 5 drops each of nitrite reagents nos. 1 and 2 to determine if nitrite is still present in medium. (See nitrate reduction under Tests and Reagents.)

Nutrient agar (meat extract agar)

1. According to the concentration of agar desired, i.e., 1.5% or 2%, soak 15 or 20 g agar in 1000 ml meat extract broth 15 min.
2. Dissolve agar **either** by careful heating over flame **or** on electric plate, **or** by autoclaving.
3. Adjust reaction to pH 7.4-7.6.
4. Dispense in tubes or bottles, as desired.
5. Sterilize 25 min at 15 psi.

Difco or BBL nutrient agar, 31 g desiccated medium dissolved in 1000 distilled water, is same as formula.

For water analysis, use without sodium chloride.

Nutrient gelatin

| Beef extract | 3 g |
| Peptone | 5 g |

Gelatin   120 g
1. Add ingredients to 1000 ml distilled water and heat until dissolved (at 50 C).
2. Sterilize at 121 C for 15 min.

BBL and Difco dehydrated products have similar formulas. Use 128 g commercial product in 1000 ml distilled water.

Organic acid media—Kauffmann-Petersen[43]

Base medium

Peptone (Bacto)   10 g
0.1N NaOH   8.5 ml
Distilled water   1000 ml

1. Dissolve ingredients in distilled water. **Add,** as indicator, 12 ml bromthymol blue solution (0.2%). It is prepared as follows:

Bromthymol blue   1 g
0.1N NaOH   25 ml
Distilled water   475 ml

2. Add 1% of following substances to separate portions of base medium:

D-Tartrate   sodium potassium tartrate, cp
L-Tartrate   tartaric acid, levorotatory
i-Tartrate   tartaric acid, inactive
Sodium citrate
Mucate   mucic acid
Adjust pH to 7.4 with 5N NaOH.

3. Sterilize (3-4 ml amounts in small tubes) at 121 C for 15 min.

4. For addition of mucic acid, sterilize portion of basal medium at 121 C for 15 min. Weigh mucic acid aseptically and add to basal medium while still hot. Add 5N or 10N NaOH in sufficient amount to bring mucic acid in solution and to adjust final pH to 7.4.

5. Distribute media in small tubes, 3-4 ml/tube, and incubate for sterility. Inoculate with loop from 20 hr broth culture. Incubate at 37 C for 14 d. Readings at 1, 2, 5, and 14 d are made both from color reaction and from addition of 0.5 ml of saturated aqueous lead-acetate solution added to D-, L-, i-tartrate and citrate tubes. Mucate tube is judged only by color reaction.

With all organic acids, positive results are characterized by change from blue to greenish yellow to white. The first 4 give only minimal precipitate with lead acetate. Unchanged blue color and large amount of precipitate on addition of lead acetate signifies negative result.

Dehydrated organic acid base medium (KP), containing peptone and bromthymol blue, is commercially available (Difco).

Oxidation-fermentation (OF) medium—Hugh-Leifson[44]

Peptone   2 g
Sodium chloride   5 g
Dibasic potassium phosphate   0.3 g
Agar   3 g
Bromthymol blue,   3 ml
  1%, **aqueous** solution

1. Dissolve ingredients in 1000 ml distilled water.
2. Adjust pH to 7.1, distribute **basal** medium in small test tubes, 3-4 ml per 13 × 100 mm tube, and sterilize at 121 C for 15 min.
3. Add glucose or other carbohydrates, as needed, to final concentration of 1% to each tube. A 10% solution of carbohydrate in distilled water, sterilized by Seitz filtration, can be used for this purpose.
4. Two tubes of medium are inoculated; to one tube add a layer of sterile melted petrolatum (0.3-0.5 cm). Acid formation in tube without petrolatum seal only indicates **oxidative utilization** of carbo-

hydrate employed. Acid formation in both tubes indicates **fermentation** reaction. No acid in either tube indicates lack of carbohydrate utilization by either method.

OF medium is available in dehydrated form (OF basal medium [BBL, Difco]).

Oxidation-fermentation medium (SB no. 15, CDC). This is a special OF medium used at the Center for Disease Control.

Distilled water   100 ml
Bacto casitone   0.2 g (0.2%)
Bacto agar   0.3 g (0.3%)
Phenol red   0.003%*†

Basal medium without carbohydrate. Adjust to pH 7.3 before addition of agar. Tube in 15 × 125 mm tubes, cotton plugs, 6 ml per tube. Autoclave 15 lb, 15 min. While base is melted, add *Seitz* filtered carbohydrate to final dilution of 1% (i.e., 0.6 ml of 10% carbohydrate solution to 6 ml base). Twirl to mix and allow to solidify; do not slant. Do not add carbohydrate before autoclaving.

Procedure

1. Inoculate tubes of medium with needle by stabbing 4 times approximately 1.25 cm below surface with growth from young infusion agar slant culture.
2. Incubate at 35-37 C and observe daily for 7 d for acid production.
3. To determine oxidation-fermentation characteristics of pure culture, inoculate 2 tubes of OF basal medium containing 1% dextrose. Overlay 1 tube with sterile petrolatum jelly. Incubate at 35-37 C.
4. Acid formation in open tube only indicates oxidative utilization of dextrose. Acid formation in both open and closed tubes indicates fermentative utilization of dextrose. No acid in either tube indicates nonutilization of dextrose.

Pectate medium[45,46]

Yeast extract   0.5 g
Distilled water   100 ml

1. Add:
   1N Sodium hydroxide   0.9 ml
   Calcium chloride ($CaCl_2 \cdot 2H_2O$),   0.6 ml
     10% solution
   Bromthymol blue 0.2% solution   1.25 ml
   Sodium polypectate no. 24 (California   3 g
     Fruit Growers Exchange)
2. Add pectate slowly and stir between additions.
3. Heat until pectate dissolves. Stir constantly. Medium will be bluish green.
4. Distribute in small test tubes, and sterilize at 121 C for 15 min. Color should now be yellowish green (pH 6.4). Allow tubes to cool upright. Do not reheat medium.
5. Inoculate by stabbing deep into column. Incubate at 37 C for 7 d. Observe for evidence of liquefaction.

Penicillinase media

1. To each 10 ml trypticase soy broth, tryptose citrate broth, brain-heart infusion broth, or other liquids used for blood cultures add, with sterile precautions, just prior to inoculation, 0.1 ml penicillinase (50,000 U/ml concentrated).
2. Do not reheat or store.

---

*0.003% Phenol red equivalent to 0.2 ml 1.5% aqueous solution to 100 ml volume.
†Personal communication from Dr. Robert Weaver, Center for Disease Control Special Bacteriology Laboratory, 1978.

Peptone water

| Bacto-peptone (Difco) | 20 g |
| Sodium chloride | 5 g |

1. Dissolve ingredients in 1000 ml distilled water by gentle heating.
2. For cholera work, pH 7.8-8.2 is favorable.
3. Ewing[10] recommends leaving pH unadjusted and states that peptone (Difco) can be replaced by 10 g Bacto-Tryptone, 15 g casitone (Difco), or 15 g trypticase (BBL).
4. Sterilize at 121 C for 15 min.

Pertussis media. See **Jones-Kendrick charcoal agar** and **Bordet-Gengou agar.**

Phenylalanine agar—Ewing-Davis-Reavis[47]

Yeast extract	3 g
DL-Phenylalanine	2 g
or	
L-Phenylalanine	1 g
Disodium phosphate	1 g
Sodium chloride	5 g
Agar	12 g

1. Dissolve in 1000 ml distilled water.
2. Tube and sterilize at 121 C for 10 min and allow to solidify in slanted position (long slant).

BBL or Difco phenylalanine agar, dehydrated, has the same composition.

Phenylethyl alcohol medium

Trypticase	15 g
Phytone	5 g
Sodium chloride	5 g
β-Phenylethyl alcohol	2.5 g
Agar	15 g

1. Dissolve ingredients in 1000 ml distilled water. Final reaction should be pH 7.3 ±. Medium is available in dehydrated form.

To prepare blood plates, add 5% defibrinated blood to cooled sterile medium.

This medium is not to be depended on for determination of hemolytic reactions, since atypical reactions may be observed. Usual blood agar plates may be made in parallel to determine degree of inhibition provided by phenylethyl alcohol medium and for determination of hemolysis.

A "brown-sugar" appearance is characteristic of dehydrated product and therefore is not an indication of deterioration.

Phenylketonuria (PKU) test materials

Demain medium,[48] modified by Guthrie-Susi[49]

1.
Dextrose	10 g
K_2HPO_4	30 g
KH_2PO_4	10 g
NH_4Cl	5 g
NH_4NO_3	1 g
Na_2SO_4	1 g
Glutamic acid	1 g
Asparagine	1 g
L-Alanine	0.5 g
Salt solution	10 ml

2. Salt solution is made as follows:

$MgSO_4 \cdot 7H_2O$	10 g
$MnCl_2 \cdot 4H_2O$	1 g
$FeCl_3 \cdot 6H_2O$	1 g
$CaCl_2$	0.5 g
Distilled water	1000 ml

3. Dextrose, 10% solution:

| Dextrose | 10 g |
| Distilled water | 100 ml |

   Sterilize by filtration.

4. Agar, 3%

| Agar | 3 g |
| Distilled water 100 ml | |

Place 100 ml 3% agar in bottle. Autoclave 15 min at 121 C.

5. Components listed under 1 are dissolved in 900 ml distilled water.
6. Dispense 90 ml vol of medium solution into each of ten 8 oz prescription bottles and sterilize by autoclaving.
7. Add 10 ml 10% dextrose (sterile) to each bottle of 90 ml medium.
8. Mix 100 ml medium (now containing dextrose) with 100 ml 3% agar that has been previously melted and then cooled to 55 C in water path.

Spore suspension

1. Grow *Bacillus subtilis* (ATCC 6051) overnight on heart infusion agar medium (Difco).
2. Transfer to potato infusion agar medium (Difco) in bottles. Inoculate heavily. Incubate 1 wk at 30 C. After spores are noted (microscopically), scrape off growth and wash off into 0.9% NaCl. Wash 3 times with 0.9% NaCl by centrifuging. (Guthrie and Susi specify 11,000 rpm in Several model SS3 centrifuge.)
3. Suspend spores in distilled water at an absorbance of 0.9, measured at 550 nm in colorimeter.
4. Dispense 0.3 ml spore suspension into each of a number of small screw-capped vials. Dry at 60 C on shaking machine. Store in refrigerator with cap tightly closed.
5. When needed, add 1 ml Demain medium to vial, scrape dried material off glass wall with sterile plastic stick, and add to 200 ml culture medium.

*β-2-Thienylalanine**

1. Make up 0.01M solution. Mol wt is 174; use 1.74 g in 1000 ml distilled water.
2. Pipet 0.3 ml into each of a number of screw-capped vials, dry, and store at room temperature.
3. When needed, rinse vial with 2 ml medium and transfer to 200 ml Demain medium (final concentration: 1.5×10^{-5}M; i.e., 2.6 mg/L medium).

Complete medium

1. Combine medium, agar, β-2-thienylalanine, and spore powder just before use.
2. Mix well by pouring back and forth and use immediately.

The PKU test procedure is described under Tests and Reagents.

NOTE: PKU test kits are available from BBL and Difco, containing spore suspension, Demain medium ready made, and β-2-thienylalanine solution as well as special filter paper, plastic tray, and control disks needed.

The components of the kit are also available separately, as well as the PKU test agar (Demain) in dehydrated form. Follow manufacturer's instructions for preparation and use of materials.

Phenolphthalein broth. See **Glucose phenolphthalein broth.**

"Phosphatase" agar (phenolphthalein phosphate agar). See *Staphylococcus.*

Plate count agar. See **Tryptone glucose yeast agar.**

Preservative solutions for stools

Banxgang-Eliot[50] solution

Sodium citrate	10 g
Sodium deoxycholate	5 g
Sodium chloride	9 g
Disodium phosphate (0.067M sol)	3 ml

1. Dissolve ingredients in 1000 ml distilled water.
2. Titrate to neutrality to litmus with 1N sodium hydroxide.

_____

*Calbiochem, Los Angeles, Calif.

3. Add 2 ml 1N sodium hydroxide, dispense in bottles, and autoclave.
4. Add sufficient phenol red to medium to give it a distinct color.

Buffered glycerol

Sodium chloride, USP	4.2 g
Dipotassium phosphate, anhydrous	3.1 g
Monopotassium phosphate, anhydrous	1 g
Glycerol, USP	300 ml

1. Dissolve sodium chloride and phosphates in 700 ml distilled water, add glycerol, and adjust to pH 7.2, using phenol red as indicator.
2. Place in specimen bottles, filling bottles less than one-half full with fluid.
3. Sterilize 30 min at 15 psi.

Pseudomonas agar

Medium A

Proteose-peptone no. 3 (Difco)	20 g
Maltose	10 g
Dipotassium phosphate	1.5 g
Magnesium sulfate	0.73 g
Agar	15 g

1. Dissolve ingredients in 1000 ml distilled water.
2. Adjust to pH 7.2 if necessary.
3. Tube and autoclave 15 min at 15 psi. Slant to obtain deep butt.

The medium is available in dehydrated form as **Pseudomonas agar F** (Difco). It is useful for enhancement of fluorescein production by *P. aeruginosa*.

Medium B

Peptone (Bacto)	20 g
DL-Alanine	2 g
Sodium citrate	10 g
Potassium sulfate	8.6 g
Potassium chloride	1.4 g
Magnesium sulfate	1.4 g
Agar	15 g
Distilled water	1000 ml

Preparation is identical to that of medium A. **Pseudomonas agar P** (Difco), available in dehydrated form, duplicates formula. Medium is useful for detection of pyocyanin by *P. aeruginosa* strains.

Rapid fermentation test for Neisseria gonorrhoeae. See *Neisseria*, Chapter 76.

Rogosa agar, selective. See *Lactobacillus*, Chapter 77.

Salmonella-Shigella agar. See **SS** agar, below.

Sanders agar

Trypticase *or* tryptone	10 g
Sodium chloride	5 g
Sodium thiosulfate	0.6 g
Ferrous ammonium sulfate	0.4 g
Phenol red	0.018 g
Agar	15 g

1. Suspend ingredients in 1000 ml distilled water. Dissolve by heating. Autoclave 15 min at 121 C.

Dehydrated medium is available from BBL and Difco.

Sanders agar and broth are used for "screening" colonies of enteric organisms. Agar can be used for fermentation studies, applying carbohydrate-impregnated disks.

Sanders booster broth (enrichment)

Tryptose *or* Biosate	20 g
Sodium phosphate	1 g
Sodium chloride	5 g
Lactose	1 g
Sucrose	1 g
Bromcresol purple	0.008 g

1. Dissolve ingredients in 1000 ml distilled water. Distribute 2 ml amounts into small tubes (13 ×

100 mm) and autoclave at 15 psi (121 C) for 15 min.

Dehydrated medium is available from BBL and Difco.

Selenite F medium—Leifson

Tryptone *or* polypeptone	5 g
Lactose	4 g
Sodium hydro-selenite, anhydrous	4 g
Combination of monosodium and disodium phosphate	10 g

1. Dissolve ingredients in 1000 ml distilled water by gentle heating.
2. Adjust reaction to pH 7.0-7.1.
3. Place 8-10 ml quantities in large test tubes so that column of fluid is 5-7 cm high.
4. Sterilize in flowing steam 30 min.

The commercially made dehydrated selenite-F media are recommended. Follow manufacturer's instructions: avoid excessive heating, sterilize in flowing steam, and **do not autoclave;** tube in sterile tubes.

Sellers agar[51]

Sodium chloride	2 g
Sodium nitrate	1 g
Sodium nitrite	0.35 g
D-Mannitol	2 g
L-Arginine	1 g
Yeast extract	1 g
Magnesium sulfate	1.5 g
Dipotassium phosphate	1 g
Gelysate (BBL) *or* Peptone (Difco)	20 g
Bromthymol blue	0.04 g
Phenol red	0.008 g
Agar	13.5 g

1. Dissolve in 1000 ml distilled water. Heat to dissolve and boil 1 min.
2. Autoclave 10 min at 121 C. Cool in slanted position to obtain 3 in. slants and 1.5 in. butts.
3. Just before inoculation add 0.15 ml sterile 50% aqueous solution of dextrose. Let it run down glass opposite slant.
4. Stab butt and streak slant with inoculum.
5. Incubate at 35-37 C for 24 h.
6. Note reactions; use ultraviolet light to determine fluorescence of slant; also note presence of about 1.25 cm yellow band at junction of slant and butt.

The medium is available in dehydrated form from BBL and Difco.

Semisolid enteric medium[52, 53]

Thiotone	10 g
Beef extract	3 g
Sodium chloride	5 g
Agar	4 g
Gelatin	80 g
Sodium citrate	2 g
L-Cystine	0.2 g
Ferrous ammonium sulfate	0.2 g

1. Suspend ingredients in 1000 ml distilled water.
2. Heat over boiling water until gelatin dissolves.
3. Boil about 2 min.
4. Dispense medium in 13 × 100 mm test tubes. Regular 16 or 18 mm test tubes may be used.
5. Sterilize in autoclave at 118 C for 15 min.
6. Medium should be inoculated by stabbing center to one-third or one-half depth of medium.

Commercial dehydrated media duplicate formula.

SF medium—Hajna-Perry

Tryptone *or* trypticase	20 g
Sodium chloride	5 g
Dextrose	5 g
Dipotassium phosphate	4 g

Monopotassium phosphate	1.5 g
Sodium azide	0.5 g
Bromcresol purple solution, 0.4%	8 ml

1. Dissolve in 1000 ml distilled water.
2. Place in 10 ml quantities in test tubes and sterilize in autoclave at 15 psi for 15 min.

Desiccated commercial products are used by dissolving 36 g in 1000 ml distilled water.

Simmons citrate agar

Sodium chloride	5 g
Magnesium sulfate	0.2 g
Ammonium dihydrogen phosphate	1 g
Dipotassium phosphate	1 g
Sodium citrate	2 g
Agar (washed vigorously for 3 d)	20 g

1. Dissolve in 1000 ml distilled water.
2. Add 40 ml 1:500 bromthymol blue indicator solution.
3. Sterilize at 121 C for 15 min and slant (1 inch butt, 1.5 inch slant).

Commercial dehydrated products are satisfactory.

Sodium acetate agar[54]

Sodium acetate	2 g
Magnesium sulfate	0.1 g
Sodium chloride	5 g
Monoammonium phosphate	1 g
Dipotassium phosphate	1 g
Bromthymol blue	0.08 g
Agar	20 g

1. Suspend ingredients in 1000 ml cold distilled water. Heat to boiling to dissolve. Distribute in 13 × 100 ml tubes, about 3 ml/tube.
2. Autoclave 15 min at 121 C. Cool in slanted position to obtain 10 mm butt and 30 mm slant.

Medium supports growth of high percentage of *E. coli* strains but not of *Shigella*. Latter are unable to utilize acetate. Dehydrated Difco product duplicates above formula.

Sodium azide agar. Add to each 100 ml blood agar before pouring, 2 ml 1% solution sodium azide in distilled water. Difco azide blood agar base with blood added may be used.

Sodium chloride broth, 6.5%

1. Mix 1000 ml infusion broth (heart or brainheart infusion broth) and 6 g sodium chloride.
2. Sterilize by autoclaving, 15 psi for 15 min.

Sodium malonate broth—Leifson, modified by Ewing[1]

Yeast extract	1 g
Ammounium sulfate	2 g
Dipotassium phosphate	0.6 g
Monopotassium phosphate	0.4 g
Sodium chloride	2 g
Sodium malonate	3 g
Glucose	0.25 g
Bromthymol blue	0.025 g

1. Dissolve ingredients in 1000 ml distilled water by heating.
2. Sterilize at 121 C for 15 min.
3. Positive result is indicated by change of indicator from green to Prussian blue.

Difco's malonate broth can be used, with addition of 1 g yeast extract and 0.25 g glucose.

SS (Salmonella-Shigella) agar

Beef extract	5.0 g
Peptone	5.0 g
Lactose	10.0 g
Bile salts mixture	8.5 g
Sodium citrate	8.5 g
Sodium thiosulfate	8.5 g
Ferric citrate	1.0 g

Agar	13.5 g
Brilliant green	0.00033 g
Neutral red	0.025 g

Dissolve ingredients (or commercial dehydrated product according to manufacturer's instructions) in 1000 ml cold distilled water. Heat to boiling to dissolve completely. **Do not sterilize in autoclave.**

Standard methods agar. See Tryptone glucose yeast agar.

Taurocholate gelatin agar medium. See *Vibrio cholerae* medium, below.

TCBS agar. See *Vibrio cholerae* media, below.

Tartrate agar—Jordan

Peptone (trypticase or Bacto)	10 g
Sodium potassium tartrate	10 g
Sodium chloride	5 g
Agar	15 g
Phenol red	0.024 g
Distilled water	1000 ml

Final pH 7.6.

1. Dispense in tubes, about 10 ml/tube, and sterilize at 121 C for 10 min. Cool tubes in upright position.
2. Inoculate by stabbing deep into column of medium with straight wire. Incubate at 37 C for 24 h.

Tarshis media. See Media for mycobacteria.

Tellurite medium

Peptone (proteose-peptone no. 3 or trypticase)	20 g
Dextrose	2 g
Sodium chloride	2 g
Agar	15 g

1. Mix ingredients in 1000 ml distilled water. Boil 1 or 2 min.
2. Sterilize 15 min at 15 psi.
3. To each 100 ml sterile melted agar, cooled to about 50 C, add, under sterile conditions:
   a. Tellurite blood solution (Difco)   5 ml
      or
   b. Sterile human serum   5 ml
      Potassium tellurite, 1%, pH 9-9.5   1 ml
4. If solution a is used, heat mixture at 75-80 C until it has appearance of "chocolate agar," cool to about 50 C, and distribute in sterile tubes or plate as desired. Inoculate medium preferably same day as prepared.
5. If mixture b is used, pour completed medium into plates (20 ml/plate) without additional heating.

Basic medium is available commercially indehydrated form as proteose-peptone no. 3 agar (Difco) and trypticase tellurite agar base (BBL).

TGY agar

Tryptone	5 g
Glucose	1 g
Yeast extract	5 g
K_2HPO_4	1 g
Agar	15 g
Distilled water	1000 ml

1. Adjust pH to 6.8-7.0 and tube 5 ml in 15 × 125 mm tubes.
2. Autoclave at 121 C for 15 min and slant.
3. Medium is used for temperature studies.

Tetrathionate broth[2]

Iodine solution

Iodine	6 g
Potassium iodide	5 g
Distilled water	20 ml

1. Dissolve 5 g potassium iodide in 20 ml distilled water by grinding in mortar.
2. Add slowly and with constant grinding 6 g iodine.
3. Keep in dark glass-stoppered bottle.

Basal medium

Peptone (polypeptone or proteose)	5 g
Bile salts	1 g
Calcium carbonate	10 g
Sodium thiosulfate	30 g
Distilled water	100 ml

1. Mix ingredients of basal medium in distilled water and dissolve by heating to boiling.
2. Tube in 10 ml quantities and sterilize at 15 psi for 15 min.
3. **Prior to use,** add 0.2 ml iodine solution (1) to each tube (containing 10 ml basal medium).

BBL and Difco desiccated tetrathionate broth base may be used.

Tetrathionate broth with brilliant green—Kaufmann
1. For each 100 ml broth described under tetrathionate (2) above add 1 ml 1:100 aqueous solution brilliant green "certified," just before sterilizing.
2. Prepare medium in same manner as tetrathionate broth.

Thayer-Martin medium.[55-57] This is a highly **selective** and the **recommended medium** for isolation and cultivation of *N. gonorrhoeae* and *N. meningitidis* from conspicuously contaminated sites (female and male gonorrhea, nasopharyngeal cultures for meningococcal carrier state). It inhibits most saprophytic neisseriae, gram-positive contaminants, gram-negative organisms, and yeasts. The **complete medium,** with antibiotics incorporated, should **not** be used for organisms other than the 2 species listed. It should **not** be used alone for spinal fluid cultures (meningitis), since it will inhibit organisms other than *N. meningitidis* (*N. lactamicus* is not inhibited; see Chapter 76).

Basal medium—chocolate agar
1. Prepare double-strength base by suspending 7.2 g GC agar base (BBL or Difco) in 100 ml distilled water, using 500 ml flask. Mix well. Heat with agitation and boil 1 min until completely dissolved.
2. Prepare **double-strength hemoglobin solution** by mixing 2 g hemoglobin in 100 ml distilled water. Start by mixing 2 g hemoglobin with about 3 ml water until smooth paste is achieved. Add water with constant stirring until suspension is homogeneous.
3. Sterilize GC agar base and hemoglobin solution, separately, in autoclave at 15 psi (121 C) for 15 min.
4. Cool solutions to 50 C.
5. Reconstitute IsoVitaleX enrichment (BBL), 2 ml vial, aseptically with 2 ml sterile rehydrating fluid (BBL). Shake to dissolve completely.
6. Add aseptically the hemoglobin and IsoVitaleX solution to sterile cooled GC agar base.

ALTERNATE METHOD
1. Follow steps 1-4 above.
2. Add hemoglobin solution aseptically to sterile medium.
3. Add Bacto supplement B (Difco) to concentration of 1% (10 ml/L).

Alternate method seems to be inferior to method given above using IsoVitaleX (see Martin et al.[57] who obtained distinctly better results using IsoVitaleX).

NOTE: **Basal medium,** as described (chocolate agar with IsoVitaleX [BBL]), **without antibiotics,** is a good medium for isolation of fastidious organisms.

Complete Thayer-Martin medium, selective
1. To make medium **selective**, prepare following antibiotic mixture:

Vancomycin	3000 µg
Colistin	7500 µg
Nystatin	12,500 units

2. Dissolve antibiotics in 10 ml distilled water.
3. Add 2 ml antibiotic mixture to 200 ml basal medium to give final concentration of 7.5 µg colistin, 3 µg vancomycin, and 12.5 units nystatin/ml medium.

NOTES:
1. With antibiotics added, medium is highly selective for *N. gonorrhoeae* and *N. meningitidis* and highly inhibitory for other organisms.
2. IsoVitaleX enrichment is available from BBL in dehydrated form, with rehydrating fluid (sterile) supplied. Composition of IsoVitaleX is described below.
3. Antibiotic mixture is available as V-C-N inhibitor from BBL, and as Antimicrobic vial CNV from Difco.

*IsoVitaleX enrichment.** The formula, developed by Mehl, is as follows:

Vitamin B_{12}	0.01 g
L-Glutamine	10 g
Adenine	1 g
Guanine hydrochloride	0.03 g
p-Aminobenzoic acid	0.013 g
L-Cystine	1.1 g
Dextrose	100 g
Diphosphopyridine nucleotide, oxidized (coenzyme I)	0.25 g
Cocarboxylase	0.1 g
Ferric nitrate	0.02 g
Thiamine hydrochloride	0.003 g
Cysteine hydrochloride	25.9 g
Distilled water	1000 ml

Thayer-Martin, modified (MTM) agar[58-60]

Peptone	15.0 g†
Corn starch	1.0 g†
Dipotassium phosphate	4.0 g†
Monopotassium phosphate	1.0 g†
Sodium chloride	5.0 g†
Agar	10.0 g†
Dextrose	1.5 g
Hemoglobin	10.0 g
Trimethoprim lactate	5.0 mg
IsoVitaleX enrichment	10.0 ml
VCN inhibitor	10.0 ml
Distilled water	1000 ml

The VCN inhibitor contains vancomycin to inhibit gram-positive contaminants, colistin to suppress gram-negative flora, and nystatin to inhibit growth of yeasts. Trimethoprim lactate is incorporated to reduce growth and swarming of *Proteus* organisms that may be present in some specimens. Dextrose concentration is increased to 0.25% for better growth, and agar content is increased to 2% to provide a more rigid medium suitable for mailing.

Preparation of MTM medium
1. Prepare 2% hemoglobin solution as follows:
   a. Suspend 10 g hemoglobin powder in 500 ml distilled water.
   b. Mix approximately 2 min in blender, or mix on magnetic stirrer approximately 10 min until visible clumps disappear.
   c. Filter hemoglobin solution through cotton gauze into 2 L flask.

---

*From BBL Division of BioQuest, IsoVitaleX product information, Cockeysville, Md.

†Those marked with a dagger can be substituted by adding 36 g **GC agar base.**

d. ALTERNATE METHOD:
   (1) Mix 10 g hemoglobin powder with about 125 ml distilled water.
   (2) Add glass beads to flask to facilitate mixing.
   (3) Allow to stand several hours or overnight in refrigerator, shaking flask occasionally.
   (4) Add sufficient distilled water to make total vol of 500 ml of hemoglobin solution and mix.

2. In 2 L flask, prepare agar base by suspending 36 GC medium base and 10 g agar in 500 ml distilled water. Mix thoroughly before sterilizing.
3. Sterilize both agar base and hemoglobin solutions by autoclaving at 121 C for 15 min.
4. Cool sterile solutions to about 50-56 C in water bath.
5. Reconstitute antimicrobial inhibitors with sterile distilled water and allow to stand 20 min.
6. Reconstitute enrichment supplement with sterile rehydrating fluid and shake to assure complete solution.
7. Aseptically add 10 ml enrichment supplement (IsoVitaleX), 10 ml antimicrobial inhibitors, 0.25 ml trimethoprim lactate solution (VCN) (20 mg trimethoprim/ml), and 6 ml sterile 25% dextrose solution to sterile, cooled agar base and mix gently.
8. Gently add hemoglobin solution to agar base to eliminate formation of bubbles; mix gently but thoroughly, and maintain at 50-56 C until dispensed.
9. Aseptically remove small sample of completed medium to beaker to solidify; determine pH electrometrically when sample is at room temperature. Medium should be pH 7.2 ± 0.2 at 25 C.
10. If larger volumes of medium are required, same method may be used, maintaining same ratio of components.

Preparation of stock solution of trimethoprim lactate (20 mg trimethoprim/ml)
1. Dissolve preweighed contents of 1 g bottle of trimethoprim lactate by adding 5 ml sterile distilled water to bottle; pour solution into 50 ml graduated cylinder.
2. To graduated cylinder, add sufficient sterile distilled water to make total volume of 38 ml, including small amounts of water used to thoroughly rinse bottle that contained trimethoprim lactate powder.
3. Dispense solution in 5 or 10 ml amounts into Pyrex tubes or screw-capped bottles and sterilize by autoclaving at 121 C for 15 min, *or* sterilize by filtrating through 0.22 μm membrane filter and dispense in sterile containers.
4. Store this solution, which should be stable for at least 1 y, at 6-10 C.
5. To facilitate dispersion of trimethoprim lactate in medium, it may be added to enrichment supplement before this is added to agar suspension.

Preparation of plated medium
1. Distribute 10-20 ml MTM into sterile plates, depending on size of plate.
2. Allow plates to dry several hours or overnight. Label with lot number.
3. Place convenient number of plates into plastic sleeve, and seal sleeve to prevent drying of medium.
4. Label sleeve with name and lot number of medium, preparation date, and expiration date (approximately 6 wk).
5. Store plates in inverted position in refrigerator.

6. Evaluate each new lot of plated medium (2) before placing in use.

Preparation of bottled medium
1. Dispense 6-8 ml liquid medium to convex side of almost horizontally positioned sterile 1 oz glass prescription bottle of approximately 30 ml capacity; this provides slight slant to agar.
2. Loosely apply **rubber-lined** screw cap to each bottle and allow medium to cool, bottle remaining in same position during solidification.
3. Introduce CO_2 atmosphere by placing bottles containing solidified medium upright in vacuum chamber, partially exhausting air with vacuum pump (15-17 lb negative pressure), and refilling chamber with filtered 20% CO_2–80% air mixture until chamber is at 5 lb positive pressure; this step is repeated 3 times. After third gassing, leave closed chamber at positive pressure 2-3 h before returning to atmospheric pressure and opening.
4. Tightly affix screw caps.
5. Place label on convex side (over layer of medium) of bottle that identifies it as "MTM medium (with CO_2-enriched atmosphere)" with lot number, preparation date, and expiration date (approximately 3 mo). On this label, leave space for patient identification.
6. Store in upright position.
7. Evaluate each new lot of bottled medium before placing in use.

Thioglycollate base

Trypticase	20 g
Sodium chloride	2.5 g
Dipotassium phosphate	1.5 g
Sodium thioglycollate	1 g
L-Cystine	0.3 g
Agar	0.5 g

1. Dissolve ingredients in 1000 ml distilled water by heating.
2. Final pH should be 7.2.
3. For fermentation studies add 10 g carbohydrate to medium, except for starch and inulin, 4 g.
4. Add 1 ml 0.1% solution resazurin to 1000 ml medium.
5. Dispense in test tubes, filling them half full and using about 15 ml in 6 × ¾ in. tubes.
6. Sterilize by autoclaving at 118-121 C (12-15 psi) for 15 min.
7. Determine acid production by adding 1 ml 0.04% solution bromcresol purple to inoculated tube after desired incubation period (in the case of clostrida, 48 h).

Medium should not be used until it has cooled to room temperature. Prepared medium should be stored in dark at room temperature, **not in refrigerator**. It may be used until not more than one-third of column of liquid has been oxidized, as shown by indicator. After prolonged storage, boil medium for a few minutes and cool before use.

Thioglycollate medium, without dextrose or indicator, BBL, in dehydrated form can be substituted.

Thioglycollate gelatin medium. See Media for anaerobes, CDC (Thiogel).

Thioglycollate medium—Brewer, modified, without indicator

Trypticase	20 g
Dextrose	6 g
Sodium chloride	2.5 g
L-Cystine	0.25 g
Sodium sulfite	0.1 g
Sodium thioglycollate	0.5 g
Agar (dissolved in 250 ml distilled water)	0.7 g

1. Add ingredients to 750 ml 2% polypeptone in water.
2. Fill high columns of liquid into large test tubes.
3. Sterilize in autoclave 20 min at 15 psi.
4. Store at room temperature.
5. Before use heat to 80 C for a few minutes and let cool.

Medium may be purchased commercially as thioglycollate medium, Brewer, without indicator.

Medium is recommended for blood culture bottles.

Thioglycollate medium, "fluid thioglycollate." Medium is used for cultivation of anaerobes and for sterility testing. It also is useful for growth of many aerobic and microaerophilic organisms.

Trypticase	15 g
L-Cystine	0.5 g
Dextrose	5 g
Yeast extract	5 g
Sodium chloride	2.5 g
Sodium thioglycollate	0.5 g
Reazurin	0.001 g
Agar	0.75 g
Distilled water	1000 ml

Commercial products. Difco product contains casitone instead of trypticase and 0.3 ml thioglycollic acid instead of sodium salt.

1. Sterilize in autoclave 15 min at 15 psi.
2. Store at room temperature, not in refrigerator.

Thioglycollate medium, motility

"Fluid thioglycollate," dehydrated, (BBL or Difco)	29.5 g
Agar	4 g

1. Dissolve in 1000 ml distilled water.
2. Tube and place in autoclave at 15 psi for 15 min.

Thyrosine agar. See *Nocardia*, Chapter 77.

Tinsdale base and enrichment.[61-63] Base has the following composition:

Proteose-peptone no. 3 (Difco)	2 g
Sodium chloride	0.5 g
Agar	2 g
Distilled water	100 ml

1. Adjust to pH 7.4 and sterilize 15 min at 121 C.
2. Cool base and add aseptically the following, in the order named[61]:

Bovine serum	10 ml
0.1N NaOH	6 ml
L-Cystine, 0.4%, in 0.1N HCl	6 ml
Potassium tellurite, 1%, aqueous	3 ml
Sodium thiosulfate, 2.5%, anhydrous	1.7 ml

Both base and enrichment can be obtained commercially.*

1. Use **45 g** dehydrated base in **1000 ml** distilled water.
2. Heat to dissolve completely; sterilize 15 min at 121 C.
3. Cool to 50-55 C and add 15 ml rehydrated Tinsdale enrichment to **each 100 ml** base.
4. Dispense in Petri dishes, after thorough mixing, in about 15 ml amounts.
5. Store at 4 C.

Inoculate to obtain discrete colonies; also, during streaking, stab through surface of medium several times. Incubate at 37 C and examine at 24 and 48 h.

Todd-Hewitt broth[64]
1. To every 450 g fat-free minced beef add 1 L water.
2. Stir mixture well.
3. Place in cold overnight.

4. Then heat to 85 C and maintain at this temperature 30 min.
5. Filter while still hot through suitable paper, any loss from evaporation being made up with distilled water.
6. Add peptone to give 2%.
7. Adjust reaction to pH 7.
8. To each liter of medium then add:

Sodium bicarbonate	2 g
Glucose	2 g
Sodium chloride	2 g
Sodium phosphate (Na$_2$HPO$_4$ · 12 H$_2$O)	1 g

9. Boil broth 15 min.
10. Filter while hot, through paper, bottle, and autoclave 10 min at 115 C.
11. Final pH is 7.8; medium does not require any further adjustment, but its pH should be checked.
12. For type identification, use Difco Neopeptone or Evans peptone.

Medium is available commercially in dehydrated form.

Transport for anaerobes. See **Media for gram-negative anaerobes.**

Transport medium—Amies.[65] Medium is patterned after Cary-Blair modification of Stuart transport medium. Incorporating charcoal in medium obviates necessity of using charcoal-impregnated swabs.

Sodium chloride	8 g
Potassium chloride	0.2 g
Calcium chloride	0.1 g
Magnesium chloride	0.1 g
Monopotassium phosphate	0.2 g
Disodium phosphate	1.15 g
Sodium thioglycollate	1 g
Charcoal	10 g
Agar	3.6 g

1. Suspend ingredients in 1000 ml distilled water. Heat to boiling to dissolve completely.
2. Dispense hot medium, to within 0.5 cm of top, into small screw-capped vials (6-8 ml capacity).
3. Screw caps on tightly and autoclave vials 15 min at 15 psi (121 C). Invert vials just before medium solidifies to distribute charcoal evenly.

Medium is available in dehydrated form from Difco.

Transport medium—Cary-Blair[66, 67]

Sodium thioglycollate	1.5 g
Disodium phosphate (Na$_2$HPO$_4$)	1.1 g
Sodium chloride	5 g

1. Suspend ingredients in 991 ml distilled water.
2. Add 5 g agar; heat only until agar is dissolved.
3. Cool to 45-50 C. Add 9 ml fresh 1% aqueous solution of calcium chloride (CaCl$_2$). Adjust pH to 8.4.
4. Dispense immediately in 7 ml amounts into 9 ml sterilized screw-capped vials. Steam in autoclave with caps loose at 100 C for 15 min if still liquid, or for 25 min if solidified.
5. Cool vials at room temperature and then tighten caps.
6. If vials are to be stored prior to use, to prevent evaporation place transparent plastic collars* over caps and allow to tighten.
7. Gaines[68] recommends that only buffer-treated swabs should be employed with this medium. Prepare by dipping cotton swabs into Sørenson's buffer, pH 8.1, that has been previously heated to boiling. Leave swabs in hot buffer only long enough to saturate cotton; dain excess buffer off

---

*Difco Laboratories, Detroit, Mich.

*Celon collars, Celon Co., Division of Thatcher Glass Mfg. Co., Inc., Muscatine, Iowa.

against side of beaker. Sterilize wet swabs in glassine syringe envelopes (2¼ × 6⅝ in., self-sealing) by autoclaving at 121 C for 15 min. Dry at room temperature (1 d).

Medium is available in dehydrated form from BBL.

Transport medium—Stuart[69]
1. Add, in sequence, the following:

Agar (Difco)	6 g
Distilled water	1.9 L

2. Dissolve:

Thioglycollic acid	2 ml

Adjust to pH 7.4 with 1N NaOH.
3. Add:

Sodium glycerophosphate, 20% (wt/vol)	100 ml
Calcium chloride, 1%	200 ml

Adjust to pH 7.4 with 1N HCl.
4. Add:

Methylene blue solution, 0.1%	4 ml

5. Dispense into ¼ oz screw-capped bottles, filling to capacity.
6. Sterilize in flowing steam 1 h. Volume lost during sterilization is reconstituted from 1 of the bottles. Screw caps down tightly.
7. Prepare swabs for taking specimens from absorbent cotton and applicator sticks. Boil prepared swabs in Sørensen's pH 7.4 phosphate buffer solution. (Untreated swabs impart acidity to medium.) Dip swabs into 1% water suspension of finely powdered charcoal such as Norit. (Charcoal inhibits deleterious action of fatty acids present in certain batches of agar.) Place swabs (2/tube) in cotton-stoppered test tubes, dry, and sterilize.
8. After taking specimens, insert swab into upper third of medium in small bottle. Cut off protruding portion of swab stick with scissors and screw lid on bottle tightly. If inoculated swabs are held in office or clinic for some time before sending to laboratory, they should be refrigerated. Bottles in which methylene blue redox indicator has turned blue should not be used.

Medium is available in prepared vials from several manufacturers.

Triple sugar iron medium (TSI)—Hajna

Polypeptone	20 g
Lactose	10 g
Sucrose	10 g
Dextrose	1 g
Sodium chloride	5 g
Ferrous ammonium sulfate	0.2 g
Sodium thiosulfate	0.2 g
Agar	13 g
Phenol red	0.025 g
Distilled water	1000 ml

Medium may be purchased in dehydrated form from commercial laboratories.
1. Suspend dehydrated powder, in amount specified by manufacturer, in 1000 ml distilled water and boil 1 or 2 min to ensure solution.
2. Tube in cotton-plugged tubes.
3. Sterilize at 115-118 C for 15 min (BBL) or 121 C for 15 min (Difco).
4. Cool tubes in slanted position such that slants with deep butts are formed.

NOTE: When used for *V. parahaemolyticus* culture, add additional 25 g of NaCl/L to formula.

Trypticase agar (Eugonagar)

Trypticase	15 g
Phytone	5 g
Sodium chloride	4 g
Sodium citrate	1 g

Sodium sulfite	0.2 g
L-Cystine	0.2 g
Dextrose	5 g
Agar	15 g

Final reaction will be pH 7.0±.
1. When using dehydrated medium, suspend 45.4 g BBL Eugonagar in 1 L distilled water.
2. Allow mixture to stand about 5 min and mix until suspension is uniform.
3. Heat gently with occasional agitation and boil 1 or 2 min or until solution has occurred.
4. Dispense and sterilize at 118 C (12 psi) for 15 min.

Trypticase lactose iron agar (BBL)

Trypticase	20 g
Agar	3.5 g
Lactose	10 g
Ferrous sulfate	0.2 g
Sodium sulfite	0.4 g
Sodium thiosulfate	0.08 g
Phenol red	0.02 g

Final reaction is pH 7.2.
1. When using dehydrated medium, dissolve 34.2 g in 1 L distilled water.
2. Sterilize in autoclave 25 min at 10-12 psi.

Trypticase soy agar

Trypticase	15 g
Phytone	5 g
Sodium chloride	5 g
Agar	15 g

Final reaction should be pH 7.3±.
1. When using dehydrated medium, suspend 40 g BBL powder in 1 L distilled water.
2. Allow to soak 5 min and mix thoroughly.
3. Heat gently, with occasional agitation.
4. Boil 1 or 2 min or until solution is complete.
5. Dispense, and sterilize at 118-121 C (15 psi) for 15 min when test tubes are used. If large volumes are used, time but not temperature may be increased.
6. For preparation of blood plates for hemolysis studies add 5% defibrinated blood to sterile trypticase soy agar that has previously been melted and cooled to about 45 C.

Trypticase soy broth (BBL)

Trypticase	17 g
Phytone	3 g
Sodium chloride	5 g
Dipotassium phosphate	2.5 g
Dextrose	2.5 g

1. When using dehydrated medium, suspend 30 g powder in 1 L distilled water.
2. Mix thoroughly.
3. Warm gently until solution is complete.
4. Dispense and sterilize in autoclave at not over 15 psi (121 C) for 15 min.
5. If desired, 0.5-1 g agar/L broth may be added before sterilization.

Tryptone broth. See Peptone water.

Tryptone glucose yeast (TGYA) agar (standard methods agar)

Tryptone	5 g
Yeast extract	2.5 g
Glucose	1 g
Agar	15 g

1. Mix ingredients in 1000 ml distilled water.
2. Heat to boiling to dissolve. Dispense in tubes or flasks.
3. Sterilize by autoclaving at 121 C for 15 min.

Medium is available in dehydrated form (Difco, Fisher).

Tryptone nitrate broth

Tryptone	10 g

Potassium nitrate	0.1 g

1. Dissolve ingredients in 1 L distilled water.
2. Adjust reaction to pH 9.0-9.4.
3. Distribute in 3 ml amounts in test tubes.
4. Sterilize in autoclave 15 min at 15 psi.

Tryptose agar (Difco)

Tryptose	20 g
Dextrose	1 g
Sodium chloride	5 g
Bacto-agar	15 g
Distilled water	1000 ml

1. When using dehydrated medium, dissolve 41 g desiccated medium in 1000 ml distilled water, distribute in tubes, and sterilize in autoclave 20 min at 15 psi.

Tryptose blood sodium azide broth—Pike

1. To each 100 ml beef heart infusion broth with 1% tryptose, add 2 ml 2% sterile solution of dextrose and 5 ml defibrinated rabbit blood.
2. Distribute into test tubes, 2 ml in each.
3. For use add to each tube 0.15 ml 1:1000 solution of sodium azide and 0.1 ml 1:25,000 solution of crystal violet.

Urea agar—Christensen[70]

1. *Urea concentrate:*

Peptone	1 g
Sodium chloride	5 g
Glucose	1 g
Monobasic potassium phosphate	2 g
Phenol red	0.012 g
Urea	20 g
Distilled water	100 ml

   a. Dissolve ingredients in distilled water.
   NOTE: Instead of 0.012 g phenol red, use 6 ml 1:500 solution of phenol red (prepare by adding 0.2 g phenol red to 100 ml distilled water).
   b. Adjust pH to 6.8-6.9.
   c. Filter sterilize.
2. *Agar solution*

Agar	15 g
Distilled water	900 ml

   a. Dissolve agar in distilled water.
   b. Sterilize agar solution at 15 psi for 15 min.
   c. Cool to 50-55 C.
3. Add urea concentrate (1) to agar solution (2) under sterile conditions. Mix and distribute in sterile tubes.
4. Slant to obtain deep butts.
Commercial media. Urea agar base is available commercially as dehydrated medium (to be sterilized by filtration) or as urea agar base concentrate (already sterilized). Either can be used for urea concentrate (1). Follow manufacturer's instructions.

Urease broth—Rustigian-Stuart

Urea	20 g
Monopotassium phosphate	9.1 g
Disodium phosphate	9.5 g
Yeast extract	0.1 g
Phenol red	0.01 g

1. Dissolve ingredients in 100 ml distilled water and filter sterilize (Seitz or candle filter).
2. Distribute broth in 1 or 2 ml amounts in small sterile tubes.
Medium is available commercially in dehydrated form.

• • •

Vibrio cholerae media

Transport and enrichment solutions
MONSUR PRESERVATIVE SOLUTION[71]

Trypticase or Casitone	10 g

Sodium chloride	10 g
Sodium taurocholate	5 g
Sodium carbonate	1 g
Distilled water (neutral)	1000 ml

1. Sterilize at 121 C for 20 min.
2. When cool add 0.002% potassium tellurite (1:200,000 concentration)—pH about 8.5.
3. Dispense in 25 ml amounts in 80 ml screw-capped bottles.
4. Inoculate with stool specimen.

ALKALINE PEPTONE WATER (pH 8.4-8.5)

Peptone (Bacto or equivalent)	10 g
Sodium chloride	10 g
Distilled water	1000 ml

1. Adjust pH to 8.4-8.6.
2. Dispense in 7 ml amounts into 9 ml screwcap tubes and sterilize 10 min at 121 C.

GOHAR PRESERVATIVE SOLUTION[72]

Peptone water (pH 7.8-8.0)	100 ml

1. After sterilization at 121 C for 15 min add 0.2 ml 1% aqueous solution of potassium tellurite.
2. Dispense and inoculate as with Monsur solution above.

Any of the 3 above-mentioned solutions may be tubed in small amounts, e.g., 0.5-1 ml, and used for transportation of rectal swab specimens collected from active cases.

AMIES TRANSPORT MEDIUM. See Transport Medium—Amies, above.

Media for isolation

TCBS agar medium (pH 8.6)*

Yeast extract	5 g
Peptone	10 g
Sodium citrate	10 g
Sodium thiosulfate	10 g
Oxgall	5 g
Sodium cholate	3 g
Sucrose	20 g
Sodium chloride	10 g
Ferric citrate	1 g
Bromthymol blue	0.04 g
Thymol blue	0.04 g
Agar	15 g
Distilled water	1000 ml

1. Suspend ingredients in water and heat gently to dissolve about. Boil 1-2 min.
2. Cool to about 50 C and dispense in Petri dishes.
3. Do **not** autoclave this medium.

Meat extract agar medium (nutrient agar)

Beef extract (Bacto or equivalent)	3 g
Peptone (Bacto or equivalent)	10 g
Sodium chloride	5 g
Agar (Difco or equivalent)	20 g
Dissolve water	1000 ml

1. Adjust to pH 7.6 with 1N sodium hydroxide.
2. Sterilize at 121 C for 15 min and dispense in Petri dishes.

Taurocholate gelatin agar medium[73]

Trypticase (or equivalent)	10 g
Gelatin (Bacto or equivalent)	30 g
Sodium taurocholate	5 g
Sodium chloride	10 g
Yeast extract	1 g
Agar	15 g
Distilled water	1000 ml

1. Sterilize at 121 C for 15 min and dispense in Petri dishes.

---

*Medium is available commercially in dehydrated form from BBL, Difco, and Eiken (Japan).

2. Medium can be used without addition of sodium taurocholate.

Monsur agar[71]

Trypticase (BBL or equivalent)	10 g
Sodium chloride	10 g
Sodium taurocholate	5 g
Sodium carbonate	1 g
Gelatin (Difco or equivalent)	30 g
Agar	15 g
Distilled water	1000 ml

1. Sterilize at 121 C for 20 min.
2. When cooled to about 50 C, add potassium tellurite in concentration of 0.002% (1:200,000).
3. Dispense in Petri dishes.

Final pH of medium is about 8.5.

Aronson medium

1. a. Meat extract, prepared with 3% agar content, pH 7.4-7.6
   b. Saturated alcoholic solution of basic fuchsin
   c. Sodium carbonate, 10% solution anhydrous
   d. Sucrose, 20% solution
   e. Dextrin, 20% solution
   f. Sodium sulfite, 10% solution, anhydrous
2. Melt agar (1a) and to each 100 ml add 5 ml carbonate solution (1c).
3. Sterilize in flowing steam 15 min.
4. While still hot add in order 5 ml sucrose solution (1d), 5 ml dextrin solution (1e), 0.4 ml fuchsin solution (1b), and 2 ml sodium sulfite solution (1f).
5. Boil for a few minutes, then pour in plates. Store in dark and use within 3 d.

• • •

Vibrio parahaemolyticus media

TCBS medium. See *Vibrio cholerae* media, above.

TSI agar. Triple sugar iron agar with 25 g NaCl added to formula (per liter).

TSA-3% NaCl. Trypticase soy agar (see above) with 25 g NaCl added to formula (per liter).

TSB-3% NaCl. Trypticase soy broth (see above) with 25 g NaCl added to formula (per liter).

Motility test medium and decarboxylase media. Same as described above, with 25 g NaCl added to formula (per liter).

Bromcresol purple broth

Peptone	10 g
Beef extract	3 g
Sodium chloride	5 g
NaCl	25 g*
Bromcresol purple	0.04 g

1. Dissolve ingredients in 1 L distilled water. Divide into 5 equal portions.
2. Add 2 g glucose to first portion, 1 g adonitol to second, 1 g cellobiose to third, 1 g arabinose to fourth, and 1 g sorbitol to fifth; stir to dissolve.
3. Dispense 8 ml portions into 16 × 150 mm tubes containing inverted Durham vials.
4. Autoclave 10 min at 121 C. Final pH 7.0 ± 0.2.

Wagatsuma agar (Kanagawa phenomenon)

Yeast extract	3 g
Bacto peptone	10 g
Sodium chloride	70 g
Dipotassium phosphate	5 g
Mannitol	10 g
Crystal violet	0.001 g
Bacto agar	15 g
Distilled water	1000 ml

1. Adjust to pH 8.0 (do **not** autoclave).
2. Steam 30 min and temper to 50 C.
3. Add 2 ml of suspension of freshly drawn citrated (to give approximately 0.5%) **human** red blood cells that were previously washed 3 times in physiologic saline.
4. Pour plates and allow to harden.
5. Dry plates thoroughly before use. Plates should be used as soon as possible.

• • •

Voges-Proskauer (VP) test medium. See Methyl red test medium.

Watson medium[74]

1. Prepare 0.5% sodium taurocholate broth by adding 5 g sodium taurocholate to 1000 ml broth (infusion broth).
2. Sterilize in autoclave at 121 C for 15 min.
3. Add 100 units streptokinase* for each ml medium.
4. For blood culture melt 15 ml bismuth sulfite agar and pour into 4 oz sterile bottles. Place bottles on their sides and allow agar to set.
5. Add 15 ml broth (containing 1500 units streptokinase) just before use.
6. Collect 5 ml blood from patient and let it clot.
7. After removal of expressed serum, add residual clot to broth in bottle.
8. Incubate bottle at 37 C for 6 h; afterward tilt bottle 2 min, letting broth run over surface of slope. Reincubate and examine after 12 and 24 h for *Salmonella typhi*, growth of which usually manifests itself as a thin, diffuse film showing characteristic blackening and sheen. In low-grade bacteremias, single colonies occur.

Wilson-Reilly medium. See *Vibrio cholerae*, Chapter 79.

X and V factor media[34]

X factor medium

1. Autoclave Levinthal stock 15 min at 20 psi.
2. Prepare agar by mixing 45 g proteose agar no. 3 (Difco) with 15 g Bacto agar/L water.
3. Combine 1 part sterile Levinthal stock and 1 part sterile melted agar.

V factor medium

1. Combine 1 part yeast extract and 9 parts melted proteose no. 3 agar (Difco).
2. Prepare yeast extract by emulsifying 100 g powdered brewer's yeast in 400 ml distilled water, adjusting pH to 4.6, and boiling 10 min. Filter through filter paper, adjust pH to 7.0, and sterilize by Seitz filtration. Filtrate should be transferred to sterile container with glass stopper; seal with sterile petrolatum.

Combined X and V factor medium

1. Combine 1 part yeast extract and 9 parts X factor medium.
2. Distribute media into small tubes (100 × 13 mm) and slant.
3. Pure hemin and coenzyme may be used as X and V factors.

Xanthine medium. See *Nocardia*, Chapter 77.

XL (xylose lysine) agar base—Taylor[30, 31, 75, 76]

Agar	15 g
Lactose	7.5 g
Sucrose	7.5 g
Xylose	3.75 g
L-Lysine HCl	5 g
Yeast extract	3 g

---

*Add only for use with *V. parahaemolyticus*.

*Lederle Laboratories, Pearl River, N.Y.

Phenol red, 1% solution   8 ml
1. Mix ingredients in 1000 ml distilled water.
2. Heat to dissolve; boil 1 min. Autoclave at 15 psi (121 C) for 15 min.
3. Cool to 55-60 C. Add 20 ml of the following solution:

Sodium thiosulfate	34 g
Ferric ammonium citrate	4 g
Distilled water	100 ml

4. Pour into plates.

XL agar base is **not** selective or inhibitory; it is satisfactory for quantitative counts of enteric organisms. Medium is available in dehydrated form from BBL and Difco.

XLD (xylose lysine deoxycholate) agar—Taylor[30, 31, 75, 76]

1. Prepare xylose lysine agar base. Add thiosulfate and ferric ammonium citrate, as described under XL agar base.
2. To 1000 ml complete XL agar base (sterile, cooled), add 25 ml sterile, 10% aqueous solution of sodium deoxycholate.
3. Adjust reaction to pH 6.9. Pour into plates.

XLD medium utilizes deoxycholate as inhibitor and is recommended for isolation of shigellae and other enteric pathogens.

XLBG (xylose lysine brilliant green) agar—Taylor[30,75]

1. Medium is prepared by adding 1.25 ml 1% aqueous brilliant green solution to 1 L XL agar base prior to autoclaving.
2. After autoclaving, cool to 55-60 C. Add thiosulfate–ferric ammonium sulfate solution, as described under XL agar base.
3. Adjust to pH 6.9 and pour into sterile plates.

XLBG medium is recommended for salmonellae isolation in food analysis. Both coliforms and shigellae are inhibited.

Media for mycobacteria
(George Kubica and Hugo David)

A number of different media have been proposed for the isolation of mycobacteria from clinical material. The choice of which medium to use is based as much on tradition and institutional preference as anything else. Formulations that have proved especially helpful to us are presented.

American Trudeau Society (ATS) medium, modified

Potato flour	20.0 g
Distilled water	490.0 ml
Glycerol	10.0 ml
Egg yolk	500.0 ml
1% malachite green in 50% alcohol	20.0 ml

1. Combine potato flour, water, and glycerol in 2 L flask.
2. Autoclave at 121 C for 30 min.
3. Cool to 50 C.
4. *Meanwhile:* Prepare fresh egg yolk as follows: Carefully clean fresh hen eggs.* Using aseptic technics, separate egg yolk from white. For 500 ml

---

*Fresh eggs, not more than 1 wk old, are cleaned by scrubbing with hand brush in soap solution (about 5%). After scrubbing, eggs are allowed to stand in soap solution 30 min. Rinse thoroughly in running water, then soak eggs in 70% alcohol 15 min. With well-scrubbed hands, break eggs into sterile flask and homogenize by hand shaking. Filter eggs through 4 layers of sterile gauze into sterile graduated cylinder.

egg yolk, use proportion of 1 whole egg to 11 yolks.
5. Combine homogenized egg yolk mixture with cooled potato flour water.
6. Add 20.0 ml malachite green. Mix thoroughly.
7. Dispense 5-6 ml per tube into sterile screw-cap tubes.
8. Slant and coagulate by inspissation at 85 C for 1 h.

Dubos-Middlebrook media (Tween-albumin broth and oleic acid–albumin agar)

Basal medium

Potassium acid phosphate (KH_2PO_4)	1.0 g
Diabasic sodium phosphate ($Na_2HPO_4 \cdot 12H_2O$) (or 2.5 g anhydrous Na_2HPO_4)	6.3 g
Asparagine	
For liquid media	2.0 g
For solid media	1.0 g

Heat above in 100 ml distilled water to dissolve.
1. Add 850 ml distilled water.
2. Then add:

Enzymatic digest of casein or Casitone	
For liquid media	2 g
For solid media	1 g
Ferric ammonium citrate	
For liquid media	0.005 g
For solid media	0.05 g
Magnesium sulfate ($MgSO_4 \cdot 7H_2O$) (1 ml 1% stock solution in distilled water)	0.01 g
Calcium chloride ($CaCl_2$) (1 ml 0.05% stock solution in distilled water)	0.0005 g
Zinc sulfate ($ZnSO_4$) (1 ml 0.01% stock solution in distilled water)	0.0001 g
Copper sulfate ($CuSO_4$) (1 ml 0.01% stock solution in distilled water)	0.0001 g

Adjust pH to 6.5-6.8 with HCl.

This basal medium may be used to prepare either liquid Tween-albumin medium or oleic acid–albumin agar.

For liquid Tween-albumin media

Basal medium	900 ml
Tween 80 (or 5 ml of 10% stock solution in distilled water)	0.5 ml

1. Autoclave and cool to 56 C.
2. Add:

Bovine albumin fraction V (100 ml 5% stock in 0.85% saline neutralized with NaOH and sterilized by Seitz filtration)	5 g
Glucose (10 ml 50% stock in distilled water; sterile in autoclave, 121 C/15 min)	5 g

3. Dispense as desired.

For oleic acid–albumin agar

1. Use only:

Asparagine	1 g
Enzymatic digest of casein	1 g
Ferric ammonium citrate	0.05 g
Basal medium	900 ml
Agar	11.0 g

2. Autoclave and cool to 56 C.
3. Add 100 ml of the following oleic acid–albumin complex:
   a. Dissolve 0.12 ml (0.1 g) oleic acid in 10 ml 20 N NaOH by shaking with rotary motion in small flask.
   b. Add 5 ml of this to 95 ml of **neutral** 5% solution of bovine albumin fraction V in 0.85% saline.

c. Sterilize by filtration through bacteriologic filters, either glass or Seitz.

4. Dispense as desired.

Lowenstein-Jensen egg medium, modified

1. For salt solution combine:

Monopotassium phosphate (anhydrous)	2.4 g
Magnesium sulfate · 7H$_2$O	0.24 g
Magnesium citrate	0.6 g
Asparagine	3.6 g
Glycerol (reagent grade)	12.0 ml
Distilled water	600.0 ml

2. Add 30.0 g potato flour.
3. Autoclave at 121 C for 30 min. Cool to room temperature.
4. Add 20.0 ml malachite green (2% aqueous solution freshly prepared).
5. Add 1000.0 ml* homogenized whole eggs.
6. Mix and pour into sterile aspirator bottle or funnel with bell attachment (test tube filling device) and dispense.
7. Place approximately 6-8 ml medium into each 20 × 150 mm sterile screw-cap test tube.
8. Slant tubes and coagulate by inspissation at 85 C for 50 min.
9. Incubate at 37 C for 48 h as sterility check.
10. Medium may be stored in refrigerator for several months if caps are tightly closed to prevent evaporation.

Middlebrook 7H-9 broth. To prepare 1 L (1000 ml) of medium:

1. Combine 900 ml distilled water with 0.5 g Tween 80 *or* 2 ml glycerol as desired. Do not use Tween 80 and glycerol together.
2. Add and dissolve the following salts in the order listed:

Ammonium sulfate (20 ml 2.5% solution)	0.5 g
Glutamic acid, monosodium salt (20 ml 2.5% solution)	0.5 g
Sodium citrate · 2H$_2$O (1 ml 10% solution)	0.1 g
Pyridoxine hydrochloride (1 ml 0.1% solution)	0.001 g
Biotin (0.25 ml 0.2% solution)	0.0005 g
Disodium phosphate (anhydrous)	2.5 g
Monopotassium phosphate (anhydrous)	1.0 g
Ferric ammonium citrate (green) (0.4 ml 10% solution)	0.04 g
Magnesium sulfate · 7H$_2$O (5 ml 1.0% solution)	0.05 g
Calcium chloride · 2H$_2$O (0.5 ml 0.1% solution)	0.0005 g
Zinc sulfate · 7H$_2$O (1 ml 0.1% solution)	0.001 g
Copper sulfate · 5H$_2$O (1 ml 0.1% solution)	0.001 g

Adjust pH of solution to 6.6 using 10% HCl.

3. Autoclave at 121 C for 20 min.
4. Allow to cool to less than 50 C and add following sterile enrichment solutions (for preparation see 6 below):

50% Glucose	4 ml
Catalase (1000 µg/ml)	2 ml
5% Bovine albumin	100 ml

5. Dispense in freshly sterilized screw-cap test tubes or other containers as desired. (Use 5 ml amounts in 20 mm diameter tubes.) Store in refrigerator. To

prevent evaporation during storage, tube caps must be securely tightened.

6. Preparation of solutions a, b, and c for step 4. (Commercial ADC contains these solutions and is a suitable substitute.)
   a. Prepare 50% glucose by dissolving 50 g glucose in 60 ml distilled water. To this add 1.0 ml 10% citric acid. Autoclave 10 min at 15 lb pressure (121 C).
   b. Add 0.02 ml catalase (technical grade) to 20 ml 0.85% NaCl in distilled water. Sterilize by membrane filtration. Prepare fresh each time needed.
   c. Mix 5.0 g bovine albumin fraction V and 95 ml 0.85% NaCl in distilled water. Adjust pH to 6.8 with either 50% NaOH or 16-19% HCl, whichever is needed. Filter-sterilize solution. Dispense in freshly sterilized screw-cap containers. Incubate at 37 C overnight to check for sterility. Place in 56 C water bath 30 min to inactivate lipase. Store at 4 C.

Commercial products. The Middlebrook 7H-9 and Dubos-Middlebrook Tween-albumin liquid media are satisfactory as supplied by commercial sources.

Prepare according to directions on label. Tube in 5 ml quantities in 20 × 150 mm sterile screw-cap test tubes. Incubate for sterility check.

Liquid media may be stored in refrigerator indefinitely, provided it is tightly capped and evaporation does not occur.

Middlebrook and Cohn 7H-10 agar, from basic ingredients. Six stock solutions may be prepared in advance. When prepared and stored as indicated, these solutions remain stable for at least a month. If precipitation or flocculation occurs in any stock solution, discard and prepare fresh solutions.

Preparation of 6 stock solutions

SOLUTION 1

Monopotassium phosphate, ACS (anhydrous)	15.0 g
Disodium phosphate, ACS (anhydrous)	15.0 g
Distilled water to make	250.0 ml

1. Autoclave at 121 C for 15 min.
2. Store this solution at room temperature.

SOLUTION 2

Ammonium sulfate, ACS	5.0 g
Monosodium glutamate (glutamic acid, monosodium salt)	5.0 g
Sodium citrate · 2H$_2$O, USP	4.0 g
Ferric ammonium citrate	0.4 g
Magnesium sulfate · 7H$_2$O, ACS	0.5 g
Biotin (in 2 ml 10% ammonium hydroxide)	5.0 mg
Distilled water to make	250.0 ml

1. Autoclave at 121 C for 15 min.
2. Store in refrigerator at 4-10 C.

SOLUTION 3

Calcium chloride · 2H$_2$O, ACS	50 mg
Zinc sulfate · 7H$_2$O, ACS	100 mg
Copper sulfate · 5H$_2$O, ACS	100 mg
Pyridoxine hydrochloride	100 mg
Distilled water to make	100 ml

Store in refrigerator at 4-10 C.

SOLUTION 4. Reagent grade glycerol. Store at room temperature.

SOLUTION 5

Aqueous malachite green, 0.01%

1. Dissolve 0.1 g malachite green in 100 ml distilled water.
2. Dilute 1:10 to make 0.01%.
3. Store at room temperature or 4-10 C **in the dark.**

---

*See ATS medium for preparation of eggs.

SOLUTION 6
Oleate-albumin-dextrose-catalase (OADC)
1. Dissolve 50 g bovine albumin fraction V in 900 ml freshly prepared saline (0.85% NaCl).
2. Add 30 ml sodium oleate prepared as follows:
   20 N NaOH   30.0 ml
   Oleic acid   0.6 ml
   Warm to 56 C and swirl gently to dissolve.
3. Adjust pH to 7.0 with 4% NaOH.
4. Heat in water bath at 56 C for 1 h.
5. Add 40 ml sterile 50% solution of dextrose prepared as follows:
   a. To 30 ml of boiling distilled water, add 25 g dextrose (glucose). Stir to dissolve.
   b. Add distilled water to make 50 ml total volume.
   c. Autoclave 10 min at 121 C.
6. Add 0.02 ml technical catalase.*
7. Sterilize by membrane filter. To facilitate this process, use prefilter with sterilizing membrane (0.45 μm) and filter while albumin is still warm.
8. Dispense in sterile screw-cap tubes in 20 ml or other convenient amounts.
9. Incubate 24 h at 35-37 C. If sterile, mixture is ready for use.
10. Store in refrigerator in air-tight containers. Do not freeze.

NOTE: If it is inconvenient to prepare solution 6, commercially available OADC is acceptable substitute.

Preparation of 800 ml completed media from 6 stock solutions (or 4 "batches" of 200 ml each)
   Distilled water   680.0 ml
   Solution 1   20.0 ml
   Solution 2   20.0 ml
   Solution 3   0.8 ml
   Solution 4   4.0 ml
1. Adjust pH to 6.6 by adding approximately 0.4 ml 6 N HCl. Check on pH meter.
2. Add 2.0 ml of solution 5.
3. Divide into 4 equal parts of 180 ml each.
4. To each 180 ml, add 3.0 g agar.
5. Autoclave at 121 C for 10 min.
6. Cool to 56 C (for drug media, cool to 50-52 C).
7. Add to each 180 ml flask:
   a. Solution 6   20.0 ml
   b. If catalase is not in OADC, prepare sterile solution containing 1000 μg/ml and add 0.4 ml (see footnote, previous page)
   c. For drug media, add sterile drug.
8. Mix gently but thoroughly and dispense into Petri dishes, (20 ml per dish or 5-6 ml per quadrant in 4-section dish). **Media must be cooled and dispensed within 1 h after autoclaving.**
9. Allow to solidify at room temperature **in the dark.**

Preparation of 7H-10 agar from commercial base. Check bottle label for this reference, "Acta Tuberc. Scand. 38:66, 1960." This reference on label indicates that bottle contains correct ingredients.

NOTE: Experience has shown that boiling basal medium before autoclaving results in medium of inferior quality. This result may be avoided by preparing medium in 200 ml amounts and autoclaving 10 min.

To prepare 200 ml complete medium follow these directions precisely:
1. Suspend 3.8 g* Middlebrook 7H-10 basal medium in 180 ml freshly distilled water and add 1.0 ml reagent grade glycerol.
2. Swirl base into suspension and sterilize in autoclave 10 min at 121 C.
3. Remove medium from autoclave **as soon as** pressure will allow and place in water bath at 50-56 C.
4. As soon as cooled to 50-56 C, add 20 ml OADC enrichment.
5. For drug media, cool to 50-52 C and then add required amount of drug.
6. Dispense **within 1 h after autoclaving.**
7. Allow to solidify at room temperature **in the dark.**

NOTE: When autoclaved medium is allowed to stand more than 1 h in water bath, a precipitate begins to form. Experience has shown that this practice should be avoided. Pour as soon as possible. Always check medium when taking it out of autoclave. It should be clear and transparent. If precipitate is present, it may be due to (1) sterilization temperature within autoclave being reached too rapidly to dissolve base in 10 min, (2) poor quality basal medium, and/or (3) dirty glassware.

CAUTION: Never autoclave 7H-10 medium base and store in refrigerator for future use. Heat required to melt it results in overheating and medium of poor quality.

For best results do not prepare in lots of more than 400 ml.

Sodium chloride tolerance. Control and sodium chloride medium should be prepared from same "batch" of basal medium. Use one of the following:

American Trudeau Society (ATS)
1. Divide 500 ml distilled water-glycerol-potato flour into 2 equal portions of 250 ml each.
2. To 1 portion add 25.0 g sodium chloride.
3. Autoclave, cool, and add 250 ml egg yolk and 10 ml malachite green to each portion.
4. Tube and inspissate as directed for ATS.

Lowenstein-Jensen (LJ)
1. Divide 600 ml salt-solution-glycerol into 2 equal portions of 300 ml.
2. To each portion add 15.0 g potato flour.
3. To 1 portion add 40.0 g sodium chloride (this is 5% NaCl final concentration in completed medium).
4. Second portion is control medium.
5. Autoclave, cool, and add 500 ml homogenized egg and 10 ml malachite green to each portion.
6. Tube and inspissate as directed for LJ.

Media and reagents for anaerobes—Center for Disease Control (CDC) usage[77, 78]
(V. R. Dowell, Jr.)

The following instructions for preparing, storing, and performance testing of various media are from *Media for isolation, characterization and identification of obligately anaerobic bacteria* (Dowell, V. R., Jr., Lombard, G. L., Thompson, F. S., and Armfield, A. Y., Atlanta, 1977, U. S. Department of Health, Education, and Welfare, Public Health Service). All of these media are now available commercially.

These media and instructions pertain to the procedures included in *Laboratory methods in anaerobic bacteriology* (Dowell, V. R., Jr., and

---

*Catalase is inactivated by Seitz and sintered glass filters. If membrane filter sterilization is unavailable, omit catalase from solution 6 and add it to sterile completed medium. To prepare sterile catalase, add 0.02 ml catalase to 20 ml 0.85% saline: this solution contains 1000 μg/ml. Sterilize by membrane filter. To each 100 ml completed medium, add 0.2 ml sterile catalase solution.

---

*Calculated from directions on label for formula in Acta Tuberc. Scand.

Hawkins, T. M., CDC Laboratory Manual, Atlanta, 1977, U.S. Department of Health, Education, and Welfare, Public Health Service, Center for Disease Control) and are described here in Chapter 70.

Media preparation is important in the cultivation of fastidious anaerobic bacteria. The following precautions should be closely observed:

1. Avoid excessive heating. Autoclave media no longer than 15 minutes.

2. Prepare media from recently opened bottles or use preweighed packets of dehydrated media.

3. Store media in the dark at room temperature in tightly sealed tubes. Biochemical media in cotton-plugged tubes should be stored in the refrigerator to prevent evaporation.

4. Do not use media containing reducing agents that have been stored longer than 14 days under aerobic conditions.

Plating media, anaerobic[77]

Anaerobe blood agar (BA), CDC. This blood agar (BA)[77] is an enriched, nonselective medium that supports the growth of essentially all types of obligately anaerobic bacteria found in clinical materials. It also supports good growth of most aerobic, facultatively anaerobic, and microaerophilic bacteria found in clinical materials if incubated appropriately.

Trypticase (BBL)	15.0 g
Phytone (BBL)	5.0 g
Sodium chloride	5.0 g
Agar	20.0 g
Yeast extract (Difco)	5.0 g
Hemin	5.0 mg
Vitamin K_1 (3 phytylmenadione)	10.0 mg
L-Cystine	400.0 mg
Distilled water	1000.0 ml
Blood (sheep), defibrinated	50.0 ml

1. Dissolve by heating in 1000 ml distilled water:

Trypticase soy agar (BBL)	40.0 g
Agar (additional)	5.0 g
Yeast extract (Difco)	5.0 g
Hemin*	5.0 mg
L-Cystine*	400.0 mg
Vitamin K_1 (3 phytylmenadione)†	10.0 mg

2. Adjust pH to 7.5.
3. Autoclave at 121 C for 15 min.
4. Cool to 48-50 C in water bath.
5. Add 50 ml sterile, defibrinated sheep blood.
6. Mix and dispense in 20 ml quantities into sterile 15 × 100 mm plastic Petri dishes.
7. After medium solidifies, place plates in cellophane bags and store in refrigerator at 4 C.

Performance testing. This medium should support good growth of fastidious and slow-growing anaerobes and of other common obligately anaerobic bacteria. This medium should also support typical pigment production by *Bacteroides melaninogenicus* and a typical double zone of hemolysis around colonies of most *Clostridium perfringens*. The colonies of *Fusobacterium necrophorum* are nonhemolytic on this medium because it contains sheep blood.

---

*In small beaker, dissolve hemin and L-cystine in 5 ml 1N NaOH before adding to other ingredients.

†Add vitamin K_1 from stock alcoholic solution containing 1 g of 3 phytylmenadione (1 CN, Cleveland, Ohio) plus 99 ml absolute ethanol.

Anaerobe blood agar with kanamycin and vancomycin (KVA), CDC. KVA[77] is used for selective isolation of obligately anaerobic gram-negative bacteria. It is especially useful for selective isolation of *Bacteroides* species. Essentially all other bacteria found in clinical specimens, including obligately anaerobic gram-positive bacteria, are inhibited by the medium.

Trypticase (BBL)	15.0 g
Phytone (BBL)	5.0 g
Sodium chloride	5.0 g
Agar	20.0 g
Yeast extract (Difco)	5.0 g
Hemin	5.0 mg
Vitamin K_1 (3 phytylmenadione)	10.0 mg
L-Cystine	400.0 mg
Distilled water	1000.0 ml
Blood (sheep), defibrinated	50.0 ml
Kanamycin	100.0 mg
Vancomycin	7.5 mg

1. Dissolve by heating in 1000 ml of distilled water:

Trypticase soy agar (BBL)	40.0 g
Agar (additional)	5.0 g
Yeast extract (Difco)	5.0 g
Hemin*	5.0 mg
L-Cystine*	400.0 mg
Vitamin K_1 (3 phytylmenadione)†	10.0 mg

2. Adjust pH to 7.5.
3. Autoclave at 121 C for 15 min.
4. Cool to 48-50 C in water bath.
5. Add 50 ml sterile defibrinated sheep blood, 100.0 mg, base activity, of kanamycin (Bristol Laboratories), and 7.5 mg, base activity, of vancomycin (Eli Lilly & Co.).
6. Mix and dispense into 15 × 100 mm plastic Petri dishes, 20 ml per plate.
7. After medium solidifies, place plates in cellophane bags and store in refrigerator at 4 C.

Performance testing. This medium should support good growth of obligately anaerobic gram-negative bacteria (e.g., *Bacteroides fragilis, Fusobacterium mortiferum*) and inhibit the growth of facultatively anaerobic bacteria (e.g., *Escherichia coli, Proteus mirabilis, Staphylococcus aureus*) and gram-positive obligate anaerobes (e.g., *Clostridium perfringens, Peptostreptococcus anaerobius*).

Anaerobe blood agar with paromomycin and vancomycin (PVA), CDC. This medium (PVA)[77] is similar to CDC anaerobe blood agar with kanamycin and vancomycin (KVA) except that paromomycin is substituted for kanamycin and the blood is laked by freezing and thawing before it is added to the medium. The PVA is especially useful for isolating *Bacteroides melaninogenicus, Fusobacterium necrophorum, Fusobacterium nucleatum*, and other fastidious, obligately anaerobic non-sporeforming gram-negative bacilli from mixed populations.

Trypticase (BBL)	15.0 g
Phytone (BBL)	5.0 g
Sodium chloride	5.0 g
Agar	20.0 g
Yeast extract (Difco)	5.0 g
Hemin	5.0 mg
L-Cystine	400.0 mg
Vitamin K_1 (3 phytylmenadione)	10.0 mg
Distilled water	1000.0 ml

---

*In small beaker, dissolve hemin and L-Cystine in 5 ml 1N NaOH before adding to other ingredients.

†Add vitamin K_1 from alcoholic solution containing 1 g of 3 phytylmenadione (ICN, Cleveland, Ohio) plus 99 ml absolute ethanol.

Blood (laked, defibrinated sheep)   50.0 ml
Paromomycin (Parke Davis & Co.)   100.0 mg
Vancomycin (Eli Lilly & Co.)   7.5 mg

1. Dissolve by heating in 1000 ml distilled water:
   Trypticase soy agar (BBL)   40.0 g
   Agar (additional)   5.0 g
   Yeast extract (Difco)   5.0 g
   Hemin*   5.0 mg
   L-Cystine*   400.0 mg
   Vitamin K₁ (3 phytylmenadione)†   10.0 mg

2. Adjust pH to 7.5.
3. Autoclave at 121 C for 15 min.
4. Cool to 48-50 C in water bath.
5. Add 50 ml of sterile, laked defibrinated sheep blood, 100.0 mg paromomycin (Parke Davis & Co.), and 7.5 mg, base activity, of vancomycin (Eli Lilly & Co.).
6. Mix and dispense into 15 × 100 mm plastic Petri dishes, 20 ml per plate.
7. After medium solidifies, place plates in cellophane bags and store in refrigerator at 4 C.

Performance testing. PVA medium should support typical colony growth of appropriate strains of *Bacteroides melaninogenicus, Fusobacterium mortiferum,* and *Fusobacterium nucleatum* and should inhibit growth of *Proteus mirabilis, Escherichia coli, Staphylococcus aureus,* and *Clostridium perfringens.*

Anaerobe blood agar with phenethylalcohol (PEA), CDC. This medium[77] is used for selective isolation of anaerobic bacteria from mixed populations containing rapidly growing gram-negative bacteria such as spreading *Proteus* spp. and other members of the family *Enterobacteriaceae.* Phenethylalcohol (0.25%) inhibits growth of gram-negative facultatively anaerobic bacteria, but most gram-negative and gram-positive obligately anaerobic bacteria will grow on it.

Trypticase (BBL)   15.0 g
Phytone (BBL)   5.0 g
Sodium chloride   5.0 g
Agar   20.0 g
Yeast extract (Difco)   5.0 g
Hemin   5.0 mg
Vitamin K₁ (3 phytylmenadione)   10.0 mg
L-Cystine   400.0 mg
Distilled water   1000.0 ml
Blood (sheep), defibrinated   50.0 ml
Phenethylalcohol   2.5 g

1. Dissolve by heating in 1000 ml distilled water:
   Trypticase soy agar (BBL)   40.0 g
   Agar (additional)   5.0 g
   Yeast extract (Difco)   5.0 g
   Hemin*   5.0 mg
   L-Cystine*   400.0 mg
   Vitamin K₁ (3 phytylmenadione)†   10.0 mg
   Phenethylalcohol   2.5 g

2. Adjust pH to 7.5.
3. Autoclave at 121 C for 15 min.
4. Cool to 48-50 C in water bath.
5. Add 50 ml sterile, defibrinated sheep blood and mix.
6. Dispense into sterile 15 × 100 mm plastic Petri dishes, 20 ml per plate.
7. Allow medium to solidify, place plates in cellophane bags, and refrigerate at 4 C.

Performance testing. This medium should support good growth of obligately anaerobic bacteria (e.g., *Bacteroides fragilis, Bacteroides melaninogenicus, Clostridium perfringens, Peptostreptococcus anaerobius*) and should inhibit growth of facultatively anaerobic gram-negative bacteria (e.g., *Proteus mirabilis, Escherichia coli*). Facultatively anaerobic gram-positive bacteria (staphylococci, streptococci, etc.) grow on PEA also.

Stiff anaerobe blood agar (stiff BA), CDC. Stiff BA[77] is used to decrease the swarming of clostridia so that microorganisms in mixed populations can be isolated in pure culture.[78] Essentially all types of obligate anaerobes will grow on it, but their colonies will be somewhat smaller than on regular CDC anaerobe blood agar.

Trypticase (BBL)   15.0 g
Phytone (BBL)   5.0 g
Sodium chloride   5.0 g
Agar   40.0 g
Yeast extract (Difco)   5.0 g
Hemin   5.0 mg
Vitamin K₁ (3 phytylmenadione)   10.0 mg
L-Cystine   400.0 mg
Distilled water   1000.0 ml
Blood (sheep, defibrinated)   50.0 ml

1. Dissolve by heating in 1000 ml distilled water:
   Trypticase soy agar (BBL)   40.0 g
   Agar (additional)   25.0 g
   Yeast extract (Difco)   5.0 g
   Hemin*   5.0 mg
   L-Cystine*   400.0 mg
   Vitamin K₁ (3 phytylmenadione)†   10.0 mg

2. Adjust pH to 7.5.
3. Autoclave at 121 C for 15 min.
4. Cool to 48-50 C in water bath.
5. Add 50 ml sterile, defibrinated sheep blood.
6. Mix and dispense into sterile 15 × 100 mm plastic Petri dishes, 20 ml per plate.
7. After medium solidifies, place plates in cellophane bags and store in refrigerator at 4 C.

Performance testing
1. This medium should support the growth of all sporeforming and non-sporeforming obligate anaerobes commonly found in clinical materials and of most aerobic, facultatively anaerobic, and microaerophilic bacteria found in clinical materials if incubated appropriately.
2. Stiff BA should decrease the swarming of *Clostridium septicum, Clostridium tetani,* and other clostridia so that pure culture isolates can be obtained from mixed populations.

Lombard-Dowell (LD) agar, Lombard-Dowell (LD) bile agar, Lombard-Dowell egg yolk agar (EYA), and Lombard-Dowell (LD) esculin agar. See **Presumpto quadrant plate media, below.**

Lombard-Dowell (LD) deoxyribonucleic acid (DNA) agar, CDC. This medium[77] is used to test the ability of obligately anaerobic bacteria to hydrolyze (depolymerize) deoxyribonucleic acid (DNA) by means of deoxyribonuclease activity. The LD-DNA agar is prepared by supplementing LD agar with DNA and toluidine blue to serve as an indicator of DNA hydrolysis. This medium shows promise as an aid in presumptive identification of clostridia.

----

*In small beaker, dissolve hemin and L-cystine in 5 ml 1N NaOH before adding to other ingredients.
†Add vitamin K₁ from stock alcoholic solution containing 1 g of 3 phytylmenadione (ICN, Cleveland, Ohio) plus 99 ml absolute ethanol.

----

*In small beaker, dissolve hemin and L-Cystine in 5 ml 1N NaOH before adding to other ingredients.
†Add vitamin K₁ from stock alcoholic solution containing 1 g of 3 phytylmenadione (ICN, Cleveland, Ohio) plus 99 ml absolute ethanol.

Trypticase (BBL) 5.0 g
Yeast extract (Difco) 5.0 g
Sodium chloride 2.5 g
Sodium sulfite 0.1 g
L-Tryptophan 0.2 g
Vitamin K$_1$ (3 phytylmenadione) 10.0 mg
Agar 20.0 g
Distilled water 1000.0 ml
L-Cystine 0.4 g
Hemin 10.0 mg
Deoxyribonucleic acid (polymerized) 1.25 g
Toluidine blue (0.25% aqueous solution) 25.0 ml

1. Mix all ingredients except hemin and L-cystine.
2. Dissolve hemin and L-cystine in 5 ml 1N NaOH before adding to other ingredients.
3. Add vitamin K$_1$ from stock solution containing 1 g of 3 phytylmenadione plus 99 ml absolute ethanol, 0.1 ml/100 ml medium.
4. After ingredients are dissolved, adjust pH of medium to 7.5. Autoclave medium at 121 C for 15 min.
5. Allow medium to cool to 48-50 C and dispense 20 ml into plastic 15 × 100 mm Petri dishes. If quadrant Petri dishes are used, dispense 5 ml medium per quadrant.
6. Place plates of solidified medium in cellophane bags and store in refrigerator at 4 C.

Inoculation, incubation, and interpretation of reactions. Place 1 or 2 drops of cell supension or broth culture on each quadrant of Presumpto Plate, and streak ¾ of medium with capillary pipet. Incubate plate in anaerobic system such as anaerobic glove box or anaerobic jar at 35 C for 48 h. DNase is an extracellular enzyme that hydrolyzes DNA. If DNase is produced, plate is characteristically pink to violet around colonies, and clear blue elsewhere. An alternate method is to flood plate with 1N hydrochloric acid. Unhydrolyzed DNA is precipitated, causing medium to become cloudy. If organism being tested produces DNase, there will be a clear zone around it, indicating DNA hydrolysis.

Performance testing. Appropriate strains of *Clostridium perfringens* and *Clostridium sporogenes* should exhibit the following reactions on LD-DNA agar when tested as described above:

Organism	DNA hydrolysis
C. perfringens	+
C. sporogenes	−

Lombard-Dowell (LD) glucose agar, CDC. This medium[77] is used in detecting fermentation of glucose and stimulation of growth by glucose as part of a procedure for presumptive identification of anaerobic bacteria. Various aerobic, facultatively anaerobic, microaerophilic, and obligately anaerobic bacteria will grow on the medium when incubated under conditions appropriate for them. LD glucose is prepared by supplementing LD agar with glucose and bromthymol blue indicator.

Trypticase (BBL) 5.0 g
Yeast extract (Difco) 5.0 g
Sodium chloride 2.5 g
Sodium sulfite 0.1 g
L-Tryptophan 0.2 g
Vitamin K$_1$ (3 phytylmenadione) 10.0 mg
Agar 20.0 g
Distilled water 1000.0 ml

L-Cystine 0.4 g
Hemin 10.0 mg
D-Glucose 6.0 g
Bromthymol blue (1% aqueous solution)* 2.0 ml

1. Mix all ingredients except hemin and L-cystine.
2. Dissolve hemin and L-cystine in 5 ml 1N NaOH before adding to other ingredients.
3. Add vitamin K$_1$ from stock solution containing 1 g of 3 phytylmenadione plus 99 ml absolute ethanol, 0.1 ml/100 ml medium.
4. After ingredients are dissolved, adjust pH of medium to 7.5. Autoclave medium at 121 C for 15 min.
5. Allow medium to cool to 48-50 C, and dispense in 20 ml quantities into plastic 15 × 100 mm Petri dishes. If quadrant Petri dishes are used, dispense 5 ml medium per quadrant.
6. Place plates of solidified medium in cellophane bags and store in refrigerator at 4 C.

Inoculation, incubation, and interpretation. Place 1 or 2 drops of cell suspension or broth culture on each quadrant of Presumpto Plate, and streak ¾ of medium with capillary pipet. Incubate plate in anaerobic system such as anaerobic glove box or anaerobic jar at 35 C for 48 h. Glucose stimulation is determined by comparing degree of bacterial growth on LD glucose agar with that on plain LD agar and record as I (growth less than LD agar control), E (growth equal to), or S (growth greater than on LD agar control). Fermentation of glucose is indicated by acid production or yellow color. Because some bacteria are capable of reducing indicator, it may be necessary to flood quadrant with a few drops of dilute bromthymol blue solution† to determine if acid was produced.

Performance testing. If plates of LD glucose medium are inoculated with appropriate strains of *Clostridium innocuum* and *C. tetani* and incubated anaerobically at 35 C for 48 h, the following results should be obtained:

Organism	Glucose fermented	Growth stimulated by glucose
C. innocuum	+	+
C. tetani	−	−

Lombard-Dowell (LD) milk agar, CDC. LD milk agar[77] is used to test the ability of obligately anaerobic bacteria to hydrolyze milk proteins. The medium is prepared by supplementing LD agar with powdered skimmed milk. This medium shows promise as an aid in the identification of clostridia.

Trypticase (BBL) 5.0 g
Yeast extract (Difco) 5.0 g
Sodium chloride 2.5 g
Sodium sulfite 0.1 g
L-Tryptophan 0.2 g
Vitamin K$_1$ (3 phytylmenadione) 10.0 mg
Agar 20.0 g
Distilled water 1000.0 ml
L-Cystine 0.4 g

---

*Bromthymol blue (1% aqueous solution). Dissolve 1 g bromthymol blue in 20 ml 0.1N sodium hydroxide. Add 80 ml distilled water.
†Dilute bromthymol blue solution is prepared by adding 3 drops 1% bromthymol blue solution to 30 ml distilled water in dropping bottle.

Hemin	10.0 mg
Skim milk, powdered	50.0 g

1. Mix all ingredients except hemin and L-cystine.
2. Dissolve hemin and L-cystine in 5 ml 1N NaOH before adding to other ingredients.
3. Add vitamin K_1 from stock solution containing 1 g of 3 phytylmenadione plus 99 ml absolute ethanol, 0.1 ml/100 ml medium.
4. After ingredients are dissolved, adjust pH of medium to 7.5. Autoclave medium at 121 C for 15 min.
5. Allow medium to cool to 48 C, and dispense 20 ml into plastic 15 × 100 mm Petri dishes. If quadrant Petri dishes are used, dispense 5 ml medium per quadrant.
6. Place plates of solidified medium in cellophane bags and store in refrigerator at 4 C.

Inoculation, incubation, and interpretation of results. Place 1 or 2 drops of cell suspension or broth culture on each quadrant of Presumpto Plate, and streak ¾ of medium with capillary pipet. Incubate plate in anaerobic system such as anaerobic glove box or anaerobic jar at 35 C for 48 h. Digestion of milk proteins is indicated by a clear zone around growth of organism. If milk is not digested, medium remains cloudy.

Performance testing. If appropriate strains of *Clostridium sporogenes* and *Clostridium perfringens* are tested on LD milk agar as described above, the following reactions occur:

Organism	Milk digested
C. sporogenes	+
C. perfringens	−

Lombard-Dowell (LD) neomycin egg yolk agar (NEYA), CDC. LD neomycin egg yolk agar[77] is a selective and differential medium useful in selective isolation and presumptive identification of certain neomycin-resistant, obligately anaerobic bacteria. It is especially useful in selective isolation and presumptive identification of clostridia. The neomycin egg yolk agar allows one to detect lecithinase, lipase, and proteolytic activities of those bacteria that grow on it. It can also be used for performing the Nagler test for presumptive identification of *Clostridium perfringens* using type A *C. perfringens* antiserum. The medium is prepared by supplementing LD egg yolk agar used in Presumpto Quadrant Plate described by Dowell and Lombard[79] with neomycin.

LD egg yolk agar base:

Trypticase (BBL)	5.0 g
Yeast extract (Difco)	5.0 g
Sodium chloride	2.5 g
Sodium sulfite	0.1 g
L-Tryptophan	0.2 g
L-Cystine*	0.4 g
Hemin*	10.0 mg
Vitamin K_1 (3 phytylmenadione)†	10.0 mg
D-Glucose	2.0 g
Na_2HPO_4	5.0 g
$MgSO_4$ (5% aqueous solution)	0.2 ml
Agar	20.0 g
Distilled water	900.0 ml

---

*In small beaker, dissolve hemin and L-cystine in 5 ml 1N NaOH before adding to other ingredients.

†Add vitamin K_1 from stock solution containing 1 g vitamin K_1 (3 phytylmenadione, ICN, Cleveland, Ohio) plus 99 ml absolute ethanol.

Egg yolk suspension (Difco)	100.0 ml
Neomycin sulfate (Eli Lilly & Co.)	100.0 mg

1. Mix ingredients for base and dissolve by heating.
2. Adjust pH to 7.4.
3. Autoclave at 121 C for 15 min.
4. Cool to 55-60 C in water bath.
5. Add 100 ml egg yolk suspension (warmed to 55-60 C) to base and mix.
6. Add aseptically (from stock solution) 100 mg neomycin sulfate and mix.
7. Dispense 20 ml quantities neomycin egg yolk agar into 15 × 100 mm plastic Petri dishes and allow to solidify.
8. Place plates in cellophane bags and store in refrigerator at 4 C.

Performance testing. This medium should inhibit growth of most facultatively anaerobic gram-negative bacilli. It should support good growth of appropriate stock strains of *Clostridium perfringens*, *Clostridium sporogenes*, and *Clostridium tertium*, and should react as follows with these microorganisms after 48 h incubation in anaerobic system at 35 C.

Organism	Growth	Lecithinase	Lipase	Proteolysis
C. perfringens	+	+	−	−
C. sporogenes	+	−	+	+
C. tertium	+	−	−	−
E. coli	−	NA	NA	NA

Lombard-Dowell (LD) starch agar, CDC. This medium[77] is used in detecting the ability of obligately anaerobic bacteria to hydrolyze starch. It is prepared by supplementing LD agar with soluble starch. The LD starch agar promises to be an aid in the identification of non-sporeforming gram-negative anaerobes and clostridia.

Trypticase (BBL)	5.0 g
Yeast extract (Difco)	5.0 g
Sodium chloride	2.5 g
Sodium sulfite	0.1 g
L-Tryptophan	0.2 g
Vitamin K_1 (3 phytylmenadione)	10.0 mg
Agar	20.0 g
Distilled water	1000.0 ml
L-Cystine	0.4 g
Hemin	10.0 mg
Soluble starch	5.0 g

1. Mix all ingredients except hemin and L-cystine.
2. Dissolve hemin and L-cystine in 5 ml 1N NaOH before adding to other ingredients.
3. Add vitamin K_1 from stock solution containing 1 g of 3 phytylmenadione plus 99 ml absolute ethanol, 0.1 ml/100 ml medium.
4. After ingredients are dissolved, adjust pH of medium to 7.5. Autoclave medium at 121 C for 15 min.
5. Allow medium to cool to 48-50 C and dispense in 20 ml quantities into plastic 15 × 100 mm Petri dishes. If quadrant Petri dishes are used, dispense 5 ml medium per quadrant.
6. Place plates of solidified medium in cellophane bags and store in refrigerator at 4 C.

Inoculation, incubation, and interpretation of reactions. Place 1 or 2 drops of cell suspension or broth culture on each quadrant of Presumpto Plate, and streak ¾ of medium with capillary pipet. Incubate plate in anaerobic system such as anaerobic glove box or anaerobic jar at 35 C for 48 h. After incubation, add iodine solution (such as Gram's iodine) to medium. A blue color indicates that unhydrolyzed starch is still present. If no blue appears, all the starch has been hydrolyzed. It is important that the reaction be read immediately after iodine is added because blue color formed with starch may fade.

Performance testing. Appropriate strains of *Clostridium perfringens* and *Clostridium sporogenes* tested as described above on LD starch agar should react as follows:

Organism	Starch hydrolysis
C. perfringens	+
C. sporogenes	−

Modified McClung Toabe egg yolk agar (EYA), CDC. McClung Toabe egg yolk agar was designed as a differential plating medium to aid in the isolation and identification of clostridia. The modified medium, EYA,[77] supports the growth of various non-spore forming obligate anaerobes as well as the clostridia, and allows one to detect lecithinase, lipase, and proteolysis of cultures.

Trypticase (BBL)	40.0 g
Na_2HPO_4	5.0 g
NaCl	2.0 g
$MgSO_4$ (5% solution)	0.2 ml
D-Glucose	2.0 g
Agar	25.0 g
Yeast extract (Difco)	5.0 g
Distilled water	900.0 ml
Egg yolk suspension (Difco)	100.0 ml

1. Heat above ingredients to mix and dissolve them.
2. Adjust pH to 7.4.
3. Autoclave at 121 C for 15 min.
4. Cool to 60 C in water bath.
5. Add aseptically 100 ml Difco egg yolk suspension.*
6. Mix and dispense 20 ml aseptically into 15×100 mm plastic Petri dishes.
7. After medium solidifies, place plates in cellophane bags and store in refrigerator at 4 C.

Performance testing. *Clostridium tertium, Clostridium perfringens,* and *Clostridium sporogenes* are suitable microorganisms for performance testing of EYA. All of these bacteria should grow well on EYA. Typical strains of these bacteria react as follows:

Organism	Lecithinase	Lipase	Proteolysis
C. perfringens	+	−	−
C. sporogenes	−	+	+
C. tertium	−	−	−

Presumpto Quadrant Plate media (Lombard-Dowell)[79]

Lombard-Dowell (LD) bile agar. LD bile agar[77] is one of the 4 media in the Presumpto Quadrant Plate that Dowell and Lombard discuss in the context of identifying bacteroides and fusobacteria.[79] This medium, because of its bile content (2.0% oxgall), is both a selective and a differential medium useful in identifying bacteroides and fusobacteria. It also promises to

aid in identifying other obligate anaerobes, e.g., the gram-positive cocci. Some organisms (e.g., *Bacteroides fragilis, B. thetaiotaomicron, B. vulgatus, B. distasonis, Fusobacterium mortiferum, F. arium*) grow well on LD bile agar, whereas others (e.g., *B. corrodens, F. Necrophorum, F. nucleatum*) do not. *B. fragilis* produces a characteristic insoluble precipitate in LD bile agar, which apparently is not produced by other *Bacteroides* or *Fusobacterium* species.

Trypticase (BBL)	5.0 g
Yeast extract (Difco)	5.0 g
Sodium chloride	2.5 g
Sodium sulfite	0.1 g
L-Tryptophan	0.2 g
L-Cystine*	0.4 g
Hemin*	10.0 mg
Vitamin K_1 (3 phytylmenadione)†	10.0 mg
D-Glucose	1.0 g
Oxgall (Difco)	20.0 g
Agar	20.0 g
Distilled water	1000.0 ml

1. Mix above ingredients and dissolve by heating.
2. Adjust pH to 7.5.
3. Autoclave at 121 C for 15 min.
4. Cool to 48-50 C in water bath.
5. Dispense in 5 ml quantities aseptically into plastic quadrant plates (Presumpto Plate) and allow to solidify.
6. Place Presumpto Plates in cellophane bags and store in refrigerator at 4 C.

Performance testing. Stock strains of *Bacteroides fragilis, Fusobacterium mortiferum,* and *Fusobacterium necrophorum* are suitable for testing the performance of LD bile agar. These microorganisms should react as follows:

Organism	Growth	Precipitate in medium surrounding growth
B. fragilis	E	+
F. mortiferum	E	−
F. necrophorum	I	−

E = Equal or greater than growth on LD agar control.
I = Less than growth on LD agar control.

Lombard-Dowell (LD) agar, CDC. LD agar[77] is one of the media in the Presumpto Quadrant Plate described by Dowell and Lombard for identification of bacteroides and fusobacteria.[79] This medium supports the growth of a variety of non-sporeforming and spore-forming obligate anaerobes, including fastidious microorganisms such as *Bacteroides melaninogenicus* and *Fusobacterium necrophorum.* A number of aerobic, facultatively anaerobic, and microaerophilic bacteria encountered in clinical specimens will also grow on it if incubated in appropriate environment. LD agar is used for detecting degree of growth, indole production, and catalase activity of *Bacteroides* and *Fusobacterium* species in the presumptive identification procedure of Dowell and Lombard.

Trypticase (BBL)	5.0 g
Yeast extract (Difco)	5.0 g
Sodium Chloride	2.5 g

---

*Temperature of egg yolk suspension should be approximately 60 C before it is added to other ingredients. If yolks of whole eggs are used (2 yolks/L medium), eggs should be free of antibiotics, and shells of eggs should be properly decontaminated before eggs are broken to remove yolks. Shells can be decontaminated by immersing eggs in beaker of 95% ethanol 1 h.

*In a small beaker, dissolve the hemin and L-cystine in 5 ml of 1N NaOH before adding them to the other ingredients.
†Add the vitamin K_1 from a stock solution containing 1 g of vitamin K_1 (3 phytylmenadione (ICN, Cleveland, Ohio)) plus 99 ml of absolute ethanol.

Sodium sulfite	0.1 g
L-Tryptophan	0.2 g
L-Cystine*	0.4 g
Hemin*	10.0 mg
Vitamin K$_1$ (3 phytylmenadione)†	10.0 mg
Agar	20.0 g
Distilled water	1000.0 ml

1. Mix above ingredients and dissolve by heating.
2. Adjust pH to 7.5.
3. Autoclave at 121 C for 15 min.
4. Cool to 48-50 C in water bath.
5. Dispense aseptically in 5 ml quantities into quadrant plastic dishes (Presumpto Plate) and allow to solidify.
6. Place Presumpto Plates in cellophane bags and store in refrigerator at 4 C.

Performance testing. Appropriate stock strains of *Bacteroides fragilis, B. thetaiotaomicron,* and *Fusobacterium necrophorum* are suitable for testing LD agar. These microorganisms should react as follows on the medium when tested as described by Dowell and Lombard[79]:

Organism	Degree of growth	Indole	Catalase
B. fragilis	Moderate	−	+
B. thetaiotaomicron	Moderate	+	−
F. necrophorum	Moderate	+	−

Lombard-Dowell (LD) egg yolk agar (EYA). LD egg yolk agar[77] is one of the Presumpto Quadrant Plate differential media by Dowall and Lombard for presumptive identification of bacteroides and fusobacteria.[79] This medium was designed to support the growth of both non-spore-forming and sporeforming obligate anaerobes and allows the detection of lecithinase, lipase, and proteolytic activity of bacteria. Fastidious microorganisms such as *Bacteroides melaninogenicus* and *Fusobacterium necrophorum* grow well on it. It is useful in the identification of clostridia and non-spore-forming gram-positive anaerobes as well as *Bacteroides* and *Fusobacterium* species.

Base:

Trypticase (BBL)	5.0 g
Yeast extract (Difco)	5.0 g
Sodium chloride	2.5 g
Sodium sulfite	0.1 g
L-Tryptophan	0.2 g
L-Cystine*	0.4 g
Hemin*	10.0 mg
Vitamin K$_1$ (3 phytylmenadione)†	10.0 mg
D-Glucose	2.0 g
Na$_2$HPO$_4$	5.0 g
MgSO$_4$ (5% aqueous solution)	0.2 ml
Agar	20.0 g
Distilled water	900.0 ml
Egg yolk suspension (Difco)	100.0 ml

1. Mix ingredients for base and dissolve by heating.
2. Adjust pH to 7.4.
3. Autoclave at 121 C for 15 min.
4. Cool to 55-60 C in water bath.
5. Add 100 ml egg yolk suspension (Difco) to base and mix. NOTE: Temperature of egg yolk suspen-

sion should be approximately 55-60 C before it is added.
6. Dispense in 5 ml quantities aseptically into quadrant plastic dishes (Presumpto Plate) or in 20 ml quantities into 15 × 100 mm plastic Petri dishes and allow medium to solidify.
7. Place plates in cellophane bags and store in refrigerator at 4 C.

Performance testing. This medium should support good growth of appropriate stock strains of *B. fragilis, F. necrophorum, C. perfringens,* and *C. sporogenes* and should react as follows with these microorganisms:

Organism	Lecithinase	Lipase	Proteolysis
B. fragilis	−	−	−
F. necrophorum	−	+	−
C. perfringens	+	−	−
C. sporogenes	−	+	+

Lombard-Dowell (LD) esculin agar. LD esculin agar[77] is one of the Presumpto Quadrant Plate media described by Dowell and Lombard for identification of bacteroides and fusobacteria.[79] This medium supports the growth of a variety of non-spore-forming and spore-forming obligate anaerobes. Most obligate aerodes, facultative anaerobes, and microaerophiles found in clinical materials will grow on it also if incubated in an appropriate atmosphere. The LD esculin agar is used in detecting esculin hydrolysis, H$_2$S production, and catalase activity as described by Dowell and Lombard in the above publication.

Trypticase (BBL)	5.0 g
Yeast extract (Difco)	5.0 g
Sodium chloride	2.5 g
L-Tryptophan	0.2 g
L-Cystine*	0.4 g
Hemin*	10.0 mg
Vitamin K$_1$ (3 phytylmenadione)†	10.0 mg
Esculin	1.0 g
Ferric citrate	0.5 g
Agar	20.0 g
Distilled water	1000.0 ml

1. Mix above ingredients and dissolve by heating.
2. Adjust pH to 7.5.
3. Autoclave at 121 C for 15 min.
4. Cool to 48-50 C in water bath.
5. Dispense in 5 ml quantities aseptically into quadrant plastic dishes (Presumpto Plate) and allow to solidify.
6. Place Presumpto Plates in cellophane bags and store in refrigerator at 4 C.

Performance testing. Appropriate stock strains of *B. fragilis, B. melaninogenicus sp. asaccharolyticus,* and *F. mortiferum* are suitable for testing LD esculin agar. They react as follows:

Organism	Growth	Esculin hydrolysis	H$_2$S	Catalase
B. fragilis	+	+	−	+
B. melaninogenicus ss. asaccharolyticus	+	−	−	−
F. mortiferum	+	+	+	−

---

*In small beaker, dissolve hemin and L-cystine in 5 ml 1N NaOH before adding to other ingredients.
†Add vitamin K$_1$ from stock solution containing 1 g vitamin K$_1$ (3 phytylmenadione, ICN, Cleveland, Ohio) plus 99 ml absolute ethanol.

---

*In small beaker, dissolve hemin and L-cystine in 5 ml 1N NaOH before adding to other ingredients.
†Add vitamin K$_1$ from stock solution containing 1 g vitamin K$_1$ (3 phytylmenadione, ICN, Cleveland, Ohio) plus 99 ml absolute ethanol.

Differential media

NOTE: **For interpretation of reactions in differential media see Table 72-3.**

Anaerobic carbohydrate fermentation medium base (CHO medium base)* CDC. The CHO medium base[77] is used as a basal medium in preparing various carbohydrate fermentation media used by the Anaerobe Section, Center for Disease Control, to aid in the characterization and identification of anaerobic bacteria. Also, a tube of the CHO base medium, without added carbohydrate, is inoculated with each culture tested to serve as a control for the carbohydrate fermentation media used.

Tryptone (Difco)	15.00 g
Yeast extract (Difco)	7.00 g
L-Cystine	0.25 g
Sodium chloride	2.50 g
Ascorbic acid	0.10 g
Sodium thioglycollate	0.50 g
Bromthymol blue	0.01 g
Agar	0.75 g
Distilled water	1000.00 ml

1. Suspend 26 g dehydrated base (Difco 0841) in 1000 ml distilled water.
2. Heat to boiling 1-2 min to dissolve ingredients.
3. Dispense in 7 ml quantities into 15 × 90 mm screw-cap tubes.
4. Autoclave at 121 C for 15 min.
5. Adjust final pH of medium to 7.5 ± 0.1 at 25 C after autoclaving.
6. Pass tubes with caps loose into anaerobic glove box containing 85% N_2, 10% H_2, and 5% CO_2.
7. Fasten caps securely and remove from glove box.
8. Store in refrigerator or at ambient temperature.

Performance testing. If appropriate strains of the microorganisms are used, the CHO base should support moderate growth (but no acid production as evidenced by a change in the color of the bromthymol blue indicator from blue-green, pH 7.0, to yellow, pH 6.0) of *Bacteroides fragilis, C. perfringens, C. sporogenes, C. tatani,* and *F. necrophorum.*

Anaerobic carbohydrate fermentation media, CDC. The carbohydrate fermentation media[77] are used in various combinations to aid in the characterization and identification of anaerobic bacteria. The media are prepared by supplementing Carbohydrate Fermentation Medium (CHO) Base (Difco 0841) with the appropriate carbohydrate. The fermentation media are suitable for testing non-sporeforming anaerobes and clostridia for fermentation.

Basal medium (CHO base). Same as CHO medium base, above.

Carbohydrate to final concentration of 0.6% with all except starch, 0.25%.

1. Suspend 26 g Difco (0841) dehydrated CHO base in 1000 ml distilled water.
2. Heat to boiling 1-2 min to dissolve ingredients.
3. Autoclave at 121 C for 15 min.
4. To **900** ml sterile basal medium cooled to 45-50 C, aseptically add 100 ml sterile aqueous carbohydrate solution (Table 72-1).
5. Mix well and dispense aseptically in 7 ml quantities into 15 × 90 mm screw-cap tubes. (Final pH of medium should be 7.0 ± 0.1 at 25 C).
6. With caps loose, pass tubes of medium into anaerobic glove box so that atmosphere of approximately 85% N_2, 10% H_2, 5% CO_2 replaces air in tubes.

---

*CHO Medium Base, Code 0841, Difco Laboratories.

Table 72-1. Preparation of anaerobic carbohydrate fermentation media (CDC)[77]

Carbohydrate	Concentration of stock solution* (%)	Amount of carbohydrate added to 900 ml CHO base	Final concentration of carbohydrate (%)
D-Glucose	6.0	100 ml	0.6
D-Maltose	6.0	100 ml	0.6
D-Mannitol	6.0	100 ml	0.6
D-Mannose	6.0	100 ml	0.6
D-Xylose	6.0	100 ml	0.6
Glycerol	6.0	100 ml	0.6
Lactose	6.0	100 ml	0.6
L-Arabinose	6.0	100 ml	0.6
Rhamnose	6.0	100 ml	0.6
Salicin	6.0	100 ml	0.6
Starch	2.5	100 ml	2.25
Sucrose	6.0	100 ml	0.6
Trehalose	6.0	100 ml	0.6

*Sterile aqueous carbohydrate solution sterilized by filtration.

Table 72-2. Reactions of representative anaerobes in carbohydrate fermentation media (CDC)[77]

	C. tetani	*C. tertium*	*B. vulgatus*	*P. acnes*
Fermentation of:				
Arabinose	−	−	+	−
Glucose	−	+	+	+
Glycerol	−	−	−	+
Lactose	−	+	+	−
Maltose	−	+	+	−
Mannitol	−	+	−	+
Mannose	−	+	+	+
Rhamnose	−	−	+	−
Salicin	−	+	−	−
Sucrose	−	+	+	−
Trehalose	−	+	−	−
Xylose	−	+	+	−
Starch hydrolysis	−	+	+	−

7. Fasten caps securely so that they are airtight and remove tubes from glove box.
8. Store in refrigerator at 4 C or at ambient temperature.

Performance testing. If appropriate strains are used and if the cultures are tested as described by Dowell and Hawkins,[77] the results in Table 72-2 should be obtained.

Chopped meat (CM) medium. The chopped meat medium presently used in the CDC Anaerobe Section[77] is supplemented with vitamin K_1 and hemin, and L-cysteine is added as a reducing agent instead of iron filings. This medium supports the growth of most nonsporeforming and sporeforming obligate anaerobes associated with human and animal infections. It is useful as a holding medium for cultures, for sporulation of clostridia, for proteolysis of clostridia, and for toxin production by certain clostridia such as *Clostridium novyi* type A. It is also used for preservation of clostridial cultures by freezing.

a. Lean ground beef   500.0 g
   Distilled water   1000.0 ml
   Sodium hydroxide (1N solution)   25.0 ml
b. Trypticase (BBL)   30.0 g
   Yeast extract (Difco)   5.0 g
   K$_2$HPO$_4$ 5.0 g
   L-Cysteine   0.5 g
   Hemin (1% solution)*   0.5 ml
   Vitamin K$_1$ (1% alcoholic solution)†   0.1 ml

1. Obtain fresh, lean beef.
2. Remove excess fat and connective tissue and grind in meat grinder (fine grind).
3. Mix 500 g meat with 1000 ml distilled water and 25 ml 1N NaOH.
4. Heat to boiling while stirring.
5. After mixture has cooled, refrigerate overnight at 4 C.
6. After refrigeration, skim remaining fat off surface of mixture.
7. Filter mixture through 2 layers of gauze. Retain meat particles and liquid filtrate.
8. Add enough distilled water to filtrate to give final volume of 1000 ml.
9. Add all ingredients in 2 above to liquid except L-cysteine.
10. Heat until ingredients dissolve completely.
11. Cool to less than 50 C and add L-cysteine. Mix to dissolve it completely.
12. Adjust pH of broth to 7.4.
13. Wash meat particles several times with distilled water to remove excess NaOH and spread thinly on clean towel to partially dry.
14. Dispense about 0.5 g meat particles with small scoop into 15 × 90 mm screw-cap tubes.
15. Add 7 ml enriched broth filtrate to each tube.
16. Autoclave tubes at 121 C for 15 min.
17. After tubes cool and with caps loose, pass them into anaerobic glove box so that atmosphere of approximately 85% N$_2$, 10% H$_2$, 5% CO$_2$ replaces air in tubes.
18. After caps are tightened securely, remove tubes from glove box.
19. Store CM tubes in refrigerator at 4 C or at ambient temperature.

Performance testing. Appropriate strains of *Clostridium tetani*, *Clostridium sporogenes*, *Bacteroides melaninogenicus*, and *Fusobacterium necrophorum* are suitable for testing the performance of CM medium. This medium should support good growth of all of these from a small inoculum (e.g., 0.01 ml of 24-48 h LD broth culture diluted to 10^{-3}) if used properly. Typical *C. sporogenes* should exhibit proteolysis of meat particles.

Chopped meat glucose (CMG) medium, CDC. The CMG medium as used at CDC[77] is prepared by supplementing chopped meat medium (CM) with glucose. This is an excellent enrichment broth medium and supports the growth of non-sporeforming and sporeforming obligte anaerobes. Many aerobes, facultative anaerobes, and microaerophiles will grow in it. It is also used to demonstrate clostridial toxins, for sporulation of clostridia, and as a holding medium for anaerobe cultures.

---

*The 1% hemin solution is prepared by dissolving 1 g hemin in 5 ml 1N NaOH and diluting to 100 ml with distilled water.
†The 1% alcoholic vitamin K$_1$ solution is prepared by dissolving 1 g vitamin K$_1$ (3 phytylmenadione, ICN, Cleveland, Ohio) in 99 ml absolute ethanol.

Ingredients. Same as CM medium with D-glucose, 3 g, added.

Preparation. Same as CM medium. Add 3 g D-glucose at step 9.

Performance testing. Appropriate strains of *C. septicum*, *C. tetani*, *C. sporogenes*, *B. melaninogenicus*, and *F. necrophorum* are suitable for testing the performance of CMG medium. This medium should support good growth of all of these microorganisms from a small inoculum (e.g., 0.01 ml of 10^{-3} dilution of 24-48 h LD broth culture) if used properly. Both *C. tetani* and *C. sporogenes* should produce characteristic spores in CMG, and *C. sporogenes* should exhibit proteolysis in it. Also the *C. septicum* and *C. tetani* cultures should exhibit typical toxin production in CMG as demonstrated by mouse toxicity and mouse toxin neutralization tests.

Chopped meat glucose starch (CMGS) medium, CDC. CMGS[77] is used primarily for selective isolation of *Clostridium botulinum* from mixed microbial populations by means of a spore selection technic (heat or ethanol treatment) and for demontsrating clostridial toxins. It is also an excellent holding medium for clostridium cultures because it supports spore production and can be used in demonstrating proteolysis and indole production by clostridia.

a. Lean beef   500.0 g
   Distilled water   1000.0 ml
   Sodium hydroxide (1N solution)   25.0 ml
b. Trypticase (BBL)   30.0 g
   Yeast extract (Difco)   5.0 g
   K$_2$HPO$_4$ 5.0 g
   D-Glucose   3-0 g
   Soluble starch   2.0 g

1. Obtain fresh lean beef.
2. Remove excess fat and connective tissue and grind in meat grinder (fine grind).
3. Mix 500 g ground beef with 1000 ml distilled water and 25 ml 1N NaOH.
4. Heat to boiling while stirring to mix.
5. After mixture has cooled, refrigerate overnight at 4 C.
6. After refrigerator, skim remaining fat off surface of mixture.
7. Filter mixture through 2 layers of gauze. Retain meat particles and liquid filtrate.
8. Add enough distilled water to filtrate to give final volume of 1000 ml.
9. Add all ingredients in 2 above to filtrate.
10. Heat until ingredients are dissolved.
11. Adjust pH of broth to 7.4.
12. Add the following to 15 × 143 mm screw-cap tubes:
    a. Pinch of iron filings,
    b. Approximately ¾ inch of meat particles,
    c. Approximately 2½ inches (7 ml) broth filtrate.
13. Autoclave at 121 C for 15 min.
14. After tubes cool and with caps loose, pass them into anaerobic glove box so that atmosphere of approximately 85% N$_2$, 10% H$_2$, 5% CO$_2$ replaces air in tubes.
15. After caps are tightened securely, remove tubes from glove box.
16. Store CMGS tubes in refrigerator at 4 C or at ambient temperature if necessary.

Performance testing. This medium should support good growth and toxin production by appropriate strains of *Clostridium botulinum* types A, B, C, D, E, F, and G. The medium should also support good growth and toxin production by appropriate strains of *C. septicum*, *C. perfringens*, and *C. tetani*.

Esculin broth, CDC. Used in detecting esculin hydrolysis by sporeforming and non-sporeforming anaerobes.[78]

Heart infusion broth (Difco)	25.0 g
Esculin	1.0 g
Agar	1.0 g
Distilled water	1000.0 ml

1. Combine above ingredients and dissolve by heating. Allow to boil 1-2 min.
2. Adjust pH to 7.0.
3. Dispense in 7 ml quantities into 15 × 90 mm screw-cap tubes.
4. Autoclave at 121 C for 15 min.
5. After tubes cool, with caps loose, pass them into anaerobic glove box so that atmosphere of approximately 85% N_2, 10% H_2, 5% CO_2 replaces air in tubes.
6. Fasten caps securely and remove tubes from glove box.
7. Store tubes of medium in refrigerator at 4 C or at ambient temperature.

Performance testing. The medium should react as following with appropriate strains of *B. Fragilis* and *C. tetani*:

Organism	Growth	Esculin hydrolysis
B. fragilis	Moderate	+
C. tetani	Moderate	−

Hydrogen sulfide (H_2S) semisolid medium, CDC. The H_2S semisolid medium, as its name implies, is a semisolid medium used in detecting hydrogen sulfide (H_2S) production by anaerobic bacteria. It is useful in characterizing non-sporeforming and sporeforming anaerobes. Since it is a semisolid medium, motility of microorganisms can also be detected in it.

Trypticase (BBL)	10.0 g
Yeast extract (Difco)	5.0 g
Lead acetate (10% aqueous solution)	2.0 g
Agar	2.0 g
D-Glucose	5.0 g
Distilled water	1000.0 ml

1. Mix above ingredients and heat to dissolve. Allow to boil 1-2 min.
2. Adjust pH to 7.2.
3. Dispense in 7 ml quantities into 15 × 90 mm screw-cap tubes.
4. Autoclave at 121 C for 15 min.
5. After tubes cool and with caps loose, pass them into anaerobic glove box so that atmosphere of approximately 85% N_2, 10% H_2, 5% CO_2 replaces air in tubes.
6. Fasten caps securely and remove tubes from glove box.
7. Store in refrigerator at 4 C or at ambient temperature if necessary.

Performance testing. Appropriate strains of *Bacteroides fragilis* and *Clostridium sordellii* should react as follows:

Organism	H_2S produced	Motility
B. fragilis	−	−
C. sordellii	+	+

Indole-nitrite medium, CDC. Indole-nitrite medium* is used in the CDC Anaerobe Section to test the

---

*BBL Indole-Nitrite Medium (No. 11299).

ability of anaerobic bacteria to produce indole and reduce nitrates. It is useful as an aid in characterizing both non-sporeforming and sporeforming anaerobes. Although most of the common obligate anaerobes grow quite well in indole-nitrite medium, some, such as *Bacteroides corrodens*, *Eubacterium lentum*, and *Actinomyces israelii*, may grow poorly in it without added supplements such as hemin or normal rabbit serum.

Trypticase (BBL)	20.0 g
Disodium phosphate	2.0 g
D-Glucose	1.0 g
Agar	1.0 g
Potassium nitrate	1.0 g
Distilled water	1000.0 ml

1. Suspend 25 g dehydrate indole-nitrite medium (BBL 11299) in 1000 ml distilled water.
2. Heat with frequent mixing and boil 1 min to dissolve ingredients completely.
3. Adjust pH to 7.2 ± 0.1.
4. Dispense in 7 ml quantities into 15 × 90 mm screw-cap tubes.
5. Autoclave at 121 C for 15 min.
6. After tubes cool and with caps loose, pass them into anaerobic glove box so that atmosphere of approximately 85% N_2, 10% H_2, 5% CO_2 replaces air in tubes.
7. Tighten caps securely and remove tubes from glove box.
8. Store in refrigerator at 4 C or at ambient temperature.

Performance testing. Appropriate strains of *C. Perfringens*, *Propionibacterium acnes*, and *B. fragilis* should react as follows:

Organism	Growth	Indole production	NO_3 reduced
C. perfringens	Abundant	−	+
P. acnes	Moderate	+	+
B. fragilis	Moderate	−	−

Lombard-Dowell (LD) broth medium, CDC. LD broth medium[77] is used to prepare bacterial suspensions to be used in inoculating other media and as a basal medium for preparing other differential media such as LD broth medium with glucose, LD broth medium with lactate, LD broth medium with threonine, etc. It supports moderate growth of most common anaerobes.

Trypticase (BBL)	5.0 g
Yeast extract (Difco)	5.0 g
Sodium chloride	2.5 g
L-Tryptophan	0.2 g
Sodium sulfite	0.1 g
L-Cystine*	0.4 g
Hemin† (1% solution)	1.0 ml
Vitamin K_1‡ (1% solution)	1.0 ml
Distilled water	1000.0 ml
Agar	0.7 g

1. Combine above ingredients except L-cystine.
2. Dissolve L-cystine in 5 ml 1N NaOH and add it to other ingredients.

---

*Dissolve L-cystine in 5.0 ml 1N NaOH.
†For 1% stock solution, dissolve 1 g hemin in 20 ml 1N NaOH and add distilled water to make final volume of 100 ml.
‡For 1% stock solution, suspend 1 g vitamin K_1 in 99 ml absolute ethanol.

Table 72-3. Interpretation of reactions given in differential media for identification of anaerobes (CDC procedures)*

Medium	Purpose	Record
Chopped meat	**Proteolysis:** Digestion usually does not become apparent for several days.	1+B = sl black on edge of few particles 2+B = black on edge of most particles 3+B = ½ meat black 4+B = all meat black S = "sooty black" on tube D = digestion G = gas
Fermentation base	**Control for fermentation media**	G = gas IR = indicator reduction†
Fermentation media	**Utilization of carbohydrates**	A = acid (pH 6.0 or lower) − = no change IR = indicator reduction†
Thiogel	**Gelatin liquefaction:** Place cultures and control in beaker of cold water in refrigerator. Check for lequefaction as soon as control is solid.	+ = liquefaction − = no liquefaction
Iron milk	**Proteolysis**	C = clot G = gas D = digestion
Indol-nitrite	**Indol production:** Extract with 1 dropperfull xylene. Add 1 dropperfull Ehrlich's reagent.	+ = red with Ehrlich's − = no red with Ehrlich's
Indol-nitrite	**Nitrate reduction‡:** Add 1 dropperfull solution A, ½ dropperfull solution B. If no color, add Zn dust.	+ = red with A and B − = red with Zn (may be slow) NO_2+ = red with Zn
H_2S	**H_2S production in lead acetate medium**	+ = obvious black color tr = slight black color − = no black color
Urea	**Urease production:** If phenol red indicator is reduced, add a few drops dilute phenol red to culture last day of reading.	+ = deep red color − = no color IR = indicator reduction
Motility	**Motility**	+ = motile − = nonmotile
Esculin	**Esculin hydrolysis:** Add 1 dropperfull 1% ferric ammonium citrate. Read immediate reaction.	+ = brownish black − = no color change
PYG agar	**Gas production**	+ = bubbles of gas − = growth with no gas
Infusion agar slant	**Catalase:** Expose slant to air 30 min before testing. Add about 1 ml 3% H_2O_2 to growth on slant. Gas evolution indicates presence of catalase.	− = no gas 4+ = bubbling to top of tube 3+ = immediate, many bubbles 2+ = delayed, considerable bubbles

*From Dowell, V. R., Jr., and Hawkins, T. M.: Laboratory methods in anaerobic bacteriology, CDC Laboratory Manual, Atlanta, 1977, U. S. Department of Health, Education, and Welfare, Public Health Service, Center for Disease Control.

†Some clostridia will reduce indicator. If this occurs, prepare dilute solution of bromthymol blue (BTB), using 2-3 drops 1% aqueous BTB/30 ml water in 30 ml dropping bottles. Put diluted indicator solution in depressions of plastic spot plates. With capillary pipet, add a few drops of culture to indicator in spot plate and observe color. Record as acid or negative.

‡Some bacteria reduce nitrate (NO_3) to nitrite (NO_2); others reduce nitrite to other products (N_2O, NH_2OH, NH_3). In nitrate test, solutions A (sulfanilic acid) and B (dimethyl-alpha-napthylamine) are used to indicate presence of nitrite (NO_2 + A + B = red color). Three types of reactions may be observed:

$$NO_3 \xrightarrow[\text{(Bacterial reduction)}]{\text{Nitratase}} NO_2; \text{ add A and B; red color} = + \text{ (Bacteria reduced nitrate)}$$

$$NO_3 \xrightarrow[\text{(Nonbacterial reduction)}]{\text{Zinc}} NO_2; \text{ with A and B; red color} = - \text{ (Bacteria did not reduce nitrate)}$$

$$NO_3 \xrightarrow{\text{Nitratase}} NO_2 \xrightarrow[\text{(Bacterial reduction)}]{\text{Dehydrogenases}} \text{Other end products; add A, B, Zn; no color} = NO_2+; \text{bacteria reduced } NO_2$$

Glucose is added to nitrate medium to serve as hydrogen donor. In agar-containing medium, nitrate reduction by zinc dust frequently takes place very slowly, sometimes requiring 15 min or more. **Any** development of red color after zinc is added is sufficient to indicate that "culture is nitrate negative"; i.e., that zinc is reducing nitrate in medium.

Table 72-3. Interpretation of reactions given in differential media for identification of anaerobes (CDC procedures)—cont'd

Medium	Purpose	Record	
		1+	= delayed, few bubbles
		tr	= few bubbles
Thioglycollate	**Growth characteristics and control for 20% bile broth**	G	= gas
		Describe growth	
20% Bile in thioglycollate	**Growth in presence of 20% bile:** Compare to growth in thioglycollate broth.	S	= stimulated
		N	= no change
		I	= inhibited
Chopped meat-dextrose	**Toxin testing on clostridia only**		

3. Heat to dissolve ingredients stirring constantly. Allow to boil 1 min.
4. Adjust pH to 7.4 ± 0.1.
5. Dispense in 7 ml quantities into 15 × 90 mm screw-cap tubes.
6. Autoclave at 121 C for 15 min.
7. After tubes cool and with caps loose, pass them into anaerobic glove box so that atmosphere of approximately 85% N_2, 10% H_2, 5% CO_2 replaces air in tubes.
8. Tighten caps securely and remove tubes from glove box.
9. Store tubes of medium in refrigerator at 4 C or at ambient temperature.

Performance testing
1. Fermentable carbohydrate content of LD medium must be low enough so that growth of anaerobic bacteria in it does not produce sufficient acid to cause aberrant fermentation reactions in micro-method or conventional systems inoculated with LD broth cell suspensions.
2. LD medium should support moderate growth of appropriate strains of *Bacteroides fragilis*, *Fusobacterium necrophorum*, and other fastidious anaerobes, and of nonfastidious species such as *Clostridium perfringens* and *Clostridium tertium*.
3. LD medium should contain only trace amounts (if any) of volatile or nonvolatile fatty acids when tested with gas-liquid chromatography as described by Dowell and Hawkins.[78]

Lombard-Dowell (LD) medium with glucose, CDC. Used in studying metabolic products of anaerobic bacteria by gas-liquid chromatography.

Same ingredients as LD broth medium with 1% D-glucose added.
1. Suspend all ingredients in **900** ml distilled water (steps 1-4 under LD broth).
2. Autoclave at 121 C for 15 min. Cool.
3. Add aseptically 100 ml sterile filter sterilized 10% aqueous D-glucose (wt/vol) solution. Swirl to mix.
4. Dispense in 7 ml quantities into 15 × 90 mm screw-cap tubes.
5. Loosen caps and pass into glove box (85% N_2, 10% H_2, 5% CO_2).
6. Tighten caps securely and remove tubes from glove box.
7. Store in refrigerator at 4 C or at ambient temperature.

Performance testing. Using appropriate strains of representative anaerobes such as *B. fragilis*, *F. necrophorum*, *P. acnes*, and *C. perfringens*, typical metabol-

ic products should be found in the LD glucose broth cultures with gas-liquid chromatography. Uninoculated LD glucose broth should show only trace amounts (if any) of volatile and nonvolatile acids when tested with gas-liquid chromatography.

Lombard-Dowell broth medium with lactate (LD lactate), CDC. The LD lactate medium is used in studies of the ability of anaerobic bacteria to utilize lactic acid. It is especially useful in differentiating closely related non-sporeforming gram-negative anaerobes. LD lactate is the same medium as LD broth medium, with sodium lactate syrup, 60%, 12.5 ml, added.

Performance testing
1. The LD lactate medium should contain only trace amounts, if any, of volatile and nonvolatile acids (except for lactic acid) when tested with gas-liquid chromatography.[78]
2. Appropriate strains of *Fusobacterium necrophorum* and *Bacteroides fragilis* tested in the LD lactate medium should react as follows:

Organism	Significant decrease in height of lactic acid peak
F. necrophorum	+
B. fragilis	−

Lombard-Dowell broth medium with threonine (LD threonine), CDC. The LD threonine medium is used in studies of the ability of anaerobic bacteria to utilize the amino acid threonine to produce increased amounts of propionic acid. This test is especially useful for differentiating closely related non-spore-forming gram-negative anaerobes. The medium is the same as LD broth medium, with the addition of 3 g DL threonine.

Performance testing
1. The LD threonine medium should contain only trace amounts, if any, of volatile and nonvolatile acids when tested with gas-liquid chromatography.[78]
2. Appropriate strains of *Fusobacterium necrophorum* and *Bacteroides fragilis* tested in the LD threonine medium should react as follows:

Organism	Significant decrease in height of propionic acid peak
F. necrophorum	+
B. fragilis	−

Iron milk medium, CDC. Iron milk is a differential medium used in determining the ability of anaerobic bacteria to react in various ways with the ingredients of whole milk (e.g., gas production, blackening, cogulation, and digestion of milk proteins). This medium is especially useful in characterization studies and in differentiating closely related Clostridium species.

Whole, nonhomogenized milk.

1. Place a few iron filings in bottom of 15 × 90 mm screw-cap tubes.
2. Add 7 ml whole, nonhomogenized milk to each tube.
3. Autoclave at 121 C for 15 min.
4. After tubes cool and with caps loose, pass them into anaerobic glove box so that atmosphere of approximately 85% N_2, 10% H_2, 5% CO_2 replaces air in tubes.
5. Tighten caps securely and remove tubes from glove box.
6. Store tubes of medium in refrigerator at 4 C or at ambient temperature.

Performance testing

1. Whole milk should contain no inhibitory substances or antibiotics.
2. Appropriate strains of *Clostridium perfringens*, *Clostridium sporogenes*, and *Fusobacterium necrophorum* tested in the iron milk medium should react as follows:

Organism	Coagula-tion	Gas	Diges-tion	Black-ening
C. perfringens	+	+	−	−
C. sporogenes	−	+	+	+
F. necrophorum	−	−	−	−

Motility medium, CDC. This medium is used in detecting motility of non-sporeforming and sporeforming anaerobes. Since it contains no added fermentable carbohydrate, it is also a suitable medium in which to **ship anaerobe isolates** to a distant laboratory.*[78]

Motility medium (Difco)	16.0 g
Nutrient broth	4.0 g
Sodium chloride	1.0 g
Distilled water	1000.0 ml

1. Combine above ingredients and dissolve by heating. Allow to boil 1-2 min to dissolve ingredients completely.
2. Distribute in 7 ml quantities into 15 × 90 mm screw-cap tubes.
3. Autoclave at 121 C for 15 min.
4. After tubes cool, and with caps loose, pass them into anaerobic glove box so that atmosphere of approximately 85% N_2, 10% H_2, 5% CO_2 replaces air in tubes.
5. Tighten caps securely and remove tubes from glove box.
6. Store in refrigerator at 4 C or at ambient temperature if necessary.

Performance testing. Appropriate strains of *Bacteroides fragilis*, *Clostridium perfringens*, and *Clostridium sordellii* should behave as follows in the motility medium:

Organism	Growth	Motility
B. fragilis	Moderate	−
C. perfringens	Moderate	−
C. sordellii	Abundant	+

*This medium contains a final concentration of 0.4% agar.

Peptone-yeast extract (PY) broth, CDC. The PY broth is used as a control medium in gas-liquid chromatography analysis of the metabolic products produced in peptone-yeast extract-glucose (PYG) broth cultures of anaerobic bacteria.

Peptone (Difco)	20.0 g
Yeast extract	10.0 g
Cysteine-HCl	0.5 g
Resazurin solution*	4.0 ml
Salt solution†	40.0 ml
Distilled H_2O	1000.0 ml

1. Suspend above ingredients in water and mix.
2. Adjust pH to 7.2.
3. Dispense in 7 ml quantities into 15 × 90 mm screw-cap tubes.
4. Autoclave at 121 C for 15 min.
5. After tubes cool and with caps loose, pass them into anaerobic glove box (85% N_2, 10% H_2, 5% CO_2).
6. Tighten caps securely and remove from glove box.
7. Store in refrigerator at 4 C or at ambient temperature.

Performance testing. Uninoculated PY should show only trace amounts, if any, of volatile and nonvolatile fatty acids when tested with gas-liquid chromatography.

Peptone-yeast extract-glucose (PYG) broth, CDC. PYG broth is used in examining metabolic products of anaerobic bacteria with gas-liquid chromatography.[78] PYG medium is prepared by supplementing the PY base with 10 g D-glucose/L.

Performance testing. Uninoculated PYG medium should show only trace amounts, if any, of volatile or nonvolatile acids when tested with gas-liquid chromatography as described by Dowell and Hawkins,[78] and PYG broth cultures of appropriate strains of control microorganisms such as *Bacteroides fragilis*, *Fusobacterium necrophorum*, and *Clostridium perfringens* should have characteristic metabolic products when tested with gas-liquid chromatography.

Thiogel medium. Thiogel medium (BBL) is used in testing the ability of obligately anaerobic bacteria to hydrolyze gelatin. It supports excellent growth of most commonly encountered anaerobes, non-sporeformers as well as clostridia.

Trypticase (BBL)	17.0 g
Phytone (BBL)	3.0 g
D-Glucose	6.0 g
Sodium chloride	2.5 g
Sodium thioglycollate	0.5 g
Agar	0.7 g
L-Cystine	0.25 g
Sodium sulfite	0.1 g
Gelatin	50.0 g
Distilled water	1000.0 ml

*Resazurin solution—11 mg resazurin in 44 ml distilled H_2O.
†Salt solution:

$CaCl_2$	0.2 g
$MgSO_4$	0.2 g
K_2HPO_4	1.0 g
KH_2PO_4	1.0 g
$NaHCO_3$	10.0 g
NaCl	2.0 g

Mix $CaCl_2$ and $MgSO_4$ in 300 ml distilled H_2O until dissolved. Add 500 ml H_2O and swirl liquid slowly while adding remaining salts. Continue swirling until all salts dissolve. Add 200 ml H_2O and store in refrigerator.

1. Suspend 90 g dehydrated Thiogel Medium (BBL) in 1000 ml distilled water that has been preheated to 50 C.
2. Mix and allow to stand 5 min.
3. Heat with frequent mixing and boil 1 min.
4. Dispense in 7 ml quantities into 15 × 90 mm screw-cap tubes.
5. Autoclave at 118 C for 15 min.
6. After tubes cool and with caps loose, pass them into anaerobic glove box so that atmosphere of approximately 85% N_2, 10% H_2, 5% CO_2 replaces air in tubes.
7. Tighten caps securely and remove tubes from glove box.
8. Store tubes of medium in refrigerator at 4 C or at ambient temperature if necessary.

Performance testing. Appropriate strains of *Bacteroides fragilis*, *Clostridium perfringens*, and *Clostridium sordellii* should react as follows[78]:

Organism	Growth	Gelatin hydrolysis
B. fragilis	Abundant	−
C. perfringens	Abundant	+
C. sordellii	Abundant	+
Uninoculated control	−	−

Enriched thioglycollate (THIO) medium, CDC. This is an excellent growth medium for most sporeforming and non-sporeforming anaerobes and serves various purposes in the isolation and identification of anaerobes. It is especially useful for cultivation of non-sporeforming anaerobes. THIO is prepared by supplementing Thioglycollate medium without indicator (BBL-0135C) with hemin and vitamin K_1 both of which are heat stable and are autoclaved in the medium with the other ingredients.

Trypticase (BBL)	17.0 g
Phytone (BBL)	3.0 g
D-Glucose	6.0 g
Sodium chloride	2.5 g
Sodium thioglycollate	0.5 g
Agar	0.7 g
L-Cystine	0.25 g
Sodium sulfite	0.1 g
Hemin (1% solution)*	0.5 ml
Vitamin K_1 (1% solution)†	0.1 ml
Distilled water	1000.0 ml

1. Weigh out 30 g Thioglycollate medium without indicator (BBL 0135C) and suspend in 1000 ml distilled water.
2. Add 0.5 ml 1% hemin solution and 0.1 ml 1% vitamin K_1 solution.
3. Heat to dissolve ingredients completely. Boil at least 1-2 min.
4. Dispense in 7 ml quantities into 15 × 90 mm screw-cap tubes.
5. Autoclave at 121 C for 15 min.
6. After tubes cool and with caps loose, pass them into anaerobic glove box so that atmosphere of approximately 85% N_2, 10% H_2, 5% CO_2 replaces air in tubes.
7. Fasten caps securely so that they are airtight and remove tubes from glove box.

*Hemin solution is prepared by dissolving 1 g hemin in 5 ml 1N NaOH and diluting to 100 ml with distilled water.

†Vitamin K_1 solution is prepared by dissolving 1 g vitamin K_1 (3 phytylmenadione, ICN, Cleveland, Ohio) in 99 ml absolute ethanol.

8. Store enriched THIO tubes in refrigerator at 4 C or at ambient temperature if necessary.

Performance testing. If used as described by Dowell and Hawkins[78] this medium should support good growth of essentially all commonly isolated anaerobes from clinical materials including appropriate strains of *C. perfringens*, *B. fragilis*, *B. melaninogenicus ssp. asaccharolyticus*, and *F. necrophorum*.

Urea semisolid medium, CDC. Urea semisolid medium is used in detecting the ability of anaerobic bacteria to hydrolyze urea. It is especially useful as an aid in differentiating *Clostridium bifermentans* and *Clostridium sordellii*, two very closely related bacteria. *C. sordellii* actively hydrolyzes urea, but *C. bifermentans* is urease negative. Most other obligately anaerobic bacteria (with a few exceptions, e.g., *Bacteroides corrodens*) do not hydrolyze urea.

a. Thioglycollate without glucose or indicator (Difco 0432-01)	9.6 g
Yeast extract (Difco)	0.8 g
Distilled water	400.0 ml
b. Urea broth (Difco)	15.5 g
Distilled water	50.0 ml

1. Combine ingredients listed under 1 above, dissolve by heating, autoclave at 121 C, and cool to about 60 C.
2. Mix urea broth and water (2 above) and sterilize by filtration.
3. Combine solutions 1 and 2 aseptically and mix. This is the urea semisolid medium.
4. Dispense medium aseptically in 7 ml quantities into 15 × 90 mm screw-cap tubes.
5. Pass tubes with caps loose into anaerobic glove box so that atmosphere of approximately 85% N_2, 10% H_2, 5% CO_2 replaces air in tubes.
6. Tighten caps securely and remove tubes from glove box.
7. Store tubes of medium in refrigerator at 4 C or at ambient temperature if necessary.

Performance testing. Appropriate strains of *C. sordellii* and *C. bifermentans* tested in the urea semi-solid medium as described by Dowell and Hawkins[78] should react as follows:

Organism	Urease production
C. bifermentans	−
C. sordellii	+

Anaerobic agar slants

Anaerobe blood agar (BA), CDC.[77] Same as BA (listed under anaerobic plating media), slanted in 15 × 90 mm screw-cap tubes, 5 ml/tube, to obtain long slant with short butt. Medium is useful in preparing cell suspension for inoculation of differential media.

Chopped meat (CM) agar. Same as CM broth medium[77] (listed under anaerobic plating media), with 15 g agar/1000 ml medium added. Agar is added to 1000 ml broth; boil to melt agar, and mix. Dispense into 15 × 90 mm screw-cap tubes the following: (1) Approximately ½ inch meat particles and (2) About 5 ml cooked meat broth agar. Autoclave at 121 C for 15 min. Allow to cool in slanted position. With caps loose, place tubes in anaerobic glove box (continue as described under CM broth).

CM agar is used to demonstrate spore production by *Clostridium* species that do not sporulate readily. The cultures are incubated anaerobically at 30 C and checked with a microscope for spores at weekly intervals for up to 3 wk.

Heart infusion agar. Heart infusion agar slants are used in the CDC Anaerobe Section for detecting catalase activity of anaerobes and for cultivation of anaerobic bacteria prior to lyophilization.

Beef heart, infusion from	500 g
Bacto-tryptose	10 g
Sodium chloride	5 g
Bacto-agar	15 g

1. Suspend 40 g Heart infusion agar (Difco) in 1000 ml distilled water and mix.
2. Dissolve ingredients by heating.
3. Adjust pH to 7.5.
4. Dispense in 5 ml quantities into 15 × 90 mm screw-cap tubes.
5. Autoclave at 121 C for 15 min.
6. Remove from autoclave and slant tubes at angle to give long slant with short butt.
7. Pass tubes with caps loose into anaerobic glove box so that atmosphere of approximately 85% N_2, 10% H_2, 5% CO_2 replaces air in tubes.
8. Fasten caps securely so that they are airtight and remove them from glove box.
9. Store heart infusion agar slants in refrigerator at 4 C.

Performance testing. This medium should support the growth of various common anaerobes* such as *Clostridium perfringens, Clostridium sporogenes, Clostridium tertium,* and *Propionibacterium acnes* without additional supplements. Appropriate strains of these grown on heart infusion agar slants should exhibit the following catalase reactions when flooded with 3% hydrogen peroxide:

Organism	Catalase reaction
Uninoculated control slant	–
C. perfringens	–
C. sporogenes	–
C. tertium	–
P. acnes	4+

Lombard-Dowell (LD) agar. LD agar[77] is a solid medium prepared by supplementing LD broth, presently used with the API and Minitek miniaturized systems in identifying anaerobic bacteria[80] with additional agar. Since it contains no added carbohydrate and is supplemented with hemin, it is an excellent medium for detecting the catalase activity of *Bacteroides fragilis.* It is also an excellent medium in which to grow various non-sporeforming and sporeforming anaerobes in preparation for inoculating other media or for storage by freezing or lyophilizing cell suspensions. LD agar is prepared like LD broth, with 15 g agar added, and after autoclaving, slanting tubes to give long slant and short butt. After 48 h incubation in anaerobic system at 35 C, *B. fragilis* should give 3-4+ catalase activity.

Reagents used in CDC anaerobic procedures[78]

Bromthymol blue 1%. Dissolve 1 g bromthymol blue in 20 ml 0.1N sodium hydroxide. Add 80 ml distilled water.

Buffered dilution water
1. Stock phosphate buffer solution:

---

*In order to grow certain fastidious anaerobes in this medium it is necessary to supplement it with other ingredients such as blood, hemin, vitamin K, etc. If blood is added, medium is not satisfactory for catalase test.

KH_2PO_4	32 g
Distilled water	500 ml

   a. Adjust pH to 7.2 (usually requires about 175 ml 1N sodium hydroxide.)
   b. Add distilled water to make total of 1000 ml.
2. Working buffered dilution water:

Stock phosphate buffer solution	1.25 ml
Distilled water to make	1000 ml

   a. Dispense in 450 ml amounts in 32 oz prescription bottles or in 9 ml amounts in 16 × 150 mm screw-cap tubes for dilution blanks.
   b. Autoclave at 121 C for 15 min.

Carbol fuchsin 1%
1. Dissolve 1 g basic fuchsin in 10 ml 95% alcohol. Add 5 ml phenol and 85 ml distilled water.
2. Dilute 1:2 with 95% alcohol for use.

Ehrlich's reagent for indol testing. Dissolve 4 g paradimethylaminobenzaldehyde in 380 ml 95% ethyl alcohol and add 80 ml concentrated hydrochloric acid.

Nitrate B. Dissolve 5 g dimethyl-α-naphthylamine in 1000 ml 5N acetic acid.

Phenol red, 1%. Dissolve 1 g phenol red in 30 ml 0.1N sodium hydroxide. Add 70 ml distilled water.

Trypsin, 1%. Dissolve 1 g trypsin 1:250 (Difco) in 100 ml distilled water. Store in refrigerator. Prepare fresh weekly.

Vaspar. Melt together equal portions (wt/wt) Vaseline and paraffin. Mix. Dispense in screw-cap Erlenmeyer flask, and autoclave at 121 C for 30 min.

Vitamin K–hemin solution
1. Stock hemin solution
   a. Dissolve 50 mg hemin in 1 ml 1N sodium hydroxide. Add 100 ml distilled water.
   b. Autoclave at 121 C for 15 min.
2. Stock menadione solution

Menadione	100 mg
95% Ethyl alcohol	20 ml

   Sterilize by filtration.
3. Working vitamin K–hemin solution. Add 1 ml sterile menadione solution to 100 ml sterile hemin solution.
4. For use add 1 ml vitamin K–hemin solution/100 ml sterile medium or 0.08 ml/8 ml tubed medium.

Ferric ammonium citrate 1%. Dissolve 1 g ferric ammonium citrate in 100 ml distilled water.

Gelatin diluent

Gelatin	2 g
Na_2HPO_4	4 g
Distilled water	1000 ml

1. Adjust to pH 6.2 with HCl.
2. Dispense into screw-cap bottles and autoclave at 121 C for 15 min.

Methylene blue indicator

$NaHCO_3$	400 g
Glucose	100 g
Methylene blue chloride	trace

1. Mix thoroughly.
2. Immediately before use, mix about 2 g indicator and about 8 ml tap water in test tube. Mixture should be light blue when oxidized and colorless when reduced.

Nitrate A. Dissolve 5 g sulfanilic acid in 1000 ml 5N acetic acid.

Media for gram-negative anaerobes—Wadsworth methodology
(Sydney M. Finegold)

The following media and instructions pertain mostly to procedures described in *Wadsworth*

Anaerobic Bacteriology Manual (Sutter, V. L., Vargo, V. L., and Finegold, S. M., ed. 2, Los Angeles, 1975, The Regents of the University of California) and reflect the technics of the Anaerobic Bacteriology Laboratory of the Wadsworth Veterans Hospital, Los Angeles.

Preparation of transport systems[81]
Transport tubes

Media (**PRAS**)* described below are used in tubes recommended for transport of clinical specimens.

Agar (PRAS)

Ionagar 2 (Oxoid)	2.00 g
Resazurin solution	0.40 ml
L-Cysteine hydrochloride	0.05 g
Distilled water	100.00 ml

1. Put ingredients (except cysteine) into flask with glass beads and boil until indicator is colorless.
2. Cool medium while gassing with carbon dioxide.
3. Add cysteine. When dissolved, adjust pH to 7.2-7.5 with 20% sodium hydroxide while medium is still warm.
4. Cap flask with rubber stopper, pass into anaerobic chamber,* and dispense 3.0 ml into screw-capped tubes (Pyrex no. 9826).
5. Stopper tubes with recessed butyl rubber stoppers (A. H. Thomas no. 8748) and cap loosely with plastic screw caps.
6. Remove from chamber and autoclave at 118 C (12 lb) for 15 min.

Broth—PY medium (PRAS)

Peptone	1.00 g
Yeast extract	1.00 g
Resazurin solution	0.40 ml
Distilled water	100.00 ml
L-Cysteine hydrochloride	0.05 g
VPI salts solution (see below)	4.00 ml

1. Put ingredients (except cysteine) into flask with glass beads and boil until indicator is colorless.
2. Cool to 45 C while gassing with carbon dioxide.
3. Add cysteine. When dissolved, adjust pH to 6.8 with 20% sodium hydroxide.
4. Cap flask with rubber stopper, pass into anaerobic chamber, and dispense 1.0 ml into screw-capped tubes (Pyrex no. 9826).
5. Stopper tubes with recessed butyl rubber stoppers (A. H. Thomas no. 8748) and cap loosely with plastic screw caps.
6. Remove from chamber and autoclave at 118 C (12 lb) for 15 min.

VPI salts solution formula

Calcium chloride (anhydrous)	0.2 g
Magnesium sulfate	0.2 g
Dipotassium phosphate	1.0 g
Monopotassium phosphate	1.0 g
Sodium bicarbonate	10.0 g
Sodium chloride	2.0 g
Distilled water	1.0 L

Cary and Blair transport medium, modified (PRAS)

Cary and Blair Medium (BBL)	2.5 g
Calcium chloride, 1% solution	1.8 ml
Resazurin solution	0.8 ml

L-Cysteine hydrochloride	0.1 g
Distilled water	198.0 ml

1. Put ingredients into flask with glass beads and heat or steam until agar is dissolved.
2. Gas out with carbon dioxide while cooling.
3. Add cysteine, dissolve, adjust so that final pH is 8.4, and continue gassing with **nitrogen.**
4. Tube in roll tubes while gassing with nitrogen and stopper with butyl rubber stoppers.
5. Steam in media press 15 min on 3 successive days.

Anaerobic "mini-jar"[83]

Sterile 1 dram vial for specimen
35 mm Metal film container with neoprene seal
Approximately 1 g pad of grade 0 steel wool
2 Dram vial of acidified copper sulfate solution

1. Dissolve 25 g cupric sulfate in 500 ml distilled water.
2. Slowly add 1.6 ml concentrated sulfuric acid, then 1.0 ml Tween 80 and mix thoroughly.
3. Saturate steel wool with copper sulfate solution and shake out excess moisture.
4. Aseptically place specimen in sterile 1 dram vial, replace cap **loosely,** and place in film container.
5. Place steel wool pad in film container and tighten lid.

Culture media[81, 84]

Most of the media suggested for use are available in dehydrated form and are prepared according to the directions of the manufacturer. Supplements are listed for each medium where enrichment is advisable or required.

Media used for biochemical tests and fermentation reactions are prereduced, anaerobically sterilized (PRAS), are prepared as described in the VPI Anaerobe Laboratory Manual,[82] and are supplemented with vitamin K_1 and hemin.* The use of thioglycollate-based medium recommended by CDC[77, 78] is an acceptable alternative to the use of PRAS media.

Bacteroides bile esculin agar (BBE)[84a]

Trypticase soy agar	40 g
Oxgall	20 g
Esculin	1 g
Ferric ammonium citrate	0.5 g
Hemin solution (5 mg/ml)	2 ml
Gentamicin solution (40 mg/ml)†	2.5 ml
Distilled water	1000 ml

1. Adjust pH to 7.0.
2. Heat to dissolve. Dispense in 100 ml bottles.
3. Autoclave at 121 C for 15 min.
4. Cool to 50 C and pour plates.

Bile broth

Tests for stimulation or inhibition of growth by bile are done by using PRAS PYG medium containing 2% dehydrated oxgall (equivalent to 20% bile) and **0.1% sodium desoxycholate.** Thioglycollate 135 C can be used to prepare 20% bile broth by adding 0.5 ml 40% oxgall to 10 ml thioglycollate medium. This medium must be used in conjunction with a control medium, thioglycollate 135 C without bile.

---

*PRAS = prereduced, anaerobically sterilized. For details, see VPI Anaerobe Laboratory Manual.[82] These media are commercially available.

---

*Ready-made media are available from Scott Laboratories, Fiskeville, R.I., and Gibco Diagnostics, Madison, Wisc.

†Garamycin injectable (Schering Laboratories) may be used.

Blood agar. The term blood agar as used here refers to Brucella blood agar (described below).

Brucella blood agar. Brucella agar is supplemented **after** autoclaving with vitamin K_1 (10 μg/ml) and 5% sheep blood.

Brucella broth. Brucella broth is used in broth dilution susceptibility tests. It is supplemented after autoclaving with Fildes enrichment (5%) and vitamin K_1 (0.1 μg/ml).

Egg yolk agar

Proteose peptone No. 2	40.0 g
Na_2HPO_4	5.0 g
KH_2PO_4	1.0 g
NaCl	2.0 g
$MgSO_4$	0.1 g
Glucose	2.0 g
Hemin solution (5 mg/ml)	1.0 ml
Agar	20.0 g
Distilled water	1000.0 ml

1. Mix well, adjust pH to 7.6.
2. Boil to dissolve.
3. Dispense 20 ml/tube.
4. Autoclave at 118 C (12 lb) for 15 min.
5. Cool to 50 C.
6. Add 2 ml oxoid egg yolk emulsion per tube.
7. Mix and pour plates.

Kanamycin-vancomycin blood agar[85]
1. Brucella agar to which 100 μg/ml kanamycin based activity is added before autoclaving.
2. Vancomycin (7.5 μg/ml) along with vitamin K_1 (10 μg/ml) and 5% sheep blood are added aseptically after autoclaving.
3. Commercial injectable antibiotics cannot be used.
4. Laboratory standard of kanamycin is available from Bristol Laboratories, Syracuse, N.Y., and of vancomycin from Eli Lilly and Co., Indianapolis, Ind.

Kanamycin-vancomycin laked blood agar
1. Brucella agar to which 75 μg/ml kanamycin base activity is added before autoclaving.
2. Vancomycin (7.5 μg/ml) along with vitamin K_1 (10 μg/ml) and laked blood (5%) are aseptically added after autoclaving.
3. Laked blood is prepared by freezing whole blood overnight and then thawing. See note above about antibiotics.

Neomycin blood agar[85]
1. Brucella agar to which 100 μg/ml neomycin base activity is added before autoclaving, and vitamin K_1 (10 μg/ml) and 5% sheep blood are added aseptically after autoclaving.
2. Commercial injectable antibiotics cannot be used.
3. Laboratory standard or bulk powder is available from The Upjohn Co., Kalamazoo, Mich.

Neomycin-vancomycin blood agar.[85] Prepare as for neomycin blood agar and add vancomycin (7.5 μg/ml) after autoclaving. See notes on antibiotics in neomycin blood agar and kanamycin-vancomycin blood agar.

Phenylethyl alcohol blood agar.[81, 86] Prepare as directed by manufacturer and supplement with vitamin K_1 (10 μg/ml) after autoclaving.

Thioglycollate, supplemented
1. Use thioglycollate 135 C; prepare and autoclave as directed.
2. Fill tubes ⅔ to ¾ full.
3. Supplement with vitamin K_1 (0.1 μg/ml) and sodium bicarbonate (1 mg/ml) in conjunction with one of the following:
   a. Hemin (5 μg/ml), THCK formulation
   b. Normal rabbit or horse serum (10% vol/vol)

   c. Peptic digest of sheep blood, Fildes enrichment (BBL) (5% vol/vol)
4. Thioglycollate should be boiled or steamed 10 min to drive off dissolved oxygen and then cooled prior to addition of supplements. (Hemin can be added prior to autoclaving.)

Urea broth. Prepare urea broth (Difco) as directed. Sterilize by filtration and dispense into sterile screw-capped tubes.

Solutions and reagents[81]

Antitoxin: *C. perfringens* type A. Used in egg yolk–Nagler test. Available from Wellcome Reagents Division, Burroughs Wellcome Co.

Egg yolk emulsion. Used in prepartion of egg yolk agar plates. Available from Oxoid Industries, Inc.*

Ehrlich's reagent. Used in conventional indole tests. To prepare, dissolve 1 g paradimethylaminobenzaldehyde in 95 ml 95% ethyl alcohol, then slowly add 20 ml concentrated hydrochloric acid. Store in dark bottle and refrigerate when not in use.

Ferric ammonium citrate. Used as 1% aqueous solution to test for esculin hydrolysis. Keep in dark bottle.

Fildes enrichment. Used as supplement for thioglycollate medium. It is added just prior to using medium. Available from BBL.

Hemin solution. Used as medium supplement in final concentration of 5 μg/ml. To prepare, dissolve 0.5 g hemin in 10 ml commercial ammonia water (or 1N sodium hydroxide), bring volume to 100 ml with distilled water, and autoclave at 121 C for 15 min. Stock solution = 5 mg/ml.

Kanamycin stock solution. Dissolve 1 g kanamycin base activity in 10 ml sterile phosphate buffer, pH 8.0. Final concentration, 100,000 μg/ml. Store in refrigerator for up to 1 y. Can be autoclaved.

McFarland Standard. See Chapter 70.

Nessler's reagent. Prepare Nessler's compound, A.P.H.A. (Harleco) according to manufacturer's directions. Store in dark bottle.

Nitrate reagents

Solution A:

Sulfanilic acid	0.5 g
Glacial acetic acid	30.0 ml
Distilled water	120.0 ml

Solution B:

1,6-Cleve's acid (5-amino-2-naphthalenesulfonic acid)	0.2 g
Glacial acetic acid	30.0 ml
Distilled water	120.0 ml

Oxgall (40%). Dissolve 40 g oxgall in 100 ml distilled water. Autoclave at 121 C for 15 min. Store in refrigerator.

Paradimethylaminocinnamaldehyde. Used as 1% solution dissolved in 10% (vol/vol) concentrated hydrochloric acid to saturate filter paper for spot indole test. Store in dark bottle and refrigerate when not in use. Reagent can be purchased from Aldrich Chemical Co.

Resazurin. Used as Eh indicator in PRAS media. Dissolve 1 tablet (Allied Chemical no. 506) in 44 ml distilled water. Store stock solution at room temperature.

Sodium bicarbonate. Used as medium supplement in final concentration of 1 mg/ml. To prepare, dissolve 2 g in 100 ml distilled water and filter sterilize. Stock solution = 20 mg/ml. For use, add 0.5 ml to 10 ml medium.

Vancomycin stock solution. Dissolve 75 mg vancomycin base activity in 5 ml 20N HCl; add 5 ml sterile

---

*K. C. Biologicals, Inc., Lenexa, Kan.

distilled water. Final concentration is 7500 μg/ml. Store in refrigerator up to 1 mo or in freezer (-20 C) up to 1 y.

Vitamin K_1 solution. Used as medium supplement in final concentration of 0.1 μg/ml for liquid media and 10.0 μg/ml for agar media. To prepare, weigh out 0.2 g vitamin K_1 (Nutritional Biochemical Corp.) on small piece of sterile aluminum foil and aseptically add to 20 ml absolute ethanol in sterile tube or bottle. Stock solution = 10 mg/ml. Stock solution can be further diluted for use in sterile distilled water. Store solutions in refrigerator in tightly closed container, protected from light.

Biochemical tests and miscellaneous procedures—Wadsworth methodology[81]

Antibiotic disk identification.[87] Use actively growing culture in supplemented thioglycollate medium as inoculum source. Moisten swab and distribute inoculum evenly over surface of brucella blood agar plate. Place the following antibiotic disks on the plate*: Kanamycin, 1000 μg; colistin, 10 μg; and vancomycin, 5μg. An SPS (sodium polyanethol) disk can be also used for *P. anaerobius* identification.† Incubate anaerobically 48 h. Measure and record zones of inhibition: less than 10 mm = resistant; equal to or greater than 10 mm = sensitive.

Bile. Inoculate tube of PRAS PYG containing 2% commercial dehydrated oxgall (equivalent to 20% bile) and 0.1% sodium desoxycholate, as well as control tube of PRAS PYG. Incubate and compare growth in 2 tubes. Observe bile broth for inhibition (less growth than in control; not necessarily total inhibition), no inhibition, or stimulation of growth. An alternative to use of PRAS media is thioglycollate.

Catalase. Cultures on egg yolk agar (or other non-selective medium that does not contain blood) are **exposed to air at least 30 min.** Drop 3% hydrogen peroxide on growth and observe for evolution of bubbles. Alternatively, growth may be removed to a drop of H_2O_2 on glass slide and observed for evolution of bubbles. If subcultures are to be made, this should be done prior to exposure of plate to air.

Egg yolk plate reactions[81]

Lecithinase. A positive lecithinase reaction is indicated by an opaque zone in the medium around the colonies.

Lipase. A positive lipase reaction is indicated by an iridescent sheen on the surface of the growth (observed under oblique light). This reaction may be delayed. Therefore plates should be kept 1 wk before being discarded as negative.

Nagler reaction. Prior to inoculating an egg yolk agar plate, swab ½ of plate with *Clostridium perfringens* type A antitoxin and allow to dry. Streak inoculum across both halves of plate, starting on half without antitoxin. Incubate 24-48 h and observe. Inhibition of lecithinase production on half of plate containing antitoxin indicates positive reaction. This antitoxin is not specific for *C. perfringens*, but is an α-toxin inhibitor. Other species produce α-toxin (a lecithinase) will also give a positive Nagler reaction. These are *C. bifermentans*, *C. sordellii*, and *C. paraperfringens*.

Esculin hydrolysis.[81] Inoculate tube of peptone yeast esculin broth. After good growth is obtained, add a few drops of 1% ferric ammonium citrate solution. A positive reaction is indicated by development of black color. Alternatively, tube may be observed under longwave ultraviolet light (365 nm). Loss of fluorescence indicates positive reaction.

Fermentation of carbohydrates.[81] Tubes of peptone yeast (PY) broth containing various carbohydrates are inoculated. After good growth is obtained, pH is determined using pH meter equipped with long, thin electrode. Interpretation is as follows: pH 5.5 and below = acid, 5.6-6.0 = weak acid, and above 6.0 = negative, providing pH in PY is 6.2 or higher. If pH in PY is 6.1 or less, lower the values for interpretation accordingly. Uninoculated tubes from each batch of medium should be gassed with CO_2 and incubated along with inoculated tubes. Ordinarily pH of such uninoculated tubes will be 6.2-6.4. Occasionally carbohydrate broths such as arabinose and xylose would have pH of 5.8 or 5.9. Therefore pH of less than 5.4 would be acid and 5.4-5.6 or 5.7 would be weak acid production.

Gelatin liquefaction.[81] Test after good growth is observed by refrigerating inoculated gelatin tube along with uninoculated tube of gelatin until uninoculated tube has solidified (usually ½ to 1 h). Remove tubes to room temperature and invert. Positive reaction is indicated if inoculated tube fails to solidify. Weak reaction is indicated when inoculated tube begins to become liquid in approximately half the time required for control (uninoculated) tube to liquefy.

Growth tests.[81] Growth of some anaerobic isolates will be enhanced by addition of supplements, e.g., bile, Fildes enrichment, or Tween 80. If isolate fails to grow well in PRAS PYG, supplements should be added, using PYG as basic medium. After 48-72 h incubation, growth in tubes containing supplements is compared with growth in PYG. If one of the supplements enhances growth, it should be added to each tube required for biochemical tests before inoculation. Same growth test principle can be appied if thioglycollate medium is used as base for determining fermentation and biochemical reactions.

Indole production

Spot test. Remove loopful of growth from **pure** culture on blood agar plate that must contain tryptophan. **Do not** test different isolates picked from same culture plate; this can cause false-positive reactions because indole is a diffusible product. Smear growth on filter paper that has been saturated with 1% paradimethylaminocinnamaldehyde in 10% (vol/vol) concentrated hydrochloric acid. A positive reaction is indicated by immediate development of blue color around growth. Negative reactions give no color change or pinkish color. Late color development should be disregarded.[88]

Tube test. Remove approximately 2.0 ml culture from indole-nitrite medium or chopped meat broth and put into tube for testing. Add 1.0 ml xylene, shake well, and let stand at least 2 min. Slowly add 0.5 ml Ehrlich's reagent down side of tube. Development of pink or fuchsia ring within 10-15 min is positive reaction; yellow ring is negative.

Meat digestion. Test is read in chopped meat glucose. Positive reaction is indicated by disintegration and gradual disappearance of meat particles, leaving flocculent sediment in tube.

Milk. Observe for development of clot in 2-4 d. Observe for gas and digestion up to 3 wk. Tube will gradually become clear as digestion takes place. This may occur with or without clot formation. Determine pH at the end of the incubation period.

Motility. Prepare hanging drop slide from 4-6 h

---

*BioQuest (BBL), Cockeysville, Md. 21030. Note that these disks are not the same as those used in the Kirby-Bauer susceptibility test.

†Personal communication from Dr. S. M. Finegold, May 1979.

thioglycollate medium culture. Observe under high-dry magnification.

Nitrate reduction.[81] Put 1.0 ml test culture from indole-nitrite medium (BBL) into separate tube. (Also remember to remove 2.0 ml for indole test before testing for nitrate.) Add 0.2 ml nitrite reagent A and 0.2 ml nitrite reagent B. Development of pink to red color indicates nitrate has been reduced to nitrite. If no color develops in a few minutes, add small amount of zinc dust and wait 15 min. Development of red color indicates that nitrate was not reduced. If no color develops, nitrate was reduced beyond nitrite (positive test) and remaining portion of indole-nitrate culture should be tested for ammonia by adding a few drops for Nessler's reagent. Deep orange color indicates a positive reaction.

Spores.[81] Spores can be observed in stained preparations (Gram or spore stain) made from solid or broth medium. Some commonly encountered species (e.g., *C. perfringens* and *C. ramosum*) sporulate poorly, and spores are rarely seen. Heat tests are often used if spores cannot be demonstrated in stained smears. Growth from chopped meat slant or other solid medium should be suspended in 2 tubes of starch broth, being careful not to touch loop to sides of tubes above level of medium; at same time, subculture to BAP for anaerobic incubation to check viability. Place 1 tube of starch broth in water bath at 80 C, with water level above level of medium in tube. Place tube containing equal amount of water and thermometer in water bath at same time. Leave starch tube in bath 10 min after tube of water has reached 80 C. Remove starch tube and incubate with unheated tube. Observe for growth (up to 10 d). Growth in both tubes indicates positive test. If growth is questionable on visual inspection, both tubes should be subcultured.

SPS disk inhibition test.[89] This test is used for **presumptive** identification of *Peptostreptococcus anaerobius*. Size of zone of inhibition at 48 h ≥ 12 mm.

Procedure
1. Heavily streak test organism on anaerobic blood agar plate.
2. Place disks containing 20 μl 5% SPS on confluent part of inoculum.
3. Incubate 48 h in anaerobic jar. Examine for zone of inhibition. Zone size ≥ 12 mm. Report as presumptive *P. anaerobius*.
   NOTE: Some strains of *P. prevotii* and *P. magnus* will show a decreased amount of growth around disk, but growth is clearly visible up to disk.

Preparation of disks
1. SPS solution:
Sodium polyanethol sulfonate (SPS)	5 g
Distilled water	100 ml
   Sterilize by autoclaving or by filtration.
2. Disks—sterile blank ¼ in. disks (Difco or Schleicher & Schuell). Add 20 μl sterile 5% SPS solution to each disk with sterile 20 μl pipet. Allow disks to dry at room temperature.
3. Storage
   SPS solution: refrigerator
   Disks: room temperature
4. Expiration:
   SPS solution: 3 mo
   Disks: 1 mo

Starch hydrolysis. Add few drops of Gram's iodine to culture in starch broth. Observe immediately. If no color is seen, starch has been hydrolyzed. If blue-black color is seen, starch is still present and reaction is recorded as negative. This color disappears rapidly, but initial blue-black color is still an indication that starch is present.

Urease. Scrape growth from egg yolk agar or other solid medium. Make heavy suspension in 0.5 ml sterile urea broth. Incubate and observe up to 24 h aerobically. Bright red color indicates positive reaction. With heavy inoculum, urease production usually will be evident within 15-30 min. If indicator has been reduced, add Nessler's reagent to determine ammonia production. Presence of ammonia indicates positive reaction.

Media for Mycoplasma

See Chapter 81 for media for Mycoplasma.

Media for fungi

Beef extract agar[90]
Sodium chloride	5 g
Beef extract (Difco), sugar free	3 g
Peptone	10 g
Agar	25 g

1. Dissolve ingredients in 1000 ml distilled water; adjust to pH 7.6.
2. Autoclave in tubes 15 min at 121 C. Slant.

Beef extract, sugar free, is available commercially (Difco).

Beef extract broth[90]
1. Prepare in same manner as beef extract agar but omit agar. Heat ingredients to dissolve in 900 ml distilled water. Adjust to pH 7.2. Tube in 18 × 150 mm tubes, 10 ml/tube. Autoclave at 121 C for 15 min.
2. For use in fermentation tests add 100 ml indicator solution before tubing and sterilizing.

Indicator solution
Bromthymol blue	0.04 g
Distilled water	100 ml

1. Add small amount of 1N NaOH to make alkaline solution (blue). Let stand overnight.
2. After dye is in solution, add 1N hydrochloric acid until exact neutral point is reached and 1 drop of either acid or base causes complete change in color.

Stock sugar solutions
1. Make **separate** solutions (20 g/100 ml distilled water) of dextrose, maltose, sucrose, and lactose.
2. Sterilize each solution by filtration or autoclaving (**10 min** at 117 C, 12 psi).
3. Add 0.5 ml sugar solution aseptically to a beef extract broth tube (final concentration 1%). Four tubes of broth, 1 of each sugar, are used.

NOTE: Beef extract agar is used for purification of *Candida* species for use in sugar fermentation tests. Beef extract broth is used for carbohydrate fermentation tests and for preparing inoculum for sugar assimilation test.

Cornmeal agar
1. Heat 40 g yellow cornmeal in 500 ml distilled water 1 h at 65 C.
2. Dissolve 15 g agar in 500 ml distilled water by boiling.
3. Mix 2 solutions. Dispense into tubes or flasks.
4. Sterilize in autoclave 25 min at 15 psi.

BBL cornmeal agar without dextrose, 21 g dissolved in 1000 ml distilled water, may be employed.

Difco cornmeal agar with dextrose, 19 g dissolved in 1000 ml distilled water, may be used instead of above formula.

Cryptococcus selective agar (*Guizotia* extract agar). See Chapter 103.

Emerson agar[91]
Beef extract	4 g
Gelysate	4 g
Sodium chloride	2.5 g
Yeast extract	1 g

Dextrose	10 g
Agar	20 g
Distilled water	1000 ml

1. Suspend ingredients in distilled water, allow to stand 5 min, and mix thoroughly.
2. Heat, with occasional agitation, and boil 2 min to ensure solution.
3. Dispense and sterilize at 118-121 C for 15 min.

Littman medium[92]

Oxgall	15 g
Gelysate or peptone	10 g
Dextrose	10 g
Agar	16 g
Crystal violet	0.01 g
Distilled water	1000 ml

1. Suspend ingredients in distilled water. Allow to stand 5 min.
2. Mix until uniform suspension is obtained.
3. Heat with occasional agitation.
4. Boil 2 min.
5. Dispense, and sterilize by autoclaving at 118 C (12 psi) for 15 min. Final pH should be 7.0 ±.
6. Cool to 46 C.
7. Add 30 units streptomycin/ml medium (see **note**).
8. For best results, isolation plates should be made with about 30 ml medium/plate. Plates should be allowed to stand, preferably about 6 h, before using.

NOTE: Littman medium should be used **without** streptomycin when presence of *Nocardia asteroides* or any other organisms having sensitivity to streptomycin is suspected.

Malt extract agar

1. Dissolve 20 g agar in 800 ml distilled water by boiling.
2. Dissolve 25 g malt extract in 200 ml distilled water.
3. Mix 2 solutions. Distribute into bottles or tubes.
4. Sterilize in autoclave 30 min at 15 psi.

Difco malt agar, 45 g dissolved in 1000 ml distilled water, is same as this medium.

Mycophil agar

Phytone	10 g
Dextrose	10 g
Agar	16 g
Distilled water	1000 ml

Final reaction should be pH 7.0 ±.

1. When using commercial medium, suspend 36 g BBL dehydrated medium in 1 L distilled water. Allow to stand 5 min and mix thoroughly.
2. When suspension is uniform, heat with occasional agitation, and boil about 2 min.
3. Dispense and sterilize at 118 C (12 psi) for 15 min.

Mycosel agar. See Selective mycology agar.
Mycobiotic agar. See Selective mycology agar.

Potato dextrose agar

1. Cook 200 g peeled and diced potatoes in 500 ml distilled water. Filter through cotton; make up voulme to 1000 ml with distilled water.
2. Add:

| Agar | 15 g |
| Glucose | 20 g |

   Dissolve by heating and sterilize at 15 psi for 15 min.

Dehydrated medium

1. Suspend 39 g BBl or Bacto potato dextrose agar in 1000 ml cold distilled water.
2. Boil 1 or 2 min to dissolve. Sterilize in autoclave 20 min at 15 psi. Final reaction is pH 5.6.
3. Label of each package of Bacto potato dextrose agar specifies quantity of sterile tartaric acid (10%

solution) that is to be added to each 100 ml sterile melted medium to adjust reaction to pH 3.5.
4. Add tartaric acid to medium, Mix well, and pour plates.
5. Medium should never be heated after acid has been added, since heating in acid state will hydrolyze agar and destroy its ability to solidify.

Rice medium

| White rice | 8 g |
| Distilled water | 25 ml |

1. Place rice and water in 250 ml flask.
2. Autoclave at 121 C for 15 min.

Sabouraud agar I

Agar	15 g
Peptone or neopeptone	10 g
Dextrose	40 g

1. Dissolve agar in 100 ml distilled water by heating.
2. While hot add peptone and dextrose.
3. Boil until dissolved. Adjust reaction to pH 5.0-5.5.
4. Distribute into bottles or tubes.
5. Sterilize in autoclave 30 min at 15 psi.

Difco, BBL, and Case Sabouraud dextrose agars are reliable desiccated products.

Sabouraud dextrose agar with streptomycin and penicillin added (50 units antibiotic/ml agar, added **after** autoclaving) is useful in culturing specimens in which bacterial contamination interferes with isolation of fungi.

Addition of cycloheximide* (0.5 mg/ml) will inhibit the growth of many saprophytic fungi.

Sabouraud agar II. This differs from above formula in that it contains maltose instead of dextrose.

Selective (Sabouraud) mycology agar

Phytone (BBL)	10 g
or	
Soytone (Difco)	10 g
Dextrose	10 g
Agar	15 g
Cycloheximide*	0.5 g
Chloramphenicol†‡	0.05 g

1. Dissolve ingredients in 1000 ml distilled water.
2. When suspension is uniform, heat with frequent agitation and bring to boil.
3. Dispense and sterilize at 12 psi (118 C) for 15 min.
4. Cool and use at once. Remelt not more than 1 time. **Avoid overheating at any time.**

The medium, in dehydrated form, is available as Mycosel Agar (BBL), Mycobiotic agar (Difco).

Trichophyton differential media

Basal media

CASEIN AGAR

Dextrose	40 g
MgSO$_4$	0.1 g
KH$_2$PO$_4$	1.8 g
Agar	20 g
Casein, 10%, acid hydrolyzed, vitamin free	25 ml

For the casein Casamino acids, vitamin free (Difco), 2.5 g, can be substituted.

1. Suspend ingredients in cold distilled water.
2. Heat to boiling to dissolve completely.
3. Distribute in tubes or flask. Autoclave at 15 psi (121 C) for 12 min. Allow tubes to cool in slanted position.

Casein agar is available in dehydrated form as Trichophyton agar no. 1 from Difco.

---

*Actidione, The Upjohn Co., Kalamazoo, Mich.
†Chloromycetin, Parke, Davis & Co., Detroit, Mich.
‡Gentamicin can be used instead of chloramphenicol. Final concentration should be 4 μg/ml medium.

AMMONIUM NITRATE AGAR

Dextrose	40 g
MgSO$_4$	0.1 g
KH$_2$PO$_4$	1.8 g
Agar	20 g
NH$_4$NO$_3$	1.5 g

Prepare as casein agar.

Ammonium nitrate agar is available as Trichophyton agar no. 6 from Difco.

Differential media
STOCK SOLUTIONS
1. Thiamine solution

| Thiamine hydrochloride | 10 mg |
| Distilled water, pH 4-5 | 1000 ml |

2. Inositol solution

| *i*-Inositol | 250 mg |
| Distilled water 100 ml | |

3. Nicotinic acid solution

| Nicotinic acid | 10 mg |
| Distilled water | 100 ml |

4. Histidine solution

| L-Histidine | 150 g |
| Distilled water | 100 ml |

Autoclave all solutions at 121 C for 10 min. Store in refrigerator.

Thiamine-casein agar, inositol-casein agar, thiamine-inositol-casein agar, and nicotinic acid–casein agar are prepared by adding aseptically 2 ml sterile stock solution of vitamin to **separate** 100 ml melted portions of casein agar. Histidine–ammonium nitrate agar is prepared by adding 2 ml sterile stock histidine solution to 100 melted ammonium nitrate agar.

The differential media are available in dehydrated form from Difco (Trichophyton agars nos. 2, 3, 4, 5, and 7).

Wort agar

Maltose, technical	12.75 g
Malt extract (Difco)	15 g
Dextrin (Difco)	2.75 g
Glycerol	2.35 g
Dipotassium phosphate	1 g
Ammonium chloride	1 g
Bacto-peptone	0.78 g
Bacto-agar	15 g

1. When using commercial medium, suspend 50 g Bacto wort agar in 1000 ml cold distilled water.
2. Boil few minutes to dissolve.
3. Distribute into tubes or flasks as desired and sterilize in autoclave 15 min at 15 psi.
4. Final reaction is pH 4.8.
5. Because of the high acidity of the medium, the heating process should be completed in as short a period of time as possible. Excessive heating of this acid medium causes a breaking down of the agar, resulting in inability to solidify properly when cool. Normally medium prepared from Bacto wort agar is soft and is ideal for plating purposes. However, if a medium of solidity satisfactory for streaking is desired, it can be prepared by using 60 g Bacto wort agar/1000 ml water.

Additional media for fungi are described in Chapters 101-104.

TESTS AND REAGENTS
Bacitracin test for group A streptococci

Disks saturated with a solution of bacitracin, 1 U/ml, inhibited approximately 97% of group A streptococci, whereas most other hemolytic streptococci grow uninhibited. The test is per-

formed by placing a disk on a heavily inoculated part of a blood agar plate. The bacitracin test is a **presumptive** procedure; final identification of group A streptococci depends on serologic grouping (Lancefield procedure) or fluorescent antibody grouping.

Preparation of disks:[93, 94*]

1. Cut filter paper disks, 6 mm in diameter, with paper punch.
2. Autoclave and then saturate with saline solution of bacitracin containing 1 U/ml.
3. Dry disks rapidly and store in refrigerator.

For further details of the bacitracin test, see Streptococci, Chapter 76.

Benzidine test

See *Staphylococcus,* Chapter 76.

Bile-esculin test

See *Streptococcus,* Chapter 76. See also esculin test, this chapter.

Coagglutination tests

See Chapter 74.

β-D-Galactosidase (ONPG) test[95–97]

Reagents
1. 1M Monosodium phosphate solution, pH 7

| NaH$_2$PO$_4 \cdot$ H$_2$O | 6.9 g |
| Distilled water | 45 ml |

   a. Dissolve salt in water. Add 3 ml NaOH, 30% solution
   b. Adjust to pH 7. Add distilled water to bring volume to 50 ml. Store at 4 C.
2. 0.0133M   o-Nitrophenyl-β-D-galactopyranoside† (ONPG), buffered:

| ONPG | 80 mg |
| Distilled water, 37 C | 15 ml |

   a. Dissolve ONPG in water. Add 5 ml 1 M NaH$_2$PO$_4$ solution (above).
   b. Solution should be colorless. Store in refrigerator.
   c. Just before use warm portion of buffered ONPG to 37 C.

Procedure. In original procedure a lactose-glucose-SH$_2$ medium was used. However, triple sugar iron (TSI) or Kligler iron agar (KIA) slants can be used with equal results. Culture is inoculated onto TSI slants and is incubated 18 h at 35-37 C.

1. Make heavy suspension of loopful of growth in 0.25 ml sterile saline.
2. Add 1 drop toluene to each tube and shake well, to liberate enzyme.
3. After addition of toluene and shaking, let tubes stand 15 min at 37 C. Add 0.25 ml buffered 0.0133M ONPG to each suspension. Incubate in water bath at 37 C. Read after 1, 2, and 24 h incubation. Positive reaction is indicated by development of stable yellow color.

β-D-Galactosidase (ONPG), Lowe[98] test

1. Prepare ONPG solution:

| ONPG | 0.6 g |

---

*Available as Taxo A disks from BBL, Division of BioQuest, Cockeysville, Md.; as Bacitracin differentiation disks from Difco Laboratories, Detroit, Mich.
†Available from Calbiochem, Los Angeles, or Sigma Chemical Co., St. Louis.

0.01M Na$_2$HPO$_4$ solution*   100 ml
Dissolve ONPG (o-nitrophenyl-β-D-galactopyran-
oside) in phosphate solution at room temperature
(pH 7.5). Sterilize by filtration. Store in refrigerator and protect from light.

2. Prepare ONPG broth:
   ONPG solution (above)   25 ml
   Peptone water   75 ml
   Add ONPG solution to peptone water aseptically.
   Place 2.5 ml vol into sterile tubes. Incubate 24 h at
   37 C for sterility. Broth is stable 1 mo, if refrig-
   erated.

3. Incubate tube of ONPG broth 18-24 h. Appearance of yellow color (o-nitrophenol) indicates
   β-D-galactosidase activity. If heavy inoculum is
   used, test will be positive in 3-6 h. Do not read
   after 24 h.

Principle. Lactose fermentation requires 2 enzymes: β-galactosidase (an intracellular, induced
enzyme) and a permease. When the permease is
lacking, the organism, potentially capable of fermenting lactose, is unable to do so, since the
lactose cannot enter the cell. The test is used to
detect potential lactose fermenters (either "late
fermenters" or "nonfermenters" in ordinary media). If such organisms are cultivated on lactose-
containing media, some of them give rise to
mutants that have permease, and thus delayed
fermentation of lactose may occur. In the ONPG
test, development of β-galactoside permease
mutants is encouraged (the enzyme is induced by
growth of lactose-containing media). The presence of β-galactosidase can be demonstrated
by using o-nitrophenyl-β-D-galactopyranoside
(ONPG), which is attacked by β-galactosidase,
releasing a yellow compound, o-nitrophenol.

When an organism is tested simultaneously for
β-galactosidase and lactose fermentation, the following situations may occur:

Result	β-Galactosidase	Lactose
A	+	+
B	+	−
C	−	−

In A both permease and β-galactosidase are
present. In B the organisms possess β-galac-
tosidase but not permease. In C neither β-ga-
lactosidase nor permease is produced.

Late lactose–fermenting strains of *E. coli, Klebsiella*, and *Citrobacter* are ONPG positive, as are
some lactose-variable or nonfermenters, e.g.,
Serratia, Vibrio, and *Aeromonas*. The nonlactose fermenters (*Salmonella, Proteus*, and
Pseudomonas) are ONPG negative. Late lactose–
fermenting *Shigella* (*S. sonnei, S. dysenteriae* 1,
S. boydii 9), *Yersinia pestis*, and *Y. pseudotuberculosis* are ONPG positive. Although the test is
not recommended as a substitute for the routine
lactose fermentation test, it is useful in differentiating *Salmonella* (ONPG negative) from

*0.01M Na$_2$HPO$_4$ (dibasic sodium phosphate). Add
1.419 g sodium phosphate, dibasic, anhydrous, to
1000 ml distilled water.

Citrobacter[99] and *Arizona* (both ONPG positive)
and also for determining the status of certain organisms other than *Enterobacteriaceae*.

Bile solubility test

1. Inoculate trypticase soy or brain-heart infusion
   broth with organism to be tested.

Preparation of bile

1. Bile may be obtained from abattoir. It is collected
   in sterile bottle.
2. Filter through sterile filter paper.
3. Place in 5 ml quantities in sterile ampules.
4. Seal in flame.
5. Sterilize in autoclave at 15 psi for 30 min.
6. If precipitate forms after a time, it can be removed
   by centrifuging bile and decanting supernatant
   fluid.
7. Filter about 5 ml original culture through sterile
   filter paper or make suspension of 1 of the colonies
   in 5 ml sterile saline.
8. Add 0.5 ml sterile bile. Incubate for 10-30 min at
   37 C.
9. Examine by means of hanging drop.
10. Pneumococci dissolve.

**Sodium taurocholate or sodium deoxycholate solu-
tions.** Solutions of pure bile salts are preferable to ox
bile because former may be sterilized and concentration better controlled. Note that heat-killed pneumococci are not bile soluble. Sodium taurocholate or
sodium deoxycholate is used in 10% solution for bile
solubility test.

Leifson technic[100]

1. Make 10% sodium deoxycholate solution with
   1:50,000 Merthiolate as preservative.
2. Add 2 drops this solution to 1 ml 24 h broth culture
   or saline suspension of test organism.
3. Prepare control of 1 ml culture and 2 drops sterile
   saline solution.
4. If organism is pneumococcus, solution clears or
   organisms are dissolved at once.
5. Examine, however, for at least 10 min before calling test negative.

CDC* method

1. Use 24-48 h broth culture. Broth should contain
   0.5% dextrose to support adequate growth of
   pneumococci.
2. Prepare Gram stain to check for purity.
3. Add 1 drop phenol red indicator to broth culture.
4. If acid, neutralize with 2-3 drops 1N NaOH. (In
   acid medium, sodium deoxycholate may form a
   precipitate and/or gel that interferes with reading
   of test.)
5. Place 0.5 ml neutralized broth culture in each of
   2 small, **clear** test tubes (12 × 75 mm).
6. To 1 tube add 0.5 ml of 2% sodium deoxycholate.
7. To other tube add 0.5 ml physiologic saline.
8. Place in 37 C incubator 10 min. If tube with
   sodium deoxycholate has not cleared, reincubate
   and examine at intervals for up to 1 h.

Alternate method

1. Scrape some of growth from blood agar plate into
   1-2 ml physiologic saline.
2. Shake well or mix with pipet to obtain smooth
   suspension.
3. Proceed with test as described above.

S. pneumoniae is readily soluble in deoxycholate
whereas streptococci are not.

*Center for Disease Control, 1976.

Lauryl sulfate test—Bayliss[101]
1. To 0.9 ml culture add 0.1 ml 2% sodium lauryl sulfate.
2. Incubate 30 min at 37 C.
3. Pneumococci will dissolve in this time.

Colony solubility test (bile)

See pneumococci, Chapter 76.

Bile solubility distinguishes pneumococci from viridans (α, greening) streptococci. Check new batch of bile solution with a known strain of of *S. pneumoniae* (soluble) and *S. faecalis* (not soluble).

Bile tolerance

The test is used to determine resistance to bile of various organisms (streptococci and others). Inoculate 10% and 40% bile agar plates (see Media). Incubate 48 hours. Growth indicates resistance to bile.

S. faecalis will grow both on 10% and 40% bile agar, *S. salivarius (hominis)* on 10% only, whereas *S. mitis* will not grow on either.

Buffers, Sørensen

Sørensen buffer solutions, used to prevent major pH changes in various culture media, are prepared from sodium and potassium phosphates. They can be prepared from anhydrous salts or purchased prepared from commercial sources. Two solutions are needed:

1. Solution A: 15 M Na_2PO_4. Dissolve 9.464 g salt, previously dried at 130 C, in distilled water to make 1 L.
2. Solution B: 15 M KH_2PO_4. Dissolve 9.073 g salt, previously dried at 110 C, in distilled water to make 1 L.
3. To obtain buffers at pH values indicated, mix solutions A and B as shown:

Solution A	Solution B	pH
0.25 ml	9.75 ml	5.29
0.5 ml	9.5 ml	5.59
1 ml	9 ml	5.91
2 ml	8 ml	6.24
3 ml	7 ml	6.47
4 ml	6 ml	6.64
5 ml	5 ml	6.81
6 ml	4 ml	6.98
7 ml	3 ml	7.17
8 ml	2 ml	7.38
9 ml	1 ml	7.73
9.5 ml	0.5 ml	8.04

CAMP test

See *Streptococcus*, Chapter 76.

Beta (β)-lactamase tests

See **determination of β-lactamase production,** Chapter 87.

Carbohydrate fermentations

See Fermentations.

Catalase test

The test **should not** be performed with colonies **grown on blood agar** (red blood cells give positive test).

Test is performed with culture grown on infusion agar slant or with single colonies from plates.

1. Pour 1 ml 3% solution hydrogen peroxide over slant, or pick colony and mix it with 1 drop 30% hydrogen peroxide on clean glass slide.
2. Positive catalase test is evidenced by appearance of bubbles (catalase-producing organisms will liberate oxygen from peroxide).
3. Use **Nichrome** wire, since platinum sometimes causes bubbling.
4. Streptococci and pneumococci are negative, whereas staphylococci and micrococci are catalase-positive.

Catalase test for anaerobes

See Table 72-3.

Citrate utilization

1. "Citrate utilization" in text, unless otherwise stated, refers to test performed with **Simmons citrate agar.**
   a. Inoculate Simmons citrate agar by streaking surface of slant with saline suspension of young agar slant culture.
   b. Incubate and observe 3 d.
   c. Indicator turns blue when citrate is utilized.

Certain organisms (e.g., *E. coli*) are unable to utilize sodium citrate as a sole source of carbon, whereas others (*Enterobacter aerogenes*) can do so. Hence the ability to grow in a synthetic medium containing nitrogen in the form of sodium–ammonium phosphate and carbon as sodium citrate serves to differentiate among such organisms (Simmons citrate agar).

2. Use **Christensen citrate agar** for testing utilization of citrate in presence of organic nitrogen.
   a. Inoculate slant and incubate at 37 C for 7 d.
   b. Red color developing in medium indicates positive test.

Citrate utilization in the presence of organic nitrogen (Christensen citrate agar) is another differential characteristic. Shigellae are unable to do so, whereas many strains of anaerogenic, nonmotile *E. coli* strains utilize the citrate and will grow on this medium.

Coagulase test

The coagulase test is discussed in the section on staphylococci (Chapter 76).

Counterimmunoelectrophoresis

Counterimmunoelectrophoresis (CIE) is an immunologic technic for the **detection** of **soluble antigens** or **antibodies** in various fluids. The presence of detectable bacterial antigen has been shown to correlate well with the presence of disease and other laboratory findings suggestive of infection. CIE has been used widely for detection of bacterial antigens in cerebrospinal fluid, serum, and urine. The technic has also been used to detect bacterial antigens in synovial and empyema fluid, sputum, and artificial media, and to detect specific antibodies in serum. Since soluble antigen is being detected, a positive CIE result may be obtained on a specimen that is negative by both Gram stain and culture. This has been observed, e.g., in patients with partially treated meningitis.

The methodology of CIE is based on the fact that most soluble bacterial antigens are negatively charged in slightly alkaline (pH 8.2-8.6) media. Under the same conditions, antibody (usually rabbit IgG) is neutral or only slightly charged. In CIE, two opposing wells are placed in an agarose gel-coated slide: One well is filled with the fluid to be tested for antigen, and the other is filled with specific antibody. An electric field is placed across the slide such that the antigen, which is pulled toward the positive electrode, will enter a zone of reaction between the two wells. The antibody, which is carried toward the negative electrode by the normal flow of buffer (electroendosmosis), also enters the zone of reaction. The resulting **antigen-antibody complex** forms a **precipitin line** between the two wells. By varying the antibody, the presence and identity of bacterial antigen can be determined. Conversely, the presence of specific antibody can be determined by using a known preparation of antigen.

CIE has now been successfully employed for the detection of numerous microbial antigens in various body fluids. The following antigens have been detected: *S. pneumoniae, Neisseria meningitidis* (group B antigen poorly detected), *Haemophilus influenzae* type b, *Pseudomonas aeruginosa, Klebsiella pneumoniae, E. coli* K-1, and groups B and D streptococci. In addition, *Toxoplasma* and *Pneumocystis*, as well as *Cryptococcus* antigen, also have been detected.

The most useful application of CIE at this time is in the diagnosis of meningitis (primarily pneumococcal, meningococcal, and haemophilus).

CIE can also be used for identification and typing of clinical isolates.

For a detailed discussion and description of technic, refer to Anhalt et al.,[102] Feigin et al.,[103] and Rytel.[104]

See also Goldschmidt's discussion in Chapter 74 of this work.

Cytochrome oxidase

See Oxidase tests.

Decarboxylase test

See *Enterobacteriaceae*, Chapter 79.

Deoxyribonuclease (DNase) test[105]

Certain species of a number of gram-positive bacteria (staphylococci, *Bacillus*) as well as some gram-negative organisms produce extracellular deoxyribonucleases (DNase). Among the *Enterobacteriaceae*, it seems that all *Serratia* strains possess DNase.[106] Some strains of *Proteus vulgaris, Enterobacter liquefaciens, Vibrio* species, and some *Aeromonas* isolates also give this reaction. Among the staphylococci, coagulase-positive strains seem to be uniformly DNase positive.

1. Streak DNase test medium with organism(s) to be tested.
2. Incubate overnight.
3. After growth has been obtained, flood plate with 1N HCl.
4. DNase-positive cultures show distinct clear zone around streak.

Endotoxin test (Limulus assay)

See cerebrospinal fluid, Chapter 75.

Enzyme-linked immunoassays—ELISA, etc.

See Chapter 74.

Esculin hydrolysis

1. Inoculate esculin (slant) medium on slant with 1 drop of 24 h infusion broth culture. Incubate at 35-37 C.
2. Observe daily up to 7 d for esculin hydrolysis. Esculin in medium will fluoresce under UV light of Wood's lamp. When esculin is hydrolyzed, medium turns reddish black and no longer fluoresces.

Fermentations and oxidations

1. If carbohydrate broths with Andrade indicator are used (recommended method),[10] inoculate lightly and incubate at 37 C.
2. Examine daily 4-5 d. Red color indicates acid production. Gas formation can be seen in inverted insert vials.
3. Make certain that insert vials are filled with medium **before** inoculation.
4. Gas formed collects in sealed end (top) of inverted tube.

Many commercial broth media are available for fermentation studies (mainly using phenol red or bromcresol purple for indicator). They are satisfactory and should be handled as the medium described above. In the presence of acid, both indicators change to yellow.

It is important to remember that gas cannot be produced without acid formation. The color of the indicator therefore is always changed to the acid color when gas bubbles are present. If gas bubbles are observed without color change, either the vial in the liquid medium is too large and did not fill up during sterilization, or the solid medium broke for some other reason such as drying. In any event, such bubbles are the result of some technical error and are not due to gas formation by the bacteria.

If semisolid or solid media are used, acid production is indicated by change in color of the medium; gas production is shown by formation of bubbles.

For practical purposes it is enough to test gas formation in dextrose only. If an organism, especially **Enterobacteriaceae**, forms gas from this carbohydrate, it may be considered a gas-former. This permits simplification of laboratory procedures, especially when fermentation vials are employed. Vials are difficult to clean and often get lost during the cleaning procedures. Should vials be used, they must be put in dextrose only; the other carbohydrate media are tubed without them. An exception, naturally, is work with water and milk.

The ability of a particular organism to ferment carbohydrates and the way in which it does so depend on the enzymes it possesses. Generally, pyruvic acid is considered as the key compound formed during the process. Different species or strains may convert pyruvic acid into a large variety of end products: organic acids, alcohols, hydrogen, CO_2, acetylmethyl carbinol, etc.

Anaerobic breakdown (**fermentation**) of a variety of substances results in the production of acid (with or without gas formation). Some organisms break down carbohydrates or other substances by **oxidation** (aerobic breakdown), and the usual fermentation or sugar tests will be negative.

Triple sugar iron agar (TSI) can be used to differentiate fermentative from nonfermentative bacteria. A TSI reaction of acid butt with or without an acid slant is indicative of a fermenter. No change of the butt and slant of a TSI or slight alkalinization of the slant is indicative of an oxidizer or nonutilizer of sugars. Occasionally an oxidizer will show slight acidity on the slant of a TSI. In cases where the TSI reaction is doubtful, to determine if the organism is oxidative or fermentative (or neither, in respect to a particular substance), proceed with **oxidation-fermentation test.**

Carbohydrates, alcohols, glucosides, and other fermentable carbon compounds are employed (commonly termed sugars). Those most often used are arabinose, rhamnose, and xylose (pentoses); dextrose (glucose), galactose, fructose (levulose), and mannose (hexoses); sucrose, lactose, trehalose, maltose, and cellobiose (disaccharides); raffinose (trisaccharide); starch, glycogen, inulin, and dextrin (polysaccharides); glycerol, erythritol, adonitol, sorbitol, mannitol, and dulcitol (alcohols); and salicin and esculin (glucosides). Inositol (benzine derivative) is also used.

The base medium used for fermentation tests is a sugar-free medium (peptone water, trypticase, or tryptone broth) to which the desired substrate is added (either in the laboratory or prepared commercially). Such a simple medium is adequate for enteric organisms and other bacteria. However, fermentations for neisseriae, streptococci, and corynebacteria should be done in rich media (add serum or ascitic fluid or use CTA medium); *Haemophilus* organisms need X and V factors added.

Fermentations, rapid

See Rapid methods, below.

Fermentations-micromethods

Several miniaturized, multiple-test systems are now available that greatly simplify identification of enterobacteria and other organisms.

Compared to conventional tests, the "mini kits" require far smaller amounts of material and yield results in less time. The variety of kits includes a system containing a series of cupules (microtubes) with dehydrated substrates that are inoculated by capillary pipet with a suspension of cells (API); a multicompartmental plastic tube containing various agars inoculated with a wire (Enterotube); a card containing dried substrates inoculated with a broth suspension of organisms (Inolex); a variety of substrates on paper disks (Minitek); a series of reagent-impregnated paper strips placed in small tubes containing suspensions of organisms (Pathotec); and a combination of 4 glass tubes with reagents in agar for a total of 14 conventional biochemical tests (RB). Several of the systems utilize computer-base (numerical) identification schemes; one of the systems (API) employs a sophisticated "profile recognition pattern" based on results obtained with more than 50,000 enteric strains, allowing computer-assisted calculation of the likelihood value of results. The numerical and computer-assisted systems have greatly improved identification of these organisms, recognition of unusual or aberrant strains, and are most helpful in epidemiologic studies. The systems represent a major advantage over conventional methodologies in the clinical laboratory.

The **micro** and **miniaturized systems** are discussed in considerable detail in Chapter 74.

Fibrinolysin

Fibrinolysin is an active substance, produced by some bacteria, notably streptococci pathogenic for humans, which dissolves human fibrin.
1. Inoculate nutrient agar plate containing 10% plasma, heated 10 min at 56 C.
2. Incubate 48 h at 37 C and observe for zones of clearing surrounding colonies. This indicates formation of fibrinolysin.

Food utensil and food equipment surface examination—materials and reagents[107]

1. Sterile Petri dishes, 15 × 100 mm
2. Sterile 1 ml pipets (milk dilution pipets preferred)
3. Sterile cotton swabs on 3 inch wood applicator sticks (Swab sticks are sterilized in envelope or glass container in such a manner that removal of 1 swab stick will not contaminate remaining sticks. In an envelope place end of stick toward one corner so that corner may be torn to expose only 1 or 2 sticks each time.)
4. Screw-capped swab bottle 23 × 70/80 mm *or* 16 × 100 mm screw-capped test tubes (Cork or rubber stoppers may be used, but screw caps are preferred. **Cotton plugs are NOT satisfactory.**)
5. Standard methods agar (**tryptone glucose yeast extract agar**)
6. Phosphate buffer stock solution:
   a. Dissolve 34 g potassium dihydrogen phosphate (KH_2PO_4) in 500 ml distilled water.
   b. Adjust pH to 7.2 with 1N NaOH solution.
   c. Make up to 1 L with distilled water.
7. Sodium thiosulfate, 10%:
   a. Dissolve 100 g $Na_2S_2O_3 \cdot 5H_2O$ in 1 L distilled water.

b. Filter and store stock solution in cool dark place, e.g., refrigerator.

8. Buffered distilled water:

Phosphate buffer stock solution	1.25 ml
Sodium thiosulfate, 10% (store in refrigerator)	5 ml
Tween 80 or Tween 20*	10 g
Asolectin† (weigh rapidly—very hygroscopic)	4 g
Distilled water to make 1 L	

   a. Adjust this solution so that pH will be 7.1-7.3 after sterilization.
   b. When hot water alone is used as sanitizing rinse and chlorine and/or quaternary ammonium compounds are known **not** to be used for sanitizing, the neutralizing agents thiosulfate, Asolectin, and Tween may be omitted from rinse solutions.

9. Swab vials: Distribute diluted solution above in swab vials in amount that will provide exactly 1 ml after sterilization, for each utensil examined. We add 4.1 ml to each vial to obtain 4 ml in each vial. Sterilize at 121 C for 20 min with vial caps slightly loosened.

Galactosidase test

See β-D-Galactosidase (ONPG) test.

Gas-liquid chromatography

See Chapter 74.

Gelatin liquefaction

1. a. Use nutrient gelatin medium for aerobes and thioglycollate gelatin medium for anaerobes.
   b. Nutrient gelatin medium should be incubated at 20 C.
   c. After 24 and 48 h, 1 wk, 2 wk, and 3 wk, put tubes in refrigerator for 30 min.
   d. If medium does not solidify, gelatin has been decomposed.
2. Alternate procedure (CDC, 1976)
   a. Medium is 12% Bacto-gelatin in heart infusion broth at pH 7.4. Tube 5 ml in 16 × 125 mm screw-cap tubes. Autoclave at 121 C for 15 min.
   b. Inoculate with 4 drops of 24 h infusion broth culture. Incubate at 35-37 C.
   c. Check for liquefaction daily by placing tube in refrigerator along with uninoculated control. Tests are read for liquefaction as soon as control hardens. Tests are held up to 14 d before being reported as negative.

Gluconate oxidation

Gluconate is converted by some organisms (such as *Pseudomonas aeruginosa*) to 2-ketogluconate. The latter can be detected by appearance of a reducing substance in the medium after adding a copper salt solution (such as Benedict [see below]) to the medium.

1. Inoculate gluconate broth (or use prepared gluconate tablet‡) heavily with culture to be tested. Incubate overnight at 37 C.
2. Add Benedict qualitative solution. Mix and boil 10 min. Brown, tan, or orange precipitate indicates positive reaction.
3. Cowan and Steel[108] recommend, as an alternative, the addition of 1 Clinitest tablet (Ames) in place

---

*Atlas Powder Co., Wilmington, Del.
†Assoc. Concentrates, Division American Lecithin Co., Inc., Long Island, N.Y.
‡Key Scientific Products Co., Los Angeles.

---

of Benedict reagent. Observe for formation of colored precipitate.

Benedict solution, qualitative

$CuSO_4 \cdot 5H_2O$	1.73 g
Sodium citrate	17.30 g
Na_2CO_3 (anhydrous)	10 g
Distilled water	to 100 ml

1. To 60 ml water, add carbonate and sodium citrate. Dissolve.
2. To 20 ml water, add copper sulfate and let it dissolve.
3. Add copper sulfate solution to first solution, with constant stirring.
4. Adjust volume with water to 100 ml.
5. Store at room temperature; do not refrigerate, since it will crystallize.

Hemolysin test for V. cholerae and V. El Tor biotype

See *Vibrio cholerae*, Chapter 79.

Hemolysis

Blood agar plates are used to study the ability of bacteria to hemolyze blood.

1. Incubate plates for 24 and 48 h.
2. Poured plates give most reliable results.
3. Add bacterial suspension or liquid culture to blood agar while it is still liquid (temperature must be as low as possible) and pour plates.
4. Allow to solidify and incubate 24 h, then observe for hemolysis; if no hemolysis has occurred, reincubate for another 24 h.

Hippurate test

1. Inoculate hippurate broth and incubate 24 h at 35 C. Centrifuge medium to pack cells.
2. Transfer 0.8 ml of clear supernate to small test tube. Add 0.2 ml reagent (2 ml concentrated hydrochloric acid, 98 ml distilled water, and 12 g ferric chloride, $FeCl_3 \cdot 6H_2O$). Mix well.
3. Observe after 15 min for precipitation.

The test is based on the ability of certain bacteria to hydrolyze sodium hippurate to benzoate. The ferric chloride precipitates both the hippurate and the benzoate. The hippurate is more readily soluble in excess. The concentration of hippurate in the medium is critical (it must be 1%). Include uninoculated tube of medium as control. The presence of a **permanent** precipitate after 15 min indicates positive test (presence of benzoate).

Hippurate rapid test

See Rapid methods.

Hydrogen sulfide production
Recommended method[1]

1. Use triple sugar iron agar (TSI) medium.
2. Stab butt and streak slant of medium. Incubate at 37 C.
3. Observe daily 7 d for blackening caused by hydrogen sulfide.

Lead acetate paper method

For certain fastidious organisms (**not** *Enterobacteriaceae*), the **lead acetate paper** method can be used.*

---

*Lead acetate paper strips are available from American Indicator Paper Co., Chicago.

1. Dissolve 10 g lead acetate, neutral, in 50 ml boiling distilled water.
2. Immerse strips of filter paper, about 2½ × ¼ in., in this solution.
3. Dry in incubator and store in well-stoppered bottles.
4. Inoculate broth cultures or slants containing peptone favorable to production of hydrogen sulfide, such as thiopeptone or proteose-peptone no. 3.
5. Insert strip of lead acetate paper between plug and neck so that it reaches into tube but does not touch medium. Incubate.
6. Observe paper for evidences of blackening or browning, which indicate H_2S formation.

The TSI method is recommended for *Enterobacteriaceae* and other nonfastidious organisms. The lead acetate method is to be used with *Brucella* (and other fastidious organisms), in a semiquantitative way, by replacing the papers with new ones each day for 4 days.

In the TSI test, thiosulfate is reduced to hydrogen sulfide in the presence of a hydrogen donor by bacteria possessing a specific enzyme, as follows:

$$Na_2S_2O_3 + 2H^+ \rightarrow H_2S + Na_2SO_3$$

The H_2S produced will react with the iron (ferrous sulfate) in the medium to give a black precipitate of ferrous sulfide.

Other methods utilize the black discoloration by H_2S of lead acetate, ferric citrate, etc.

Indole test

The test distinguishes bacteria capable of producing indole from tryptophan (depending on the presence of the enzyme tryptophanase) from those unable to do so.

Inoculate **peptone water** or 2% tryptone broth from an overnight slant or broth culture; incubate at 37 C for 48 h.

Kovacs method[1]

Reagent

Pure amyl *or* isoamyl alcohol	150 ml
Para-dimethylaminobenzaldehyde	10 g
Concentrated pure hydrochloric acid	50 ml

1. Dissolve aldehyde in alcohol and add acid slowly.
2. Reagent should be prepared in small quantities.
3. Store in refrigerator when not in use.

Procedure

1. Add 0.5 ml reagent to culture and shake gently. Deep red color develops in presence of indole.

Ehrlich's method

Reagent

Ethyl alcohol, 95%	95 ml
Para-dimethylaminobenzaldehyde	1 g
Hydrochloric acid, conc.	20 ml

1. Dissolve aldehyde in alcohol and then slowly add acid. Dry aldehyde should be light straw in color.
2. Ehrlich's reagent should be prepared in small quantities and stored in refrigerator when not in use.

Procedure

1. Incubate tryptone broth culture at 35-37 C for 48 h.

2. Add 1 ml xylene to culture and shake vigorously to extract indole. Allow to stand 1-2 min for xylene extract to layer on top.
3. Add 0.5 ml Ehrlich's reagent down side of tube. It should form layer between broth and xylene. If indole is present, red ring will develop just below xylene layer.

NOTE: Tests for indole production with either Ehrlich's or Kovacs reagents may be made after 24 h incubation, but all negative tests should be repeated on separate 48 h broth culture.

Indole paper strip method—Weil-Saphra[109]

The method can be used with lysine-iron agar slants (or other media rich in tryptophan, such as trypticase soy agar). Do **not** use TSI or Kligler agar.

1. Saturate paper strips, approx. 2½ × ¼ in., with Kovacs reagent (see above).* Dry strips in incubator; store in well-stoppered bottle.
2. Insert strip between plug or stopper and neck so that it reaches into tube but does not touch inoculated medium.
3. Incubate overnight. Positive reaction is indicated by appearance of red coloring on strip. **All negative tests for indole obtained by this method should be retested by conventional methods.**

NOTE: **Oxalic acid paper** can be used in place of paper strip impregnated with Kovacs reagent. Impregnate filter paper strips (1 × 6 cm) with hot saturated aqueous oxalic acid solution. Dry at 50-60 C and store in tightly closed container.

Indole rapid tests

See Rapid methods.

Indophenol oxidase

See Oxidase tests.

KCN test

See *Enterobacteriaceae*, Chapter 79.

β-Lactamase tests

See Chapter 87.

Lactic acid (in CSF)

See Cerebrospinal fluid, Chapter 75.

Limulus assay (Limulus amebocyte lysate assay for endotoxin)

See Cerebrospinal fluid, Chapter 75.

Malonate utilization[1]

1. Inoculate sodium malonate broth from young agar slant or broth culture (preferably with 3 mm loopful of broth culture).
2. Incubate at 37 C for 48 h.
3. Positive test is evidenced by change from green to Prussian blue in medium.

The test is used in differentiation of salmonellae and *Arizona* strains and is also of value in other areas of the *Enterobacteriaceae* family.

---

*Weil and Saphra recommend the following reagent:

Para-dimethylaminobenzaldehyde	5 g
Methyl alcohol	50 ml
Phosphoric acid, reagent grade	10 ml

Methyl red test

1. Inoculate tubes of methyl red–Voges-Proskauer medium and incubate **2 d.**
2. To each 5 ml medium add 5 drops freshly prepared solution of methyl red.
3. Red color indicates positive reaction.
4. Methyl red solution is prepared by dissolving 0.1 g methyl red in 300 ml 95% ethyl alcohol. Dilute to 500 ml with H_2O.

Test is based on final hydrogen ion concentration (acidity) reached by culture in broth containing dextrose after **2 d** incubation at 37 C. Test will be positive if pH is 4.5 or lower and negative if pH is above 4.5.

Micromethods

See Fermentations-micromethods, this chapter, and Chapter 74.

Milk reactions

1. Inoculate bromcresol purple milk or anaerobic iron milk.
2. Record formation of acid, gas, clotting, and peptonization.

Milk contains galactose, lactose, casein, and a small amount of dextrose and salts. If acid is produced, the color of the indicator changes; if much acid is produced, a clot is formed. Rennet produces a clot also that afterward contracts and expresses a clear whey. If proteolytic enzymes are produced, the clot is peptonized.

Miniaturized methods

See Chapter 74.

Motility

Motility can be examined microscopically by the dark-field technic or by hanging drop preparation.

Hanging drop method

1. Use young (6-24 h), actively growing 25 C broth culture. Place 1 loopful of culture in center of a no. 1 cover slip. On each corner of cover slip put small drop of immersion oil. Invert cover slip over concavity of depression slide. Examine with high dry (4 mm) objective, if possible. If this magnification is inadequate, use oil immersion, taking care not to crack cover slip.
2. In hanging drop preparation, motility must be differentiated from brownian movement and flow of fluid caused by pressure on cover slip. In true motility, organisms change position with respect to each other, whereas in brownian movement and fluid flow they may appear quite active but remain in same relative position to other organisms or debris in field.

A more reliable and recommended method is inoculation of **semisolid media.** Several motility media are listed; for *Enterobacteriaceae* and other nonfastidious organisms use motility test medium.

Semisolid agar method

1. Take small amount of growth on straight needle from 18-24 h infusion agar slant culture or plate.
2. Inoculate once to a depth of only ¼- ½ in. in middle of tube.
3. Incubate at 35-37 C and examine daily up to 7 d. Motile organisms will spread out into medium from site of inoculation.

Nitrate reduction

For aerobic organisms use nitrate medium; inoculate by stabbing into column. For anaerobes use anaerobic nitrate broth or indol-nitrite broth. Incubate nitrate medium 24 h at 37 C; anaerobic medium, for 48 h.

1. Prepare following reagents[1]:
   a. Dissolve 8 g sulfanilic acid in 1000 ml 5N acetic acid.
   b. Dissolve 5 g α-naphthylamine in 1000 ml 5N acetic acid.
2. Just before use, mix equal parts of a and b; add 0.1 ml mixture to culture. Development of red color in 1-3 min indicates reduction of nitrate to nitrite (positive test).
3. **Negative tests should be confirmed by adding minute amount of zinc dust to culture. Development of red color proves presence of unreduced nitrate.**

Nitrate reduction can be accomplished by certain bacteria; it can be shown by detecting the presence of one of the breakdown products (such as nitrite, nitrous oxide, etc.) or by proving the disappearance of nitrate from the medium. If $-NO_3$ is reduced to $-NO_2$, the sulfanilic acid in acetic acid solution added will bring about the formation of nitrous acid (nitrite + acetic acid), which in turn will diazotize the sulfanilic acid to a diazonium salt. The addition of α-naphthylamine results in its coupling with the diazo compound to form a red or purple dye.

The Center for Disease Control (*CDC Laboratory Methods in Special Medical Bacteriology,* 1976) recommends the following reagents:

Nitrite test reagents
Solution 1
Glacial acetic acid	100.0 ml
Distilled water	250.0 ml
Sulfanilic acid	2.8 g

Solution 2
Glacial acetic acid	100.0 ml
Distilled water	250.0 ml
Dimethyl-α-naphthylamine	2.1 ml

Alternate reagent
Solution 1
Glacial acetic acid	30.0 ml
Distilled water	120.0 ml
Sulfanilic acid	0.5 g

Solution 2
Glacial acetic acid	30.0 ml
Distilled water	120.0 ml
1,6-Cleve's acid (5-amino-2-naphthalenesulfonic acid)	0.2 g

1. Add water to Cleve's acid and warm with frequent shaking until most of compound is dissolved. Almost all of compound will dissolve in reasonably warm water. Do not boil.
2. Filter solution, cool, and then add acetic acid.
3. Use same procedure with reagent 1 and filter if necessary.
4. Store reagents in refrigerator.

Procedure
1. To 48 h nitrate broth culture add 0.25 ml nitrite reagent 1 and 0.25 ml nitrite reagent 2.
2. Observe for red color developing within 1-2 min. Red color indicates presence of nitrites. If no red color develops it may mean that (1) nitrate in medium has not been reduced or (2) it has been reduced beyond nitrite state to some other compound or to nitrogen, as detected in gas insert

vials. To determine which has taken place, add a little powdered zinc to tube. If nitrates are still present they will be reduced by zinc, and red color will develop in 5-10 min.

For a further discussion of the nitrate reduction test, see footnote for Table 72-3.

ONPG test

See β-D-Galactosidase test.

Optochin

Optochin (ethylhydrocupreine hydrochloride) inhibits the growth of pneumococci, whereas greening streptococci grow in its presence. Disks impregnated with Optochin are placed on blood plate inoculated heavily with suspected organisms. A large, 15-30 mm zone of inhibition is seen with pneumococci after overnight incubation, whereas no zone or 10 mm zone is seen with streptococci.

Preparation of Optochin disks[110]*

1. Sterilize disks of filter paper 8 mm in diameter by dry heat at 160 C for 1½ h. Then add to each disk 0.02 ml 1:400 solution Optochin; dry them at 37 C.
2. Solution can be kept in refrigerator for some weeks. It is unaffected by autoclaving. Do not sterilize disks with added solution, since considerable loss of potency occurs. Disks prepared as just described, stored in screw-capped bottles in refrigerator, were found to remain stable 9 mo. Commercially prepared disks are available (Difco, BBL).

For further details of the procedure, see Pneumococcus, Chapter 76.

Organic acid utilization

See Organic acid media.

Oxidase tests

The members of the genus *Neisseria* and some other bacteria (notably *Pseudomonas*) and yeasts possess an oxidizing enzyme that, in the presence of air, acts on certain aromatic amines to produce colored compounds.

Performance of the test is described under *Neisseria gonorrhoeae*.

Oxidase tests for Neisseria

NOTE: Oxidase reagent is toxic, and care should be taken to protect skin from direct contact.

Method 1

Reagent. 0.5-1.0% dimethyl-*p*-phenylenediamine hydrochloride. Prepare fresh each day in distilled water.

Test
1. With capillary pipet or platinum wire loop,† drop oxidase reagent on suspected colonies on Thayer-Martin (TM) plates or in Transgrow bottles.
2. If growth is sparse, remove colony for subculturing

before applying oxidase reagent to colony site where color changes will be observed.
3. *Positive oxidase reaction:* colonies will develop pink color progressing to maroon, dark red, and finally black in 5-30 min.

NOTE: Oxidase reaction may be slower in a Transgrow bottle than on a Thayer-Martin plate.

Method 2: Kovacs' test[111]

Reagent. 0.5-1.0% solution tetramethyl-*p*-phenylenediamine hydrochloride. Store for no more than 1 wk at 4-10 C.

Test
1. Moisten strip of filter paper with oxidase reagent.
2. With sterile loop,* remove portion of suspected colony from TM plate or Transgrow bottle and rub on moistened filter paper.
3. *Positive oxidase reaction:* area where bacteria are deposited on filter paper will turn dark purple within 10 s.
4. *Delayed positive oxidase reaction:* color change takes 10-60 s to develop. This reaction is not typical of *Neisseria* strains; such cultures should be reexamined using fresh young subculture.

NOTE: Kovacs' filter paper method 2 is more sensitive than method 1.

Impregnated disks for the oxidase test are available commercially (Taxo N disk, BBL; Oxidase disk, Difco; Pathotec-CO test paper, Warner-Chilcott). These are **not** recommended for work with the gonococcus but may be used with gram-negative rods.

Cytochrome oxidase (indophenol oxidase)† test for differentiation of Enterobacteriaceae and other gram-negative organisms–Ewing-Johnson modification[112]

1. Grow culture on nutrient agar slants 18-20 h.
2. Prepare following reagents:
   a. Dissolve 0.1 g α-naphthol in 10 ml ethyl alcohol, 95%.
   b. Dissolve 0.1 g *p*-aminodimethylaniline oxalate in 10 ml distilled water.
3. After incubation introduce 2-3 drops each reagent into tubes and tilt them so that reagents are mixed and flow over entire slants. Positive results are indicated by **intense blue color** within **30 s** (maximum, 60 s). All *Enterobacteriaceae* give negative result, whereas *Pseudomonas, Alcaligenes, Aeromonas,* and *Vibrio* give positive reactions.

Oxidation-fermentation (OF) test— Hugh-Leifson[44]

The test is used to differentiate microorganisms that break down carbohydrates oxidatively, rather than fermentatively (see **Fermentations**). It is useful in distinguishing many gram-negative oxidative rods (e.g., *Pseudomonas,* Mimeae) or those that do not utilize dextrose in either way (*Alcaligenes,* etc.) from the *Enterobacteriaceae,* which are fermentative. Performance of the test is described under oxidation-fermentation medium; see also Fermentations and oxidations, above.

---

*Available as Taxo P disks from BBL, Division of BioQuest, Cockeysville, Md.; as Optochin disks from Difco Laboratories, Detroit, Mich.
†Wire loops made of iron-containing wire (e.g., nichrome, chromel) may cause false-positive reactions.

---

*Wire loops made of iron-containing wire (e.g., nicrome, chromel) may cause false-positive reactions.
†The test was called cytochrome oxidase in the United States until about 1965; since then the 2 designations are used interchangeably.

Phenylalanine test—Ewing-Davis-Reavis[47]

1. Inoculate slant of phenylalanine agar.
2. Incubate 4 h or 18-24 h at 37 C.
3. Prepare reagent by dissolving 1 g ferric chloride in 10 ml distilled water.
4. After incubation let 4-5 drops of reagent run down over growth. Green color forming in syneresis fluid and in the slant proves the formation of phenylpyruvic acid.

See also Rapid methods.

Phenylketonuria (PKU) inhibition assay[49,113,114]*

Phenylketonuria is an inborn (congenital) metabolic defect characterized by the absence of the enzyme phenylalanine hydroxylase and the subsequent failure to metabolize phenylalanine, which is present in most proteins. In infants with this defect, phenylalanine accumulates in the blood and phenylketones are excreted in the urine. Phenylalanine accumulating in the blood results in brain damage and mental retardation. If phenylketonuria can be detected early enough and if the infant is placed on a low-phenylalanine diet, brain damage and mental retardation can be prevented.

Although other tests are available (e.g., ferric chloride test, fluorometric procedure), the Guthrie PKU test has been widely employed. It is based on the finding that β-2-thienylalanine inhibits the growth of *Bacillus subtilis* in a minimal medium; however, when phenylalanine is added, the inhibition of *B. subtilis* is prevented. Blood from a heel puncture is placed on filter paper disks that in turn are placed on the culture medium containing β-2-thienylalanine and *B. subtilis*. If the test disk is impregnated with blood containing phenylalanine, a zone of growth will be seen on incubation. Control disks impregnated with known amounts of phenylalanine are also used, and the growth zone around the test disk(s) is compared to that shown by the control disks.

A zone comparable to that produced by the 4 mg/100 ml control disk is considered "presumptive positive."

Specimens
1. Obtain fresh blood by heel puncture. Apply immediately to thick filter paper (Schleicher & Schuell no. 903). Let it air dry. Spot should have diameter of about ⅜ in. Number individual filter paper with pencil for identification purposes.
2. Place filter paper on metal screening and autoclave 3 min at 15 psi. Punch out disk (¼ in. in diameter) from center of blood spot.

Medium, inoculum, and β-2-thienylalanine. See Phenylketonuria (PKU) test materials.

Controls
1. Obtain outdated blood from blood bank and assay it for phenylalanine content (spectrophotometric method).

2. Add L-phenylalanine to various aliquots of blood to obtain final concentrations of 2, 4, 6, 8, 10, 12, and 20 mg/100 ml.
3. Place blood on filter paper and let it air dry (same as specimens). Control disks can be kept in desiccator under refrigeration.
4. Autoclave controls simultaneously with unknown specimens.
5. Punch out disk from each spot for use.

Assay procedure
1. Demain medium, with *B. subtilis* spore suspension and β-2-thienylalanine added, is poured into Pyrex baking dish or plastic tray. Allow agar to cool and solidify. It is important that tabletop be perfectly level, since it ensures agar layer uniformly thick.
2. Place dish over pattern sheet with printed grid to facilitate arrangement of disks. Up to 100 unknown disks and 7-10 control disks can be accommodated. (Some workers prefer to use 4 control disks of 4 mg/100 ml each instead of 1.) Place disks on agar with aid of forceps.
3. Cover tray and incubate overnight at 35-37 C for 16-18 h.
4. Read results by comparing growth zones around unknown disks with those around control disks. Any unknown specimen showing zone corresponding in size to that produced by 4 mg/100 ml control disk is reported as presumptive positive. Such specimen should be confirmed by phenylalanine fluorometric procedure.

NOTES
1. Specimens should be collected before infant is discharged from hospital (4-5 d of age).
2. In case commercial kits (BBL or Difco) are used for PKU test, carefully follow manufacturer's recommendations and instructions.

Phosphatase test

See *Staphylococcus,* Chapter 76.

Pigment production

Two media, *Pseudomonas* agar P (also known as "Tech" agar) and agar F ("Flo" agar), were developed to enhance formation of the water soluble pigments pyocyanin and pyoverdin (fluorescein) produced by some *Pseudomonas* species. The correct peptones are most important (for description, see Media).

1. Inoculate surface of slants with 1 drop of 24 h broth culture. Do not inoculate butt of agar. These pigments are colorless in anaerobic atmosphere.
   a. Incubate slants at 35-37 C and examine after 24 h and up to 7 d. Pigment will usually be seen by 72 h.
   b. Pyoverdin may be demonstrated by ultraviolet (UV) light from Wood's lamp in darkened room. This type of illumination is not required to detect other pigments.
2. Interpretation of pigments
   a. Colors appearing in P medium vary with strains studied. Predominantly pyocyanin-producing strains of *Pseudomonas aeruginosa* give pigment ranging from light aqua to dark blue or green. With strains producing mainly pyorubin, color ranges from light pink to dark maroon. Strains producing both pigments show a variety of color, including many shades and mixtures of reds and blues.
   b. On F medium, pigment most frequently observed is pyoverdin. This pigment is fluorescent and of greenish yellow color. Some

---

*From Guthrie and Whitney[114] and PKU test, Product information, BBL, Division of BioQuest, Cockeysville, Md.

strains of *Pseudomonas aeruginosa* also produce a small amount of pyocyanin, giving medium bright green appearance. Yellowish pigments formed usually after 72 h that are not fluorescent under UV light are produced by many bacteria and should be ignored. Pyoverdin may be produced in greater amounts by incubation at 25 C. *Pseudomonas aeruginosa* may also produce dark brown pigment.

Sodium hippurate test

See Hippurate test, Hippurate hydrolysis, Rapid methods, this chapter; *Streptococcus,* Chapter 76.

"String" test

See *V. cholerae,* Chapter 79.

Temperature studies

1. Inoculate 3 tubes of **TGY** medium (see Media) with 1 drop each of 24 h broth culture.
2. Incubate 1 tube at 25 C, 1 tube at 37 C, and 1 tube at 42 C for 18-24 h.
3. Read tubes for comparative growth at different temperatures.

Transformation assay

See *Acinetobacter,* Chapter 79.

Urease production

Christensen urea agar—recommended method
1. Inoculate by heavily streaking surface of slant.
2. Incubate at 37 C and examine at 2 h, 4 h, and after overnight incubation.
3. Observe negative tubes 4 d to detect delayed reactions.
4. Positive reaction is indicated by red color in medium.

Urea broth
1. Inoculate heavily and incubate at 37 C.
2. Observe at frequent intervals for 24 h.

Test is used to determine ability of some bacteria to split urea into ammonia and CO_2 by means of enzyme urease. If urea is split to form ammonia, medium becomes alkaline and indicator turns red.

See also Rapid methods.

Voges-Proskauer test

Inoculate tubes of methyl red–Voges-Proskauer medium and incubate 48 h. Then carry out one of the methods below.

Recommended procedure

Reagent (O'Meara, modified by Ewing[1])

Potassium hydroxide	40 g
Creatine	0.3 g
Distilled water	100 ml

1. Dissolve alkali in water; add creatine. Prepare reagent frequently and refrigerate when not in use. If refrigerated, reagent can be used 2-3 wk.[1]

Procedure
1. Add 1 ml reagent to 1 ml culture. Mix by gentle shaking; place tubes in water bath 4 h at 37 C or at room temperature 4 h. Shake tubes occasionally.
2. Development of delicate eosin-pink color indicates positive test.

Test depends on ability of certain bacteria to produce acetylmethylcarbinol (acetoin) from glucose. Under al-

kaline conditions it is oxidized to diacetyl, which reacts with guanidino compounds present in broth to give red-colored complex.

Alternate test (Coblentz method)

Reagents
1. Reagent A. 5% alpha naphthol in 95% ethanol. (Keeps 1 mo at room temperature.)
2. Reagent B. 0.3% creatine in 40% KOH. (Keeps 2 wk at room temperature. 40% KOH is stable indefinitely.)

Culture
1. Inoculate 2 ml buffered peptone glucose broth (MR-VP broth) heavily by scraping growth from 18-24 h infusion agar culture with loop. In case of organisms that grow lightly, such as *Listeria,* use capillary pipet and wash off entire growth from slant, using MR-VP broth as suspending medium.
2. Incubate broth culture at 35-37 C for 6 h.

Procedure
1. Add 0.6 ml reagent A to culture. Shake gently.
2. Add 0.2 ml reagent B. Shake vigorously.
3. Observe 5-10 min, shaking occasionally. Positive = pink to cherry red color. Negative = no color change.

RAPID METHODS

A large number of "rapid" and micromethods have been developed in the last 20 years in an attempt (1) to shorten the time needed for completion of characterization tests and (2) to reduce the amount of media and substrates used and to simplify the technics involved, e.g., to economize on material and labor.

Cowan and Steel[108] classify these tests into 3 groups: the **multitest** media, in which 2 or more reactions can be observed simultaneously; the **micromethods,** in which the volume of reagents is reduced and the inoculum correspondingly made heavier; and the **"mini-tests,"** in which the reagents and/or media are contained in impregnated disks or tablets.

The multitest media include media such as Kligler iron agar (KIA), triple sugar iron agar (TSI), Sellers medium, Gillies composite media (mainly used in England), and others.

The micromethods are of 2 kinds. In the first type, a heavy inoculum is grown in a small volume of medium. Weaver's[115] methods include a number of tests used in diagnostic bacteriology. In the second type, such as Clarke and Cowan's[116] procedures, water or saline suspensions of living organisms are added to the test substrate. The organisms do not multiply and only preformed enzymes are detected, whereas in the first type induced enzymes are also detected.

Multitests use prepared, ready-made substrates and reagents (tablets, disks, etc.). Many **miniaturized** tests are available. See Fermentations-micromethods, this chapter, and Chapter 74.

Most of these methods are in reality not rapid methods, since most of them do require pure subcultures; tests that could be applied to colonies (preferably on isolation plates) would be more aptly named **rapid tests.** The slide coagulase test (see staphylococci), the oxidase disk test (see above), and the catalase test are examples.

A few rapid methods are described below. See also Chapter 74.

Fermentations, rapid methods

See McDade and Weaver[117] for aerobes and Kaufman and Weaver[118] for anaerobes.

Bergquist-Searcy micromethod[119]

This method is useful for rapid detection of acid and gas formed by aerobes.

1. Add phenol red broth, 0.3 ml, containing 1% added carbohydrate, to 6 × 50 mm culture tubes.
2. Invert in each tube of medium a microcapillary tube (1.4 × 10 mm), sealed at 1 end. Stopper tubes with plastic foam and autoclave at 121 C (15 psi) for 5 min.
3. Inspect microcapillary tubes after autoclaving; they should be completely filled with media.
4. Inoculate each tube with single, isolated colonies from initial plating medium.
5. Incubate at 37 C in constant-temperature aluminum block.

Acid production is detectable within 2 h; gas formation is evidenced by gas bubble in capillary tube.

Hippurate hydrolysis, rapid[120]

Use. The ability of certain organisms to hydrolyze sodium hippurate to benzoic acid and glycine is used in the identification of streptococci. In this 2 h rapid test, the glycine is detected by the development of a purple color when a solution of ninhydrin is added.

Reagents

1. 1 g Sodium hippurate in 99 ml distilled water (1% solution). Dispense in 0.4 ml portions in 13 × 100 screw-top tubes and freeze at −20 C until used.
2. 3.5 g Ninhydrin in mixture of 50 ml acetone and 50 ml butanol (1:1 solution).

Procedure

1. Thaw 1 tube sodium hippurate solution for each test.
2. Pick large loopful of streptococcal colony from blood agar and emulsify in sodium hippurate tube.
3. Incubate 2 h in temperature block at 37 C.
4. After incubation, add 0.2 ml ninhydrin solution and incubate in temperature block 10 more minutes.
5. Remove from temperature block and observe.

A purple color (gentian violet) is **positive,** indicating the ability of the organism to hydrolyze hippurate. This is a very deep purple color for group B streptococcus, but some group D (enterococcus) will give a weaker positive reaction. No color change is a **negative** reaction.

Indole tests, rapid
Arnold-Weaver test[121]

1. Inoculate very heavily 0.4 ml amounts of tryptone broth (peptone water), containing tryptophan, with pure culture from slant or plate.
2. Incubate at 37 C for 2 h.
3. Add Kovacs reagent (see above); shake gently.

Red color in reagent layer indicates formation of indole.

Indole spot test—Vracko-Sherris[122]

1. Place no. 1 Whatman filter (9 cm) into cover of Petri dish. Moisten with 1 ml 5% solution of *p*-dimethylaminobenzaldehyde in 10% aqueous HCl.
2. Smear colonies from overnight growth on blood agar plate over small area of moist filter paper.

Presence of indole is indicated by development of brown-red to purple-red color within 20 s. White-yellow color indicates absence of indole. Same test can be performed on loopfuls of peptone water fluid culture (containing pure culture).

Disadvantages

1. Test cannot be performed if growth is taken from media lacking tryptophan (such as MacConkey, EMB, or Mueller-Hinton). Organism must be grown on blood agar base, trypticase soy agar, or chocolate agar.
2. Colonies can be used only if separated by at least 5 mm from all others or if taken from pure culture.

Advantages

1. Many tests can be performed on piece of impregnated filter paper.
2. Individual cultures can be examined on several occasions during day.

Interpretation. The test is somewhat less sensitive, when done on colonies on solid media, than the 48 hour standard test, but seems to be of value with the lactose-fermenting *Enterobacteriaceae* and with spreading *Proteus* organisms. Some difficulties have been experienced with fresh isolates of *Proteus vulgaris;* also, some indole-positive strains are being found to be negative on first tests from tryptophan-containing solid media. With *Proteus,* therefore, a negative test is always checked with a tube indole test. The test was found to be reliable for lactose-fermenters.[123]

Phenylalanine microtest[124]

1. Prepare small tubes (6 × 50 mm) with 0.3 ml 0.2% aqueous L-phenylalanine. Sterilize by autoclaving.
2. Inoculate tubes with single colonies; incubate in constant-temperature aluminum block at 37 C.
3. Add 2 drops 8% solution of $FeCl_3$ after 60 min to tube.

Immediate development of green color indicates conversion of substrate to phenylpyruvic acid. All *Proteus* and *Providence* strains give positive reactions.

Voges-Proskauer test, rapid
Rapid indirect test[125]

1. Inoculate 0.2 ml MR-VP broth with no more than 1 colony (from MacConkey agar or EMB).
2. Incubate 4-6 h at 37 C.
3. Add 2 drops creatine (0.5% aqueous solution), 3 drops α-naphthol (5% in 95% ethyl alcohol), and 2 drops KOH (40% solution in distilled water).

Appearance of pink to red color within 15 min indicates presence of acetylmethylcarbinol.

Rapid direct test[125]

This test can be done on colonies from MacConkey plates but not EMB, since the color of the resulting suspension interferes with the reaction. The test is less reliable than the indirect method.

1. Prepare dense suspension of pink or red colonies from overnight MacConkey agar plate in 2 drops creatine (0.5% aqueous solution).
2. Add 3 drops α-naphthol (as above), shake, add 2 drops KOH (as above). Shake.

Appearance of pink to red color in 15 min is considered positive test.

The authors cited routinely do a direct VP test on all lactose-fermenting colonies from MacConkey agar. If negative, they are further tested after 4-6 h by the indirect method. Slow fermenters or lactose nonfermenters are subcultured onto TSI agar slants and the organism tested directly from the TSI slant if the slant is acid. If the slant is alkaline, the indirect test is performed.

Urease test, rapid

From differential tubes (TSI, etc.)

1. Inoculate **very heavily** 0.5 ml amounts of Stuart-Rustigian urea broth with growth from slant.
2. Place tube in water bath at 35-36 C.

Urea is hydrolyzed rapidly by *Proteus*, with release of ammonia. This is indicated by color change of medium (reddening, in 15 min-2 h).[126] Others recommend reading the test in 30 min.

From single-colony isolates[127]

1. Impregnate glass fiber strips (5 × 30 mm) with 50 μl 15% aqueous urea solution, dry at room temperature, and store in Petri dishes.
2. Elute urea from strip in 5 ml ammonia-free distilled water (10 min at 37 C).
3. Inoculate urea eluate with single-colony isolate.
4. Incubate 5 min in heating block at 37 C.
5. Add 1 ml sodium hypochlorite and 1 ml sodium phenate–sodium nitroprusside reagent.
6. Incubate additional 5 min at 37 C.

Ammonia production, due to urease activity, is indicated by formation of blue dye in presence of sodium phenate and sodium nitroprusside (Berthelot reaction). According to Bergquist and Searcy,[127] all strains of *Proteus* give this reaction.

Prepared, ready-made substrates and reagents

"Rapid substrate" tablets (for indole, urease, gelatin, and Voges-Proskauer test) that can be used with sterile water and obviate the need for preparing and storing a large variety of media were described by Hoyt and Pickett.[128] Filter paper strips or disks containing carbohydrates with or without nutrient medium were devised by numerous workers (e.g., see Sanders et al.,[129] described under "screening of stool cultures"). Clark and Steel[130] described the use of disks impregnated with substrates, which are placed on the fully grown lawn culture on nutrient agar. After incubation (ranging from 1-2 h) reagents are added to the disk to react with the enzyme products to form a colored compound, or a second disk containing the reagent is superimposed on the first disk after the incubation period for enzyme action.

A large variety of commercially prepared impregnated disks, tablets, and strips is available. Some have been used with reasonable success; others have not yet been sufficiently evaluated.*

It should be clearly understood that pure cultures (or well-isolated single colonies) must be used.

The use of controls with any of the above methods (as well as with the standard methods) is mandatory. Uninoculated blanks and known cultures should be employed to control the sensitivity and specificity of reactions.

For **miniaturized, multi-test micromethods**, see Fermentations-micromethods, this chapter, and a detailed discussion in Chapter 74.

---

*Carbohydrate disks: Taxo carbohydrate disks from BBL, Division of BioQuest, Cockeysville, Md.; Bacto differentiation disks from Difco Laboratories, Detroit, Mich.
Tablets: Fermentation tablets from Key Scientific Products Co., Los Angeles.
Reagents and/or substrates: Pathotec strips, for cytochrome oxidase, urease, phenylalanine deaminase, lysine decarboxylase, indole, Voges-Proskauer, and citrate tests from General Diagnostics Division, Warner-Chilcott Laboratories, Division of Warner-Lambert Pharmaceutical Co., Morris Plains, N.J.; X and V factor strips for *Haemophilus* identification from BBL, Difco. Key substrate tablets from Key Scientific Products Co. For Optochin, bacitracin, and oxidase disks see standard tests.

REFERENCES

1. Ewing, W. H., and Davis, B. R.: Media and tests for differentiation of Enterobacteriaceae, 1970 (reprinted 1977), Atlanta, U.S. Dept. of Health, Education, and Welfare, Center for Disease Control.
2. Gorski, T. W., and Ritzert, R. W.: Appl. Environ. Microbiol. 34:242, 1977.
3. Trabulsi, L. R., and Ewing, W. H.: Public Health Lab. 20:137, 1962.
4. Venkatraman, K. V., and Ramakrishnan, C. S.: Indian J. Med. Res. 29:681, 1941.
5. Cowan, S. T.: Cowan and Steel's manual for identification of medical bacteria, ed. 2, Cambridge, 1974, Cambridge University Press.
6. Center for Disease Control: Diarrheal disease caused by *Campylobacter fetus* subspecies jejuni, Memorandum from Director, Bureau of Laboratories, Center for Disease Control, Aug. 7, 1978.
7. Waterborne Campylobacter gastroenteritis—Vermont, Morbid. Mortal. Weekly Rep. 27(25):207, June 23, 1978.
8. Campylobacter enteritis—Colorado, Morbid. Mortal. Weekly Rep. 27(27):226, July 7, 1978.
9. Veron, M., and Chatelain, R.: Int. J. Syst. Bacteriol. 23:122-134, 1973.
10. Ewing, W. H.: Enterobacteriaceae—biochemical methods for group differentiation, PHS pub. no. 734, Atlanta, 1960, Communicable Disease Center.
11. McBride, M. L., and Girard, K. F.: J. Lab. Clin. Med. 55:153, 1960.
12. Gonococcus—procedures for isolation and identification, PHS pub. no. 499, Atlanta, 1960, Communicable Disease Center, Venereal Disease Branch.

13. King, E. O.: Identification of unusual pathogenic gram-negative bacteria, Atlanta, 1964, Communicable Disease Center.
14. Mackey, N., and Sandys, B.: Br. Med. J. **2**:1286, 1965.
15. Ellner, P. D., Stoessel, C. J., Drakeford, E., et al.: Am. J. Clin. Pathol. **45**:502, 1966.
16. Hebert, G. A., and Jones, G. L., editors: Legionnaires': the disease, the bacterium and methodology, Atlanta, 1978, U.S. Dept. Health, Education, and Welfare, Public Health Service, Center for Disease Control.
17. Edwards, P. R., and Ewing, W. H.: Identification of Enterobacteriaceae, ed. 2, Minneapolis, 1962, Burgess Publishing Co.
18. Moeller, V.: Acta Pathol. Microbiol. Scand. **36**:158, 1955.
19. Falkow, S.: Am. J. Clin. Pathol. **29**:598, 1958.
20. Panja, G., and Ghosh, S. K.: Indian Med. Gaz. **78**:55, 1943.
21. DiSalvo, J.: Med. Tech. Bull. **9**:191, 1958.
22. McClung, L. S., and Toabe, R.: J. Bacteriol. **53**:139, 1947.
23. Elek, S.: Br. Med. J. **1**:493, 1948.
24. King, E. O., Frobisher, M., Jr., and Parsons, E. I.: Am. J. Public Health **39**:1314, 1949.
25. Hermann, G. J., Moore, M. S., and Parsons, E. I.: Am. J. Clin. Pathol. **29**:181, 1958.
26. Feeley, J. C., Gorman, G. W., Weaver, R. E., et al.: J. Clin. Microbiol. **8**:320, 1978.
27. Fildes, J.: Br. J. Exp. Pathol. **1**:129, 1920.
28. Fildes, J.: Br. J. Exp. Pathol. **2**:16, 1921.
29. Hajna, A. A.: Public Health Lab. **13**:83, 1955.
30. Taylor, W. I., and Harris, B.: Am. J. Clin. Pathol. **44**:476, 1965.
31. Taylor, W. I., and Harris, B. G.: Am. J. Clin. Pathol. **48**:350, 1967.
32. Jones, G. L., and Kendrick, P. L.: Health Lab. Sci. **6**:40, 1969.
33. Moeller, V.: Acta Pathol. Microbiol. Scand. **34**:115, 1954.
34. Alexander, H.: The Hemophilus group. In Dubos, R., editor: Bacterial and mycotic infections of man, ed. 3, Philadelphia, 1958, J. B. Lippincott Co.
35. Lenert, T. F., and Hobby, G. L.: Proc. Soc. Exp. Biol. Med. **65**:235, 1947.
36. von Haebler, T., and Miles, A. A.: J. Pathol. Bact. **46**:245, 1938.
37. Stokes, E. J.: Clinical bacteriology, ed. 2, London, 1960, Edward Arnold (Publishers) Ltd.
38. Edwards, P. R., and Fife, M. A.: Appl. Microbiol. **4**:46, 1956.
39. Bearns, R. E., and Girard, F. K.: Am. J. Med. Tech. **25**:120, 1959.
40. Mueller, J. H., and Hinton, J.: Proc. Soc. Exp. Biol. Med. **48**:330, 1941.
41. Mueller,, J.: Immunol. **37**:103, 1939.
42. Naylor, P. G. D.: J. Med. Lab. Tech. **17**:184, 1960.
43. Kauffmann, F., and Petersen, A.: Acta Pathol. Microbiol. Scand. **38**:481, 1956.
44. Hugh, R., and Leifson, E.: J. Bacteriol. **66**:24, 1953.
45. Starr, M. P.: Phytopathology **37**:291, 1947.
46. Davis, R. B., and Ewing, W. H.: J. Bacteriol. **88**:16, 1964.
47. Ewing, W. H., Davis, B. R., and Reavis, R. W.: Public Health Lab. **15**:153, 1957.
48. Demain, A. L.: J. Bacteriol. **75**:517, 1958.
49. Guthrie, R., and Susi, A.: Pediatrics **32**:338, 1963.
50. Banxgang, E. N., and Eliot, C. P.: Am. J. Hyg., Sec. B **31**:16, 1940.
51. Sellers, W.: J. Bacteriol. **87**:46, 1964.
52. Edwards, P. R., and Bruner, D. W.: U. Kentucky, Circular 54, 1942.
53. Hajna, A. A.: Public Health Lab. **8**:36, 1950.
54. Trabulsi, L. R., and Ewing, W. H.: Public Health Lab. **20**:137, 1962.
55. Thayer, J. D., and Martin, J. E.: Public Health Rep. **79**:49, 1964.
56. Thayer, J. D., and Martin, J. E.: Public Health Rep. **81**:559, 1966.
57. Martin, J. E., Billings, T. E., Hackney, J. F., et al.: Public Health Rep. **82**:361, 1967.
58. Martin, J. E., Armstrong, J. H., and Smith, P. B.: Appl. Microbiol. **27**(4):802-805, 1974; Williams, W. J., Snyder, H. A., and Farmer, A. D.: Public Health Lab. **29**:99, 1971.
59. Center for Disease Control: Protocol for evaluation of modified Thayer-Martin (MTM) medium plates, Atlanta, 1975, U.S. Dept. of Health, Education, and Welfare, Center for Disease Control.
60. Center for Disease Control: Protocol for evaluation of modified Thayer-Martin (MTM) medium bottles by consumers, Atlanta, 1975, U.S. Dept. of Health, Education, and Welfare, Center for Disease Control.
61. Tinsdale, G. F. W.: J. Pathol. Bacteriol. **59**:461, 1947.
62. Moore, M. S., and Parsons, E. I.: J. Infect. Dis. **102**:88, 1958.
63. Billings, M.: Master's thesis, University of Michigan, 1955.
64. Todd, E. W., and Hewitt, L. F.: J. Pathol. Bact. **35**:973, 1932.
65. Amies, J.: Can. J. Public Health **56**:27, 1965.
66. Cary, S. G., and Blair, E. B.: J. Bacteriol. **88**:96, 1964.
67. Gaines, S., Ul Haque, S., Pamiom, W., et al.: Am. J. Trop. Med. **14**:136, 1965.
68. Gaines, S.: Newsletter, Clin. Diag. Microbiol. A.S.M. **1**:3, 1967.
69. Stuart, R. D., Toshach, S. R., and Patsula, T. M.: Can. J. Public Health **45**:73, 1954.
70. Christensen, W. B.: J. Bacteriol. **52**:461, 1946.
71. Monsur, K. A.: Bull. W.H.O. **28**:387, 1963.
72. Gohar, M. A., and Makkawi, M.: J. Trop. Med. Hyg. **51**:95, 1948.
73. White, J. D., and McGavran, M. H.: J.A.M.A. **194**:294, 1965.
74. Watson, K. C.: Am. J. Trop. Med. **5**:131, 1956.
75. Taylor, W. I.: Am. J. Clin. Pathol. **44**:471, 1965.
76. Taylor, W. I., and Schelhart, D.: Am. J. Clin. Pathol. **48**:356, 1967.
77. Dowell, V. R., Jr., Lombard, G. L., Thompson, F. S., and Armfield, A. Y.: Media for isolation, characterization and identification of obligately anaerobic bacteria, Atlanta, 1977, U.S. Department of Health, Education, and Welfare, Public Health Service, Center for Disease Control.
78. Dowell, V. R., Jr., and T. M. Hawkins, T. M.: *Laboratory methods in anaerobic bacteriology,* CDC laboratory manual, Atlanta, 1977, U.S. Department of Health, Education, and Welfare, Public Health Service, Center for Disease Control.
79. Dowell, V. R., Jr., and Lombard, G. L.: Presumptive identification of anaerobic nonsporeforming gram-negative bacilli, Atlanta, 1977, U.S. Department of Health, Education, and

Welfare, Public Health Service, Center for Disease Control.

80. Stargel, M. D., Thompson, F. S., Phillips, S. E., J. Clin. Microbiol. **3:**291-301, 1976.
81. Sutter, V. L., Vargo, V. L., and Finegold, S. M.: Wadsworth anaerobic bacteriology manual, ed. 2, Los Angeles, 1975, The Regents of the University of California.
82. Holdeman, L. V. Cato, E. P., and Moore, W. E. C., editors: Anaerobe laboratory manual, ed. 4, Blacksburg, Va., 1977, Anaerobe Laboratory, Virginia Polytechnic Institute and State University.
83. Attebery, H. R., and Finegold, S. M.: Am. J. Clin. Pathol. **53:**383-388, 1970.
84. Finegold, S. M., Sugihara, P. T., and Sutter, V. L.: Use of selective media for isolation of anaerobes from humans. In Shapton, D. A., and Board, R. G., editors: Isolation of anaerobes, New York, 1971, Academic Press, pp. 99-108.
84a. Livingston, S. J., Kominos, S. D., and Yee, R. B.: J. Clin. Microbiol. **7:**448, 1978.
85. Finegold, S. M., Miller, A. B., and Posnick, D. J.: Ernährungsforschung **10:**517, 1965.
86. Dowell, V. R., Jr., Hill, E. O., and Altemeier, W. A.: J. Bacteriol. **88:**1811, 1964.
87. Sutter, V. L., and Finegold, S. M.: Appl. Microbiol. **21:**13-20, 1971.
88. Sutter, V. L., and Carter, W. T.: Am. J. Clin. Pathol. **58:**335-338, 1972.
89. Graves, M. H., Morevo, J. A., and Kocka, F.: Appl. Microbiol. **27:**1131, 1974.
90. Ajello, L., Georg, L. K., Kaplan, W., and Kaufman, L.: Laboratory manual for medical mycology, Public Health Service pub. no. 994, Atlanta, 1963, Communicable Disease Center.
91. Emerson, R. L., Whiffen, A. J., Bohonos, N., and DeBoer, C.: J. Bacteriol. **52:**357, 1946.
92. Littman, D.: Science **106:**109, 1947.
93. Maxted, W. R.: J. Clin. Pathol. **6:**224, 1953.
94. Levinson, M. L., and Frank, P. F.: J. Bacteriol. **69:**284, 1955.
95. LeMinor, L., and Ben Hamida, F.: Ann. Inst. Pasteur **102:**267, 1962.
96. Lubin, A. H., and Ewing, W. H.: Public Health Lab. **22:**83, 1964.
97. Costin, I. D.: Zentralbl. Bakteriol. (Orig.) **200:**49, 1966.
98. Lowe, G. H.: J. Med. Lab. Tech. **19:**21, 1962.
99. Pickett, M. J., and Goodman, R. E.: Appl. Microbiol. **14:**178, 1966.
100. Leifson, E.: J.A.M.A. **104:**213, 1935.
101. Bayliss, M.: J. Lab. Clin. Med. **28:**748, 1943.
102. Anhalt, J. P., Kenny, G. E., and Rytel, M. W.: Detection of microbial antigens by counter-immunoelectrophoresis, Cumitech no. 8, Washington, D.C., 1978, American Society for Microbiology.
103. Feigin, R. D., Wong, M., Shackelford, P. G., et al.: J. Pediatr. **89:**773, 1976.
104. Rytel, W. M.: Public Health Lab. **36:**15, 1978.

105. DiSalvo, J.: Med. Technol. Bull. **9:**191, 1958.
106. Martin, W. J., and Ewing, W. H.: Can. J. Microbiol. **13:**616, 1967.
107. Procedure for the bacteriological examination of food utensils and/or food equipment surfaces, no. 1631. Technical Information Bull. no. 1. Cincinnati, 1967, Food Sanitation Section, U.S. Public Health Service.
108. Cowan, S. T., and Steel, K. J.: Manual for the identification of medical bacteria, Cambridge, 1965, Cambridge University Press.
109. Weil, A. J., and Saphra, I.: Salmonellae and shigellae, Springfield, Ill., 1953, Charles C Thomas, Publisher.
110. Bowers, E. F., and Jeffries, L. R.: J. Clin. Pathol. **8:**58, 1955.
111. Kovaes, N.: Nature **178:**703, 1956.
112. Ewing, W. H., and Johnson, J. G.: Int. Bull. Bact. Nomen. Taxon. **10:**223, 1960.
113. Guthrie, R., and Tieckelman, H.: Proceedings of the London Conference on the Scientific Study of Mental Deficiency, London, 1962, May & Baker.
114. Guthrie, R., and Whitney, S.: Phenylketonuria, Children's Bureau pub. no. 419, Washington, D.C., 1964 (rev. 1965), Dept. Health, Education, and Welfare.
115. Weaver, R. H.: Am. J. Med. Technol. **20:**14, 1954.
116. Clarke, P. H., and Cowan, S. T.: J. Gen. Microbiol. **6:**187, 1952.
117. McDade, J. J., and Weaver, R. H.: J. Bacteriol. **77:**65, 1959.
118. Kaufman, L., and Weaver, R. H.: J. Bacteriol. **79:**119, 1960.
119. Bergquist, L. M., and Searcy, R. L.: Am. J. Med. Technol. **28:**337, 1962.
120. Hwang, M., and Ederer, G.: J. Clin. Microbiol. **1:**114-115, 1975.
121. Arnold, W. M., and Weaver, R. H.: J. Lab. Clin. Med. **33:**1334, 1948.
122. Vracko, R., and Sherris, J. C.: Am. J. Clin. Pathol. **39:**429, 1963.
123. Sherris, J. C.: Personal communications, 1968-1969.
124. Bergquist, L. M., and Searcy, R. L.: Am. J. Clin. Pathol. **39:**544, 1963.
125. Barry, A. L., and Feeney, K. L.: Appl. Microbiol. **15:**1138, 1967.
126. Simmons, J. M., and Gentzkow, C. J.: Medical and public health laboratory methods, Philadelphia, 1955, Lea & Febiger.
127. Bergquist, L. M., and Searcy, R. L.: J. Bacteriol. **85:**954, 1963.
128. Hoyt, R. E., and Pickett, M. J.: Am. J. Clin. Pathol. **27:**343, 1957.
129. Sanders, A. C., Faber, J. E., and Cook, T. M.: Appl. Microbiol. **5:**36, 1957.
130. Clark, P. H., and Steel, K. J. In Gibbs, B. M., and Skinner, F. A., editors: Identification methods for microbiologists, Part A, New York, 1966, Academic Press.

73

QUALITY CONTROL IN THE MICROBIOLOGY LABORATORY

Charles T. Hall

The purpose of a microbiology laboratory quality control program is to assure the physician, the patient, and the laboratorian of the **validity** and **preciseness** of all cultural and serologic determinations performed in that laboratory. The Clinical Laboratories Improvement Act of 1967 stimulated the development of quality control programs, but the concept of quality control is not new; it has been an integral part of the chemistry and diagnostic immunology laboratory for a number of years. What laboratorian would think of running a glucose determination without first calibrating the automated system against an aqueous reference standard, incorporating a serum standard to establish the effect of the serum matrix, and then incorporating a previously analyzed serum control at specified intervals to maintain an ongoing check on the system? What serologist would run a VDRL test without incorporating a reactive, weakly reactive, and nonreactive serum in the run? Unfortunately quality control in the microbiology laboratory has lagged behind that in other disciplines. Over the years the microbiologist has prepared media for use at the bench with only cursory examination, if any, of its growth capabilities.

On December 31, 1968, regulations were published in the *Federal Register* that were applicable to clinical laboratories involved in the interstate traffic of human specimens. These regulations were mandatory for laboratories, and thus the impetus for quality control came from a regulatory program administered by the Center for Disease Control (CDC), Atlanta. More than 10 years later the administration of the regulatory program is in a transitory phase; the responsibility of administering and implementing the program is being transferred to the various state governments. In addition the scope of the regulatory program apparently will be expanded to include many laboratories heretofore excluded from compliance with federal regulations. The many implications of the redelegations of authority to the state as opposed to a uniform, centralized federal program are at this time unclear, as are the identity and role of a federal agency to coordinate state activities.

Despite these many questions it is very probable that state government personnel will be involved in the implementation of a national program that will be composed of 50 individually administered but comparable state programs. It is with this distinct possibility in mind that sections of a CDC Laboratory Examination Checklist (CDC 3.1010, dated October 1977) are included in this chapter. It is possible, in fact probable, that the checklist will have been revised extensively before this edition is printed. Nevertheless the checklist is valuable in revealing to the laboratorian what might be expected of a clinical laboratory.

Documentation of quality control measures performed within a laboratory must be available to laboratory examiners. Several logs may have to be kept for recording maintenance data, temperatures, and control values relating to specific specimens in the accession records. The failure to record the results of controls often causes embarrassment to the laboratorian because there is no way to substantiate that laboratory findings for specific patients on a given date were valid determinations.

Too often the standard method of analysis used in a laboratory has never been printed in a Standard Operating Procedural Manual (SOPM) and made available to the technical staff. Even more often the typed page bearing the standard method has been marked with cryptic pencilled notes modifying the procedure, changing concentrations, substituting components, and increasing times of reaction. None of the added information is documented with regard to its influence on the test results, and none of it can be traced to a specific individual in the laboratory.

The SOPM containing only those tests performed in the laboratory should be available at each station in the laboratory at all times. The technical supervisors should review the SOPM

Text continued on p. 1478.

DEPARTMENT OF HEALTH, EDUCATION, AND WELFARE
PUBLIC HEALTH SERVICE
CENTER FOR DISEASE CONTROL
ATLANTA, GEORGIA 30333

GENERAL
Laboratory Examination Checklist — CLIA '67 — CDC

Code No.

Examiner(s)

Name of Laboratory

Interviewee(s)

Address

Date(s) of examination

NOTE TO EXAMINER:

For each item marked with an *, mark "No" if there is no record to confirm that the laboratory is actually applying the standard. A record is REQUIRED; however, if a laboratory CLAIMS IT APPLIES THE STANDARD but has no record, indicate under comment space.

PERSONNEL POLICIES CFR 74.52 405.1315(f) (1)		NO (Code)	COMMENT
1. The laboratory maintains current personnel records for each employee			
	Director	☐ 90000	
	Technical Supervisor	☐ 90019	
	General Supervisor	☐ 90020	
	Technologist	☐ 90021	
	Technologist Trainee	☐ 90022	
	Cytotechnologist	☐ 90023	
	Technician	☐ 90024	
	Technician Trainee	☐ 90025	
2. Personnel records include a complete resume of each employee's			
	Training	☐ 90001	
	Experience	☐ 90002	
	Duties	☐ 90003	
	Dates of employment	☐ 90004	
SPECIMENS ACCESSION RECORDS CFR 74.53 405.1316(f)			
3. Daily accession records on specimens are maintained		☐ 90005	
4. The accession records contain the following:			
	Laboratory number or other identification	☐ 90006	
	Name or identification of person from whom specimen was taken	☐ 90007	
	Name or identification of person who submitted the specimen	☐ 90008	
	Date the specimen was collected	☐ 90009	
	Date the specimen was received in the laboratory	☐ 90010	
	Type of test performed	☐ 90011	
	Results of test or cross reference to results	☐ 90012	
	Date of test completion	☐ 90013	
	Condition of unsatisfactory specimens when received	☐ 90014	
5. The laboratory report is sent promptly to client		☐ 90015	
6. The name of the laboratory actually performing the examination is indicated in the report to the client		☐ 90016	
7. Reports include the usual range of values for good health, where indicated		☐ 90017	
8. A list of analytical methods employed by the laboratory and the basis for the usual range of values for good health is made available to the client		☐ 90018	

CDC 3.1010
10-77

GENERAL

CDC laboratory examination checklist (1977)—general

	BACTERIOLOGY	Code No.
DEPARTMENT OF HEALTH, EDUCATION, AND WELFARE PUBLIC HEALTH SERVICE CENTER FOR DISEASE CONTROL ATLANTA, GEORGIA 30333	LABORATORY EXAMINATION CHECKLIST—CLIA '67 – CDC	Examiner(s)
Name of Laboratory		Interviewee(s)
Address		Date(s) of examination

NOTE TO EXAMINER:
  a) *For each item marked with an* *, *mark "No" if there is no record to confirm that the laboratory is actually applying the standard. A record is required; however, if a laboratory CLAIMS IT APPLIES THE STANDARD but has no record, indicate under comment column.*
  b) *The examiner must check each block to the left of the question or specific item to indicate if the item is available or used in this laboratory.*

PREVENTIVE MAINTENANCE CFR 74.20(a) 405.1317(a)(1)		NO	CODE	COMMENT
1. Each equipment item is tested periodically for proper operation	Autoclaves	* ☐	01000	
	Incubators	* ☐	01001	
	Fluorescent Microscope	* ☐	01002	
	Biosafety Cabinet	* ☐	01003	
2. Each equipment item is subjected to preventive maintenance	Autoclaves	* ☐	01004	
	Incubators	* ☐	01005	
	Fluorescent Microscope	* ☐	01006	
	Biosafety Cabinet	* ☐	01007	
3. Records document remedial actions taken for detected defects		☐	01008	
TEMPERATURES CFR 74.20(b) 405.1317(a)(2)	Incubators	* ☐	01009	
4. Temperatures are monitored each day of use	Refrigerators	* ☐	01010	
	Water Baths	* ☐	01011	
	Heat Blocks	* ☐	01012	
	Freezers	* ☐	01013	
☐ STERILIZATION CFR 74.20(b)405.1316(d) 5. Each sterilization cycle includes a device to assure proper performance or a recording thermometer is used		☐	01014	
6. Each autoclave is checked monthly with spores to assure proper performance		* ☐	01015	
STANDARD OPERATING PROCEDURE MANUAL (SOPM) CFR 74.20(d)(e)(f) 405.1317(a)(4)(5)(6) 7. The bacteriology section has an SOPM		☐	01016	
8. The SOPM is in bacteriology work bench area		☐	01017	
9. The SOPM has a supervisor's written attestation that SOPM is current		☐	01018	
10. The supervisor's review of the SOPM is dated		☐	01019	
11. The SOPM includes only those procedures currently in use		☐	01020	
12. All changes in procedures are documented (description of change and date) in the SOPM and have the written approval (initials and date) of the supervisor		☐	01021	

13. For each procedure, if offered by the lab, the bacteriology SOPM includes the following:

PROCEDURE	Instructions NO (Code)	COMMENT	PROCEDURE	Instructions NO (Code)	Reagents NO (Code)	COMMENT
☐ Biopsy culture	☐ 01023		☐ Antimicrobial susceptibility	☐ 01042	☐ 01043	
☐ Blood culture	☐ 01024		☐ Antisera	☐ 01044	☐ 01045	
☐ Bone marrow culture	☐ 01025		☐ Capsule stain	☐ 01046	☐ 01047	
☐ Bronchial washing culture	☐ 01026		☐ Catalase test	☐ 01048	☐ 01049	
☐ Cerebrospinal fluid culture	☐ 01027		☐ Coagulase test	☐ 01050	☐ 01051	
☐ Ear culture	☐ 01028		☐ Discs	☐ 01052		
☐ Eye culture	☐ 01029		☐ Ferric chloride test	☐ 01054	☐ 01055	
☐ Genital tract culture	☐ 01030		☐ Flagella stain	☐ 01056	☐ 01057	
☐ Joint fluid culture	☐ 01031		☐ Gram stain	☐ 01058	☐ 01059	
☐ Mouth culture	☐ 01032		☐ Indole test	☐ 01060	☐ 01061	
☐ Naso-pharyngeal culture	☐ 01033		☐ Methyl red test	☐ 01062	☐ 01063	
☐ Paracentesis culture	☐ 01034		☐ Methylene blue stain	☐ 01064	☐ 01065	
☐ Prostate culture	☐ 01035		☐ Nitrate test	☐ 01066	☐ 01067	
☐ Skin culture	☐ 01036		☐ Oxidase test	☐ 01068	☐ 01069	
☐ Stool culture	☐ 01040		☐ Spore stain	☐ 01070	☐ 01071	
☐ Wound culture	☐ 01041		☐ Strips	☐ 01072		
☐ Sputum culture	☐ 01037		☐ Tellurite reduction test	☐ 01074	☐ 01075	
☐ Throat culture	☐ 01038		☐ Voges-Proskauer test	☐ 01076	☐ 01077	
☐ Urine culture	☐ 01039		☐ Identification system (commercial) ☐ 01078		☐ 01079	

CDC 3.1005 8-77   BACTERIOLOGY – Page 1 of 4 pages

CDC laboratory examination checklist (1977)—bacteriology

Continued.

MATERIALS CFR 74.20(c) 405.1317 (a)(3)		NO (Code)		COMMENT	
14. The following are labeled (identity, titer or concentration, recommended storage, preparation or expiration date)	Antimicrobials	☐ 01080			
	Antisera	☐ 01081			
	Control Organisms	☐ 01082			
	Media (tubes, plates, kits)	☐ 01083			
	Disc	☐ 01084			
	Strips	☐ 01085			
	Reagent Solutions	☐ 01086			
15. Materials in use are "in-date", reactive, and not deteriorated	Antimicrobials	☐ 01087			
	Antisera	☐ 01088			
	Control Organisms	☐ 01089			
	Media (tubes, plates, kits)	☐ 01090			
	Disc	☐ 01091			
	Strips	☐ 01092			
	Reagent Solutions	☐ 01093			

TESTING OF REAGENTS CFR 74.20(a) 405.1317(a)(1) 405.1317(b)(1)

		Positive Reaction NO (Code)	Negative Reaction NO (Code)	Written Q.C. NO (Code)	COMMENT
16. The following reagents (in use as individual biochemical tests or as a part of a commercial system) are tested each day of use to demonstrate a positive and negative biochemical reaction	Catalase	*☐ 01094	*☐ 01095	*☐ 01096	
	Coagulase	*☐ 01097	*☐ 01098	*☐ 01099	
	Ferric Chloride	*☐ 01100	*☐ 01101	*☐ 01102	
	Indole	*☐ 01103	*☐ 01104	*☐ 01105	
	Methyl red	*☐ 01106	*☐ 01107	*☐ 01108	
	Nitrate	*☐ 01109	*☐ 01110	*☐ 01111	
	Oxidase	*☐ 01112	*☐ 01113	*☐ 01114	
	Voges-Proskauer	*☐ 01115	*☐ 01116	*☐ 01117	
17. The following disc and/or strips are tested when each new vial is opened and each week of use to demonstrate positive and negative biochemical reactions.	Bacitracin	*☐ 01118	*☐ 01119	*☐ 01120	
	Optochin	*☐ 01121	*☐ 01122	*☐ 01123	
	ONPG	*☐ 01124	*☐ 01125	*☐ 01126	
	X	*☐ 01127	*☐ 01128	*☐ 01129	
	V	*☐ 01130	*☐ 01131	*☐ 01132	
	XV	*☐ 01133	*☐ 01134	*☐ 01135	
18. The following antisera are tested when each new vial is opened and each month of use to demonstrate positive and negative agglutination reactions	E. Coli	*☐ 01136	*☐ 01137	*☐ 01138	
	Hemophilus	*☐ 01139	*☐ 01140	*☐ 01141	
	Herella	*☐ 01142	*☐ 01143	*☐ 01144	
	Salmonella	*☐ 01145	*☐ 01146	*☐ 01147	
	Shigella	*☐ 01148	*☐ 01149	*☐ 01150	
	Streptococcal	*☐ 01151	*☐ 01152	*☐ 01153	

STAINS CFR 74.21(a) 405.1313(b)(1)(i)

19. The following stains are tested each day of use to demonstrate expected staining characteristics.	Capsule	*☐ 01154		*☐ 01156	
	Flagella	*☐ 01157		*☐ 01159	
	Methylene Blue	*☐ 01160		*☐ 01162	
	Spore	*☐ 01163		*☐ 01165	
20. Gram stain is tested when prepared and each week of use to demonstrate expected staining characteristics (positive and negative reactions)		*☐ 01166	*☐ 01167	*☐ 01168	

21. Each batch of the following media, if used by the lab, is tested for the following characteristics

GROWTH MEDIUM	Support Growth No (Code)	Sterility No (Code)	Written Q.C. NO (Code)	COMMENT
Blood Agar	*☐ 01169	*☐ 01170	*☐ 01171	
Brain Heart Infusion Agar/Broth	*☐ 01172	*☐ 01173	*☐ 01174	
Chocolate Agar	*☐ 01175	*☐ 01176	*☐ 01177	
Heart Infusion Agar	*☐ 01178	*☐ 01179	*☐ 01180	
Motility	*☐ 01181	*☐ 01182	*☐ 01183	
Mueller Hinton	*☐ 01184	*☐ 01185	*☐ 01186	
Nutrient Agar/Broth	*☐ 01187	*☐ 01188	*☐ 01189	
Thioglycollate Broth	*☐ 01190	*☐ 01191	*☐ 01192	
Tryptic Soy Agar/Broth	*☐ 01193	*☐ 01194	*☐ 01195	
Todd Hewitt Broth	*☐ 01244	*☐ 01246	*☐ 01247	

CDC laboratory examination checklist (1977)—bacteriology—cont'd

21. (Continued) Each batch of the following media, if used by the lab, is tested for the following characteristics:

SELECTIVE MEDIUM	Support Growth NO (Code)	Inhibits Growth NO (Code)	Sterility NO (Code)	Written Q.C. NO (Code)	COMMENT
Azide Blood Agar	*☐ 01196	*☐ 01197	*☐ 01198	*☐ 01199	
Eva Broth (6.5% NaC1)	*☐ 01200	*☐ 01201	*☐ 01202	*☐ 01203	
GN Broth	*☐ 01204	*☐ 01205	*☐ 01206	*☐ 01207	
Potassium Cyanide (KCN)	*☐ 01208	*☐ 01209	*☐ 01210	*☐ 01211	
Loeffler's	*☐ 01212	*☐ 01213	*☐ 01214	*☐ 01215	
Pai	*☐ 01216	*☐ 01217	*☐ 01218	*☐ 01219	
Phenyl Ethyl Alcohol (PEA)	*☐ 01220	*☐ 01221	*☐ 01222	*☐ 01223	
Pseudomonas Agar	*☐ 01224	*☐ 01225	*☐ 01226	*☐ 01227	
Selenite F Broth	*☐ 01228	*☐ 01229	*☐ 01230	*☐ 01231	
Sodium Azide Agar	*☐ 01232	*☐ 01233	*☐ 01234	*☐ 01235	
Tetrathionate Broth	*☐ 01236	*☐ 01237	*☐ 01238	*☐ 01239	
Thayer Martin Agar	*☐ 01240	*☐ 01241	*☐ 01242	*☐ 01243	
Transgrow	*☐ 01248	*☐ 01249	*☐ 01250	*☐ 01251	

BIOCHEMICAL MEDIUM	Positive Control NO (Code)	Negative Control NO (Code)	Sterility NO (Code)	Written Q.C. NO.(Code)	
Arginine dihydrolase	*☐ 01584	*☐ 01585	*☐ 01586	*☐ 01587	
Carbohydrate Media (CTA)					
Adonitol	*☐ 01252	*☐ 01253	*☐ 01254	*☐ 01255	
Arabinose	*☐ 01256	*☐ 01257	*☐ 01258	*☐ 01259	
Dulcitol	*☐ 01260	*☐ 01261	*☐ 01262	*☐ 01263	
Glucose (Dextrose)	*☐ 01264	*☐ 01265	*☐ 01266	*☐ 01267	
Inositol	*☐ 01268	*☐ 01269	*☐ 01270	*☐ 01271	
Lactose	*☐ 01272	*☐ 01273	*☐ 01274	*☐ 01275	
Maltose	*☐ 01276	*☐ 01277	*☐ 01278	*☐ 01279	
Mannitol	*☐ 01280	*☐ 01281	*☐ 01282	*☐ 01283	
Raffinose	*☐ 01284	*☐ 01285	*☐ 01286	*☐ 01287	
Rhamnose	*☐ 01288	*☐ 01289	*☐ 01290	*☐ 01291	
Salicin	*☐ 01292	*☐ 01293	*☐ 01294	*☐ 01295	
Sorbitol	*☐ 01296	*☐ 01297	*☐ 01298	*☐ 01299	
Sucrose	*☐ 01300	*☐ 01301	*☐ 01302	*☐ 01303	
Xylose	*☐ 01304	*☐ 01305	*☐ 01306	*☐ 01307	
Carbohydrate Media (Diff.)					
Adonitol	*☐ 01308	*☐ 01309	*☐ 01310	*☐ 01311	
Arabinose	*☐ 01312	*☐ 01313	*☐ 01314	*☐ 01315	
Dulcitol	*☐ 01316	*☐ 01317	*☐ 01318	*☐ 01319	
Glucose (Dextrose)	*☐ 01320	*☐ 01321	*☐ 01322	*☐ 01323	
Inositol	*☐ 01324	*☐ 01325	*☐ 01326	*☐ 01327	
Lactose	*☐ 01328	*☐ 01329	*☐ 01330	*☐ 01331	
Maltose	*☐ 01332	*☐ 01333	*☐ 01334	*☐ 01335	
Mannitol	*☐ 01336	*☐ 01337	*☐ 01338	*☐ 01339	
Raffinose	*☐ 01340	*☐ 01341	*☐ 01342	*☐ 01343	
Ramnose	*☐ 01344	*☐ 01345	*☐ 01346	*☐ 01347	
Salicin	*☐ 01348	*☐ 01349	*☐ 01350	*☐ 01351	
Sorbitol	*☐ 01352	*☐ 01353	*☐ 01354	*☐ 01355	
Sucrose	*☐ 01356	*☐ 01357	*☐ 01358	*☐ 01359	
Xylose	*☐ 01360	*☐ 01361	*☐ 01362	*☐ 01363	
Carbohydrate Media (OF Util.)					
Adonitol	*☐ 01364	*☐ 01365	*☐ 01366	*☐ 01367	
Arabinose	*☐ 01368	*☐ 01369	*☐ 01370	*☐ 01371	
Dulcitol	*☐ 01372	*☐ 01373	*☐ 01374	*☐ 01375	
Glucose (Dextrose)	*☐ 01376	*☐ 01377	*☐ 01378	*☐ 01379	
Inositol	*☐ 01380	*☐ 01381	*☐ 01382	*☐ 01383	
Lactose	*☐ 01384	*☐ 01385	*☐ 01386	*☐ 01387	
Maltose	*☐ 01388	*☐ 01389	*☐ 01390	*☐ 01391	
Mannitol	*☐ 01392	*☐ 01393	*☐ 01394	*☐ 01395	
Raffinose	*☐ 01396	*☐ 01397	*☐ 01398	*☐ 01399	
Ramnose	*☐ 01400	*☐ 01401	*☐ 01402	*☐ 01403	

Continued.

CDC laboratory examination checklist (1977)—bacteriology—cont'd

21. (Continued) Each batch of the following media, if used by the lab, is tested for the following characteristics

BIOCHEMICAL MEDIUM	Positive Control NO (Code)	Negative Control NO (Code)	Sterility NO (Code)	Written Q.C. NO (Code)	COMMENT
Salicin	*☐ 01404	*☐ 01405	*☐ 01406	*☐ 01407	
Sorbitol	*☐ 01408	*☐ 01409	*☐ 01410	*☐ 01411	
Sucrose	*☐ 01412	*☐ 01413	*☐ 01414	*☐ 01415	
Xylose	*☐ 01416	*☐ 01417	*☐ 01418	*☐ 01419	
Citrate	*☐ 01420	*☐ 01421	*☐ 01422	*☐ 01423	
DNase Test Agar	*☐ 01424	*☐ 01425	*☐ 01426	*☐ 01427	
Gelatin	*☐ 01428	*☐ 01429	*☐ 01430	*☐ 01431	
Kligler's Iron Agar	*☐ 01432	*☐ 01433	*☐ 01434	*☐ 01435	
Litmus Milk	*☐ 01436	*☐ 01437	*☐ 01438	*☐ 01439	
ONPG	*☐ 01580	*☐ 01581	*☐ 01582	*☐ 01583	
SIM	*☐ 01440	*☐ 01441	*☐ 01442	*☐ 01443	
Tinsdale	*☐ 01444	*☐ 01445	*☐ 01446	*☐ 01447	
Triple Sugar Iron Agar (TSI)	*☐ 01448	*☐ 01449	*☐ 01450	*☐ 01451	
Urease Agar/Broth	*☐ 01452	*☐ 01453	*☐ 01454	*☐ 01455	
SELECTIVE/BIOCHEMICAL MEDIUM					
Bile Esculin Agar	*☐ 01456	*☐ 01457	*☐ 01458	*☐ 01459	
Bismuth Sulfite Agar	*☐ 01460	*☐ 01461	*☐ 01462	*☐ 01463	
Brilliant Green Agar	*☐ 01464	*☐ 01465	*☐ 01466	*☐ 01467	
Cystine Tellurite Agar	*☐ 01468	*☐ 01469	*☐ 01470	*☐ 01471	
Desoxycholate Agar	*☐ 01472	*☐ 01473	*☐ 01474	*☐ 01475	
Eosin Methylene Blue Agar (EMB)	*☐ 01476	*☐ 01477	*☐ 01478	*☐ 01479	
Hektoen Agar	*☐ 01480	*☐ 01481	*☐ 01482	*☐ 01483	
Lysine Decarboxylase Broth/agar	*☐ 01484	*☐ 01485	*☐ 01486	*☐ 01487	
Lysine Iron Agar	*☐ 01488	*☐ 01489	*☐ 01490	*☐ 01491	
MacConkey Agar (MAC)	*☐ 01492	*☐ 01493	*☐ 01494	*☐ 01495	
Malonate Broth	*☐ 01496	*☐ 01497	*☐ 01498	*☐ 01499	
Mannitol Salt Agar	*☐ 01500	*☐ 01501	*☐ 01502	*☐ 01503	
Ornithine Decarboxylase Agar	*☐ 01504	*☐ 01505	*☐ 01506	*☐ 01507	
Pfizer Selective Enterococcus	*☐ 01508	*☐ 01509	*☐ 01510	*☐ 01511	
Salmonella-Shigella	*☐ 01512	*☐ 01513	*☐ 01514	*☐ 01515	
Staph No. 110	*☐ 01516	*☐ 01517	*☐ 01518	*☐ 01519	
Streptococcus Fecalis Broth	*☐ 01520	*☐ 01521	*☐ 01522	*☐ 01523	
Tellurite Glycine Agar	*☐ 01524	*☐ 01525	*☐ 01526	*☐ 01527	
Vogel Johnson Agar	*☐ 01528	*☐ 01529	*☐ 01530	*☐ 01531	
Xylose Lysine Desoxycholate (XLD)	*☐ 01532	*☐ 01533	*☐ 01534	*☐ 01535	

COMMERCIAL SYSTEMS					SYSTEM
Each commercial system in use is tested each shipment with sufficient known organisms to give at least one positive and one negative biochemical response for each constituent.	*☐ 01536	*☐ 01537	*☐ 01538	*☐ 01539	API
	*☐ 01540	*☐ 01541	*☐ 01542	*☐ 01543	Enterotube
	*☐ 01544	*☐ 01545	*☐ 01546	*☐ 01547	Mini-Tek
	*☐ 01548	*☐ 01549	*☐ 01550	*☐ 01551	Oxy-Ferm
	*☐ 01552	*☐ 01553	*☐ 01554	*☐ 01555	R/B
	*☐ 01556	*☐ 01557	*☐ 01558	*☐ 01559	Other

SUSCEPTIBILITY TESTING CFR 74.21 405.1317(b)(1)

	NO (Code)	Zone NO (Code)	Limits NO (Code)	Within Limits NO (Code)	COMMENT
22. Antimicrobials are tested each day os use with:					
S. aureus (ATCC25923)	*☐ 01560	*☐ 01561	*☐ 01562	*☐ 01563	
E. coli (ATCC25922)	*☐ 01564	*☐ 01565	*☐ 01566	*☐ 01567	
P. aeruginosa (ATCC27853)	*☐ 01568	*☐ 01569	*☐ 01570	*☐ 01571	
23. Automated antimicrobial instrument is calibrated with a filter each day of use.	*☐ 01572		*☐ 01573	*☐ 01589	

	NO (Code)	
24. A written statement of quality control for antibiotic susceptibility testing is available.	☐ 01590	

RECORDS CFR 74.50 74.54(a) 405.1316 405.1316(g)

25. Records of observations are made concurrently with the performance of each step in the examination of specimens.	☐ 01574	
26. Records are retained at least two (2) years:		
Accession	☐ 01575	
Control	☐ 01576	
Equipment maintenance	☐ 01577	
Observations of each step of specimen testing	☐ 01578	
Reports to clients	☐ 01579	

CDC 3.1005 8-77   BACTERIOLOGY — Page 4 of 4 Pages

CDC laboratory examination checklist (1977)—bacteriology—cont'd

ANAEROBIC BACTERIOLOGY

LABORATORY EXAMINATION CHECKLIST — CLIA '67 — CDC

DEPARTMENT OF HEALTH, EDUCATION, AND WELFARE
PUBLIC HEALTH SERVICE
CENTER FOR DISEASE CONTROL
ATLANTA, GEORGIA 30333

Code No.

Examiner(s)

Name of Laboratory

Interviewee(s)

Address

Date(s) of examination

NOTE TO EXAMINER:

a) For each item marked with an *, mark "No" if there is no record to confirm that the laboratory is actually applying the standard. A record is REQUIRED: however, if a laboratory CLAIMS IT APPLIES THE STANDARD but has no record, indicate under comment space.

b) The examiner must check each block to the left of the question or specific item to indicate if the item is available or used in this laboratory.

PREVENTIVE MAINTENANCE CFR 74.20(a) 405.1317(a)(1)		NO (Code)	COMMENT
1. Each equipment item is tested periodically for proper operation	Anaerobic jar Autoclave Biosafety cabinet	*☐ 01600 *☐ 01601 *☐ 01602	
	Gas chromatograph Incubator Glove box	*☐ 01603 *☐ 01604 *☐ 01605	
2. Each equipment item is subjected to preventive maintenance	Autoclave Biosafety cabinet Gas chromatograph	*☐ 01607 *☐ 01608 *☐ 01609	
	Incubator Glove box	*☐ 01610 *☐ 01611	
3. Records document remedial actions taken for detected defects		☐ 01613	
TEMPERATURES CFR 74.20(b) 405.1317(a)(2)			
4. Temperatures are monitored each day of use	Incubators Refrigerators Water baths Heat blocks Freezers	*☐ 01614 *☐ 01615 *☐ 01616 *☐ 01617 *☐ 01618	

STANDARD OPERATING PROCEDURE MANUAL (SOPM) CFR 74.20(d)(e)(f) 405.1317(a)(4)(5)(6)	
5. The anaerobic bacteriology section has an SOPM	☐ 01619
6. The SOPM is in the anaerobic bacteriology work bench area	☐ 01620
7. The SOPM has a supervisor's written attestation that the SOPM is current	☐ 01621
8. The supervisor's review of the SOPM is dated	☐ 01622
9. The SOPM includes only those procedures currently in use	☐ 01623
10. All changes in procedures are documented (description of change and date) in the SOPM and have the written approval (initials and date) of the supervisor	☐ 01624

11. For each procedure, if offered by the lab, the syphilis serology SOPM includes the following:

PROCEDURE	Instructions NO (Code)	PROCEDURE	Instructions NO (Code)	Reagents NO (Code)	COMMENT
☐ Identification protocol ☐ Isolation protocol ☐ Specimen collection protocol ☐ Specimen handling protocol	☐ 01625 ☐ 01626 ☐ 01627 ☐ 01628	☐ Antimicrobial suscep ☐ Catalase test ☐ Flagella stain ☐ Gram stain	☐ 01629 ☐ 01631 ☐ 01633 ☐ 01635	☐ 01630 ☐ 01632 ☐ 01634 ☐ 01636	
		☐ Indole test ☐ Nitrate test ☐ Spore stain ☐ Identification system	☐ 01637 ☐ 01639 ☐ 01641 ☐ 01643	☐ 01638 ☐ 01640 ☐ 01642 ☐ 01644	

MATERIALS CFR 74.20(c); 405.1317(a)(3)		NO (Code)	COMMENT
12. The following are labeled (identity, titer or concentration, recommended storage, preparation or expiration date)	Antimicrobials Control Organisms Media (tube, plate, & kit) Reagent solutions	☐ 01645 ☐ 01646 ☐ 01647 ☐ 01648	

CDC 3.1005-2 10-77

ANAEROBIC BACTERIOLOGY — Page 1 of 3 Pages

Continued.

CDC laboratory examination checklist (1977)—anaerobic bacteriology

MATERIALS CFR 74.20(c); 405.1317(a)(3)		NO (Code)		COMMENT
13. Materials in use are "in-date", reactive and not deteriorated	Antimicrobials	☐ 01649		
	Control organisms	☐ 01650		
	Media (tube, plate, & kit)	☐ 01651		
	Reagent solutions	☐ 01652		

TESTING OF REAGENTS CFR 74.20(a) 405.1317(a)(1) 405.1317(b)(1)		Positive Reaction NO (Code)	Negative Reaction NO (Code)	COMMENT
14. The following reagents are tested each day of use to demonstrate positive and negative biochemical reactions	Catalase	*☐ 01653		
	Ferric ammonium citrate	*☐ 01655		
	Indole	*☐ 01657		
	Nitrate	*☐ 01659		

STAINS CFR 74.21(a) 405.1317(b)(1)(i)				
15 The following stains are tested each day of use to demonstrate expected staining characteristics	Capsule	*☐ 01661		
	Flagella	*☐ 01663		
	Spore	*☐ 01665		
16. Gram stain is tested when prepared and each week of use to demonstrate positive and negative reactions		*☐ 01667	*☐ 01668	

MEDIA CFR 74.21(a); 405.1317(b)(i)

17. Each batch of the following media, if used by the laboratory, is tested for the following characteristics

GROWTH MEDIUM	Support Growth NO (Code)	Sterility NO (Code)	Written Q.C. NO (Code)	COMMENT
Blood agar	*☐ 01669	*☐ 01670	*☐ 01671	
Chopped meat broth	*☐ 01672	*☐ 01673	*☐ 01674	
Egg-yolk agar lecithinase	*☐ 01675	*☐ 01676	*☐ 01677	
Egg-yolk agar lipase	*☐ 01678	*☐ 01679	*☐ 01680	
Peptone yeast broth	*☐ 01681	*☐ 01682	*☐ 01683	
Motility	*☐ 01684	*☐ 01686	*☐ 01687	
Stuart transport	*☐ 01685	*☐ 01688	*☐ 01689	
Thioglycollate	*☐ 01690	*☐ 01692	*☐ 01693	

SELECTIVE MEDIUM	Support Growth NO (Code)	Inhibits Growth NO (Code)	Sterility NO (Code)	Written Q.C. NO (Code)	COMMENT
Phenylethyl alcohol agar (PEA)	*☐ 01694	*☐ 01695	*☐ 01696	*☐ 01697	

BIOCHEMICAL MEDIUM	Positive Control NO (Code)	Sterility NO (Code)	Written Q.C. NO (Code)	COMMENT
Carbohydrate Media				
Adonitol	*☐ 01698	*☐ 01700	*☐ 01701	
Arabinose	*☐ 01702	*☐ 01704	*☐ 01705	
Dulcitol	*☐ 01706	*☐ 01708	*☐ 01709	
Glucose (Dextrose)	*☐ 01710	*☐ 01712	*☐ 01713	
Inositol	*☐ 01714	*☐ 01716	*☐ 01717	
Lactose	*☐ 01718	*☐ 01720	*☐ 01721	
Maltose	*☐ 01722	*☐ 01724	*☐ 01725	
Mannitol	*☐ 01726	*☐ 01728	*☐ 01729	
Raffinose	*☐ 01730	*☐ 01732	*☐ 01733	
Ramnose	*☐ 01734	*☐ 01736	*☐ 01737	
Salicin	*☐ 01738	*☐ 01740	*☐ 01741	
Sucrose	*☐ 01742	*☐ 01744	*☐ 01745	
Trehalose	*☐ 01746	*☐ 01748	*☐ 01749	
Xylose	*☐ 01750	*☐ 01752	*☐ 01753	
Mannose	*☐ 01754	*☐ 01756	*☐ 01757	
Glycerol	*☐ 01758	*☐ 01760	*☐ 01761	
Esculin agar	*☐ 01762	*☐ 01764	*☐ 01765	
Gelatin	*☐ 01766	*☐ 01768	*☐ 01769	
Lead acetate	*☐ 01770	*☐ 01772	*☐ 01773	
Milk digestion	*☐ 01774	*☐ 01776	*☐ 01777	
Starch	*☐ 01778	*☐ 01780	*☐ 01781	
Urea	*☐ 01782	*☐ 01784	*☐ 01785	

CDC 3.1005-2 10-77   ANAEROBIC BACTERIOLOGY – Page 2 of 3 Pages

CDC laboratory examination checklist (1977)—anaerobic bacteriology—cont'd

MEDIA (Cont'd)
17. Each batch of the following media, if used by the lab, is tested for the following characteristics (Cont'd)

COMMERCIAL SYSTEM	Positive Control NO (Code)		Sterility NO (Code)	Written Q.C. NO (Code)	SYSTEM	COMMENT
Each commercial system in use is tested each shipment with sufficient known organisms to give at least one positive and one negative biochemical reaction for each constituent	* ☐ 01786 * ☐ 01790 * ☐ 01794		* ☐ 01788 * ☐ 01792 * ☐ 01796	* ☐ 01789 * ☐ 01793 * ☐ 01797	API Minitek Other	

RECORDS CFR 74.50, 74.54(a) 405.1316 405.1316(g)	NO (Code)	COMMENT
18. Records of observations are made concurrently with the performance of each step in the examination of specimens	* ☐ 01798	

19. Records are retained at least two years
                Accession
                Control
                Equipment maintenance
                Observations of each step of
                  specimen testing
                Reports
	* ☐ 01799
	* ☐ 01800
	* ☐ 01801
	
	* ☐ 01802
	* ☐ 01803	

CDC laboratory examination checklist (1977)—anaerobic bacteriology—cont'd

DEPARTMENT OF HEALTH, EDUCATION, AND WELFARE
PUBLIC HEALTH SERVICE
CENTER FOR DISEASE CONTROL
ATLANTA, GEORGIA 30333

MYCOBACTERIOLOGY
LABORATORY EXAMINATION CHECKLIST—CLIA '67—CDC

Code No.

Examiner(s)

Name of Laboratory

Interviewee(s)

Address

Date(s) of examination

NOTE TO EXAMINER:

a) *For each item marked with an* *, *mark "No" if there is no record to confirm that the laboratory is actually applying the standard. A record is required; however, if a laboratory CLAIMS IT APPLIES THE STANDARD but has no record, indicate under comment column.*

b) *The examiner must check each block to the left of the question or specific item to indicate if the item is available or used in this laboratory.*

PREVENTIVE MAINTENANCE CFR 74.20(a) 405.1317(a)(1)		NO	CODE	COMMENT
1. Each equipment item is tested periodically for proper operation	Autoclaves	*☐	01825	
	Incubators	*☐	01826	
	Fluorescent Microscope	*☐	01827	
	Biosafety Cabinet	*☐	01828	
2. Each equipment item is subjected to preventive maintenance	Autoclaves	*☐	01830	
	Incubators	*☐	01831	
	Fluorescent Microscope	*☐	01832	
	Biosafety Cabinet	*☐	01833	
3. Records document remedial actions taken for detected defects		☐	01835	
TEMPERATURES CFR 74.20(b) 405.1317(a)(2)				
4. Temperatures are monitored each day of use	Incubators	*☐	01836	
	Refrigerators	*☐	01837	
	Water Baths	*☐	01838	
	Heat Blocks	*☐	01839	
	Freezers	*☐	01840	
STERILIZATION CFR 74.20(b) 405.1316(d)				
5. Each sterilization cycle includes a device to assure proper performance or a recording thermometer is used		☐	01841	
6. Each autoclave is checked monthly with spores to assure proper performance		*☐	01842	
STANDARD OPERATING PROCEDURE MANUAL (SOPM) CFR 74.20(d)(e)(f) 405.1317(a)(4)(5)(6)				
7. The mycobacteriology section has an SOPM		☐	01843	
8. The SOPM is in the mycobacteriology workbench area		☐	01844	
9. The SOPM has a supervisor's written attestation that SOPM is current		☐	01845	
10. The supervisor's review of the SOPM is dated		☐	01846	
11. The SOPM includes only those procedures currently in use		☐	01847	
12. All changes in procedures are documented (description of change and date) in the SOPM and have the written approval (initials and date) of the supervisor		☐	01848	

13. For each procedure, if offered by the lab, the mycobacteriology SOPM includes the following:

PROCEDURE	Instructions NO (Code)	Reagents NO (Code)	PROCEDURE	Instructions NO (Code)	Reagents NO (Code)
☐ Biopsy culture	☐ 01849		☐ Acid fast stain	☐ 01857	☐ 01858
☐ Bronchial washing culture	☐ 01850		☐ Arylsulfatase test	☐ 01859	☐ 01860
☐ Joint fluid culture	☐ 01851		☐ Catalase test	☐ 01861	☐ 01862
☐ Sputum culture	☐ 01852		☐ Drug susceptibility	☐ 01863	☐ 01864
☐ Stool culture	☐ 01853		☐ Niacin test	☐ 01865	☐ 01866
☐ Urine culture	☐ 01854		☐ Nitrate reduction test	☐ 01867	☐ 01868
☐ Concentration technique	☐ 01855	☐ 01856	☐ Tellurite reduction	☐ 01869	☐ 01870
			☐ Tween 80 Hydrolysis	☐ 01871	☐ 01872
			☐ Flurochrome stain	☐ 01873	☐ 01874

MATERIALS CFR 74.20(c) 405.1317(a)(3)		NO	(CODE)	COMMENT
14. The following are labeled (identity, titer or concentration, recommended storage, preparation or expiration date)	antimicrobials	☐	01875	
	control organisms	☐	01876	
	media (tubes, plates)	☐	01877	
	reagent solutions	☐	01878	
	strips	☐	01879	

CDC 3.1005-2
10-77

Mycobacteriology — Page 1 of 2

CDC laboratory examination checklist (1977)—mycobacteriology

MATERIALS CFR 74.20(c) 405.1317(a)(3)

15. Materials in use are "in-date", reactive and not deteriorated		NO	(CODE)	COMMENT
	antimicrobials	☐	01880	
	control organisms	☐	01881	
	media (tubes, plates)	☐	01882	
	reagent solutions	☐	01883	
	strips	☐	01884	

16. The following reagents are tested each day of use with an acid fast organism which produces a positive biochemical response

	NO (Code)	Written Q.C. NO (Code)		NO (Code)	Written Q.C. NO (Code)
Arylsulfatase	*☐ 01885	*☐ 01886	Nitrate reduction	*☐ 01891	*☐ 01892
Catalase	*☐ 01887	*☐ 01888	Tellurite reduction	*☐ 01893	*☐ 01894
Niacin	*☐ 01889	*☐ 01890	Tween 80 hydrolysis	*☐ 01895	*☐ 01896

STAINS CFR 74.21(a) 405.1317(b)(1)(i)

	(+) React. NO (Code)	(−) React. NO (Code)	Written Q.C. NO (Code)
17. Stains for acid fast organisms are tested each day of use with a known acid fast bacterium	*☐ 01897		*☐ 01898
18. Fluorochrome stains are tested each day of use with a known acid fast and non-acid fast organism	*☐ 01899	*☐ 01900	*☐ 01901

19. Each batch of the following media, if used by the lab, is tested for the following characteristics

MEDIUM	Expected Growth NO (Code)	Sterility NO (Code)	Written Q.C. NO (Code)	COMMENT
Lowenstein-Jensen	*☐ 01902	*☐ 01903	*☐ 01904	
Petragnani	*☐ 01905	*☐ 01906	*☐ 01907	
7H10 agar	*☐ 01908	*☐ 01909	*☐ 01910	
7H9 agar	*☐ 01911	*☐ 01912	*☐ 01913	

RECORDS CFR 74.50 74.54(a) 405.1316 405.1316(g)

	NO	(Code)
20. Records of observations are made, concurrently with the performance of each step in the examination of specimens	☐	01914

21. Records are retained at least 2 years:	NO (Code)		NO (Code)		NO (Code)
Accession	☐ 01915	Equipment maintenance	☐ 01917	Reports	☐ 01919
Control	☐ 01916	Observation of each step of specimen testing	☐ 01918		

CDC 3.1005-2
10-77

Mycobacteriology — Page 2 of 2

CDC laboratory examination checklist (1977)—mycobacteriology—cont'd

DEPARTMENT OF HEALTH, EDUCATION, AND WELFARE
PUBLIC HEALTH SERVICE
CENTER FOR DISEASE CONTROL
ATLANTA, GEORGIA 30333

MYCOLOGY
LABORATORY EXAMINATION CHECKLIST — CLIA '67 — CDC

Code No.
Examiner(s)
Interviewee(s)
Date(s) of examination

Name of Laboratory

Address

NOTE TO EXAMINER:

a) For each item marked with an *, mark "No" if there is no record to confirm that the laboratory is actually applying the standard. A record is REQUIRED; however, if a laboratory CLAIMS IT APPLIES THE STANDARD but has no record, indicate under comment space.

b) The examiner must check each block to the left of the question or specific item to indicate if the item is available or used in this laboratory.

		NO	(CODE)	COMMENT
PREVENTIVE MAINTENANCE CFR 74.20(a) 405.1317(a)(1)				
1. Each equipment item is tested periodically for proper operation	Autoclaves	* ☐	02000	
	Incubators	* ☐	02001	
	Fluorescent Microscope	* ☐	02002	
	Biosafety Cabinet	* ☐	02003	
2. Each equipment item is subjected to preventive maintenance	Autoclaves	* ☐	02005	
	Incubators	* ☐	02006	
	Fluorescent Microscope	* ☐	02007	
	Biosafety Cabinet	* ☐	02008	
3. Records document remedial actions taken for detected defects		☐	02010	
TEMPERATURES CFR 74.20(b) 405.1317(a)(2)				
4. Temperatures are monitored each day of use	Incubators	* ☐	02011	
	Refrigerators	* ☐	02012	
	Water Baths	* ☐	02013	
	Heat Blocks	* ☐	02014	
	Freezers	* ☐	02015	
STERILIZATION CFR 74.20 (b) 405.1316(d)				
5. Each sterilization cycle includes a device to assure proper performance or a recording thermometer is used		☐	02016	
6. Each autoclave is checked montlhy with spores to assure proper performance		* ☐	02017	
STANDARD OPERATING PROCEDURE MANUAL (SOPM) CFR 74.20(d)(e)(f)				
7. The mycology section has an SOPM 405.1317(a)(4)(5)(6)		☐	02018	
8. The SOPM is in the mycology work bench area		☐	02019	

9. For each procedure, if offered by the lab, the mycology SOPM includes the following:

Procedure	Instructions No (Code)	Procedure	Instructions No. (Code)	Reagents No (Code)	Comment
☐ Abscess culture	☐ 02020	☐ Carbohydrate assimilation	☐ 02038	☐ 02039	
☐ Biopsy culture	☐ 02021	☐ Carbohydrate fermentation	☐ 02040	☐ 02041	
☐ Blood culture	☐ 02022	☐ Germ tube test	☐ 02042	☐ 02043	
☐ Bone marrow culture	☐ 02023	☐ Giemsa stain	☐ 02044	☐ 02045	
☐ Bronchial wash culture	☐ 02024				
☐ Cerebrospinal fluid culture	☐ 02025	☐ Gram stain	☐ 02046	☐ 02047	
☐ Ear culture	☐ 02026	☐ India ink preparation	☐ 02048	☐ 02049	
☐ Eye culture	☐ 02027	☐ KOH (potassium hydroxide)			
☐ Hair culture	☐ 02028	preparation	☐ 02050	☐ 02051	
☐ Joint fluid culture	☐ 02029	☐ Lactophenol cotton blue preparation	☐ 02052	☐ 02053	
☐ Mouth culture	☐ 02030	☐ Modified acid fast stain	☐ 02054	☐ 02055	
☐ Nail culture	☐ 02031	☐ Nitrate test	☐ 02056	☐ 02057	
☐ Pleural fluid culture	☐ 02032	☐ PAS stain	☐ 02058	☐ 02059	
☐ Skin culture	☐ 02033				
☐ Sputum culture	☐ 02034				
☐ Throat culture	☐ 02035	☐ Wright's stain	☐ 02060	☐ 02061	
☐ Urine culture	☐ 02036	☐ Identification system(commercial)	☐ 02062	☐ 02063	
☐ Vaginal culture	☐ 02037				

	NO	(Code)	
10. The SOPM has a supervisor's written attestation that SOPM is current	☐	02066	
11. The supervisor's review of SOPM is dated	☐	02067	
12. The SOPM includes only those procedures currently in use	☐	02068	

CDC 3.1004 10-77

MYCOLOGY — Page 1 of 3 Pages

CDC laboratory examination checklist (1977)—mycology

	No	(Code)	Comment
13. All changes in procedures are documented (description of change and date) in the SOPM and have the written approval (initials and date) of the supervisor	☐	02069	

MATERIALS CFR 74.20(c) 405.1317(a)(3)

14. The following are labeled (identity, titer or concentration, recommended storage, preparation or expiration date).		No	(Code)	
	Antisera	☐	02070	
	Control organisms	☐	02071	
	Media (tubes, plates, kits)	☐	02072	
	Reagents-solutions	☐	02073	
	Reagents-strips	☐	02074	
	Stains	☐	02075	

15. Materials in use are "in-date", reactive, and not deteriorated				
	Antisera	☐	02077	
	Control organisms	☐	02078	
	Media (tubes, plates, kits)	☐	02079	
	Reagents-solution	☐	02080	
	Reagents-strips	☐	02081	
	Stains	☐	02082	

TESTING OF REAGENTS CFR 74.20(a) 74.21 405.1317(a)(i) 405.1317(b)(i)

16. The following reagents are tested each day of use to demonstrate positive and negative biochemical reactions		Positive Reaction No. (Code)	Negative Reaction NO (Code)	Written Q.C. No (Code)	Comment
	Nitrate	*☐ 02084	*☐ 02085	*☐ 02086	
	Plasma (germ tube)	*☐ 02087	*☐ 02088	*☐ 02089	

17. Each batch of the following media, if used by the lab, is tested for the following characteristics

MEDIUM	Expected Growth No (Code)	Selectivity and Biochem reactions No (Code)	Sterility No. (Code)	Written Q.C. No (Code)	Comment
Ammonium nitrate basal medium	*☐ 02090	*☐ 02091	*☐ 02092	*☐ 02093	
Ammonium nitrate basal medium + histidine	*☐ 02094		*☐ 02095	*☐ 02096	
Blood agar base	*☐ 02097		*☐ 02098	*☐ 02099	
Brain heart infusion agar	*☐ 02100		*☐ 02101	*☐ 02102	
Brain heart infusion agar with antibiotics	*☐ 02103	*☐ 02104	*☐ 02105	*☐ 02106	
Brain heart infusion agar with blood	*☐ 02107		*☐ 02108	*☐ 02109	
Wickerham broth	*☐ 02110		*☐ 02111	*☐ 02112	
Casein basal medium	*☐ 02113		*☐ 02114	*☐ 02115	
Casein basal medium + inositol	*☐ 02116		*☐ 02117	*☐ 02118	
Casein basal medium + inositol + thiamin	*☐ 02119		*☐ 02120	*☐ 02121	
Casein basal medium + thiamin	*☐ 02122		*☐ 02123	*☐ 02124	
Casein basal medium + nicotinic acid	*☐ 02125		*☐ 02126	*☐ 02127	
Casein	*☐ 02128		*☐ 02129	*☐ 02130	
Chlamydospore agar	*☐ 02131	*☐ 02132	*☐ 02133	*☐ 02134	
Corn meal with tween 80	*☐ 02135	*☐ 02136	*☐ 02137	*☐ 02138	
Corn meal without tween 80	*☐ 02139	*☐ 02140	*☐ 02141	*☐ 02142	
Dermatophyte test media (DTM)	*☐ 02143		*☐ 02144	*☐ 02145	
Fermentative sugars					
Dextrose	*☐ 02146	*☐ 02147	*☐ 02148	*☐ 02149	
Maltose	*☐ 02150	*☐ 02151	*☐ 02152	*☐ 02153	
Sucrose	*☐ 02154	*☐ 02155	*☐ 02156	*☐ 02157	
Lactose	*☐ 02158	*☐ 02159	*☐ 02160	*☐ 02161	
Galactose	*☐ 02162	*☐ 02163	*☐ 02164	*☐ 02165	
Xylose	*☐ 02166	*☐ 02167	*☐ 02168	*☐ 02169	
Raffinose	*☐ 02170	*☐ 02171	*☐ 02172	*☐ 02173	
Cellobiose	*☐ 02174	*☐ 02175	*☐ 02176	*☐ 02177	
Trehalose	*☐ 02178	*☐ 02179	*☐ 02180	*☐ 02181	
Inositol	*☐ 02182	*☐ 02183	*☐ 02184	*☐ 02185	
Melibiose	*☐ 02186	*☐ 02187	*☐ 02188	*☐ 02189	
Dulcitol	*☐ 02190	*☐ 02191	*☐ 02192	*☐ 02193	
Francis glucose cystine blood agar	*☐ 02194		*☐ 02195	*☐ 02196	
Gelatin	*☐ 02197	*☐ 02198	*☐ 02199	*☐ 02200	
Littman agar	*☐ 02201	*☐ 02202	*☐ 02203	*☐ 02204	
Loeffler's medium	*☐ 02205	*☐ 02206	*☐ 02207	*☐ 02208	
Malt extract broth	*☐ 02209	*☐ 02210	*☐ 02211	*☐ 02212	

CDC 3.1004 10-77   MYCOLOGY — Page 2 of 3 Pages

CDC laboratory examination checklist (1977)—mycology—cont'd   *Continued.*

MEDIUM	CHARACTERISTICS				
	Expected Growth No (Code)	Selectivity and Biochem reactions No (Code)	Sterility No (Code)	Written Q.C. No (Code)	Comment
Milk	*☐ 02213		*☐ 02214	*☐ 02215	
Mycosel	*☐ 02216	*☐ 02217	*☐ 02218	*☐ 02219	
Mycobiotic agar	*☐ 02220	*☐ 02221	*☐ 02222	*☐ 02223	
Mycophil agar	*☐ 02224	*☐ 02225	*☐ 02226	*☐ 02227	
Oxidative sugars media					
Dextrose	*☐ 02228	*☐ 02229	*☐ 02230	*☐ 02231	
Lactose	*☐ 02232	*☐ 02233	*☐ 02234	*☐ 02235	
Galactose	*☐ 02236	*☐ 02237	*☐ 02238	*☐ 02239	
Maltose	*☐ 02240	*☐ 02241	*☐ 02242	*☐ 02243	
Sucrose	*☐ 02244	*☐ 02245	*☐ 02246	*☐ 02247	
Raffinose	*☐ 02248	*☐ 02249	*☐ 02250	*☐ 02251	
Cellobiose	*☐ 02252	*☐ 02253	*☐ 02254	*☐ 02255	
Trehalose	*☐ 02256	*☐ 02257	*☐ 02258	*☐ 02259	
Inositol	*☐ 02260	*☐ 02261	*☐ 02262	*☐ 02263	
Melibiose	*☐ 02264	*☐ 02265	*☐ 02266	*☐ 02267	
Dulcitol	*☐ 02268	*☐ 02269	*☐ 02270	*☐ 02271	
Xylose	*☐ 02272	*☐ 02273	*☐ 02274	*☐ 02275	
Potato dextrose agar	*☐ 02276		*☐ 02277	*☐ 02278	
Rice agar	*☐ 02279	*☐ 02280	*☐ 02281	*☐ 02282	
Sabouraud broth	*☐ 02283		*☐ 02284	*☐ 02285	
Sabouraud dextrose agar	*☐ 02286		*☐ 02287	*☐ 02288	
Sabouraud dextrose agar with chloramphenicol	*☐ 02289	*☐ 02290	*☐ 02291	*☐ 02292	
Sabouraud dextrose with chloramphenicol and cyclohexamide	*☐ 02293	*☐ 02294	*☐ 02295	*☐ 02296	
Starch agar	*☐ 02297	*☐ 02298	*☐ 02299	*☐ 02300	
Thioglycollate broth	*☐ 02301		*☐ 02302	*☐ 02303	
Tyrosine agar	*☐ 02304	*☐ 02305	*☐ 02306	*☐ 02307	
Urea agar	*☐ 02308	*☐ 02309	*☐ 02310	*☐ 02311	
Xanthine agar	*☐ 02312	*☐ 02313	*☐ 02314	*☐ 02315	

COMMERCIAL SYSTEMS	Positive Control NO (Code)	Negative Control NO (Code)	Sterility NO (Code)	Written Q.C. No (Code)	System	COMMENT
Each commercial system in use is tested each shipment with sufficient known organisms to give at least one positive and one negative biochemical response for each constituent	*☐ 02316	*☐ 02317	*☐ 02318	*☐ 02319	API	
	*☐ 02320	*☐ 02321	*☐ 02322	*☐ 02323	Mini-Tek	
	*☐ 02324	*☐ 02325	*☐ 02326	*☐ 02327	Uni-Tek	
	*☐ 02328	*☐ 02329	*☐ 02330	*☐ 02331	Other	

STAINS CFR 74.21(a) 405.1317(b)(1)(i)

18. Following stains are tested each day of use to demonstrate expected staining characteristics	No (Code)	Written Q.C. No (code)	COMMENT
Acid fast stain with 3% acid (HCl) alcohol)	*☐ 02332	*☐ 02333	
Modified Kinyoun's acid fast stain (with 1% aqueous H_2SO_4)	*☐ 02334	*☐ 02335	
Periodic acid Schiff stain	*☐ 02336	*☐ 02337	
Wright's	*☐ 02338	*☐ 02339	
Giemsa	*☐ 02340	*☐ 02341	

19. Gram stain is tested when prepared and each week of use to demonstrate positive and negative reactions	Positive Reaction NO (Code)	Negative Reaction NO (Code)	Written Q.C. NO (Code)	COMMENT
	*☐ 02342	*☐ 02343	*☐ 02344	

RECORDS CFR 74.50 74.54(a); 405.1316; 405.1316(g)

	No. (Code)
20. Records of observations are made, concurrently with the performance of each step in the examination of specimens	☐ 02345
21. Records are retained at least 2 years	
Accession records	☐ 02346
Copy of final report to client	☐ 02347
Equipment maintenance records	☐ 02348
Control records	☐ 02349
Records of observation of each step of specimen testing	☐ 02350

CDC 3.1004 10-77

MYCOLOGY — Page 3 of 3 pages

CDC laboratory examination checklist (1977)—mycology—cont'd

DEPARTMENT OF HEALTH, EDUCATION, AND WELFARE
PUBLIC HEALTH SERVICE
CENTER FOR DISEASE CONTROL
ATLANTA, GEORGIA 3033J

PARASITOLOGY

Laboratory Examination Checklist — CLIA '67 — CDC

Code No.

Examiner(s)

Name of Laboratory

Interviewee(s)

Address

Date(s) of examination

NOTE TO EXAMINER:

a) For each item marked with an *, mark "No" if there is no record to confirm that the laboratory is actually applying the standard. A record is REQUIRED; however, if a laboratory CLAIMS IT APPLIES THE STANDARD but has no record, indicate under comment space.

b) The examiner must check each block to the left of the question or specific item to indicate if the item is available or used in this laboratory.

TEMPERATURE CFR 74.20(b) 405.1317(a)(2)	NO	(Code)	COMMENT
1. Temperatures of refrigerators, in which specimens are stored, are monitored each day of use	*☐	03000	

STANDARD OPERATING PROCEDURE MANUAL SOPM CFR 74.20(d)(e)(f) 405.1317(a)(5)(6)	NO	(Code)	
2. The Parasitology section has an SOPM	☐	03001	
3. The SOPM is in the Parasitology work bench area	☐	03002	
4. The SOPM has a supervisor's written attestation that SOPM is current	☐	03017	
5. The supervisor's review of SOPM is dated	☐	03018	
6. The SOPM includes only those procedures currently in use	☐	03019	
7. All changes in procudures are documented (description of change and date) in the SOPM and have the written approval (initials and date) of the supervisor	☐	03020	

8. For each procedure, if offered by the lab, the parasitology SOPM includes the following:

PROCEDURE	Instructions NO (Code)		Reagents NO (Code)	Controls NO (Code)
☐ Blood and tissue parasite preparations	☐	03003	☐ 03004	
☐ Cellulose tape preparation	☐	03006		
☐ Concentration procedures of fecal specimens	☐	03008	☐ 03009	
☐ Direct microscopic examination of fecal specimens (wet mounts)	☐	03010	☐ 03011	
☐ Macroscopic examination of fecal specimens	☐	03012		
☐ Staining procedures	☐	03014	☐ 03015	☐ 03016

MATERIALS CFR 74.20(c) 405.1317(a)(3)	NO	(Code)	COMMENT
9. The following are labeled (identity, titer or concentration, recommended storage, preparation or expiration date)			
Controls	☐	03021	
Reagents	☐	03022	
Stains	☐	03023	
10. Materials in use are "in-date", reactive, and not deteriorated			
Controls	☐	03024	
Reagents	☐	03025	
Stains	☐	03026	

CONTROL PROCEDURES 74.21(b) 405.1317(b)(i)(ii)	NO	(Code)	
11. The laboratory has a reference collection of parasites: (slides, photographs, or gross specimen are acceptable)			
Blood and tissue parasites	☐	03027	
Helminth eggs	☐	03028	
Helminth larvae	☐	03029	
Protozoan cysts	☐	03030	
Protozoan trophozoites	☐	03031	
12. An ocular micrometer which has been calibrated by the laboratory is available	*☐	03032	
13. The following stains are tested with each new batch, and once per month of use:			
Alum cochineal stain	*☐	03033	
Azure A	*☐	03034	
Buffered methylene blue	*☐	03035	
Carmine stain	*☐	03036	
Chlorazol Black E stain	*☐	03037	
Delafield's hematoxylin	*☐	03038	
Giemsa stain	*☐	03040	
Hematoxylin stain	*☐	03041	

CDC 3.1003 10-77   PARASITOLOGY — Page 1 of 2 pages

CDC laboratory examination checklist (1977)—parasitology

Continued.

13. (Continued) The following stains are tested with each new batch, and once per month of use:	NO	(Code)	COMMENT
Modified Heidenhain	*☐	03043	
Quensel's stain	*☐	03044	
Reynold's stain	*☐	03045	
Semichon acetic carmine	*☐	03046	
Thionin stain	*☐	03047	
Trichrome stain	*☐	03048	
RECORDS CFR 74.50 74.54(a) 405.1316; 405.1316(g) 14. Records of observations are made, concurrently with the performance of each step in the examination of specimens	☐	03049	
15. Records are retained at least 2 years			
Accession	☐	03051	
Copy of final report to client	☐	03052	
Observations of each step of specimen testing	☐	03054	
Stain control	☐	03055	

CDC laboratory examination checklist (1977)—parasitology—cont'd

DEPARTMENT OF HEALTH, EDUCATION, AND WELFARE
PUBLIC HEALTH SERVICE
CENTER FOR DISEASE CONTROL
ATLANTA, GEORGIA 30333

VIROLOGY
Laboratory Examination Checklist — CLIA '67 — CDC

Code No.

Examiner(s)

Name of Laboratory

Interviewee(s)

Address

Date(s) of examination

NOTE TO EXAMINER:

a) For each item marked with an *, mark "No" if there is no record to confirm that the laboratory is actually applying the standard. A record is REQUIRED; however, if a laboratory CLAIMS IT APPLIES THE STANDARD but has no record, indicate under comment space.

b) The examiner must check each block to the left of the question or specific item to indicate if the item is available or used in this laboratory.

		NO (Code)	COMMENT
PREVENTIVE MAINTENANCE CFR 74.20(a) 405.1317(a) (1)			
1. Each equipment item is tested periodically for proper operation:	Autoclave(s)	*☐ 04000	
	Freezer(s)	*☐ 04001	
	Incubator(s)	*☐ 04002	
	Fluorescent microscope(s)	*☐ 04003	
	Biosafety cabinet(s)	*☐ 04004	
	Refrigerator(s)	*☐ 04007	
2. Each equipment item is subjected to preventive maintenance	Autoclave(s)	*☐ 04008	
	Freezer(s)	*☐ 04009	
	Incubator(s)	*☐ 04010	
	Fluorescent microscope(s)	*☐ 04011	
	Biosafety cabinet(s)	*☐ 04012	
	Refrigerator(s)	*☐ 04015	
3. Records document remedial actions taken for detected defects		☐ 04016	
TEMPERATURES CFR 74.20(b) 405.1317(a)(2)			
4. Temperatures are monitored each day of use:	Incubators	*☐ 04017	
	Refrigerators	*☐ 04018	
	Water baths	*☐ 04019	
	Heat blocks	*☐ 04020	
	Freezers	*☐ 04021	
STERILIZATION CFR 74.20(b) 405.1316(d)			
5. Each sterilization cycle includes device to assure proper performance OR a recording thermometer is used:		☐ 04022	
6. Each autoclave is checked monthly with spores to assure proper performance.		* ☐ 04023	
STANDARD OPERATING PROCEDURE MANUAL (SOPM) CFR 74.20(d)(e)(f) **405.1317(a)(4)(5)(6)**			
7. The virology section has an SOPM		☐ 04024	
8. The SOPM is in virology work bench area:		☐ 04025	
9. The SOPM has a supervisor's written attestation that the SOPM is current:		☐ 04056	
10. The supervisor's review of the SOPM is dated.		☐ 04057	
11. The SOPM includes only those procedures currently in use.		☐ 04058	
12. All changes in procedures are documented (description of change and date) in the SOPM and have the written approval (initials and date) of the supervisor:		☐ 04059	

13. For each procedure, if offered by the lab, the virology SOPM includes the following:

PROCEDURE	Instructions NO (Code)	Reagents NO (Code)	Controls NO (Code)	PROCEDURE	Instructions NO (Code)	Reagents NO (Code)	Controls NO (Code)
☐ Orthomyxovirus	☐ 04026	☐ 04027	☐ 04028	☐ Pox virus	☐ 04041	☐ 04042	☐ 04043
☐ Myxovirus—Paramyxovirus	☐ 04029	☐ 04030	☐ 04031	☐ Adenovirus	☐ 04044	☐ 04045	☐ 04046
☐ Reovirus	☐ 04032	☐ 04033	☐ 04034	☐ Togavirus-Rubella	☐ 04047	☐ 04048	☐ 04049
☐ Picornavirus	☐ 04035	☐ 04036	☐ 04037	☐ Rhinovirus	☐ 04050	☐ 04051	☐ 04052
☐ Herpesvirus	☐ 04038	☐ 04039	☐ 04040	☐ Arbovirus	☐ 04053	☐ 04054	☐ 04055

CDC 2.1007
10-77

VIROLOGY — Page 1 of 4 pages

CDC laboratory examination checklist (1977)—virology

Continued.

MATERIALS CFR 74.20(c) 405.1317(a)(3) 14. The following are labeled (identity, titer or concentration, recommended storage, preparation or expiration date):		NO (Code)	COMMENT
	Antigens	☐ 04060	
	Antisera	☐ 04061	
	Control organisms	☐ 04062	
	Reagent solutions	☐ 04063	
	Tissue cultures	☐ 04064	
	Reagents dehydrated	☐ 04065	
15. Materials in use are "in-date", reactive, and not deteriorated			
	Antigens	☐ 04066	
	Antisera	☐ 04067	
	Control organisms	☐ 04068	
	Reagent solutions	☐ 04069	
	Tissue cultures	☐ 04070	
	Reagents dehydrated	☐ 04071	
TESTING OF REAGENTS CFR 74.22(b) 405.1317(b)(2)(ii) 16. Each new lot of the following is tested concurrently with one of known acceptable reactivity before being placed in routine use:			
	Antigen	*☐ 04072	
	Antisera	*☐ 04073	
	Complement	*☐ 04075	
	Hemolysin	*☐ 04076	

ISOLATION SYSTEMS CFR 74.21(c) 405.1317(b)(1) (iii) 17. FOR THE SERVICES OFFERED.	a. At least one of the following isolation systems is available	b. Uninoculated host system control is included with each run of specimens	
ORTHOMYXOVIRUS	NO (Code)	NO (Code)	
a. Influenza A & B: Primary monkey kidney cell culture and/or embryonated eggs	☐ 04077	*☐ 04078	
b. Influenza C: Embryonated eggs	☐ 04079	*☐ 04080	
MYXOVIRUS-PARAMYXOVIRUS			
a. Parainfluenza: Primary monkey kidney	☐ 04081	*☐ 04082	
b. Respiratory Syncytial Virus (RSV): Primary monkey kidney or established cell lines	☐ 04083	*☐ 04084	
c. Mumps: Embryonated eggs or primary monkey or human kidney cells or established cell lines	☐ 04085	*☐ 04086	
d. Measles: Primary monkey or human kidney or established cell lines	☐ 04087	*☐ 04088	
REOVIRUS Primary monkey kidney or established cell lines	☐ 04089	*☐ 04090	
PICORNAVIRUS			
a. Polio and ECHO: Primary or established cell lines	☐ 04091	*☐ 04092	
b. Coxsackie: Primary or established cell lines and suckling mice	☐ 04093	*☐ 04094	
HERPESVIRUS			
a. Herpes simplex: Embryonated eggs, primary or diploid cell cultures	☐ 04095	*☐ 04096	
b. Cytomegalovirus (CMV) diploid cell cultures	☐ 04097	*☐ 04098	
c. Varicella Zoster, (Chicken pox): primary or diploid cell cultures	☐ 04099	*☐ 04100	
POX VIRUS Embryonated eggs and primary or established cell lines	☐ 04101	*☐ 04102	
ADENOVIRUS Established cell cultures	☐ 04103	*☐ 04104	
TOGAVIRUS-RUBELLA Primary green monkey kidney cell culture or established cell lines	☐ 04105	*☐ 04106	
RHINOVIRUS Human diploid cell lines or primary embryonic kidney	☐ 04107	*☐ 04108	

CDC 3.1007
10-77

VIROLOGY — Page 2 of 4 pages

CDC laboratory examination checklist (1977)—virology—cont'd

ISOLATION SYSTEMS (Continued) 17. FOR THE SERVICES OFFERED	a. At least one of the following isolation systems is available	b. Uninoculated host system control is included with each run of specimens	COMMENT
ARBOVIRUS Suckling mice, duck embryo tissue culture, and established cell line (½-day-old mice may be used in limited situations)	NO (Code) ☐ 04109	NO (Code) *☐ 04110	

IDENTIFICATION SYSTEMS CFR 74.21(c) 74.22(a) 405.1317(b)(1)(iii) 405.1317(b)(2)(i) 18. FOR THE SERVICES OFFERED	a. At least one of the following identification systems is available	b. The following controls are included with each run	
		1)Positive	2)Negative
	NO (Code)	NO (Code)	NO (Code)
ORTHOMYXOVIRUS (Influenza) Hemagglutination inhibition (HI), Complement fixation (CF), Hemadsorption-inhibition test (HAdI) Neutralization or Fluorescent antibody (FA)	☐ 04167	*☐ 04111	*☐ 04112
MYXOVIRUS-PARAMYXOVIRUS a. Parainfluenza: HAdI, CF, HI, Neutralization or FA	☐ 04168	*☐ 04113	*☐ 04114
b. Respiratory Syncytial Virus (RSV): CF, Neutralization or indirect FA	☐ 04169	*☐ 04115	*☐ 04116
c. Mumps: HAdI, Neutralization, HI or CF	☐ 04170	*☐ 04117	*☐ 04118
d. Measles: Neutralization, HI, CF or FA	☐ 04171	*☐ 04119	*☐ 04120
REOVIRUS HI, CF or Neutralization	☐ 04172	*☐ 04121	*☐ 04122
PICORNAVIRUS a. Polio and ECHO: Neutralization, CF, HI or FA	☐ 04173	*☐ 04123	*☐ 04124
b. Coxsackie: Neutralization. CF, HI or FA	☐ 04174	*☐ 04125	*☐ 04126
HERPESVIRUS a. Herpes simplex: Neutralization, CF, Passive hemagglutination test, HI, Immunodiffusion or FA	☐ 04175	*☐ 04127	*☐ 04128
b. Cytomegalovirus (CMV): Cytopathic effect (CPE), CF, or Neutralization	☐ 04176	*☐ 04129	*☐ 04130
c. Varicella-zoster: Neutralization, CF, Passive hemagglutination test, HI or Immunodiffusion	☐ 04177	*☐ 04131	*☐ 04132
POX VIRUS Neutralization, CF, HI, Precipitation in agar gel or Passage with temperature challenge (Vaccinia 40°C, Variola 36° C)	☐ 04178	*☐ 04133	*☐ 04134
ADENOVIRUS Characteristic CPE, Retention of infectivity after exposure to ether or chloroform, Group-specific antigenicity, CF, Neutralization, or HI.	☐ 04179	*☐ 04135	*☐ 04136
TOGAVIRUS-RUBELLA HI, Neutralization, CF or indirect FA	☐ 04180	*☐ 04137	*☐ 04138
RHINOVIRUS Neutralization	☐ 04181	*☐ 04139	*☐ 04140
ARBOVIRUS Inactivation by sodium desoxycholate, Inactivation by ethyl ether or chloroform to distinguish from enterovirus, Neutralization, CF or HI	☐ 04182	*☐ 04141	*☐ 04142
RABIES VIRUS Microscopic examination of mouse brain for Negri bodies and Rabies virus antigen with fluorescent ~~antigen~~ antibody or cross-protection test	☐ 04183	*☐ 04143	*☐ 04144

CDC laboratory examination checklist (1977)—virology—cont'd

Continued.

IDENTIFICATION SYSTEMS FOR THE SERVICES OFFERED (Continued)	NO (Code)	
The components of tests are controlled as follows:		
Complement Fixation Tests		
19. Hemolysin titrated with each new cell batch	*☐ 04145	
20. Complement titrated each time test performed.	*☐ 04146	
21. Serum/complement control included each time test performed.	*☐ 04147	
22. Tissue antigen/complement control included each time test performed	*☐ 04148	
23. Antigen/complement control included each time test performed.	*☐ 04149	
24. Buffer/complement control included each time test performed.	*☐ 04150	
25. Red cell control included each time test performed	*☐ 04151	
Hemagglutination-Inhibition Tests		
26. Antigen titrated each time test performed.	*☐ 04152	
27. Serum/cell/buffer control included each time test performed.	*☐ 04153	
28. Cell/buffer control included each time test performed.	*☐ 04154	
Neutralization Tests		
29. TCD 50 determined each time test performed.	*☐ 04155	
30. Positive and negative control included each time a new vial of antisera is reconstituted.	*☐ 04184	
31. Cell culture control included each time test performed.	*☐ 04157	
32. Serum toxicity control included each time test performed (when serum testing only).	*☐ 04158	
Hemadsorption-Inhibition Tests		
33. A cell culture control is included with the Hemadsorption-Inhibition test each time tests are performed.	*☐ 04159	
RECORDS CFR 74.50; 74.54(a); 405.1316; 405.1316(g)		
34 Records of observations are made concurrently with the performance of each step in the examination of specimens.	☐ 04160	
36. Records are retained at least 2 years.		
Accession	☐ 04162	
Control	☐ 04163	
Copy of final report to client	☐ 04164	
Equipment maintenance	☐ 04165	
Observations of each step of specimen testing	☐ 04166	

CDC laboratory examination checklist (1977)—virology—cont'd

DEPARTMENT OF HEALTH, EDUCATION, AND WELFARE
PUBLIC HEALTH SERVICE
CENTER FOR DISEASE CONTROL
ATLANTA, GEORGIA 30333

DIAGNOSTIC IMMUNOLOGY
Syphilis Serology
LABORATORY EXAMINATION CHECKLIST – CLIA '67 – CDC

Code No.

Examiner(s)

Name of Laboratory

Interviewee(s)

Address

Date(s) of examination

NOTE TO EXAMINER:

a) For each item marked with an *, mark "No" if there is no record to confirm that the laboratory is actually applying the standard. A record is REQUIRED; however, if a laboratory CLAIMS IT APPLIES THE STANDARD but has no record, indicate under comment space.

b) The examiner must check each block to the left of the question or specific item to indicate if the item is available or used in this laboratory.

PREVENTIVE MAINTENANCE CFR 74.20(a) 405.1317(a)(1)		NO (Code)	COMMENT
1. Each equipment item is tested periodically for proper operation	Automated Analyzers Fluorescent Microscopes Heat Blocks	*☐ 11000 *☐ 11001 *☐ 11002	
	Incubators Rotators Water Baths	*☐ 11003 *☐ 11004 *☐ 11005	
2. Each equipment item is subjected to preventive maintenance	Automated Analyzers Fluorescent Microscopes Heat Blocks	*☐ 11006 *☐ 11007 *☐ 11008	
	Incubators Rotators Water Baths	*☐ 11009 *☐ 11010 *☐ 11011	
3. Records document remedial actions taken for detected defects		☐ 11012	
TEMPERATURES CFR 74.20(b) 405.1317(a)(2) 4. Temperatures are monitored each day of use	Incubators Refrigerators Water baths	*☐ 11013 *☐ 11014 *☐ 11015	
	Heat blocks Freezers Ambient	*☐ 11016 *☐ 11017 *☐ 11018	
STANDARD OPERATING PROCEDURE MANUAL(SOPM) CFR 74.20(d)(e)(f) 405.1317(a)(4)(5)(6) 5. The syphilis serology section has an SOPM		☐ 11019	
6. The SOPM is in the syphilis serology work bench area		☐ 11020	
7. The SOPM has a supervisor's written attestation that the SOPM is current		☐ 11054	
8. The supervisor's review of the SOPM is dated		☐ 11055	
9. The SOPM includes only those procedures currently in use		☐ 11056	
10. All changes in procedures are documented (description of change and date) in the SOPM and have the written approval (initials and date) of the supervisor		☐ 11057	

11. For each procedure, if offered by the lab, the syphilis serology SOPM includes the following:

PROCEDURE	Instructions NO (Code)	Reagents NO (Code)	Controls NO (Code)	PROCEDURE	Instructions NO (Code)	Reagents NO (Code)	Control NO (Code)
☐ VDRL (qualitative)	☐ 11021	☐ 11022	☐ 11023	☐ RPR, 18 mm circle card (quantitative)	☐ 11036	☐ 11037	☐ 11038
☐ VDRL (quantitative)	☐ 11024	☐ 11025	☐ 11026	☐ ART (qualitative)	☐ 11039	☐ 11040	☐ 11041
☐ VDRL, CSF (qualitative)	☐ 11027	☐ 11028	☐ 11029	☐ ART (quantitative)	☐ 11042	☐ 11043	☐ 11044
☐ VDRL, CSF (quantitative)	☐ 11030	☐ 11031	☐ 11032	☐ FTA-ABS	☐ 11045	☐ 11046	☐ 11047
☐ RPR, 18mm circle card (qualitative)	☐ 11033	☐ 11034	☐ 11035	☐ USR	☐ 11048	☐ 11049	☐ 11050
☐ Reagent Parallel Testing	☐ 11114			☐ RST	☐ 11051	☐ 11052	☐ 11053

MATERIALS CFR 74.24(c) 405.1317(a)(3)		NO (Code)	COMMENT
12. The following are labeled (identity, titer or concentration, recommended storage, preparation or expiration date)	Antigens Controls Conjugate Sorbent Kits	☐ 11058 ☐ 11059 ☐ 11060 ☐ 11061 ☐ 11062	

CDC 3.1002 10-77   SYPHILIS SEROLOGY (Page 1 of 3)

CDC laboratory examination checklist (1977)—syphilis serology

Continued.

MATERIALS (Continued)

		NO (Code)	COMMENT
13. Materials in use are "in-date," reactive, and not deteriorated	Antigens	☐ 11063	
	Controls	☐ 11064	
	Conjugate	☐ 11065	
	Sorbent	☐ 11066	
	Kits	☐ 11067	

CONTROL PROCEDURE CFR 74.22(c) 405.1317(b)(2)(iii)

☐ **NON-TREPONEMAL TEST (Manual)**

		NO (Code)
14. The mechanical rotator is checked prior to each test run	USR 180 rpm ±2	*☐ 11068
	VDRL 180 rpm ±2	*☐ 11069
	RST 130 rpm	*☐ 11070
	RPR 95-110 rpm	*☐ 11071

15. The needle is checked prior to each test run

TEST	REAGENT	NEEDLE GAUGE	NO DROPS DELIVERED PER ML OF REAGENT	
VDRL (qualitative)	Antigen suspension	18	60 ±2	*☐ 11072
VDRL (quantitative)	Antigen suspension	19	75 ±2	*☐ 11073
VDRL	0.9 percent saline	23	100 ±2	*☐ 11074
VDRL (CSF)	Sensitized Antigen Suspension	21 or 22	100 ±2	*☐ 11075
USR	0.9 Percent saline	18	60 ±2	*☐ 11076
RPR (qualitative)	Antigen suspension	20	60 ±2	*☐ 11077

16. Antigen used for:

	NO (Code)
a. VDRL is used on the day of preparation only	☐ 11079
b. CSF VDRL is sensitized before use	☐ 11080
c. VDRL is prepared in a 30 ml round bottle with a ground glass stopper with a flat inner bottom surface of approximately 35 mm diameter	☐ 11081

17. a. Slides used for the VDRL or USR are:

	VDRL NO (Code)	USR NO (Code)	
2 X 3 inch with 2 paraffin or ceramic rings approximately 14 mm in diameter for serum tests	☐ 11082	☐ 11083	
2 x 3 inch with concavities measuring 16 mm in diameter and 1.75 mm in depth for spinal fluid tests (VDRL only)	☐ 11084		
b. Cards used for RPR card test are approximately 18 mm in diameter	☐ 11085		

18. Controls of graded reactivity are included with each test run of:

Test	Non React.		Wkl. React.		React.	
	No	(Code)	No	(Code)	No	(Code)
VDRL (qualitative)	*☐	11116	*☐	11117	*☐	11118
VDRL (quantitative)	*☐	11119	*☐	11120	*☐	11121
VDRL (CSF)	*☐	11122	*☐	11123	*☐	11124
USR	*☐	11125	*☐	11126	*☐	11127
RPR (qualitative)	*☐	11128	*☐	11129	*☐	11130
RST (qualitative)	*☐	11131	*☐	11132	*☐	11133

19. Each of the following materials is tested concurrently with one of known reactivity prior to being placed in routine use

Test	Control		Antigen	
	No	(Code)	No	(Code)
VDRL (qualitative)	*☐	11134	*☐	11135
VDRL (quantitative)	*☐	11136	*☐	11137
VDRL (CSF)	*☐	11138	*☐	11139
USR	*☐	11140	*☐	11141
RPR (qualitative)	*☐	11142	*☐	11143
RST (qualitative)	*☐	11144	*☐	11145

CDC laboratory examination checklist (1977)—syphilis serology—cont'd

		NO (Code)	COMMENT
☐ NON-TREPONEMAL TEST (Automated)			
20. Controls of graded reactivity are included with each test run	Reactive Non-Reactive	*☐ 11091 *☐ 11092	
21. Each of the following materials is tested concurrently with one of known reactivity prior to being placed in routine use	Antigens Controls	*☐ 11093 *☐ 11094	
TREPONEMAL TESTS			
22. The following controls are included each time the FTA-ABS test is performed	Reactive control serum in diluent Reactive control serum in sorbent Minimally reactive control in serum	*☐ 11095 *☐ 11096 *☐ 11097	
	Non-specific serum control in diluent	*☐ 11098	
	Non-specific serum control in sorbent	*☐ 11099	
	Non-specific staining control in diluent	*☐ 11100	
	Non-specific staining control in sorbent	*☐ 11101	
23. Each of the following test components is tested concurrently with one of known reactivity prior to being placed in routine use	Antigen Controls Sorbent Conjugate	*☐ 11102 *☐ 11103 *☐ 11104 *☐ 11105	
RECORDS CFR 74.50; 74.54(a); 405.1316; 405.1316(g) 24. Record of observations are made concurrently with the performance of each step in the examination of specimens		☐ 11106	
25. The following records are retained at least 2 years	Accession Equipment Maintenance Control Observations of each step of performance Copy of final report to client	☐ 11108 ☐ 11109 ☐ 11110 ☐ 11111 ☐ 11113	

CDC laboratory examination checklist (1977)—syphilis serology—cont'd

DEPARTMENT OF HEALTH, EDUCATION, AND WELFARE PUBLIC HEALTH SERVICE CENTER FOR DISEASE CONTROL ATLANTA, GEORGIA 30303	DIAGNOSTIC IMMUNOLOGY **Non-Syphilis Serology** LABORATORY EXAMINATION CHECKLIST – CLIA '67 – CDC	Code No.
Name of Laboratory		Examiner(s)
		Interviewee(s)
Address		Date(s) of examination

NOTE TO EXAMINER:

a) For each item marked with an *, mark "No" if there is no record to confirm that the laboratory is actually applying the standard. A record is REQUIRED; however, if a laboratory CLAIMS IT APPLIES THE STANDARD but has no record, indicate under comment space.

b) The examiner must check each block to the left of the question or specific item to indicate if the item is available or used in this laboratory.

PREVENTIVE MAINTENANCE CFR 74.20(a) 405.1317(a)(1)	NO	(Code)	COMMENT
1. Each equipment item is tested periodically for proper operation			
Automated Analyzers	*☐	12000	
Densitometer	*☐	12001	
Electrophoresis Power Supply	*☐	12002	
Fluorescent Microscopes	*☐	12003	
Incubators	*☐	12004	
Radioisotope Counting Equipment	*☐	12005	
Spectrophotometer	*☐	12006	
Automatic Pipettors	*☐	12007	
Automatic Dilutors	*☐	12008	
2. Each equipment item is subjected to preventive maintenance			
Automated Analyzers	*☐	12009	
Densitometers	*☐	12010	
Electrophoresis Power Supply	*☐	12011	
Fluorescent Microscopes	*☐	12012	
Incubators	*☐	12013	
Radioisotope Counting Equipment	*☐	12014	
Spectrophotometer	*☐	12015	
Automatic Pipettors	*☐	12016	
Automatic Dilutors	*☐	12017	
3. Records document remedial actions taken for detected defects	☐	12018	
TEMPERATURES CFR 74.20(b) 405.1316(d)			
4. Temperatures are monitored each day of use			
Incubators	*☐	12019	
Refrigerators	*☐	12020	
Water Baths	*☐	12021	
Heat Blocks	*☐	12022	
Freezers	*☐	12023	
STANDARD OPERATING PROCEDURE MANUAL (SOPM) CFR 74.20(d)(e)(f) 405.1317(a)(4)(5)(6) 5. The non-syphilis serology section has an SOPM	☐	12025	
6. The SOPM is in the non-syphilis serology work area	☐	12026	

7. For each procedure, if offered by the laboratory, the non-syphilis serology SOPM includes the following:

	Instructions NO (Code)	Reagents NO (Code)	Controls NO (Code)	Calibration NO (Code)
☐ Alpha-1-antitrypsin	☐ 12027	☐ 12028	☐ 12029	☐ 12030
☐ Anti-deoxyribonuclease (ADNase)	☐ 12031	☐ 12032	☐ 12033	
☐ Anti-mitochondrial antibody	☐ 12034	☐ 12035	☐ 12036	
☐ Anti-nuclear antibodies (ANA)	☐ 12037	☐ 12038	☐ 12039	
☐ Anti-parietal cell antibody	☐ 12040	☐ 12041	☐ 12042	
☐ Anti-skeletal muscle antibody	☐ 12043	☐ 12044	☐ 12045	
☐ Anti-smooth muscle antibody	☐ 12046	☐ 12047	☐ 12048	
☐ Anti-streptococcal hyaluronidase (ASH)	☐ 12049	☐ 12050	☐ 12051	
☐ Anti-streptolysin O (ASO) Titer	☐ 12052	☐ 12053	☐ 12054	
☐ Anti-thyroglobulin antibodies	☐ 12055	☐ 12056	☐ 12057	
☐ Anti-toxoplasmosis antibody	☐ 12058	☐ 12059	☐ 12060	
☐ Brucella agglutination	☐ 12064	☐ 12065	☐ 12066	
☐ Carcinoembryonic antigen assay (CEA)	☐ 12067	☐ 12068	☐ 12069	☐ 12070
☐ Ceruloplasmin	☐ 12071	☐ 12072	☐ 12073	☐ 12074
☐ Coccidioidomycosis, Precipitin	☐ 12075	☐ 12076	☐ 12077	

CDC 3.1016 10-77   Page 1 of 4 pages

CDC laboratory examination checklist (1977)—non-syphilis serology

STANDARD OPERATING PROCEDURE MANUAL (SOPM) — Continued

PROCEDURE	Instructions NO (Code)	Reagents NO (Code)	Controls NO (Code)	Calibrations NO (Code)
☐ Anti-streptolysin O (ASO) Screen	☐ 12078	☐ 12079	☐ 12080	
☐ Complement, (Total Serum C′ and C′ 3 and components)	☐ 12081	☐ 12082	☐ 12083	☐ 12084
☐ C-reactive protein (CRP)	☐ 12085	☐ 12086	☐ 12087	
☐ Febrile agglutinations	☐ 12088	☐ 12089	☐ 12090	
☐ Fluorescent Antibody	☐ 12061	☐ 12062	☐ 12063	
☐ Glucose-6 Phosphate Dehydrogenase (G-6-PD)	☐ 12095	☐ 12096	☐ 12097	
☐ Haptoglobin	☐ 12098	☐ 12099	☐ 12100	☐ 12101
☐ Hepatitis B antigen (HB$_S$Ag)	☐ 12102	☐ 12103	☐ 12104	☐ 12105
☐ Hepatitis B antibody (HB$_S$Ab)	☐ 12106	☐ 12107	☐ 12108	☐ 12109
☐ Heterophile antibodies (Presumptive titer)	☐ 12110	☐ 12111	☐ 12112	
☐ Heterophile with absorptions (Differential)	☐ 12113	☐ 12114	☐ 12115	
☐ Histoplasma agglutination	☐ 12116	☐ 12117	☐ 12118	
☐ Immunoelectrophoretic procedures	☐ 12119	☐ 12120	☐ 12121	
☐ Infectious Mononucleosis (Screen)	☐ 12122	☐ 12123	☐ 12124	
☐ Latex — fixation (RA)	☐ 12125	☐ 12126	☐ 12127	
☐ Latex — fixation (LE)	☐ 12128	☐ 12129	☐ 12130	
☐ Leptospira agglutination	☐ 12131	☐ 12132	☐ 12133	
☐ Macroglobulins by ultra centrifugation	☐ 12134	☐ 12135	☐ 12136	☐ 12137
☐ Mucoprotein (seromucoid)	☐ 12138	☐ 12139	☐ 12140	
☐ *Mycoplasma pneumoniae* CF test	☐ 12141	☐ 12142	☐ 12143	
☐ Ox cell hemolysin test	☐ 12144	☐ 12145	☐ 12146	
☐ Q-Fever, agglutination titer	☐ 12147	☐ 12148	☐ 12149	
☐ Q-Fever, complement fixation	☐ 12150	☐ 12151	☐ 12152	
☐ Radioallergo Sorbent test (RAST Test)	☐ 12153	☐ 12154	☐ 12155	☐ 12156
☐ Reagent Parallel Testing	☐ 12157			
☐ Rubella HI antibody	☐ 12160	☐ 12161	☐ 12162	
☐ Serum Specific proteins (IgG; IgA; IgM; IgD, IgE)	☐ 12163	☐ 12164	☐ 12165	☐ 12166
☐ Sheep cell agglutination test for RA	☐ 12167	☐ 12168	☐ 12169	
☐ Streptococcus MG agglutination	☐ 12170	☐ 12171	☐ 12172	
☐ Thyroid auto-antibodies	☐ 12173	☐ 12174	☐ 12175	
☐ Trichina agglutination	☐ 12176	☐ 12177	☐ 12178	
☐ Toxoplasmosis agglutination	☐ 12179	☐ 12180	☐ 12181	
☐ Tularemia agglutination	☐ 12182	☐ 12183	☐ 12184	

	NO (Code)	COMMENT
8. The SOPM has a supervisor's written attestation that the SOPM is current	☐ 12185	
9. The supervisor's review of the SOPM is dated	☐ 12186	
10. SOPM includes only those procedures currently in use	☐ 12187	
11. All changes in procedures are documented (description of change and date) in the SOPM and have written approval (initials and date) of the supervisor	☐ 12189	

MATERIALS CFR 74.20(c) 405.1317(a)(3)

12. The following are labeled (identity, titer or concentration, recommended storage, preparation or expiration date)		NO (Code)	
	Antigens	☐ 12190	
	Antisera	☐ 12191	
	Calibrators	☐ 12192	
	Cell Suspensions	☐ 12193	
	Complement	☐ 12194	
	Conjugates	☐ 12195	
	Controls	☐ 12196	
	Diluents and Buffers	☐ 12197	
	Hemolysin	☐ 12198	
	Immunodiffusion Plates	☐ 12199	
	Kits	☐ 12200	
	Stains	☐ 12201	
13. Materials in use are "in-date", reactive and not deteriorated			
	Antigens	☐ 12203	
	Antisera	☐ 12204	
	Calibrators	☐ 12205	
	Cell Suspensions	☐ 12206	
	Complement	☐ 12207	
	Conjugates	☐ 12208	
	Controls	☐ 12209	
	Diluents and Buffers	☐ 12210	
	Hemolysin	☐ 12211	
	Immunodiffusion Plates	☐ 12212	
	Kits	☐ 12213	
	Stains	☐ 12214	

CDC 3.1016　10-77　　　　　　　Page 2 of 4 pages

Continued.

CDC laboratory examination checklist (1977)—non-syphilis serology—cont'd

CONTROL PROCEDURES CFR 74.22(a)(b) 405.1317(b)(2)(i)

14. Each qualitative test is controlled as follows: A positive and a negative control is included with each test run; each new lot of reagent and each new lot of control is compared, prior to routine use, with one of known reactivity.

TESTS	Positive Control NO (Code)	Negative Control NO (Code)	Reagent Comparison NO (Code)	COMMENT
Anti-mitochondrial antibody	*□ 12216	*□ 12217	*□ 12218	
Anti-nuclear antibodies (ANA)	*□ 12220	*□ 12221	*□ 12222	
Anti-parietal cell antibody	*□ 12224	*□ 12225	*□ 12226	
Anti-skeletal muscle antibody	*□ 12228	*□ 12229	*□ 12230	
Anti-smooth muscle antibody	*□ 12232	*□ 12233	*□ 12234	
Anti-streptolysin O (ASO) screen	*□ 12236	*□ 12237	*□ 12238	
Anti-thyroglobulin antibodies	*□ 12240	*□ 12241	*□ 12242	
Coccidioidomycosis , Precipitin	*□ 12244	*□ 12245	*□ 12246	
C-reactive protein (CRP)	*□ 12248	*□ 12249	*□ 12250	
Febrile agglutinations	*□ 12252	*□ 12253	*□ 12254	
Glucose-6 Phosphate Dehydrogenase (G-6-PD)	*□ 12256	*□ 12257	*□ 12258	
Hepatitis B antigen (HB$_S$Ag)	*□ 12260	*□ 12261	*□ 12262	
Hepatitis B antibody (HB$_S$Ab)	*□ 12264	*□ 12265	*□ 12266	
Infectious Mononucleosis (Screen)	*□ 12268	*□ 12269	*□ 12270	
Latex – fixation (RA)	*□ 12272	*□ 12273	*□ 12274	
Latex – fixation (LE)	*□ 12276	*□ 12277	*□ 12278	
Leptospira agglutination	*□ 12280	*□ 12281	*□ 12282	
Macroglobulins by ultra centrifugation	*□ 12284	*□ 12285	*□ 12286	
Radioallergo Sorbent Test (RAST Test)	*□ 12288	*□ 12289	*□ 12290	

15. Each quantitative test is controlled as follows: A positive control of graded reactivity and a negative control is included with each test run; each new lot of reagent and each new lot of control is compared, prior to routine use, with one of known reactivity.

TESTS	Positive Control NO (Code)	Negative Control NO (Code)	Reagent Comparison NO (Code)	COMMENT
Alpha-1-antitrypsin	*□ 12292		*□ 12294	
Anti-deoxyribonuclease (ADNase)	*□ 12296		*□ 12298	
Anti-nuclear antibodies (ANA)	*□ 12300	*□ 12301	*□ 12302	
Anti-parietal cell antibody	*□ 12304	*□ 12305	*□ 12306	
Anti-skeletal muscle antibody	*□ 12308	*□ 12309	*□ 12310	
Anti-smooth muscle antibody	*□ 12312	*□ 12313	*□ 12314	
Anti-streptococcal hyaluronidase (ASH)	*□ 12316		*□ 12318	
Anti-streptolysin O (ASO) titer	*□ 12320		*□ 12322	
Anti-thyroglobulin antibodies	*□ 12324	*□ 12325	*□ 12326	
Anti-toxoplasmosis antibody	*□ 12328	*□ 12329	*□ 12330	
Brucella agglutination	*□ 12332	*□ 12333	*□ 12334	
Carcinoembryonic antigen assay (CEA)	*□ 12336			
Ceruloplasmin	*□ 12340			
Complement, (Total Serum C′ and C′3 and components)	*□ 12348			
Febrile agglutinations	*□ 12352	*□ 12353	*□ 12354	
Fluorescent antibody	*□ 12356	*□ 12357	*□ 12358	
Glucose-6 Phosphate Dehydrogenase (G-6-PD)	*□ 12364	*□ 12365	*□ 12366	
Haptoglobin	*□ 12368			
Heterophile antibodies (Presumptive Titer)	*□ 12380	*□ 12381		
Heterophile with absorptions (Differential)	*□ 12384	*□ 12385		
Histoplasma agglutination	*□ 12388	*□ 12389	*□ 12390	
Immunoelectrophoretic Procedures	*□ 12392			
Latex – fixation (RA)	*□ 12400	*□ 12401	*□ 12402	
Mucoprotein (seromucoid)	*□ 12404	*□ 12405	*□ 12406	
Mycoplasma pneumoniae CF test	*□ 12408	*□ 12409	*□ 12410	
Ox Cell hemolysin test	*□ 12412	*□ 12413		
Q-fever, agglutination titer	*□ 12416	*□ 12417	*□ 12418	
Q-fever, complement fixation	*□ 12420	*□ 12421	*□ 12422	
Rubella HI antibody	*□ 12428	*□ 12429	*□ 12430	
Serum specific proteins (IgG; IgA; IgM; IgD; IgE)	*□ 12432			
Sheep cell agglutination test for RA	*□ 12436	*□ 12437	*□ 12438	
Streptococcus MG agglutination	*□ 12440	*□ 12441	*□ 12442	
Thyroid auto-antibodies	*□ 12444	*□ 12445	*□ 12446	
Trichina agglutination	*□ 12448	*□ 12449	*□ 12450	
Toxoplasmosis agglutination	*□ 12452	*□ 12453	*□ 12454	
Tularemia agglutination	*□ 12456	*□ 12457	*□ 12458	

CDC 3.1016
10-77

Page 3 of 4 pages

CDC laboratory examination checklist (1977)—non-syphilis serology—cont'd

☐ COMPLEMENT FIXATION TESTS		NO (Code)	COMMENT
16. Hemolysin titrated with each new cell batch		*☐ 12460	
17. Complement titrated each time test performed		*☐ 12461	
18. Serum complement control included each time test performed		*☐ 12462	
19. Tissue antigen-complement control included each time test performed		*☐ 12463	
20. Antigen-complement control included each time test performed		*☐ 12464	
21. Buffer-complement control included each time test performed		*☐ 12465	
22. Red cell control included each time test performed		*☐ 12466	
HEMAGGLUTINATION-INHIBITION TESTS (RUBELLA AND OTHER VIRAL SEROLOGY)			
23. Antigen titrated each time test performed		*☐ 12467	
24. Serum/cell/buffer control included each time test performed		*☐ 12468	
25. Cell/buffer control included each time test performed		*☐ 12469	
NEUTRALIZATION TESTS (VIRAL SEROLOGY)			
26. TCD 50 determined each time test performed		*☐ 12470	
27. Cell culture control included each time test performed		*☐ 12472	
28. Serum toxicity control included each time test performed (when serum testing only)		*☐ 12473	
HEMABSORPTION-INHIBITION TESTS (VIRAL SEROLOGY)			
29. A cell culture control is included with the Hemabsorption-Inhibition test each time tests are performed		*☐ 12474	
RADIOIMMUNOASSAY TESTS			
30. Counting equipment is checked for background stability each day of use		*☐ 12476	
31. Counting equipment is checked with a radioactive standard each day of use		*☐ 12477	
32. Manufacturer's directions for commercial kits are followed by bench personnel OR changes have been validated by this laboratory for the following:	Carcinoembryonic antigen assay (CEA)	*☐ 12478	
	Immunoglobulin (IgE)	*☐ 12479	
	Hepatitis B Antigen (HB$_S$Ag)	*☐ 12480	

33. Established limits are available for each control for the following:		ESTABLISHED LIMITS NO (CODE)	WRITTEN COURSE OF ACTION NO (CODE)	REMEDIAL ACTION DOCUM. NO (CODE)
	Carcinoembryonic antigen assay (CEA)	*☐ 12481	*☐ 12502	☐ 12503
	Immunoglobulin (IgE)	*☐ 12482	*☐ 12504	☐ 12505
	Other:	*☐ 12506	*☐ 12507	☐ 12508
IMMUNODIFFUSION TESTS				
34. Established limits are available for each control for the following:	Alpha-1-antitrypsin	*☐ 12484	*☐ 12509	12510
	Ceruloplasmin	*☐ 12485	*☐ 12511	12512
	Complement	*☐ 12486	*☐ 12513	12514
	Haptoglobin	*☐ 12487	*☐ 12515	12516
	Serum Specific Protein: IgA	*☐ 12488	*☐ 12517	☐ 12518
	IgD	*☐ 12489	*☐ 12519	☐ 12520
	IgG	*☐ 12490	*☐ 12521	☐ 12522
	IgM	*☐ 12491	*☐ 12523	☐ 12524
	IgE	*☐ 12492	*☐ 12525	☐ 12526

RECORDS CFR 74.50; 74.54(a); 405.1316; 405.1316(g)		NO (CODE)	
35. Records of observation are made, concurrently with the performance of each step in the examination of specimens		☐ 12495	
37. Records are retained at least 2 years	Accession records	☐ 12497	
	Control records	☐ 12498	
	Copy of final report to client	☐ 12499	
	Equipment maintenance records	☐ 12500	
	Records of observations of each step of specimen testing	☐ 12501	

CDC laboratory examination checklist (1977)—non-syphilis serology—cont'd

annually, and such reviews should be signed by the director of the laboratory. All notations, additions, or deletions entered in the SOPM should be initialed by the technical supervisor and the director.

Accession records constitute a great source of error in laboratories because it is here that the information specifically identifying the patient, the requesting physician, the date, the type of specimen, and the test requested is replaced by an identifying laboratory code number. Errors made in transferring this data result in delays, confusion, and in some instances misleading information. In designing clerical procedures it is imperative that the necessity for transferring information from one record to another be held to a minimum or at least that provision be made for minimal opportunity for error.

In the checklists on the following pages, which are representative of those used by laboratory examiners, many of the questions imply that the inquiry is dictated by regulations and that failure to satisfy all of the detailed statements constitutes noncompliance with those regulations. In numerous instances this is not the case. Nonconformance to many of the items listed might elicit a recommendation from the examiner but not an edict. In perusing the checklists consider the relative merit of each item for improving laboratory services rather than just whether it is required to meet the minimum criteria of a regulatory program.

MEDIA

The "quality control of media" as practiced in today's laboratory is more accurately described as the "evaluation of media." Quality control implies that a medium under study conforms to a predetermined standard. The purchase of preplated and tubed media has become the rule rather than the exception, and the laboratorian therefore has little direct control over the formulation of media. Since microbiologic media may contain such indefinable or irreproducible constituents as agar, peptone, meat extract, yeast extract, bile salts, and gelatin, it is not surprising that even in the hands of the manufacturer quality control of media is relative; that is, the medium conforms to a formulation rather than meeting the precise specifications of a standard. For assurance that a medium was prepared according to a prescribed formulation the average laboratory must rely on the integrity of the manufacturer. In any case this assurance of strict adherence to a formula does not ensure the growth characteristics of the finished medium. The laboratorian must first select an appropriate medium for a particular situation and then establish the growth characteristics of that medium under routine conditions.

Selection

Each clinical specimen that comes to the microbiology laboratory for analysis is inoculated on a variety of media, each of which has been chosen for its ability to enhance recovery of certain etiologic agents. These media vary in mode of action (Fig. 73-1), some selecting out certain types of organisms at the expense of others, some differentiating one group of organisms from another by some physiologic characteristic, and still other enriched media assuring growth of most bacteria but relying on the skills of the laboratorian to physically separate representative

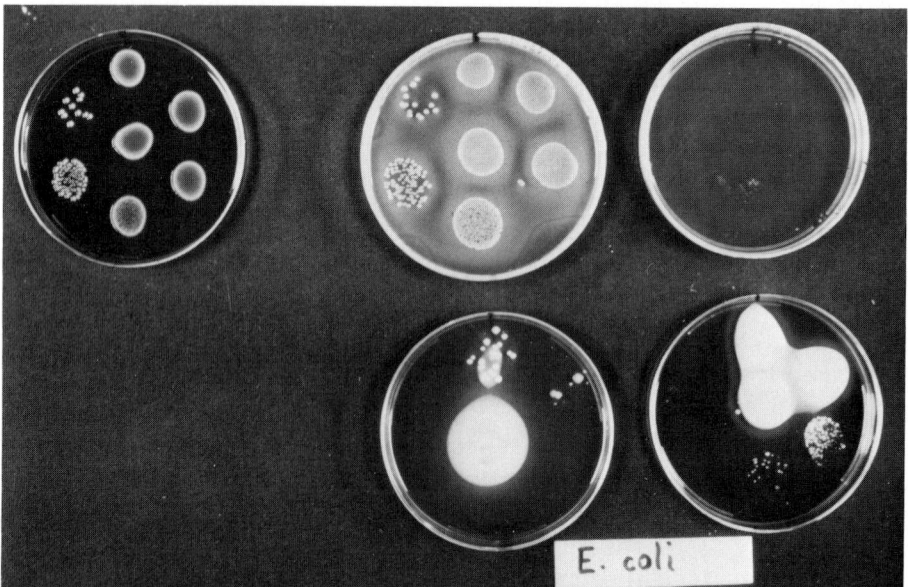

Fig. 73-1. Tenfold dilutions of standardized suspension of *Escherichia coli* placed drop by drop on several recovery media. *Top, left to right:* Sheep blood agar, MacConkey agar, Salmonella-Shigella agar. *Bottom, left to right:* Xylose-lysine-deoxycholate agar, Hektoen agar.

colonies of the mixed population. In the laboratory it is the usual practice to select a battery of media from these 3 general types and to inoculate the routine clinical specimens on these media.

The choice of isolation media is extremely important because in making this selection from many alternatives the laboratorian is predetermining the limits or capabilities of the laboratory. Lack of an appropriate recovery medium can frustrate the efforts of a well-trained staff in an otherwise adequately equipped laboratory. The selection of media for routine isolation procedures should be based on a thorough understanding of the mode of action of the medium,[1,2] a review of the current literature for evidence of practicality, stability, and reliability, and finally a documented in-house study of the medium under the specific demands of the daily routine. The new medium should be used routinely in the laboratory and evaluated in parallel with the current procedures before it is selected as a replacement for a long used and proved medium.

Preparation

In recent years the average laboratory has become increasingly dependent on commercially available preplated and pretubed media. A medium is prepared in the laboratory only in those rare instances when it is not available commercially or when an unexpected etiologic agent is encountered. A supply of dehydrated media is kept in most laboratories for such an eventuality. It is ironic, however, that in many laboratories media preparation is relegated to the least experienced personnel, who have little understanding of the task or of the implications of any technical errors made. For this reason the subject of media preparation is discussed in some detail.

Storage

The medium should be stored properly as soon as it is delivered to the laboratory, and the date of receipt should be recorded on the label. Unless the label states that the medium should be refrigerated, the unopened bottle is stored at a temperature below 25 C in an area of low humidity and out of direct sunlight. The medium should not be stored near autoclaves, drying ovens, Arnold steam sterilizers, or other sources of heat or steam.

Weighing

When preparing to weigh out media check the dates on the bottles. Use the oldest stock of medium first. Do not open a new lot of medium until the previous lot has been exhausted or unless when examined closely the old lot appears to have taken up moisture or darkened in color. If there is not enough of the old lot of powdered medium to fill the request, do not mix the new lot with the old. Keep the lots separate and distinct. The blending of 2 lots may produce a gradual transition from a good medium to an inferior one,

which cannot be discerned at the bench. If necessary prepare a small second batch from the new lot to satisfy the request. **Date the bottle of the new lot when it is opened the first time.**

Use a balance and weights that are frequently checked for accuracy. Dehydrated media, being very hygroscopic, should be weighed quickly but accurately in a room with low humidity. The bottle should be closed tightly and the powdered medium on the weighing paper put into solution as quickly as possible. Return the stock bottle to storage.

Dissolution

Use only borosilicate glassware that has been thoroughly washed and rinsed with pure water USP (either distilled or deionized). Do not use water suspected of containing chlorine, copper, lead, or detergents. A quick spot check for residual detergents can be made by running a drop of pH indicator down the inside surface of a piece of glassware and observing whether there is an alkaline color reaction. The distilled water should be tested frequently for conductivity. Resistance determinations performed on an osmometer should read 0.5 Mohms or higher. After 1 drop saturated KCl is added to 50 ml water the pH should be between 5.5 and 7.0.

Before applying heat to dissolve dehydrated media, **read the label.** Some media (e.g., urea broth, urea agar) must not be subjected to temperatures above 55 C, but powdered media suspended in distilled water may be boiled to assure complete dissolution and even distribution of the ingredients. The medium should be stirred to avoid scorching any undissolved medium in the bottom of the flask. Swirling of the medium during heating should be performed with caution because some media, particularly those containing agar, may foam and overflow. To avoid overflow prepare the medium in a flask no smaller than 2½ times the volume of the medium. Prolonged heating of the medium should be avoided; bringing it to the boiling point usually is sufficient to completely dissolve the ingredients. The bulk medium should be dispensed into screw-capped tubed (tops left loose) or into appropriate flasks for sterilization.

Sterilization

Read the label. Many media cannot withstand the rigorous conditions of sterilization in an autoclave. In some cases the media must be sterilized by filtration. However, some media are so selective that they do not require heat or filter sterilization (e.g., Salmonella-Shigella agar, desoxycholate citrate agar, bismuth sulfite agar, tetrathionate broth, selenite broth). The selective activity of these media is destroyed during autoclaving.

Filtration

A liquid is passed through a sterile material with pores so small that bacteria and even viruses can be physically held back, permitting the collection of a biologically sterile substrate. Filtration can be influenced by electrical charges on the filter and pH of the substrate as well as by the properties of a mechanical sieve. Depending on the filter used, it can be a more complex operation than simple straining of a substrate. Numerous filters of different types and varying pore sizes are available to the microbiologist. The Berkefeld and Chamberland filters, which are made from diatomaceous earth and unglazed porcelain, respectively, are used now only rarely. Although retrievable, these filters have been largely replaced by synthetic membranes of cellulose esters and asbestos pads, which are cheap and disposable and do not require exhaustive maintenance and cleaning.

The asbestos pads (Seitz filters) are available in 2 porosities: fine and extra fine, designated type serum 1 and type serum 3, respectively. While effective, the asbestos filter pad does have some disadvantages. Filtration with asbestos pads often causes the substrate to become alkaline. Fortunately a well-buffered medium is not markedly influenced by this type of filter. The asbestos filter has also been shown to release cations (i.e., primarily calcium and magnesium ions) into the substrate. The presence of these ions could influence the substrate by chelative effects. The asbestos pad has 2 other disadvantages: it cannot be used to filter small volumes of substrate without absorbing a large portion of the substrate, and foaming can be a problem when the Seitz filter is used. Consideration must be given to the fact that asbestos filter pads may introduce subtle changes into the substrate being sterilized.

The membrane filter (Millipore Corp., Bedford, Mass.) is probably the most widely used filter system in the laboratory today. It is composed of cellulose esters, which possess good wet strength and can be used with the Swinny hypodermic adaptor on a syringe or for sterilizing large volumes of medium. The membrane filters are available in various pore sizes, but the HA type (0.45 μm) and the GS type (0.22 μm) are most widely used. The membrane filter differs from asbestos pads and other filter systems in that it relies primarily on pore size to hold back contaminating bacteria. In contrast diatomaceous earth, porcelain, and asbestos filters use electrical charges to entrap the bacteria against the walls of the comparatively large pores.

Autoclaving

The medium must be sterilized without excessive and prolonged cycles. Overautoclaving a medium is in some respects a more grievous error than understerilization. Routine sterility checks on the medium will reveal an unsterile medium; however, a medium whose biochemical characteristics have been altered by excessive autoclaving can produce countless problems in routine use at the bench. Selective or differential characteristics of the medium might be reduced, or conversely the medium could demonstrate an increased inhibitory characteristic that could influence its ability to recover bacteria. It is advisable to preheat media, particularly larger volumes, to avoid lag time in reaching sterilization temperatures. Volumes of media exceeding 1 L require additional time at sterilization temperature.

It is important that the autoclave be functioning properly and that the sterilization cycle recommended by the manufacturer be adhered to strictly. The autoclave should be placed on a preventive maintenance program and examined at specified intervals. Efficiency of the autoclave must be monitored, that is, how long it takes to reach sterilization temperature and how long it takes to "come down." Either of these factors can contribute to oversterilization of a medium. The autoclave may have clogged and rusted pipes that need to be replaced. Temperature and pressure gauges should be checked during preventive maintenance.

For monitoring efficiency the autoclave should be fitted with a thermocouple within the chamber and connected to a recording device. In the small laboratory that does not have a thermocouple system the cycle should be monitored by observing the temperature gauge. Pressure gauges are generally inefficient and give low readings. Any adjustments in regulating the flow of steam should be monitored on the temperature scale. The temperature and time should be recorded for each run in a log. The recording chart from the thermocouple serves as a record for each run.

As a backup system to the thermocouple or temperature gauge the sterilization system should be monitored by incorporating a biologic indicator into a run at least once a month. For wet loads a suspension in broth (e.g., Kilit autoclave control, BBL, Division of BioQuest, Cockeysville, Md.) is satisfactory, but for dry loads it is best to include a control composed of spores on a dry piece of filter paper (e.g., Spordex strips, American Sterilizer Co., Erie, Pa.; Attest ampules, 3M Company, Medical Products Division, St. Paul, Minn.). The organism used for high-temperature sterilization is *Bacillus stearothermophilus*. Ampules or strips may be placed in a test pack or in a tube or envelope. If a tube is used it should be laid on its side uncapped. One tube should be placed on the front bottom shelf (coolest part of the chamber) in addition to other spots if the autoclave or the load is large. The date of use and results of these controls should be recorded in a log.

Spore strips should be stored under the conditions specified by the manufacturer. They are usually sealed in a plastic bag and stored at 4 C in a refrigerator. Spore strips should not be stored in a freezer because the sublimation of residual moisture in the strip during freezing increases the spores' resistance due to the effects of this freeze-drying. This increased resistance can influence sterility determinations, particularly in ethylene oxide sterilizers where a certain amount of residual moisture must be present for the gas to function properly.

Systems other than bacterial spore suspensions are available for monitoring heat sterilization systems. The concept is based on the use of chemical temperature indicators and reliance on the specific melting points of certain chemical compounds to demonstrate that specified temperatures have been attained (e.g., succinic anhydride, mp 119.6 C; acetanilide, mp 113-114 C). The disadvantage in using melting points is that although the temperature has been attained the length of exposure remains unknown. Autoclave indicator tape that is heat sensitive and undergoes a color change at an appropriate time and temperature is available from the 3M Company. Still another means of checking the efficiency and even distribution of heat in an oven or autoclave is to place Browne's tubes (Albert Browne, Ltd., Chancery Street, Leicester, England) at various points in the chamber. These tubes are of 3 types: type I responds to 121 C at 15 minutes, type II to 115 C at 15 minutes, and type III to 160 C at 60 minutes. It should be emphasized, however, that none of the chemical temperature indicators should be used to the total exclusion of the bacterial spore system. The incorporation of the chemical indicator into the chamber for each run is recommended, but the biologic spore system should be used at least monthly.

Storage

Unless specified otherwise, prepared media should be stored at 2-8 C. One notable exception is thioglycollate broth, which should be stored at room temperature out of direct sunlight because atmospheric gases are more soluble in liquids at refrigerator temperature. It is important that atmospheric oxygen not be dissolved in the thioglycollate medium because the metabolites will be oxidized and become organic peroxides, which might be particularly toxic in subsequent utilizations involving anaerobiosis.

The most common detrimental effect of storage is dehydration. Dehydration should not be a problem with liquid or solid media kept in well-sealed, screw-capped containers but is very likely to occur with plated media, particularly in the small laboratory where certain media are used only occasionally and must be stored for prolonged periods. With media that are selective to begin with, this inadvertent concentration of inhibitory substances becomes a real problem. Plating media should be stored in the refrigerator in sealed plastic bags and removed from storage only a short time before use.

All media should be brought to room temperature before they are used. Refrigerated tubes of carbohydrate media containing inverted Durham tubes should be warmed to room temperature immediately before use, and tubes showing trapped bubbles of atmospheric gases should be discarded.

Addition of enrichments

Enrichments to be added to basal media must be checked for sterility. In most instances enrichments are heat labile and should not be subjected to temperatures in excess of 50 C. The basal medium should be cooled to 45-50 C before aseptic addition of the enrichment. Cold enrichment should not be added to agar media because agar lumps may be formed. A medium is easily homogenized if the enrichment is prewarmed to at least room temperature, and preferably to 37 C, before it is added to the medium with gentle swirling. Vigorous mixing should be avoided. For chocolatized agar the blood should be added to the basal medium, which is at 80-85 C.

The most common enrichment for culture media is blood. The species of animal from which the blood is obtained can affect the selectivity of the medium in recovering bacteria and can influence the hemolytic activity expressed by some bacteria. If an agar plate is enriched with sheep blood, *Haemophilus influenzae* cannot be recovered from the plate. Updyke[3] found that most group D streptococci were α-hemolytic in sheep blood but β-hemolytic in rabbit, horse, and human blood agar.

Outdated human blood from a blood bank should not be used as an enrichment without extensive preliminary examination. Blood containing oxalate or citrate is toxic to members of the genus *Streptococcus*. If the transfusion bag contains these anticoagulants, a bag containing a full unit of blood should be chosen in order to assure maximum dilution of these chemical substances. Moreover the donor blood might contain residual antibiotics (e.g., penicillin) to which streptococci are highly susceptible. In addition human donor blood may contain elevated levels of antistreptolysin O, which could hinder the expression of β-hemolytic activity by β-hemolytic streptococci. Finally, the presence of added glucose in the blood (e.g., Alsever's solution), with the resulting production of acid, would tend to inhibit hemolysin production by the streptococci, negating a very important identification criterion. Thus the choice of human blood places an increased quality control burden on the laboratorian.

Testing for sterility

All batches of medium should be checked for sterility, and sterility control is even more essential for plated media and for those tubed media prepared by breaking into an already sterile medium to add one or more filter-sterilized sugars or other heat-labile enrichments under aseptic conditions. However, in checking media for sterility the microbiologist is placed in a dilemma. The sterility of a batch of medium can be determined only by incubating the entire collection of plates or tubes under prescribed conditions. Unfortunately, having undergone prolonged conditions of incubation the medium may no longer be acceptable as a routine growth medium. As a compromise a representative portion (at least 5%) of each new batch should be incubated under conditions approximating those for predicted use. Ideally the medium should be held for 3-5 days, although gross contamination would probably be evident after 18-24 hours. Some of the plates should be incubated at room temperature to detect contaminating psychrophilic bacteria. Media likely to be incubated for long periods, such as those used in the cultivation of *Mycobacterium tuberculosis*, should be proved free of contaminating slow growers.

Selective media, because they are inhibitory to many organisms, pose special problems. Even gross contamination may not be detected by the methods described above. In routine use contamination of selective media is often recognized because the picking of well-isolated colonies to noninhibitory media repeatedly gives rise to mixed populations. Inoculation of a small portion of the selective medium suspected of being contaminated into a large volume of sterile broth (to dilute the inhibitory substances in the selective medium) will permit detection of heavy contamination and will partially solve this problem.

Sterility testing is seldom helpful in those infrequent instances of isolated single-colony contamination that occur while plates are being poured or tops tilted to facilitate drying. This sporadic contaminant is difficult to detect before the plate is inoculated with a specimen. If heavy growth of a particular colonial type begins suddenly halfway through a streaked population, the possibility must be considered that the abrupt appearance of the colonial type resulted from a

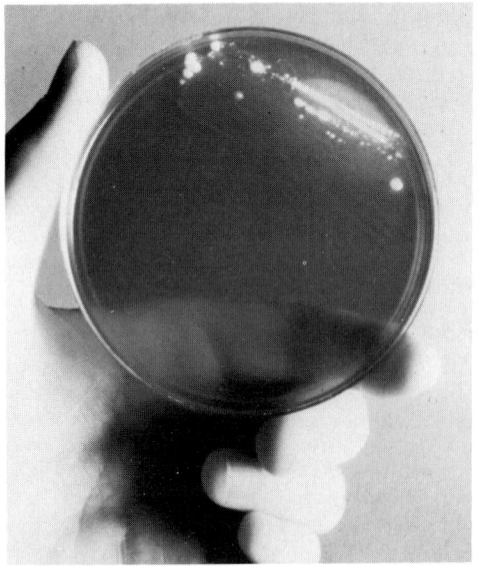

Fig. 73-2. Strain of *Salmonella paratyphi* B streaked on new plate of Salmonella-Shigella agar to evaluate growth capabilities of medium.

contaminating microcolony. Under such circumstances a request for resubmission of the specimen is indicated, or at the very least the report should indicate a questionable result.

Evaluation

The initial step in evaluating new batches of media is the gross visual observation. Comparison of the new batch with that in current use can reveal deficiencies quickly and without the needless expenditure of other resources. A new batch of plate medium that is not as red or as green or as blue as previous batches may indicate a significant shift in pH or possibly a weighing error during preparation. Check the pH at room temperature using a pH meter standardized with buffer at pH 7.0. Plating media may be checked with a surface electrode, or the medium can be macerated in clean glassware and the electrodes inserted into the medium. The pH of the medium must fall within ±0.2 unit of the value specified by the manufacturer. A medium containing a faint turbidity but proving to be sterile may have lost a nutrient essential to the recovery of some bacteria. In such instances the medium should be discarded, or at the very least the growth characteristics should be tested with a variety of organisms.

It is common practice in the microbiology laboratory to evaluate a new batch of medium by streaking representative plates with a positive and a negative control culture. As can be seen in Fig. 73-2, *Salmonella paratyphi* B inoculated on a new batch of Salmonella-Shigella (SS) agar and incubated overnight grows on the medium. This widely used quality control measure reveals very little about the quality of the new batch because the growth observed may constitute recovery of only 1 organism in hundreds or thousands. The evaluation of a selective medium is not as simple as recovery of the positive control and total inhibition of the negative control.

Variations in laboratory media are not uncommon but generally are too subtle to be detected by the microbiologist's all-or-nothing approach to quality control. The growth characteristics of a medium are best measured by using 10-fold dilutions of an optically adjusted suspension of a stock culture. By using a standardized suspension the laboratorian can establish the sensitivity of the medium for recovering or inhibiting chosen organisms. An even better measure is to run the medium in parallel with a nonselective medium that serves as a basis for comparison (Fig. 73-3).

Almost invariably different lots of Salmonella-Shigella (SS) agar will totally inhibit *Escherichia coli* but not without a substantial inhibition of the enteric pathogens. In Fig. 73-4 it can be observed that some lots of SS agar recover approximately one-tenth the number of organisms recovered on a nonselective blood agar plate when inoculated with *Salmonella paratyphi* B. Note that some lots recover only a hundredth of the number recovered on the nonselective plate. In contrast the same SS media (Fig. 73-5) recover only a thousandth of the number of *Shigella boydii* recovered with the reference blood medium.

Variations have been observed in other enteric media. A number of samples of xylose-lysine-deoxycholate (XLD) agar plated with 10-fold dilutions of optically adjusted suspensions of *Salmonella typhi*, *Shigella sonnei*, *Shigella boydii*, and *Escherichia coli* showed striking variations.

The various samples of XLD media were found to recover numbers of salmonella and shigellae comparable to those recovered on a blood agar medium. Variations observed primarily in the failure to produce blackened colonies indicative of the hydrogen sulfide–producing strains of *Salmonella*. These lots of media also demonstrated a tendency to produce yellow colonies of salmonellae that became characteristically red only after 36-48 hours of incubation at 37 C. However,

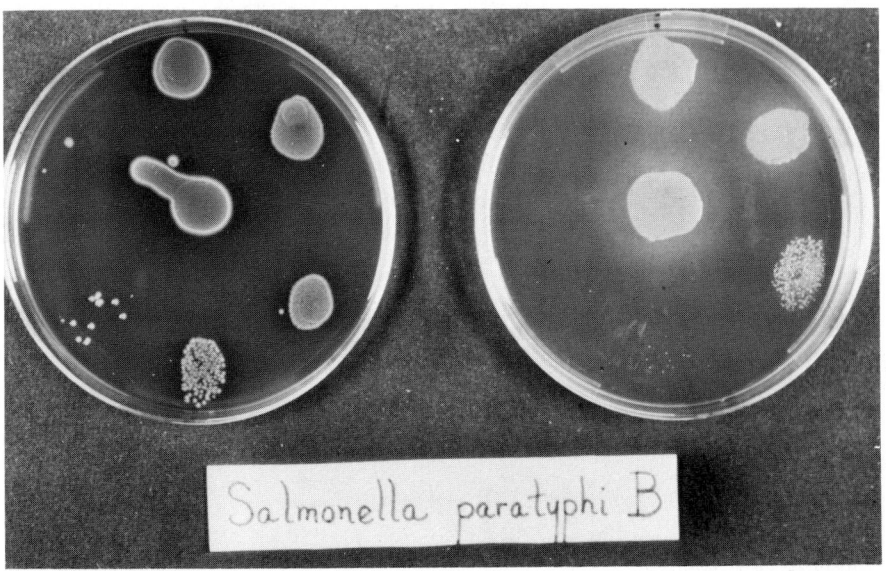

Fig. 73-3. Tenfold dilutions of suspension of *Salmonella paratyphi* B plated on sheep blood agar plate (*left*) and Salmonella-Shigella (SS) agar. Note inhibitory characteristic of SS agar.

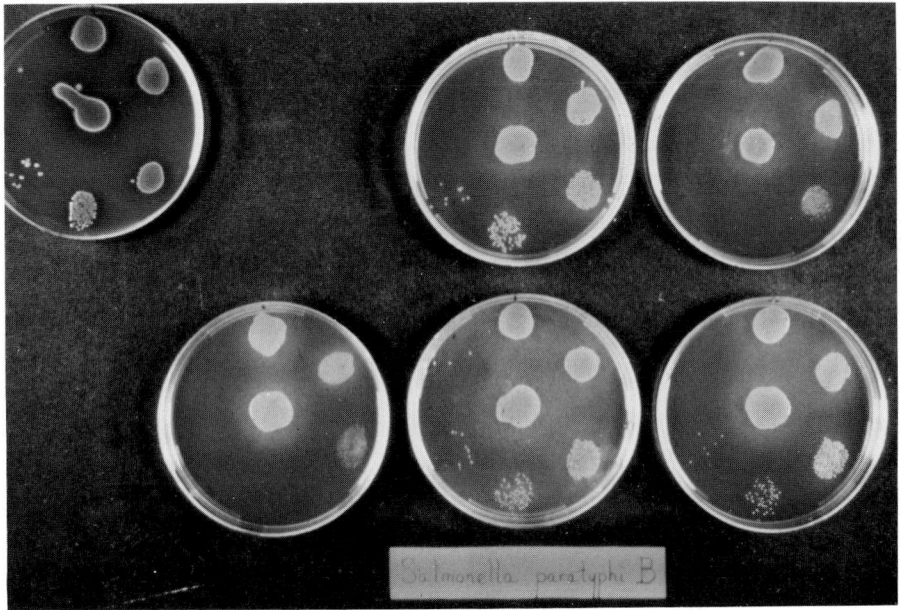

Fig. 73-4. Variations in recovery of *Salmonella paratyphi* B on 5 different samples of SS agar using sheep blood agar plate (*upper left*) as basis of reference.

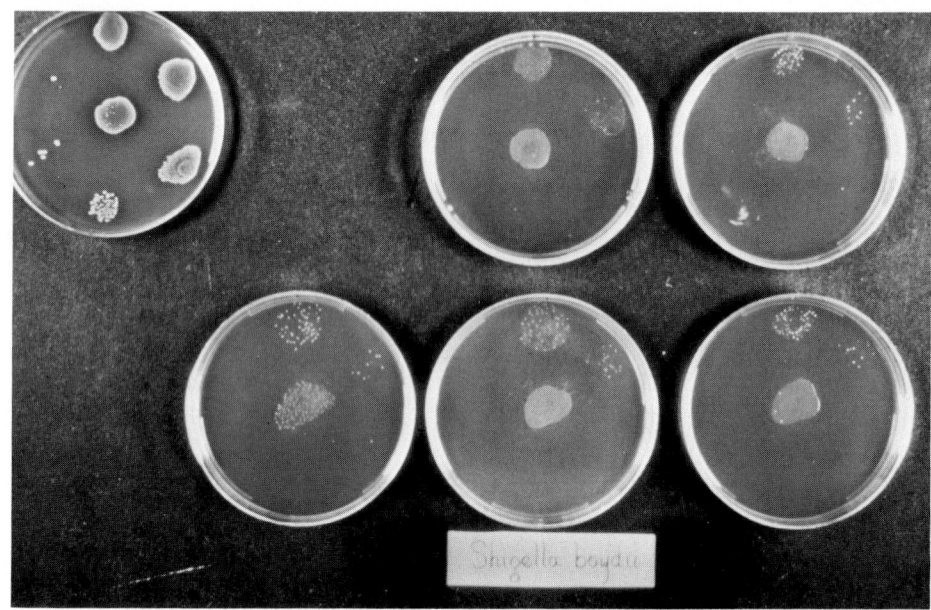

Fig. 73-5. Thousandfold inhibition of *Shigella boydii* on SS agar with sheep blood agar plate used as basis of reference.

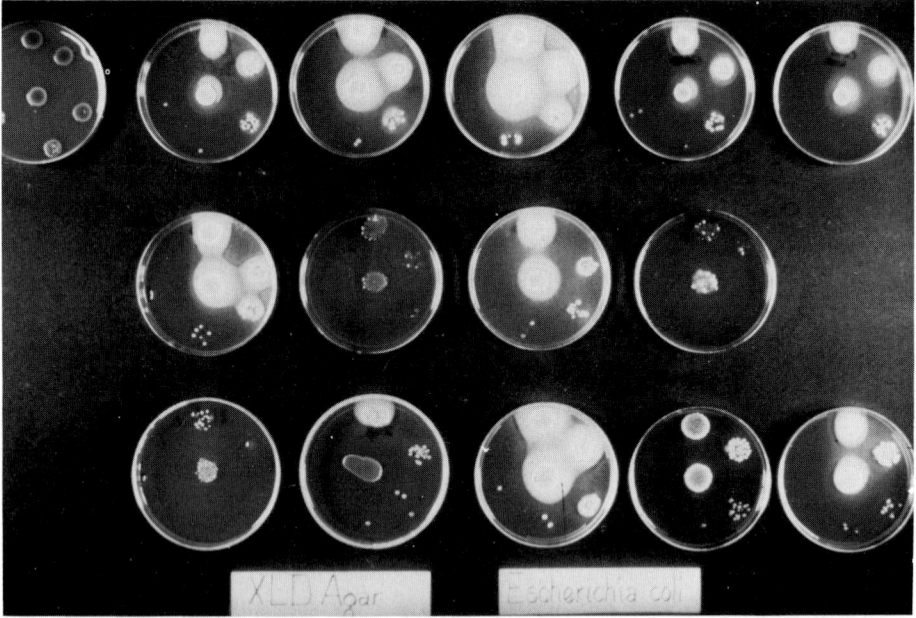

Fig. 73-6. Variations in inhibition of *Escherichia coli* obtained on lots of xylose-lysine-deoxycholate (XLD) agar and on sheep blood reference plate (*upper left*). In addition note that isolated colonies on plates 2 and 4 of middle row were more characteristic of *Shigella* than *E. coli.*

the greatest variation noted with the XLD medium was in its inhibitory capacity for *Escherichia coli* and in the growth of atypical colonies of *E. coli* whose morphology was more characteristic of shigellae than of coliforms. Such variations can be seen in Fig. 73-6.

A satisfactory alternative, described by Blaze-vic et al.,[4] to the cumbersome dilution method described above is to prepare a 1:10 dilution in broth of a suspension of test culture(s) equivalent in turbidity to the McFarland 0.5 standard and to streak plates with this suspension with an 0.001 ml calibrated loop to obtain isolated colonies.

The primary concern regarding enriched

media is sterility. The major difficulty encountered with enriched media is contamination rather than selection or inhibition of inoculum. Nevertheless the possibility exists that a critical supplement may have been omitted during preparation. For this reason enriched media should be monitored with the most fastidious organisms for which the medium was designed. For example, supplemented chocolate agar should be tested with both *Neisseria gonorrhoeae* and *Haemophilus influenzae*, since the important growth factors in this medium are different for each of these organisms. Inactivation of the V factor by overheating would result in failure of the medium to support the growth of *H. influenzae* but would not affect its ability to isolate *N. gonorrhoeae*.

In summary, the quality control system for evaluating media should measure the ability of a medium to recover small numbers of the organisms to be cultured on it, and for selective media the additional capacity to inhibit comparatively large numbers of competing commensal organisms.

Biochemical test media should be controlled with 2 or more organisms so that the accuracy of both positive and negative results is determined. When fermentation media containing polysaccharides are tested it must be kept in mind that in quality control tests the breakdown of these carbohydrates into glucose during the preparation of media could falsely indicate a specific fermentation but without providing a clue that it is fermentation of glucose rather than the sugar(s) put into the medium. Maltose is the sugar most often implicated in erroneous determinations, either because poor quality maltose was used initially or because the maltose was broken down during sterilization. Therefore an organism that attacks the polysaccharide and one that does not possess the trait should be used in parallel. The method of inoculation and the inoculum size should be those used routinely in performing the biochemical test.

In recent years **commercial identification systems** (e.g., API, Analytab Products, Plainview, N.Y.; Minitek, BBL, Division of BioQuest, Cockeysville, Md.; Enterotube, Oxi/Ferm, Roche Diagnostics, Nutley, N.J.; Inolex, Inolex Biochemical Div., Wilson Pharmaceutical & Chemical Corp., Glenwood, Ill.; R/b, Corning Medical Diagnostic, Roslyn, N.Y.; Pathotec, General Diagnostics, Morris Plains, N.J.; Bactec, Johnston Laboratories, Cockeysville, Md.; TD3, Grand Island Biological Co., Grand Island, N.Y.) have replaced the classical media in numerous laboratories. Each new shipment of these systems should be checked with enough known organisms to give at least one positive and one negative biochemical response for each constituent.

During those early years of bacteriology testing, particularly enteric bacteriology, one of the major faults of the laboratorian was the failure to pick enough isolated colonies to assure isolation of the enteric pathogen. There was some justification for this hesitancy to select numerous colonies because each colony represented an additional workload on subsequent days and the classical identification methods were cumbersome. When packaged identification systems became commercially available it was hoped that additional colonies would be selected for characterization because identification became simpler. Results of proficiency testing surveys indicate that the problem of insufficient characterization of mixed bacterial populations persists, not because of additional workload but because costs of newer systems do not permit the increased characterization of isolates. The laboratorian must consider this problem in designing the protocol for the laboratory manual and in selecting the appropriate media. It may be necessary in some instances to consider the implementation of a screening procedure between the primary isolation medium and the inoculation of biochemical media or packaged identification systems.

A log should be kept of all media tested, including the date tested, control or lot number, stock organism used, results of testing, and the name of the person doing the testing. The logs should be easily available to the laboratory staff so that any questions arising about the quality or performance of a particular lot of medium can be answered.

REAGENTS

All stains and reagents used in detecting and identifying microbial agents should be tested periodically for proper reactivity with appropriate media and stock organisms possessing known characteristics. The frequency of the reagent check varies with the stability of the reagent in question. Some relatively unstable reagents (e.g., catalase, coagulase, ferric chloride, indole, methyl red, nitrate, oxidase, Voges-Proskauer) would warrant testing each day they are used to demonstrate a positive and negative biochemical reaction.

The Gram stain should be tested when prepared, and once each week it is used to demonstrate the expected staining characteristics. Less frequently used stains (e.g., capsule flagella and spore) should be tested each day they are used with appropriate stock strains.

Results of these control tests should be recorded in a log. Each entry in the log should be dated and initialed by the staff member performing the evaluation.

ANTISERA

In the clinical laboratory, antisera are widely used to establish the serologic group and type of certain etiologic agents. These antisera should be used in conjunction with cultural, biochemical, and morphologic characteristics to identify bacteria. In numerous laboratory situations rapid

presumptive identification is attempted by
the agglutination of uncharacterized isolated
colonies growing on primary isolation media
(e.g., non-lactose-fermenting colonies of gram-
negative rods on MacConkey agar). These presumptive identifications are often invalid as a result of specific serologic reactions with antigens
common to more than one bacterium. Furthermore normal antibody levels present in the laboratory animal before immunization may persist in
the grouping or typing antisera even after routine
adsorption procedures. These normally residing
antibodies are free to react with a multitude of
bacteria and can confuse the identification of the
etiologic agent. The manufacturer's directions for
use of the antiserum should be followed exactly,
with particular attention to specified precautions
in the use of the serum. The use of these antisera
for direct testing for the purpose of presumptive
identification requires exhaustive pretesting and
adsorption of the antiserum to assure specificity
of reactions.

If antisera are to be used exclusively as a
confirmatory step in the identification of organisms, for reasons of time and economics, they
need only be periodically tested. It is a difficult
task to maintain enough smooth *Salmonella* serotypes to check *Salmonella* antisera thoroughly. If
an occasional organism biochemically resembles
Salmonella or *Shigella* but does not agglutinate
in the appropriate antiserum, it should be standard procedure to send it to a reference laboratory for complete identification. Should this happen with any frequency, however, the antisera
should be subject to prompt quality control testing.

As soon as they arrive in the laboratory antisera
should be dated and if lyophilized the date of
rehydration marked on the label. Antisera must
be stored at refrigerator temperature and should
be examined each time they are used for clarity
or indications of contamination or deterioration.
The reactivity of a new antiserum should be
established before initial use with appropriate
control cultures and checked at monthly intervals
thereafter. Monospecific antisera (e.g., group A
Streptococcus, *Shigella* group A, *E. coli* 0127:B8)
should be checked with positive and negative
control organisms. The negative control organisms should be selected for their ability to
challenge the specificity of the antisera. A group
C *Streptococcus*, *Shigella* group B, and *E. coli*
026:B6 would serve as suitable controls for the
above antisera. Polyvalent or multispecific antisera should be checked with control organisms
representing each major group of antigens. Fluorescent antibody conjugates must be checked
each time they are used with control cultures that
would conceivably cross react with poorly adsorbed conjugates (e.g., *Neisseria gonorrhoeae*
conjugate with *Neisseria meningitidis* organisms; group A *Streptococcus* conjugate with
group C and G streptococci).

ANTIBIOTICS

A detailed discussion of the performance and
quality control of antimicrobial susceptibility
testing is presented in Chapter 87. However,
some points should be reemphasized. Only those
antibiotic powders approved for laboratory in
vitro diagnostic procedures should be used for
dilution testing or as controls for antibiotic as-

Table 73-1. Acceptable zone size ranges for the disk diffusion antibiotic susceptibility test
of modified Bauer-Kirby-Sherris-Turck[7]*

Antimicrobial agent	Disk content	E. coli (ATCC 25922)	S. aureus (ATCC 25923)	P. aeruginosa (ATCC 27853)
Ampicillin	10 μg	15-20	24-35	
Carbenicillin	100 μg	24-29	NA	19-25†
Cephalothin	30 μg	18-23	25-37	
Chloramphenicol	30 μg	21-27	19-26	
Clindamycin	2 μg	NA	23-29	
Erythromycin	15 μg	NA	23-30	
Gentamicin	10 μg	19-26	19-27	16-22†
Kanamycin	30 μg	17-25	19-26	
Methicillin	5 μg	NA	17-22	
Neomycin	30 μg	17-23	18-26	
Penicillin G	10 U	NA	26-37	
Polymyxin B	300 U	12-16	NA	13-18†
Streptomycin	10 μg	12-20	14-22	
Tetracycline	30 μg	18-25	19-28	
Tobramycin	10 μg	18-26	19-29	19-25
Trimethoprim-sulfamethoxazole	1.25 μg 23.75 μg	24-32	24-32	
Vancomycin	30 μg	NA	15-19	

*From Blazevic, D. J., Hall, C. T., and Wilson, M. E. In Balows, A., coordinating editor: Practical quality control procedures for
the clinical microbiology laboratory, Cumitech no. 3, Washington, D.C., 1976, American Society for Microbiology.
†Modified ranges recommended by C. Thornsberry, Bacteriology Division, CDC, Atlanta.

says. Therapeutic preparations are not suitable because they may contain preservatives or carrier substances and may possess varied solubility characteristics depending on the salt synthesized during manufacture. Powders should be desiccated and stored at refrigerator temperature. When highly concentrated stock solutions of antibiotics are prepared they should be stored in small aliquots at −20 C or below. Once thawed, any unused portion must be discarded. Organisms possessing known minimum inhibitory concentrations should be used as controls when dilution tests are run.[5]

Antibiotic disks for susceptibility testing should be stored with a desiccant at −14 C or below if possible; if space is at a premium at least all penicillins and cephalosporins should be kept in the refrigerator in a tight container with a desiccant. After disks are removed from the freezer or refrigerator they should be allowed to come to room temperature before the container is opened. Exposure of cold disks to warm and humid room conditions produces moisture of condensation in the vial and causes the antibiotic to leach out of the disk with an appreciable loss of reactivity in the disk. Disks must not be used after the expiration date indicated by the manufacturer.

The disks should be checked with organisms of known susceptibility each day susceptibility tests are run.[6] *E. coli* (ATCC 25922) and *Staphylococcus aureus* (ATCC 25923) should be tested with the disks routinely used for gram-negative bacilli and gram-positive cocci, respectively. In addition *Pseudomonas aeruginosa* (ATCC 27853) should be used to test carbenicillin, gentamicin, and tobramycin. Zone sizes to be obtained with these organisms are listed in Table 73-1.

If appropriate zone sizes are not observed with the control strains the tests should be repeated. Failure to obtain the indicated zone sizes can be due to deficiencies in the antibiotic disks or in the Mueller-Hinton plates or to failure to follow exactly the directions for the standardized disk diffusion method of Bauer et al. as modified by the National Committee for Clinical Laboratory Standards (NCCLS).[8]

The quality control procedures recommended by the NCCLS should be followed precisely. However, by comparing the zone sizes of certain antibiotics each day with the acceptable zone size ranges for *E. coli*, *S. aureus*, and *P. aeruginosa* control organisms (Table 73-1), it is possible to detect **trends** and probable **sources of error** quickly and without great effort.

1. The zone sizes observed for most antibiotic control disks either exceed or are barely within the upper limits of the acceptable zone size ranges in Table 73-1.

Corrective action: carefully check the density of the control suspensions and routine specimens against the BaSO$_4$ turbidity standard. Numerous large zone sizes suggest too light an inoculum.

2. Zone sizes of most of the antibiotic control disks either fail to or barely reach the minimum limits of the acceptable zone size ranges in Table 73-1.

Corrective action: adjust the control and routine suspensions to the BaSO$_4$ turbidity standard more carefully. Small zone sizes suggest too heavy an inoculum.

3. Zone sizes for *S. aureus* and *E. coli* controls for tetracycline approach or exceed the acceptable zone size range, while zone sizes for lincomycin, erythromycin, gentamicin, and to some degree kanamycin are too small.

Corrective action: check the pH of the medium. The abnormally wide zone for tetracycline and the small zones for the other antibiotics suggest a low (acidic) pH. Replace the medium.

4. Opposite of situation 3: zones are too small for tetracycline and too large for lincomycin, erythromycin, and the aminoglycosides.

Corrective action: check the pH of the medium. These zone sizes suggest an excessively alkaline pH. Replace the medium.

5. Zone sizes too small for *P. aeruginosa* (ATCC 27853) with disks impregnated with the aminoglycosides (e.g., gentamicin, kanamycin, amikacin).

Corrective action: the medium probably contains too high levels of cations or too heavy an inoculum of *Pseudomonas*. Rerun the controls and be particularly careful to adjust the bacterial suspension to the BaSO$_4$ turbidity standard. Should small zone sizes with the *Pseudomonas* culture persist, excessive levels of cations must be present and the medium will have to be replaced. All new batches of Mueller-Hinton agar should be evaluated for excessive or deficient levels of cations.

6. Abrupt and dramatic change in zone size patterns with the stock strains more than likely involving the control strain of *S. aureus*.

Corrective action: rerun the susceptibility tests with fresh strains of the quality control cultures. It is easy to contaminate the control strains during inoculation. It is especially important to monitor results daily and to replace the control stock slants weekly from frozen or lyophilized stock collections. In some laboratories it is routine practice to transfer the control strains in broth at daily intervals to maintain an active and fresh inoculum. When strains of *P. aeruginosa* are transferred over prolonged periods they develop increased resistance to carbenicillin. *S. aureus* (ATCC 25923) poses a special problem because the control culture may inadvertently be contaminated with a wild strain, which will result in a gradual and subtle shift in characteristics. All control cultures should be replaced at specified intervals instead of replacing only those cultures that have produced obviously deviant results.

STOCK CULTURE COLLECTION
Selection

How large a stock culture collection must a laboratory maintain? This is a difficult question to answer. Most certainly, no one stock size is suitable for all laboratories. As a general rule of thumb a laboratory should maintain a positive and negative control for each culture medium, biochemical reaction, and serologic determination performed. Therefore the mission of the laboratory strongly influences the complexity of its services and indirectly the number of positive and negative controls it must maintain. Even in the large reference laboratory the judicious selection of bacteria that possess a diversity of metabolic processes can minimize the total number of control strains.

Other factors must be considered in the selection of stock cultures in addition to the number required. The strains used to evaluate media, antisera, and reagents must be stable in their reactivity. The reactions of the stock strains must be reproducible and predictable.

Sources

Quality control stock cultures may be obtained from a variety of sources:

1. The American Type Culture Collection (ATCC), Rockville, Md.

2. Bactrol Disks (Difco Laboratories, Detroit) and Bact-Chek Disks (Roche Diagnostics, Hoffmann-LaRoche, Nutley, N.J.). For small laboratories the commercial disk is an excellent source of cultures. These disks require no maintenance and are inexpensive. Nevertheless they must be supplemented with other more fastidious organisms, so disks are only a partial solution.

3. Proficiency test programs. Proficiency test specimens to be used as stock cultures must be carefully selected. Often atypical strains may be submitted to participants in proficiency testing programs because they challenge the capabilities of the laboratory staff. Strains isolated in proficiency testing surveys should be withheld from stock collections until the organism's identity and biologic characteristics are confirmed by the testing agency.

4. Departments of Health. These agencies should not be called on as primary sources of stock cultures. However, occasional requests for standard strains or organisms of special medical significance may be honored by these laboratories.

5. Routine isolates within the laboratory. It has long been recognized that fresh clinical isolates differ subtly from laboratory-oriented stock strains that have been carried on artificial media for countless transfers. On primary isolation fresh clinical isolates may demonstrate feeble motility, produce initial scanty growth, require the presence of elevated levels of CO_2, demand serum supplements, demonstrate capsular materials that block serologic reactions, and on occasion demonstrate feeble enzyme metabolic activity. While it may be advisable to check new lots of media, reagents, and antisera with fresh clinical isolates, the transient nature of these character-istics must be taken into account when the organisms are used in quality control studies.

Maintenance

A number of methods can be used to maintain a stock culture collection. Some methods are simple and quite inexpensive; others are quite complex and require extensive preparation of materials and manipulation of expensive equipment. Generally the simpler the technic the shorter the shelf-life of the culture. Nevertheless an adequate stock culture collection can be maintained at relatively little expense and can require a minimum of the laboratory personnel's time.

Before any storage program is implemented certain important factors must be considered that can exert adverse effects on the culture collection: (1) media containing fermentable carbohydrates should not be used, (2) selective media should never be used, (3) cultures should not be allowed to dry out (tightly closed screw-capped tubes or paraffin seals should be used), (4) temperature-sensitive organisms such as *Neisseria gonorrhoeae* and *N. meningitidis* should not be refrigerated but can be quick-frozen for long-term maintenance, and (5) stock cultures recommended as controls should not be used daily for longer than 1 week but must be drawn at no more than weekly intervals from frozen or lyophilized stocks or from a supply of commercial culture control dishes stored as recommended by the manufacturer.

Lyophilization is the most reliable method for maintaining stock culture collections. The greatest benefit of lyophilization, aside from prolonged viability of bacteria, is the retention of the immunologic and physiologic traits of the isolate. Too often the subtleties of the primary isolate are lost on repeated subculture, and in time the stock culture bears only a strong resemblance to its original form. A general description of lyophilization apparatus and details of the technic are given by Bartlett.[9]

In the modern laboratory one of the most common methods of preserving cultures is storing them in the **freezer.** After the initial expense the system is relatively efficient and requires little maintenance. Unfortunately the system is not without an Achilles heel, the power outage, which can destroy the collection. The freezer must be monitored continuously and an automatic alarm system must be installed. If the freezer is used a concurrent, alternate storage system should be considered.

In preparation for storage in the freezer, growth from young plates or agar slants is harvested in 3-5 ml sterile, defibrinated rabbit or sheep blood (suspensions may also be made in broth containing 15% glycerol). The suspensions should be dispensed in small volumes into small screw-capped vials to protect against sublimation of the ice during storage at subzero temperatures. Other suitable vials requiring little storage space are cotton-plugged Durham tubes (inverted tubes used in fermentation media) placed in screw-capped salve or cold cream jars available from pharmacies. The vials should be quick-frozen in a dry ice–ethanol bath and stored at temperatures below −40 C. The freezer section in most household refrigerator-freezer combination units rarely exceeds −20 C. In fact, the temperature usually ranges from −5 to −15 C, depending on the accumulation of ice in the freezer section. Storing stock cultures in these units is not recommended because the viability of frozen cultures is appreciably shortened under these conditions. It goes without saying that the self-defrosting refrigerator-freezer unit is **not** recommended for maintaining frozen reagents or cultures in the laboratory.

For the sake of convenience stock strains are often stored on culture media. These media must be chosen carefully for their ability to maintain viability and stability of organisms over long periods without permitting extensive growth or metabolic activity. The following media have been found useful (their formulations are given in the second edition of the *Manual of Clinical Microbiology*).[10]

1. CTA. Cystine-trypticase agar (CTA) **without** carbohydrates is a semisolid agar that will support growth for long periods at room temperature. Organisms should be checked for viability every 2-3 months by subculture to an appropriate growth medium.

2. Soybean casein digest agar deeps. Many organisms such as staphylococci and *Enterobacteriaceae* may be maintained for years by stabbing them into a tube of soybean casein digest agar. After the organisms are incubated overnight at 35 C the tube should be sealed with a paraffin-coated cork; then the top should be dipped into melted paraffin to seal it. For subculture the paraffin seal is broken, a small amount of growth is removed aseptically, and the tube is resealed in the original manner for further storage. Working cultures of these same organisms may be maintained for at least a month on soybean casein digest slants at room temperature.

3. Blood or chocolate agar slants. Fastidious organisms (pneumococci and streptococci) may be maintained on blood agar slants in screw-capped tubes in the refrigerator. These cultures should be transferred every 2 weeks to a blood agar plate to check viability and morphology and then to a fresh blood agar slant. *H. influenzae* may be stored in the same manner on chocolate agar slants. *N. gonorrhoeae* is best maintained by daily or every-other-day subculture to fresh chocolate agar. Since this organism does not survive repeated subculturing, it is best to use each new isolate as a quality control strain.

4. Cooked meat medium. Cooked meat medium is an excellent maintenance medium for anaerobes and facultative anaerobes. After incubation overnight the cultures should be stored at room temperature in closed containers. Although the medium can maintain organisms for very long

periods, the cultures should be checked for viability every 2-3 months.

As with most cultures the major concern of the laboratorian is to prevent drying of the stock cultures during storage. A time-honored process for preventing moisture loss from a culture is to overlay the slant with sterile mineral oil, sealing in the moisture and suppressing additional growth by excluding oxygen. Screw-capped tubes are preferable to cotton-plugged tubes because of the possibility of getting oil on the cotton plugs.

Among the bacteria, as a rule, only the heavy growing, nonfastidious organisms are well adapted to this technic. Weiss[11] reported that the genera that survived well on oil-sealed cultures were *Achromobacter*, *Bacillus*, most of the *Enterobacteriaceae*, *Flavobacterium*, *Micrococcus* (some species), *Proteus*, *Pseudomonas*, *Sarcina*, *Serratia*, *Streptococcus*, and *Vibrio* (saprophytic forms). On the other hand, Weiss was unsuccessful in preserving cultures of *Azotobacter*, *Lactobacillus*, *Mycobacterium*, *Rhodospirillum*, and *Salmonella*.

The culture should be inoculated on heart infusion agar prepared as short slants in screw-capped tubes. After appropriate incubation the slants should be covered to a depth of 1 cm above the top of the slant with the sterile mineral oil so that no medium remains exposed. The white mineral oil or liquid petrolatum (heavy medicinal grade) can be sterilized by heating it to 170 C for 1 hour in a drying oven or autoclaving it at 121 C for 1 hour and then at 110 C for 1 hour to drive off any entrapped moisture. The oiled cultures are stored at the same temperature used for unsealed cultures. The bacteriologic loops used in the transfer of growth from oil-covered slants should be carefully flame sterilized after use. To avoid splattering any residual growth adhering to the loop, the loop should be stabbed into a flask containing sand and alcohol before it is heated in the burner.

Yeasts and fungi may be stored in sterile distilled water in the refrigerator or at room temperature for long periods. Well-sporulated cultures of fungi may also be maintained by the oil overlay technic and stored at room temperature or in the refrigerator.

For long-term storage of **mycobacterial cultures**[12] growth in Middlebrook 7H-9 broth is dispensed into small vials with rubber stoppers attached by a crimped metal cap. The vials should be placed in a −70 C freezer. Immersion in a dry ice–ethanol bath is not necessary. To retrieve the culture the authors recommend rapid thawing of the vial in a 37 C water bath. After it is used for subculturing the thawed stock culture can be returned to the −70 C freezer. Kubica (personal communication) reports that no appreciable loss in viable count was observed after 5 transfers with subsequent refreezing each time. A satisfactory alternative to frozen broth is the storage of Lowenstein-Jensen slants at −20 C. Kubica reports that this method was successful with strains of *Mycobacterium tuberculosis* and *M. bovis* (un-published data). A widely used method for maintaining stock cultures of mycobacteria is the storage of Lowenstein-Jensen slants at room temperature in the dark.[13] If this procedure is used the cultures must be transferred to fresh media every 3 months.

Table 73-2 lists appropriate storage conditions for various organisms used in quality control.

EQUIPMENT

The proper functioning of equipment is a critical responsibility in the laboratory. All equipment should be checked routinely, and major pieces of equipment should be included in a preventive maintenance program requiring periodic, scheduled examinations. Routine preventive maintenance may be performed in-house by knowledgeable members of the laboratory staff, but in some laboratories preventive maintenance programs are contracted to commercial firms, which provide specially trained personnel to periodically examine and adjust equipment.

A list of the equipment in the laboratory, the serial numbers, and the dates of purchase should be maintained in the laboratory. The list should also include the number to call for emergency service, the routine maintenance to be performed, the frequency with which the maintenance should be performed, the date of last service, the service performed, and the initials of the individual performing the maintenance. Laboratories subject to the Clinical Laboratories Improvement Act (CLIA) of 1967 are required by regulation to maintain an equipment log containing this information.

The **temperature** of controlled temperature spaces such as incubators, refrigerators, freezers, water baths, and heating blocks should be recorded at the beginning of each day, noted at the time of use, and checked again at the end of the day. Temperature charts should be attached to each piece of equipment and daily readings retained for an appropriate length of time. Laboratories subject to federal regulations (CLIA 1967) must retain all records for a minimum of 2 years. An internal thermometer immersed in glycerol or a large volume of water should always be kept in incubators and refrigerators.

The contents of refrigerators should be checked monthly, and outdated reagents and materials should be discarded. The interior of the refrigerator should be cleaned at the time of the monthly inventory. The freezer compartment should be defrosted at least every 3 months and more often if accumulations of ice indicate the need.

Autoclaves and hot-air ovens should contain an **indicator tape** or a **recording thermometer** in each sterilizing run to assure that the system is working properly. At least once each month the autoclave should be checked with a spore suspension or spore strip in addition to the routine tape or color indicator included in each run.

The **pH meter** should be adjusted with a stan-

Table 73-2. Methods of maintenance for quality control cultures*

Organism	Maintenance
Enterobacteriaceae, nonfermenters, staphylococci	TSA agar deeps at room temperature CTA Cooked meat Quick-freezing; storage at <-40 C Lyophilization
Streptococci (including pneumococci), *Listeria*	Blood agar slants (4-8 C) Blood agar plates (subculture *twice weekly*) CTA Cooked meat Quick-freezing; storage at <-40 C Lyophilization
Haemophilus influenzae	Chocolate slants (4-8 C) Chocolate plates (subculture twice weekly) Quick-freezing; storage at <-40 C Lyophilization
Neisseria gonorrhoeae, N. meningitidis	Chocolate agar (subculture every other day) Quick-freezing; storage at <-40 C
Corynebacterium diphtheriae	Cooked meat Quick-freezing; storage at <-40 C Lyophilization
Bordetella pertussis	B-G agar (4-8 C) Quick-freezing; storage at <-40 C Lyophilization
Yeasts	Sterile distilled water (4-8 C or room temperature)
Fungi	Sterile soil (4-8 C) Overlay with sterile mineral oil (4-8 C or room temperature)
Mycobacterium spp.	Lowenstein-Jensen medium (25 C in dark) Freezing at -70 C

*From Blazevic, D. J., Hall, C. J., and Wilson, M. E. In Balows, A., coordinating editor: Practical quality control procedures for the clinical microbiology laboratory, Cumitech no. 3, Washington, D.C., 1976, American Society for Microbiology. Code: TSA, trypticase soy agar; B-G, Bordet-Gengou.

dard pH 7.0 buffer solution each time it is used. If it is being used for a range below pH 6.0, the meter should also be calibrated with a standard pH 4.0 buffer as well. The buffer should be examined for evidence of bacterial or fungal growth and discarded at the first indication of contamination or turbidity. The temperature of the room must be compensated for in adjusting the meter.

The **analytical balance** should be checked at least once each week with certified weights. The weights should never be touched with the fingers but handled with forceps at all times. The weights must be stored in a dry environment; however, they should not be stored in the presence of caustic drying agents. The balance should be thoroughly cleaned monthly. In the interim the pans and chamber must be swept clean of any dropped materials after each use.

Brushes and bearings should be checked in **centrifuges** every 6 months during the routine preventive maintenance examination. Settings of revolutions per minute (rpm) marked on the face of the rheostat control should be checked each month by recording the tachometer readings achieved at each rheostat setting.

MYCOLOGY

Because mycologic and bacteriologic procedures are based on the same basic concepts (i.e., recovering an etiologic agent and identifying it by biochemical and serologic technics) little can be added in this text that has not been previously discussed. However, the selectivity of a primary recovery medium may be a more critical decision in the mycology laboratory than in its bacteriology counterpart. The comparative slowness of growth by some pathogenic fungi increases the possibility of overgrowth by bacteria and fungi that grow more rapidly. Thus the quality control evaluation of selective mycologic media must measure their recovery of small numbers of probable etiologic agents while simultaneously determining whether they inhibit relatively large numbers of competing commensal organisms.

Carbohydrate fermentation and assimilation tests pose particular problems to the mycologist. Because the identification of yeasts can require interpretation of weak or delayed reactions of fermentation and assimilation tests, the presence of trace amounts of contaminating sugars in media tends to confuse identification procedures. Just as in the bacteriology laboratory, old or impure reagents such as maltose contaminated by glucose degradation products can produce confusing biochemical characterizations of isolates. For this reason all mycologic carbohydrate media should be checked with stock strains to assure the correct reactivity of the media. This carbohydrate evaluation can be achieved with 2 stock strains: *Cryptococcus laurentii*, which utilizes all the common sugars needed to identify yeasts, and *Torulopsis glabrata*, which utilizes only glucose and trehalose. Failure of *C. laurentii* to produce acid in a particular fermentation tube or to assimilate a particular sugar suggests that the sugar was omitted from the medium. Conversely, utilization of a sugar other than glucose and trehalose by *T. glabrata* suggests that the medium was improperly prepared or that the intended carbohydrate substrate had deteriorated to a fermentable derivative.

PARASITOLOGY

In the clinical laboratory the direct microscopic examination of a wet mount and an iodine-stained preparation is the procedure most widely used for parasitologic examinations. Recently the collection of polyvinylalcohol (PVA) specimens has gained favor, and the PVA smears are being used to supplement the wet mount. Parasitology in the clinical laboratory is for the most part a visual science with diagnosis depending on results of microscopic observations. It should not be surprising that quality control measures are primarily directed to the care and proficient use of the microscope. Every laboratory in which parasitologic examinations are made should have a reference collection of parasites to which the staff can refer as an aid in processing clinical specimens. This reference collection may consist of prepared slides or gross material from which slides can be made. In addition photographs or projection slides should be available for reference purposes. This reference collection should include representative samples of blood parasites, helminth eggs and larvae, and protozoan cysts and trophozoites. Because size is a very important criterion in differentiating some parasites, the ocular for any microscope used for parasitic examinations should contain an ocular micrometer calibrated to that microscope. It is recommended that the calibration calculations be taped to the base of the microscope or entered conspicuously in a log at the bench.

Iodine solutions for wet mounts of fecal material should be prepared fresh every 10-14 days and kept at proper concentration. Permanent stains (e.g., trichrome, hematoxylin, Giemsa, modified Heidenhain) should be tested immediately after preparation and once a month thereafter.

SYPHILIS SEROLOGY

In any serologic procedure all new lots of reagents should be tested in parallel with old lots. This parallel evaluation must be completed in time to permit any defective new lot to be replaced. Only "in-date" reagents may be used at the bench in performing routine diagnostic tests.

In those tests requiring rotation of the test slides the mechanical rotator must be checked before each test run. The speed of rotation is critical in the test: too slow rotation lowers the sensitivity of the test; too fast increases the sensitivity and in addition may cause reactants from one test to spill over into another test. Exceeding the prescribed time for rotation also increases the sensitivity of the test. The prescribed times and speeds of rotation are shown in Table 73-3.

Dropping needles for delivering antigen into the rings or wells must be checked before each test run to assure that the proper volumes of reagent are added, as shown in Table 73-4.

Calibrated needles used for dropping antigen or reagent in the tests should be cleaned after each use in conformance with the recommendations of the manufacturer. VDRL and USR test syringes and delivery needles should be rinsed with distilled water and then with ethanol and dried with acetone. The RPR needle is coated with silicone, and vigorous cleaning with water,

Table 73-3

Test	Rpm*	Time (min)	Diameter circle of rotation (in.)
Unheated serum reagin (USR)	180 ± 2	4	¾
Venereal Disease Research Laboratory (VDRL)	180 ± 2	4	¾
Reagin screen test (RST)	130	6	¾
Rapid plasma reagin (RPR)	95-100	8	¾
Syphla-Chek	180 ± 2	6	Unspecified

*Revolutions per minute can be determined easily by counting taps of rotating shelf against pencil held loosely in fingers while observing sweep second hand on wall clock.

Table 73-4

Test	Reagent	Needle gauge	No. drops/ml
VDRL (qualitative)	Antigen suspension	18	60 ± 2
VDRL (quantitative)	Antigen suspension	19	75 ± 2
VDRL	Saline, 0.9%	23	100 ± 2
VDRL (CSF)	Sensitized antigen suspension	21 or 22	100 ± 2
USR	Antigen suspension	18	45 ± 1
RPR (qualitative)	Antigen suspension	20	60 ± 2
RST (qualitative)	Antigen suspension	Dropper	60 ± 2
Syphla-Chek	Antigen suspension	Calibrated needle	60 ± 2

alcohol, and acetone is not recommended. This needle should be flushed with distilled water and blown dry. To protect the silicone coating and to preserve the calibration of the RPR needle, do not wipe the needle dry with a towel. The disposable calibrated needle in the Syphla-Chek kit resembles the RPR needle and, although it is not specifically stated in the manufacturer's instructions, rinsing with water and blow drying should not impair delivery characteristics of the needle. The needle in the RST kit is fixed permanently to the antigen dispenser. The manufacturer recommends that the needle be wiped clean with tissue paper at the end of the day and the plastic protective cover replaced over the tip of the needle to assure continued proper delivery.

If too many drops per milliliter are delivered by the appropriate needle the opening of the tip is too small. The VDRL, USR, and Syphla-Chek needles can be adjusted to deliver larger drops by reaming out the tip with a sharp-pointed instrument such as the sharpened end of a triangular file. Conversely, if too few drops are delivered the opening of the tip is too large. This can be remedied by pressing the tip together slightly or by filing the edges of the needle inward.

The tips of the delivery needles must be carefully protected. If needles are dropped on the floor, in the sink, or to the bottom of wash beakers, they should be set aside for recalibration. Needles should be checked **each day** before they are used and adjustments made if necessary.

Each new lot of cardiolipin antigen (VDRL) or antigen suspension (RPR [18 mm circle] card and USR) should be checked in parallel with a standard reagent or lot of proved reactivity to verify that the new lot is of acceptable reactivity. Parallel tests should be run on different days with different reference specimens of graded reactivity (reactive, weakly reactive, and nonreactive) for each test period. A permanent record of these results should be maintained. Because standard reagents are not currently available for the RST or Syphla-Chek tests the laboratorian should compare new lots with lots currently being used. The new lot must give identical reactivity patterns with the current lot to be considered an acceptable replacement.

Assuming that the new antigen is found to be of good quality and standard reactivity, the routine test should include control serums of graded reactivity each time the serologic procedure is performed. The pattern of reactivity of the antigen suspension must be reestablished each day. If the pattern is not acceptable the routine testing must be postponed until optimal reactions are obtained. Results of all controls must be recorded daily, and these records must be readily retrievable to substantiate the validity of a run.

All serologic tests for syphilis should be performed in strict compliance with the methodologies in the 1969 *Manual of Tests for Syphilis*[14] or the brochure accompanying the commercial reagent. No modification or variation should be introduced into the procedure. Slide flocculation tests for syphilis are affected by room temperatures. **For reliable and reproducible results, tests should be performed within the temperature range 23-29 C (73-85 F). At lower temperatures test reactivity is decreased; at higher temperatures test reactivity is increased.**

For further details see Chapter 106.

DIAGNOSTIC IMMUNOLOGY

The technologic advances of recent years have given rise to a variety of new methodologies in diagnostic immunology. The time-honored complement fixation and flocculation tests have been augmented by chromatographic and radiometric procedures. Because of the increased complexity of immunologic determinations, quality control must be discussed in general terms. Regardless of the method, however, certain control measures are necessary in any immunologic determination. A preventive maintenance program should be set up in all laboratories for equipment used in these various procedures (e.g., automated analyzers, densitometers, fluorescence microscopes, incubators, radioisotope counting equipment, spectrophotometers, automatic pipetters, and automatic diluters) with regular and scheduled examinations by a trained technical staff. Permanent records should be kept of all equipment and entries made of any deficiencies, the date they were found, the corrective action taken, the initials of the repairman, and the date of the next scheduled examination.

Temperatures of all controlled-temperature spaces (e.g., incubators, water baths, refrigerators, heat blocks, and freezers) should be recorded each day. These records should be retained for at least 2 years and in such a form as to permit cross-referencing with test results on a given day.

Each run of qualitative tests must be accompanied by a positive and negative control; before it is used each new lot of reagent or control is compared with one of known reactivity. Each run of quantitative tests must contain a positive control of graded reactivity and a negative control. The pattern of reactivity of the graded controls must show the reagents in the test to be of good quality and of standard reactivity. Each component of the test system must be subject to a control measure, and the performance of that component should be shown to be within acceptable limits.

In radioimmunoassay tests counting equipment should be checked for background stability and also with a radioactive standard each day it is used.

VIROLOGY

In comparison with other disciplines in microbiology, virology is a relatively new science. For this reason virology testing is not as standardized as that of other disciplines. With a few notable exceptions standards do not exist for reagents. Methodologies are quite diverse and subject to the innovativeness of the laboratorian. For these reasons much of the responsibility for quality control falls on the laboratory director and the technical supervisor in the laboratory.

The development of a standard operating procedural manual (SOPM) for the laboratory is very important. In virology as in all other biologic sciences the work-up of a specimen is not predetermined by the laboratorian but is dictated by the etiologic agent. The anatomic site of the infection suggests the isolation system to be used to recover the viral agent. The SOPM should specify the host systems to be used in isolating the most probable etiologic agents from various specimens. The manual should clearly delineate the alternatives available to the laboratorian at each step in the isolation and identification procedure and specify the approved method for each determination.

An uninoculated host system must be included in each run of specimens for viral isolation. Sometimes a granularity within the host system may be suggestive of a virus, but attempts to recover the agent may be unsuccessful. The presence of the uninoculated control is an excellent basis for comparison. Conversely the recovery of a virus in the uninoculated host system could indicate a general laboratory contamination with a virus or the contamination of a particular cell line.

For serologic procedures used in the diagnosis of viral diseases the quality control measures should be the same as those used in the routine diagnostic immunology laboratory.

SELF-IMPROVEMENT PROGRAMS

In the preceding text the implementation of quality control procedures in the laboratory has been emphasized. The evaluation of reagents, proper maintenance of equipment, control of test conditions, strict adherence to written protocol, and incorporation of controls into the system provide increased assurance that the laboratory will function properly. It must be recognized, however, that these precautions fail to take into account the skill of the laboratory personnel or the adequacy of the test procedure itself. Every laboratory should participate in a self-assessment program to evaluate its total performance.

Laboratory performance can be evaluated by submitting specimens of predetermined identities or reactivities to the laboratory personnel for analysis. Essentially all evaluation or proficiency testing programs are based on this premise, whether the specimens be administered by an outside agency or by someone from within the laboratory itself.

External proficiency testing programs (i.e., specimens submitted and results evaluated by an outside agency) have become widely used in recent years. These programs are conducted by several organizations (College of American Pathologists, Center for Disease Control, American Association of Bioanalysts, and numerous state, county, or city health departments). Generally it is acknowledged that proficiency testing specimens submitted openly to laboratories from an external source receive special handling and more than mere routine examination. For this reason the external proficiency testing program has been criticized as an invalid method for evaluating laboratory performance. No one can deny that the programs have been abused, and for this reason external programs are more nearly a measure of the best a laboratory can perform. Nevertheless the external proficiency testing program has much to offer the laboratorian: (1) if an erroneous result occurs despite special handling in the laboratory a profound problem exists with regard to that determination and corrective actions should be investigated, (2) performance of the laboratory can be compared against that of a peer population using the same methodology on comparable test material, and (3) the laboratorian can compare the accuracy of the routine procedure used in that laboratory against a variety of methods used by the other participants.

The in-house or **internal proficiency testing program** should not be viewed as an alternative but rather an adjunct to an externally administered program. In some respects the in-house program has definite advantages over the external program. An internal program is much cheaper to implement because most programs are simply the resubmission of randomly selected routine specimens into the daily workload for reanalysis. Since it is administered from within, the specimens can be directed to specific members of the staff. Quite often the specimens can be integrated (without knowledge of the staff) into the daily workload and be processed in the routine fashion. By the simple expediency of splitting the sample it is possible to determine reproducibility of laboratory results by individual or between individuals. Despite these advantages it must be recognized that in-house proficiency testing programs have obvious shortcomings. The specimens selected for resubmission into the laboratory have been preselected by the laboratory routine, and all subsequent results are biased. If the initial screening procedure is inherently insensitive, the results of the in-house proficiency testing program can only confirm to the laboratorian that the test system is functioning at the usual level of insensitivity or worse. Only by participation in an external program can the relative sensitivity of the screening procedure be established.

The results of both external and internal proficiency testing programs should be reviewed critically by the laboratory director and technical supervisors. On the basis of these results the adequacy of the procedure should be reaffirmed. In addition deficiencies in performance by staff members should be defined and corrective training implemented.

• • •

Use of trade names is for identification only and does not constitute endorsement by the Public Health Service or by the U.S. Department of Health, Education, and Welfare.

REFERENCES

1. Manual of dehydrated culture media and reagents, ed. 9, Detroit, 1953, Difco Laboratories.
2. BBL manual of products and laboratory procedures, ed. 5, Cockeysville, Md., 1968, BioQuest, Division of Becton-Dickinson and Co.
3. Updyke, E. L.: Public Health Rep. **15:**78, 1957.
4. Blazevic, D. J., Hall, C. T., and Wilson, M. E. In Balows, A., coordinating editor: Practical quality control procedures for the clinical microbiology laboratory, Washington, D.C., 1976, Cumitech 3.
5. Washington, J. A., II., and Barry, A. L.: Dilution test procedures. In Lennette, E. H., Spaulding, E. H., and Truant, J. P., editors: Manual of clinical microbiology, ed. 2, Washington, D.C., 1974, American Society for Microbiology.
6. Blazevic, E. J., Koepcke, M. H., and Matsen, J. M.: Am. J. Clin. Pathol. **57:**592, 1974.
7. Bauer, A. W., Kirby, M. M., Sherris, J. C., and Turck, M.: Am. J. Clin. Pathol. **45:**493, 1966.
8. National Committee for Clinical Laboratory Standards: Performance standards for antimicrobial disk susceptibility tests, Villanova, Pa., 1975, The Committee.
9. Bartlett, R. C.: Medical microbiology: quality cost and clinical relevance, New York, 1974, John Wiley & Sons.
10. Vera, H. D., and Dumoff, M.: Culture media. In Lennette, E. H., Spaulding, E. H., and Truant, J. P., editors: Manual of clinical microbiology, ed. 2, Washington, D.C., 1974, American Society for Microbiology.
11. Weiss, F. A. Maintenance and preservation of cultures. In Conn, H. J., editor: Manual of microbiological methods, Society for American Bacteriologists, New York, 1957, McGraw-Hill Book Co.
12. Kim, T. H., and Kubica, G. P.: Appl. Microbiol. **25:**956, 1973.
13. Morton, H. E.: Maintenance and use of stock cultures in microbiological quality control. In Prier, J. E., Bartola, J. F., and Friedman, H., editors: Quality control in microbiology, Baltimore, 1975, University Park Press.
14. U.S. Department of Health, Education and Welfare: Manual of tests for syphilis, 1969 revision, PHS publ. no. 411, Washington, D.C., 1969, U.S. Government Printing Office.

74

INSTRUMENTATION, AUTOMATION, AND MINIATURIZATION

Millicent C. Goldschmidt

Since the seventh edition of this text was published there has been rapid growth in the numbers of instrumented and noninstrumented procedures applicable to the more rapid detection, identification, characterization, and antibiotic susceptibility testing of clinically important microorganisms. Creative collaboration between microbiologists and engineers has produced intriguing and imaginative instrumentation and degrees of automation based on such diverse technics as light scattering, chromatography, immunoassays, luminescence, and radioactivity. The miniaturization of many biochemical and immunologic technics and their emergence in commercially available kits has also occurred within this time.

In addition many instruments are now produced that mechanize such routine procedures as pipetting, diluting, plating, and staining of specimens.

The term **mechanization** usually refers to instrumented procedures performing a series of steps that do not involve interpretation of results and that substitute mechanical operation for a manual task. **Automation** refers to the controlled operation of an apparatus or system by mechanical or electronic devices, which includes independent observation and decision making. Since there are also semiautomated instruments, it is in many instances difficult to describe the various procedures using such terminology. There are probably no truly automated instruments. Even the most sophisticated, such as the AMS-Automicrobic system, require some manual activity (i.e., insertion of paks into the instrument). To resolve this situation, if the procedure under discussion is "commonly" referred to in the literature as mechanized, semiautomated, or automated, these terms will be used.

This chapter deals with many of the concepts involved with these instruments and with several miniaturized approaches to microbiologic analyses, with particular attention to their usefulness in the clinical laboratory. The emphasis is on technics involving available instrumentation or kits, although promising methods are also briefly mentioned. The instruments and kits mentioned do not imply endorsement by the author or the editors; they are used merely as illustrations of the technics under discussion and should be considered in that light. The lists of similar instruments and manufacturers (if given) are also not complete. For example, chromatography and electrophoresis instruments are available from most of the major manufacturers of scientific equipment, although only a few are mentioned.

The population explosion in instrumentation has also resulted in an even greater "explosion" in the literature. Every new technic has in turn generated many articles. For example, thousands of papers each year are published in the field of chromatography alone. The references listed should serve merely as a guide in providing both a background for some of the concepts and indicating comparisons of the various technics based on data reported from various microbiology laboratories.

Several journals usually carrying pertinent articles and reviews include the *Journal of Clinical Microbiology, Applied and Environmental Microbiology, Analytical Biochemistry, Microbiological Reviews, CRC Publications,* the *Journal of Chromatography,* and *Journal of Physics E: Scientific Instruments.* In addition the journal *Analytical Chemistry* has published fundamental and application reviews annually since 1949. They cover many areas of instrumentation and technics of importance to microbiologists. Several good books and reviews have also been published[1-10] (see especially Prier et al.,[4] Goldschmidt and Fung,[5] Isenberg and MacLowry,[8] and Mitruka[10]). Two international symposia have been held on rapid methods and automation (Sweden, 1973, and England, 1976). The proceedings of the first meeting and abstracts of both have been published.[11-13] The *Index Medicus, Chemical Abstracts,* and *Biological Abstracts* are good sources of current information. Many articles have been computerized by these and other groups for customized literature searches, which are available through cooperative library systems.

Contributions to automation and miniaturization have come from varied sources, including clinical and medical microbiologists, armed forces and space programs, various industries, and other scientific (applied and basic) laboratories. Their common aims include the mechanization and automation of routine laboratory procedures, rapid detection and characterization of microorganisms or reaction systems, and miniaturization of test systems. Some of these technics have been perfected; others are still in their infancy. The journals *Analytical Chemistry* and *Science* annually publish detailed guides to scientific instruments.

ROUTINE LABORATORY PROCEDURES

Mechanization or automation of routine procedures such as plating, diluting, and counting undoubtedly free the laboratory worker for more important tasks; it is not surprising therefore to find increasing instrumentation in this area. The number of specimens or tests actually performed in the laboratory should indicate the usefulness of the instruments described below. Laboratories with heavy work loads would benefit greatly from several of them.

Sample preparation

In addition to various **blenders,** an instrument named the Stomacher (A. J. Seward & Co., England; Dynatech Laboratories, Alexandria, Va.) "massages" a disposable bag containing specimen and diluent. There are several models based on the sample/diluent capacity (models 80, 400, and 3500). The shear forces created when 2 reciprocating paddles pulverize the sample release microorganisms from sputum, swabs, tissue biopsies, or food. Emswiller et al.[14] found this instrument useful because of the time and labor saved with the sterile disposable bags. Andrews et al. [15,16] compared several methods of sample preparation of foods including submersion, blending, and "stomaching." They found that the effectiveness of the Stomacher was "food specific" and recommended an in-house trial by individual laboratories before use. Laboratories dealing with solid specimens such as tissues or food will find this instrument most helpful.

Plating, streaking, and inoculation

An automatic benchtop **agar sterilizer,** the Agar-Matic, is available (New Brunswick Scientific Co., Edison, N.J., model AS 3 [3 L capacity] and model AS 20 [20 L capacity]). All ingredients are placed in the sterilizing vessel. Sterilization time, maintenance, and dispensing temperatures are adjustable. A dispensing valve and pump facilitate the sterile transfer of desired amounts of agar or other solutions into suitable containers (e.g., Petri plates, flasks). An accessory, the Pour-Matic, is a self-stacking carousel-type unit that fills Petri plates. Thus a complete closed system (the in-house plate preparation system) is possible from sterilization to Petri plate (Fig. 74-1).

The 3 models of the Manostat Mediamatic System (Manostat Corp., New York) can be used in concert, individually, or with other instruments. Together they can fill, stack, and label up

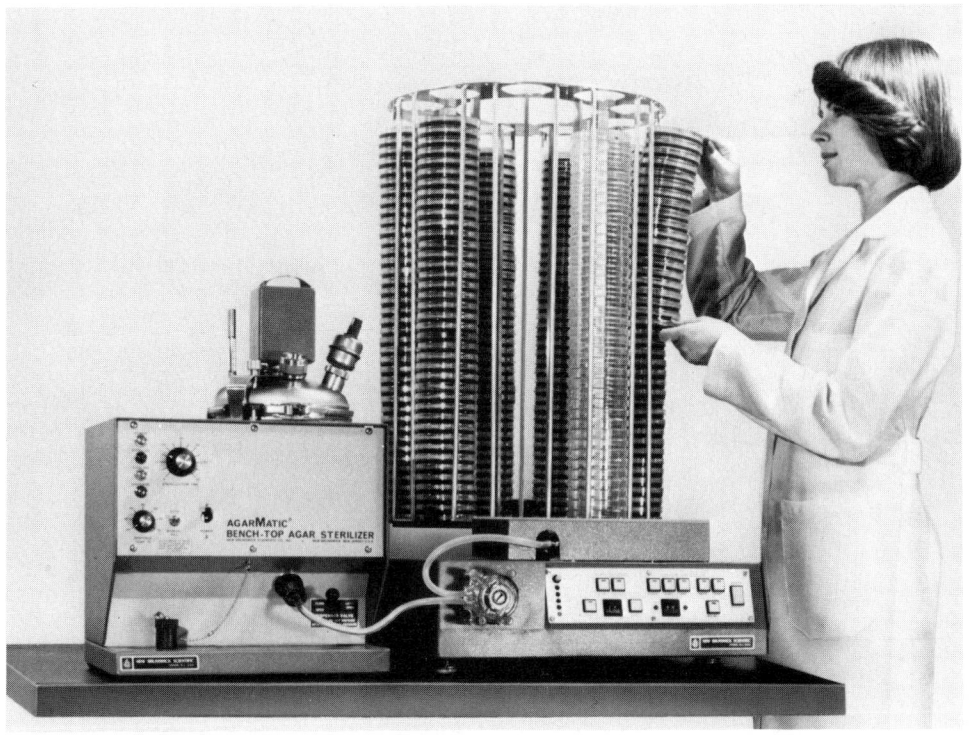

Fig. 74-1. In-house Plate Preparation System, semiautomated closed system that includes automatic benchtop agar sterilizer, dispensing valve and pump, and self-stacking carousel-type unit that fills and stacks Petri plates. (Courtesy New Brunswick Scientific Co., Edison, N.J.)

to 1200 Petri plates per hour. A similar instrument, the Petrimat (Bellco Glass, Vineland, N.J.) also fills and stacks up to 600 plates per hour. All of these instruments have had good reports from users. Many companies market adjustable peristaltic pumps that can be used with sterile tubing to fill Petri plates or flasks (e.g., Valveless Electric Dispenser model P-350, Kraft Apparatus, Mineola, N.Y.).

Two interesting instruments are available for **automated streaking** of agar plates. The Autostreaker (Tomtec Co., Orange, Conn.) streaks plates for either isolation or quantitation. It can streak up to 10 different types of media from 1 inoculum source as well as sort, label, and stack the plates for the desired incubator. An oscillat-

ing head spreads a given amount of inoculum on a spinning plate. Tilton and Ryan[17] indicated that agar plates with well-separated colonies and accurate colony counts were produced; dilutions are prepared manually. Laboratories doing many plate counts on different media will benefit from this instrument. Héden[11] discusses a semiautomated method in which standardized agar blocks are cut, carried, encased, and inoculated. This instrument might be more difficult to manipulate.

In 1971 Campbell[18] introduced the concept of adding inoculum to agar plates in the form of an Archimedes spiral. This instrumentation was further developed,[19,20] and a semiautomated instrument employing this principle, the Spiral

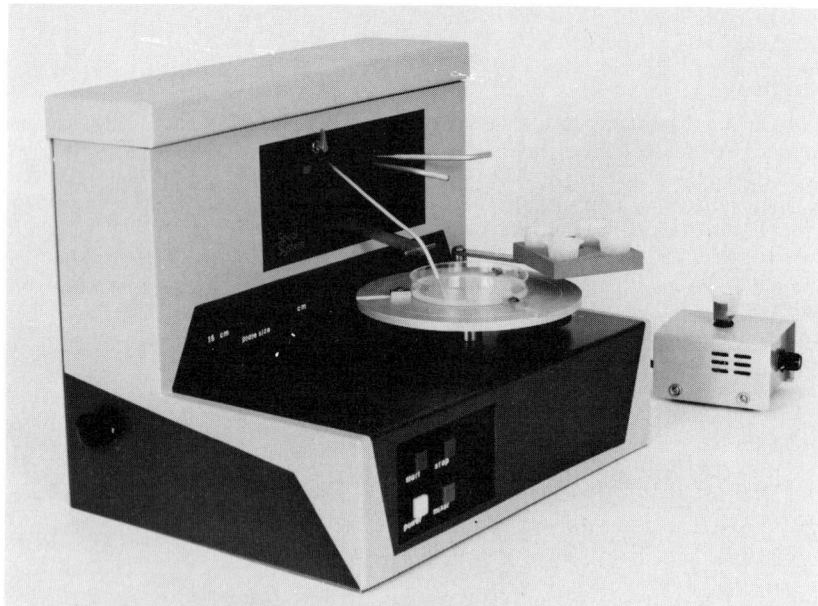

Fig. 74-2. Spiral Plater, model B, an instrument that adds decreasing volume of liquid in an Archimedes spiral to solid medium in revolving Petri plate. (Courtesy Spiral Systems Marketing, Bethesda. Md.)

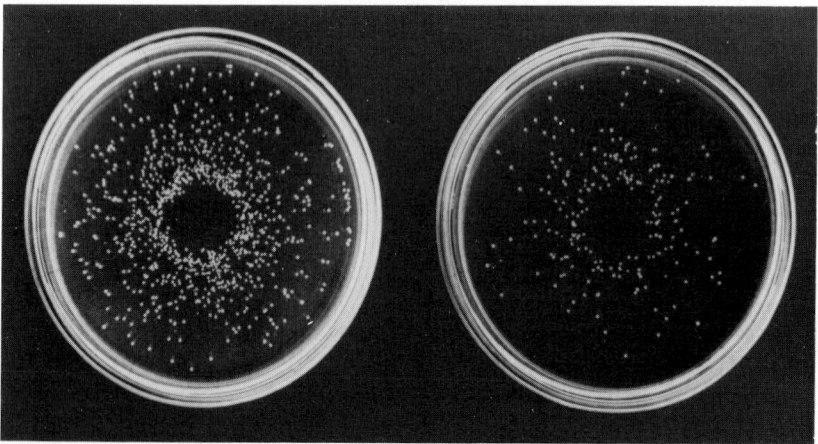

Fig. 74-3. Appearance of colonies plated by Spiral Plater. (Courtesy Spiral Systems Marketing, Bethesda, Md.)

Plater (Spiral Systems Marketing, Bethesda, Md.) has been recommended for adoption as an official first action for foods and cosmetics by the Association of Official Analytical Chemists[21] (Fig. 74-2).

The unique feature incorporated in this instrument is **automatic sample dilution** during the streaking procedure. A progressively decreasing amount of sample is deposited on a rotating plate in the form of an Archimedes spiral. When the colony count is divided by the volume that is dispensed in a given area the bacterial concentration can be determined. On a standard agar plate (100 × 15 mm) a gradient dilution of 10,000:1 can be made using a total inoculum of 35 μl. About 50 samples per hour can be plated with this instrument. Fig. 74-3 shows the distribution of colonies on the plate after incubation. This instrument has been favorably evaluated when compared with the standard methods for determining numbers of viable microorganisms in foods[22] and in large-scale studies on the varied microbial ecology of humans.[23] This instrument conserves media and preparation time, since dilution blanks and many plates are not needed. Occasionally the stylus becomes clogged but is easily cleaned.

Several instruments are also available for the manual streaking of plates, such as a motorized turntable (Fig. 74-4) (Fisher Scientific Co., Pittsburgh).

In 1959 Steers et al. developed an **inoculum-replicating apparatus (Steers replicator)** for routine testing of bacterial susceptibility to antibiotics and bacteriophages.[24] It is basically a head containing needle or needlelike projections in a fixed pattern. Similar devices have been semiautomated.[25] The Replicator multiple inoculator (Cathra, Toronto) accommodates 36 samples of inoculum, which can be transferred to the surface of a Petri plate via a head containing 1 or 3 mm "rods." The AIM-4 system (Axford International, Denver) is similar; however, its Petri plates have a raised grid to prevent spreading, and the needles on the inoculator head are disposable. Wiberg described a floating-loop replica-plating device for inoculating agar surfaces.[26] A computer-controlled prototype automatic cell inoculator (Cyclops) was described by Sevastopoulos et al. that delivers 10^{-9} L drops of liquid cell suspensions (containing approximately an average of 1 bacterium) in adjustable square arrays of evenly spaced rows and columns on a standard agar plate.[27] This instrument was used in studying a large number of mutants of *Escherichia coli*.

Colony counting

There are several "automated" instruments that perform colony counts on Petri plates. These include the Petriscan (American Instrument Co., Silver Spring, Md.), The Automatic Colony Counter model 480 (Fisher Scientific Co., Pittsburgh), the 3M Automated Colony Counter (Curtin Matheson Co., Houston), and the Biotran II model C11A (Fig. 74-5) (New Brunswick Scientific Co., Edison, N.J.). The latter has a TV camera and a videoscanner and can be adapted to count bacteriophage plaques. It can be modified for observation of tissue culture flasks as well. It has been used in experiments involving the Ames *Salmonella* microsome mutagenicity test.[28] The Fisher counter has been favorably compared with standard plate counts.[29] The 3M counter gave lower counts than manual reading when used to evaluate manufacturing grade milk, but

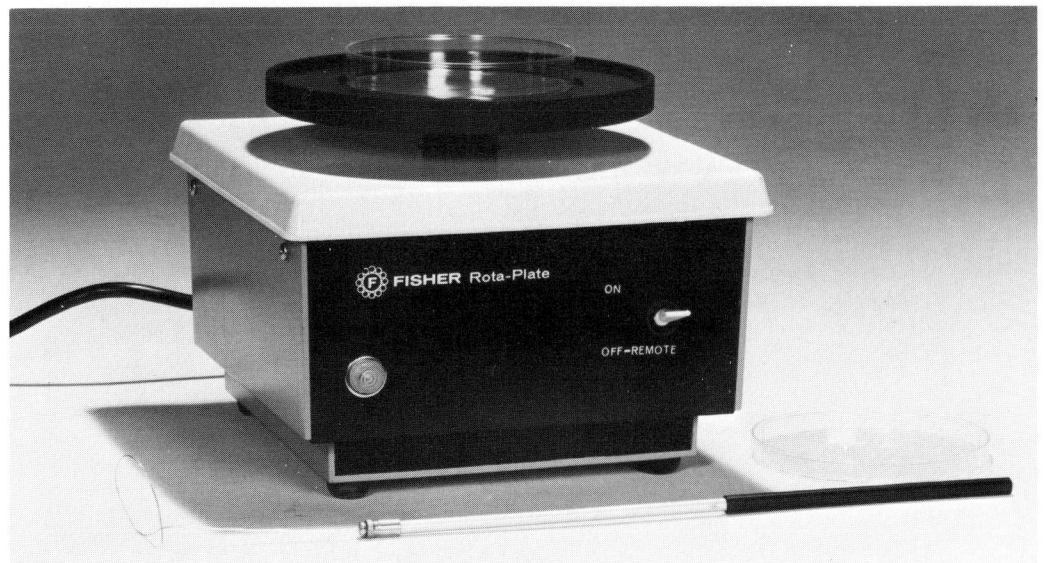

Fig. 74-4. ROTA-PLATE turntable, aid for manual streaking of plates. (Courtesy Fisher Scientific Co., Pittsburgh, Pa.)

this could be overcome with appropriate correction factors.[30]

An instrument with a calibrated circular grid arrangement for manual use and a Laser Bacteria Colony Counter model 500A (Fig. 74-6) to be used with a spiral plater is also available (Spiral Systems Marketing, Bethesda, Md.). The latter produces a spiral inward scan of the Petri plate starting from the perimeter to determine the cell concentration from the annular area containing a preselected number of colonies. It can also be used to determine total plate count of either "spiral" or "standard" plates. Both the manual and the laser colony counters have been favorably evaluated.[21-23] Laboratories with a heavy work load in this area would do well to investigate these systems.

Pipetting, diluting, harvesting, and reading

Some instruments that have long been used in chemistry laboratories have now found their way into various areas of microbiology. Many com-

panies market **manual pipetting instruments.** An example is the Pipetman (Rainin Instrument Co., Brighton, Mass.), which has 4 sizes of continuously adjustable digital microliter pipets and uses disposable tips. Automated **dilutors** and **pipetters** are available that dilute liquid specimens (e.g., buffers, antigens, antibiotics, cells, vitamins). Sykes and Evans[31] reported an automated instrument that would fill 64 cups in an assay plate with antibiotic solutions. Another automatic dilutor was described for vitamin and antibiotic assays.[32] An adaptable system for timed aseptic sampling of microbial cultures has been developed by Newman[33] for sampling various types of containers anaerobically, aerobically, or from cultures stored under refrigeration. Microtiter instrumentation, including an automated susceptibility testing system that combines various dilutions of antibiotics with different media and organisms, has a manual reader (Dynatech Laboratories, Alexandria, Va.). Other systems include Micromedic (Micromedic, Philadelphia),

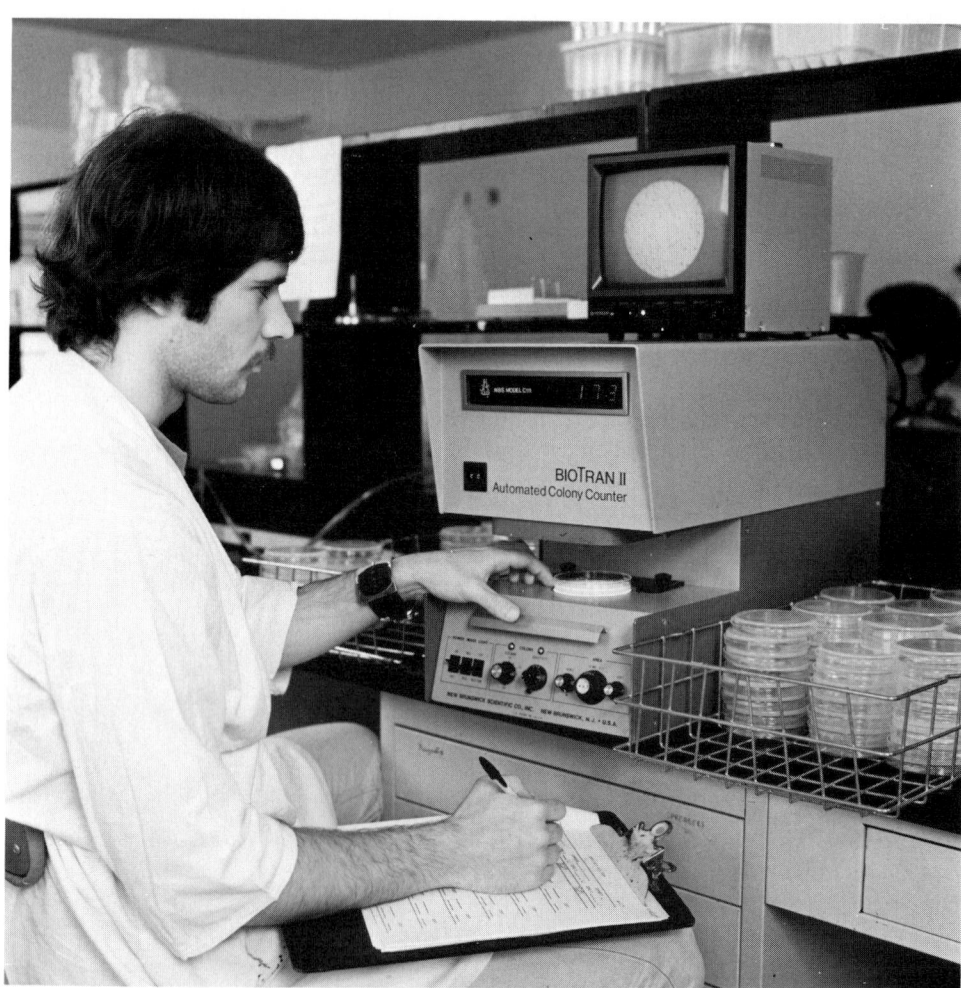

Fig. 74-5. Biotran II, semiautomated colony counter with videoscanner. Instrument can be adapted to count plaques or to observe growth in tissue culture flasks. (Courtesy New Brunswick Scientific Co., Edison, N.J.)

Bioreactor (Biomedica, Geneva, Switzerland), Medimixes (Tinbro Chemical Co., New Haven, Conn.), Brinkman Instruments, (Westbury, N.Y.), and the Autotiter system (Canalco Co., Rockville, Md.). One of the newest is the PRIAS system (Packard Instrument Co., Downers Grove, Ill.). Designed for radioimmune assays or other liquid scintillation assays, it measures the samples and reagents, premixes them, and delivers them according to a computer-programmed sequence. The use of Microtiter instrumentation is increasing in clinical microbiology laboratories.

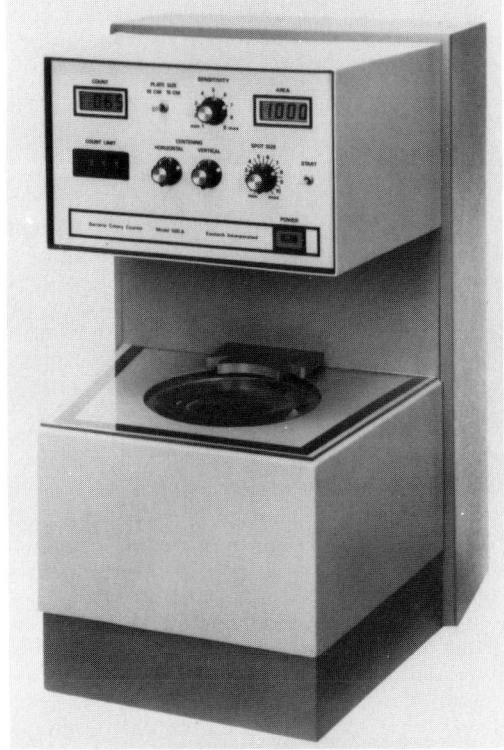

Fig. 74-6. Laser Bacteria Colony Counter (model 500A). Instrument uses laser beam in spiral scan moving inward from perimeter. It can be used to read plates prepared from Spiral Plater (Fig. 75-1) or with plates streaked in conventional manner. (Courtesy Spiral Systems Marketing, Bethesda, Md.)

Automated **washers** and **harvesters** include Illacon (Tonbridge, England) and Microbiological Associates (Walkersville, Md.) instruments. Some of these systems have been evaluated.[34] A computer-programmed **dispenser, incubator,** and **sampler** that can handle up to 600 small tubes is available (Science Spectrum, Santa Barbara, Calif.). **Dipping probe colorimeters** (Brinkman Instruments, Westbury, N.Y.) were used with phenol red solutions of known pH: the percent transmission scale could then be correlated and calibrated in terms of relative pH. It was then used in an automated system for continuous pH monitoring.[35] A **fiber optics colorimeter** has also been developed to make color determinations in microtiter plates; automated and semiautomated systems have been described.[36, 37] The PRP 8 computer photometer (Carl Zeiss, New York) is programmable for various enzymatic analyses. Two systems, the Repliscan and AIM-4, have semiautomated reading devices and are discussed in the section on diagnostic kits (see Miniaturized systems). Many instrument manufacturers market programmable spectrophotometer systems that include accessories such as sample dispensing units and automatic data processing capabilities (Gilford Instruments, Oberlin, Ohio).

Staining machines

Long the workhorses of cytology and histology laboratories, automated and semiautomated stainers are at last being produced for the microbiology laboratory and herald a new era in staining. The Microstainer II (Cooke Laboratory Products, Alexandria, Va.) can perform many types of staining reactions including the Gram, acid-fast, Giemsa, and Wright stains. An earlier model has been favorably evaluated when compared with manually prepared slides by Fung[38] and by Ryan et al.[39] Staining is 7-8 times faster than the manual procedure, and reagents are easily replenished or changed. The Honeywell HMS 360 slide stainer (Honeywell Test Instruments Division, Denver) can process up to 360 slides per hour (Fig. 74-7); stain interpretations are 3.4% more accurate compared with conventional technics and are completed in half the time.[40] If laboratories routinely stain a great

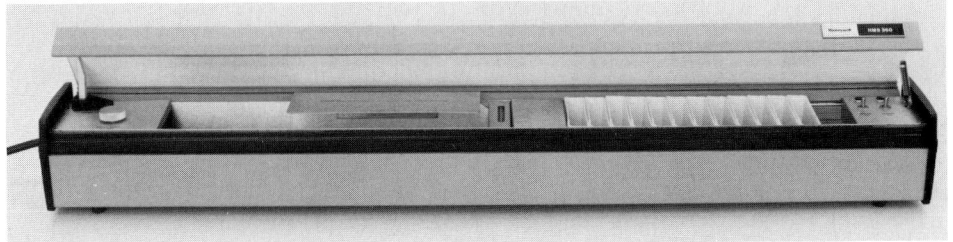

Fig. 74-7. HMS 360 Slide Stainer, device for automatically staining and processing microscope slides. It can be used for Gram or other staining procedures. (Courtesy Honeywell, Test Instruments Division, Denver).

number of slides, staining machines would be very helpful. They are easy to operate and have great flexibility. Stains are particularly easy to change on the Microstainer as the bottles containing the staining solutions "snap" in and out.

PHYSICAL METHODS OF DETECTION AND CHARACTERIZATION

The physical properties of cells (e.g., size, shape, color, electrical charge) have been used to detect and characterize microorganisms. Several interesting instruments are available for these procedures.

Particle counting and electrical measurements

As early as 1962 the Coulter Counter (Coulter Electronics Co., Hialeah, Fla.) was being evaluated for use in determining bacteriuria.[41] Several similar instruments are available based on the same concept.

In **particle counting** procedures of this type, particles (e.g., bacteria, leukocytes) suspended in an electrically conducting fluid are individually pulled through a small orifice. At that instant the current flux is altered; this in turn causes a voltage pulse that can be electronically detected. Depending on the instrument, the size and number of particles can be determined and recorded by computer, which can then calculate the number of particles, the size or sizes, as well as the number of particles in any particular size range. The computer can also be directed to record only specific size ranges. For example, the lectin concanavalin A agglutinates *Streptococcus faecium* but not *S. sanguis*. The Celloscope (A. B. L. Ljundberg & Co., Stockholm) was used to quantitate this reaction using an 100 μm orifice.[42] Gall et al.[43] indicated that a pulse-height analyser, modified to measure bacterial sizes, could be used to detect **bacteriuria** and determine **antibiotic susceptibility**. Rapid identification of freshly isolated urinary pathogens by agglutination with homologous antisera could also be detected with this instrument.

When the enterotoxins produced by *Vibrio cholera* and *Escherichia coli* are added to cells of Chinese hamster ovary cells in tissue culture the adhesiveness of the cells increases and less are found floating freely in the medium. The aspirated culture fluid was counted in a Coulter Counter and compared with control cultures. Using this system a simple, sensitive quantitative **assay for the enterotoxins** was developed that could detect toxin even in 100- to 200-fold diluted culture fluids.[44] Curby and Gall discussed the practical and theoretical application of this technic in rapidly detecting bacteriuria and antibiotic susceptibility of microorganisms.[45] The Coulter Counter has also been used in estimating the ploidy levels in large conidial populations of *Verticillium albo-atrum* and *V. dahliae*.[46] Goldschmidt and Wheeler used changes in electrical measurements to determine the presence of microorganisms in urine.[47, 48] All of these

particle-counting instruments require that the operator have some training. They can be used as rapid presumptive screening procedures.

Martens and Morton discuss in detail the uses of **automatic image analysis** in microbiology.[49] These instruments scan images and convert optical information into electrical signals representing image brightness profiles found along the scan lines. The profiles are then processed for the desired information and displayed on a television screen. These instruments can thus count, measure individual or multiple features, sort and classify according to chosen parameters, and even measure the motion of objects. The number of bacteria or other cell types in a sample can be counted, and certain features such as nuclear areas can be measured. The effects of antibiotics, growth factors, or other compounds on microorganisms can be rapidly assessed. Available instruments include the πMC system (Millipore Corp., Bedford, Mass.) and the Omnicron Pattern Analysis system (Bausch & Lomb, Analytical Systems Division, Rochester, N.Y.). These instruments are somewhat more complex to operate and require a fair amount of training. Although not mentioned in the literature as yet, this would be an excellent procedure to detect the effects of cholera and *E. coli* heat-labile enterotoxins on tissue culture cells. The cells change shape after exposure to the toxins.

Light measurement

When a beam of light (the incident ray) passes through a cell suspension at a certain angle (the incident angle) the light can be absorbed, reflected, refracted, or diffracted. The amount of light or angle of the emergent ray can be quantitatively detected by a photomultiplier tube and translated into various units. The intensity, wavelength, and angle of the incident beam can be manipulated.

These types of measurements are by far the most common among microbiologic procedures and range from simple turbidimetric detection to complex laser beam light-scattering spectrophotometry. Semiautomated and automated instrumentation is available in these areas.

The Autobac instruments (Charles Pfizer, Groton, Conn.), the MS-2 (Abbott Laboratories Diagnostic Division, Dallas), and the Automicrobic system (Vitek Systems, subsidiary of McDonnell-Douglas Corp., St. Louis) are examples of commercially available instruments using turbidimetric and light-scattering measurements with a fixed-angle beam.

Autobac-1 and Autobac-MTS

The Autobac-1 (Fig. 74-8) is a semiautomated instrument using light-scattering photometry in growth or inhibition studies. The Autobac-MTS is a retrofitted Autobac-1 that also has the capacity for MIC determinations. Pure cultures of microorganisms are dispensed into a liquid and adjusted to a predetermined turbidity before be-

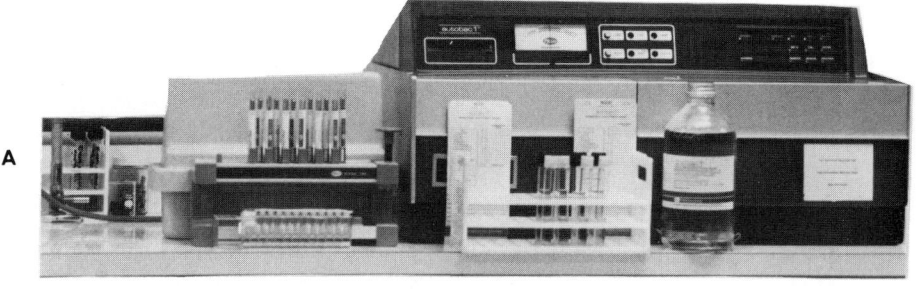

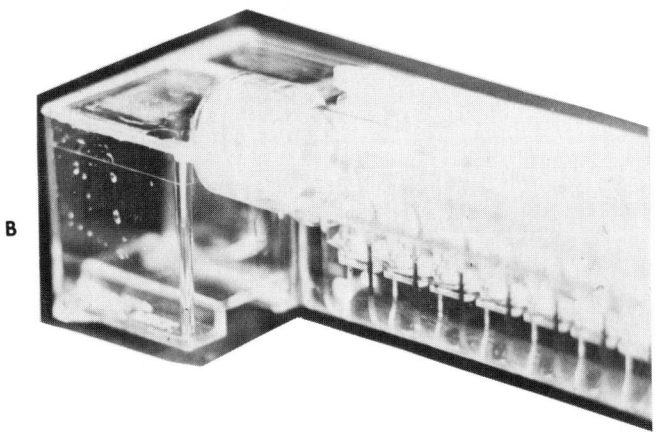

Fig. 74-8. Autobac-1, semiautomated system used mainly for antibiotic susceptibility testing based on light-scattering photometry. **A,** New revised Autobac instrument. **B,** Autobac cuvette. (Courtesy Pfizer Diagnostics Division, Groton, Conn.)

ing added to the specially designed cuvette containing 13 cells; 1 cell serves as a control. The cuvettes contain a growth medium and elution disks containing antibiotics. The concentration of antibiotics in the disks is adjusted to give interpretations comparable to those used in the Bauer-Kirby and MIC determinations. Results are recorded at designated periods (3-5 hours) during incubation. Antibiograms are usually obtained by that time. Excellent descriptions of Autobac-1 are given by Praglin[50] and McKie.[51]

Favorable reports were issued by a group of collaborative laboratories when Autobac-1 was compared with the standard methods for antibiotic susceptibility and minimal inhibitory concentration (MIC).[52-55] The instruments are in clinical use, primarily for **antibiotic sensitivity tests and MIC determinations,** but other uses are also being developed. For example, urine specimens could be reliably screened for *Enterobacteriaceae* at 4 hours when 0.2 ml urine was added to 1.5 ml broth in a cuvette cell. It was not initially reliable for gram-positive cocci, *Pseudomonas,* and yeasts in that time period.[56] Ngui-Yen and Smith[57] used the Autobac-1 for presumptive identification of several yeasts based on carbon assimilation studies. Using the Autobac-1 to generate both antibiogram and susceptibility patterns to various inhibiting

agents (e.g., organic and inorganic compounds, dyes, antineoplastic agents) Sielaff et al. reported **presumptive identification** of organisms on the same day[58, 59] finding 95-97% agreement with conventional (manual) methods. Only cuvettes made by the manufacturer can be used in the instruments.

MS-2 system

The MS-2 system (Fig. 74-9) uses light-emitting diode photodetectors to monitor turbidity every 5 minutes in each cuvette position. The 11-cell cuvette cartridge can be loaded with appropriate antibiotic elution disks or other compounds and appropriate controls. The top of the cuvette is filled with a freshly inoculated pure culture. When log phase growth starts the culture is automatically transferred into the test chambers.

Kinetic analysis data are generated by a programmed microprocessor and can be printed, displayed on a television screen, or stored for future reference. Applications include the effects of growth inhibition (e.g., **antibiotic** susceptibility testing), MIC determinations, and studies of bioassay technics. A 90-95% accuracy and reproducibility of susceptibility and MIC determination has been reported by several groups. The antibiotic concentration on the disks was com-

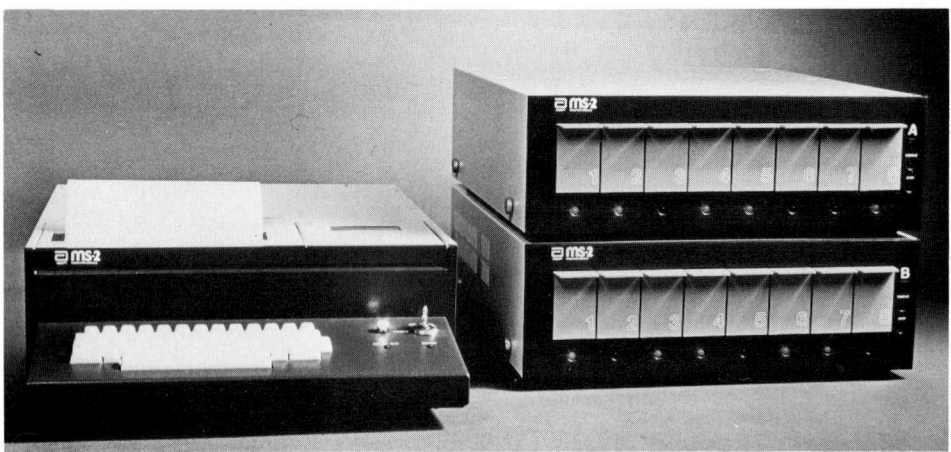

Fig. 74-9. MS-2, semiautomated Microbiology Testing System that monitors turbidity every 5 min and generates kinetic analysis data. It is mainly used for antibiotic sensitivity determinations. Results can be printed out. (Courtesy Abbott Laboratories, Diagnostic Division, Dallas).

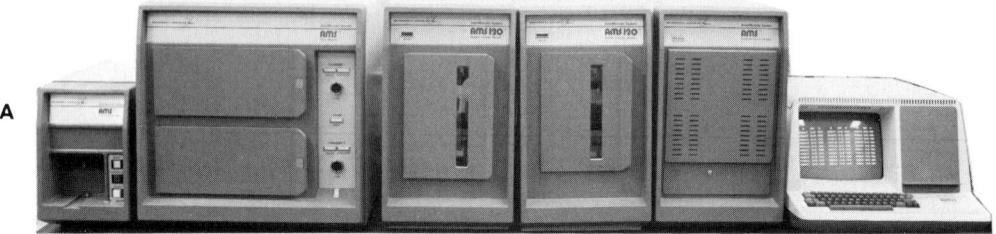

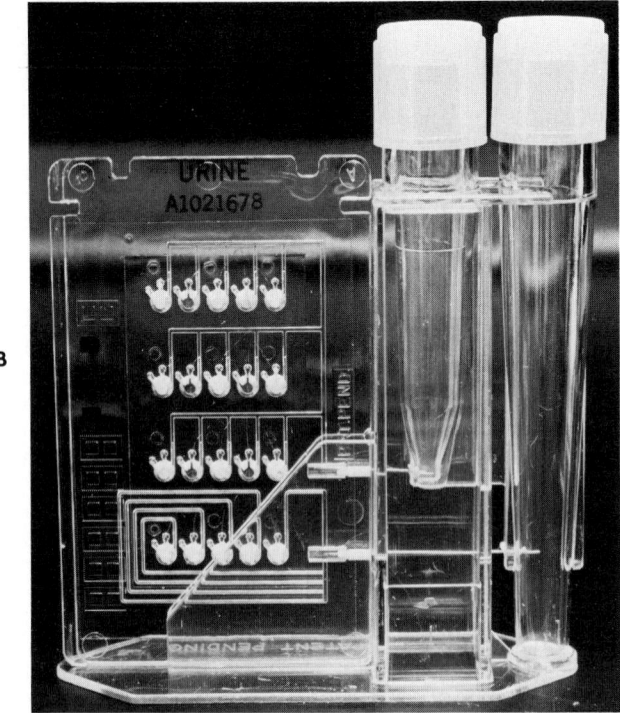

Fig. 74-10. AMS-Automicrobic System. **A,** Automated instrument based on turbidimetric detection of growth in highly selective media. It is used for detection and characterization of organisms present in urine. **B,** Plastic "Identipak" for urine cultures with inoculating tubes in place. (Courtesy Vitek Systems, Hazelwood, Mo., subsidiary of McDonnell-Douglas Corp., St. Louis.)

parable to that in the standard Bauer-Kirby and MIC methods.[60-62] The antibiotic susceptibility patterns generated could also quickly reveal delayed drug activity, bacteriolytic action, and even the emergence of mutants.[63] This instrument is also marketed for industrial use by Akro-Medic Engineering (Denville, N.J.). They have named it the RSBA (*rapid sequential bacteriological analyzer*). Only cuvettes supplied by the manufacturer can be used in the instrument. Operation of the instrument is not difficult. Clinical use of the instrument, together with additional applications (e.g., urine screening), is expected shortly.

AMS (Automicrobic System)

This is an automated, combined **detection-enumeration-identification-antibiotic susceptibility** testing system (Fig. 74-10). It is the first system to bypass the requirement for primary isolation; it directly addresses the specimen. A small disposable cuvette (Identi-pak) has 20 wells that contain specific selective media. The wells are inoculated pneumatically after 2 diluting and dispensing steps. Since the wells contain freeze-dried media that are highly differential and selective for specific microorganisms, pure cultures are not required as an inoculum. Theoretically only 1 species of organism will grow in a designated well. Some wells contain nonselective media to determine the microbial concentration (enumeration) and growth. The paks are scanned every hour by an electro-optical system employing light-emitting diodes. Although primarily derived to test urine, the instrument also performs antibiotic susceptibility, MIC determinations, and biochemical reactions with pure cultures (*Enterobacteriaceae* at this time). Only cuvettes supplied by the manufacturer can be used in the instrument. Printouts of interim and final status reports are prepared by the computer-programmed module, which also controls a visual display screen. When this system was evaluated and compared with conventional methods by several groups, an accuracy of 90% or higher was found.[64-69a] This instrument seems to be well accepted by technologists in the laboratories that have evaluated it.

Differential III system

This programmable instrument (Science Spectrum, Santa Barbara, Calif.) (Fig. 74-11) detects light scattered from a bacterial suspension. The cuvette containing the sample is irradiated by a vertically polarized helium-neon laser beam. An array of detectors lying in a plane at the same radial distance from the specimen measures the scattered intensity at different selected angles (from 28-134°) relative to the incident beam; earlier instruments (Differential I and II) had 1 rotating detector. Differential light-scattering patterns are produced. Characteristic shifts in the patterns have been used to detect sensitivity to antimicrobial agents and other compounds.[70] This instrument therefore does not monitor growth effects only but is sensitive to morphologic changes in size, shape, or size distribution when treated cells are compared with controls. The instrument was designed to rapidly determine MICs in 90 minutes. It contains a carousel that holds up to 10 cuvettes, a keyboard for entering information, a printer, and an extensive programmable microprocessor system that can convert MIC data into the classic "sensitive" or "resistant" results. The computer can also store, analyze, and report monthly antibiograms and various epidemiologic statistics and even perform routine analyses for other instruments. Wyatt has published 2 excellent discussions of differential light-scattering methods applied to microbiology.[70,71] The instrument has been used in bioassays for drug residues in food-producing

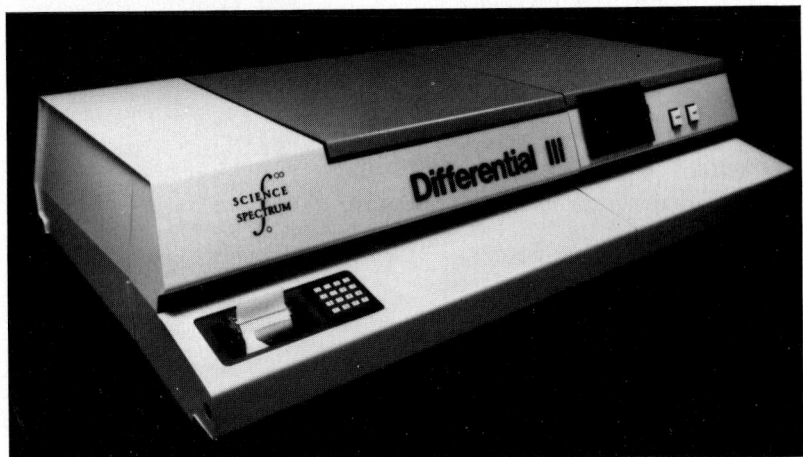

Fig. 74-11. Differential III, laser beam spectrophotometer that can be used to determine minimal inhibitory concentrations of antibiotics and to detect morphologic changes in size, shape, or size distribution. (Courtesy Science Spectrum, Santa Barbara, Calif.)

animals.[72] Possible uses include the detection of bacteria in blood or urine specimens, identification of the organisms in pure cultures, and quantitation of synergistic action of 2 or more drugs. As with most instruments some operator training is necessary. The cuvettes are inexpensive and may be obtained from many sources. FDA approval for clinical laboratory use is pending.

Miscellaneous instruments

Laser beam spectophotometry has been used to detect microbial contamination of bovine serum albumin and other pharmaceuticals[73] and to quantitate immunoglobulins.[74] A semiautomated turbidimetric method using continuous-flow systems has been described for microbiologic, vitamin, and antibiotic susceptibility assays.[75]

Chromatography

Chromatographic procedures are used to separate components of a mixture based on their differential characteristics when partitioned between 2 phases. One phase, usually a solid, is stationary, while the other (mobile phase) moves across it. The mobile phase can be a liquid (**liquid chromatography,** LC) or a gas (**gas chromatography,** GC). In GC the stationary phase can be a solid (**gas-solid chromatography,** GSC) or a liquid (**gas-liquid chromatography,** GLC). Partitioning can also occur with liquid-liquid phases (**liquid-liquid chromatography,** LLC).

Among methods used to isolate compounds, chromatographic procedures are probably the most valuable. These technics are unsurpassed for separating complex mixtures of very small amounts of samples. However, ancillary technics such as mass spectroscopy are often necessary for final identification. Automated and semiautomated instruments are available and have found their place in the microbiology laboratory, particularly in the detection and characterization of microbial end products and cellular components from anaerobes and other microorganisms. It is a useful tool in the field of **chemotaxonomy**[76] (discussed later in this chapter).

Gas-liquid chromatography

Many of the reports in the literature referring merely to gas chromatography are really referring to GLC systems. Mitruka has edited a book extensively covering the applications of gas chromatography to microbiology;[77] it should be consulted for extensive discussions of theory, selection of gases and columns, as well as other aspects.

The sample or derivatives made from the sample must be sufficiently volatile to be analyzed by this technic. There are 3 main modules to a gas chromatograph: (1) a heater volatilizes the sample so it can be carried by the gaseous mobile phase (usually inert gases) over (2) the separation

column (the stationary phase, held on an inert support) while (3) a detector continuously monitors the gas and detects the sample in various ways as it leaves the column. It sends a signal that is duly amplified and recorded. The types of column materials and supports are very specialized and depend on the types of compounds being analyzed. Detectors range from **flame ionization detectors, thermionic detectors,** and **electron capture detectors** to infrared or ultraviolet group-specific detectors. The type of detector ultimately used depends on the type of compounds usually monitored routinely in individual laboratories. Flame ionization, thermal conductivity, or electron capture detectors are most commonly used in microbiology. The detectors and columns are located in "ovens" kept at specified (usually programmable) temperatures. The length of time before various compounds emerge from the column depends on their differential affinity for the stationary phase. Those with little affinity are swept out fairly quickly, while those with greater affinity are retained for selectively longer periods.

Chromatographic procedures are delicate, critical, and fairly difficult to master. Even the heat from a hand holding an injection syringe or the method of injection might make a difference in the results. Fortunately many companies offer automatic equipment including everything from sample preparation and automated sample injection to dedicated computer systems that sequen-

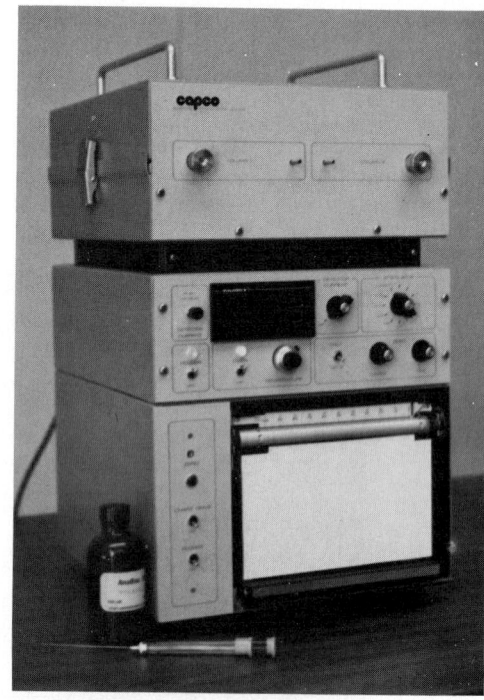

Fig. 74-12. Anaerobic Identification System, model 700. Instrument designed mainly for identification of anaerobes based on gas-liquid chromatography methodology. (Courtesy Clinical Analysis Products, Sunnyvale, Calif.)

tially program the oven temperatures, compute component concentrations from the raw data, and print out the results. Companies producing automated equipment include Varian Associates (Palo Alto, Calif.), Perkin-Elmer (Norwalk, Conn.), Hewlett-Packard (Avondale, Pa.), Packard Instruments (Downers Grove, Ill.), and Beckman Instruments (Fullerton, Calif.). However, the automated instruments are quite expensive and fairly complex.

Several companies market **semiautomated gas-liquid chromatographs** specifically designed for the microbiology laboratory. They include the Bacterial ID system, 700 series (Chemical Data Systems, Oxford, Pa.), the CAPCO Anaerobe Identification system model 700 (Clinical Analysis Product Corp., Sunnyvale, Calif.) (Fig. 74-12), and the model 400 series Anaerobe Chromatograph (Antek Instruments, Houston). The Virginia Polytechnic Institute (VPI) *Anaerobe Laboratory Manual*[78] contains detailed information on the **identification of anaerobes by GLC.** A description of methodology employed for identification of acid metabolic products of anaerobic bacteria as used at the Center for Disease Control follows.

Gas-liquid chromatography in identification of acid metabolic products of anaerobes*

Numerous reports in the literature have emphasized the importance of determining the metabolic products (particularly organic acids) of anaerobic bacteria as an aid to their classification and identification. Practical procedures, using gas liquid chromatography (GLC), are now available which allow rapid identification of metabolic products in a clinical microbiology laboratory. The GLC procedures can be performed with a relatively inexpensive chromatograph (available from various scientific instrument manufacturers).

The information provided by GLC examination allows more rapid and accurate identification of anaerobes with fewer differential tests. This actually results in decreasing the costs for accurate identification of these bacteria.

Rapid and accurate identification of anaerobic bacteria is quite important in the management of patients, particularly those with life-threatening infections. Therapy required for some infections caused by anaerobic bacteria may be quite different from that for infections caused by facultative or aerobic microorganisms. Also, treatment of infections caused by certain anaerobic bacteria must sometimes be radical, and its effectiveness decreases with delay.

A. **Identification of volatile acids.** This procedure allows the identificaion of a number of volatile acids that are soluble in ether (e.g., acetic, propionic, iso-

*From Dowell, V. R., Jr., and Hawkins, T. M.: Laboratory methods in anaerobic bacteriology, CDC laboratory manual, Department of Health, Education and Welfare, Atlanta, 1977, Center for Disease Control.

butyric, butyric, isovaleric, valeric, isocaproic, and caproic acids), but pyruvic, lactic, and succinic acids are not detected. These nonvolatile acids are identified by the examination of methyl derivatives (section B).

1. Inoculate 8 ml tubes prereduced peptone–yeast extract–glucose (PYG) medium with few drops (0.05-0.1 ml) actively growing broth culture.
2. Incubate under anaerobic conditions for 48 h or until adequate growth is obtained.
3. Acidify cultures to pH 2.0 or below by adding 0.1-0-2 ml 50% vol/vol aqueous H_2SO_4.
4. Transfer 4.0 ml acidified culture to 16×125 mm screwcap tube. (Save remainder of culture for methylation procedure, if necessary.)
5. Add 1 ml ethyl ether, tighten cap, and mix by inverting tube gently about 20 times.
6. Centrifuge briefly in clinical centrifuge (1500-2000 rpm) to break ether-culture emulsion.
7. Place ether-culture mixture in freezer (-10 C or lower) and leave until aqueous portion (bottom) is frozen. Pour off ether layer into small (13×100 mm) screwcap tube, add anhydrous $MgSO_4$ to equal about one-half the volume of ether extract, tighten cap, and let stand at least 10 min to allow removal of water from extract. (Extracts not chromatographed on day of preparation should be held in freezer to prevent evaporation of ether.)
8. Inject 14 μl into column.
9. Identify volatile acids by comparing elution times of products in extracts with those of known acids chromatographed on same day.
10. Examine tube of uninoculated PYG medium in same manner, since some lots of peptone and yeast extract have been shown to contain significant quantities of these acids. Medium should be as free of contaminating acids as possible; however most will contain trace amount of acetic acid.

B. **Analysis of methylated products.** This is required if no volatile acids are detected or if only acetic acid is detected. Currently either of 2 methods may be used for the preparation of methyl derivatives.
   1. *Boron trifluoride–methanol method*
      a. Transfer 1 ml acidified culture to 13×100 mm screwcap tube.
      b. Add 1 ml boron trifluoride–methanol (14% vol/vol) and let stand at room temperature for at least 4 h (preferably overnight), or heat in waterbath at 100 C for 5 min or at 70 C for 30 min.
      c. Add 0.5 ml chloroform and mix by inverting tube gently about 20 times. It may be necessary to centrifuge tube slowly to break emulsion in chloroform layer.
   2. *Methanol method*
      a. Transfer 1 ml original acidified culture to 13×100 mm screwcap tube.
      b. Add 2 ml methanol and 0.4 ml 50% H_2SO_4 (vol/vol). Place tube in 55 C water bath for 30 min or hold overnight at room temperature.
      c. Add 1 ml distilled water and 0.5 ml chloroform. Mix by inverting tube gently about 20 times. It may be necessary to centrifuge tube slowly to break emulsion in chloroform layer.

Regardless of method used to prepare methyl derivatives, chloroform extracts are all tested in manner shown below.
1. Fill syringe with chloroform extract after placing tip of needle beneath aqueous layer.

2. Wipe off outside of needle with clean tissue and inject 14 μl chloroform extract into column. After testing about 15-20 methylated samples, recondition column by injecting 14 μl methanol.
3. Do analyses of chloroform extracts with same column and conditions as used for volatile acids.
4. Identify methylated acids by comparing elution times of products in extracts with those of known methylated acids.
5. Test uninoculated medium by 1 of methods described above to detect presence of nonvolatile acids (especially lactic and succinic acid). If these acids are present in any amount, corrections must be made or medium discarded.

C. **Chromatographs, equipment, and supplies**
1. CDC recommends Beckman model GC2A chromatograph (Beckman Instruments, Silver Spring, Md.) (thermal conductivity), with 6-f × ¼ in. stainless steel column (Resoflex LAC-1-R-296 standard concentration [P], Burrell Corp., Pittsburgh), and a Beckman 10-in. laboratory potentiometer recorder.
2. The VPI manual[78] recommends the CAPCO Anaerobe Identification system model 700 (Clinical Analysis Products, Sunnyvale, Calif.) with Supelco (Bellefonte, Pa.) 1000 column packing preferred.

   Other thermal conductivity instruments are available from Fisher Scientific (Pittsburgh), Hewlett-Packard (Avondale, Pa.), and Varian Associates (Palo Alto, Calif.).

D. **Standard solutions.** (Standards for volatile acids, nonvolatile acids, and alcohols are available from CAPCO.)
1. Volatile acid standard. To 100 ml distilled water add:

Acetic	0.057 ml
Propionic	0.075 ml
Isobutyric	0.092 ml
Butyric	0.091 ml
Isovaleric	0.127 ml
Valeric	0.125 ml
Isocaproic	0.126 ml
Caproic	0.126 ml

   Prepared standard solution contains about 1 mEq each acid depending on purity of reagent. To use, acidify 4 ml standard and proceed as for culture.
2. Nonvolatile acid standard. To 100 ml distilled water add:

Pyruvic acid	0.068 ml
Lactic acid (85%)	0.084 ml
Succinic acid	0.06 g

   Prepared standard contains about 1 mEq each acid depending on purity of reagent. To use, methylate 1 ml standard and proceed as for culture.

E. Approximate elution time for standard acids in minutes:
1. Volatile acids:

Acetic	4.5
Propionic	6.0
Isobutyric	6.5
Butyric	8.5
Isovaleric	10.0
Valeric	13.0
Isocaproic	17.0
Caproic	20.0

2. Nonvolatile acids:

Methyl-pyruvate	3.0
Methyl-lactate	3.5
Methyl-succinate	12.0

For more details on gas-liquid chromatography consult the VPI anaerobe manual,[78] Wadsworth anaerobe manual,[79] Moss,[80] and the Symposium on Applications of Gas and High-Pressure Chromatography in Microbiology (1977).[81]

• • •

Microbial analyses by GLC can be done using whole cells, extracts of cells or culture fluids, or head space gases. The literature abounds with reports.[77] In addition **body fluids** such as synovial and serous fluids and pus often contain compounds derived from microbial or viral infections. Analyses of synovial fluid specimens for bacterial metabolites showed differences between arthritis caused by staphylococci, streptococci, or gonococci from those due to traumatic arthritis.[82] Gorbach et al. used GLC to identify short-chain fatty acids characteristic of anaerobes in specimens of serous fluid and pus. They reported an excellent correlation between GLC data and conventional methods of identification.[83] Tuberculous meningitis and *Haemophilus influenzae* type B meningitis can be detected in cerebrospinal fluid by GLC with a frequency pulsed–modulated electron capture detector.[84] Nord diagnosed anaerobic infections by GLC.[85] Bricknell et al. reported that GLC could be used directly to assay bacterial metabolites and products in dental plaque.[86] Viruses, viral products, and changes in host fluids induced by viruses have been reported.[77] Hayward and Jeavons, using **head space–GLC**, could detect 10^5 or greater milliliters *Escherichia coli* and *Proteus mirabilis* in urine within 3-5 hours by the production of specific metabolites in special media.[87] Head space–GLC has also been used to detect volatile fatty acids and alcohols produced by *Bacteroides fragilis*, *Clostridium perfringens*, and *Propionibacterium acnes*.[88] In several cases nonvolatile compounds have been pyrolized ("thermal fragmentation") before entering the gas chromatograph. **Pyrolysis** can be used for all components. Sometimes a temperature as high as 1300 C has been used to analyze *Bacteroides fragilis* and to distinguish species of *Salmonella*.[89,90] Here the sample to be pyrolized is applied to a wire and the wire heated. Special types of ferromagnetic wires can be used that only heat to certain temperatures and then stabilize (curie-point pyrolysis). Excellent reproducibility has been obtained in discriminating between strains of oral streptococci.[91] The Viking Lander Biology Instrument contained gas chromatographic equipment to help investigate the possibilities of life on Mars. One experiment involved pyrolysis–gas chromatography.[92]

Although identification patterns are obtainable with GLC using standards and so on, the absolute identification of compounds is not possible. Mass spectrometers have been combined with gas chromatography for this purpose (GCMS). In the mass spectrograph the sample is ionized either with an electron beam or a charged reagent gas.

The excess energy imparted to the compound results in its fragmentation, and the fragment weights are measured in the instrument and recorded. Every individual compound has a different fragmentation pattern (although similar chemical groups give similar fragmentations). Structure can therefore be determined. Even the position of an isotope within a molecule present in a complex mixture can be determined at nanogram levels. Ryhage has an excellent discussion of this procedure.[93] These systems have been automated (Finnigan Instruments Corp., Palo Alto, Calif.). Identification of amino sugars in the lipopolysaccharides of various organisms has been reported with this technic[94] as well as the identification of the genus *Pityrosporum*.[95] Again, these procedures require a fair amount of training and probably would be used in special instances.

Liquid chromatography

Other important methods of chromatographic analysis of nonvolatile or thermally unstable compounds include variations of liquid chromatography. In these procedures nonvolatile compounds are separated by their relative affinities for a solid substrate. Often the mobile phase concentration (the mobile strength) must be increased to elute substances that are strongly retained. Automated liquid chromatographs with solvent programmers are available to generate many gradient shapes (Varian Associates, Palo Alto, Calif.). Detectors are usually visible or ultraviolet light photometers. The 4 basic modes of liquid chromatography include partition (normal and reversed phase), absorption, ion exchange, and steric exclusion. The first 3 are the most widely used. High-speed or high-performance liquid chromatography (HPLC) procedures have only recently been utilized by microbiologists.[96] Again, learning the basic technology, operating the instruments at maximum efficiency, and determining the proper packing materials and solvents requires in-depth training. This procedure has been used to rapidly identify mycotoxins (rubratoxins)[97] and to quickly determine the concentration of various antibiotics (cephalothin, 5-fluorocytosine, amphotericin B, and tetracycline) in biologic fluids.[98] High-performance steric exclusion chromatography has been used to rapidly purify avian myeloblastosis virus and hamster melanoma virus from plasma proteins and tissue culture media. The time required for column purification was 5 minutes.[99] This procedure has much potential for detection of viruses in sewage and so on. Since many aflatoxins and related mycotoxins cannot be analyzed by GC or GC/MS, the combination of liquid chromatography with mass spectroscopy has been successfully employed.[100] If a molecule is derivatized, for example tagged with a strongly ultraviolet absorbing group, HPLC detection is much easier. These instruments have particular application in testing laboratories that must certify pharmaceuticals or foods to be either free of toxic or other substances or within acceptable levels. Peanut butter, for example, must be tested for aflatoxin concentration, and this method can be used.

Thin-layer chromatography

In thin-layer chromatography thin layers of absorbent are applied to a suitable backing material such as glass, polyester fiber, or aluminum foil. The compound is spotted with a capillary pipet close to 1 edge on 1 side of the layer. After drying the plate is placed in a development tank (developing module) and the mobile phase (the solvent) is drawn through the layer by capillary action. Both ascending and descending TLC (depending on the direction of the solvent flow) have been used. There are presently over 10,000 publications documenting the separation of compounds by TLC. The technic, as in all chromatography, is based on differential affinities of the applied mixture so that the compounds are moved at different rates by the solvent and hence can be separated from each other. The procedures are fairly simple. Manual equipment is not expensive. Miniaturization of the technic onto microscope slides has been reported.[101] Several semiautomated instruments are marketed for this procedure.

The Chromatape system (J. T. Baker Chemical Co., Phillipsburg, N.J.), designed primarily for the clinical chemical laboratory but applicable to microbiologic specimens, places the sample on a movable tape, receives the solvent, starts and stops the development, passes the flexible tape through an oven and through a scanning densitometer, and records the results. In LC the detector is rigidly connected to the chromatographic module. Thin-layer chromatography, however, can be performed in a separate chamber, allowing for greater flexibility in both modules. Automated densitometers and automated elution systems are available from various chromatography equipment companies (Autoscanner, Helena Laboratories, Beaumont, Texas; Eluchron, CAMAG, Basel, Switzerland). The detectors usually scan in 4 basic modes: transmission (usually visible light), remission (usually visible light), fluorometry (UV excitation and visible light emitted), and fluorescence quenching (background UV excitation and emitted light from background attenuated by fluorescent quenching). Identification and differentiation of various species of *Mycobacterium* has been reported using TLC of extracted lipids.[102] Aflatoxin B-1 and aflatoxin-like substances also have been identified by this procedure.[103] Several of the densitometers can be used to scan electrophoretic material as well.

Affinity chromatography

This is a special type of absorption chromatography in which the stationary phase has a biologic affinity for the substance being isolated from a mixture. One of the components of a reversibly reacting system is coupled to the insoluble matrix (e.g., Sepharose and its derivatives, Pharmacia Fine Chemicals, Piscataway, N.J.). Thus antigen-antibody, enzyme-inhibitor, enzyme-substrate, hormone-carriers, or other biologic systems can be employed. After the unbound substances have washed through the column, changing experimental conditions cause the attached material to desorb from the column. This "biologic amplification" procedure is rapid. However, the choice of reagents and preparation of phases may be complex. Various types of manual and semiautomated detectors can be used on the effluent. Specific antibodies have been isolated by automated affinity chromatography equipment. These procedures are presently not in routine laboratory use.

Field-flow fractionation

Field-flow fractionation is "single-phase" chromatography. This elution method depends on the separation of macromolecules and particulate species as they move horizontally on a "carrier fluid" through a ribbonlike channel or column. An external gradient (force field) is applied at right angles to this flow, interacting with the carrier fluid and forcing it against the far wall. If the compound in the carrier fluid reacts strongly with the field it will be tightly compressed in a layer against the wall. If it reacts lightly it will not be as tightly bound and will expand. Once the layer has formed, the flow moves the substance downstream. Substances near the center of the channel (not bound as tightly) will be swept out, and those that are more tightly bound will be retained longer. This procedure has been used to quickly separate viruses and proteins.[104] However, it is quite complex. It may be used in a reference laboratory or a virus laboratory but probably will not become a routine procedure in most laboratories unless automation occurs in the future.

Other chromatographic procedures

The Centichrome (Ivan Sorvall, Norwalk, Conn.) is a chromatographic device to be used with the Sorvall centrifuge for liquid chromatography. Centrifugal force packs the slurry (stationary phase) into a glass column. Sample and solvent are applied at the top of the column in a second operation. Centrifugation forces the sample to migrate down through the stationary phase. A special tool aids in extruding the chromatogram from the column. This is a simple procedure and could be used in the clinical laboratory.

Electrophoresis

A particle in solution will move when subjected to an externally applied electric field. The direction and rate will depend on several parameters. These include the surface charge and the type of particle. Thus different particles can be separated by this method. A good discussion on the electrophoretic mobility of microorganisms is given by Richmond and Fisher.[105]

A large number of companies market electrophoretic equipment, including Pharmacia Fine Chemicals (Piscataway, N.J.), Millipore Corp. (Acton, Mass.), Ortec (Oakridge, Texas), Helena Laboratories (Beaumont, Texas), and Gelman Instruments (Ann Arbor, Mich.). Because of the many variables there are no completely automated systems. Some of the detectors have been automated, however, such as the Corning 720 Fluorometer/Densitometer (Corning Glass Works, Corning, N.Y.) and Quick Quant II autoscanner (Helena Laboratories). Many publications are found in the literature on this subject, and the procedures are becoming more visible in the clinical laboratories.

An adaptation of this technic, **isoelectric focusing,** has been used in microbiology. Ampholytic molecules in the electric field migrate in a pH gradient to the region where the pH is equal to the isoelectric points of the molecules. Thus, for example, proteins can be separated and become "focused" or concentrated at pH corresponding to their isoelectric points. There are numerous variations on the types and shapes of support materials, polyacrylamide or agarose films or gels, slabs, disks, and so on. In a procedure referred to as **isotachophoresis** the UV detection of complex proteins is aided by the use of non-UV-absorbing "spacers" consisting of proteins that have mobilities in the same range. Some electrophoretic technics are simple; others are more complex. *Haemophilus influenzae* produces a bactericidal factor that is active against other species of *Haemophilus* and several genera of *Enterobacteriaceae*. This factor has been partially purified by polyacrylamide gel electrophoresis.[106] Isoelectrofocusing technics showed that a carbenicillin-resistant strain of *Pseudomonas aeruginosa* was resistant due to increased β-lactamase activity.[107]

However, one of the electrophoretic methods easily applicable to the routine of the clinical microbiology laboratory is that of **counterimmunoelectrophoresis** (CIE or CIEP). The methods used are relatively simple, and commercially prepared "slides" are available (Millipore Biomedica, Acton, Mass.; Gelman Instruments, Ann Arbor, Mich.). Wells are cut opposite each other in a gel medium and filled with solutions of antibodies or antigens. These are placed in a relationship both to the electrical field and to each other so that they migrate toward the center when the voltage is applied. The negatively charged antigen moves toward the anode side of the gel, and the "neutral" antibody moves toward the cathode by "osmophoresis." The 2 meet in a zone in the middle, and precipitin bands form at the correct concentrations. This procedure has proved very useful; it is discussed further in this chapter (see Immunoelectrophoretic technics).

ELECTROCHEMICAL INSTRUMENTATION
Impedance

Impedance represents the total "opposition" (actually a vector sum) of a circuit element to the flow of the sinusoidal alternating current in an electric circuit containing resistance, inductance, and capacitance (the latter 2 are the "reactive" part of the circuit). More simply it can be described as the ratio of the sinusoidal voltage to the sinusoidal current when a sinusoidal alternating current is applied to a circuit and there is a linear time response to the event (impedance = voltage/current). Therefore the presence of organisms or their end products in a circuit will alter the voltage current relationship and thus also change the impedance.[48] In measuring impedance or other electrical characteristics the physiologic event is placed between measuring electrodes in such a way that any changes that alter the current density distribution between the electrodes can be manifested as a change in impedance. Impedance measurements have long been used in physiology. These instruments thus have a source of sinusoidal alternating current, bipolar or tetrapolar electrodes, amplification systems, and a detector to recover or record the signal (voltmeter, null indicator, oscilloscope, or phase-sensitive circuit). There are several reviews and articles in this area.[48,108,109]

The instruments are not difficult to use and the procedure is rapid. An impedance instrument, the Bactobridge (distributed in the United States by H. E. M. Research, Rockville, Md.), is based on Ur's work.[110] Cady et al.[109,111,112] have developed another instrument, the Bactometer (Bactomatic, Palo Alto, Calif.*), with 2 models, the 32 and the more automated M 120 (Fig. 74-13). The latter is microprocessor controlled. It can handle up to 400 samples at a time and provide a printed copy of the results. Both of these instruments are based on the principle that microorganisms convert substrates (complex molecules) into simpler "electrically active" end products that change the impedance of the culture compared with a sterile control. Thus organisms can be detected in biologic fluids such as urine[113] and milk or food products such as beer and vegetables.[112] Other uses would include determination of biochemical and antibiotic susceptibility patterns and lymphocyte activation and metabolism.[114] Impedance measurements may eventually have much usefulness in the clinical microbiology laboratory. They are slower than some of the immunologic methods (such as ELISA) but do not require purified inocula when used as a presumptive screen of specimens. Some training is required for operation of these instruments, but they are not difficult to use.

Goldschmidt and Wheeler used a method simi-

---

*This company is no longer in operation. Based on the success of the tests to date, however, this type of technology should shortly appear in other instruments now in planning stages.

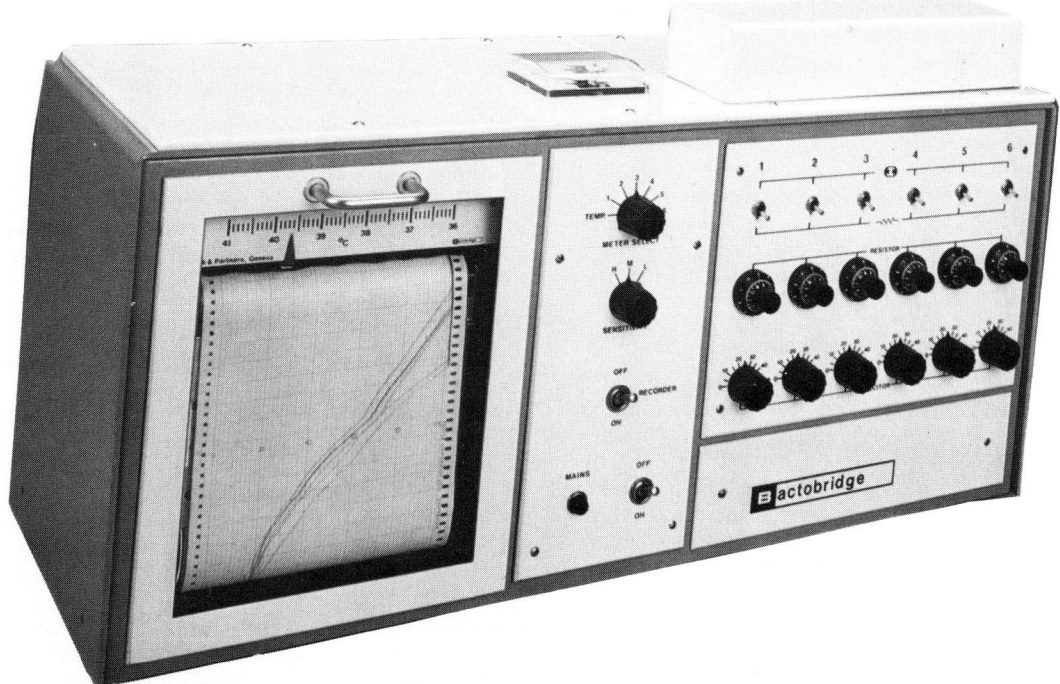

Fig. 74-13. The 6-channel integrated Bactobridge, based on electrical impedance changes. Interchangeable cell blocks are plugged in for measurement. (Courtesy HEM Research, Rockville, Md.)

lar to the impedance systems to rapidly (within 15 minutes) determine the presence of microorganisms in urine specimens in the absence of growth.[47,48]

Ion-sensitive electrodes

Gas and ion-sensitive electrodes are being used more frequently in the clinical and industrial microbiology areas. Wilkins et al.[115] have developed a compact multichannel electrochemical microbial detection unit in which appropriate electrodes detect hydrogen production, register an increase in voltage, and record the results on a strip-chart recorder. They propose its use for the detection of microorganisms in water or urine. The procedure can detect 10^6 organisms in 1 hour and 10^2 in 5 hours after incubation at 35 C. Bacterial cultures have been continuously monitored for pH, growth, CO_2, and NH_3 production by in situ ion-sensitive electrode probes.[115a] Electron probes are simple to use, and many can be connected to existing digital pH/mV meters. Measurements are rapid, and the methods are fairly sensitive. They have great potential for rapid determination of various end products. A wide range of these electrodes are available (Orion Research, Cambridge, Me.; Beckman Instrument Co., Fullerton, Calif.; Corning Glass Works, Corning, N.Y.) These electrodes have been used for on-line monitoring of fermentation as well. Ion-sensitive electrodes are available for many biologically important end products including ammonia, amino groups, hydrogen, oxygen, nitrate, nitrite, sulfides, thiols, and urea. Buck extensively reviewed this field.[116] These electrodes would make good detectors for various chromatographic procedures. Ion-sensitive electrode monitoring of antibiotic susceptibility is another possibility.

Gabridge[117] used an oxygen electrode to study the effect of *Mycoplasma pneumoniae* on tracheal organ cultures. Instrumentation exists for various monitoring procedures ranging from fluoride monitors for on-line analysis of potable water (Electronic Instrument, Richmond, Surrey, England) to those suitable for clinical analysis of glucose.[118]

Enzyme–ion-sensitive electrode probes

Recently enzymes have been combined with ion-sensing electrodes for even more sensitive analyses. Bowers and Carr[119] have reviewed applications of immobilized enzymes in analytical chemistry. Controlled substrate diffusion through a thin layer of catalyst (the enzyme) produces end products that can be detected by ion-sensitive electrode sensors. Enzyme–ion sensitive electrode analysers for glucose are commercially available (Yellow Springs Instrument Co., Yellow Springs, Ohio; Technicon Corp., Tarrytown, N.Y.; Corning Glass Works, Corning, N.Y.). "Catalinks" (Miles Laboratory, Elkhart, Ind.) is actually used as a subsystem for flow analyzers. In a semiautomated glucose analyzer (Hoffman-LaRoche, Nutley, N.J., model 5410)

the enzymatic reaction (glucose → glucuronic acid) is detected by a sensor containing the enzyme glucose oxidase layered on a platinum electrode. The electron acceptor is hexacyanoferrate, which is reoxidized at the platinum electrode.[120] A semipermeable membrane separates the sensor from the solution. This reaction has also been developed for a chemiluminescence analyzer (see below, Bioluminescence and Chemiluminescence).

Going a step farther, Reichnitz et al. have produced a glutamine-selective membrane electrode that uses living bacterial cells. A strain of *Sarcina flava* is held at the surface of an ammonia-sensing electrode (Orion 95-10) by a dialysis membrane.[121] The bacteria function as a catalyst to enzymatically convert glutamine to NH_3. A change in measured potential is noted within 5 minutes. Response to other amino acids was negligible. This is a novel concept but probably pioneers the development of other similar sensors. Bioelectrochemical fuel cells formed by an oxygen cathode and a platinum bioanode in a glucose-utilizing suspension of *Saccharomyces cerevisiae* has been reported. Appropriate combination of bacterial strains with ion- or gas-sensing elements should produce bacterial electrodes of both fundamental and practical significance. In general ion-sensitive and enzyme–ion-sensitive probes should find a role in rapid identification and detection methods. Probably those combining microorganisms in the probes are the least practical for long-term use.

Luminescent reactions

In some enzymatic reactions the electrons in the products absorb enough energy to be raised to a higher level (an electronically excited state), which is usually unstable. As these products return to the ground levels (relaxation) the "excess" energy is rapidly emitted as light (photons). Luminescence reactions are very sensitive, and as little as $10^{-15}M$ can be determined in some cases. Seitz and Neary have published an excellent review on bioluminescent and chemiluminescent reactions.[122]

Bioluminescence

Bioluminescent reactions refer to those luminescent systems involving enzymes derived from living organisms. A classic example is the reaction of adenosine triphosphate (ATP) with luciferin-luciferase, an extract of firefly lanterns. Luciferase in a bioluminescent bacterium, *Photobacterium fischeri*, has been used to measure flavin mononucleotide (FMN) and reduced nicotinamide adenine mononucleotide (NADH) and to monitor pollutants. Several coelenterates also have bioluminescent systems. When the enzyme and other necessary factors (e.g., inorganic ions such as magnesium or calcium) are in excess, the amount of light produced is proportional to the substrate concentration. Thus quantitative determinations are possible.

The ATP–firefly luciferin-luciferase luminescent reaction has been used in the clinical laboratory to detect and quantitate the presence of microorganisms in urine and potable water supplies. However, according to various reports almost all naturally occurring nucleotides and most nucleoside triphosphate compounds can be determined by this reaction. Many enzymes can also interfere with the procedure such as adenylate kinase, nucleoside diphosphate kinase, ATPase, and DNA and RNA polymerases. The first 2 enzymes are present in crude firefly extract, and thus the reaction is not specific for ATP. In addition the amount of ATP per bacterial cell varies with the species and previous treatment of the organisms. Thus much care must be taken to ensure enzyme purity. The luciferin is removed during this purification procedure. It is available commercially, however, and only a few micrograms are needed. With the above comments in mind, the method can probably be used as a rapid screening procedure to detect the presence of microorganisms in various body fluids or water supplies, but it is not too accurate. An evaluation of this method in detecting bacteriuria indicated an 89% agreement between ATP assay and routine culture methods (using 10^5 organisms per milliliter as indicative of a positive bacteriuria). However, 27% false-negatives were also found.[123] Microbial growth in soils was also determined by this method.[124]

Chemiluminescence

Chemiluminescence reactions involve chemical rather than biologic reactions. They are much the same as bioluminescent reactions in that electrons are similarly excited and emit light as they return to a lower level. Here, however, the reactions also require electron transfer, singlet oxygen, or the decomposition of peroxides. This leads to some very interesting adaptations to microbiologic assay systems. One of the classic reactions involves light production when alkaline solutions of luminol interact with hydrogen peroxide in the presence of various metal ions such as nickel, iron, cobalt, and manganese. The concentration of iron porphyrin compounds in microorganisms is more constant than ATP concentration and seems to be less affected by previous conditions. Therefore in an excess of luminol and hydrogen peroxide, light production is proportional to the concentration of metal ions and hence to the concentrations of microorganisms. In practice, cells and luminol are put into a light-tight reaction cell, and the injection of H_2O_2 initiates the reaction. Other applications include the analysis of glucose. Glucose + glucose oxidase $\rightarrow$ gluconic acid + H_2O_2; H_2O_2 + luminol + ferricyanide (metal ions) produces luminescence. The glucose oxidase has been immobilized and used as a monitoring system in flow-through systems (see also the section on ion-sensitive electrodes).[119] Nitrogenous compound such as proteins can also be detected by chemiluminescence reactions. The compounds are pyrolyzed and oxidized to NO_2. R-N + $O_2 \rightarrow NO$;

$NO + O_3 \rightarrow NO_2^*$ (*indicates the electronically activated state); $NO_2^* \rightarrow NO_2$ + light.

NADH can also be determined by chemiluminescence systems by chemically coupling NADH oxidation via methylene blue to the formation of H_2O_2. The experimental and theoretical limits of the use of chemiluminescent detection of bacteria has been discussed.[125]

Several manual and semiautomated instruments are marketed for luminescent reactions. They have in common a system for mixing the reacting ingredients, a light-tight container, and a detector. A phototube or photomultiplier tube can be used as a detector. Liquid scintillation systems are probably the most sensitive of the instruments. In the simpler instruments detectors are usually coupled to digital or analog meters. Rapid-scan spectrometers have been used. Several luminescent photometers on the market include the Lab-Line ATP-photometer (Melrose Park, Ill.), the ATP photometer (SAI Technology Co., San Diego, Calif.), the Chem-Glow Photometer (American Instruments Co., Silver Spring, Md.), and the Luminescence Biometer (DuPont, Wilmington, Del.). The FDA has recently withdrawn approval of the use of the Luminescence Biometer for detection of bacteriuria. Picciolo et al. reported on a semiautomated instrument, the Vitatect IIs (Vitatect Corp., Alexandria, Va.), which uses the firefly luciferin-luciferase assay to detect ATP.[126] The reaction system filters and treats the samples on a movable filter tape. The tape can be washed or extracted and the necessary reagents added. The tape is wound on reels and moves across the surface of the phototube, which measures the intensity of the reaction. The Technicon AutoAnalyzer has also been used to detect small numbers of organisms by a chemiluminescent reaction involving luminol.[127] The Pico-Lite system (Packard Instruments, Downers Grove, Ill.) is microprocessor controlled to detect several bioluminescence or chemiluminescence reactions. A thermal printer (optional) can provide hard copy. Liquid scintillation spectrometers can also be used.

Antek Instruments (Houston) markets several nitrogen detectors based on the luminescent measurement of excited NO_2 after pyrolysis and ozone exposure. Gas, liquid, or solid samples can be analyzed after pyrolysis. The detector can also be coupled to a gas chromatograph (model 705) to identify those peaks containing nitrogen (Fig. 74-14).

An interesting adaptation is the activation of the chemiluminescent reactions by H_2O_2, which is produced by peroxidase (see below, enzyme-linked immunosorbent assays). **Chemiluminescent immunoreactions** are thus possible and have been reported.[128,129] Here antibodies have been conjugated (horseradish peroxidase or other enzymes such as glucose oxidase[130]) and in some cases immobilized on a polymeric support such as Aclar 33C.[128] The hydrogen peroxide thus generated activates the chemiluminescent reaction.

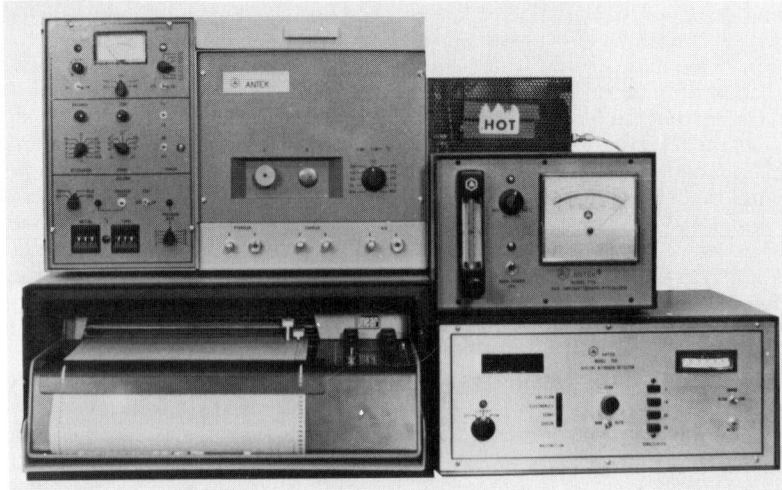

Fig. 74-14. Model 750, Gas-Liquid Chromatograph coupled with microprocessor-controlled nitrogen detector based on chemiluminescent reaction. (Courtesy Antek Instruments, Houston.)

Leukocytes increase their oxidative metabolism and produce a chemiluminescent reaction following phagocytosis. This reaction can be measured in liquid scintillation counters.[131,132] The relationships of group B streptococcal opsonins in human and rabbit serum were assessed by neutrophil chemiluminescence.[131] Sodium fluoride could stimulate the oxidative metabolism of polymorphonuclear leukocytes in the absence of phagocytosis and result in detectable chemiluminescence.[133] These sensitive methods show much promise both for the rapid detection of microorganisms, for the chemical amplification of enzyme and immunologic reactions, and for gaining insight into the interactions of leukocytes with microorganisms.

Calorimetry

Heat is a well-known byproduct of most chemical, physical, and biologic interactions. The amount of heat that is produced can be quantitated and related to the rate of the reaction under observation. Calorimetry can measure whole-body heat production (respiration) or microgram substrate reactions (microcalorimetry) of various biologic systems. Spink and Wadsö[134] published an excellent review covering the use of calorimetry as an analytical tool in biochemistry and biology; a section on microbiology is included. These procedures have increasing application to various areas of clinical microbiology as well as basic studies on microbial pathogenesis. Equipment requires some training and special work areas in some cases.

Calorimetric studies are particularly applicable to tissue, soil, and cell suspensions and do not disturb the system under investigation. The instrument systems include a reaction chamber or vessel that is thermally insulated from the environment by various means. If heat is absorbed or evolved in the reaction a temperature change

occurs, which is measured by means of thermodetectors (thermocouples) in the vessel or its walls. The voltage changes reflect the temperature differences. Semiautomated flow-through microcalorimetry instrumentation is available (LKB, Rockville, Md.) (Fig. 74-15). It can be used to study enzyme-substrate interactions, metabolic reactions (e.g., metabolism of glucose by microorganisms), enzyme-inhibitor reactions, the effects of various antibiotics on bacteria, and growth rates.[135-137] Flow-microcalorimetry has also been used in the hygienic control of polluted waters. Heat production was proportional to the metabolic activity of the heterotrophic aquatic populations.[138] Fermentation processes such as fungal production of novobiocin and cellulase have been monitored by in situ dynamic calorimetry. This method could determine the efficiency and physiologic state of the cells during fermentation.[139]

Photoacoustic spectroscopy

Photoacoustic spectroscopy is another approach to using heat production to determine metabolic activity and identification of compounds. It is based on an effect described by Alexander Graham Bell in the 1880s when a gas in an enclosed cell was periodically illuminated by light. The energy absorbed by the gas was converted into kinetic energy, which in turn gave rise to pressure changes. A microphone converted these pressure changes into sound. Recently Rosencwaig[140] has used this principle in photoacoustic or "opticoacoustic" spectroscopy of solids (PAS). A solid sample (e.g., blood smear, plant materials, microorganisms) is placed in a closed cell containing a gas and a pressure-sensitive microphone. The sample is then discontinuously illuminated with a light source, which is usually monochromatic (such as a laser beam), set at a desired frequency. Absorbed light

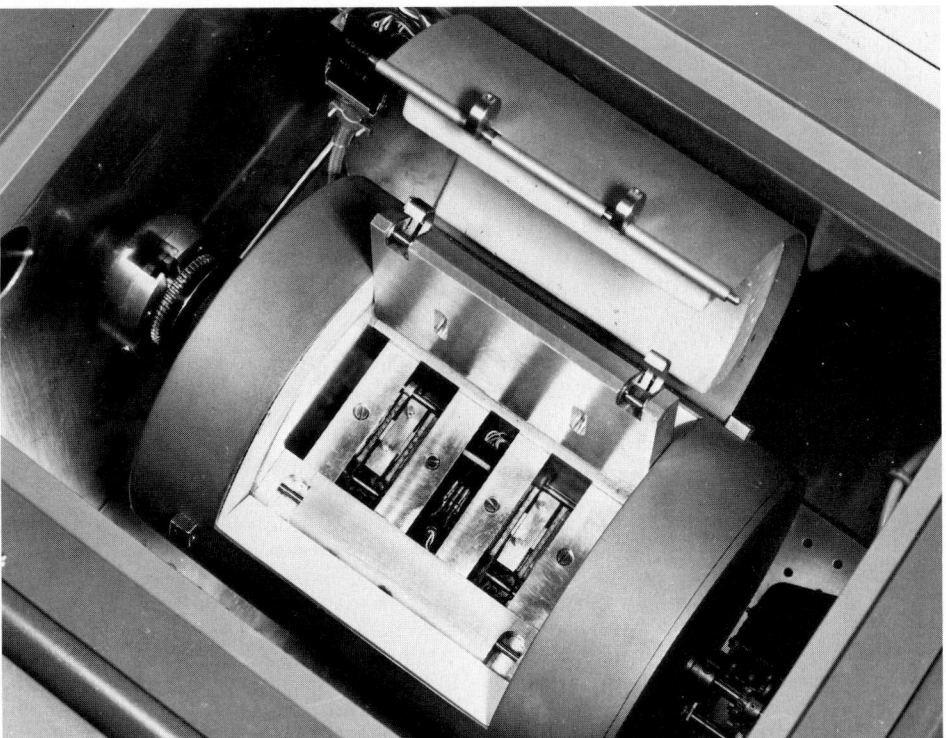

Fig. 74-15. Batch Microcalorimeter for microcalorimetry studies of various exothermic reactions. (Courtesy LKB Instruments, Rockville, Md.)

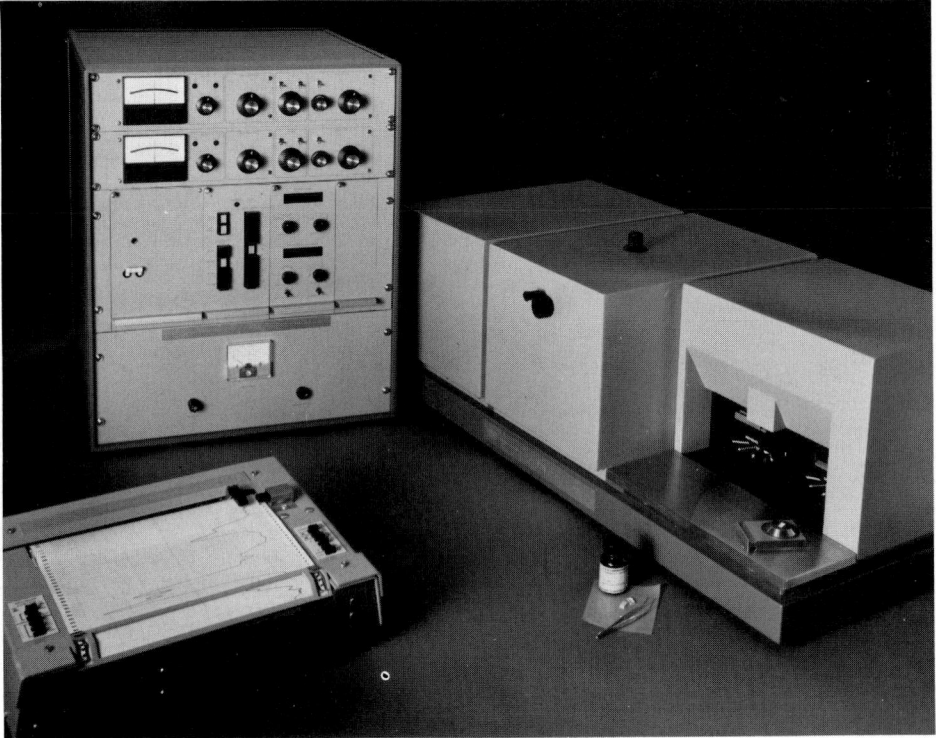

Fig. 74-16. Photoacoustic Spectrometer, model R-1500. Spectrum is obtained similar to atomic absorption spectrum when laser beam intermittently irradiates specimen in gas-filled tube containing detector. (Courtesy Gilford Instrument Labs, Oberlin, Ohio.)

is converted into heat energy, causing pressure changes in the gas, which are then detected by the microphone. The sound waves are converted to electrical signals and recorded. The magnitude of the response is proportional to the amount of heat given off by the sample. Therefore PAS spectra are similar to optical absorption spectra. Since only the absorbed light is converted to sound, light scatter is not a problem.[140,141] The Gilford R-1500 Photoacoustic Spectrometer (Gilford Instrument Co., Oberlin, Ohio) (Fig. 74-16) can be used for automatic scanning in the visible, ultraviolet, and near-infrared ranges (240-2500 nm). This technic has been used to study β-carotene, various membranes, and the mechanism of resistance to heavy metals.[142,143] It has been used as a adjunct to gas chromatography with an infrared laser radiation source. The effluent gas is irradiated and the photoacoustic spectrum is obtained. As little as 20 pg compound has been detected.[144] These procedures are fairly complex but hold promise for rapid determinations in the clinical laboratory. This method appears more sensitive than other infrared-chromatography combinations, although the use of a Fourier transform infrared (FT-IR) spectrometer with GC also seems to have speed and sensitivity.[145]

Radioactive technics

Substrates containing radioactive elements such as ^{14}C, ^{125}I, or ^{32}P have been used in micro-

biology to study metabolic pathways, detect microorganisms, and tag radioimmune assays (see below). Scintillation or Geiger counters and radiospirometers can be used to detect radioactivity.

Since CO_2 is the most common end product of carbohydrate metabolism, $^{14}CO_2$ from radiolabeled substrates such as glucose has been used to rapidly detect the presence of microorganisms in blood and various foods. Earlier reviews have covered the detailed use of this technic.[5,7,10] Two radiometric experiments were incorporated in the biology instrument aboard the Viking Lander. One measured the release of $^{14}CO_2$ from labeled organic compounds and the other measured ^{14}C incorporation into cellular components.[92]

The Bactec (Johnston Laboratories, Cockeysville, Md.), an instrument designed for $^{14}CO_2$ detection, is widely used for **detection of bacteria in blood cultures.** Several models with varying degrees of automation are available (Fig. 74-17). The amount of liberated $^{14}CO_2$ can be correlated with the presence of microorganisms and is translated into a "growth index." The Bactec has also been used with ^{14}C-glucose, -maltose, and -fructose and (unlabeled) ONPG to identify various species of *Neisseria*. When compared with conventional methods and fluorescent antibody technics in 1 experiment the labeled substrate utilization by resting cells was the more reliable method.[146] It has also been employed for de-

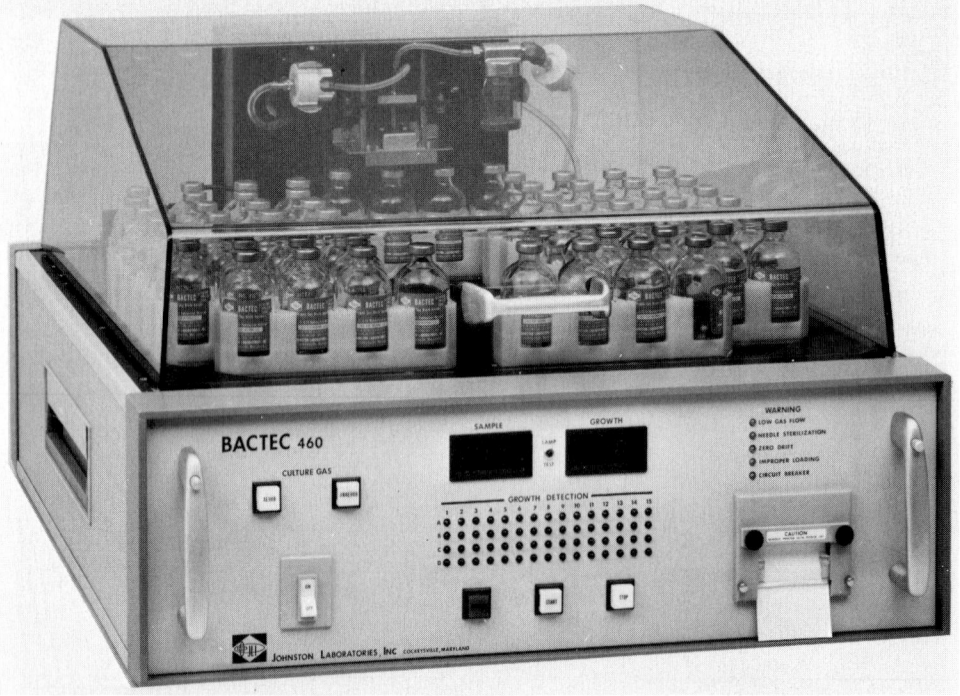

Fig. 74-17. Bactec model 460. Semiautomated instrument based on radiometric detection of $^{14}CO_2$ released by microbial utilization of ^{14}C-substrate. It has capacity for automatic sampling at predetermined intervals and can print out results. (Courtesy Johnston Laboratories, Cockeysville, Md.)

termining the susceptibility of yeast isolates to amphotericin B[147] and sterility testing of pharmaceuticals.[148] Since the synthesis of urease by *Proteus* converts ^{14}C-urea to $^{14}CO_2$ and ammonia, and since gentamicin inhibits this organism, the production of $^{14}CO_2$ can also be used to assay the amount of this antibiotic in serum. The Bactec assay for gentamicin levels in serum was compared with both a radioimmune assay procedure[149] and the traditional agar diffusion bioassay.[150] It was a more reliable procedure than either of the others.

The ^{14}C-radiospirometer was used to study the effects of chemical contaminants on microbial communities.[151] A summary of instrumentation for detection and characterization outlining procedures, instruments, principles, and comments appears in Table 74-1.

IMMUNOLOGIC TECHNICS FOR DETECTION AND CHARACTERIZATION

Immunologic technics have long been used as rapid detection methods for substances capable of provoking an antigenic response either by themselves or coupled to other molecules. Agglutination, precipitation complement fixation, and similar reactions form the basis of these tests. Good discussions on the applications of basic immunologic reactions to various areas of microbiology have been published.[5,10,11] These technics have been enhanced by conjugation with fluorescent compounds, radioactive elements, and enzymes. Mechanized and semiautomated instrumentation exists for many of these procedures (see introduction above for additional books and reviews on subject).

Immunoelectron microscopy

The transmission and scanning electron microscopes and the electron microprobe have been used to rapidly detect immunologic reactions, particularly those involving viruses.[152-155] In these procedures virus and antibody are incubated together, prepared for electron microscopy, and observed in the usual manner. A "halo" of antibodies will be seen around the virus particles if a positive reaction has occurred. Scanning electron microscopes (Bioprobe) and electron microprobes (Autoprobe) have been automated (Etec Corp., Hayward, Calif.). The Mecca system (Tracor Northern, Middleton, Wis.) provides automated x-ray analysis with its electron microprobe and scanning electron microscope.

Fluorescent technics

When some compounds are illuminated with light from 200-800 nm, the molecules become electronically excited and some electrons are raised to a higher energy state. When they again return to the "ground" level some of this energy is emitted as light at a longer wavelength than the incident one. If the time from excitation to emission is less than 10^{-4} seconds it is called fluorescence; if greater than 10^{-4} seconds (and often lasting up to several seconds) it is called **phosphorescence.** Note the similarity of fluorescence to luminescence; the main difference between the two lies in the method of excitation. Fluorescence staining technics are several magnitudes more sensitive than visual or chromogenic procedures and are capable of detecting concentrations as low as 10^{-8} to 10^{-10} g/ml. Under controlled conditions the amount of fluorescence emitted is proportional to the concentration of the emitting compound. Nonimmunologic generalized fluorescent staining procedures have been used to detect microorganisms and various compounds such as proteins, nucleic acids, and amines. Fluorescein, fluorescein isothiocyanate (FITC), 1-anilino-8-naphthalene sulfonic acid and fluorescamine have been used in these methods.[156-159] Flow microfluorometry (FMF) has been used to characterize bacterial growth rates and analyze individual cells for changes in protein and nucleic acid content at a rate of several thousand cells per second.[160,161] Thiamine has been assayed using manual and semiautomated fluorometric technics.[162] The Virometer, an instrument based on reflection fluorescence, can visually detect and size viruses.[163] Many manual and semiautomated fluorescence spectrometers are marketed.

Immunofluorescent reactions are highly sensitive and specific technics for rapid detection and identification of microorganisms. Viruses in particular can be easily identified by immunofluorescent reactions.

Immunofluorescence light microscopy and immunofluorescence reactions

Immunofluorescent procedures are routinely performed in many laboratories, and a microscope with fluorescent capabilites is a common sight. The FTA-ABS (fluorescent treponemal antibody, absorbed) test is used to detect *Treponema pallidum* antibody. Some false-positive reactions have been obtained from patients with lupus or rheumatoid factor.[164] Although several methods have been proposed, there are no presently approved immunologic detection methods for gonococcal antibodies. A correlation exists between the presence of antibody-coated bacteria and kidney infections, since bacteria from bladder infections are usually not coated. Immune fluorescence can detect these differences.[165] *Rickettsia*, *Legionella pneumophila* (the bacterium causing Legionnaires' disease), *Treponema pallidum*, and various viruses have also been identified in tissues and in other preparations by these methods.[166-170] Many more tests are reported in the literature. For a detailed discussion see Chapter 70.

Miniaturized or automated immunofluorescence reactions

Various methods for immunologic procedures involving fluorescence have been miniaturized or semiautomated for identification of various microorganisms including streptococci, gonococci, viruses, *Rickettsia, Pseudomonas,* salmonellae, and *Treponema.*[171-176] Mishuck and Roberts published an excellent discussion on several such instruments, including the AMB SeroMatic system, Aerojet Automated Bioassay system, flying spot laser scanning systems, and the "FAST" (fluorescent antibody staining technics) instument initially developed for the Army.[175] Ultraviolet spectrophotometers, fluorometers, and other detectors are used in these systems.

Other immunologic technics

Mechanized and semiautomated instruments are available for many other immunologic technics such as microcomplement fixation for toxoplasmosis[177] and automated photometers and nephelometers for detection of viruses and syphilis-specific antibodies.[178-181] The AutoAnalyzer system (Technicon Co., Tarrytown, N.Y.) has been adapted for hemagglutination, complement fixation, and the reagin test for syphilis (automated reagin test, ART). The Beckman Immunochemistry Analyzer in combination with a fixed volume diluter, a fixed volume dispenser, and an immunochemistry kit measures the change in light scattering from precipitin reactions. Centrifugal fast analyzers have been used in various immunological analyses.[182] Another interesting procedure, spin immunoassay, involves the detection of free radical groups by electron-spin resonance instrumentation. The free radical groups are immobilized by the interaction with antibody, and a flat curve is obtained rather than the sharp peaks characteristic of the nontreated controls.[183]

These technics range from fairly easy (miniaturized microtiter techniques) to difficult (electron-spin resonance immunoassays). Again the type of laboratory specimens most commonly encountered should dictate the type of instrumentation employed.

Immunoelectrophoretic technics; counterimmunoelectrophoresis

The combination of electrophoretic and immunologic technics results in a simple, rapid, and sensitive method for the detection and quantitation of many substances. The principles of this procedure were discussed earlier. Terms describing these procedures include **counterimmunoelectrophoresis** (CIE or CIEP), **immunoelectro-osmophoresis** (IEOP), and **immunoelectrophoresis** (IE or IEP). Penn and Batya have published a book on the interpretation of immunoelectrophoretic patterns.[184]

Electroimmunoassay procedures are sometimes termed **rocket immunoelectrophoresis** because of the final shape of the precipitin bands. This procedure was used to monitor polysaccharide production during the growth of *Streptococcus pneumoniae* type 2. Results were obtained in 3-4 hours as compared with 18-24 hours with standard methods.[185] **Immunoelectro-osmophoresis** has been used to identify antigenic groups of streptococci.[186] The authors report that the method is safe, specific, economical, and rapid.

Counterimmunoelectrophoresis (CIE) was used to detect *Clostridium perfringens* enterotoxin in human fecal samples and the antitoxin in sera within 1 day of reported illness.[187] CIE is successfully used in the diagnosis of bacterial meningitis. According to Colding and Lind,[188] compared with direct microscopy and culture CIE detected 55% of the etiologic agents, direct microscopy 77%, and culture 85%. However, a combination of direct microscopy and CIE led to a detection rate of 85%, and results were obtained within an hour.[188] The quality and specificity of the sera are important factors in the accuracy of these tests. Cross-reactions have been observed. Smaron[189] reports that from 10^5 to 10^7 colony-forming units (CFU) per milliliter were necessary to detect antigens of (1) group A, B, C, and D streptococci and *Neisseria meningitidis* group B (10^7 CFU/ml), (2) *Haemophilus influenzae* group B and *N. Meningitidis* group A and C (10^6 CFU/ml, and (3) *Streptococcus pneumoniae* (10^5 CFU/ml). Detailed procedures for detection of microbial antigens are given by Anhalt et al.[190] (See also Chapter 72.)

Rapid identification of blood culture isolates using CIE was reported using antisera for pneumococcal, meningococcal, *Klebsiella, H. influenzae* antigens, and staphylococcal teichoic acid antigens. Specific identification of 91% of the cultures containing either pneumococci, *Klebsiella, Haemophilus,* or meningococci was verified 24 hours earlier than by culture methods.[191] There are numerous other reports of this technic in the rapid identification of viruses, antibodies to *Treponema pallidum,* and enterotoxins.

In summary, immunoelectrophoretic technics are rapid, sensitive, and relatively easy to perform. Although no automated instrumentation exists, commerical kits are available (Hyland Laboratories, Costa Mesa, Calif.). The kit contains a disposable electrophoresis base unit with foil electrodes, a sponge, prepunched agar gel plates, barbital buffer solution, and a power supply.[192]

Immunoamplification technics

Enzyme-linked immunoassays and **radioimmunoassays** are 2 important technics that have greatly amplified the sensitivity of immunologic detection systems. The 2 methods compare favorably with each other in terms of sensitivity. They are more sensitive than immunofluorescence, hemagglutination, and complement-fixation technics. However, the radioimmunoassays require complex instrumentation (e.g., Geiger or scintillation counters). In addition the use of radionuclides such as ^{125}I and ^{14}C requires special permits, and rigid safety precautions must be followed in the use and disposal of these materials.

Enzyme-linked immunoassays, on the other hand, do not require complex instrumentation. The methods are simpler and easier to perform. The reagents are more stable and less expensive, and the procedures do not require elaborate safety precautions. For these reasons the enzyme-linked systems will probably find wide acceptance. **Coagglutination** procedures (see below) will probably also be widely used.

Enzyme-linked immunoassay procedures

Terms describing enzyme-linked immunoassay procedures include enzyme-immunoassay (EIA), enzyme-linked immunosorbent assay (ELISA), enzyme-linked immunocytochemical technic (ELICT), enzyme-multiplied immunoassay technic (EMIT), immunoperoxidase technic (IP or IPT), and conjugated-immunoglobulin technic (CIT). The most common term is ELISA (pronounced "Lisa"). Micro-ELISA tests are also performed. Several good articles and reviews are available[193,194]; in fact, an entire supplement to the *Journal of Infectious Diseases* is devoted to this subject,[193] and an excellent review appeared in the *Bulletin of the World Health Organization*.[195] Although peroxidase is the most common enzyme used, alkaline phosphatase, glucose oxidase, lysozyme, and β-galactosidase have also been employed.[196] Synthetic disaccharides have been used to elicit highly specific antibodies against 63 subgroups of salmonellae for these reactions.[197] The method can detect, among others, heat-labile *Escherichia coli* enterotoxin,[198] Epstein-Barr virus antigens,[199] capsular antigen of *Haemophilus influenzae* type b in clinical preparations,[200] and hepatitis A antigen in the stool (and antibody to this antigen in sera).[201] Aflatoxin was localized by ELICT.[202]

Compared with the usual hemagglutination assay, ELISA was more sensitive in detecting higher concentrations of IgG and IgM reacting with 0 antigens of *Escherichia coli* in the sera of patients with pyelonephritis. Sera of patients with asymptomatic bacteriuria did not react as strongly to these antigens. Different strains of *E. coli* not usually recovered from urinary tract infections elicited very little reaction.[203]

Instead of tube assays these technics have been miniaturized and performed in microplates. Antibodies to *Legionella pneumophila* (Legionnaires' disease organism),[204] *Salmonella* antigens,[205] staphylococcal enterotoxin A,[206] and hepatitis B antigen[207] were among those so adapted. Both macro-ELISA and micro-ELISA were used in detecting several parasitic infections. The micromethod was more sensitive than the macromethod, and both were more sensitive than immunofluorescence technics.[208]

These tests have been semiautomated. Saunders and Clinard[209] used an automatic pipetter and performed 96 tests in 30-60 minutes. They think it is applicable to large-scale screening of sera to detect animal diseases. "Hepanostika," a kit for hepatitis B surface antigen based on a ELISA system, is available (Organon Scientific Development Group, Atlanta). This kit can be further automated by using multichannel pipetters to add conjugate, substrate, and H_2SO_4 to develop this reaction.[210] It compares favorably with RIA. Leinikki and Passila discuss a quantitative semiautomated ELISA for the determination of virus antibodies that is controlled by a programmable calculator.[211] A colorimeter capable of reading results from micro-ELISA tests in microtiter plates has been described. It is capable of reading 96 specimens in approximately 5 minutes and is as accurate as a conventional spectrophotometer.[212] In an interesting adaptation of ELISA, antigens or antibodies were linked to magnetic polyacrylamide-agarose beads instead of microtiter plates. Peroxidase, glucose oxidase, or alkaline phosphatase was then conjugated to these beads. Magnets fixed to a rack were used to immobilize the beads during washing procedures. This eliminated centrifugation and excess handling. The best results were obtained with alkaline phosphatase.[213] The authors stress the need to individually determine the best enzyme for the desired antibody-antigen system.

Immunoelectrodiffusion methods have been linked with ELISA reactions. The precipitated immune complexes are taken up by the enzyme-conjugated antibodies specific to the immunoglobulins of each class. Termed ELIEDA (**enzyme-linked immunoelectron diffusion assay**), the method is very sensitive and specific. It has been used to explore humoral immunity in aspergillosis.[214]

A ciguatoxin assay has been developed using the ELISA technic. Since β-galactosidase is absent from fish tissues, this enzyme can be used in in the ELISA assay and applied directly to pieces of fish to determine the presence of the toxin.[215]

Radioimmunoassay

The concept underlying the second major amplification technic, radioimmunoassay (RIA), is discussed in detail in Volume I. If ^{14}C is used a Geiger or scintillation counter is necessary. For ^{125}I a gamma counter or scintillation counter is used. Occasionally ^{3}H and ^{57}Co are used. The β-radiation they emit can be also counted in a liquid scintillation counter. Here, for example, the x-radiation from the ^{125}I decay is turned into light in the scintillation module. The light pulse is detected by a photomultiplier tube, amplified, and recorded. Radioactive iodine is popular because it binds easily to tyrosine and sulfur-containing amino acids. When conjugated to an antigen or antibody the immunospecificity and the radioactivity of the radionuclide allow highly precise, rapid, quantitative analyses. Therefore these technics are more sensitive than immunofluorescence or competitive protein-binding methods. Radioimmunoassays have also been combined with precipitin reactions (**radioimmunoprecipitation,** RIP) and electrophoretic

Table 74-1. Instrumentation for detection and characterization

Procedure	Instrument	Principle	Comments
Methods of detection not requiring growth			
Particle counting	Coulter Counter	Bacteria in electrically conducting fluid alter current flux, which is translated into counts	Range of procedures; counting single cells; observation of agglutination reactions
Automatic image analysis and scanning	Omnicron pattern analyzer	Optical information is converted into electrical signals representing image brightness profiles	Counting bacteria; observing morphologic features ± inhibitors; TV display screen
Differential light scattering	Laser beam spectrometer Polar nephelometer	Photomultiplier tube detector converts light scattering into concentration curves	Detects microbial contamination if sufficient organisms (10^4) present; sensitive to morphologic changes
Luminescence	Simple photometers to complex detectors (Vitatect IIs), Pico-Lite	Light-emitting reactions (bio- and chemiluminescence) proportional to concentration of organisms present; based on presence of ATP, porphyrin, nitrogen	Rapid methods; porphyrin- or nitrogen-based procedures more stable and accurate than ATP
Impedance	Bactobridge	Presence of organisms based on altered relationships between voltage-current in impedance circuit	Presence of organisms or their products alter impedance compared with control; can monitor growth or inhibition also
Photoacoustic spectroscopy	Photoacoustic spectrometer	Laser beam chops light, absorbed light converted to heat, gas impinging on microphone, sound waves turned into electrical signal	Photoacoustic spectrum is characteristic of compound; complex procedure; similar to optical absorption spectra; rapid
Methods of detection requiring growth			
Nephelometry and turbidity	Simple measurements; photometers to complex semiautomated instrumentation such as the Autobac-1, Autobac-MTS, MS2, AMS-Automicrobic system, and laser beam spectrophotometers	Light-emitting diode photodetectors detect scattered light or turbidity resulting from growth of various organisms	Procedure can be used for growth inhibition studies as well. MS2 has kinetic data analysis capability (see also characterization and identification sections below)
Radiometric procedures	Bactec; various scintillation counters, Geiger and gamma counters	Detection of radionuclides from tagged substrates (e.g., production of $^{14}CO_2$ from ^{14}C-glucose or other compounds such as ^3H, ^{125}I, ^{57}Co	Detects growth of organisms isolated from various sources; also can be used for inhibition studies.
Chromatography	Simple thin-layer to complex gas chromatographs	Separation of components based on differential characteristics when partitioned between 2 phases	Detection of microbial end products and cellular constituents; pyrolysis, derivitization of nonvolatile compounds also possible
Ion-sensitive electrodes	Electrodes connected to detector such as pH meter	Production of volatile compounds such as H_2, CO_2, NH_3 (and pH) changes during growth can be measured	Rapid and sensitive method to detect growth or utilization of substrates
Calorimetry	Calorimeter, microcalorimeter	Detection of heat absorbed or evolved in various reaction systems during growth	Heat produced or absorbed proportional to growth or metabolic activity

Table 74-1. Instrumentation for detection and characterization—cont'd

Procedure	Instrument	Principle	Comments
Methods of identification and characterization			
Physical			
Nephelometry and turbidity	Laser beam spectrometer (Differential I, II, III)	Measurement of light scattering at different angles produces characteristic recognition patterns	Light-scattering patterns will change depending on growth conditions; inhibitory compounds change patterns diagnostically; sensitive method
	Autobac-1	Detects antibiotic susceptibilities based on differences in light scattering at a fixed angle	Can be used with growth-promoting and assimilation studies (e.g., fungi) and identification procedures
	MS2	Detects antibiotic susceptibilities based on kinetic (turbidimetric) data analyses obtained every 5 min	Can be used for other test systems also
	AMS-Automicrobic system	Turbidity detection of growth in selective media yields presumptive identification	Pure inoculum not necessary; presently for urine cultures but capabilities for other body fluids possible; antibiotic susceptibilities and other inhibition studies also possible
Calorimetry	See above	See above	Growth or lack of growth on various substrates yields characteristic identification patterns
Chromatography	See above	See above	Characteristic metabolites can be presumptively identified by comparison with known compounds
Mass spectroscopy	Mass spectrometer	Ionization of specimen results in fragmentation; fragment weights and patterns recorded to determine actual structure	Identification of characteristic metabolites in various fluids; usually used in conjunction with gas chromatography procedures
Electrophoresis	Electrophoresis instrumentation	Particles in solution move in electrical field depending on type of particle and surface charge	Identification of characteristic metabolites and cell constituents
Electron spin resonance and nuclear magnetic resonance	ESR and NMR instruments	Free radical groups are detected by electron spin and resonance detection	Characteristic curves obtained of metabolites having free radical groups or groups capable of detection by these procedures
Immunologic			
Immunoelectron microscopy	Transmission electron, scanning electron, and microprobe microscopes	Antibody-antigen reactions appear as "halo" of antibodies around antigen	Used particularly for rapid detection of viruses
Fluorescent technics	Fluorescent microscope, UV spectrophotometer, fluorimeter	Antibodies or antigens with fluorescent tag can be visualized either in situ or otherwise	Rapid detection of bacteria, fungi, viruses, or their products
Immunoelectrophoretic technics (e.g., counterimmunoelectrophoresis, electroimmunoassays)	Electrophoresis equipment	Precipitin reactions occur at proper concentrations, which are reached as antigens and antibodies move toward each other in electric field	Rapid detection of antigens *or* antibodies

Continued.

Table 74-1. Instrumentation for detection and characterization—cont'd

Procedure	Instrument	Principle	Comments
Immunoamplification technics			
Enzyme-linked immunoassays	Multichannel titrators	Enzyme is linked to antigen or antibody (which is immobilized); addition of enzyme substrate elicits reaction	Very sensitive detection system; likely will be used widely because ease of test and relatively inexpensive reagents
Radioimmunoassay	Geiger, gamma, or scintillation counters	^{125}I, ^{14}C, ^{3}H, ^{57}Co bound to antibody or antigen complex is detected and indicates that reaction occurred	Immunospecificity and radioactivity allow high precision and rapid analyses. Expensive reagents and equipment necessary
Coagglutination reactions (can also be coupled with ^{125}I or fluorescein)	Coulter counter, scintillation counter, fluorometer, or visual	Cowan-1 strain of *Staphylococcus aureus* contains protein A, which binds to immunoglobulin G (through Fc portion); Fab site can react with homologous antigen and agglutination reaction occurs	Rapid, sensitive method; pure cultures not necessary; detection possible on primary isolation plate; commercial source of protein A available also
Bacteriophage	Automated colony counter	Bacteriophage covalently bound to antigen or to antibody	No plaques formed if antigen-antibody reaction has occurred

technics (electroimmunodiffusion, **radioimmunoelectrophoresis,** and **radioimmunoelectrophoretic binding**). Initially developed for hormone analyses in the clinical chemical laboratory, the methodology has been successfully applied to numerous microbiologic studies.

Many kits are available from commercial sources for these assays. In addition automated and semiautomated equipment is available. The PRIAS system (Packard Instruments, Downers Grove, Ill.) is a newer one and consists of 3 independent units that can be used separately or combined to form a complete integrated system for radioassays of various types. The sample preparation system provides automated diluting and pipetting. The automatic γ- counting system was designed specifically for radioimmunoassays but can be used with other assays involving γ- counting as well. The liquid scintillation counting system has preset counting for ^{3}H, ^{125}I, and ^{14}C. Counting and data analysis are automated and programmed. A semiautomated instrument, "Concept 4" (Micromedic Systems, Horsham, Pa.), provides prepackaged and premeasured reagents in preloaded racks and automates the procedure after the sample is added. Auto-Assay (Salt Lake City) offers an RIA automatic instrument with a reusable antibody chamber and an automated flow-through system.

There are many reports on the use of this procedure in microbiology. Among the many viruses detected by this procedure are arboviruses,[216] measles,[217] herpes simplex,[218] and hepatitis viruses.[219] Bacteria,[220] fungi, and their products have also been identified by this procedure. They include group B streptococci,[221] *Fusobacterium polymorphum*,[222] cholera toxin and cholera toxin antibodies,[223] staphylococcal enterotoxins,[224, 225] meningococci,[226] *Candida* antibodies,[227] and the M antigen of histoplasmin.[228] Gentamicin serum levels[229] and netilmicin[230] have also been assayed by this procedure and detected in sera. Aminoglycoside-^{125}I RIA kits for gentamicin, tobramycin, and amikacin are available (Diagnostic Products Corp., Los Angeles). "Immunobeads" (BIO-RAD Laboratories, Richmond, Calif.), lyophilized micron-sized hydrophilic particles covalently bound to highly purified antibodies, can have radionuclides or enzymes bound to them for further amplification procedures.

Other immunoamplification technics
Coagglutination

The Cowan-1 strain of *Staphylococcus aureus* (ATCC 12598) is very rich in protein A on the outer surface and can bind immunoglobulin G (IgG) nonspecifically through the Fc portion of the immunoglobulin molecule. This leaves the Fab sites free to react with the homologous antigen. The reaction is visualized by the clumping or agglutinating reaction with staphylococci on a glass slide, in a tube, or directly on an agar plate. For example, after streaking for isolation, colonies of salmonellae could be identified directly on the Petri plate by detecting this reaction after a suspension of staphylococci conjugated with specific antisalmonella IgG antibodies is added. The procedure is very simple and does not require complex instrumentation or hazardous chemicals. It should become a routine screening technic in the clinical laboratory and could replace counterimmunoelectrophoresis and slide agglutination tests.

The Phadebact streptococcus test (Pharmacia Fine Chemicals, Piscataway, N.J.) is based on this technic and allows identification of groups A, B, D, and G β-hemolytic streptococci. However, this strain of staphylococci is available from the American Type Culture Collection (Rockville, Md.), and the conjugation reactions with IgG are not too difficult to perform.[231] The Phadebact gonococcus test has been favorably evaluated.[232] Coagglutination has been used for the detection of rubella-specific immunoglobulin M antibodies,[233] toxoplasmosis,[234] and influenza virus.[235]

Protein A has been purified from *Staphylococcus aureus* and coupled with fluorescein isothiocyanate (FITC), a fluorescent molecule, without any loss of biologic activity (Pharmacia Fine Chemicals). The freeze-dried preparation is stable for 2 years at below 8 C. Thus immune reactions involving FITC-protein A-IgG-antigen can now be detected by a more sensitive fluorescent marker. Innumerable semiautomated or manual spectrophotometers with fluorescent capabilities can be used to detect these reactions.

Other adaptations of this method include fluorescein-conjugated staphylococcal protein A complexed to antibodies[236] and ^{125}I-conjugated staphylococcal protein A coupled to antibody or antigen to detect type A human influenza virus. It was found to be 10-20 times as sensitive as hemagglutination inhibition tests and complement fixation tests.[237] Radioimmunoassays of C-type virus polypeptide have been improved by coupling ^{125}I with the staphylococcal protein A conjugate.[238]

Bacteriophage amplification

Bacteriophage can be covalently bound to antigens. On reaction with specific antibody the phage is no longer infectious and no plaques will appear.[194]

Liposome amplification

If a liposome containing a marker is labeled with antigen and reacted with specific antibody and complement, the bilayer is disrupted and the marker is released.[194]

Immunoaffinity chromatography

Cyanogen bromide–activated Sepharose and bromelain-extracted hemagglutinin were prepared. Antisera were run through the column, and the antibodies were fractionated according to their affinity. Thus antisera in rabbits prepared against several closely related influenza A_3 strains could be ordered in the degree of antigenic similarity of the hemagglutinins.[239]

MINIATURIZED SYSTEMS

Since 1947 when Weaver and colleagues first started adding concentrated inocula to different kinds of media in minute tubes and other containers, miniaturized systems and rapid detection methods have gained steadily in popularity.[240] A great variety of kits that cover many different procedures are available commercially. These range from enumeration of organisms in urine specimens and determination of antibiotic susceptibilities to more complex identification systems based on biochemical and immunologic characteristics. A detailed comparison of all major systems discussed in this section is shown in Table 74-2.

Increased use of discardable plastic items paved the way for the development of disposable multiwelled dishes of various shapes and sizes such as microtiter plates, wheels, plastic "cards," trays, or the multisectioned AIM-4 Petri dishes. Several reviews have covered the use of microtiter plates and other miniaturized microbiologic technics.[5,241,242] Many of these systems contain dehydrated media in wells or prepared solid media in tubes or ready-made substrates in disks, tablets, or strips. If purchased in 100-unit lots they are usually cheaper than conventional tubed media. Most kits are convenient to use and substantially reduce the amount of time spent in routine preparation and disposal procedures. Some of the tests are more rapid than others (e.g., Micro-ID can be read as early as 4 hours compared with 18-24 hours for most of the others). In addition identification charts, computer-aided data analyses of varying complexity, and toll-free information services are usually available from the manufacturers. The clinical laboratory has greatly profited from miniaturized methods, and the majority of kits are geared toward identification of organisms of medical and veterinary importance. This includes organisms isolated from clinical specimens, foods, and the environment. Identification procedures include those for *Enterobacteriaceae*, other aerobic and anaerobic gram-negative and gram-positive organisms, and yeasts. The presumptive detection of bacteriuria, MIC determinations, and enzyme screens have also been miniaturized.

These kits are not a panacea for the diagnostic ills that may befall a laboratory. Good microbiology laboratory procedures still need to be stressed including quality control procedures as well as sterile isolation and transfer technics. Staining reactions and colonial characteristics should coincide with the biochemical data. It is necessary to follow the manufacturers' directions **exactly** and interpret color reactions according to their schemes. A red reaction might indicate a positive result in 1 kit and a negative result in another. Some kits are presumptive screens only and do not replace conventional methods.

Smith[244] writes, "The accuracy of identification of cultures depends on correct biochemical results, obviously, but also on the identification scheme provided by the manufacturer. Most such schemes (for *Enterobacteriaceae*), where used, depend on key reactions such as H_2S and indole production for identification. If these key reactions are correct, but some other reactions incorrect, it is still possible to arrive at a correct identification. For example, a urease and phenylalanine deaminase positive, H₂S negative culture is probably *Proteus vulgaris* or *P. mirabilis*, and the V-P reaction is unimportant. Conversely, however, an erroneous key reaction may very quickly lead to an incorrect identification, even if the other test results are correct.

These biochemical reactions are usually based on standard methods covered elsewhere in this text. Some important modifications are discussed as well as the methods, efficacy, and accuracy of the tests.

Identification of *Enterobacteriaceae*

Probably over 50% of the organisms isolated from blood and urine specimens in the hospital microbiology laboratory are members of the *Enterobacteriaceae*. It is no surprise that the majority of kits either are primarily designed for this group or include it. Presently at least 9 identification kits are marketed for these organisms; the major ones are discussed in detail. A comparison of methods is included at the end of the section.

r/b Enteric differential system

This agar-based method (Corning Medical Diagnostics, Roslyn, N.Y.) is probably closest to conventional tests. Up to 14 biochemical reactions are available. The system, named after its inventors (Rollender and Beckford) includes 4 tubes, 2 basic and 2 "expanders," each with a constriction near the lower end to prevent mixing and diffusion of the ingredients. These are inoculated by touching a needle (the last ¼ inch is bent back on itself) to an isolated colony and inoculating the bottom of the tube. The upper slant is streaked as the needle is withdrawn. The second tube and optional expander(s) are similarly inoculated without flaming the needle in between tubes or touching another colony. After 18-24 hour incubation at 35-37 C, results are recorded and compared with the *Enteric Analyzer*, an identification guide furnished by the manufacturer. Laboratory evaluations indicate an overall accuracy of 90-99%.[245-248] Over 2000 clinical isolates were identified by this system without any difficulty.[248] About 13% of these were atypical strains. The motility test was the most unreliable but did not result in misidentification.

Enterotube II

This system (Roche Diagnostics, Nutley, N.J.) consists of a plastic shell containing 12 compartments (providing 15 tests) and a special integrated inoculating needle that can be touched to an isolated colony and pulled lengthwise through the tube, thus inoculating all of the compartments. After 18-24 hour incubation the biochemical reactions are compared with those in a manual (*Enterotube II Computer Coding and Identification System*) containing identification keys and numerical codes. This represents a large data base using either a binomial computer system or a 4-digit reference number. Both are available from the manufacturer. A toll-free phone line and consultation laboratory service is also available. The test is easy to perform but has a short shelf life (3-5 months) and is fairly inflexible. However, it has been evaluated by several laboratories and has proved 91-98% accurate.[249-251] Maloway et al. bypassed primary isolation and inoculated Enterotube with broth from positive blood culture bottles. Of 200 isolates 189 were correctly identified within 18 hours (95%) by this method.[252]

Minitek

This system (BioQuest, Cockeysville, Md.) is quite flexible. It allows the investigator to select the desired tests from a battery of 34 cartridges, each of which contains paper disks impregnated with either a biochemical or a reagent. Ten selected cartridges at a time are placed in a dispenser that drops the disks into a sterile 12-well plastic tray. Two additional disks can be added manually by a single-cartridge dispensing unit if desired. An isolated colony is suspended in 1.0 ml Minitek inoculum broth. A pipet or Minitek pipette is used to add 0.05 ml suspension to each well; mineral oil is then added. The plates can be incubated aerobically in a humidified atmosphere provided by a moistened sponge in a container, a "humidor," or anaerobically in a suitable anaerobic chamber. A color comparator card is available to help interpret the results. A toll-free phone line is also available for consultation. Good agreement (91-100%) with conventional systems was reported.[253-255] Cox and Mercuri reported rapid confirmation of suspect *Salmonella* species with this method.[256] Although used most often for enteric organisms, the variety of tests allows identification of a wide range of organisms including *Yersinia enterocolitica*,[257] *Haemophilus*,[258] and other organisms.[259] Because of its broad application it is mentioned under other categories in this section.

API

The API system (Analytab Products, Plainview, N.Y.) consists of a series of miniaturized identification kits for gram-negative aerobes, anaerobes, yeasts, and yeastlike fungi. **API 20E** is used for the identification of *Enterobacteriaceae*, nonfermentative gram-negative rods, and other gram-negative rods (see below). The **API 50E** plate, used for research purposes or in-house use only, is an expanded 20E card and is used to identify the same organisms as the API 20E. A **10S** card is used as a presumptive preliminary screen for possible enteric organisms. All of these kits use the same basic procedure and format consisting of cupules in a plastic strip or plate.

The API 20E system (Fig. 74-18) consists of 20 cupules with a preset battery of 21 biochemical tests that are highly useful for the identification

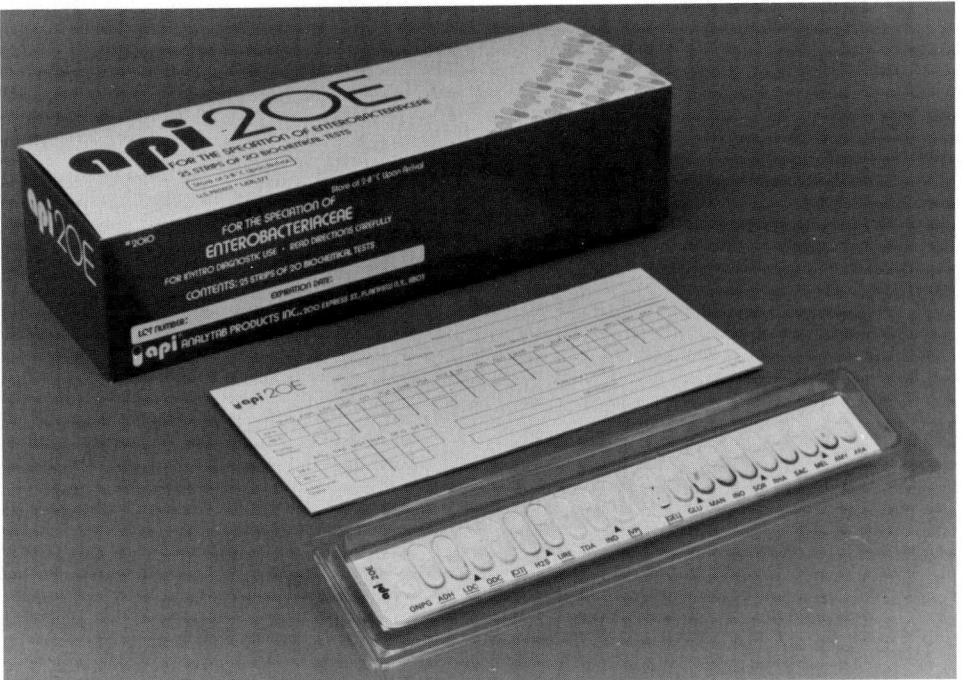

Fig. 74-18. API 20E. Miniaturized diagnostic kit for biochemical identification of *Enterobacteriaceae.* Individual cupules contain dehydrated substrates and other biochemicals. (Courtesy Analytab Products, Plainview, N.Y.)

of *Enterobacteriaceae* in 18-24 hours. Nitrate reduction can also be done in the glucose cupule, but the oxidase reaction is not done on the strip. The small cupules contain dehydrated media and substrates. A loopful of bacteria is suspended in 5 ml sterile saline and drawn up into a Pasteur pipet. The cupules are then carefully filled. Mineral oil is added to 4 designated cupules. The strips are housed in moistened small plastic chambers and incubated for 18-24 hours after the addition of reagents to 3 cupules. The results, expressed as a 7-digit profile (for *Enterobacteriaceae* and other gram-negative bacteria), are compared with the API Analytical Profile Index. To identify other gram-negative rods and nonfermenters additional testing includes nitrate reduction, gas production, growth on MacConkey's agar, OF glucose, and motility media. These are then used to generate a 9-digit profile number. The company offers a complimentary computer service by either telephone or direct computer access. A toll-free information service and reference laboratory is also available.

The system has been favorably evaluated in North America,[260-262] Europe,[263] and Japan.[264] The API 20E system is by far the most widely used micromethod for the identification of *Enterobacteriaceae* in the United States.[265] It has the largest computer data base with which to compare the reaction of unknown bacteria; the base is continually updated. The API 50E is not sold commercially but is used in-house to increase the data base and is also available to microbiologists

for research purposes. Cox et al.[362] found that both the API-50 and conventional methods were negative after 48 hours with some slower-growing organisms. Since strips are routinely incubated in nonsterile moistened small plastic containers, dehydration and spore contamination sometimes cause problems of interpretation. For this reason, Analytab Products suggests that API strips not be incubated for lengthy periods. For laboratories wishing to use fewer initial tests there is an API presumptive screen (API 10), which correctly identifies 96% of the isolates to the genus level.[267] In a comparison of the API 20E, Enterotube, and r/b systems, using results of the College of American Pathologists Survey (including 4 species of *Enterobacteriaceae*, i.e., *Serratia marcescens, Proteus stuartii, Klebsiella pneumoniae,* and *Citrobacter freudii*), Marymont et al.[265] noted that API 20E arrived at the correct identifications (to both genus and species) significantly more often than any other method including conventional methods. Washington[266] stated in 1976 that "API currently represents the most complete and most accurate kit for speciation of *Enterobacteriaceae.*" Holmes et al.[261] were able to identify 88% of 206 strains (many atypical), compared with 94% by conventional methods, and suggested some improvements. Other workers cited 82-96% accuracy.[260-262, 268, 269, 361] No differences in results were noted when the API 20E was inoculated with 4-6 hour tryptic soy broth cultures (from positive blood cultures containing gram-negative bacilli) compared with the recommended method of inoculation.[270] The API 20E was also used to study the effect of plasmids on the biotypes of *Escherichia coli* K-12 strains.[271]

Entero-Set

The former Inolex and Auxotab sets are now marketed as the Entero-Set (Fisher Scientific Co., Orangeburg, N.Y.). The kit consists of plastic cards with 10 or 20 capillary molded compartments containing a bulge in the middle (where anaerobic conditions exist) and a small air hole at the end to displace the air after inoculating. Thus with reazurin as an indicator various degrees of oxidation-reduction can be observed. The reagents are impregnated on a filter paper layer sandwiched between the top and bottom of the compartment.

Several methods are available. The 3-hour determination of organisms in a positive blood culture bottle requires 2-3 centrifugations. The first sediments the blood, the second pelletizes the cells and removes the culture broth. If the pellet is still oxidase positive a third centrifugation is required. The pellet is resuspended to a turbidity matching a McFarland no. 5 standard, and 5 drops are added to each compartment. In the 7-hour technic an isolated colony is added to prewarmed broth and incubated for 3-4 hours until the turbidity matches a McFarland no. 3 standard. After centrifugation the pellet is resuspended in saline to a turbidity equivalent to a McFarland no. 5 standard and the card is inoculated. In the 24-hour technic an isolated colony is resuspended in 2 ml saline and the card is inoculated. The cards are incubated in individual plastic containers. If many specimens are to be tested, centrifugation can be tedious and time consuming. The system is based on the presence of preformed enzymes to obtain the desired reactions, and the directions must be followed **exact-ly**. Too few cells or dead or starved cells can cause poor results. Earlier workers had difficulty with these tests.[243] The system has been improved and the accuracy greatly increased, but dead or starved cells can still give positive results with some tests.[272, 273] Thioglycollate and other media that sometimes contain a small amount of agar should not be used with these kits. The agar pelletizes with the cells and tends to clog the capillaries. Other problems involve difficulty in obtaining enough inoculum when pelletizing to reach the required turbidity.

PathoTec

The PathoTec rapid ID test system (General Diagnostics Division, Warner-Lambert, Morris Plains, N.J.) is a flexible diagnostic kit. There are 12 different reagent-impregnated strips available. The test is based on enzymatic reactions with heavy suspensions of organisms placed in small tubes. A different strip is added to each tube. Since results are obtained within 4 hours, sterility is not a factor. In some cases such as the cytochrome oxidase test the colony can be rubbed directly on the strips. A numeric system and consultation are available. The strips are stable for 1-2 years if kept dry. Goldschmidt and Fung,[5] and Cox et al.[243] have reviewed this technic including reports of its use dating from 1965. The overall accuracy ranged from 80-100%, depending on the strips employed. The citrate and lysine strips were the least dependable in the hands of some workers. Smith et al.[274] compared this system with standard tube methods using 471 cultures of *Enterobacteriaceae*. They reported 94-96% accuracy in 4910 comparisons of individual tests and concluded that it was a flexible and accurate method. This system can also be used for *Haemophilus*, facultative gram-positive cocci, anaerobes, and gram-negative nonfermenters.[243]

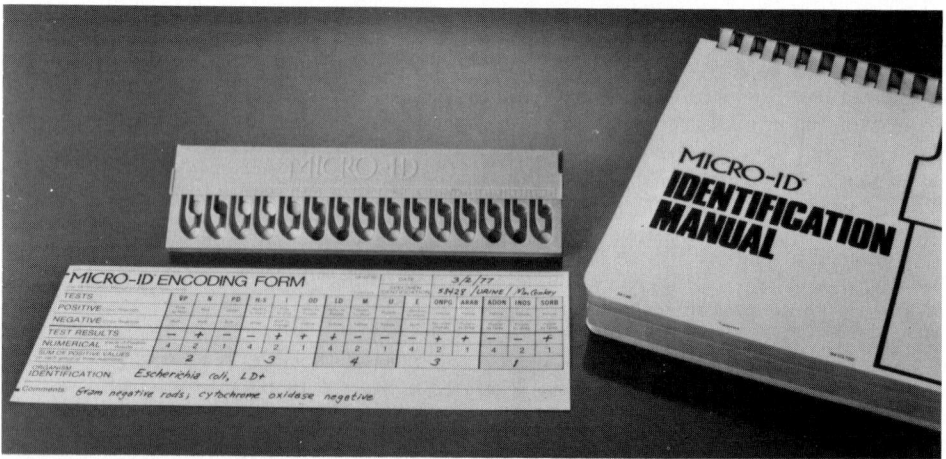

Fig. 74-19. Micro-ID 4-h identification system for 30 enteric organisms. Unit is inoculated and incubated upright for 4 h, rotated to moisten upper disks, and results identified by use of manual. (Courtesy General Diagnostics Division of Werner-Lambert Co., Morris Plains, N.J.)

Micro-ID

The Microbiological Identification (Micro-ID) system (General Diagnostics) is an extension of the PathoTec reagent-impregnated strip system described above. This system consists of a hard molded plastic tray with 15 "reaction chambers" and a hinged cover (Fig. 74-19). The first 5 chambers contain a substrate and a reaction disk; the remaining 10 contain a single "substrate-detection" disk. The surface of the tray is covered with a clear plastic tape. As with the PathoTec system, sterility is not necessary, as a concentrated suspension of organisms is used that has a minimal turbidity matching a 0.5 McFarland standard (usually several colonies in 3-5 ml saline). Approximately 0.2 ml suspension is added to the inoculation wells at the top of the tray. The cover is closed, and the tray is incubated in an upright position. The organism will wet the bottom disks but not the reaction disks, which are located in an area above the substrate disks in the first 5 chambers. After 4-hour incubation KOH is added to the Voges-Proskauer chamber only. The unit is rotated clockwise 90° to wet the upper reaction disks, and the reactions are read and interpreted according to the manufacturer's instructions. This system has less flexibility than PathoTec, as there is no choice of tests unless portions of the tray are deliberately not inoculated. The unopened pouches are sealed in foil and must be kept refrigerated until needed and used before an expiration date. In addition this system is recommended for use only with 18- to 24-hour cultures of gram-negative, cytochrome oxidase–negative organisms. Cox reported a 98% agreement with conventional methods when the Micro-ID system was used with *Enterobacteriaceae* freshly isolated from foods.[275] A 98.5% agreement was reported when over 350 fresh clinical isolates and 50 stock cultures were tested.[276] These authors also noted that stock cultures required a higher inoculum. Other workers reported a 96% correlation with organisms isolated from blood and urine.[277]

MicroDilution system (MDS)

The manufacturer (Micro Media Systems, Campbell, Calif.) markets several systems: Micro-ID, MIC/ID, and MMS identification systems. To avoid confusion with the Micro-ID system of General Diagnostics, the term MDS is used here. The identification panels consist of plastic trays with wells, each containing 100 μl **frozen** media containing various biochemicals, antibiotics, or other antimicrobial agents. Several colonies are suspended in 0.5 ml brain-heart infusion (BHI) broth and incubated 4-6 hours at 37 C.

The inoculum (0.05 ml) is pipetted into 9 ml sterile water containing 0.02% Tween 80. The inoculum is poured into the "seed trough." In the Quad panels the seed trough has 4 different compartments, 1 for each of the 4 organisms. The Combo and MIC panels have only 1 compart-ment. The inoculum for these are prepared in the same manner, but a volume of 25 ml is used. The pronged lid (transfer lid) on the seed trough is used to transfer the inoculum to the panel. The prongs pick up approximately 5 μl inoculum. The lid is lifted from the seed tray and placed on the panel. The inoculum is pulled off the prongs by capillary action when they touch the media in the panel. Some of the wells must be covered with plastic. Directions also include punching holes in the plastic over some of the wells. Panels are incubated in a non-CO_2 incubator for 18 hours at 35 C.

The 4 sections of the Enteric Quad panel each contain 20 biochemicals, thus allowing 4 separate aerobic, gram-negative, and dextrose-fermenting bacterial rods to be identified on the same plate. The Enteric Combo panel combines 20 bio-chemicals (21 identification tests) with several dilutions of 9 antibiotics and 2 other antimicrobial agents for simultaneous identification and MIC interpretation of 1 organism. The Strep Quad panel for gram-positive aerobes is similar in design and function to the Enteric Quad panel and contains 16 biochemicals. The Strep Combo panel combines 15 biochemicals and several dilutions of 8 antibiotics and 2 other antimicrobial agents for the simultaneous identification and MIC interpretation of 1 organism. The gram-positive MIC panel (for 1 organism) contains several dilutions of 9 antibiotics and 2 other antimicrobial agents. The gram-negative urinary tract infection MIC panel contains dilutions for 11 antibiotics and 3 other antimicrobial agents and is used for a single organism. It is multi-purpose as it can be used for MIC determinations with all gram-negative and gram-positive organisms isolated from urinary tract infections as well as gram-negative organisms isolated from any other site. An anaerobe MIC panel containing dilutions of 6-10 antibiotics is undergoing final evaluation. Sterility and growth control wells are provided with all MIC panels. The identification tests are read against an indirectly lighted background and the antibiotics and antimicrobial agents against a dark background. A data interpretation manual, *Biotype Code Book,* is provided by the manufacturer, as is a toll-free phone line consultation with a computer data-based information retrieval system. Reference laboratory service is also available.

Borchardt and Gibson[278] indicated a 98% agreement of the MDS Enteric Quad system (MMES) with conventional methods. They felt that this system had significant advantages in several aspects including ease of inoculation, interpretation, and cost. Johnson[279] also felt the MMES was a good system. Aldridge et al.[268] reported a 90% identification when 373 organisms were tested by this procedure. However, they also reported that only 74% of the plates had sufficient numbers of colonies to produce the required density. This could pose a problem with this method. The antimicrobial susceptibility data appear to have a good correlation with conventional methods.

AIM-4

This system (Axford International, Markham, Ontario) allows simultaneous identification and MIC susceptibility testing of up to 37 organisms at a time. Although discussed briefly in the section on instrumentation, it is also included here because it is possible to use the system manually. A total of 21 biochemicals are individually added to special Petri plates and solidified with agar. The plate is partitioned into 37 diamond-shaped sections by plastic dividers. At present similarly divided plates containing antimicrobials must be made by the investigator pending FDA approval for distribution in the United States. Isolated colonies are suspended in Micron Broth (provided by the manufacturer), assigned a number, and added to the inoculator well plate. Up to 37 organisms can be added per well plate. A replicator head with disposable pins transfers the organisms to the plates. This can be performed manually. However, the manufacturer sells a semiautomated instrument with a rotating turntable for this purpose. After overlaying 3 of the plates with mineral oil the plates are incubated for 18 hours. Another instrument greatly aids pattern analysis: buttons corresponding to color changes (or growth for antibiotic plates) can be entered in the instrument, which then processes the data and prints identity, biochemical reactions, and breakpoint MIC susceptibility. The AIM-4 data can be interpreted by other computer systems. The manufacturer provides update and enlargement of memory base within a year of purchase. No in-use data have yet been published. This system is for *Enterobacteriaceae* and gram-negative non-glucose-fermenters only.

MORLOC

Although the MORLOC system (Biotrol Co., Jamaica, N.Y.) is a lesser known system, users claim that it appears to be as accurate (96%) as the API system with more reproducibility and less cost and is easier to use.[280,281] Six doughnut-shaped disks (Bioloops) are contained on a flat, flexible card 2½ in. square. The card is placed in a Petri dish containing moistened filter paper. A saline suspension is prepared from an overnight triple sugar iron (TSI) slant and added by Pasteur pipet to the center of the disks. The Bioloops contain a growth medium and the components *m*eliobiose, *O*NPG, *r*hamnose, *l*ysine, *o*rnithine, and *c*itrate (hence the name of the test). The heavy inoculum provides results after overnight incubation, as both growth and preformed enzymatic activity are present. A 3-digit "numeric signature" is formed using a 4-2-1 coding system. The reactions on TSI and MacConkey media provide supplementary tests. Occasionally arabinose, sorbitol, motility, and urea tests are also needed. The manufacturer provides an interpretation system.

Metatec S-4

Metatec S-4 (Biotrol Co.) is a test strip containing 4 reagents (urea, ONPG, tryptophan deaminase, and indole) for rapid (3 hours or less) identification of enteric organisms in stool cultures. An isolated colony is picked from the plates and added to 0.3 ml saline in a small tube. The strip is dropped in and incubated.

Repliscan

This system was mentioned earlier in the section on instrumentation. The "repliplates" represent a miniaturized system in which 36 different organisms can be replicated on 1 plate. Several antibiotic and 16 different biochemical plates are available. Colonies are first incubated in broth; each culture is pipetted into an individual well in the inoculum holder. A replicator head transfers the cultures to the plates. After 18-24 hour incubation 32 plates are oriented in a special carrier tray so that the same organism is simultaneously scanned on all plates through viewing windows. Light-sensitive diodes signal results to the computer, which scans the data bank and prints sensitivity and identity data.

Comparison of technics and kits

There are several reports and reviews of the systems used in the identification of the *Enterobacteriaceae*.[5,240-244] In a comparison of the MMES (MDS) system with the API 20E Aldridge et al. found both systems performed equally well.[268] Johnson also compared MMES (MDS) with API 20E and found them equivalent but thought the API system was easier to use.[279] Of over 300 organisms identified by API 20E and conventional methods, 95% or higher were also correctly identified by the Micro-ID system.[276,282] Hayek and Willis[262] compared Enterotube and API 20E to conventional methods and reported that Enterotube identified 93% of these correctly, while API 20E identified 100%. The results of a study of 390 organisms by 3 separate hospital microbiology laboratories comparing API 20E and r/b with each other and with conventional tube methods were interesting.[283] There were no significant differences in the ability of the 3 methods to identify these organisms to genus and species. However, the ability of the system to reproduce the same results on different occasions was 61% for r/b, 45% for API 20E, and 60% for the conventional methods, pointing out a "limited usefulness of these systems for biochemical biotyping." Combined use of the Micro-ID system with the Autobac-1 offered final culture and susceptibility results within 24 hours for urine specimens as well as preliminary results for blood cultures in 4 hours after detection. The Micro-ID system identified 96% of 166 isolates compared with API 20E profiles.[277] Guthertz and Okoluk[284] compared the ability of several tests to identify members of *Enterobacteriaceae* to the genus and species level. They reported that agreement with conventional methods included

93% for PathoTec, 94% for both API 20E and Inolex (now Entero-Set), and 97% for Minitek. API 20E and Minitek were superior for speciation.

The 3-hour Entero-Set was used in conjunction with the Bactec instrument for rapid detection and identification of organisms in blood cultures.[285] The authors found that the Entero-Set successfully identified the majority of the *Enterobacteriaceae* and indicated the presence of nonfermenters such as *Pseudomonas* and *Acinetobacter* species. They cautioned that this rapid test should only be considered presumptive. Blood cultures should always be streaked for isolation, since occasionally more than 1 organism may be present. In a comparison of API 20E and the r/b system in identifying 373 strains of *Enterobacteriaceae* from poultry and meat products, the agreement in classification between the 2 systems was found to be 59%. API classified 82% of the isolates and the r/b system 72% when compared with conventional methods rather than each other. The *Klebsiella-Enterobacter-Serratia* group gave the most trouble.[268a] The authors concluded that these kits were less efficient with isolates from food products compared with the high degree of accuracy found with clinical isolates.

The usefulness of the *Enteric Analyzer,* the manual provided by Corning Medical Diagnostics for use with the r/b system, was evaluated using biochemical results obtained from r/b, Minitek, and conventional methods. With this manual conventional methods were 77% accurate, r/b 74% accurate, and Minitek 60.5%. The analyzer does not consider delayed reactions, and this probably accounted for the low percentages.[286]

Identification of nonfermentative and other gram-negative rods

Several systems are available for the identification of nonfermenting gram-negative organisms (e.g., *Pseudomonas, Moraxella, Alcaligenes, Acinetobacter,* and *Bordetella*) as well as non-*Enterobacteriaceae* fermenters (e.g., *Yersinia enterocolitica, Vibrio, Aeromonas*).

Oxi/Ferm

This kit is similar in construction to the Enterotube and is also marketed by Roche Diagnostics (Nutley, N.J.). One plastic tube contains 8 individual compartments, each containing a separate substrate; in all, 9 tests can be done. An integrated inoculating needle is used to touch the colonies. The media are inoculated when the needle is pulled back through the center of the tube. It is reinserted into the last 3 compartments and broken off. A trypticase soy (TS) plate is inoculated at the same time, and both are incubated at 37 C for 48 hours. An oxidase test is done and together with the other tests forms a 4-digit number, the "ID Value." Supplemental tests are suggested for organisms having the same ID Value. Fifty different ID Values are provided, but only 10 correspond to a single species or genus. The other 40 (80%) require from 1-9 supplemental tests, since 2-6 possible organisms have identical initial ID Values. Organisms that cannot grow on the TS plate are not considered identifiable by the Oxi/Ferm procedure.

Shayegani et al.[287] evaluated this system and reported that it was only 41% accurate at the species level and 60.4% at the genus level. *Pseudomonas* and *Acinetobacter* species were identified correctly, but 27% of the organisms included in the identification guides were misidentified and 16.7% were not listed. They concluded that it could not be used in the reference laboratory. Other evaluations gave higher (43-98%) correlations.[288-292] When reproducibility of the method was evaluated on duplicates of 200 clinical isolates at 2 different times by 2 different workers, 75% of the results were identical, while 18% were identified as the same species but with different ID Values. The arginine dihydrolase and N_2 gas production were the 2 tests with the greatest discrepancies.[293]

When the time involved in identification was compared with conventional methods the Oxi-Ferm actually took longer due to the required 48-hour incubation period followed by the suggested supplemental tests.[289]

API 20E

Although the API 20E system was originally designed for identification of *Enterobacteriaceae,* it is now used also for other gram-negative rods by adding several other tests and when needed incubating for 36-48 hours. In a study involving 221 nonfermenting isolates[294] the biochemicals were in close agreement with conventional method results, but only 50% of the isolates were correctly identified to the genus level and only 22% to species and biotype. When the expected level of identification was based on the API *Analytical Profile Index* and reaction chart 43% of the isolates included in the API system were identified. Similar to the comments on the Oxi/Ferm system, the authors thought the API 20E to be useful in the clinical laboratory but not accurate enough for a reference laboratory. Dowda[295] obtained better results (see Comparative investigations below).

Uni-N/F Tek

Uni-N/F Tek (Corning Medical Diagnostics, Roslyn, N.Y.) is an identification system for gram-negative nonfermenters (N/F) consisting of 2 tubes and a wheel with 12 wells (Fig. 74-20). Each well contains a different substrate or reagent. Since the bulk of nonfermenters in the clinical laboratory are *Pseudomonas* species, the 2 tubes act as a preliminary screen for these organisms. One is incubated at 42 C to observe growth and pigment (pyocyanin) production at that temperature, and the other (GN/F tube), constricted in the middle, screens for fluorescence,

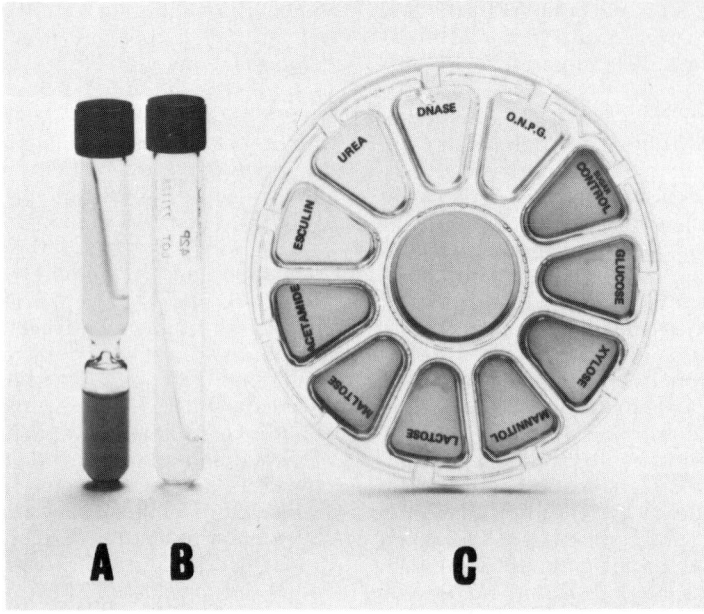

Fig. 74-20. Uni-N/F Tek System for identification of nonfermenters consists of 2 tubes and a wheel. Tubes are preliminary screens. **A,** GN/F tube is constricted in middle and screens for fluorescence, glucose fermentation, and N₂ production. **B,** Tube is incubated at 42 C and screens for growth and pigment (pyocyanin) production. **C,** Wheel contains other diagnostic substrates. (Courtesy Corning Medical Diagnostics, Roslyn, N.J.)

glucose fermentation, and N₂ production. If *Pseudomonas* species are not present a heavy suspension of cells from the GN/F tube is prepared in 2 ml sterile distilled water; 1 drop is added to each of the 12 wells. The medium in the center well is designed to detect H₂S production and should be deeply stabbed. Supplemental tests are suggested when necessary. Identification is by a simple logic scheme and a computerized coding system. Toll-free technical assistance is available. This system has been favorably evaluated. Using this procedure reaction patterns of 718 nonfermenting oxidase-positive gram-negative rods were compared with those generated by conventional procedures, with 86% identified in 24 hours. This included 23 species. *Pseudomonas aeruginosa* (87%) and both *Acinetobacter calcoaceticus* var. *antitratus* and *P. maltophilia* (95% each) were correctly identified.[296] This system appears to be more accurate than the Oxi/Ferm on the basis of initial evaluations. The GN/F tube used in this system is also marketed separately by Corning as a UNI-OF glucose tube, 1 of 6 carbohydrate tubes for oxidation and fermentation test (O-F) in a single reaction tube.

Other systems

Micro Media Systems will be marketing an MDS system for gram-negative urinary tract infection MIC panel to be used with all gram-negative organisms from any body site. The procedures have been discussed in the section on kits for *Enterobacteriaceae*. The Minitek sys-

tem can also be used to identify this group of organisms.

Comparative investigations

Dowda[295] compared the Oxi/Ferm and the expanded API 20E systems in identifying 176 commonly encountered oxidase-positive or nonfermenting gram-negative rods. API 20E identified 61% without computer assistance from API and 25% more (total of 86%) after consultation, with 14% misidentified, not identified completely, or not identified at all. Oxi/Ferm correctly identified 75% initially and an additional 19% after supplemental testing; 4.5% were misidentified. Three other comparisons of these 2 systems indicated that they were about equal in their ability to identify this group of organisms and had the same degree of reproducibility. Oxi/Ferm and API 20E usually need some supplemental tests and computer consultation. Most of the misidentification or other difficulties occurred with atypical organisms.[292,297,298] Oxi/Ferm, Minitek, and the expanded API 20E were compared with conventional methods by Bannister et al.[299] Using 150 organisms they found that the API 20E had an 88% agreement, Minitek 80%, and Oxi/Ferm 87%. All easily identified *Pseudomonas aeruginosa*, but more variation was found with the non-*P. aeruginosa* organisms. They also noted that API was unable to speciate 8% of the organisms, Minitek 9%, and Oxi/Ferm 21%. In summary it appears that there is a rather remarkable variation in the reported accuracy of these kits to identify this group of organisms. Reports ranging from 40-98% correlation are difficult to assess. Suggested supplemental tests are very often necessary, sometimes extending the actual time of testing beyond that of conventional methods. Laboratories contemplating the use of any of these systems would be well advised to first conduct fairly extensive testing in parallel with conventional methods.

Anaerobe identification kits
API 20 anaerobe system (API 20A)

The basic API system and the inoculation procedures have been previously described. The anaerobic API system has 16 carbohydrate-containing cupules, with the 4 others containing gelatin, esculin, urea, and a medium for indole production. Several colonies from a purified culture are suspended in 4 ml API anaerobic suspension medium (Lombard-Dowell medium), keeping conditions as anaerobic as possible. The final density should be equivalent to the no. 1 McFarland standard. The tubes are inoculated aerobically (unless an anaerobic chamber or glovebox is used) and then incubated anaerobically either in a glovebox or anaerobe chamber (a gas atmosphere of 85% N_2, 10% H_2, and 5% CO_2 is recommended). A GasPak anaerobic jar (B-D Laboratories, East Rutherford, N.J.) containing a special API convertor rack that will hold several strips can also be used. In addition other types of anaerobe jars or large glass tubes are available from most scientific supply houses. Palladium catalysts and appropriate gas mixtures are necessary with these chambers. Two blood agar plates should also be streaked, 1 incubated anaerobically and the other aerobically or in a candle jar. Explicit directions on the procedure are given and should be followed. The same bacterial suspension should also be used to inoculate supplemental media such as egg yolk agar, medium for GLC analysis, and a holding medium such as chopped-meat broth. After a 24- to 48-hour incubation at 37 C the tests are read in accordance with the directions supplied by the manufacturer. Rapid growers such as *Clostridium perfringens* can be identified in 24 hours, while more fastidious anaerobes require 48 hours. In 1973 Starr et al.[300] evaluated 104 cultures with this system using an anaerobic glove box. They found a 91% agreement with the conventional methods employed by the Center for Disease Control. When GLC and various supplementary tests were used, slightly higher agreement (93%) was obtained. They also used Ehrlich reagent (instead of Kovac's) for the indole test. The tests for nitrate reduction and H_2S production caused the greatest discrepancy. Other evaluations also indicated correlations of 71-99%.[301,302] A later publication[303] reported the results of 2 modifications of the API 20 procedure. In one mineral oil was added to strips containing the API basal medium and the trays were incubated aerobically. In the other a modified

Viande-Levure medium containing Tween 80, hemin, and vitamin K_3 was used as the inoculating medium. These modifications and the recommended API incubation procedures were compared with the prereduced anaerobically sterilized (PRAS) medium routinely used at the Virginia Polytechnic Institute (VPI) anaerobe laboratory.[78] The overall agreement with the VPI procedure was 83.2% for the aerobic and mineral oil procedure, 98.5% for the Viande-Levure medium, and 91.7% for the recommended API method.

Minitek

The Minitek system has also been used to identify anaerobes. It has been favorably compared (94-100%) with conventional methods for lactobacilli and a variety of anaerobes.[301,304,305] Stargel et al[305] suggested a modification of the manufacturer's procedure to include the use of Lombard-Dowell broth and an inoculum equivalent to a McFarland no. 5 standard. They reported that at 48 hours the modified Minitek procedure agreed satisfactorily with the conventional tests, which took 5-7 days.

MDS system

The Micro Media system for anaerobes is an anaerobe MIC only panel. The details of this system have been previously discussed. The trays are thawed and reduced in a glove box (1-2 hours) or GasPak system (3-4 hours) before being inoculated. A culture grown anaerobically overnight (turbidity greater than a no. 1 McFarland standard) is diluted 1:10 and used as the inoculum. Serial dilutions of 6-10 antibiotics are included in the panel, which is incubated anaerobically for 48 hours. Results are obtained by using the identification manual provided by the manufacturer. An extensive data base and a toll-free telephone line are available. The manufacturer also will identify "problem" organisms sent in by system users. This system is in the final field-testing stage, and results thus far agree well with conventional data.

Comparative reports on anaerobe kits

Moore et al.[306] compared 130 known anaerobic organisms with the API 20A system, the CDC conventional (thioglycolate supplemented with hemin and vitamin K_1) medium, and the VPI-PRAS medium. The API 20A was read at 1 and 2 days; CDC medium at 1, 2, and 7 days; and the PRAS at 3 weeks. The organisms included gram-positive non-spore-forming rods, clostridia, cocci, and gram-negative rods. A total of 2600 tests was performed. There was 80% agreement between all systems. API agreed with CDC 91% of the time and 85% with PRAS. CDC and PRAS agreed with each other 85%. The authors concluded that the miniaturized API 20A system could be used in the clinical laboratory. Hansen and Stewart compared API 20A and Minitek with conventional methods and found the Minitek slightly better. API 20A ranged from 70.8% (positive reactions) to 99.4% (negative reactions), while Minitek had a 97.1% correlation with positive reactions and a 100% correlation with negative reactions.[301]

Thus it appears that the Minitek and API 20A systems can be used to accurately identify a wide variety of anaerobic bacteria. The Micro Media system has yet to be evaluated. Laboratories that are not equipped with GLC or VPI equipment will find these methods rapid and reproducible.

Identification of gram-positive organisms
MDS

As mentioned above, a Micro-ID strep identification panel is available. The Strep Quad Panel contains 4 sets of 16 reagents and allows simultaneous testing of 4 organisms. The panel differentiates Lancefield group A, B, and D from each other and from micrococci and staphylococci. It also speciates group D organisms. Coding is based on a 7-digit biotype. An extensive data base and toll-free consultation also aid in identification. The Strep Combo Panel, awaiting FDA approval will contain 1 set of 15 biochemicals, 8 antibiotics (some serially diluted), and 2 antimicrobials. Thus MIC, antibiotic sensitivities, and biochemical reactions may be determined at the same time.

Streptex Streptococcus test[306a]

This procedure (Wellcome Reagents, Greenville, N.C.) is a rapid latex test for identification of Lancefield A, B, C, D, F, and G streptococci. In this system an enzyme (obtained from cultures of *Streptomyces griseus*) is used to extract the group-specific cell-wall carbohydrate. Antigen in the resulting extract is identified using polystyrene latex particles that have been coated with group-specific antibodies. These latex particles agglutinate strongly in the presence of homologous antigen and remain in smooth suspension in the absence of homologous antigen. Pure cultures growing on solid media or in broth may be identified using this system. In addition streptococci growing in mixed cultures on primary isolation media can be reliably grouped providing they are present in sufficient numbers. This is a distinct advantage over the Phadebact Streptococcus test.

Phadebact Streptococcus test

This procedure (Pharmacia Diagnostics, Piscataway, N.J.) involves a coagglutination reaction between *Staphylococcus aureus* Cowan I (ATCC 12598) bound with specific antibody to either Lancefield group A, B, D, or G β-hemolytic streptococci. The concept behind the procedure and its broad applications have been discussed in detail (see Immunologic technics for detection and identification). Colonies from a sheep blood agar plate that have characteristic hemolytic and morphologic characteristics are transferred to 2

ml Todd-Hewitt broth and incubated overnight at 37 C. The lyophilized antibody-conjugated staphylococcal cells (the "reagent") are reconstituted in buffer solution (provided by the manufacturer), and a drop of each is placed 30 mm apart on a clean, dry slide. A drop of the streptococcal culture to be identified is added to each of the 4 reagent drops. The slide is rocked gently (with 10-15 "tilts") at a 45° angle for 1 minute. Visible coagglutination occurs within 1 minute in a positive reaction. The slide is read against a transilluminated background within 3 minutes. Several groups have reported excellent results with this method.[307, 308] Leland et al. used this technic to identify group B organisms in supernatant from 6-hour mixed cultures.[231] Slifkin et al. removed isolated colonies from agar plates and mixed them with buffer and reagent. A minimum of 5 colonies was needed to coagglutinate 5-15 μl reagent.[309] They correctly identified 127 of 129 primary isolates by this procedure. *Streptococcus pneumoniae* will coagglutinate with group C reagent. Other weak agglutinations can also occur. As mentioned earlier, antibodies to other microorganisms (e.g., bacteria, viruses) can be bound to this strain of *Staphylococcus aureus* for coagglutination reactions.

A Staph-Strip for coagulase testing is available (Biotrol Co., Jamaica, N.Y.). The strip is impregnated with premeasured lyophilized rabbit plasma. A strip is placed into a small tube containing 0.5 ml physiologic saline. A loopful of a 16-24 hour pure culture is spread on the wall of the tube away from the strip. The almost empty loop is dipped into the fluid and used to mix the staphylococcal culture on the wall. Coagulation should occur immediately or within 1-2 hours. It is sometimes necessary to push the culture down in the liquid if coagulation does not occur within few minutes.

Identification of yeasts

Several companies market kits for identification of some of the medically important yeasts and yeastlike fungi, including members of *Candida*, *Cryptococcus*, *Geotrichum*, *Torulopsis*, *Rhodotorula*, and *Saccharomyces*.

API 20C

This kit is similar to the other API kits previously described. It contains 20 cupules with dehydrated substrates for assimilation reactions. A glass vial or bottle of yeast basal medium agar is provided with the kit. After the agar is melted and held in a water bath at 50-55 C for at least 10 minutes, it is inoculated with an isolated colony (minimum diameter 2 mm) from a Sabouraud agar plate. Enough cells are suspended evenly in the agar to increase the turbidity only slightly. This is an important step in the procedure. Too light or too heavy a suspension can lead to false results. Each cupule on the strip is then inoculated using a Pasteur pipet, with the fermentation tubes only filled to the lower margin and overlaid with paraffin and the assimilation tubes filled completely. The strips are then incubated at (preferably) 30 C and read after 24, 48, and 72 hours. Identification charts and a *Profile Index* are provided by the manufacturer. Various evaluations of this kit indicated a 94-98% agreement with conventional methods for the fermentation and assimilation results.[310–312] However, several workers stressed the need for additional tests (e.g., microscopic morphology, nitrate utilization, germ tube formation, growth on corn meal agar) and suggested the addition of nitrate assimilation or reduction tests and urease in place of some reagents presently included.[310, 312] Some difficulty was encountered in adding the paraffin to the tubes so that no air was trapped. This kit will also identify *Trichosporon* and *Prototheca*.

Uni-Yeast-Tek System

This kit consists of a "wheel" and 2 tubes. The sealed round plastic plate ("wheel") has a center well (with cornmeal—Tween agar for mycelium and chlamydospore production) and 10 peripheral wells containing biochemical indicators and reagents for assimilation, fermentation, urea, and nitrate tests. One tube contains a glucose-beef extract medium to promote germ tube formation in 2 hours at 35-37 C, while the other contains a sucrose assimilation medium (Fig. 74-21). Growth from an 18- to 24-hour pure culture grown on Sabouraud agar is added to a tube containing 5 ml sterile distilled water and adjusted to a density of just below a 1+ on the

Wickerham turbidity card provided with the kit. A density corresponding to 70% transmission at 540 nm can also be used (about 10^6 cells/ml). One drop suspension is added to each peripheral well through the channels in the edge. Both tubes are inoculated, and an isolated colony is "scratched" (standard Dalmau cut) and then streaked on the surface of the center well. A flame-sterilized coverslip is then placed over the cut. The plates are incubated in an upright position for 7 days at 25 C and examined at daily intervals. A checkerboard chart of expected reactions is provided. A toll-free consultation service is also available. The incubation period was extended to 10 days by some investigators. This system has been very favorably evaluated and had an accuracy of 99%.[310] Another study reported a 92% correlation at 72 hours, 96% after 1 week, and 97% after 2 weeks.[313] Bacterial contamination and yeasts altered by previous exposure to antifungal agents can present some problems, but these would also be encountered by conventional methods.

Micro-Drop yeast identification test system

This kit (Clinical Sciences, Whippany, N.J.) aids in the identification of *Candida, Cryptococcus, Torulopsis,* and *Trichosporon.* It includes reagents for 12 carbohydrates (fermentation and assimilation), urea, nitrate utilization, and vials of a "yeast identification" agar. Medium for germ tube production and cornmeal agar for morphology and chlamydospore production are not provided in the kit. Vials of agar are melted and cooled at 45 C. Isolated colonies no older than 24-72 hours, are transferred by swab into a tube

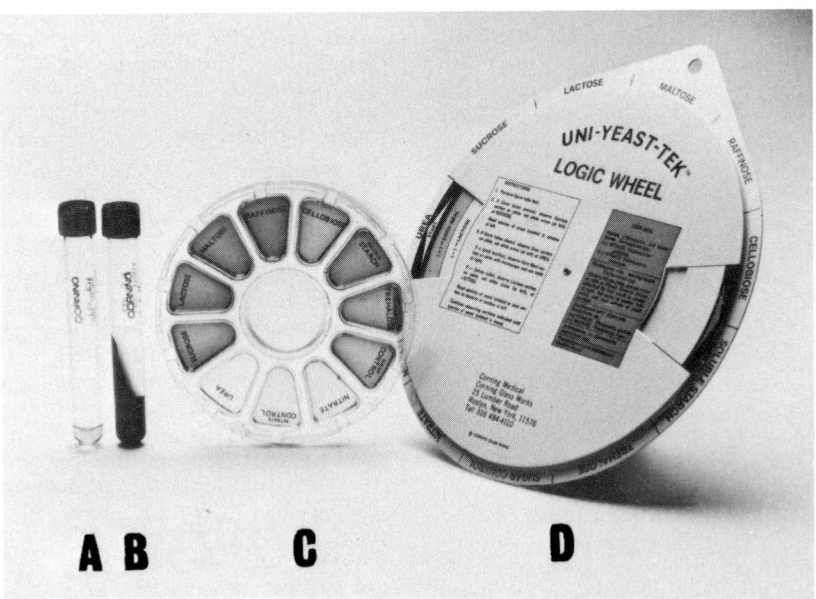

Fig. 74-21. Uni-Yeast-Tek System for identification of yeastlike fungi consists of 2 tubes and a wheel. **A,** Glucose-beef extract medium for germ tube formation. **B,** Medium for sucrose assimilation. **C,** Wheel contains other diagnostic substrates. **D,** Identification aid provided by manufacturer. (Courtesy Corning Medical Diagnostics, Roslyn, N.J.)

containing 5 ml sterile saline and adjusted to a turbidity that just almost obliterates the lines on the provided Wickerham turbidity card. Alternatively a 25-30% transmission at 540 nm can be used. Using a sterile pipet 1.5 ml suspension is evenly suspended in the agar vial. Sixteen wells in the reaction plate are then filled with 1 ml seeded agar according to specific directions, and certain wells are left empty. Assimilation tests cannot be performed in close proximity to the fermentation tests, as false-positive reactions will result. Following a suggested outline 1 drop appropriate control or substrate reagent is placed on the agar surface in the designated well. The reaction plate is covered and incubated without inversion at room temperature (25-28 C). Directions concerning appropriate times to read different reactions and data interpretation sheets (including tables and charts) are provided by the manufacturer. The MD system gave assimilation results within 48 hours, but only 83% of the identifications were accurate,[310] and in several cases it was possible to miss a reaction unless frequent observations were made. Difficulties often arose with the reagent dispensers including crystallization of sugars and various mechanical manipulations.

Minitek

The Minitek impregnated reagent disks have been successfully used in a modified auxanographic carbon assimilation technic completed in 3.3 days compared with 5 days for the Wickerham broth method. It was also more accurate and more reproducible.[314]

Multi-test systems

This system (Randolph Biologicals, Houston) includes 3 plates for the identification of yeasts and some other fungi. A 3 × 5 plastic plate with 24 wells is filled with agar containing Wickerham medium plus various carbohydrates for assimilation studies, urea, nitrate, a birdseed medium for *Cryptococcus*, cyclohexamide well, and various controls. Colonies are picked from an isolation plate and suspended to a density comparable to a +1 on a Wickerham turbidity card. Two drops are used to inoculate the wells. The plates are incubated at 30 C for 1-8 days. The MT-YX plate is an expanded yeast plate containing 18 carbohydrates for assimilation studies, nitrate detection medium, birdseed agar, and controls. The MT-M (multitest mycology) plate has 16 carbohydrate substrates for yeasts, 4 media for dermatophytes, and 4 for *Nocardia*. The MT-Y (multitest yeast) plate has 2 sets of 12 reagents, permitting either 2 different organisms to be identified simultaneously or an unknown and a control. It contains 7 carbohydrates for assimilation, urea, nitrate, cyclohexamide, birdseed agar, and controls. These systems were favorably evaluated.[315] The MT-DN system is similar to MT-Y, containing reagents for identification of dermatophytes and *Nocardia*.

Microstix

This kit (Ames Co., Elkhart, Ind.) contains radiation-sterilized "sticks" in transparent envelopes, a dropping bottle of rehydration fluid, and self-sealing pouches. A pad of cellulose containing dehydrated Nickerson medium in alginate is bonded to the end of a clear plastic strip. The pad is moistened with a few drops of rehydration fluid; a swab containing the specimen is rolled on the surface. The stick is placed in one of the self-sealing pouches and incubated for 24 hours at 37 C. A bismuth indicator in the medium turns brown if *Candida* species are present. The number of brown spots could be roughly correlated with the number of cells. Other yeasts such as *Torulopsis glabrata* will grow but may not cause color change.[316] In 27 severely ill patients suspected of harboring *Candida* 100% agreement was found. In 72 different clinical specimens giving positive results with this test, 51 were *Candida* and 21 were other yeasts.[317] Another study reported good agreement with conventional methods when 425 patients were screened.[318] Both studies recommended microscopic confirmation of germ tube production, chlamydospore formation, and so on, for definitive identification. This method appears to be a fairly accurate and rapid presumptive screen.

Other technics

Segal and Ajello[319] used filter paper disks impregnated with carbohydrates (Difco Laboratories, Detroit; Key Scientific Products, Los Angeles) in the rapid identification of yeasts. Saturated cell suspensions were streaked on plates containing a basal agar medium and indicator. The disks were placed via a dispenser. Approximately 94% of the isolates were correctly identified in 72 hours compared with 2 weeks for conventional methods.

Comparative studies

In a comparison of API 20C, Micro-Drop and Uni-Yeast-Tek (UYT) systems with conventional procedures[310] the API was found to be 94% in agreement, Micro-Drop 84%, and Uni-Yeast-Tek 99%. The API and Micro-Drop required the most manipulation. The Uni-Yeast-Tek plate appeared to be the easiest to use and the most accurate. In a similar study[320] the Randolph MTM plate and the API 20C were 92% accurate and Uni-Yeast-Tek 99%. Ngui-Yen and Smith[57] prepared 11 carbohydrate disks and appropriate controls for assimilation studies in the Autobac-1. They used 218 strains of *Candida* and *Torulopsis* to compare Autobac-1, API 20C, and UYT with conventional methods. They found a 95% correlation with UYT, 93% with API 20C, and 95% with the Autobac-1.[57] The Autobac-1 could detect changes in growth as early as 12 hours.

In summary, the miniaturized kits for identification of yeasts (and a few other medically important fungi) appear to be both rapid and accurate and can be safely used in place of conventional methods. However, morphologic studies and other supplemental tests should not be neglected with those tests that do not identify at the species level.

Identification of *Neisseria gonorrhoeae*

Miniaturized and rapid tests for the identification of *N. gonorrhoeae* are needed.

Microcult-GC

The Microcult-GC (Ames Co., Elkhart, Ind.) is a miniaturized culture system in which a modified Thayer-Martin medium is absorbed on a porous cellulose matrix and dried. The medium is rehydrated before use and inoculated with clinical specimens. It is incubated in a foil pouch with a tablet that releases CO_2. This system has been evaluated by several laboratories with mixed results depending on the source of the specimen.[321-324] When specimens were plated on both Thayer-Martin and the Microcult-GC system more positive cultures were detected by the conventional method, especially from anal and tonsillar specimens.[321,322] However, the predictive tests with Microcult-GC were 90-95% accurate for urethral and vaginal smears.[322] Therefore this system is a good **presumptive** test in venereal disease clinics with a relatively high prevalence of gonorrhea.

Minitek

The Minitek system was compared with the conventional system of carbohydrate degradation patterns in cystine-tryptophan-peptone (CTA) agar for the detection of *N. gonorrhoeae*. Minitek correctly identified 98% of the strains.[325] Morse and Bartenstein[326] developed a suspending medium containing proteose peptone no. 3 (Difco Laboratories, Detroit) and $NaHCO_3$ for use with the Minitek carbohydrate disks in differentiating between *N. gonorrhoea*, *N. meningitidis*, and *N. lactamica*. More isolates of *N. gonorrhoeae* were identified with this system than with the conventional CTA media, and a positive identification could be made in less than 1 hour. By 4 hours 91% of the isolates could be identified.

Other systems

Valu[327] placed carbohydrate disks (Difco) on Thayer-Martin plates that had been previously streaked with a pure culture. There was a 100% correlation compared with the conventional carbohydrate fermentation in CTA tubes.[327] In addition results were obtained in 24 hours. A gonococcus coagglutination kit is also available.[232]

Comparative studies

The results of an investigation comparing Minitek, Bactec, and a direct fluorescence antibody (FA) technic with the conventional CTA procedure indicated that FA was 95% accurate, Minitek 98%, and Bactec 100% (when a growth index of 30 was used with the Bactec; a growth index of 20 gave positive readings for maltose, which could lead to misidentification of the organisms).[325]

Thus it appears that the Microcult-GC can be used as a rapid, presumptive screen for urethral or vaginal specimens but not for the anal canal or tonsils. Direct smears are also necessary. The Minitek system appears to be excellent for rapid and accurate identification of *Neisseria*. The Bactec instrument needs further evaluation for *Neisseria* characterization.

Brucellosis detection
Brewer Diagnostic Kit

The manufacturers of the Rapid Plasma Reagin (RPR) Card Test (Hynson, Wescott, and Dunning, Baltimore) have adapted their general method to the detection of brucellae antibodies. Stained buffered whole-cell suspensions of *Brucella abortus* and the test serum are mixed on a card (similar to the card used for RPR tests) and rocked slowly for 4 minutes. If an agglutination reaction occurs the test is considered positive. Correlation of 95.3% has been reported.[328] However, false-positive reactions were a problem. The method is recommended as a **presumptive** screen, but the conventional method (tube agglutination) appears to be more accurate (see Serology).

Bacteriuria

Several kits are available for the detection of bacteria in urine.

Microstix-3

The Microstix-3 (Ames Co., Elkhart, Ind.) has 3 bands. One is impregnated with N-(1-naphthyl)-ethylene diamine, which turns red in the presence of organisms that can convert nitrate to nitrite. The other 2 bands contain culture medium zones that detect gram-negative colonies and give total numbers after a 12-hour incubation. The strip is moistened with urine and incubated in a sterile cellophane envelope. A Microstix-nitrite single-reagent strip is also available as a presumptive "dip-and-read" test for bacteriuria.

Bacturcult

The Bacturcult (Wampole Laboratories, Cranbury, N.J.) consists of a small screw-capped plastic tube that has the inner surface coated with a special nutrient, allowing for presumptive detection. A midstream specimen is collected directly into the tube until it is almost full. The urine is then poured out and the cap replaced snugly. The cap is loosened before incubation at 35-40 C for 18-24 hours or 32-48 hours at 20-25 C. The medium contains phenol red as a pH indicator. Lactose fermenters such as *E. coli* and enterococci turn the tube yellow; *Klebsiella*, staphylococci, and streptococci turn it rose to orange; and *Proteus* and *Pseudomonas* turn it bright magenta. A "counting strip" (circle divided by lines into quarters) provides an approximation of the colony count.

Dip'n Count

Dip'n Count (Royal Scientific, Buffalo, N.Y.) is double-sided dip slide encased in a screw-capped tube (the cap is the handle of the slide). One side contains cystine-lactose-electrolyte-deficient (CLED) agar medium, and the other side has MacConkey agar medium similar to Oxoid and Uricult systems used in England.[329] The slide is immersed in a sterile container containing a midstream urine sample, drained, and returned to its tube. The number of colonies is counted on the CLED medium, while Mac-Conkey medium is used for identification. The tube is incubated in an upright position (cap side up) for 16-24 hours at 37 C.

Comparison of methods

Opinions about the efficacy of these "slides," "strips," and "sticks" vary. Bailey[330] thought the Microstix strip was a simple and convenient method of screening urine specimens (and obtaining a semiquantitative count) and that it could correctly predict 10^5 or more gram-negative organisms in 84% of the samples and over 10^5 gram-positive organisms in 72% of the cases. He suggested culturing a specimen containing 10^4 organisms. Winter,[331] on the other hand, thought both Microstix and Bacturcult produced too many false-negative results and that direct counting was more accurate. Edwards et al.[329] thought the Oxoid and Uricult dip slides (comparable to the Dip'n Count slides) were good presumptive screens.

A dip-incubate-read test (Microstix-3) (Miles Laboratories, Elkhart, Ind.) was recently reported[332] consisting of a small plastic strip with 3 selective "paper culture" areas and 2 polymeric overlay areas for culture, which form an agarlike surface when rehydrated by urine. The paper areas are reported to provide presumptive identification of *Streptococcus faecalis*, *Proteus*, and *Pseudomonas* species. The polymeric overlay areas provide total and gram-negative populations after a 22-24 hour incubation period. Correlation was 90% or greater.

Many of the instruments and immunologic technics mentioned earlier probably are more accurate for the detection of urinary tract infections. It appears that these "dip" methods could be used (with great caution) in physicians' offices or in small clinics. Acidified urine samples or the presence of antibacterial agents or certain types of medication may affect the results of the test. If there is more than 1 type of organism present in the urine specimen the color changes might also be incorrect.

Antimicrobial susceptibility testing

For a detailed discussion of susceptibility testing see Chapter 87. Only brief reference is made here to some miniaturized methods that have recently appeared.

MDS

MDS are (frozen) test panels (Micro Media Systems, Campbell, Calif.) for determining the minimum inhibiting concentration (MIC) of antimicrobial drugs against gram-positive and gram-negative organisms. A detailed description of the trays and procedures for their use are found under the MDS section on miniaturized kits for *Enterobacteriaceae*. The panels contain various clinically appropriate dilutions of each antimicrobial agent sequentially added to the wells of the trays along with control wells for growth and sterility. Barry et al.[333] have reported the results of a thorough collaborative study by 3 clinical laboratories located near 3 Micro Media distribution centers in California, Oregon, and Ohio. These panels were compared with standard broth "macrodilution" MIC assay and in 1 laboratory also to MICs obtained using the Dynatech MIC 2000 system (Cooke). Different lots of the MDS microdilution panels prepared in different parts of the country gave essentially the same results, thus indicating important standardization and reproducibility factors available nationwide. The MDS panels and the Dynatech MIC 2000 microtiter trays gave equivalent results. Both tended to have MICs that were 1 doubling dilution lower than the standard method with the gram-negative organisms but equivalent MIC dilutions when gram-positive organisms were used. These discrepancies were further explored by putting the same antibiotic solutions in tubes and microtrays. Similar results were obtained. The MICs in the macrodilution system were again about 1 doubling dilution higher with the gram-negative organisms and equivalent with the gram-positive organisms. Panels that were 60 days old performed as well as fresh ones. The investigators concluded that the **frozen** MDS microdilution MIC test panels were a satisfactory and convenient substitute for the standard microdilution MIC method and that the ability to have standardized and reproducible frozen panels available was helpful.

Sensititre

"Sensititre" are (lyophilized) test panels (Gibco Diagnostics, Lawrence, Mass.) for determining the minimum inhibitory concentration (MIC) of antimicrobial drugs against gram-positive and gram-negative organisms. Three standard plates are available: one for gram-positive organisms, one for gram-negative organisms, and one for organisms isolated from urinary tract infections. Dried stabilized antimicrobials are prepared in multiwell polystyrene plates to give 2-fold dilutions after addition of broth; drug-free controll wells are also included. Each plate is sealed with aluminum foil and contained in a foil pouch. A final organism density of approximately 10^5 colony-forming units is prepared from a pure culture of the organism. Mueller-Hinton broth is recommended for testing the majority of rapidly growing aerobic bacteria (supplied by Gibco). The final inoculum (50 μl) is then added by either using an 8-channel micropipet, which can be purchased from the manufacturer, or an ordinary microliter pipet. After inoculation the plate is sealed with an adhesive seal and incubated overnight at 35 C.

The advantage of this system over MDS is that plates are stored at room temperature and retain potency for 1 year from date of manufacture. Thus they are easily employed in the clinical microbiology laboratory that determines MICs infrequently. The system was favorably evaluated by Phillips et al.[333a]

Autobac, MS-2, and AMS

These systems are discussed in the section on physical methods of detection and characterization in this chapter.

ABAC system (API-1)

This antibiotic susceptibility testing system (Fig. 74-22) was developed in Europe (Intertechnique, Plaisir, France) and is currently being modified in the United States (Analytab Products, Plainview, N.Y.). The system consists of a rotor-cuvette containing lyophilized medium, antimicrobial agents (and controls) located in 36 chambers ("microtube") along the periphery, and an automated instrument including a centrifuge, photometer, and printer. The inoculum is placed in the center, and hydrostatic pressure fills the spokes. The cap fits down into the center and blocks any flow from the spokes back into the center. The capped rotor-cuvette is then placed on the instrument and spun briefly; centrifugal force then inoculates the outer microtubes via connecting capillaries. Several different rotor-cuvettes contain a variety of substances. Capabilities exist for MIC and antibiotic susceptibility determinations for gram-positive and gram-negative organisms. Differential media for identification could also be used.

MIC-2000 microtube plate system

Antibiotic susceptibility of staphylococci was determined with this system (Cooke Laboratories, Alexandria, Va.) within 4 hours using tetrazolium salts to provide a definitive end point.[334] In this procedure the microtube plate system has been utilized for simultaneous identification and susceptibility testing. An MIC-2000 dispenser was used to fill the 96 wells; 71 contained dilutions of antimicrobial agents and the remainng 25 contained various substrates. The MIC-2000 inoculator was used to add 10^5-10^6 bacteria per milliliter to each well; the plates were incubated for 16-18 hours. A 96% agreement between conventional identification methods and the MIC-2000 system was found. The MIC and standard antibiotic susceptibility tests were also in good agreement.[335] An 80-microtube plate was similarly filled with 20 biochemicals and 7 dilutions of 8 antimicrobial agents to obtain simultaneous identification and antimicrobial susceptibility data.[336]

Text continued on p. 1544.

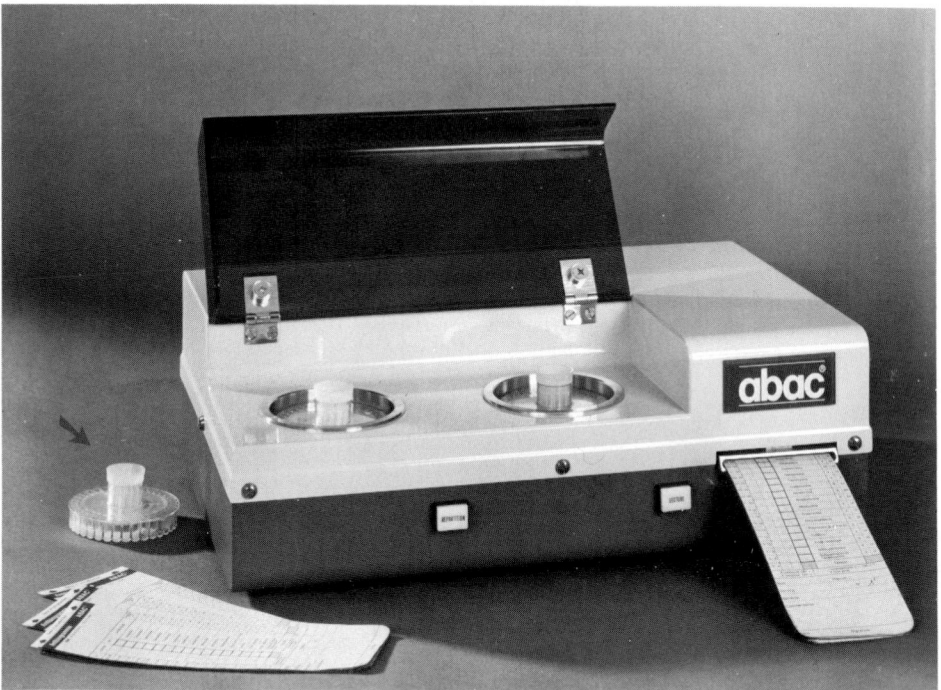

Fig. 74-22. ABAC (API-1), antibiotic sensitivity-testing instrument using photometer to detect turbidity changes. Marketed by Intertechnique, Plaisir, France. Rotor on left (*arrow*) contains lyophilized antibiotics and media. (Courtesy Analytab Products, Plainview, N.Y.)

Table 74-2. Comparison of miniaturized methods

System	Number of tests available*	Type of media	Inoculation procedure	Incubation time
r/b	8-14 B	Agar tubes	Inoculating needle	18-24 h
Enterotube II	15 B	Agar in 1 multicompartmented shell; 12 compartments	Integrated inoculating needle with kit	18-24 h
Minitek	34 B	Dehydrated paper disks	Broth suspension, pipet	18-24 h
API				
20E	20 B	Contain dehydrated media in cupules on plastic strips or plates	Saline suspension added by Pasteur pipet	18-24 h
50E	50 B			48 h
10S	10 B			18-24 h
20A	20 B		Lombard-Dowell medium suspension added by Pasteur pipet	24-48 h
20C	20 B	Cupules contain media for assimilation studies only	Yeast basal medium agar suspension added by Pasteur pipet	24-72 h
Entero-Set	10-20 B	Paper layer containing biochemicals between plastic in capillary compartments	Centrifugation, first for blood or rapid method, resuspending pellet, Pasteur pipet into capillaries	3-18 h
PathoTec	12 B	Reagent-impregnated paper strips	Strips placed into heavy suspension or suspension rubbed on strips	4 h
Micro-ID	15 B	Reagent-impregnated disks	Saline suspension of colonies pipetted into reaction chambers	4 h
MDS				
Enteric Quad	19 B	Either media or appropriately diluted antibiotics or other antimicrobial agents for MIC determinations are placed in wells in plastic panels and then frozen	Complex; diluted inoculum placed in "seed-trough," multipronged lid transfers inoculum from trough to panel; process not difficult after proper dilution achieved	18-24 h
Enteric Combo	19 B			
	9 A, 2 M			
Gram-negative rod combo	24 B			
	11 A, 3 M			
Strep Quad	16 B			
Strep Combo	15 B			
	8 A, 2 M			
Gram-negative MIC	9 A, 2 M			
Gram-negative urinary tract infection MIC panel	11 A, 3 M			

*A, antibiotics; B, biochemicals; M, antimicrobials. Some biochemical wells can be used for more than 1 test (e.g., MDS gram

Ease of reading and interpreting results	Type of identification aids	Organisms identified	Comments
irly simple	*Enteric Analyzer,* toll-free consultation and reference laboratory	*Enterobacteriaceae*	Two tubes with 8 tests, expandable to 14 tests with 2 other tubes
latively easy	Coding manual, *Enterotube II Computer Coding and Identification System;* toll-free hotline information and consultant laboratory service available also	*Enterobacteriaceae* and oxidase-negative, nonfermentative gram-negative bacteria	Short shelf life (3-5 mo); only 15 tests; inflexible arrangement
sy	"Coder" toll-free hotline for consultation	Wide-range aerobes, anaerobes, nonfermenters, yeasts	Very flexible (user decides tests to be used), good for *Neisseria,* anaerobes
ir; hard to differentiate veak positive from negaive	API Analytical Profile Index; free computer service either by telephone direct use of computer system; reference laboratory also available	*Enterobacteriaceae* and nonfermentative gram-negative rods and other gram-negative rods	Occasionally there is some dehydration; tedious to fill cupules
		Possible enteric pathogens	Preliminary screen only
		Any anaerobes	Adaptable to various anaerobic incubating devices
r; inoculation procedure lifficult		Yeasts and yeastlike fungi including *Trichosporon* and *Prototheca*	Long shelf life; not sterile; no longer than 48-72 h necessary
ficult due to initial versimplification of harts	Codon, *Entero-trak* identification manual, toll-free computer consultation	*Enterobacteriaceae*	12 mo stability at room temperature; formerly called Auxotab and Inolex; incubation of inoculum required; broth causes false readings
irly simple	Guide provided by manufacturer	*Enterobacteriaceae* and other bacteria	Flexible, rapid, depends on enzymes; sterility not a problem; strips have 1-2 y shelf life
quires care in developng color reactions	Differentiation checkerboard in Micro-ID identification manual; 5-digit octal number system; toll-free hotline consutation and reference service also available	*Enterobacteriaceae* only	Trays **must** be refrigerated until used; incubated vertically
sitives and negatives asily identifiable, but eading antimicrobial suseptibilities may be rather omplex; dark background s needed for antibiotic and ntimicrobial susceptibilies and diffused light background for biohemicals	Instructions provided by manufacturer; "Biotype Code Book—2nd Edition" identification manual is available; hotline, consultation with computer data base; reference laboratory service also available	Aerobic, gram-negative rods; dextrose fermenting bacteria only	Panels delivered frozen; must be stored at -20 C or colder; Quad panel for 4 organisms; Combo panel for 1 organism and MIC; panels can be refrigerated and read later; color change may occur on freezing; directions for discarding are given; CO_2 incubator cannot be used; enriched media needed for *Haemophilus* and *Streptococcus pneumoniae*
		As above but will also eventually include nonfermenters	
		Gram-positive aerobic streptococci only	
		Gram-negative aerobic bacteria	
		All gram-negative and gram-positive organisms isolated from urinary tract as well as gram-negative organisms from any site	
			This panel replaces gram-negative MIC panel

ative rod Combo has 24 biochemicals but actually performs 30 tests).

Continued.

Table 74-2. Comparison of miniaturized methods—cont'd

System	Number of tests available*	Type of media	Inoculation procedure	Incubation time
Anaerobe MIC	6-10 A			
Sensititre				
Gram-positive MIC	11 A	Appropriate concentrations of lyophilized antimicro-bials for MIC	Complex; diluted inoculum placed in test panel with multichannel inoculator; process not difficult after proper dilution achieved	18-24 h
Gram-negative MIC	9 A			
Urinary tract MIC	6 A, 3 M			
AIM-4	25 B, vari-ous A	Agar in multisectioned Petri plate; 1 compound per plate	Suspension of organisms into cartridge plate; multi-head replicator inoculates up to 37 organisms per Petri plate	18 h
Repliscan	16 B, various A may be selected	Individual agar plates for each compound	Similar to AIM-4; 36 differ-ent organisms per Petri plate are added	18 h
MORLOC	8 B	Dehydrated media impreg-nated on doughnut-shaped disks (Bioloops)	Cell suspension added to center of Bioloops with Pasteur pipet	18-24 h
Metatec S-4	4 B	Dehydrated reagents on paper strip	Strip added to heavy sus-pension in small tube	1-3 h
Oxi/Ferm	9 B	Agar in 8 multicompart-mented tubes	Integrated inoculating nee-dle with kit	48 h
Uni-N/F Tek	17 B	Agar in 2 tubes, one con-stricted GNF tube; 12 wells filled with solid media in wheel-shaped plate	Inoculate 2 tubes, first; if no *Pseudomonas* use heavy suspension from GNF; 1 drop from tube into wells; stab through center well	24-48 h
Phadebact *Streptococcus* test	4 B	Todd-Hewitt broth	Glass slides and reconsti-tuted reagent and buffer plus 1 drop 24 h culture of streptococci	1 min
Streptex streptococcus test	6 B	Solid or broth media	Enzyme extraction followed by addition of extract and polystyrene latex particles to glass tile	2 min

Ease of reading and interpreting results	Type of identification aids	Organisms identified	Comments
		Anaerobes	In final evaluation stages
ading of antimicrobial wells relatively easy with viewbox available from manufacturer	Instructions given by manufacturer	Gram-positive aerobic bacteria, gram-negative aerobic bacteria, gram-positive and gram-negative organisms isolated from urinary tract	Panels stored at room temperature; 1 y expiration date; enrichment needed for fastidious organisms
ear-cut	Computer data-base machine data processor and inoculator available; MIC data processed	*Enterobacteriaceae* and gram-negative non-glucose-fermenters	Test could be run manually; easier with instruments for inoculation and data processing; disposable replicator pins on multihead
n be read manually; however, instrumentation should be used; fairly easy to read	Positive and negative readings by light-sensitive diodes interpreted by Repliscan unit; single- or multiple-reading units are available	Gram-negative bacteria; optional gram-positive sensitivity testing	Data bank and update available from manufacturer
nple	Three-digit number, numerical system for positive reactions; supplementary tests suggested; identification interpretation provided by manufacturer	*Enterobacteriaceae*	Supplemental test needed as 2-5 organisms may have same numerical signature
irly easy		Enteric organisms isolated from feces	MORLOC useful for complete identification
irly easy interpretation; more difficult with weak reactions	Coded 4-digit number system (ID Value) manual provided by manufacturer with suggested supplemental tests; computer identification data available	Oxidative-fermentative gram-negative rods	Organisms unable to grow on supplementary trypticase soy agar plates are not identifiable by this method; up to 34 conventional supplemental tests suggested
irly easy	Information supplied by manufacturer and toll-free technical information service; Simple logic scheme, computerized coding system	Nonfermenting gram-negative rods (oxidase +)	Excellent for identification of *Pseudomonas*
ery good	Directions from manufacturer	*Streptococcus* Lancefield groups A, B, D, G	Specific antibodies bound to surface of S. *aureus* Cowan I (ATCC 12598) coagglutinate homologous streptococci; store at 2-8 C; 1 mo shelf life when reconstituted
ery good	Directions from manufacturer	*Streptococcus* Lancefield groups A, B, C, D, F, and G	Store at 2-8 C; latex suspensions and freeze-dried enzyme will retain potency 1 y from date of last test by Wellcome; reconstituted extraction enzyme will retain potency for at least 6 mo

Continued.

Table 74-2. Comparison of miniaturized methods—cont'd

System	Number of tests available*	Type of media	Inoculation procedure	Incubation time
Uni-Yeast-Tek system	12 B	Sterile solid media; sealed wheel-shaped plate with 11 wells and tube containing liquid medium for germ tube test	Pasteur pipet suspension into 10 outer wells, streak from another colony on middle well, and use another colony to inoculate tube	1-7 d (or longer)
Micro-Drop yeast identification system	16 B	Liquid reagents and biochemicals added to seeded solidified medium in wells from reagent dispensers	Seeded agar added to wells by pipet; addition of reagent to solidified agar is sometimes difficult to regulate	18-48 h (or longer)
Microstix-*Candida*	1 B	Dehydrated reagent on strip	Strip is moistened and surface rubbed with swab	24 h
Multitest systems				
Multitest expanded yeast plate (MT-YX)	24 B including 3 controls	Solid media in wells	Broth suspension added by pipet to wells	1-7 d
Multitest mycology plate (MT-M)	24 B			1-14 d
Multitest yeast plate (MT-Y)	2 sets 12 B			1-7 d
Multitest dermatophyte plate (MT-DN)	2 sets 12 B			1-14 d
Microcult-GC test	1	Dehydrated medium on porous cellulose matrix	Inoculated with clinical specimen after rehydration	24-48 h
Brucellosis test card	1	Stained whole cells of *Brucella abortus*	Sera mixed with antigen on special "card"	Few min
ABAC (API-1)	16	Mueller-Hinton or eugonic broth and antimicrobial agents	Inoculum into center well; centrifugal force fills microtubes at edges of "wheel"	18-24 h
API-ZYM	20	Dehydrated chromogenic enzyme substrates	Cell suspension fills wells	Depends on rapidity of enzyme system ± 1 h

Ease of reading and interpreting results	Type of identification aids	Organisms identified	Comments
..sy to use and interpret	"Logic wheel" identification provided by manufacturer, toll-free consultation is available	Medically important yeast-like fungi	Uninoculated plate stored at 2-8 C, plates incubated at 25 C, tube at 35-37 C for 2 h
..equent observations must be made between 18-24 h for some isolates; time consuming, some reactions not clear-cut, some indicator may fade after 48 h	Interpretation tables and flow chart provided by manufacturer	Yeastlike fungi	Manufacturer does not provide corn meal agar for morphology and chlamydospore production or medium for germ tube production test with kit; reaction vials stable for 3 mo; storage at 2-8 C is necessary
..irly simple	None; presence of brown spots indicates positive test	*Candida* species	Will pick up other yeasts on occasion; *Torulopsis glabrata* will appear in 48 h with no color change; presumptive *Candida* screen from saliva and urine
..irly simple	Information from manufacturer; manual and checkerboard color chart	Yeastlike fungi	Corn meal agar and germ tube medium not included; assimilation media only; prior starvation required for *Trichophyton*
		Yeastlike fungi, *Trichophyton*, dermatophytes, *Nocardia*	
		Yeastlike fungi	Corn meal agar and germ tube medium not included; assimilation media only; 12 in duplicate for 2 cultures on same plate
		Dermatophytes and *Nocardia*	Corn meal agar and germ tube medium not included; assimilation media only; 12 in duplicate for 2 cultures on same plate; shelf life 6 mo at 4-8 C
..elatively simple	None needed	*Neisseria gonorrhoea*	Medium is stable at room temperature for a long time
..elatively simple	Comparison with control; microscopic observation	*Brucella abortus* detects antibodies	False-positive reactions may occur; however, method may serve as presumptive screen
..hotometric determinations machine interpreted	Instrument interpretation; API data bank access (eventually)	Various organisms, both gram-positive and gram-negative	Lyophilized compounds, shelf life 1 y at room temperature; instrument probably necessary for optimum results; not available yet in U.S.
..olor reactions relatively simple to interpret	Directions from manufacturer; see API above for additional services	Various organisms, aerobes, anaerobes	Methods have great potential as adjuncts to rapid identification; strips should be stored in dark, below 30 C

Other systems using microtiter plates

Microtiter plates containing freeze-dried reagents for a modified hemaglutination inhibition test for rubella antibodies have been favorably evaluated by a collaborative study involving 6 laboratories.[337] Microtiter plates can also be used as the solid support system in an enzyme-linked immunosorbent assay test for hepatitis B surface antigen.[210]

It appears that miniaturization of the technics for MIC, biochemical identification, and antibiotic susceptibilities can be performed simultaneously in microtiter plates. The reports indicate that these systems are accurate, reproducible, and easy to perform. The capability of obtaining simultaneous data in these 3 areas is very important and will be most helpful to the clinical microbiologist, the physician, the patient, and the epidemiologist.

Enzyme strip tests

The ability of microorganisms to utilize carbohydrates and other substrates has long been used as a method of identification. Rapid and miniaturized methods for using specific bacterial enzymes as adjuncts to speciation are being investigated. These systems hold much promise. Maddocks and Greenan[338] reported a rapid method for identifying bacterial enzymes by detecting the fluorescent methylumbelliferone released from nonfluorescent substrates by specific enzymatic activity. n-Acetyl-β-D-glucosaminidase, n-acetyl-β-D-galactosaminidase, and β-D-galactosidase were among the enzymes detected. Bradbury[339] described methods for the rapid detection of β-D-glucosidase and phosphatase to help characterize cultures of *Mycoplasmatales*. The fluorogenic tests could be read in less than 1 hour compared with several days for the conventional tests. Watson[340] discussed the use of aminopeptidase activity as a method of identifying bacteria, fungi, and parasites. He was able to distinguish closely related species and even strains of the same species using the enzymatic liberation of fluorescent β-naphthylamine (β-NA) from a nonfluorescent L-amino acid-β-naphthylamide. Profiles were obtained on 26 compounds. These substrates are available from a number of manufacturers (Mann Research Laboratories, New York; Sigma Chemical Co., St. Louis; Nutritional Biochemicals, Cleveland). Watson used these tests to identify many species of fungi, such as *Aspergillus*, *Candida*, *Fusarium*, *Mucor*, and *Saccharomyces*. He also could distinguish between closely related strains of *Neisseria* and some *Enterobacteriaceae*.

API-ZYM

These enzyme-substrate strips are presently used in Europe and the United States, mostly for research purposes but will no doubt have an important place in the ever increasing armamentarium that is available to microbiologists seeking to identify microorganisms. The strip, similar to other API strips (see above), contains chromogenic substrates for 19 different tests. Substrates for glucosidase, peptidases, lipases, α- and β-galactosidase, fucosidase, manosidase, alkaline phosphatase, and esterases are available. It is hoped that multiple enzyme profiles will eventually produce diagnostic schemata based on these reactions. A data base is slowly being established. Reports on the API-ZYM strips indicate that this procedure can be as useful as the Entero-Set and the umbelliferone methods. They have been used for *Streptococcus faeceium*, *S. mutans*, *S. sanguis*, *S. miteor*, *S. milleri*, *Staphylococcus aureus*, coagulase-negative strains of *S. aureus*, *Pseudomonas aeruginosa*, *Proteus*, *Klebsiella*, *Escherichia coli*, and *Serratia*.[341] The API-ZYM test could clearly distinguish between genera and species of gram-negative anaerobes encountered in human infections. Both type species and clinical isolates were tested.[342] The authors reported that these methods appear to be simple and reliable identification aids. D'Amato et al.[343] have successfully used chromogenic enzyme profiles in experimental API strips to separate *Neisseria gonorrhoea* and *N. meningitidis* from each other and from other genera and species tested within 4 hours. The aminopeptidases were important, as was n-γ-glutamyl-β-naphtylamide. They felt that enzymatic analyses were a reproducible and rapid method for identifying *neisseria* species.

Immunologic test kits

Although not all are directly involved with the detection of microorganisms, these kits can be used to monitor the concentration of immunoglobulins, antigens, and various proteins that may be indicative of a disease state and to follow treatment. Many kits are available; 3 are reported here as examples of their variety.

Crypto-LA kit

This kit (International Biological Laboratories, Cranbury, N.J.) is a rapid test system to aid in the diagnosis of cryptococcosis. It is based on a rapid latex agglutination procedure to detect the presence of *Cryptococcus neoformans* **antigen** in serum or cerebrospinal fluid.

M Partigen immunodiffusion plates

These immunodiffusion plates (Behring Diagnostics, Somerville, N.J.) are used for the quantitative determination of plasma proteins. Protein standards and dilutions are added to the wells according to directions, and the plates are incubated for 50 hours at room temperature with the lids tightly closed. The diameter of the precipitin rings can be measured and a curve constructed to measure concentrations. In all, 19 separate plates are available to determine various components including transferrin, albumin, Gc globulin, and so on.

Fiax system

The Fiax test kit (International Diagnostic Technology, Santa Clara, Calif.) is an aid for determining the concentrations of immunoglobulins G, A, and M in serum. Diluted serum samples are reacted with excess fluorescent-labeled class-specific antibodies (e.g., IgA and IgM). The unreacted class of fluorescent antibody, which could be IgG in this case, binds to the immunochemically active surface of a plastic shallow spoonlike "stick" (StiQ-Sampler), and the concentration is determined fluorometrically. Separate StiQ-samplers can be prepared for IgA and IgM determinations. The manufacturer markets a Fiax model 100 fluorometer and Fiax model 110 microcomputer to convert the signals from the fluorometer into a print-out of results. Similar systems could be adapted for microbiology.

Removawell strip system

The system (Dynatech Laboratories, Alexandria, Va.) consists of an Immulon plastic strip with 8 flat-bottomed wells. They are made of the same plastic that is used for the 96-well microELISA plate and are in the same format as the microtiter plates. The wells can be separated and used singly or in groups. This allows great flexibility in assembling a "customized" system to simultaneously screen for a small number of antigens or antibodies by the ELISA or other procedures. Disposable or reusable holders are also available for use with these strips.

COMPUTER-AIDED DATA INTERPRETATION

It is inherent in the nature of scientific workers to attempt the (sometimes) impossible in creating order out of chaos. Microbiologists interested in identification and taxonomy are no different but have a more difficult task confronting them. Through the years identification of microorganisms has been based on many different parameters, including morphologic and biochemical characteristics, deoxyribonucleic acid–based composition, and gas chromatographic patterns. Recently antibiograms and enzymatic data have been used. As detection methods have become more sophisticated and sensitive, different aspects have been revealed that help to further clarify interrelationships between organisms.

When the vacuum tube was replaced by the transistor many new vistas opened for laboratory workers. Computers and calculators, now less expensive and more efficient, became the keepers and guardians of many kinds of functions including programming instruments, calculating results, and storing data on tapes, disks, bubbles, or other exotic elements. Complex computations and comparisons of raw data with stored information have greatly influenced the ability of microbiologists to make rapid presumptive and confirmed identifications. In the past few years the increased access to multiple data banks has given impetus to both identification systems and numerical taxonomy studies. The earlier sections of this chapter often refer to computer-generated programs and data-based information used for identification purposes.

It is necessary to distinguish between "identification" and "numerical taxonomy." A list of distinguishing characteristics based on various parameters is used to "officially" establish the identity of an organism. Numerical taxonomists sort these organisms into larger groups based on their similarities employing, among other methods, probability estimates, numerical clustering, and mathematical construction of keys based on serologic, biochemical, and other characteristics. The mathematical basis for these numerical concepts is fairly complex. Thus identification and taxonomy are interrelated to a certain degree.

Computer-aided identification

Balows and Isenberg[344] have discussed automation and standardization of biotyping and their roles in the clinical microbiology laboratory. In many cases numerical taxonomy studies have aided in the identification of microorganisms as well as clarifying their generic relationships. Gyllenberg and Niemalä[345] thought that a continuous interaction between identification and classification systems is necessary for constant updating and readjustment of the reference framework used in these procedures. Kelley and Kellog,[346] for example, developed a computer program based on a Bayesian probalistic model to be used as a rapid and precise aid in identifying unknown anaerobic bacteria. A Wang 2200C computer system used in conjunction with an accessory, the Micrologger, has been programmed to compare data obtained from replicate plate methods for antibiotic susceptibility and biochemical characteristics with stored information to identify members of the *Enterobacteriaceae.*[346a] Sielaff et al.[58] developed a computer program based on data from the Autobac-1 instrument to identify bacteria solely on the basis of their sensitivity to various antimicrobial agents. These included the salts of heavy metals, organic compounds, dyes, and antineoplastic agents. However, great caution must be used in interpreting data based on these types of tests. The ability of microorganisms to not only develop resistance to many compounds but to transfer the genetic information for these capabilities to other organisms by various means (e.g., via plasmids, bacteriophages) is well known. Even though Sielaff et al. were not using compounds commonly encountered by microorganisms, transferrable resistance developed to a compound that, for example, involves permeability; receptor site alterations may also simultaneously change sensitivity to other seemingly unrelated compounds. Organisms damaged by previous exposure to antimicrobial agents or other deleterious substances may also give erroneous results in such systems.

Drucker[76] used computer-stored data to identify organisms using their GLC "fingerprints." Mitruka[77] suggested excellent identification capabilities if GLC and mass spectrometry were coupled with the computer to provide an analysis of the mass spectra based on an extensive data base. Mandel and Wade[347] also thought that gas chromatographic data would provide rapid and reproducible data for the identification of microorganisms. The use of enzymatic analyses has also been proposed.[343]

In short, any of the systems yielding data in some distinctive parameter could be computer correlated with existing data for identification purposes. Most of the identification systems used with miniaturized kits employ computer bases. Some companies (i.e., Pfizer Diagnostics) envision having a few central computer stations for correlating data derived from their Autobac instruments. Laboratory computer terminals would interface with these stations using an automatic dialer coupled with a WATS line. Accumulated laboratory data would be fed to the central computer as desired and identification profiles generated and returned to the individual laboratory in minutes. (In fact, direct access to the Analytab Products computer base is available to API 20E, 20C, and 20A system users utilizing the laboratories' own computer terminals.) It is hoped that there will be no blackouts or electronic "gremlins" involved at crucial moments, as all data could be wiped at the unexpected "blink" of a transistor. Noncomputerized manuals should be available for backup.

Numerical taxonomy

As previously mentioned, the concepts behind numerical taxonomy are complex, involving mathematical formulations and statistical analyses. Mitruka[10] has an excellent discussion on the subject. Drucker[76] discusses the use of clustering and linkage methods when using gas liquid chromatography data in numerical taxonomy. Canonical variate analysis has been used with pyrolysis-gas-liquid chromatography.[348] Cluster analyses were used in a computerized flexible approach to phenotypic feature frequency calculations.[349] This approach was also used in numerical taxonomy studies on bacteria that could metabolize hydrocarbons in Arctic aquatic ecosystems.[350] Gyllenberg[351] used 3 different independent taxonomic principles and indicated that they produced almost identical conclusions. Lechevalier[352] discussed the role of lipids in bacterial chemotaxonomy and predicted future use of physicotaxonomic data in this field.

Probablistic methods have also been used in numerical taxonomy.[353,354] According to Mitruka,[10] "there appears to be no method a priori in a biological system of determining whether a probablistic matrix will operate successfully or whether an empirical trial is needed."

Key construction is usually based on the formulation of groups based on similar characteristics based on various parameters such as biochemical activities, serologic reactions, morphologic markers, toxin production, and so on. Established classification guides such as *Bergey's Manual of Determinative Bacteriology*,[355] *Identification of Enterobacteriaceae*,[356] and other recognized identification schemes are the basis for many of the computer-programmed numerical taxonomic keys. Sometimes the distinguishing characteristics themselves are not inherently stable. The presence of plasmids or bacteriophages can introduce genetic information that changes the biochemical or other characteristics of the organisms. For example, the genetic capabilities for the production of several toxins in some of the clostridial species is carried by different temperate bacteriophages. If bacteriophage 3C integrates into the bacterial genome of a nontoxogenic strain (HS-37), type C botulinum toxin is subsequently produced by this strain (now said to be "lysogenic" for bacteriophage 3C) and is classified as *Clostridium botulinum* type C. If strain HS-37 becomes lysogenic for type D bacteriophage, type D toxin is produced and the bacterium is classified as *Clostridium botulinum* type D. When strain HS-73 becomes lysogenic for bacteriophage NA-1, novyi type A toxins are produced and the organism is classified as *Cl. novyi* type A.

New and more sensitive probes will continue to improve classification and reveal new taxonomic relationships. The computer will play an important role in these processes.

FUTURE PREDICTIONS

Mechanization and semiautomation of the preparative aspects of microbiology will continue to aid laboratories with large work loads. Balows[357] thinks that detection times have significantly decreased due to instrumented procedures. In theory, in the not too distant future the use of pure cultures may no longer be necessary even for determining antimicrobial susceptibilities. Rapid separation by 1 or more physical procedures could be combined with image analysis or flow microfluorometry, which can monitor growth rates and analyze individual cells for changes in the presence of various antimicrobial agents; growth-stimulating effects could also be determined.

Capabilities already exist (AMS system) for identification of mixed cultures by turbidometric procedures based on growth responses to specialized media. Immunologic amplification technics such as ELISA could detect antigens of organisms in clinical specimens and substitute for growth in selected systems. The use of sera or other body fluids with this type of "immunologic instrumentation" could quickly indicate the causal agent in frank disease and recognize asymatomatic infections or carrier states. Similarly, microbial "pollution" of foods, pharmaceutical preparations, water supplies, and so on, can be detected and monitored by various immunologic and other amplification systems. Clinical laboratories, health maintenance organizations, public health laboratories, pharmaceutical companies, and food processing industries (from slaughter houses to canneries) will probably employ these systems. Impedance and radiometric procedures will probably eventually be replaced by immunologic methods for rapid detection if there is enough demand for purified reagents to make these tests sufficiently reproducible, reliable, and readily available at reasonable cost. The accuracy achieved in immunologic procedures or in any assay system obviously depends on the purity of the reagents and the sensitivity of the detection system. Chromatography technics singly or in combination with mass spectroscopy or other detection systems will continue to be used for ancillary procedures, separation of compounds, and as a tool for taxonomic studies. Acoustic microscopy, still in its infancy, should develop into an important aid in many areas of microbiology. Focused sound beams can differentiate internal structures on the basis of elastic and other mechanical properties. Microorganisms show little contrast optically and must be stained, while acoustic imaging can be used to reveal morphologic information in unstained cells and tissues. It is expected that this technic will be used to detect antigen-antibody reactions, growth stimulation and inhibition, substrate utilization, and morphologic changes during differentiation and growth.

The skyrocketing cost and increased complexity of instrumentation may well limit its usefulness in the smaller laboratory. Down time and repair costs are always important factors. As a result kits may prove to be both important backup factors, if not the mainstays, of many laboratories. Some of the technics and immunologic reactions available in miniaturized form are quite rapid and accurate. Again, pure cultures are not necessarily required for some of the technics. For example, organisms in mixed broth cultures can be identified by coagglutination reactions. Thus rapid test systems and kits are here to stay. Combinations of antibiotic susceptibilities and biochemical characteristics will become more common (no doubt some automated instruments will adopt these procedures also). In fact, kits may become even more miniaturized into waferlike elements, while enzymatic profiles and similar rapid reactions will become more prevalent. Microbiologists will continue to borrow from biochemical and biophysical technics.

Recently Eastman Kodak scientists have utilized some of the solid-phase technology used in photographic films and have developed a simplified and rapid (7 minutes) semiautomated analytical technic for the detection of several clinically important compounds.[358] Using a wafer 1 cm² in area and 0.1 mm thick they have miniaturized many of the tests presently used in analyzing serum. Individual tests incorporated in separate wafers are available for glucose, blood urea nitrogen, amylase, bilirubin, and triglycerides. The wafer base is a transparent plastic material, and the reagent layer coated on top of the base is a hydrophilic polymer such as gelatin or agarose. The top layer, an isotropically porous spreading layer, consists of cellulose acetate pigmented with TiO_2 (0.1 mm thick). When serum is added the spreading layer distributes it evenly and rapidly over the surface of the wafer. When the reagent layer is hydrated the chemical reaction is initiated, and the resultant colored products can be measured through the bottom plastic layer by reflection densitometry. The applications of this type of system both to kits and to semiautomated instrumentation for microbiology are obvious.

It should be kept in mind, however, that good laboratory practices include proper quality control methods and sterile technics. Microorganisms previously exposed to antimicrobial agents or other deleterious conditions may have aberrant reactions. The ability of plasmids and bacteriophages to transfer genetic material from 1 organism to another could result in different immunologic, enzymatic, and antibiotic susceptibility patterns. Correlation of results between different types of technics is sometimes difficult. Many kits are good presumptive screens, and more definitive methods are necessary for exact enumeration or species determination.

Which instruments, miniaturized methods, or computer systems should be used? These choices ultimately must be determined by the laboratory's needs and resources. The types of specimens or routine procedures most frequently encountered will ultimately dictate the final decisions. For example, Cox et al.[359] thought that many kits that are accurate and approved for clinical specimens are not necessarily the most suitable for the microbiologic analysis of food. The acceptance of instruments or kits by governmental bodies (e.g., FDA) or other official groups (e.g., AOAC) will also play a role in this selection process. Industrial laboratories monitoring fermentation procedures may well use ion-sensitive electrode systems as well as computer-controlled processing and monitoring equipment. Pharmaceutical companies concerned about particulate matter might use a Coulter Counter. Microbiologists working in the field or in the military need compact instrumentation or rapid noninstrumented analyses. Developing countries that are struggling to improve health care will benefit greatly from the rapid test kits and miniaturized procedures.

Computers will continue to be irreplaceable adjuncts in programming, analyzing, summarizing, and reporting all types of data. Imagination, creativity, and ingenuity coupled with the capabilities of computers will refine even further many of the present technics as well as play important roles in inventing new ones.

REFERENCES

1. Johnston, H. H., and Newsom, S. W. B., editors: Rapid methods and automation in microbiology, Forest Grove, Ore., 1977, International Scholarly Book Services.
2. Board, R. G., and Lovelock, D. W., editors: Some methods for microbiological assay, The Society for Applied Bacteriology Technical Series, vol. 8, New York, 1975, Academic Press.
3. Sharpe, A. N., and Clark, D. S., editors: Mechanizing microbiology, Springfield, Ill., 1978, Charles C Thomas, Publisher.
4. Prier, J. E., Bartola, J., and Friedman, H., editors: Modern methods in medical microbiology: systems and trends, Baltimore, 1976, University Park Press.
5. Goldschmidt, M. C., and Fung, D. Y. C.: J. Food Prot. **41**:201, 1978.
6. Goldschmidt, M. C., and Fung, D. Y. C.: Food Technol. **33**:63, 1979.
7. Goldschmidt, M. C.: J. Am. Assoc. Adv. Med. Instr. **5**:63, 1971.
8. Isenberg, H. D., and MacLowry, J. D.: Ann. Rev. Microbiol. **30**:483, 1976.
9. Gall, L. S., and Curby, W. A.: Instrumented approach to microbiological analysis of body fluids, C. R. C. Uniscience Series, West Palm Beach, Fla., 1979, Chemical Rubber Co.
10. Mitruka, B. M.: Methods of detection and identification of bacteria, West Palm Beach, Fla., 1976, Chemical Rubber Co.
11. Héden, C.-G., and Illeni, T., editors: Automation in microbiology and immunology, New York, 1975, John Wiley & Sons.
12. Héden, C.-G., and Illeni, T., editors: New approaches to the identification of microorganisms, New York, 1975, John Wiley & Sons.
13. Second international symposium on rapid methods and automation in microbiology, New York, 1976, Learned Information (Europe).
14. Emswiller, B. S., Pierson, C. J., and Kotula, A. W.: Food Technol. **31**:40, 1977.
15. Andrews, W. H., Wilson, C. R., Poelma, P. L., and Romero, A.: Appl. Environ. Microbiol. **33**:65, 1977.
16. Andrews, W. H., Wilson, C. R., Poelma, P. L., et al.: Appl. Environ. Microbiol. **33**:89, 1978.
17. Tilton, R. C., and Ryan, R. W.: J. Clin. Microbiol. **7**:298, 1978.
18. Campbell, J. E.: Clin. Lab. Forum **3**:2, 1971.
19. Gilchrist, J. E., Campbell, J. E., Donnelly, C. B., et al.: Appl. Microbiol. **25**:244, 1973.
20. Donnelly, C. B., Gilchrist, J. E., Peeler, J. T., and Campbell, J. E.: Appl. Environ. Microbiol. **32**:21, 1976.
21. Gilchrist, J. E., Donnelly, C. B., Peeler, J. T., and Campbell, J. E.: J. Assos. Off. Analyt. Chem. **60**:807, 1977.
22. Jarvis, B., Lach, V. H., and Wood, J. M.: J. Appl. Bacterol. **43**:149, 1977.
23. Briner, W. W., Wunder, J. A., Blair, D. W., et al. In Sharpe, A. N., and Clark, D. S., editors: Mechanizing microbiology, Springfield, Ill., 1978, Charles C Thomas, Publisher.
24. Steers, E., Foltz, L. L., and Graver, B. S.: Antibiot. Chemother. **9**:307, 1959.
25. Hill, I. R. In Baillie, A., and Gilbert, R. J., editors: Automation, mechanization and data handling in microbiology, New York, 1970, Academic Press.
26. Wiberg, J. S.: J. Appl. Bacteriol. **43**:433, 1977.
27. Sevastopoulos, C. G., Wehr, C. T., and Glaser, D. A.: Proc. Natl. Acad. Sci. USA **74**:3485, 1977.
28. Brusick, D. J.: Pharmaceut. Technol. **2**:37, 1978.
29. Fruin, J. T., and Clark, W. S., Jr.: J. Food Prot. **40**:552, 1977.
30. LaGrange, W. S., Moon, N. J., and Reed, W.: J. Food Prot. **40**:744, 1977.
31. Sykes, D. A., and Evans, C. J. In Board, R. G., and Lovelock, D. W., editors: Some methods for microbiological assay, The Society for Applied Bacteriology Technical Series, vol. 8, New York, 1975, Academic Press.
32. Palmer, G. H., and Hamilton, P. In Board, R. G., and Lovelock, D. W., editors: Some methods for microbiological assay, The Society for Applied Bacteriology Technical Series, vol. 8, New York, 1975, Academic Press.
33. Newman, P. B.: J. Appl. Bacteriol. **41**:497, 1976.
34. Barbaree, J. M., Habas, J., Rossing, P. H., and Dobbins, J. F.: Appl. Environ. Microbiol. **34**:484, 1977.
35. Castronovo, F. P., Jr.: J. Nucl. Med. **14**:341, 1973.
36. Ruttenberg, E. J., Brusi, B. J., and Steerenberg, P. A.: J. Clin. Microbiol. **3**:541, 1976.
37. Clem, T. R., and Yolken, R. H.: J. Clin. Microbiol. **7**:55, 1978.
38. Fung, D. Y. C.: J. Milk Food Technol. **38**:262, 1975.
39. Ryan, R. W., Sedgwick, A. K., and Tilton, R. C.: Health Lab. Sci. **10**:82, 1973.
40. Beaman, K. D., Vaccaro, J. A., and Mack, J. C.: Annual Meeting, American Society for Microbiology, abstract, 1978, p. 302.
41. Truant, J. P., Brett, W. A., and Merckel, K. E.: Henry Ford Hosp. Med. Bull. **10**:359, 1962.
42. Orstavik, D.: Acta Pathol. Microbiol. Scand. (B) **85**:47, 1977.
43. Gall, L. S., Baum, J. M., and Curby, W. A.: Annual Meeting, American Society for Microbiology, abstract, 1978, p. 302.
44. Nozawa, R. T., Yokota, T., and Kuwahara, S.: J. Clin. Microbiol. **7**:479, 1978.
45. Curby, W. A., and Gall, L. S.: Public Health Lab. **35**:118, 1977.
46. Typas, M. A., and Heal, T. B.: J. Gen. Microbiol. **101**:177, 1977.
47. Wheeler, T. G., and Goldschmidt, M. C.: J. Clin. Microbiol. **1**:25, 1975.
48. Goldschmidt, M. C., and Wheeler, T. G. In Schlessinger, D., editor: Microbiology—1975, Washington, D.C., 1976, American Society for Microbiology.
49. Martens, A. E., and Morton, R. A. In Héden, C.-G., and Illeni, T., editors: Automation in microbiology and immunology, New York, 1975, John Wiley & Sons.
50. Praglin, J., Curtiss, A. C., Longhenry, D. K., and McKie, J. E., Jr.: In Héden, C.-G., and Illeni, T., editors: Automation in microbiology and immunology, New York, 1975, John Wiley & Sons.
51. McKie, J. E., Jr., Borovoy, R. J., Dooley, J. F., et al. In Héden, C.-G., and Illeni, T., editors: Automation in microbiology and immunology, New York, 1975, John Wiley & Sons.
52. Thornsberry, C., Gavan, T. L., Sherris, J. C., et al.: Antimicrob. Ag. Chemother. **7**:466, 1975.
53. Gavan, T. L., Baker, C. N., Schoenknecht, F. D., and Yu, P. K. W.: Annual Meeting, American Society for Microbiology, abstract, 1978, p. 311.
54. Stager, C. E., and Wende, R. D.: Annual Meeting, American Society for Microbiology, abstract, 1978, p. 311.
55. Tilton, R. C., Kwasnik, I., and Ryan, R.: Ann. Clin. Lab. Sci. **8**:70, 1978.

56. Hale, D. C., and Matsen, J. M.: Annual Meeting, American Society for Microbiology, abstract, 1978, p. 301.
57. Ngui-Yen, J. H., and Smith, J. A.: J. Clin. Microbiol. **7**:118, 1978.
58. Sielaff, B. H., Johnson, E. A., and Matsen, J. M.: J Clin. Microbiol. **3**:105, 1976.
59. Sielaff, B. H., Buck, G. E., and Matsen, J. M.: Annual Meeting, American Society for Microbiology, abstract, 1977, p. 52.
60. Spencer, H. J., Welaj, P., Vannest, R., et al.: Annual Meeting, American Society for Microbiology, abstract, 1978, p. 311.
61. Stockert, J. E., Wilborn, R. C., and Fekete, N. M. G.: Annual Meeting, American Society for Microbiology, abstract, 1977, p. 56.
62. McCarthy, L. R., Sherris, J. C., and Anhalt, J. P.: Annual Meeting, American Society for Microbiology, abstract, 1978, p. 311.
63. Thornsberry, C., McCarthy, L. R., and Sherris, J. C.: Annual Meeting, American Society for Microbiology, 1978, p. 297.
64. Sonnenwirth, A. C.: J. Clin. Microbiol. **6**:400, 1977.
65. Aldridge, C., Jones, P. W., Gibson, S., et al.: J. Clin. Microbiol. **6**:406, 1977.
66. Isenberg, H. D., Telenson, M., Washington, J., II, et al.: Annual Meeting, American Society for Microbiology, abstract, 1978, p. 302.
67. Marso, E. L., Cue, J., Oshima, C., et al.: Annual Meeting, American Society for Microbiology, abstract, 1978, p. 301.
68. Madden, J., Higbee, J., and Johnson, R.: Annual Meeting, American Society for Microbiology, abstract, 1978, p. 302.
69. Smith, P. B., Gavan, T. L., Isenberg, H. D., et al.: J. Clin. Microbiol. **8**:657, 1978.
69a. Isenberg, H. D., Gavan, T. L., Sonnenwirth, A., et al.: J. Clin. Microbiol. **10**:226, 1979.
70. Wyatt, P. J. In Norris, J. R., and Ribbons, D. W., editors: Methods in microbiology, vol. 8, New York, 1973, Academic Press.
71. Wyatt, P. J. In Amsterdam, D., editor: Handbook on disease methodology, vol. 1, New York, 1978, Marcel Dekker.
72. Wyatt, P. J., Sher, M. G., and Phillips, D. T.: J. Ag. Food Chem. **25**:1086, 1977.
73. Wertheimer, A., Seligman, E. B., Jr., Hochstein, H. D., and Parshall, D.: Annual Meeting, American Society for Microbiology, abstract, 1977, p. 266.
74. Miller, J., Moon, I., and Reynoso, G.: Annual Meeting, American Society for Microbiology, abstract, 1977, p. 81.
75. Berg, T. M., DenBerger, J. M., and Behagel, H. A. In Board, R. G., and Lovelock, D. W., editors: Some methods for microbiological assay, The Society for Applied Bacteriology technical series, vol. 8, New York, 1975, Academic Press.
76. Drucker, D. B. In Norris, J. R., editor: Methods in microbiology, vol. 9, New York, 1976, Academic Press.
77. Mitruka, B. M., editor: Gas chromatographic applications in microbiology and medicine, New York, 1975, John Wiley & Sons.
78. Holdeman, L. V., Cato, E. P., and Moore, W. E. C., editors: Anaerobe laboratory manual, ed. 4, Blacksburg, Va., 1977, Virginia Polytechnic Institute and State University.
79. Sutter, V. L., Vargo, V. L., and Finegold, S. M.: Wadsworth anaerobic bacteriology manual, ed. 2, Berkeley, Calif., 1975, University of California Press.
80. Moss, C. W.: Publ. Health Lab. **33**:81, 1975.
81. Mårdh, P.-A., and Grubb, R., editors: Acta Pathol. Microbiol. Scand. (B) **259** (suppl.):1, 1977.
82. Brooks, J. B., Kellogg, D. S., Alley, C. C., et al.: J. Infect. Dis. **129**:660, 1974.
83. Gorbach, S. L., Mayhew, J. W., Bartlett, J. G., et al.: J. Clin. Invest. **57**:478, 1976.
84. Edman, D. C., Converse, J. D., Brooks, J. B., and Craven, R. B.: Annual Meeting, American Society for Microbiology, abstract, 1978, p. 303.
85. Nord, C.: Acta Pathol. Microbiol. Scand. (B) **259** (suppl.):55, 1977.
86. Bricknell, K. S., Grinero, V., Carlton, D., and Newman, M. G.: Annual Meeting, American Society for Microbiology, abstract, 1978, p. 292.
87. Hayward, N. J., and Jeavons, T. H.: J. Clin. Microbiol. **6**:202, 1977.
88. Larsson, L., Mårdh, P.-A., and Odham, G.: J. Clin. Microbiol. **7**:23, 1978.
89. Ericsson, I., Larsson, L., and Mårdh, P.-A.: Acta Pathol. Microbiol. Scand. (B) **259**(suppl.):43, 1977.
90. Emswiller, B. S., and Kotula, A. W.: Appl. Environ. Microbiol. **35**:97, 1978.
91. Stack, M. V., Donoghue, H. D., and Tyler, J. E.: Appl. Environ. Microbiol. **35**:45, 1978.
92. Adelson, H. E., Brown, F. S., Clausen, O. W., et al.: Publ. no. 21020-6003-RU-00, NASA contract no. NAS-1-9000, Redondo Beach, Calif., 1975, TRW Systems Group.
93. Ryhage, R.: Q. Rev. Biophys. **6**:311, 1973.
94. Teece, R., Bowser, D. V., and Somani, S. M.: Annual Meeting, American Society for Microbiology, abstract, 1978, p. 23.
95. McGinley, K. J., Leyden, J. J., Webster, G. F., and Labows, J. N.: Annual Meeting, American Society for Microbiology, abstract, 1978, p. 320.
96. Mårdh, P.-A., and Grubb, R., editors: Acta Pathol. Microbiol. Scand. (B) **259** (suppl.) 1977.
97. Unger, P. D., and Hayes, A. W.: J. Chromatog. **153**:115, 1978.
98. Nilsson-Ehle, I.: Acta Pathol. Microbiol. Scand. (B) **259** (suppl.):61, 1977.
99. Darling, T., Albert, J., Russell, P., et al.: J. Chromatog. **131**:383, 1977.
100. McFadden, W. H., Bradford, D. C., Games, D. E., and Gower, J. L.: Am. Lab. **9**:55, 1977.
101. Sherma, J., Klopping, K. E., and Getz, M. D.: Am. Lab. **9**:66, 1977.
102. Sehrt, I., Käppler, W., and Lange, A.: Z. Erkr. Atmungsorgane. **143**:203, 1975.
103. Purchio, A.: Mycopathol. **58**:13, 1976.
104. Giddings, S. C., Yang, F. J., and Myers, M. N.: J. Virol. **21**:131, 1977.
105. Richmond, D. V., and Fisher, D. J. In Rose, A. H., and Tempest, D. W., editors: Advances in microbial physiology, vol. 9, New York, 1973, Academic Press.
106. Venezia, R. A., Matusiak, P. M., and Robertson, R. G.: Antimicrob. Ag. Chemother. **11**:735, 1977.
107. Labia, R., Guionie, M., Masson, J.-M., et al.: Antimicrob. Ag. Chemother. **11**:785, 1977.
108. Ur, A., and Brown, D. F. J. In Héden, C.-G., and Illeni, T., editors: New approaches to the identification of microorganisms, New York, 1975, John Wiley & Sons.
109. Cady, P. In Sharpe, A. N., and Clark, P. S., editors: Mechanizing microbiology, Springfield, Ill., 1978, Charles C Thomas, Publisher
110. Ur, A., and Brown, D. F. J.: Biomed. Eng. **9**:18, 1974.

111. Cady, P., Dufour, S. W., Lawless, P., et al.: J. Clin. Microbiol. **7:**273, 1978.

112. Cady, P., Hardy, D., Martins, S., et al.: J. Food Prot. **41:**277, 1978.

113. Throm, R., Specter, S., Strauss, R., and Friedman, H.: J. Clin. Microbiol. **6:**271, 1977.

114. Peters, J. E., Kahn, W. N., and Best, J. T.: Annual Meeting, American Society for Microbiology, abstract, 1978, p. 62.

115. Wilkins, J. R., Young, R. N., and Boykin, E. H.: Appl. Environ. Microbiol. **35:**214, 1978.

115a. Ladenson, J. H., Huebner, M., and Marr, J. J.: Analyt. Biochem. **63:**56, 1975.

116. Buck, R. P.: Anal. Chem. **46:**28R, 1974.

117. Gabridge, M. G.: J. Clin. Microbiol. **3:**560, 1976.

118. Llenado, R. A., and Rechnitz, G. A.: Anal. Chem. **45:**826, 1973

119. Bowers, L. D., and Carr, P. W.: Anal. Chem. **48:**545A, 1976.

120. Mor, J.-R., and Guarnaccia, R.: Anal. Biochem. **79:**319, 1977.

121. Rechnitz, G. A., Riechel, T. L., Kobos, R. K., and Meyerhoff, M. E.: Science **199:**440, 1978.

122. Seitz, W. R., and Neary, M. P. In Glick, D., editor: Methods of biochemical analysis, vol. 23, New York, 1976, John Wiley & Sons.

123. Alexander, D. N., Ederer, G. M., and Matsen, J. M.: J. Clin. Microbiol. **3:**42, 1976.

124. Paul, E. A., and Johnson, R. L.: Appl. Environ. Microbiol. **34:**263, 1977.

125. Miller, C. A., and Vogelhut, P. O.: Appl. Environ. Microbiol. **35:**813, 1978.

126. Picciolo, G. L., Chappelle, E. W., Thomas, R. R., and McGarry, M. A.: Appl. Environ. Microbiol. **34:**720, 1977.

127. Oleniacz, W. S., Pisano, M. A., and Rosenfield, M. H. In Technicon Symposium: Automation in analytical chemistry, vol. 1, New York, 1966, Mediad.

128. Halmann, M., Velan, B., and Sery, T.: Appl. Environ. Microbiol. **34:**473, 1977.

129. Puget, K., Michelson, A.M., and Avrameas, S.: Anal. Biochem. **81:**447, 1977.

130. Bostick, D. T., and Hercules, D. M.: Anal. Chem. **47:**447, 1975.

131. Hemming, V. G., Hall, R. T., Rhodes, P. G., et al.: J. Clin. Invest. **58:**1379, 1976.

132. Nelson, R. D., Herron, M. J., Schmidtke, J. R., and Simmons, R. L.: Infect. Immun. **17:**513, 1977.

133. Harvath, L., Amirault, H. J., and Anderson, B. R.: J. Clin. Invest. **61:**1145, 1978.

134. Spink, C., and Wadsö, I. In Glick, D., editor: Methods of biochemical analysis, vol. 23, New York, 1976, John Wiley & Sons.

135. Beezer, A. E.: Biochem. Soc. Trans. **4:**570, 1976.

136. Mårdh, P.-A., Andersson, K. E., Rippa, T., and Wadsö, I.: Scand. J. Infect. Dis. **9**(suppl.):12, 1976.

137. Lloyd, D., Phillips, C. A., and Statham, M.: J. Gen. Microbiol. **106:**19, 1978.

138. Tiefenbrunner, F.: Zentralbl. Bakteriol. [Orig. B] **161:**519, 1976.

139. Mov, D. G., and Cooney, C. L.: Biotechnol. Bioeng. **18:**1371, 1976.

140. Rosencwaig, A.: Anal. Chem. **47:**592A, 1975.

141. Pao, Y., editor: Optoacoustic spectroscopy, New York, 1977, Academic Press.

142. Oda, S., Sawada, T., and Kamada, H.: Anal. Chem. **50:**865, 1978.

143. Rosencwaig, A., and Pines, E.: Biochem. Biophys. Acta **493:**10, 1977.

144. Kreuzer, L. B.: Anal. Chem. **50:**597A, 1978.

145. Coffey, P., Mattson, D. R., and Wright, J. C.: Am. Lab. **10:**126, 1978.

146. Strauss, R. R., Holderbach, J., and Friedman, H.: J. Clin. Microbiol. **7:**419, 1978.,

147. Hopfer, R. L., and Gröschel, D.: Antimicrob. Ag. Chemother. **11:**277, 1977.

148. Sloane, P. S.: Annual Meeting, American Society for Microbiology, abstract, 1978, p. 205.

149. Jacobs, P. F., Burdash, N. M., West, M. A., and Buchner, P. A.: Annual Meeting, American Society for Microbiology, abstract, 1978, p. 296.

150. Gunn, B. A., Brown, S. L., Otey, C. S., et al.: Annual Meeting, American Society for Microbiology, abstract, 1978, p. 300.

151. Johnson, B. T., and Romanenko, V. I.: Annual Meeting, American Society for Microbiology, abstract, 1978, p. 209.

152. Milne, R. G., and Luisoni, E. In Maramorosch, K., and Koprowski, H., editors: Methods in virology, vol. 6, New York, 1977, Academic Press.

153. Hughes. J. H., Gnau, J. M., Hilty, M. D., et al.: J. Med. Microbiol. **10:**203, 1977.

154. Mebus, C. A., and Newman, L. E.: Am. J. Vet. Res. **38:**553, 1977.

155. Faulkner, G. P., Shirodaria, P. V., Follett, E. A., and Pringle, C. R.: J. Virol. **20:**487, 1976.

156. Weigele, M. D., Bernado, S., and Leimgruber W.: Biochem. Biophys. Res. Comm. **54:**899, 1975.

157. Undenfriend, S., Stein, S., Bohlen, P., et al.: Science **178:**871, 1972.

158. Smith, B. J., and Bailey, J. M.: Annual Meeting, American Society for Microbiology, abstract, 1978, p. 213.

159. Mayfield, C. I.: Microsc. Acta **78:**295, 1976.

160. Paau, A. S., Cowles, J. R., and Oro, J.: Can. J. Microbiol. **23:**1165, 1977.

161. Bailey, J. E., Fazel-Makjlessi, J., McQuitty, D. N., et al.: Science **198:**1175, 1977.

162. Defibaugh, P. W., Smith, J. S., and Weeks, C. E.: J. Assoc. Off. Anal. Chem. **60:**522, 1977.

163. Hirschfeld, T., Block, M. J., and Mueller, W.: J. Histo. Cytochem. **25:**719, 1977.

164. Pien, F. D., Markowitz, H., McKenna, C. H., and Schroeter, A. L.: J. Am. Vener. Dis. Assoc. **3:**20, 1976.

165. Thomas, V. L., Forland, M., and Shelokov, A.: Proc. Soc. Exp. Biol. Med. **148:**1198, 1975.

166. Al-Samarri, H. T., and Henderson, W. G.: Br. J. Vener. Dis. **53:**1, 1977.

167. Pederson, C. E., Jr., Bagley, L. P., Kenyon, R. H., et al.: J. Clin. Microbiol. **2:**121, 1976.

168. Chandler, F. W., Hicklin, M. D., and Blackmon, J. A.: N. Engl. J. Med. **297:**1197, 1977.

169. Murphy, F. A., Buchmeier, M. J., and Rawls, W. E.: Lab. Invest. **37:**502, 1977.

170. Emmons, R. W., and Riggs, J. L. In Maramorosch, K., and Koprowski, H., editors: Methods in virology, vol. 6, New York, 1977, Academic Press.

171. Ormsbee, R., Peacock, M., Philip, R., et al.: Am. J. Epidemiol. **103:**261, 1977.

172. Lamy, M. E., Favart, A. M., Burtonboy, G., and Arana, A.: J. Clin. Microbiol. **6:**66, 1977.

173. Munson, T. E., Schrade, J. P., Bisciello, N. B., Jr., et al.: Appl. Environ. Microbiol. **31:**514, 1976.

174. Standard, P. G., and Kaufman, L.: J. Clin. Microbiol. **3:**191, 1976.

175. Mishuk, E., and Roberts, M.: In Héden, C.-G., and Illeni, T., editors: Automation in microbiology and immunology, New York, 1975, John Wiley & Sons.

176. Hambie, E. A., Larsen, S. A., Felkner, M., et al.: J. Clin. Microbiol. **5:**167, 1977.

177. Ruitenberg, E. J., Buys, J., and Meeuwsen, F.: Zentralbl. Bakteriol. [Orig. A] **233:**561, 1975.

178. Drescher, J., and Desselberger, O.: Arch. Virol. **50:**97, 1976.
179. Sire, J., Denoyel, G. A., Colle, A., and Manuel, Y.: Pathol. Biol. (Paris) **25:**425, 1977.
180. Klagge, E., and Kortung, H. J.: Z. Hautkr. **52:**651, 1977.
181. Arndt-Jovin, D. J., Ostertag, W., Eisen, H., et al.: J. Histochem. Cytochem. **24:**332, 1976.
182. Burtis, C. A., Tiffany, T. O., and Scott, C. D. In Glick, D., editor: Methods of biochemical analysis, vol. 23, New York, 1976, John Wiley & Sons.
183. Leute, R., Ullman, E. F., and Goldstein, A.: J.A.M.A. **221:**1231, 1972.
184. Penn, G. M., and Batya, J.: Interpretation of immunoelectrophoretic patterns, Chicago, 1978, American Society of Clinical Pathologists.
185. Maigetter, R. Z., Mancinelli, R. J., King, J. J., et al.: Annual Meeting, American Society for Microbiology, abstract, 1978, p. 109.
186. Bergogne-Berezin, E., and Slim, A.: Ann. Biol. Clin. (Paris) **34:**415, 1976.
187. Naik, H. S., and Duncan, C. L.: J. Clin. Microbiol. **7:**337, 1978.
188. Colding, H., and Lind, I.: J. Clin. Microbiol. **5:**405, 1977.
189. Smaron, M. F.: Annual Meeting, American Society for Microbiology, abstract, 1978, p. 308.
190. Anhalt, J. P., Kenny, G. E., and Rytel, M. W.: Detection of microbial antigens by counterimmunoelectrophoresis. In Gavan, T. L., editor-coordinator: Cumitech 8, Washington, D.C., 1978, American Society for Microbiology.
191. Waters, C. A., Fossieck, B. E., and Parker, R. H.: Annual Meeting, American Society for Microbiology, abstract, 1978, p. 307.
192. Thompson, N. L., and Ellner, P. D.: J. Clin. Microbiol. **7:**493, 1978.
193. Sever, J. L., and Madden, D. L., editors: Enzymelinked immunosorbent assay for infectious agents, J. Infect. Dis. **136**(suppl.), 1977.
194. Blaedel, W. J., and Boguslaski, R. C.: Anal. Chem. **50:**1026, 1978.
195. Bidwell, E. D., et al.: Bull. WHO **54:**129, 1976.
196. Ternynck, T., and Avrameas, S.: Immunochemistry **14:**767, 1977.
197. Svenungsson, B., and Lindberg, A. A.: Acta Pathol. Microbiol. Scand. (B) **86:**35, 1978.
198. Yolken, R. H., Greenberg, H. B., Merson, M. H., et al.: J. Clin, Microbiol. **6:**439, 1977.
199. Granlund, D. J., and Andrese, A. P.: Int. J. Cancer **20:**495, 1977.
200. Crosson, F. J., Jr., Winkelstein, J. A., and Moxon, E. R.: Annual Meeting, American Society for Microbiology, abstract, 1978, p. 294.
201. Mathiesen, L. R., Feinstone, S. M., Wong, D. C., et al.: J. Clin. Microbiol. **7:**184, 1978.
202. Lawellin, D. W., Grant, D. W., and Joyce, B. K.: Appl. Environ. Microbiol. **34:**88, 1977.
203. Akerlund, A. S., Ahlstedt, S., Hanson, L. A., et al.: Int. Arch. Allergy Appl. Immunol. **55:**458, 1977.
204. Farshy, C. E., Klein, G. C., and Feeley, J. C.: J. Clin. Microbiol. **7:**327, 1978.
205. Sippel, J. E., Mammay, H. K., Weiss, E., et al.: J. Clin. Microbiol. **7:**372, 1978.
206. Saunders, G. C., and Bartlett, M. L.: Appl. Environ. Microbiol. **34:**518, 1977.
207. Wolters, G., Kuijpers, L. P., Kačaki, J., and Schurs, A. H. W. M.: J. Infect. Dis. **136**(suppl.):311, 1977.
208. Ruitenberg, E. J., and van Knapen, F.: J. Infect. Dis. **136** (suppl.):267, 1977.
209. Saunders, G. C., and Clinard, E. H.: J. Clin. Microbiol. **3:**604, 1976.
210. Vandervelde, E. M., Cohen, B. J., and Cossart, Y. E.: J. Clin. Pathol. **30:**714, 1977.
211. Leinikki, P. O., and Passila, S.: J. Infect. Dis. **136** (suppl.):294, 1977.
212. Clem, T. R., and Yolken, R. H.: J. Clin. Microbiol. **7:**55, 1978.
213. Guesdon, J.-L., and Avrameas, S.: Immunochemistry **14:**443, 1977.
214. Pinon, J. M., Gorse, J. P., and Dropsy, G.: Mycopathologia **60:**115, 1977.
215. Berger, L. R., and Berger, J. A.: Annual Meeting, American Society for Microbiology, abstract, 1978, p. 194.
216. Parikh, G. C., Sorenson, T. C., and Duvall, C. S. In Héden, C.-G., and Illeni, T., editors: Automation in microbiology and immunology, New York, 1975, John Wiley & Sons.
217. Amesse, L. S., and Payne, F. E.: Annual Meeting, American Society for Microbiology, abstract, 1978, p. 261.
218. Kalimo, K. O., Marttila, R. J., Ziola, B. R., et al.: J. Med. Microbiol. **10:**431, 1977.
219. Bradley, D. W., Maynard, J. E., Hindman, S. H., et al.: J. Clin. Microbiol. **5:**521, 1977.
220. Benbough, J. E., and Martin, K. L.: J. Appl. Bacteriol. **41:**47, 1976.
221. Wilkinson, H. W.: J. Clin. Microbiol. **7:**194, 1978.
222. Sandford, B. A., and Smith, K. O.: J. Immunol. Methods **14:**313, 1977.
223. Ceska, M., Effenberger, F., and Grossmüller, F.: J. Clin. Microbiol. **7:**209, 1978.
224. Orth, D. S.: Appl. Environ. Microbiol. **34:**710, 1977.
225. Robern, H., Gleeson, T. M., and Szabo, R. A.: Can. J. Microbiol. **24:**436, 1978.
226. Zollinger, W. D., and Mandrell, R. E.: Infect. Immun. **18:**424, 1977.
227. Huang, S. Y., Berry, C. W., and Newman, J. J.: Annual Meeting, American Society for Microbiology, abstract, 1978, p. 322.
228. Reiss, E., Hutchinson, H., Pine. L., et al.: J. Clin. Microbiol. **6:**598, 1977.
229. Comer, J. B., Cunha, B. A., and Chow, M.: Annual Meeting, American Society for Microbiology, abstract, 1978, p. 300.
230. Ryan, R. W., Kwasnik, I. M., Lentnek, A., and Tilton, R. C.: Annual Meeting, American Society for Microbiology, abstract, 1978, p. 300.
231. Leland, D. S., Lachapelle, R. C., and Wlodarski, F. M.: J. Clin. Microbiol. **7:**323, 1978.
232. Menck, H.: Acta Pathol. Microbiol. Scand. (B) **84:**139, 1976.
233. Handsher, R., and Fogel, A.: J. Clin. Microbiol. **5:**588, 1977.
234. Chantler, S., Devries, E., Allen, P. R., and Hurn, B. A.: J. Immunol. Methods **13:**367, 1976.
235. Zalan, E., and Wilson, C.: Arch. Virol. **56:**177, 1978.
236. Ades, E. W., Phillips, D. J., Shore, S. L., et al.: J. Immunol. **117:**2119, 1976.
237. Wise, J. A., Brown, J. P., and Foy, H. M.: Annual Meeting, American Society for Microbiology, abstract, 1978, p. 243.
238. Deshayes, L., Levy, D., Fournier, G., and Gilly, L.: Compt. Rendus (series D) **286:**435, 1978.
239. Van Wyke, K. L., and Eckert, E. A.: Annual Meeting, American Society for Microbiology, abstract, 1978, p. 243.
240. Bachman, B., and Weaver, R. H.: J. Bacteriol. **54:**28, 1947.
241. Hartman, P. A.: Miniaturized microbiological methods, New York, 1968, Academic Press.

242. Fung, D. Y. C., and Hartman, P. A.: In Héden, C.-G., and Illeni, T., editors: Automation in microbiology and immunology, New York, 1975, John Wiley & Sons.

243. Cox, N. A., McHan, F., and Fung, D. Y. C.: J. Food Prot. **40**:866, 1977.

244. Smith, P. B.: Performance of six bacterial identification systems, Atlanta, 1977, Center for Disease Control.

245. Brenner, D. J., and Balows, A.: J. Clin. Microbiol. **2**:235, 1975.

246. O'Donnell, E. D., Kaufman, F. J., Longo, E. D., and Ellner, P. D.: Am. J. Clin. Pathol. **53**:145, 1970.

247. Brown, W. J.: Am. J. Med. Technol. **39**:272, 1973.

248. Isenberg, H. D., Smith, P. B., Balows, A., et al.: Appl. Microbiol. **27**:575, 1974.

249. Wust, J., and Kayser, F. H.: Pathol. Microbiol. **40**:316, 1974.

250. Isenberg, H. D., Scherber, J. S., and Cosgrove, J. D.: J. Clin. Microbiol. **2**:139, 1975.

251. Finlayson, M. H., and Gibbs, B.: S. Afr. J. Lab. Clin. Med. **20**:1219, 1974.

252. Malowany, M. S., Mikkelsen, G., Kittick, J., et al.: Annual Meeting, American Society for Microbiology, abstract, 1978, p. 307.

253. Kiehn, T. E., Brennan, K., and Ellner, P. D.: Appl. Microbiol. **28**:668, 1974.

254. Hansen, S. L., Hardesty, D. R., and Myers, B. M.: Appl. Microbiol. **28**:798, 1974.

255. Cox, N. A., and Williams, J. E.: Poult. Sci. **55**:1968, 1976.

256. Cox, N. A., and Mercuri, A. J.: J. Appl. Bacteriol. **41**:389, 1976.

257. Chester, B., and Evans, G. L.: Annual Meeting, American Society for Microbiology, abstract, 1978, p. 252.

258. Back, A. E., and Oberhofer, T. R.: J. Clin. Microbiol. **7**:312, 1978.

259. Slifkin, M., and Pouchet, G. R.: Annual Meeting, American Society for Microbiology, abstract, 1977, p. 50.

260. Smith, P. B., Tomfohrde, K. M., Rhoden, D. L., and Balows, A.: Appl. Microbiol. **22**:928, 1972.

261. Holmes, B., Wilcox, W. R., and Lapage, S. P.: J. Clin. Pathol. **31**:22, 1978.

262. Hayek, L. J., and Willis, G. W.: J. Clin. Pathol. **29**:158, 1976.

263. Nord, C.-E., Lindberg, A. A., and Dahlback, A.: Med. Microbiol. Immunol. **159**:211, 1974.

264. Sakazaki, R.: J. Gen. Microbiol. **46**:407, 1975.

265. Marymont, J. H. III, Marymont, J. H., Jr., and Gavan, T. L.: Am. J. Clin. Pathol. **70**:539, 1978.

266. Washington, J. A. II: Human Pathol. **7**:151, 1976.

267. Robertson, E. A., and MacLowry, J. D.: J. Clin. Microbiol. **1**:515, 1975.

268. Aldridge, K. E., Gardner, B. B., Clark, S. J., and Matsen, J. M.: J. Clin. Microbiol. **7**:507, 1978.

268a. Cox, N. A., and Mecuri, A. J.: J. Food Prot. **41**:107, 1978.

269. Washington, J. A. II, Yn, P. K. W., and Martin, W. J.: Appl. Microbiol. **22**:267, 1971.

270. Blazevic, D. J., Trombley, C. M., and Lund, M. E.: J. Clin. Microbiol. **4**:522, 1976.

271. Liberman, D. F., and Kovacic, S.: Annual Meeting, American Society for Microbiology, abstract, 1978, p. 304.

272. Rhoden, D. L., Tomfohrde, K. M., Smith, P. B., and Balows, A.: Appl. Microbiol. **26**:215, 1973.

273. Braune, L. M., and Kocka, F. E.: Med. Microbiol. Immunol. **161**:189, 1975.

274. Smith, P. B., Rhoden, D. L., and Tomfohrde, K. M.: J. Clin. Microbiol. **1**:359, 1975.

275. Cox, N. A., Mecuri, A. J., Carson, M. O., and Tanner, D. A.: J. Food Prot. (In press.)

276. Edberg, S. C., Atkinson, B., Chambers, C., et al.: Annual Meeting, American Society for Microbiology, abstract, 1978, p. 305.

277. Davies, T. J., Janda, W. M., Kaplan, R. L., and Morello, J. A.: Annual Meeting, American Society for Microbiology, abstract, 1978, p. 302.

278. Borchardt, K. A., and Gibson, J.: Health Lab. Sci. **14**:5, 1976.

279. Johnson, J. E.: Annual Meeting, American Society for Microbiology, abstract, 1978, p. 290.

280. Amsterdam, D., Phillips, S. B., and Richter, M. W.: J. Clin. Microbiol. **4**:160, 1976.

281. Branson, D.: Am. J. Med. Technol. **42**:267, 1976.

282. Stuver, J. C., and Matsen, J. M.: Annual Meeting, American Society for Microbiology, abstract, 1978, p. 271.

283. Rutherford, I., Moody, V., Gavan, T. L., et al.: J. Clin. Microbiol. **5**:458, 1977.

284. Guthertz, L. S., and Okoluk, R. L.: Appl. Environ. Microbiol. **35**:109, 1978.

285. Koka, F. E., and Morello, J. A.: J. Infect. Dis. **131**:456, 1975.

286. Shayegani, M., Hubbard, M. E., Hiscott, T., et al.: J. Clin. Microbiol. **2**:186, 1975.

287. Shayegani, M., Lee, A. M. and McGlynn, D. M.: J. Clin. Microbiol. **7**:533, 1978.

288. Nadler, H., George, H., and Barr, J.: Annual Meeting, American Society for Microbiology, abstract, 1978, p. 290.

289. Timm, J. H., Hall, M. K., and Washington, J. A. II: Annual Meeting, American Society for Microbiology, abstract, 1978, p. 303.

290. Smith, P. B., Hill, E. O., and Isenberg, H. D.: Annual Meeting, American Society for Microbiology, abstract, 1978, p. 304.

291. Isenberg, H. D., and Sampson-Scherer, J.: J. Clin. Microbiol. **5**:336, 1977.

292. Rinehart, S. L., and Oberhofer, T. R.: Annual Meeting, American Society for Microbiology, abstract, 1978, p. 303.

293. McHale, K. M., Teplitz, M. G., and Gavan, T. L.: Annual Meeting, American Society for Microbiology, abstract, 1978, p. 304.

294. Shayegani, M., Maupin, P. S., and McGlynn, D. M.: J. Clin. Microbiol. **7**:539, 1978.

295. Dowda, H.: J. Clin. Microbiol. **6**:605, 1977.

296. Barnishan, J., and Ayres, L.: Annual Meeting, American Society for Microbiology, abstract, 1978, p. 290.

297. Snyder, J., Vincent, S., Hoyng, C., et al.: Annual Meeting, American Society for Microbiology, abstract, 1978, p. 304.

298. Otto, L. A., Aspin, M. M., and Blachman, U.: Annual Meeting, American Society for Microbiology, abstract, 1978, p. 303.

299. Bannister, E. R., West, M. E., Buchner, P. A., et al.: Annual Meeting, American Society for Microbiology, abstract, 1978, p. 303.

300. Starr, S. E., Thompson, F. S., Dowell, V. R., Jr., and Balows, A.: Appl. Microbiol. **25**:713, 1973.

301. Hansen, S. L., and Stewart, B. J.: J. Clin. Microbiol. **4**:227, 1976.

302. Nadaud, M., and Cancet, B.: Zentralbl. Bakteriol. [Orig. A] **237**:530, 1977.

303. Essers, L., and Haralambie, E.: Zentralbl. Bakteriol. [Orig. A] **238**:394, 1977.

304. Gilliland, S. E., and Speck, M. L.: Appl. Environ. Microbiol. **33**:1289, 1977.

305. Stargel, D., Thompson, F. S., Philips, S. E., et al.: J. Clin. Microbiol. **3**:291, 1976.

306. Moore, H. B., Sutter, V. L., and Finegold. S. M.: J. Clin. Microbiol. **1**:15, 1975.
306a. Burgard, L., Cole, B., and Sonnenwirth, A.: Abstracts, Annual Meeting, American Society for Microbiology, Abstract C 166, 1979, p. 337.
307. Arvilommi, H.: Acta Pathol. Microbiol. Scand. (B) **84**:79, 1976.
308. Hahn, G., and Nyberg, I.: J. Clin. Microbiol. **4**:99, 1976.
309. Slifkin, M., Engwall, C., and Pouchet, G. R.: J. Clin. Microbiol. **7**:356, 1978.
310. Bowman, P. I., and Ahearn, D. G.: J. Clin. Microbiol. **4**:49, 1976.
310a. Zwadyk, P., Jr., Tarlton, R. A., and Proctor, A.: Am. J. Clin. Pathol. **67**:269, 1977.
311. Roberts, G. D., Wang, H. S., and Hollick, G. E.: J. Clin. Microbiol. **3**:302, 1976.
312. Burgard, L. E., and Sonnenwirth, A. C.: Annual Meeting, American Society for Microbiology, abstract, 1976, p. 29.
313. Cooper, B. H., Johnson, J. B., and Thaxton, E. S.: J. Clin. Microbiol. **7**:349, 1978.
314. Mickelson, P. A., McCarthy, L. R., McGinnis, M. R., and Propst, M. A.: Annual Meeting, American Society for Microbiology, abstract, 1976, p. 29.
315. Quadri, H. S. M., and Nichols, C. W.: Am. J. Med. Tech. **44**:368, 1978.
316. Davies, R. R., and Savage, M. A.: J. Clin. Pathol. **28**:750, 1975.
317. Berdicevsky, I., Ben-Aryeh, H., Glick, D., and Gutman, D.: Oral Surg. **44**:206, 1977.
318. Rindt, W., and Weigerding, A.: Med. Klin. **72**:598, 1977.
319. Segal, E., and Ajello, L.: J. Clin. Microbiol. **4**:157, 1976.
320. Quadri, S. M. H., Stager, C. E., Quadri, S. G. M., and Weyman, L.: Annual Meeting, American Society for Microbiology, abstract, 1978, p. 286.
321. Olmos, L., Bergues, J. P., Ellena, V., et al.: Dermatologica **155**:224, 1977.
322. Nielsen, A. O., and Andersen, K. E.: Sex. Transm. Dis. **4**:15, 1977.
323. Judson, F. N.: Sex. Transm. Dis. **4**:22, 1977.
324. Bowden, J. V., Krizmanic, D. L., and Hammock, S. L.: Annual Meeting, American Society for Microbiology, abstract, 1978, p. 279.
325. Buchner, P. A., Burdash, N. M., Manos, J. P., and Alexander, M. M.: Annual Meeting, American Society for Microbiology, abstract, 1978, p. 280.
326. Morse, S. A., and Bartenstein, L.: J. Clin. Microbiol. **3**:8, 1976.
327. Valu, J. A.: J. Clin. Microbiol. **3**:172, 1976.
328. Russell, A. O., Patton, C. M., and Kaufmann, A. F.: J. Clin. Microbiol. **7**:454, 1978.
329. Edwards, B., White, R. H. R., Maxted, H., et al.: Br. Med. J. **2**(5969):463, 1975.
330. Bailey, R. R.: NZ Med. J. **82**:331, 1975.
331. Winter, C. C.: J. Urol. **114**:755, 1975.
332. Meek, J. V., Strenkoski, L. F., Widomski, M. J., and Chapman, D. J.: Annual Meeting, American Society for Microbiology, abstract, 1978, p. 287.
333. Barry, A. L., Jones, R. N., and Gavan, T. L.: Antimicrob. Ag. Chemother. **13**:61, 1978.
333a. Phillips, I., Warren, C., and Waterworth, P. M.: J. Clin. Pathol. **31**:531-535, 1978.
334. Kroemer, G., Brückler, J., and Blobel, H.: Zentralbl. Bacteriol. [Orig. A] **239**:42, 1977.
335. Harris, E. E., Venturini, D. R., and Allen, S. D.: Annual Meeting, American Society for Microbiology, abstract, 1978, p. 289.
336. Kilgore, J. G., Byron, B., and Mertens, B. F.: Annual Meeting, American Society for Microbiology, abstract, 1978, p. 289.
337. van Weemen, B., and Kacaki, J.: J. Hyg. (Camb.) **77**:31, 1976.
338. Maddocks, J. L., and Greenan, M. J.: J. Clin. Pathol. **28**:686, 1975.
339. Bradbury, J. M.: J. Clin. Microbiol. **5**:531, 1977.
340. Watson, R. R. In Norris, J., editor: Methods in microbiology, vol. 9, New York, 1976, Academic Press.
341. Humble, M. W., King, A., and Phillips, I.: J. Clin. Pathol. **30**:275, 1977.
342. Tharagonnet, D., Sisson, P. R., Roxby, C. M., et al.: J. Clin. Pathol. **30**:505, 1977.
343. D'Amato, R. F., Eriquez, L. A., Tomfohrde, K. M., and Singerman, E.: J. Clin. Microbiol. **7**:77, 1978.
344. Balows, A., and Isenberg, H. D., editors: Biotyping in the clinical microbiology laboratory, Springfield, Ill., 1978, Charles C Thomas, Publisher.
345. Gyllenberg, H. G., and Niemelä, T. K. In Héden, C.-G., and Illeni, T., editors: New approaches to the identification of microorganisms, New York, 1975, John Wiley & Sons.
346. Kelley, R. W., and Kellog, S. T.: Appl. Environ. Microbiol. **35**:507, 1978.
346a. Filburn, B., Houston, F., Shull, V., et al.: Abstract, Annual Meeting, American Society for Microbiology, Abstract 304, 1978.
347. Mandel, R. J., and Wade, T. J. In Prier, J. E., Bartola, J., and Friedman, H., editors: Modern methods in medical microbiology, Baltimore, 1976, University Park Press.
348. Macfie, H. J. H., Gutteridge, C. S., and Norris, J. R.: J. Gen. Microbiol. **104**:67, 1978.
349. Walczak, C. A., Johnson, R., and Krichevsky, M. I.: Annual Meeting, American Society for Microbiology, abstract, 1978, p. 90.
350. Horowitz, A., Krichevsky, M. I., and Atlas, R. M.: Annual Meeting, American Society for Microbiology, abstract, 1978, p. 208.
351. Gyllenberg, H. G.: Arch. Immunol. Ther. Exp. (Warsz) **24**:1, 1976.
352. Lechevalier, M. P.: CRC Crit. Rev. Microbiol. **5**:109, 1977.
353. Bowie, I. S., Hill, L. R., and Lapage, S. P.: Second International Symposium on Rapid Methods and Automation in Microbiology, New York, 1976, Learned Information (Europe) Ltd, abstract, p. 91.
354. Johnson, R., Rogosa, M., Gherna, R. L., and Jackson, C.: Annual Meeting, American Society for Microbiology, abstract, 1978, p. 290.
355. Buchanan, R. E., and Gibbons, N. E., editors: Bergey's manual of determinative bacteriology, ed. 8, Baltimore, 1974, Williams & Wilkins Co.
356. Edwards, P. R., and Ewing, W. H.: Identification of *Enterobacteriaceae*, ed. 3, Minneapolis, 1972, Burgess Publishing Company.
357. Balows, A.: In Johnston, H. H., and Newsom, S. W. B., editors: Rapid methods and automation in microbiology, Forest Grove, 1977, International Scholarly Book Services.
358. Cassatt, B.: Analyt. Chem. **50**:695A, 1978.
359. Cox, N. A., and Mercuri, A. J.: J. Food Protect. **40**:709, 1977.
360. Cox, N. A., Mecuri, A. J., and McHan, F. In Second International Symposium on rapid methods and automation in microbiology, New York, 1976, Learned Information (Europe), p. 163.

75

COLLECTION AND CULTURE OF SPECIMENS AND GUIDES FOR BACTERIAL IDENTIFICATION

Alex C. Sonnenwirth

In this section methods are described for the collection, handling, and cultivation of specimens from clinical material as well as certain procedures and guides for the identification of bacteria.

Primary culture methods to be used usually depend on the site from which the specimen was obtained and, in certain instances, on the specific disease or organism suspected. The routine methods outlined for every specimen are recommended, regardless of special requests. When special procedures are ordered, these should be carried out in addition to the routine methods. In general, specimens from **sites normally sterile** are cultured on a variety of highly nutrient liquid and solid media to ensure the growth of any bacteria present. Specimens from **sites with a normal flora** are also cultured on such media, but in addition, selective and differential methods and media are used, which greatly increase the chance of recovering known pathogens. In the case of special surveys (detection of staphylococcal or meningococcal carriers or of diphtheria bacilli) it is permissible to use only selective methods for the one organism or group of organisms in question. In addition, when searching for certain organisms (such as *Mycobacterium, Leptospira*, etc.), it is necessary to use specialized procedures and media regardless of the site from which the specimen was taken.

COLLECTION OF SPECIMENS— GENERAL RULES

The success of bacteriologic procedures depends to a great extent on the manner in which the specimens are obtained and the promptness with which they are taken to the laboratory. Such procedures are more often than not made valueless by lack of care and faulty methods used in collection and handling of specimens. The following rules should be observed:

1. **Label** all specimens with the patient's name, the time, and date of collection. A request form, signed by the individual collecting the sample, should state the name and age of the patient, the number of the room or ward, the **nature** of the specimen and the **site** from which it was obtained, the clinical diagnosis and duration of the illness, and the **test** required.[1]

2. Obtain specimens, if at all possible, **before** antibiotics or antimicrobial agents are administered. If antibiotics or chemotherapeutic agents have been administered, inform laboratory (note on requisition). Often a purulent cerebrospinal fluid will reveal no bacterial pathogens on smear or culture when an antibiotic has been given within the previous 24 h.

3. Because the skin, intestinal tract, mucous membranes, etc. all have a population of the normal microbial flora, it is necessary to utilize **special procedures** to distinguish etiologic agents from members of the normal flora. Matsen and Ederer[2] recommend the following approaches:

   a. Clean the area with disinfectant (i.e., 70% alcohol and 2% iodine in case of skin preparation for blood culture).

   b. Culture specifically for organisms known to be etiologic agents (e.g., group A streptococci in throat).

   c. Bypass areas with normal flora (e.g., use suprapubic aspiration for urine specimen when culturing for anaerobes, or transtracheal aspiration instead of sputum).

   d. Quantitate culture results (e.g., quantitative urine cultures).

In a similar vein, Lipsky and Plorde[3] succinctly state that most specimens for bacterial culture represent 1 of 3 areas: (1) **deep closed body areas**, (2) **deep communicating body areas**, or (3) **superficial body surfaces.**

(a) Those specimens from deep areas, **normally sterile,** are the most satisfactory (circulating blood, pleura, peritoneum, joint, etc.). Careful skin preparation is needed.

(b) Those specimens from deep areas that communicate with the surface (endocervix, bladder, fistulas) **may be contaminated by normal flora.** Bypass of the area may be needed (see *3c* above).

(c) Specimens from superficial body surfaces (skin, mucous membranes) are the most unreliable, since these sites are **heavily contaminated** with normal flora. Here one needs to restrict the search to a specific etiologic agent (*Salmonella, Shigella, Yersinia enterocolitica* in stool, *Neisseria gonorrhoeae* in urethra).

4. Send specimens to the laboratory as soon as possible. *Neisseria meningitidis* is very sensitive to temperature changes; therefore spinal fluid should be delivered while still warm. If it cannot be cultured immediately, incubate at 37 C. Specimens for the culture of *Neisseria gonorrhoeae* should be either plated at the bedside or placed in special transport medium (Stuart). The same holds for eye swabs.

5. **Tissue.** Deliver in dry, **sterile,** wide-mouth, screwcap bottle or plastic container without addition of water or saline; send without delay. Obviously, no formalin should be added.

6. **Use sterile containers** without transport medium or preservative for the collection of **urine, sputum,** and **cerebrospinal fluid.** Collect **stool** in a sterile bedpan[4] and place a suitable portion of it in a clean waxed carton or screwcapped bottle for immediate delivery to laboratory. If stool cannot be processed immediately, it should be placed in preservative solution or transport medium (see stool examination). **Sputum** should be collected in a sterile, glass, screwcapped bottle or in sterile disposable plastic containers. Do not use paper containers.

7. For material from the **throat, nose, eye, ear, wounds, abscesses,** or **rectum,** use cotton-tipped or, preferably, Dacron-tipped* or calcium alginate–tipped† applicator sticks. Some workers recommend placing the inoculated cotton applicator sticks into a tube containing a few drops of infusion broth to prevent drying. Others justifiably object to the broth because multiplication of bacteria may take place, contaminants rapidly outgrowing the significant organisms; for brief periods, a few drops of sterile physiologic saline may be used to prevent drying out of the swab.‡

As a general rule, clinical material should be cultured immediately, since many anaerobes die very rapidly on exposure to oxygen. Use aspirated material instead of swabs where possible. (See below, Anaerobic culture.)

Cotton wool has been shown to inhibit certain bacteria, probably due to fatty acids present in the cotton. For this reason, specimens on dry cotton-tipped swabs should not be used. Dacron swabs require no broth, saline, or other transport media because the bacteria dry rapidly on the inert, nonwettable fiber; such swabs can be kept dry in a tube or envelope for several days without loss of viability of *Streptococcus pyogenes* group A organisms, especially if **silica gel** is incorporated into the container before autoclaving.[5] For this reason, Dacron swabs are preferred for throat swabs. For further discussion see swabs for specimens (below).

8. Handling of swabs
   a. Swabs used in conjunction with screw-capped transport media are usually placed in transport vial and broken off just below the rim of the vial. Care should be taken that the portion of the swab that has been handled is removed.
   b. Swabs in large tubes. Some workers break off the portion of the applicator that has been handled and drop the swab into the tube. Such swabs are awkward to manipulate in the laboratory; it is preferable to let ½ in. of the swab handle project through the plug at the top of the tube. The top can then be flamed. Certain commercially available swab-tube assemblies (disposable) circumvent this difficulty by having a plastic cap that covers the end of the swab and also serves as the closure cap for the tube, thus eliminating handtouching of the swab itself.

   The tubes containing swabs may be plugged with cotton or closed with a stainless steel cap (Morton culture tube closure).

   Numerous disposable, presterilized swab-tube assemblies are available.*

9. For obtaining nasopharyngeal specimens, cotton- or alginate-tipped 28-gauge Ni-chrome wire is recommended in place of the wooden stick. Flexible nasopharyngeal swabs, calcium alginate–tipped, are commercially available.

10. **Blood** should be collected in sterile bottles containing broth or sterile tubes containing anticoagulant. **Bone marrow** preferably

---

*Dacron polyester bulk, Sears, Roebuck & Co.; Dacron swabs, Econ Microbiological Laboratories, Minneapolis; Scientific Products, Evanston, Ill.
†Colab Laboratories, Inc., Chicago Heights, Ill.
‡Disposable Cepti-Seal Culturette swabs, Scientific Products, Evanston, Ill.

---

*Falcon Plastics, Division of BioQuest, Los Angeles, Calif.; Calgiswab Kit, Colab Laboratories, Chicago Heights, Ill.; Trans-Cul; Handi-swab; Culture Caddy. Most of these contain small amounts of Stuart or Amies holding medium.

should be collected in sterile tubes; however, since the specimen often clots, sterile tubes containing nonbactericidal anticoagulant (see blood culture) are preferred.

11. Delay between collection and culturing. A number of **transport media,** including **anaerobic collection and transport systems** (see below), are available for prolonging the survival of organisms. If any appreciable delay is expected between collection and culturing, swabs should be placed in transport medium vials.

Send specimens to the laboratory as early in the day as possible, Whenever immediate attention is required (dark-field examination for spirochetes, spinal fluid culture, etc.), notify the laboratory in advance.

12. **All specimens for culture should be carefully examined upon receipt.** Leaking containers or soaked cotton plugs are dangerous to the nurses and laboratory staff, and the introduction of contaminating organisms may lead to a false diagnosis. Contaminated or leaking containers should be autoclaved or incinerated, and another specimen should be requested.

Swabs for specimens. The use of cotton- vs. Dacron- or calcium alginate–tipped swabs was briefly discussed under collection of specimens above.

Many conflicting claims have been made about the value of various materials other than cotton for use on swabs. In this regard, the data of Ellner and Ellner[6] are instructive, even when it is taken into consideration that their work was done with saline suspensions of bacteria and not with clinical specimens where the organisms might have been protected by serum, pus, mucus, or other body fluids. Their data show very poor survival of *Haemophilus influenzae,* streptococci (group A, β-hemolytic), *Corynebacterium diphtheriae,* and *N. gonorrhoeae* on untreated cotton, calcium alginate, Dacron, Fortrel (a polyester fiber), and PVA cotton (cotton treated with polyvinyl alcohol) swabs. The best survival, up to 120 h with all organisms listed (except *N. gonorrhoeae,* 21 h), was obtained with untreated cotton swabs in Stuart transport medium. The poor survival of streptococci on Dacron swabs observed by Ellner and Ellner is in contrast to the findings of Hollinger and Rantz[7] that group A streptococci survive well on dry filter paper or on dry Dacron swabs. No comparison was made with the specially treated swabs recommended for use in Stuart transport medium.

In view of these conflicting findings, it is strongly recommended that whenever any delay is expected between obtaining specimen and its culturing, swabs of specimens be placed in transport medium except when proved dry transport sets such as Dacron swab–silica gel sets for throat swabs are available.

ANAEROBIC CULTURE COLLECTION AND TRANSPORT

Generally, specimens from areas normally sterile (deep closed body areas and deep communicating areas, i.e., blood, pericardial, peritoneal, pleural, and joint fluids, transudates, transtracheal aspirates, abscesses, pus aspirated

from deep wounds, and surgical specimens obtained from normally sterile areas) also are cultured anaerobically. Specimens from superficial body areas (e.g., drain site, throat, nose, skin, mouth, urethra, colostomy material, and vaginal swab) or from areas easily contaminated by normal flora (urine, sputum) are not usually cultured anaerobically.

For those to be anaerobically cultured, special collection and transport containers are needed, since it is necessary to keep exposure of specimens to atmospheric oxygen as low as possible.

Several types of vials,* gassed out with O_2-free CO_2 or N_2, are commercially available; aspirated specimen is injected through rubber stopper (after expelling all air bubbles from syringe) and the specimen is transported to laboratory without exposure to oxygen. Swab outfits* in gassed-out tubes, with or without prereduced and anaerobically sterilized transport media, are also available.

Anaerobic collection methods and transport are further discussed in considerable detail below (see "Anaerobic infections and anaerobic cultures," this chapter) and in Chapters 70, 72, and 82; for the Bio-Bag system, see Chapter 86 (Collection).

For an evaluation of 7 transport systems for aerobes and anaerobes (Culturette,† Trans-Cul‡ with Stuart transport medium, Trans-Cul with Amies,‡ Handiswab,§ Securline‖ with modified Amies medium or with Amies medium, and Culture-Caddy¶), see Ederer and Christian.[8]

TRANSPORT MEDIA

Delay during the transmission of specimens from source to laboratory most noticeably affects delicate organisms that survive poorly over a period of 24-48 hours (*N. gonorrhoeae, Haemophilus pertussis, Trichomonas vaginalis, Shigella* sp.) and anaerobes. Stuart[9] described a transport medium that has proved most valuable in preserving specimens in transit. It is used to provide a convenient, simple, and reliable method for transport of swab specimens from patient to laboratory. Good results have been obtained in recovering the organisms listed, in addition to pneumococci, β-hemolytic (pyogenic) streptococci, *H. influenzae,* and *Haemophilus vaginalis,* for a 24 h transport. Recovery diminishes afterward, but most of the sturdier organisms can be cultured even after 72 h.

Stuart medium ** is essentially a nonnutrient,

*Bioquest (BBL), Cockeysville, Md.; Gibco Diagnostics, Madison, Wis.; Scott Laboratories, Fiskeville, R.I.
†Marion Scientific Corp., Medi/Flex Division, Rockford, Ill.
‡Toluca Industries Corp., North Hollywood, Calif. 91605.
§Fisher Scientific Co., St. Louis, Mo. 63132.
‖Precision Dyamics Corp., Burbank, Calif. 91504.
¶Wilson Diagnostics, Inc., Glenwood, Ill. 60425.
**Stuart medium: BBL, Division of BioQuest, Cockeysville, Md.; Difco Laboratories, Detroit, Mich.

NOTICE TO CARRIER

This package contains LESS THAN 50 ml OF AN ETIOLOGIC AGENT, N.O.S., is packaged and labeled in accordance with the U.S. Public Health Service Interstste Quarantine Regulations [42 CFR, Section 72.25 (c) (1) and (4)], and MEETS ALL REQUIREMENTS FOR SHIPMENT BY MAIL AND ON PASSENGER AIRCRAFT.

This shipment is EXEMPTED FROM ATA RESTRICTED ARTICLES TARIFF 6-D [see General Requirements 386 [d(1)] and from DOT HAZARDOUS MATERIALS REQULATIONS [see 49 CFR, Section 173.386(d) (3)]. SHIPPER'S CERTIFICATES, SHIPPING PAPERS, AND OTHER DOCUMENTATION OR LABELING ARE NOT REQUIRED.

Date _____

Signature of shipper _____

Address _____

semisolid, highly reductive preparation that inhibits self-destructive enzymatic reactions within the cells and also prevents the effects of oxidation, thus maintaining the specimen at "status quo." No multiplication of the organisms occurs. The medium should be used with specially prepared swabs: (1) Boil absorbent cotton-tipped applicator sticks in Sørensen phosphate buffer and then dip in a 1% suspension of finely powdered charcoal. The coating and boiling of the swabs are necessary for destroying or neutralizing any inhibitory substances in the agar and cotton. (2) Instead of cotton, calcium alginate can be used to tip the swabs. It has some advantage in that, if preferred, it can be dissolved completely in a variety of solutions (e.g., Ringer), permitting complete recovery of organisms.

The **Cary-Blair transport medium†** has proved to be a satisfactory and effective means for the collection and transport of fecal material. **Amies transport medium‡** employs charcoal in the medium, thus obviating the need for charcoal-impregnated swabs.

The various transport media are available in dehydrated form and also as prepared kits. The latter include anaerobic kits.

The swab-vial kits are recommended for office use when immediate delivery to the clinical laboratory is not always feasible or in situations in which culturing must unavoidably be delayed.

SHIPPING OF SPECIMENS

Sometimes it becomes necessary to submit specimens or cultures to a reference laboratory, requiring mailing.

1. Place fecal specimens for shipping or specimens held for laboratory examination for enteric patho-

---

†Cary-Blair transport medium: BBL, Division of Bio-Quest.
‡Amies transport medium: Difco Laboratories.

MEDICAL MATERIALS

CONFORMS WITH FEDERAL STANDARD
49 CFR 173, 387; 42 CFR 72.25 (c);
AND *NIH GUIDE*, FEBRUARY 10, 1975.

gens in a preservative solution. Use approximately 1 g fecal material in 10 ml preservative. Add sufficient phenol red to impart a definite color. If the indicator is yellow upon receipt of the specimen, the material is usually unsuitable for isolation work.

Transport media (Stuart, Cary-Blair, Amies; see media) are increasingly used for collection, holding, or shipping fecal specimens, since they are more convenient to handle and assure better recovery of fecal organisms than the preservative solutions. Stuart medium is preferred for specimens on swabs.

2. Specimens may have to be shipped in the frozen state (in particular, for virus isolation). Spinal fluid, stools, tissue, throat washing, and rectal swabs for such purpose must be frozen immediately and shipped on dry ice.

3. A culture of an isolated organism may be mailed on a slant.

The *Federal Register* (vol. 37, no. 127, June 30, 1972) contains the Interstate Quarantine Regulation on etiologic agents, which lists a number of packaging and labeling requirements.

This regulation requires that a label (Fig. 75-1) be attached to each shipment (size 2 × 4 in., red print, white background). The required packaging of etiologic agents is shown in Fig. 75-2.

In addition, because of demands by the Airline Pilots Association and the Air Transport Association (1975-1977), the CDC now recommends that 2 labels (see boxed material) be securely attached to **all** shipments of etiologic agents (regardless of size, volume, or number of agents).

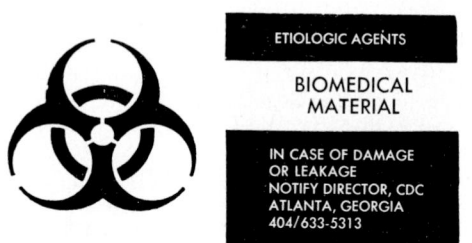

Fig. 75-1. Shipping label (red and white) for bacteriologic material. (From Code of Federal Regulations, Section 72.25, Part 72, Title 42, revised July 31, 1972.)

For details of procedures and problems involved in obtaining, handling, and shipping microbiological specimens see Huffaker (Center for Disease Control, 1974).[10]

EXAMINATION OF SPECIMENS

It is important to examine every specimen **macroscopically** upon receipt in the laboratory. Swabs that smell of antiseptic and sputum specimens that in reality are nothing but saliva are not suitable specimens. Rectal swabs should contain a specimen of stool, clearly seen. Portions of the specimen containing blood or pus should be noted and, if possible, used for culture.

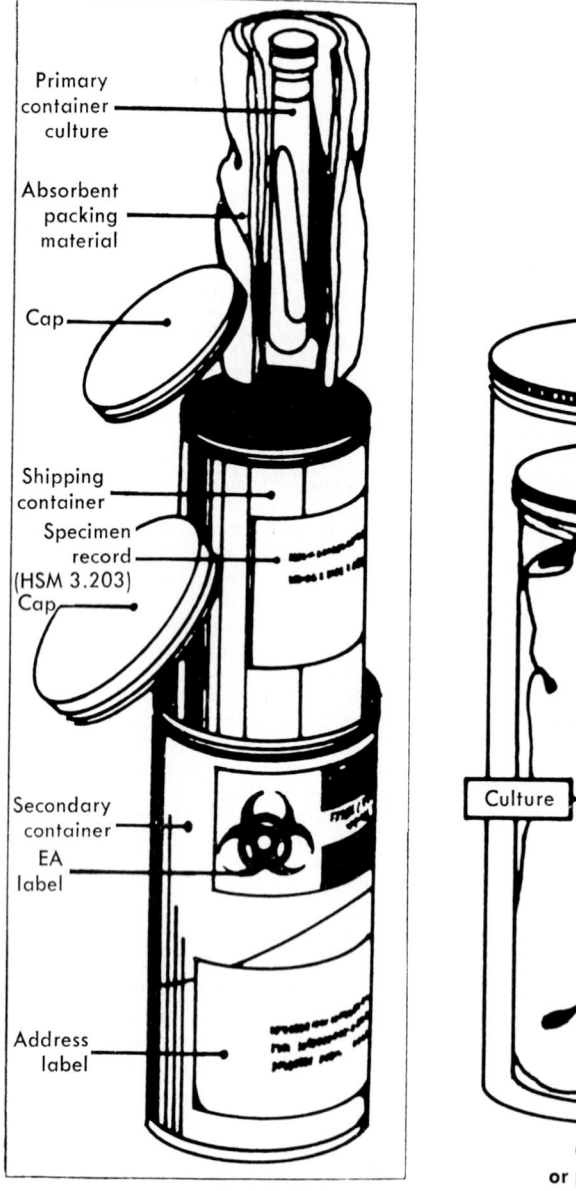

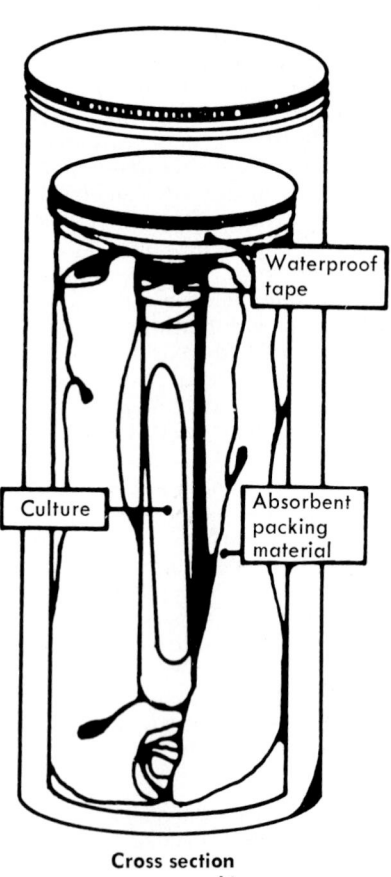

Primary
container
culture

Absorbent
packing
material

Cap

Shipping
container

Specimen
record
(HSM 3.203)
Cap

Secondary
container
EA
label

Address
label

Waterproof
tape

Culture

Absorbent
packing
material

**Cross section
or proper packing**

Fig. 75-2. Packaging for shipment of bacteriologic material. (From Code of Federal Regulations, Section 72.25, Part 72, Title 42, revised July 31, 1972.)

Microscopic examination of gram-stained smears is imperative and, if possible, should precede culture to determine the proportion of different species in the specimen; if fungi are seen, cultures with mycologic media should also be performed. (Stool specimens are not Gram stained or wet mounted; Gram stain should be done in case of suspected enterocolitis for staphylococci; for wet mount see discussions on parasitology.)

Direct smears serve as a guide for possible need of special media, control of quality of certain specimens (e.g., sputum), and as a check on cultural results (e.g., if organisms are seen on smear that do not grow on culture, a discrepancy exists that must be resolved, possibly by repeat or anaerobic culture).

Gram stain. Prepare **Gram stain;** also acid-fast or Giemsa stain or both, if necessary.

Wet-mount procedure

1. Place loopful of material on clean glass slide and cover with coverglass. It is advisable to ring coverslip with petrolatum to prevent drying and streaming. It is important that material to be examined should not be too thick; occasionally it will be necessary to dilute it with loopful of saline.
2. Examine with bright-field or dark-field microscope (for **technic of dark-field examination,** see *Treponema*).
3. Same method may be used for examination of cultures.

Hanging-drop preparation (Fig. 75-3). Organisms in the living state can be examined by using hanging drop method; clinical specimens or cultures can be used. The procedure is mainly used to determine motility of microorganisms, but dark-field examination is more reliable. **In any case, final decision about motility of most bacteria should be made by growing them in semisolid motility medium.**

1. Hanging-drop slide should be fat-free and lint-free. Clean ⅞ in. coverglass, taking care not to touch glass with fingers.
2. Place small quantity of petrolatum around edge of coverglass.
3. Pick up loopful of material to be examined and place it in center of coverglass. Take care not to take too large a loopful, since it will touch hanging-drop slide and give a false appearance when examined.
4. Pick up coverglass with the hanging-drop slide by inverting hanging-drop slide over coverslip so that loopful of material is in center of concavity of slide. Then invert again so that coverslip is on top.
5. Place preparation on microscope stage and move it until drop is directly under 16 mm objective.
6. Remove Abbé condenser, use plane surface of mirror, shut off most of light by manipulating mirror, and focus up until edge of drop is distinctly in focus.
7. Move slide until edge of drop is in center of microscopic field.
8. Change to 4 mm objective and concave surface of mirror, lower objective until it touches slide, adjust light, then focus up very slowly until drop comes into view. By focusing for edge of drop, worker has definite line for which to look. Bacteria are too pale to afford good medium for focusing.
9. Take care not to turn fine adjustment of microcope too far objective might crash into coverglass of preparation and break it. There is no way of sterilizing objective without injury and since preparation contains living bacteria, there is danger of contamination.

INOCULATION AND INCUBATION

Ideally, the proper media should be inoculated with all specimens as soon as they arive in the laboratory, but this is not always feasible. It has already been pointed out that spinal fluids, eye swabs, and specimens suspected of harboring *N. meningitidis* and *N. gonorrhoeae* must be handled without delay. On the other hand, it is possible to refrigerate specimens like swabs from wounds or the urogenital tract and samples of sputum or feces for 2-3 hours. Urine specimens may be refrigerated for 24 hours. Gastric washings for *Mycobacterium tuberculosis* and resected lung tissue should be processed on arrival.

For anaerobic cultures, follow procedures described in Chapters 70, 72, 82 and 86.

For most organisms, 35-37 C is the optimal growth temperature.* It will be seen, however, that for certain organisms, initial incubation is more favorable at different temperatures; e.g., *Leptospira*, when cultured in Fletcher medium, should be incubated at 30 C. For certain differential methods (enterococci), 45 C is preferred. In the absence of a number of incubators, a water bath can be used for incubation of such cultures. Cotton-plugged tubes should not be used in the water bath, since on prolonged cultivation condensation from the water bath cover may wet and contaminate the cotton plugs. Ideal-

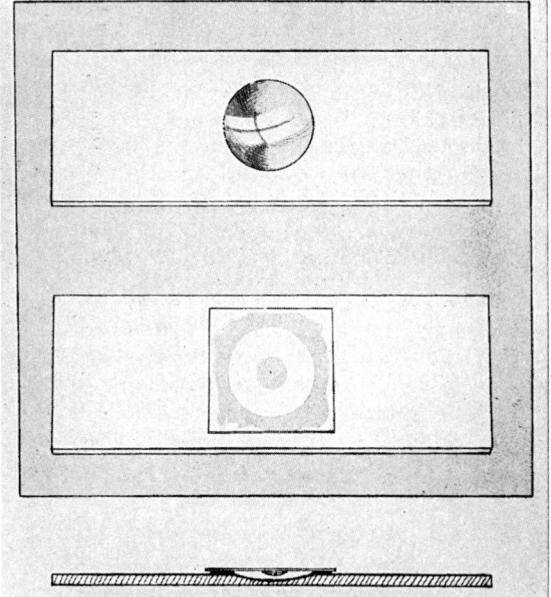

Fig. 75-3. Preparing hanging-drop specimen.

*See incubators, Chapter 68, for discussion of optimal temperatures.

ly, all cultures should be incubated in air plus 5-10% carbon dioxide, as well as anaerobically, if indicated. Exceptions are stool and urine, cultures of which are incubated in air only.

In small laboratories it may not be practicable to incubate all cultures in CO_2; however, cultures for gonococci, meningococci (spinal fluid), and *Brucella* **must** be incubated under increased carbon dioxide tension.

For anaerobic methods and CO_2 incubation see Chapter 70.

Although speed is of the essence in the clinical laboratory, it should be remembered that not all organisms grow after overnight incubation. *Actinomyces, Nocardia, Haemophilus*, neisseriae, brucellae, some pasteurellae, etc. require more than 18-24 hours incubation. Certain organisms such as greening streptococci (*Streptococcus mitis*, etc.) will grow rapidly in sputum or throat cultures but may take 1-2 weeks to grow in blood cultures taken from patients with subacute bacterial endocarditis (SBE). Rules should be established regarding the length of time after which a culture can be regarded as negative. Blood cultures (broth) are customarily kept for at least 1 week, with adequate subculturing. Agar plates should be kept at least 48 at proper incubation temperature before discarding. *Brucella* cultures (Castañeda) should be kept 30 days. Mycobacteria should be kept 3 weeks on 7H-10 medium and at least 8 weeks on other media.

On the other hand, it is important to inspect cultures **as soon** and **as often** as possible. If a culture is started at 4 AM, it should be inspected at midmorning and again at 4 PM. Cultures started at 8 AM should be inspected, if at all possible, at 8 PM.[11]

SELECTION OF MEDIA FOR PRIMARY CULTURES

Primary culture media. These are media used for the general cultivation of bacteria from clinical specimens or samples. Many organisms have very complex nutritional requirements, and for this reason a great number of media have been designed for meeting the special requirements of fastidious organisms. For general use the following are recommended:

Medium	*Purpose*
Blood agar*	General purpose
Brucella blood agar	*Brucella;* anaerobes
MacConkey or eosin methylene blue (EMB) agar	Gram-negative organisms (e.g., enteric bacteria)
Mannitol salt or Staph. 110 agar	*Staphylococcus aureus*
Heart infusion or brainheart infusion broth	General purpose
Thioglycollate broth or chopped (cooked) meat medium	Anaerobes (secondary medium)

*Prepared from blood agar base, heart infusion agar, or trypticase, tryptic or tryptone soy broth and agar with addition of 5-10% blood.

These media will give good results in the primary cultivation of bacteria. It should be emphasized that blood agar is the medium of choice for primary general medium because it will support the growth of most fastidious pathogens. It also serves as a differential medium, serving for the detection of hemolysis. Use media free of fermentable substances such as dextrose or sodium azide, since these media cause false readings of hemolysis.

In the primary isolation of pathogens it is frequently desirable to employ **differential media,** which contain an indicator system visibly changed as the result of metabolic activities and allow observation of differential reactions, permitting presumptive identification of bacterial species. **Selective media** are also used. These are nutritionally adequate for some bacteria; they contain inhibitor(s) capable of suppressing the growth of certain organisms but allowing (selecting) the growth of one or more desired types.

Numerous chemical substances are employed as inhibitors, e.g., dyes, bile salts, and, increasingly, antibiotics. **Media containing antibiotics** take advantage of the selective antimicrobial activity of certain antibiotics and are most useful for the selective isolation of certain species from mixed cultures. Several antibiotic-containing media are described in the section on **media** and are also discussed in the various succeeding chapters.

Differential and selective media. The following media are used for gram-negative enteric organisms (stool):

Eosin–methylene blue agar (EMB)
MacConkey agar
Deoxycholate agar
Deoxycholate-citrate agar (DCA)
Salmonella-Shigella agar (SS)
Bismuth sulfite agar (BS)
Xylose lysine deoxycholate (XLD) agar
Hektoen enteric agar (HE)

The first of these inhibits gram-positive organisms and contains an indicator that distinguishes bacteria that ferment lactose rapidly from those that do not attack the sugar. The next two inhibit somewhat the growth of *Escherichia coli*, whereas *Salmonella* and *Shigella* strains grow well. The DCA, SS, and XLD media are highly selective. The majority of coliform bacteria are inhibited on these, whereas the strains of *Proteus* that develop are prevented from swarming, *Salmonella* and *Shigella* growing uninhibited. Bismuth sulfite medium is used for isolation of *Salmonella*. XLD medium supports growth of shigellae and offers differential diagnostic characteristics (see also Table 75-3 in "Stool culture," below).

Specific indications. The following media are used for isolation of **specific organisms,** as listed.

N. gonorrhoeae and *meningitidis:* Thayer-Martin medium, chocolate agar (CO_2 incubation)

Table 75-1. Clinical specimens and media for primary isolation

Type of specimen	Aerobic BA/CO₂	Anaer. BA	Anaer. NBA	Anaer. LKV	MAC	BIS	SS	XLD	CHOC/CO₂	TM/CO₂	Thio Suppl.	GN	Gram stain
Abscess	X	X	X	X	X						X		X
Antrum	X	X	X	X	X						X		X
Autopsy	X										X		
Bile, gallbladder	X	X	X	X	X	X	X		X		X	X	X
Body fluids (pleural, pericardial, peritoneal, etc.)	X				X						X		X
Cervical	X	X	X	X	X				X	X	X		X
Cord	X				X						X		X
Ear, nose, sinus (head)	X	Sinus only			X				X		X		X
Eye, cornea, conjunctiva	X				X				X		X		X
Gonococcus (GC only)										X			
Joint fluid	X	X	X	X	X						X		X
Nasopharyngeal	X	X	X		X				X		X		X
Pelvic	X			X	X				X	X	X		X
Prostatic	X				X				X	X	X		X
Exudate, deep wound	X	X	X	X	X						X		X
Root canal					X				X		X		
Sinus (other than nasal)	X	X	X		X				X		X		X
Spinal fluid (CSF)	X	X	X		X	X	X		X		X		X-2
Sputum, bronch. tracheal—5	X				X			X	X		X		X
Stool, rectal swab†					X	X	X	X				X	
Throat, pharynx‡	X				X								X
Tissue	X	X	X	X	X				X		X		X
Transtracheal aspiration	X	X	X	X	X				X		X		X
Urethral	X				X				X	X			X
Urine—quantitative	X				X								X
Uterine	X	X	X	X	X				X	X	X		X
Vaginal	X				X				X	X			X

*Anaer, anaerobic; BA, blood agar; NBA, neomycin blood agar; LKV, laked kanamycin-vancomycin agar; MAC, MacConkey; BIS, bismuth sulfite agar; SS, *Salmonella-Shigella* agar; XLD, xylose lysine deoxycholate agar; CHOC, chocolate agar; TM, Thayer-Martin agar; Thio suppl, supplemented thioglycollate; GN, gram-negative broth. CO₂, incubate in CO₂, 5-10%. Some laboratories use sheep blood agar plate with *Staphylococcus* streak (*S. aureus* culture known to produce deoxyribonuclease) instead of chocolate agar plate (for isolation of *Haemophilus influenzae*).
†For *Vibrio* sp., *Yersinia enterocolitica*, and *Campylobacter* sp., see detailed instructions for **stool.**
‡Inoculate TM and chocolate plates if meningococcus, supraglottic edema, gonorrhea, or epiglottitis is suspected. If diphtheria is suspected, see detailed outline.

Bordetella pertussis: Bordet-Gengou or Jones-Kendrick charcoal agar

Gram-negative anaerobes: Antibiotic-containing media: neomycin, kanamycin, vancomycin, paromomycin, see media

Clostridia: Selective medium containing neomycin, etc.; see Chapter 84

H. influenzae: Blood agar plate, cross-streaked with staphylococci or saturated with reduced diphosphopyridine nucleotide (DPNH); or add XV factor strip (commercially available) if blood-free medium is used or V strip (containing DPNH) if chocolate or blood agar is used

Leptospira: Fletcher medium

Francisella tularensis: Cystine dextrose blood agar

Brucella: Brucella broth and agar, trypticase soy broth and agar (CO_2 incubation)

C. diphtheriae: Tinsdale medium (recommended—do not use plates if stored longer than 3 d!); Loeffler serum medium, tellurite blood agar

Staphylococci: Mannitol salt agar, tellurite glycine agar, Staphylococcus 110 agar

M. tuberculosis: Lowenstein-Jensen, ATS medium, 7H-10 medium (recommended)

Fungi and yeasts: Sabouraud dextrose agar, brain-heart infusion agar, selective medium with cycloheximide and chloramphenicol.

See media, Chapter 72, for specific media for isolation of *Campylobacter, Vibrio cholerae,* and *Vibrio parahaemolyticus.* See also "Stool culture," below.

Enrichment media. In these media the nutritional environment is adjusted so that the growth of a certain bacterial type in a mixed inoculum is selectively enhanced by supplying additional nutritional requirements; they may also suppress undesirable organisms by means of inhibitors. *Salmonella* may be enriched from feces, urine, sewage, etc. by the use of **tetrathionate, selenite,** or **GN** broths.

Selection of media for primary isolation from various clinical specimens is shown in Table 75-1.

Throughout this section a variety of satisfactory media will be described and recommended for the isolation and identification of the organisms discussed. The media just listed as well as those listed throughout the text are the ones recommended in clinical work; they reflect my personal preferences and do not necessarily include many media used successfully by other workers. Equivalent media can be substituted as long as the rationale for their use is kept in mind (see also Cumitech no. 9[11a] for collection and processing).

CULTURE OF SPECIMENS
Blood

Blood cultures are of extreme importance for the diagnosis of bacteremia and prognosis of certain infections. Almost all known pathogens and various organisms usually considered harmless have been cultured from the blood.[12] Blood cultures should be obtained **before** antibiotic or chemotherapeutic therapy is instituted. The number of cultures taken is of some importance; in subacute bacterial endocarditis it has been found that 3-4 cultures taken at convenient intervals in 24 hours are preferable to taking as many as a dozen cultures around the clock at 2-hour intervals. A single blood culture should never be depended on to eliminate the possibility of bacteremia. The stage of the disease is also important. For example, in typhoid fever positive blood cultures can be obtained usually in the first week of the disease, the organisms disappearing from the blood by the end of the second week.

Bartlett and others'[13,14] observations and guidelines to **timing** and **number** of **blood cultures** in adults are as follows:

1. In severe life-threatening clinical septicemia, obtain two 10 ml samples by separate venipuncture (preferably one from each arm). Collect immediately **before** starting treatment.

2. In suspected subacute bacterial endocarditis (SBE) or low-grade intravascular infection, obtain 3-4, but no more than four 10 ml samples within the first 24 hours at intervals spaced no closer than 1 hour. These should include 2 collected at the earliest sign of a febrile episode.

3. In suspected bacteremia of unknown origin in patients already on antibiotic therapy, if therapy cannot be suspended for a few days, draw 4 to 6 cultures within the first 48 hours. Take cultures immediately **before** the next dose of antimicrobial agent if the patient is receiving intermittent parenteral therapy.

In some institutions, limits are imposed—no more than 5 or 6 blood cultures will be accepted during any one episode.

In the case of infants, 1-2 ml samples of blood are usually collected. Two blood cultures usually suffice for diagnosing sepsis of the newborn. Volume of blood drawn from small children should be determined by the physician.

With pyogenic organisms, when the classic syndrome of **septicemia** is present (chills, fever, shock), there is usually little trouble in isolating the organism. The difficulties are more pronounced when the causative organism is present only in small numbers or appears only intermittently (subacute bacterial endocarditis, brucellosis).

A great variety of methods is recommended for blood cultures. Regardless of the method used, there are certain precautions and rules that must be observed:

1. Care must be taken to eliminate skin organisms from the culture.

2. Care must be taken to eliminate air organisms from the culture.

3. Both aerobic and anaerobic methods of culture should be used.

4. Since many of the species that can be found in bacteremia are fastidious and grow with difficulty in culture media, rich and highly nutrient media should be used.

5. Too little blood will not contain enough bacteria to obtain a good growth.

Anticoagulant. Clotting of blood should be prevented either by addition of blood to large volumes of nutrient medium or by addition of an anticoagulant. Citrate and oxalate have been commonly used; however, it has been known for some time that both are toxic for many bacteria. Heparin, which is not toxic, cannot be autoclaved.

The best anticoagulant presently available for blood cultures is **sodium polyanethol sulfonate** (SPS; originally known as Liquoid), an autoclavable synthetic substance, which also inactivates certain aminoglycoside and polypeptide antibiotics, as well as leukocytes, and has anticomplementary activity.[13] Its use was suggested first by von Haebler and Miles in 1938,[15] but it was not until later that controlled trials of its use were undertaken. Many bacteria survive at room temperature for 6 hours and an additional 18 hours at 5 C (except *Neisseria*) in collection tubes of SPS blood,[16] a marked improvement over survival in citrated blood. Finegold et al.[17] found SPS, final concentration 0.5%, to be strikingly beneficial in blood cultures (broth) in terms of increased numbers of positives and more rapid growth. It was not beneficial in pour plate cultures and was detrimental in membrane filter cultures.

SPS can be used either (1) in collection tube as anticoagulant,* by adding 5 ml blood to 1 ml 0.3% sterile SPS solution,[16] thus allowing transport of blood to the laboratory where broth bottles (without added Liquoid) can be inoculated and, if so desired, pour plates can be prepared; or (2) in broth bottles for blood culture with blood inoculated directly into bottles at bedside (see Liquoid broth, in **Media,** final concentration of SPS 0.05%).

Sodium amylosulfate (SAS) recently has been recommended for replacement of SPS in blood cultures, mainly because of the inhibitory activity of SPS on anaerobic cocci, especially *Peptostreptococcus anaerobius* (a medium-dependent effect). In large trials, SAS was no better than SPS, and there was a hint of some inhibition by SAS of certain gram-negative organisms (e.g., *Klebsiella pneumoniae*).[18,19]

Media; blood culture bottles. In general, 1 aerobic and 1 anaerobic blood culture bottle is used with each blood specimen. Each bottle has 50 ml of broth media with 0.025% sodium polyanethol sulfonate as an anticoagulant and 5-10% CO_2 in the atmosphere; commercial bottles also have a vacuum.

Recently, bottles with 100 ml medium have become available.

Each 50 ml medium bottle receives 5 ml of patient's blood (to give a dilution of 1 ml blood to 9 ml of broth); each 100 ml medium bottle, therefore, receives 10 ml of blood.

The **aerobic blood culture bottle** contains a broth medium that will support the growth of essentially all aerobic and facultative bacteria. Such media include **tryptic** or **trypticase soy**

---

*Available from Becton, Dickinson & Co., Rutherford, N.J. as a Vacutainer tube.

broth, **Columbia broth, brain heart infusion broth,** and **Brucella broth.** Filtered air is allowed to enter this bottle (**venting;** see below), and it is subcultured routinely on the first and fifth to seventh days of incubation.

The **anaerobic blood culture bottle** media may include **Columbia broth** with 0.05% cysteine, **Schaedler broth, prereduced brain-heart** infusion broth, **Thio broth,** or tryptic or trypticase soy broth. This bottle is **not** vented and is subcultured routinely on the second and fifth to seventh days of incubation.

The use of prereduced (supplemented) anaerobic media (bottles) does not result in significant increase in isolation of anaerobes, but may impair recovery of facultatives and aerobes.

For isolation of *Legionella pneumophila,* use agar slant and broth bottle (modifications of Feeley and associates' method) as described by Edelstein et al.[19a]

Osmotic stabilizers. Media with added 10-30% sucrose in blood culture bottle have been recommended for recovery of small numbers of microorganisms or for recovery of cell wall damaged bacteria in patients receiving antimicrobial therapy. While some studies found better recovery in such **hypertonic** sucrose media, others failed to note beneficial effects.[20, 21]

Skin preparation and obtaining blood culture specimen

The preparation of skin prior to venipuncture must be done with utmost care; rigid antiseptic technic is required to guard against contamination from the skin and air.

Materials
1. Blood culture bottles (2; one marked "aerobic," other marked "anaerobic")
2. 70% Alcohol
3. 2% Tincture of iodine
4. Tourniquet
5. Four sterile 4 × 4's
6. Clamp
7. Plastic syringe (12 cc)

Procedure[13]
1. a. Assemble and prepare equipment.
   b. Label **each** culture bottle (name and patient identification).
   c. Complete and fill out requisition.
2. Apply tourniquet and select optimal venipuncture site.
3. Release tourniquet and proceed to prepare skin.
4. Prepare skin as follows:
   a. Vigorously cleanse skin with a 70% alcohol–soaked gauze.
   b. Then swab concentrically with 2% tincture of iodine–soaked gauze.
   c. Allow to dry.
   d. Once skin is disinfected, cover site with sterile gauze.
   e. Venipuncture site **should not** be probed unless fingers are similarly decontaminated or sterile gloves are worn.
   f. NOTE: In known cases of hypersensitivity to iodine, skin is **vigorously** prepared exclusively with 70% isopropyl alcohol or ethyl alcohol.

5. Remove black screwtops and swab diaphragm tops of culture bottles with alcohol. Allow to dry.
6. Replace tourniquet.
7. With plastic syringe and needle, withdraw 10 ml of blood.
8. a. Without changing needles, distribute blood between aerobic and anaerobic culture bottles by adding 5 ml to each. NOTE: Changing needle may serve as a source of contamination.
   b. Replace black tops.
   c. Do **not** vent either blood cluture bottle.
   d. Mix contents of bottle by **gently** tilting bottle 2 to 3 times.
9. Deliver bottles to the laboratory immediately. A completed requisition must accompany each set of bottles.

NOTE: Some workers[22] prefer to use larger volumes of blood for culture, i.e., 10 ml of blood for bottle containing 100 ml medium; in such case, it is necessary to withdraw 20 ml of blood and to distribute 10 ml into each of two 100 ml blood culture bottles.

Alternative procedure 1. Follow steps 1-4 and 6-7 under **Procedure**. Draw blood into **sterile** Vacutainer tube (or inoculate Vacutainer tube with syringe) containing 3.4 ml of 0.35% SPS in saline.* Mix gently but well and transport to laboratory where blood will be withdrawn from tube and distributed between aerobic and anaerobic blood culture bottle.

Alternative procedure 2. This method[23] uses commercially available blood culture bottles under vacuum. The bottles are used with a commercial **blood collecting unit** rather than a syringe and hypodermic needle for venipuncture. (For collecting from an infant, a needle and syringe may be necessary.)

1. Clean site for venipuncture as described under **Procedure**, step 4.
2. Remove cotton-filtered shield (save) from needle of blood collecting unit and perform venipuncture. Unclamp hemostat and allow blood to flow into needle.
3. Reclamp hemostat and uncover anaerobic bottle. Insert free needle into this bottle and unclamp tubing, allowing blood to reach mark that indicates addition of 5 ml. Reclamp.
4. Remove needle from anaerobic bottle and insert into aerobic bottle. Allow to flow to mark. Clamp.
5. Remove needle from patient's arm and cover needle with sterile cotton-tipped filter that was saved when first removed. Unclamp hemostat and allow air to flow through filter into bottle until vacuum is filled.
6. Remove needle, wash both bottle tops with alcohol, and replace caps for cleanliness.
7. Send to laboratory immediately.

Problems encountered collecting specimen using alternative procedure 2.

1. If needle is inserted into bottle before tubing is clamped, vaccuum will be lost.
2. Use of unfiltered needle for ventilation with vacuum bottles can be source of contamination if surface air is pulled into bottle.
3. Commercial collecting unit is more expensive than disposable syringe and needle; also, it requires more education of personnel to technic than does syringe method.
4. Blood must flow to end of tubing before inserting needle into anaerobic bottle, or air will be introduced into system.

5. Vacuum will create problem when adding blood to bottle from needle and syringe. Care must be taken not to introduce unsterile air into bottle. Also, there is a chance of allowing entire 10 ml to be pulled into 1 bottle.
6. Aerobe bottle must be entered last in order that it be ventilated without reentry.

Pour plate: alternative procedure 3. Follow description under alternative procedure 1. In addition to distributing blood into aerobic and anaerobic bottle, prepare agar **pour plates** also. This allows counting the number of colonies/ml blood.

The value of making pour plates has been questioned; the method is most valuable if common skin organisms such as *Staphylococcus epidermidis* are grown. Enumeration of the colonies may be useful for ruling out contamination. If, in a pour plate, there are 5 or more colonies all of the same species and no other growth, contamination is unlikely.

1. Melt 2 tubes blood agar base.
2. Keep agar in water bath between 44 and 46 C. Agar at this temperature will remain liquid but will not be hot enough to kill bacteria that may be present in patient's blood. If agar is too hot, it will coagulate blood added to it, giving "chocolate" agar instead of undissolved or uncoagulated blood.
3. Using all sterile precautions, transfer 1 ml unclotted blood to each tube of blood agar base and rotate both immediately between palms of hands. To prevent contamination with air bacteria, flame mouth of tube, flame pipet (not hot enough to coagulate blood), hold tube in slanting position, and allow blood to flow into agar.
4. Flame mouth of tube; pour mixture into sterile Petri dishes and allow to harden.
5. Incubate plates and liquid media at 35-37 C in CO_2.

Alternative procedure 4: membrane filter technic. See Chapter 70.

Penicillinase—addition to blood culture. If patient receives penicillin at the time the blood culture is obtained, it may be necessary to add penicillinase to the blood culture to neutralize the effect of penicillin. However, many authorities believe that the addition of penicillinase increases the chance of contamination; furthermore, if the blood is sufficiently diluted (1:10 or more), the inhibitory effect of penicillin is thereby reduced to the point of no consequence.

Special procedures

BRUCELLOSIS. If *Brucella* is suspected, it is advisable to incubate aerobic bottle in 5-0% CO_2 atmosphere (candle jar, etc.) In this case, rubber diaphragm should be removed with aseptic precautions and a sterile cotton plug substituted. If possible, Castañeda bottles (see *Brucella*, Chapter 67) should be used.

LEPTOSPIROSIS. If *Leptospira* is suspected, eject from syringe at bedside (using unclotted, noncitrated blood) 0.05-0.1 ml blood into 15 ml Fletcher medium. Organisms are present in blood during first week of illness.

For animal inoculations employed and other details, see *Leptospira*.

TULAREMIA. To culture *F. tularensis*, inoculate 4 cystine glucose blood agar slants and 1 nutrient agar slant with 0.5 ml blood (unclotted) at bedside. Incubate 10 days at 37 C. Organism will grow only on cystine glucose blood agar slants.

---

*B-D Vacutainer tube no. S3208 XF308, Becton Dickinson & Co., Rutherford, N.J.

RAT-BITE FEVER. Two organisms may cause rat-bite fever. *Streptobacillus moniliformis* usually grows as "cotton balls" in thioglycollate medium. *Spirillum minus* cannot be grown, but its presence can be demonstrated by mouse and guinea pig inoculation. Organism does not remain viable for long after blood is drawn so that inoculation of animals should be done almost immediately.

1. Inject intraperitoneally 3 mice and 1 guinea pig. It is important to determine that animals are free of naturally occurring spirilla.
2. Inject guinea pig with 2 ml patient's blood, and mice with 1 ml.
3. Examine once a week for minimum of 4 wk as follows:
   a. Tap peritoneum of mouse with capillary pipet or syringe and needle and examine blood with dark-field microscope for spirilla.
   b. Obtain about 2 ml blood from guinea pig's heart, collecting in anticoagulant; centrifuge defibrinated blood and examine supernatant fluid under dark field.
4. For control, heat patient's blood to 52 C for 1 h and inject 3 mice and 1 guinea pig at same time when unheated blood above is injected.
5. Examine animals injected with heated blood in same manner as other animals. No organisms should be found.

TYPHOID FEVER. When blood culture is ordered expressly for isolation of *Salmonella typhi*, use bile broth or Watson taurocholate-streptokinase broth. Use of latter medium results in higher rate of isolation of *S. typhi*. Watson procedure (described under Watson medium) uses blood clot for culture instead of whole blood and has been found very useful.

Detection of fungi in blood cultures. Roberts and Washington,[24] using a biphasic medium consisting of brain-heart infusion broth and a brain-heart infusion agar slant (in addition to blood culture bottles usually employed), showed that detection of fungemia is significantly improved by the use of this biphasic system.

Radiometric detection of bacteremia. See Chapter 74.

Incubation of blood cultures and atmospheric conditions: venting. It has been demonstrated,[25,26] that when unvented vacuum blood culture bottles are used, the growth of *Pseudomonas* and of yeasts is delayed and their recovery is decreased. When vacuum bottles are vented, delayed and decreased recovery of Bacteroidaceae occurs in the vented bottles. Therefore it is now generally accepted[13] that 2 vacuum blood culture bottles are to be used and that one of these ("aerobic" bottle) should be **vented** by puncturing the diaphragm with a sterile cotton-plugged needle. The needle should be removed when the pressure has equilibrated to avoid loss of CO_2 (i.e., vent only long enough to release the vacuum but not to lose CO_2).

Venting aerobic blood culture bottle
1. This procedure must be done **before** any blood culture is placed in incubator.
2. Vent aerobic bottle, but not anaerobic bottle.

MATERIALS
1. Sterile needle with sterile cotton plug
2. Cotton pledget soaked in 70% alcohol

PROCEDURE
1. With cotton pledget soaked in 70% alcohol, wipe top of rubber diaphragm on aerobic bottle.
2. Allow alcohol to dry to avoid injection of alcohol into blood culture bottle.
3. Remove needle container from tube and carefully remove plastic cap. Remove protective sleeve from needle (top plugged with cotton). **Be careful not to contaminate needle.**
4. Aseptically insert needle into alcohol-sterilized top of aerobic bottle.
5. Let needle remain in bottle for about 5-10 s until atmospheric equilibration is accomplished. There may be an audible "hiss" from bottle as this occurs.
6. **Remove needle** from aerobic bottle.
7. **Mark aerated bottle with** a "**V**" and put "**V**" on back of requisition with your initials and time vented.
8. **Then** place blood culture set and requisition into incubator (35-36 C).

Examination and subculture of blood cultures

Remove bottles for inspection gently from the incubator without disturbing sedimented blood layers. Examine under bright light (by visual inspection) blood cultures daily throughout the first week of incubation. Before examination do not shake blood cultures, thus allowing for inspection of appearance of medium.

When a blood culture is positive, the growth may assume one of several different appearances.

Streptococci may grow initially only in the thioglycollate medium, with "cotton ball" colonies seen on top of the red cell layer; the upper broth layer may be clear. Beta-hemolytic streptococci or other hemolytic organisms cause marked hemolysis, and the medium is **turbid**. Staphylococci may produce a coagulum in the broth; the broth is turbid and gross colonies may develop. Aerobic gram-negative rods (enterics) produce turbidity, and **gas bubbles** due to dextrose fermentation may be seen. Some *Bacteroides* species may produce a **foul odor**, whereas *Clostridium* species produce a considerable amount of gas.

Negative cultures usually remain clear, but some cloudiness may occur after prolonged incubation.

Appearance should never be taken as a reliable guide; **sampling of the culture** should be carried out with subcultures and Gram stain made. If blood cultures with agar slants are used, colonies will usually appear on the slant; however, in some cases there may be growth in the broth but not on the slant.

Subculture

Regardless of visual appearance, every blood culture bottle, aerobic or anaerobic, should be sampled, ideally after overnight incubation, and again after 5-7 days if the culture appears negative ("blind" subculture).

If evidence of growth is seen, mix the contents of the bottle, decontaminate rubber diaphragm of bottle with 70% alcohol, and aspirate 0.5-1.0 ml of contents with syringe and needle.

Whenever contents are aspirated (evidence of growth or "blind" subculture), inoculate (1) an enriched agar medium (i.e., chocolate agar) to allow for growth of *Neisseria gonorrhoeae* of *Haemophilus influenzae*, and (2) a blood agar plate (freshly prepared or prereduced) for anaerobic incubation. The chocolate plate should be incubated under 3-5% CO_2. A Gram stain should also be prepared; if gram-negative rods are seen, inoculate a MacConkey agar or EMB agar plate also.

Subculture plates should be incubated for 48 hours before being discarded. If organisms have been seen in the Gram stain of original bottles but have not been grown, keep plates another 48-72 hours.

It is generally believed that incubation of 7 days is sufficient for the routine procedure.[13] In cases of suspected subacute bacterial endocarditis,[27] fungemia, or brucellosis, blood cultures are usually held for 2-4 weeks.

Preliminary and final report. A "preliminary report" of **growth** or **no growth** at 2 or 3 days after start should be issued by the laboratory. **Telephoned report should be given when evidence of growth is found and Gram stain confirms it.** Final reports should be made after 7 days' subcultures are negative for 48 hours.

It has been pointed out that blood culture media sometimes contain small numbers of dead organisms (often *Bacillus* sp.), with subsequent lack of growth after "positive" Gram stain.[13] In such case, reincubate culture for 2 hours and repeat Gram stain.

Gram stain findings of blood culture bottle contents.

If Gram stain of broth culture shows organisms at any time, proceed as follows:

1. If gram-positive cocci are seen, place Optochin disk (Chapter 76) on heavily inoculated portion of blood agar plate before incubation. This will aid in rapid identification of pneumococci, which are inhibited by this agent, whereas greening streptococci, similar in colonial appearance, are not.
2. If gram-negative rods are seen, in addition to chocolate plate, inoculate eosin–methylene blue or MacConkey agar plate.

Note also that often anaerobes (anaerobic and microaerophilic streptococci, micrococci, *Bacteroides*) will be found in the blood stream,[28] and these will not grow on aerobic blood plates but will be present on properly incubated anaerobic blood plates. If gram-positive rods are seen, particularly those that are slender, diphtheroid-like in appearance, streak McBride or tryptose plate in addition to blood agar. Incubate plates at 37 C and determine on growth whether they may be *Listeria*. Large, blunt-ended bacilli (gram positive) may be *Bacillus* or *Clostridium*.

NOTE:

1. If stain is positive, **call physician immediately** and report positive blood culture and Gram stain findings.
2. Appropriate **biochemicals** can be done directly from blood culture broth to speed

up identification of organism; for gram-negative rods, API strip or similar kit can be inoculated. Streak out control plate to ascertain that organism was present in pure culture; 10-15% of positive blood cultures are polymicrobial (i.e., have more than 1 species present).

3. **Antibiotic sensitivity.** Preliminary diffusion (disk) tests can be performed directly from a positive blood culture bottle; while the inoculum will not be standardized, results can sometimes be read in 6-8 hours and may be of considerable importance to the clinician (and the patient). Reports should indicate that the results are **preliminary** and that the test will be repeated and confirmed under standardized conditions. Use control plate (as in 2 above) for ruling out mixed culture.

In certain instances, e.g., bacterial endocarditis, it is often important to determine sensitivity by broth or agar dilution to obtain minimum inhibitory concentration (MIC) and/or minimum bactericidal concentration (MBC) of the organism.

Some workers advocate placing positive blood culture broth into a small (4 ml) tube of trypticase soy broth (TSB) and incubating for 4 hours (for standardization) before performing sensitivity test. Direct sensitivity test from blood culture broth should be confirmed with pure isolates and standard procedures.

Processing of subcultures

1. **If gram-positive aerobic cocci are present:**

a. *Staphylococci.* Be cautious if nonhemolytic, noncoagulase-forming staphylococci are found. They may be contaminants. For rapid differentiation, the coagulase test and hemolysis on blood agar are satisfactory.

b. *Streptococci.* Make preliminary differentiation according to growth and hemolysis on blood agar plates. For rapid differentiation of β-hemolytic organisms, use bacitracin disks and serologic classification; inoculate bile-esculin medium, and test for heat resistance and salt tolerance (growth at 45 C; in 6.5% NaCl medium or in 0.1% methylene blue milk; bile-esculin positive).

α-Hemolytic streptococci must be tested with Optochin disk or for bile solubility and dextran formation from 5% sucrose.

c. *Pneumococci.* These are Optochin-sensitive and bile-soluble organisms. Salt, 6.5%, and heat-tolerant, methylene blue–reducing organisms may be enterococci.

2. **If gram-negative cocci are present:**

a. They may be mutants or variants of gram-positive organisms. These grow well on blood agar plates and show typical reactions if not changed too much.

b. Meningococci grow well under aerobic conditions, whereas gonococci grow better in CO_2 atmosphere. Both give positive oxidase reactions.

3. **If gram-negative rods are present:**

a. If gram negative rods, which grow well under aerobic conditions, are present, use colonies from MacConkey or eosin–methylene blue plates for biochemical testing (Chapter 79).

b. *Brucella abortus* grows on tryptose agar only in

CO_2 atmosphere, whereas other brucellae grow well on this medium in a normal atmosphere.

4. **If gram-positive bacilli are present:** if gram-positive bacilli are present, aerobic sporeformers may or may not be indicative of contamination.

a. See *Bacillus*, Chapter 77.

b. Anaerobic gram-positive organisms are classified as sporeformers (*Clostridia*) and "others" (Chapters 84 and 85).

c. For *Listeria*, see Chapter 77.

Examination of pour plates (from alternative procedure no. 3)

1. Examine plates at 24 h from CO_2 atmosphere. Look for subsurface colonies.
2. Count colonies and record number of organisms per milliliter.
3. Gram stain, subculture, and identify isolates.
4. Reincubate negative plates for 3 d before discarding as negative.

Contaminants

Staphylococcus epidermidis, diphtheroids (*Corynebacterium* sp., *Propionibacterium* sp.), and *Bacillus* sp. are usually considered contaminants; they may not necessarily be such. If isolated from more than 2 cultures of the same patient, taken at separate times and from separate locations, they should not be dismissed without considering SBE—clinical probabilities must be taken into account. The laboratory cannot state that a particular isolate is a contaminant. It should advise the physician of probabilities, but the physician must make the final decision on the significance of the isolate.

Pseudosepticemia

Episodes of (false-positive) pseudosepticemia have been reported. Two outbreaks were traced to contamination of penicillinase added to blood culture media; in others, contaminated commercial culture media and contaminated aqueous benzalkonium used for skin antisepsis were implicated.[29-31]

Stock culture

It is recommended that all significant organisms isolated from blood cultures be preserved as stock cultures for 2-3 months, to allow for retesting if the patient fails to respond to therapy, comparison with later isolates, and for more extensive susceptibility, biochemical or serologic testing, if needed.

Organisms found in bacteremia[32]

This is **not** a complete list of organisms ever found in blood cultures; it only illustrates the relative frequency of occurrence of various bacteria in blood cultures.

Common
E. coli
Klebsiella
Enterobacter
Proteus
Pseudomonas aeruginosa
Bacteroides fragilis, other *Bacteroides*
Group D *Streptococcus* (enterococcus)
Staphylococcus aureus
Staphylococcus epidermidis
Streptococcus pneumoniae (pneumococcus)
Corynebacterium, Propionibacterium
    (aerobic and anaerobic "diphtheroids")
Streptococcus, α- and β-hemolytic

Less common
Citrobacter
Providencia
Serratia
Aeromonas
Yeasts: *Candida* and *Torulopsis*
Acinetobacter
Clostridium perfringens
Clostridium septicum[33, 34]
Salmonella
Neisseria meningitidis
Neisseria gonorrhoeae
Listeria
Yersinia enterocolitica[35]
Haemophilus influenzae
Edwardsiella
Actinobacillus
Campylobacter (Vibrio) fetus
Erwinia
Enterobacter agglomerans
Bacillus sp.
Fusobacterium
Leptospira
Anaerobic streptococci (*Peptococcus,*
    Peptostreptococcus)
Brucella
Pseudomonas maltophilia

Rare
Shigella
Pasteurella multocida
Francisella tularensis
Streptobacillus moniliformis

NOTE: Recently the isolation of *Legionella pneumophila* from blood has been reported.[19a]

Septicemia associated with contaminated intravenous fluids[36, 37]

Septicemia may occur in any patient receiving intravenous (IV) therapy; however, rapid onset of severe clinical symptoms of septicemia in an otherwise not seriously ill patient who has received IV therapy for only a short period of time and has no other obvious site of infection should raise a strong suspicion of intrinsic contamination of the IV fluid. Currently the great majority of septicemias related to IV therapy are probably due to extrinsic or in-use contamination; however, in the event that intrinsic contamination of IV fluid is suspected as the cause of a patient's symptoms, the following measures are recommended:

1. Discontinue IV fluid system entirely, including removal of cannulae or needles. **This is the single most important therapeutic step.** Indicate nature of fluid and exact lot number on patient's chart.
2. Draw 2 blood cultures from 2 **independent** sites.
3. Administer appropriate antibiotic therapy. Or-

ganisms that are often associated with intrinsic contamination are frequently resistant to cephalothin and ampicillin.

4. Place sterile closure on end of delivery-set tubing, wrap suspect IV system in clean plastic bag, and send it to laboratory for immediate culture: (a) Aseptically withdraw 20 cc of fluid from IV line; use 1 cc to prepare pour plate, and place rest in blood culture bottle; incubate plate and blood culture bottle aerobically at 35-37 C. (b) If IV bottle or bag is more than half full of fluid, aseptically drain to no more than half full. Aseptically add to bottle an equal volume of double-strength brain-heart infusion broth enriched with 0.5% beef extract, and incubate bottle aerobically at 35-37 C. (c) Perform all laboratory procedures in as clean an area as possible, preferably in laminar-flow hood, and **monitor working area with settling plates.**

5. **Nature of solution and exact lot number should be recorded on laboratory requisition or other permanent laboratory record.**

6. **Identify, segregate, and save all bottles of implicated lot number.**

7. **Notify local or state health authorities and Food and Drug Administration (FDA) immediately.**

Contamination of fluids by gram-negative bacilli can be detected rapidly by using the **Limulus** in vitro endotoxin assay.[38] For details, see **Limulus** assay under cerebrospinal fluid, below.

Blood and plasma from blood bank

There are no reliable figures regarding the proportion of contaminated blood bank blood used for transfusion. It is, however, well documented that, rarely, serious and sometimes fatal transfusion reactions are due to the use of blood or plasma contaminated with a variety of microorganisms. According to the 1977 Technical Manual of the American Association of Blood Banks (AABB),[39] blood should be examined routinely to detect evidence of bacterial contamination; unusual color or the presence of hemolysis are cause for suspicion. **If bacteria are suspected to be the cause of a transfusion reaction, both the blood from the bag and blood from the patient should be cultured.**

While routine sterility testing is no longer required,[40] culture may be desirable when abnormal donor bloods/components are noted on inspections, or in case of transfusion reaction.

1. Use total sample of no less than 10 ml of blood.

2. Employ for culture fluid thioglycollate or thioglycollate broth medium 10 times volume of sample of blood.

3. Add blood to one or more test vessels in a ratio of blood to medium of 1 to 10 for each vessel; mix thoroughly, incubate 7-10 days at 30-32 C. Examine visually for growth every workday during test period.

4. Subculture at least 1 ml from each vessel on third, fourth, or fifth day in same culture medium. Incubate subculture for 7-9 days at 30 to 32 C; examine for growth every day.

Organisms found in blood or plasma bottles are various *Pseudomonas* species (some of which are capable of growth at refrigerator temperature), *Citrobacter freundii*, various other enteric organisms, and *Achromobacter* species. Many of the organisms are capable of growth at refrigerator temperatures.

Cerebrospinal fluid

Bacteriologic examination of spinal fluid (CSF) is necessary in any case of suspected meningitis.

In acute bacterial meningitis, there is an increased **white cell count** (several hundred to 50,000/cu mm, usually a few thousand) with polymorphonuclears predominating and the fluid usually **purulent; CNS glucose** is reduced (usually less than 40 mg/100 ml), with **protein** being elevated (100 or more mg/100 ml).

In addition to the **Gram stain** and **culture** of CSF, to be always performed, there are now a number of technics available for speeding up and improving the diagnosis of suspected meningitis.

Rapid technics
Counterimmunoelectrophoresis (CIE)

Countercurrent immunoelectrophoresis has been recently established as a useful technic for rapid diagnosis (within 1 hour) and management of bacterial meningitis due to *H. influenzae*, type b, *Streptococcus pneumoniae*, and *N. meningitidis*, groups A, C, and D.[41] For details see Chapter 74.

Lactic acid determinations in CSF

The concentration of lactic acid in cerebrospinal fluid can be determined by gas-liquid chromatography (GLC)[42-45] and by enzymatic measure of lactic acid.[43] Both methods have been used successfully; for a thorough discussion of results obtained with GLC, see Brook et al.[42]

Kits for the chemical determination of lactate levels are available from Boehringer-Mannheim Co. and Dow Chemical Co.

Detection of cryptococcal antigen

Diagnosis of cryptococcal meningitis may be made with the latex agglutination test for the detection of cryptococcal antigen in cerebrospinal fluid. For details see Chapter 107.

Limulus assay (Limulus amoebocyte lysate assay for endotoxin)*

Gram-negative bacteria contain complex lipopolysaccharide molecules (endotoxin) in the outer membrane of their cell envelope. These endotoxins also cause fever in experimental animals, such as the rabbit, and are also known as "pyrogens." Since endotoxins can cause severe and often fatal complications if present in the bloodstream, special care must be taken to ensure that parenteral and other injectable biologic products are endotoxin-free.[46] Injection into rab-

---

*Contributed by M. Goldschmidt, Ph.D.

bits produces a temperature rise that can be correlated with the concentration of endotoxin. This is the classic assay for detecting endotoxin. However, animal tests are expensive, time consuming, and not too sensitive.

A less costly, rapid, and much more sensitive test is the **Limulus amoebocyte lysate assay.** When an aqueous extract of blood cells (amoebocytes) from the horseshoe crab, *Limulus polyphemus,* is reacted with lipopolysaccharide-containing material at 37 C, an enzyme (a protease) is activated that causes a protein in the extract (or "lysate") to polymerize and form a firm gel or clot. As little as 1 pg/ml of endotoxin can be detected by this very sensitive system.

Horseshoe crabs are bled and the amoebocytes washed by centrifugation and resuspension. Lysis occurs after the washed amoebocytes are agitated overnight at 25 C in pyrogen-free distilled water.[47] After centrifugation to get rid of the debris, the supernatant ("lysate" or "extract") can be lyophilized or frozen and stored at −20 C. The lysate is available commercially from several sources.*

In the test either 0.1 ml of endotoxin standard or "unknown" are mixed with 0.1 ml of lysate and incubated 1 hour at 37 C. If a positive reaction has occurred, the gel that has formed will not break apart when the tube is gently inverted. Positive and negative controls are necessary. A spectrophotometer can also be used to more exactly quantitate the results based on turbidity changes. The tests have also been performed on slides. All of these procedures are easy to perform and take no special skill. It is absolutely imperative that all glassware, syringes, pipets, etc. be totally pyrogen free; commercial grade "pyrogen-free" materials may not be usable for this test.

Sullivan et al. have presented an excellent and detailed discussion of the Limulus amoebocyte lysate assay.[48] Levin and Bang were among the first to study the system and recognize its potential.[49] This assay system has been used to detect pyrogen in parenteral and biologic products.[50] The lysate will also react with endotoxin still bound to gram-negative bacteria. As a result, many workers have investigated its efficacy in detecting gram-negative bacteremia, especially those caused by anaerobes, and endotoxin.[51-53] It has also been used to detect endotoxin in dental plaque and periodontal disease.[54,55] A word of caution, however; the Limulus lysate method is not necessarily specific for lipopolysaccharide as isolated peptidoglycan material from various gram-positive bacteria such as *Staphylococcus aureus, S. epidermidis,* and *Streptococcus pyogenes* (group A) also react with the lysate (through at much higher concentrations).[56] In addition, human plasma contains an inhibitor that must either be removed by chloroform extraction

or diluted. According to Sullivan et al.,[48] there is also a poor correlation between the acutal presence of lipopolysaccharide in the blood and numbers of organisms in the blood or even with the actual presence of a bacteremia per se. The test, however, will indicate if lipopolysaccharide is present. Owing to its high sensitivity, it will continue to be useful but should be used with caution.

The Limulus assay has been successfully applied in the diagnosis of **gram-negative** bacterial meningitis.[57,58]

Capsular swelling and precipitin tests on cerebrospinal fluid

Alexander[59] described a capsular swelling test and a precipitin test to be performed on spinal fluid for the diagnosis of *H. influenzae* meningitis.

Capsular swelling (Quellung) test
1. Mix loopful (3 mm) spinal fluid with loopful of diagnostic *H. influenzae* typing antiserum on coverslip.
2. Add methylene blue to color drop lightly.
3. Invert preparation on hollow ground slide or flat slide and seal with oil or petrolatum.
4. Examine under oil immersion. In positive test, swelling of the capsule is visible. (For description of Quellung phenomenon, see discussion on pneumococci.)

Precipitin test. The test is useful when the organisms are numerous. When no organisms can be demonstrated, the procedure is usually negative.
1. Layer 1 cm column of spinal fluid in precipitin tube (50 × 6 mm) with capillary pipet onto equal amount of diagnostic antiserum.
2. In positive test, white ring appears at interface of fluids. Both fluids must be crystal clear.

The same Quellung and precipitin test can be performed on spinal fluid for detection of *N. meningitidis* (meningococcus).

Fluorescent antibody technics

For an evaluation of FA technics in the diagnosis of meningitis see Fox et al.[60]

Bacteriologic examination

It is advantageous for the cerebrospinal fluid specimen to arrive in the laboratory in a sterile screwcap centrifuge tube. These tubes (commercially available) keep contamination to a minimum for both carrier and specimen.

Spinal fluids should **always** get emergency handling and should **never** wait for other cultures to be processed. The carrier should place the specimen in the hands of the person in charge of processing the culture and not in the refrigerator or on the bench.

Collect spinal fluid in 2 sterile tubes, 1 for culture and 1 for **cell count** and chemical analysis. Fluid should arrive in laboratory still warm; if it cannot be examined immediately, place it in the **incubator** for examination within 1 h.
1. Note and record color and presence of turbidity or clot.

---

*Woods Hole Marine Biological Laboratory, Woods Hole, Mass.; Microbiological Associates, Besthesda, Md.; and Difco Laboratories, Detroit, Mich.

2. Centrifuge specimen at about 3000 rpm for 10 min.
3. Transfer supernatant fluid to separate clean container (can be used for serologic or chemical examination).
4. Use sediment for **smears** and **cultures,** as described below.
5. If specimen is clotted, remove small pieces of clot onto slides for staining and add some sterile glass beads to remainder and shake vigorously to break clot before centrifuging.
6. If specimen was not turbid and no visible sediment is left after centrifugation, use bottom 1-2 ml portion of spinal fluid in centrifuge tube after removing excess supernatant liquid.
7. Save unused portion of specimen and incubate overnight at 35-37 C for reexamination next day.

Perform smear and staining, and microscopic examination immediately when fluid is cloudy.

Culture

1. Streak sediment or bottom portion of fluid on 2 sheep blood agar, a chocolate agar, and MacConkey agar (or EMB) plate.
2. Inoculate tube of trypticase soy broth (TSB) and tube of thioglycollate medium.
3. Incubate 1 blood agar plate, chocolate agar plate, and TSB tube in CO_2 atmosphere (candle jar, etc.), 1 blood agar plate anaerobically, and MacConkey in air, all at 35-37 C.

The Co_2 blood plate should be cross streaked with a staphylococcal culture (or a V factor strip, available commercially, should be placed in the area of heavy inoculum) to ensure rapid growth of *H. influenzae.*

For **membrane filter technic,** see Chapter 70.

Additional cultures

If yeast are suspected, inoculate, in addition to above media, a heart infusion agar for 35 C incubation and 2 Sabouraud dextrose agar slants, 1 to be incubated at 35 C, the other at room temperature.

If tuberculosis is suspected and if spinal fluid is not contaminated with other organisms, it may be cultured directly on media favorable for growth of *M. tuberculosis.*

1. Inoculate thioglycollate broth tube with 0.2-0.5 ml spinal fluid and observe for growth after overnight incubation at 37 C.
2. If no growth occurs, proceed with culture for *M. tuberculosis.* Meanwhile keep specimen in incubator.
3. If growth does occur in thioglycollate medium, spinal fluid should be digested and decontaminated before use as inoculum for mycobacterial media (Chapter 78).
4. If animal inoculation is desired, inject guinea pig.

Direct smear and microscopic examination

1. Use clean, flamed slides for smears from sediment.
2. Make **Gram stain** of smears. Examine stained smears very carefully because they serve as guides for special media, and finding of organisms and their preliminary description is a most useful guide to treatment that is urgent. **Direct sensitivity testing** should be performed if enough organisms are seen on stained smear. Stain also serves as check on cultural results: if organisms are seen that do not grow, discrepancy exists. However, it should be remembered that antibiotic administration **prior** to obtaining CNS fluid will

interfere with successful culture. When fluid is turbid with white cells, mainly polymorphonuclear leukocytes, organism is likely to be *N. meningitidis,* pneumococci, *H. influenzae,* or *Listeria.* No effort should be spared in searching for organisms resembling one of these.

NOTE: Cellular response in spinal fluid should be carefully noted. Polymorphonuclear leukocytosis is usually seen when etiologic agent is pyogenic organism. When monocytes predominate, fungal, tuberculous, viral, or leptospiral meningitis should be considered.

3. If gram stain is negative:
   a. Do **India ink** preparation (see *Cryptococcus,* below).
   b. Do acid-fast stain if requested (see Chapter 78).

Examination of stains

Neisseria meningitidis. In direct smears it is often difficult to detect presence of *N. meningitidis* because of debris and cells present. Organisms are gram-negative diplococci with adjacent sides flattened. If no organisms are seen in Gram-stained smear and meningococcal meningitis is suspected, make a methylene blue–stained smear from centrifuged specimen. In such preparations, presence of biscuit-shaped diplococci can sometimes be detected.

Pneumococci. These organisms appear as large, gram-positive lancet-shaped diplococci. Frequently, capsule is seen as clear, narrow halo surrounding organisms. If diagnostic sera are available, Quellung test may be used for rapid identification.

Haemophilus influenzae. *H. influenzae* is difficult to detect in direct smears. Organisms are minute gram-negative coccobacilli that often have a tendency to string out into long threadlike rods. They are gram-negative and take stain very lightly and so are frequently obscured by debris or taken for debris. Quellung test with *H. influenzae* antisera performed directly on spinal fluid allows rapid identification of these organisms. For problems with ampicillin-resistant *H. influenzae,* see Chapter 79 (*Haemophilus*).

Other gram-negative rods. When gram-negative rods are seen in smears from spinal fluid, organisms other than *H. influenzae* should also be considered. Enteric organisms also occur in meningitis. Enteric organisms will grow rapidly on any medium, whereas *Bacteroides* will grow only anaerobically.

Listeria. Listeria are small, regular, gram-positive rods that occur singly, in pairs, or V shapes, and are (occasionally) stained unevenly or partially decolorized; they strongly resemble diphtheroid organisms. On occasion they are more coccoid than bacillary in morphology. However, on culture they assume typical gram-positive bacillary appearance. **Any "diphtheroid" isolated from spinal fluid should be suspected as *Listeria monocytogenes* until proved otherwise.**

Cryptococcus neoformans. In direct smears stained by Gram method these organisms appear as very large oval bodies appearing almost black. In methylene blue-stained smears these organisms appear more typical and show large oval, budding cells. If such forms are seen or if Cryptococcus is suspected, it is imperative to perform an **India ink preparation.** Mix portion of sediment or drop of spinal fluid with drop of India ink on slide, under coverslip, and examine under oil-immersion objective for oval, sometimes single-budding bodies surrounded by wide capsule that appears as clear halo around each cell. (See also *Cryptococcus* latex test for antigen-detection, Chapter 107.)

Leptospira. In the past few years it has become evident that as many as 10% of so-called aseptic meningitides may be caused by various *Leptospira* species. *Leptospira* does not stained with simple dyes like gentian violet. Culture methods, sometimes animal inoculation, and serologic proof of antibody formation are necessary for diagnosis.

Achromobacter (Acinetobacter) (Mima-Herellea) and Flavobacterium species. These have also been isolated from meningitis; they cannot be identified on smears beyond being gram-negative rods. Both grow well on usual laboratory media.

Pasteurella multocida. Organism is small gram-negative rod and appears as pleomorphic coccobacillus in spinal fluid stains. It has been confused with meningococci or *H. influenzae* in smears.

Examination of cultures

Examine cultures daily for evidence of growth. Proceed with identification, using methods described under blood and in the appropriate sections on the organisms suspected. Keep all negative cultures for 7 days before discarding.

Microorganisms found in meningitis

The following is **not** an exhaustive list of all organisms ever found in CSF, but it indicates the general frequency of their isolation from CSF.

H. influenzae (most frequent in infants and children)
N. meningitidis
Streptococcus pneumoniae
Staphylococci, streptococci, enterococci; group **A** plus **B** β-hemolytic streptococci
L. monocytogenes
Cryptococcus neoformans
Enteric organisms—*E. coli*, frequent in the newborn; *Pseudomonas, Proteus, Serratia; Edwardsiella tarda* (Sonnenwirth and Kallus[61])
P. multocida
Yersinia enterocolitica (Sonnenwirth[38])
Bacteroides sp.
M. tuberculosis
Propionibacterium acnes[67]
Achromobacter (*Acinetobacter*) (Mima-Herellea group)
Leptospira
Flavobacterium

For an exhaustive review of bacterial meningitides see Swartz and Dodge;[63] see also *Cerebrospinal meningitis control* (WHO).[64]

Viruses (see section on viral and reckettsial diseases) are also involved in meningitides as well as various **fungi.**

Parasites such as *Toxoplasma gondii* and soil-type amebas, *Naegleria* sp., and *Hartmanella-Acanthamoeba* sp. have also been found in human meningitis (Chapter 97).

For **anaerobic meningitis,** see Feldman[65] and O'Grady et al.;[66] for a review of **chronic meningitis,** see Ellner and Bennett.[67]

Bone marrow

In some instances of infections giving negative blood cultures it is possible to isolate the offending organism from the bone marrow. Diseases in which such isolations have been reported include typhoid fever, brucellosis, and histoplasmosis. Whenever bone marrow is taken for microscopic examination, it has been suggested that it also be cultured. Inoculate a blood agar and a chocolate agar plate (incubate in CO_2), a tube of thioglycollate broth, and, if enough material is available, a *Brucella* agar slant for *Brucella* and a Sabouraud dextrose agar slant for fungi.

M. tuberculosis has been recovered from the bone marrow by inoculating an aseptically handled aspirate directly into at least 5 times its volume of Tween-albumin broth or Middlebrook 7H-9 broth. The broth is incubated at 37 C in an atmosphere of 2.5% CO_2, and smears of the broth are made weekly. When and if acid-fast organisms are seen on smear, the broth is streaked onto egg media or 7H-10 agar. If no acid-fast organisms are seen after 4 wk, streak broth onto solid medium at weekly intervals for 4 wk before discarding.

For the technic of marrow biopsy see Heinle et al.[68]

The usefulness of bone marrow culture for isolation of *Salmonella typhi* has been reemphasized by Gilman et al.[69] and Vaisrub.[70] Tu et al.[71] and Greene et al.,[72] on the other hand, find the usefulness of bone marrow cultures highly limited.

Throat and nasopharyngeal specimens

The **normal** throat contains a multitude of microorganisms, among them greening streptococci, *Neisseria catarrhalis* and other species, coagulase-negative, occasionally coagulase-positive staphylococci, *H. influenzae* and *Haemophilus haemolyticus*, pneumococci, β-hemolytic streptococci other than group A, corynebacteria, and yeasts. After antibiotic therapy, coliform and other gram-negative organisms can be found (in particular after penicillin) in increased numbers.

Throat cultures are done primarily for the diagnosis of exudative tonsillitis or pharyngitis. Although some physicians insist on identification of all organisms in throat cultures, only group A streptococci and sometimes *Neisseria gonorrhoeae* are **common** causes of pharyngitis. When gonorrhea is suspected, specific request should be made and the specimen should be plated on a selective agar such as Thayer-martin medium.

In the United States, *Corynebacterium diphtheriae* should only be looked for when requested; if the laboratory is not equipped to deal with this organism, specimens should be sent to a reference laboratory. **Toxigenicity** testing of *C. diphtheriae* should only be done by laboratories competent in this area. For many laboratories this means the specimen should be sent to a reference laboratory such as a city or state public health laboratory. Treatment of suspected diphtheria should be instituted **immediately.** Diagnosis must be established on clinical grounds rather than waiting for laboratory results. Laboratory results are confirmatory.

Reporting. Routine throat cultures (without any other specific requests) are reported as "negative for group A streptococci" or "group A streptococci present"; other organisms are not identified.

Special requests. If the physician has special requests related to a throat culture, they should be specifically stated. Examples would be suspected **diphtheria, epiglottitis (*H. influenzae*)** (however, both diphtheria and epiglottitis are **clinical** diagnoses, and waiting for laboratory results may prove fatal to the patient), **peritonsillar** or **retropharyngeal abscess, whooping cough,** or **gonorrhea.**

Culture. Sheep blood agar plates should be used for culture. There is a debate about the optimal atmosphere for incubation. I use pour plates incubated aerobically in my laboratory. A recent study[73] concluded that aerobic plates are satisfactory for detecting group A streptococci as long as the agar is stabbed. However, some authors[74,75] feel that anaerobic incubation, agar overlay, or pour plates give an improved yield; theoretically, they should, because the streptolysins are more active anaerobically. The quality of the blood agar plates is probably as important as the method of incubation used.

Use of **special selective media** for screening throats has been suggested. The data on use of gentamicin blood agar plates is controversial, but a recent paper[76] suggests that trimethoprim-sulfamethoxazole combination gives an improved yield of group A streptococci.

How important is it to identify hemolytic streptococci as being group A? Physicians have usually 3 options when dealing with upper respiratory infections: (1) some ignore laboratory services altogether and treat with antibiotics on a "blanket" basis; (2) some ask for throat cultures and want to know if β-hemolytic streptococci are present, then treat accordingly; and (3) a small number want to know whether these are group A streptococci and are willing to wait 18-24 hours for this information.

Grouping can be done using bacitracin disks (presumptive grouping), staphylococcal coagglutination, latex agglutination, or immunofluorescent staining. The Lancefield method is too slow and costly. Some studies suggest that placing a bacitracin disk on the heavy part of the **initial** inoculum gives 85-90% correlation with standard grouping procedures, although one study showed only about 60% agreement. It should be recognized that, at best, using pure culture, the bacitracin method is only 95% accurate.

Obtaining throat culture

In order to avoid contamination with the saliva and normal flora of the mucous membranes, the swab should be carefully inserted through the mouth with the aid of a strong light, with the tongue depressed. Rub the swab over each ton-

sillar area and the posterior pharynx. Any area with exudate should also be touched. Do not contaminate the swab by touching the tongue and lips. Return swab to tube and inoculate onto blood agar plate as soon as possible. Broth, 0.5 ml, in the collecting tube may be used to prevent drying; however, it permits the overgrowth of contaminating organisms and interferes with estimation of the number of β-hemolytic streptococci present.

If **diphtheria** is suspected, **lift edge of membrane and swab underneath it** to reach deeply located diphtheria organisms.

To obtain specimens from throat: Use sterile cotton- or Dacron-tipped applicators. See discussion of swabs and collection tubes, Chapter 70 collection of swabs, earlier in this chapter.

To obtain specimens from nasopharynx: Use chrome or stainless steel wire applicators (B.&S. 28-gauge). Dip 7 in. length of wire in collodion and then cover tip with small bit of cotton. Bend other end into large loop. Sterilize in pairs in plugged tubes. Sterilized wire applicators are commercially available.

Throat and nasopharyngeal cultures
Routine culture

Diphtheria culture. See below.
β-hemolytic streptococci[77,78]

1. **Medium.** Blood of choice is defibrinated sheep blood. It is preferable to rabbit, horse, or human blood. Sheep blood also contains a factor that inhibits the growth of *H. haemolyticus*, an organism that can be mistaken for β-hemolytic streptococci. Blood agar base, available commercially from numerous manufacturers, is recommended for preparation of base medium. Add blood to a concentration of 5%; if hematocrit of sheep blood is low, use 7-10% blood.

2. Streak sheep blood agar plate with loopful of broth from collecting tube or, preferably, inoculate with swab a small area of surface of plate (about one-sixth). Streak inoculum over plate with wire loop. Make a few **stabs** into agar with loop to allow for observation of subsurface hemolysis under reduced O_2 tension. Incubate at 35-37 C anaerobically if possible, or under 3-5% CO_2 atmosphere (candle jar).

3. **Pour plate.** If streak plate can be incubated anaerobically, pour plate is not necessary. In laboratories where anaerobic cultures cannot be readily prepared, **blood agar pour plate is highly useful for detection of β-hemolytic streptococci** if there are relatively few of these organisms present. If streak plate alone is used, β-hemolytic streptococci will be found only if they are present in large numbers. Broth for pour plate can be prepared by immersing swab into tube containing 10 ml trypticase soy broth. Twirl vigorously against side of tube to obtain as much material in suspension as possible.

   a. From capillary pipet add 1 drop broth suspension to tube of melted trypticase soy agar. Melted agar should be cooled to 48-50 C.

   b. Add 0.8-1 ml blood. Tube blood in 1 ml amounts in sterile tubes and store in refrigerator. Simply pour 1 tube of blood into inoculated agar after flaming mouth of tube.

   c. Mix blood, inoculum, and agar well. It is important that blood and inoculum be evenly distributed throughout agar.

  d. Pour mixture into sterile Petri dish. Incubate at 35-37 C for 18-24 h. If no β-hemolytic colonies are found, reincubate for another 18-24 h.

Examination of plates. Normal flora of throat should be taken into consideration when examining blood agar plates inoculated with specimens from throat or nasopharynx.

Streak plate. If incubated anaerobically, β-hemolytic streptococci yield large zones of hemolysis and grow better than in air. Many throat commensals that produce large colonies in air will show minute colonies when incubated anaerobically. Examine plates with hand lens, by transmitted light, and note presence or absence of β-hemolytic colonies. If such colonies are present, make Gram stain of a colony. Subculture on blood agar if it is a streptococcus and test with bacitracin disk for presumptive differentiation (screening) of group A, or other methods (see above, *Grouping*).

Whether plate is incubated in CO_2 atmosphere or in air, procedure is similar to that described above. In any case, it is important to subculture the suspected colony to obtain pure culture for bacitracin test and grouping procedure.

Pour plate. Examine plate for β-hemolytic colonies. If found, fish out with straight needle, make Gram stain, and culture as above for further identification.

  NOTE: The type of hemolysis (α or β) can be best observed with dissecting microscope or with the 16 mm objective of standard miscroscope. When observed under 2× magnification, area around deep β-hemolytic colonies is totally devoid of intact red blood cells. Area around α-hemolytic colonies shows intact but discolored red cells. Sometimes an outer zone of complete hemolysis surrounds the discolored area.[78]

Meningococci may be isolated on streak blood agar plates incubated in CO_2 or air. Incubation for approximately 72 h is necessary for aerobic growth of these organisms. They will appear as small, gray, raised, slightly mucoid, nonhemolytic colonies, smears from which will show typical gram-negative, biscuit-shaped cocci in pairs and irregular clusters. Colonies may be identified as *Neisseria* by oxidase reactions; since other *Neisseria* also give a positive reaction, suspected colonies should be tested by slide agglutination with polyvalent meningococcal antiserum. If results are positive, fermentation reactions should be carried out for final identification.

If nasopharyngeal culture is carried out specifically for isolation of *N. meningitidis*, streak swabs on Thayer-Martin agar and incubate 24-48 h in CO_2 atmosphere.

Fluorescent antibody technics for group A β-hemolytic streptococci

See Chapter 70.

Examination for diphtheria

Current views tend to place the responsibility for diagnosing diphtheria on the clinician. The laboratory is charged with the task of bacteriologic confirmation, which takes 2-3 days even when the most advanced methods are used. The risk to the patient in delaying administration of antitoxin is extremely great and cannot be made dependent on laboratory findings. "It is safer to err on the side of an occasional needless serum treatment than to lose time which can make the difference between recovery and death."[79]

Nevertheless, the methods used in the laboratory should be accurate and as rapid as possible; examination for diphtheria is requested not only in the acutely ill patient but also in the convalescent case, the healthy carrier, and occasionally in skin or wound diphtheria.

Staining of throat swab smears for diphtheria should be made with Loeffler methylene blue or Albert stain. Smears of throat swabs cannot be depended on for the identification of *C. diphtheriae*. Although the morphology of the organism is characteristic, other corynebacteria occur in the throat that are indistinguishable from the diphtheria bacillus. Unless the bacteriologist has a great deal of experience in reading diphtheria slides, the error may be too great. If organisms resembling *C. diphtheriae* are seen on the original smear, this should be reported to the physician as "organisms morphologically resembling *Corynebacterium diphtheriae* seen."

The diagnosis of diphtheria depends on the isolation of the organism and performance of a virulence test for proof of toxin production by the organism. The media used most often are various **tellurite** media (tellurite-chocolate blood), **Loeffler's serum slant,** and a later modification of tellurite medium, the **Tinsdale medium.** Whenever a culture for diphtheria is made, a blood agar plate should also be streaked for isolation of β-hemolytic (group A) streptococci; infections caused by these streptococci are often difficult to distinguish from diphtheria. In addition to the Tinsdale medium, the following tellurite media are in use: dextrose-proteose no. 3 medium (Difco) with tellurite blood solution, Mueller tellurite base (Difco) enriched with Mueller tellurite serum, and trypticase tellurite agar (BBL).

Moore and Parsons[80] reported their experience with a modified **Tinsdale** tellurite medium for the primary isolation of *C. diphtheriae* and *C. ulcerans*. This medium has the unique ability of distinguishing these 2 organisms from all others grown from nose and throat specimens. The 2 organisms grow as gray-black colonies surrounded by a distinct dark brown halo. The authors believe that especially those inexperienced in work with the diphtheria organism can isolate it more reliably from this medium than from Loeffler slants or tellurite media.

Method 1, recommended procedure

1. Streak specimen to 2 Tinsdale medium (modified) plates. Do not use plates if they have been stored longer than 3 d.
2. Incubate 24 h.
3. Examine for smooth, gray-black, shiny, convex surface colonies. *Gravis* and *mitis* stains produce intense dark brown halos, often after 24 h. *Minimus* and other small colony types often require 48 h. *C. ulcerans* produces halos characteristic of *C. diphtheriae.* Diphtheroids produce light gray to black colonies without halos even on prolonged incubation. β, α, and nonhemolytic streptococci, staphylococci, neisseriae, pneumococci, klebsiellae, *Haemophilus*, and escherichiae produce no halos around colonies on this medium. Stabbing of

medium with inoculating wire or swab at time of inoculation accentuates darkening of medium by *C. diphtheriae* and gives presumptive evidence of presence of this pathogen within 12-14 h. Suspicious colonies can be fished directly from plate and used for virulence testing (either in guinea pig or preferably on Elek-King agar diffusion virulence test medium*). *C. ulcerans* occurs rarely and has to be differentiated by biochemical means.

4. Streak blood agar plate (for streptococci).
5. Streak specimen on Loeffler serum agar also. Examine as in method 1. In laboratories with restricted facilities, 2 Tinsdale plates will suffice. In larger laboratories, additional medium should be employed.

Method 2, alternate procedure. Cultures on Loeffler serum should be made from throat, and from each side of nose.

1. Incubate at 37 C for 24 h or less, preferably 12-18 h.
2. Make smears from typical dew-drop, gray colonies, and stain with Loeffler methylene blue or other stain for granules. Look for organisms morphologically similar to diphtheria bacillus.
3. If these are found, plate on blood agar, using streak method of inoculation, and making culture in such way as to give distinct colonies.
4. Incubate at 37 C for 24 h.
5. Examine colonies microscopically to determine whether they have characteristics of diphtheria bacillus. Margins are lacelike and irregular. Colonies are small, grayish, and granular and turn blood brown.
6. Make smear from part of one of these colonies to determine morphologic similarity to diphtheria bacilli.
7. If organism appears to be diphtheria bacillus, transplant to tubes of Loeffler blood serum medium. Make several transplants from different colonies.
8. Incubate at 37 C for 24 h or until good growth is obtained.
9. Make smear and stain with Loeffler methylene blue or other granule stain to determine whether organism growing on culture is same as one selected.
10. Add about 2 ml sterile physiologic saline (0.85% sodium chloride) to slant of Loeffler if pure culture is obtained.
11. Loosen growth from slant by means of platinum or Nichrome loop so that living organisms are suspended in saline.
12. Inject 1 ml into abdominal cavity of guinea pig.
13. Tag guinea pig. Record number of pig and laboratory identification of culture on record sheet.
14. If organism isolated was true diphtheria bacillus, guinea pig will die within 4 d.
15. Diphtheria in guinea pig is accompanied by area of inflammation and necrosis of tissue at point of inoculation and congestion in adrenal glands so that they appear inflamed and enlarged.
16. If no true diphtheria bacilli are present, guinea pig will not become ill.
17. **For other toxicity tests, see** *C. diphtheriae*, **Chapter 77.**

Fluorescent antibody test for rapid diagnosis of diphtheria. Whitaker et al.[81] employed diphtheria antitoxin conjugated with fluorescent dye for rapid diagnosis of diphtheria.

1. Smear pharyngeal swabs on slides, air dry, fix in acetone 10 min and then stain with drop of diphtheria antitoxin conjugate.
2. After 30 min staining, wash off excess dye, place coverslip on slide, and examine under fluorescence microscope. If there are any toxin-producing diphtheria organisms in smear, antitoxin combines with toxin and organisms fluoresce.

The method has not been particularly successful and is not generally used.

Diagnosis of pertussis

Many laboratories are not equipped for isolation of *Bordetella pertussis;* specimens may have to be collected and transported to a central laboratory for this service.

Collection and transport. The likelihood for positive isolation is 95% in the first week of the disease (catarrhal stage), and less than 50% in the fourth week of disease.

Procedure recommended by Center for Disease Control*

1. To obtain specimen, immobilize patient's head and gently pass swab (Teflon tubing with cotton wad, or flexible wire with cotton) through nostril into nasopharynx. If entry cannot be gained through either nostril, enter through mouth.
2. Emulsify swab material in 0.25-0.50 ml 1% Casamino Acids (CAS) solution, sterile, pH 7.2.[82] Material can be held for no longer than 2 h. If time needed is longer for delivery to laboratory, place swab in transport medium such as Stuart's or inoculate charcoal agar slant. Jones and Kendrick[83] devised a blood-free medium for transport and growth of *B. pertussis* (see Media, Chapter 72). The CDC recommends transporting on **Jones-Kendrick charcoal agar slant;** inoculate surface of slant with swab used for collection.
3. From CAS solution, swab is used to streak 2 Bordet-Gengou agar plates (one with and one without penicillin). Incubate at 35 C; growth may take 48 h or longer. Fluorescent antibody (FA) staining can be performed from suspension of suspected colonies; also perform slide agglutination test with absorbed serum, or biochemical tests. With swab, also prepare smears for direct FA staining (see below); stain with *B. pertussis* and normal rabbit conjugates.
4. From Jones-Kendrick charcoal slant, receiving laboratory should do (1) FA stain, (2) subculture to Bordet-Gengou medium, and (3) continue to incubate slant as received.

Procedure for direct FA staining of B. pertussis

1. Emulsify either a colony or nasopharyngeal swab in CAS broth.
2. Make 2 smears on slide with loopful or small drop of emulsified material.
3. **Allow to air dry.**
4. **Heat fix by gently passing through flame 3 times.**
5. Place on flat surface and add drop of *B. pertussis*

---

*For agar diffusion virulence test, see Elek-King medium. It is also available from Difco Laboratories as KL virulence agar and KL virulence enrichment.

*Proficiency Testing Summary, Bacteriology 1, 1978, Summary Analysis, Center for Disease Control, Atlanta.

conjugate and drop of normal rabbit conjugate to remaining smear.

6. Leave in moist chamber 30 min.
7. Tap off excess conjugate and rinse in 1 container PBS, pH 7.6.
8. Transfer to clean PBS and leave 10 min.
9. Air dry or gently blot dry.
10. Place drop of mounting fluid on smear and coverslip.
11. Examine under fluorescence microscope that is equipped with appropriate filters.
12. Read for very small, brightly stained organisms that may occur singly or in small groups. There should be no staining with normal rabbit conjugate.

Inoculation of Bordet-Gengou plates
1. For inoculation of Bordet-Gengou plate, place 1 drop of 1000 unit penicillin/ml solution on surface of plate (If Bordet-Gengou medium contains penicillin [0.5 units/ml finished medium], there is no need for this step.) Pass swab through drop and then streak plate with sterile loop. It is important to rub swab with inoculum into penicillin solution: suspension then serves for streaking. Penicillin is used to inhibit growth of many of commensal organisms normally present in nasopharynx. Pertussis organism is not inhibited by penicillin.
2. Incubate plates 4-5 d and examine for presence of colonies resembling mercury droplets. Identify organism by agglutination with specific antiserum* and staining reaction.

Cough plates. Cough plates are not used as widely as before; their description is included here because they are still used in some areas outside the United States.
1. Hold plate containing Bordet-Gengou medium a few inches in front of patient's mouth and induce him to cough on plate. Incubate plate aerobically at 37 C for 4 or 5 d. To prevent drying of medium, keep plate in moist atmosphere. This may be accomplished by placing plate on piece of heavy wire mesh or perforated metal over a flat container of water, keeping plate covered with inverted glass vessel.
2. Colonies of *B. pertussis* usually appear in 2-5 d. They are small, gray-white, hemispherical, opaque "mercury droplets." Quantity of blood in medium is too great to make reading of zone of hemolysis distinct enough to be of diagnostic value.
3. Digestion of hemoglobin will be noted.

Vincent's angina

Vincent's angina is an inflammatory condition of the mouth, pharynx, gums, or tonsils (frequently simulating diphtheria), which is most likely caused by a number of organisms normally present in these areas: *B. melaninogenicus*, "fusiform" organisms (*Fusobacterium nucleatum*, *F. necrophorum*, and probably others), *Borrelia vincentii*, and other spiral organisms. In Vincent's angina these organisms are present in enormous numbers, and diagnosis is usually made by microscopic examination of a smear made from the lesion. Gram, methylene blue, or dilute carbol fuchsin stains will show clearly the

*Difco Laboratories, Detroit.

abundance of spirochetal and fusiform organisms. The fusiform organisms are tapered at both ends and are thin. *B. vincentii* cells are thin, with open coils and pointed ends; under dark field they show very active serpentine movement.

Cultures are not usually done, since they are of no value in this condition.

Lower respiratory tract specimens:
I. Sputum

The reliability of sputum cultures (for the etiologic diagnosis of lower respiratory tract infections) has been challenged repeatedly, both because of lack of specificity and of sensitivity.[3] In pneumococcal pneumonia (with bacteremia), the pneumococcus has been recovered from the sputum in 50% to 94% of cases.[84,85]

The potential pathogen that may be recovered may also be obscured by heavy overgrowth of oropharyngeal contaminants. While repeated washing of sputum and/or quantitative culture of sputum has been advocated in order to remove oropharyngeal contamination, such attempts have not been successful.

Accordingly, **expectorated sputum, nasopharyngeal aspirates,** and **bronchoscopy aspirates** are regarded as inevitably contaminated to some degree with the normal flora of the oropharynx. Interpretation of cultures of expectorated sputum and nasopharyngeal and bronchscopic aspirates should be based therefore on direct microscopy (gram stain for cell types and numbers, as well as for bacteria) and semiquantitative culture results, together with clinical correlations.[86]

Sputum scoring. It is now generally agreed (Bartlett et al.[86]) that sputum should first be examined by Gram stain and scored to determine if the specimen is contaminated with upper respiratory material.

Select a purulent portion of sputum and transfer to a clean Petri dish. Prepare Gram stain and examine first for the presence of leukocytes and squamous epithelial cells.[86] Table 75-2 shows a composite of the scoring systems of Murray and Washington[87] and Geckler et al.[88]

Table 75-2. Classification of sputum specimens based on presence of leukocytes and squamous epithelial cells*

Group	Cells (no./field)†	
	Leukocytes	Squamous epithelial cells
6	<25	<25
5	>25	<10
4	>25	10-25
3	>25	>25
2	10-25	>25
1	<10	>25

*From Bartlett, J. G., Brewer, N. S., and Ryan, K. J.: Laboratory diagnosis of lower respiratory tract infections, Cumitech No. 7, (Washington, J. A., coord. ed.), Washington, D.C., 1977, American Society for Microbiology.
†×100 magnification.

Bartlett et al.,[86] concurring with Geckler et al.,[88] recommend that sputa in groups 1, 2, and 3 not be cultured, or that they be cultured only by specific request. Finegold et al.[89] state that it is reasonable to reject sputum specimens with both more than 10 epithelial cells and less than 25 leukocytes per high-power (100×) field. Van Scoy[90] found that specimens with more than 25 leukocytes per field yield reliable data; it appears that the number of polymorphonuclear leukocytes is more important in indicating adequate sputums than the number of epithelial cells.

If a sputum is adjudged to be unsatisfactory, it is put in the refrigerator and an additional specimen is requested.

NOTE: (1) **Scoring is irrelevant for specimens submitted for acid-fast (AFB) or fungus cultures.** (2) **Anaerobic cultures should not be done on expectorated sputum.**

Sputum culture

The handling of sputum specimens varies in many institutions, depending on local facilities. Some laboratories will **start** culture but not work it up if Gram stain scoring reveals unsatisfactory quality of sputum specimen. The usefulness of sputum cultures depends on how carefully they are collected, on whether the laboratory rejects poor specimens, and on whether the specimens are handled properly in the laboratory. **Blood cultures** should be done in all patients suspected of having pneumonia. Some feel that **selective medium for pneumococci** (5 μg/ml of gentamicin in blood agar plates) is a good way to increase the yield of pneumococci and may be better than mouse inoculation; however, it should be remembered that gentamicin will inhibit other organisms that may be pathogens.

In an average hospital, approximately 50% of the cases of pneumonia are pneumococcal, 10% are due to gram-negative rods (often hospital acquired), 7-8% are due to *Staphylococcus aureus*, 2-2½% are due to *Haemophilus influenzae* (therefore they should be looked for in the sputum), and the remaining 30-35% are caused by viruses, mycoplasmas, anaerobes, *Legionella*, or have no etiology established.

For culture, sputum should be collected in sterile glass or disposable plastic container. Do not use paper cups.

1. The major problem confronting the diagnostic laboratory in regard to sputum culture is the neglect and carelessness with which sputum collection is treated; as a result, the number of sputum specimens submitted for culture that are, in fact, nothing but saliva, is astonishing. Purulent or mucopurulent material is needed for sputum culture, and it should be obtained on awakening if possible. Deep coughing followed by expectoration will result in adequate material as long as the patient is productive of sputum. (See "Sputum scoring," above).

2. Sputum should be collected before antimicrobial therapy is commenced.

3. Specimen should be cultured as soon as possible. It is permissible to refrigerate for 1-3 h if immediate culture cannot be done.

4. **For isolation of** *Mycoplasma pneumoniae*, sputum should be collected in sterile container. Throat swabs placed in 3 ml transport medium* are also used for culture of *M. pneumoniae*. The organism can be recovered from specimens frozen at −70 C. See also *Mycoplasma*, Chapter 81.

Microscopic examination

1. **Scoring** for leukocytes and epithelial cells: see "Sputum scoring," above.
2. Prepare **Gram stain** from purulent or bloody flecks. This allows early presumptive diagnosis of staphylococcal pneumonia and pneumonia caused by gram-negative aerobic organisms (*Klebsiella, E. coli,* etc.). Pneumococcal pneumonia cannot be diagnosed with certainty in stained preparations because pneumococci look very much like streptococci.
3. A Quellung reaction may be performed on the sputum for pneumococci or *Haemophilus*. "Omniserum," a polyvalent pneumococcus antiserum (available from Statens Seruminstitut, Copenhagen, Denmark) has been used successfully for identification of pneumococci in specimens.
4. Make acid-fast or auramine-rhodamine stain if requested.
5. Look for **fungal elements,** both in wet preparation and stained smear.

Sputum culture procedures

Isolation of M. tuberculosis. See Chapter 78.
Pathogenic fungi and yeasts. See Chapter 103.
Legionella pneumophila (Legionnaires' disease bacterium). See **transtracheal aspirate** and **pleural effusion,** below.
Preparation of cultures. Cultures should be prepared from purulent, mucopurulent, or bloody material and not from saliva. Cultures of **sputum** in cases of **acute bacterial infections** of respiratory tract are performed as follows:

1. Inoculate 1 blood agar plate and 1 MacConkey or EMB agar plate. Some workers also inoculate a chocolate agar plate (for *Haemophilus*).
2. Incubate blood agar and chocolate agar in 3-10% CO_2 and other media in air, all at 35-37 C.

In cases of suspected **lung abscess, bronchiectasis,** and **empyema,** transtracheal aspirates should be cultured anaerobically.

Yersinia pestis. If examining for *Y. pestis,* culture on 3% salt agar in addition to blood agar.

Inoculation. Assuming that sputum specimens have been screened to determine if they are adequate, it is important to have a consistent way of streaking plates in a reproducible manner so that some (semi-) quantitative estimate of the number of colonies can be given. This is estimated by the number of colonies growing in various parts of the streak.[86] Such systems allow the recognition of predominant organisms, thereby limiting workup to those organisms that qualify as "**predominant.**"

Examination of blood agar plate. Look for small, shiny, greening, transparent, flat colonies with depressed centers and raised edges. They are most likely **pneumococci;** identify by Optochin test or, to speed

_____

*Bovine albumin, 0.5%, in trypticase soy broth, pH 7.2.

and simplify the identification of pneumococci, use the **spot bile test**[91] (see also Chapter 76, pneumococci). Greening streptococci are often mistaken for pneumococci. Many strains of *H. influenzae* will grow on the primary plate. Look particularly for minute colonies growing clustered around larger colonies (usually staphylococci). Gram-staining reveals very small gram-negative rods. The organism should be identified as described under *Haemophilus*.

Klebsiella pneumoniae grows very well both on the blood agar plate and the EMB and MacConkey agar plate. Typical strains show large mucoid colonies; the organism is nonmotile and many strains ferment lactose. Capsular swelling tests with specific antisera should be used for serologic identification.

Neisseria meningitidis should be identified because it may cause pneumonia. In general, it is important that the physician give his or her impression of the type of the infection in the patient, as this may help direct the laboratory's initial culture activities and interpretation of results.

Legionella pneumophila (Legionnaires' disease bacterium) does **not** grow on blood agar (see transtracheal aspirate and pleural fluid, below).

S. aureus is increasingly found as the cause of acute pneumonia. Coagulase tests should be performed.

In **chronic infections** (bronchitis, emphysema, asthma) mixed cultures are usually found. It is doubtful whether routine cultures yield any valuable information in such cases.

The MacConkey or MacConkey eosin–methylene blue (EMB) plate is included in the sputum culture because it will suppress the gram-positive organisms and will yield usually pure cultures of *Klebsiella* or other similar organisms. Sensitivity tests can then be performed on the isolated organisms without having to purify the culture.

Pneumonias caused by gram-negative bacilli are increasing; the etiologic agents involved are *Pseudomonas*, *E. coli*, *Klebsiella-Enterobacter* (*Aerobacter*), and *Proteus* species.

Workup and reporting

Assuming that the specimen was of good quality, it is reasonable to workup, identify, and report the predominant (aerobic) organisms only. There is some risk involved here, unless "predominant" is defined and consistently applied. It is possible to count organisms and to define as predominant all those that result in growing at least 10 (or more) colonies in first streak area, at least 5 (or more) in second streak area, but less than 5 in third streak area—**as long as all sputum plates are consistently inoculated in the same manner.**[86] The results of the Gram stain (and scoring) should always be included in the report.

NOTE: Murray et al.[93] recommend that the **routine** identification of yeasts recovered from **sputum and bronchial washings** not be done. However, all yeasts should be examined for production of urease, and those that are urease positive should be identified so that *Cryptococcus neoformans* will be detected.

II. Transtracheal aspirate[94–96]

The **transtracheal aspirate** (also known as **infralaryngeal aspirate**) is a specimen obtained by procedures that bypass the upper respiratory flora. A needle is inserted below the larynx and a catheter is passed through the needle; 3-4 ml of sterile saline are injected, causing the patient to cough. Material is then aspirated back into the syringe. In most instances, there should not be any oropharyngeal or nasopharyngeal microorganisms in such specimens. The specimen should be cultured both **aerobically** and **anaerobically** and should be Gram stained.

For **anaerobic** culture, use anaerobic blood culture agar plate (see Chapter 72, media for anaerobes), and antibiotic-containing selective anaerobic plates if available (e.g., LKV or similar type), as well as thioglycollate broth. Incubate anaerobic set of media in anaerobic jar or "glove box" (see Chapters 70 and 82).

III. Pleural effusion

Pleural effusions or **empyema fluid** should be Gram stained and should be cultured aerobically and anaerobically. **Anaerobic cultures** of transtracheal aspirates and pleural material are particularly important for diagnosing **anaerobic pleuropulmonary infections**[95] as occur in patients who aspirate.

IV. Bronchoscopy and tracheostomy material

Bronchoscopy specimens are usually contaminated with oropharyngeal material as are **endotracheal tubes** and material obtained from suction through a tracheostomy. These specimens should **not** be cultured anaerobically. Gram stains should be done and the results correlated with the culture results.

Legionella pneumophila (Legionnaires' disease bacterium) culture

Legionnaires' disease pneumonia may resemble *Mycoplasma* or chlamydial pneumonia. Sputum specimens are poor candidates for isolation of *Legionella pneumophila*, and either **tissue, transtracheal aspirate**, or **pleural fluid** should instead be used; recently isolation of the organism from blood has been reported[19a] (see "Blood culture," above). The Center for Disease Control (CDC) currently recommends use of Feeley-Gorman (FG) cysteine and ferric pyrophosphate agar and charcoal yeast extract agar (CYE) plates[92] (see media, Chapter 72). If the materials are not available for these media, Mueller-Hinton agar with extra IsoVitaleX supplementation (2%) can be used, although it is not as efficacious as the F or CYE media. Legionnaires' pneumonia is usually diagnosed by serologic tests, although **direct immunofluorescence** has allowed diagnosis in several cases and culture alone has allowed diagnosis of a few cases.

For isolation of *Legionella*, plates must be held 14 days before discarding; the organisms may appear in 3-5 days. They may be **presumptively** identified by the slow growth, and lack of growth on blood agar at 42 C and at room temperature. In tissue sections or in material from lungs, the organisms are best stained with a modification of the **Dieterle silver impregnation stain**[92,97] (see Chapter 71) or by **direct fluorescent staining** (see FA staining, Chapter 70).

Initial processing and media inoculation.[92] The initial preparation, media inoculation, and subculturing of colonies suspected of containing *Legionella* (Legionnaires') must be performed in a biologic safety hood. Personnel must wear masks and gloves when culturing.

A. **Liquid specimens** (pleural fluid and transtracheal aspirate) require no special preparation before being inoculated directly on media. Inoculate both FG and CYE agars in 2 spots. Leave 1 spot undisturbed and streak the other with a bacteriologic loop for isolated colonies.

B. **Solid specimens** (lung, spleen, liver) should be processed (ground) as follows:
1. Grind 1 part tissue in 9 parts phosphate buffered saline, pH 7.2, to prepare 10% suspension.
2. Decant **portion** of 10% suspension into sterile, screwcapped test tube and freeze at -70 C.
3. Then inoculate both FG and CYE agars in 2 spots with 10% suspension. Leave 1 spot undisturbed and streak other with loop for isolation.
4. **Also,** prepare 1/50 dilution of 10% tissue suspension as follows:
   a. Add 0.1 ml 10% tissue suspension to 4.9 ml phosphate buffered saline, pH 7.2. Mix.
   b. Then inoculate FG and CYE agars with 0.1 ml suspension (0.2%). Spread inoculum over entire surface of each medium with sterile glass rod.

C. Incubation
1. Place FG and CYE plates into **candle jar.** Do not use CO_2 incubator as CO_2 concentration must be only 2½%.
2. Place **moist towel** in jar before closing.
3. Incubate at 35 C for 2 wk.

For **direct fluorescent antibody test** (FA), see FA staining, Chapter 70.

Culture examination. Examine all cultures both macroscopically and microscopically each day for 2 wk. Keep paper towel in candle jar moist!

FG agar. Examine this medium macroscopically with fluorescent desk lamp, allowing light to pass through agar. In areas of heavy inoculum, confluent growth will be visible in 2-3 d, and there will be distinctive brownish darkening of colonies and surrounding agar. In areas of light inoculum, colonies of *Legionella pneumophila* should appear in 4-5 d as white pinpoint dots. These colonies will increase in diameter after longer incubation. Examine heavy growth in dark with longwave (366 nm) ultraviolet light (Woods' lamp). A butter yellow color should be detectable in 4- to 5-day growth. Examine colonies suspected to be *Legionella* microscopically by placing plates on stage of dissecting microscope and illuminating one side of plate with light source held at slightly greater than 10° angle to horizontal. *Legionella* colonies will have cut-glass texture.

CYE agar. Examine plates in same manner described for FG plates. *Legionella* colonies will appear in 3-5 d. Young colonies have slight cut-glass texture that is rapidly lost after additional incubation. Browning of agar is not observable on this medium.

Identification of *Legionella pneumophila.* Process in safety hood. Wear mask and gloves!
1. Presumptive identification
   a. Pick colonies with a characteristic cut-glass appearance.
   b. Subculture colonies suspected of being *Legionella* to both a *Legionella* growth-supporting

medium (FG) and also to a non-*Legionella* growth-supporting medium (tryptose blood agar plate). Blood agar plate does not contain L-cysteine required for growth of *Legionella pneumophila*.
   c. Incubate media at 36 C in 2½% CO_2 (candle jar with moist towel) for 5 d.
   d. Examine plates daily for growth.
   e. Test cultures that grow on *Legionella* growth-supporting agar but not on blood agar for **definitive identification** of *Legionella*. Cultures that grow on blood agar are not *Legionella pneumophila*.
2. Definitive identification
   a. Direct fluorescent antibody (FA) test
      (1) Prepare suspension of suspect *Legionella pneumophila* colonies in 1% neutral formalin to give light turbidity (McFarland no. 1 or 2).
      (2) Prepare smears on double-ring slide that has been alcohol flamed.
      (3) Air dry and heat fix.
      (4) Perform direct FA staining (see Chapter 70).
   b. If direct FA test is positive, submit isolate to CDC for confirmation. Mail isolate to CDC on slant of FG or CYE medium. If slants of these media are not available, then prepare slants of Mueller-Hinton agar containing 1% hemoglobin and 2% IsoVitaleX (MH-IH agar).

Component A	
Mueller-Hinton agar	38 g
Distilled water	490 ml
Component B	
Hemoglobin powder	10 g
Distilled water	490 ml
Component C	
IsoVitaleX	20 ml

      (1) Prepare components A and B separately, and autoclave at 121 C for 15 min.
      (2) Cool to 50 C, mix together, and hold at 50 C in water bath.
      (3) Prepare component C by adding 10 ml sterile distilled water to each of two 10 ml vials of IsoVitaleX.
      (4) Add contents of both vials to A-B mixture.
      (5) Check pH of medium and adjust as needed to final pH of 6.9.
      (6) Dispense 8 ml into sterile 16 × 125 sterile screwcap tubes and slant.

For further details, see "*Legionella,*" Chapter 79.

Urine

The diagnosis and treatment of urinary tract infections requires urine cultures. Catheterization of the bladder has been implicated as a definite risk in infecting the urinary tract; therefore, "clean-voided, midstream" specimens are preferred. Since the urethra is contaminated with bacteria, especially near its external orifice, it is important to secure proper specimens to eliminate contamination.

Collection

Clean-voided specimen
Materials
Five or more sterile gauze squares
Tincture of green soap

Warm water
Wide-mouth receptacle for collection
Set of graphic instructions, preferably reinforced orally
Procedure
1. Patient removes all undergarments and washes hands thoroughly.
2. *Female:* "Spreads herself" holding both sides of labia back with one hand. *Male:* Retracts foreskin before washing head of penis.
3. Clean exposed area with 1 sponge wet with green soap passed from front to back. Discard sponge. Wash 3 more times with soap in same manner, discarding sponges with each backward stroke. Use 1 wet sponge to remove soap.
4. Patient voids and catches urine in container.
5. Fill container half full and give to attendant without holding top of container.
6. Specimen is capped by attendant and time of collection written on label.

Suprapubic aspiration
Occasionally, suprapubic aspiration of the bladder may be necessary, and is performed by the physician. It involves direct puncture of the bladder through the abdominal wall with a needle and syringe.
Materials
3% Iodine and 70% alcohol
1½ inch 19 to 20-gauge needle
20 ml syringe
Container for urine or rubber stopper for needle if specimen is kept in syringe
Procedure
1. Check and schedule patient with full bladder before procedure is attempted.
2. Paint skin of patient with iodine and allow to dry. Area covered is from point in midline about ⅓ distance from symphysis pubis to umbilicus.
3. Pass needle through skin into bladder maintaining negative pressure on syringe after inserting through skin.
4. Place urine in container or insert needle into sterile rubber stopper and record time of collection.
5. Take directly to laboratory.

Indwelling catheter[98]
Procedure
1. Clean catheter with alcohol sponge; puncture directly with needle and syringe.
2. Aspirate urine.
NOTE: Silicone catheter will leak if punctured.

Transport and storage

Urine is an excellent culture medium, and bacteria will multiply rapidly if specimen is left at room temperature for any appreciable time. For this reason, urine specimens should be transported to the laboratory immediately after obtained and should be processed within 1 hour; or, they should be refrigerated at 4 C (up to 24 hours) until culture can be performed. Failure to follow these instructions will lead to erroneous results.

Any specimen received more than 2 hours after collection without evidence of refrigeration should not be cultured; request new specimen.

Properly handled urine specimens will usually yield a biphasic distribution of colonies. Most specimens will contain either less than 1000 organisms/ml or more than 100,000/ml. If too many specimens contain organisms between 1000-100,000/ml, it is likely that the results are due to improper handling that allows multiplication of contaminants; finding more than 1 organism (in large numbers), many epithelial cells, or many lactobacilli points to contamination.

General principles of urine culture

1. Quantitative evaluation of urine by means of bacterial counts has been accepted as a routine procedure. Counts of 100,000 organisms/ml urine are generally regarded as indicative of infection (see below). Quantitation is done by culture, but a rapid tentative report may be obtained by doing a **Gram stain** on the undiluted specimen (see below). Counts from culture can be obtained using a **calibrated loop, pipet dilution,** or a **pour plate** method. The pour plate procedure is the reference method and can be used to control the accuracy of either the calibrated loop or pipet dilution method.

2. Centrifugation of urine and culturing of sediment for bacteria are definitely not recommended.

3. The following organisms can frequently be found in normal urine: yeasts, coliforms, coagulase-negative staphylococci, enterococci, diphtheroids, greening streptococci, *Proteus* sp.

Organisms found in infected urine are *Salmonella, Shigella, N. gonorrhoeae,* β-hemolytic streptococci, *E. coli, Klebsiella, Enterobacter, Serratia, Pseudomonas* sp., *Proteus* sp., enterococci, coagulase-positive staphylococci, *M. tuberculosis, Alcaligenes* sp., *Haemophilus* sp.

For an excellent review of urinary tract infections and their detection, see Kunin's manual[99]; for a brief but authoritative summary, see Barry et al.[98]

Screening methods

In the past few years a large number of screening procedures (many available commercially as kits) have been devised for the detection of "clinically significant bacteriuria" (100,000 organism/ml or higher), especially in cases of asymptomatic bacteriuria. A very large number of publications pertaining to the evaluation of these methods can be found in the literature. Generally the screening methods have not proved acceptable as substitutes for careful culture methods. Some, as indicated below, can be used for **screening** as long as their limitations are known and taken into account.

Microscopy. Gram-stained smears are prepared (1) from the centrifuged sediment and examined with oil-immersion lens; finding of more than 5 bacteria/oil-immersion field is considered a positive test (10^5 organisms/ml),[100] or (2) from uncentrifuged urine, based on the principle that bacteria must be present in the urine in a concentration of 100,000/ml before there is a chance of demonstration by staining.[101]

Triphenyltetrazolium chloride test (TTC).[102] The test depends on the respiratory activity of growing bacteria; when present in "significant" numbers, actively metabolizing bacteria will reduce the reagent to a pink-red precipitate of triphenylformazan in 4 hours. A commercially prepared kit is available.

Nitrite test—Griess.[103] The test is based on the ability of most urinary pathogens to reduce nitrate to nitrite, which can be detected by a simple diazotization reaction. Smith et al.[104] modified the test by adding nitrate to the urine and incubating it for 1 hour at room temperature; Sleigh[105] recommends incubation at 37 C for 4 hours. A commercial kit based on the Griess test principle is available.

Filter paper strip technic—Ryan et al.[106] A filter paper strip of definite dimensions was found by Ryan et al. to convey a standard inoculum of urine to the culture medium. A commercial kit incorporating their technic is available. It consists of a 2 × 1.3 cm rectangular sealed plastic dish filled with trypticase soy agar and sterile strips of filter paper with a perforated mark 1 cm from one end. The filter strip is dipped in urine to the perforated mark; this area of the strip is applied to the surface of the unsealed culture medium and then removed. The dish is resealed with its tape and incubated at 37 C for 12-18 hours. Growth of 3 or more colonies per culture indicates significant bacteriuria.

Electronic counter method. Quantitative estimates of bacteria in urine can be obtained by utilizing the Coulter counter. For details of the procedure and its problems, refer to Truant et al.[107,108]

Glucose test paper. See Schersten et al.[109]

Agar-coated slide method. See Cohen and Kass.[110]

Paddle or dip-slide culture kits. A number of commercially prepared types (Oxoid dip-slide, Uricult-Orion, Dip 'n Count—Royal Scientific) are available. They generally consist of a flat paddle coated on each side with agar media (usually one selective and the other nonselective). The paddle is dipped in the urine, removed, and after reinsertion into its sterile container, is incubated. Rough quantitative estimates of viable counts can be obtained. While Ellner and Papachristos[111] advocate the use of a dip-slide method for routine use in general hospitals, many workers feel that the method is not economical or useful in a clinical laboratory. Organisms are difficult to purify for susceptibility testing (Bartlett).[112]

Coated tube or cylinder culture kits. Bacturcult (Wampole Diagnostics) is one example of a sterile disposable tube coated with a nutrient indicator culture medium on the inner wall. The urine is poured into the container and then decanted. The tube is sealed and incubated.

Automated screening tests. Two instruments (Autobac-Pfizer, and MS-2/Abbott) are currently being evaluated for screening of urines, i.e., detecting levels up to 10^5 colonies/ml in 4-5 hours (positive), with those having lower levels being reported as negative.

Evaluation of screening tests

Opinion is divided concerning the value of some of these tests. Sacks and Abramson[100] pooled the results of many investigators and listed their findings as follows: The Griess test identifies only about ⅔ of urine specimens with 100,000 bacteria/ml; the 4-hour method (Sleigh) identifies about 90% of positive cases. The TTC test, also requiring 4-hour incubation, identifies about 80% of cases. Both Griess and TTC tests have low sensitivity as indicators of bacteriuria due to gram-positive cocci. Gram stain on uncentrifuged specimens identifies about 90% of cases, with ca 10% false positive results.

Kunin[113] emphasizes the value of microscopic examination and states that neither of the chemical methods (nitrite or TTC) is superior to or as rapid as microscopic studies. The chemical methods, according to Kunin, detect 70-90% of significant bacteriuria with a false-positive and false-negative test rate of 5-10%.

Two evaluations of the filter paper technic (Honeywell et al.[114] and Parker et al.[115]) found 93% and 95% correlation with standard quantitative counts (at the level of 10^5 bacteria/ml).

Thus the microscopic technics, when performed by skilled individuals, are acceptable as rapid screening tests. The filter paper technic, which requires incubation of 12-18 hours, seems to be a reasonably reliable screening test as an office procedure; identification and antibiotic sensitivity tests can be carried out on the colonies grown. Most workers do not recommend the chemical tests; even those that do, emphasize the need for standard culture procedures and sensitivity tests after the screening tests. All available screening methods fail to detect more than 60% of the urine specimens with counts between 10,000 and 100,000 bacteria/ml, which may be associated with urinary infections.

Both the **dip-slide** and the **coated tube type** kits are useful in physicians' offices and can also be used for large-scale screening studies of bacteriuria.[99]

Automated urine culture: detection, enumeration, and identification of bacteria and yeasts

The Vitek (McDonnell-Douglas) Automicrobic System (AMS) is the first automated instrument with a miniaturized selective/differential media system that addresses directly the specimen, bypassing the pure culture/agar plate concept. For details, see Sonnenwirth,[116] Aldridge et al.,[117] and Smith et al.[118]; also Chapter 74.

Quantitative urine culture methods

Studies by Kass,[119] Sanford, MacDonald, Beeson, and others reveal that significant clinical bacteriuria is indicated by the presence of 100,000 organisms/ml or more in a clean-voided urine. A count of less than 1000/ml is generally not considered indicative of infection, whereas counts between 10,000 and 100,000 are suggestive of infection and the count should be repeated on a fresh specimen.

Quantitative urine cultures on voided specimens furnish valuable information regarding the number of organisms and their significance.

Standardized, calibrated loop inoculation[98, 120]

This method is based on use of a calibrated loop to inoculate a known volume of urine on agar plates. After streaking and incubation, the colonies grown are counted.

Loop needed. Standard platinum dilution loop calibrated to deliver 0.001 ml (Scientific Products, no. N2075-2; or Arthur H. Thomas Co., no. 7011-J20).

Procedure

1. Flame and cool loop.
2. Hold vertically and immerse loop just below surface of urine specimen. Move loop straight up and down.
3. Withdraw loop and use loopful of urine to inoculate each agar plate with straight line down center of plate.
4. Streak plate for isolation with regular loop by series of streaks at 90° angle through original line.

Inoculate 1 blood agar and 1 MacConkey (or EMB) agar plate. Sodium azide or phenyl–ethyl alcohol–blood agar can be used for isolation of gram-positive organisms from mixed cultures containing such gram-negative organisms as *Proteus.*

If suspected typhoid carriers are examined: Inoculate, in addition to plates listed, 1 tube of selenite broth. Subculture, after overnight incubation, on MacConkey or eosin–methylene blue plate.

If leptospirae are suspected: See Chapter 80.

If tubercle bacilli are suspected: See Chapter 78.

Alternative loop inoculation procedure[98]

1. Apply 1 loopful of urine to 1 quadrant of agar plate in V-shaped, 2-3 cm long pattern.
2. Spread inoculum over half of plate with bent glass rod ("hockey stick"), bent wire, or another loop.
3. Then streak over other half of plate by 3 to 4 quadrant streaking technic.

Incubation and examination of plates. After incubation overnight at 35-37 C, count colonies on blood agar plates (total count) and on MacConkey or EMB plate (for gram-negative rod count). Each colony represents 1000 organisms/ml in the specimen; **multiply each count** by 1000 to give the number of bacteria per milliliter of urine.

Proceed with identification and reporting according to guidelines described in interpretation and workup, below. There have been scattered reports of *Staphylococcus aureus* and *Klebsiella ozaenae* as well as other *Klebsiella* strains from urine specimens that require CO_2 for growth.[121,122] For this reason, some workers recommend incubation of MacConkey plates in CO_2 (not only from urine culture, but other cultures as well, e.g., sputum), which is similar to CO_2 incubation of blood plates.

Care and quality control of calibrated loops[98]

1. When loops are not in use, insert them into test tubes and hold in place with cork stoppers for protection. After flaming of loop, it is imperative to let it cool in air before use.
2. Volume delivered by calibrated loops changes with use due to damage, incinerated material add-on, and corrosion. Inspect loops regularly to ascertain that loop is still round and weld is intact. Check delivery volume at least once a month.[98]
   a. Prepare stock solution by adding 0.75 g Evans blue dye to 100 ml distilled water. Filter through no. 40 Whatman filter paper and keep in stoppered bottle at room temperature.
   b. Prepare accurate 1:500, 1:1000, 1:2000, and 1:4000 dilutions of stock solution. Determine their absorbances in a spectrophotometer at 600 nm. Plot absorbance on a linear scale against the concentration of dye.
   c. Check delivery of loop by transferring 10 loopfuls stock solution to 10 ml distilled water. Rinse loop in distilled water, flame and cool between each loopful. Determine absorbance of this solution in spectrophotometer; it should correspond to that of 1:1000 dilution on standard curve within ± 20%. If error is greater, loop should be replaced or appropriate correction be made in colony counts using that loop.[98]
3. Another method for checking accuracy of loops is by comparison with counts by pour-plate procedure.

Pipet dilution method

1. Shake specimen well to ensure even distribution of organisms.
2. Prepare 1:10 dilution of urine by adding 1 ml urine to 9 ml water blank. Prepare 1:100 dilution by adding 1 ml of 1:10 dilution to 9 ml water blank. Mix dilutions thoroughly.
3. Measuring between lines of serologic pipet (0.2 ml or 1 ml), pipet 0.1 ml of 1:10 dilution to center of blood agar and 0.1 to MacConkey or EMB plate.
4. Pipet 0.1 ml of 1:100 dilution to center of blood agar plate.
5. Spread inoculum evenly over plates with loop or sterile glass spreader and incubate plates 18-24 h at 35 C. A turntable can be used to evenly spread inoculum.

This technic does not give adequate separation of colonies in 10^5 col/ml or higher range.

Pour plate method

1. Shake specimen well to ensure even distribution of organisms.
2. Prepare 1:100 dilution of urine as in pipet dilution procedure or by adding 0.1 ml urine to 9.9 ml water blank. Prepare 1:1000 dilution by pipetting 1 ml of 1:100 dilution to 9.0 ml water blank.
3. Add 1.0 ml of 1:100 dilution to 20 ml melted blood agar base cooled to approximately 45 C. Mix well.
4. Flame lip of tube containing agar-specimen mixture and pour into sterile Petri dish.
5. Wipe lip of tube with disinfectant-soaked cotton.
6. Repeat steps 3-5 with 1:1000 dilution of specimen.
7. Allow agar to solidify and incubate plates overnight.

Determination of colony count

1. Use of 2 dilutions allows determination of both high and low counts. Total counts are determined on noninhibitory media such as blood agar plates. MacConkey (EMB) plate is used to estimate number of enteric gram-negative rods and as basis for identification.
2. Count colonies on all noninhibitory plates containing 30-300 colonies and calculate number of organisms per milliliter of undiluted urine. If both dilutions contain colonies in countable range, use average of 2 results for total counts.
3. To determine total counts per milliliter of undiluted urine, multiply count obtained by dilution. In each method listed, plate count of lowest dilution is multiplied by 100 and highest dilution by 1000.

Simplified spread plate method[123]

In this method, no urine dilutions are prepared. Instead, sterile USP dropper delivering 20 drops/ml or 2 drops/0.1 ml is used.

1. Draw small quantity of urine into sterile dropper. Hold dropper vertically and allow excess urine to drain from outside. Discard 2 drops urine.
2. Holding dropper vertically, allow 2 drops urine to fall from distance of about 1 in. onto surface of trypticase soy agar plate.
3. Spread urine immediately with L-shaped sterile glass rod over entire surface of plate.
4. Incubate 24 h; count colonies. Number of colonies on plate multiplied by 10 equals number of bacteria per milliliter urine.

The method allows accurate counts up to 3000/ml and is primarily for use in screening children suspected of having pyelonephritis. In adults, dilutions of urine (as described above) should be used.

Interpretation and workup

A. Clean-voided specimen, Foley and indwelling catheter

1. Identify organisms on counts under 10,000 only when patient is currently on therapy or when specimen is taken by bladder puncture, unless specifically requested.
2. Identify organisms from 10,000-100,000 counts. Hold culture for sensitivity if special request is made by physician.
3. Do antibiotic sensitivity and identification on counts greater than 100,000/ml.
4. Designate predominant organism in mixed infection of greater than 100,000/ml.
5. Since mixed infections can occur, 2 gram-negative rods in specimen would be identified but 3 gram-negative rods would probably indicate gross contamination and new specimen would be requested.

B. Catheterized specimen

1. Identify up to 3 organisms if they are present in 1000/ml or greater number.

Identification

Identify potential pathogens at least to generic level,[98] but preferably to species, especially when there is a difference in antimicrobial susceptibility within the genus (e.g., *Pseudomonas* or *Proteus*).

Rapid screening tests and/or various miniaturized kits (API, Minitek, Enterotube, Micro-ID, etc.) can be used for identification of common urinary tract pathogens.

Antimicrobial susceptibility

Direct sensitivity testing of urine is not recommended except in cases of clinical emergency. Isolates should be tested if the physician requests it.

Anaerobic urine culture

Voided urine should never be cultured anaerobically because of the inevitable presence of anaerobes of the normal flora of the urethra and the surrounding areas.[89] Anaerobic urinary tract infections are exceedingly rare; if there is clinical or radiologic evidence of anaerobic infection, or the Gram stain suggests presence of anaerobes in the urine, obtain specimen by *suprapubic aspiration*.[98]

Urinary catheter tip culture

There is a general agreement in the literature[124] that the practice of culturing the tip of a **urinary catheter** after it is removed is an exercise in futility because the catheter tip is contaminated as it is removed from the urethra. It is strongly recommended that urinary catheter tips **should not** be submitted for culture and that instead a urine specimen should be cultured.

"Stone" (calculus) culture (kidney, bladder)

Nemoy and Stamey[125] recommend that stones recovered by needle aspiration at time of surgery should be cultured. They recommend that the stone be washed 4 times with sterile saline and then be crushed in sterile mortar (with sterile pestle) with 5 ml sterile saline until pulverized. Culture mixture by quantitative procedure (like urine); identify organism grown. They demonstrated that urea-splitting organisms are deeply embedded in the stone.

Autopsy material

During the course of an autopsy the surface of the organs becomes grossly contaminated. The outside of the organs should be seared with a red hot spatula; hold it on the area until the tissue is thoroughly dry.

Blood culture. Silver and Sonnenwirth (1969)[126] described a practical and efficacious method for obtaining significant postmortem blood cultures. They found that the most effective method is that in which a sterile puncture is made **through the closed chest cavity prior to removal of the bowel:** Reflect skin covering thorax. Sear third intercostal space adjacent to and to left of sternum with red hot spatula. Insert sterile 18-gauge needle (with attached syringe) through seared area and directly adjacent and perpendicular to sternum so that it enters right ventricle. Withdraw approximately 10 ml blood and inoculate into proper media as described under blood culture.

Leptomeninges. If dura is intact after removal of calvaria, it may be reflected from cerebral hemisphere and cultures of leptomeninges taken with swab or pipet without searing of surface. Otherwise, leptomeninges must be seared with heated spatula, which may kill organisms immediately beneath it. To obtain viable organisms, swab or pipet should be inserted through seared area and directed through subarachnoidal space into adjacent unheated, uncontaminated region.

Culture as described under pus. Add chocolate agar plate (incubate under CO_2).

Cerebrospinal fluid. Take with lumbar puncture needle and syringe. Puncture may be made on ventral surface of spinal column through intervertebral disk in lower thoracic region, or cisternal puncture may be made at base of skull.

Heart valves from cases of bacterial endocarditis. Obtain small piece of friable vegetation, using sterile forceps and scissors. Wash vegetation by passing it through 5 or 6 tubes of sterile saline solution. Transfer washed vegetation to tube of thioglycollate broth. Crush against side of tube with sterile glass rod. Make smears by crushing ground-up vegetation between 2 glass slides. Stain by Gram method. See also preparation of tissues for culture.

If gram-positive cocci are seen, streak 2 blood agar plates with 1 loopful of valve suspension. Streak 2 blood infusion agar plates with some macerated vegetation; incubate 1 set of plates in CO_2, another in anaerobic jar.

If gram-negative cocci are seen, streak some crushed vegetation onto chocolate agar plate. Inculate plate and broth culture 48 h in carbon dioxide or candle jar; also prepare 1 blood agar plate for anaerobic culture.

Intestinal material and gallbladder cultures. If typhoid fever is suspected, material should be taken from ileum. In dysentery, colon should be cultured.

Sear small area at site selected, and with hot iron perforate intestine. Insert sterile swab into opening and rotate swab against intestinal mucosa. Transfer material thus obtained ot tube of sterile selenite broth. Rub swab against side of tube until cloudy suspension results.

Streak loopful of original suspension onto Mac-Conkey or EMB agar plates and several loopfuls onto SS agar and bismuth sulfite plate. After overnight incubation, proceed with examination of lactose nonfermenting colonies.

Always prepare Gram stains from autopsy material (except intestinal specimens) as well as acid-fast stains, if required. Examine fluids for yeasts and fungi (see discussion on cerebrospinal fluid) by coverslip preparation or India ink (if *Cryptococcus* is suspected).

If possible, a portion of the original tissue should be frozen; it may serve as a guarantee against breakage or contaminated media. **Cultures for fungi** should be included whenever autopsy material is cultured.

Tissues from premature infants, aborted fetuses, and young babies autopsied as a result of an infectious process should always be examined for *Listeria*.

Preparation of tissues for culture. Tissue for culture should be ground into a fine suspension to allow for recovery of small numbers of organisms. Use sterile tissue grinder, such as the Ten Broeck grinder, made of heavy-walled Pyrex glass with sterile saline or broth. Some workers use sterile 60-mesh aluminum oxide to facilitate grinding. After tissue is ground into suspension, the latter is left to settle; the supernatant fluid is then used for inoculation of various media or inoculation of animals.

Brewer and Weed[127] have noted that some microbiologic information can be obtained even when a body has been embalmed.

Virus isolation

In fatal cases of central nervous system disease where viral etiology is suspected, it may be advisable to obtain postmortem specimens.[89]

1. Collect blood specimen by cardiac puncture; separate serum and refrigerate it.
2. Remove entire brain and refrigerate (do not freeze).
3. Tie off at both ends a 3-inch segment of descending colon.
4. Obtain aliquots of various other tissues (e.g., in respiratory disease, collect lung tissue and tracheobronchial swab).

Place all items in steps 2-4 into sealed sterile containers and refrigerate. Send all such specimens to virus reference laboratory (state, federal, university) as soon as possible.

See also section on viral and rickettsial diseases.

Tissue, biopsy material, abscesses, ulcers, fistulas, sinuses·

1. **Specimen container for tissue:** screwcap, widemouth, sterile bottle or sterile plastic container should be used.
2. **Container for closed abscess or purulent drainage material:** to allow for anaerobic culture, **closed abscesses** should be aspirated with syringe and needle and material should be injected into **anaerobic transport** tube. Purulent material may contain actinomycotic **granules;** inspect pus for presence of granules (*Actinomyces, Nocardia*) and perform Gram stain. Swabs are **not** adequate for collection.

Sinus tract. Curette with sterile curette so as to include portion of wall of tract or lesion. Purulent material from sinus cavity should not be collected on swabs—these are not adequate.[127] If possible, **aspirate** material and inject it into anaerobic transport tube.

Surgical specimens. Lymph nodes should be cultured, in addition to histologic examination. Spleen, when removed, should be cultured—study any granulomatous lesions or abscesses. Portion of tissue material may be refrigerated or frozen for further studies (if routine studies are unsuccessful). Tissue should be **ground** into fine suspension for culture (see preparation of tissues for culture under **autopsy material**).

Culture procedure. Generally, it is important to use rich media for detection of possible fastidious organisms (blood agar, chocolate agar, anaerobic media, heart infusion broth) and also to employ differential and selective media (MacConkey agar, media for fungi or mycobacteria). Incubation should be (1) air with 3-5% CO_2 and (2) under anaerobic conditions (for list of specimens to be cultured anaerobically, see **anaerobic infections,** below, and also Chapter 82).

In some institutions, granulomatous lesions, both caseous and noncaseous, are cultured for mycobacteria, *Brucella,* fungi, and general bacteria.[127] *Listeria monocytogenes,* as well as *Yersinia enterocolitica,* occasionally can be recovered only after **cold enrichment** (storage in buffer at 4 C for 1-3 wk). See *Listeria,* Chapter 77 and *Yersinia,* Chapter 79.

Microscopic examination. Gram stain (and acid-fast stain, if indicated or requested) of materials should be performed.

If mycotic elements are seen (or fungal infection is suspected), proceed with methods described in Chapter 103.

If tuberculosis is suspected, collect as much pus as possible and some tissue scrapings for processing and inoculation as described under mycobacteria (Chapter 78).

Legionnaires' disease (Legionella pneumophila). Lung biopsy specimens may be cultured for Legionnaires' disease bacterium (see above, "Lower respiratory tract specimens").

Liver abscess. For details, consult Palmer,[128] Lazarchik et al.,[129] and Sabbaj et al.[130]

Brain abscess. For a detailed review, see Louvois.[131]

Anaerobic infections and anaerobic cultures

Because anaerobic bacteria, under proper circumstances, can invade and cause disease in any organ or region of the body, **all body fluids and tissues from sites not contaminated with normal flora should be cultured anaerobically.** On the other hand, because anaerobic bacteria are normal inhabitants of the oral cavity, gastrointestinal tract, genitourinary orifices, and skin, certain specimens ordinarily **should not be cultured anaerobically:** (1) throat or nasopharyngeal swabs, (2) sputum or bronchoscopic specimens, (3) feces or rectal swabs, (4) voided or catheterized urine, (5) vaginal or cervical swabs not collected by visualization via a speculum, (6) material from superficial wounds or abscesses not collected properly to exclude surface contaminants, and (7) material from abdominal wounds obviously contaminated with feces, such as contamination from an open intestinal fistula.

Aspirated materials and biopsied specimens are preferred for the isolation of anaerobes. These should be processed immediately or placed in anaerobic tubes or vials containing an oxygen-free gas for transport to the laboratory.[132,133]

If swab specimens are collected, one should use either a transport system with oxygen-free gas or tubes of prereduced, anaerobically sterilized (PRAS) transport medium, such as Cary-Blair. Many transport systems suitable for collection and transport of clinical specimens are now available commercially from various companies.

Culture collection and transport. For details, see "Anaerobic culture collection and transport," this chapter.

Anaerobic methods. For detailed discussion of anaerobic methods (roll tube or VPI method, anaerobic jars, anaerobic glove box), inoculation, processing, incubation, etc., see anaerobic methods, Chapters 70 and 82.

Media, reagents, and biochemical procedures for anaerobes. See Chapter 72.

Initial culture

The Center for Disease Control (CDC) recommends for initial culture of all types of clinical material (except blood)[134]:

1 tube enriched thioglycollate broth
1 tube chopped meat dextrose medium
2 blood agar plates (If clostridia are suspected, inoculate 1 egg yolk agar (EYA) plate.)
1 kanamycin-vancomycin-menadione blood agar plate and/or phenylethyl alcohol blood agar

The Wadsworth group[132] recommends as a minimum inoculation of:

1 enriched blood agar
1 kanamycin-vancomycin laked blood agar
1 phenylethyl alcohol blood agar
1 liquid medium (supplemented thioglycollate or chopped meat broth)

For further recommendations, including use of *Bacteroides* bile esculin agar (BBE), see Chapters 82 and 86.

NOTE 1: **Direct Gram stain is essential for an immediate presumptive diagnosis of anaerobic infection and is also important for quality control** (all of the different morphologic types seen should be recovered in culture).

NOTE 2: **Whenever anaerobic culture is performed, it is absolutely necessary to also culture for aerobic (with or without CO$_2$) incubation.**

For further details, see Chapter 82.

Bite wounds: human and animal[135]

There is a wide variety of aerobic and anaerobic bacteria isolated from both human and animal bite wounds. Practically all such wounds have aerobic or facultative organisms isolated from them; at least half of them also contain anaerobes.

Most organisms in these wounds are derived from the normal oral flora. In human bites, group A streptococci, *Staphylococcus aureus*, and *Eikenella corrodens* are usually associated with infection.

In dog bites, an unidentified gram-negative rod has been associated recently with serious infections (bacteremia).[136]

Another often isolated organism from animal bites is *Pasteurella multocida*.

Culture: When feasible, aspirate material (pus); otherwise collect with swab. Transport aspirate or swab in anaerobic containers. Plate on MacConkey agar, phenylethyl blood agar, enriched blood agar, incubated aerobically; a chocolate agar plate incubated in 10% CO$_2$; blood agar plate, kanamycin-vancomycin laked blood agar with hemin and vitamin K$_1$, incubated anaerobically. A liquid medium, enriched thioglycollate broth, should also be used.

Material from serous cavities

Pleural, synovial, pericardial, and peritoneal fluid should be collected in anaerobic transport containers.

Centrifuge fluid specimen (2500 rpm 20-30 min), remove supernatant aseptically, and smear and culture sediment.

Inoculate 2 blood agar plates, selective anaerobic media (see anaerobic infections and cultures above), 1 MacConkey, Endo, or eosin–methylene blue (EMB) plate, thioglycollate broth, and brain-heart infusion broth. Incubate 1 blood agar plate and selective anaerobic media anaerobically, the other plates aerobically.

If *Neisseria gonorrhoeae* is suspected (joint fluid), inoculate chocolate agar or Thayer-Martin agar (incubation in 3-5% CO$_2$).

If anticoagulant is needed, use SPS (see "Blood culture," above) or a preservative-free heparin solution.[89]

Wounds

In the ordinary infected wound the methods of culture described under **Tissue,** etc. may be sufficient. In postoperative, hospital-acquired infections the organisms usually found are staphylococci, various gram-negative enteric organisms, and more rarely, hemolytic streptococci. However, anaerobes are also often involved.

Selective and general anaerobic media (see anaerobic infections and cultures, above) should always be used for the culture of **deep** wounds. Often, the flora of infected wounds consists of a mixture of many aerobic and anaerobic organisms that have to be isolated and grown in pure cultures. A careful Gram stain performed on the clinical specimen will often serve as a guide to the appropriate media and procedures to be followed.

Skin

Superficial wound
1. Clean surface with 70% alcohol.
2. Swab or aspirate areas as deep as possible; avoid surface of lesion, if possible.
3. Transport swab or aspirate in transport medium.

Decubiti or burns
1. Punch biopsy is recommended for quantitative culture.[137] Otherwise, collect material on swabs.
2. Inoculate blood agar, MacConkey agar, thioglycollate broth; if foul smelling or gas present, culture anaerobically, also.

Petechiae
1. Meningococci (and occasionally other pathogens) can be cultured from material taken from petechiae.
2. For detection of Rickettsia, see Chapter 95.

Deep lesion, closed abscess. See **anaerobic infections and anaerobic cultures,** above. For a detailed review of the bacteriology and management of cutaneous abscesses, see Meislin et al.[138]

Smear for Mycobacterium leprae. See Chapter 78, Mycobacteria.

Fungi. See methods in mycology, Chapter 103.

Vesicles. Examine for viruses. See Chapter 92.

Staphylococcus epidermidis, "diphtheroids" (*Corynebacterium, Propionibacterium*), and micrococci are usually found on the skin. *S. aureus* is the only "pathogen" that commonly is found on the skin. Occasionally *C. diphtheriae* causes ulceration, often indistinguishable from anthrax. Cultures in such cases should include media for selective isolation of the diphtheria organism (see discussion of throat and nasopharyngeal cultures).

Catheter tips

Urinary tract catheter, Foley. See urine, above.

Intravenous (IV) catheter. Maki et al.[139] recommend a **semi-quantitative culture technic** for identifying infection due to IV catheters. This technic distinguishes infection ($\geq$15 colonies) from contamination and is more specific in diagnosis of catheter-related septicemia than culture of the catheter in broth.
1. Place catheter segment on surface of a 100 mm 5% sheep blood agar plate. While downward pressure is exerted with flamed forceps, roll catheter (or smear if it is bent) back and forth across surface at least 4 times. After this, immerse segment in trypticase soy broth.
2. Incubate plate and broth at 35-37 C. Subculture broths (turbid or without apparent growths) after 72 h onto blood agar plates.
3. Count all colony types appearing on primary plates. Identify all organisms from primary plates and broths.

Mouth

Microbial infections that may occur in the mouth, although some quite rarely, include tuberculosis, syphilis, gonorrhea, nocardiosis, actinomycosis, kala-azar, yaws, candidiasis, her-pes simplex, etc. Consult the appropriate chapter for the collection and culture of specimens for these cases. Cultivation and enumeration of lactobacilli from saliva or the determination of acidogenic properties of the salivary flora are not established methods for determining the caries activity rate of the individual patient. Cultivation of material from the gums yields no useful information in the case of periodontitis. Cultivation of the root canal (periapical region) is useful only just prior to final filling of the root canal; for a review of root canal, socket, and periapical abscess cultures, see Grossman[140] and Nolte.[141]

Cultures of periapical region. To culture the periapical region through the root canals with the tooth in position, proceed as follows:

1. Isolate tooth with rubber dam.
2. Sterilize coronal surface with 3% tincture of iodine.
3. Remove filling with sterile instruments.
4. Remove filling in root canal with sterile instruments.
5. Cleanse and dry canal with sterile cotton and insert sterile paper points slightly moistened with sterile saline solution to absorb any moisture oozing into canal; remove points and drop them into tube of glucose ascites medium (brain-heart infusion with *p*-aminobenzoic acid, 0.05 g/L, and 10% ascitic fluid).*
6. If no moisture oozes in, pass sterile, fine broach or pick through canal and drop it into tube of medium.

Cultures of gums. Smears may be made from the gums. Allow to dry and stain for spirochetes and bacteria.

For a discussion of the normal bacterial flora of the mouth, and the role of anaerobes in dentoalveolar infections, see Finegold[142] and Burnett et al.[143]

Eye examination

Specimens should be obtained under aseptic conditions and before antibiotic therapy. Collect materials from conjunctivitis, blepharitis, and hordeola (styes) on sterile swabs, surgical instruments, or sterile platinum loop.

Do not take smears and cultures within 4 hours after irrigation or instillation of disinfectant solutions or ophthalmic medications. Medications may contain antibacterial preservatives; local anesthetics tend to flush organisms from the conjunctival sac.

Scrapings, usually taken with a small platinum spatula and fixed on microscope slides, should be stained with Giemsa stain and examined for eosinophils and inclusion bodies and for trachoma, inclusion conjunctivitis, and other virus infections. Smears of secretions stained with Gram stain are important for selection of suitable culture media. Swabs with exudate should be used for inoculation of media.

---

*Available from Difco Laboratories in prepared tubes.

Specimens

The film technic is designed particularly for the ophthalmologist in private practice, whereas the combined film and culture technic is designed for the clinic.

Smear technic

Material required. Two stains are necessary. The Gram stain gives all information needed in conjunctivitis of bacterial origin. Polymorphonuclear (PMN) leukocytes in the Gram stain usually mean that the process is bacterial; however, PMNs can also be found in inclusion conjuctivitis. Finding of mononuclear cells suggests nonbacterial etiology. Giemsa stain gives the information required in trachoma and in inclusion conjunctivitis (inclusion blennorrhea and swimming-pool conjunctivitis) and also enables the eosinophilia of vernal conjunctivitis to be determined.

Giemsa stain. Fix scrapings (on glass slide) in methyl alcohol 10 min. Stain overnight in incubator at 37 C with Giemsa stain diluted 1 drop to each ml neutral distilled water. Decolorize in 95% alcohol twice for total decolorizing time of 5 s. Dry in air and examine.

If rapid diagnosis is required, the following technic may be used: Fix 1 min with Wright stain. Dilute fixative with equal number of drops of neutral distilled water and allow solution to remain 4 min. Transfer to dilute Giemsa and stain 15 min or longer. Decolorize in alcohol. Dry in air.

Procedure. Make 4 preparations from each case, 2 epithelial scrapings and 2 secretion smears. Place 1 epithelial scraping and 1 secretion smear in absolute methyl alcohol. Stain secretion smears with Gram stain. If it gives satisfactory information, discard other slides.

Culture technic

Procedure. Cultures are taken most satisfactorily from the lower cul-de-sac, with care to avoid lashes and lid margin. In chronic blepharoconjunctivitis, take cultures also from lid margins and inner canthus. Incubate at 37 C.

Inoculation of a variety of media is recommended to increase chances of isolating etiologic agent. Relatively large inocula are generally most productive, unless material is frankly purulent.

Although it is not possible to predict precisely the species that may be isolated, the majority of specimens can be successfully cultured with a minimum of carefully selected media. Besides those suggested below, others may be used as indicated by Gram-stained preparation, clinical observations, and tentative diagnosis.

These media may be inoculated with swabs or with aliquots of the secretion using sterile wire loop:
1. Blood agar plate, for isolation of organisms.
2. Chocolate agar plate, incubated in an atmosphere containing about 10% carbon dioxide, for possible presence of *N. gonorrhoeae, Haemophilus,* meningococci, and other pathogens.
3. Serum tellurite agar or Loeffler slant is particularly useful for isolation of *C. diphtheriae,* streptococci, pneumococci, *H. influenzae,* and certain yeasts and molds.
4. Thioglycollate medium. It is used as an enrichment culture for assurance that organisms present in small numbers, which may fail to appear on the original isolation plates, will not go undetected. (For eye areas other than conjunctiva, include anaerobic blood agar.)
5. Trypticase soy broth, with sterile serum or with sterile defibrinated animal blood added, is also popular as an enrichment medium for rapid growth and detection of fastidious organisms in as litttle as 4-6 h. It is especially useful when specimen contains few bacteria. If no growth appears on plates, isolation or sensitivity test plates should be streaked from thioglycollate medium and/or trypticase soy broth.
6. Mycosel agar and Sabouraud dextrose agar for isolation and cultivation of fungi.

Saprophytic organisms found in the eye include *Corynebacterium xerosis, Corynebacterium pseudodiphtheriticum, S. epidermidis,* and *Propionibacterium.* "Pathogens" include *N. gonorrhoeae, Haemophilus* sp., pneumococci, *Streptococcus pyogenes, Staphylococcus aureus,* Chlamydia of inclusion conjunctivitis, *Pseudomonas aeruginosa, Proteus* sp., *E. coli,* fungi, anaerobes, and *Moraxella lacunata.*

Acute and subacute conjunctivitis

Haemophilus and pneumococci are most often found, along with *S. aureus* and certain gram-negative enteric organisms. *N. gonorrhoeae* is often found in ophthalmia neonatorum if preventive measures are not used.

Pseudomembraneous conjunctivitis

C. diphtheriae, and, more rarely, *S. pyogenes* are most often involved.

Lacrimal conjunctivitis

Lacrimal conjunctivitis is secondary to infection of the lacrimal sac and does not respond to treatment of the conjunctiva. The prognosis is most favorable in the newborn in whom the lacrimal stenosis usually heals spontaneously. In adults the condition usually requires either removal of the sac or one of the more physiologic operations that restore drainage into the nose. The chronic conjunctivitis that follows dacryocystectomy is usually nonbacterial and probably results from the disturbance in lacrimal function.

The most common agents in lacrimal conjunctivitis are, in order of frequency: *S. pneumoniae, H. influenzae,* and *S. pyogenes.*

Vernal conjunctivitis

The constant finding of eosinophilic cells in the conjunctival secretion is of diagnostic importance. The eosinophils are typically fragmented and the eosinophilic granules widely scattered. The finding of scattered eosinophilic granules, even though but few cells are present, is extremely suggestive of vernal conjunctivitis and is particularly useful in doubtful cases in which the clinical signs of the disease are not fully developed. A number of subclinical cases that have the subjective but not the objective signs of the disease yield positive microscopic findings. Scrapings from the upper tarsal conjunctiva are the most instructive.

Bacteria in conjunctivitis

Cultures of 2160 patients with conjuctivitis, by Nicholas and Goolden[144] showed that the most common "pathogenic" organism recovered was *S. aureus* (in 14.6% of the cases). The most frequently recovered organism was *S. epidermidis* (albus, coagulase negative), 47.8%. The next most frequent isolates were *Corynebacterium*, 13.4%; *S. viridans*, 8.6%; and *Pseudomonas*, 1.4%. Other organisms (*Moraxella, Klebsiella,* pneumococcus, Mimeae, *Proteus, Haemophilus*) were recovered with less than 1% frequency.

Infective corneal ulceration

Infective corneal ulceration may be due to almost any bacterial organism. The infection is usually introduced through a small corneal abrasion. Cocci or gram-negative rods are involved most often: *P. aeruginosa* causes a very severe infection.

Ulcerative blepharitis

Chronic infection of the eyelids and eyelash follicles is most often due to *S. aureus.*

Viral and fungal eye infections

For a detailed discussion see the review of Birge.[145] A number of viral agents as well as bedsoniae are involved in eye infections. For technics of obtaining specimens and isolation see section on viral and rickettsial diseases, Chapter 92 and 95.

In addition to the more common fungal pathogens, *Cladosporium trichoides* and *Neurospora sitophilia* (a red bread mold) are known to be involved in eye infection. For obtaining specimens, etc. see section on mycology.

Microbiology of contact lens

Contact lenses have been shown to be involved in eye infections. The most flagrant bacterial offender seems to be *P. aeruginosa.* It is present in tap water and a number of solutions used by contact lens wearers. *Candida, Aspergillus, Cephalosporium,* and many other so-called benign fungi have been implicated. Adenovirus infections, especially epidemic keratoconjuctivitis, seem to occur more frequently among contact lens wearers.

Contact lens containers, especially the sponge material on which the lenses rest, have been shown to be contaminated with bacteria and fungi.

If infection occurs in contact lens wearers, as shown by corneal ulcer, cultures and scrapings should be taken and proper treatment should be instituted.

For further details see Theodore[146] and Winkler and Dixon.[147]

Material from ear, mastoid, and paranasal sinuses

To cultivate organisms in furuncles of the **external auditory canal,** the skin should be cleansed with alcohol, and pus picked up with a sterile swab. Inoculate blood agar plate, chocolate agar, EMB, or MacConkey plates, and also thioglycollate broth.

In **otitis media** the otologist collects the material by tympanocentesis, taking care that the needle tip (used for aspiration) does not get in contact with the speculum or the auditory canal.[148] Inoculate **both** aerobic (blood agar, EMB or MacConkey, and chocolate agars) and anaerobic media (anaerobic blood agar, thioglycollate broth-enriched or chopped meat, kanamycin-vancomycin laked blood agar, and PEA) with aspirated material.

Pus from chronic otitis media yields only aerobes in ca. 40% of patients, mixed aerobes and anaerobes in about 50%, and only anaerobes in a few patients. The most common isolate usually is *Pseudomonas aeruginosa,* followed by *Staphylococcus aureus* and *Proteus* spp. Most common anaerobes are *Peptococcus* and *Peptostreptococcus* followed by *B. fragilis* and *B. melaninogenicus.*[148]

The bacteriology of **chronic mastoiditis** is similar to that of otitis media, and it commonly involves anaerobes.[142]

Acute sinusitis (suppurative) involves pneumococci, staphylococci, and streptococci. Occasionally *Haemophilus influenzae, Bacteroides,* and *Klebsiella* are isolated from serious infections.

Genital tract:
I. Female genital tract—cervical, urethral, uterine, and vaginal specimens

In **acute infections** of the genital areas (urethritis, cervicitis, vulvovaginitis in children) specimens are usually examined and cultured for *N. gonorrhoeae.* Other organisms implicated in these infections are β-hemolytic streptococci, *E. coli* and other coliform organisms, *S. aureus,* and anaerobic streptococci. In **acute vaginitis,** β-hemolytic streptococci, *Corynebacterium (Haemophilus) vaginalis,* and often the yeast *Candida albicans* and the protozoan *T. vaginalis* are found. In **puerperal sepsis** and **septic abortion,** group A β-hemolytic streptococci, clostridia, enteric organisms, anaerobic streptococci, and *bacteroides* are often found.

In **chronic infections,** the organisms most often involved are *N. gonorrhoeae, Trichomonas vaginalis,* and *Candida albicans* (vaginal discharge); *Listeria monocytogenes* and *Vibrio fetus* have also been isolated. Ulcers, chancres, and sores can be due to syphilis, *Haemophilus ducreyi,* or the agent of lymphogranuloma venereum.

Examination of specimens from females is complicated by the occurrence of a large variety of bacteria in the normal vagina. It is important to obtain material with the least possible contamination.

The normal vaginal flora (during childbearing years) consists predominantly of lactobacilli, *S.*

epidermidis, and corynebacteria, with a variety of anaerobes (*Bacteroides,* anaerobic cocci) also present in about 70% of women. Other bacteria of lower incidence are viridans streptococci, enterococci, group B streptococci, nonpathogenic neisseriae, enteric bacilli, *Acinetobacter* sp., *Haemophilus (Corynebacterium) vaginalis* and *Mycoplasma* spp. In the postmenopausal years the flora remains about the same, the only significant difference being the greater incidence of gram-negative bacilli, other than *E. coli,* in postmenopausal women.

The normal urethra usually contains some contaminants from the external mucous membranes of the genital organs, such as staphylococci, corynebacteria, enteric bacilli, enterococci, *Haemophilus (corynebacterium) vaginalis, Acinetobacter,* and various *Candida* sp.

The vulva has a mixture of skin organisms and other bacteria descending from the vagina.

Isolation of *Neisseria gonorrhoeae*— female genital tract*

General recommendations[148a]

1. To diagnose gonorrhea in women, specimens should be obtained from the **endocervical** and **anal canals** and inoculated separately onto **Modified Thayer-Martin (MTM)** (Thayer-Martin medium with 2% agar, 0.25% dextrose, and 5 μg/ml trimethoprim lactate)[149-151] medium in culture plates, bottles, or other suitable container. In a screening situation, only culture specimens from the endocervical canal are recommended. The combination of a positive oxidase reaction of typical colonies containing typical gram-negative diplococci grown on this medium provides sufficient criteria for *presumptive identification* of *Neisseria gonorrhoeae.* (See below for criteria for confirmatory identification of isolates, especially those obtained from nonanogenital sites.)

2. **Tests of cure** are recommended for all women treated for gonorrhea. For test of cure, culture specimens should be obtained from both the endocervical and the anal canals, inoculated on MTM medium, and interpreted as in no. 1 above.

3. **Oropharyngeal specimens** (inoculated on MTM medium) should be obtained from all patients suspected of having disseminated gonococcal infection or pharyngeal gonococcal infection. Once pharyngeal gonococcal infection has been demonstrated, at least 2 pharyngeal specimens should be obtained after treatment in order to document cure.

4. **Gram-stained or fluorescent antibody-stained smears (of specimens) are not recommended for the diagnosis of gonorrhea in women** except as an adjunct to cultures. Although Gram-stained smears from the endocervical canal may be quite specific if examined by well-trained personnel, they are not adequately sensitive to rule out gonorrhea.[152]

5. **Gram-stained or fluorescent antibody-stained smears are not recommended** as a test of cure in women.

Collection of specimens[148a]

Endocervical canal (choice site for culture):
1. Moisten speculum with warm water; do *not* use any other lubricant.
2. Remove excessive cervical mucus, preferably with cotton ball held in ring forceps.
3. Insert sterile cotton-tipped swab into endocervical canal; move swab from side to side; allow 10-30 seconds for absorption of organisms onto swab.

Anal canal (rectal GC culture):
NOTE: This specimen can easily be obtained without using anoscope.
1. Insert sterile cotton-tipped swab approximately 1 in. into anal canal.
2. Move swab from side to side in anal canal to sample crypts; allow 10-30 seconds for absorption of organisms onto swab.

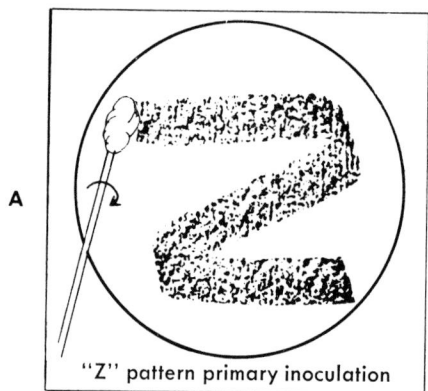

"Z" pattern primary inoculation

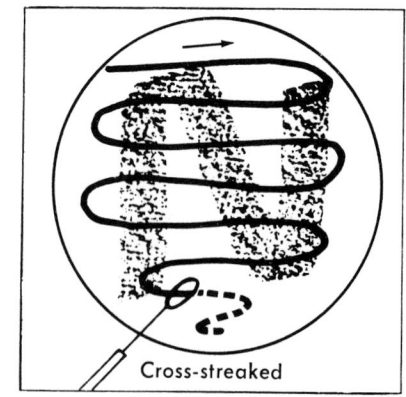

Cross-streaked

Fig. 75-4. Method for inoculation of modified Thayer-Martin (MTM) medium in round or rectangular plate. **A,** Roll swab in large Z pattern. **B,** Cross-streak **immediately** with sterile loop or tip of swab. (From Criteria and techniques for the diagnosis of gonorrhea, Atlanta, 1977, Center for Disease Control, Venereal Disease Control Division.)

---

*Based on *Criteria and techniques for the diagnosis of gonorrhea,* Center for Disease Control, Venereal Disease Control Div., Atlanta, undated (received 1977).

Urethra or vagina:
Cultures are indicated when endocervical culture is not possible; e.g., hysterectomy patients and children.
URETHRA
1. Strip urethra toward orifice to express exudate.
2. Use sterile loop or cotton swab to obtain specimen.

Urethral cultures in women should not be collected until at least 1 hour after urinating. Stimulate discharge by pressure and massaging of urethra against pubic symphysis through vagina. If no discharge is obtained, insert a thin alginate swab into distal urethra for ca. 2 cm and rotate gently.[152]

VAGINA. Use speculum to obtain specimen from posterior vaginal vault or obtain specimen from vaginal orifice if hymen is intact.

Oropharynx:
The oropharynx is a common local source for disseminated gonococcal infection. Swab posterior pharynx and tonsillar crypts with cotton-tipped applicator.

Blood or synovial fluid:
Culture of blood or synovial fluid on enriched broth medium (such as trypticase soy broth supplemented with 1% IsoVitaleX, 10% horse serum, and 1% glucose) is a recommended procedure in **special situations** such as suspected **gonococcal arthritis** or **septicemia**.

Conjunctiva:
Specimens from conjunctiva should be inoculated on MTM medium and chocolate agar supplemented with 1% IsoVitaleX. Identification of *Neisseria gonorrhoeae* should include sugar fermentation or fluorescent antibody technics.

Inoculation and incubation of media

Modified Thayer-Martin medium (MTM) in plates:
Medium should be at room temperature before inoculation. **Do not place** inoculated culture medium in refrigerator or expose it to extreme temperatures.
1. Roll swab in large "Z" pattern on MTM medium in round or rectangular plate (Fig. 75-4, *A*).
2. Cross-streak immediately with sterile wire loop or tip of swab, *in clinical facility,* Fig. 75-4, *B.* (If cross-streaking has inadvertently been omitted in clinical facility, it should be done in laboratory before incubation.)
3. Place culture in CO_2-enriched atmosphere (e.g., candle jar) within 15 minutes. (Be sure to relight candle each time jar is opened.) Deliver to laboratory as soon as possible for incubation.
4. Begin incubation of plates within few hours (the sooner the better) at 35-36 C.

If plate is inoculated in laboratory (see note below), place plate immediately in CO_2 incubator (35-36 C) or in candle jar (smokeless white candle); incubate at 35-36 C. The burning candle will generate about 3% CO_2 before extinction.

NOTE: In hospitals, specimens may be submitted on swab in holding medium (e.g., Culturette) a short time after obtained from patient. Inoculate **immediately** to MTM plate, Transgrow bottle, or other available system (Jembec, etc.).

Do not leave specimens suspected of harboring gonococci at room temperature or in incubator (35 C), unless in Transgrow or other transport medium.[89]

CO_2-generating tablets[153, 154]:
Several systems* now use a CO_2-generating tablet to create a CO_2-enriched atmosphere in an enclosed container (e.g., special plastic bag). Care must be taken that:
1. The tablet is dry and used before the expiration date.
2. The tablet is placed within the chamber immediately after the MTM medium is inoculated.
3. The medium is sufficiently moist to create the humid atmosphere necessary for release of CO_2.
4. The chamber is tightly sealed or closed before incubation.

Modified Thayer-Martin medium in bottles—with a 10% CO_2 atmosphere (Transgrow)[149, 150]†
1. Inoculate specimens on surface of medium as follows.
   CAUTION: Keep neck of bottle in upright position to prevent CO_2 loss.
   a. Remove cap of bottle only when ready to inoculate medium.
   b. Soak up all excess moisture in bottle with specimen swab and then roll swab from side to side across medium, starting at bottom of bottle.
   c. Tightly cap bottle immediately to prevent loss of CO_2.
2. When possible, incubate bottle in upright position at 35-36 C for 16-18 hours before sending to laboratory, and note this on accompanying request form. Resultant growth usually survives prolonged transport and is ready for identification on arrival at laboratory. (If incubator is not available, store culture at room temperature [25 C or above] 16-18 hours before subjecting it to prolonged transport and/or extreme temperatures.)
3. Package **incubated** culture bottle and request form in suitable container to prevent

---

*Gono-Pak, Ames Co. (Div. of Miles Laboratories), Elkhart, Ind.; Jembec, Flow Labs, Rockville, Md.; Gibco Diagnostics, Columbus, Ind.; and others.
†Baltimore Biological Lab., Cockeysville, Md.; Difco Labs., Detroit, Mich.

breakage, and immediately send to central bacteriologic laboratory by postal service or other convenient means.

4. In the laboratory, examine preincubated bottles immediately for *Neisseria gonorrhoeae;* incubate other bottles at **35-36 C** for 24-28 hours and examine. Bottles received with loose caps should be incubated in candle jar or CO_2 incubator; leave cap loose.

NOTE: Adjust incubator to 35 C, because some strains of *N. gonorrhoeae* may not grow well at 37 C.

Choice of media. The Center for Disease Control recommends MTM medium in plates as the medium of choice. Bottled MTM, a selective medium for the transport and cultivation of *N. gonorrhoeae,* is recommended only when specimens cannot be delivered to the laboratory or incubator on the day they are taken. Validity of culture results depends on proper technics for obtaining, inoculating, and handling specimens.

Shelf-life and storage of media. The storage life of MTM medium in plates, not sealed to prevent drying, and stored at room temperature, is only 2 weeks. MTM medium in plates sealed in plastic and refrigerated has a shelf-life of 4-6 weeks. MTM medium in bottles, when refrigerated, has a shelf-life of 3 months. All media should be stored according to the directions supplied by the manufacturer.

Direct smears. If purulent exudate from the endocervix or urethra is present and the Gram stain is positive, there is a strong presumption of gonorrheal diagnosis. The sensitivity of the endocervical smear, however, is only about 60% when done by trained microbiologists. Therefore culture must be performed on specimens from the cervix.[152]

The direct Gram stain report should state the presence and amount of pus cells (polymorphonuclear cells) and epithelial cells, and should indicate the morphology, or numbers of all bacteria seen.

In a typical case of acute gonococcal urethritis, the report might read: "3+ pus cells, 1+ epithelial cells, 3+ gram-negative intracellular diplococci." A stain from a poorly collected specimen, on the other hand, might state: "2+ pus cells, 2+ squamous epithelial cells, 3+ gram-negative rods, 2+ gram-negative cocci, 2+ gram-positive cocci." In this case the mixed flora and epithelial cells indicate vaginal contamination; the report does not support or refute the diagnosis of gonococcal infection.[152]

Gram staining and specific fluorescent antibody staining (see Chapter 70) of smears from *conjunctivae, joint fluids,* or *skin lesions* can be used as an *adjunct* in the diagnosis of gonococcal infections of these sites, particularly when partial therapy may prevent cultural recovery of organisms.

Culture media for Neisseria gonorrhoeae

"Chocolate agar" with commercial peptones and yeast extract was used for many years for the isolation of *N. gonorrhoeae.*

The introduction of a selective medium in 1964 by Thayer and Martin,[151] utilizing the antibiotics polymyxin B and ristocetin to suppress the growth of contaminating organisms, provided a major new impetus to the cultural diagnosis of gonorrhoeae. Thayer and Martin[155] later improved the medium by replacing the antibiotic supplements with a new antimicrobic solution of sodium colistimethate, nystatin, and vancomycin (V-C-N inhibitor; BBL, Cockeysville, Md.; and Difco Labs, Detroit). In addition, Thayer and Martin replaced the yeast extract with a chemically defined additive. The medium allows growth of *N. gonorrhoeae* and *N. meningitidis,* but inhibits other neisseriae and suppresses *Pseudomonas* and *Proteus* sp.

A modification of Thayer-Martin medium (**MTM**) for transport and growth purposes was introduced by Lester and Martin[149,150] in 1971. This formulation contained twice as much agar as the former and increased concentration of glucose. The unit (called "Transgrow") consists of a bottle containing MTM medium slant with a carbon dioxide atmosphere to maximize the recovery of the fastidious *Neisseria* during transit to the microbiology laboratory from physicians' offices, clinics, public health laboratories, etc. A further selectivity of Transgrow was obtained by the inclusion of trimethoprim lactate to inhibit the "spreading" property of *Proteus;* preincubation of Transgrow prior to transport is required for optimal results. (For MTM medium composition and preparation, see media, Chapter 72).

A medium known as **New York City (NYC)** medium was introduced in 1973 by Faur et al.[156, 157] It contains 4 antimicrobials (colistin, vancomycin, trimethoprim lactate, and nystatin or amphotericin) and is capable of initiating and supporting luxuriant growth of pathogenic *Neisseria;* it is also very selective.

In 1974, Martin, Armstrong, and Smith[157] introduced a compact, economical carbon dioxide–generating system to replace the cumbersome candle jar extinction procedure. They reported success using a citric acid–sodium bicarbonate tablet with cultures incubated in polyethylene plastic bags at 35-37 C.

Humidity in the bag catalyzed generation of carbon dioxide. Their trials found the new system to be as equally effective as the candle jar method using the modified Thayer-Martin medium to recover gonococci.

Another development has been a rectangular plastic plate that contains a small well to accommodate a CO_2-generating tablet (Jembec plate). The CO_2-generating tablet sealed in a plastic pouch and the plate provide a CO_2 environment enclosure.

Symington[153] compared Amies charcoal transport medium Jembec chambers with "Neigon" plates (modified Thayer-Martin medium) and Jembec chambers with plates of modified NYC transport medium. There was no significant difference between the 3 systems for the first 2 days in transit; however, after 3 days in transit, the Jembec-NYC medium chambers were significantly better than the other systems.

In 1977, Martin and Lewis[158] modified the MTM medium by raising the vancomycin concentration from 3 μg/ml to 4 μg/ml, and replacing the nystatin with anisomycin (for more effective inhibition of yeasts). The medium is known as the **ITM** (improved Thayer-Martin medium) or **ML** (Martin-Lewis medium).

Examination of plates and identification

Primary gonococcus colonies appear **translucent, raised,** finely granular, and moderately convex with lobate margins. They are usually **mucoid** and vary in size from punctiform to 5 mm in diameter, depending on the medium and the crowding on the plate.

The gonococcal colonies appear usually as pure growth on the selective TM, MTM, or NYC medium, with most neisseriae, other gram-negative and gram-positive contaminants, and yeasts being almost totally inhibited. Gonococcal growth is slightly inhibited in the first 16 hours but not after 48 hours. The colonies range from punctiform to 5 mm in diameter. In Transgrow bottles, colonial growth may or may not be typical.

If TM, MTM, NYC, or chocolate agar medium is used, **presumptive identification** of *N. gonorrhoeae* is made by observing typical colonial morphology, obtaining a positive **oxidase** reaction (see oxidase test, Chapter 72 and *Neisseria,* Chapter 76), and demonstrating the characteristic gram-negative diplococci in a smear made from the oxidase-positive colony.

NOTE: Sugar fermentation or fluorescent antibody reactions should be used to confirm **presumptive identification** of *Neisseria gonorrhoeae* in all cases of isolates obtained from other than anal or genital sites. In addition, suger fermentation or fluorescent antibody reaction should be used for specific identification of organisms isolated on MTM medium from the anogenital sites in situations where gonococcal infection appears unlikely (e.g., in low-prevalence populations), and in special social, medicolegal, and research situations.

Definitive identification (**confirmation**) of presumptive positive colonies is made by sugar "**fermentations**" (CTA base) or **rapid nongrowth carbohydrate degradation** (4 hour "fermentation") test; see Chapter 76, *Neisseria gonorrhoeae.* Glucose is the only sugar fermented by *N. gonorrhoeae* (with the production of acid, but not gas). Presumptive positive colonies may also be definitively identified by the **direct fluorescent antibody staining** procedure. If FA method is used with satisfactory anti–*N. gonorrhoeae* conjugate, sugar tests are not needed (see also FA procedures, Chapter 70, and *Neisseria,* Chapter 76).

The direct FA method is unsuitable for use as a "test of cure," since it stains dead gonococci present in the specimen.

Recently a **coagglutination** procedure has been introduced for the confirmatory identification of gonococci[159] (Phadebact Gonococcus Test, Pharmacia Diagnostics, Piscataway, N.J.). This serologic test, as well as a latex agglutination test, is currently being evaluated as are **counterimmunoelectrophoresis** and the **ELISA** (enzyme-linked immunosorbent antibody) technic.

For further details on identification, see the section on *N. gonorrhoeae,* Chapter 76.

An excellent and detailed source of information is the World Health Organization's 1978 report, *Neisseria gonorrhoeae and gonococcal infections.*[160]

Cultures of other organisms from female genital tract

Media selective for gonococci are usually employed when examining specimens from the female genital tract; however, a number of other organisms may be involved in acute or chronic infections of the genital areas. Specific cultures should be performed depending on **suspected diagnosis** or specific **area** involved.

Amniotic fluid. Use MacConkey or EMB, blood agar, anaerobic blood agar, and/or selective anaerobic media, thioglycollate-enriched or chopped meat broth.

Cervix. Unless request is for "G.C. only" (or "*N. gonorrhoeae* only," or "gonococcus only"), use in addition to gonococcal medium, blood agar, and MacConkey or EMB agar plate. See also *Haemophilus (Corynebacterium) vaginalis* (below).

Vagina. Same as for cervix. *Trichomonas, Candida albicans,* and *H. (Corynebacterium) vaginalis* are commonly involved in vaginitis. Perform **wet mount** for *Trichomonas;* look for actively motile flagellates.

Vaginal cuff. Specimens from vaginal cuff infections should be handled and treated as anaerobic (abscess) specimens.

Uterine materials (lochia, placenta), vulva (Bartholin's abscess). Same as for cervix.

Vulvar abscess, cul de sac. Add anaerobic media.

Listeria monocytogenes

This is an organism involved in chronic infection of the female genital tract and in abortions and is discussed in Chapter 77.

Campylobacter (Vibrio) fetus

This also is possibly involved in abortions. See stool examination, below; also Chapter 79.

Haemophilus (Corynebacterium) vaginalis

The frequent isolation from cervical and vaginal material of a gram-negative pleomorphic bacillus, *H. vaginalis*, has been described since the 1950s.[161-169] The organism produces characteristic small (1-2 mm), discrete, puffball aggregations dispersed throughout the upper 75% of fluid thioglycollate column. It grows under CO_2 on sheep blood agar as minute, colorless, transparent colonies, frequently surrounded by a clear zone of hemolysis. It does **not** grow on Mac-Conkey agar, in peptone, or in infusion broth medium. Starch agar medium supports its growth (several formulae are in use); **V (vaginalis) agar**[170] (Greenwood et al.) has been used for successful isolation from a mixed flora.

V (vaginalis) agar[170]

The medium consists of Columbia agar base (BBL) with 1% proteose peptone no. 3 (Difco) added. To the autoclaved and cooled medium add 5% human blood (preserved with citrate phosphate dextrose solution).

Inoculated plates are incubated at 35 C for 48 hours in a candle jar (ca. 3% CO_2) lined with water-saturated paper towel. After incubation, plates are examined for colonies showing diffuse β-hemolysis. Such colonies are subcultured on a plate of chocolate agar (for purity check, do Gram stain and oxidase and catalase tests) and a V agar plate (inoculum for biochemical tests). For details, see *Haemophilus vaginalis*, Chapter 79.

The exact role of *H. vaginalis* in various genital infections has not been completely clarified, but a significant association has been claimed for its occurrence with leukorrhea or vaginitis[168]; however, some authors[169] consider it to be part of the normal vaginal flora.

The taxonomic status of *H. vaginalis* is unclear. It apparently does not require either factor X or V; some workers have found it to be gram variable, and the suggestion has been made to place it in the genus *Corynebacterium*. (See *Corynebacterium vaginalis*, Chapter 77.)

Gardner and Dukes[161] demonstrated that *H. vaginalis* parasitizes the surfaces of vaginal epithelial cells. In wet mount, such cells present a distinctive granular effect. The term "**clue cell**" has been coined to describe these cells. Dunkelberg[162] found that Gram stains and wet mounts of vaginal smears, when observed specifically for **epithelial** cells with an overlay of large numbers of small gram-negative bacilli and equally dense bacterial masses next to the epithelial cells, were highly efficient in diagnosing the presence of *H. vaginalis*.

For salient features of the organism, factors affecting isolation and identification, and a detailed review, see Greenwood and Pickett,[171] Bailey et al.,[172] and Dunkelberg[167]; see also Chapters 77 (*Corynebacterium*) and 79 (*Haemophilus*).

Haemophilus ducreyi ("soft chancre," chancroid)[173]

Chancroid is a specific ulcerative genitoinfectious disease caused by *Haemophilus ducreyi*, a small gram-negative bacillus. Characteristic inguinal adenopathy often accompanies the genital lesion but systemic spread does not otherwise occur. Chancroid is transmitted by sexual contact, but its incidence is much lower in women than in men (5-10% of reported incidence).

H. ducreyi is a fine, short (1-2 μm) nonspore-forming nonacid-fast, gram-negative bacillus with rounded ends. In smears from primary lesions, it is most commonly observed singly or in small clusters along strands of mucus, whereas in bubo aspirate the organisms form no definite pattern.

H. ducreyi is fastidious but can be cultured on special media incorporating human or rabbit blood or blood products. Hammond et al.[174] recently have successfully isolated *H. ducreyi* on chocolate agar +1% IsoVitaleX (Baltimore Biological Laboratory) enrichment (CA plate), and on the same chocolate agar made selective by addition of vancomycin, 3 μg/ml (CA + V plate).

Smears[175]
1. Cleanse lesion with sterile saline and dry with gauze swabs.
2. Collect serous exudate from undermined border of ulcer on cotton-tipped applicator and carefully roll (in one direction) onto glass slide. This technic is essential to preserve morphologic integrity of organisms.
3. Stain with Gram's stain; Barritt's modification of Pappenheim's Pyronin Methyl Green Stain may be preferable.[176] With Barritt's modifications, pus cells stain bluish green and bacteria, a brilliant red. Smears prepared from bubo aspirate may reveal typical gram-negative coccobacilli as the sole flora.

Culture. The organism is fastidious, and culture may not be warranted as a routine diagnostic measure in some clinical settings but should be employed in environments where chancroid is seen commonly. Method 1 (below) is the simplest and most efficacious culture method.

METHOD 1 (Hammond et al.[174])
1. Cleanse ulcer base with gauze pad moistened in normal saline.
2. Sample ulcer base with cotton swab moistered in saline. Streak surface of CA (chocolate agar, see media, Chapter 72) and/or chocolate agar with vancomycin (3 μg/ml).
3. Incubate at 33 C in 5-10% CO_2 in presence of saturated water vapor atmosphere in CO_2 incubator. Growth on CA and CA + V media is slow, colonies being observed 2-9 d after inoculation (a median of 4 d is required to achieve sufficient growth for recognition).

METHOD 2[175]
1. Inoculate material into serum surrounding fresh clot (3 ml of patient's or other human blood is used). Inactivation of serum at 56 C for 30 min is essential for growth of laboratory strains, but may be omitted for clinical isolates.

2. Clean ulcers. Collect serous exudate from ulcer margin with platinum loop.

3. After 72 h incubation at 35 C, examine by stained smear and subculture onto Bacto-nutrient agar 1.5%, containing 5% human blood. After incubation in candle jar at 35 C for 48 h, *H. ducreyi* appear as slightly gray colonies 2-5 mm in diameter with rough surface texture.

Calymmatobacterium; Donovanosis (granuloma inguinale)[173]

Donovanosis is a specific chronic granulomatous disease that usually affects the genitalia. The name granuloma inguinale, though widely used, is inappropriate for this condition. "Granuloma" is a nonspecific term, and its use may cause confusion with lymphogranuloma venereum (LGV), although this confusion is more marked when the term "granuloma venereum" is used. "Inguinal" is inappropriate, since the inguinal region is involved in only a minority of cases and is usually secondary to genital infection.

The role of sexual contact is controversial; the disease is more commonly reported in men (male:female ratio, 2.3:1).

Although rare in most western countries, only 51 cases being reported in the United States in fiscal year 1974 (July 1, 1973 to June 30, 1974), donovanosis is very common in New Guinea, India, the Caribbean, and many other tropical or subtropical environments. In West New Guinea, up to 25% of some populations were infected in the 1920s, and 23.5% of male patients attending one urban VD clinic in 1972 had donovanosis. In India, 5.3% of patients attending a venereal disease clinic had this disease.

The infectious agent is *Calymmatobacterium (Donovania) granulomatis*, a gram-negative bacterium measuring 1.5 μm by 0.7 μm. In tissue smears the bacteria appear enclosed in vacuolar compartments in large histiocytic cells or occasionally in polymorphonuclear leukocytes or plasma cells.[177] The bacteria reproduce in multiple foci within these cells until the vacuole contains 20-30 organisms, which mature and are then liberated when the infected cell ruptures.

Sites. The genitalia are involved in 90% of cases, the inguinal region in 10%, the anal region in 5-10%, and distant sites in 1-5%. Lesions are limited to the genitalia in approximately 80% of cases and to the inguinal region in less than 5%. Unilateral lesions are more common than bilateral ones. In the man, lesions most commonly occur on the prepuce or glans and in the woman, lesions on the labia are the most common. The most common distant sites infected are on the head (mouth, lips, throat, face), but involvement of the liver, thorax, and bones has also been reported.

Diagnosis. The clinical presentation is highly suggestive of the diagnosis in most cases. However, the diagnosis is readily confirmed by a **stained crush preparation** from the lesion. The sensitivity of this test is closely related to the manner in which it is performed.

1. Spread piece of clean granulation tissue from lesion against slide to be examined.
2. Air dry and stain with Wright's or Giemsa's stain.

Donovan bodies (Figs. 75-5 to 75-7) appear as clusters of blue- or black-staining organisms with a "safety pin" appearance (from bipolar chromatin condensation) in the cytoplasm of large mononuclear cells. Histologic examination of biopsied tissue is a less reliable diagnostic procedure, since the pathognomonic Donovan bodies are infrequently seen.

Culture on chick chorioallantoic membrane is not feasible as a routine diagnostic measure. Granuloma inguinale has been treated successfully with tetracyclines, streptomycin, and chloramphenicol; penicillin is not effective.

Lymphogranuloma venereum (LGV)[173, 178, 179]

Lymphogranuloma venereum (LGV) is a systemic sexually transmitted disease that may be produced by a number of closely related **Chlamydia.** Primary inoculation may occur at any anatomic site involved in intimate contact. Regional lymphadenitis develops in the nodes draining this site and the disease disseminates further via the lymphatic system. Progression of the disease may produce chronic buboes, elephantiasis, fistulae, and strictures.

The causative organism has been grown on chick embryo yolk sac, but this method is unsatisfactory for routine diagnosis.

The Frei skin test has been the most widely used test. It becomes positive 12-40 days after appearance of the primary lesion and usually re-

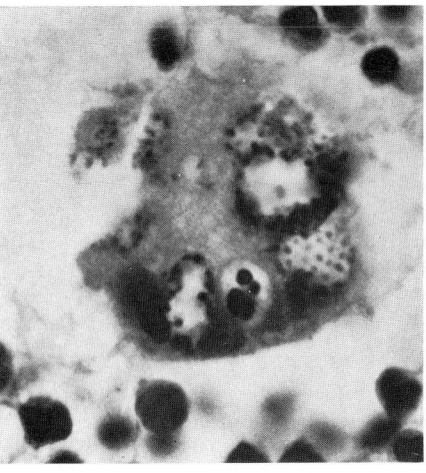

Fig. 75-5. Black male. Biopsy section of granulating lesions of glans penis. Diagnosis is granuloma inguinale. Pathognomonic cell containing encysted Donovan bodies. (Stained with hematoxylin and eosin; ×2280.) (From Pund, E. R., and Greenblatt, R. B.: Arch. Path. **23**:244, 1937.)

mains so for life. However, it is less than 70% sensitive—frequently negative even in advanced stages of infection. Furthermore, it is nonspecific and frequently reacts in individuals who have been infected with any chlamydial organisms.

The LGV complement-fixation test (LGV-

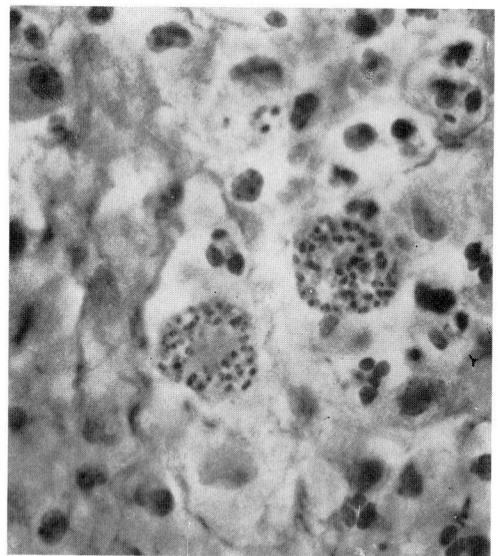

Fig. 75-6. Pathognomonic cell of granuloma inguinale containing encysted Donovan bodies. (Stained by Dieterle silver method.) (Courtesy E. R. Pund and R. B. Greenblatt.)

CFT) is 90-95% sensitive and becomes positive earlier than the Frei Test (usually within 1-3 weeks). It is nonspecific, but can be titrated, which enhances its value. However, neither the Frei test nor the LGV-CFT is of great value alone and certainly of no value as a screening test.

The immunofluorescence[180] and neutralization test[181] are specific for LGV but are not widely available and have had limited evaluation.

In the presence of the clinical syndrome, a 4-fold rise in titer of the complement-fixation test is diagnostic. However, this test has usually risen to a stable titer by the time most patients present for diagnosis, and may not decline significantly for several months.

Syphilis (*Treponema pallidum*)

1. The organism is **not** cultivable.
2. For demonstration of organism, see Chapters 80 (dark-field) and 106 (FA method).
3. For serologic methods, see Chapter 106.

Mycoplasma

Mycoplasmas are often found in cases of nonspecific urethritis and cervicitis and are discussed in Chapter 81.

Nongonococcal urethritis (NGU)

Nonspecific urethritis is widespread; it accounts for 45-60% of cases among men and probably 60-70% among women. The term NGU includes all cases of urethritis **not** due to *N. gonorrhoeae*. Agents associated with NGU are

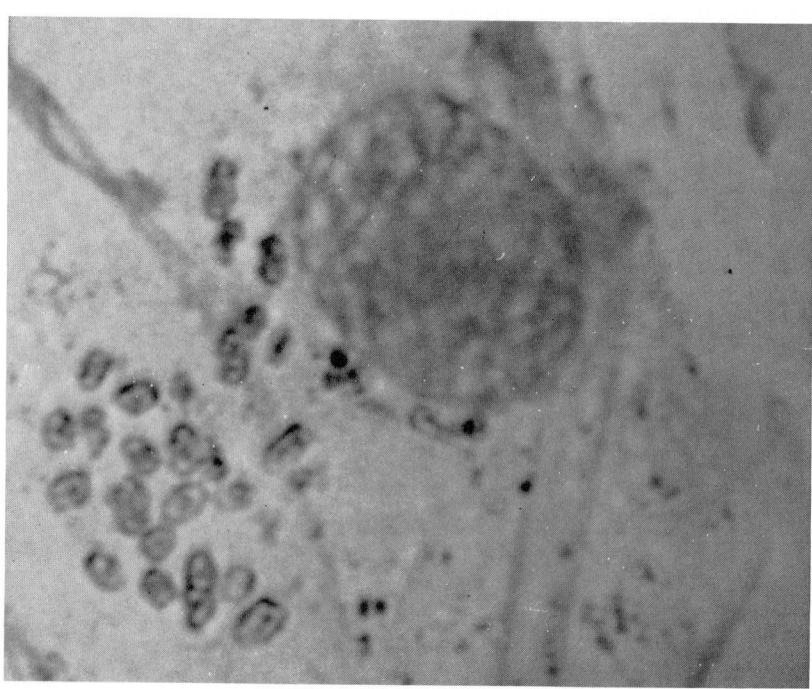

Fig. 75-7. Donovan bodies from spreads of lesion (greatly magnified). (From Gradwohl, R. B. H., Benitez Soto, L., and Felsenfeld, O.: Clinical tropical medicine, St. Louis, The C. V. Mosby Co.)

Chlamydia trachomatis, Mycoplasma hominis, T-mycoplasma, *Herpes hominis,* cytomegalovirus, *Candida albicans,* and *Trichomonas vaginalis.* Of these, *C. trachomatis* is involved in a large proportion of NGU cases. Diagnosis of *C. trachomatis* infection is made by **tissue culture** in McCoy cells[182] and gram-stained smear of exudate (neutrophils, absence of gram-negative diplococci).

For further details on NGU, see references 182-189.

II. Male genital tract—urethra, testes, epididymis, prostatic fluid
Isolation of Neisseria gonorrhoeae— recommended procedures in men[148a]

1. **Microscopic demonstration** of typical gram-negative, intracellular diplococci on smear of a **urethral exudate** constitutes sufficient basis for a diagnosis of gonorrhea. Prepare smear by **rolling** swab on slide. **Do not** rub swab on slide because microscopic morphology will be distorted (see direct smear, below).

2. When gram-negative diplococci cannot be identified on direct smear of urethral exudate, or when urethral exudate is absent, a **culture specimen** should be obtained from anterior urethra and inoculated on MTM medium. The combination of positive oxidase reaction of typical colonies containing typical gram-negative diplococci grown on this medium provides sufficient criteria for presumptive identification of *Neisseria gonorrhoeae.*

3. In homosexual men, additional culture specimens should be obtained anal canal and oropharynx and should be inoculated on MTM medium.

4. Tests of cure are recommended for all men treated for gonorrhea and all sites that were infected before therapy should be retested. This is accomplished by inoculating a culture specimen from these sites on MTM medium; cultures should be obtained and interpreted as in item 2 above.

5. Pharyngeal gonococcal infection (see oropharyngeal specimens of female genital tract, above).

6. Fluorescent antibody staining of smears of urethral exudates is **not** recommended in men.

7. A negative Gram stain of urethral exudates should **not** be accepted as evidence of cure.

Direct smear (urethral exudate). In acute gonorrhea, groups of intracellular gram-negative, kidney-shaped diplococci with flattened, opposed margins are seen within polymorphonuclear leukocytes, with few if any other types of organisms present. Such findings correlate highly with a confirmed diagnosis of acute gonorrhea **in the male.**

The Gram stain report should indicate the presence and amount of pus cells (polymorphonuclear leukocytes) and the morphology, staining, and numbers of bacteria seen.

Collection of specimens
Urethra. A culture is indicated when Gram stain of urethral exudate is not positive, in tests of cure, or as a test for asymptomatic urethral infection.

Use sterile bacteriologic wire loop to obtain specimen from anterior urethra by gently scraping mucosa. An alternative to loop is sterile calcium alginate urethral swab that is easily inserted into urethra.

Anal canal. This culture can be taken in the same manner as for women (see "Female genital tract").

Oropharynx. This culture can be taken in the same manner as for women (see "Female genital tract").

Special situations. Culture of **blood** or **synovial fluid** on enriched broth medium (such as trypticase soy broth supplemented with 1% IsoVitaleX, 10% horse serum, and 1% glucose) is a recommended procedure in special situations such as suspected gonococcal arthritis or septicemia. Specimens from **conjunctiva** should be inoculated on MTM medium and chocolate agar supplemented with 1% IsoVitaleX. Identification of *Neisseria gonorrhoeae* should include sugar fermentation or fluorescent antibody technics.

Gram staining and **specific fluorescent antibody staining** of smears from **conjunctivae, joint fluids,** or **skin lesions** can be used as an adjunct in the diagnosis of gonococcal infections of these sites, particularly when partial therapy may prevent cultural recovery of organisms.

Sugar fermentation of fluorescent antibody reactions should be used to confirm presumptive identification of *Neisseria gonorrhoeae* **in all cases of isolates obtained from other than anal or genital sites.** In addition, sugar fermentation or fluorescent antibody reaction should be used for specific identification of organisms isolated on MTM medium from the anogenital sites in situations where gonococcal infection appears unlikely (e.g., in low-prevalence populations), and in special social, medicolegal, and research situations.

Inoculation, incubation, choice of media, examination of plates, and identification. See "Isolation of *N. gonorrhoeae* from female genital tract," above.

Other organisms

In addition to media for gonococci, add blood agar plate, MacConkey or EMB agar, thioglycollate, or prereduced heart infusion broth or chopped meat broth.

Prostatic fluid. Physician obtains secretion for smear and culture by digital massage through rectum. Use sterile tube anaerobic transport medium.

Epididymis and testes. Procedure is same as for prostatic fluid.

• • •

Chancroid, donovanosis, LGU, mycoplasma, syphilis, H. vaginalis, nongonococcal urethritis (NGU): See "Cultures of other organisms from female genital tract," above.

Gastric contents and vomit

(a) Examination of gastric lavage for mycobacteria. See Chapter 78.
(b) Occasionally vomit is examined for the presence of food-poisoning organisms. *S. aureus, Salmonella,* and *Shigella* are most often implicated. The specimen should be streaked on blood agar (incubate anaerobically if possible), selective media for *Salmonella* and *Shigella,* and a tube of thioglycollate broth. If *S. aureus* is isolated, it is necessary to determine whether it is an enterotoxin-producing strain. Facilities for toxicity tests and bacteriophage typing are available at public health laboratories. The vomit may be examined for *Clostridium botulinum* toxin by filtering it and injecting it into mice; controls should be protected by clostridial antitoxins (see Chapter 84). *Salmonella* is more readily isolated from stool than from vomit.

Bile

1. Collect several milliters in sterile container (aspirate with syringe during surgery, through nasogastric tube from duodenum, or from postoperative drainage site).
2. Plate out bile on aerobic and anaerobic blood agar, and eosin–methylene blue to MacConkey agar plate and inoculate tube of thioglycollate broth.
3. Incubate 24-48 h or until growth is obtained.
4. Proceed in usual manner for differentiation of bacteria present (especially search for *Salmonella* and/or *Clostridium*).

Stool examination
Acute diarrhea[189a]

Diarrheal illness is one of the most common disorders of man. Diarrheas can be grouped as follows:

1. Drug-induced diarrhea. Antimicrobial agents (clindamycin, lincomycin, probably others), antimetabolites, and thyroid replacement may cause diarrhea. It may vary from mild to severe colitis with pseudomembrane formation. The drug should be discontinued; if diarrhea persists 1 week after discontinuation, continue workup.

2. Common source diarrhea ("food poisoning"). Common source diarrhea involves a history of other persons with similar illness following a common exposure.

When such food-borne disease is suspected and none of those involved has a fever, a toxin-mediated illness should be suspected. With very short incubation (2-4 hours), **staphylococcal food poisoning** is probable.

When onset is later than 12-16 hours after ingestion, suspect *Clostridium perfringens* or other toxigenic bacteria.

If patient(s) has fever, likely causative agents

are *Salmonella* or *Shigella;* perform stool cultures (and food cultures).

Special procedures (media) are to be used for stool culture of *Vibrio parahaemolyticus* (to be suspected during summer months when the patient has eaten improperly cooked seafood), *Vibrio cholerae, Yersinia enterocolitica,* and *Campylobacter fetus* (methods are described below).

It is highly important that the laboratory be apprised of patient's history and any suspicion the physician may entertain concerning patient's exposure.

Fecal leukocytes in diarrhea: microscopic examination of stool[190-195]

Numerous workers[190-192] have emphasized that, in addition to history, the presence or absence of fecal polymorphonuclear or mononuclear leukocytes is a highly important point in the evaluation of patients with diarrhea.

The test can be easily performed in the physician's office, emergency room, or laboratory.[190]

1. Place small fleck of mucus (or if mucus is not present, drop of liquid stool) on glass microscope slide with wooden applicator stick and mix thoroughly and carefully with approximately equal volume of Loeffler methylene blue (found in laboratories where reticulocyte staining is done).
2. Place coverslip on mixture, and after 2 or 3 min, identify leukocytes under "high dry" objective of light microscope in patients with colitis.[190]

Fecal leukocytes are produced by bacteria that invade the colonic mucosa, i.e., infection caused by *Salmonella, Shigella, Yersinia,* and invasive *E. coli.* Other disorders (involving mucosal inflammation) positive for fecal leukocytes are ulcerative colitis and antibiotic-associated colitis. Fecal leukocytes are usually **not** present in the stools of those with diarrhea secondary to toxigenic bacteria, parasites, and viruses.

Patients with positive fecal leukocytes should have stool cultures for *Shigella* and *Salmonella,* and blood cultures should be obtained in those with high fever.

The usual bacterial causes of fecal leukocytes are invasive *E. coli, Shigella,* and *Salmonella;* however, only the latter 2 are identified by the routine diagnostic laboratory.

In the **absence of fecal leukocytes,** agents involved may be toxin producers (*Staphylococcus,* toxigenic *E. coli, Vibrio cholerae*), or those capable of inducing lesions in small bowel mucosa (viruses, *Giardia lamblia*); these may cause watery diarrhea without leukocytes in stools. If *Vibrio, Campylobacter,* or *Yersinia* infection is suspected, order stool culture specifically for the organism(s) suspected, **in addition** to routine stool culture.

For parasite examinations of stools, see Chapter 100.

Collection of material

Stool examinations are not complete if they do not include both bacteriologic and parasitologic studies.

Only fresh or properly preserved material may be used. Many pathogenic organisms such as entamebae, shigellae, etc. can be recovered from specimens only if the specimens have been cultured or fixed within a few minutes after the stool has been passed. If specimens must be shipped or held for some time before plating, it is imperative that they be placed in a **preservative solution** or **transport medium.**

Both stool and fecal material collected from the intestines may be examined.

Fresh stool specimens. In hospitals the nurses usually collect fresh stool specimens and deliver them immediately to the laboratory. In clinics the technician is often responsible for the collection of the stools. The patient is asked to come to the laboratory in the morning and instructed to collect the stool on a cardboard tray fitted into the toilet.

Stokes[196] recommends that **bedpans for collecting specimens for culture should be sterile** to prevent accidental contamination by bacteria from another sample of feces. Some laboratories supply the patients with half-pint ice cream cardboard cartons or wide-necked bottles and ask them to obtain the specimens directly in these. Fecal material must never be permitted to dry before plating.

It should be remembered that certain enteric organisms (*Shigella*) decrease in number rather rapidly after the specimen is voided. It is desirable to plate specimens as soon as obtained. **Freshly passed stools** are the ideal material for the examination of enteric infections. In diarrheal diseases it is imperative to obtain specimens in the acute stage of the disease.

Rectal swabs. In chronic bacillary dysentery, immediate plating of swabs taken directly from lesions during proctoscopy is the most satisfactory method of isolating *Shigella*. Often, as in the case of outbreaks of enteric disease, stool specimens may not be readily obtainable; **rectal swabs** are the most practical method of obtaining material for culture under such circumstances. Insert swab beyond rectal sphincter and rotate. Swab should either be immediately plated or placed in preservative solutions.

Preservative solutions. Edwards and Ewing[196a] recommend the use of buffered glycerol-saline solution or the solution of Banxgang and Eliot (buffered saline–sodium citrate–sodium deoxycholate). Phenol red is added to these solutions to impart a distinct color; if, on arrival in the laboratory, the suspension of stool has a distinct yellow color, it should be discarded, since it indicates acid conditions unfavorable to dysentery bacilli. Approximately 1 g feces should be added to 10 ml preservative and thoroughly emulsified.

Transport media. The Amies or Cary-Blair transport medium is recommended.

Stool specimens for viral examinations. Stool specimens and rectal swabs for virus isolation must be frozen immediately after obtained and kept frozen at all times prior to their inoculation (at -20 C or preferably at -70 C). No preservative should be added.

Methods for parasitologic examinations. See Chapter 100.

Media for stool culture

The intestinal tract of humans harbors a large number and variety of microorganisms. Many of these are anaerobic (*Bacteroides*, anaerobic streptococci, clostridia); these are not encountered in cultures since stool cultures are always incubated aerobically. The reason for this is that the pathogens searched for in enteric infections are all capable of aerobic growth. Of the aerobic organisms, *E. coli* is numerically the most prominent. Other gram-negative enteric organisms found in the normal intestine are members of the Klebsiella-Enterobacter (*Aerobacter*) group, *Citrobacter* (formerly *Escherichia*) *freundii*, *Proteus* sp., *P. aeruginosa*, and *Alcaligenes faecalis*; occasionally, *Serratia* and *Aeromonas*. In addition, various streptococci (mostly enterococci), staphylococci, and yeasts (mainly *Candida*) are present.

• • •

Established etiologic agents that are the subject of search in most enteric infections are various members of the genera *Salmonella*, *Arizona*, *Shigella*, and *Vibrio*, as well as the parasites *Entamoeba*[199] and *Giardia*.[200]

Newer agents of gastrointestinal infections are:

Yersinia enterocolitica[201]

Vibrio parahaemolyticus[202]

Enterotoxigenic and enteropathogenic *E. coli*

Campylobacter fetus[206]

Clostridium difficile (pseudomembranous colitis)[207]

Viruses (enteroviruses, reovirus, rotavirus, Norwalk agent, calcivirus, etc.)[208-210]

Rarely a fulminating diarrhea, caused by large numbers of coagulase-positive staphylococci, has been demonstrated (staphylococcal enteritis or pseudomembranous enterocolitis).

Isolation and preliminary identification of *Salmonella* and *Shigella*

A great variety of media has been devised for the isolation of salmonellae and shigellae from stool specimens. Eosin–methylene blue (EMB) agar, Endo agar, and other early preparations inhibit gram-positive organisms and contain indicators that distinguish bacteria that ferment **lactose** rapidly from those that do not attack this sugar. The colonies that attack lactose form colored colonies, whereas those that do not form colorless colonies. Bile salts are added to MacConkey agar and deoxycholate (DA) agar. These are **differential** media. (*Salmonella* and *Shigella*

Table 75-3. Enteric differential and selective media*

Medium	Gram-positive bacteriostatic agent	Fermentable carbohydrate	Indicator	Colony color		Inoculation	Incubation
				Fermenter	Nonfermenter		
Enteric differential media							
EMB agar	Eosin Y Methylene blue	Lactose† Sucrose	Eosin Y Methylene blue	Red Black with sheen	Colorless	Loopful or less	18-24 h 35 C
MacConkey agar	Crystal violet Bile salts	Lactose	Neutral red	Red	Colorless	Loopful or less	18-24 h 35 C
Desoxycholate agar	Bile salts	Lactose	Neutral red	Red	Colorless	Loopful or less	18-24 h 35 C
XLD agar	Bile salts	Xylose Lactose Sucrose	Phenol red and H_2S indicator	Yellow	Pink to red	Loopful	18-24 h 35 C
Enteric selective media							
Desoxycholate-citrate agar	Bile salts	Lactose	Neutral red	Red	Colorless	Large loopful or swab	18-24 h 35 C
Hektoen enteric agar (HE)	Bile salts	Salicin Lactose Sucrose	Bromthymol blue and H_2S indicator	Yellow orange	Green or blue-green	Loopful	18-24 h 35 C
Bismuth sulfite agar (BS)	Brilliant green	Glucose	Bismuth sulfite	N/A‡	N/A‡	Heavily with swab	24-48 h 35 C

*From Rhoden, D. L., and Hermann, G. J.: Isolation and identification of *Enterobacteriaceae* in the clinical laboratory, Center for Disease Control, Atlanta, 1974.
†Levine EMB agar contains lactose only.
‡Not applicable. H_2S-producing salmonellae produce black colonies, and other noninhibiting organisms produce brown or greenish colonies.

organisms do not ferment lactose; however, lactose-fermenting *Salmonella* **do** occur. See Chapter 79 for a discussion of biochemically atypical *Salmonella* under *Enterobacteriaceae*—preliminary examination of cultures.) See Table 75-3.

NOTE: Reliance on MacConkey agar and deoxycholate citrate agar alone for *Salmonella* isolation will result in missing lactose-fermenting *Salmonella;* bismuth sulfite agar is useful for such strains.

Among the **differentially selective** media are the deoxycholate citrate agar (DCA) of Leifson, *Salmonella-Shigella* agar (SS), xylose lysine deoxycholate agar (XLD), Hektoen enteric agar (HE), bismuth sulfite medium of Wilson and Blair, and Kauffmann brilliant green agar. These media inhibit the majority of coliform organisms (*Escherichia, Klebsiella,* and *Enterobacter*) and *Proteus* species, permitting the growth of most strains of *Salmonella* and *Shigella.* Those *Proteus* strains that grow are prevented from swarming. This is accomplished by the use of various inhibitory substances: brilliant green and selenium salts inhibit the growth of coliforms, sodium citrate favors the growth of salmonellae over coliforms, etc. Among the differential characteristics of these media in addition to lactose (or xylose, sucrose, salicin) fermentation, is the use of sulfite, which is reduced to sulfide by many salmonellae and gives a black color to the colony in the presence of iron salts (bismuth sulfite agar and others).

Enrichment media contain various chemicals that temporarily inhibit the growth of coliforms but permit *Salmonella* or *Shigella* organisms to multiply. The most widely used enrichment media are **selenite broth, tetrathionate broth,** and **GN broth.** The enrichment media are subcultured after 6-18 hours on one or more differential or selective media. All the media discussed are available commercially in dehydrated form.

Stool culture

Culture for Salmonella and Shigella
1. Inoculate 1 plate of differential (less selective) medium. MacConkey agar and eosin–methylene blue agar plate are satisfactory. This plate will allow an estimate of total gram-negative flora; it also allows examination for (enteropathogenic) *E. coli* strains. These media should be inoculated lightly.
2. Inoculate 1 plate of selective-differential medium. XLD, SS, or HE agar is preferred; deoxycholate citrate agar is also satisfactory. Inoculate this plate by adding small portion of feces or drop of heavy suspension of feces from enrichment medium. Streak with loop over surface of plate.
3. Inoculate bismuth sulfite agar plate heavily by streaking; this is best available medium for detection of *S. typhi.* For *Salmonella* **other than typhi, brilliant green agar** is an excellent medium. If culture is made from suspected healthy carrier of *S. typhi,* it is advisable to also prepare poured bismuth sulfite plate. Use 5 ml heavy broth suspension of stool to which are added about 20 ml melted and cooled bismuth sulfite agar.

4. Inoculate tube of GN, selenite, or tetrathionate enrichment medium with about 1 g feces (or leave swab overnight in enrichment medium tube). After 6-18 h, **but not later,** transfer loopful to EMB or MacConkey plate **and** XLD or SS plate and bismuth sufite plate or to XLD or SS and brilliant green plate.

No single medium can be used for all purposes; the number of media used will depend on the facilities of the laboratory. However, there is a certain minimum standard that must be used to obtain any meaningful results. Always use the following:

1. MacConkey or EMB agar, **and**
2. XLD, HE,* or SS, **and**
3. Bismuth sulfite agar, **and**
4. GN **or** selenite enrichment broth

Brilliant green agar should be added to above for isolation of largest possible number of *Salmonella* (other than *S. typhi*).

Additional platings

For enteropathogenic or enterotoxigenic E. coli: In addition to above plates, inoculate a blood agar or plain infusion agar plate; always use MacConkey or EMB; often pure cultures are obtained.

For staphylococci: Inoculate a highly selective medium like mannitol salt agar or Staphylococcus medium 110; some workers prefer 5% sheep blood agar or PEA (phenyl-ethyl alcohol) blood agar plate for comparative purposes, i.e., establishing predominant organism(s).

For Vibrio cholerae, V. parahaemolyticus, Yersinia enterocolitica, Campylobacter (Vibrio) fetus: See below.

Special methods of stool examination

Special methods may be used for the control of **carriers** or for **special surveys.** These methods are applicable in closed communities such as military establishments, mental hospitals, etc., and during outbreaks of diseases caused by certain organisms. After the organism has been identified, the special methods serve as specialized examinations of contacts and carriers.

Typhoid bacilli. Examine postcathartic stools in cases without diarrhea. Use stools of patients with diarrhea.
1. Inoculate 1 tube selenite-F and 1 tube tetrathionate broth with stool. Incubate 24 h at 37 C.
2. Have ready bismuth sulfite agar melted and cooled to 45 C. Make emulsion of stool in saline. Place 1 drop emulsion in 1 sterile Petri dish and 0.5 ml emulsion in second. Pour agar into both Petri dishes and mix well. Allow to harden and incubate 48 h.
3. Streak from selenite-F 1 SS plate or 1 DCA plate; from tetrathionate fluid streak bismuth sulfite plate after enrichment fluids have been incubated. Incubate plates.
4. Let enrichment fluids stand at room temperature 24 h more and then repeat streaking *(3)* and incubating.

---

*King and Metzger[211] reported that Hektoen enteric agar (HE) was superior to SS agar in terms of recovery of *Salmonella* and *Shigella.*

Salmonella

1. Inoculate 1 tube selenite-F and 1 tube tetrathionate broth and incubate. Streak 2 MacConkey plates or deoxycholate agar plates and 2 brilliant green agar plates. Incubate.
2. On second and third days plate from selenite-F tube and tetrathionate broth to 1 plate deoxycholate agar and 1 plate brilliant green agar.
3. Incubate.

Shigella

1. Collect specimens by means of swab and also collect postcathartic stools.
2. Using swab, streak SS agar or DA plate. Streak sectors on surface of medium. Incubate.
3. Using stools, streak 2 plates each of (a) either MacConkey agar **or** deoxycholate agar medium, (b) eosin–methylene blue, and (c) XLD agar or DCA plate **or** SS agar. Incubate.
4. If organisms do not grow on SS agar, DCA, or XLD agar, use other 2 plates in triplicate.

Appearance of organisms on various media

For orientation, the appearance of various enteric organisms on the media used for platings is here described. The descriptions are based on commercially available media. (For *Vibrio*, *Yersinia*, and *Campylobacter*, see below.)

MacConkey agar. Isolated colonies of coliform bacteria are brick red and may be surrounded by a zone of precipitated bile. This reaction is due to the action of the acids, produced by fermentation of lactose, on the bile salts and the subsequent absorption of neutral red. Typhoid, paratyphoid, and dysentery bacilli do not ferment lactose and do not greatly alter the appearance of the medium. These colonies, in reality giving an alkaline reaction, are uncolored and transparent. When growing in proximity to coliform bacteria, they have the appearance of clearing the areas of precipitated bile. On plates that are not overcrowded the differentiation is exceptionally distinct. A plate crowded with coli will appear red and opaque, yet if not too crowded, typhoid or other lactose nonfermenting organisms may easily be detected by transmitted light. On such plates they will appear as small transparent areas against the red background. A plate showing discrete colonies is to be desired for isolation purposes.

Eosin–methylene blue agar (EMB). *E. coli* colonies usually show a dark center and have a greenish metallic sheen. Occasionally variants are observed that have no metallic sheen; some coliforms may form mucoid colonies. Colonies of *Enterobacter (Aerobacter)* are usually larger, mucoid, brownish in center, and not as dark as *E. coli*. Metallic sheen is observed only occasionally. *Salmonella* and *Shigella* species form translucent, colorless colonies.

Deoxycholate agar (DA). Coliform organisms are red; *Enterobacter (Aerobacter)* colonies are pale with pink centers; *Salmonella* and *Shigella* are colorless; *Proteus* colonies are large and colorless.

Deoxycholate citrate agar (DCA). On deoxycholate citrate agar the growth of coliform bacteria is inhibited or greatly suppressed. **Salmonella** and **Shigella** organisms grow quite unrestricted. Occasionally, however, coliform strains are encountered that persist on deoxycholate citrate agar. Such strains, if present in large numbers, produce acid from the lactose, precipitate the bile salt, and give an opaque red medium that makes it difficult to detect the pathogens. Organisms that grow on deoxycholate citrate agar but

do not ferment lactose produce colorless, raised colonies. *S. typhi* produces translucent colonies with a bluish cast. Other *Salmonella* colonies are large and opaque and may possess a brownish center. *Shigella* produces opaque, ground-glass appearing colonies with even margins. Coliform organisms that persist on deoxycholate citrate agar form raised, even, red colonies that are often surrounded by a red halo of precipitated bile salt.

Most **Proteus** strains are inhibited.

Salmonella-Shigella agar (SS). *Shigella*, *Salmonella*, and other organisms not fermenting lactose form opaque, transparent, or translucent uncolored colonies, which generally are smooth. The few lactose-fermenting organisms that may develop on the medium are readily differentiated by the formation of a red color in the colony. At times, isolated coliform colonies may not show a definite red color, being pink or nearly colorless with a pink center. Occasionally an aerogenes type will develop a characteristic large, white or cream-colored, opaque, and mucoid colony. Some *Proteus* and *Salmonella* types may, under certain conditions, produce black-centered colonies.

Lactose-fermenting *Salmonella* (rare), *Arizona* (about half of strains), and *Citrobacter* grow as black-centered red colonies on SS agar.

Bismuth sulfite (Wilson-Blair) agar

Streak or smear plate. The typical discrete surface typhoid colony is black and is surrounded by a black or brownish black zone, which may be several times the size of the colony. By reflected light, preferably daylight, this zone exhibits a distinctly characteristic metallic sheen (Fig. 75-8). Plates heavily seeded with typhoid may not show this reaction except possibly near the margin of the mass inoculation. In these congested areas, typhoid frequently appears as small light green colonies.

Pour plate. Well-isolated subsurface typhoid colonies are circular, jet black, and well defined. The size of the black colony may vary from 1-4 mm in diameter, depending on the particular strain, length of incubation, and position of the colony in the agar. Only those colonies growing very close to the surface or on the surface will show a decided black, metallic sheen. Plates containing typhoid too numerous to permit the development of individual colonies give a black plate or a plate dotted with black areas. Plates with about 300-1000 typhoid colonies will exhibit this appearance. When typhoid colonies develop in a plate in still larger numbers, typical blackening does not occur, and the appearance is that of a negative plate.

Ordinarily typhoid will develop well-isolated colonies showing typical round, jet black colonies, with or without sheen, from either the 5 ml or 1 drop inoculation of cotton-filtered fecal suspension, using the pour plate method. However, the typhoid organisms developing from the specimens containing large numbers of typhoid may be so numerous that the blackening cannot occur typically, and the plate may appear dotted black or greenish gray.

Colonies other than S. typhi. *S. schottmuelleri* B and *S. enteritidis* grow luxuriantly upon Bacto-Bismuth Sulfite Agar, forming black surface and subsurface colonies slightly more moist but otherwise similar to those produced by *S. typhi*.

S. paratyphi A, *S. typhimurium*, *S. cholerae-suis*, and *Proteus morganii* develop on Bacto-Bismuth Sulfite Agar, yielding flat or only slightly raised green colonies.

Generally the members of the dysentery group other than Flexner and Sonne are inhibited. The Flexner and Sonne strains that do develop on this medium produce

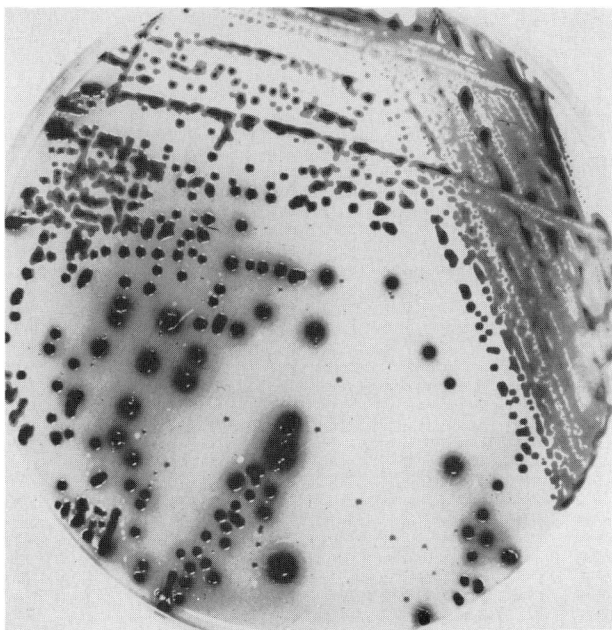

Fig. 75-8. Bismuth sulfite plate with salmonellae.

brownish raised colonies with depressed centers and exhibit a craterlike appearance.

E. coli is usually completely inhibited. Occasionally a strain will be encountered that will develop small black, brown, or greenish glistening surface colonies. This color is confined entirely to the colony itself and shows no metallic sheen. Likewise a few strains of *E. aerogenes* may develop on this medium, forming raised, mucoid colonies. These may exhibit a silvery sheen, appreciably lighter in color than that produced by typhoid.

Brilliant green agar (Kauffmann). Inoculation with heavy suspensions of stools or other materials suspected of containing *Salmonella* usually results in an almost pure culture of these organisms. Growth of other bacteria is almost completely inhibited. Following incubation at 37 C for 18-24 h the plates are examined for typical *Salmonella* colonies. These appear as slightly pink-white opaque colonies surrounded by a brilliant red medium. The few lactose- or sucrose-fermenting organisms that may develop on the medium are readily differentiated by the formation of a yellow-green colony surrounded by an intense yellow-green zone. Bacto-Brilliant Green Agar is highly recommended for the isolation of *Salmonella*. However, **it is not suitable for the isolation of** *S. typhi* or *Shigella* **organisms.** Some strains of *S. typhi* will develop on this medium, forming colonies identical to other *Salmonella*. Some strains of *Proteus* may also grow, forming red colonies.

Xylose lysine deoxycholate agar (XLD).[212] The rationale of the medium is described by Taylor. Xylose is fermented rapidly by all enterics **except** shigellae, *Providencia*, and *Edwardsiella*. Thus a xylose medium would allow the recognition of xylose late fermenters or nonfermenters. However, *Salmonella* and *Arizona*, which ferment xylose rapidly, would resemble the coliforms. To allow for their differentiation, the lysine decarboxylation reaction is utilized. Since both salmonellae and *Arizona* sp. decarboxylate lysine, lysine was added to the medium, allowing the organism to exhaust the xylose, attack the lysine, and revert to an alkaline

pH that mimics the *Shigella* reaction. Lactose and sucrose are added so that lysine-positive coliforms will produce acid in excess. An H_2S indicator is also incorporated for rapid presumptive identification of salmonellae, *Arizona*, and *Edwardsiella* (Asakusa and Bartholomew, "biotype 1483-59"). *Escherichia, Enterobacter (Aerobacter), Klebsiella, Citrobacter, Proteus*, and *Serratia* species produce **opaque, yellow** colonies. *Shigella, Providencia,* H_2S-negative *Salmonella (paratyphi* A, *cholerae-suis,* etc.) grow as **red** colonies. *Salmonella, Arizona*, and *Edwardsiella* sp. produce **black-centered red** colonies. Some *Pseudomonas* and *Proteus rettgeri* may produce red colonies. **Do not read later than 24 h;** incubation for more than 24 h may result in misleading colony appearance.

Hektoen enteric agar.[211] Rapid lactose-fermenters (coliforms) are moderately inhibited. When present, colonies are bright colored, orange to salmon-pink. *Shigella* is more green than *Salmonella* and shows larger colonies than on SS agar. The periphery of colonies is often lighter than central portion. *Salmonella* forms blue to blue-green colonies, varying in size. Most colonies have black centers (H_2S producers). Most strains of *Proteus* are inhibited. *P. mirabilis* may produce dark-centered, greenish colonies somewhat similar to *Salmonella*, but smaller. *Proteus* strains not producing H_2S resemble *Shigella* but are smaller. In general, colonies of *Proteus* have a more glistening or watery appearance than do *Salmonella* or *Shigella*.

Arizona colonies are similar to those of *Salmonella*, whereas *Citrobacter* is usually inhibited. When present, colonies are small and bluish green. Most *Pseudomonas* strains are inhibited. When present, colonies are very small, flat, and green to brown in color.

Preliminary examination and screening of stool cultures for *Salmonella* and *Shigella*[193, 214–224, 226]

The procedures described here refer **only** to stool cultures. All Enterobacteriaceae must be

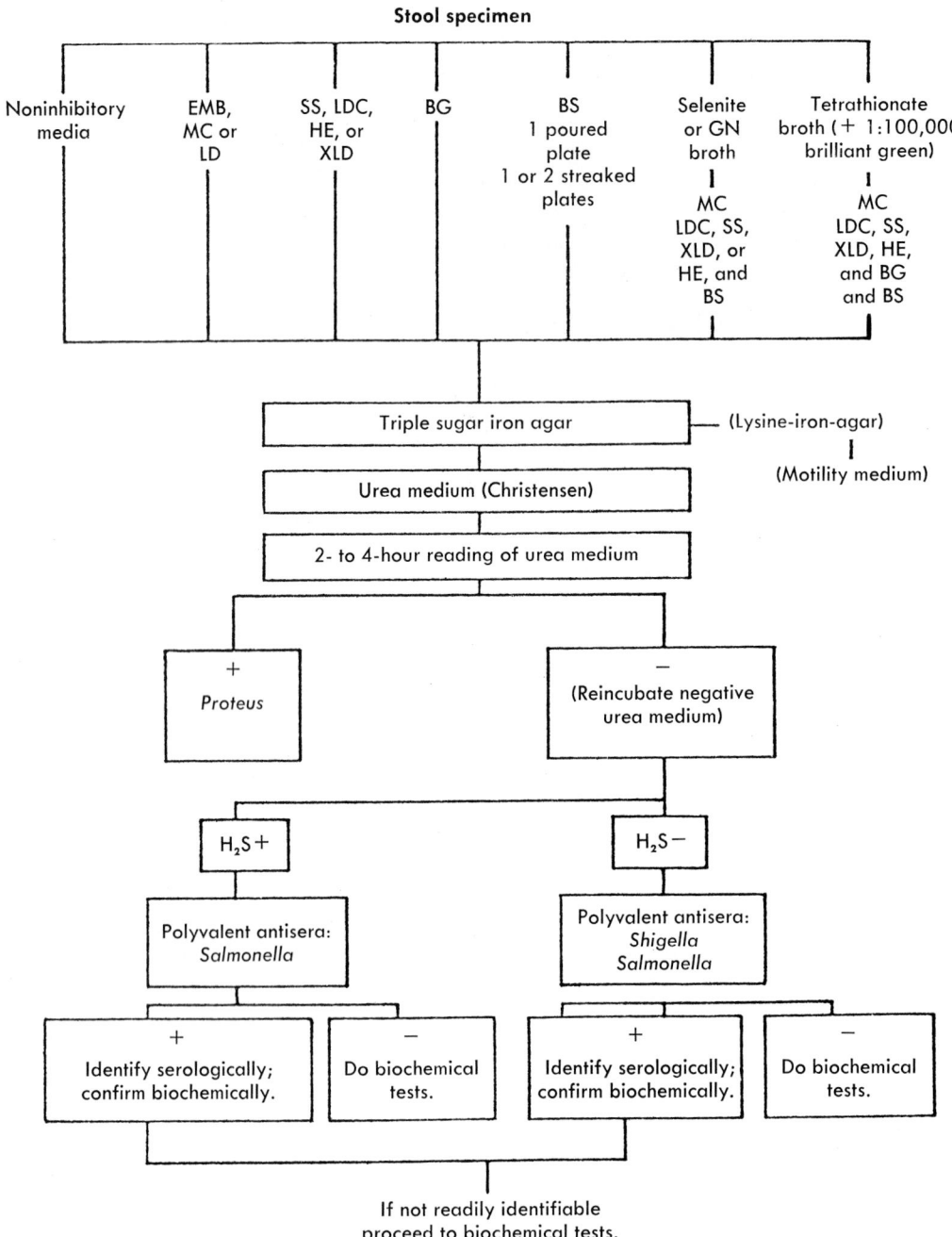

Fig. 75-9. Isolation and preliminary identification of *Salmonella* and *Shigella. EMB,* Eosin methylene blue agar; *MC,* MacConkey agar; *LD,* Leifson's desoxycholate agar; *LDC,* Leifson desoxycholate citrate agar; *SS,* Shigella-Salmonella agar; *BS,* bismuth sulfite agar; *BG,* brilliant green agar; *XLD,* xylose lysine desoxycholate agar; *HE,* Hektoen enteric agar. (From Ewing, W. H.: Isolation and identification of *Salmonella, Shigella,* Atlanta, 1974, Center for Disease Control.)

further identified if they are isolated from any other part of the body (Chapter 79). For a flowsheet summarizing Ewing's recommended procedures for isolation and preliminary identification of *Salmonella* and *Shigella,* see Fig. 75-9.)

The organisms requiring identification are, in general, *Salmonella, Arizona, Shigella,* and in certain cases, enteropathogenic *E. coli* (**see also** *Y. enterocolitica, Vibrio,* **and** *Campylobacter,* **below**).

Oxidase test. This test, rapidly and easily performed (see Chapters 72 and 79), immediately divides organisms into **oxidase positives** (*Vibrio* ssp., *Aeromonas, Campylobacter*) and **oxidase negatives** (all *Enterobacteriaceae*).

Lactose fermentation **alone** is not acceptable for defining or identifying groups of Enterobacteriaceae, since groups known as lactose-fermenters contain strains that are late fermenters or nonfermenters and groups known as lactose nonfermenters, such as *Salmonella,* contain a few strains that ferment lactose. However, this characteristic is still useful enough to allow screening by differential and selective media. On lactose-containing plating media (MacConkey; EMB, which also contains sucrose; deoxycholate, SS agar, and XLD agar), lactose-fermenting coliforms usually produce typically shaped, **colored** colonies. Color depends on indicator used: colonies are red to pink on MacConkey, deoxycholate, and SS agar; yellow on XLD agar. On the more selective media, growth of the coliforms is greatly inhibited. On DCA agar coliforms that persist form even, **red** colonies; on bismuth sulfite *E. coli* forms small black, brown, or greenish colonies, whereas *Enterobacter aerogenes* forms raised, gray, mucoid colonies.

Lactose nonfermenters or late fermenters, such as *Salmonella, Shigella, Proteus,* etc., usually produce **colorless** colonies with typical appearance on the lactose-containing plates; on bismuth sulfite agar most salmonellae appear as black colonies, with or without metallic sheen surrounding them, or sometimes as smaller greenish colonies. On brilliant green agar, salmonellae appear as slightly pink-white, opaque colonies surrounded by a brilliant red medium.

Thus it is important to be familiar with the appearance of these organisms on the plating media used. It should be kept in mind, however, that atypical colonies may also appear, especially on selective media.

The media should be examined after 18-24 hours incubation. EMB, MacConkey, and XLD plates can be discarded if nothing but typical coliform colonies are seen.

The more selective media (deoxycholate citrate, SS, bismuth sulfite, brilliant green) should be examined next. These will show much less growth, if any, of the typical coliforms (lactose-fermenting colonies) and occasionally may be sterile. If no colonies resembling *Shigella* or *Salmonella* are found, these plates should be reincubated for another 24 hours.

NOTE:

1. *Shigella* organisms will not grow on bismuth sulfite and brilliant green agar; *S. typhi* will not grow on brilliant green agar. Other salmonellae will grow on both bismuth sulfite and brilliant green agar.

2. *Arizona* strains (about half of which ferment lactose promptly) present a distinct problem. On MacConkey and SS agar some produce colonies that resemble those of *E. coli,* whereas others produce colorless colonies. When inoculated into triple sugar iron (TSI) agar, they may give typical acid slant/acid butt reaction (see below), usually

with H_2S production but sometimes without it, and thus would be discarded. To circumvent this difficulty, it is strongly suggested, especially if no *Salmonella* or *Shigella* are detected, to pick *Salmonella*-like colonies (black, green, or brownish) from bismuth sulfite plates into lysine iron agar (LIA) slants. Salmonellae and *Arizona* strains regularly decarboxylate lysine **and** produce H_2S. Therefore all cultures showing alkaline or neutral reactions in the slant and butt of LIA agar with H_2S production are to be followed up with biochemical and serologic tests.

3. **Enrichment broth.** As stated earlier, transfers should be made from selenite or other enrichment broths after no more than 16 hours to a MacConkey **and** SS or XLD and bismuth sulfite **or** brilliant green agar plate (however, *S. typhi* will not grow on the latter).

Isolation of colonies

Colonies other than those of frank coliforms and any atypical colonies must be "picked" and isolated to examine their biochemical and antigenic characteristics. Whereas *Shigella* and *Salmonella* ordinarily produce colonies of a typical aspect on selective media, their appearance may be altered by growth in close association with other organisms. Thus even persons of long experience in enteric bacteriology may be misled by colony appearance.

It is always advisable to pick 2 representatives of **each** type of colony that appears on the plates **except frank coliforms.** Examination of the plates with a Quebec colony counter has been found very helpful in distinguishing the various colony types. **The greatest care should be exercised in picking colonies if pure cultures are to be obtained.** Use a straight needle and touch only the center of the selected colony. Avoid touching the surface of the agar if possible.

Colonies should be picked with a straight needle and planted on **TSI (triple sugar iron agar)** slants. First stab to the bottom of the butt; then streak the needle over the slant so as to produce sufficient surface growth. If medium is available, it is strongly advised to also inoculate **lysine iron agar (LIA)** at this stage. Inoculate LIA with straight wire **immediately** after inoculating TSI medium (**do not** go back to colony), by stabbing the butt **twice** and then streaking the slant as thoroughly as possible. If more inoculum is needed after TSI inoculation, it is advised to touch the spot where the stab was made in the TSI medium with the tip of the wire.

Ewing[222] recommended suspending a strip of filter paper previously impregnated with Weil-Saphra reagent over inoculated tubes of LIA medium (see indole paper strip technic, Chapter 72). In this manner, information about indole production can be obtained by the tme the LIA and TSI reactions are read. **Caution:** All negative tests for indole obtained by paper strip method should be retested by standard method.

Inoculate from **same** colony a slant of **Christen-**

sen urea agar. Inoculate heavily on slant only. *Proteus* cultures will produce a marked alkalinity in the urea medium in 2-4 hours (the medium turns red). Any colony that produces this reaction is a urease producer (*Proteus*) and can be excluded from consideration in the search for *Salmonella* or *Shigella*. Colonies that do not show the reaction should be incubated overnight. Certain colon organisms produce varying degrees of alkalinity after 24-72 hours incubation. *Salmonella* and *Shigella* cultures give negative urease tests.

Multiple test systems ("minikits")

Recently, several **miniaturized, multiple test systems** have been developed that greatly simplify identification of enterobacteria. Compared to conventional tests, the **"mini kits"** require far smaller amounts of material and yield results in less time.

The variety of kits includes, among others, a system containing a series of cupules (microtubes) with dehydrated substrates that are inoculated by capillary pipet with a suspension of cells (API); a multicompartmental plastic tube containing various agars inoculated with a wire (Enterotube); a card containing dried substrates inoculated with a broth suspension of organisms (Micro-ID); a variety of substrates on paper disks (Minitek); a series of reagent-impregnated paper strips placed in small tubes containing suspensions of organisms (Pathotec); and a combination of 4 glass tubes with reagents in agar for a total of 14 conventional biochemical tests (R-B).

Most of the systems use computer-based (numeric) identification schemes; the first system to do so (API) now employs a sophisticated "profile recognition pattern" based on results obtained with more than 50,000 enteric strains, allowing computer-assisted calculation of the likelihood value of results. The numeric and computer-assisted systems have greatly speeded up and improved identification of these organisms, recognition of unusual or aberrant strains, and are most helpful in epidemiologic studies. The systems represent a major advantage over conventional methodologies in the clinical laboratory. For details of the systems, see Chapter 74.

Examination of cultures

The TSI tubes are incubated overnight. They should be closed with a cotton plug or loose, metal closure but not with tight rubber or cork stoppers. Those that show an acid reaction, yellow slant and yellow butt throughout, can be discarded unless H_2S is produced (by *Arizona*, rare *Salmonella*, and *Proteus vulgaris*, see below). They contain organisms that rapidly ferment lactose or sucrose or both; such organisms are not *Salmonella* or *Shigella*. All tubes showing an alkaline slant (red) and acid butt (yellow), with or without gas formation or blackening, are held for

further study unless they show rapid urease formation on urea agar, in which case they can be discarded. (**NOTE: See also reactions of** *Yersinia enterocolitica, Pasteurella pseudotuberculosis, Vibrio,* **and** *Aeromonas,* **below, and in Chapter 79**).

Some *Arizona* organisms, which produce typical black colonies on bismuth sulfite agar, may show acid slant and acid butt in TSI (with H_2S and gas production). This is the situation in which the LIA tube will furnish valuable information. If the Lia tube shows an alkaline reaction throughout (alkaline slant, purple, with alkaline or neutral butt, with or without H_2S), that is evidence of **decarboxylation of lysine**, positive with all *Salmonella* and *Arizona,* and the isolate should be followed up with further biochemical and serologic tests. *Proteus* is eliminated by urease test or by **lysine deamination** shown by red slant and yellow (acid) butt in LIA medium.

Alternatively, one could perform a lysine decarboxylase test on all H_2S-positive organisms. This, however, is inconvenient, and use of lysine iron agar is recommended for early presumptive differentiation.

Occasionally colonies will be encountered that will give an **alkaline reaction throughout in the TSI medium** (slant and butt red). These are organisms (*Alcaligenes* or *Pseudomonas* sp.) that do not ferment any of the 3 sugars present. Such organsisms are sometimes picked from plates because they are lactose nonfermenters. These should be discarded.

Typical coliform organisms that rapidly ferment sucrose or lactose, the *Proteus* organisms, and those giving alkaline reactions throughout the TSI medium can thus be eliminated from further work. The remainder of the TSI tubes must be examined further by biochemical and serologic methods to determine whether they contain *Shigella, Salmonella,* or other organisms.

Edwards and Ewing[191] recommend inoculation of TSI agar slant on the first day with overnight incubation and the discarding of those that show an acid reaction throughout. In their outline the urease test is performed on the second day on those TSI tubes that show an acid butt and an alkaline slant. The inoculation of the Christensen urea agar slant at the time when the TSI tube is inoculated may result in some waste of material but, in the case of rapidly positive urease reaction, it eliminates *Proteus* organisms the same day.

The reactions on TSI agar and LIA agar are described below; a more detailed description is given in Chapter 79.

Brief summary and outline of preliminary identification of cultures. The following should be thoroughly examined as possible *Shigella, Arizona,* or *Salmonella* organisms. The methods are those described by Edwards and Ewing,[191] Ewing,[214] and Martin et al.[216] and are highly recommended. See also below for a schema with flowsheet and tables for differentiation of

Salmonella, Shigella, and *Arizona* groups from stool.

Acid slant, acid butt in TSI. Such organisms are not *Salmonella* or *Shigella.* If H_2S is present, organism is either *Citrobacter, Proteus,* or *Arizona.* The latter gives an alkaline reaction (alkaline slant and butt) in LIA agar, usually with H_2S production. Alternatively, perform a lysine decarboxylase test. **Phenylalanine deaminase–positive** organisms are either *Proteus* (urease positive) or *Providencia* (urease negative).

Rapid urease production on Christensen urease agar. Discard; organisms are *Proteus* strains.

Slow urease production (24-72 h). Discard; *Salmonella* and *Shigella* do not produce urease.

Alkaline slant, acid butt in TSI

H_2S-positive, gas produced. Organisms giving this reaction may be *Salmonella, Proteus, Citrobacter,* certain types of *Arizona,* or *Edwardsiella. Proteus* organisms should be eliminated by rapid urease production on Christensen urea agar.

Organisms producing **no** alkalinization of the urea agar and producing gas and H_2S with an alkaline slant and acid butt should be examined as follows:

1. Perform agglutinations with polyvalent and somatic (O) group *Salmonella* antisera. Use growth from TSI slant. Suspensions that agglutinate with the polyvalent serum should then be tested with the O group *Salmonella* sera. A culture that is agglutinated in a typical manner by polyvalent serum and by one or more of the O grouping sera may be reported as a probable *Salmonella,* if preliminary biochemical examination indicates that it is a member of the genus. **Results should be confirmed by extended biochemical tests** (Table 79-16). Cultures that fail to react with polyvalent serum should be tested with **Vi** serum, especially if the reaction of the culture in the TSI agar resembles that produced by *S. typhi. (S. typhi* produces no gas, and some strains at least produce insufficient H_2S to blacken the TSI agar.) Testing with **Vi** serum is described below.

2. Proceed with the following essential tests: indole, methyl red, Voges-Proskauer, Simmons citrate, motility, lysine decarboxylase, lactose, sucrose, salicin, adonitol. Others such as KCN and ONPG (β-galactosidase) are helpful. These tests and reagents are discussed in Chapters 72 and 79. In the differentiation of *Salmonella* and *Citrobacter,* the primary tests are KCN and lysine.

For practical purposes, **any culture that ferments lactose, sucrose, salicin, or adonitol or that produces indole in amounts detectable in the usual tests (with very few exceptions) can be excluded from the genus.** Likewise, methyl red–negative and Voges-Proskauer–positive organisms are not *Salmonella;* **neither are salmonellae capable of growing in KCN broth.** Most salmonellae are citrate positive (exceptions: *S. paratyphi* A, *S. typhi, S. sendai, S. pullorum, S. gallinarum,* and a few other types).

3. If the organism fails to agglutinate in polyvalent serum (and with Vi serum), it should be subjected to the biochemical tests listed above and, in addition, to those listed in Table 79-16. If the organism cannot be eliminated from the genus *Salmonella* by these tests, it should be sent to a reference laboratory.

H_2S-negative, gas not produced. Organisms giving this reaction may be *Salmonella* (some cultures of *S. typhi*), *Shigella, Proteus,* or *Providencia. Proteus* is eliminated by urease reaction, *Providencia* by phenyl-

alanine test; both are eliminated by **lysine deamination** reaction (red slant over yellow butt) in LIA agar.

1. Use polyvalent *Shigella* group antisera (A, B, C, D). A prompt, complete reaction in one of the polyvalent sera is **presumptive** evidence that the organism is a *Shigella* type. **Such cultures must be confirmed biochemically. Cultures that do not react with the grouping antisera but appear to be *Shigella* in the TSI medium** should be suspended in physiologic saline solution. Heat at 100 C for ½ h, cool, and retest.

2. Proceed with the following tests: motility, lactose, sucrose, glucose, salicin, adonitol, indole, Simmons citrate agar, methyl red, and Voges-Proskauer.

Any motile organism can be eliminated as *Shigella*; fermentation of lactose or sucrose in **24** h, a positive citrate test, utilization of salicin or adonitol, or growth in KCN broth excludes a culture from the genus *Shigella.* Shigellae do not form gas except for certain variants of *Shigella flexneri* 6; these sometimes form enough gas to become apparent in TSI agar. Do not eliminate the culture from examination because there is no evidence of H_2S production.

3. As mentioned before, certain *Salmonella* cultures form no gas or H_2S. For this reason, *Salmonella* agglutinations should be carried out. Cultures that fail to agglutinate with polyvalent serum should be tested with **Vi** serum. If the culture reacts with Vi serum, a portion of the suspension should be heated in boiling water bath 20 min and, after cooling, again should be tested with the O sera and Vi serum. After boiling, *S. typhi* cultures should react with D serum; and *S. paratyphi* C cultures, which also may contain **Vi** antigen, should react with C_1 serum. Cultures that react with Vi serum and that, after heating, react with *Salmonella* group D serum may be reported as *S. typhi,* after which the H antigens should be identified and biochemical tests performed. Cultures that continue to agglutinate in Vi serum after heating and that are not agglutinated by the O grouping sera may be presumed to contain O antigens related to those of the Bethesda-Ballerup organisms *(Citrobacter).*

H_2S-negative, gas produced

1. Some *Salmonella* types, mentioned earlier, may give this reaction in TSI agar. Perform agglutinations and biochemical tests as described above.

2. Certain biochemical variants of *S. flexneri* 6 produce some gas in TSI agar. Examine as for *Shigella.*

3. Some *Providencia* strains (phenylalanine positive) form gas but not H_2S.

H_2S-positive, no gas produced

1. Production of H_2S eliminates the culture from consideration as *Shigella.*

2. Certain cultures of *S. typhi* usually produce a small amount of H_2S but no gas in TSI agar. Anaerogenic (no gas forming) strains of other *Salmonella* also occur; therefore such cultures should be examined as described above for *Salmonella.*

Lysine iron agar reactions. Always use lysine iron (LIA) agar in conjunction with TSI or Kligler iron agar. The medium is not a substitute for the standard decarboxylase test medium.

Alkaline slant, alkaline butt (purple), H_2S not produced.[222] This reaction indicates decarboxylation of

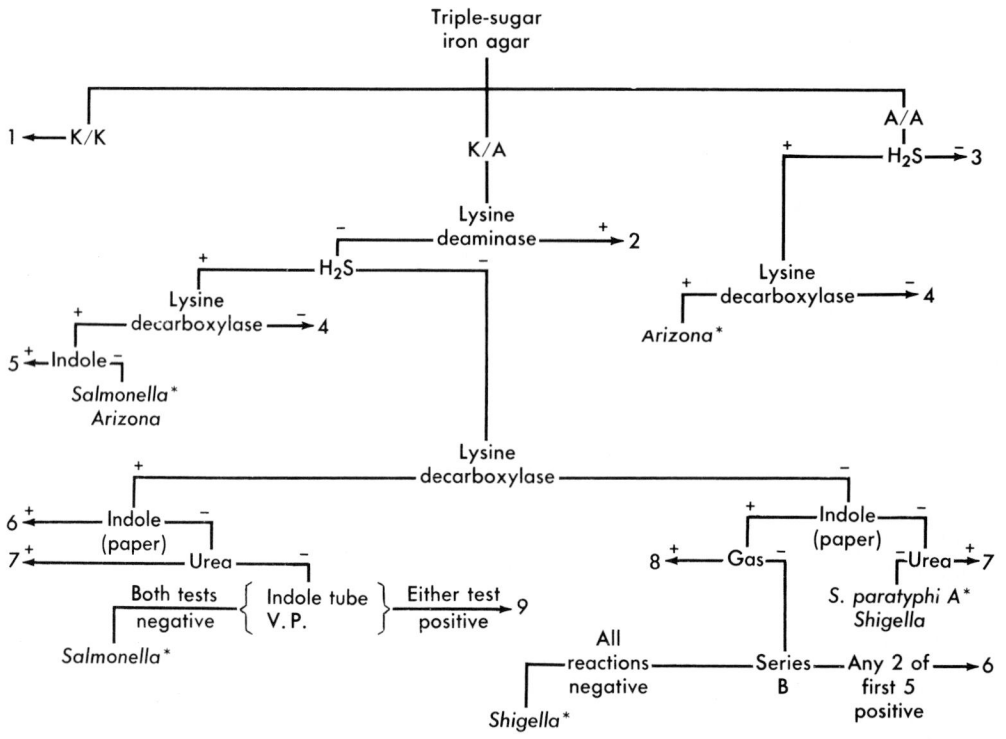

Fig. 75-10. Schema for differentiation and recognition of *Shigella, Salmonella,* and *Arizona* group in stool cultures. Symbols: K/K = alkaline slant, alkaline butt; K/A = alkaline slant, acid butt; A/A = acid slant, acid butt (triple-sugar iron agar); + = positive reaction; − = negative reaction; * = confirm by agglutination test with appropriate antisera and biochemical series A (Table 75-4) and, in the case of *Shigella,* biochemical series B (Table 75-5). ←or→ = discard. Probable identities of discards are: **1,** not an Enterobacteriaceae; **2,** *Proteus* or Providence group; **3,** *Escherichia coli, Klebsiella-Enterobacter,* or H_2S^- *Citrobacter;* **4,** *Citrobacter;* **5,** *Edwardsiella;* **6,** *E. coli;* **7,** Proteus (lysine decarboxylase reaction may be equivocal); **8,** *E. coli, Proteus,* Providence group, etc.; and **9,** *E. coli, Klebsiella, Hafnia, Serratia,* etc. (From Johnson, J. G., Kunz, L. J., Barron, W., and Ewing, W. H.: Appl. Microbiol. **14:**212, 1966.)

lysine. Such organisms can be *Escherichia,* some *Salmonella* or *Arizona* strains, *Klebsiella, E. aerogenes, E. hafniae,* or *Serratia.*

Alkaline slant, alkaline butt, H_2S produced. This reaction is given by most *Salmonella* and *Arizona* strains and by *Edwardsiella.*

Alkaline slant, acid butt (yellow), no H_2S produced. Organism may be *Shigella,* rare *Salmonella,* rare *Citrobacter,* or *Enterobacter cloacae.*

Alkaline slant, acid butt, H_2S produced. Reaction normally given by *S. paratyphi A* or *C. freundii.*

Deamination of lysine (red slant over acid butt, yellow). Reaction indicates *Proteus* sp. or *Providencia* sp. and is very characteristic for these 2 groups.

See Table 79-14 for a summary of TSI and LIA agar reactions.

Schema for differentiation of Shigella, Salmonella, and Arizona group in stool cultures—Johnson-Kunz-Barron-Ewing[225]

Among the conventional methodologies for recognition of *Salmonella* and *Shigella* is the useful and practical procedure devised by Johnson et al.,[225] based on the use of triple sugar iron agar (TSI) and lysine iron agar (LIA). Fig. 75-10 illustrates the reactions and the subsequent tests employed.

NOTE: The authors of the procedure have recently ceased to use it and have adopted a multiple test system (API) for identification of gram-negative rods. The method is reproduced here for those laboratories continuing to use conventional methodologies.

The flowsheet (Fig. 75-10) and Tables 75-4 and 75-5 are based on the criteria and taxonomic system of Ewing[222-223] (see Enterobacteriaceae, Chapter 79). The tests and media, with few exceptions, are based on the methods of Edwards and Ewing[196a] and Ewing[222, 223] described in this volume (Chapter 72, Tests and reagents, and Chapter 79, Enterobacteriaceae).

The tests in Tables 75-4 and 75-5 are predicated on the use of standard methods and **not** on rapid methods or micromethods or on prepared, ready-made substrates or reagents.

It should be pointed out that the schema will not necessarily identify all aberrant or atypical strains. A small number of *Salmonella* strains are indole positive; such strains will usually give strong agglutination reactions with the proper *Salmonella* antisera (Sonnenwirth[227]). They should not be eliminated because of the

Table 75-4. Biochemical series A for confirmation of *Salmonella* and *Shigella**

Test or substrate	Salmonella (majority)	S. para-typhi A	S. typhi	Arizona group	Edwards-iella	Citro-bacter	Shigella†
Gas from glucose	+	+	−	+	+	+	−‡
Lactose	−	−	−	D	−	D	−§
Sucrose	−	−	−	−	−	D	−§
Mannitol	+	+	+	+	−	+	D
Salicin	−	−	−	D	−	D	−
Dulcitol	+	+	− or (+)	−	−	D	D
Lysine decarboxylase	+	−	+	+	+	−	−
Motility	+	+	+	+	+	+	−
Gelatin	−	−	−	(+)	−	−	−
Urea	−	−	−	−	−	D	−
H₂S	+	−	+W	+	+	+	−
Indole	−	−	−	−	+	−	D
Methyl red	+	+	+	+	+	+	+
Voges-Proskauer	−	−	−	−	−	−	−
Citrate (Simmons)	+	+	−	+	−	+	−
Malonate	−	−	−	+	−	D	−

*From Johnson, J. C., Kunz, L. J., Barron, W., and Ewing, W. H.: Appl. Microbiol. **14:**212, 1966.

Symbols: + = positive; − = negative; (+) = delayed; D = different biochemical types; +W = weak.

†Use biochemical series B to differentiate between *Shigella* and anaerogenic, lac- nonmotile strains of *E. coli* (A-D biotypes).

‡Certain biotypes of *S. flexneri* 6 produce gas (these are indole negative).

§*S. sonnei* ferments lactose and sucrose slowly.

Table 75-5. Biochemical series B for differentiation of *Shigella* and aberrant (anaerogenic, nonmotile, lactose-negative) *E. coli**

Test or substrate	Shigella	Escherichia coli
Acetate	−	+ (rare −)
Mucate	−	+ (rare −)
Xylose	−†	+ (rare −)
Salicin	−	+, −
Motility	−	+, −
Citrate	−	− (very rare −)

*From Johnson, J. C., Kunz, L. J., Barron, W., and Ewing, W. H.: Appl. Microbiol. **14:**212, 1966.

Symbols: − = negative reaction; +, − = may be either positive or negative; usually 2 or more of the first 4 reactions are positive with *E. coli*.

†Some shigellae ferment xylose. However, the most commonly occurring types do not.

positive indole reaction but should be submitted to a reference laboratory for verification and final identification. All atypical or not easily identifiable strains should be submitted to the proper reference laboratories.

• • •

Fecal examination for "predominant organisms" or "total flora." Douglas et al.[228] pointed out that under certain circumstances such as in patients with cancer or other debilitating diseases it is important to be able to specifically and rapidly identify a number of Enterobacteriaceae in addition to *Salmonella* and *Shigella*. The so-called "nonpathogens" (coliforms, etc.) most frequently are secondary invaders in a host with depressed immune responses due to radiation, immunosuppressive drugs, or the disease itself.

Their simplified biochemical routine includes:

Day 1—TSI agar, urea agar

Day 2—Screening agglutinations with *Salmonella* or *Shigella* antisera as indicated by TSI/urea combination, MR-VP broth (2 tubes), Simmons citrate, motility agar tube, phenylalanine agar, KCN broth, decarboxylase broths (lysine, arginine, ornithine, control with no amino acid)

They were able to identify 93% of all slow or nonlactose-fermenting strains of Enterobacteriaceae within 48 hours after inoculation into these biochemicals. For further details see Douglas.[228]

• • •

Comments regarding preliminary examination of stool cultures:

1. No **final** identification of *Salmonella* or *Shigella* organisms can or should be made on biochemical or serologic grounds alone. **Both** procedures must be used.

2. If biochemical confirmation and polyvalent agglutination have been done, grouping and typing of the organism should be carried out. See Enterobacteriaceae, Chapter 79.

3. Certain cultures that are agglutinated by polyvalent *Salmonella* antisera may give aberrant biochemical results. This may mean that the organism is a rare *Salmonella* strain, an *Arizona*, or a *Citrobacter*. Further biochemical tests (as described under Enterobacteriaceae) should be carried out and the culture should be submitted to a reference laboratory.

4. Organisms that agglutinate in polvalent *Shigella* antisera must be confirmed biochemically, since some organisms of other groups agglutinate in certain *Shigella* antisera. The same holds true for *Salmonella* agglutinations.

5. If an organism shows biochemical characteristics of the *Salmonella* group but fails to agglutinate in polyvalent serum, further biochemical tests should be carried out. If the organism cannot be excluded from the

genus *Salmonella*, it should be sent to a reference laboratory.

6. Fermentation of certain substrates may be delayed from 24 h to many days. Cultures should be examined periodically to detect any fermentation. Salicin, sucrose, and lactose tubes should, if possible, be plugged after the first 24 h with cork stoppers sterilized by soaking in hot paraffin. This will reduce the time necessary for fermentation to become apparent. Cultures should be incubated, if indicated, for 30 d for observation of fermentation before being discarded as negative. However, reports should not be delayed for unduly long periods.

7. *Yersinia enterocolitica, Y. pseudotuberculosis, Vibrio* ssp., and *Aeromonas* have been isolated from stool. See below and Chapter 79.

Screening for enteropathogenic and enterotoxigenic *Escherichia coli*

The rationale and value of **serotyping** of "enteropathogenic" *E. coli* has been seriously questioned; however, there is no agreement on the total abandonment of this procedure.

Tests for **toxigenicity** (toxin production) or **invasive potential** of *E. coli* strains presently require tissue culture and animal inoculation methods (Y-1 Mouse adrenal cell test, HeLa cell test, Sereny test, infant mouse test).

For serotyping and pathogenicity tests, see *E. coli*, Chapter 79.

Alternate methods for stool culture and screening for Salmonella and Shigella

The methods preferred and recommended are the ones described earlier. A number of alternate methods are listed below to illustrate various approaches, especially in attempting to shorten the time for preliminary identification of organisms. None of the procedures has met with widespread approval.

Sanders-Okabe method.[218,219] Sanders and Okabe devised a booster broth designed to screen colonies of enteric organisms and to enhance growth for inocula of subcultures (for determination of lactose or sucrose fermentation). Initial culture is the same as in the recommended method. The Sanders booster broth* is warmed to 37 C and is used usually in 2 ml quantities. Three nonlactose-fermenting colonies selected from a differential plate such as deoxycholate, MacConkey, or *Salmonella-Shigella* agars are inoculated into 3 tubes each of the broth. The inoculated tubes are placed in a 37 C water bath for 2 h. Tubes showing acid are discarded. Tubes remaining alkaline are then studied.

The procedure is as follows.

1. 0.15 ml broth from each tube is inoculated into 25 ml Sanders agar, melted, cooled to 43 C, and the mixture poured into plates for carbohydrate and H₂S tests.
2. The authors recommend that aliquots of the broth be used for indole tests with Kovacs reagent, for serology, and for hanging-drop studies.
3. The booster broth cultures may also be conveniently used for other inoculations. For example, trypticase agar base may be stabbed for detection of motility (without time-consuming mi-

croscopic studies, which may be less reliable for determining lack of motility) and for maintenance of cultures.

Inoculation of a urease medium, such as urea agar slants, may be conveniently done concurrently with the Sanders agar plate so that results will be available at the same time as the fermentation reactions.

The Sanders agar contains an iron salt indicator added to phenol red base for detection of fermentation and sulfide reactions. It can be used with paper disks impregnated with various carbohydrates. Four paper disks, one each of dextrose, lactose, mannitol, and sucrose, are applied to Sanders plates inoculated as described above. The plates are incubated and examined after 6-8 h incubation for appearance of yellow (acid) zones and for bubbles or splits in the agar due to gas formation. Evidence of sulfide production is obtained from blackening around the periphery of yellow zones. A final reading should be made at 24 h.

Rapid screening method for *Salmonella* and *Shigella*—Bicknell-Butt-Mattman[221]

1. Dissolve in 1000 ml distilled water by heating:

Beef extract	1 g
Proteose-peptone no. 3	10 g
Sodium chloride	5 g
Lactose	10 g
Dextrose	1 g
Sodium thiosulfate	0.3 g
Yeast extract	0.3 g
Bromcresol purple	0.015 g
Agar	3 g

2. Distribute into small test tubes.
3. Autoclave at 15 psi for 10 min.
4. Preheat to 37 C in water bath before use.
5. Pick colonies simultaneously to Kligler tubes, urea broth, and to above medium.
6. Fasten lead acetate paper between plug and inner mouth of latter tubes to detect H₂S production.
7. Read results after 3½ h incubation at 37 C in **water bath**.

• • •

Isolation and preliminary identification of *Vibrio cholerae*

For a description of *V. cholerae*, see Chapter 79.

Naked eye examination of specimen. The stool is rice-watery as a rule; i.e., it is a whitish fluid containing flakes of epithelium without any fecal matter, alkaline in reaction, and emitting a peculiar fishy smell. It may be bile-stained or rarely tinged with blood.

Microscopic examination. A flake disintegrated on a slide, fixed, and stained with dilute carbolfuchsin shows short, comma-shaped vibrios, sometimes arranged in fish-in-stream manner; spirochetes are longer and pale-stained in large numbers, and there are a few desquamated columnar epithelial cells. No pus cells and red blood cells as a rule are found. Vibrios may be absent or there may be very few.

Stool collection and culture. The methods given are those of Ewing et al.,[229,230] Balows et al.,[212] and the World Health Organization.[231]

Collect stool specimens within the first 24 hours of the disease. Rectal swabs can be used during the acute phase; during convalescence,

---

*BBL, Cockeysville, Md.

swabs are not reliable (unless used after a purge). If specimens cannot be cultured immediately or must be transported, inoculate alkaline peptone water (pH 8.4) and transport medium (Monsur or Gohar). Plate separate sets of plates as described below.

1. Streak out 1-2 loopfuls of stool on **nutrient agar** (meat extract agar) **with 0.5 NaCl**; inoculate lightly; also inoculate **taurocholate gelatin** agar (moderate inoculum) and **TCBS agar** or Monsur agar (inoculate heavily). Incubate 16-24 h at 35-37 C.
2. Place 1-2 loopfuls of stool specimen into 0.5-1 ml **alkaline peptone water** (pH 8.4). Incubate 6-8 h at 37 C. Streak out set of plates as described above (second set of plates).

Identification. (1) Examine plates directly and by oblique lighting for iridescent colonies, zones of gelatin liquefaction, colonies with dark centers (Monsur agar), and yellow colonies (TCBS agar). (2) Pick suspect colonies to Kligler iron agar (KIA) and also to lysine iron (LIA) slants. Touch only the top central portion of the colonies with inoculating wire. (3) Incubate 18-24 hours.

Do **presumptive agglutination** tests with polyvalent antiserum and with Ogawa and Inaba antisera on isolates that give reactions typical of *V. cholerae* on KIA and LIA media.

KIA reactions of *V. cholerae* are: alkaline (K) slant, acid (A) in the butt, and no gas and no H_2S produced (K/A $^-$).

LIA reactions: K/K$^-$ or K/N$^-$ (N = neutral or alkaline).

TSI reactions: A/A.

Oxidase test: positive.

Decarboxylase activity: lysine +, arginine −, ornithine +.

For further biochemical characteristics see *Vibrio*, Chapter 79.

NOTE: Regardless of the outcome of the serologic tests, a subculture of a suspected isolate should be submitted immediately to the state health department and the specimen should be accompanied by a clinical history, if possible. The director of laboratories, state health department, **should be alerted by telephone that the culture is being submitted to the state health department laboratory.**

Isolation and preliminary identification of *Vibrio parahaemolyticus**

Vibrio parahaemolyticus is a marine microorganism, the identity of which was established by Sakazaki et al. in 1963.[197] It is an enteropathogenic, halophilic (salt-loving), gram-negative, facultative anaerobe occurring in most of the marine waters of the world.[232]

In the summer of 1971, *V. parahaemolyticus*

---

*Adapted from Twedt, R. M.: Isolation and identification of *Vibrio parahaemolyticus*. In FDA Bacteriological Analytical Manual, Association of Official Analytical Chemists, Publ., Washington, D.C., 1978.

was recovered from both patients and contaminated foods (steamed crabs and crab salad) in the United States. Since then, additional outbreaks have occurred in several states.[198]

NOTE: **All media must contain at least 3% NaCl unless other concentrations are specified.**

Initial culture. Stools, rectal swabs, or vomitus specimens in outbreaks should be obtained. Specimens must be obtained at the earliest opportunity because the carrier state is short-lived.

1. If transit time is much beyond 8 h:
   a. Place stool specimens in Cary-Blair transport medium.
   b. In laboratory, streak loopful onto TCBS agar (see *Vibrio* media, Chapter 72) in addition to other enteric media employed.
   c. Incubate at 35 C for 24-48 h.
   (Do not discard plates as negative before 48 h.)
2. If transit time is 8 h or less:
   a. Place stool specimen in alkaline peptone water.
   b. After 8 h incubation, streak loopful onto TCBS agar.
   c. Incubate at 35 C for 24-48 h.
3. Rectal swab specimen:
   a. Sample specimen (preferably polyester fiber–tipped swab) contained in 7 ml medium (see *1a* or *2a*, above) by streaking loopful onto TCBS agar and other enteric agars.
   b. Incubate plates at 35 C for 24-48 h.

Appearance of *V. parahaemolyticus* on TCBS agar plates
1. Colonies are round, 2-3 mm in diameter, with green or blue centers.
2. *V. alginolyticus* colonies appear larger and yellow.
3. Coliform, *Proteus*, and enterococci, if present, appear as small and translucent colonies.

Identification. Perform **oxidase test:** the organism is oxidase positive.

Pick, with needle, 2 or more typical or suspicious colonies, if present, from TCBS agar plates onto the following media:

TSI agar slant
1. Streak slant and stab butt.
2. Incubate overnight at 35 C.
3. *V. parahaemolyticus* produces alkaline slant and acid butt; no gas is produced and culture growth on TSI slant is negative for H_2S. This is typical *Shigella*-like reaction.

TSB (trypticase soy broth with 3% NaCl) and TSA (trypticase soy agar slant with 3% NaCl)
1. Inoculate TSB and TSA; and incubate overnight at 35 C.
2. Use these cultures as source of inoculum for other tests, Gram stains, and microscopic examinations.
3. *V. parahaemolyticus* is a gram-negative, pleomorphic organism exhibiting curved or straight rods with **polar** flagella.

Motility test medium
1. Inoculate tube of motility test medium by **stabbing** column of medium to depth of approximately 5 mm.
2. Incubate 24 h at 35 C.

3. Diffuse circular growth from line of stab constitutes positive test.
4. *V. parahaemolyticus* is motile.
Salt trypticase broth (STB), halophilism
1. Using TSA slant culture, inoculate 4 tubes STB base (A71) containing 0%, 6%, 8%, and 10% NaCl, respectively.
2. Incubate at 35 C for 24 h.
3. *V. parahaemolyticus* will grow well in 6% and 8% NaCl concentrations, but will not grow or will grow poorly in 0 and 10% NaCl.

According to Twedt,[232] a minimal screening list of characteristics that would assure the **presumptive** presence of *V. parahaemolyticus* should include the following:

1. Morphology: Gram-negative curved asporogenous rod
2. TSI appearance: Alkaline slant/acid butt, gas negative, H_2S negative
3. Hugh-Leifson test: Glucose-O/F positive, gas negative
4. Cytochrome oxidase: Positive
5. Arginine dehydrolase test: Negative
6. Lysine decarboxylase test: Positive
7. Halophilism test: 0% NaCl negative; 6%, 8% NaCl positive; 10% NaCl negative or poor
8. Growth at 42 C: Positive
9. Voges-Proskauer test: Negative
10. Sucrose fermentation: Negative

For further biochemical identification and tests, see *Vibrio*, Chapter 79.

• • •

Isolation and preliminary identification of *Yersinia enterocolitica*[*233–239]

Yersinia enterocolitica occurs in animate and inanimate environments, including fecal material, foodstuffs, and water. The organisms have been isolated in specimens from swine, dogs, rabbits, chinchillas, cows, sheep, horses, deer, cats, beavers, raccoons, various birds, and oysters, as well as nonchlorinated well water. The most common form of clinical infection in humans is acute **gastroenteritis** with abdominal pain and nonbloody diarrhea. Fever may be present. The second most common clinical manifestation is a syndrome of **pseudoappendicitis, mesenteric lymphadenitis,** or ileitis. Other forms of illness include arthritis, septicemia, meningitis, and urinary tract infection.

Stool culture for *Y. enterocolitica*
Routine procedure
1. Inoculate 1 plate of MacConkey (1 loopful) and 1 plate of SS agar (2 loopfuls) with stool. Incubate plates at **25 C,** since *Y. enterocolitica* grows more readily on plates at 25 C than at 35 C.

***

*Based on Hawkins, T. M., and Brenner, D. J.: Isolation and identification of *Yersinia enterocolitica*, Atlanta, 1978, Center for Disease Control; and Sonnenwirth, A. C.: Mt. Sinai J. Med. **43:**736, 1976.

2. In some laboratories the above 2 plates are inoculated as part of the routine stool culture; i.e., Mac Conkey and other enteric agars are inoculated and incubated at 35 C, with the 2 plates described in step 1 added to each stool culture, and incubated separately at room temperature, i.e., 22-25 C.
Cold enrichment. *Y. enterocolitica* proliferates at 4-5 C and presumably outgrows other enteric flora. The recovery of *Y. Enterocolitica* is much more satisfactory using the **cold enrichment** technic than by direct plating of specimens. If possible, all sample material should be **refrigerated** from time of collection.
Greenwood et al.[237] and Weissfeld and Sonnenwirth[238] have shown that *Y. enterocolitica* can be eventually recovered by cold enrichment from feces specimens that do not yield the organism on direct 35 C or 25 C culture.
1. Place rectal swab or swab dipped in feces in test tube containing 5 ml of 0.067M phosphate buffered saline (PBS), pH 7.6, and hold tubes at 4-5 C.
The 0.067M PBS is prepared by mixing 8.5 g NaCl with 120 ml of 0.067M KH_2PO_4 and 880 ml of 0.067M Na_2HPO_4.
   a. Perform routine culture, as above (0 day culture).
   b. Hold cold enrichment specimens at 4-5 C for 3 wk. Plate specimens on MacConkey and SS agar plates after **7, 14,** and **21** d of enrichment. Incubate plates at 25 C.

The stool culture methodology for *Y. enterocolitica* is shown in Table 75-6.

Examination of plates and subcultures

1. Plating media for isolation of *Y. enterocolitica* should be incubated at 25 C for 48 hours. Colony size will vary with the medium and temperature. On plates incubated at 35 C, colonies are usually pinpoint in size at 24 hours of incubation but are 1-3 mm in size after 48 hours. Other enteric plating media such as EMB, XLD, Hektoen enteric, and brilliant green phenol red should **not** be used for isolating *Y. enterocolitica*. On EMB agar, growth may be poor, and some strains produce a metallic sheen like *E. coli*. On Hektoen agar, sucrose and salicin are fermented, and on XLD the sucrose and xylose are fermented so that *Y. enterocolitica* colonies look like coliforms. Brilliant green is inhibitory to *Y. enterocolitica*.
   a. On MacConkey agar, typical colonies are 1-2 mm in diameter after overnight incubation and up to 3 mm after 48 hours. Typical colonies are a light pink to peach color. It is helpful to examine MacConkey plates under a dissecting microscope with oblique transmitted light.
   b. Typical colonies grown on SS agar are similar in color to those grown on MacConkey's agar but slightly smaller. After 48 hours of incubation the colonies are smooth and colorless, resembling *Shigella*. Not all *Y. enterocolitica* stains will grow on SS agar.
2. Pick typical colonies from plating media to triple sugar iron agar (**TSI**), **urea,** and 2 tubes of **motility** medium for presumptive identification. Incubate 1 motility tubes at **25 C** and remaining media at **35 C.**

Table 75-6. Isolation of *Yersinia enterocolitica*

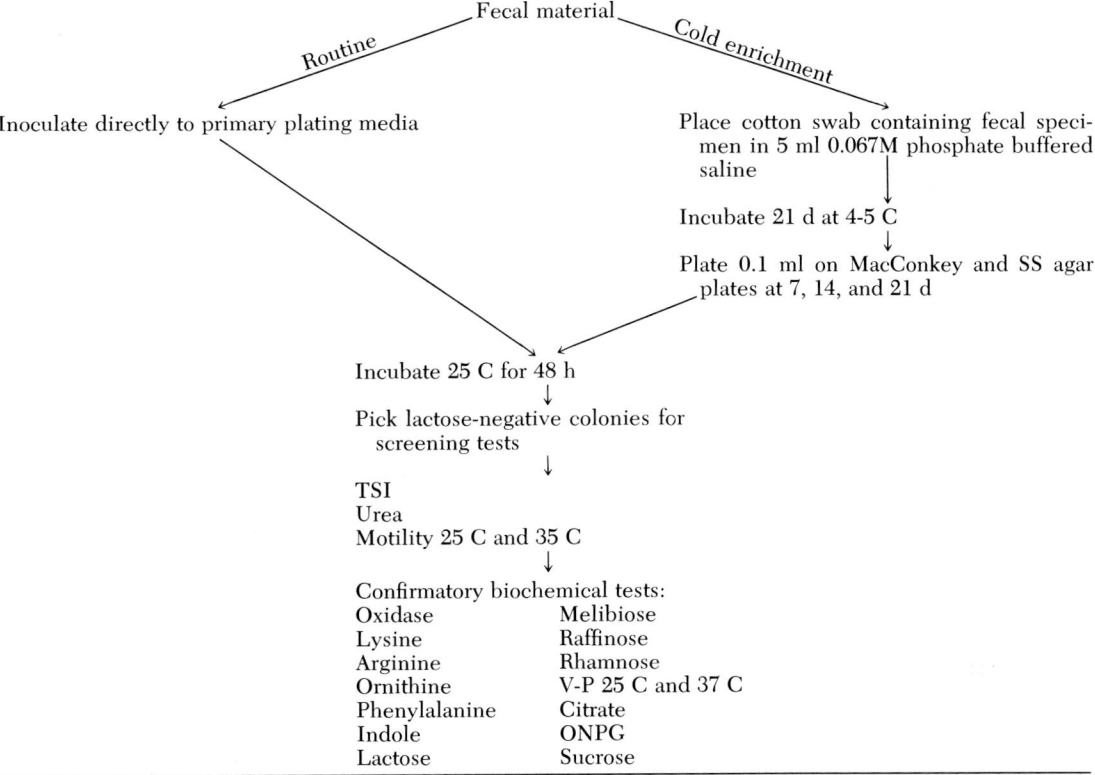

From Hawkins, T. M., and Brenner, D. J.: Isolation and identification of *Yersinia enterocolitica*, Atlanta, 1978, Center for Disease Control.

On TSI, typical reactions are acid butt, acid slant (due to fermentation of sucrose) with no gas or H_2S. However, 2 biogroups of *Y. enterocolitica* are sucrose negative. These strains will give an acid butt, alkaline slant TSI reaction.

Y. enterocolitica are urea positive in 3-24 hours, and most strains are motile at 25 C, but very few are motile at 35 C.

Isolates on TSI slants should be Gram stained, since some gram-positive organisms can give the same TSI reaction. *Y. enterocolitica* are gram-negative rods that may be coccoid when incubated at 25 C.

3. Isolates resembling *Y. enterocolitica* in the screening media should be tested in the confirmatory biochemicals listed under *Yersinia*, Chapter 79.

• • •

Isolation and identification of *Campylobacter fetus* ssp. *jejuni*[241–246]

Until recently, *C. fetus* ssp. *jejuni* was thought to be only an unusual cause of systemic infection.

_____
*Based on Diarrheal disease caused by *Campylobacter fetus* subspecies *jejuni*, Atlanta, Aug. 7, 1978 memorandum from Director, Bureau of Laboratories, Center for Disease Control.

Since technics have been developed that permit isolation from feces,[243,244] however, the organism has proved to be a common cause of enteritis in Europe and Africa.[245] Two outbreaks were reported in the United States during the first half of the summer of 1978.[241,246]

The symptoms of enteritis caused by *C. fetus* ssp. *jejuni* include diarrhea, abdominal pain or cramps, malaise, headache, fever, and vomiting. The stools may be watery or mucosanguineous.

Collection and transport of clinical specimens. Obtain feces or rectal swabs from individuals with diarrhea. If these can not be transported within 4 hours, the rectal swabs or swabs containing feces are immersed in Cary Blair transport medium in screwtop vials.

Inoculation, incubation, and primary examination of plates

1. Use rectal swabs or swab specimens of feces to inoculate area, approximately 1-1¼ in. (2.540-3.175 cm) in diameter, of surface of plate of selective medium (blood agar base no. 2—Oxoid, with 7% lysed horse blood and 3 antimicrobials, i.e., vancomycin, 10 μg/ml, polymyxin B, 2.5 I μ/ml, and trimethoprim, 5 μg/ml; see **media,** Chapter 72). Then streak plate to obtain isolated colonies.

2. Incubate plates at **42-43 C** in anaerobic jar (**catalyst removed);** evacuate to 15 in. (38.1 cm) Hg twice, and refill each time with either of the following gas mix-

tures: (1) 10% carbon dioxide, 10% hydrogen, and 80% nitrogen; or (2) 5% carbon dioxide, 10% hydrogen, and 85% nitrogen. (If facilities for gasing out an anaerobic jar are not available, a disposable GasPak hydrogen–carbon dioxide generator, **without catalyst,** may be substituted. Not all strains of *C. fetus* ssp. *jejuni* grow as well when GasPak generators are used, and some strains may not grow at all. *C. fetus* ssp. *jejuni* is a microaerophile, not a strict anaerobe.)

3. Examine plates after 24, 48, and 72 h of incubation. Colonies of *C. fetus* ssp. *jejuni* are usually detectable by 24 h. The colonies vary from pinpoint, glossy-appearing colonies to those that spread over entire surface of the agar.

Since *C. fetus* ssp. *jejuni* is an **oxidase-positive** organism, the oxidase test is used to screen suspect colonies. This is done by removing a portion of each colony selected and testing it for oxidase on filter paper by Kovacs' technic (see *oxidase test*, Chapter 72).

Microscopic characteristics. *C. fetus* ssp. *jejuni* is a gram-negative rod that is motile by a polar flagellum. Characteristically, it is a slender, curved rod; it may have a single curve or form an "S" or a spiral. These forms are observed best in 18- to 24-hour cultures. In older cultures, coccoid forms may predominate. In wet mounts observed by dark-field microscopy, *C. fetus* ssp. *jejuni* is readily distinguished from the usual enteric gram-negative rods by its smaller size and tumbling or darting motility.

Identification. *C. fetus* ssp. *jejuni* may be identified on the basis of the following characteristics:

Oxidase	+
Catalase (done on slide or blood-free medium)	+
TSI, acid slant or butt	−
H_2S (TSI or SIM)	−
Acid from glucose (broth fermentation or OF medium)	−
Nitrate reduction	+
Motility (wet mount)	+
Growth in *Brucella* broth*	
at 25 C	−
at 35 C	+
at 42 C	+

Subcultures of the initial isolate will usually grow at 42 C in a candle jar. If agar media are incubated in room air, there will be no growth or very scant growth.

For further differentiation, see *Campylobacter*, Chapter 79.

• • •

SPECIMENS AND DATA FLOW: REQUISITIONS, RECORDS, REPORTS

While computerization has made some inroads in the microbiology laboratory,[247–248a] the great majority of hospital microbiology laboratories are still handling much of their data flow manually.

Requisition; presumptive and final reports. The physician's order, usually transcribed by ward clerk or nurse, is entered onto a microbiology laboratory requisition form. The form also includes information that may be of importance in performing the appropriate culture methods.

Two forms in use at the Jewish Hospital of St. Louis are shown in Fig. 75-11. The forms (on NCR multicopy forms) are also used as (a) a work card in the laboratory; (b) 1 copy is sent out as a presumptive (preliminary) result report; (c) the original serves as a final report; and (d) the last copy serves as the charge card. In this manner, transcription is held to a minimum and errors are minimized.

NOTE: The requisition requests information about the patient's demographic status, but it also asks for specimen source and nature (the word "pus" alone is not acceptable—source must be given), pertinent diagnosis (physician's suspicions or special requests are also entered here), listing of antibiotics patient is receiving, time of collection, and name of physician ordering test.

When the specimen, accompanied by requisition, arrives in the laboratory, it is usually registered in an acquisition (log) book and given a number.

Media and tests performed during the culture process are entered on **work card** (either requisition copy itself or separate work card) or workbook. **Presumptive** (preliminary) and **final** identifications are then placed on requisition (or a separate report form) and returned to patient's record.

An antimicrobial susceptibility (sensitivity) report form is shown in Fig. 75-12. The results are directly entered on the 3-part form; one part is sent to patient's chart, another is sent to data processing for monthly (or bimonthly) computer-generated summary, and the third part is retained in the laboratory file.

Copies of the reports are kept in the laboratory files for intervals usually prescribed by the government (anywhere from 2-7 years).

Emergency reports ("panic values"). In life-threatening test results it is imperative that the physician be notified immediately because the tests may indicate (1) an immediate hazard to the patient (e.g., meningitis), or (2) public health hazard or threat to other hospital patients or staff (e.g., salmonellosis).

A list ("panic list") modified from Duckworth[240] and in use in our laboratory, is shown in Table 75-7.

Note that the list is headed by positive blood cultures—all of which are immediately reported to physician, by telephone, as are the other findings on the list.

IDENTIFICATION OF BACTERIA

It is necessary to differentiate between **taxonomy, nomenclature,** and **identification.**[249] A

---

*If *Brucella* broth is not available, fluid thioglycollate medium may be substituted.

A

B

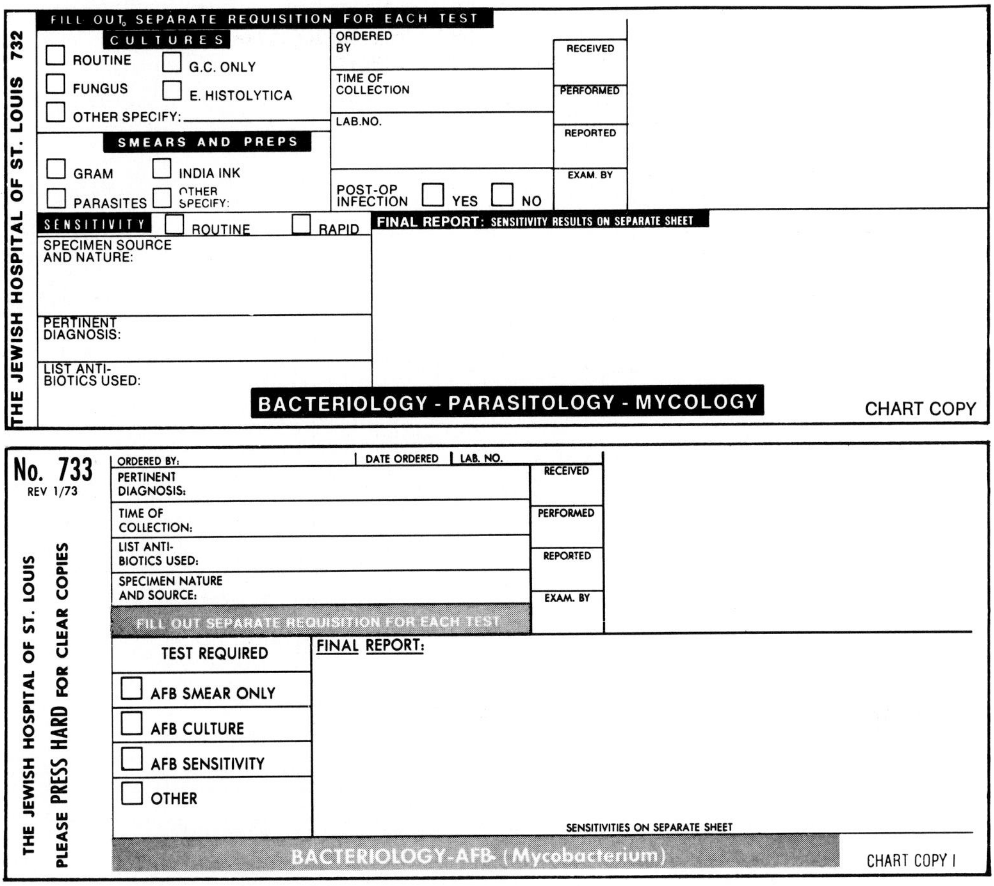

THE JEWISH HOSPITAL OF ST. LOUIS 732

FILL OUT SEPARATE REQUISITION FOR EACH TEST

CULTURES

☐ ROUTINE ☐ G.C. ONLY

☐ FUNGUS ☐ E. HISTOLYTICA

☐ OTHER SPECIFY:

SMEARS AND PREPS

☐ GRAM ☐ INDIA INK

☐ PARASITES ☐ OTHER SPECIFY:

SENSITIVITY ☐ ROUTINE ☐ RAPID

ORDERED BY

TIME OF COLLECTION

LAB.NO.

POST-OP INFECTION ☐ YES ☐ NO

RECEIVED

PERFORMED

REPORTED

EXAM. BY

FINAL REPORT: SENSITIVITY RESULTS ON SEPARATE SHEET

SPECIMEN SOURCE AND NATURE:

PERTINENT DIAGNOSIS:

LIST ANTIBIOTICS USED:

BACTERIOLOGY - PARASITOLOGY - MYCOLOGY

CHART COPY

No. 733

REV 1/73

THE JEWISH HOSPITAL OF ST. LOUIS

PLEASE PRESS HARD FOR CLEAR COPIES

ORDERED BY: | DATE ORDERED | LAB. NO.

PERTINENT DIAGNOSIS:

TIME OF COLLECTION:

LIST ANTIBIOTICS USED:

SPECIMEN NATURE AND SOURCE:

RECEIVED

PERFORMED

REPORTED

EXAM. BY

FILL OUT SEPARATE REQUISITION FOR EACH TEST

TEST REQUIRED

☐ AFB SMEAR ONLY

☐ AFB CULTURE

☐ AFB SENSITIVITY

☐ OTHER

FINAL REPORT:

SENSITIVITIES ON SEPARATE SHEET

BACTERIOLOGY-AFB- (Mycobacterium)

CHART COPY I

Fig. 75-11. Combined requisition and report forms used in Bacteriology Division of the Jewish Hospital, St. Louis. **A**, Bacteriology, parasitology, and mycology form. **B**, AFB (mycobacteriology) form. Size of form is 18.5 × 8 cm (7⅜ × 3¼ in); 1 original, 4 copies.

Table 75-7. Emergency reports ("panic list")

Finding	*Possible effect*
Positive blood culture	Septicemia
Any indication of *Clostridium* on wound culture	Septicemia, gangrene
Any positive cerebrospinal fluid, Gram stain or culture	Meningitis
Any positive TB smear or culture	Public health implications; nosocomial infection
Any positive *Salmonella, Shigella,* or *Yersinia* culture	Public health implications; nosocomial infection
Any positive **systemic** fungus culture	Sepsis, disseminated systemic mycoses
β-Hemolytic streptococci in all cultures	Rheumatic fever, rheumatism, heart disease, glomerulonephritis (group A, β-hemolytic); pediatric disease (group B)
Any positive joint, bone, pericardial, pleural, peritoneal, or thoracentesis fluid	Septic arthritis, pericarditis, empyema, peritonitis
All positive newborn cultures or nursery cultures of infants	Neonatal sepsis and death; nursery epidemics
Eye—*Pseudomonas, Staphylococcus aureus,* or pure culture of any organism	Serious eye damage or blindness
Any organism with unusual antimicrobial susceptibility	Resistance to treatment; nosocomial infections; public health implications
Any significant findings in nosocomial surveillance	Spread of nosocomial infection
Nosocomial infection	Spread of nosocomial infection

Modified from Duckworth, J. K.: Med. Lab. Obs. **9**:35, 1977.

THE JEWISH HOSPITAL OF ST. LOUIS – DIVISION OF MICROBIOLOGY
MICROBIAL SENSITIVITY REPORT

PATIENT _____ ROOM _____ PHYSICIAN _____ LAB. # _____

ADDRESS _____ PRELIM. REPORT _____ FINAL REPORT _____

EXAMINED BY _____ CHECKED BY _____

SPECIMEN OBTAINED: _____

SENSITIV. PERFORMED: _____ REPORTED: _____

SENSITIVITY REG.: _____ RAPID _____

TUBE DILUTION _____ DISK _____ MIXED FLORA TESTED _____

TUBE DILUTION SENSITIVITY		
Antimicrobial Agent	MIC ★	MBC ★★

★MIC – MIN. INHIB. CONC.   ★★MBC – MIN. BACTERIC. CONC.

I – INTERMEDIATE
R – RESISTANT
S – SENSITIVE

CODE	SPECIMEN	CODE	ORGANISM	CODE	ORGANISM	CODE	ANTIBIOTIC	RESULT
	Abd. Drain		To Be Identified:	51	Neisseria:	05	Ampicillin	
	Abd. fluid		Rod	51	sp.	07	Chloramphenicol	
	Abscess		Coccus	52	gonorrhoeae (G.C.)	09	Tetracycline	
	Amniotic fluid			53	Meningococcus	15	Cephalothin	
	Bile	29	Acinetobacter calcoaceticus var. anitratus (Herellea)	55	Pasteurella:	17	Penicillin	
	Blood					19	Methicillin	
	Bone Marrow	30	Acinetobacter calcoaceticus var. Iwoffi (Mima)	04	Proteus:	49	Clindamycin	
	Bronch. Wash			06	P. morganii	23	Erythromycin	
	Burnsite	31	Aerococcus	06	P. vulgaris	29	Gentamicin	
	Cervix	32	Achromobacter sp.	05	P. mirabilis	53	Tobramycin	
	Conjunctiva	33	Arizona	12	Providencia	51	Trimethoprim/ — Sulfamethoxazole	
	Cornea	34	Aeromonas					
	C S F	35	Alcaligenes	13	Pseudomonas aerug.	03	Sulfisoxazole	
	Ear	36	Bacillus sp.	14	Pseudomonas sp.:	25	Nitrofurantoin	
	Eye	37	Bacteroides			27	Nalidixic Acid	
	Fistula			09	Salmonella	31	Carbenicillin	
	Lochia	39	Brucella		group:	37	Ticarcillin	
	Lymph Node	08	Citrobacter	10	Serratia	55	Amikacin	
	Nail	26	Clostridium perfr.	11	Shigella	13	Kanamycin	
	Nasal Sinus	27	Clostridium sp.:		group:	59	Cefamandole	
	Nasoph. Swab			16	Staph. aureus (coag pos.)	61	Cefoxitin	
	Nose	40	Corynebacterium:	17	Staph. epiderm.(coag.neg.)	01	Colistin	
	Pharynx			19	Strep., beta hem., gr. A	47	Polymyxin B	
	Pericardial fluid	01	E. coli			35	Nafcillin	
	Peritoneal Fluid	02	Enterobacter:	19	Strep., beta hem., non-A	37	Oxacillin	
	Pleural Fluid					39	Cloxacillin	
	Rectal Swab			19	Strep. beta hem. gr.:	41	Dicloxacillin	
	Skin					43	Vancomycin	
	Sputum	41	Edwardsiella	20	Enterococcus ("S. Faecalis"–gr. D Strep Enterococc.)	45	Cephaloridine	
	Stool	42	Flavobacterium			21	Lincomycin	
	Throat	43	Fusobacterium (incl. B. fundulif.)	21	Strep. alpha (viridans)	11	Streptomycin	
	Trach. Aspir.					33	Neomycin	
	Urethra	44	Haemophilus:	22	Streptococcus pneumoniae (pneumococcus)			
	Urine Cath.							
	Urine CVS	45	Haemoph. vagin.	23	Strep. anaerob.			
	Urine-Kidney	03	Klebsiella	23	Cocci., anaerob.			
	Ulcer			24	Strep. gr. D. (non-enterococc.)			
	Uterine Cult.	47	Listeria					
	Vaginal Swab	48	Micrococcus	25	Capnophilic Streptococcus (CO₂ Depend)			
	Wound	49	Moraxella:					
	Hand - - Finger - - Wrist			57	Escherichia sp.			
	Thigh - - Foot - - Toe			59	Yersinia enterocolitica			
	Appendix							
				61	Yersinia, other			

For Details of Culture Results,
See
Regular Bacteriology Report Form.

Form 343-001   Rev. 3/79   MICROBIAL SENSITIVITY REPORT

WHITE: CHART
PINK: LAB.
YELLOW: E.D.P.

Fig. 75-12. Antimicrobial sensitivity report used in the Microbiology Division of the Jewish Hospital, St. Louis. Size of form is 21 × 27 cm (8 × 11 in); original, to chart; first copy, to laboratory; second copy, to computer.

taxonomic scheme is a system of classification that can be established for a group of related organisms, using any kind of designation (places, names, numerals, letters of alphabet, etc.) for the different serologic types, biotypes, etc. that make up the group. Nomenclature is concerned with naming the units with the correct specific names that are subject to certain internationally accepted rules (International Code of Nomencla-

ture of Bacteria and Viruses). Identification of an unknown isolate requires determination of certain of its characteristics and the comparison of these with characteristics of known bacteria. In this manner it is possible to identify the unknown with one of the known organisms and state that it is different from all other knowns (Cowan and Steel[249]). Once identified, it then can be given its proper name, depending on the classification adopted. The usual and most logical procedure for identification is to determine a certain number of major characteristics and then to perform certain additional tests to lead to the identification of the unknown. The kinds and numbers of tests to be performed, of course, depend on available information based on knowledge of classification and nomenclature. The nomenclature and classification used in this text is based, to a considerable extent, on the eighth edition of *Bergey's Manual of Determinative Bacteriology*.[250]

However, considerable effort has been made to list synonyms for many species or genera and to use classification systems developed in the years after publication of the eighth edition of *Bergey's Manual* and to point out evidence available for reclassifying or regrouping certain organisms. Both taxonomy and nomenclature are subject to change; new evidence of biochemical, physiologic, and other characteristics, sometimes subject to many differences of opinion among expert workers, are used for making such changes. The identity of an organism must be judged by the **spectrum** of its biochemical and physiologic properties and not by a single characteristic. From the practical point of view, the major and overriding concern is the use of **essential tests** and the delimitation of a manageable number of such tests to allow for identification **within a reasonable time and with accuracy.**

In the clinical laboratory a large number of bacteria isolated are usually of the "routine" variety, so called because they are seen quite often. Their characteristics are rather familiar and can usually be identified rapidly and without difficulty. For purposes of identification, certain tests and characteristics can be given more weight than others if they have important differential value: the urease and phenylalanine deaminase tests in the case of *Proteus-Providencia* organisms, the coagulase test for staphylococci, etc. (Cowan and Steel[249]). Others are "nonroutine," i.e., are seen less often and require considerably more tests for accurate identification. The mark of a good worker and reliable laboratory is the extent to which unusual organisms are recognized as "not fitting" the definition of frequently seen organisms, the willingness to undertake further work for identification, and the conscientiousness displayed in submitting such unusual organisms to reference laboratories equipped for accurate identification (State Health Departments or the Center for Disease Control, which accepts cultures submitted through the state departments).

Considerable controversy, not yet resolved, accompanies any discussion of the scope and depth of bacterial identification, e.g., to what extent one should identify an isolate in terms of genus, species, or variety. Also, should all organisms isolated from a clinical specimen be identified?

This writer agrees with Steel's[251] statement: "In identification, speed is imperative and sec-ond only in importance to accuracy." It is more useful to report **rapidly** that a gram-negative rod, sensitive to certain antibiotics and resistant to others, has been isolated (from a clinically significant site such as blood or spinal fluid) than to delay the report until exact identification of the organism can be provided. In my laboratory this practice is followed (emergency, presumptive, or preliminary report) with accurate identification following the original report.

In addition, is is most important to be familiar with the normal or indigenous biota (flora) of ordinarily nonsterile body sites; for instance, greening streptococci and neisseriae are normally present in the throat and need not be further identified. However, β-hemolytic streptococci from the same site should be further characterized as to their antigenic group. Whenever organisms involved in transmissible and notifiable infectious disease are encountered, definitive identification should be made; also, when "nonroutine" organisms, which do not conform to the characteristics established for "routine" organisms, are encountered, accurate identification should be attempted. Many instances of infections due to "opportunist" or "nonpathogenic" organisms have been established because definitive identification was performed.

In the past few years the debate about the scope and depth of bacterial identification, cost benefits and priorities, evaluation of specimen quality, and in general, the constraints under which the microbiology laboratory is functioning, have been explored, among others, by Bartlett,[252,253] the College of American Pathologists,[254] Balows,[255] Kunz,[248] and Sonnenwirth.[1]

Despite the widely divergent views, it is now generally agreed that the following are needed:

1. Criteria for rejection of specimens (e.g., quality of sputum, number of types of organisms in a given urine specimen). Do **not** throw away any specimen until discussed with physician!

2. Consensus on extent of identification.

Finegold et al.[89] lean heavily toward definitive identification; it is also necessary to remember that level of testing and of sophistication in identification depends on size of laboratory and availability of manpower, equipment, and reagents.[1] Still, **any** laboratory claiming to do clinical microbiology testing must have the capability for detecting and isolating as well as presumptively identifying the more common organisms, or it must know when and how to refer specimens or cultures for the benefit of the patient.

Mutation, variation, and dissociation

The laboratory worker attempting to identify bacteria must be familiar with certain changes that may occur during the cultivation and isolation of bacteria in the laboratory and with the steps to be undertaken to minimize or reverse such changes.

The repeated transfer, on artificial media, of a

pure bacterial culture may result in the appearance of a mixture of colony types with various new properties. The emergence of such colonies is due to 2 processes, common to all living organisms: **mutation** and **selection** (new genotypes), and **phenotypic variation,** e.g., physiologic adaptation. The appearance of a **rare** mutant (new genotype) may result in its selection, i.e., it will grow faster than the parent strain. Phenotypic variation, on the other hand, usually involves all the cells in the culture.

Many of the inheritable changes occurring in bacteria are **adaptations,** e.g., increased ability to fit in a new environment. Antibiotic-resistant mutants, selected during growth in the presence of the antibiotic, are a typical example of genetic adaptation. **Dissociation,** on the other hand, is a term applied to the appearance of a new kind of colony type, without any obvious adaptive advantage. Changes occurring as the result of dissociation may so extensively alter cultural and other characteristics as to deprive the culture of its usefulness in the diagnostic laboratory. One of the best known changes is the S→R dissociation. This involves the disappearance of the original, virulent, smooth (S) colony isolate and appearance of the rough (R) type.

Smooth (S) colonies, among pneumococci and salmonellae, possess a specific surface antigen and are virulent. Avirulent mutants, which lack such antigen(s), are rough. The smooth pneumococcus colony is associated with the possession of a capsule; loss of the capsule results in transition to the rough (R) form. The smooth cells of certain Enterobacteriaceae will form a mucoid (M) colony if a capsule is produced.

Other alterations may include loss of type-specific antigen, phase variations, e.g., a shift from 1 antigenic type (phase 1) to another (phase 2), and changes in biochemical reactions (fermentations, pigment formation, etc.). Biochemical mutants may appear among cells on an inoculated plate; the emergence of a mutant progeny within a single colony (mutant subclone) is shown by the appearance of a **sectored** colony when grown on differential media. **Papillae** may appear in nonfermenting colonies after prolonged incubation; these are fermenting mutants arising after prolonged growth of the colony.

Dissociation occurring in a stock culture may give rise to an occasional R-type colony or may produce a culture that is predominantly R-type with no S-type colony or only an occasional one. Furthermore, individual colonies may show different degrees of roughness, which are designated RS or SR.

Once a culture has dissociated to the R type it is difficult and sometimes impossible to induce the reverse change, R → S. One should attempt to find S colonies by plating the culture and examining under the dissecting microscope (see next paragraph). Any S colonies found may then be transferred to fresh media, replated, and resected until the culture is again in a stable,

smooth state. Under certain circumstances this can be done with the aid of anti-R sera to suppress the rough forms.

The appearance of colonies is best studied using a low-power microscope with oblique illumination, which may be achieved by placing the mirror on the table top between the microscope and the illuminating lamp. The lamp is then directed at the mirror, and the latter is so placed that the beam of light reaches the microscope stage at an angle, or a hand-held magnifier can be used. Under these conditions, differences between S, R, and RS (partly rough) colonies are accentuated. When difficulty is experienced in identifying R-types by appearance, advantage may be taken of the fact that R cells agglutinate more readily in saline or in 1:1000 **acriflavine** than do the S-type cells. Kauffman states, with reference to the Enterobacteriaceae, that none of these criteria is entirely reliable.

S → R dissociation may be avoided by the following:

1. Careful selection of S-type colonies each time a subculture is made
2. Infrequent subcultures
3. Growth of stock cultures on carbohydrate-poor media
4. Storage of stock cultures, after preliminary incubation at 37 C, in the refrigerator at 5 C
5. Lyophilization (the most satisfactory method) or freezing

It should be emphasized that the "normal" form is characteristic of each species. In certain cases, e.g., *B. anthracis* and many clostridia, R-types are normal and S-types are atypical.

Many other dissociations have been described, such as H → O (motile to nonmotile), V → W (loss of Vi antigen in *S. typhi* and certain other *Salmonella* species), appearance of P (phantom), M (mucoid), and D (dwarf) colonies. In addition, there are changes in antigenic, nutritional, and biochemical characteristics that are not accompanied by changes in colony morphology. When one desires to suppress dissociation, he should take steps to reduce the rate of multiplication and hence the possibility for mutation. At the same time one should be familiar with the normal colony form of each organism and be able to select it from among a number of mutants.

Identification procedures

The identification of bacteria is accomplished using the following criteria and procedures.

Cultural characteristics. Growth on primary cultures affords important clues to the rapid recognition (and often presumptive identification) of many frequently encountered bacteria by taking into account (1) colonial morphology (see Fig. 75-13), (2) growth on simple, complex, differential, or selective media, (3) growth rate, (4) aerobic or anaerobic growth, and (5) microscopic characteristics such as staining properties, Gram stain, acid-fastness, shape—rod or coccus, and size.

Gram stain. When performed carefully, a Gram stain can assign the organism to either 1 of 2 groups: the

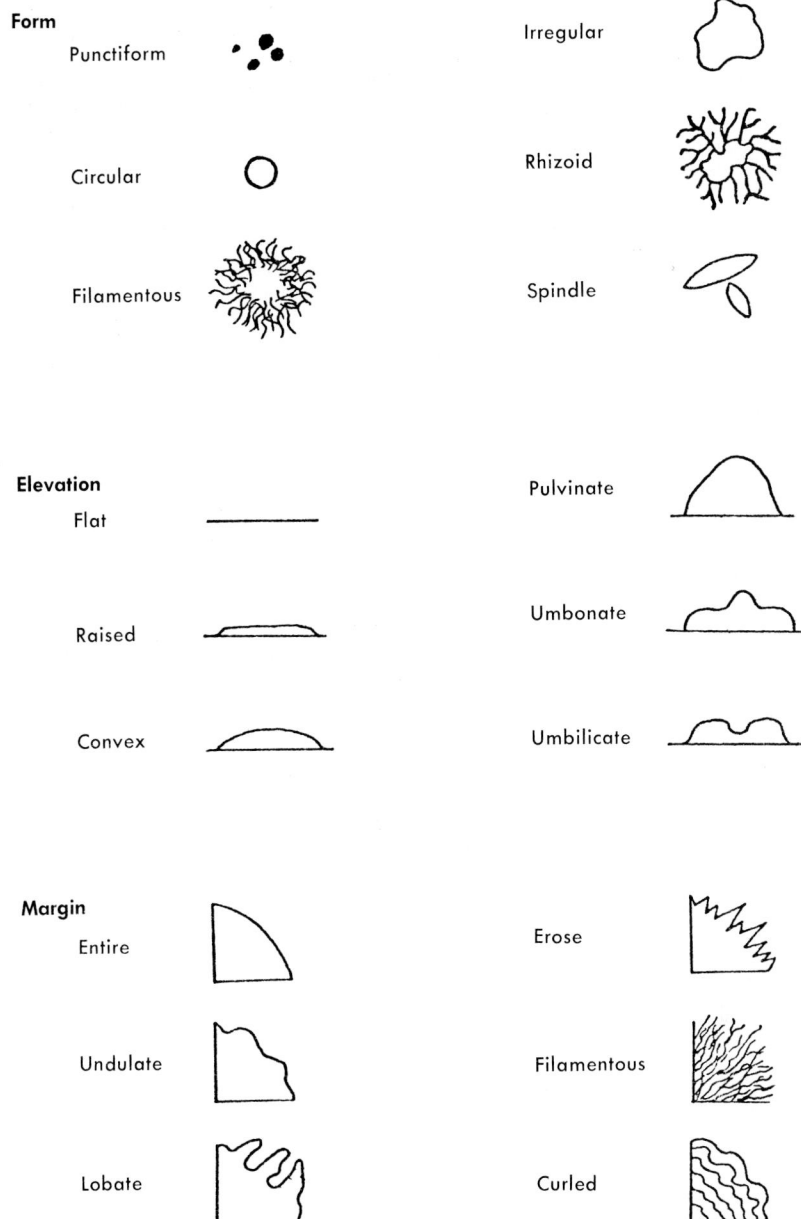

Fig. 75-13. Colony characteristics and description of bacterial colonies.

gram-positive or gram-negative. It should be remembered that age affects the staining: gram-positive organisms tend to lose this characteristic as they age. Use young cultures, preferably 24 h old or younger (see "cellular morphology," below).

Acid fastness. This is characteristic of mycobacteria and of some nocardiae.

Colony characteristics

1. Colony surface: smooth, rough, rugose (wrinkled), contoured (an irregular, smoothly undulating surface like that of a relief map), granular (fine, medium, coarse), papillate, dull, glistening
2. Optical characteristics
   a. Opaque: not allowing light to pass through
   b. Translucent: allowing light to pass through without allowing complete visibility of objects seen through colony
   c. Opalescent: resembling color of an opal
   d. Iridescent: exhibiting changing rainbow colors in reflected light
   e. Dull: not glossy or glistening
   f. Glistening: glossy, not dull
3. Consistency
   a. Butyrous: growth of butterlike consistency
   b. Viscid: growth follows needle when touched and withdrawn
   c. Membranous: growth thin, coherent, like a membrane

d. Brittle: growth dry, friable under platinum needle
4. Emulsifiability: homogenous, granular or membranous suspension
5. Pigmentation of growth: white, buff, light yellow, straw yellow, deep yellow, pink, red, etc.

Growth characteristic on heart infusion agar slant
1. Degree of growth*: very light, light, moderate, heavy
2. Color: soluble and nonwater soluble pigments
3. Opacity: translucent, semiopaque, opaque
4. Growth: moist, wet, dry, dull, glistening, wrinkled, runny, confluent

Growth characteristics in heart infusion broth
1. Degree of growth*: very light, light, moderate, heavy
2. Turbidity: uniform, granular, homogenous
3. Pellicle: ring, surface
4. Sediment: smooth, rough, granular, flocculent, stringy or ropey (sediment on shaking rises as coherent swirl)

Cellular morphology (stained)
1. Shape: cocci, coccoid, coccoid-bacillary, filaments, commas, spirals, pleomorphic, rods, etc.
2. Axis: straight or curved
3. Size
   a. *Overall:* minute, small, medium, large
   b. *Length:* short, medium, long, filaments
   c. *Breadth:* thin, medium, thick
4. Sides: parallel, ovoid (bulging), concave, irregular
5. End: rounded, truncate, concave, pointed, feathery
6. Arrangement: singly, pairs, chains, tetrads, palisading, groups, clusters, packets, chinese letters, etc.
7. Pleomorphic forms: variation in size and shape, clubs, citron, filamentous, branched, fusiform, giant swollen forms, shadow forms
8. Spores: central, terminal, subterminal, round, oval, swelling or not swelling the rod
9. Staining (Gram): negative, positive, variable; evenly, irregularly, unipolar, bipolar, beaded, barred, variation in depth, granules

Biochemical and physiologic characteristics
Some of the primary criteria and tests useful for identification are listed below; for details, see Chapter 72.

Motility. Perform hanging-drop or dark-field examination; or, preferably, inoculate semisolid motility agar.

Catalase test. This is an important and easily performed procedure. It cannot be performed on colonies grown on blood-containing media.

Oxidase test. This is an important test used for identification of neisseriae and for separation of gram-negative (aerobic and facultative) rods. It can be performed either by flooding portion of a plate with the reagent, mixing colony portion with reagent, by the use of oxidase test papers, or by the Ewing-Johnson modification (cytochrome oxidase test, also known as the indophenol oxidase test).

Bile solubility plate test. This can be used for the rapid differentiation of pneumococci (soluble) from greening streptococci (insoluble).

Optochin. Optochin inhibition also differentiates pneumococci.

Carbohydrate utilization. **Fermentation vs. oxidation.** The oxidation-fermentation (OF) test is a most important step in the preliminary identification of many organisms that are not obvious fermenters ("late fermenters" or nonfermenters). Among the aerobic gram-negative rods the Enterobacteriaceae, *Pasteurella* sp., *Aeromonas* sp., *Vibrio,* and *Actinobacillus* sp., are fermentative, whereas *Pseudomonas* sp., *Flavobacterium* sp., and *Herellea* sp. are oxidative (utilization of glucose). Certain other organisms are neither glucose oxidizers nor fermenters (see Chapter 72).

Coagulase test. This is used for characterization of staphylococci.

Other tests such as phenylalanine deaminase, urease, H_2S production, citrate utilization, indole production, decarboxylases, and the Voges-Proskauer test are very useful for characterization of gram-negative rods and other organisms. Several of these can be performed rapidly by using various test papers, microtechnics, or multiple test systems.

A number of other tests are utilized for definitive identification and are discussed in the following chapters.

Hemolysis: *Reactions on blood agar.** Hemolytic reactions and colony morphology usually are determined on primary plates. If not possible (mixed culture, etc.) or not done, the culture to be identified should be plated on a blood agar plate containing 5% defibrinated **rabbit** or **sheep** blood. The tables on identification of unusual pathogenic gram-negative rods (see Chapter 79) are based on the use of rabbit blood, and there may be some minor differences in hemolytic reactions between the 2 types of blood.

Streak blood agar plate carefully to obtain well-isolated colonies. Stab agar several times with edge of loop while streaking plate to produce some reduced oxygen tension, which may enhance hemolysis reactions. Incubate plate overnight at 35-37 C.

Besides the well-known α (alpha) and β (beta) hemolysis (see Streptococci, Chapter 76), there are other hemolytic reactions that seem to be fairly consistent for many different species of bacteria. These reactions are rather difficult to describe, and the factors producing them are not known.

1. β-**hemolysis** is the same as that described for the streptococci, except that the total destruction of all red cells within the hemolytic area is not important as for the streptococci. Some organisms show little hemolysis surrounding individual colonies, but show marked hemolysis in the stabs. For example, *Listeria monocytogenes* will show very weak hemolytic action under the streaks and usually none at all under isolated colonies. In the stabs this organism will show a very distinct, narrow, clear zone of β-hemolysis at 24 h. Other organisms show a well-defined zone of hemolysis extending out from the heavy portion of the streak. β-Hemolysis usually has a very sharp and well-defined edge. The zones in this case seem to be devoid of hemoglobin and appear colorless. A typical exception to this would be *Haemophilus vaginalis,* which, after 3 to 4 d incubation under 5% CO_2 would show wide but incomplete zones of β-hemolysis. Even on prolonged incubation the hemolytic action would never become completely clear nor would the edge of the zone become well defined.

Though the terms "alpha," "alpha prime," and

---

*Degree of growth: dysgonic = very light growth; eugonic = moderate to heavy growth.

*From Laboratory methods in special medical bacteriology—techniques, Atlanta, June 1976 (reprinted Jan. 1977), Bacteriology Training Branch, Center for Disease Control.

"beta" have been worked out with exactitude for the streptococci, the same terms may be adapted to the action of other organisms with perhaps less stringent rules.

2. **Lysis:** The term lysis is used when the red blood cells have been lysed but the hemoglobin has not been decolorized (destroyed) as in the β-hemolysis. The edge of the zone here is not well defined. Some organisms may lyse the whole area of the plate; some may produce lysis only under the heavy portion of the streak. Well-isolated colonies never show any action on the blood.

3. **Greenish lysis:** Same general action as with lysis, except the lysed area has a greenish tinge.

4. **α-Hemolysis:** Pronounced greening under heavy growth and around well-isolated colonies, usually without a lysed area. Some organisms show this only on prolonged incubation. These usually show α-hemolysis around stabs and faintly under heavy growth in 24 h. These organisms usually, but not always, grow very lightly. There is no lysis of red cells.

5. **Browning of blood:** Blood turns dark brown and completely opaque under heaviest growth. Well-isolated colonies of some strains may show α-hemolysis.

6. **Lavender-green (L-G):** This reaction is shown only by very proteolytic organisms. Plate is usually completely lysed, and under areas of heavy growth, blood agar shows lavender and green colorations. Typical examples for this type of reaction can be seen by proteolytic organisms such as *Pseudomonas aeruginosa, Pseudomonas maltophilia, Aeromonas hydrophila, Serratia marcescens, Flavobacterium meningosepticum*, etc.

7. **Brown pigments** may be formed that differ from browning of blood. Blood remains clear, and clear brown pigment diffuses from heavy portions of growth.

8. **Zones of inhibition of lysis:** Some organisms will exhibit unusual effect where blood immediately surrounding isolated colony is unchanged by zone of lysis that occurs outside this protected area.

9. **Compacted cells:** A characteristic of several organisms is seen where well-isolated colony has very narrow zone of lysis immediately surrounding colony and, beyond this, "compacted" and narrow, dense band of red cells.

10. **No action on blood:** Blood agar plate remains unchanged.

Serologic identification. Use known antisera to identify unknown isolate.

Pathogenicity (virulence) tests

Information gained by use of some or all the foregoing principles allows placing the unknown organism into a known family or genus; by further use of certain tests it can then be identified as to species, after comparing results of the tests with characteristics of already known genera or species. This can be done by using a dichotomous key, such as Skerman's *A Guide to the Identification of the Genera of Bacteria*,[256] which poses a series of questions (characteristics) answerable in the affirmative or negative. For clinical work the dichotomous key is not very suitable because its use is laborious and time

consuming. Instead, various flow charts and tables are used extensively for listing essential characters and also variable reactions, thus allowing rapid scanning of available information. For example, Cowan and Steel[249] use diagnostic tables that employ the step-by-step or progressive method in which a few fundamental characters are first determined (first-stage tables). Afterward, a number of additional tests are performed, listed in additional second- or sometimes third-stage tables. Others employ punch card sorting systems by transferring characteristics of a genus or species, as described in reference sources, to master cards that are then compared with a card (or cards) bearing the characteristics and reactions of the unknown organism (see Schneierson and Amsterdam[257]). Olds[258] devised an information sorter that allows rapid sorting of essential information recorded for a certain number of medically important organisms and its comparison with information obtained about an unknown isolate. Attempts were made by Dybowski et al.[259] to use a computer for bacteriologic diagnosis.

For a comprehensive review of attempts to use the computer for classification and identification, see Krichevsky,[260]; also see Friedman et al.[261]

In this chapter (see below) 2 guides are used to allow preliminary and presumptive placement of an unknown isolate into a larger group (genus or family) and to indicate the selected characteristics and reactions most likely to be useful for its identification. Detailed tables and descriptions listing the reactions of various families, genera, and certain species (included in the specific headings for each group of organisms) are to be consulted for definitive identification. If necessary, use also the most recent edition of *Bergey's Manual of Determinative Bacteriology*.

Initial steps for identification

The importance of **pure culture** usage cannot be overemphasized. It is practically impossible to correctly identify mixed cultures. When "fishing" (picking) colonies for various tests, it is absolutely essential that extreme care be exercised in obtaining material from well-isolated **single** colonies. For inexperienced workers it is recommended that at all steps (fermentation tests, etc.) a control plate be streaked with the inoculum used for the various tests to check for purity.

The **initial steps** for identification of bacteria are as follows:

1. Examine isolated colonies on primary overnight plate cultures, preferably with hand lens by reflected and transmitted light. Note number of colonies; record any distinctive features, hemolysis, spreading if any, pigment formation, colony characteristics, and ascertain whether one or more types of colonies are present.

2. Pick a single colony of each type, make Gram stains of them, and examine under microscope. It should be remembered that the morphology of bacterial cells is not absolutely constant and that their microscopic appearance can be altered by

slight changes in the composition of the medium in which they are grown. Organisms seen in infected body fluids may look different when cultured on blood agar.

After Gram staining, transfer remains of colony examined, **or another exactly like it,** into medium that is likely to give good growth for further tests.

3. Examine liquid media, tubes or flasks, and note whether turbid; some organisms will grow throughout medium, giving even turbidity. Others grow mainly in bottom of tube and sediment can be noted. Pellicle formation and granular growth should be noted. Make Gram stain of loopful of culture. Always make subcultures on plates from liquid media.

Mixed cultures. Occasionally plate cultures may be overgrown by spreading gram-negative organisms (*Proteus* sp.) that may interfere with isolation of gram-

positive organisms. In broth cultures both gram-positive and gram-negative organisms may be present, and it may be necessary to isolate them separately since both kinds usually will grow on blood agar cultures.

Isolation of gram-negative organisms that grow well on ordinary media: Broth culture or mixed culture from plate should be streaked on EMB, MacConkey, or deoxycholate agar plates. Enteric organisms will grow well, whereas most gram-positive organisms will be inhibited. Spreading of *Proteus* may be inhibited by raising agar content of blood plates to 5% or by using Naylor medium (Lemco medium)[262] that has proved satisfactory. It has the advantage of containing no inhibitory substances and allows the growth of all but the most fastidious pathogens.

Separation of gram-positive cocci from gram-negative organisms: Potassium tellurite, sodium azide, and phenylethyl alcohol are very helpful in separating

Table 75-8. Growth on primary plate cultures*

Blood agar (aerobic) after overnight incubation			
Colonies 1 mm or more in diameter		2. No growth on MacConkey medium‡	Group A (β-hemolytic) streptococci
Gram positive cocci	Staphylococci		*S. pneumoniae* (pneumococcus)
	Micrococci		*Streptococcus viridans*
	(Streptococci)	Gram-positive cocci in clumps	(Staphylococci)
Gram-negative cocci	*Neisseria*		Micrococci
Gram-positive rods	*Corynebacterium*	Gram-negative cocci	*Neisseria*
	Bacillus	Gram-positive rods	*Corynebacterium*
Gram-negative rods			*Lactobacillus*
1. Growth on MacConkey agar	Enterobacteriaceae including *Yersinia; Aeromonas, Vibrio, Flavobacterium, Acinetobacter*		*Nocardia*
			Erysipelothrix
			Listeria
	Pseudomonas (Brucella, Pasteurella, Actinobacillus)		
2. No growth on MacConkey agar‡	*(P. multocida,* few other *Pasteurella* sp., *Haemophilus)*	Gram-negative rods	*Haemophilus*
			Brucella†
			Pasteurella†
			Bordetella†
Colonies less than 1 mm in diameter			
Gram-positive cocci in pairs or chains (short)			
1. Growth on MacConkey medium	Enterococci *(Streptococcus* group D)		
	Streptococci of groups B, C, G		

Blood agar (anaerobic +10% CO_2) after overnight incubation (no equivalent growth on aerobic culture)			
Colonies about 1 mm or spreading		Gram-positive rods	*Lactobacillus*
Gram-positive rods	*Clostridium*		*Corynebacterium*
Colonies minute§			*Actinomyces*
Gram-positive cocci	Anaerobic streptococci		*Eubacterium*
	Anaerobic micrococci	Gram-negative rods	*Bacteroides*‖
Gram-negative cocci	*Veillonella*		*Fusobacterium*

*Modified from Stokes, E. J.: Clinical bacteriology, ed. 3, London, 1968, Edward Arnold, Ltd.
†These organisms often require special media and conditions for primary isolation; occasionally they will grow on the media shown above. *Brucella abortus* does not grow on primary isolation without CO_2; *Francisella tularensis* usually does not grow on ordinary media; *P. multocida* does not grow on MacConkey agar.
‡No growth on MacConkey agar: sensitive to bile salts.
§Many of these small colonies fail to appear for several days. Some may prove to be microaerophilic, not true anaerobes.
‖Occasionally 1 mm or larger.

Table 75-9. A simplified guide to the presumptive recognition of common groups of bacteria*

1. Aerobic cultures
   A. Gram-positive cocci
      1. Catalase positive
         a. Arranged in clusters, large colonies: *Staphylococcus* (perform coagulase test); dextrose fermented anaerobically
         b. In pairs, fours, or small clusters; use dextrose oxidatively or not at all: *Micrococcus*
      2. Catalase negative
         a. Short and long chains and even pairs; fermentative (anaerobic) utilization of sugars: *Streptococcus*
            NOTE: β-hemolytic streptococci may belong to pyogenes or enterococcus group; α-hemolytic streptococci may belong to viridans or enterococcus group; nonhemolytic streptococci (γ) may be viridans or enterococcus group
            (1) Pyogenes group: Usually, but not always, β-hemolysis; do not grow at 45 C; do not survive 30 min at 60 C; serologic groups A, B, C, F, G, H, K, L, M, O; Lancefield grouping or fluorescent antibody technic; most group A strains sensitive to bacitracin
            (2) Viridans group: α-hemolysis or none; not soluble in bile; not inhibited by Optochin; usually grow at 45 C (*Aerococcus* group of Cowan and Steel[249] included here)
            (3) Enterococcus group: Some β-hemolytic, others α- or γ-; grow in 0.1% methylene blue milk, in 6.5% NaCl, and at pH 9.6; grow at 45 C and survive 30 min at 60 C; usually grow on MacConkey agar; bile-esculin positive
            (4) Usually lancet shaped, pairs, single or short chains, bile soluble, inhibited by Optochin, α-hemolysis, no growth at 45 C, virulent for mouse: Pneumococci (*Streptococcus pneumoniae*)
         b. Primarily clumps and tetrads, no acid from dextrose anaerobically: *Aerococcus*
   B. Gram-negative cocci, mostly in pairs
      1. *Neisseria* (**all oxidase positive**)
         a. No growth at 22 C or on nutrient agar; growth on modified Thayer-Martin agar (MTM)
            (1) Requires enriched medium, acid from dextrose and maltose; agglutination by antimeningococcal serum: *N. meningitidis*
            (2) Requires enriched medium, acid from dextrose only: *N. gonorrhoeae*
         b. Growth on MTM; ferments glucose, maltose, and **lactose**: *N. lactamicus*
         c. Growth at 22 C and on nutrient agar; light inoculum yields no growth on MTM
            (3) Grows on ordinary media, no acid from dextrose, maltose, sucrose, or lactose: *N. (Branhamella) catarrhalis*
            (4) Yellow pigment, no acid from dextrose, maltose, sucrose, or lactose: *N. flavescens*
            (5) Grow well on ordinary media; acid from dextrose and maltose; Pharyngeal group
      2. Rule out *Acinetobacter* (former *Mima-Herellea* group, *Achromobacter, B. anitratum*) (see *C, 1, e*)
   C. Gram-negative rods
      1. Grow well on ordinary media, including MacConkey agar[†]
         a. **Fermentative,[‡] oxidase negative,[§]** nitrate reduced to nitrite
            (1) Lactose usually fermented,[‖] phenylalanine deaminase not produced
               (a) Voges-Proskauer, citrate, urease, and H₂S negative, indole and methyl red positive: *Escherichia*
               (b) V-P and citrate positive, grow in KCN, indole negative, urease positive or delayed, motile: *Enterobacter;* nonmotile: *Klebsiella*
               (c) H₂S and citrate positive, lysine decarboxylase not produced, V-P, urease, and indole negative, grows in KCN: *Citrobacter*
               (d) Lysine decarboxylase and H₂S produced, malonate positive, no growth in KCN, lactose prompt or delayed: *Arizona* (use specific antisera)
            (2) Lactose usually not fermented,[‖] phenylalanine deaminase not produced
               (a) H₂S, citrate, and lysine decarboxylase positive, indole, V-P, urease, and KCN negative: *Salmonella* (exceptions—no gas, little H₂S: *S. typhi* and others) (use specific antisera); β-galactosidase and malonate positive: *Arizona*
               (b) H₂S, citrate, V-P, and urease negative, nonmotile, usually no gas; *Shigella* (or nonmotile *Escherichia*); some *Shigella* sp. ferment lactose slowly
               (c) V-P and citrate positive, urease delayed positive, motile, pigment often formed, especially at room temperature: *Serratia*
               (d) H₂S, indole, lysine, and methyl red positive; urease, V-P, citrate, and KCN negative; most sugars (except glucose and maltose) not fermented: *Edwardsiella*

---

*Based on data from Buchanan and Gibbons,[250] Cowan and Steel,[249] Edwards and Ewing,[196, 223–226] Kalz,[263] Weaver et al.,[264] Weaver,[265] and Brenner et al.[266]

†Some do not grow on MacConkey agar; exceptions listed.

‡O-F medium; fermentation observable in TSI medium.

§Cytochrome (indophenol) oxidase test.

‖Lactose is valuable in the case of prompt fermenters (on differential plates overnight or in 24-48 hr in fermentation media); some strains of the groups listed show delayed or no fermentation of lactose. See Enterobacteriaceae.

¶Usually no change in TSI medium or on carbohydrate-containing differential plate media.

Continued.

Table 75-9. A simplified guide to the presumptive recognition of common groups of bacteria—cont'd

(3) Phenylalanine deaminase produced
  (a) Urease positive: *Proteus*
    (i) H$_2$S positive, indole positive: *P. vulgaris*
    (ii) H$_2$S positive, indole negative: *P. mirabilis*
    (iii) H$_2$S negative, citrate negative: *P. (Morganella)*[266] *morganii*
    (iv) H$_2$S negative, citrate positive: *P. (Providencia)*[266] *rettgeri*
  (b) Urease negative: *Providencia*
b. **Fermentative, oxidase negative,** growth on MacConkey, usually on SS (exceptions); motile at 20 to 25 C but not 35 C; urease positive, phenylalanine negative: *Yersinia pseudotuberculosis, Yersinia enterocolitica*
c. **Fermentative, oxidase positive**
  (1) Catalase positive, nitrate reduced, usually motile, arginine dehydrolase produced: *Aeromonas*
  (2) Cells spiral or comma shaped, motile, fermentative, lysine and ornithine decarboxylase produced: *Vibrio* (identify *V. cholerae* with specific antisera, biochemical tests); *V. parahaemolyticus*
  (3) **No growth on MacConkey:** See *Pasteurella (multocida, urea, etc.); Cardiobacterium*
  (4) Grows on MacConkey: *Pasteurella haemolytica*
d. **Oxidative utilization of sugars** (OF medium, no fermentation)¶
  (1) Oxidase positive, no gas, motile, **grow on MacConkey,** SS, and cetrimide agar, many have soluble pigments (green or yellow): *Pseudomonas* spp.
  (2) Oxidase positive (or variable), **growth variable on MacConkey agar,** oxidative or no utilization of sugars, yellow pigment, no reduction of nitrate: *Flavobacterium*
  (3) Oxidase negative, grow on MacConkey agar, malonate negative, nonmotile, no reduction of nitrate, no decarboxylases, 10% lactose, citrate positive, majority lactose positive: *Acinetobacter* (other former names and groups: *Achromobacter anitratus, B. anitratus, Mima-Herellea* group)
  (4) **No growth on MacConkey agar,** oxidase negative: *Pseudomonas mallei*
e. **Carbohydrates not attacked** (no oxidation or fermentation, OF medium)
  (1) Oxidase positive, grows on MacConkey and cetrimide agar, nitrate reduced to nitrite, urease negative, no decarboxylases, motile: *Alcaligenes*
  (2) Oxidase positive, nonmotile, **usually no growth on MacConkey agar (exceptions),** penicillin sensitive, citrate and urease negative: *Moraxella*
  (3) Oxidase negative, grows on MacConkey agar:
    (a) *Achromobacter (lwoffii), Acinetobacter lwoffii*[249]

(b) *Pseudomonas maltophilia*
(c) *Bordetella parapertussis*
  (4) Oxidase positive, grows on MacConkey, microaerophilic, slow growth: *Campylobacter (Vibrio) fetus*
2. Some grow on ordinary media, others need enriched media; **fermentative, no gas produced, oxidase** usually positive, nitrate reduced, catalase positive: *Pasteurella*
3. **Slow growth,** pleomorphic cells, nonmotile, **fermentative,** no gas, often polar staining, oxidase and catalase variable, slow coagulation of milk, no decarboxylases: *Actinobacillus;* grow on MacConkey, **oxidase positive:** *A. lignieresi, A. equuli;* no growth on MacConkey, **oxidase negative:** *A. actinomycetemcomitans;* **oxidative,** no growth on MacConkey, oxidase negative: *P. mallei*
4. **Some requirement of special media** (no growth on MacConkey) and conditions, no capsule, nonmotile: *Brucella* (members of this group have to be differentiated by CO$_2$ requirement, H$_2$S production, dye inhibition test, and agglutination tests)
5. **No growth or poor growth without special factors in media;** capsule variable, nonmotile
  a. Require factors X and/or V: *Haemophilus;* characteristic satellitism along *Staphylococcus* streak or other colonies, no growth on plain agar, encapsulated strains identified by type-specific antisera: *H. influenzae;* grows on plain agar along a *Staphylococcus* streak or other colonies providing factor V: *H. parainfluenzae; H. ducreyi* cultivation rare; *H. aphrophilus*
  b. Do not require factors X and/or V, growth improved by addition of serum or ascitic fluid, sugars not attacked, **oxidase positive:** *Moraxella;* **oxidase-negative:** *C. (Haemophilus) vaginalis*
6. **Primary isolation best on complex media with blood:** oxidase positive; shows characteristic colonies on Bordet-Gengou agar, agglutination by specific antiserum: *Bordetella pertussis* (rough variant of *B. pertussis* grows on ordinary media); *B. parapertussis* and *B. bronchiseptica* grow on MacConkey agar, closely related antigenically
7. **No growth on ordinary media;** requires special media (cystine-glucose-blood agar): *Francisella tularensis*
8. Grow best on enriched media, crescent-shaped or spiral cells (long screws or portions of a turn): *Spirillum* (various species); no growth on artificial media: *S. minus* and *S. volutans*
D. Gram-positive rods
1. **Catalase positive, no spores** formed, no growth on MacConkey agar
  a. Nonmotile, arranged in Chinese figures, stain unevenly with bands and granules: *Corynebacterium;* toxin production, fermentative: *C. diphtheriae* and *C. ulcerans;* other corynebacteria and "diphtheroids" differentiated by biochemical and toxigenicity tests, some fermentative, others do not attack sugars at all

Table 75-9. A simplified guide to the presumptive recognition of common groups of bacteria—cont'd

b. Motile (at 20 but usually not at 37 C), short, "diphtheroid"-like rods, often narrow zone of β-hemolysis: *Listeria monocytogenes* (use biochemical and pathogenicity tests)

c. Motile, do not attack sugars, indole and nitrate reduction negative, long rods, some form filaments and coccoid bodies in broth: *Kurthia*

2. **Catalase negative, no spores** formed
a. Nonmotile, frequently form long filaments, usually no growth in litmus milk, fermentative (dextrose, lactose), H₂S in butt of TSI agar, nonbranching: *Erysipelothrix*
b. Form chains, grow better on tomato juice agar, H₂S negative in butt of TSI agar: *Lactobacillus*

3. **Acid fast,** no branching, no spores
a. Nonmotile, no branching, no hyphae: *Mycobacterium*
(1) Special media required, slow gowth: *M. tuberculosis* (distinguish by biochemical and cultural characteristics); **nontuberculous mycobacteria** (formerly **atypical**) (use cultural characteristics, pigment formation, physiologic and biochemical tests)
(2) Rapid growth: "saprophytes" (nonpathogens)

4. Nonmotile, some branching, some acid fast; hyphae, but no true conidia produced, oxidative: *Nocardia*

5. Catalase positive, spores formed, many motile: *Bacillus*
a. Characteristic colonies, nonmotile, usually nonhemolytic: *B. anthracis* (use biochemical differentiation)

II. Anaerobic cultures
A. Gram-positive cocci
1. Occurring mainly in clusters but also in pairs: *Peptococcus* (gas chromatography, biochemical reactions)
2. Mainly in pairs and chains: *Peptostreptococcus* (identification by gas chromatography and biochemical reactions)

B. Gram-negative cocci
1. In irregular masses, small cocci: *Veillonella, Acidaminococcus, Megasphaera*
C. Gram-negative rods
1. Usually nonmotile of varying sizes and shapes, nonsporeforming, often foul smelling, cells greater than 0.6 μm, do not produce butyric acid: *Bacteroides*
2. Some with pointed ends, effuse colonies; many very pleomorphic, produce butyric acid: *Fusobacterium*
3. Motile, polar flagella, curved: *Butyrivibrio, Succinimonas*
4. Spiral organisms: *Treponema, Borrelia*
D. Gram-positive rods, no spores
1. Vegetative mycelium produced, which fragments; true branching, non-acid-fast: *Actinomyces* (Identified by cultural and biochemical characteristics; catalase negative; slow-growing, dry, crumbly colonies on solid media, resembling tubercle bacillus colonies; in fluid medium granules adherent to walls of tube; unstained preparation of crushed granule shows typical clubs; must be differentiated from anaerobic "diphtheroids" and lactobacilli)
2. No catalase or indole produced, no spores: *Bifidobacterium*
3. Catalase and indole positive, nitrate reduced, gas from glucose: produce propionic acid: *Propionibacterium*
4. Nonmotile, nonbranching, do **not** ferment lactose, produce butyric acid: *Eubacterium*
E. Gram-positive rods, spores formed; some species may appear gram-negative
1. Motile and nonmotile, forming endospores that distort the cells, some species microaerophilic; catalase negative: *Clostridium* (Many members of this genus are saprophytes but some highly pathogenic for man and animals; differentiation by gas-liquid chromatography, biochemical reactions, pathogenicity tests, and specific toxins)

---

gram-positive cocci from cultures containing gram-negative organisms. On such media, gram-positive cocci grow uninhibited; gram-negative organisms are either inhibited or grow with much smaller colonies than usual. Spreading usually does not occur.

Use of fluorescent antibody (FA) technics. As described earlier (Chapter 70), FA technics have been developed for the identification and detection of a great number of bacterial, fungal, etc. species. At the time of writing, FA technics were not used as extensively as would be expected because of the following limitations.

Availability of labeled antisera. Although a large number of labeled antisera are commercially available, many are not, and the average laboratory is not equipped to do its own labeling and quality control, assuming that the proper unlabeled antisera are at hand. In addition, the quality and reliability of commercially available labeled antisera leave much to be

desired. Many are diluted almost to titer and are inadequate, sometimes useless.

Availability of equipment. FA equipment is becoming simpler and sturdier, and its price is correspondingly competitive. However, it still represents considerable investment.

Availability of trained personnel. It cannot be overemphasized that reliable FA work requires reliable, knowledgeable, and trained personnel.

Guides for identification

Tables 75-8 and 75-9 are presented as aids to guide the initial steps of identification. Table 75-8 indicates to which group (genus, family) a bacterium is likely to belong when all that is known about it is the appearance of its growth on the primary plate cultures (blood agar, MacConkey agar plates, aerobic or anaerobic, Gram staining, and coccal or rod-shaped).

Table 75-8 is no substitute for further careful tests; it is intended only as a general guide. Table 75-9 is a more detailed guide, in which selected, additional characters are listed to enable the laboratory worker to recognize the main groups of commonly occurring organisms. The list is not a determinative key, but it is intended to serve as a first step in the identification procedure. Once the group has been determined, reference should be made to the specific headings for each group of organisms in this text. Final identification depends on specific tests described for each genus or species, usually grouped in tables that include the results of the tests. The guide does not include all the important bacteria; some of the less common and unusual forms are described in the text.

REFERENCES

1. Sonnenwirth, A. C.: Ann. Intern. Med. **89**(part 2):785, 1978.
2. Matsen, J. M., and Ederer, G. M.: Hum. Pathol. **7**:297, 1976.
3. Lipsky, B. A., and Plorde, J. J.: Postgrad. Med. **64**:80, 1978.
4. Stokes, E. J.: Clinical bacteriology, ed. 4, London, 1975, Edward Arnold (Publishers).
5. Hosty, T. S., Johnson, M. B., Freear, M. A., et al.: Health Lab. Sci. **1**:163, 1964.
6. Ellner, P. D., and Ellner, C. J.: J. Bacteriol. **91**:905, 1966.
7. Hollinger, N., and Rantz, L. A.: Pediatrics **24**:1112, 1959.
8. Ederer, G. M., and Christian, D. L.: Am. J. Med. Technol. **41**:27, 1975.
9. Stuart, R. D.: Public Health Rep. **74**:431, 1959.
10. Huffaker, R. H., editor: Collection, handling and shipment of microbiological specimens, Atlanta, 1974, Department of Health, Education, and Welfare, Center for Disease Control.
11. Sherris, J.: Relevance in clinical bacteriology, presented at the American Society of Microbiology meeting, May 1, 1967, New York.
11a. Isenberg, H. D., Shoenknecht, F. D., and Graevenitz, A. V.: Collection and processing of bacteriological specimens. Cumitech no. 9, Washington, D.C., 1979, American Society for Microbiology.
12. Sonnenwirth, A. C., editor: Bacteremia, laboratory and clinical aspects, Springfield, Ill., 1973, Charles C Thomas, Publisher.
13. Bartlett, R. C., Ellner, P. D., and Washington, J. A. II: Blood cultures, Cumitech no. 1, (Sherris, J. C., coord. ed.), Washington, D.C., 1974, American Society for Microbiology.
14. Bartlett, R. C.: Contemporary blood culture practices. In Sonnenwirth, A. C., editor: Bacteremia: laboratory and clinical aspects, Springfield, Ill., 1973, Charles C Thomas, Publisher.
15. von Haebler, T., and Miles, A. A.: J. Pathol. **46**:245, 1938.
16. Ellner, P. D., and Stoessel, C. J.: J. Infect. Dis. **116**:238, 1966.
17. Finegold, S. M., Ziment, I., White, M. L., et al.: In Hobby, G. L., editor: Antimicrobial agents—1967, Ann Arbor, Mich., 1968, American Society for Microbiology.
18. Dorn, G. L., Haynes, J. R., and Burson, G. G.: J. Clin. Microbiol. **3**:251 and 258, 1976.
19. Hall, M. M., Warren, E., Ilstrup, D. M., and Washington, J. A. II: J. Clin. Microbiol. **3**:212, 1976.
19a. Edelstein, P. H., Meyer, R. D., and Finegold, S. M.: Lancet, April 7, 1979, p. 750.
20. Rosner, R. In Sonnenwirth, A. C., editor: Bacteremia: laboratory and clinical aspects, Springfield, Ill., 1973, Charles C Thomas, Publisher, pp. 61-75.
21. Washington, J. A. II, Hall, M. M., and Warren, E.: J. Clin. Microbiol. **1**:79, 1975.
22. Hall, M. M., Ilstrup, D. M., and Washington, J. A. II: J. Clin. Microbiol. **3**:643, 1976.
23. Laboratory methods in clinical bacteriology, Atlanta, 1976, Center for Disease Control.
24. Roberts, G. D., and Washington, J. A., II: J. Clin. Microbiol. **1**:309, 1975.
25. Gantz, N. M., Swain, J. L., Medeiros, A. A., et al.: Lancet **2**:1174, 1974.
26. Knepper, J. G., and Anthony, B. F.: Lancet **2**:285, 1973.
27. Cannady, P. B., and Sanford, J. P.: Negative blood cultures in infective endocarditis: a review, South. Med. J. **69**:1420-1423, 1976.
28. Sonnenwirth, A. C.: Incidence of intestinal anaerobes in blood cultures. In Balows, A., DeHann, R. M., Dowell, V. R., and Guze, L. B., editors: Anaerobic bacteria: role in disease, Springfield, Ill., 1974, Charles C Thomas, Publisher.
29. Faris, H. M., and Sparling, F. F.: J.A.M.A. **219**:76, 1972.
30. Noble, R. C., and Reeves, S. A.: J.A.M.A. **230**:1002, 1974.
31. Kaslow, R. A., Mackel, D. C., and Mallison, G. F.: J.A.M.A. **236**:2407, 1976.
32. Sonnenwirth, A. C.: Bacteremia—extent of the problem. In Sonnenwirth, A. C., editor: Bacteremia: laboratory and clinical aspects, Springfield, Ill., 1973, Charles C Thomas, Publisher.
33. Alpern, R. J., and Dowell, V. R., Jr.: J.A.M.A. **209**:385, 1969.
34. Koransky, J. R., Stargel, M. D., and Dowell, V. R., Jr.: Am. J. Med. **66**:63, 1979.
35. Sonnenwirth, A. C.: Ann. N.Y. Acad. Sci. **174**(art. 2):488-502, 1970.
36. Center for Disease Control: Morbidity and Mortality Weekly Report **22**(13):115, 1973.
37. Maki, D. G., Rhame, F. S., Goldman, D. A., et al.: The infection hazard posed by contaminated intravenous infusion fluid. In Sonnenwirth, A. C., editor: Clinical and laboratory aspects of bacteremia, Springfield, Ill., 1973, Charles C Thomas, Publisher.
38. Jorgensen, J. H., and Smith, R. F.: Appl. Microbiol. **26**:521, 1973.
39. American Association of Blood Banks: Technical manual, ed. 7, Washington, D.C., 1977, The Association.
40. American Association of Blood Banks: Standards for blood banks and transfusion services, ed. 8, Washington, D.C., 1977, The Association.
41. Shackelford, P. G., Campbell, J., and Feigin, R. D.: J. Pediatr. **85**:478, 1974.
42. Brook, I., Bricknell, K. S., Overturf, G. D., and Finegold, S. M.: J. Infect. Dis. **137**:384, 1978.
43. Controni, G., Rodriguez, W. J., Hicks, J. M., et al.: J. Pediatr. **91**:379, 1977.
44. Controni, G., Rodriguez, W. J., Deane, C., et al.: Clin. Proc. Child. Hosp. Natl. Med. Center **31**:194, 1975.
45. Hurd, C. A., Fennema, K. J., and Blazevic, D. J.: Am. J. Med. Technol. **44**:11, 1978.

46. Elin, R. J., and Wolff, S. M.: Ann. Rev. Med. **27**:127, 1976.
47. Jorgensen, J. H., and Smith, R. F.: Appl. Microbiol. **26**:43, 1973.
48. Sullivan, J. D., Jr., Valois, F. W., and Watson, S. W. In Bernheimer, A. W., editor: Mechanisms in bacterial toxinology, New York, 1976, John Wiley & Sons.
49. Levin, J., and Bang, F. B.: Bull. Johns Hopkins Hosp. **115**:337, 1964.
50. Cooper, J. F., Levin, J., and Wagner, H. N.: Lab. Clin. Med. **78**:138, 1971.
51. Sonnenwirth, A. C., Yin, E. T., Sarmiento, B. S., and Wessler, S.: Am. J. Clin. Nutr. **25**:452, 1972.
52. Levin, J.: N. Engl. J. Med. **228**:1297, 1973.
53. Garibaldi, R. A., Allman, G. W., Larsen, D. H., et al.: Infect. Dis. **128**:551, 1973.
54. Shapiro, L., Lodato, F. M., Jr., Courant, P. R., and Stallard, R. E.: J. Periodontol. **43**:591, 1972.
55. Fine, D. H., Tabek, L., Salkind, A., and Oshrain, H.: J. Periodontol. Res. **13**:127, 1978.
56. Wildfever, A., Heymer, B., Schleifer, K. H., and Haferkamp, O.: Appl. Microbiol. **28**:867, 1974.
57. Nachum, R., Lipsey, A., Siegel, S. E. N. Engl. J. Med. **289**:931, 1973.
58. Ross, S. et al.: J.A.M.A. **233**:1366, 1975.
59. Alexander, H.: The Hemophilus group. In Dubos, R., and Hirsch, J. G., editors: Bacterial and mycotic infections of man, ed. 4, Philadelphia, 1965. J. B. Lippincott Co.
60. Fox, H. A., Hagen, P. A., Turner, D. J., et al.: Pediatrics **43**:44, 1969.
61. Sonnenwirth, A. C., and Kallus, B.: Am. J. Clin. Pathol. **49**:92, 1968.
62. Graber, C. D., Higgins, L. S., and Davis, J. S.: J.A.M.A. **192**:956, 1965.
63. Swartz, M. N., and Dodge, P. R.: N. Engl. J. Med. **272**:898, 1965.
64. World Health Organization Study Group: Cerebrospinal meningitis control, WHO Tech. Rep. Ser. no. 588, Geneva, 1976.
65. Feldman, W. E.: Am. J. Dis. Child. **130**:880, 1976.
66. O'Grady, L. R., and Ralph, E. D.: Am. J. Dis. Child. **130**:871, 1976.
67. Ellner, J. J., and Bennett, J. E.: Medicine **55**:341, 1976.
68. Heinle, E. W., Jensen, W. N., and Westerman, M. P.: Am. Rev. Respir. Dis. **91**:701, 1965.
69. Gilman, R. H., et al.: Lancet **1**(7918):1211, 1975.
70. Vaisrub, S.: J.A.M.A. **233**:1196, 1975.
71. Tu, K., Bartholomew, W. R., and Wicher, K.: Am. Soc. Microbiol. Abstr., 1973.
72. Greene, W. H., Schimpff, S. C., et al.: Am. J. Clin. Pathol. **60**:404, 1973.
73. Murray, P. R., Wold, A. D., Schreck, C. A., and Washington, J. A.: J. Clin. Microbiol. **4**:54, 1976.
74. McGonagle, L. A.: Health Lab. Sci. **11**:61, 1974.
75. Dykstra, M. A., McLaughlin, J. C., and Bartlett, R. C.: J. Clin. Microbiol. **9**:236, 1979.
76. Kurzynski, T. A., and Meise, C. K.: J. Clin. Microbiol. **9**:189, 1979.
77. Wannamaker, L. W.: A method for culturing beta-hemolytic streptococci from the throat, New York, 1965, American Heart Association.
78. Moody, M. D.: Public Health Lab. **26**:165, 1968.
79. Pappenheimer, A. M.: The diphtheria bacilli and the diphtheroids. In Dubos, R., editor: Bacterial and mycotic infections of man, ed. 3, Philadelphia, 1958, J. B. Lippincott Co.
80. Moore, M. S., and Parsons, E. I.: J. Infect. Dis. **102**:88, 1958.
81. Whitaker, J. A., Nelson, J. D., and Fink, C. W.: Pediatrics **27**:214, 1961.
82. Pitman, B. In Lennette, E. H., Spaulding, E. H., and Traunt, J. P., editors: Manual of clinical microbiology, ed. 2, Washington, D.C., 1974, American Society for Microbiology.
83. Jones, G. L., and Kendrick, P. L.: Health Lab. Sci. **6**:40-45, 1969.
84. Barrett-Connor, E.: Am. Rev. Respir. Dis. **103**: 845-848, 1971.
85. Drew, W. L.: J. Clin. Microbiol. **6**:52-55, 1977.
86. Bartlett, J. G., Brewer, N. S., and Ryan, K. J.: Laboratory diagnosis of lower respiratory tract infections, Cumitech no. 7, (Washington, J. A., coord. ed.), Washington, D.C., 1977, American Society for Microbiology.
87. Murray, P. R., and Washington, J. A.: Mayo Clin. Proc. **50**:339, 1975.
88. Geckler, R. W., Gremillion, D. H., McAllister, C. K., and Ellenbogen, C.: J. Clin. Microbiol. **6**:396, 1977.
89. Finegold, S. M., Martin, W. J., and Scott, E. G.: Bailey and Scott's diagnostic microbiology: a textbook for the isolation and identification of pathogenic microorganisms, ed. 5, St. Louis, 1978, The C. V. Mosby Co.
90. Van Scoy, R. E.: Mayo Clin. Proc. **52**:39, 1977.
91. Hawn, C. V., and Beebe, E.: J. Bacteriol. **90**:549, 1965.
92. Jones, G. L., and Hebert, G. A.: "Legionnaires"—the disease, the bacterium, and methodology, Atlanta, May 1978 (rev. Oct. 1978), Center for Disease Control.
93. Murray, P. R., Van Scoy, R. E., and Roberts, G. D.: Mayo Clin. Proc. **52**:42, 1977.
94. Bartlett, J. G.: Am. Rev. Respir. Dis. **115**:777, 1977.
95. Bartlett, J. G., and Finegold, S. M.: Am. Rev. Respir. Dis. **110**:56-77, 1974.
96. Bartlett, J. G., Rosenblatt, J. E., and Finegold, S. M.: Ann. Intern. Med. **79**:535-540, 1973.
97. Van Orden, A. E., and Greer, P. W.: J. Histotechnol. **1**:51-53, 1977.
98. Barry, A. L., Smith, P. B., and Turck, M.: Laboratory diagnosis of urinary tract infections, Cumitech no. 2, (Gavan, T. L., coord. ed.), Washington, D.C., 1975, American Society for Microbiology.
99. Kunin, C. M.: Detection, prevention and management of urinary tract infections: a manual for the physician, nurse, and allied health worker, ed. 2, Philadelphia, 1974, Lea & Febiger.
100. Sacks, T. G., and Abramson, J. H.: J.A.M.A. **201**:1, 1967.
101. Rehm, A.: Ohio Med. J. **60**:139, 1964.
102. Simmons, N. A., and Williams, J. D.: Lancet **1**: 1377, 1962.
103. Griess, P.: Ber. Deutsch. Chem. Gesellsch. **12**: 426, 1879.
104. Smith, L. G., Thayer, W. R., Malta, E. M., and Utz, J. P.: Ann. Intern. Med. **54**:66, 1961.
105. Sleigh, J. D.: Br. Med. J. **1**:765, 1965.
106. Ryan, W. L., Hoody, S., and Luby, R.: J. Urol. **88**:838, 1962.
107. Truant, J. B., Breit, W. A., and Merkel, K. E.: Henry Ford Hosp. Med. Bull. **10**:359, 1962.
108. Truant, J. P., Merckel, K. F., and Swieczkowski, D. In Kass, E. H., editor: Progress in pyelonephritis, Philadelphia, 1965, F. A. Davis Co.
109. Schersten, B., Dahlquist, A., Fritz, H., et al.: J.A.M.A. **204**:113, 1968.
110. Cohen, S. N., and Kass, E. H.: N. Engl. J. Med. **277**:176, 1967.

111. Ellner, P. D., and Papachristos, T.: Am. J. Clin. Pathol. **63**:516, 1975.
112. Bartlett, R.: Personal communication, March 1979.
113. Kunin, C. M.: Ann. Rev. Med. **17**:383, 1966.
114. Honeywell, K., Dalton, H. P., and Mendelow, H.: Am. J. Med. Technol. **32**:207, 1966.
115. Parker, R. H., Croft, G. F., and Hoeprich, P. D.: Am. J. Med. Sci. **254**:836, 1967.
116. Sonnenwirth, A. C.: J. Clin. Microbiol. **6**:400, 1977.
117. Aldridge, C., Gibson, J., Lanham, M., et al.: J. Clin. Microbiol. **6**:406, 1977.
118. Smith, P. B., Gavan, T. L., Isenberg, H. D., et al.: J. Clin. Microbiol. **8**:657, 1978.
119. Kass, E. H.: Ann. Intern. Med. **56**:46, 1962.
120. Hoeprich, P. D.: J. Lab. Clin. Med. **56**:899, 1960.
121. Thomas, M.: Br. Med. J. **2**:830, 1977.
122. Barker, J., Brookes, G., and Johnson, T.: Br. Med. J. **1**:300, 1978.
123. Hinkle, N. H., Partin, J. C., and West, C. D.: Am. J. Dis. Child. **100**:333, 1960.
124. Gross, P. A., Harkany, L. M., Barden, G. E., and Kerstein, M.: J.A.M.A. **228**:72-73, 1974.
125. Nemoy, N. J., and Stamey, T. A.: J.A.M.A. **215**:1470, 1971.
126. Silver, H., and Sonnenwirth, A. C.: Am. J. Clin. Pathol. **52**:433, 1969.
127. Brewer, N. S., and Weed, L. A.: Hum. Pathol. **7**:141, 1976.
128. Palmer, E.: J.A.M.A. **231**:192, 1975.
129. Lazarchik, J., Souzae Silva, N. A., Nichols, D. R., and Washington, J. A., II: Mayo Clin. Proc. **48**:349, 1973.
130. Sabbaj, J., Sutter, V., and Finegold, S. M.: Ann. Intern. Med. **77**:627, 1972.
131. Louvois, J.: J. Antimicrob. Chemother. **4**:395, 1978.
132. Sutter, V. L., Vargo, V. L., and Finegold, S. M.: Wadsworth anaerobic bacteriology manual, ed. 2, Los Angeles, 1975, Wadsworth Hospital Center, Veterans' Administration, and the Department of Medicine, University of California at Los Angeles School of Medicine.
133. Wilkins, T. D., and Jimenez-Ulate, F.: J. Clin. Microbiol. **2**:441-447, 1975.
134. Dowell, V. R., Jr., and Hawkins, T. M.: Laboratory methods in anaerobic bacteriology. DHEW publ. no. (CDC)-78-8272, Atlanta, 1978, U.S. Department of Health, Education and Welfare, Public Health Service, Center for Disease Control.
135. Goldstein, E. J. C., Citron, D. M., Wield, B., et al.: J. Clin. Microbiol. **8**:667, 1978.
136. Butler, T., Weaver, R. E., Ramani, T. K. V., et al.: Ann. Intern. Med. **86**:1, 1977.
137. Krizek, L. J., and Robson, M. C.: Am. J. Surg. **130**:579, 1975.
138. Meislin, H. W., Lerner, S. A., Graves, M. H., et al.: Ann. Intern. Med. **87**:145, 1977.
139. Maki, D. G., Weise, C. E., and Sarafin, H. W.: N. Engl. J. Med. **296**:1305, 1977.
140. Grossman, L. I.: Endodontic practice, ed. 8, Philadelphia, 1974, Lea & Febiger.
141. Nolte, W.: Oral microbiology, ed. 3, St. Louis, 1977, The C. V. Mosby Co.
142. Finegold, S. M.: Anaerobic bacteria in human disease, New York, 1977, Academic Press.
143. Burnett, G. W., Scherp, H. W., and Schuster, G. W.: Oral microbiology and infectious disease, ed. 4, Baltimore, 1976, The Williams & Wilkins Co.
144. Nicholas, J. P., and Goolden, E. B.: Arch. Ophthalmol. **74**:639, 1966.

145. Birge, H. L.: Am. J. Med. Sci. **246**:239, 1963.
146. Theodore, F. H.: Eye Ear Nose Throat Mon. **46**:382, 1967.
147. Winkler, C. H., and Dixon, J. M.: Arch. Ophthalmol. **72**:817, 1964.
148. Brook, I., and Finegold, S. M.: J.A.M.A. **241**:487, 1979.
148a. *Criteria and technique for the diagnosis of gonorrhea*, Atlanta, undated (received 1977), Center for Disease Control, Venereal Disease Control Division.
149. Martin, J. E., and Lester, A.: HSMHA Health Rep. **86**:30-33, 1971.
150. Williams, W. J., Synder, H. A., and Farmer, A. D.: Public Health Lab. **29**:99-101, 1971.
151. Thayer, J. D., and Martin, J. E., Jr.: Public Health Rep. **79**:49-57, 1964.
152. Kellogg, D. S., Jr., Holmes, K. K., and Hill, G. A.: Laboratory diagnosis of gonorrhea, Cumitech no. 4, (Marcus, S., and Sherris, J. C., coord. ed.), Washington, D.C., 1976, American Society for Microbiology.
153. Symington, D. A.: J. Clin. Microbiol. **2**:498, 1975.
154. Martin, J. E., Jr., Armstrong, J. H., and Smith, P. B.: Appl. Microbiol. **27**:802, 1974.
155. Thayer, J. D., and Martin, J. E., Jr.: Public Health Rep. **81**:559-562, 1966.
156. Faur, Y. C., Weisburd, M. H., Wilson, M. E., and May, P. S.: Health Lab. Sci. **10**:44, 1973.
157. Faur, Y. C., Weisburd, M. H., and Wilson, M. E.: Health Lab. Sci. **10**:55 and **10**:61, 1973.
158. Martin, J. E., Jr., and Lewis, J.: Public Health Lab. **35**:53, 1977.
159. Danielsson, D., and Kronvall, G.: Appl. Microbiol. **27**:368-374, 1974.
160. World Health Organization Scientific Group: *Neisseria gonorrhoeae* and gonococcal infections, WHO Technical Report Series, no. 616, Geneva, 1978, World Health Organization.
161. Gardner, H. L., and Dukes, C. D.: Am. J. Obstet. Gynecol. **69**:962, 1955.
162. Dunkelberg, W. E.: Am. J. Obstet. Gynecol. **91**:998, 1965.
163. Edmunds, P. N.: J. Obstet. Gynaecol. Br. Comm. **66**:917, 1959.
164. Park, C. H., Fauber, M., and Cook, C. B.: Am. J. Clin. Pathol. **49**:590, 1968.
165. Edmunds, P. N.: J. Pathol. Bacteriol. **79**:273, 1960.
166. Dukes, C. D., and Gardner, H. L.: J. Bacteriol. **81**:277, 1961.
167. Dunkelberg, W. E.: J. Am. Vener. Dis. Assoc. **4**:69, 1977.
168. Pheifer, T. A., Forsyth, P. S., Durfee, M. A., et al.: N. Engl. J. Med. **298**:1429, 1978.
169. McCormack, W. M., Hayes, C. H., Rosner, B., et al.: J. Infect. Dis. **136**:740, 1977.
170. Greenwood, J. R., Pickett, M. J., Martin, W. J., and Mack, E. G.: Health Lab. Sci. **14**:102, 1977.
171. Greenwood, J. R., and Pickett, M. J.: Clin. Microbiol. **9**:200, 1979.
172. Bailey, R. K., Voss, J. L., and Smith, R. F.: Clin. Microbiol. **9**:65, 1979.
173. Hart, G.: Chancroid, donovanosis, and lymphogranuloma venereum, Atlanta, 1975, Center for Disease Control.
174. Hammond, G. W., Lian, C. J., Wilt, J. C., and Ronard, A. R.: J. Clin. Microbiol. **7**:39, 1978.
175. Borchardt, K. A., and Hoke, A. W.: Arch. Dermatol. **102**:188, 1970.
176. Barrit, M. M.: Br. Med. J. **1**:254, 1943.
177. Dodson, R. F., Fritz, G. S., Hubler, W. R., Jr. et al.: J. Invest. Dermatol. **62**:611, 1974.
178. Schachter, J.: J. Infect. Dis. **120**:372, 1969.

179. Abrams, A. J.: J.A.M.A. **205**:199, 1968.
180. Nichols, R. L., and McComb, D. E.: J. Exp. Med. **120**:639, 1964.
181. Graham, D. M., and Layton, J. E. In Nichols, R. L., editor: Trachoma and related disorders, Amsterdam, 1971, Excerpta Medica.
182. Gordon, F. B., and Quan, A. L.: Proc. Soc. Exp. Biol. Med. **118**:354, 1965.
183. Kaufman, R. E., and Wiesner, P.: N. Engl. J. Med. **291**:22, 1175-1177, 1974.
184. Jacobs, N. F., and Kraus, S. J.: Ann. Intern Med. **82**:12, 1975.
185. Schachter, J., Hanna, L., Hill, E. C., et al.: J.A.M.A. **231**:1252-1255, 1975.
186. Jacobs, M. F., Arum, E. S., and Kraus, S. J.: Ann. Intern. Med. **86**:314, 1977.
187. Mardh, P., Ripa, T., Svensson, L., and Westrom, L.: N. Engl. J. Med. **296**:1377-1379, 1977.
188. Grayston, J. T., and San-pin, W.: J. Infect. Dis. **132**:87, 1975.
189. Holmes, K. K., Handsfield, H. H., Wang, S.P. et al.: N. Engl. J. Med. **292**:1199-1205, 1975.
190. Satterwhite, T. K., and Dupont, H. L.: J.A.M.A. **236**:2662, 1976.
191. Harris, J. C., Dupont, H. L., and Hornick, R. B.: Ann. Intern. Med. **76**:697, 1972.
192. Pickering, J., Dupont, H. L., Olarte, J., et al.: Am. J. Clin. Pathol. **68**:562, 1977.
193. Willmore, J. G., and Shearman, C. H.: Lancet **2**:200-206, 1918.
194. Graham, D.: Lancet **1**:51-55, 1918.
195. Anderson, J.: Lancet **2**:998-1002, 1921.
196. Stokes, E. J.: Clinical bacteriology, ed. 2, London, 1960, Edward Arnold (Publishers).
196a. Edwards, P. R., and Ewing, W. H.: Identification of Enterobacteriaceae, ed. 3, Minneapolis, 1972, Burgess Publishing Co.
197. Sakazaki, R., Iwanami, S., and Fukumi, H.: Jpn. J. Med. Sci. Biol. **16**:161-188, 1963.
198. Barker, W. H., Weaver, R. E., Morris, G. K., and Martin, W. T.: Epidemiology of *Vibrio parahaemolyticus* infection in humans. In Schlessinger, D., editor: Microbiology 1974, Washington, D.C., 1975, American Society for Microbiology.
199. Krogstad, D. J., Spencer, H. C., and Healy, G. R.: N. Engl. J. Med. **298**:262, 1978.
200. Wolfe, M. S.: N. Engl. J. Med. **298**:319, 1978.
201. Black, R. E., Jackson, R. J., Tsai, T., et al.: N. Engl. J. Med. **298**:76, 1978.
202. Barker, W. H.: Lancet **1**:551, 1974.
203. Gangarosa, E. J., and Merson, M. H.: N. Engl. J. Med. **296**:1210, 1977.
204. Rosenberg, M., Koplan, J. P., Wachsmuth, I. K., et al.: Ann. Intern. Med. **86**:714, 1977.
205. Sack, D. A., and Sack, R. B.: Infect. Immun. **11**:334, 1975.
206. Lauwers, S., De Boech, M., and Butzler, J. P.: Lancet **1**:604, 1978.
207. Bartlett, J. G., Chang, T. W., Gurwith, M., et al.: N. Engl. J. Med. **298**:531, 1978.
208. Chrystie, I. L., Totterdell, B. M., and Banatrala, J. E.: Lancet **1**:1176, 1978.
209. Parrino, T. A., Schreiber, D. S., Trier, J. S., et al.: N. Engl. J. Med. **297**:86, 1977.
210. McSwiggan, D. A., Cubitt, D., and Moore, W.: Lancet **1**:1215, 1978.
211. King, S., and Metzger, W. I.: Appl. Microbiol. **16**:577 and 579, 1968.
212. Taylor, I.: Am. J. Clin. Pathol. **44**:471, 1965.
213. Balows, A., Hermann, G. J., and DeWitt, W. E.: Health Lab. Sci. **8**:167-175, 1971.
214. Ewing, W. H.: Public Health Lab. **27**:19, 1969.
215. Ewing, W. H.: Differentiation of Enterobacteriaceae by biochemical reactions, Atlanta, 1968, National Communicable Disease Center.
216. Martin, W. J., Ewing, W. H., McWhorter, A. C., and Ball, M. M.: Public Health Lab. **27**:61, 1969.
217. Kubica, G. P., and Vestal, A. L.: Tuberculosis—laboratory methods in diagnosis, Atlanta, 1960, Communicable Disease Center.
218. Sanders, A. C., and Okabe, K.: U. S. Armed Forces Med. J. **4**:1053, 1953.
219. Sanders, A. C., and Okabe, K.: Public Health Lab. **12**:12, 1954.
220. Sanders, A. C., Faber, J., and Cook, T.: Appl. Microbiol. **5**:36, 1957.
221. Bicknell, A. K., Butt, F., and Mattman, L. H.: Am. J. Public Health **42**:437, 1952.
222. Ewing, W. H.: Isolation and identification of Enterobacteriaceae: principles and practice, Atlanta, 1966, Communicable Disease Center.
223. Ewing, W. H.: Differential reactions of Enterobacteriaceae, Atlanta, 1966, Communicable Disease Center.
224. Ewing, W. H.: Enterobacteriaceae: taxonomy and nomenclature, Atlanta, 1966, Communicable Disease Center.
225. Johnson, J. C., Kunz, L. J., Barron, W., and Ewing, W. H.: Appl. Microbiol. **14**:212, 1966.
226. Ewing, W. H.: Revised definitions for the family Enterobacteriaceae: its tribes and genera, Atlanta, 1967, Communicable Disease Center.
227. Sonnenwirth, A. C.: Unpublished observations, 1969.
228. Douglas, G. W., O'Connor, C., and Young, V. M.: Am. J. Clin. Pathol. **45**:497, 1966.
229. Ewing, W. H., Davis, B. R., and Martin, W. J.: Outline of methods for the isolation and identification of *Vibrio cholerae*, Atlanta, 1966, Communicable Disease Center.
230. Ewing, W. H., Tomfohrde, K. M., and Nando, P. J.: API Species **2**:10, 1979.
231. WHO Bacterial Diseases Unit: Guidelines for the laboratory diagnosis of cholera, Geneva, 1974, World Health Organization.
232. Twedt, R. M.: Isolation and identification of *Vibrio parahaemolyticus*. In FDA bacteriological analytical manual, Washington, D.C., 1978, Association of Official Analytical Chemists, Publ.
233. Sonnenwirth, A. C.: Mt. Sinai J. Med. **43**:736-745, 1976.
234. Morris, G. K., and Feeley, J. C.: Bull. WHO **54**:79-85, 1976.
235. Highsmith, A. K., Feeley, J. C., and Morris, G. K.: Health Lab. Sci. **14**:253-260, 1977.
236. Darland, D., Ewing, W. H., and Davis, B. R.: The biochemical characteristics of *Yersinia enterocolitica* and *Yersinia pseudotuberculosis*, DHEW publ. no. (CDC)-75-8294, Atlanta, 1974, Center for Disease Control.
237. Greenwood, J. R., Flanigan, S. M., Pickett, M. J., and Martin, W. J.: J. Clin. Microbiol. **2**:559, 1975.
238. Weissfeld, A. S., and Sonnenwirth, A. C.: Abstracts of the Annual Meeting of the American Society for Microbiology, abstr. C(H)70, 1979, p. 358.
239. Hawkins, T. M., and Brenner, D. J.: Isolation and identification of *Yersinia enterocolitica*, Atlanta, 1978, Center for Disease Control.
240. Duckworth, J. K.: Med. Lab. Obs. **9**:35, 1977.
241. Waterborne *Campylobacter* gastroenteritis (Vermont), Morbidity and Mortality Weekly Report **27**(25):207, June 23, 1978.
242. King, E. O.: J. Infect. Dis. **101**:119, 1957.

243. Butzler, J. P., Dekeyser, P., Detrain, M., and De-haen, F.: J. Pediatr. **82**:493-495, 1973.

244. Skirrow, M. B.: Br. Med. J. **2**:9-11, 1977.

245. *Ca..ipylobacter* enteritis, Lancet **2**:135-136, 1978.

246. *Campylobacter* enteritis (Colorado), Morbidity and Mortality Weekly Report, **27**(27):226, July 7, 1978.

247. Kunz, L. J.: Hum. Pathol. **7**:169, 1976.

248. Kunz, L. J.: Conventional methods, speciation, and the computer. In Lorian, V., editor: Significance of medical microbiology in the care of patients, Baltimore, 1977, The Williams & Wilkins Co.

248a. Isenberg, H. D., and McLowry, J. D.: Annu. Rev. Microbiol. **30**:483, 1976.

249. Cowan, T., and Steel, K. J.: Manual for the identification of medical bacteria, Cambridge, 1965, Cambridge University Press.

250. Buchanan, R. E., and Gibbons, N. E.: Bergey's manual of determinative bacteriology, ed. 8, Baltimore, 1974, The Williams & Wilkins Co.

251. Steel, K. J.: The practice of bacterial identification. In Symposium of the Society of General Microbiology, no. 12, 1962, Society of General Microbiology, p. 405.

252. Bartlett, R. C.: Medical microbiology: quality, cost, and clinical relevance, New York, 1974, John Wiley & Sons.

253. Bartlett, R. C.: Medical microbiology: how fast to go—how far to go. In Lorian, V., editor: Significance of medical microbiology in the care of patients, Baltimore, 1977, The Williams & Wilkins Co.

254. Dolan, C., et al., editorial board: Proceedings of the 1975 Aspen conference in microbiology, Chicago, 1977, College of American Pathologists.

255. Balows, A., editor: Clinical microbiology: how to start and when to stop, Springfield, Ill., 1975, Charles C Thomas, Publisher.

256. Skerman, V. B. D.: A guide to the identification of the genera of bacteria, ed. 2, Baltimore, 1967, The Williams & Wilkins Co.

257. Schneierson, S. S., and Amsterdam, D.: Am. J. Clin. Pathol. **42**:328, 1964.

258. Olds, R. J.: In Gibbs, B. M., and Skinner, F. A., editors: Identification methods for microbiologists, pt. A, New York, 1966, Academic Press.

259. Dybowski, W., Franklin, D. A., and Payne, L. C.: J. Clin. Pathol. **17**:197, 1964 (Abst.).

260. Krichevsky, M. I., editor: Computer-aided determinative bacteriology, Int. J. Syst. Bacteriol. **24**:493, 1974.

261. Friedman, R. B., Bruce, D., MacLowry, J., and Brenner, V.: Computer-assisted identification of bacteria, Am. J. Clin. Pathol. **61**:395, 1973.

262. Naylor, P. G.: J. Med. Lab. Tech. **17**:184, 1960.

263. Kalz, G. G.: Principles and practice of diagnostic bacteriology. In Dubos, R., editor: Bacterial and mycotic infections of man, ed. 3, Philadelphia, 1958, J. B. Lippincott Co.

264. Weaver, R. E., Tatum, H. W., and Hollis, D. G.: The identification of unusual pathogenic gram-negative bacteria, Atlanta, April 1978 (rev.), Center for Disease Control.

265. Weaver, R. E.: Gram-negative organisms: an approach to identification, Atlanta, Nov. 1977, Center for Disease Control.

266. Brenner, D. J., Farmer, J. J., III, Hickman, F. W., et al.: Taxonomic and nomenclature changes in Enterobacteriaceae, Atlanta, 1977, Center for Disease Control.

76

GRAM-POSITIVE AND GRAM-NEGATIVE COCCI

Alex C. Sonnenwirth

Micrococci and staphylococci

The term "micrococci" is applied to a large variety of gram-positive and mostly catalase-positive cocci, some of which are saprophytes, widely distributed in nature, whereas others are parasitic and potentially pathogenic. They occur in pairs, small clusters, tetrads, or packets. Although there is considerable disagreement regarding their classification and nomenclature,[1] the 2 genera *Staphylococcus* and *Micrococcus* are generally recognized and separated on the ability of *Staphylococcus* to grow and produce acid from glucose anaerobically and its susceptibility to lysis by lysostaphin (*Micrococcus* is negative in both of these tests). Variability in these characteristics has been reported by several workers (undoubtedly due to lack of uniformity in methodology). The International Subcommittee on Taxonomy of Staphylococci and Micrococci[2] has recommended adoption of a standard method for distinguishing these organisms by the anerobic utilization of carbohydrates. Accordingly, if the **standard** test is used (for medium see *Micrococcus* below) those organisms that utilize glucose fermentatively (anaerobically) and are lysed by 1μ/ml lysostaphin endopeptidase are designated as *Staphylococcus* and those that do not at all produce acid from glucose, or do so oxidatively (aerobically) only, are designated as *Micrococcus*. *Bergey's Manual* (ed. 8[3]) includes additionally the genus *Planococcus* in the *Micrococcaceae* and the genera *Aerococcus*, *Pediococcus*, and *Leuconostoc* in the family *Streptococcaceae*, whereas the International Subcommittee on the Nomenclature of Staphylococci and Micrococci[4] places *Aerococcus* in the *Micrococcaceae* (the genus to include *Pediococcus*, and *Gaffkya*). *Planococcus* and *Leuconostoc* are not further discussed here because they do not occur in human infections.

Facklam and Smith[5] have suggested a practical scheme usable in clinical microbiology:

I. Cytochrome enzymes present: Strong catalase (strong bubbling of hydrogen peroxide) —*Micrococcaceae*
  A. Nonmotile
    1. Acid from glucose anaerobically, lysed by lysostaphin—*Staphylococcus*
    2. No acid from glucose anaerobically, not lysed by lysostaphin—*Micrococcus*
  B. Motile, usually yellow brown pigment— *Planococcus*
II. No cytochromes present: Catalase reaction usually negative—*Streptococcaceae*
  A. Gas from glucose aerobically—*Leuconostoc*
  B. No gas from glucose aerobically
    1. Acid from glucose anaerobically, mostly chains and pairs—*Streptococcus*
    2. Mainly tetrads and clumps, acid not formed from glucose anaerobically— *Aerococcus*

The genera *Staphylococcus*, *Micrococcus*, *Streptococcus* (most strains), and *Aerococcus* are aerobic or facultative, while *Peptococcus* and *Peptostreptococcus* are anaerobic (see Chapter 83).

For differential characteristics of micrococcaceae, see Fig. 76-1.

Catalase test and benzidine test for differentiation of Micrococcaceae from Streptococcaceae

The **catalase test** consists of flooding the growth on the surface of a blood-free agar medium with 3% hydrogen peroxide and observing any vigorous bubbling.[5]

In some cases, however, release of oxygen from hydrogen peroxide is not catalase mediated (e.g., aerococci). Also, some strains of *Micrococcaceae* (*Micrococcus mucilaginosus*, formerly *Staphylococcus salivarius*) do not decompose hydrogen peroxide.

The **benzidine test** (Deibel and Evans[6]) can be used for differentiating *Micrococcaceae* from the *Streptococcaceae* when the catalase test may be unsatisfactory or unusable.

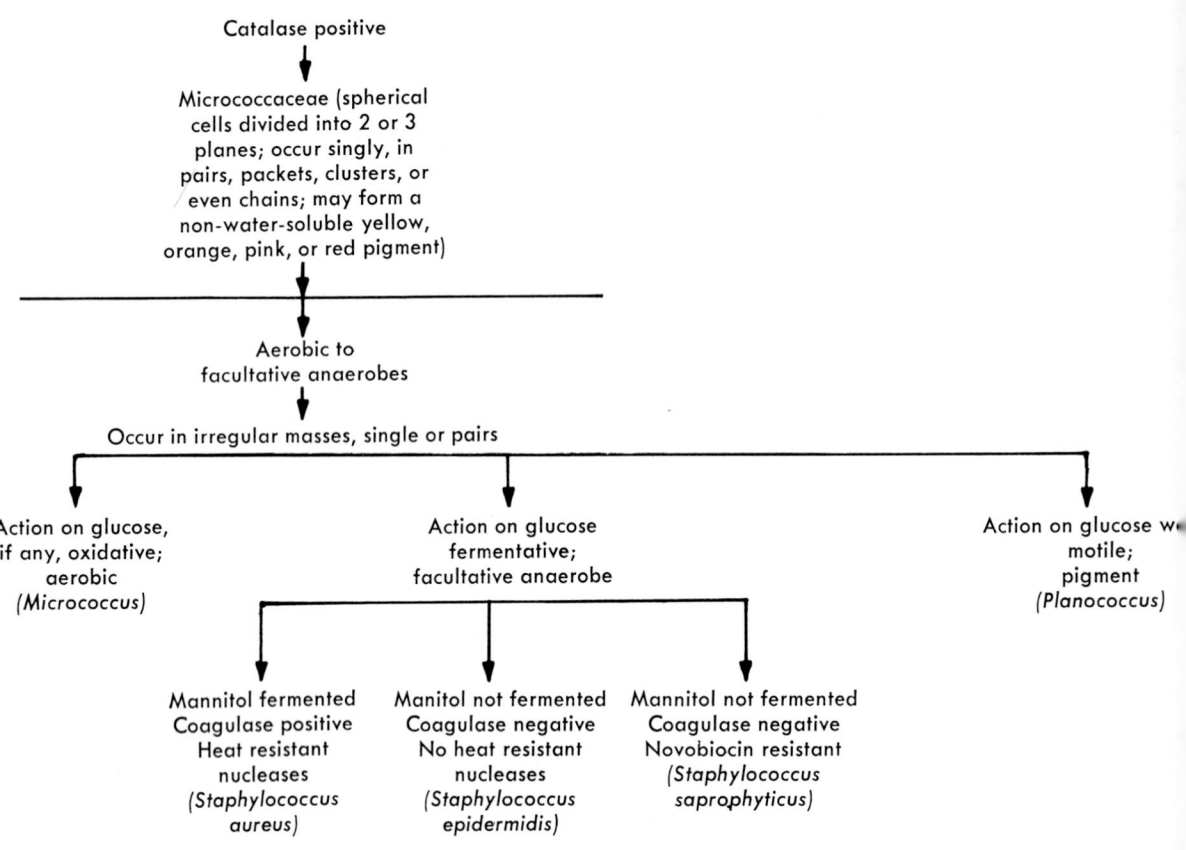

Fig. 76-1. Differential characteristics of organisms in the family Micrococcaceae. (Based on data from *Bergey's Manual*, ed. 8,[3] Facklam and Smith,[5] and ICSB Subcommittee.[4])

Catalase reagent and test

See tests and reagents, Chapter 72.

Benzidine reagent and test [6]

Reagent

1. Benzidine dihydrochloride   1 g
   Glacial acetic acid   20 ml
   Partially dissolve benzidine in acetic acid.
2. Distilled water   30 ml
   Add to benzidine solution. Heat gently.
   Cool.
3. 95% ethyl alcohol
   Add to benzidine solution; Mix.
   Reagent can be held at least 1 mo if refrigerated.

Procedure

1. Flood 24-48 h culture plate with benzidine solution.
2. After all colonies (growth) have been covered or contacted by reagent, add equal vol 5% hydrogen peroxide.
3. Positive benzidine test is evidenced by appearance of deep green or bluegreen color.

All the *Micrococcaceae* yield a positive benzidine test for cytochrome enzymes, whereas *Aerococcus* and other streptococci do not.[5]

STAPHYLOCOCCUS
S. aureus, S. epidermidis, S. saprophyticus

Staphylococci are spherical organisms (cocci), 0.8-1+ μm in size, occurring singly, in pairs, but more commonly in clusters that resemble bunches of grapes. The cocci form a designlike arrangement in smears from solid media. They grow well on blood-free basal media (tryptose, meat infusion, etc.) and are gram positive and catalase positive. The colonies are confluent, circular, with unbroken edges, and opaque, and they may be white, yellow, or orange. Glucose is attacked fermentatively, and the organisms are facultative anaerobes (grow in air as well as anaerobically). Many strains are hemolytic on blood agar.

Although responsible for a number of often severe diseases in humans (see "Pathogenicity of staphylococci"), it should be noted that staphylococci are present in the permanent bacterial flora of the skin and the nasopharynx of humans. Potentially pathogenic forms (*Staphylococcus aureus*) are carried in the nose, on the skin, or on various mucous membranes by 20-40% of all individuals in the absence of overt disease.

The Subcommittee on the Taxonomy of Staphylococci and Micrococci, at its 1975 session,[7] agreed to recognize a simplified scheme for identification of staphylococci and recommended in human clinical situations the identification of 3 species, i.e., *S. aureus*, *S. epidermidis*, and *S. saprophyticus* (for other schema, see Kloos

Table 76-1. Differentiation of staphylococci[7]

Character	S. au-reus	S. epi-dermi-dis	S. sap-rophyti-cus
Key			
Coagulase	+	−	−
Sucrose, acid (aerobically)	+	+	+
Trehalose, acid (aerobically)	+	−	+
Mannitol, acid (aerobically)	+	−	+
Phosphatase	+	+	−
Novobiocin	S	S	R

S, sensitive; R, resistant.

and Schleifer[8] and Oeding and Digranes[9]).

Differential characteristics of the 3 species are shown in Table 76-1.

S. epidermidis and *S. saprophyticus* are **coagulase negative;** the former does not form acid (aerobically) from trehalose and mannitol, while the latter is usually phosphatase negative and resistant to novobiocin. *S. aureus* is **coagulase positive,** produces acid aerobically from trehalose and mannitol, produces thermostable nuclease, and (most strains) deoxyribonuclease and phosphatase.[10]

Based on Baird-Parker's work,[11-13] the 3 *Staphylococcus* species have been further subdivided into biotypes[1] (*S. aureus*, biotypes A-F[14], *S. epidermidis*, biotypes 1-4; and *S. saprophyticus*, biotypes 1-4); however, for clinical purposes only differentiation into the 3 species is of importance.

Pathogenicity of staphylococci

S. aureus causes localized abscesses such as boils, carbuncles, and furuncles in addition to impetigo, pyelitis, and cystitis as well as serious infections such as septicemia, meningitis, osteomyelitis, pneumonia, and endocarditis. It is involved in a major proportion of hospital-acquired wound infections and outbreaks of infections in the nursery, in the form of pemphigus, conjunctivitis, septic spots, and paronychia. It is commonly found in mothers' breast abscesses. Enterotoxin-producing strains of *S. aureus* may be isolated from food, vomitus, and feces in food-poisoning outbreaks. Staphylococcal enteritis (pseudomembraneous enterocolitis), a relatively rare but extremely dangerous complication, usually develops after prolonged antibiotic therapy accompanied by emergence of resistant strains.

S. epidermidis is less virulent but can cause stitch abscesses and mild urinary tract infection after instrumentation. It is also involved in endocarditis, bacteremia, and occasionally in infections after cardiac surgery.

S. saprophyticus resembles *S. epidermidis* but is somewhat distinctive by its resistance to novobiocin. It is now considered by some workers to be a common cause of acute urinary tract infection, especially in young women (outpatients)[15]; however, only a small number of patients were found to yield over 10[4] coagulase-negative staphylococci per milliliter in pure culture in a study by Williams et al.[16]

Isolation, identification, and assessment of virulence of staphylococci

The isolation of staphylococci can be readily accomplished by using commonly accepted bacteriologic procedures. Their identification and assessment of virulence, on the other hand, are somewhat controversial. A multitude of media and a need for various fermentation and pathogenicity tests have been advocated. Major sources of information on staphylococci are Cohen's *The Staphylococci*[17] and Jeljaszewicz's *Staphylococci and Staphylococcal Diseases.*[18]

Recommended media for isolation and identification

It should be remembered that when a specimen from an infectious process is delivered to the laboratory, the causative organism is not known and therefore initial culture of any specimen must be carried out on a number of media, as used for various specimens, including anaerobic medium for the complete diagnostic routine. Many of the media listed below are specifically for staphylococci and are to be used in conjunction with the usual media employed for isolation and differentiation of bacteria from clinical specimens, unless the study concerns itself solely and specifically with staphylococcus problems.

Dwarf forms of *S. aureus*, menadione- or thiamine-requiring strains. *S. aureus* growing as dwarf colonies on usual media has been reported by a number of investigators. Recently Acar et al.[19] reported on dwarf strains (isolated from human infections) that require menadione or thiamine to grow normally.

There are situations where it may be necessary to use enriched medium (chocolate agar with IsoVitaleX or brain-heart agar with IsoVitaleX; see Media) with added menadione to assure detection and isolation of deficient strains: (1) when *S. aureus* is seen on Gram stain and culture is negative, (2) with cultures from patients with known *S. aureus* infections who are receiving antibiotic therapy, or (3) with patients who have chronic staphylococcal infections (especially osteomyelitis).

Blood agar. Any good blood agar base (blood agar base, heart infusion agar, tryptone soy agar, Columbia agar, trypticase soy agar) plus 5-10% blood is recommended. In case outdated human blood bank blood is used the following test should be carried out:

Pour several blood agar plates with blood from new bottle and streak them with group A β-hemolytic streptococcus strain. If organism does not grow, do not use new bottle of blood because it probably contains inhibitory amounts of antibiotics.

Sheep blood (available commercially) is recommended mainly because sheep cells are lysed by α-toxin, considered to be the most important staphylococcal toxin, whereas human red cells are lysed by δ-lysin.[20]

Broth. Heart infusion, tryptone soy, and trypticase soy broths are satisfactory media for the isolation and cultivation of staphylococci. For blood cultures commercially available blood culture outfits are recommended, consisting of a bottle of sterile broth and the necessary equipment for taking a sample.

Mannitol salt agar.[21] This medium should be used in addition to blood agar when contamination with other bacteria is expected, for example, in fecal specimens from suspected staphylococcal enteritis or in specimens from wound infections. Because of the high content of sodium chloride (7.5%) and the presence of mannitol and phenol red in this medium, *S. aureus* will appear as a yellow colony surrounded by a yellow zone, whereas other staphylococci usually form a small colony in a red or purple zone, and other organisms, including gram-negative organisms, are usually completely inhibited.

As a routine procedure a blood agar plate, a broth tube, and, depending on the specimen, a mannitol salt agar plate are usually satisfactory for the isolation of staphylococci.

A number of other media are available.

Tellurite glycine agar. Tellurite glycine agar is a medium containing glycine, lithium chloride, and potassium tellurite as selective agents. Coagulase-positive staphylococci produce black colonies, whereas coagulase-negative staphylococci or other organisms fail to produce visible growth in 24 h or form gray colonies.

Staphylococcus medium no. 110 and Chapman-Stone agar. These high salt content media containing mannitol and gelatin[22,23] are now used less frequently than before, since gelatin liquefaction is no longer considered a differential test in classification.

Mannitol neomycin agar.[24] Mannitol neomycin agar may be used to advantage for isolation and identification of staphylococci. The medium consists of trypticase soy agar (1 L), mannitol (10 g), neomycin sulfate (0.0005 g), phenol red (0.0025 g), and defibrinated sheep blood (50 ml). This medium inhibits coagulase-negative staphylococci and micrococci but not coagulase-positive staphylococci, *Streptococcus*, *Proteus*, *Pseudomonas*, or *Candida*.

Phenolphthalein phosphate ("phosphatase") agar.[25] Blood agar base with 0.01% phelolphthalein phosphate added aseptically to the molten medium is a useful screening medium for coagulase-positive organisms. **Phosphatase**, which is constantly found in such staphylococci, splits off the phenolphthalein. When exposed to strong ammonia, coagulase-positive colonies become deep pink. However, it should be noted that some staphylococci produce phosphatase but not coagulase. The medium is prepared by adding 1 ml 1% filtered, sterile solution of phenolphthalein diphosphate (pentasodium salt) to 100 ml melted blood agar base. After incubation and growth, preferably at 30 C, invert agar plate over Petri dish lid (glass) or other container filled with 0.880 sp. gr. ammonia.

Phenylethyl alcohol agar. See Media, Chapter 72.

Primary culture—specimens from pathologic conditions

The procedures below include only methods specific for staphylococci; they are to be used in conjunction with other media used for various specimens.

All specimens except blood culture and feces. Use blood agar plate and tube of broth and make Gram stain. Streak plates carefully, crosshatching to secure well-isolated colonies. If initial Gram stain shows large numbers of gram-negative rods, use mannitol salt agar. Inoculate heavily but crosshatch carefully. Incubate blood plates for 16-24 h and mannitol salt agar plates for 24-48 h.

Feces. Make Gram stain. If large numbers of gram-positive cocci in clusters are seen, make immediate preliminary report and proceed with the culture.

Use mannitol salt agar plate and blood agar plate.

Blood. Use routine blood culture as described in Chapter 75.

Examination of primary cultures

Blood agar plate. Smooth, round, opaque, moist, shiny, domed, "oil paintlike" colonies 5-7.5 cm in diameter grow within 18-24 h after inoculation.[26] Contrary to earlier beliefs calling for the presence of hemolysis and pigment to be present to warrant further investigation, any staphylococcus-like colony showing gram-positive cocci in clusters on smear may be potentially pathogenic, even in the absence of hemolysis or pigment or both. Therefore do **not** discard the plate if no pigmented, hemolytic colonies are present. If more than 1 type of staphylococcus-like colony is present (i.e., 1 hemolytic and the other nonhemolytic, or 1 pigmented and another nonpigmented), both types must be examined further.

Older colonies of staphylococci become umbonate, and as autolysis of the center develops, multiple papillae are formed.[24] Diphtheroid, streptococcus, and occasionally yeast colonies may resemble staphylococci so that microscopic examination may be necessary. Streptococci can be distinguished from staphylococci with the aid of the **catalase reaction**, which is consistently negative in streptococci and positive in staphylococci (with rare exceptions).

Mannitol salt agar. Select an isolated staphylococcus-like colony surrounded by a yellow zone (indicating mannitol fermentation). If none is present select any other isolated staphylococcus-like colony and proceed as under Blood agar plate.

If poor growth is found on original mannitol salt agar plate, reincubate overnight.

Broth culture. Transfer to blood plate and mannitol salt agar plate and continue as under Blood agar plate.

Criteria for identification and assessment of virulence: *S. aureus*

Coagulase test. The most important single in vitro test and the one presently considered as the most significant in the differentiation of potentially pathogenic and nonpathogenic staphylococci is the **coagulase test.** Fermentation of mannitol, hemolysis, and pigmentation, criteria formerly held in high esteem, are not presently accepted as valid criteria for distinguishing *S. aureus* from other staphylococci. However, coagulase-negative staphylococci are also known to have been implicated in disease. Unless a particular study is centered solely on staphylococcus problems, always report both coagulase-positive and coagulase-negative colonies found.

As a rule, all staphylococcus-like colonies showing gram-positive cocci in clusters must be coagulase tested regardless of pigmentation and presence or absence of hemolysis.

Since the coagulase test is accepted as a practical criterion for identifying *S. aureus*, it is necessary to deal briefly with the rationale of the test and to point out a number of pitfalls and limitations that should be familiar to the laboratory worker.

The ability of certain staphylococci to clot (citrated or oxalated) plasma of certain mammalian species has been known since the beginning of the twentieth century. The extracellular or **"free" coagulase** (released into the medium), **detected by the coagulase tube test,** interacts with a plasma factor (coagulase reacting factor, CRF) to produce an active principle, thrombokinase-like in action; fibrinogen is clotted and converted to fibrin.[27] CRF, unlike thrombokinase, does not require calcium for its formation. **"Bound" coagulase** (clumping factor) is detected by the **coagulase slide test;** it is not found in culture filtrates and it does not require CRF. The 2 tests correlate well; **however, a negative slide test should be checked with a tube test.**

Rabbit plasma (citrated) is recommended for testing staphylococci from human sources.

False clotting. Several organisms other than *S. aureus* are known to clot citrated plasma, such as strains of *Pseudomonas aeruginosa, Serratia marcescens,* and especially strains of enterococci (*Strep. faecalis*). These organisms most often clot the plasma not by coagulase activity but by utilization of citrate, thereby releasing the calcium, which is then available for the normal physiologic clotting (Bayliss and Hall).[28] For this reason the use of plasma rendered incoagulable by oxalate, heparin, or EDTA (ethylenediamino tetraacetate) is advocated by some workers.

False-negative coagulase test. Some *S. aureus* strains produce so much fibrinolysin that the clot formed by coagulase cannot be observed (read test after 1 h!). Also some strains produce small amounts of coagulase, and overnight incubation may be needed.

Tube tests. Several methods are available.

1. Emulsify single colony from 24 h blood agar culture in 1 ml citrated rabbit plasma (diluted 1:5 with physiologic saline). Incubate at 37 C in water bath and examine for clotting at 1, 2, 4, 8, and 24 h. Set up known positive and negative controls. Any degree of clotting is accepted as coagulase activity (standard method recommended by International Subcommittee[2]). Facklam and Smith[5] state that test should **not** be incubated overnight and it **should** be read at 4 h.
2. Add human blood bank or fresh rabbit plasma to heart infusion or soy broth in 10% concentration. Dispense aseptically in 1 ml amounts in sterile tubes ("plasma broth").[25]

Because of individual variations that may occur in various batches of plasma, batch should be tested with coagulase-positive strains before being put into routine use.

Lyophilized commercial plasma. Several workers have reported[29] that the lyophilized commercial products are much more uniform than plasma selected at random. For smaller laboratories, in particular, the use of desiccated plasma is much more advantageous than that of fresh plasma. The manufacturer's directions should always be followed if commercial dried plasma is used. It has been found that although inoculation of a broth tube with an isolated colony, incubation for 2-4 h, and subsequent use of this broth culture in the reconstituted plasma is an effective way of performing the test, single colonies emulsified in 0.2 ml brain-heart infusion and immediately mixed with plasma solution in a tube will also give satisfactory results.

Slide test.[30] One of the fastest and easiest means of performing the coagulase test is a slightly modified version of the slide method. After a little practice with known cultures, the laboratory worker should be able to attain a 99% correlation of this method with the conventional tube test. The test detects bound coagulase.

1. Using wax pencil, draw circles of about ¾ in. diameter on inside of bottom of plate.
2. Place small drop of water in each circle.
3. Emulsify loopful of *Staphylococcus* growth in water to appearance of milk.
4. After emulsions are prepared, add small drop of coagulase plasma to each.
5. Gently rock plate for about 1 min.

Positive cultures form small flocs or masses readily visible without a microscope. Negative tests must be repeated by the tube method.

Pigment formation. As pointed out earlier, the presence or absence of pigment is not a valid single criterion for pathogenicity of staphylococci; however, there is still sufficient correlation between coagulase production and pigment formation to make pigment formation significant. Incubation at 35-37 C does not enhance pigment formation, whereas incubation at room temperature or growth on milk agar is useful for pigment production. Spreading a colony on white filter paper and allowing it to dry is a simple and satisfactory way of detecting pigment.[26]

If there are no isolated colonies but only mass growth of *Staphylococcus*-like organisms, proceed as above but at the same time streak onto a fresh blood agar plate to be sure the culture is pure. If it proves not to be a pure culture, repeat all of the above tests from an isolated colony.

Agar slant. From all coagulase-positive isolates prepare nutrient agar slant, incubate overnight, and then store in refrigerator for possible bacteriophage typing (see below).

Deoxyribonuclease (DNase) activity determination. The deoxyribonuclease activity determination was first described by Weckman and Catlin.[31] DNase activity seems to be correlated with coagulase activity. DNA (2 mg/ml) is incorporated into trypticase soy agar with 0.8 mg anhydrous calcium chloride per milliliter.[32] The bottom side of each agar plate of this medium is divided into 4 squares, and each strain to be tested is streaked onto a square. After growth occurs the plate is flooded with normal hydrochloric acid. Cultures producing DNase show a zone of clearing around the streaks, the unaffected medium appearing cloudy.

Thermostable nuclease production.[33] This is a supportive test to be used with weaker (2+) coagulase reactions. It entails a color change from blue to bright pink.

1. Prepare microslides by spreading 3 ml toluidine blue–deoxyribonucleic acid agar on surface of each microscope slide. When agar has solidified, cut 2 mm diameter wells (10-12 per slide) in agar and remove agar plug by aspiration.
2. Add approximately 0.01 ml heated sample (15 min in boiling water bath) of broth cultures used for coagulase test to well on prepared slide.
3. Incubate slides in moist chamber 4 h at 35 C. Positive reaction is development of bright pink halo extending at least 1 mm from periphery of well.

Toluidine blue –DNA agar[34]

Deoxyribonucleic acid (DNA)	0.3 g
Agar	10 g
Calcium chloride (anhydrous)	1.1 mg
Sodium chloride	10 g
Toluidine blue O	0.083 g
Tris(hydroxymethyl)aminomethane	6.1 g

1. Dissolve the tris(hydroxymethyl)aminomethane in 1 L distilled water and adjust pH to 9.0.
2. Add remaining ingredients except toluidine blue O and heat to boiling to obtain complete solution of DNA and agar.
3. Dissolve toluidine blue O in this solution and dispense in smaller portions in rubber-stoppered flasks. Sterilization is not necessary.

The medium is stable at room temperature for as long as 4 mo and remains satisfactory even after several melting cycles.

A similar method utilizing Petri plates rather than microslides, is described by Zarzour and Belle[10] and Lachica et al.[34]

Lysostaphin susceptibility[33]

1. Transfer isolated colony from agar plate by inoculating loop to 0.2 ml phosphate saline buffer and emulsify.

2. Transfer half of suspended cells to another tube (13 × 100 mm) and mix with 0.1 ml phosphate saline buffer as control.
3. Add 0.1 ml lysostaphin (Schwarz/Mann Research Lab., Orangeburg, N.Y.), dissolved in 0.02 M phosphate buffer containing 1% NaCl, to original tube to give concentration of 25 γm lysostaphin/ml.
4. Incubate both tubes at 35 C for not more than 2 h.

If turbidity clears in test mixture, test is considered positive. If clearing has not occurred in 2 hours, test is negative. *S. aureus* is generally positive.

For a method using lysostaphin incorporated in agar, see Kloos and Schleifer.[8]

Other tests. A number of other tests for staphylococci have been described (see below).

Classification and reporting

In routine work all coagulase-positive staphylococci should be designated as *aureus*, regardless of hemolysis or pigmentation. If a hemolytic or pigmented but coagulase-negative strain is present, at least 3 colonies should be tested for coagulase production. If coagulase negative, test for oxidative or fermentative utilization of glucose; if oxidative (or does not utilize glucose at all), it is *Micrococcus;* if fermentative, it is *S. epidermidis.* Report should state "Staphylococcus aureus" or "coagulase-positive staphylococci"; "S. epidermidis" or "coagulase-negative staphylococci" is also adequate.

Bacteriophage typing (see below) is the most reliable and final test in identifying *S. aureus* strains. It has no diagnostic or therapeutic significance and should be used only in epidemiologic and research studies.

Antibiotic sensitivity tests

The antibiotic sensitivity pattern (antibiogram) does not identify strains as well as bacteriophage typing, but it is a guide to therapy and as such is an important clinical laboratory test. The method used depends mainly on the available resources and work force of a particular laboratory. Although the tube dilution method is considered more accurate, it is also time consuming and expensive. The disk method is more rapid and easier to perform; automated methods also are used (see Chapter 87).

Emergence of *S. aureus* strains resistant to various antimicrobial agents is a considerable problem facing the clinician. Penicillinase-producing strains are resistant to penicillin (about 80% of strains responsible for hospital-acquired staphylococcal infection and 35-50% of community strains); resistance to erythromycin and tetracycline is also common. The availability of semisynthetic penicillins (not susceptible to penicillinase), such as methicillin, oxacillin, cloxacillin, and sodium nafcillin, makes it mandatory that antibiotic susceptibility testing also include such agents.

β-Lactamase detection. High levels of resistance of penicillin with many organisms correlate with the presence of β-lactamase (see Chapter 87).

Methicillin-resistant strains of *S. aureus*, many of which are also resistant to cloxacillin, oxacillin, nafcillin, and the cephalosporins and are involved in serious infections, have been found in Europe, England, and the United States; recently, gentamicin-resistant strains have also appeared.

Bacteriophage typing[35, 36]

Bacteriophage typing is essential in the detection of sources of nursery epidemics and other outbreaks and for controlling such events. It is based on the susceptibility of *S. aureus* to infection by various bacterial viruses (bacteriophages) that are specific for staphylococci. Phage typing can prove 2 strains to be identical or different. The saving of cultures (on agar slants for a period of 1-3 mo under refrigeration) will enable any hospital in the event of an outbreak to submit these cultures to a state or regional laboratory performing phage typing. Phage typing is **not** recommended as a routine procedure and should be restricted to epidemiologic investigations.

The set of basic phages in use (minimum number), used for typing *S. aureus*, is as follows[33, 37, 38]:

Group I	29, 52, 52A, 79, 80
Group II	3A, 3B, 3C, 55, 71
Group III	6, 7, 42E, 47, 53, 54, 75, 77, 83A
Group IV	42D
Miscellaneous	81, 187

Coagulase-negative staphylococci can also be studied with typing phages: Van Boven et al.[39] developed a set of 18 phages for typing *S. epidermidis*. For details, see Van Boven.[40]

An authoritative publication on methods of typing is that of Blair and Williams.[37]

Additional tests for staphylococci

Coagulase-plate method[41]
1. Mix rabbit or human plasma with nutrient agar in concentration of 12-15% (vol/vol) of plasma at 46 C.
2. Pour mixture into Petri dishes and allow to solidfy.
3. Make spot inoculation and incubate 12-18 h or overnight.
4. Coagulase production is indicated by development of opacity around spots.
5. If organism is strongly proteolytic or fibrinolytic, clot may be lysed, and opacity disappears after prolonged incubation.

Egg yolk opacity test[42]
1. Add 5 parts fresh hen egg yolk to 100 parts digest or infusion broth.
2. Add 2 g/dl kieselguhr after thorough stirring.
3. Mix, allow to stand 30 min, and then filter through filter paper pulp.
4. Add 1% glucose and filter through Seitz pad, pH 7.2.
This will be usable for at least 4 wk.
5. Inoculate 2 tubes, each containing 1 ml glucose yolk broth. To one add 1 drop, or about 0.03 ml,

antitoxin (Burroughs Wellcome & Co., Tuckahoe, N.Y.), 250 U/1.9 ml.
6. Incubate 3 days at 37 C in covered water bath.
Opacity in broth and absence in broth containing antitoxin is positive result (EYP). Absence of opacity in both is negative (EYN).

Hyaluronidase production. Methods of determining hyaluronidase production are complex and exacting. Hyaluronic acid substrate must be produced from either synovial fluid or umbilical cords. The commercial product is unsatisfactory.[43-46]

Toxin production (agar plate method)[47]
1. Inoculate 1.25% (soft) agar plates, pH 7.2, with heavy inoculum and place in jars above excess of $CaCO_2$.
2. Run down side of jar sufficient HCl to give 20% atmosphere of CO_2; close jar at once. Incubate 48 h.
3. Cut agar into small pieces and suck through conical Buchner funnel to break it up.
4. Filter through paper in wide Buchner funnel.
5. After final sterilization through Seitz filter, bring to pH 7.0-7.2.
6. Add a few drops chloroform.
7. Cover surface of filtrate with layer of sterile mineral oil.

Toxin production (embryonate egg method)[48]
1. Inoculate chorioallantoic sac of 12-day chick embryo with 0.1 ml 10^{-3} dilution of 18 h broth culture of staphylococcus.
2. Incubate inoculated embryos at 37 C for 2-3 days. Approximately half of these will die.
3. Pool relatively clear allantoic fluid of surviving embryos and centrifuge to remove bacterial cells.
4. Preparations can be frozen in dry ice chamber without loss of activity. At refrigerator temperature activity gradually decreases.

Alpha hemolysin production in broth cultures[49]
1. Grow staphylococci in nutrient broth for 48 h in air containing 30% CO_2.
2. Obtain clear supernatant fluids by centrifuging cultures at 4000 rpm for 15 min.
3. Make doubling dilutions using physiologic saline as diluent.
4. To each 1 ml dilution add 1 ml 2.5% suspension in saline of rabbit washed red cells.
5. Prepare control tube with 0.02 ml commercial staphylococcus antitoxin (Burroughs Wellcome & Co., Tuckahoe, N.Y.) added to lowest dilution of supernate. This control is used with each experiment.
6. Read after 1 h incubation in water bath at 37 C.
7. Reciprocal of highest dilution producing 50% hemolysis is activity in hemolytic units/ml.

Leukocidin production and test[50]
1. Obtain human blood cells by venipuncture. Wash in saline, using narrow centrifuge tube for final washing so as to concentrate leukocytes.
2. Dilute toxin prepared according to Panton et al.[47] (above)—1:2 and 1:8, using saline as diluent.
3. Incubate equal vol cells and filtrate for 1 h in Wright pipet.
4. After thoroughly washing in and out of pipet, mix contents in proportions of 2 vol toxin-cell mixture with 1 vol fresh human serum and 1 vol staphylococcus suspension.
5. Incubate 20 min and again wash out contents.
6. Thoroughly stir drop with platinum loop and make film from loopful of mixture.
7. Allow to dry and stain with blood stain. No fixative is needed if Wright stain is used. If Giemsa stain

is used, slides must be fixed by allowing methyl alcohol to remain in contact with films for 5 min preliminary to staining.

When leukocidin is strong, all phagocytes are destroyed in both 1:4 and 1:116 dilutions. Well-stained lymphocytes are present.

Such toxins usually produce clots. Films of clots show masses of almost basophil cell debris entangling normal lymphocytes.

Weak leukocidins produce partial or almost complete destruction of leukocytes at 1:4 and little action at 1:16. Some filtrates have no destructive effect at all. Control films without toxin must be run at same time as test.

Δ-Lysin (leukocidin) production[51, 52]

Highest yields of Δ-lysin are obtained when staphylococci are grown on cellophane.

1. Place sheets of ordinary wrapping cellophane, cut to fit, in sterile Petri dish with a little water to keep them moist.
2. Sterilize in autoclave at 5-10 psi for 10 min. Do not allow sheets to dry or become overheated to prevent wrinkling and loss of efficiency.
3. Place sterilized sheets aseptically on freshly poured, undried nutrient agar plates (Lemco peptone).
4. Inoculate with 3 drops broth culture and distribute over entire surface with spreader.
5. Incubate plates at 37 C for 24-48 h in 20-30% CO_2 atmosphere.
6. To harvest lysin, wash staphylococci off cellophane with saline, using 1.5-2 ml/sheet.
7. Allow these thick suspensions of organisms to stand at 4 C for 3 h or overnight. Then remove cocci by centrifugation.

Test for Δ-leukocidin

1. Collect human blood according to method of Miller and Ackerman,[53] collecting about 10 ml in siliconized tube containing 0.1 ml heparin (10 mg/ml) and 1 ml 6% dextran solution in saline.
2. Mix and incubate 30 min at 37 C at 30° angle.
3. Remove supernatant fluid, using Pasteur capillary pipet. This fluid contains thrombocytes, polymorphonuclear leukocytes, some lymphocytes, and red blood cells.
4. Drop 0.5 ml supernatant fluid into siliconized tube containing 7 ml Hanks solution.
5. Centrifuge 2 min at 500 rpm.
6. Remove sediment using capillary pipet and place 1 drop on glass slide.
7. Add 1 drop broth prepared for Δ-leukocidin and cover with coverglass.
8. Incubate control without added toxin at 37 C for 15 min.
9. Examine under low and high magnification.

Δ-Leukocidin will burst polymorphonuclear leukocytes, whereas lymphocytes, monocytes, and control polymorphonuclears remain rounded and may even demonstrate motility. Coverslips may be slipped off and slide and covers dried in air, later to be fixed and stained for examination.

Necrotoxin determination (rabbit skin test)[54]

1. Give intradermal doses of 0.2 ml toxin. If filtrates are strongly α-hemolytic, use in 1:20 dilution. This gives area of necrosis 1.5-2 cm in diameter, indicating strong necrotoxin.
2. Use feebly hemolytic filtrates in 1:5 and 1:20 dilutions. The 1:5 dilution is usually feebly positive, whereas 1:20 dilution is usually negative, including weak necrotoxin. When 1:5 dilution is negative, make subsequent test with undiluted toxin.

Always take fresh rabbits and test up to 6 filtrates simultaneously on same animal.

Virulence in rabbits (IV).[55] Intravenous injection of 0.1-0.5 ml culture of strain of S. aureus recently isolated from suppurative focus generally proves fatal in 24-48 h. Postmortem examination shows hemorrhages and bloody exudations on serous membranes and parenchymatous degeneration of glandular organs. Cocci can be recovered from bloodstream.

Intravenous injection of similar dose, about 0.01-0.05 ml, gives rise to pyemia, accompanied by loss of weight and general weakness, proving fatal in 1-6 wk. Disseminated abscesses are found especially in the kidneys. Endocarditis and osteomyelitis are seen less frequently. S. albus is usually much less pathogenic. Strains recently isolated from suppurative foci may cause death on intravenous injection of 1-2 ml of a 24 h broth culture. Strains isolated from saprophytic sources are nonpathogenic unless given in large doses, when death occurs apparently from toxemia.

Virulence in mice (IV).[56] Give to each of 10 albino mice, by intravenous route, 0.05 ml overnight infusion broth culture of strain to be tested. If 50% or more of mice die within 2 days after inoculations, then disease in patient from whom strain was obtained is likely to prove severe.

MICROCOCCUS

Micrococci are gram-positive, catalase-positive, nonmotile cocci that occur in pairs, irregular clusters, or tetrads. They utilize sugars oxidatively or not at all, are aerobic, do not coagulate plasma, and fail to ferment glucose anaerobically (Fig. 76-1.)

The organisms are usually saprophytes and present in air, dust, water, and on the skin. Although micrococci are usually described as being of relatively little importance in human disease, some strains have been implicated in soft tissue abscesses, septicemia, endocarditis, and meningitis.

In the clinical laboratory micrococci are often mistaken for coagulase-negative staphylococci; aerobic utilization or no utilization of glucose by the method described below should suffice for separation (as long as the organism is catalase positive and a gram-positive coccus).

Test for separation of Staphylococcus from Micrococcus[2, 11]*(Subcommittee method)

Inoculum. Grow gram-positive and catalase-positive cocci for 24 h at 37 C on tryptone yeast extract agar (Difco tryptone, 1.0; Difco yeast extract, 0.1; agar, 1.5; quantities are given as % wt/vol).

Medium. Difco tryptone, 1.0; Difco yeast extract, 0.1; glucose, 1.0; Difco agar, 0.2, and bromcresol purple, 0.004 (quantities are given as % wt/vol). Adjust pH to 7.0. Dispense in 10 ml amounts into 16 × 120 mm tubes. Sterilize by autoclaving for 20 min, 115 C.

Test. If stored, steam medium for 10-15 min (to remove dissolved oxygen); cool in iced water. Inoculate duplicate tubes heavily with a long wire loop so that inoculum reaches bottom of tubes. Cover 1 tube of pair

---

*The test is based on the oxidation-fermentation (O-F) test of Hugh and Leifson, described in Chapter 72, but utilizes a richer medium.

with 25-30 mm layer of sterile mineral (paraffin) oil. Incubate at 37 C for 5 days.

Interpretation. (1) If the indicator changes to yellow throughout both tubes, acid is produced fermentatively (anaerobically) and the organism is a *Staphylococcus*. (2) If acid is produced only in the unsealed (aerobic) tube (oxidative utilization of glucose) or no change occurs in either tube (no utilization), the organism is a *Micrococcus*.

In the clinical laboratory the test is of importance if gram-positive, catalase-positive cocci are isolated, under clinically significant circumstances, which cannot be identified unequivocally as *S. aureus* or *S. epidermidis*.

ANAEROBIC STAPHYLOCOCCI AND MICROCOCCI

See Chapter 83.

Streptococci

Streptococci belong to the family *Streptococcaceae*, genus *Streptococcus* (*Bergey's Manual*, ed. 8[3]). The family also includes, among others, the genus *Aerococcus*.

STREPTOCOCCUS

Streptococci are spherical or ovoid cells, arranged in short or long **chains** or in **pairs.** They are nonmotile and non-spore-forming. Some species form capsules. They are gram positive, benzidine and catalase negative, and, with the exception of *S. pneumoniae*, not soluble in bile. Growth on artificial media is slight. Various carbohydrates are split fermentatively with the production of lactic acid (the **facultative** streptococci are **homofermentative,** while **anaerobic** streptococci are **heterofermentative** and do not produce lactic acid).

Most species fail to liquefy gelatin. Several species produce characteristic change in media containing blood. Most species are facultatively anaerobic, but some are obligate anaerobes (see Chapter 83). Many species are parasitic to humans or animals and form an important part of the normal flora, whereas other species are highly pathogenic.

Morphology and staining

The cells are spherical or ovoid, occur as short or long chains or in pairs but never in packets, vary greatly in size, and are 0.5-1 μm in diameter. The cells are gram positive, some species decolorizing easily.

Colonies

Small grayish and delicate opalescent colonies are visible on blood agar plates, usually within 18-24 h. They are round with smooth or slightly corrugated edges. Minute hemolytic streptococci of groups F and G form tiny colonies. Variants of the same strain may show different colony forms.

Among group A hemolytic streptococcus strains the differentiation is into matt, glossy, and mucoid colonies.

Pathogenicity

Streptococci cause a wide variety of diseases in both humans and animals and continue to be among the commonest causes of bacterial infections of humans. In general the hemolytic species are the most pathogenic. Among Lancefield's serologic groups, group A strains are predominantly pathogenic for humans, being the most usual cause of pharyngitis and septic lesions; they are also responsible for acute rheumatic fever and acute nephritis. Over 80% of streptococcal infections in humans are caused by strains of group A streptococci; about 15% are caused by strains of group B, C, D, F, and G. Nonhemolytic streptococci, both viridans and enterococci, are often disease inducing in humans and are responsible for most cases of subacute bacterial endocarditis (SBE). Anaerobic streptococci are a frequent source of severe infections. For human infections caused by groups other than A (*S. pyogenes*) or D (enterococci) see Reinarz and Sanford[57] and Moellering et al.[58]; for infections caused by group B streptococci see Anthony and Okāda,[59] Wilkinson,[60] and Patterson[61]; for a study of streptococcal bacteremias see Duma et al.[62]

Excellent reviews are Wannamaker and Matsen's *Streptococci and Streptococcal Diseases*,[63] and, for β-hemolytic streptococci, that of Breese.[64]

Classification

Systems for the nomenclature of streptococci are based on (1) changes produced in blood (hemolytic activity), (2) serologic grouping (antigen analysis), and (3) physiologic characteristics. In addition a common usage nomenclature has also developed. Table 76-2 summarizes the relationships among the various systems of streptococcal nomenclature.

Classification based on changes produced in blood. Brown[65] described 3 different types of reaction on blood agar plates: (1) the α **(viridans)** type, which produces a greenish discoloration and partial hemolysis of the red cells surrounding the colony, although an outer clear zone may develop on preservation of the cultures in the refrigerator; (2) the β **(hemolytic)** type, which produces a clear zone of hemolysis about the colony with no intact red cells and no further extension of the area on refrigeration; and (3) the γ **(nonhemolytic)** type, which does not affect the red blood cells in the medium.

Classification based on antigen analysis. Lancefield[66-69] has shown that hemolytic streptococci can be differentiated serologically by means of the precipitin reaction into distinct and sharply defined groups, based on the fact that the strains of each group contain a group-specific carbohydrate, the so-called C substance. Those of major medical importance are groups A, B, C, F, G, and

Table 76-2. Relationships among various systems of streptococcal nomenclature*

Serologic group	Hemolytic activity	Physiologic species	Common usage
A	β	S. pyogenes	β-Hemolytic streptococci (**pyogenic**)
B	β, γ	S. agalactiae	β-Hemolytic streptococci
C	β	S. equisimilis	β-Hemolytic streptococci
		S. zooepidemicus	
		S. equi	
C	α	S. dysgalactiae	
D	α, β, γ	S. faecalis	(Group D) **enterococci**
		S. faecium	Fecal streptococci
		S. durans	
D	α, γ	S. bovis	(Group D) **nonenterococci**
		S. equinus	
		S. avium†	
E	β	S. infrequens	
F	β	S. anginosus	Minute-colony streptococci
G	β	S. anginosus	Minute-colony streptococci
		—	Large-colony streptococci
H†	α	S. sanguis	Viridans streptococci
K†	α, γ	S. salivarius	Viridans streptococci
L	β	—	
M	β	—	
N	α, γ	S. lactis	**Lactic** streptococci
		S. cremoris	
		S. diacetylactis	
O†	α	—	
P	β	S. infrequens	
Q†	α	S. avium	
R	α	S. suis (II)	
S	α	S. suis (I)	
T	α	—	
U	β	S. infrequens	
V	β	S. infrequens	
Proposed group	β	S. iniae	
—	α, γ	S. pneumoniae	**Pneumococcus**
—	α, γ	S. mutans	**Viridans** streptococci
		S. uberis	
		S. sanguis (I)	
		S. sanguis (II) } S. mitior	
		S. mitis	
		S. MG (intermedius) } S. milleri	
		S. anginosus (constellatus)	
		S. salivarius	
		S. morbillorium	
		S. acidominimus	

*Modified from Wilkinson, H. W.: Pathogenesis and identification of streptococci. In Clinical Microbiology Newsletter **1**(9):1, 1979.
† Groups H, K, and O are now more commonly classified as viridans, and Q as a subtype of Group D streptococci; hence the double inclusion of species names. Not all group H strains speciate as *S. sanguis*. Not all *S. sanguis* are serologic group H. The same situation applies to group K and *S. salivarius*.

D. Groups E, F, H, K, and O are found in humans but are less often pathogenic.

Classification based on physiologic characteristics. With the aid of a number of physiologic and biochemical tests, streptococci can be divided into a number of groups (previously designated **pyogenic, viridans, enterococococcus,** and **lactic**). Table 76-4 shows the presumptive identification of streptococci and Table 76-5 lists additional characteristics based on physiologic findings. It may be noted that there are relationships between the serologic groups and the physiologic characteristics. Thus **determining hemolytic activity is the most important step in the presumptive identification of streptococci.**

• • •

The *screening, presumptive, and confirmatory tests* used for classification and identification are described on pp. 1645-1650.

• • •

Hemolytic* (pyogenic) streptococci

Group A. These streptococci contain the group A carbohydrate component described by Lancefield. They are subdivided into serologic types by precipitin reactions. Group A streptococci, producing β-hemolysis in blood agar plates, form 2 types of hemolysins: **streptolysin O** and **streptolysin S.** The latter is oxygen stable and thus is responsible for surface hemolysis, whereas streptolysin O, oxygen labile, lyses only in subsurface (deep) colonies. Antibodies to streptolysin O develop in patients recovering from streptococcal disease (ASO test, Chapter 107). They are susceptible to bacitracin, do not hydrolyze hippurate, do not give a positive CAMP reaction, and do not hydrolyze bile-esculin or grow in 6.5% NaCl broth.

They usually do not grow on 10% and 40% bile agar, no growth occurs at pH 9.6, in 6.5% NaCl broth, at 45 C, nor do they survive 60 C for 30 minutes. They do hydrolyze arginine, form acid in litmus milk, and ferment maltose, trehalose, and salicin but not glycerol, mannitol, or sorbitol. The large majority of streptococcal infections in humans are caused by strains of group A (*S. pyogenes*). For **fluorescent antibody technics** used in their identification see Chapter 70.

Group A streptococci have been further subdivided into serologic types based on type-specific protein, the so-called M antigen.[70-74] Griffith[75] developed a slide agglutination technic and designated the first 30 types according to the predominant antigen present in strains freshly isolated from human infections. For type differentiation in group A, Lancefield employs the precipitin test[66-69] with acid extracts of the streptococci—the so-called M fraction—and immune rabbit sera. The results of this method have been shown to parallel those obtained with the specific agglutination and mice-protection tests. The precipitin reaction depends on the M antigen alone, whereas agglutination may be due to either M or another protein antigen, the T antigen. One or more T antigens occur in most strains of group A streptococci; the distribution is independent of the distribution on the type-specific M antigen. A particular streptococcus strain almost always possesses only a single M protein[76]; therefore the precipitin test gives the more specific reaction. New types have been identified in various laboratories from time to time since Griffith's classification, and at least 55 M types are now recognized.

For the epidemiologic study of streptococcal infections, identification of the serologic group and type of streptococci is needed.

NOTE: Group A streptococci that are **α-hemolytic** (**not** β-hemolytic) have on occasion been isolated from infections in humans.[77] The organism is usually narrowly β-hemolytic in pour plates but not on surface growth either aerobically or anerobically.

Non-β-hemolytic streptococci should be grouped (to determine whether they are group A) if (1) there is an outbreak of acute rheumatic fever and no group A β-hemolytic organisms can be isolated from acutely ill patients, and (2) if the laboratory chooses to group all streptococci from serious infections, e.g., endocarditis.

Group B. In the past these β-hemolytic streptococci were found mostly in cattle (bovine mastitis) and have been rarely implicated in human infections. In the last decade, however, the reported frequency of group B infections in humans has increased.[59-61,78] They have been isolated from infections in diabetics, from septicemia, empyema, arthritis, and meningitis. The organisms are found in about 5% of normal human throats; they have been isolated from the vagina, vulva, and genitourinary tract. Butter and de Moor[79] found that approximately 10% of healthy individuals act as carriers of group B streptococci, and 9% of parturient women and newborn infants carry the organism in the throat or in the vagina, on the nipples, and on the umbilicus (carrier rates of up to 25% have now been reported). **Meningitis of the newborn** due to group B streptococci has been increasing, and it is now (1978) the leading cause of meningitis during the first 2 months of life in several geographic regions.[59-61,80-83]

The organism can often be presumptively recognized on blood agar plates because of the β-hemolysis, often accompanied by a "double zone hemolysis" (especially when embedded in the blood agar)[57] and because of the size of the colonies that are considerably larger than those of group A streptococci.

The term *S. agalactiae* has been applied to these organisms; serologic types Ia, Ib, Ic, II, II/Ic, and III are known, with about 2% of strains being nontypeable.[84]

Group B streptococci are β-hemolytic and are usually resistant to **bacitracin** (although occasional strains are susceptible to bacitracin). They hydrolyze **hippurate** and give a positive **CAMP** reaction. They do **not** hydrolyze **bile esculin** medium, and some strains tolerate **6.5% NaCl broth,** especially after 48 hours' incubation. They grow on 40% bile agar, and are heat sensitive (no growth at 45 C).[85]

NOTE: About 2% of group B streptococci are **nonhemolytic**[84]; these can be identified with (1) immunofluorescence, (2) presumptively the CAMP test, or (3) hippurate test, and (4) as a confirmatory test, the capillary precipitin (Lancefield) test; other serologic tests available are counterimmunoelectrophoresis, latex agglutination, and coagglutination.

Group C. These streptococci produce β-hemolysis on blood agar plates (larger zone of hemolysis than group A); they are **bacitracin** resistant, do **not** hydrolyze hippurate or bile-esculin, do **not** give a CAMP reaction, and do

---

*The term "hemolytic" generally is used to denote β-hemolytic streptococci.

not grow in 6.5% NaCl broth. They produce in glucose broth a final pH between 4.5-5.4. Some strains of group C *(S. equisimilis)* grow on 10% bile agar, but very few grow on 40% bile agar. They can be further differentiated into 4 groups. One of these subgroups *(Streptococcus equi)* ferments neither trehalose nor sorbitol, another (Animal C, *S. zooepidemicus*) ferments sorbitol but not trehalose, a third *(S. equisimilis)* ferments trehalose but not sorbitol, and the fourth *(Streptoccus dysgalactiae)* ferments trehalose; fermentation of sorbitol is variable. Colonies of the typical *S. equi* type are large, honey colored, and of viscous consistency.

Group C strains	Trehalose	Sorbitol
S. equisimilis	+	−
S. zooepidemicus	−	+
S. equi	−	−

Group F. Organisms in this group grow slowly on blood agar plates, forming minute, pinpoint, transparent colonies surrounded by a narrow zone of β-hemolysis. They are identical to the strains described by Long and Bliss[86] as "**minute hemolytic streptococci.**" They produce a final pH of 4.8-5.2 in glucose broth, do not hydrolyze sodium hippurate or bile-esculin, are bacitracin resistant, CAMP negative, 6.5% NaCl negative, do not reduce methylene blue in milk, and do not grow on either 10% or 40% bile agar. None ferment sorbitol, but some strains ferment trehalose. They ferment lactose and salicin. This group has been found in cultures from the human throat.

Group G. A final pH of 4.4-5.2 is produced in glucose broth. Organisms in this group do not hydrolyze sodium hippurate, do grow on 10% bile agar but not on 40% bile agar, and do not reduce methylene blue in milk. Trehalose and lactose but not sorbitol are fermented. They are bacitracin resistant and CAMP, bile, hippurate, and 6.5% NaCl negative. Organisms from matt colonies of groups C and G resemble each other in fermenting trehalose but not sorbitol and in producing fibrinolysin and streptolysin O. On blood agar plates they form a wide zone of β-hemolysis. Among the large colony type there are at least 3 serologic types. The small colony strains all appear to belong to one type. Most group G strains have been isolated from humans, monkeys, or dogs.

Group H. The original group H streptococci were described by Hare[87] as narrow-zone β-hemolytic colonies, with a tendency to throw off nonhemolytic variants. No soluble hemolysin is produced. Among the nonhemolytic strains 2 serologic types were established. Most strains of *S. sanguis,* producing α-hemolysis according to White and Niven,[88] possess H antigen; however, both the validity of the species designation and their placement in the pyogenic group has been questioned by Rosebury.[89,90] Cowan and Steel[91] list the organism as producing α-hemolysis and

remark that extracts of some strains do not react with H antisera. Group H is now more commonly classified as **viridans.**[92] The organism was originally isolated from heart valve vegetations in cases of subacute bacterial endocarditis.

Viridans group

Streptococci that form colonies surrounded by a zone of α-hemolysis, showing the characteristic green discoloration, or are nonhemolytic, are referred to as the **viridans** group. Although they are serologically ungrouped, a few represent immunologically distinct varieties. They do **not** hydrolyze bile esculin or hippurate, do not give positive CAMP reactions, and do not grow in 6.5% NaCl broth. Some of the strains are susceptible to bacitracin, but they are still viridans streptococci.

Occasional α- or nonhemolytic group B streptococci (see Group B above) can be presumptively identified as such because they hydrolyze hippurate and give positive CAMP reactions and do not react in bile-esculin tests. This identification should be confirmed by serogrouping.

Viridans streptococci usually grow at 45 C but not at pH 9.6 or in 0.1% methylene blue.

Most species do not grow on 40% bile agar; some may grow on 10% bile agar.

S. salivarius ferments inulin and raffinose and forms large, mucoid colonies (levan) on 5% sucrose or raffinose agar; it is usually nonhemolytic (γ) on blood agar.

S. mitis, usually α-hemolytic, does not ferment inulin; it usually (but not always) ferments raffinose. *S. uberis* (bovine mastitis) and *S. thermophilus* (from milk and milk products) grow at 45 C and survive at 60 C for 30 min, whereas *S. salivarius* and *S. mitis* do not survive at 60 C.

Serologic groups H, K, and O (Table 76-2) are now more commonly classified as viridans; not all group H strains speciate as *S. sanguis,* and not all *S. sanguis* are serologic group H. The same is true of group K and *S. salivarius* (Wilkinson).[92]

Viridans streptococci are constantly present in the human mouth and throat and are often found in the intestines of humans and animals; they are the commonest cause of **subacute bacterial endocarditis (SBE) in humans.**

The organisms also occur in infections following instrumentation in patients with damaged endocardium or heart valves, in brain abscess, and liver abscess.

S. mutans,[93,94] often requiring increased CO_2, nonhemolytic on surface of blood agar, hydrolyzing esculin (20-50% of strains), and producing extracellular glucan (dextran) in 5% sucrose broth and 5% sucrose agar is often involved in subacute bacterial endocarditis.

S. milleri,[95] synonymous with *S. MG (intermedius)* and *S. anginosus (constellatus),* has been recently noted for the high frequency of its involvement in clinically significant suppurative, pyogenic infections (abscesses, peritonitis, cholangitis, empyema, often with gastrointestinal source). Isolation of the organism from blood cultures should serve as a signal to look for a suppurative process.

• • •

For identification and differentiation ("speciation") of viridans streptococci, see Table 76-5. They are identified as to species usually only when isolated from serious infections (blood cultures, etc.).

• • •

Some workers, especially in England, have in the past included *Diplococcus pneumoniae (pneumococcus)* among the streptococci; the International Subcommittee on the Taxonomy of Streptococci and Pneumococci finally recommended in 1967 that *Streptococcus pneumoniae* is the correct term rather than *Diplococcus pneumoniae*.[96] *S. pneumoniae* is discussed in detail below.

• • •

Lactic group

Group N is found in dairy products and on certain plants and is considered nonpathogenic. These organisms grow well at 10 C, reduce methylene blue, and grow on 10% and 40% bile agar. The organisms possess the group N specific polysaccharide.

Group D streptococci: enterococci and nonenterococci

Group D streptococci possess a common polysaccharide antigen. Some members of the group are β- or α-hemolytic, others are not. Generally they do not produce a filtrable hemolysin.

Group D streptococci are divided into 2 groups: enterococci and group D nonenterococci.

Group D enterococcal streptococci ("enterococci"). These organisms are bile-esculin (BE) and 6.5% NaCl positive. An occasional strain will hydrolyze hippurate, but generally any strain that is BE positive is a group D streptococcus (for exceptions see bile-esculin test), and if it tolerates 6.5% NaCl it is an enterococcus. They do **not** give positive CAMP reactions.

Enterococci produce a final pH of 4.2-4.8 in glucose broth; grow freely on 10% and 40% bile agar, in 6.5% salt broth, at 45 C, at pH 9.6, and in 0.1% methylene blue milk; and are heat resistant, most strains withstanding a temperature of 60 C for 30 minutes. They usually but not always ferment trehalose, sorbitol, and mannitol; always ferment lactose and salicin; and decarboxylate tyrosine.

Species of group D **enterococci** (*Bergey's Manual*, ed. 8[3]) are:
1. *Streptococcus faecalis* with:
   a. ssp. *faecalis* (not hemolytic)
   b. ssp. *liquefaciens* (not hemolytic, gelatin liquefied)
   c. ssp. *zymogenes* (β-hemolytic on blood agar)

2. *Streptococcus faecium* (previously with var. *durans*[97])

S. faecalis and its varieties tolerate 0.04% tellurite, ferment sorbitol and glycerol, and reduce tetrazolium.

S. faecium, as described, is distinguished by fermentation of arabinose and melibiose and inability to ferment melezitose and inositol. It also grows at 50 C (*S. faecalis* does not). It is either α- or β-hemolytic, and it fails to reduce litmus milk.

Enterococci are found mainly in the intestinal tract, the genitourinary tract, and saliva. Although they are normal commensals, they are often implicated in disease (SBE, urinary tract infections, etc.). Their relative resistance to several antibiotics, including penicillin, makes their identification imperative.

Group D "nonenterococcal" streptococci. These organisms produce positive results **only** in the BE test. They do **not** tolerate 6.5% NaCl or hydrolyze hippurate or give positive CAMP reactions, and they are usually nonhemolytic. They are susceptible to penicillin, whereas the enterococci are resistant. Patients with nonenterococcal group D infections can be managed as if they had a viridans streptococcal infection, but patients with systemic enterococcal infections must be treated with combined antibiotic therapy if the causative organisms are to be eradicated.

Group D **nonenterococcal** streptococci (*Bergey's Manual*, ed. 8[3]) are *S. bovis* (ferments lactose, α or γ reaction on blood agar) and *S. equinus* (does not ferment lactose, usually γ, occasional α reaction on blood agar).

Prevalence of *S. bovis* in fecal cultures from patients with carcinoma of the colon was reported by Klein et al.,[98] who noted the possible association in patients with *S. bovis* endocarditis and colonic carcinoma. The same association (*S. bovis* endocarditis in patients with carcinoma of the colon) was also noted by Levy et al.[99] *S. bovis* is a normal habitant of the mouth, has been identified in human feces, and is an important cause of bacterial endocarditis.[100]

S. equinus is not a significant pathogen in humans; when encountered it can be distinguished from *S. bovis* because of its failure to grow in litmus milk and to form acid in lactose broth.[101]

• • •

Group D strains can be differentiated by physiologic tests as follows:

Group D strains	6.5% NaCl	Arginine	Pyruvate
S. faecalis	+	+	+
S. faecium	+	+	−
S. bovis	−	−	−

Satellite streptococci

Satellite streptococci (nutritionally deficient organisms that grow on blood agar only around other bacteria) have been described from cases of endocarditis.[102] Since it is recognized that nutritionally variant streptococci exist,[103, 104] blood agar plates used for subculture of blood culture or other broth culture should be streaked with staphylococci, especially when organisms seen in Gram stains of broth fail to grow on solid media.[105]

Anaerobic streptococci

See Chapter 83.

Isolation and identification of streptococci

Most specimens come from throat (tonsils and oropharynx), nose, and vaginal secretions, sputum, pus, skin lesions, blood, and spinal fluid of patients. For collection of specimens, swabs, and transport media, see Chapter 63.

Microscopic. Look for gram-positive cocci, arranged in long or short chains.

Cultural. In general the streptococci may be cultivated on blood agar media for primary isolation and for subsequent identification.

The primary isolation of streptococci from uncontaminated material such as blood, cerebrospinal fluid, etc. is carried out on blood agar and in trypticase soy broth or brain-heart infusion broth.

Microaerophilic as well as other streptococci grow well in thioglycollate broth. For the isolation of enterococci Difco's **bile-esculin** medium (containing 40% bile, i.e. 40 g oxgall per liter) is recommended. **Sodium azide blood** plate and **phenylethyl alcohol** plate are excellent media for the isolation of streptococci from contaminated material.

Most enterococci grow on Endo agar, whereas other streptococci do not grow.

Streaked plates. With each specimen, inoculate plates of 5-7% defibrinated blood agar medium. Streak inoculum carefully; make several **stabs** in the agar to demonstrate subsurface hemolysis.

Often the laboratory may not achieve the proper hemolysis because incorrect blood media have been used. *A Method for Culturing β-Hemolytic Streptococci from the Throat* by Wannamaker (American Heart Association)[106] lists the major factors involved as follows:

1. **Blood: Sheep blood** should be used; it is preferable to rabbit, horse, or human blood. (If outdated human blood bank blood is used each unit of blood must be checked for toxicity of the anticoagulant, residual antibiotic, and elevated ASO titers by growing a known group A streptococcus on streak and pour plates prepared with the blood tested.) Sheep blood contains a factor that inhibits the growth of *Haemophilus haemolyticus*, whose colonies can be mistaken for β-hemolytic streptococci. Use **defibrinated** (not citrated) blood.

2. **Medium:** Blood agar base, available from several manufacturers, should be used. Avoid media containing glucose or other fermentable carbohydrate, which may alter the type of hemolysis produced. Add 5-7% defibrinated sheep blood; mix and add 15-20 ml amounts of blood agar mixture into Petri dishes. The layer of blood agar should be approximately 6 mm thick.

If **horse blood** is used, more *Haemophilus* organisms will produce lysis; with **rabbit blood** α-hemolysis is rather poor. Human blood should be avoided, since a large variety of organisms will produce hemolysis.

Incubate plates anaerobically, if possible; otherwise use candle jar (3-5% CO_2).

Pour plates. Tilt the plate carefully to distribute the inoculum evenly. (For preparation of pour plate see Chapter 75).

Hemolysis. Streaked (and poured blood) agar plates are used. Determine **hemolysis** microscopically in the *stabbed* area of blood agar plate: This is the most important initial determination.

NOTE: It should be remembered that the type of hemolysis seen on blood plates is not adequate to characterize streptococci. β-Hemolytic streptococci may be group A (which is sensitive to penicillin) or group D (enterococci, relatively resistant to penicillin and other antibiotics). Greening streptococci may be viridans, enterococcus, or any other group. Nonhemolytic (γ) streptococci may belong to a variety of groups, including enterococci. All isolates should be adequately tested for final identification. In most laboratories the **bacitracin** test (for group A organisms) and the use of bile-esculin medium, 6.5% sodium chloride broth, hippurate hydrolysis, and CAMP test are entirely feasible and should be performed. For differentiation of greening streptococci from pneumococci see bile and Optochin tests (*Pneumococcus,* below).

Broth media. For serologic group or type identification and for the production of hemolysin, Todd-Hewitt medium[107] is satisfactory. For type identification of group A strains. Difco Neopeptone and Evans peptone are suitable.

Enrichment media. For the isolation of streptococci from throat cultures containing only small numbers of the organisms, Pike enrichment medium[108] may be employed.

For selective media employed for group A streptococci see Throat culture, Chapter 75.

Media for biochemical tests. Sugar fermentation tests, when needed, are carried out in peptone water, cystine trypticase base, or extract broth with 1% test sugar.

Examination of plates for β-hemolytic colonies. See Throat and nasopharyngeal culture, Chapter 75.

Streptococcal groups and species to be identified; antimicrobial susceptibilities

Table 76-3 lists those streptococci that should be identified in **all** clinical laboratories (Wilkinson[92]); reasons for this requirement are based on information needed for antimicrobial treatment of patients.

While it has been stated generally that group A

streptococci do not need to be tested for antimicrobial susceptibility (at this time, 1978, they are still sensitive to penicillin), it has recently been urged (Drapkin et al.[109]) that *all* streptococci isolated from patients with serious infections be grouped serologically and tested for antibiotic susceptibilities, especially if therapy with antibiotics other than penicillin is considered.

Group A streptococci resistant to clindamycin, tetracycline, and erythromycin have been reported.[109]

Group B streptococci seem to be somewhat more resistant to antimicrobials than other β-hemolytic streptococci, and group D enterococci are known for their resistance to penicillin and other antimicrobials.

Some viridans streptococci, also generally thought to be sensitive to penicillin, have lately displayed relative resistance to penicillin in vitro,[110] especially in patients who have received long-term penicillin prophylaxis.

The need for species identification may not be evident; however, the question of relapse versus reinfection and evaluation of possible therapeutic failure may require identification. Similarly, antimicrobial susceptibility determination (including minimum inhibitory concentration, MIC, and minimum bactericidal concentration, MBC) of penicillin G should be performed for the selection of appropriate therapy in serious viridans streptococcal infections.

For the occurrence of antimicrobial-resistant strains of *Streptococcus pneumoniae*, see *Pneumococcus,* below.

Identification

Standard, definitive identification.[98, 111] The best method for identifying the streptococci is by growing isolated pure colonies of the infecting organism, extracting the group carbohydrate, and demonstrating a **serologic reaction** (Lancefield) between the extracted antigen and specific grouping antiserum. The Center for Disease Control recommends the serologic grouping procedure as the method of choice. However, this method of growing and extracting the organism is time consuming, and the cost of obtaining specific potent antisera makes the method unacceptable for some laboratories.

NOTE: In addition to the Lancefield procedure there are a number of other procedures: **immunofluorescence,**[113, 114] **coagglutination,**[115-117] **latex agglutination,**[118, 119] **counterimmunoelectrophoresis,**[120, 121] and **capillary precipitation** (for pneumococci).[122] All of these procedures are described in this volume (see Chapters 70, 72, 74, and this chapter).

Alternative methods for identification.[92, 112] Laboratories not performing serologic grouping should consider an alternative method based on the following determinations.

Table 76-3. Minimal extent of streptococcal identification required in clinical laboratory*

Identify	Reason
Group A	Treat to prevent rheumatic fever
Group B	More resistant to antimicrobics than other β-hemolytic streptococci
Group D enterococcus	Resistant to several antimicrobics, including penicillin
Streptococcus pneumoniae	To distinguish from normal flora; antibiotic-resistant strains occur
Viridans group	Relative resistance to penicillin may occur (see text)

*Modified from Wilkinson, H. W.: Pathogenesis and identification of Streptococci, Clin. Microbiol. Newsletter 1(9):1, 1979.

Table 76-4. Presumptive identification of streptococci based on physiologic findings*

Hemolysis	Beta	Beta	Beta	Alpha, beta, none	Alpha, none	Alpha, none	Alpha
Bacitracin susceptibility	+	−†	−†	−	−	−†	±
Hippurate hydrolysis or CAMP reaction	−	+	−	−	−	+	−
Bile-esculin hydrolysis	−	−	−	+	+	−	−
Tolerance to 6.5% NaCl	−	±	−	+	−	−	−
Optochin susceptibility or bile solubility	−	−	−	−	−	−	+
Presumptive identification	Group A	Group B	Beta hemolytic not group A, B, or D	Group D enterococci	Group D not an enterococcus	Viridans	Pneumococci

*From Facklam, R. R.: Isolation and identification of streptococci. III. Center for Disease Control, Atlanta, 1977.
† Exceptions occasionally occur.

Table 76-5. Additional differential characteristics of streptococcal groups

	Hemolytic streptococci	Viridans streptococci	Enterococci	Lactic group*
Serologic group	A, B, C, E, F, G, H, K, L, M, O	Ungrouped	D	N
Antibiotic sensitivity	Usually sensitive	May be resistant	More resistant than others	—
Growth in 0.1% methylene blue in milk	—	—	+	+
Growth in broth at pH 9.6	—	—	+	—
Growth in 40% bile blood agar	− †	±	+	+
Growth on 10% bile blood agar	− †	±	+	+
Growth at 10 C	—	—	+	+
Growth at 45 C	—	+	+	—
Survive 60 C for 30 min	—	—	+	±

*No known pathogenic propensities.

† Rare exceptions (group B grows both on 10% and 40% bile agar; some group C and G strains grow on 10% bile agar).[91]

Table 76-6. Key to identification of viridans streptococci (α or γ)*†

Test	Clinical isolate
Acid formed in mannitol and lactose broths	
Hippurate hydrolyzed, glucans not produced on sucrose agar or broth	S. uberis
Hippurate not hydrolyzed, glucans produced on sucrose agar and broth	S. mutans
Acid formed in lactose but not mannitol broth	
Acid formed in inulin broth	
Glucans (dextrans) produced on both sucrose agar and broth, NH_3 split from arginine, α-hemolytic	S. sanguis I
Glucans (levans) produced on sucrose agar only, no NH_3 from arginine, nonhemolytic	S. salivarius
Acid not formed in inulin broth	
Esculin hydrolyzed	Streptococcus MG-intermedius‡
Esculin not hydrolyzed	
Acid formed in raffinose broth	S. sanguis II
Acid not formed in raffinose broth	S. mitis
No acid formed in mannitol or lactose broth	
Hippurate hydrolyzed	S. acidominimus
Hippurate not hydrolyzed	
Esculin hydrolyzed, growth in 40% bile broth, litmus milk reduced weakly	S. anginosus-constellatus‡
Esculin not hydrolyzed, no growth in 40% bile broth, litmus milk not reduced	S. morbillorium

*From Facklam, R. R.: Physiological differentiation of viridans streptococci, J. Clin. Microbiol. **5:**184, 1977.

† Not β-hemolytic. Extracts do not react with group B or D antisera. Occasional positive reaction on bile-esculin or methylene blue milk. Growth in 6.5% NaCl or at 10 C is rarely observed.

‡ Streptococcus MG and S. anginosus are classified by some workers as S. milleri.[95]

1. **Bacitracin** susceptibility
2. Determination of the presence of the **CAMP factor** or hydrolysis of **sodium hippurate**
3. Hydrolysis of **esculin** in the presence of 40% bile (bile-esculin, BE, test)
4. Tolerance to 6.5% NaCl broth

For suspected pneumococci, perform Optochin or bile solubility tests. Table 76-4 summarizes presumptive identifications based on physiologic findings, and Table 76-5 lists additional characteristics.

The formulas for the media, description of the tests, and analyses of results follow below. These tests, when run properly with adequate controls, will accurately identify more than 95% of the pathogenic streptococci from clinical material. The resulting identifications are, however, **presumptive,** and reports should indicate this fact.

• • •

For presumptive identification see Table 76-4; for identification of viridans streptococci see Table 76-6. Also, use key A for β-hemolytic streptococci and key B for non-β-hemolytic streptococci. Additional characteristics are listed in Table 76-5.

The following keys are based on the use of

standard tests, described below under "Screening, presumptive and confirmatory tests." **Table 76-4 should be used in conjunction with the keys.** When the organism is producing α-hemolysis or is nonhemolytic (γ) and species identification is desired, proceed to "Identification of viridans streptococci" and Table 76-5 below.

A. Key for β-hemolytic streptococci

Bacitracin negative
Bile esculin (BE) negative

CAMP negative and/or sodium hippurate negative	β-hemolytic streptococcus, not group A or B
CAMP positive and/or sodium hippurate positive	Group B

BE positive

CAMP negative, 6.5% NaCl positive	β-hemolytic, group D enterococcus

For further identification see key for non-β-hemolytic treptococcus.

Bacitracin positive

CAMP negative	Group A streptococcus
CAMP positive, sodium hippurate positive, sometimes less surface and stab hemolysis	Group B
CAMP positive, sodium hippurate negative	Group B
CAMP positive	Group A or B

B. Key for non-β-hemolytic streptococci

Bile-soluble, optochin +, α-hemolytic	*S. pneumoniae*
Bile-negative, optochin −, α- or γ-hemolytic	
Bile esculin (BE) positive	
6.5% NaCl positive	Group D enterococcus
Further identification only if from blood culture	
Mannitol positive, tetrazolium reduced (sometimes β-hemolytic)	*S. faecalis*
Mannitol positive, tetrazolium not reduced	*S. faecium*
6.5% NaCl negative	Group D nonenterococcus
Lactose positive, litmus milk acid	*S. bovis*
Lactose negative, litmus milk negative	*S. equinus*
BE negative	
CAMP and/or hippurate positive	Group B nonhemolytic streptococcus
CAMP test negative	"*S. viridans*"; for further speciation see Identification of viridans streptococci and Table 76-6

Identification of viridans streptococci (α or γ; non-β-hemolytic)

Identification of viridans streptococci is usually done on isolates from blood cultures (also heart valves and other circulatory isolates), spinal fluid, and serious infections.

Media
  1% Mannitol
  1% Lactose
  1% Inulin
  1% Raffinose
  1% Esculin
  Moeller's arginine and control (add layer of mineral oil after inoculation)
  40% Bile broth
  Litmus milk
  Sodium hippurate test
  Sucrose broth
Interpretation of results
1. 1% broth of mannitol, lactose, inulin, esculin, raffinose. Positive reaction: indicator change from purple to yellow (acid production). Readings made daily for 3 days.
2. Arginine and control. Incubate 3 days at 35 C before reading. Positive reaction is recorded when the indicators turn to a violet to reddish violet. Control tube should be yellow, indicating growth in base and acid reaction.
3. 40% bile broth. Examine 3 days for growth.
4. Litmus milk. Examine daily for 3 days for reaction of acid production (A, pink color), reduction of indicator (N, white color) and clot (C).
5. Hippurate hydrolysis. See separate description of rapid hippurate test (*Rapid methods*, Chapter 72). Rapid test is inoculated with loopful of organism from blood agar plate.
6. Sucrose broth. Examine daily for 3 days for increase in viscosity.
7. Tetrazolium plates. Positive reduction: brick-red colonies within 3 days.

Key for identification of "viridans" streptococci. See Table 76-6.

Screening, presumptive, and confirmatory tests for streptococci

The tests and reactions listed below are of major importance in the examination and identification of facultative streptococci.

Hemolysis

See Isolation and identification above.

Bacitracin differentiation test

Maxted[123] reported that group A streptococci are more sensitive to bacitracin than are the other β-hemolytic streptococci and that this sensitivity can be used for the selection of group A strains. He suggested the use of filter paper strips dipped in a 5 U/ml solution of bacitracin. These paper strips are then dehydrated and placed on the surface of inoculated blood agar plates as in the usual disk sensitivity test. A modified method, eliminating dehydration of the impregnated filter paper, has been found to work equally well. A sterile filter paper disk is dipped into a 1 U/ml solution of bacitracin and the wet disk placed immediately on the surface of the inoculated blood agar. Group A streptococci show a zone of inhibition, whereas the growth of most other serologic groups is not inhibited (however, some strains of groups B, C, and G are inhibited). This test is now widely used for the **presumptive differentiation** of group A streptococci. (Bacitracin differentiation disks are commercially available from Difco Laboratories, Detroit, and as Taxo A disks from BBL, Division of BioQuest, Cockeysville, Md. The commercially available disks contain 0.02-0.04 U/disk of bacitracin. **Do not confuse this test with the bacitracin susceptibility test disk.**)

Jelinkova and Rotta[124] point out certain limitations of the test. There are some group A strains that display relatively low sensitivity to bacitracin. Increasing the concentration of bacitracin to detect all the group A strain, the test becomes positive for some strains of groups C and G. Using 0.7 U bacitracin disks, they obtained an inhibition ring of at least 5 mm around the disk, but they also found some C and G group strains giving the same result. They state that the reliability of the test in routine work depends on the source of the material to be tested. In testing material for human streptococcal disease, its reliability is high (90-95%). In examining carriers (in whom C and G strains are frequent) it is less reliable, and when used to test strains from animal sources its reliability is quite low (because of occurrence of group L stains, some of which are sensitive to bacitracin).

In general it has been found that the results of the test are in close conformity with those of serologic grouping of acute upper respiratory tract infection cultures. Whenever possible all β-hemolytic streptococci should be grouped by the precipitin method or other serologic method available, after initial bacitracin screening.

Center for Disease Control criteria for bacitracin test. Facklam,[125] based on Center for Disease Control (CDC) procedures, summarized the bacitracin test as follows:

1. **Use differential disks, not susceptibility disks.** Be sure to purchase **differential** (0.04 U), not **sensitivity** disks. Disks sold and used for bacitracin sensitivity testing have too high concentration of bacitracin to accurately differentiate between group A and nongroup A streptococci.
2. **Use heavy inoculum.** Heavy inoculum of pure culture is advisable because if inoculum is too light, non-group A streptococci will appear to be susceptible to bacitracin.
3. **Use pure culture.** Placing differential disk on primary plates inoculated with throat swabs has shown only 70% accuracy of identification for group A streptococci. The test is designed for use with pure cultures, not mixed cultures (see also Throat and Nasopharyngeal culture, Chapter 75).
4. **Use only β-hemolytic streptococci.** The test is designed for differentiating β-hemolytic streptococci. Hemolysis must be correctly determined before this differential test can be reliable. Many α-hemolytic streptococci, including pneumococci, are sensitive to bacitracin differential disk. Lots of commercial disks may vary; therefore each new lot of disks obtained should be tested with known strains of group A and non-group A

streptococci. Disks should be tested with control strains biweekly to determine reliability of disks.
5. **Interpret any zone size as positive.** The following criteria should be used to read the tests: (a) **any** zone of inhibition, regardless of diameter, means culture is positive; (b) no zone of inhibition (growth right up to edge of disk) means culture is resistant; (c) zone size requirements are stated in the literature, and one manufacturer, in a technical bulletin, implies that a zone size is necessary for presumptive identification of group A streptococci. The originator of the test (Maxted) did **not** specify that zones should be a certain size. No experimental data are available to show that zone diameters must be measured in order to differentiate group A from non-group A streptococci.

False-positives are potentially less harmful than false-negatives. By requiring zones of 10 mm or more for presumptive identification of group A streptococci, at least one group of investigators increased error of test by 10% (false-negatives).

The users of differential disks should realize that the bacitracin disk inhibits the growth of some strains of β-hemolytic streptococci other than group A. Therefore the report should be as follows: (a) "**presumptive β-hemolytic group A by bacitracin,**" or (b) "**β-hemolytic streptococci, not group A by bacitracin.**"

In a recent CDC series,[112] more than 99% of group A streptococci were susceptible to Taxo A disks (bacitracin disk, BBL). About 6% of group B streptococcal strains were susceptible; this error can be eliminated, however, by using a physiologic test (see CAMP and hippurate tests below) to presumptively identify group B streptococci.

The greatest source of error in the bacitracin test is the susceptibility of the β-hemolytic non-group A, B, or D streptococci. Group C and G streptococci are occasionally (7.5%) susceptible to bacitracin and are thus erroneously presumptively identified as group A by the bacitracin test. The potential error of the bacitracin test caused by the susceptibility of the viridans streptococci (7.8%) can be eliminated by correctly identifying the hemolytic activity of the strains.

CAMP test[111, 125-129]

The CAMP test, developed by Christie et al.,[125] depends on synergistic hemolysis between *Staphylococcus aureus* β-toxin and a streptococcal factor (CAMP factor, CAMP protein[111]) on sheep blood agar or ox blood agar; human blood agar **cannot** be used for this purpose.[129]

When a staphylococcus is inoculated as a streak across a plate and the streptococcus is inoculated at a right angle but **not** touching, the lytic zone assumes an **arrowhead** shape; the tip points toward the staphylococcus. The CAMP test is a test for the presumptive identification of β-hemolytic group B streptococci.

Procedure
1. Using inoculating needle, streak *Staphylococcus aureus* CDC #695 in 1 single straight line across center of blood agar plate (Fig. 76-2).

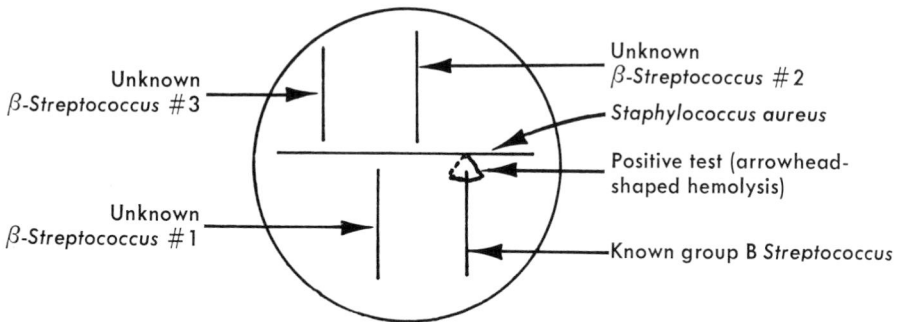

Fig. 76-2. CAMP test procedure (see text).

2. Inoculate positive control (Group B, β-streptococcus CDC #617) in single straight line (2-3 cm) at 90° angle to staphylococcus streak. **Do not touch staphylococcus with streptococcus.**
3. Inoculate unknown test organism as described in 2. Up to 3 unknowns may be used on each plate.
4. Place plate in CO_2 at 37 C (candle jar or CO_2 incubator), **not** anaerobically.
5. Positive readings may occur at 5-6 h of incubation.
6. Positive CAMP test produces zone of hemolysis (arrowhead shape) between staphylococcus and streptococcus.
7. False-positive results will occur if unknown is not *Streptococcus*. Some *S. epidermidis* will give false-positive test.
8. Confirm all CAMP positive, β-hemolytic streptococci by Lancefield procedure, coagglutination, or latex agglutination.
9. Send report out as follows: "Group B β-hemolytic streptococci (by CAMP test procedure); to be confirmed."

NOTE: Recently a **CAMP-disk** procedure has been described by Wilkinson.[128]

Bacitracin-negative, CAMP-positive, β-hemolytic streptococci can be reported as presumptive group B streptococci.

Bacitracin-positive, CAMP-positive, β-hemolytic streptococci are either group A or group B. The bacteriologist must decide which organism the unknown strain resembles most. This can be done by examining the hemolytic activity. Group B streptococci show much **less** surface and stab hemolysis of the blood agar than do the group A streptococci. Bacitracin-positive, CAMP-positive group A (10%) and group B (6%) streptococci occur quite frequently, thereby making it necessary for bacteriologists to familiarize themselves with the difference in their hemolytic activity.[112]

Bacitracin-positive, CAMP-negative, β-hemolytic streptococci are presumptive group A streptococci. Bacitracin-negative, CAMP-negative, β-hemolytic streptococci are β-hemolytic streptococci not group A or B.[112]

Nonhemolytic group B streptococci are CAMP positive; therefore nonhemolytic streptococci that are bile-esculin negative and CAMP positive can be presumptively identified as nonhemolytic group B streptococci.[112]

Hippurate hydrolysis test[130, 131]

See Hippurate test, Chapter 72, and Hippurate rapid test in Rapid methods, Chapter 72.

All strains of group B and some strains of group D produce hydrolysis of this compound.

Bile-esculin (BE) test[112, 132–134]

Medium
1. Add 23 g nutrient agar to 400 ml H_2O, mix well, heat until colloidal.
2. Add 40 g oxgall to 400 ml H_2O, mix well, heat into solution.
3. Add 0.5 g ferric citrate to 100 ml H_2O, mix well, heat into solution.
4. Combine solutions 1, 2, and 3, mix well, heat to 100 C for 10 min.
5. Sterilize in autoclave at 121 C for 15 min. (This is base medium.)
6. Cool to 50 C.
7. Add 1 g esculin to 100 ml H_2O, heat gently to dissolve, and sterilize by filtration (Seitz or Millipore).
8. Aseptically add sterile esculin solution to base medium, mix well, dispense into 16 × 125 mm screwcap tubes, and slant tubes.

Dehydrated medium (Difco) can be resuspended, tubed and autoclaved, slanted, and used with excellent results.

BE medium will identify group D streptococci. All group D streptococci (includes all enterococci) will blacken the BE slant, usually within 48 hours. Most non-group D streptococci do not blacken the medium.

Not all group D streptococci are enterococci (penicillin resistant). *S. bovis* and *S. equinus* are group D species, but they are not enterococci.

S. bovis (BE positive) is found in a significant number of group D infections and is penicillin sensitive; therefore further tests are needed to adequately differentiate the enterococci from nonenterococci. A streptococcus that gives a positive BE reaction should be reported as a "presumptive group D streptococcus by BE hydrolysis." The BE test does not differentiate enterococci from nonenterococci; thus a positive BE test should **not** be reported as presumptive identification of enterococci.

NOTE: (1) Some viridans streptococci (about

10%) will give positive BE reactions. (2) The source of the inoculum influences the result of the BE test. False-positive tests are obtained occasionally depending on the medium used, a matter currently not well understood (personal communication, Facklam, November 1978).

Salt-tolerance test (6.5% NaCl test)[112]

Medium

Heart infusion broth	25 g
NaCl	60 g
Dextrose	1 g
Indicator (1.6 g bromcresol purple in 100 ml ethanol)	1 ml
Distilled water	1000 ml

Mix reagents, dissolve, mix, dispense in suitable tubes (15 × 125 mm screwcap), and autoclave at 15 lb pressure for 15 min.

Positive reaction is recorded when indicator changes from purple to yellow or when growth is obvious even though indicator does not change.

Enterococci (S. faecalis and its varieties zymogenes and liquefaciens; S. faecium) will usually give heavy growth and an indicator change within 24 hours. Some enterococcal strains take 48 hours, and some will grow with no accompanying indicator change even after 72 hours.

About 80% of group B streptococci will also grow in this medium, and some change the indicator. Beta groups A, C, G, and F usually do not grow in the medium. The α-hemolytic, nongroupable streptococci (viridans), such as S. mitis, S. sanguis, S. salivarius, S. mutans, and S. MG, do not grow in 6.5% NaCl medium, nor do group D species S. bovis and S. equinus.

A positive BE test and positive growth in 6.5% NaCl broth confirm the presence of enterococci. Even if serologic reactions are determined, growth in 6.5% NaCl broth should be used to confirm that the group D streptococcus is an enterococcus.

Salt-tolerant, β-hemolytic strains other than groups B and D streptococci occur very rarely. Salt-tolerant group A streptococci occur occasionally. Strains that give positive salt-tolerance tests and that are not presumptive group B (hippurate) or presumptive group D (BE) streptococci should be tested for purity by streaking the growth from the salt-tolerance test medium onto a blood agar plate and comparing the morphology with that of the original strain. If the morphology differs, a Gram stain and a catalase test should be performed.

Optochin test

See Pneumococcus, below, and Optochin test, Chapter 72.

Media for physiologic tests for streptococci[112]

Trehalose and sorbitol broths
1. Heart infusion broth, 22.5 g in 900 ml distilled water
2. Trehalose or sorbitol, 10 g in 100 ml distilled water

3. One-ml indicator (1.6 g bromcresol purple in 100 ml 95% ethanol)

Add 1, 2, and 3 together, dispense in 3 ml amounts in 13 × 100 mm screwcap tubes. Sterilize in autoclave for 10 min at 121 C.

Positive reaction is recorded when indicator changes from purple to yellow.

Moeller's decarboxylase media for arginine hydrolysis
1. Peptone (Orthana special), 5 g
2. Beef extract, 5 g
3. Bromcresol purple, same as above, 0.625 ml
4. Cresol red (0.2%, prepared by grinding 0.5 g cresol red powder to a fine powder, adding 26.2 ml 0.01 N NaOH, and diluting to 250 ml with distilled water), 2.5 ml
5. Pyridoxal, 5 mg
6. L-Arginine, 10 g (if DL-arginine is used, add 20 g)
7. Distilled water, 1,000 ml

Adjust pH to 6.0-6.5 and dispense in 3 ml amounts in 13 × 100 mm screwcap tubes. Sterilize in autoclave for 10 min at 121 C. Immediately after inoculation add layer (about 10 mm) of sterile mineral oil.

Positive reaction is recorded when indicators turn to a violet to reddish violet. Yellow color is not a positive reaction; this only indicates acid reaction, not deamination.

Pyruvate broth
1. Tryptone, 10 g
2. Yeast extract, 5 g
3. K_2HPO_4, 5 g
4. NaCl, 5 g
5. Sodium pyruvate, 10 g
6. Bromthymol blue, 0.04 g
7. Distilled water, 1,000 ml

Check pH; adjust to pH 7.1-7.4, if necessary. Dispense in 13 × 100 mm screwcap tubes; sterilize by autoclaving 15 min at 121 C.

Positive reaction is recorded when indicator changes from green to definite yellow. Yellow-green indicates weak reaction and should be regarded as negative utilization of pyruvate.

Serologic methods for streptococci
Extraction procedures*

For **grouping** streptococci it is necessary to prepare **extracts** of the organism. This is accomplished by partially disintegrating the cell wall with the subsequent release of the soluble C substance (carbohydrate). It is necessary that the released C substance should not be antigenically altered; i.e., it should retain its serologic specificity and reactivity. Several methods of extracting the **group** antigens from streptococci have been described. They differ considerably in complexity and effectiveness.

The **Lancefield hot acid technic**[66–74] is considered the standard technic with which all others should be compared. Unfortunately, it is relatively complex and time consuming. However, if group A and B streptococci are to be **typed,** the Lancefield technic must be used. It is the only technic that extracts the protein-type antigens as well as the carbohydrate (groups A, B,

---

*Abridged and modified from Facklam, R. R.: Isolation and identification of streptococci, Atlanta, 1977, Center for Disease Control.

C, F, and G) and teichoic acid (groups D and N) antigens from streptococci.

The **Fuller** hot formamide technic[135] is also relatively complex and, like the Lancefield technic, extracts all **group** antigens. This technic destroys the protein-**type** antigens of group A and B streptococci, and thus the formamide extracts cannot be used to type these streptococci.

Rantz and Randall's autoclave technic[136] is relatively simple to perform, and although less group antigen is extracted, it can be used very effectively in identifying the streptococci by serologic procedures.

Maxted's *Streptomyces albus* enzyme extraction technic[137] is easy to perform and works very well with the β-hemolytic group A, B, C, F, and G streptococci. This technic does **not** perform well with the group D streptococci. Most group D strains are not extracted by the *S. albus* enzyme.

Watson's *S. albus*-lysozyme enzyme extraction technic[138] has an advantage over the other 2 enzyme extraction technics in that it extracts group D streptococci as well as the β-hemolytic group A, B, C, F, and G streptococci. Unfortunately, the reagents for this technic are more costly than those for any of the other technics.

The effectiveness of all extraction technics depends largely on the quality of the antisera used in the precipitin test. With potent, specific antisera all technics work well within the limits of the tests described above. Test strains of streptococci should be available for quality control testing of each new lot of commercial antisera. Some have been notoriously poor. The Lancefield, Fuller, Rantz and Randall, and Watson technics can be used to extract and identify the group A, B, C, D, F, and G streptococci with good antisera.

• • •

Preparation of antisera

1. Prepare antigen for grouping sera by growing culture in 200 ml Todd-Hewitt broth from young culture for 16-18 h. Plate culture to test for purity, centrifuge, and resuspend cells in 10 ml 0.85% saline; add formalin (0.4%) and leave suspension in refrigerator for 24 h. Test for nonviability of organisms. To prepare grouping sera, immunize rabbits with suspension (diluted 20 times with saline) by injecting 1 ml intravenously each day for 5 successive days in first week, 2 ml each day for 5 successive days in third week, and 4 ml in fifth week. Five days after last injection bleed from ear and test by capillary pipet precipitin method. If satisfactory precipitin reaction is obtained with extracts of strains of homologous group, bleed rabbits. Test sera with homologous and heterologous streptococci for specificity and titer. Usually group antibodies appear sooner than type antibodies.

2. To prepare antigen for **type-specific sera** of group A streptococci grow culture in 400 ml Todd-Hewitt broth (with Neopeptone) for 16-18 h. Then centrifuge culture and resuspend cells in 100 ml 0.85% saline. Heat in water bath at 56-60 C for 30 min. Add Merthiolate to 1:10,000 final concentration. Prepare type-specific sera by injecting rabbits with above suspension, following schedule used for preparation of group sera;

0.25 ml each day for 5 successive days in first week, 0.5 ml in third week, and 1 ml in fifth week. The non-type-specific antibodies have to be removed by absorption with killed suspension of heterologous type streptococcus. In some cases better antisera are obtained if streptococci are disintegrated by vigorous mechanical shaking with very small glass beads.

• • •

Streptococcal antisera and control extracts are commercially available. **Quality control** performed in the clinical laboratory of such antisera is essential.

Lancefield's hot acid extraction (modified from Lancefield[67])[112]

1. Strains for extraction are grown in 30 ml Todd-Hewitt (or other suitable) broth. Broth is inoculated and incubated overnight at 35-37 C.
2. Pack cells by centrifugation.
3. Discard supernatant fluid; save cells.
4. Add 1 drop 0.04% **metacresol purple*** and about 0.3 ml 0.2N **HCl** to sedimented cells. Mix well and transfer to Kahn tube. If suspension is not a definite pink (pH 2.0 to pH 2.4), add another drop or so 0.2N HCl. HCl is made up in 0.85% NaCl.
5. Place in boiling water bath for 10 min, shaking tube several times.
6. Remove from water bath and pack cells by centrifugation.
7. Decant supernatant into clean Kahn tube; discard sediment.
8. Neutralize extract by adding 0.2N **NaOH** (made up in distilled water) drop by drop until it is slightly purple (pH 7.4 to 7.8). Deep purple indicates pH is too high. Adjust back to light purple with 0.2N HCl because too high pH may cause nonspecific cross-reactions. Try to avoid having to readjust.
9. Clarify by centrifugation and decant supernatant fluid into small screwcap vial. Store at 4 C. To preserve extract, prepare 1:100 dilution of Merthiolate solution in 1.4% Na borate, and dilute up to 1:500. Add 1 drop 1:500 solution to extract.
10. React with grouping antisera.

Fuller's hot formamide extraction[112, 135]

1. Strains for extraction are grown in 5 ml Todd-Hewitt or other suitable broth. Broth is inoculated and incubated overnight at 35-37 C.
2. Pack cells by centrifugation.
3. Discard supernatant fluid; save cells.
4. Add 0.1 ml formamide; mix by shaking.
5. Place in oil bath at 150 C for 15 min.
6. Cool. Add 0.25 ml acid-alcohol. Acid-alcohol is made with 95 parts anhydrous (100%) alcohol and 5 parts 2N HCl. Shake tube to mix.
7. Centrifuge and decant supernatant to small tube; keep supernatant.
8. Add 0.25 ml acetone; shake tube to mix.
9. Centrifuge and discard supernatant fluid; keep precipitate.
10. Add 1 ml saline and 1 drop phenol red indicator to precipitate. Shake and neutralize with trace of sodium carbonate powder. If after shaking a part

---

*Metacresol purple: grind 200 mg powder in mortar with 26.7 ml N/50 NaOH. Dilute above mixture to 500 ml with distilled H_2O for working solution.

does not dissolve, centrifuge and neutralize supernatant.

11. React with grouping antisera.

Rantz and Randall's autoclave extraction[112, 136]

1. Cells for extraction are grown in 30 ml Todd-Hewitt or other suitable broth. Broth is inoculated and incubated overnight (16-24 h) at 35-37 C.
2. Pack cells by centrifugation.
3. Discard supernatant fluid; save cells.
4. Add 0.5 ml 0.85% NaCl solution. Shake to suspend cells.
5. Autoclave tube and cells for 15 min at 121 C.
6. Centrifuge to sediment cellular debris.
7. Decant supernatant fluid into clean sterile container; discard sediment.
8. React with grouping antisera.

Maxted's *Streptomyces albus* **enzyme extraction method**[112, 137]

1. Strains for extraction are grown on blood agar plate, 16-24 h at 37 C.
2. Pipet 0.25 ml enzyme solution (*Streptomyces albus* enzyme; available commercially) into small test tube, 12 × 75 mm or smaller.
3. Scrape large loopful of growth from blood agar plate and suspend in enzyme solution.
4. Place in 45 C water bath until solution is clear (about 90 min).
5. Cool to room temperature and centrifuge for 10 min at 2,000 rpm.
6. Decant into clean container.
7. React with grouping antiserum.

S. albus enzyme should be resuspended in volume according to manufacturer's suggestions. Aliquots should be stored at −20 to −70 C until used.

Watson's *S. albus*-**lysozyme enzyme extraction**[112, 138]

1. Strains for extraction are grown on blood agar plate. Agar is inoculated and incubated overnight (16-24 h) at 35-37 C.
2. Prepare enzyme mixture as follows. Place 5 mg/ml lysozyme in distilled water. Convenient vol is 25 mg in 5 ml distilled water, since *S. albus* enzyme is prepared to be resuspended in 5 ml distilled water. Use 5 ml lysozyme solution to resuspend *S. albus* enzyme. Centrifuge solution to clarify and store in 0.5 ml quantities in 10 × 75 mm cork-stoppered tubes at −20 C.
3. Remove growth from blood agar plate with sterile swab and transfer to enzyme solution (0.5 ml). Mix swab with solution and squeeze it against side of tube to remove as much moisture as possible. Discard swab.
4. Incubate enzyme-cell mixture in water bath at 45-50 C for 90 min.
5. Centrifuge to clarify and decant into clean container.
6. React with grouping antisera.

Group precipitin test

Ring method[66-69]

1. Pipet 0.1 ml undiluted serum into 100 × 8 mm tubes and add, without mixing, equal vol of extract to be tested.
2. Include as controls tubes containing similar vol of each extract and saline, of saline and each serum, and of homologous extract and serum.
3. Record presence of ring formation after test has stood for 10 min at room temperature or in water bath at 37 C. If no ring formation occurs with any group sera, incubate successively for 2 h in water bath at 37 C and store overnight at 5 C before recording final results.

Capillary method[112, 139-141]

1. Dip the capillary tube* into serum and allow serum to run 1.0 cm up into capillary; wipe outer side of capillary with piece of cotton gauze or blotting paper.
2. Dip tip of capillary into extract of strain, which is allowed to run up 1.0 cm into capillary to give equal vol extract and serum. If air bubble separates serum and extract, discard tube and repeat.
3. Wipe tube carefully.
4. Push capillary into strip of Plasticine, the forefinger being placed over top of capillary while this is being done so that column of serum remains on the extract, until small plug fills opening. Do not let reactants mix.
5. **Invert** tube and insert gently into Plasticine-filled groove of rack.
6. After 5-10 min examine with bright light against dark background. White cloud or ring at center of column represents positive result. Strong reaction appears in 5 min; weaker reaction develops more slowly. Since after 30 min reaction may fade or false-positive may appear, examine capillary tubes at frequent intervals between 10 and 30 min.

The Center for Disease Control (CDC) recommends the **capillary method,** and the layering of the antigen (extract) over the antiserum (rather than vice versa as Lancefield originally recommended).[112]

Type precipitin test.[70-74] Technic of capillary tube method is same as that for group precipitin test; use **type-specific antisera.**

1. Incubate rack of capillary tubes for 2 h at 37 C and examine.
2. Then leave in refrigerator overnight and reexamine.

Group precipitin tests may be performed in most well-equipped clinical laboratories. **Typing** is performed only for special purposes, usually in reference laboratories.

Coagglutination and latex agglutination

Coagglutination is discussed in Chapter 74; see also Burgard, Cole, and Sonnenwirth for a comparison of coagglutination and latex agglutination[119] and also references 115 to 118.

Reagents are commercially available for both tests (coagglutination, Streptococcus Phadebact test, Pharmacia Diagnostics; Streptococcus latex test, Streptex, Burroughs Wellcome) and are most useful.

Counterimmunoelectrophoresis

For details, see Chapter 72.

Immunofluorescence

For details, see Chapter 70.

---

*Vaccine capillary tubes, Kimble borosilicate glass, both ends open and lightly fire-polished. Tubes to be bulk packed. Absorbance 1.20-2 mm (in 50 lb lots).

STREPTOCOCCUS PNEUMONIAE— PNEUMOCOCCI*

Pneumococci, *Streptococcus* (formerly *Diplococcus*) *pneumoniae*, are oval or spherical organisms measuring $0.6\text{-}0.8 \times 1$ μm. They may occur singly, often in pairs, or in short chains, the chains showing the pair formation. In fresh specimens and often in cultures they show a capsule that surrounds the single organism, the pair, or the chain. They are **lancet shaped,** arranged along the long axis, and gram positive. Pinpoint, distinct colonies are formed. On blood agar they show a zone of greening, and the colonies (especially when young) are indistinguishable from those of greening streptococci. *S. pneumoniae* is soluble in bile, sensitive to Optochin (ethylhydrocupreine hydrochloride) and highly virulent to mice. Viridans streptococci are insoluble in bile, resistant to Optochin, and much less virulent to mice.

S. pneumoniae is a common cause of lobar pneumonia and meningitis and is associated with inflammations of the upper respiratory tract; many patients with pneumococcal pneumonia have pneumococcus bacteremia, and the organism is also prominent in infections of the middle ear, eye, or mastoid. The pneumococcus has also been occasionally isolated from appendicitis[110] and enteritis.[142] There are now 84 recognized serologic types of pneumococci, but only a small number of types (i.e., types 1, 3, 4, 7, 8, 12) account for the majority of human infections.

Both virulence and serologic type are dependent on the capsule of the organism (M— mucoid, capsulated form). The nonencapsulated form is designated as S and the true rough form as R.

The organism is found in the throat and respiratory tract secretions of many normal individuals (30-60% of healthy adults).

Isolation and identification

Good growth is obtained on blood agar plates (trypticase agar with 5% sheep blood). Incubate plates in CO_2 incubator or candle jar (some strains **require** CO_2); rarely, obligately anaerobic strains of pneumococci are encountered.[143]

At 24 hours the colonies are round, transparent, small, and surrounded by narrow α-hemolysis (greening); they resemble colonies of *S. viridans*, but by 48 hours they are quite characteristic, with a dense center and a raised margin, showing a concentric ring appearance. Some strains (e.g., type 3) have large mucoid colonies and resemble droplets of oil on the surface of the agar.

For identification the following tests are carried out, depending on availability of materials: Optochin, bile solubility, mouse virulence, capsular swelling reaction (Quellung), and precipitation.

Bergey's Manual, ed. 8[3]: family Streptococcaceae, genus *Streptococcus*, based on International Subcommittee on Streptococci and Pneumococci recommendation (1967).[96]

Optochin (ethyl-hydrocupreine) test

Bowers and Jeffries[144] reported that when sterile filter paper disks or strips saturated with Optochin* are placed on the surface of blood agar plates inoculated with pneumococci, a large zone (15-30 mm) of inhibition is obtained. Greening streptococci (98%) are not inhibited or show a very small zone of inhibition. The test correlates very well with bile solubility; it can be performed on overnight primary cultures or on pure cultures.

Procedure[145]
1. Streak surface of half of blood agar plate with 1-3 suspected colonies.
2. With flamed forceps place Optochin disk in center of inoculated area.
3. Incubate at 37 C for 18-24 h in CO_2 incubator or candle jar.
4. Measure zone of inhibition in millimeters including diameter of disk.
   a. If 6 mm disk is used: positive = zone of inhibition 14 mm or greater; negative = no zone of inhibition; doubtful = any zone of inhibition less than 14 mm.; test with bile solubility.
   b. If 10 mm disc is used: positive = zone of inhibition 16 mm or greater; negative = no zone of inhibition; doubtful = any zone of inhibition less than 16 mm.
   c. Typical streptococci and positive Optochin test are indicative of *S. pneumoniae.* Cultures giving doubtful Optochin test may be α-hemolytic streptococci or *S. pneumoniae.* These cultures should be tested by bile solubility test, Quellung test, or agglutination tests. If bile soluble but give small zones of Optochin sensitivity, identify as pneumococcus.

Bile solubility

For the **tube test** see Chapter 72, Bile solubility test.

Bile colony (plate) solubility test

The colony (plate) solubility test is adaptable for the rapid identification of pneumococcus-like colonies. Add a small drop of 10% aqueous deoxycholate reagent to the suspected colonies on blood agar. Pneumococcus colonies are lysed in approximately 5 min. Green-producing streptococcus colonies are not lysed. Do not float the colony away by forceful addition of the deoxycholate reagent. The test is easier to read if the deoxycholate reagent is allowed to be absorbed into the media (usually within 20 min).[146]

Hawn and Beebe[147] and Glasgow and Coene[148] modified the procedure by placing a 4 mm loopful of sterile 2% aqueous sodium deoxycholate over each colony. The latter found a 95% correlation with the Optochin test.

Capsular swelling reaction (Neufeld "Quellung" reaction)

This was the most important test used for the identification and type determination of pneu-

---

*Optochin disks, Difco Laboratories, Detroit; Taxo P disks, BBL, Division of BioQuest, Cockeysville, Md.

mococci before the antibiotic era. Therapy was then dependent on the administration of type-specific antiserum, and it was obviously necessary to determine the exact serologic type of the isolate.

The test is useful for **rapid identification** of the organism in spinal fluid, sputum, throat swabs in a few drops of broth, primary cultures, and mouse peritoneal fluid (see note on antisera, below).

The method was first described by Neufeld and was later modified by Sabin. The word "Quellung" means the swelling of the capsule of the pneumococcus when it comes in contact with its homologous serum.

Procedure[145]
1. Place drop of material to be tested (spinal fluid, sputum, etc.) or of light suspension of young culture on slide.
2. Near it place drop of methylene blue.
3. At third spot, near others, place drop of specific antiserum.
4. Using sterile loop or applicator stick, mix stain and organism suspension; then mix serum into drop of stained organisms.
5. Cover with No. 1 coverslip and examine with oil-immersion objective after 10-15 min. If negative, reexamine after another 10-15 min.
6. In presence of specific antiserum, **capsule** of organism appears to be **considerably larger** than in preparation with heterologous antiserum.

The test may be done on body fluids such as spinal fluid, sputum, etc., and hence permits rapid, specific diagnosis. It may also be done on young cultures from broth or solid media. However, if cultures are used care must be taken to have a suspension of less than 50 organisms per oil-immersion field. Larger numbers of organisms may dissipate the antibody to such an extent that capsular swelling is not apparent (Fig. 76-3).

The principle of the test has been extended to typing of *Haemophilus influenzae, Klebsiella*, and *Neisseria meningitidis* organisms (with their specific antisera).

NOTE: An omnivalent serum, reacting with all pneumococcal types, has been prepared[149] and is available as "Omniserum" from the Statens Seruminstitut, Copenhagen. Various pools and individual type antisera are available from the same source as well as from Difco Laboratories, Detroit.

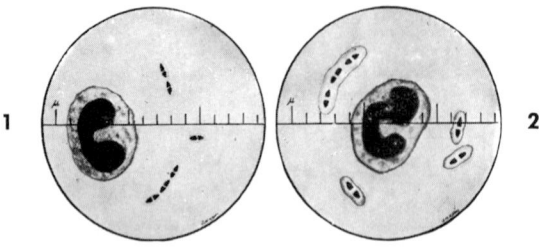

Fig. 76-3. Neufeld reaction showing, **1,** negative and, **2,** positive results. Note size of swollen capsules on **2** as compared with the leukocyte.

For a definitive review of the Quellung reaction, see Austrian.[150]

Capillary precipitin typing[151]

This test, not requiring microscopic examination, has been recently designed for typing pneumococci. The test is as specific as the Neufeld test.

Procedure
1. Pneumococci are cultured in Todd-Hewitt broth under CO_2 at 37 C for 16 h.
2. Two ml aliquots of bacterial suspension are transferred to disposable glass culture tubes (12 × 75 mm). Culture tubes are placed in water bath at 100 C for 5 min and then cooled in tap water.
3. Centrifuge tubes at maximum speed (clinical centrifuge) for 5 min.
4. Discard sediment and test supernatant.
5. Dip capillary pipet (N-51A glass, Kimble Glass Co., Vineland, N.J., absorbance 0.7-1.0 mm, 14 cm long) into antiserum until column about 15 mm is drawn in by capillary action. Wipe pipet with tissue paper and dip into supernatant (pneumococcal antigen solution) until about 15 mm column is drawn in.
6. Invert pipet until column of air is present at each end. Insert vertically in Plasticine holder so that serum is on top of column.
7. Read with naked eye against black background with tungsten light bulb or fluorescent light, immediately after antigen is mixed with antiserum and again after 30 min, in same manner as streptococcal extracts are read (see Streptococcus, group precipitin capillary method).

Detection of pneumococcal antigen

Counterimmunoelectrophoresis (CIE) has been used to detect pneumococcal antigen in spinal fluid, etc. See Counterimmunoelectrophoresis, Chapter 72.

Precipitation test. Filtrates of sputum, cerebrospinal fluid, urine, and pleural exudate may contain pneumococcus precipitinogen in the absence of the organisms because of autolysis of the bacteria. Such substances may be found also in the peritoneal cavity of mice.

The fluid suspected of containing pneumococcus precipitinogen can be used for precipitation reactions in the same manner as streptococcal extracts.

Mouse virulence

The pneumococcus is virulent for the mouse. It can be isolated from mixed cultures by injecting a mouse intraperitoneally, waiting until the mouse dies, and staining and culturing the peritoneal fluid and heart blood of the mouse (or tapping the peritoneum as soon as the mouse appears ill). An important exception is type 14 pneumococcus, which is not virulent for the mouse. Another use of mouse inoculation is the differentiation of pneumococci from greening stepto-cocci that are avirulent for the mouse.

Procedure
1. Pick up mouse by tail, using right hand.
2. Then grasp mouse by nape of neck with thumb and index finger of left hand. (This can be done more easily if mouse is holding on to edge of table or wire of its cage with its front feet.) Maintaining

this position, turn mouse over, pulling its tail down center of palm toward wrist. Hold tail and left hind leg down with little finger. With middle and ring fingers hold loose skin of its back tightly.

3. Locate soft depression near right hip of mouse. Swab this area with iodine.

4. Inject 1-1.5 ml pathologic material intraperitoneally into soft spot, using syringe and intradermal needle (about 0.6 cm long).

5. After 4-6 h, or sooner if mouse appears ill, hold mouse in same position and tap abdomen. Use capillary dropper with fine yet not flexible end. Insert this into abdomen of mouse and withdraw fluid for typing or culture or both (Fig. 76-4).

Antibiotic susceptibility of pneumococci

For some time after the introduction of antibiotics, pneumococci were sensitive to many commonly used antibiotics. Since 1963 several reports appeared describing the appearance of pneumococcal strains resistant to tetracycline.[152, 153] In 1967[154] a pneumococcal strain resistant to both erythromycin and lincomycin was reported, as well as several strains relatively resistant to penicillin (in Australia and New Guinea).[155] A few such strains with moderately increased penicillin resistance have been also reported from the United States[156-160] and elsewhere.[161-163] S. pneumoniae strains with much greater resistance to penicillin and other antibiotics were discovered in 1977 in South Africa[164, 165] and Minnesota (1 strain).[166]

Culture surveys in several South African communities demonstrated that antibiotic-resistant pneumococci have at least 5 resistance patterns: (1) penicillin resistance only (minimal inhibitory concentration [MIC] = 0.5-4 μg/ml); (2) penicillin and tetracycline (MIC = 16-64 μg/ml) resistance; (3) penicillin, tetracycline, and chloramphenicol (MIC = 16-32 μg/ml) resistance; (4) penicillin and chloramphenicol resistance; and (5) penicillin, tetracycline, chloramphenicol, erythromycin (MIC = 8-64 μg/ml),

and clindamycin (MIC = >128 μg/ml) resistance (strains in group 5 are called "multiply resistant.") Several of the multiply-resistant pneumococci have also developed resistance to rifampin (MIC = >4 μg/ml). All resistant isolates are additionally resistant to aminoglycosides, cephalosporins, carbenicillin, and ampicillin.

Because pneumococci have been considered universally susceptible to penicillin, it has been recommended that they not be subjected to antimicrobial susceptibility tests.[168] However, in 1970 Sonnenwirth,[169] and more recently others,[170, 171] have recommended routine screening of pneumococci for antimicrobial resistance, since the above findings are of grave potential importance.

Using a 10 unit (U) penicillin disk (in the Kirby-Bauer disk diffusion test) Cooksey et al.[170] recommend that any pneumococcal isolate from meningitis with a zone size of less than 35 mm (with the 10 U penicillin disk) should be regarded potentially penicillin resistant and an MIC should be performed.

Gartner and Michaels[160] use the 1 μg oxacillin disk to screen for moderately penicillin-resistant strains and the 10 U penicillin disk to detect markedly resistant strains (such as those reported from South Africa). By their procedure, the mean diameter of zones of inhibition for **nonresistant** pneumococcal strains around the oxacillin disk is about 26 mm, for the 10 U penicillin disk 45 mm.

Thornsberry (Center for Disease Control) recently used a 1 μg oxacillin disk for screening pneumococcal strains (personal communication, December 1978). Strains with an inhibition zone of 20 mm or more with the oxacillin disk are considered sensitive, while those with a zone of 12 or less mm are considered resistant; those with zones of 13-19 mm are doubtful. MICs are performed on the latter 2 categories.

Jacobs and Koornhof,[171] using a 5 μg methicillin disk, recommend MICs for strains with inhibition

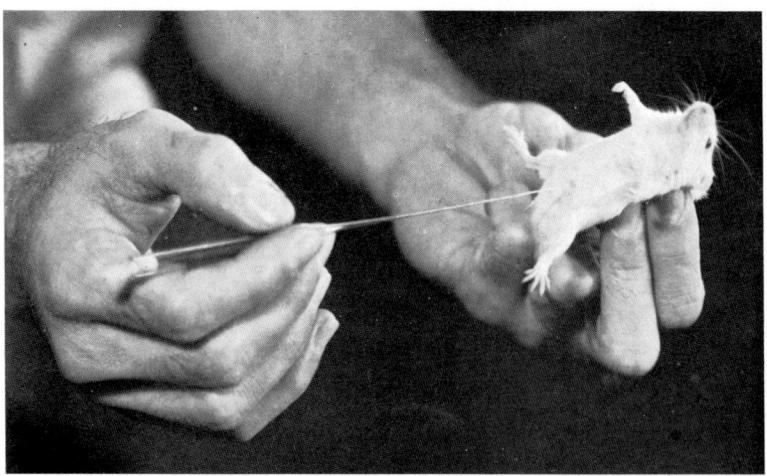

Fig. 76-4. Correct method of holding a white mouse for intraperitoneal injection.

Table 76-7. Some characteristics of Aerococcus and Streptococcus*

Differential tests	Aerococcus viridans	Viridans streptococci	Group D enterococcus
Glucose fermentation†	−	+	+
Streptococcus group D reaction	−	−	+
Bile-esculin reaction	V	−	+
Grows in 6.5% NaCl broth	+	−	+
Grows in 40% fresh bile broth	+	V	+
Growth at 10 C	+‡	−	+
Growth at 45 C	−	V	+
Hydrolysis of hippurate§	+	−	−
Hydrolysis of arginine	−	V	+
Anaerobic growth‖	−	+	+

* Based on data from Bergey's Manual, ed. 8,[3] and Facklam.[5]
† Many exceptions.
‡ In anaerobic medium.
§ Some exceptions.
‖ International Subcommittee media.

zones of less than 25 mm around the methicillin disk; they state that in their hands methicillin was superior to penicillin G in screening for intermediate penicillin resistance.

AEROCOCCUS

Aerococcus (classified as genus IV of the family Streptococcaceae in *Bergey's Manual*, ed. 8,[3] but as part of the family Micrococcaceae by the International Subcommittee on Nomenclature of Micrococcaceae[4]) is thought to be primarily an airborne contaminant, widely distributed in the hospital environment, and also commonly found on raw and processed vegetables and in meat-curing brines.[5,172]

Colman,[173] and Parker and Ball[174] isolated aerococcus-like organisms from blood cultures of patients with subacute bacterial endocarditis (SBE) and from urine cultures of patients with urinary tract infections.

Organisms previously described as *Gaffkya tetragena* and *G. homari* seem to be similar to or identical with *Aerococcus*.[5]

Aerococci are gram-positive cocci with a strong tendency toward **tetrad** and **clump** formation. They are negative in the benzidine test (unlike *Staphylococcus* and *Micrococcus*). They do not produce acid from glucose in anaerobic culture, while *Streptococcus* usually does.

The organism produces small colonies on blood agar with α-hemolysis, very similar to many streptococci; however, the greening may be delayed for 48 hours.

Most strains hydrolyze hippurate, tolerate 6.5% NaCl, 40% fresh bile broth, and pH 9.6; some also blacken bile-esculin medium. Thus they resemble enterococci in some respects, but they do not possess the group D antigen, do not grow at 10 or 45 C, and do not hydrolyze arginine. Also they are considerably more sensitive to antibiotics than are the enterococci. See Table 76-7 for comparison of differential characteristics of *Aerococcus* and *Streptococcus*.

Neisseriae

The family *Neisseriaceae* consists (according to *Bergey's Manual*, ed. 8[3]) of the genera *Neisseria* and *Branhamella* (gram-negative cocci), *Moraxella* (plump, gram-negative rods in pairs or short chains), and *Acinetobacter* (gram negative, rod-shaped when actively growing but nearly coccal when in stationary phase, predominantly in pairs or short chains).

This taxonomic arrangement has been disputed, and it has been strongly suggested that *Acinetobacter* be removed from the family (possibly by creating a new family for it). In his extensive review of the 4 genera, Henriksen[175] points out that *Neisseria*, *Branhamella*, and *Moraxella* share a number of characteristics; they are obligate parasites on mucous membranes of warm-blooded animals, while *Acinetobacter* is saprophytic or an opportunistic pathogen.

Species in the genera *Neisseria*, *Branhamella*, and *Moraxella* are **oxidase positive**, while *Acinetobacter* organisms are **oxidase negative**. Finally, genetic evidence (homology) points to very close relationships between *Moraxella* and *Branhamella* (B. catarrhalis, B. ovis, and B. caviae) but little or no homology between these 2 genera and *Neisseria* or *Acinetobacter*.

Members of *Neisseria* and *Branhamella* are discussed below; for *Acinetobacter* and *Moraxella* see Chapter 79.

NEISSERIA AND BRANHAMELLA

The organisms in the genus *Neisseria* are gram-negative cocci occurring singly but often in pairs with **adjacent slides flattened**; they are nonmotile, catalase and oxidase positive, aerobic or facultatively anaerobic, and attack sugars by oxidation (O-F test) or not at all. For differential characteristics of Neisseriae see Table 76-8.

Branhamella are similar, but they do not produce acid from carbohydrates and they grow on ordinary media without blood.

Table 76-8. Differential characteristics of Neisseriae*

| Organism | Acid production from carbohydrate[†] | | | | | | Growth | | |
| | Oxidase | Glucose | Maltose | Sucrose | Lactose (or ONPG)[‖] | Fructose (levulose) | MTM[‡] 35-36 C | Nutrient agar[§] | |
								35-36 C	22-25 C
N. gonorrhoeae	+	+	−	−	−	−	+	−	−
N. meningitidis	+	+	+	−	−	−	+	−(+)[¶]	−
N. lactamica	+	+	+	−	+[#]	−	+	+(−)[**]	−(+)
N. sicca	+	+	+	+	−	+	−	+	+
N. mucosa[††]	+	+	+	+	−	+	−	+	+
N. subflava[‡‡]	+	+	+	−[§§]	−	−[§§‖]	−	+(−)	+(−)
N. flavescens[††]	+	−	−	−	−	−	−	+	+
Branhamella (Neisseria) catarrhalis	+	−	−	−	−	−	−(+)	+(−)	+(−)
Moraxella osloensis (Mima polymorpha var. oxidans)	+	−	−	−	−	−	−(+)		

*Slightly modified from Procedures for use by the laboratory in the isolation and identification of *Neisseria gonorrhoeae*, Atlanta, 1975 (reprinted 1977), Center for Disease Control, Venereal Disease Training Branch.

†In CTA base; or in rapid carbohydrate degradation (fermentation) test, used primarily with *Neisseria* species growing on MTM.

‡Modified Thayer-Martin medium.

§NaCl-free nutrient agar inoculated with single drop of broth culture.

‖o-Nitrophenyl-β-galactoside; β-galactosidase test.

¶(+), Few positive, late.

#Most strains will produce acid in 48 h in CTA-lactose.

**−, Few negative.

††Reduces nitrate to gas.

‡‡Yellow pigmentation on Loeffler's serum medium.

§§Strains formerly classified as *N. perflava* are positive.

‖Strains formerly classified as *N. flava* are positive.

Neisseria meningitidis (meningococcus)[3, 176, 177]

The meningococci occur in pairs of gram-negative cocci, the adjacent sides of which are usually flattened, producing the biscuit or reniform shape. They produce acid from **glucose** and **maltose** but not from sucrose (Table 76-8).

The colonies are nonpigmented, smooth, and nonhemolytic; the organism is **oxidase** positive. They grow well on chocolate agar, Thayer-Martin or modified Thayer-Martin medium, or blood agar; 3-10% CO_2 atmosphere greatly enhances the growth; after 20 hours on blood agar, colonies are larger than 1 mm. Some strains fail to grow without added CO_2; for this reason it should always be added. Usually there is no growth at room temperature (22 C). The organisms cause **meningitis, meningococcemia,** and other infections.

The normal habitat of meningococci is the human nasopharynx. Carrier rates are variable in different age groups and geographic locations. Carrier rates of 25-30% have been found without clinical disease.

On the basis of antigenic differences, 4 serologic groups of meningococci have been recognized, i.e., A, B, C, and D (earlier designated as I, II, IIα, and IV). Slaterus in 1963[178] recognized 3 additional serologic types, which he designated as X, Y, and Z. Hollis et al.[179] in 1968 confirmed the occurrence of these serotypes in the United States and recommended that they be designated as E, F, and G groups. The groups are based on agglutination reactions with immune sera. Groups A and C are encapsulated; capsular swelling has not been demonstrated with group B organisms. Polyvalent and (some) type-specific antisera are commercially available.

For a detailed review of the serology of the meningococcus, see Vedros.[180]

Detection and isolation

Blood cultures. Blood cultures are important in the diagnosis of meningococcemia; they are positive in approximately one half of the cases of meningococcal meningitis, if taken early in the disease.

Blood should be inoculated into both solid and liquid media; add 5-10 ml blood to 50 ml tryptose phosphate or infusion broth. Spread 0.1 ml blood over the surface of a chocolate agar or blood agar plate. Incubate cultures at 37 C in a candle jar or carbon dioxide jar (5-10%). Inspect cultures for 7 days before discarding as negative.

In overwhelming infections it is sometimes possible to recognize gram-negative diplococci in blood smears. In cases with early petechial rash the organisms may be demonstrated by smear or culture.

Spinal fluid. It is preferable to inoculate plates by letting spinal fluid drop on the surface of chocolate and blood agar plates (incubate in 3-5% CO_2). Do not use Thayer-Martin medium (with antibiotics incorporated) for spinal fluid culture. Inoculate in addition a tube of brain-heart or heart infusion broth. Incubate 2-3 ml spinal fluid in a sterile tube at 37 C overnight and repeat culture from this tube. Occasionally the incubated spinal fluid yields a positive culture when the initial cultures are negative.

Perform cell count and smear on another portion of spinal fluid. A marked polymorphonuclear pleocytosis is the usual finding.

Stain the centrifuged sediment with methylene blue (also Gram stain) and examine with oil immersion for intracellular or extracellular diplococci.

See fluorescent antibody staining, below.

Nasopharyngeal swab. For detection of carriers and in cases of suspected meningococcal infection, nasopharyngeal culture should be performed. The use of a flexible wire swab and of the modified Thayer-Martin (MTM) medium with incorporated antibiotics (see Media) allows recovery of meningococci (and gonococci) with comparative ease.

Petechiae. Cultures of petechial hemorrhages often grow meningococci. Use MTM and blood agar plates.

Rectum. Meningococci may be isolated from the rectum. Use MTM medium.[181]

Cervix. Occasionally recovered from cervix on MTM (when sampling done for N. gonorrhoeae).

Fluorescent antibody (FA) staining. FA microscopy provides a rapid and relatively sensitive method for detecting N. meningitidis in smears of spinal fluid sediments.[176] However, as with other serologic procedures, various cross-reactions occur with FA. Some antisera are available commercially (Difco, Detroit; Burroughs-Wellcome, Research Triangle Park, N.C.).

See also Chapter 75 (Spinal fluid) and Chapter 70 (FA technics).

Counterimmunoelectrophoresis. See Spinal fluid (Chapter 75) and Counterimmunoelectrophoresis (Chapters 72 and 74) for detection of meningococcal antigen.

Quellung reaction and precipitin test. As described under Spinal fluid (Chapter 75), a "Quellung" or precipitin test can be performed on the spinal fluid with specific meningococcal antiserum, if large numbers of organisms are present. The precipitin test is occasionally positive even when no organisms are demonstrable in the smear.

Identification and differentiation

Oxidase test. This test should be performed on colonies as described in Chapter 72.

Differentiation from other neisseriae. N. meningitidis is differentiated by growth characteristics, serologic tests, and acid production from various substrates. N. meningitidis produces acid from glucose and maltose and does not grow at 22 C or on nutrient agar (extremely rare exceptions) (Table 76-8).

For fermentation tests use semisolid crystine-trypticase agar (CTA) with appropriate carbohydrate (0.5-1%) and indicator,* or **preferably** the rapid carbohydrate degradation (nongrowth "fermentation" test); see Neisseria gonorrhoeae, below, for detailed description.

Comments

1. Lactose-fermenting neisseriae are being isolated in increasing numbers. They also ferment glucose and maltose, grow on TM and MTM (Thayer-Martin, modified Thayer-Martin) medium, and thus may be easily mistaken for N. meningitidis. See Neisseria lactamicus (below).

Practically all N. lactamicus strains to date have been recovered from carriers and only rarely has it been implicated in meningitis[182]; for this reason it is advisable to test lactose in addition to the other carbohydrates.

2. Rarely, asaccharolytic (acid not produced from the usual carbohydrates) neisseriae have been isolated from cases of meningitis. After mouse passage[183] or by quantitative genetic transformation,[184] some of these have been shown to be atypical N. meningitidis strains.

Enzymatic profile (API) procedure for differentiation. A different approach has recently been reported by D'Amato et al.,[185] who use chromogenic substrates to establish enzymatic profiles for a rapid and economical system for the identification of N. meningitidis and N. gonorrhoeae.

Radiometric procedure for differentiation of meningococci. See discussion of radiometric procedure under Neisseria gonorrhoeae, below.

Minitek procedure for meningococcci. See Neisseria gonorrhoeae, below.

Serologic identification. Prepare saline with 0.1% potassium cyanide added to inhibit the autolytic process. Emulsify colonies to be examined in small amounts of cyanide-saline. Add an amount of polyvalent meningococcal antisera (or, if available, group-specific antisera A, B, C, and D) and observe for agglutination. Controls should include normal serum diluted 1:50 and a saline suspension of the organism. Neither of these should show agglutination.

The **tube agglutination** test is somewhat more reliable than the **slide agglutination** test. In the tube agglutination test shake the suspension and incubate at 37 C for 2 hours in a water bath.

Capsular swelling (Quellung reaction) can also be performed with polyvalent or type-specific antiserum. In the **slide agglutination test** normal rabbit serum should be used as a control instead of the immune serum in any positive agglutination reaction, since some strains of N. meningitidis agglutinate spontaneously in normal rabbit serum. Antigenic cross-relations exist among various neisseriae and group B and also between groups A and C.

---

*The medium is available as CTA prepared tubes with indicator and carbohydrates from BBL, Division of BioQuest, Cockeysville, Md.

Antibiotic susceptibility of meningococci

Sulfonamide-resistant strains of *N. meningitidis* have appeared in 1963 in the United States.[186] Since then, resistance to sulfonamide has become widespread; a large proportion (>65%) of group C isolates and many group B isolates are resistant (not inhibited by 1 mg/100 ml sulfadiazine).

For antibiotic sensitivity testing of meningococci, it is preferable to use agar plates into which an antibiotic or chemotherapeutic agent (such as sulfonamide) has been incorporated. Agar plate dilution sensitivities with sulfonamides can be performed by the method of Frank et al.[187] (Mueller-Hinton agar is used, and the sensitivity is expressed as mg sulfonamide/100 ml) or the method of Feldman.[188]

Bennett et al.[188a] have described a disk test for the sulfonamide testing of meningococci. Consult their publication for details.

See also Chapter 87 of this work.

Resistance to penicillin has not been encountered as of this writing. While it is presently the drug of choice in the treatment of meningococcal disease, it is not successful in the prophylactic treatment of carrier. Most of the (sulfadiazine-resistant) strains in carriers can be eradicated with rifampin or minocycline.

Neisseria gonorrhoeae (gonococcus)[181,189,190]

Neisseria gonorrhoeae is the cause of a number of contagious inflammatory conditions such as urethritis, prostatitis, pharyngitis, proctitis, cervicitis and salpingitis of adults, vulvovaginitis of children, and ophthalmia of the newborn and adults.

The diagnosis of gonorrhea is strongly suggested by the finding of gram-negative diplococci in the stained exudate of suspected gonococcal infection obtained from defined loci. The gonococcus appears in the exudate as a diplococcus with contiguous sides, flattened or slightly concave, resembling a pair of kidney beans and measuring 0.6-1 μm in diameter. Microorganisms that may confuse the microscopic diagnosis of gonorrhea are staphylococci, streptococci, enterococci, diphtheroids, coliforms, *Achromobacter*, *Acinetobacter* (Mima-Herella sp.), and other species of *Neisseria*. These organisms when found singly or in pairs may closely resemble the gonococcus. Old staphylococcal cells are prone to stain red by the Gram method and may be confused with the gonococcus. Certain gram-negative diplobacilli are particularly difficult to distinguish from gonococci. Staining smears with methylene blue greatly multiplies the difficulty of microscopic identification of the gonococcus and is not recommended as a laboratory procedure.

Smears taken during the first 4 or 5 hours of penicillin therapy show gonococcal forms that progressively enlarge and decrease in stainability until none can be detected. Similar morphologic changes are observed during therapy with other antibiotics but not during sulfonamide treatment.

The diagnosis of gonorrhea **in men** is made on the basis of characteristic clinical symptoms and can be confirmed by demonstrating microscopically (direct smear) intracellular, gram-negative diplococci in the pus cells of the urethral discharge. When gram-negative diplococci cannot be identified in the direct smear or there is no exudate, culture should be performed.

Stained smears are of little value in gonorrhea in women except as an adjunct to the culture.

• • •

For details of specimen collection, staining and microscopy, transport media, isolation of *N. gonorrhoeae*, and a detailed review of culture media for *N. gonorrhoeae*, see Genital tract, part I (female) and part II (male), in Chapter 75.

• • •

For a detailed review of the physiology and metabolism of *N. gonorrhoeae*, see Morse (1979)[191]; for an overview of the organism, infections caused by it, and procedures for its isolation and identification, see the World Health Organization's *Neisseria gonorrhoeae and gonococcal infections* (1978)[192] and the volume edited by Roberts, *The Gonococcus* (1977).[193]

Cultivation

The gonococcus grows best under aerobic conditions, at pH 7.2-7.6, at a temperature of 35-36 C. Some strains do not grow satisfactorily at 37-38 C, and in general growth is not initiated at 20-25 C. Most strains require an atmosphere containing from 2-10% CO_2 (candle jar, CO_2 jar, or CO_2 incubator) to initiate development. Although gonococci grow well on the moist 1-1.5% agar, excessive moisture as produced by syneresis of the agar is undesirable, especially for primary isolation, because it favors bacterial spreaders that easily overgrow the more slowly growing gonococci.

As pointed out in detail in Chapter 75 (Genital tract), selective media such as Thayer-Martin (TM), modified Thayer-Martin (MTM), New York City (NYC) medium, or Lester-Martin medium should be used for isolation of gonococci (and of meningococci from mixed flora) instead of the earlier GC agar medium or chocolate agar.

Incubation of inoculated plates. Plates are placed in an air-tight container such as a vacuum desiccator, large pickle jar, or suitable tin canister as soon after inoculation as possible. A moistened paper towel or gauze should be placed within the jar to supply maximum humidity. A short, thick, smokeless candle fixed to a Petri dish bottom is lighted and placed on top of the agar plates. The lid is placed on the jar, and if it is not a tight fit Plasticine may be used to effect a seal. The burning candle will generate about 3% carbon dioxide before extinction, an adequate amount to stimulate growth of the gonococcus.

The incubator should be adjusted to 35-36 C,

since many strains of gonococci do not grow well at 37.5 C.

If available, incubate in CO_2 incubator.

Examination of plates. Primary gonococcus colonies appear translucent, raised, finely granular, and moderately convex with lobate margins. They are usually mucoid; after 20 hours in a CO_2 jar or candle jar, colonies are 1-2 mm in size.

The gonococcal colonies appear usually as pure growth on the selective (MTM) medium, with most neisseriae, other gram-negative and gram-positive contaminants, and yeasts being almost totally inhibited.

Crawford et al.[194] recently reported that gonococci that require arginine, hypoxanthine, and uracil form atypical small colonies.

Identification of N. gonorrhoeae
Presumptive identification

If TM, MTM, or NYC (selective) medium is used, **presumptive identification** of *N. gonorrhoeae* is made by (1) observing typical colonial morphology, (2) obtaining a positive **oxidase reaction** (see below), and (3) demonstrating the characteristic gram-negative diplococci in a smear made from the oxidase-positive colony.

Oxidase test. Members of the genus *Neisseria* possess an oxidizing enzyme that, in the presence of air, acts on certain aromatic amines to produce colored compounds. The color changes produced by indicators in contact with colonies are readily observed. If nonselective media are used the reaction often aids in finding an obscure gonococcus colony that would have been otherwise overlooked by microscopic examination.

The oxidase test is **not** confirmatory for gonococci, since the other species of *Neisseria* possess this enzyme together with a few other bacteria and yeast. When 1% aqueous solution of dimethyl-*p*-phenylenediamine is added to a suspected colony the colonies of gonococci turn **pink**, then **purple**. The reagent **kills** the gonococci within a few minutes but does not modify their morphologic and staining characteristics.

All members of the genus *Neisseria*, as well as certain bacteria and yeasts occasionally found in the flora of the urethra and cervix, also can produce oxidase. Nevertheless, positive oxidase reaction, coupled with typical colonial characteristics that show the presence of gram-negative diplococci resembling the gonococcus, constitutes presumptive cultural evidence that should be confirmed by sugar fermentation or FA technic (for circumstances requiring confirmation, see Genital tract, Chapter 75).

Gram stain. Make smear from oxidase-positive colony; look for characteristic gram-negative diplococci.

Definitive identification (confirmation)

1. Definitive identification (confirmation) of presumptive positive colonies is made by determining acid production from carbohydrates in **CTA base** or **preferably** by the **rapid carbohy-**

drate degradation (4-hour "fermentation") **tests**; *N. gonorrhoeae* produces acid only from glucose (no gas is produced); see Table 76-8.

A few strains do not produce acid from glucose or do so weakly even on adequate medium[3]; subculture repeatedly or add 10% ascitic fluid or inactivated rabbit serum to the CTA medium to aid growth and breakdown of sugar.

2. Confirmation of presumptive positive colonies may also be done by the **direct fluorescent antibody staining procedure.** If FA method is used with satisfactory anti-*N. gonorrhoeae* conjugate, sugar tests are not needed.

The direct FA method is unsuitable for use as a "test of cure," since it stains dead gonococci present in the specimen.

3. For other technics, e.g., coagglutination, enzymatic profiles, see below.

A. Carbohydrate "fermentation" tests*:
I. Cystine trypticase agar† base (CTA)

The medium to which the carbohydrates are added must be free of sugars and readily support the growth of freshly isolated gonococci. If serum enrichment is added, it should be inactivated at 56 C for 30 minutes. Rabbit serum is more suitable than sheep or horse serum because of their strong maltase activity.

Cystine trypticase agar (CTA) is used as a basic medium for "fermentation" tests. Although this medium without serum enrichment will support growth of practically all gonococci, some strains do not grow or grow poorly. Tubes of the CTA medium containing, respectively, 1% reagent grade glucose, maltose, sucrose, and lactose, are utilized in the fermentation test.

When identification of other species of *Neisseria* is to be made, as for *catarrhalis, sicca,* etc., fructose medium must be prepared also (Table 76-8).

Procedure

1. Inoculate "fermentation" medium from growth on Thayer-Martin plate (TM, MT, etc.) purification plate, or 0.2% starch CTA medium (see below). Only surface of sugar tubes need be inoculated, since gonococcus will not grow well below surface. Rather heavy inoculum should be used.

2. Tubes are incubated at 35 C in CO_2 (2-10%) atmosphere with loose caps, and examined for acid production (indicator changes from red to yellow) after 24-48 h. Frequently 18-48 h incubation is sufficient.

3. Growth must have occurred in tubes and must be pure culture. Gram-stained smear of growth will establish purity of culture.

Kellogg states that it is necessary to "inoculate . . . cell suspension onto the surface of the CTA fermentation tube media . . . **tighten tube caps,** and incubate at 36 C in an environment without CO_2."[195] The reason for this is given as the lack of uniformity in all laboratories pertaining to loose

---

N. gonorrhoeae (and other neisseriae) attack sugars by oxidation or not at all.

†Same as cystine tryptic digest of casein.

screwcaps, which seemed to contribute to erratic results. Sometimes strains of *N. gonorrhoeae* will not perform properly in CTA regardless of the CO_2 situation.

The Center for Disease Control has now obviated this problem by using a rapid "fermentation" procedure; see below (Kellogg, personal communication, February 1976).

II. Rapid "fermentation" tests[196-198] (nongrowth carbohydrate degradation test)[189]

The tests discussed here are mainly based on the work of Kellogg and Turner[199] and Brown (1974,[196] 1976,[197] 1977[198]).

NOTE: **The rapid tests require a purification plate step (transfer plate).** Single colonies of the organism to be tested should be picked to one (or more) chocolate agar (GC base or VCN[198]) plate(s) and heavily streaked to result in heavy growth for the tests. Incubate the plate(s) for no more than 18 hours. Do **not** test colonies directly from TM medium. Despite the purification step, the procedure allows confirmatory identification 28 hours after colony has been streaked for purification (overnight incubation, 4-hour reading for test).

Modified rapid fermentation test (MRFT) for confirmation of Neisseria gonorrhoeae[196*]

Equipment
1. Water bath (37 C)
2. Bacteriologic loop (3 mm)
3. Waterproof marking pen
4. Test tube rack
5. Rubber bulb for Pasteur pipets
6. Glassware:
    Sterile screwcap bottle (150-200 ml)
    10 × 75 mm glass tubes
    Sterile screwcap glass tubes (or sterile plastic tubes with tight caps), 20 ml or greater, for storage of 20% carbohydrate preparations
    1 ml pipets graduated in 0.1 ml
    Disposable Pasteur pipets (5¾ in long with a 1-mm bore)

Reagents
1. Buffer-salt solution (BSS), pH 7.0. Dissolve:

Dipotassium hydrogen phosphate (K_2HPO_4)	0.04 g
Potassium dihydrogen phosphate (KH_2PO_4)	0.01 g
Potassium chloride (KCl)	0.8 g
Distilled water	100.0 ml
Phenol red (1% aqueous solution)	0.2 ml

    This solution may be stored at 5 C in sterile screwcap bottle for up to 8 wk while being used.
2. Concentrated carbohydrate solutions (20%)— glucose, maltose, sucrose, fructose, and lactose. These solutions may be stored in 5 or 10 ml amounts (in sterile screwcap tubes or sterile plastic tubes with tight caps) in freezer for up to 6 mo. Once these solutions have been thawed and appropriate amounts have been removed for test-

ing, remainder may be stored at 5 C for up to 8 wk. Check visually for contamination before each use.

Preparation of specimens
1. With waterproof marker label cell suspension tube (10 × 75 mm) for each culture to be tested.
2. With 1 ml pipet accurately measure 0.3 ml BSS and place in cell suspension tube.
3. Add two 3 mm loopfuls of **pure** culture of suspected *N. gonorrhoeae* from **purification** (transfer) chocolate agar **plate.**
4. Prepare homogeneous suspension by mixing well with Pasteur pipet.

Test procedure
1. All reagents should be at room temperature when used. Label fermentation tube (10 × 75 mm) for each carbohydrate to be tested with each culture. Place fermentation tubes in line behind suspension tube in test tube rack.
2. With 1 ml pipet add 0.1 ml BSS to each fermentation tube.
3. With Pasteur pipet add 1 drop (0.04 ml) carbohydrate to its labeled fermentation tube.
4. With another Pasteur pipet add 1 drop (0.04 ml) from cell suspension tube to each fermentation tube.
5. Shake each tube gently by hand to mix contents. Incubate rack of tubes in 37 C water bath. No tube caps or covers are needed.

One carbohydrate, glucose, will identify *N. gonorrhoeae*, but maltose must also be used to rule out *N. meningitidis*. In addition, test either sucrose or fructose as negative reaction control. Lactose may be tested to further distinguish *N. lactamica* from *N. meningitidis*. Test each new lot of reagent (BSS or carbohydrates) with known cultures of *N. gonorrhoeae*.

Reading results
1. Some strains of *N. gonorrhoeae* start to react in 15-30 min. Others take 3-4 h. Read fermentation reaction after **4 h** of incubation. **Do not** read results **after** tests have incubated **overnight** because of possible contamination.
2. Read and report as follows:
    a. Positive for *N. gonorrhoeae*—phenol red indicator in only glucose fermentation tube turns from red to yellow. Some strains of *N. gonorrhoeae* may cause indicator to turn gold instead of yellow.
    b. Negative for *N. gonorrhoeae*—(1) phenol red indicator in glucose fermentation tube remains unchanged, regardless of any color change in any of other fermentation tubes, or (2) indicator in glucose tube turns yellow and indicator in one or more of other fermentation tubes turns yellow. In latter case, results are indicative of organism other than *N. gonorrhoeae*.
3. Reactions of *Neisseria* sp. **commonly** isolated on Thayer-Martin (TM) medium:

	Glucose	Maltose	Lactose	Sucrose
N. gonorrhoeae	+	–	–	–
N. meningitidis	+	+	–	–
N. lactamicus	+	+	+	–

The MRFT procedure was compared with the standard CTA and the Mueller-Hinton agar (MHA) slant[197] methods and was shown to have greater sensitivity than the other 2 methods; results could be obtained with it within 4 hours as compared with overnight for the other 2 methods.[197]

---

*Based on Current Item 242 (Robinson, R. Q.), Atlanta, March 4, 1974, Center for Disease Control, Bureau of Laboratories.

*Modified rapid fermentation test (MRFT)—
improved*[198]

In this improved modification Brown describes
the preparation of previously prepared, labeled
reagents in economic quantities and their storage
at −20 or −70 C. This eliminates the need for
mixing reagents at the time of testing; the procedure also eliminates the need for preparation
of the suspension tube, allowing direct inoculation of the fermentation tubes from the 18-24
hour (purification) chocolate agar plate with
approximately one-half to full 3 mm loopful of
suspected organisms.

Do **not** use colonies grown on TM medium as
purification plate.

Materials
1. Frozen tubes with BBS (buffer-salt solution) +
   lactose, BBS + sucrose, BBS + maltose, and
   BSS + dextrose (for preparation of BSS, see MRFT
   test, above). Each frozen tube contains 0.1 ml
   BSS and, respectively, 0.04 ml lactose, maltose,
   sucrose, and glucose.

Procedure
1. For each isolate of *Neisseria* to be tested, thaw
   1 set of tubes to room temperature (BSS +
   glucose, BSS + maltose, BSS + sucrose, BSS +
   lactose).
2. Prepare **heavy** suspension of *Neisseria* cells by
   adding 1 loopful from **pure culture on chocolate
   agar** to each of 4 fermentation tubes. Deposit
   inoculum onto top side of tilted tube, then mix
   vigorously with loop into BSS containing carbohydrate. **Flame loop** between each transfer to prevent carryover of carbohydrate.
3. Place inoculated tubes in 37 C water bath.
4. Read and interpret as MRFT test, above. Reactions in this improved MRFT are actually faster
   (when tubes stored frozen are employed) than in
   earlier MRFT procedure; many strains can be
   read in 15-20 min, while *N. meningitidis* and
   N. lactamicus react with maltose and lactose
   within 2 h.

If pure culture is older than 24 h or was grown on
Thayer-Martin (TM) medium for purification, limited or
negative reactions may occur. Many strains of *N.
lactamicus* seem to lyse early (less than 24 h) and thus
make it impossible to obtain acceptable inoculum.

*B. Confirmation of Neisseria gonorrhoeae
by fluorescent antibody methods**[200]

If fluorescent antibody confirmation of a culture is required, prepare a **thin** smear for staining on a slide having a 6 mm diameter etched
circle. Place a loopful of distilled water in the
area of the circle, lightly touch a loop or needle
to the suspected colony, emulsify the material
in the water, and spread as thinly as possible over
the etched circle and the surrounding area; or
prepare in 0.5 ml sterile distilled water a slightly
opalescent suspension of the suspected colony
and spread a small loopful over the etched circle.
Air dry the smear. (Smears may be prepared from

---

* From Procedures for use by the laboratory in the iso-
lation and identification of *Neisseria gonorrhoeae*,
Atlanta, 1975 (reprinted 1977), Center for Disease
Control, Venereal Disease Training Branch.

a colony and stained with fluorescein-labeled
conjugate up to 15 minutes after the colony has
been treated with oxidase reagent.)

Fluorescent antibody staining technic
1. Thoroughly air dry smear.
2. Place full 3 mm loopful of anti-*Neisseria gonorrhoeae* conjugate evenly over specimen **within
   6 mm circle** and incubate at room temperature for
   5 min in moisture chamber to prevent drying.
3. Gently rinse smears in running distilled water.
   Air dry or blot gently with clean bibulous paper.
4. Mount with coverslip, using mounting medium
   of 9 parts glycerine and 1 part carbonate-bicarbonate buffer, pH 9.0.
5. Examine smears with fluorescence microscope
   fitted with 10× ocular and 100× oil-immersion
   objective, BG-12 primary filter, and Corning 3-72
   (3387) or equivalent secondary filter (GG9).
6. Gonococci appear as yellow-green diplococci.

Use a positive urethral smear or a smear prepared from a known fresh isolate of gonococci as
a positive staining control. Use a smear of
Neisseria meningitidis as a negative staining control and a smear of a boiled suspension of *Enterobacter cloacae* as a nonspecific staining control.
(Smears may be stored in the freezer for use as
controls.)

When purchasing conjugate, specify those
"Tested by the Center for Disease Control (CDC)
and found to meet CDC specifications." Each
new lot of conjugate should be evaluated before
use with known fresh isolates of *N. gonorrhoeae*
and fresh isolates of *N. meningitidis* and with
smears of a boiled suspension of *E. cloacae*.

C. Other identification procedures

Enzymatic profiles. See discussion of D'Amato
et al.[185] under *Neisseria meningitidis:* differentiation from other neisseriae, this chapter.

Coagglutination. A coagglutination procedure
has recently been introduced (Phadebact Gonococcus test, Pharmacia Diagnotics, Piscataway,
N.J.) based on Danielsson and Kronvall's
report.[200 a] The test is presently under evaluation.[201] For a discussion of the coagglutination
principle, see Chapter 74; also Streptococci,
this chapter.

Detection of *N. gonorrhoeae* by coagglutination of broth culture sediments has been reported
by Lue and Ellner.[202]

**Counterimmunoelectrophoresis (CIE) and en-
zyme-linked immunosorbent antibody technic
(ELISA) for detection of N. gonorrhoeae antigen.**
Both procedures are presently being evaluated
for the detection of (small numbers of) gonococci;
see Lue and Ellner.[202]

Radiometric procedure. The radiometric detection method (see Bactec instrument, Chapter 74)
has been adapted to the identification of *Neisseria.* Strauss et al.[203] reported that the radiometric procedure is more rapid (3 hours) than the
CTA procedure and more accurate than either the
CTA or the fluorescent antibody test (FA), while
Appelbaum and Lawrence[204] reported 100%

correlation between the radiometric (Bactec) and other methods (CTA, FA) for gonococci and other miscellaneous *Neisseria* but found a major problem with meningococci in the Bactec procedure (fructose levels falsely high in 45% of *N. meningitidis* strains tested).

Minitek procedure. The Minitek system (Baltimore Biological Laboratory, BBL, Cockeysville, Md.) has been evaluated for the identification of *Neisseria* by Morse and Bartenstein,[205] Reddick,[206] and Appelbaum and Lawrence.[204] The Minitek system allows identification of most isolates (90-97%) in 4 hours; it seems somewhat better suited for the identification of meningococci than for gonococci[204] but can be used for both.

Antibiotic susceptibilities of N. gonorrhoeae: penicillin resistance and penicillinase (β-lactamase) production

Until 1976 antibiotic susceptibility testing of gonococci was said to be mostly of epidemiologic value[189] and when needed should be performed by the agar dilution procedure.[207] From 1955 to 1965 there was, in fact, a relentless increase in the number of gonococcal strains (from 0.6% to 42%) that required more than 0.05 U/ml penicillin for growth inhibition.

Since the increase was not due to penicillinase production, and penicillin in increased dosage still remained the most effective treatment modality even for most resistant strains encountered until 1976 (resistance of 1 μg/ml to penicillin), there was little need for performance of susceptibility testing of gonococci in the clinical microbiology laboratory.

In 1976,[207] several strains of highly penicillin-resistant gonococci that acquired the ability to produce penicillinase were isolated in the United States from patients who did not respond to penicillin treatment; similar strains were found in England[208] and in 15 other countries.[209]

These strains can be tested for **susceptibility** with the Kirby-Bauer procedure, using a 10-U penicillin disk with the gonococcus on a chocolate agar plate[189]; zones of inhibition of less than 20 mm suggest a penicillinase-producing strain. Submit such a strain to a reference laboratory (usually state laboratory). For details of the **susceptibility test** see Chapter 87.

Several tests are available for rapid detection of β-lactamase production by gonococci (and other bacteria), i.e., rapid iodometric, acidometric, and chromogenic cephalosporin tests. For detailed descriptions see Chapter 87 (**β-lactamase tests**).

Presently (1979) it is recommended that all isolates be retained from patients who are culture positive for *N. gonorrhoeae* 3-7 days after treatment with penicillin or ampicillin and that a penicillin disk diffusion test be performed on all such treatment failure isolates; if available, a β-lactamase test should also be performed. Penicillin-resistant, penicillinase-producing

strains should be submitted to a state laboratory for confirmation.

Isolation and purification of N. gonorrhoeae from mixed cultures

When the highly selective Thayer-Martin (TM), modified Thayer-Martin (MTM), or NYC medium is used, most of the procedures described below are usually not needed.

For those who may be using other less selective or nonselective media,* a detailed description of examination and purification technics is given.

Cultures may be inspected for "typical" colonies of gonococci at end of 24 h; however, negative plates should be returned to incubator for total of about 48 h incubation. Negative report for gonococci should never be made after only 24 h of incubation.

On chocolate agar, colonies of gonococci are usually opaque, grayish white, raised, finely granular, glistening, slightly convex (sometimes with crest), and if colony is not too small, with lobate margins. Almost all strains will be found to be mucoid. Size of colony may be from 1-4 mm in diameter. There is much variation in colonial morphology and size. This variation is influenced by amount of surface moisture and age of medium. Large numbers of colonies on plate, either gonococci or contaminants, will cause colonies to be small. Differences in particular gonococcus strain or contaminated "mixed" colonies will influence size and colonial morphology. Only firsthand experience in observing colonies of gonococci will make apparent to worker the meaning of "typical colonies."

Plates showing no typical colonies of gonococci after 24 h are returned to incubator. Those plates with suspected colonies are subjected to oxidase test and purification measures.

Plates showing suspected or typical colonies of gonococci are examined first. If there are relatively large numbers of typical colonies, oxidase reagent may be applied by medicine dropper to segment of plate. Plate should be inclined by allowing it to rest against Petri dish cover. In this way drop of oxidase reagent will flow over suspected colonies and collect in bottom of dish. Typical colonies that are well isolated from contaminants and other gonococcus colonies should be reserved for purification procedures.

Inspection of colonies for purity and morphology may be greatly facilitated by means of hand lens or dissecting microscope of 10-30 magnification. Frequently, tiny contaminating colonies lying adjacent to or even as part of gonococcal colony may be seen and avoided. Selected colonies can be fished while under microscopic observation. One to 3 such isolated colonies are picked up with inoculating needle or small loop (1 mm). Some workers prefer to flatten needle tip in shape of spatula.

As each colony is removed from agar surface, tiny drop or loopful of oxidase reagent is applied to colony site where color change will be observed in agar. Colony is then introduced into tube containing about 0.3 ml trypticase soy broth (BBL). Colony is best emulsified by rubbing it aginst wet wall of tube. After picking up and emulsifying several colonies, smear is prepared on glass slide from loopful of suspension and heat-fixed for Gram staining.

---

*Laboratories in the United States are now using selective media; some laboratories outside the United States are using nonselective media.

If microscopic examination reveals gram-negative diplococci typical of gonococcus, purification plate is prepared by inoculating fresh chocolate agar plate with drop of suspension prepared as above and streaking it out. Purification plates are incubated for 24-48 h in candle jar at 35 C.

An alternative method, provided single, well-isolated characteristic colony can be fished from plate, is to inoculate surface of tube of CTA semisolid medium containing 0.2% starch. After incubation for 24-48 h, surface growth is examined microscopically for gram-negative typical diplococci. Fermentation media can then be inoculated from this culture.

On plates showing no suspected or typical colonies of gonococci, entire agar surface is flooded with oxidase reagent and tilted to allow drainage. These plates are observed carefully for several minutes. When secretion contains very few gonococci or when there is crowding by contaminants, colonies of gonococci may be small, few in number, and easily overlooked by macroscopic inspection. Any colony turning pink should be fished immediately and emulsified in 0.5 ml broth to stop toxic action of reagent. Since plate has been flooded with reagent, picked colony will be contaminated and must undergo purification if stained smear reveals gram-negative diplococci.

Plates that show no oxidase-positive colonies are reported negative for gonococcus.

Unsatisfactory cultures may be encountered when plates are covered by "spreaders" or when large numbers of staphylococci, coliform organisms, diphtheroids, or yeast may overgrow more slowly growing gonococcus. When such condition prevails, culture should be reported "unsatisfactory" and new culture requested.

Certain colonies of microorganisms as noted above may react in varying degree of oxidase reagent. Color changes of indicator are atypical and reaction time delayed. Colonial characteristics of these organisms usually serve to differentiate them from colonies of gonococci.

Certain gram-negative rods give positive oxidase test and on casual microscopic examination appear to be diplococci. These so-called "diplobacilli" are less likely to be confused with gonococcus if one recalls that cell axis of gonococcus parallel to plane of division is greater than axis perpendicular to line of fission. Where microscopic examination of organisms leaves doubt as to their being diplococci or diplobacilli, sugar fermentation of purified culture must be made. (Confusion occasionally arises when oxidase-positive diplococci are isolated from urethritis that do not give typical reactions of *Neisseria*. Diplococcal forms predominate on solid media, whereas in liquid media rods and filaments are formed. For discussion of these organisms see *Moraxella* and *Acinetobacter*, Chapter 79.)

Other Neisseriae

For identification refer to Table 76-8. These neisseriae usually grow at room temperature and can be identified by biochemical reactions; they usually do **not** grow on selective media (TM, TMT).

Branhamella (Neisseria) catarrhalis often agglutinates in normal horse serum or saline, grows at room temperature and on plain nutrient agar, but does not produce acid from the usual carbohydrates; its colony is grayish white, friable,

and granular. Occasional strains grow on MTM medium (Table 76-8).

N. flavescens has yellow pigmentation when first isolated and grows on plain nutrient agar; it has been isolated from a limited epidemic of meningitis.

N. subflava (formerly *N. perflava* and *N. flava*) usually produces small greenish to yellowish colonies, often wrinkled or hard.

The organism formerly known as *N. haemolysans* is oxidase and catalase negative; the genus designation *Gemella* has been assigned to it. In *Bergey's Manual*, ed. 8,[3] it is included in the family Streptococcaceae.

Neisseria lactamicus

As mentioned earlier under meningococci, *N. lactamicus*, sp. nov.,[182] strains are isolated in increasing numbers. The characteristics of the organism are shown in Table 76-8.

Hollis et al.[182] in 1969 compared these lactose-utilizing strains with a large number of *N. meningitidis* and other species of *Neisseria*, and they considered the differences among them significant enough to warrant designation of a new species. The organism is found mostly in the nasopharynx of humans; on a few occasions it has been isolated from spinal fluid, blood, genital sites, tracheal aspirate, lung tissue, etc.[210] It is considered of little clinical importance.

N. lactamicus is positive for β-D-**galactosidase** activity, is **oxidase positive**, and in the O-F medium of King (0.5% Casitone [Difco], 0.3% agar, 0.003% aqueous phenol red, pH 7.3, and 1% carbohydrate) demonstrates fermentative activity, unlike other neisseriae that are oxidative. It produces acid from glucose, maltose, and lactose and grows on TM medium; individual strains vary in their ability to grow on nutrient agar at both 25 C and 37 C.

The organism is serologically distinct from the *N. meningitidis* serogroups A, B, C, D, X, Y, or Z.

Anaerobic gram-negative cocci

See Chapter 83.

Mimeae

The designations *Mima* and *Herellea* were formerly used to denote certain gram-negative, motile or nonmotile, aerobic, nonsporulating rods that grow well on meat extract media, producing smooth, white, convex colonies.

They are mentioned here because on solid media they appear predominantly as diplococcal forms and were occasionally confused with neisseriae. In liquid culture, rods and filaments are abundant.

For detailed discussion see *Moraxella* and *Acinetobacter*, Chapter 79.

REFERENCES

1. Baird-Parker, A. C.: Ann. N.Y. Acad. Sci. **236**:7, 1974.
2. International Subcommittee on Taxonomy of

Staphylococci and Micrococci: Int. Bull. Bacteriol. Nomen. Taxon. **15**:109, 1965.

3. Buchanan, R. E., and Gibbons, N. E.: Bergey's manual of determinative bacteriology, ed. 8, Baltimore, 1974, The Williams & Wilkins Co.

4. Baird-Parker, A. C.: International Subcommittee on Taxonomy of Staphylococci and Micrococci: Int. J. Syst. Bacteriol. **21**:161, 1971.

5. Facklam, R. R., and Smith, P. B.: The gram-positive cocci, Human Pathol. **7**:187, 1976.

6. Deibel, R. H., and Evans, J. B.: J. Bacteriol. **79**:356, 1960.

7. International Subcommittee on the Taxonomy of Staphylococci and Micrococci, Int. J. Syst. Bacteriol. **26**:333, 1976.

8. Kloos, W. F., and Schleifer, K. H.: J. Clin. Microbiol. **1**:82-88, 1975.

9. Oeding, P., and Digranes, A.: Acta Pathol. Microbiol. Scand. (B) **85**:136-142, 1977.

10. Zarzour, J. Y., and Belle, E. A.: J. Clin. Microbiol. **7**:133, 1978.

11. Baird-Parker, A. C. In Gibbs, B. M., and Skinner, F. A., editors: Identification methods for microbiologists, part A, New York, 1966, Academic Press.

12. Baird-Parker, A. C.: J. Gen. Microbiol. **30**:409, 1963.

13. Baird-Parker, A. C.: J. Gen Microbiol. **38**:363, 1965.

14. Hajek, V.: Maršálek. Zbl. Bakt. Hyg. I. Acta (A) **217**:176, 1971.

15. Wallmark, G., Arremark, I., and Telander, B.: J. Infect. Dis. **138**:791, 1978.

16. Williams, D. N., Lund, M. E., and Blazevic, D. J.: J. Clin. Microbiol. **3**:556-559, 1976.

17. Cohen, J. O., editor: The staphylococci, New York, 1972, Interscience, John Wiley & Sons.

18. Jeljaszewicz, J., editor: Staphylococci and staphylococcal diseases, Stuttgart, 1976, Gustav Fischer Verlag.

19. Acar, J. F., Goldstein, F. W., and Lagrange, P.: J. Clin. Microbiol. **8**:142, 1978.

20. Marks, J., and Vaughn, A.: J. Pathol. Bateriol. **62**:597, 1950.

21. Chapman, G. H.: J. Bacteriol. **50**:201, 1945.

22. Chapman, G. H.: J. Bacteriol. **51**:409, 1946.

23. Chapman, G. H.: Food Res. **13**:100, 1948.

24. Greer, J. E., and Menard, N.: Am. J. Public Health **49**:685, 1959.

25. Blair, J. E., Borman, E. K., Bynoe, E. T., et al.: Hospital acquired staphylococcal disease: recommended procedures for laboratory investigation, Atlanta, 1958, United States Department of Health, Education and Welfare, Public Health Service.

26. Smith, I. M.: Staphylococcal infections, Chicago, 1958, Year Book Medical Publishers.

27. Morse, S. I., In Dubos, R., and Hirsch, J. G., editors: Bacterial and mycotic infections of man, ed. 4, Philadelphia, 1965, J. B. Lippincott Co.

28. Bayliss, B. G., and Hall, E. R.: J. Bacteriol. **89**:101, 1965.

29. Turner, F. J., and Schwartz, B. S.: Bacteriol. Proc. 1956, p. 55.

30. Cadness-Graves, B., Williams, R., Harper, G. J., and Miles, A. A.: Lancet **1**:736, 1943.

31. Weckman, N., and Catlin, J.: J. Bacteriol. **73**:747, 1957.

32. DiSalvo, J. W.: Med. Tech. Bull. **9**:191, 1958.

33. Bennett, R. W. In FDA bacteriological analytical manual, Washington, D.C., 1978, Association of Official Analytical Chemists, Publ.

34. Lachica, R. V. V., Genigeorgis, G., and Hoeprich, P. D.: Appl. Microbiol. **21**:585-587, 1971.

35. Anderson, E. S., and Williams, R. E. O.: J. Clin. Pathol. **9**:94, 1956. Also reprinted in Selected materials on staphylococcal disease, Atlanta, 1958, United States Department of Health, Education and Welfare, Communicable Disease Center.

36. Subcommittee on the Phage Typing of Staphylococci: Int. J. Syst. Bacteriol. **21**:165, 167, 171, 1971.

37. Blair, J. E., and Williams, R. E. O.: Bull. WHO **24**:771, 1961.

38. Smith, P. B.: Bacteriophage typing of *S. aureus*. In Cohen, J. O., editor: The staphylococci, New York, 1972, Interscience, John Wiley & Sons.

39. Van Boven, C. P. A., Verhoef, J., and Winkler, K. C.: Antonie van Leeuwenhoek **35**:232, 1969.

40. Van Boven, C. P. A. : Phage typing of *Staphylococcus epidermidis*. In Jeljaszewicz, J., editor: Staphylococci and staphylococcal disease, Stuttgart, 1976, Gustav Fischer Verlag.

41. Lack, C., and Wailling, D.: J. Pathol. Bacteriol. **68**:431, 1954.

42. Adler, V., Gillespie, W., and Herdan, G.: J. Pathol. Bacteriol. **66**:205, 1953.

43. McClean, D., Rogers, H. J., Williams, B. W., and Hale, C. W.: Lancet **1**:355, 1943.

44. Schwabacker, H., Cunliffe, A. C., Williams, R. E. O., and Harper, G. J.: Br. J. Exp. Pathol. **26**:124, 1945.

45. Burnet, F.: Aust. J. Exp. Biol. Med. Sci. **26**:71, 1948.

46. Oakley, C., and Warrack, H.: J. Pathol. Bacteriol. **63**:45, 1951.

47. Panton, P., Valentine, F., and Dix, V.: Lancet **2**:1180, 1931.

48. Jones, M.: J. Bacteriol. **51**:789, 1946.

49. Anderson, K.: J. Clin. Pathol. **9**:257, 1956.

50. Panton, P., and Valentine, F.: Lancet **1**:506, 1932.

51. Marks, J., and Vaughan, A.: J. Pathol. Bacteriol. **62**:597, 1950.

52. Jackson, A., and Little, R.: Can. J. Microbiol. **3**:101, 1957.

53. Miller, R. P., and Ackerman, G. A.: Am. J. Clin. Pathol. **32**:100, 1959.

54. Panton, P., and Valentine, F.: Lancet **1**:506, 1932.

55. Wilson, G. S., and Miles, A. A.: Topley and Wilson's principles of bacteriology and immunity, ed. 4, Baltimore, 1955, The Williams & Wilkins Co.

56. Smith, I., Beals, P., and Hansenclever, H.: Bacteriol. Proc. 1957, p. 90.

57. Reinarz, J. A., and Sanford, J. P.: Medicine **44**:81, 1965.

58. Moellering, R. C., Watson, B. K., and Kunz, L. J.: Am. J. Med. **57**:239, 1974.

59. Anthony, B. F., and Okada, D. M.: Annu. Rev. Med. **28**:355, 1977.

60. Wilkinson, H. W.: Annu. Rev. Microbiol. **32**:41, 1978.

61. Patterson, M. J., and Hafeez, A. E. B.: Bacteriol. Rev. **40**:774, 1976.

62. Duma, R. J., Weinberg, A. N., Medrek, T. F., and Kunz, L. J.: Medicine **48**:87, 1969.

63. Wannamaker, L. W., and Matsen, J. M., editors: Streptococci and streptococcal diseases, New York, 1972, Academic Press.

64. Breese, B. B.: Am. J. Dis. Child. **132**:502, 612, 1978.

65. Brown, J. H.: Monogr. Rockefeller Inst. Med. Res. no. 9, 1919.

66. Lancefield, R. C.: J. Exp. Med. **47**:481, 1928.

67. Lancefield, R. C.: J. Exp. Med. **57**:571, 1933.

68. Lancefield, R. C.: J. Exp. Med. **78**:465, 1943.

69. Lancefield, R. C.: J. Exp. Med. **96**:83, 1952.

70. Lancefield, R. C.: J. Exp. Med. **47**:91, 1928.

71. Lancefield, R. C.: J. Exp. Med. **71**:521, 1940.

72. Lancefield, R. C.: J. Exp. Med. **71**:539, 1940.

73. Lancefield, R. C.: J. Exp. Med. **84**:449, 1946.

74. Lancefield, R. C.: J. Exp. Med. **96**:71, 1952.

75. Griffith, F.: J. Hyg. **25**:385, 1926; **26**:369, 1927; **27**:113, 1928; **35**:542, 1934; **35**:23, 1935.

76. WHO Expert Committee: Streptococcal and staphylococcal infections, WHO Tech. Rep. Ser. 394, 1968.

77. James, L., and McFarland, R. B.: N. Engl. J. Med. **284**:750, 1971.

78. Eickhoff, T., Klein, J. O., Daly, A. K., et al.: N. Engl. J. Med. **271**:1221, 1964.

79. Butter, M. N., and Moor, C. E. de: Antonie van Leeuwenhoek **33**:439, 1967.

80. Lazarus, J. M., Sellers, D. P., and Marine, W. M.: N. Engl. J. Med. **272**:46, 1965.

81. Van Peenen, P. F. D.: N. Engl. J. Med. **272**:486, 1965.

82. Hood, M., Janney, A., and Dameron, G.: Am. J. Obstet. Gynecol. **82**:809, 1961.

83. Baker, C. J.: J. Infect. Dis. **136**:137, 1977.

84. Wilkinson, H. W.: J. Clin. Microbiol. **7**:176, 1978.

85. Colman, G.: J. Gen. Microbiol. **50**:149, 1968.

86. Long, P. H., and Bliss, E. A.: J. Exp. Med. **60**:619, 1934.

87. Hare, R.: J. Pathol. Bacteriol. **41**:499, 1935.

88. White, J. C., and Niven, C. F.: J. Bacteriol. **51**:717, 1946.

89. Rosebury, T. In Dubos, R., and Hirsch, J. G., editors: Bacterial and mycotic infections of man, ed. 4, Philadelphia, 1965, J. B. Lippincott Co.

90. Rosebury, T.: Microorganisms indigenous to man, New York, 1962, McGraw-Hill Book Co.

91. Cowan, T., and Steel, K. J.: Manual for the identification of medical bacteria, Cambridge, 1965, Cambridge University Press.

92. Wilkinson, H. W.: Clin. Microbiol. News **1**(9):1, 1979.

93. Facklam, R. R.: Int. J. Syst. Bacteriol. **24**:313-319, 1974.

94. Neef, L. I., Chretien, J. H., Delaha, E. C., and Garagusi, V. F.: J.A.M.A. **230**:1298, 1974.

95. Murray, H. W., Gross, K. C., Masur, H., and Roberts, R.: Am. J. Med. **64**:759, 1978.

96. International Subcommittee on Streptococci and Pneumococci: Int. J. Syst. Bacteriol. **17**:281, 1967.

97. Deibel, R. H.: Bacteriol. Rev. **28**:330, 1964.

98. Klein, R. S., Recco, R. A., Catalano, M. T., et al.: N. Engl. J. Med. **297**:800, 1977.

99. Levy, B. S., von Reyn, C. F., Arbeit, R. D., et al.: N. Engl. J. Med. **298**:572, 1978.

100. Ravreby, W. D., Bottone, J. J., and Keusch, G. T.: N. Engl. J. Med. **289**:1400, 1973.

101. Facklam, R. R.: Appl. Microbiol. **23**:1131, 1972.

102. McCarty, L., and Bottone, E.: Am. J. Clin. Pathol. **61**:585, 1974.

103. Carey, R., Brause, B., and Roberts, R.: Ann. Intern. Med. **87**:150, 1977.

104. Washington, J.: Ann. Intern. Med. **87**:793, 1977.

105. Nadel, S. M., Jackson, J. W., and Ploth, D. W.: J.A.M.A. **241**:2294, 1979.

106. Wannamaker, L. W.: A method for culturing beta-hemolytic streptococci from the throat, New York, 1965, American Heart Association.

107. Todd, E. W., and Hewitt, L. F.: J. Pathol. Bacteriol. **35**:973, 1932.

108. Pike, R. M.: Proc. Soc. Exp. Biol. Med. **57**:186, 1944.

109. Drapkin, M. S., Karchmer, A. W., and Moellering, R. C.: J.A.M.A. **236**:263, 1976.

110. Hussey, H. H.: J.A.M.A. **236**:1388, 1976.

111. Bernheimer, A., Linder, R., and Avigad, L. S.: Infect. Immun. **23**:838, 1979.

112. Facklam, R. R.: Isolation and identification of streptococci, parts I-III, Atlanta, 1977, Center for Disease Control.

113. Moody, M. D., Siegel, A. C., Pittman, B., and Winter, C. C.: Am. J. Public Health **53**:1083-1092, 1963.

114. Romero, R., and Wilkinson, H. W.: Appl. Microbiol. **28**:199-204, 1974.

115. Rosner, R.: J. Clin. Microbiol. **6**:23-26, 1977.

116. Slifkin, M., Engwall, C., and Pouchet, G. R.: J. Clin. Microbiol. **7**:356-360, 1978.

117. Szilagyi, G., Mayer, E., and Eidelman, A. I.: J. Clin. Microbiol. **8**:410-412, 1978.

118. Lue, Y. A., Howit, I. P., and Ellner, P. D.,: J. Clin. Microbiol. **8**:326-328, 1978.

119. Burgard, L., Cole, B., and Sonnenwirth, A.: Abstracts Ann. Meeting Am. Soc. Microbiol. Abstr. C 116, p. 337, 1979.

120. Fenton, L. J., and Harper, M. H.: J. Clin. Microbiol. **8**:500-502, 1978.

121. Hill, H. R., Riter, M. E., Menge, S. K., et al.: J. Clin. Microbiol. **1**:188-191, 1975.

122. Russell, H., Facklam, R. R., Padula, J. F., and Cooksey, R.: J. Clin. Microbiol. **8**:355-359, 1978.

123. Maxted, W. R.: J. Clin. Pathol. **6**:224, 1953.

124. Jelinkova, J., and Rotta, J.: Int. J. Syst. Bacteriol. **17**:297, 1967.

125. Christie, R., Atkins, N. E., and Munch-Petersen, E.: Aust. J. Exp. Biol. Med. Sci. **22**:197, 1944.

126. Darling, C. L. J.: Clin. Microbiol. **1**:171, 1975.

127. Fuchs, P. C., Christy, C., and Jones, R. N.: J. Clin. Microbiol. **7**:232, 1978.

128. Wilkinson, H. W.: J. Clin. Microbiol. **6**:42, 1977.

129. Gubash, S. M.: J. Clin. Microbiol. **8**:480, 1978.

130. Ayers, S. H., and Rupp, P.: J. Infect. Dis. **30**:388, 1922.

131. Facklam, R. R., et al.: Appl. Microbiol. **27**:107, 1974.

132. Facklam, R. R.: Appl. Microbiol. **26**:138, 1973.

133. Facklam, R. R.: Appl. Microbiol. **20**:245, 1970.

134. Facklam, R. R., et al.: Appl. Microbiol. **27**:107, 1974.

135. Fuller, A. T.: Br. J. Exp. Pathol. **19**:130, 1938.

136. Rantz, L. A., and Randall, E.: Stanford Med. Bull. **13**:290, 1955.

137. Maxted, W. R.: Lancet **2**:255, 1948.

138. Watson, B. K., et al.: J. Clin. Microbiol. **1**:274, 1975.

139. Swift, H. F., Wilson, A. T., and Lancefield, R. C.: J. Exp. Med. **78**:127, 1943.

140. Greenblatt, J. J., Eichmann, K., Braun, D., et al.: J. Infect. Dis. **124**:387, 1971.

141. Harrell, W. K., and George, J. R.: Appl. Microbiol. **23**:1047, 1972.

142. Mills, J., Orenstein, W., and Cohen, S. N.: Am. J. Dis. Child. **126**:244, 1973.

143. Yatabe, J. A. H., Baldwin, K. L., and Martin, W. J.: J. Clin. Microbiol. **6**:181, 1977.

144. Bowers, E. F., and Jeffries, L. R.: J. Clin. Pathol. **8**:58, 1955.

145. Laboratory methods in clinical bacteriology, Atlanta, 1976, Center for Disease Control.

146. Salinger, A., and Geraghty, S.: Public Health Lab. **14**:136, 1956.

147. Hawn, C. V., and Beebe, E.: J. Bacteriol. **90**:549, 1965.

148. Glasgow, L. A., and Coene, D. H.: J. Pediatr. **71**:574, 1967.

149. Lund, E., and Rasmussen, P.: Acta Pathol. Microbiol. Scand. **68**:458, 1966.
150. Austrian, A.: Mt. Sinai J. Med. **43**:699, 1976.
151. Russell, H., Facklam, R. R., Padula, J. F., and Cooksey, R.: J. Clin. Microbiol. **8**:355, 1978.
152. Turner, G. C.: Lancet **2**:1292, 1963.
153. Schaffner, W., Schreiber, W. M., and Koenig, M. G.: N. Engl. J. Med. **274**:451, 1966.
154. Kislak, J. W.: N. Engl. J. Med. **276**:852, 1967.
155. Hansman, D., Glasgow, H., Sturt, J., et al.: N. Engl. J. Med. **284**, 175-177, 1971.
156. Naraqi, S., Kirkpatrick, G. P., and Kabins, S. G.: J. Pediatr. **85**:671-673, 1974.
157. Paredes, A., Taber, L. H., Yow, M. D., et al.: Pediatrics **58**:378-381, 1976.
158. Mace, J. W., Janik, D. S., Sauer, R. L., et al.: J. Pediatr. **91**:506-507, 1977.
159. Iyer, P. V., Kahler, J. H., and Jacobs, N. M.: Pediatrics **61**:157-158, 1978.
160. Gartner, J. C., and Michaels, R. H.: J.A.M.A. **241**:1707, 1979.
161. Dixon, J. M. S., Lipinski, A. E., and Graham, M. E. P.: Can. Med. Assoc. J. **117**:1159-1161, 1977.
162. Howes, V. J., and Mitchell, R. G.: Br. Med. J. **1**:996, 1976.
163. Ahronheim, G. A., Reich, B., and Marks, M. I.: Am. J. Dis. Child. **133**:187-191, 1979.
164. Jacobs, M. R., Koornhof, H. J., Robins-Browne, R. M., et al.: N. Engl. J. Med. **299**:735-740, 1978.
165. Morbid. Mortal. **26**:285, 1977; **27**:1, 1978.
166. Morbid. Mortal. **26**:345, 1977.
167. Morbid. Mortal. **27**:1, 1978.
168. Finland, M.: N. Engl. J. Med. **284**:212-214, 1971.
169. Sonnenwirth, A. C. In Frankel, S., Reitman, S., and Sonnenwirth, A. C., editors: Gradwohl's clinical laboratory methods and diagnosis, ed. 7, St. Louis, 1970, The C. V. Mosby Co., ch. 64.
170. Cooksey, R. C., Facklam, R. R., and Thornsberry, C.: Antimicrob. Agents Chemother. **13**:645, 1978.
171. Jacobs, M. R., and Koornhof, H. J.: J. Antimicrob. Chemother. **4**:481, 1978.
172. Evans, J. B., and Kerbaugh, M. A.: Health Lab. Sci. **7**:76, 1970.
173. Colman, G.: J. Clin. Pathol. **20**:294, 1967.
174. Parker, M. T., and Ball, L. C.: J. Med. Microbiol. **9**:275, 1976.
175. Henriksen, S. D.: Ann. Rev. Microbiol. **30**:63-83, 1976.
176. Catlin, B. W. In Lennette, E. H., Spaulding, E. H., and Truant, J. P., editors: Manual of clinical microbiology, Washington, D.C., 1974, American Society for Microbiology.
177. Cheever, S. F. In Dubos, R., and Hirsch, J. G., editors: Bacterial and mycotic infections of man, ed. 4, Philadelphia, 1965, J. B. Lippincott Co.
178. Slaterus, K. W.: Antonie van Leeuwenhoek **29**:265, 1963.
179. Hollis, D. G., Wiggins, G. L., and Schubert, J. H.: J. Bacteriol. **95**:1, 1968.
180. Vedros, N. A.: Serology of the Meningococcus. In Bergan, T., and Norris, J. R., editors: Methods in microbiology, vol. X, New York, 1978, Academic Press.
181. Thayer, J. D.: Public Health Lab. **26**:85, 1968.
182. Hollis, D. G., Wiggins, G. L., and Weaver, R. E.: Appl. Microbiol. **17**:71, 1969.

183. Kippax, P. W., Saeed, N., and Pamplin, W. A. V.: J. Clin. Pathol. **21**:440, 1968.
184. Bøvre, K.: Acta Pathol. Microbiol. Scand. **76**:148, 1969.
185. D'Amato, R. F., Eriquez, L. A., Tomfohrde, K. M., and Singerman, E.: J. Clin. Microbiol. **7**:77, 1978.
186. Millar, J. W., Siess, E. E., Feldman, H. A., et al.: J.A.M.A. **186**:139, 1963.
187. Frank, P. F., Wilcox, C., and Finland, M.: J. Lab. Clin. Med. **35**:188, 1950.
188. Feldman, H. A.: Meningococcal disease. In Beeson, P. B., and McDermott, W., editors: The Cecil-Loeb textbook of medicine, ed. 14, New York, 1975, W. B. Saunders Co., pp. 330-336.
188a. Bennett, J. V., Camp, H. M., and Eickhoff, T. C.: Appl. Microbiol. **16**:1056, 1968.
189. Kellogg, D. S., Jr., Holmes, K. K., and Hill, G. A.: Laboratory diagnosis of gonorrhea, Cumitech 4, (Marcus, S., and Sherris, J. C., coord. ed.), Washington, D.C., 1976, American Society for Microbiology.
190. Johnson, T. W.: Gonorrhea. In Hoeprich, P. D., editor: Infectious diseases, New York, 1972, Harper & Row, Publishers.
191. Morse, S. A.: Sex. Trans. Dis. **6**:28, 1979.
192. WHO Scientific Group: *Neisseria gonorrhoeae* and gonococcal infections, WHO Tech. Rep. Ser. 616, 1978.
193. Roberts, B., editor: The *Gonococcus*, New York, 1977, John Wiley & Sons.
194. Crawford, G., Knapp, J., and Holmes, K. K.: Clin. Res. **25**:156A, 1977.
195. Kellogg, D. S.: *Neisseria gonorrhoeae* (gonococcus). In Lennette, E. H., Spaulding, E. H., and Truant, J. P., editors: Manual of clinical microbiology, ed. 2, Washington, D.C., 1974, American Society for Microbiology, pp. 124-129.
196. Brown, W. J.: Appl. Microbiol. **27**:1027, 1974.
197. Brown, W. J.: Health Lab. Sci. **13**:54, 1976.
198. Brown, W. J.: Health Lab. Sci. **14**:172, 1977.
199. Kellogg, D. S., and Turner, E. M.: Appl. Microbiol. **25**:50-52, 1973.
200. Peacock, W. L., Welch, B. G., Martin, J. E., Jr., and Thayer, J. D.: Public Health Rep. **83**:337-339, 1968.
200a. Danielsson, D., and Kronvall, G.: Appl. Microbiol. **27**:368, 1974.
201. Barnham, M., and Glynn, A. A.: J. Clin. Pathol. **31**:189, 1978.
202. Lue, Y. A., and Ellner, P. D.: Sex. Trans. Dis. **5**:14, 1978.
203. Strauss, R. R., Holderbach, J., and Friedman, H.: J. Clin. Microbiol. **7**:419, 1978.
204. Appelbaum, P. C., and Lawrence, R. B.: J. Clin. Microbiol. **9**:598, 1979.
205. Morse, S. A., and Bartenstein, L.: J. Clin. Microbiol. **3**:8, 1976.
206. Reddick, A.: J. Clin. Microbiol. **2**:72, 1975.
207. Morbid. Mortal. **25**:307, 1976.
208. Percival, A., Corkill, J. E., Arya, O. P., et al.: Lancet **2**:1379-1382, 1976.
209. Morbid. Mortal. **26**:153, 1977.
210. Hollis, D. G., Wiggins, G. L., Weaver, R. F., et al.: Ann. N. Y. Acad. Sci. **174**:444, 1970.

77

GRAM-POSITIVE BACILLI

Alex C. Sonnenwirth

Corynebacteria

The genus *Corynebacterium*, including non-sporeforming **gram-positive rods** (*C. diphtheriae*, the causative agent of diphtheria, and a number of usually nonpathogenic organisms indigenous to man and animals), was for many years included in the family Corynebacteriaceae in the sixth and seventh editions of *Bergey's Manual of Determinative Bacteriology*. In the eighth edition[1] the family is not recognized, and instead a "Coryneform Group of Bacteria" is described (*Bergey's Manual*,[1] Part 17, "Actinomycetes and Related Organisms"). The group includes the genera *Corynebacterium*, *Arthrobacter* (with the related genera *Brevibacterium* and *Microbacterium*, the latter 2 as genera of uncertain standing), *Cellulomonas*, and *Kurthia*.

The **anaerobic corynebacteria** (diphtheroids), previously described as *C. acnes*, *C. granulosum*, and *C. avidum*, are now excluded and are described under the genus *Propionibacterium* (Chapter 85).

The genera *Listeria* and *Erysipelothrix*, for many years also part of the family Corynebacteriaceae, are now described as genera of uncertain affiliation in the family *Lactobacillaceae* (*Bergey's Manual*,[1] Part 16, "Gram-positive, Asporogenous, Rod-Shaped Bacteria"); the genus *Lactobacillus* (family Lactobacillaceae) is also included in Part 16.

CORYNEBACTERIUM

The genus *Corynebacterium* is now divided into 3 sections[1]: (I) human and animal parasites and pathogens, (II) plant pathogenic corynebacteria, and (III) "nonpathogenic" corynebacteria.

Sections II and III (the latter composed of many ill-defined and poorly characterized organisms most commonly isolated from water, soils, and air) are not discussed further here. Section I organisms are described in detail below.

Organisms in the genus *Corynebacterium* are aerobic and facultatively anaerobic, pleomorphic rods. Many of the strains appear to be widely distributed in nature, whereas others are associated with the body surfaces and tissues of man and animals. Corynebacteria other than *C. diphtheriae* and a closely associated species, *C. ulcerans*, are chiefly important in man to the extent that they may confuse the diagnosis of diphtheria. Characteristically the organisms in this genus show angular and palisade (picket fence) arrangements of cells and often show club-shaped swellings.

They are nonmotile (except for some plant pathogens that are motile), do not form spores, do not usually show branching, and are catalase positive (with few exceptions). Sugars are utilized fermentatively or not at all. Most corynebacteria characteristically show a beaded or banded appearance ("metachromatic granules") when suitably stained.

Corynebacterium diphtheriae

For obtaining specimens, choice of media to be used in examination for diphtheria, and the fluorescent antitoxin test for rapid identification of *C. diphtheriae* see discussion of Throat and nasopharyngeal specimens in Chapter 75.

C. diphtheriae rods occur singly or in palisade formation and vary greatly in dimensions: 0.3-0.8 μm in breadth and 1-8 μm in length. They are straight or slightly curved, are frequently swollen at one or both ends, and do not stain uniformly but have granules or bars of more deeply staining properties.

The organisms are usually pleomorphic and may show a variety of forms (e.g., clubbed, granular, barred, wedge shaped, and solid staining). Direct smears from the throat show much less pleomorphism; the organisms are usually shorter and stain more uniformly than those grown in culture.[2]

Colony appearance

Tinsdale medium (recommended). *C. diphtheriae* and *C. ulcerans* produce typical smooth, gray-black, shiny, convex colonies, with dark brown halos around the colonies after 24-48 h incubation. Most diphtheroids produce no halos. If there is no growth after 24 h, reincubate plates for another 24 h.

Tellurite medium. Staphylococci and streptococci are generally inhibited, whereas diphtheria bacilli develop black or grayish black colonies in 18-24 h. Occasionally a strain of *Staphylococcus* is encountered that grows on this medium, producing black colonies. These, however, may be readily recognized as cocci by microscopic examination. Confirmation of typical colonies is made by microscopic examination of the cells and by testing their fermentation reactions. The morphology of *C. diphtheriae* grown on tellurite medium varies somewhat from that obtained on Loeffler medium. On the selective medium the organisms are generally club shaped, many are barred, and only a few show the bipolar staining characteristic of *C. diphtheriae* on Loeffler medium. Confirmation may be made by transferring the black suspected colony to Loeffler medium on which typical morphology can be demonstrated as soon as there has been sufficient growth.

Loeffler serum agar slant. After 24 h incubation at 37 C the colonies are about 1 mm in diameter, circular, with smooth surface and entire edge. They are creamy, easily emulsifiable in water or saline, and convex with a slightly raised center. After 48-72 h incubation the colonies enlarge, the center becomes more raised, and the periphery remains flat and appears more transparent than the center, giving the "poached-egg" appearance.[3]

Blood agar. Colonies are small with a matt appearance; some strains are hemolytic (*C. diphtheriae*, type *mitis*).

Cystine tellurite medium (recommended). Colonies appear grayish black (gunmetal gray).

Identification

From suspected colonies prepare Gram and methylene blue stains to eliminate organisms other than corynebacteria. The organisms are usually pleomorphic with many granules. For workers with experience and in an epidemic situation, it usually suffices to rely on colonial morphology and microscopic appearance in order to make a preliminary report and to carry out virulence and biochemical tests afterward. However, when single cases are investigated and the worker does not have sufficient experience with the diphtheria bacillus (as is the case in most parts of the United States), fermentation reactions and virulence (toxigenicity) tests are essential to rule out diphtheroids (or atoxigenic diphtheria strains). As already discussed under throat and nasopharyngeal specimens, no diagnosis should be made on the basis of a throat swab stained with methylene blue or Gram stain. Colonies on Tinsdale medium are suggestive, but fermentation reactions and toxigenicity testing are still essential.

Suspected colonies should be transferred to obtain pure cultures. **Virulence (toxigenicity) tests** are the critical diagnostic tests; fermentation tests will eliminate some diphtheroids.

C. diphtheriae is nonmotile, forms no spores, and is catalase positive. It ferments glucose and maltose, with acid but no gas. Some *mitis* types (see below) ferment sucrose; distinction from *C. xerosis* may be made by the ability of the *mitis* strain to produce toxin and by hemolysis. *Gravis* types, in addition, ferment starch and dextrin. *C. ulcerans* liquefies gelatin, whereas *C. diphtheriae* does not. Use Christensen urea agar for urease test; if positive, test further because *C. ulcerans* is toxigenic.

Fermentation tests can be carried out in Cystine trypticase agar (CTA medium; BBL, Division of BioQuest, Cockeysville, Md.) or Cystine tryptic agar (Difco Laboratories, Detroit) containing the appropriate carbohydrate. Table 77-1 lists the reactions of corynebacteria. Growth and fermentation occur more promptly if the carbohydrate is incorporated into Hiss serum water.

Hiss serum water. Mix 1 part serum (horse, sheep, ox) with 3 parts distilled water. Add 5 ml 0.2% solution phenol red/100 ml mixture. Incorporate various sugars in the proportion of 1%. Sterilize in steamer for 20 min each day on 3 successive days. **An alternate method** is to prepare peptone-water-sugar media such as phenol red carbohydrate media and add, with sterile precautions, 0.5 ml sterile rabbit or human serum to each 10 ml medium.

Deoxyribonuclease activity. An interesting observation was reported by Diamond and Judson (1967).[6] According to their findings, all *C. diphtheria* strains (toxigenic **and** nontoxigenic) contain an enzyme that depolymerizes deoxyribonucleic acid. This was demonstrated on DNase agar (Difco). No other corynebacteria gave a positive DNase reaction. The enzyme does **not** relate to toxin production but is present in the *mitis*, *intermedius*, and *gravis* types of *C. diphtheriae*.

Fluorescent antibody technic for detection of *C. diphtheriae*. Refer to fluorescent antibody technics (Chapter 60), to throat and nasopharyngeal culture (Chapter 63), and to the review of Cherry and Moody.[7] The test is not in general use; if employed, it should always be used in conjunction with standard cultural technics.

Virulence (toxigenicity) tests

Virulence of *C. diphtheriae* and *C. ulcerans* is dependent on the production of a toxin by the organism. This toxin accounts almost entirely for the clinical injury occurring in diphtheria. Nontoxigenic (non-toxin-producing) strains are encountered (especially var. *mitis*); therefore to definitively identify an isolate as a toxigenic (virulent) organism it is necessary to carry out virulence tests.

Gel-diffusion (in vitro) method. Method of Elek[8] and modification by King[9] is gel-precipitation reaction between known diphtheria antitoxin incorporated in suitable growth medium and toxin that may be liberated by organisms growing on medium.

Prepare plates of Elek-King agar diffusion medium (see Elek toxigenicity medium). Before medium cools completely, lay across the surface a sterile paper strip that was previously soaked in diphtheria antitoxin containing 500 U/ml (but see CDC comments below). Push strip into agar with sterile pair of tweezers. When agar has hardened, inoculate it with isolate (either from an overnight broth culture or agar slant) by making a single streak perpendicular to strip and extending 12-18 mm on each side of filter paper. Each plate may be inoculated with 4-6 cultures. Known positive and known negative cultures should also be inoculated to serve as controls.

Table 77-1. Differentiation of various corynebacteria*

	C. diphtheriae var. gravis	C. diphtheriae var. intermedius	C. diphtheriae var. mitis	C. ulcerans	C. xerosis	C. pseudodiphtheriticum†	C. pyogenes	C. equi‡	C. haemolyticum
Morphology	Rods, pleomorphic, short	Rods, pleomorphic, longer	Rods, barrel, clubbed, long	Rods at 4 h; coccoid at 24 h	Polar staining rods	Slender rods, clubbed	Small rods, chains may form, occasional club forms	Coccoid to long clubbed forms; some acid fast	Small, coccoid to diphtheroid forms
Catalase	+	+	+	+	+	+	-	+	-
Motility	-	-	-	-	-	-	-	-	-
Glucose	+	+§	+	+	+	-	+	-	+
Maltose	+	+	+	d‖	+	-	+	-	+
Sucrose	-	-	-	-	+	-	d‖	-	+/-
Trehalose	-	-	-	+	-	-	-	-	-
Starch	+	+	-	+	-	-	+	-	-
Nitrate reduced	+	+	+	-	+	+	+	+/-	-
Hemolysis	-	+/-	+	+	-	-	+	-	+
Urea hydrolyzed	-	-	-	+	-	+	-	+/-	-
Toxigenic	+¶	+¶	+¶	+¶	-	-	-	-	-

*Data from *Bergey's Manual*,[1] Wilson and Miles,[3] Cowan and Steel,[4] and Hermann and Weaver.[5]
†*C. hofmannii.*
‡Characteristically, pink and moist colonies.
§*Minimus* variants ferment glucose very slowly if at all.
‖d = variable.
¶Nontoxigenic strains encountered.

Positive test is shown by formation of line of whitish precipitate at 45° angle between filter paper and culture streak. Other secondary, indistinct lines may also appear later, usually at angles other than 45°; these may confuse interpretation of test (false-positive test).

Test can be performed more rapidly (giving positive results in about two-thirds of original positive diagnostic specimens) by adding 0.033% potassium tellurite (1.5 ml sterile 0.3% solution to 10 ml agar base) and 2 ml serum or serum substitute to special medium and inoculating with swab from patient or with loopful of growth on original isolation plates.

Precautions to be observed
1. Check activity of diphtheria antitoxin used. Not all lots of antitoxin are satisfactory for this test, even when they are potent toxin neutralizers.
2. Check each lot of antitoxin in gel diffusion to determine degree of secondary lines.
NOTE: Schubert and Blank[10] compared (1) Elek in vitro method,[8] (2) King modification of Elek method,[9] (3) commercial medium prepared with various animal sera, and (4) same medium used with serum substitute[10] ("virulence enrichment"). They found that original Elek method was superior to any modification. They stated that serum substitute did not perform satisfactorily and should not be used to replace serum; horse serum proved superior to rabbit serum; monkey serum was better than either.

Intradermal virulence test—Frobisher.[11] This method can be used with rabbits or guinea pigs.
1. Grow pure culture for 24 h in meat infusion broth.
2. Clip hair on back of animal. Mark 2 areas of 2 cm² with indelible pencil for each culture to be tested.
3. Inject 0.2 ml test suspension **into** skin with ½ in. needle, 26 gauge. Small bleb should appear at site of injection. Also inject suspension of known toxigenic strain (control). Store syringe containing test suspension at 4 C until reinjected into animal.
4. Inject 500-1000 U diphtheria antitoxin intravenously into rabbit (intraperitoneally into guinea pig) 5-7 h after primary injection. Immediately afterward (rabbit), or 30 min later (guinea pig), reinject animal with 0.2 ml test suspension.
5. Make preliminary readings after 24 h (guinea pig) or 48 h (rabbit). Report any positive readings at this time. Make final readings at 48 h (guinea pig) or 72 h (rabbit). First injection (5 h before antitoxin) of toxigenic strain and of known control results in central necrotic area, 5-10 mm in size, surrounded by 10-15 mm zone of redness. Second injection (after antitoxin) results in pinkish nodule, 5-10 mm, with no necrosis.

Chicken test—Frobisher et al.[12] Inject Plymouth Rock or Rhode Island strain chickens, 7-20 d old, with 50-100 U antitoxin into areolar tissue dorsally between wing insertions.

After 1 h inject about 1-2 ml bacterial growth from Loeffler or blood agar tubes into same area. Use 4 chickens, 2 protected with antitoxin and 2 unprotected.

Virulent strains usually kill both unprotected chickens within 24 h. In surviving animals, wing paralysis may indicate toxicity of culture.

Center for Disease Control comments and recommendations on toxigenicity testing

The Special Bacteriology Unit of the U.S. Center for Disease Control (CDC) has published the following summary[13] of the advantages and disadvantages of the various toxigenicity test methods.

I. **Guinea pig subcutaneous test**[14]
   A. Advantages
      1. Does not require positive and negative controls.
      2. Any diphtheria antitoxin (1000 antitoxin units [AU]) can be used.
      3. Results are easily interpreted since end point is death (necrosis only in rare instances).
   B. Disadvantages
      1. Requires use of pure cultures.
      2. Requires 10-12 ml of turbid 48-72 h heart infusion broth (HIB) culture.
      3. Requires 2 animals per culture tested.
      4. Negative animals must be observed for 1 wk.

II. **Rabbit or guinea pig intradermal test**[14]
   A. Advantages
      1. Multiple cultures can be tested on 1 animal.
      2. Any diphtheria antitoxin (500-1000 AU) can be used.
      3. Final readings may be made at 48-72 h.
   B. Disadvantages
      1. Requires use of pure cultures.
      2. Requires 0.4 ml of turbid 48-72 h HIB culture.
      3. Requires positive control.
      4. Small percentage of cultures may yield equivocal results and have to be retested by subcutaneous test.

III. **In vitro agar gel plate**[14]
   A. Advantages
      1. Mixed cultures (even original swab) may be tested.
      2. Three to four test cultures and two controls can be tested per plate.
      3. Positive results can be read in 24-48 h.
   B. Disadvantages
      1. Requires special agar medium and sterile serum.
      2. Requires positive and negative controls.
      3. Concentration of antitoxin may be critical. Antitoxin that produces secondary lines in this test must be diluted to concentration that will allow development of strong primary lines while holding development of secondary lines to minimum.
      4. Experience is required in interpreting results. If antitoxin that produces secondary lines is used, positive and negative controls should be placed next to each test strain.
      5. Negative strains should be confirmed by in vivo test.

The medium used at the CDC is as follows.
Elek toxigenicity medium (modified, CDC)[15]
Base
1. Prepare solutions as follows:

Proteose peptone (Difco)	20.0 g
Maltose	3.0 g
Lactic acid	0.7 ml
NaOH solution, 40%	1.5 ml
Distilled water	500.0 ml

   Heat to boiling, shaking constantly. Filter through Whatman (Clifton, N.J.) no. 12 filter paper.
2. Add filtrate to following solution:

Agar	15 g
NaCl	5 g
Distilled water	500 ml

3. Adjust pH to 8.0.
4. Dispense 10 ml volumes of agar base into screw-capped tubes, autoclave at 115 C for 10 min. Solution can be stored for 6 mo at room temperature.

Test plate

1. Place into scratch-free plastic or glass Petri dish:

Sterile serum	2.0 ml
Sterile 0.3% potassium tellurite	1.0 ml
Tube of melted agar base (60 C)	10.0 ml

2. Mix thoroughly by gentle rotation.
3. Saturate strip of sterile filter (Whatman no. 3, 15 × 70 mm) with diluted diphtheria antitoxin. Use 100 antitoxin unit (AU) containing dilution (see below). Allow excess antitoxin to drain. Using sterile forceps put strip in center of agar **before** agar hardens.
4. Let plate sit, top slightly open, for 1-2 h to allow excess moisture to evaporate. Inoculate (no later than 2 h) test culture by streaking it perpendicular to and on either side of strip. Do **not** touch strip with inoculum.
5. Incubate plate in inverted position at 35-36 C. Read after 1 or 2 overnight incubations (18-48 h).
6. Look for primary toxin-antitoxin line; it forms 45° angle with inoculum.
7. Positive (toxigenic) control and negative (nontoxigenic) control culture must be included on each plate.

Summary. Generally, the CDC has found KL virulence agar (Difco Laboratories, Detroit) also satisfactory.[16] **Each lot of CDC or Difco medium must be tested with toxigenic control strain.** The enrichment required for this test must also be carefully screened in a prechecked base with a positive control culture that should give a strong reaction within 36-48 hours. CDC has obtained good results with commercial rabbit serum. Difco's KL virulence enrichment can be used with the KL virulence agar but does not work well with the modified Elek medium formula.

Difco's Chapman Tellurite Solution has been found to be satisfactory with either base by CDC. The tellurite is only necessary when mixed cultures are being tested, although the black growth of the pure cultures is a good contrast to the white precipitin lines.

If the antitoxin available for the in vitro test produces secondary lines it should be diluted to 100 AU/ml; otherwise, it may be used at 200-500 AU/ml. Difco's KL antitoxin strips usually give strong primary lines and few if any secondary lines. These strips may be used with either base.

Some strains of *C. ulcerans* will give a positive in vitro toxigenicity test. Since these cultures produce both the diphtheritic exotoxin and an endotoxin, both test and control guinea pigs will die when the subcutaneous test is used, and the control spot will also be ulcerative when the intradermal test is used. The main characteristics that distinguish these organisms from *C. diphtheriae* are a positive urea reaction, negative nitrate reaction, heavy growth on Pai's medium, and microscopic morphology from Pai's or Loeffler's media.

Colorimetric tissue culture toxigenicity assay

Murphy et al.[17] have recently described a cell assay method for determining toxigenicity of *C. diphtheriae.*

Determination of toxigenicity by counterimmunoelectrophoresis

Thompson and Ellner[18] have described a method for detecting toxin production in *C. diphtheriae* cultures by counterimmunoelectrophoresis. Precipitin lines were observed in toxigenic strains in 30 minutes.

Stock toxigenic and nontoxigenic C. diphtheriae strains

The American Type Culture Collection (ATCC, Rockville, Md.) is a source for *C. diphtheriae* strains. Strain E-11913 (nontoxigenic) and strain E-13812 (toxigenic) are available from the ATCC's Educational Collection for a small fee.

For **maintenance,** grow organisms on Mueller-Hinton agar or nutrient agar slant at 35-37 C for 18-24 hours. Keep refrigerated; transfer monthly for 3 months to fresh agar slant.

For **long-term storage,** suspend growth from a fresh agar culture in *Brucella* broth containing 15% glycerol. Place 0.5 ml suspension into small (1, 2, or 5 ml) screw-capped vial. Freeze at −55 C.

Types of Corynebacterium diphtheriae

The 3 major types of *C. diphtheriae* (*gravis, mitis,* and *intermedius*) were first described by Anderson et al.[19] in 1931. They noted a difference in appearance of diphtheria bacilli when grown on heated blood agar medium containing potassium tellurite. When subcultured and tested by the usual methods, these 2 different colonies, black or gray-black, gave all the reactions of typical toxigenic *C. diphtheriae.* They were differentiated in other ways—by their power to ferment starch and glycogen, by their growth in broth, and by the production of hemolysis. It is interesting to note that in Leeds, where this study was made during a severe epidemic of diphtheria, 1 of the 2 types was isolated from the severe and fatal cases, and the other type was isolated only from mild cases. For this reason McLeod et al. called 1 type *C. diphtheriae gravis* and the other *C. diphtheriae mitis.* They noted, too, the existence of a certain number of intermediate strains, corresponding neither to the *gravis* nor to the *mitis* type. Subsequently these same workers noted that the "intermediate" strains formed a third type, with well-differentiated characteristics of its own. This type came from cases that were more severe than the cases caused by *mitis* strains but less severe than the cases caused by *gravis* strains.

The characteristics of these 3 types (on heated rabbit blood–tellurite agar) may be summarized as follows[20]:

C. diphtheriae, type gravis. Gives gray or gray-black "daisy head" colony on blood-tellurite medium, the degree of striation of surface and crenation of edge varying considerably. Ferments dextrin, starch, and glycogen (in addition to dextrose and maltose, which are fermented by all types of *C. diphtheriae*). Gives surface growth and granular deposit in broth, generally with an early (2-3 d) reversal of pH to alkaline side. Usually nonhemolytic. Stained films from 18 h cultures on Loeffler's medium (morphology of *C. diphtheriae* grown on blood-tellurite medium is quite atypical) show bacillary forms with 1 or 2 darkly staining areas, the rest of the cell staining very lightly. Metachromatic granules are rare, and when present are very small. Some 60% of *gravis* strains conform to this morphology; others may show much the same appearance as *mitis* or *intermedius* strains.

C. diphtheriae, type mitis. Gives convex, smooth, black, shining colony on blood-tellurite medium, with an entire edge. Does not ferment starch or glycogen. Determination of dextrin is variable. Gives diffuse turbidity in broth, with nongranular deposit. Surface growth is infrequent; when it occurs, it is soft. There is later a reversal of pH to alkaline side (4 to 5 d). Usually hemolytic. The bacilli stain very irregularly, and metachromatic granules are very prominent.

C. diphtheriae, type intermedius. Gives small, flat colony on blood-tellurite medium, with central, raised, black or gray-black portion, and lighter, slightly crenated periphery. Does not ferment starch or glycogen. Fermentation of dextrin is variable. Gives fine granular deposit in broth, with no surface growth. No reversal of pH. This type is consistently nonhemolytic. Morphology is characteristic, about 98% of bacilli being barred.

C. diphtheriae, type minimus. Observed by Frobisher et al.[21] during epidemic in Baltimore (1944). Ferments glucose very slowly if at all.

Other varieties of *C. diphtheriae* have also been found that differ from those described. However, the toxins produced by all types are immunologically homogenous.

The most reliable criteria for the differentiation of the 3 major types are the type of colony formed on blood-tellurite medium and the power to ferment starch and glycogen. The *mitis* type is hemolytic.

• • •

For an excellent, detailed review of *C. diphtheriae* and its relatives, concerning morphology, nutrition, metabolism, and relationships with mycobacteria and nocardia, see Barksdale.[22] The mode of action and structure of diphtheria toxin have been reviewed by Collier.[23]

Corynebacterium ulcerans

Gilbert and Stewart[24] first described this organism that resembles *C. diphtheriae* except for certain biochemical reactions. It produces diphtheriae toxin and an additional toxigenic factor.

Growth on Loeffler slant is abundant, with heavy growth after a 24-hour incubation. On Tinsdale medium the colonies are indistinguishable from those of *C. diphtheriae*. On blood agar they are 0.5-1 mm in diameter, convex, yellowish white, and opaque with matt surface. Most strains are surrounded by a small zone of hemolysis.[25] On tellurite medium the colonies are indistinguishable from those of *C. diphtheriae*.

Features differentiating *C. ulcerans* from *C. diphtheriae* are the following: urea is hydrolyzed (Christensen urea agar slant, incubated

overnight), nitrate is not reduced, and trehalose is fermented.[26] Microscopically the rods change to predominantly coccoid cells in 24 hours. *C. ulcerans* liquefies gelatin slowly at 22 C (3-4 days).

The clinical picture with *C. ulcerans* resembles diphtheria but is somewhat milder.

"Diphtheroids"

Many different organisms in this genus, present in man (skin, mucous membranes) under normal conditions and frequently contaminating blood cultures, are usually spoken of as "diphtheroids" in the clinical laboratory. They are chiefly important in that they present a problem to the inexperienced worker in distinguishing them from *C. diphtheriae*, since they morphologically resemble it. In addition, it is certain that cases of *Listeria* infections may be missed because of the superficial resemblance of *L. monocytogenes* to many diphtheroid-like organisms. Endocarditis due to various diphtheroids, especially after cardiac surgery, has been reported.[27,28] Endocarditis due to coryneform bacteria has been reviewed by Scoy et al.,[29] and serious infections caused by diphtheroids were summarized by Johnson and Kaye.[30]

A useful taxonomic schema for the identification and classification of corynebacteria (aerobic diphtheroids) from human skin has been developed by Somerville.[31] For differentiations of various corynebacteria, see Table 77-1.

Corynebacterium xerosis

The gram-positive rods show polar staining and occasional club-shaped forms. Colonies are thin, grayish, and adherent. Growth is scant and slow. Acid is formed in glucose, maltose, and **sucrose**. Occasional strains may not ferment sucrose and may create confusion with atoxigenic strains of *C. diphtheriae*. The organism is present in the normal conjunctiva.

Two cases of proved *C. xerosis* endocarditis after aortic valve replacement with a Starr-Edwards valve prosthesis have been reported.[27] Infection and colonization with *C. xerosis* have been described by Porschen et al.[32]

Corynebacterium pseudodiphtheriticum (hofmannii)

C. pseudodiphtheriticum rods are gram positive, with rounded ends, 0.3-0.5 μm × 0.8-1.5 μm in size, usually clubbed. Barred forms may be found, although polar granules are usually seen. On blood serum media the colonies are opaque, grayish to cream colored, smooth, homogeneous, and entire. The organism does **not** ferment carbohydrates and is nonpathogenic. It is found in the throat as a harmless saprophyte. It reduces nitrate and produces urease.

As described earlier, it is not always possible to distinguish *C. pseudodiphtheriticum (hofmannii)* from *C. diphtheriae* on colonial appearance. *C. pseudodiphtheriticum (hofmannii)* is usually somewhat shorter and plumper on staining than *C. diphtheriae* and shows no metachromatic granules. On tellurite plates it resembles the *mitis* type of the diphtheria bacillus. It is necessary to perform fermentation tests.

Corynebacterium pseudotuberculosis (ovis)

The organism is found in sheep, horses, and cattle, where it causes severe suppurative lesions known as "pseudotuberculosis." The colonies often are yellow in color. Acid is formed in glucose, maltose, and starch; acid formation is variable in lactose and sucrose. Urease is positive, hemolysis is variable, and a toxin is produced that is immunologically distinct from diphtheria toxin. A case of human infection was reported by Lopez et al.[33]

Corynebacterium pyogenes

The organism is related to the streptococci, considering the similarity of their cell-wall composition. It is β-hemolytic, nonmotile, does not grow on 40% bile agar, liquefies gelatin, is **catalase negative,** and ferments arabinose, glucose, lactose, maltose, and starch; acid formation is variable in sucrose (fermentations in Hiss serum water). It does not grow on ordinary agar. *C. pyogenes* has been isolated from lesions in cattle and from pathologic processes in man.[34]

Corynebacterium hemolyticum

McLean et al.[35] originally described this organism that resembles *C. pyogenes* and *C. pseudotuberculosis (ovis)* and is occasionally isolated from cases of acute pharyngitis and cutaneous lesions. Its morphology is suggestive of *C. diphtheriae,* but it grows poorly on tellurite-containing isolation media.

The hemolysis produced by *C. hemolyticum* is much more pronounced on media containing human or rabbit blood than on sheep blood agar. The organism usually grows in broth media only when a small amount of sterile serum is added. In such circumstances it ferments glucose, maltose, and lactose in 24-48 hours; most but not all strains also ferment sucrose. Unlike *C. pyogenes,* it fails to liquefy gelatin or digest milk; but it is also **catalase negative.**

Involvement of *C. hemolyticum* in brain abscess,[36] septicemia,[37] and osteomyelitis[38] has been reported.

Corynebacterium bovis

C. bovis can cause bovine mastitis and rancidity in cream. Until 1977 only 1 human case of *C. bovis* infection had been reported. In 1977, 6 cases in England (2 with central nervous system involvement, 2 with bacterial endocarditis after artificial valve replacement, 1 with chronic otitis media, and 1 with a persistent leg ulcer) were reported.[39]

Most *C. bovis* strains produce acid from glucose anaerobically using OF (oxidation-fermentation) media; almost all strains ferment glucose, fructose, maltose, and glycerol using fermentation media. *C. bovis* is **oxidase positive;** and it grows in broth with 9% NaCl.

Corynebacterium equi

C. equi has been isolated from pneumonia in foals, genital tract of horses, and submaxillary glands of swine.[1] The Center for Disease Control identified 34 isolates from human sources through 1970; Berg et al.[40] reported *C. equi* infections in neoplastic disease.

Some strains are **acid fast;** *C. equi* grows well on ordinary media with colonies being moist and typically pink. At 18-24 hours the organisms are coccoid in appearance, but in 3-5 hours of growth, rod forms predominate.

The organism does **not** produce acid from any carbohydrate in usual tests.[1] Nitrate reduction and urease production are variable, while catalase is produced by all strains.

Other corynebacteria

1. Corynebacterium aquaticum has been isolated from distilled water and named by Leifson.[41] The organism is not listed in the eighth edition of *Bergey's Manual.*[1] It has been isolated from blood, spinal fluid, and sputum; Weiner and Werthamer[42] reported its isolation from a case of septicemia.

C. aquaticum may be confused with *Listeria monocytogenes;* it produces acid from glucose **aerobically** but not anaerobically (OF medium), while *L. monocytogenes* is fermentative. It also produces acid from sucrose, maltose, and xylose in OF media; the oxidase test is negative, and catalase is produced. The organism is **motile.**

2. A new species of Corynebacterium (as yet unnamed) has been reported recently by Hande et al.[43] and Pearson et al.[44] as the cause of septicemia in 16 patients; it caused death in 3 of these patients. All the patients had predisposing illness at the time of infection.

The organism is catalase positive, but oxidase, urease, nitrate, and indole negative. When grown on blood agar (under CO_2) the isolates have a characteristic metallic sheen in 24-48 hours when viewed with reflected light. In phenol red broth with 1% carbohydrates and with a few drops of serum, it produces acid in both glucose and maltose; lactose, sucrose, mannitol, and xylose broths become alkaline. Most strains are resistant to commonly used antibiotics; however, vancomycin minimum inhibitory concentrations (MIC) were found consistently to be less than 1 μg/ml by the tube dilution method.

3. Anaerobic corynebacteria and Propionibacterium are discussed in Chapter 85.

4. Corynebacterium vaginale (Haemophilus vaginalis): this gram-variable, rod-shaped, sometimes coccobacillary organism, was originally named *Haemophilus vaginalis.* Later it was shown that it has no requirement for X or V factors; therefore it could not be a member of the genus *Haemophilus.* In 1963 the name

Corynebacterium vaginale was proposed for the organism; however, it is **catalase negative** (whereas most corynebacteria are catalase positive), and its cell wall lacks arabinose (which is present in corynebacteria). Thus the organism is likely neither *Haemophilus* nor *Corynebacterium*. In the eighth edition of *Bergey's Manual*,[1] it is placed under *Haemophilus*, because that is "the place in which readers will probably look for it."

For a detailed discussion of *C. vaginale* (*H. vaginalis*) see Chapters 75 and 79.

LISTERIA*
Listeria monocytogenes

Prior to 1950 little thought was given to *L. monocytogenes* as a pathogen for man. Only some 100 cases had been reported in the world's medical literature, and most medical bacteriology texts devoted scarcely a full page to a discussion of the bacterium. In many instances it was completely ignored or page space was granted grudgingly, since this was "a rare pathogen for man," although it often caused disease in domesticated animals, particularly sheep, goats, and cows. However, it was recognized as an interesting laboratory curiosity that produced a marked purulent conjunctivitis when instilled in the eye of a susceptible laboratory animal or a marked monocytosis when inoculated intravenously into rabbits.

Although the first recorded isolation of *L. monocytogenes* from man appeared as early as 1929,[45] a quarter century passed before the bacterium emerged as a significant pathogen. Perhaps the most important factor responsible for this emergence was the suggestion in 1952 by Seeliger[46] that the numerous cases of so-called "granulomatosis infantiseptica" observed at that time in East Germany might be due to *L. monocytogenes* rather than to a new species of bacterium, *Corynebacterium infantiseptica*, as reported by Potel.[47] Confirmation of this and subsequent demonstration by numerous investigators that *L. monocytogenes* might be an important cause of prenatal infection or death in human infants helped to stimulate an awareness of listeric infection. As a result it has become apparent that the disease is not actually rare; it is merely rarely recognized. Public health authorities regard listeriosis as a potential menace. It has also become a relatively frequent complicating factor in malignant diseases (see below).

Occurrence and pathogenicity

Listeriosis is regarded as a **zoonosis** (a disease and infection that is naturally transmitted between vertebrate animals and man). The host range is wide; it includes some 40 mammals, 20 birds, crustaceans, ticks, and fish. The disease in animals is characterized by septicemia, monocytosis, and multiple focal abscesses; involvement of the uterus and fetus and meningoencephalitis have also been described. Healthy enteric carriers seem to be common in many species, including man.

Transmission from animals to man does occur (handling of newborn calves, infected dogs, drinking of infected milk). In the United States, however, most cases occur among urban residents with few or no animal contacts. Since the extensive occurrence of *L. monocytogenes* as free-living organisms on plants and in soil has been demonstrated, it is likely that the soil and plants play a major role in transmission of the disease. Some now regard listeriosis as a **sapronosis** (man and animals contaminated from a common origin, i.e., the environment).

L. monocytogenes has been associated with a variety of disorders: **meningoencephalitis** or **meningitis, perinatal infection, septicemia, infectious mononucleosis–like syndrome, endocarditis, localized** internal or external **abscesses,** and pustular or papular **cutaneous lesions.** A study by Gray[48] of more than 400 cases of listeric infection in man showed meningitis to be the most prevalent form of the disease in the United States. Almost 50% of these patients were less than 1 month old and born apparently normal to mothers who experienced no obvious illness during pregnancy. However, many mothers could recall vague flulike symptoms accompanied by mild fever several weeks to a few days before parturition, suggesting prenatal infection resulting from low-grade or inapparent infection in the mother. If the obstetrician is aware of this possibility, cultures taken from the mother's blood during the febrile period may reveal the bacterium. Infants born to mothers who show this syndrome during pregnancy should be observed closely for at least 6 months for any sign suggestive of early meningitis.

Listeric **meningitis** in adults is often superimposed on underlying primary disorders (neoplastic diseases, diabetes, collagen diseases, organ transplants). Administration of cortisone appears to enhance susceptibility to a dangerous degree, as do immunosuppressive agents and radiotherapy.

There are no symptoms that distinguish listeric meningitis from that due to other causes. There may be an increase in the number of polymorphonuclear leukocytes in the spinal fluid, and often gram-stained smears reveal gram-positive rods. Prompt diagnosis and treatment with antibiotics is imperative if the prognosis is to be favorable.

The first case of a bacterial aortic aneurysm due to *L. monocytogenes* was reported by Navarrete-Reyna et al.[49] An association between listeriosis, as a complicating factor, and malignant disease was reported by Louria et al.,[50] whereas listeriosis complicating lymphoma was described by Simpson et al.[51] For a review of

---

*Family *Lactobacillaceae,* genus *Listeria* (Part 16, "Gram-Positive, Asporogeneous, Rod-Shaped Bacteria").[1]

infections see Kalis et al.,[52] Ascher et al. (in transplant patients),[53] Medoff et al.,[54] Gantz et al. (in immunosuppressed patients),[55] Bayer et al. (endocarditis),[56] Visintine et al. (in children),[57] and Bojsen-Moller.[58]

Perinatal septicemia, the most common form of listeric infection in Europe, is rare in the United States. It constitutes approximately 2% of all cases. Birth is usually premature, and the infant is either stillborn or born acutely ill. Mortality is high. The meconium often contains large numbers of the bacterium, which may be detected readily in stained smears.[59] Although the mother is not ill, in most instances *L. monocytogenes* may be isolated from her vagina for several weeks postpartum. This seldom has any long-lasting detrimental effect on the reproductive system.[60]

Rost et al.[61] have suggested that *L. monocytogenes* may be responsible for some cases of **habitual abortion** in women. They observed a marked rise in antibody titer against *L. monocytogenes* at the time of abortion but failed to demonstrate the actual presence of the bacterium. Treatment with tetracycline antibiotics throughout a subsequent pregnancy usually resulted in a normal full-term birth. Rappaport et al.[62] supported this suggestion by isolation of the bacterium from the cervix of some women with histories of habitual abortion. Toaff et al.[63] isolated *Listeria* from the genital tract of 3 of 60 husbands studied; the 3 had positive semen cultures. Each of their wives had repeated abortions or stillbirths. Antibiotic treatment of the husband or wife (or both) resulted in normal pregnancies. The subject was considered carefully and in detail at the Second Symposium on Listeric Infection,[64] but no conclusions were reached; the relationship, although intriguing, remains obscure.

L. monocytogenes may produce a syndrome clinically identical to infectious mononucleosis. It can be distinguished from true infectious mononucleosis only by isolation of the bacterium and the absence of heterophile antibody.

At present it is well established that listeric infection is not necessarily an acute, highly fatal disease but may be manifested by low-grade, even inapparent infections. These may pass undetected in nonpregnant subjects but often lead to grave infection of the uterine contents of the pregnant subject.

With the known high susceptibility of the gravid uterus to listeric infection it is advisable for pregnant laboratory personnel to avoid contact with suspect material.

The true incidence of listeric infection in man remains undetermined. Of the known number of confirmed cases, approximately 2000, more than four-fifths, were recorded during the years 1958-1963, reflecting a relationship between awareness and **apparent** incidence. **Actual** incidence does not appear to be greater today than in the past. This emphasizes the need for an educational program directed toward dispelling

3 important misconceptions: (1) that all small, gram-positive, diphtheroid-like rods isolated from blood, spinal fluid, ear, throat, and vaginal swabs, urine, amniotic fluid, etc. are contaminants; (2) that *L. monocytogenes* attacks only the central nervous system; and (3) that since *L. monocytogenes* grows well and can be cultivated easily **after** isolation, it is always easy to isolate from infected material. This program should also emphasize that some forms of listeric infection may mimic disorders usually associated with *Mycobacterium tuberculosis* and that in stained smears of fluids and tissues the bacterium may resemble *C. diphtheriae* or, if poorly stained, *Haemophilus influenzae*. Where such a program is put into effect, listeric infections often cease to be rare.

• • •

For an exhaustive review of *L. monocytogenes*, characterization of the organism, methods for isolation, and listeric infections see Gray and Killinger,[65] Buchner and Schneiersohn,[66] Lavetter,[67] and Woodbine.[68] For a detailed biologic characterization see Wetzler et al.,[69] Killinger,[70] and Bottone and Sierra.[71]

Isolation and identification

In the following discussion, data from Gray,[64] Killinger,[70] and the exhaustive study of Wetzler et al.[69] are utilized.

L. monocytogenes is a small, gram-positive, non-sporeforming, extremely resistant, diphtheroid-like rod, with a peculiar tumbling motility when grown at 18-22 C. It is aerobic to microaerophilic and is not known to produce either endotoxins or exotoxins.

Although *L. monocytogenes* usually grows well on most commonly employed bacterial media **after** isolation, there is considerable evidence based on both naturally and artificially induced infections that initial isolation attempts may not always be successful.

In general, the technics that have proved most successful for isolation of *L. monocytogenes* stress the need for tissue maceration. This may be due to the frequent intracellular location of the bacterium. The most effective method consists of macerating suspect tissue in a mortar or Waring blender together with a few milliliters of sterile distilled water or tryptose broth. Saline should be avoided because it may have a harmful effect on the bacterium, especially if the population is low. A portion of this suspension is plated on tryptose, blood, or modified McBride agar[72] (Chapter 72) **and the remainder placed at 4 C.** Body fluids, swabs, etc. are similarly plated, and **remainder of specimen should be stored at 4 C** (swabs stored in tube with 5 ml tryptose broth).

Wetzler et al.[69] recommended holding specimens for *Listeria* culture in a diluent containing 0.5% yeast extract with 40 μg/ml potassium tellurite and storing specimen at 4 C until ready for processing. In their experience the best solid medium combination for direct *L. monocytogenes* isolation has been 5% sheep blood–trypticase soy agar with 0.5% yeast extract and a tryptose blood agar plate.

Nalidixic acid selective medium is also recommended.[73] For stock solution, add nalidixic acid to distilled water and dissolve by adding 40% sodium hydroxide drop by drop until dissolved. Adjust with distilled water to give a concentration of 10,000 μg/ml. The solution is stable and can be autoclaved at 121 C. For preparing medium, add 2 ml stock nalidixic acid solution to 200 ml clear nutrient agar (such as Oxoid blood agar base no. 2 or Difco nutrient agar). Autoclave. Pour medium into Petri dishes to give a depth of about 3 mm. Examine colonies with Gray's technic and look for characteristic bluish color (see below); gram-negative organisms usually are inhibited, but streptococci, diphtheroids, and yeasts grow.

For **other selective media,** see Woodbine.[68]

The plates are incubated at 35 C for 18-24 hours and examined with a scanning microscope or even a hand lens with the plate resting on a laboratory tripod, using obliquely transmitted illumination as described by Henry[74] and shown in Fig. 77-1. When viewed by this method,

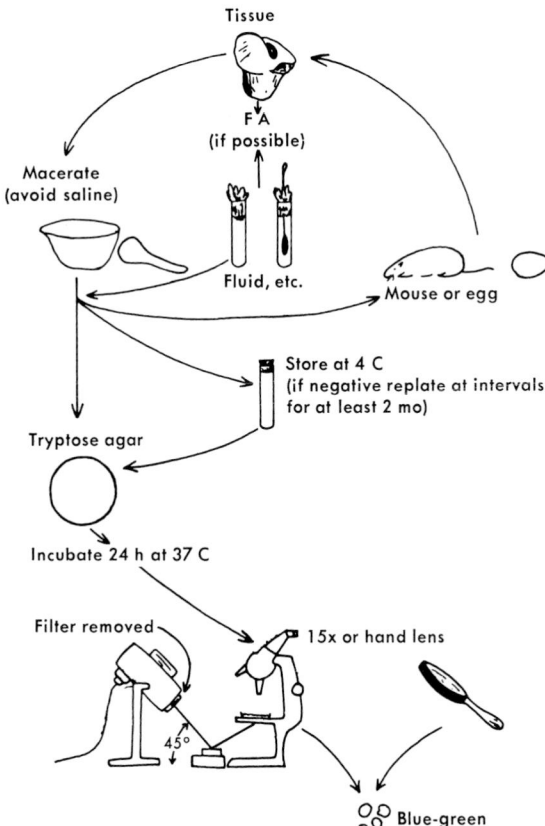

Fig. 77-1. Scheme for isolation of *Listeria monocytogenes*. (From Gray, M. L.: Ann. N. Y. Acad. Sci. **98:**686, 1962.)

18-24-hour-old smooth colonies of *L. monocytogenes* have a distinctive blue-green color. They are 0.2-0.8 mm in diameter, round with an entire margin, translucent, slightly raised with a finely textured surface, watery in consistency, and so characteristic that with a little practice they can be identified quickly even in highly contaminated cultures.[75] In spite of the black color of colonies on potassium tellurite plates, *L. monocytogenes* can be recognized by the blue-green margin at the base of the colony. Although colonies that develop on blood agar or other colored media possess essentially the same morphologic characteristics, they lack the distinctive blue-green color and cannot be distinguished as readily from other pathogens or contaminants.

Colonies on blood agar usually show a **narrow zone of β-hemolysis.** These hemolytic colonies may be mistaken for hemolytic streptococci if not carefully examined in stained smears and tested for motility at room temperature. Also, because the organism often shows palisade formation on smear and also grows well on potassium tellurite, it may frequently be mistaken for a "diphtheroid" and discarded as a contaminant. It can also be confused with enterococci because of its growth on bile-esculin agar.

Smooth colonies are composed most often of small gram-positive rods in palisade arrangement, measuring 1-2 $\times$ 0.5 μm with a few cells 6-7 μm or more in length. In smears from infected material the rods may be very short and easily mistaken for cocci.

If the initial culture fails to reveal *L. monocytogenes* after 72 hours' incubation, the refrigerated tissue suspensions, fluids, swabs, etc. should **be replated** at intervals of several days for a period of at least 2 months. Usually only a few days or a few weeks of refrigeration are required for the bacterium to appear, but there are numerous instances in which 30-50 days or more elapsed before the bacterium was isolated. Admittedly this method ("**cold enrichment**") is slow, has serious disadvantages for the diagnostician, and is cumbersome for the laboratory staff; yet it has been shown that this procedure not only enhances the probability of isolating *L. monocytogenes* by 20-90% but also that a **diagnosis of listeric infection cannot be eliminated merely by failure to isolate the bacterium on initial culture attempts.**

KCNS tryptose broth. Killinger[70] recommends that subcultures be done weekly from the cold-enriched tryptose broth suspensions into **KCNS tryptose broth.** This is prepared by adding 3.75% potassium thiocyanate (reagent grade) to tryptose phosphate broth (Difco) before autoclaving. To subculture, transfer 0.2 ml of the cold-enriched tryptose broth suspension to 5 ml of KCNS tryptose broth weekly for first month, and monthly for 4-6 months if no isolations occur earlier. Incubate subculture at room temperature for 48 hours; then inoculate loopful of KCNS tryptose broth to blood agar, tryptose agar, or modified

McBride agar plate. Incubate plates at 35 C for 24-48 hours.

The mechanism of this enhancing effect at 4 C is not understood. When it was first described by Gray et al.[76] in 1948, it was suggested that it might be related to some inhibitory factor in the bovine brain. Attempts to confirm this were unsuccessful, and during the intervening years this delayed growth has been demonstrated in all animal and human tissue and body fluids. Since *L. monocytogenes* will grow slowly at 4 C, mere multiplication may play some part in the phenomenon. However, there are indications that other still obscure factors, perhaps chemical or enzymatic or even a filtrable form of the bacterium, are responsible. Whatever the cause of this delayed growth may be, it emphasizes the need for a more effective method of isolation to avoid a possible delay in confirming a clinical diagnosis and to prevent an erroneous diagnosis when initial cultures fail to reveal the bacterium.

In an effort to overcome this difficulty, a number of investigators have suggested the inoculation of mice with suspect material for the isolation of *L. monocytogenes*. To date this has not been accepted widely in this country or Western Europe. However, it has been employed successfully for many years in the Soviet Union. By this method the bacterium has been isolated not only from human and animal sources but also from *Ixodes* ticks,[77] stream water,[78] crustaceans,[79] and silage.[80] The use of mice should be encouraged until more reliable results can be obtained with nonliving media.

Embryonating chicken eggs are highly susceptible to infection with *L. monocytogenes*. This led Dontenwill and Knothe[81] to suggest their use for attempts to isolate the bacterium. They claim that the conspicuous necrotic foci that develop on the chorioallantoic membrane 48 hours after exposure of 10-day-old eggs are almost pathognomonic. The bacterium can then be isolated easily from these eggs. This method has not been employed with material of human origin but has been used successfully to isolate *L. monocytogenes* from spinal fluid of sheep with listeric encephalitis.[82] This too may be deserving of further investigation until the present methods of isolation are improved.

The several methods presented for attempting to isolate *L. monocytogenes* are shown graphically in Fig. 77-1. Each has advantages and disadvantages, and until a simple but effective method is developed, the true incidence of this still poorly understood bacterial infection will remain obscure.

The interrelationships of various gram-positive, non-acid-fast, nonsporing rods are shown in Fig. 77-2.

Biochemical reactions and diagnostic characteristics of *L. monocytogenes* useful in the identification of suspect colonies are shown in Table 77-2. A summary of the distinctive characteristics of *L. monocytogenes* is shown in Table 77-3.

Separation of pathogenic from apathogenic L. monocytogenes. Recently Groves and Welshimer[83] found that pathogenicity of *L. monocytogenes*, with few exceptions, seems to correlate with a combination of 3 reactions. Strains that are nonhemolytic or CAMP (Chapter 76) negative and that produce acid from xylose are apathogenic. Many such strains are isolated from nonclinical sources.

Strains that are hemolytic or CAMP positive on sheep blood agar and that produce acid from rhamnose but not from xylose are pathogenic.

Some apathogenic organisms may be xylose negative and rhamnose positive.

Anton's test. Place 2-3 drops broth culture (24 h growth), or suspension of growth from tryptose slant in 5 ml distilled water, with Pasteur pipet into conjunctival sac of rabbit (or guinea pig). Do not scarify tissue. Purulent conjunctivitis develops in inoculated eye within 24-36 h if organism is *L. monocytogenes* (Fig. 77-3).

Motility test for L. monocytogenes. Most commercially available motility media are suitable for performing the test with *Listeria*. Wetzler (Table 77-2) used Motility GI Medium (Difco); I have been using successfully a **0.1% dextrose semisolid agar:**

Tryptose	10 g
NaCl	5 g
Agar	4 g
Dextrose	1 g

Add to 1000 ml distilled water; distribute in tubes so that column of about 6 cm is formed. Inoculate 2 tubes by stabbing column to about 2-3 cm depth. **Incubate**

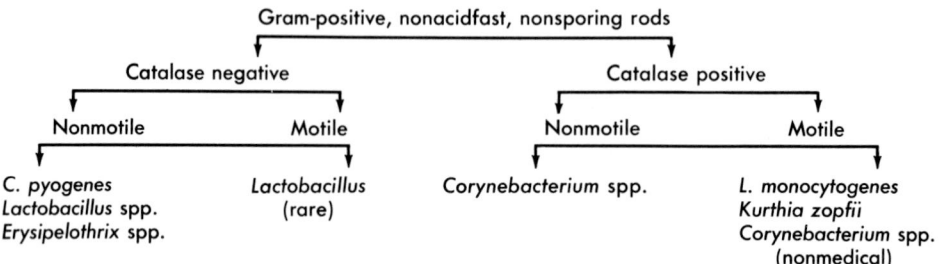

Fig. 77-2. Interrelationships of gram-positive, non-acid-fast, non-sporeforming rods. (From Wetzler, R. F., et al.: Health Lab. Sci. **5:**46, 1968.)

Table 77-2. Differential diagnostic criteria for laboratory diagnosis of *L. monocytogenes**

Reaction	*L. monocytogenes*	Reaction	*L. monocytogenes*
Catalase (3% H_2O_2)	+	Anaerogenic fermentation#	
Motility†		Glucose	+
8 C	+$_{(6-14)}$‡	Trehalose	+
20 C	+$_{(1-3)}$	Cellobiose**	+
35 C	+$_{(1-3)}$§	Mannitol**	−
OF (Hugh-Leifson), glucose	F‖	Raffinose**	−
β-D-galactosidase	+	Salicin	+
Alkaline phosphatase	+	Lactose	+
Nitrate reduction	−	Maltose	+
Hemolysis	+$_{(13\%-)}$¶	Sucrose	±
Methyl red	+	Rhamnose	+/−¶
Urease	−	Xylose	+/−¶

*Based on Wetzler et al.[69] and Groves and Welshimer.[83]
†Motility performed in Difco Motility GI Medium, 2 ml in Kahn tubes, inoculated lightly with wire to 1 cm depth.
‡Subscript = time in days.
§Motility usually absent at 35-37 C.
‖F = fermentative.
¶See separation of pathogenic from nonpathogenic *L. monocytogenes.*
#Fermentations in Difco purple broth, 1% carbohydrate; no gas.
**Filter-sterilized carbohydrate added to basal medium.

Table 77-3. Summary of distinctive characteristics of *L. monocytogenes**

Acid without gas

48 h at 35 C	3-14 d	Variable (some strains +, others −)	Completely absent, 14 days
Glucose†	Lactose	Melezitose	Raffinose†
Levulose†	Maltose	Rhamnose	Inulin
Trehalose†	Glycerol	Sucrose	Dulcitol
Salicin†	Dextrin	Sorbitol	Adonitol
Mannose		Xylose	Mannitol†
Galactose			Erythritol
Esculin			Arabinose
Amygdalin			Melibiose
Cellobiose†			Sorbose

Biochemical properties

Does not reduce nitrate† or produce indole
H_2S production: most authors give "negative" (dependent on medium?)
Catalase: positive†
Voges-Proskauer test: positive
Methyl red: positive (may be dependent on choice of peptone)†
Litmus milk acidified slowly, decolorized, no clot; bromcresol purple milk better, clear-cut acid reaction
Alkaline phosphatase: positive†

Gelatin and coagulated serum not liquefied
Starch and urea not hydrolyzed
Hemolysis: narrow, slight (partial) β or absent (may depend on species of blood); faint, translucent when present
No growth on Simmons citrate agar or in malonate
β-D-galactosidase: positive
Lysine, arginine, ornithine decarboxylase: negative
Aerobic and facultative
Bile tolerance (10%, 40%): positive

Other characteristics

Motile at room temperature (18-22 C) but usually not at 37 C†‡
Conjunctivitis (Anton's test) in rabbit, guinea pig, and mouse (Fig. 77-3): Suspend 18-24 h growth on tryptose slant in 5 ml distilled water; 2-3 drops (for rabbit) into conjunctival sac with Pasteur pipet; do not scarify†

Production of monocytosis in rabbits: 0.5 ml distilled water suspension of 18-24 h culture standardized to no. 1 tube McFarland nephelometer, IV, in average-sized rabbit may give 30% or more in 4-5 d

*Based on data from Gray[64] and Wetzler et al.[69]
†Diagnostic criteria.
‡According to Gray[64]; motile at 35 C in 1-3 d according to Wetzler.[69] See Table 77-2. **It is recommended that motility test medium be incubated at room temperature (20-22 C).**

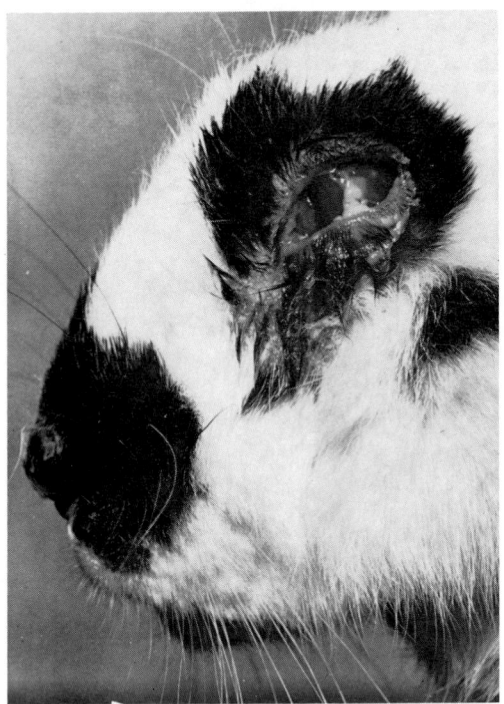

Fig. 77-3. Typical listeric conjunctivitis 9 days after instillation of *Listeria monocytogenes,* showing edema, corneal opacity, and copious purulent exudate. (From Gray, M. L., Singh, C., and Thorp, F., Jr.: Proc. Soc. Exp. Biol. Med. **89:**163, 1955.)

one tube at **20-22 C** and another at **35 C;** observe for 2-5 d (Fig. 77-4).

Motility can be observed by phase or dark-field microscopy. Use a 6-8 h broth culture incubated at 20-22 C.

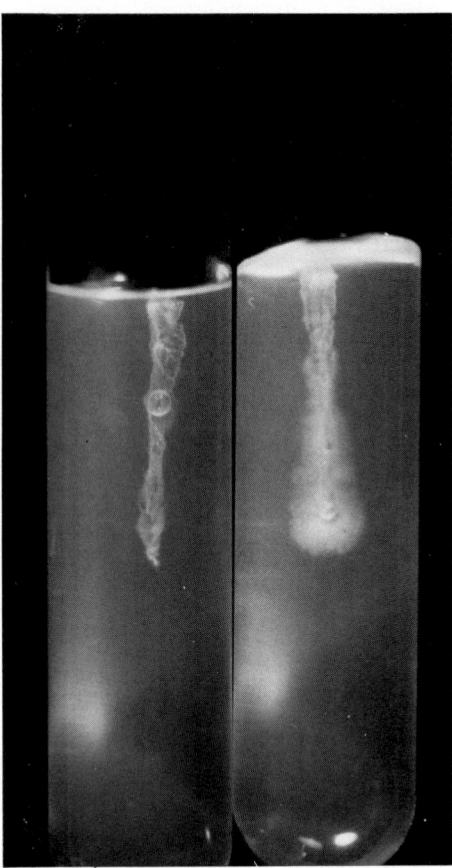

Fig. 77-4. Stab culture of *Listeria monocytogenes. Left,* Incubated at 35 C for 18 h. *Right,* Incubated at 22 C for 18 h; note motility (growth spreading from inoculum).

Serologic types of Listeria monocytogenes and serodiagnosis of listeric infections

The genus *Listeria* is divided into 4 main serologic types and 11 subtypes (7 main types according to Seeliger). Types 2 and 3 are rare; type 4b comprises approximately two-thirds of all cultures isolated in the United States, but in Europe until recently type 1 was the predominant type; in the mid-1960s, type 4b seemed to predominate also in Europe. Serotype does not seem to be related to host species or disease process.

For serotyping an isolated strain of *L. monocytogenes,* type-specific (somatic O and flagellar H) antisera are used. For the methods of preparing antisera and a detailed discussion of the serofactors see Gray and Killinger.[65] **Fluorescent antibody methods** are also used for serotyping[84,85] (see below).

Since *L. monocytogenes* is often difficult to isolate, some investigators have resorted to serologic methods for possible detection of exposure to the bacterium. However, *L. monocytogenes* shows a marked tendency not only to autoagglutinate but also to cross react with a number of commonly occurring bacteria, and serologic findings must be interpreted with considerable caution. Neter et al.[86] demonstrated by means of

the hemagglutination test that *L. monocytogenes* contains the so-called Rantz antigen, an antigen of undetermined chemical composition common to many gram-positive bacteria. This offers a possible explanation for the cross-reactions between *L. monocytogenes* and various groups of streptococci, including enterococci and *Staphylococcus aureus.*[87] It is now generally agreed that a valid titer against *L. monocytogenes* cannot be determined by any serologic test unless the serum is first absorbed by *S. aureus* and perhaps enterococci and *Bacillus subtilis.* This discredits many earlier publications reporting high titers against *L. monocytogenes* in the serum from apparently normal human and animal populations. It also dictates extreme caution in making a diagnosis of listeric infection based solely on serologic evidence.

Serologic diagnosis of listeric infection is further complicated by the well-established fact that high titers produced either by deliberate injection of antigen or as a result of naturally induced infection are usually transient and of relatively short duration. Sometimes they may persist for months, rarely years. Also some patients fail to produce detectable antibody even after severe, bacteriologically confirmed cases of the disease. For these reasons no real significance should be attached to high titers years or even months after suspected infection unless paired serum samples are available. This casts considerable doubt on a number of reports of listeric infection based only on serologic evidence. At present a **serodiagnosis** can be made only on fluctuations in titer in a series of acute and convalescent serum samples during or following a clinical course suggestive of listeric infection. In all other instances a positive diagnosis can be made **only by isolation of** L. monocytogenes.

For a discussion of the difficulties involved in the serodiagnosis of listerosis in the absence of the actual isolation of the bacterium see Gray and Killinger.[65]

Fluorescent antibody methods (FA) for identification of L. monocytogenes. Labeled antisera specific for L. monocytogenes (and for the 4 main serologic types) have been successfully used for the detection and identification of Listeria in clinical material as well as in cultures. For details see Smith et al.[88,89] and Eveland.[84,85]

Animal inoculation[65,69]

Inject 0.1 ml broth culture (18 hours, 20-25 C) intraperitoneally into each of 3 mice. The infected animals usually die between the second and fifth day. Culture heart's blood and peritoneal swabs to recover L. monocytogenes.

Antibiotic susceptibility

Fuzi[90] proposed a diagnostic test based on neomycin sensitivity for the rapid differentiation of Listeria and Erysipelothrix: Listeria strains are very sensitive to neomycin, but Erysipelothrix strains are very resistant. L. monocytogenes is usually sensitive to penicillin, chloramphenicol, tetracyclines, erythromycin, and ampicillin.[69] Resistance is usually found against sulfadiazine and other sulfonamides, polymyxin B, and oxacillin. Intermediate susceptibility or rapidly developing resistance is seen with streptomycin.

ERYSIPELOTHRIX*

Erysipelothrix rhusiopathiae is well known as the cause of the cutaneous lesion, erysipeloid, in man (usually involving the hands and fingers). It is widespread in nature, occurs in decaying and decomposing matter, and is parasitic in a number of domestic animals (swine, sheep, turkeys, ducks), wild animals, rodents, fish, etc. Erysipeloid seems to be an occupational hazard of meat and fish handlers, veterinarians, and housewives.

Systemic infections in man (endocarditis, septicemia), although not very common, have been reported. See Silberstein,[91] McCracken et al.,[92] Simerkoff and Rahal,[93] and Park et al.[94] for literature review.

The organisms are gram-positive rods, form no spores, and are not acid fast. **No catalase is produced;** sugars are utilized fermentatively. They are facultative anaerobes (microaerophilic, growing either aerobically or anaerobically) and are **nonmotile.** On primary isolation they may be gram variable; on subculture they become invariably gram positive, and filaments tend to form. They grow poorly on simple media; addition of serum and glucose improves growth.

The characteristic "lamp-brush" appearance (formation of a lateral outgrowth in gelatin stab cultures) is a diagnostic feature, but it may take 2-3 weeks and is not consistent. α-Hemolysis is produced in sheep blood agar and less often in human blood agar.

The organism can be distinguished from Listeria by its **lack of motility** both at 37 and 20 C, α-**hemolysis, absence of catalase,** and a restricted fermentation spectrum. Fuzi[90] found that whereas Listeria is very sensitive to neomycin, Erysipelothrix is regularly very resistant. Smooth forms of the organism grow better at 31-37 C, but at 37 C the rough form predominates. **Anton's test,** using Erysipelothrix, produces only a mild conjunctivitis in the rabbit eye, whereas Listeria produces a severe keratoconjunctivitis (Fig. 77-3).

Isolation, identification, and diagnostic characteristics

The organisms do not grow at 45 or 15 C. No acid or clot is produced in litmus milk within 24 hours. Lactose, glucose, galactose, and fructose are usually fermented. Rhamnose, mannitol, sucrose, dextrin, salicin, and raffinose are not fermented. No catalase, indole, or acetylmethylcarbinol (Voges-Proskauer test) is produced: the **methyl red test is negative.** When inoculated **in triple sugar iron (TSI) agar, the organism produces** H_2S **in the butt portion,** a characteristic unique to E. rhusiopathiae among similar gram-positive rods.

Swabs from local lesions usually do not yield the organism. It is recommended that a biopsy be taken and cultured for 24 hours in glucose broth, to be followed by subculture on blood agar plates. Suspect material should also be inoculated intraperitoneally into white mice. Heart's blood from the mice will yield a pure culture of Erysipelothrix in 24 hours.

Two distinct antigenic types of Erysipelothrix are known; fluorescent antibody technics have also been applied in its identification.

Susceptibility to antibiotics. The organism is sensitive to penicillin, methicillin, tetracycline, cephalosporins, clindamycin, erythromycin, ampicillin, and chloramphenicol; it is variable in respect to streptomycin and novobiocin and is resistant to sulfonamides and neomycin. Penicillin has been the therapy of choice.

KURTHIA*

The genus *Kurthia* consists of gram-positive, **motile,** non-sporeforming, **catalase-positive,** strictly aerobic[1] organisms, **which do not attack carbohydrates.** Three species are described: K.

---

*Family *Lactobacillaceae*, genus *Erysipelothrix*.[1]

*Coryneform group, genus IV, *Kurthia*.[1]

zopfii, K. variabilis, and *K. bessonii.* They are not normally regarded as pathogenic, having been found in decomposing organic matter; *K. bessonii* has been isolated from normal and diarrheic human feces. Elston,[95] however, isolated *K. bessonii* from clinical material, and recently Pancoast et al.[95a] isolated it from endocarditis.

The organisms grow well aerobically; no hemolysis is produced; the indole and Voges-Proskauer reactions are negative. No motility is observed at 35 C; however, the organism is motile at 20 C (Fig. 77-2).

K. bessonii can be distinguished from *K. zopfii* by the former's ability to liquefy gelatin.

LACTOBACILLI

The lactobacilli (*Bergey's Manual,*[1] Part 16, Gram-Positive, Asporogeneous, Rod-Shaped Bacteria, family I, *Lactobacillaceae,* genus I, *Lactobacillus*) are described here briefly because (1) they are important members of the normal flora of man (mouth, lower intestine, vagina), (2) there are apparent similarities between some "diphtheroids" and certain anaerobic forms, and (3) they rarely may be involved in disease.

Lactobacilli are **gram-positive,** straight or curved rods, often long and slender, usually occurring singly or in chains. They are facultative to anaerobic, nonmotile (rare strains are motile), non-sporeforming, and non-acid-fast. **Catalase is not produced;** sugars are attacked fermentatively. Optimal growth is attained at about pH 6. Half or more of the end product carbon from glucose metabolism is lactate.

The lactobacilli are normal inhabitants of the mouth, lower intestine, and vagina. The forms most commonly found in man are indistinguishable from those recovered from dairy and plant products.

L. casei, the most common form found in the mouth, produces a smooth colony with curved rods in curling chains. *L. acidophilus* forms small colonies with rather long and straight rods. *L. fermentum,* very common in the mouth, forms large, smooth colonies with short and straight rods.

L. bifidus, very common in intestinal contents of nursing infants and also in the mouth and vagina, shows some rudimentary branching. This group of organisms often presents similarities with *Actinomyces israelii* and has now been placed in the genus *Bifidobacterium* (*Actinomycetaceae*); see Chapter 85.

For a detailed review of indigenous lactobacilli see Rosebury[96] and Skinner and Carr[97]; for diagnostic characteristics see Cowan[4] and *Bergey's Manual.*[1]

Döderlein's bacillus is a designation given to a variety of human vaginal strains of the genus *Lactobacillus.* Rogosa and Sharpe[98] found that strains isolated from the vagina and designated as Döderlein's bacillus included *L. acidophilus, L. casei, L. fermentum, L. cellobiosus,* and *Leuconostoc mesenteroides* strains.

The **homofermentative** lactobacilli (14 species) produce lactic acid as the major product from glucose (85% or more). The **heterofermentative** (11 species) produce either some 50% end product as lactic acid, with CO_2, acetic acid, and ethanol accounting for the rest, or they produce DL-lactic acid, CO_2, and acetate.

Homofermentative species (e.g., *L. acidophilus*) do not usually produce gas from glucose, while heterofermenters usually do produce gas.

The ecology and taxonomic status of lactobacilli have recently been reviewed by London.[99]

Isolation and identification

Many lactobacilli grow poorly on blood agar plates; some grow better anaerobically. Incubation for 48 hours at 35-37 C is recommended. They are straight or curved rods, often long and slender, sometimes in chains, filaments, or palisade formation. Lactobacilli are catalase and oxidase negative and attack glucose fermentatively. They are usually identified only to genus level; when it is necessary to obtain species identification, isolates should be submitted to a reference laboratory: special media and specialized methods are used in differentiation of lactobacilli.

The organisms grow better at lower pH (tomato juice or Rogosa agar at about pH 6); this distinguishes them from *Erysipelothrix,* while the negative catalase differentiates them from most corynebacteria.

Thomas[100] described a schema for isolation and identification of lactobacilli from the genital tract based on the use of selective Rogosa agar at pH 5.4; use fresh blood agar plates also.

Rogosa agar[101]	
Trypticase	10 g
KH₂PO₄	5 g
Ammonium citrate	6 g
Salt solution (see below)	2 g
Glucose	5 ml
Sorbitan monooleate	20 g
Sodium acetate hydrate	1 g
Acetic acid	25 g
Agar	1.32 ml
	15 g

Add distilled water to 1000 ml. Final solution pH is 5.4.

Salt solution:

$MgSO_4 \cdot 7H_2O$	11.5 g
$MnSO_4 \cdot 2H_2O$	2.4 g
$MnSO_4 \cdot 4H_2O$	2.8 g
$FeSO_4 \cdot 7H_2O$	0.68 g
Distilled water, add to	1000 ml

This medium does not need autoclaving. It can be kept for 6 mo in refrigerator. The medium is also available in dehydrated form from Difco and from Oxoid Ltd.

On Rogosa agar lactobacilli grow as small white colonies; except for some yeasts and molds, no other organisms grow. On blood agar plates (fresh), preferably incubated in anaerobic jar, they appear as minute colonies. They are catalase negative, penicillin sensitive (but not always), and sulfonamide resistant. Most strains grow as microaerophiles on subculture.

From a pure culture on Rogosa agar, inoculate heavily into each of 4 MRS broths (glucose, mannitol, sucrose, salicin).

MRS carbohydrate broths[102]

Yeast extract	5 g
Peptone	10 g
Lab Lemco (Oxoid Ltd.)	10 g
Tween 80	1 ml
K_2HPO_4	2 g
Sodium acetate	5 g
Triammonium citrate	2 g
$MgSO_4 \cdot 7H_2O$	200 mg
$MNSO_4 \cdot 4H_2O$	50 mg
Bromcresol green	10 ml

Add distilled water to 1000 ml. Autoclave at 121 C for 15 min. Add sterile solution of fermentable substance (glucose, sucrose, mannitol, salicin) to give a final concentration of 2%. Adjust to **final pH of 6-6.5.** Add Durham tube to glucose broth (for gas production).

Reactions of some lactobacilli using the MRS carbohydrate broths (at pH 6.2) after 3-4 d are as follows[100]:

The homofermentatives *L. acidophilus* and *L. casei ss. rhamnosus* ferment sucrose, salicin, and glucose, with the latter also fermenting mannitol; occasional strains of *L. casei ss. rhamnosus* do not ferment sucrose.

The heterofermentatives *L. fermentii* and *L. cellobiosus* ferment sucrose and glucose (prominent gas formation occurs with glucose in both species); *L. cellobiosus* also ferments salicin.

Lactobacilli in disease

Lactobacilli are not usually considered as pathogens except for their role in dental caries. However, there is evidence in isolated reports of human endocarditis, septicemia, and meningitis due to lactobacilli. It is possible that their slow and poor growth in blood culture media and on blood agar and nutrient agar contributes to their presence in clinical specimens being frequently overlooked.

See Sharpe et al.,[103] Isenberg,[104] Tennenbaum and Warner,[105] and Bayer et al.[105a] for reports of lactobacillus infections.

Aerobic actinomycetes

NOCARDIA, STREPTOMYCES, ROTHIA, AND BACTERIONEMA

In the eighth edition of *Bergey's Manual*,[1] Part 17 ("Actinomycetes and Related Organisms") includes the **order Actinomycetales** divided into 8 families. The medically important **families** are as follows:

I. *Actinomycetaceae* (the genera *Actinomyces*, *Arachnia*, *Bifidobacterium* [all 3 described in Chapter 85], and *Bacterionema* are mostly anaerobic to facultatively anaerobic; *Rothia* grows best aerobically).

II. *Mycobacteriaceae* (aerobic, acid fast; see Chapter 78).

VI. *Nocardiaceae* (*Nocardia*, *Pseudonocardia;* obligate aerobes, some acid fast).

VII. *Streptomycetaceae* (*Streptomyces* and 3 other genera; aerobic).

The family *Dermatophilaceae* includes *Dermatophilus congolensis*, the agent of streptotrichosis, which affects sheep, cattle, horses, and to a lesser extent, goats and other animals, and rarely man.

The organisms in the families *Actinomycetaceae*, *Nocardiaceae*, and *Streptomycetaceae* are commonly referred to as actinomycetes. They are gram-positive, relatively slow-growing organisms with a definite tendency to branching; a characteristic mycelium is produced. In some genera the filaments fragment into pleomorphic cells, some of which are club shaped. These have a definite resemblance to corynebacteria and mycobacteria; some are at least partially acid fast. For many years the actinomycetes were described as fungi and were included in mycology textbooks because of their mycelial colonies and also because the chronic lesions caused by certain *Actinomyces* and *Nocardia* bear a striking resemblance to those caused by some fungi. However, consideration of their fundamental biologic properties leaves no doubt about classifying the actinomycetes as bacteria. Pine and Georg[106] list the following considerations:

1. The organisms are all of bacterial size; they lack a nuclear membrane (are prokaryotic) and mitochondria.

2. They are all sensitive to antibacterial antibiotics but are resistant to antifungal antibiotics, e.g., griseofulvin, nystatin, amphotericin B, and candicidin.

3. Their cell walls contain muramic acid, diaminopimelic acid, or lysine, which are not found in the cell walls of fungi.[107] They also lack chitin and glucans, which are characteristic of fungal cell walls.

4. Some actinomycetes can be infected by phages (actinophages).

Streptomyces species resemble fungi more than do *Nocardia* (and the anaerobic *Actinomyces*). Their filaments do not usually fragment during growth; asexual spores (conidia) are formed at the tips of the filaments (sporophores). Most are soil forms; some occur as skin contaminants, and a few are parasitic and cause disease. Many antibiotics of medical use are produced by strains of *Streptomyces;* for this reason they have been and still are studied exhaustively. The species of *Streptomyces* resemble *Nocardia* species in growth and appearance. Differentiation of these 2 genera can readily be accomplished in the reference laboratory by cell-wall analysis for the presence of diaminopimelic acid. However, for the routine clinical laboratory physiologic tests combined with microscopic observations can generally differentiate *Nocardia* from *Streptomyces*.

Differentiation of aerobic actinomycetes

The aerobic actinomycetes most often encountered in the clinical laboratory are members of the genera *Nocardia*, *Streptomyces*, and *Actinomadura*.

Generally the aerobic actinomycetes produce

Table 77-4. Differentiation of *N. asteroides, N. brasiliensis, N. caviae,* and saprophytic *Streptomyces*[*][†]

| Organism | Decomposition[‡] of: | | | Colony characteristics | Growth in lyso-zyme[‡] | Gram stain | Acid-fast stain |
	Casein	Tyrosine	Xanthine				
N. asteroides	–	–	–	Hard, brittle, heaped, chalky white to yellow to deep orange	+	Delicate gram-positive branching filaments (1 μm diameter) that break into bacillary forms of various lengths	Acid fast to partially acid fast; may lose acid fastness on SDA but usually acquire acid fastness on L-J and Middlebrook 7H10 and/or 7H11
N. brasiliensis	+	+	–	As above	+	As above	As above
N. caviae	–	–	+	As above	+	As above	As above
Streptomyces sp.	+[§]	+	±	Flat to heaped, usually covered with white, chalky growth with black-gray pigments in medium	–	Delicate, gram-positive branching filaments that break up into chains of conidia	Non-acid-fast

*From Papageorge, C., and Griffin, C.: Proficiency Testing Critique, Mycology—1975, Atlanta, 1976, Center for Disease Control.
† – = Negative; + = Positive; ± = Variable; SDA = Sabouraud dextrose agar; L-J = Lowenstein-Jensen medium.
‡For media and procedures, see *Nocardia.*
§Except colonies that only discolor medium around colony.

branched aerial hyphae, which separates them from some of the rapidly growing, pigmented *Mycobacterium* species.

Physiologic tests combined with an acid-fast stain differentiate the nocardiae from members of the genus *Streptomyces.* The tests that separate the more common nocardiae and streptomycetes are given in Table 77-4.

Actinomadura madurae (Nocardia madurae) can usually be differentiated with these physiologic tests. For confirmed analysis of some isolates a reference laboratory should perform cell-wall analysis. A culture that was isolated from a clinical specimen that was acid fast or partially acid fast should be inoculated onto 7H10 (Chapter 72) agar to observe for aerial hyphae and to repeat the acid-fast stain. Aerial hyphae usually appear on one of these culture media in 3-5 days and can be observed under the dissecting microscope.

The **Kinyoun's acid-fast stain** helps differentiate the nocardiae from the streptomycetes. The members of the genus *Streptomyces* do not stain acid fast, while hyphae of *N. asteroides, N. brasiliensis,* and *N. caviae* are acid fast to partially acid fast.

An excellent and authoritative study on the laboratory identification of clinically important aerobic actinomycetes is that of Berd.[108]

NOCARDIA

The genus *Nocardia* is composed of organisms that show slender filaments or rods, frequently swollen and occasionally branched, with a few forms producing a limited mycelium; they are **aerobic** and exhibit morphologic characteristics intermediate between the bacteria and molds. Conidia are not formed. They are **gram positive.** Some types are **partially acid fast.** Frequently moist, glabrous strains may be difficult to distinguish from atypical and saprophytic mycobacteria. The latter, however, are strongly acid fast and do **not** produce branched mycelium.

Several species can cause disease in man and animals.

Nocardiosis is an infection producing a wide variety of disease entities such as primary pulmonary infection resembling tuberculosis, cerebral abscesses, meningitis, pneumonitis, diffuse peritonitis, and subcutaneous tumorlike lesions (**mycetomas**) with multiple abscess formation. In tissues or exudates small yellow, red, or black granules may be observed. These are composed of a delicate branching mycelium that may or may not have clubs on the hyphae at the periphery. Organized granules may not be found in sputum, spinal fluid, or other exudates. Only gram-positive, branching, or bacillary forms may be present. The source of nocardiosis, in contrast to actinomycosis, is exogenous; *N. asteroides, N. brasiliensis,* and *N. caviae* exist as saprophytes in nature. When nocardiae are introduced into tissues at the time of an injury, subcutaneous infection (mycetoma) may follow. Inhalation of the organism may be followed by systemic infection. The disease is not transmissible from man to man or from animals to man.[109]

N. asteroides is the most common cause of systemic nocardiosis, whereas *N. brasiliensis* and *N. caviae*[110,111] have generally been implicated as agents of mycetoma. However, both *N. brasiliensis*[112] and *N. caviae*[110] are now known to be causative agents in systemic disease. It is possible that the relative paucity of the involvement of the latter 2 organisms is partly due to their misidentification as *N. asteroides* or *Nocardia* species. *N. asteroides* frequently produces opportunistic disease (secondary invader in immunosuppressed patients or those with malignancies of chronic debilitating diseases), but it also may be a primary pathogen, as *N. brasiliensis* and *N. caviae* also occasionally are.

For a review of nocardiosis see Murray et al.,[113] Goodman and Koenig,[114] Kurup et al.,[115] and Palmer et al.[116]; for *N. brasiliensis* infections, see the review of Berd[112]; and for *N. caviae*, see Causey.[110]

The taxonomy, occurrence, distribution, and parasitism of nocardioform bacteria have been reviewed by Goodfellow and Minnikin.[117]

Morphology

The organisms consist of delicate branching hyphae, 1 μm or less in diameter, when examined in specially prepared cell cultures. The mycelium is septate. In culture, some species are filamentous, whereas other species develop hyphae with a marked tendency to branch and fragment into bacillary and coccoid structures. Some varities may develop into diphtheroid forms.

Staining

All species are gram positive; *N. asteroides*, *N. brasiliensis*, and *N. caviae* are **acid fast** or **partially** acid fast (use of **Kinyoun stain** is recommended). They may resemble tubercle bacilli and are sometimes mistaken for such.

On the Gram stain they show branching and filamentous elements; some fragment readily into bacillary or coccoid elements.

Examination of specimens and cultivation

Microscopic, unstained preparations of scrapings and pus should be examined for **granules.** Materials should be cultured on blood agar plates, and Sabouraud glucose agar medium (with and without antibiotics) both at 37 and 22 C (room temperature); **incubate under 10% CO₂.** Sputum, spinal fluid, and other materials should be handled similarly. Always prepare Gram stain and acid-fast stain of materials.

It should be noted that although some tuberculosis digestion procedures destroy nocardiae, some, especially *N. asteroides*, often survive. **Cultures should be made of sputum and bronchial washings before and after digestion.** To be considered negative for *Nocardia*, inoculated media should be held for 3 weeks. A digestion procedure (for sputum or bronchial washing) facilitating the isolation of *Nocardia* (and also fungi) follows.

Digestion for isolation of Nocardia
1. Put specimen (sputum or bronchial washing) and equal volume of digestant (*N*-acetylcysteine without NaOH) into screw-cap, 50 ml, graduated centrifuge tube.
2. Mix on Vortex mixer for 5-10 s.
3. Add phosphate-buffered saline to 50 ml.
4. Centrifuge for 15 min at 2100 rpm. Decant supernatant.
5. Add enough penicillin to give final concentration of 20 U/ml.

Since some nocardiae grow well on tuberculosis isolation media, always examine the latter for colonies appearing earlier than those of *M. tuberculosis.*

The organisms will not grow on antibiotic-containing media (Mycosel, etc.), since they are sensitive to a number of antibiotic agents.

For demonstration of branched mycelium formation, use slide culture technic.

Slide culture for demonstration of branching (for Nocardia, Streptomyces, and Mycobacterium species)

Procedure
1. Make slide cultures in routine manner (see Mycology) using 7H10 medium.
2. Incubate slide cultures at 37 C.
3. Examine slide cultures every 2 d for 2-4 d.

Interpretation. Most *Nocardia* and *Streptomyces* species will produce aerial hyphae, which can be seen growing along the undersurface of the coverslip. *Mycobacterium* species do not produce aerial hyphae. Occasionally an aerobic actinomycete will fail to produce aerial mycelium, and it becomes necessary to examine the vegetative hyphae carefully to differentiate this organism from a *Mycobacterium* species. The vegetative hyphae of *Streptomyces* species and *Nocardia* species are rhizoid in appearance, often with much intertwining. The vegetative filaments of *Mycobacterium* species are short, do not intertwine, and are delicate in appearance. These filaments will fragment, and the growth has a featherlike appearance. Further studies are needed to differentiate *Nocardia* from *Streptomyces* species.

Growth

All species are aerobic and are cultivated readily on a wide variety of media at both room temperature and 37 C; growth is more rapid under 10% CO₂. Development is slow. Colonies are usually dry, granular, and wrinkled and exhibit a variety of pigments such as coral, cream, yellow, pink, orange, and brick red. Some colonies may resemble acid-fast bacteria. Pigmentation is stable on some media and variable on others. Some colonies are tenacious and difficult to remove from the surface of the medium, whereas others are soft, friable, and easily removed. In liquid media **surface pellicles** are usually produced, with no growth taking place in the other portions.

Identification and diagnostic characteristics

Catalase is usually produced. The organisms are not motile and form no spores or oxidase.

N. asteroides and *N. caviae* **do not** hydrolyze casein, whereas *N. brasiliensis* and *Streptomyces* species **do.** Tyrosine is decomposed by *N. brasiliensis* and *Streptomyces* species, and *N. caviae* decomposes xanthine (*Streptomyces* species are variable in this respect). See Table 77-4 for differential characteristics. Media and procedures are described below.

Casein agar[118]

A.	Skim milk	10 g
	Distilled water	90 ml
B.	Agar	3 g
	Distilled water	97 ml

Procedure
1. Autoclave A and B separately at 121 C, 15 psi for 10 min.
2. Allow to cool to 48-50 C.
3. Combine and pour into Petri dishes.

Inoculation and examination of casein medium
1. Place large fragment of actinomycete colony in center of casein agar plate.
2. Incubate at room temperature.
3. Examine plate daily for evidence of casein hydrolysis.
4. Hold plate at least **2 wk** before discarding as negative. Occasional strain of *N. brasiliensis* or *N. madurae* may require at least 2 wk to hydrolyze casein.

Interpretation. If casein is hydrolyzed, a clear zone will develop around the inoculum. *Streptomyces* species and *N. brasiliensis* will hydrolyze casein; *N. asteroides* and *N. caviae* do not hydrolyze casein.

Tyrosine or xanthine agar[119]

Basal medium (pH 7.0)

Beef extract	3.0 g
Peptone	5.0 g
Agar	15.0 g
Distilled water	1000 ml

1. Heat to bring ingredients into solution.
2. Place **100 ml** aliquots into 250 ml flasks. Sterilize by autoclaving at 15 psi for 10 min.
3. Allow medium to cool almost to solidification; at which time add 0.5 g tyrosine or 0.4 g xanthine to 100 ml basal medium. Mix well but with care to avoid bubbles.
4. Pour into X or Y compartment Petri dishes.

NOTE: It is essential that granules of tyrosine or xanthine be kept in suspension until medium solidifies. If molten agar is hot when tyrosine or xanthine granules are added, time required for medium to solidify in Petri dishes will be long enough to permit settling out of most of compound. Thus, to avoid this, molten medium is allowed to cool just short of solidification before tyrosine or xanthine is added. While agar is cooling, Petri dishes are placed in refrigerator.

Sterile solutions. Although it is not imperative to use sterile solutions of either tyrosine or xanthine, they may be prepared in the following manner:
1. To 10 ml distilled water add either 0.5 g tyrosine or 0.4 xanthine.
2. Autoclave at 15 psi for 15 min.
3. Add sterile suspension to 100 ml basal agar and pour into Petri dishes.

Inoculation and examination of tyrosine and xanthine plates
Tyrosine decomposition
1. Inoculate heavily in same manner as done with

casein agar. Positive and negative control cultures should be included.
2. Incubate at room temperature for **4 wk.** Examine every 3-4 d for clearing around colony or directly beneath it.
Xanthine decomposition
1. Inoculate heavily as done with casein and tyrosine media. Be sure to include control cultures.
2. Incubate at room temperature for **3 wk.** Examine every 3-4 d for clearing of medium around or directly beneath colony.

Lysozyme broth[120]

1. *Glycerol broth (basal medium)*

Peptone	5.0 g
Glycerol	70 ml
Distilled water	1000 ml

Divide into 2 equal aliquots and sterilize by autoclaving at 15 psi for 15 min. One aliquot will serve as control broth; it can be tubed aseptically in 5 ml amounts.
2. *Lysozyme broth*
   a. Preparation of lysozyme

   | Lysozyme | 100 mg |
   | 0.01N HCl | 100 ml |

   Sterilize by filtration.
   b. To 95 ml glycerol broth add 5 ml lysozyme solution.
   c. Mix and tube aseptically in 5 ml aliquots.

All broths and lysozyme solution can be stored in refrigerator. They should be kept in screw-cap flasks or in test tubes.

Procedure for lysozyme sensitivity test
1. Place several fragments of culture into tube of control broth (glycerol broth without lysozyme).
2. Do same with tube of broth containing lysozyme.
3. Set up control set of broths using known *Streptomyces* sp. This set of cultures indicates whether or not lysozyme is active (should have growth in control tube but not in lysozyme tube).
4. Incubate all tubes at room temperature until control tubes show good growth, at which time tests may be read and discarded.

An actinomycete may grow in the bottom of the control broth but fail to form a pellicle. Thus, look carefully for growth before agitating tubes. Most *Nocardia* isolates will form a pellicle, but examination for growth in the bottom of the tubes should be made.

Animal pathogenicity of Nocardia

Many strains of *Nocardia* differ in their capacity to initiate disease. The species pathogenic for man, which usually shows pathogenic properties for laboratory animals, is *N. asteroides.*[121]

N. asteroides is usually pathogenic in the guinea pig, but *N. brasiliensis* usually is **not** pathogenic. Intraperitoneal injection into **guinea pigs** results in a diffuse peritonitis, but death is usually due to a toxic effect.

Death of **mice** occurs on injection of *N. asteroides* in a suspension of 5% hog gastric mucin.[122]

In **rabbits,** generalized disease occurs with the production of miliary abscesses throughout the body, depending on the size of the inoculum. If the organism is injected intramuscularly or subcutaneously, only local abscesses occur.

Antimicrobial susceptibility testing of Nocardia

Conventional technics (e.g., Kirby-Bauer disk diffusion test) have given somewhat inconsistent results with *Nocardia* when compared with dilution technics; part of the difficulty lies in the necessity of preparing uniformly dispersed cultures.

Bach et al.[123] described an agar dilution technic based on the use of carefully standardized, dispersed cultures. When they used the standard Kirby-Bauer technic (Chapter 87), modified by use of cultures standardized by actual counts of the number of colony-forming units (CFU), good correlation was obtained with erythromycin, minocycline, and ampicillin disks (compared to agar dilution) but not with tetracycline.

Variations of inoculum, pH, and composition of agar media each influenced results in an agar dilution technic described by Lerner and Baum.[124]

The sulfonamides have been the accepted chemotherapy for *Nocardia* infections; minocycline and amikacin are very active in vitro.

Very few strains of *N. caviae* have been tested (see Black and McNellis[125] and Arroyo et al.[126]).

Actinomycotic mycetoma

Chronic, granulomatous localized lesions due to actinomycetes are called actinomycotic mycetomas. Such lesions are caused by a number of species of the genera *Nocardia* (see above) and *Streptomyces*.

The characteristics of actinomycotic mycetoma are swelling of the tissues followed by development of draining sinuses to the skin surface. Fibrosis of the diseased tissues follows.

Aerobic species involved in actinomycotic mycetomas, in addition to *Nocardia*, are *Streptomyces somaliensis*, *S. pelletieri*, and *A.* (*N.*) *madurae*. The latter is the cause of mycetomas all over the world, whereas the others are found in Africa and Latin America.

S. pelletieri and *A. madurae* grow best at 37 C; *S. somaliensis* at 30 C. Differentiation is based mainly on gross colony morphology and microscopic examination (*A. madurae*: chains of conidia; *S. somaliensis*: chains of spores may be present on aerial mycelium). They are all proteolytic. Aerial mycelium may be developed by *S. somaliensis* and *A. madurae*. Pathogenicity tests in mice and guinea pigs are not successful.

ROTHIA

The genus *Rothia*[1] includes organisms (common inhabitants of the normal mouth and throat) that resemble *Actinomyces* species but grow better aerobically (previously known as *Nocardia dentocariosa* or *N. salivae*). They differ significantly from members of the genera *Actinomyces* and *Nocardia*.

For isolation use enriched media (brain heart infusion or trypticase soy) with **aerobic** incubation at 37 C. Cultures in deep agar butts of these media remain viable 3-4 months at room temper-

ature. For long-term storage, lyophilization of suspensions in milk is satisfactory. Little or no growth is obtained on Sabouraud dextrose agar. In oxidation-fermentation (OF) glucose medium, *Rothia* ferments glucose, while *Nocardia* oxidizes or does not attack glucose.[1]

BACTERIONEMA

The genus, with the species *B. matruchotii*, resembles *Leptotrichia* (Chapter 86), but it is aerobic and has gram-positive branching filaments. Long, nonseptate filaments occur, with an attached "bacillus body" at one end.

For details see Slack and Gerencser[126a] and Gilmour et al.[126b]

RHODOCROUS

A heterogeneous group of gram-positive, aerobic, slightly acid-fast rods with characteristics overlapping the genera *Mycobacterium* and *Nocardia* is referred to as the **rhodocrous taxon;** the genus designations *Gordonae, Jensenia,* and *Rhodococcus* have also been proposed.[127-138]

Isolates form orange or red colonies in air at 28 C and 37 C in 3-4 days on Sabouraud dextrose agar. Microscopically the organism is pleomorphic and nonsporing, often forming a primary mycelium fragmenting into rod and coccoid elements.

It is differentiated from rapidly growing mycobacteria by only slight acid-fastness, ability to utilize sucrose as its sole carbon source, and absence of aryl sulfatase activity at 2 weeks. It is differentiated from *Nocardia* by its fragmenting or absent mycelia, acid formation from mannose, and ability to reduce nitrate and to utilize sucrose as its sole carbon source (Table 77-5).

The organisms are considered nonvirulent saprophytes. However, they have also been implicated in a few clinical isolations (pericarditis, skin lesion, pneumonia with septicemia, bronchitis).[139]

Aerobic sporeformers

BACILLUS*

Organisms in the genus *Bacillus* are rod-shaped cells, sometimes in chains, capable of producing endospores aerobically. They are gram positive; some species are gram variable. The organisms are catalase positive, **aerobic** or facultatively anaerobic, motile (some nonmotile forms do occur), and non-acid-fast. Most of the members of the genus are saprophytes and are found in the soil, dust, and decomposing materials; many are common laboratory contaminants. A few are animal, and especially insect, parasites, or pathogens. One species, *B. anthracis* (the agent of anthrax), is an important animal and human pathogen (rare in the United States).

_____
Bergey's Manual, Part 15, Family Bacillaceae, genus I, *Bacillus*.

Table 77-5. Differential characteristics of some *Bacillus* species*†

	B. cereus and B. mycoides‡ (40)§	B. anthracis (10)	B. megaterium (7)	B. subtilis (20)	B. licheniformis (2)
Gas from glucose	−	−	−	−	−
Action on blood	Beta	− or Sl Al	Beta(Ly)	Beta(Ly)	Beta
Carbohydrates					
Base used	Ferm	Ferm	Ferm	Ferm	Ferm
Glucose	A	A	A	A	A
Xylose	−	−	−(1A)	−	−,A[7]
Mannitol	−	−	A	A	A
Lactose	−(A)	−(A)	−	−	−
Sucrose	A or −	A or −	A	A	A
Maltose	A	A	A(−)	Var	A
Salicin	A	−(A,L)			
Arabinose	−	−			
Starch hydrolysis				+	+
Catalase	+	+	+(1−)	+	+
Oxidase	+(−)	+(−)	Var	Var	+,+W
Growth on or in					
Nutrient broth	+	+	+	+	+
MacConkey agar	−	−	−	−	−
SS agar	−	−	−	−	−
Simmons citrate (Alk) agar	−	−	−	− or +	+
Christensen urea agar	−(+)	−(+)	Var	+ or −	−,+7
Nitrate reduction	+	+	Var	+(−)	+
Indole	−	−	−	−	−
TSI					
Slant/butt	A(Alk)/A	A(Alk)/A	A(Alk)/A	Alk(A)/A	A/A
H₂S-Butt/paper	−/+ or −	−/+(−)	−/+	−/Var	−/+,−
MR	+(−)	Var	− or +	+(−)/+	−,+
VP	−(+)/+2	−(+)/+2	−/−	+(−)/+	+/
Gelatin hydrolysis	+ Rapid	−(W7)	+	+	+
Litmus milk	Pep or NC	Pep or NC	Var	Pep	Pep, Clt
Flagella (motile)	+(−)	NM	+	+	+
Pigment			−	−	−
Gas, anaerobic nitrate				−	+
Cell diameter	≧0.9 μm	≧0.9 μm	≧0.9 μm	<0.9 μm	<0.9 μm
Methylene blue red	+	−(L)			
Growth at 25 C; 37 C; 42 C	+;+;+(−)	+;+;+(−)	+;+;+	+;+;+	+;+;+
Esculin hydrolysis	+(−)	−(+)?	+(2−)	+	+
Fat granules	+	+	+	−	−
Spores	Oval, do not swell cell	Oval, do not swell cell	Oval, do not swell cell	Oval, do not swell cell	Oval, do not swell cell
Lecithinase	+ Wide zone	Negative or narrow zone			

*Modified from Weaver, R. E., Tatum, H. W., and Hollis, D. G.: The identification of unusual pathogenic gram-negative bacteria (E. C

†Reaction in parentheses = reaction of occasional strain; A = acid; A⁷ = acid but not before 7 days; Alk = alkaline; N = neutral; L =

= weak; +S = strong positive reaction; Sl = slight; Pep = peptonized; Peri = peritrichous; NM = nonmotile; NC = no change; Clt =

= lavender green coloration under heavy growth, indicating proteolysis; Beta = beta hemolysis under isolated colonies; Al = alpha ly

complete reduction of nitrates and nitrites; OF = oxidative fermentative carbohydrate base; Ferm = peptone–meat extract broth base;

‡Rhizoid growth.

§Number of strains given in parentheses.

B. firmus (2)	*B. pumilus* (16)	*B. alvei* (1)	*B. stearother- mophilus* (1)	*Rhodochrous group* (*Mycobacterium;* 50)	*Brevibacterium acetylicum* (11 and ATCC strain)
−	−	−	−	−	−
− or LG	Beta (−)	Ly		−	− to Al
Ferm	Ferm	Ferm	Ferm	OF	Ferm
A	A	A	A	A	A
−	−	−	−	Alk-N	−
A	A	−	−	A(Alk)	A
−	−	−	A	Alk	−
A	A	A	A	A(N-Alk)	A
A	−	A	A	Alk(N-A)	A
−	−				
−	−(A)				
	−	+W			
+	+	+		+	+
−(Kovac +)	−(+W)	+		−(+W)	+W(or −)
−	+	+	+	+(−)	+(−)
−	−	−	−	−	−
−	−	−	−	−	−
−	−(+5-7)	−	−	−(+)	−
−	−	+2	+,L	Var	−
+(NO₂+)	−	−	+	+ or −	−
−	−	+	−	−	−
A/A	Alk/A	A/A	A/A	Alk/N	A/A
−/+	−/+(−)	−/+	−/+	−/+	−/
−	Var	+	+		−(+W)
−/	Var/+	+/	−/		+(−)/
+7-14	+	+		−	+
−	−(Pep)	Clt	A,W	Alk	Pep
+	+	+	+	−	Peri
−	−	−	−	Pink, coral, yellow	Yellow(−)
<0.9 μm	<0.9 μm	<0.9 μm	<0.9 μm		
+;+;+	+;+;+	+;+;+	−;−;+,+(65 C)	+(−);+;Var	+;+;Var
−	+		+	−	+(−)
−					
Oval, do not swell cell	Oval, do not swell cell	Oval, do not swell cell; parallel in rows	Oval, swell cell	−	−

ng), Atlanta, Sept. 1972 (revised April 1978), Center for Disease Control.

positive reaction; + = positive reaction; − = negative reaction or no growth; Var = variable; +W = weak positive reaction; W
Ly = diffuse lysis of red cells extending out from heavy growth (no action by colonies probably due to alkaline products); LG
− (nitrate test) = no action on nitrates (confirmed with zinc dust); + (nitrate test) = nitrates reduced to nitrites; NO₂+ (nitrate test) =
immons citrate [Alk]) = growth as evidenced by alkaline reaction; red = reduced.

B. cereus has been implicated in food-borne disease, and it and other species (e.g., *B. subtilis, B. circulans, B. macerans*) have been involved in cases of septicemia, meningitis, and pneumonia (see Ihde and Armstrong[140] and Pennington et al.[141]).

The taxonomy and differentiation of species has been greatly clarified by Gordon et al.'s monograph[142] and the subsequent treatment of the subject by Gibson and Gordon in *Bergey's Manual*.[1]

Bacillus anthracis

The rods are gram-positive and large ($1 \times 3\text{-}10$ μm in size) with square to concave ends, often occurring in long, parallel chains (in smears of colonies). Spores are central; **the organism is nonmotile.** Spores are not formed in the living host. Typical colonies of virulent strains grown on nutrient agar for 24 hours are dull gray and flat and have the typical "medusa head" appearance. The medusa head is made up of outgrowths of chains from the margin of the colony, which curve back toward it; they give an interlacing effect. When the border of the colony is examined under the high-power objective, the parallel arrangement of the bacterial chains can be seen.

Fluorescent antibody (FA) methods can be used successfully for obtaining valuable diagnostic information rapidly. An air-dried, heat-fixed smear of the specimen should be submitted to the state public health laboratory or the Center for Disease Control, Atlanta. For details of procedure, see Cherry and Freeman[143] and Cherry et al.[144]

Brown et al.[145] summarized the characteristics of *B. anthracis*, stating that it is a gram-positive rod with few vacuoles and spores after 2 days' incubation at 30 C. The organism produces cuneiform, viscid colonies made up of long, tangled chains. When grown in broth, a stringy sediment occurs beneath a clear supernatant. *B. anthracis* is virulent for rabbits when injected subcutaneously (0.2 ml in 18-hour broth culture). The cells are susceptible to lysis by γ-phage. They emphasized that *B. anthracis*, in the opinion of many workers, is a pathogenic variety of *B. cereus* and that it is important to differentiate between the moist, nonviscid, and nonadherent colonies of the latter and those of *B. anthracis*, which are viscid and adhere to the needle or loop. For further details see Identification, below.

Isolation

Use nutrient agar and blood agar (preferably sheep blood) plates. On sheep blood agar the organism is **nonhemolytic** or only very slightly so; when hemolysis is present, it appears slowly. This serves to distinguish *B. anthracis* from the strongly β-hemolytic saprophytic *Bacillus* species. Some *B. cereus* strains, however, are also nonhemolytic.

A **selective medium,** stated to allow recovery of *B. anthracis* but not of *B. cereus*, was developed by Knisely.[146] If selective media are used, a nonselective medium (blood agar) should also be used.

The medium (PLET medium) consists of heart infusion agar (Difco) with the following additions:

Polymyxin	30 U/ml
Lysozyme	40 μg/ml
Disodium ethylenediamine tetraacetate (EDTA)	300 μg/ml
Thallous acetate	40 μg/ml

After a 24-hour incubation, *B. anthracis* colonies are smaller on the PLET medium than on plain heart infusion agar. *B. cereus* usually does not grow on PLET medium.

The excretions and secretions of infected animals and man are examined. In man the stools, urine, and pus from pustules are usually selected for the test, although the organisms may be found in the skin, intestines, spinal fluid, and lungs. Since bacteremia is a common complication of anthrax infection, blood is the material of choice. Respiratory anthrax is very rare.

In animals the modus of infection is considered in the selection of material. In living animals the hair, food, and soil on which they graze are important. In dead animals the cadaver is examined for evidence of infection, the inner organs being selected for cultures.

The examination of blood of infected animals will usually show typical anthrax bacilli even in a stained smear. Cultures on blood agar may be made for definitive diagnosis.

Use extreme caution when working with suspected *B. anthracis*. Do not create aerosols; decontaminate all areas.

Identification

Motility. Motility should be determined by a hanging-drop test using Edwards-Bruner **semisolid motility medium** in which *B. anthracis* is nonmotile. Motility test medium (see Chapter 72) with 80 g gelatin added (BBL) is satisfactory as is Motility test medium (Difco). Incubate for 4 days at 37 C.

Hemolysis. See discussion of isolation.

Sensitivity to γ-bacteriophage. This test is not practicable in the general laboratory.

Differential media. Knisely[147] described the following 2 differential media, which should aid in differentiating *B. anthracis* from *B. cereus:*

1. **PEA medium:** PEA (2-phenylethanol) is added to heart infusion agar (Difco) in a final concentration of 0.3%.
2. **CH medium:** A 10% solution of chloral hydrate (CH) is prepared, Seitz filtered, and added to heart infusion agar in a final concentration of 0.25%.

B. anthracis strains are almost completely inhibited on the PEA medium and are completely inhibited on the CH medium; but *B. cereus* and other *Bacillus* strains grow uninhibited on both media.

Growth on penicillin agar. *B. anthracis* is sensitive to penicillin, 10 U/ml, but *B. cereus* is not. Thus on 10 U/ml penicillin agar (Tryptose agar (Difco) containing 10 U penicillin/ml) there is either no growth or very slight growth of *B. anthracis*, but *B. cereus* grows well.

Salicin fermentation, growth at 45 C. In both respects *B. anthracis* is negative, but most strains of *B. cereus* grows well.

Growth on bicarbonate medium. Nutrient agar plates (Difco) with 5% sodium bicarbonate added are heavily inoculated and incubated for 24-48 hours in a **20% CO₂ atmosphere.** Virulent *B. anthracis* grows as mucoid (capsulated, smooth) colonies; avirulent strains produce rough colonies similar to those of other *Bacillus* species.

According to Knisely, results in PEA and CH medium, lack of hemolysis, and lack of motility should allow preliminary identification of *B. anthracis*. The other reactions listed (penicillin sensitivity, etc.) are useful confirmatory tests.

For differential reactions, as determined at the Center for Disease Control, see Table 77-5.

Pathogenicity studies

Inject subcutaneously 0.2 ml of 18-hour broth culture into rabbits; guinea pigs or 2- to 3-week-old mice can also be used. A gelatinous exudate appears at the site of the injection; the liver and spleen are enlarged and dark; death usually occurs in 48-96 hours. **Extreme caution should be exercised when performing animal pathogenicity tests with anthrax.**

NOTE: Any organisms suspected of being *B. anthracis* should be submitted to a public health or reference laboratory for final confirmation.

Ascoli precipitin test (antigen detection)

In advanced decomposition of animals when cultures would be almost impossible, the precipitin method of Ascoli is used. This method is a mixing of immunized rabbit serum (not available commercially in the United States) with an extract of organs under examination for the production of a precipitate.

1. Grind up organs or blood of suspected animals.
2. Suspend in saline.
3. Boil for 5 min.
4. Filter through filter paper and allow to cool.
5. Carefully stratify 0.5 ml of this extract on 0.5 ml immune serum in small test tube.
6. Allow to stand for 15 min at room temperature.
7. Define ringlike precipitate forms at junction of the 2 fluids in positive cases.
8. Always run controls with known anthrax extract and with normal serum.

Other Bacillus species

With the data of Gibson and Gordon in *Bergey's Manual*, ed. 8,[1] Gordon et al.,[142] or Wolf and Barker,[148] it is possible to distinguish a large number of *Bacillus* species by a variety of physiologic, morphologic, and biochemical characteristics.

The sugar reactions were studied in **medium with ammonium salt base.**[1,129]

Ammonium salt sugar medium[149]	
MgSO₄·7H₂O	0.2 g
KCl	0.2 g
(NH₄)₂HPO₄	1 g
Yeast extract	0.2 g
Agar	0.2 g
Distilled water	1000 ml
Bromcresol purple, 0.2% solution	4 ml

Dissolve solids by steaming in water. Add indicator. Autoclave at 115 C for 20 min. Cool medium to 60 C. Add appropriate carbohydrate as sterile solution to final solution of 1%. Distribute with aseptic cautions into sterile tubes; slant.

B. cereus seems to intergrade with *B. anthracis*. *B. cereus* is usually **motile,** except for *B. cereus* var. *mycoides,* and nonrhizoid variants, which are nonmotile. It is not pathogenic for rabbits, is not susceptible to lysis by γ-bacteriophages, is **hemolytic** on sheep blood agar, and grows at **45 C.** Colonies vary from small, smooth, shiny colonies to the spreading, large, feathery type of *B. cereus* var. *mycoides.* Most *B. cereus* strains ferment **salicin,** reduce **methylene blue** in 24 hours, and grow on PEA and CH medium.

B. subtilis is usually motile in young cultures. Agar colonies are rough, dull, opaque, and waxy.

For differential reactions (U.S. Center for Disease Control determinations) see Table 77-5; **note media used.**

Antibiotic susceptibility of Bacillus

B. anthracis is sensitive to penicillin, which is the drug of choice in anthrax.

Coonrod et al.[150] have tested strains of 6 species of *Bacillus* (**not** including *B. anthracis*) and determined the minimal inhibitory concentrations of 9 antibiotics by an agar dilution technic as well as by the Kirby-Bauer disk diffusion method. Almost all strains of *Bacillus* were inhibited by 6.2 μg/ml tetracycline, kanamycin, gentamicin, or chloramphenicol. Penicillin G, ampicillin, methicillin, and cephalothin were highly active against *B. subtilis*, less active against *B. pumilus* and *B. licheniformis*, and had little activity against *B. cereus.* They caution against applying the interpretive standards of the disk diffusion method to susceptibility testing for *Bacillus* species.

REFERENCES

1. Buchanan, R. E., and Gibbons, N. E., editors: Bergey's manual of determinative bacteriology, ed. 8, Baltimore, 1974, The Williams & Wilkins Co.
2. Smith, D. T., and Conant, N. F.: Zinsser's microbiology, ed. 12, New York, 1960, Appleton-Century-Crofts.
3. Wilson, G., and Miles, A. A.: Topley & Wilson's principles of bacteriology and immunity, ed. 5, Baltimore, 1964, The Williams & Wilkins Co.

4. Cowan, S. T.: Cowan and Steel's manual for the identification of medical bacteria, ed. 2, New York, 1974, Cambridge University Press.
5. Hermann, G. J., and Weaver, R. E. In Blair, J. E., Lennette, E. H., and Truant, J. P., editors: Manual of clinical microbiology, Bethesda, Md., 1970, American Society for Microbiology.
6. Diamond, B. E., and Judson, J. M.: Public Health Lab. **25**:193, 1967.
7. Cherry, W. B., and Moody, M. D.: Bacteriol. Rev. **29**:222, 1965.
8. Elek, S. D.: Br. Med. J. **1**:493, 1948.
9. King, E. O., Frobisher, M., Jr., and Parsons, E. I.: Am. J. Public Health **39**:1314, 1949.
10. Schubert, J. H., and Blank, B. E.: Public Health Lab. **23**:170, 1965.
11. Frobisher, M. In Diagnostic procedures and reagents, ed. 4, New York, 1963, American Public Health Association.
12. Frobisher, M., Jr., Parsons, E. I., and Tung, T.: Am. J. Hyg. **35**:381, 1942.
13. Bureau of Laboratories, Center for Disease Control: Current item no. 241: Toxigenicity testing of *Corynebacterium diphtheriae* cultures, Atlanta, Jan. 22, 1974, The Center.
14. Bodily, H. L., Updyke, E. L., and Mason, J. O., editors: Diagnostic procedures for bacterial, mycotic and parasitic infections, ed. 5, New York, 1970, American Public Health Association, ch. 5.
15. Bickham, S. T., and Jones, W. L.: Am. J. Clin. Pathol. **57**:244-246, 1972.
16. Hermann, G. J., Moore, M. S., and Parsons, E. I.: Am. J. Clin. Pathol. **29**:181-183, 1958.
17. Murphy, J. R., Bacha, P., and Teng, M.: J. Clin. Microbiol. **7**:91, 1978.
18. Thompson, N. L., and Ellner, P. D.: J. Clin. Microbiol. **7**:493, 1978.
19. Anderson, J. S., Happold, F. C., McLeod, J. W., et al.: J. Pathol. **34**:667, 1931.
20. Topley, W. W. C., and Wilson, G. S.: Principles of bacteriology and immunity, Baltimore, 1946, William Wood & Co.
21. Frobisher, M., Adams, M. L., and Kuhns, W. J.: Proc. Soc. Exp. Biol. Med. **58**:330, 1945.
22. Barksdale, L.: Bacteriol. Rev. **34**:378, 1970.
23. Collier, R. J.: Bacteriol. Rev. **39**:54, 1975.
24. Gilbert, R., and Stewart, F. C.: J. Lab. Clin. Med. **12**:756, 1927.
25. Bridson, E. Y.: J. Med. Lab. Techn. **16**:280-283, 1959.
26. Hermann, G. J., and Parsons, E. I.: Public Health Lab. **15**:34, 1957.
27. Geraci, J. E., Forth, R. J., and Ellis, H. E.: Mayo Clin. Proc. **42**:736, 1967.
28. Johnson, W. D., Cobbs, G. C., Arditi, L. I., et al.: J.A.M.A. **203**:919, 1968.
29. Scoy, R. E., Cohen, S. N., Geraci, J. E., et al.: Mayo Clin. Proc. **52**:216, 1977.
30. Johnson, W. D., and Kaye, D.: Ann. N.Y. Acad. Sci. **174**:568, 1970.
31. Somerville, D. A.: J. Med. Microbiol. **6**:215, 1973.
32. Porschen, R. K., Goodman, Z., and Rafai, B.: Am. J. Clin. Pathol. **68**:290, 1977.
33. Lopez, J. F., Wong, F. M., and Quesada, J.: Am. J. Clin. Pathol. **46**:562, 1966.
34. Barksdale, W. L., Li, K., Cummins, C. S., et al.: J. Gen. Microbiol. **16**:749, 1957.
35. McLean, P. D., Liebow, A. A., and Rosenburg, A. A.: J. Infect. Dis. **79**:69, 1946.
36. Washington, J. A., Martin, W. J., and Spiekerman, R. E.: Am. J. Clin. Pathol. **56**:212, 1971.
37. Jobanputra, R. S., and Swain, C. P.: J. Clin. Pathol. **28**:798, 1975.
38. Ceilley, R. I.: Arch. Dermatol. **113**:646, 1977.
39. Vale, J. A., and Scott, G. W.: Lancet **2**:682, 1977.
40. Berg, R., Chmel, H., Mayo, J., et al.: Am. J. Clin. Pathol. **68**:73, 1977.
41. Leifson, E.: Int. Bull. Bacteriol. Nomen. Taxon. **12**:161, 1962.
42. Weiner, M., and Werthamer, S.: Am. J. Clin. Pathol. **64**:378, 1975.
43. Hande, K. R., Witebsky, F. G., Brown, M. S., et al.: Ann. Intern. Med. **85**:423, 1976.
44. Pearson, T. A., Braine, H. G., and Rathbun, H. K.: J.A.M.A. **238**:1737, 1977.
45. Nyfeldt, A.: Compt. Rend. Soc. Biol. **101**:590, 1929.
46. Seeliger, H. P. R.: Deutsch. Med. Wochenschr. **77**:587, 1952.
47. Potel, J.: Zbl. Bakt. (Abt. 1) **158**:329, 1952.
48. Gray, M. L. In Gray, M. L., editor: Second symposium on listeric infection, Bozeman, Mont., 1963, Montana State College.
49. Navarette-Reyna, A., Rosenstein, D. L., and Sonnenwirth, A. C.: Am. J. Clin. Pathol. **43**:438, 1965.
50. Louria, D. B., Hensle, T., Armstrong, D., et al.: Ann. Intern. Med. **67**:261, 1967.
51. Simpson, J. F., Leddy, J. P., and Hare, J. D.: Am. J. Med. **43**:39, 1967.
52. Kalis, P., LeFrock, J. L., Smith, W., et al.: Am. J. Med. Sci. **271**:159, 1976.
53. Ascher, N. L., Simmons, R. L., Marker, S., et al.: Arch. Surg. **113**:90, 1978.
54. Medoff, G., Kunz, L. J., and Weinberg, A. N.: J. Infect. Dis. **123**:247, 1971.
55. Gantz, N. M., Myerowitz, R. L., Medeiros, A. A., et al.: Am. J. Med. **58**:637, 1975.
56. Bayer, A. S., Chow, A. W., and Guze, L. B.: Am. J. Med. Sci. **273**:319, 1977.
57. Visintine, A. M., Oleske, J. M., and Nahmias, A. J.: Am. J. Dis. Child. **131**:393, 1977.
58. Bojsen-Moller, J.: Acta Pathol. Microbiol. Scand. [B] **229**:1-157, 1972.
59. Alex, R.: Geburtshilfe Frauenheilkd. **20**:599, 1960.
60. Potel, J., and Alex, R.: Geburtshilfe Frauenheilkd. **16**:1002, 1956.
61. Rost, H. F., Paul, H., and Seeliger, H. P. R.: Deutsch Med. Wochenschr. **83**:1893, 1958.
62. Rappaport, F., Rabinovitz, M., Toaff, R., et al.: Lancet **1**:1273, 1960.
63. Toaff, R., Krochick, R., and Rabinovitz, M.: Lancet **2**:482, 1962.
64. Gray, M. L., editor: Second symposium on listeric infection, Bozeman, Mont., 1963, Montana State College.
65. Gray, M. L., and Killinger, A. H.: Bacteriol. Rev. **30**:309, 1966.
66. Buchner, L. H., and Schneiersohn, S. S.: Am. J. Med. **45**:904, 1968.
67. Lavetter, A., Leedom, J. M., Mathies, A. W., et al.: N. Engl. J. Med. **285**:598, 1971.
68. Woodbine, M., editor: Problems of listeriosis. Proceedings of the Sixth International Symposium, New York, 1975, Humanities Press.
69. Wetzler, T. F., Freeman, N. R., French, M. L. V., et al.: Health Lab. Sci. **5**:46, 1968.
70. Killinger, A. H. In Lennette, E. H., Spaulding, E. H., and Traunt, J. P., editors: Manual of clinical microbiology, ed. 2, Washington, D.C., 1974, American Society for Microbiology, ch. 13.

71. Bottone, E. J., and Sierra, M. F.: Mt. Sinai J. Med. N.Y. **44**:42, 1977.
72. McBride, M. E., and Girard, K. F.: J. Lab. Clin. Med. **55**:153, 1960.
73. Glencross, E. J. G. In Laboratory Methods 1, Public Health Laboratory Service Monograph Series No. 5, London, 1974, Her Majesty's Stationery Office.
74. Henry, B. S.: J. Infect. Dis. **52**:374, 1933.
75. Gray, M. L.: Zbl. Bakt. (Abt. 1) **169**:373, 1957.
76. Gray, M. L., Stafseth, H. J., Thorpe, F., Jr., et al.: J. Bacteriol. **55**:471, 1948.
77. Olsufev, N. G., and Emelyanova, O. S.: Zh. Mikrobiol. **22**:67, 1951.
78. Olsufev, N. G., Petrov, V. G., and Shlygina, K. N.: Zh. Mikrobiol. **30**:112, 1959.
79. Shlygina, K. N.: Zh. Mikrobiol. **30**:68, 1959.
80. Gray, M. L.: Science **132**:1767, 1960.
81. Dontenwill, W., and Knothe, H.: Artzl. Wochenschr. **11**:204, 1956.
82. Eveleth, D. F., Bolin, F. M., and Turn, J.: North Dakota Agric. Exp. Stat. Bull. **16**:47, 1953.
83. Groves, R. D., and Welshimer, H. J.: J. Clin. Microbiol. **5**:559, 1977.
84. Eveland, W. C.: J. Bacteriol. **85**:1448, 1963.
85. Eveland, W. C.: Health Lab. Sci. **1**:261, 1964.
86. Neter, E., Anzai, H., and Gorzynski, E. A.: Proc. Soc. Exp. Biol. Med. **105**:131, 1960.
87. Seeliger, H. P. R.: Listeriosis, ed. 2, New York, 1961, Hafner Publishing Co.
88. Smith, C. W., Marshall, J. D., Jr., and Eveland, W. C.: Proc. Soc. Exp. Biol. Med. **103**:842, 1960.
89. Smith, C. W., Metzger, J. F., and Hoggan, M. D.: Am. J. Clin. Pathol. **38**:26, 1962.
90. Fuzi, M.: J. Pathol. Bacteriol. **85**:524, 1963.
91. Silberstein, E. B.: J.A.M.A. **191**:862, 1965.
92. McCracken, A., Mauney, C. U., Huber, T. W., et al.: Am. J. Clin. Pathol. **59**:219, 1973.
93. Simerkoff, M. S., and Rahal, J. J.: Am. J. Med. Sci. **266**:53, 1973.
94. Park, C. H., Poretz, D. M., and Goldenberg, R.: South. Med. J. **69**:1101, 1976.
95. Elston, H. R.: J. Pathol. Bacteriol. **81**:245, 1961.
95a. Pancoast, S. J., Ellner, P. E., Jahre, J. A., and Neu, H. C.: Ann. Intern. Med. **90**:936, 1979.
96. Rosebury, T.: Microorganisms indigenous to man, New York, 1962, McGraw-Hill Book Co.
97. Skinner, F. A., and Carr, J. G., editors: The normal microbial flora of man, New York, 1974, Academic Press.
98. Rogosa, M., and Sharpe, M. E.: J. Gen. Microbiol. **23**:197, 1960.
99. London, J.: Annu. Rev. Microbiol. **30**:279, 1976.
100. Thomas, M. E. M. In Laboratory methods 1, Public Health Laboratory Service Monograph Series No. 5, London, 1974, Her Majesty's Stationery Office.
101. Rogosa, M., Mitchell, J. A., and Wiseman, R. F.: J. Bacteriol. **62**:132, 1951.
102. DeMan, J. C., Rogosa, M., and Sharpe, M. E.: J. Appl. Bacteriol. **23**:130, 1960.
103. Sharpe, M. E., Hill, L. R., and Lapage, S. P.: J. Med. Microbiol. **6**:281, 1972.
104. Isenberg, D.: Proc. R. Soc. Med. **70**:278, 1977.
105. Tennenbaum, M. J., and Warner, J. F.: Ann. Intern. Med. **82**:539, 1975.
105a. Bayer, A. S., Chow, A. W., Betts, D., and Guze, L. B.: Am. J. Med. **64**:808, 1978.
106. Pine, L., and Georg, L.: Int. Bull. Bacteriol. Nomen. Taxon. **15**:143, 1965.

107. Cummins, C. S., and Harris, H.: J. Gen. Microbiol. **18**:173, 1958.
108. Berd, D.: Appl. Microbiol. **25**:665, 1973.
109. Ajello, L., Georg, L. K., Kaplan, W., et al.: Laboratory manual for medical mycology, Public Health Service pub. no. 994, Atlanta, 1963, Center for Disease Control.
110. Causey, W. A.: Appl. Microbiol. **28**:193, 1974.
111. Gordon, R. E., and Mihm, J. M.: Ann. N.Y. Acad. Sci. **98**:628, 1962.
112. Berd, D.: Am. J. Clin. Pathol. **59**:254, 1973.
113. Murray, J. F., Finegold, S. M., Froman, S., et al.: Am. Rev. Respir. Dis. **83**:315, 1961.
114. Goodman, J. S., and Koenig, M. G.: Ann. N.Y. Acad. Sci. **174**(2):552, 1970.
115. Kurup, P. V., Randhawa, H. S., and Gupta, N. P.: Mycopathologia **40**:193, 1970.
116. Palmer, D. L., Harvey, R. L., and Wheeler, J. K.: Medicine (Baltimore) **53**:391, 1974.
117. Goodfellow, M., and Minnikin, D. E.: Annu. Rev. Microbiol. **31**:159, 1977.
118. Gordon, R. E., and Mihm, J. M.: J. Bacteriol. **73**:15, 1957.
119. Gordon, R. E., and Mihm, J. M.: J. Gen. Microbiol. **27**:1, 1962.
120. Gordon, R. E. In Gray, T. R. G., and Parkinson, D., editors: The ecology of soil bacteria, Liverpool, 1967, Liverpool University Press, p. 293.
121. Conant, N. In Dubos, R., editor: Bacterial and mycotic infections of man, ed. 3, Philadelphia, 1958, J. B. Lippincott Co.
122. Straus, R., Kligman, A., and Pillsbury, D.: Am. Rev. Respir. Dis. **63**:441, 1951.
123. Bach, M. C., Sabath, L. D., and Finland, M.: Antimicrob. Agents Chemoth. **3**:1, 1973.
124. Lerner, P. I., and Baum, G. L.: Antimicrob. Agents Chemother. **4**:85, 1973.
125. Black, W. A., and McNellis, D. A.: Antimicrob. Agents Chemother. **10**:346, 1970.
126. Arroyo, J. C., Nichols, S., and Carroll, G. F.: Am. J. Med. **62**:409, 1977.
126a. Slack, J. M., and Gerencser, M. A.: Actinomyces, filamentous bacteria—biology and pathogenicity, Minneapolis, 1975, Burgess Pub. Co.
126b. Gilmour, M. N., Howell, A., Jr., and Bibby, B. G.: Bacteriol. Rev. **25**:131, 1961.
127. Tsukamura, M.: J. Gen. Microbiol. **68**:15, 1971.
128. Goodfellow, M., Fleming, A., and Sackin, M.: Int. J. Syst. Bacteriol. **22**:81, 1972.
129. Jones, D.: J. Gen. Microbiol. **87**:52, 1975.
130. Tsukamura, M.: Jpn. J. Microbiol. **18**:94, 1974.
131. Tsukamura, M.: Jpn. J. Microbiol. **18**:37, 1974.
132. Tsukamura, J.: J. Gen. Microbiol. **80**:553, 1974.
133. Mordarski, M., and Szyba, K.: J. Gen. Microbiol. **94**:235, 1976.
134. Alshamaony, L., Goodfellow, M., and Minnikin, D. E.: J. Gen. Microbiol. **92**:188, 1976.
135. Alshamaony, L., Goodfellow, M., Minnikin, D. E., et al.: J. Gen. Microbiol. **92**:183, 1976.
136. Goodfellow, M., and Minnikin, D. E.: Annu. Rev. Microbiol. **31**:159, 1977.
137. Hyman, I. S., and Chaparas, D. S.: J. Gen. Microbiol. **100**:363, 1977.
138. Stottmeier, K. D., and Mallory, M. E.: Appl. Microbiol. **26**:213, 1973.
139. Haburchak, D. R., Jeffery, B., Higbee, J. W., et al.: Am. J. Med. **65**:298, 1978.
140. Ihde, D. C., and Armstrong, D.: Am. J. Med. **55**:839, 1973.
141. Pennington, J. E., Gibbons, N. D., Strobeck, J. E., et al.: J.A.M.A. **235**:1473, 1976.

142. Gordon, R. E., Haynes, W. C., and Pang, C. H.: The genus *Bacillus*, Agriculture Handbook no. 427, Washington, D.C., 1973, U. S. Department of Agriculture.

143. Cherry, W. B., and Freeman, E. M.: Zbl. Bakt. (Abt. 1) **175:**582-604, 1959.

144. Cherry, W. B., Goldman, M., Carski, T. R., et al.: Fluorescent antibody techniques in the diagnosis of communicable diseases, PHS pub. no. 729, Atlanta, 1960, United States Department of Health, Education and Welfare, Communicable Disease Center.

145. Brown, E. R., Moody, M. D., Treece, E. L., et al.: J. Bacteriol. **75:**499, 1958.

146. Knisely, R. F.: J. Bacteriol. **92:**784, 1966.

147. Knisely, R. F.: J. Bacteriol. **90:**1778, 1965.

148. Wolf, J., and Barker, A. N. In Gibbs, B. M., and Shapton, D. A., editors: Identification methods for microbiologists, Part B, New York, 1968, Academic Press.

149. Smith, N. R., Gordon, R. E., and Clark, F. E.: Aerobic spore-forming bacteria, Agr. Monograph no. 16, 1952, U. S. Department of Agriculture.

150. Coonrod, J. D., Leadly, P. J., and Eickhoff, T. C.: J. Infect. Dis. **123:**102, 1971.

78

THE MYCOBACTERIA

George P. Kubica
Hugo L. David

Changing role of the laboratory

Of the several disciplines and areas of concentration concerned with the diagnosis, treatment, and control of tuberculosis and related mycobacterioses, the bacteriology laboratory has been one of the most dramatically affected over the years. Not many decades ago the simple demonstration of acid-fast bacilli in smears was the sole bacteriologic confirmation needed to support the clinical diagnosis of tuberculosis. In the 1940s and 1950s less emphasis was placed on smears; the identification of mycobacteria and determination of their virulence for man were based on a few cultureal technics (e.g., temperature and speed of growth, pigmentation, and colony morphology) and animal pathogenicity tests.

Today the laboratory plays a far greater role in the management of the mycobacterioses. The smear is regaining prominence, and there is increased need for cultural studies and a vital need to monitor more precisely the bacteriologic change in the patient. There are 2 major reasons for the increased role of the laboratory. First, the introduction over 25 years ago of effective antituberculosis drugs precipitated 2 laboratory-related changes: (1) the problem of acquired bacterial drug resistance and the need to use and understand in vitro susceptibility tests, and (2) the need for in vitro culturing to monitor the results of chemotherapy. Second, the realization that tubercle bacilli were not the only mycobacteria pathogenic for man necessitated definition of a meaningful, clinically oriented taxonomy of the acid-fast bacilli.

Levels of laboratory service

The present-day mycobacteriology laboratory has 4 basic functions: (1) detection and isolation of mycobacteria, (2) identification of the organism isolated, (3) drug susceptibility testing, and (4) monitoring of patient response to treatment. To perform all 4 functions is time consuming, requiring reagents and facilities not routinely used in most other areas of bacteriology, and necessitates maintenance of a level of expertise attained only by regular examination of many specimens or cultures. It is possible, however, to segregate these laboratory functions into various levels of activity, some more easily learned than others, with not all levels necessarily having to be performed at the same institution. The current trend to treat tuberculosis in general hospitals and outpatient clinics, rather than in TB sanatoriums, could result in a rather even distribution of the laboratory work load of a community among personnel currently not experienced in mycobacteriology. To compensate for this, the concept of levels of services is suggested.[1,2] The function of each level is briefly as follows:

Level I
1. Collect adequate diagnostic specimens and transport to level II or III for further processing.
2. Develop expertise in preparing and examining stained smears for rapid reporting to the clinician. Use of the Clorox (sodium hypochlorite) method (described later under "Concentration methods for smears only") is strongly recommended for Level I laboratories.

Level II
1. Routinely culture all specimens.
2. Precisely identify *Mycobacterium tuberculosis*.
3. Perform susceptibility tests for first line drugs (streptomycin, isoniazid, *p*-aminosalicylic acid, ethambutol, rifampin).

Level III
1. Perform all activities of level II.
2. Provide training for levels I and II.
3. Precisely identify all clinically important mycobacteria.
4. Perform susceptibility test to all antituberculosis drugs.
5. Conduct research.

• • •

The clinical bacteriologist should become thoroughly familiar with the procedures de-

This chapter was written by Drs. Kubica and David in their private capacities. No official support or endorsement by the Public Health Service or the Department of Health, Education and Welfare is intended or should be inferred.

scribed in this chapter, so that he may decide whether the number of specimens received for mycobacteriologic examination are sufficient to warrant his maintenance of the expertise required for one of the previously listed 3 levels of service. It may be advantageous, both for the laboratory and the patient, to willingly refer some (or all) phases of the mycobacterial work to another laboratory having greater expertise in their performance.

GENERAL DESCRIPTION AND CHARACTERISTICS

The mycobacteria comprise a large group of acid-fast, alcohol-fast, aerobic or microaerophilic, non-sporeforming, nonmotile bacilli, ranging in size from $0.2-0.6 \times 1.0-10.0$ μm. Some cells may exhibit branching or filamentous growth, but only slight manipulation of cultures results in their fragmentation into rod or coccoid elements. Lipid content of the cells is high, the most characteristic components being genus-specific α-OH, branched chain fatty acids with 80 or more carbon atoms (mycolic acids). Mycobacteria grow relatively slowly; more rapidly growing strains require only 2-3 days on simple media, while most pathogens appear only after 2-6 weeks or more on complex media incubated at restricted temperatures. The genus includes species of widely divergent pathogenetic potential, ranging from frank saprophytes to obligatory parasites,

together with intermediate forms that are commonly saprophytic but possess potential pathogenicity in the appropriate situation (opportunists).

The eighth edition of *Bergey's Manual of Determinative Bacteriology*,[3] in a dramatic departure from previous editions, divides the bacteria into 19 parts, each with a vernacular name and occasionally that of a taxon. The mycobacteria fall into Part 17, Actinomycetes and Related Organisms; Order I, *Actinomycetales;* Family II, *Mycobacteriaceae;* Genus I, *Mycobacterium.*

Brief history

The first organism of the genus, described by Hansen in 1868, was the leprosy bacillus *(M. leprae).* In 1882 Koch described the mammalian tubercle bacilli. He noted the organisms to be constantly associated with disease, isolated the bacilli in pure culture, reproduced the disease in laboratory animals, and was able to recover the bacilli from the experimental disease process. The foregoing experimental requirements fulfill what we now know as Koch's postulates. Strauss and Gamelia (1891) isolated *M. avium* from fowl, while Johne and Frothingham (1895) described *M. paratuberculosis,* the causative agent of Johne's disease, a chronic enteritis of cattle and sheep. In 1896 Theobald Smith was able to subdivide the mammalian tubercle bacilli, recognizing the 2 species now called *M. tuberculosis* and *M. bovis.* In 1905 the rat leprosy bacillus was

Table 78-1. Mycobacteria recovered from vertebrates

Complex	Species	Synonyms	Complex	Species	Synonyms
Potentially clinically significant			*Usually not significant*		
TB	*M. tuberculosis* *M. bovis* *M. africanum* *M. microti**	*M. tuberculosis* var. *hominis* *M. tuberculosis* var. *bovis* *M. tuberculosis* var. *muris*		*M. bovis* BCG	
	M. kansasii *M. marinum* *M. simiae*	*M. luciflavum* *M. balnei, M. platypoecilus* *M. habana*			
MAIS	*M. szulgai* *M. scrofulaceum*	*M. marianum, M. paraffinicum*		*M. gordonae* *M. flavescens*	*M. aquae*
	M. avium *M. intracellulare* *M. xenopi* *M. ulcerans*	*M. brunense* *M. littorale* *M. buruli*	Terrae	*M. gastri* *M. nonchromo-* *genicum* *M. terrae* Wayne *M. triviale*	*M. terrae* Tsukamura *M. novum*
Fortuitum	*M. fortuitum* *M. chelonei* *M. chelonei* subsp. *abscessus*	*M. giae, M. peregrinum* *M. ranae, M. minetti* *M. borstelense* *M. abscessus* *M. runyonii*	Parafor- tuitum	*M. phlei** *M. smegmatis** *M. vaccae* *M. parafortuitum* *M. aurum* *M. neoaurum*	*M. moelleri* *M. butyricum* *M. diernhoferi*
	M. paratubercu- *losis** *M. leprae* *M. lepraemurium**	*M. johnei*			

*Species never, or rarely, found in man.

described by Stefansky, Rabinowitsch, and Dean. From 1890 to the present more than 300 species names have been ascribed to the genus *Mycobacterium*, but the vast majority of these have proved to (1) belong to other genera, (2) be illegitimate names, or (3) be synonyms of previously described species. In the early 1950s it was recognized that mycobacteria other than tubercle bacilli could cause clinical disease in man. Three early publications[4-6] focused attention on these "new microbes," and stimulated a profusion of papers that increased our knowledge about clinical and taxonomic characteristics of all mycobacteria. Runyon[7,8] provided a systematic basis for our early discussions of those then unclassified mycobacteria with a documentation of the now well-known 4 groups of Runyon. The application of numerical taxonomic methods, facilitated by computer technology, has enabled detailed analysis of thousands of strains of mycobacteria, to the end that well-defined species within each of the 4 Runyon groups are now recognized and internationally accepted.[9-11] So precise is our taxonomy of mycobacteria that such nebulous terms as "Group I," "scotochromogen," and "atypical" are only rarely tenable. For example, strains that cannot easily be equated with existing taxa may be categorized as "unidentified Group III" or "Group II scotochromogen-species unknown" until such time as more precise delineation is possible. A trend that is rapidly catching hold is the use of complex names to designate groups of organisms of common pathogenic potential for which further speciation would be of little clinical value, [3,12-14] e.g., *M. avium* complex, MAIS complex (*M. avium-intracellulare-scrofulaceum*), *M. terrae* complex, or *M. fortuitum* complex. Thus, if species or complex names are known, they should be used in preference to the undesirable group or vernacular terms. Table 78-1 lists species of mycobacteria recovered from man, some common synonyms (their use should be avoided), and some of the "complex names" currently in vogue.

SAFETY IN THE MYCOBACTERIOLOGY LABORATORY

The establishment of strict rules of conduct for personnel in the mycobacteriology laboratory is not done to frighten the technician nor to imply excessive difficulty in containment of these microorganisms. The respect afforded the acid-fast bacilli reflects a combination of factors: (1) the chronicity of the disease they may invoke, (2) the fact that specialist laboratories may encounter more strains of drug-resistant tubercle bacilli that, in the face of laboratory-acquired infection, could prove difficult to treat clinically, and (3) the multiple drug resistance of strains of potentially pathogenic mycobacteria other than tubercle bacilli that are sent to a clinical laboratory for identification.

The responsibility for laboratory safety is both an administrative and an individual one. Administratively, each laboratory employee must be properly trained in safe laboratory procedures, be apprised of especially dangerous technics requiring special care, and be prepared for unexpected accidents or emergencies. Adherence to established laboratory rules and correct use of equipment will greatly minimize the hazard of work in the mycobacteriology laboratory. Each individual must accept responsibility for proper work performance to ensure his own safety as well as that of his co-workers. The well-trained individual who can foresee potentially dangerous laboratory operations and take measures to avoid or minimize them is less likely to be injured or infected.

Most mycobacterial disease is acquired via the airborne route, with bacteria-bearing droplet nuclei (<5 μm diameter) being the major vehicle for transmission of the organisms into the primary site of implantation, which is a pulmonary alveolus. Many manipulations in the laboratory lead to the production of aerosols that if not properly controlled will produce infection. Common sources of potentially infectious aerosols include (but are not limited to) the opening of specimen containers or lyophilized vials, pipetting (especially if the last drop is forcefully expelled), flaming of loops, shaking machines and centrifuges, syringes, and animal autopsies or surgical excision of diseased tissue from a patient. The following recommendations represent attempts to minimize the danger from aerosols.

Proper laboratory layout. Ideally, a self-contained suite should be available containing all equipment needed to process specimens from date of receipt until issuance of final reports. Suggested laboratory layout is presented elsewhere.[15] Air flow in this suite should be one-pass, and unidirectional, from a clean to a less clean area. Exhaust air from this suite should pass through absolute filters for removal of all bacteria prior to discharge outside the building.

Biological safety cabinets. The single most important piece of required equipment is an effective biologic safety cabinet. No handling of untreated clinical specimens or transfer of viable mycobacterial cultures should be permitted in a laboratory lacking a biologic safety cabinet. Two general types of cabinets are in use and are satisfactory. One is a negative-pressure biologic safety cabinet drawing a minimum of 75 lineal feet of air per minute across the entire frontal opening; the other is a laminar flow bio-safety cabinet that blows bacteria-free (<0.3 μm) air over the work area.*

Ultraviolet (UV) light. Bulbs emitting UV rays of wavelength 254 nm may be mounted in the safety cabinet (as an adjunct to surface decontamination *after* work is completed) or in eye-pro-

---

*Consult Center for Disease Control, Office of Biosafety, 1600 Clifton Road, Atlanta, Georgia 30333, for information on safety cabinets and their maintenance.

tective wall units to irradiate the upper air of the laboratory suite, thereby helping to destroy droplet nuclei that escape the confines of the safety cabinet. These bulbs must be cleaned frequently (be certain the light is off) with an alcohol-soaked gauze, and their output of germicidal wavelength rays should be monitored at 3- to 6-month intervals (replace when they emit 70% or less of initial rated output).

Face masks. Because no hood is 100% effective, use of face masks capable of minimizing passage of most bacteria is recommended. Two that have been used are Bordic, Deseret Filtermask (C. R. Bard, Inc., Murry Hill, N.J.), and Aseptex or Filtron surgical masks (3M Co., St. Paul, Minn.).

Aerosol-free containers. Materials subjected to shaking or centrifugation should be placed in glass, plastic, or metal containers sealed with O-rings or with plastic or rubber-lined screw caps.

Alcohol-sand flask.[15] This may be used to clean inoculating wires, loops, or spades prior to flame sterilization. A 250-500 ml Erlenmeyer flask is half filled with washed sea sand, and the flask is then filled with 95% ethanol. Alternatively one may use commercially available Bunsen burners with glass-enclosed side-arm incinerators attached.

Disinfectants. Use of disinfectant-soaked gauze pads over the immediate work area in the safety cabinet will both minimize spattering of materials dropped from pipets, loops, etc., and effectively decontaminate such spills. In our experience, the disinfectants that retain effectiveness for a long period of time, on a wide variety of surfaces, and in the presence of organic debris are the phenolic-based products, 5% phenol, 5% saponated cresol, or 3% Lysol being especially good. The reader should consult the company brochures and other available literature before buying because some products have virtually no tuberculocidal activity (e.g., the quaternary ammonium compounds).

Personnel. Laboratory staff should be selected with care, and all should have a tuberculin skin test and chest x-ray at the time of employment. Many inherent unknown factors make it difficult to set forth a uniform procedure for surveillance testing of personnel. A recent recommendation[15] suggests the recognition of "safe" and "unknown" laboratories.

The **safe laboratory** is one in which personnel are carefully trained, all safety equipment is routinely monitored, and routine skin testing has yielded no recent converters to the tuberculin test. With such documented information, tuberculin-negative personnel need be retested no more than annually, and x-rays would be required only for symptomatic individuals.

The **unknown laboratory** has no supportive data regarding tuberculin conversion rates, routine monitoring of safety equipment, or definitive safety training program. Here tuberculin-nega-

tive employees should be retested every 4-6 months until evidence suggests that tuberculin conversion is not a problem. Tuberculin-positive personnel should have x-rays semiannually until observation of tuberculin-negative staff indicates this is not necessary (no converters found). A strict safety program should be established and safety equipment should routinely be monitored.

If an employee converts his skin test to positive, he should be referred to a physician for isoniazid preventive therapy or treatment. Under such conditions, the employee and his administrator should check laboratory procedures of all personnel and re-evaluate the efficiency of all safety equipment.

ISOLATION OF MYCOBACTERIA FROM CLINICAL MATERIAL
Collection of specimens

Definitive diagnosis of tuberculosis or other mycobacterioses in man is dependent (except for leprosy) on isolation of the offending mycobacterium in culture. For diagnostic purposes, clinical specimens should be collected before initiation of therapy, since even a few days of drug treatment may render the patient culture negative, thus leaving the bacteriologic confirmation in doubt. Optimal laboratory results are usually obtained under the following conditions:

1. Specimen containers should be clean and sterile, preferably used only once (plastic, disposable);
2. Multiple-use containers (usually glass) should be cleaned with dichromate sulfuric acid and sterilized before reuse;
3. A series of single specimens (3-5) collected on successive days is usually easier to manipulate in the laboratory and less likely to be contaminated, especially if sent by mail[16-18];
4. Specimens should be delivered to the laboratory as soon as possible;
5. If transportation to the laboratory is delayed, specimens should be refrigerated[18]; and
6. Specimen containers should be carefully sealed and packaged to avoid leakage or breakage in transit.[2, 15]

The microbiologist should provide clinical and nursing staff with instruction sheets on collection and proper transport of specimens. He should also report immediately any deviation from acceptable procedure and call attention of attending medical personnel to reasons for inadequate specimens (e.g., insufficient amount, improper packaging, excessive delay in transport, etc.). Successful cultivation of the pathogen requires the best specimen, properly collected, transported, and processed.

Sputum

Because attending personnel cannot always be present to ensure proper collection of sputum, the patient must be instructed in securing the most useful specimen. He should be told to rinse his mouth free of food and residual mouthwash or oral drugs prior to sputum collection. Nasopharyngeal discharge and saliva are **not** sputum, and patients should be told to collect only the exudative material brought up from the lungs after a deep, productive cough. The specimen should be collected only in a laboratory-approved container, clearly labeled with the patient's name or hospital number or both. Three to five single specimens (usually early morning samples) should be collected on successive days; from patients yielding strongly positive smears, 3 specimens may be enough, while suspected tuberculous patients whose bacilli are difficult to detect on smear should submit 5 or more specimens. For patients who are nonproductive or from whom mycobacteria are isolated with difficulty, collect 24 to 48-hour pooled specimens.[19]

If natural expectoration is insufficient or absent, sputum may be obtained by **nebulization technics.**[20] Inhalation of warm, aerosolized, sterile 10% sodium chloride solution is irritant enough to induce cough and production of a thin, watery "sputum" sample. Because they resemble saliva, induced sputa should be so identified on the laboratory request slip. Aerosol induction must be carried out in an isolated area with a proper exhaust system designed to protect personnel from the droplet nuclei discharged by the patient being induced.

Gastric lavage

Gastric lavage may be performed when patients are unwilling or unable to cooperate in provision of direct or induced sputum (e.g., children, patients with neurologic disorders, comatose patients), when radiologic evidence suggests tuberculosis but sputum is consistently negative, or when patients are suspected of submitting sputum other than their own. The specimen is collected early in the morning on a fasting stomach, preferably while the patient is still in bed. Using a 50 ml syringe, 20-50 ml of sterile, distilled water is passed through a disposable, plastic tubing inserted into the stomach. The collected specimen should be processed promptly because mycobacteria die rapidly in gastric washings. If delay is anticipated (e.g., transportation), neutralization may be effected by the addition of 1.5 ml 40% disodium phosphate solution[21] or 2 pH 7.4 pHydrion buffer capsules (or tablets). Although induced sputum is preferable to and singularly more productive than gastric washing, when the latter is performed 30 minutes after sputum induction, the combined procedures yield more positive cultures than either procedure alone.[22]

Urine

In order of preference, urine specimens should be collected as single, early morning, voided, midstream specimens or 12 to 24-hour pooled samples.[23] Because bacterial populations may be diluted in large volumes of urine, the processing of multiple specimens may be necessary to demonstrate the presence of mycobacteria.

Other body fluids

Pleural, pericardial, spinal, synovial, and ascitic fluids, blood, bone marrow, and pus are commonly collected by the physician using aseptic aspiration or sterile surgical procedure. If immediate handling of the specimen by the microbiologist is not possible, sterile ammonium oxalate or heparin should be added to prevent clotting. By prior arrangement with the laboratory, aseptically collected fluids (without anticoagulants) may be inoculated directly into enriched Middlebrook 7H-9 (commercial) or serum-supplemented Proskauer-Beck (commercial) liquid media, in a ratio of 1 vol fluid to 5-10 vol medium. These media are incubated at 35-37 C in an atmosphere of 5-10% CO_2 with daily shaking. Smears should be made at weekly intervals, and when acid-fast bacilli are detected, the liquid medium is streaked onto Lowenstein-Jensen egg slants and Middlebrook 7H-10 (or 7H-11) agar. If the smear is negative after 4 weeks, the liquid medium should still be streaked to solid medium at weekly intervals for another 4 weeks.

Tissues

Surgical specimens must be collected aseptically and placed in sterile containers without preservatives or fixatives. If the specimen cannot be carried immediately to the laboratory or must be transported, maintain at 5-10 C or ship in dry ice.

Demonstration of organisms in stained smear preparations

Although smear examination is the least sensitive method for detection of mycobacteria and does not permit specific identification of the observed organisms, microscopic examination is valuable in the following ways: (1) it is the easiest, most rapid procedure that can be performed, thereby providing a presumptive diagnosis of mycobacterial disease; (2) it helps identify organisms other than mycobacteria in a disease process; (3) it can confirm that culture growth is acid-fast; and (4) it may be used to follow the progress of a known tuberculous patient on chemotherapy.

It has been repeatedly demonstrated[24-27] that patients who are smear positive provide the greatest threat to the community; they are the "infectious reservoirs," the source of spread of tubercle bacilli. Conversely, the smear-negative (even if culture positive) patient, or even the smear-positive case covered by adequate chemotherapy,[27] is less likely to spread the disease to his contacts. The current trend to treat tuberculosis in general hospitals and to release patients for continued treatment on an outpatient basis[27-29] is strongly influenced by smear examination[30]; thus it behooves the general hospital or outpatient clinic laboratory (i.e., level I, discussed earlier) to attain a high level of expertise in microscopic examination of acid-fast stained smears.

Direct smear

These should be prepared **only** under a biologic safety cabinet. New, clean, unscratched slides should be used. Select from the specimen the bloody, caseous, or purulent particles, and by means of an applicator stick or bacteriologic loop, streak the sample uniformly over an area approximately 1 × 3 cm on the slide. After the smear has air dried, it should be heat fixed either on an electric slide warmer (65-75 C) for 2 hours or by passing 3 times through the blue cone of a Bunsen burner flame; do not scorch the smear.

Concentration methods for smear only

Technics here described should be used in level I laboratories that do not have biologic safety cabinets yet must prepare and examine smears for the presence of acid-fast bacilli. These procedures kill most, if not all, mycobacteria, hence if the physician also requests a culture, a second specimen from the patient should be sent to the next higher level laboratory (level II or III), where facilities for culture and handling of viable organisms are available.

Autoclave method[31]
1. Autoclave specimen 15 min at 121 C (15 psi).
2. Allow coagulated material to cool and settle.
3. Decant supernatant fluid; make smears from sediment. Although this method is used, some authors have reported autoclaving to reduce number of detectable acid-fast bacilli.[32]

Clorox method[33]
1. Add an equal volume Clorox to specimen; stopper securely.
2. Shake 10-15 min. Fill tube with sterile distilled water.
3. Centrifuge at 2000-3000 × g for 15 min.
4. Decant supernatant fluid; make smears from sediment. (Clorox will cause disintegration of bacilli if allowed to act too long, so smears should be prepared and examined promptly.)

Staining methods

A large number of staining procedures have been described, including the use of fluorochrome dyes and several cold-staining methods. Several procedures are detailed in Chapter 71. All of the technics are based on the relatively unique property of mycobacteria to retain the primary stain even after exposure to strong mineral acids or acid-alcohol, hence the term, acid-fast bacilli. The procedures detailed in Chapter 71 are the Ziehl-Neelsen stain, Kinyoun's cold stain, and fluorochrome staining with auramine O followed by counterstaining with either potassium permanganate or acridine orange. Each procedure is used successfully by the Mycobacteriology Branch at the Center for Disease Control in

Atlanta.[15] Great diligence must be exercised in the preparation and staining of smears to avoid such problems as poorly stained preparations or false-positive or false-negative reports. The following suggestions may help to avoid many problems.

1. Beware of insufficient destaining with acid-alcohol.
    a. Most mycobacteria are strongly acid-fast and are not easily decolorized
    b. Smears that are too thick are difficult to destain and, when counterstained, may obscure acid-fast bacilli.
2. Use contrasting counterstain
    a. Counterstain should not be so intense that it "hides" mycobacteria.
    b. Color-blind individuals may find fluorochrome staining procedures easier to examine.
3. Beware of false-positive smears. Common sources of acid-fast bacilli that can contribute to this problem are:
    a. Tap water and infrequently cleaned distilled water reservoirs. Check these sources from time to time to see if acid-fast bacilli can be detected.
    b. Ice-making machines; such ice is often used to facilitate passage of gastric tubes and may cause false-positive smears or cultures.
    c. Transfer of material from slide to slide in bulk-staining tanks. Stain slides individually.
    d. Transfer of "positive" flakes from thick slides to other slides via immersion oil. Don't make thick smears; carefully heat-fix smears; wipe oil immersion lens between slides; allow oil to free-fall from applicator onto smear, rather than touching applicator to slide.

Examination of smears

Careful smear examination is an essential part of today's tuberculosis control program. Training of the microscopist should emphasize the importance attached to the smear by the clinician who is considering discharge of his patient to a regimen of outpatient home treatment and possibly even to gainful employment.[27-30]

To encourage excellence in microscopic examination, it is necessary to have a good microscope and a comfortable work area. Methods for reading smears vary from laboratory to laboratory. We have had most success in examining smears by area covered, rather than by trying to establish a fixed time of examination for each smear. It is recommended that 3 longitudinal sweeps of the smear be made parallel to the length of the slide, regardless of how much time this takes. In this manner the microscopist should see 60-100 fields in 1 sweep or as many as 300 fields if he finds it necessary to examine 3 full sweeps. If the smear is moderately or heavily positive, of course, fewer fields need be examined and a report may be made even though less than 1 length of the smear has been examined.

Reporting results of smears

In order to provide clinically meaningful information, smear reports must be quantitated. A quantifiable decrease in the number of bacilli detectable in stained smears is concomitant with good response to chemotherapy, while stable or increasing bacillary numbers may suggest inadequate therapy or the emergence of drug-resistant tubercle bacilli. The method recommended by the American Lung Association[34] is commonly used.

Number of organisms seen	Report
3-9 per slide	Rare
10 or more per slide	Few
More than 1 per oil immersion field	Numerous

Recently the Mycobacteriology Branch of the Center for Disease Control has adopted a new method of smear examination reporting that provides semiquantitative reporting in roughly 10-fold increments.

Number of organisms seen	Report
None in 100 or more fields	No acid-fast bacilli found
1-9 per 100 fields	1+
1-9 per 10 fields	2+
1-9 per field	3+
10 or more per field	4+

The presence of 1 or 2 bacilli in the entire smear should not be reported unless confirmed by another smear. The microscopist might also report any deviations in normal staining characteristics of individual cells, odd cellular morphologies, or peculiar cellular arrangement if relevant.

The reader must remember that the stained smear is only presumptive evidence of mycobacterial disease. If the smear is being used just to monitor patient response to treatment of an already diagnosed disease, routine cultures need not be done. On the other hand, if precise identification of the disease agent has not been ascertained, then untreated specimens must be sent to the laboratory for culture and identification.

Demonstration of organisms by concentration and culture

Efficient digestion-decontamination procedures effectively homogenize the clinical specimens, destroy all (or most) contaminating organisms, permit survival of maximal numbers of mycobacteria, and enable ready concentration of bacilli by centrifugation or other means. Specimens that are not contaminated (e.g., surgically excised tissue or aseptically aspirated material from closed lesions) may be cultured directly without prior decontamination. All procedures for culture isolation must be carried out in a properly operating biologic safety cabinet.

Concentration methods for culture

Many concentration methods have been described, nearly all of which will kill a certain proportion of the mycobacteria in the specimen. For this reason it is necessary to follow precisely the step-wise procedures in all digestion/decontamination methods. Maximal yield of mycobacteria should be expected from use of the mildest digestants that still effectively suppress contaminants. Several of the more widely recommended digestion procedures are detailed here.

N-acetyl-L-cysteine-sodium hydroxide (NALC-NaOH) method [13, 15, 35, 36]

Prepare the volume of NALC-NaOH needed as follows:

| Volume of digestant needed (ml) | Mix indicated amounts (ml) | | Add NALC (g) |
	4% NaOH	2.9% Sodium citrate	
50	25	25	0.25
100	50	50	0.50
200	100	100	1.00
500	250	250	2.50
1000	500	500	5.00

The NaOH and sodium citrate may be prepared and sterilized (by autoclaving) in advance of mixing. Prepare only the volume of digestant actually needed, because mucolytic activity of NALC is lost on standing (use within 18-24 hours).

Sputum specimens (natural or induced)
1. Transfer about 10 ml sputum to a sterile 50 ml screw-capped centrifuge tube. Smaller tubes may be used for lesser volume specimens; however, volume of sample should not exceed one-fifth capacity of tube.
2. Add an amount of NALC-NaOH solution equal to volume of sputum. Tighten cap of tube and mix by swirling on a test tube mixer until liquefied (usually 5-20 s). Avoid extreme agitation or frothing as this will oxidize and inactivate the NALC; the centrifugal mixing afforded by the test tube mixer provides ideal mixing action.
3. Let stand for 15 min at room temperature to effect decontamination. If more active decontamination is desired, it is advisable to increase concentration of NaOH shown in preceding table to 5% or 6% rather than increasing time of exposure of specimen to digestant.
4. Fill tubes to within 1.25 cm of top with sterile distilled water or pH 6.8 phosphate buffer (0.067M). Tighten screw cap and swirl by hand to mix.
5. Centrifuge at 2000-3000 × g for 15 min using aerosol-free, sealed centrifuge cups.
6. Decant supernatant fluid into a discard can containing disinfectant, flame lip of tube, and replace cap.
7. With a sterile pipet add 1-2 ml sterile 0.2% bovine albumin fraction V (Armour Pharmaceutical Co., Scottsdale, Ariz., or Pentex, Inc., Kankakee, Ill.).* Shake gently to resuspend sediment; neutralization of this final suspension is not required.

---

*Prepare in 0.85% sodium chloride solution, adjust to pH 6.8-7.0, and sterilize by Seitz filtration.

8. For diagnostic culture, resuspended sediment (both undiluted and after a 10-fold dilution in sterile saline or water) should be inoculated onto the surface of at least 2 kinds of media (preferably an egg base, such as Lowenstein-Jensen, and an agar base, such as Middlebrook 7H-10). Dilution of resuspended sediment acts to decrease the concentration of toxic substances that may inhibit growth of mycobacteria.

9. Make a smear of undiluted sediment by spreading a drop over a 1 × 2 cm area on a clean, new microscope slide. Carefully heat-fix before staining. If sufficient sediment is available, smears may be made with sterile applicator stick or flamed inoculating loop *before* resuspension in bovine albumin solution.

10. If direct drug susceptibility tests are to be performed, two 100-fold dilutions of resuspended sediment are prepared, based on numbers of acid-fast bacilli observed on smear.

No. of acid-fast bacilli per oil immersion field	Approximate dilutions of sediment to be used as inocula
<1	Undiluted and 10^{-2}
1-10	10^{-1} and 10^{-3}
>10	10^{-2} and 10^{-4}

Gastric lavage specimens

1. Gastric lavage specimens are collected in 50 or 250 ml screw-capped tubes (depending on volume of water used for lavage).
2. If specimen is especially mucoid, 50-100 mg NALC powder is added, screw cap is tightened, and tube is mixed by hand or with a test tube mixer just prior to centrifugation.
3. After this step, or for more fluid gastric lavage specimens, centrifuge at 2000-3000 × *g* for 30 min.
4. Pour off supernatant fluid, resuspend sediment in 2-5 ml sterile distilled water, add an equal volume of NALC-NaOH solution, and proceed as for sputum.

Tissue

1. Seek advice of surgeon or pathologist regarding portion(s) of tissue most likely to be productive of positive cultures.
2. Grind tissue with sterile tissue grinder, using sterile 0.85% saline or 0.2% bovine albumin.
3. If tissue has been aseptically handled since sterile excision, homogenized material may be inoculated directly into both liquid and solid media. If there is doubt about aseptic handling of tissue, a portion may be inoculated directly to media, while another sample of the homogenate may be treated as for sputum.

• • •

Depending on the physical nature of and the care exercised in handling other specimens submitted for culture, the judicious selection and use of appropriate laboratory procedures will usually provide positive evidence of mycobacterial disease.

Zephiran–trisodium phosphate (Z-TSP) method[13,15,37]

Reagent

1. Dissolve 1 kg trisodium phosphate ($Na_3PO_4 \cdot 12H_2O$) in 4 L hot distilled water. To this add 7.5

ml conc (17%) benzalkonium chloride (Zephiran, Winthrop Laboratories, New York, N.Y.). Mix well and store at room temperature.

Procedure

1. Add to the specimen a quantity of Z-TSP equal to the volume of the specimen.
2. Tighten screw cap securely and agitate vigorously on a shaking machine for 30 min.
3. Let stand 20-30 min without further shaking.
4. Transfer to 50 ml screw-capped centrifuge tube, and centrifuge at 2000-3000 × *g* for 20 min.
5. Decant supernatant fluid, and resuspend sediment in 20 ml pH 6.6 Tamol-N neutralizing buffer (Difco Laboratories, Detroit, Mich.).
6. Centrifuge again for 20 min, and discard supernatant fluid.
7. Use a sterile capillary pipet to mix sediment, and inoculate 3 drops onto each tube or plate of medium.

Sodium hydroxide (NaOH) method[13,38]

NaOH is extremely toxic for mycobacteria as well as contaminants; therefore care must be exercised in the use of this digestion procedure, and indicated timing for each step must be strictly adhered to. The digestant, 2% to 4% NaOH (lowest concentration compatible with effective digestion and decontamination), is prepared in volume and sterilized by autoclaving. A 2.0N HCl solution may be prepared to neutralize the NaOH solution after digestion; dilute 33 ml concentrated HCl to 200 ml with water (*always* add acid to water, never the reverse) and sterilize by autoclaving. A solution of phenol red pH color indicator may be used separately or combined with the HCl solution.*

Procedure

1. Add an equal volume of appropriate NaOH solution to specimen contained in Teflon-lined, screw-capped tubes, and securely tighten caps.
2. Shake vigorously in a paint-conditioning machine or test tube mixer for 15-20 min.
3. Centrifuge specimen for 15 min at 2000-3000 × *g*.
4. Decant supernatant fluid and neutralize sediment with HCl. Either add 1 drop indicator solution, followed by dropwise addition of HCl, or use HCl–phenol red indicator. Add HCl until indicator changes from red to first persistent yellow. Resuspend sediment and inoculate desired media.

Oxalic acid method[15,39]

The oxalic acid method is especially useful when treating sputa from patients whose specimens consistently are contaminated with *Pseudomonas* species. Prepare 5% oxalic acid by dissolving 50 g oxalic acid in sufficient distilled water to make 1 L. A 4% NaOH solution together with a solution of phenol red indicator is used to neutralize the digested specimen.

Procedure

1. Add an equal volume 5% oxalic acid to speci-

---

*Hydrochloric acid–phenol red indicator: Combine 20 ml of phenol red (0.4% in 4% NaOH) and 85 ml concentrated HCl with sufficient distilled water to make 1000 ml.

men, stopper securely, and mix on a test tube mixer.

2. Let stand 30 min; shake occasionally.
3. Fill tube with sterile saline or water and centrifuge at 2000-3000 × *g* for 20 min.
4. Decant supernatant fluid and neutralize sediment with NaOH until first appearance of a persistent pink tinge in phenol red indicator.
5. Inoculate desired media.

Sulfuric acid (H₂SO₄) method[15,40]

This procedure is especially useful for thin body fluids that do not contain much tenacious organic debris. It is often recommended for urine specimens (see following). Prepare 4% sulfuric acid by *slowly* adding 40 ml concentrated H₂SO₄ to 960 ml distilled water. A 4% NaOH solution and phenol red indicator may be used for neutralization.

Procedure
1. Centrifuge entire specimen at 2000-3000 × *g* for 30 min.
2. Decant supernatant fluid; if several centrifuge tubes were used for 1 specimen, pool sediments, using 1 or 2 ml sterile distilled water, if necessary.
3. Add an equal volume H₂SO₄ to suspended sediment, mix, and let stand 15 min at room temperature.
4. Fill tube with sterile saline or water and again centrifuge at 2000-3000 × *g* for 20 min.
5. Add 1 drop phenol red indicator, and neutralize sediment with NaOH until appearance of first persistent pink tinge.
6. Inoculate desired media.

Cetylpyridinium chloride (CPC) method[41]

The CPC method was recently proposed as a means of decontaminating sputa in transit, so that, on arrival in the laboratory, the specimens need only be concentrated by centrifugation prior to inoculaton onto media. Preliminary observations suggest that this method provides a significant decrease in laboratory time required for processing, increased numbers of cultures positive for mycobacteria (especially bacilli other than *M. tuberculosis),* and less contamination than the NaCl-NaOH method. The success of this procedure centers on the use of the cationic quaternary ammonium compound, cetylpyridinium chloride as a decontaminating agent. Effective liquefaction of sputum is achieved with 2% sodium chloride. The digestant/decontaminant (CPC) solution is prepared by dissolving 10 g CPC and 20 g NaCl in 1L water. The solution is self-sterilizing and remains stable for long periods if tightly capped and stored at room temperature protected from excessive heat and light. Any crystals that form in this working solution may be dissolved with gentle heat.

Procedure
1. Collect sputa in 50 ml screw-capped centrifuge tubes.
2. Add an equal volume CPC solution, securely tighten caps, and shake by hand until specimens appear liquid.
3. Package specimens in double mailing containers[15]

and send to laboratory for processing. Specimen is thoroughly digested and decontaminated in transit.

4. On receipt in laboratory, fill each sputum container nearly to top with sterile distilled water, replace cap, and securely tighten.
5. Centrifuge at 2000 × *g* for 20 min.
6. Decant supernatant fluid and resuspend sediment in 1-2 ml sterile water, saline, or 0.2% bovine albumin fraction V (Armour Pharmaceutical Co. or Pentex, Inc.).
7. Inoculate resuspended sediment onto Lowenstein-Jensen medium. NOTE: Residual bacteriostatic activity of CPC for mycobacteria prohibits inoculation of specimens onto Middlebrook 7H-10 medium (bacteriostatic activity of CPC is neutralized by egg medium but not by Middlebrook 7H-10).

• • •

The detachment of smears of concentrated sediments from the microscope slide is rarely a problem if one is careful to clean slide with alcohol just before use and if heat fixation of smears is properly done. On occasion, however, when using digestants that contain detergents or reagents that lower the viscosity of the specimen, smears may slide off the slide during the staining process. If this is a problem, the slide surface may be covered with a thin film of a serum or albumin fixative before the smear is made. Drying and fixation of smears may then be performed as described earlier for direct smears.

Serum fixative for smears
1. Mix 25 ml sterile serum with 75 ml sterile distilled water in a sterile container.
2. Add 1 or 2 drops 1:10 solution of thimerosal (Merthiolate) as preservative and store at 5 C.
3. Dilute 1:4 with sterile distilled water before use.

Albumin fixative for smears
1. mix 50 ml egg white with 50 ml glycerol and filter through gauze into a sterile container.
2. Add a few small crystals of thymol as preservative and store at room temperature.
3. Dilute 1:4 with sterile distilled water before use.

Culture methods

Although microscopy is a valuable tool in modern day tuberculosis control programs, it does not enable precise species identification of the causative agent of mycobacterial disease. For this reason the organism must be recovered on culture medium to permit definitive diagnosis of the pathogen.

The literature is replete with different formulations of media that have been suggested for the cultivation of mycobacteria. Most of these are variations of egg-potato–base or serum-agar–base formulations, and the selection of any one medium is based as much on institutional tradition or personal experience as on any other factor. A number of variables contribute to the preparation of a good medium, including such things as purity of component ingredients, care used in preparation and sterilization, pH, exposure of final product to light, method and length of storage before use, and proper environment for incubation. Once adapted to artificial cultivation, mycobacteria are among the least fastidious of the pathogenic microroganisms; however, the need for the bacilli to accomodate to an in vitro environment following their removal from a rich, in vivo milieu often necessitates a period of adaptation. This bacillary adaptation to an extra-tissue, "test tube" existence commonly dictates the need for a richer primary isolation medium in order for the laboratory to confirm a clinical diagnosis of mycobacterial disease.

Choice of medium and media for routine diagnostic use

An ideal medium should (1) support early and luxuriant growth from small inocula, (2) permit preliminary separation of mycobacteria based on pigment production and colonial morphology, (3) suppress the growth of contaminants, (4) enable performance of reliable drug susceptibility tests, and (5) be economical and easy to prepare. No single medium meets all these requirements, but a number of them have been widely used and accepted.

Among the very popular egg-base media, the 2 most widely used are the **American Trudeau Society** (ATS) medium[15,42] and the **Lowenstein-Jensen** medium.[15] Of the agar-base media, the most popular are **Dubos oleic acid–albumin agar,**[13] **Middlebrook 7H-10** agar,[13,15] and **Middlebrook 7H-11** agar.[43] The agar-base media are commonly prepared from commercially available powdered bases and enrichments. Numerous other media are available; however, because of limited use or only passing popularity, they will not be mentioned (for Media, see Chapter 72).

Because different strains of mycobacteria may grow better on one medium than another, it is recommended that at least 2 media be used for routine diagnostic purposes.

Other factors affecting growth. Perhaps more important than the kind of medium selected for culture of mycobacteria is the actual care employed in its preparation. All glassware and equipment must be thoroughly clean and sterile (when so indicated). To ensure reproducibility of media, all reagents must be freshly prepared from chemicals of certified purity, using freshly distilled water. Media formulations and directions for preparation must be precisely followed. The media preparation room must be kept clean and free of dust and preferably should be located in an isolated area where traffic flow is minimal. Wet mopping of floors, disinfectant swabbing of counters, dust-free filters in air intakes, and UV irradiation of upper air (when room is not in use) all serve to minimize air contaminants. Strict aseptic technique must be used when adding heat-labile enrichments or drugs to media. Sterilizing capabilities of filters (Seitz, sintered glass, or membrane) and autoclaves must be monitored periodically to ensure that they are functioning properly.

Excessive light and heat must be avoided in the preparation of the various Middlebrook types of media (7H-9, 7H-10, 7H-11), to minimize chances for formation of toxic formaldehyde.[53] The addition of 0.1% L-aspartic acid (potassium salt) to the basal Middlebrook 7H-10 medium greatly enhances niacin production by *M. tuberculosis* growing on this clear agar medium.[54]

If *M. bovis* is suspected, it is advisable to enrich the medium with 0.2% pyruvate[55,56] and to omit glycerol because the latter is known to inhibit bovine tubercle bacilli.[57,58] When egg-base medium is used, the eggs should be carefully scrubbed in soap solution prior to cracking, in order to minimize carry over of contaminants from the egg shells.

Inoculation and incubation of media

A variety of methods are used for inoculating media: bacteriologic loops, disposable straws, cotton-tipped applicator sticks, and capillary and serologic pipets. Commonly the sediment is spread evenly over the surface of the medium, although when capillary pipets are used to inoculate plates of media (e.g., Middlebrook 7H-10), the inoculum often is deposited as a series of discrete drops that are touched to the medium just before they "free fall" from the pipet (this, of course, is to minimize spatter and aerosol production from free-falling droplets).

After inoculation, tubes should be incubated for at least 1 week in a slanting position to ensure even distribution of growth. Thereafter, if shelf space is needed, the tubes may be placed upright. Incubation should continue for a minimum of 8 weeks at 35-37 C, with tubes being examined weekly for evidence of growth. If the culture inoculum was derived from superficial areas of the body, incubation of a duplicate set of inoculated media should be made at 30-33 C.

The various clear agar-base media (Middlebrook 7H-10 and 7H-11) are preferably prepared in plastic Petri dishes. After inoculation they are placed into clear CO_2-permeable polyethylene bags (do not stack plates more than 6 high), media side down, and placed in an incubator in which a CO_2 concentration of 5-10% can be maintained. If a CO_2-incubator is not available, 2 alternative methods may be employed.

1. Small air-tight boxes constructed of metal or plastic can be built to fit on the incubator shelves. Inlet and outlet petcock valves may be built into the boxes, and once daily these boxes, with the inoculated plates inside, may be flushed with a compressed mixture of 10% CO_2 and 90% air.

2. "Mini" CO_2-incubators may be made using 7 × 14 in. CO_2-impermeable Mylar plastic bags.[44,45] A piece of 2½ in. square silver ducting tape may be used to affix to the Mylar bag a 1 × 1 in. square of $1/_{16}$ in. thick neoprene rubber. Six or 8 plates (stacked in 2 piles, each 3 or 4 plates high) may be placed in the bag and the bag opening closed by twisting and sealing with masking tape. A vacuum line may be constructed as shown

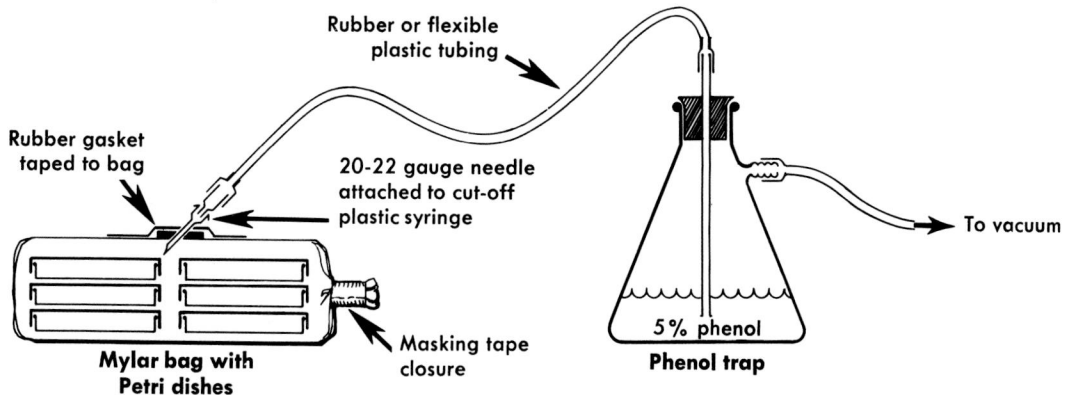

Fig. 78-1. Schematic drawing of a vacuum line to be used for evacuating air from Mylar bag "mini" CO_2 incubators.

in Fig. 78-1, using a 1 L side-arm Erlenmeyer flask, rubber pressure tubing, and the barrel of a plastic 1 ml syringe to which is attached a 20- or 22-gauge needle. By passing the needle carefully through the rubber gasket, the air may be evacuated from the Mylar bag through a reservoir of 5% phenol (a few milliliters of an antifoam solution in the reservoir prevents excessive frothing). The bag is then reinflated with a mixture of 10% CO_2 and 90% air; it is necessary that the cylinder of compressed gas be fitted with a step-down pressure gauge that will enable pressure control of 1 or 2 psi. As before, a rubber hose with attached syringe barrel and 22-gauge needle may be attached to the compressed gas and the needle inserted through the gasket to enable inflation of the bag. (These mini-Mylar bag incubators must be evacuated and refilled 3 times weekly to maintain the required CO_2 concentration.) The Mylar bags, with enclosed plates, may then be placed on the shelf of an incubator having the proper temperature for culture isolation.

The growth of most strains of mycobacteria, and especially tubercle bacilli, is stimulated by carbon dioxide. The early studies of Novy and Soule[46] on the effect of CO_2 on mycobacteria were confirmed by others.[47-50] A concentration of 10% CO_2 was shown[51] to be stimulatory for *M. tuberculosis* grown on Middlebrook 7H-10 agar. Although most attention has been directed to the CO_2 stimulation of mycobacteria growing on Middlebrook 7H-10 agar, Whitcomb et al.[52] showed a similar effect on acid-fast bacilli growing on egg-base medium.

Examination of cultures

It is essential to establish a uniform procedure for reading and recording cultural observations. Whether one employs egg- or agar-base medium (or both), it is advisable to use some type of magnification to visualize the colonies; a hand lens (3-10×), lamp magnifier, or dissecting microscope (10-50×) may be employed. With this method, young colonies may be observed at an early stage of growth, detailed morphology of mature colony forms noted, and observation of thin, transparent colony forms of some mycobacteria facilitated.[15, 59-62]

All cultures should be examined 5-7 days after inoculation and at least weekly thereafter for 8 weeks before discarding as negative; although longer incubation may yield more positive results, the low yield from such cultures is generally counteracted by the processing of more specimens from the same patient. If facilities permit, however, prolonged incubation in selected cases may be advisable.

Reporting culture results

The number of days required for colonies to appear (growth rate) and the temperature at which growth occurred must be recorded, as well as the quantity of growth. A convenient way to record amount of growth is as follows.[15]

No colonies	Negative
<50 colonies	Actual count
50-100 colonies	1+
100-200	2+
200-500 colonies (almost confluent)	3+
>500 colonies (confluent)	4+

Additional observations to record on the primary isolate would include the following.

Pigment production. The mycobacteria may be categorically placed into 3 large groups on the basis of pigment formation. These observations are best recorded on cultures having isolated colonies; hence, if growth is confluent, fresh subcultures should be prepared using inocula that will yield individual colonies.

1. *Photochromogens.* These are organisms whose colonies are white, cream, or buff (i.e., nonpigmented) when grown in the dark and that become pigmented only after light exposure.

2. *Scotochromogens.* These are organisms

whose colonies reveal yellow to orange or red pigment both in the dark and the light; the pigment may intensify if cultures are exposed to light continuously for 2 weeks.

3. *Nonphotochromogens*. These are organisms that normally are nonpigmented or at most may possess only pale pastel pigments; in either case, the pigment is unaffected by light exposure.

Colony morphology. On culture media inoculated with bacterial suspensions sufficiently diluted to yield isolated colonies, individual colony types may be observed and described and may often prove valuable in the differential identification of the cultured organism. The reader is referred to earlier publications for descriptions and photographs of mycobacterial colonies.[15,59-62]

As will be discussed later, the few simple observations of growth rate, temperature of growth, pigment, and colonial morphology enable a preliminary subgrouping of the mycobacteria that greatly facilitates the more precise identification based on a number of in vitro tests.

Demonstration of organisms by animal inoculation

With the more refined culture methods now available and the processing of multiple specimens from the same patient, it usually is not necessary to resort to animal inoculation. In rare instances animal inoculation may be a valuable adjunct to culture procedures, e.g., in sputa that are consistently contaminated on culture, in urine specimens from patients with repeatedly negative cultures but in whom tuberculosis is still suspected, and in aseptically collected body fluids in which organisms may be few in number and every attempt is being made to establish the diagnosis of tuberculosis. Specimens submitted for animal inoculation should also be inoculated onto culture medium because some organisms (mycobacteria other than tubercle bacilli and some isoniazid-resistant tubercle bacilli) may fail to produce progressive disease in laboratory animals. Except as cited previously, and as a matter of policy, specimens for animal inoculation should be discouraged or referred to reference laboratories.

Choice of animal

The guinea pig is the animal of choice whenever confirmation of a diagnosis of tuberculosis in man is needed; it is extremely susceptible to infection with tubercle bacilli and can effectively control most contaminants present in clinical specimens, thereby minimizing the need for toxic decontaminants (NaOH concentrations as low as 0.25% commonly provide sufficient decontamination of specimens for animal inoculation). Young, tuberculin-negative guinea pigs of either sex (do not mix the sexes in 1 cage), weighing 250-400 g, are recommended. Animals should have negative skin tests when tuberculin tested with 25 TU (in 0.1 ml) commercially available Tween-stabilized PPD (250 TU PPD from Panray may be diluted 1:10 in isotonic 0.067M [$^1/_{15}$M] pH 7.3 phosphate-buffered saline containing 0.005% Tween 80). Tuberculin (0.1 ml containing 25 TU) should be injected intradermally into the shaved flank of the guinea pig with a 26- or 27-gauge needle. At 24 or 48 hours after the injection the diameter of the erythematous reaction (if present) should be measured with a millimeter ruler. After animals have been inoculated with clinical material suspected of containing tubercle bacilli, a positive reaction to a repeat tuberculin testing at 4 or 6 weeks suggests a diseased animal; a 24- or 48-hour reaction measuring 10 mm or more may be used as indication that the animal is diseased and ready for autopsy. If reaction is negative, autopsy animals after 8 weeks.

Other animals and fowl (e.g., rabbits, chickens, quail) have been used in the past for differential identification of such mycobacterial species as *M. bovis* and *M. avium*. Currently available in vitro test procedures for specific identification of mycobacteria are generally easy to perform, yield highly reliable results in much less time than that required for animal tests, and are significantly less expensive to perform. For these reasons there is no longer any justification for maintaining or using diverse animal or fowl species in the clinical mycobacteriology laboratory.

Care of animals and quarters

Guinea pigs should be housed in dry, well-ventilated, well-lighted, and properly air-conditioned rooms that are frequently cleaned and disinfected. Wall- and ceiling-mounted ultraviolet lights minimize air contaminants or the rarely produced droplet nuclei containing tubercle bacilli. Separate rooms should be available for normal, noninfected animals and for infected test animals. Cages should be spacious and easily handled, cleaned, and sterilized.

Guinea pigs should be fed a vitamin C–fortified, pelletized food. Supplementing the diet with assorted vegetable greens should be discouraged because of the potentially harmful effects (e.g., diarrhea) of some greens. Only authorized personnel should be allowed in the animal quarters.

A well-equipped animal complex should include cleaning and disinfection supplies, an incinerator for disposing of carcasses, a wash basin with foot-operated controls, a shower room, separate clothes-changing room with lockers, a supply of protective clothing to be worn during inoculation and autopsy of animals, and one or more biologic safety cabinets.

Preparation of specimens for inoculation

Add to the specimen (e.g., sputum or urine) sufficient 4% sodium hydroxide to provide a final concentration of 0.25%. Mix by hand or with a test tube mixer and treat as for culturing. After centrifugation, neutralize the sediment and re-suspend it in 0.2% bovine albumin fraction V (Armour Pharmaceutical Co. or Pentex, Inc). Save a portion of this resuspended sediment in the freezer (-70 C) for reinoculation in the event that an animal dies prematurely.

Noncontaminated fluids from enclosed spaces or aseptically homogenized tissues may be in-oculated directly into guinea pigs without the initial decontamination step.

Route of inoculation

As a guard against premature death of one of the animals, inoculate at least 2 guinea pigs. As much as 2 or 3 ml resuspended sediment may be inoculated subcutaneously in the groin area. In-jection of larger volumes (up to 20 ml/animal) of sample (e.g., aseptically collected fluids or tissue homogenates) may be facilitated by distributing the inoculum into left and right inguinal and axil-lary areas and into several supra-abdominal or suprathoracic sites. Since draining abscesses may form at the site(s) of inoculation, such infected animals must be handled with care.

Results of infection

Depending on the number of tubercle bacilli injected and their virulence, the lymph nodes draining the inoculation site may become hyper-trophied (detectable by palpation) and an ulcera-tive nodule may appear within 10 to 14 days after injection. This, of itself, is strongly suggestive of tuberculosis. From this initial site the organisms move to the local and regional lymph nodes, into the lymphatic system, and thence to the vascular system where they are disseminated throughout the body. In the guinea pig the organs most ob-viously involved are the lung, spleen, and liver. Animals may be autopsied following response to tuberculin testing (mentioned earlier) or at 8 weeks after initial infection.

Autopsy and examination for disease

All autopsies should be performed only by trained professional personnel and only in a bio-logic safety cabinet. Acid-fast bacilli must be demonstrated by smear and culture before a posi-tive diagnosis is reported. Sacrifice the animals by placing in a tightly covered container with a chloroform-soaked cotton pad. Smears and cul-tures may be made from the softened caseous material from local and regional lymph nodes. Of the visceral organs, tuberculous involvement of the spleen is most easily detected; there is marked splenomegaly with or without prominent surface nodules having a gray or creamy yellow color. Raised pearly gray or dirty yellow nodules are the characteristic lung lesions commonly ob-served. Involvement of the liver is not always obvious; one may see a rough, granular, dull (not shiny) surface with or without flat, gray, or en-larged yellow caseous areas. Smears and cultures from these 3 major visceral organs, and especially from suspect lesions, must be made. If sterile

instruments and aseptic technic are employed, decontamination of material from these lesions may not be necessary prior to culture. The diffi-culty in maintaining sterile conditions during guinea pig autopsy usually mandates the con-comitant cultivation of lesional material follow-ing some decontamination procedure.

Reliability of animal tests

Other organisms (e.g., *Coccidioides immitis*, species of *Brucella* and *Salmonella*, and some streptococci) may produce pathology in the guinea pig that is indistinguishable grossly from tuberculosis.[63,64] Mycobacteria other than tuber-cle bacilli and certain drug-resistant (notably isoniazid-resistant) tubercle bacilli may be in-capable of producing disease in guinea pigs or other laboratory animals, even though they may be pathogenic for man. For these reasons, it is necessary (1) that all suspected pathologic changes in the guinea pig be confirmed by smear and culture and (2) that the guinea pig test alone not be relied on to diagnose tuberculosis.

TESTS FOR DIFFERENTIAL IDENTIFICATION OF MYCOBACTERIA

The recognition that mycobacteria other than tubercle bacilli could produce disease in man stimulated more than a decade of research aimed at developing a series of in vitro tests for the differential identification of mycobacteria. The application of computer technology to the prin-ciples of numerical taxonomy permitted the evaluation of hundreds of in vitro tests on thou-sands of strains of mycobacteria, the end result being a sound taxonomic classification for the acid-fast bacilli. One thing, more than any other, has contributed both to the definition and inter-national acceptance of the many new species in the genus *Mycobacterium*, and that has been the cooperative efforts of the International Working Group on Mycobacterial Taxonomy (IWGMT), whose members worked unselfishly toward the realization of these taxonomic goals. The work of the IWGMT has enabled the establishment of a meaningful, clinically oriented taxon-omy.[9–11,65–67,94] Subsequent individual efforts permitted the judicious selection from this array of taxonomic features of a few "key tests" capable of identifying the most commonly encountered mycobacteria in specific clinical laboratories.[68–72] With these few basic tests, it often is possible to clearly segregate the potentially pathogenic from the commonly saprophytic mycobacteria. Although precise speciation may not always be realized, the clinical microbiologist may lump organisms of common disease potential into groups or complexes,[13–15] a subdivision that, in most cases, is wholly adequate for the clinician (see Table 78-1).

The in vitro tests detailed later are those that have found wide use in the differential identi-fication of mycobacteria encountered in the United States.[2,13,15,34] For optimal results and to

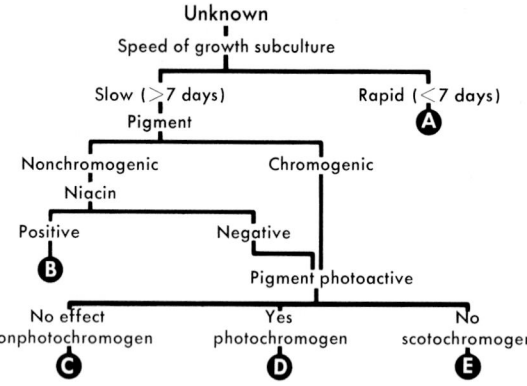

Fig. 78-2. Flow sheet for rough separation of mycobacteria. For species definition within each of groups *A-E* above, consult tables as follows: *A*, see Table 78-2; *B*, see Table 78-3; *C*, see Table 78-4; *D*, see Table 78-5; *E*, see Table 78-6.

ensure continued competence in performance and interpretation of these tests, it is recommended that they be performed primarily by laboratories that handle sufficient numbers of cultures each week to develop an innate awareness of the pitfalls, exceptions, and other idiosyncrasies of each test. For ease in performance and economy of time all the in vitro tests should be set up on a given culture at the same time, rather than by use of the dichotomous approach of measuring one test character before deciding which one to select next. Once a preliminary subdivision of the organisms has been achieved based on pigment production and speed of growth (see Fig. 78-2), it is easier to select those tests of greatest value in confirming the identity of the isolate in question. Specific identification of a given unknown should never be decided by a single test or characteristic because individual strains may deviate from anticipated results of a given taxon.[72]

Arylsulfatase

The arylsulfatase test is most valuable in the differential identification of the potentially pathogenic, rapidly growing mycobacteria (the *M. fortuitum* complex) that commonly are positive within 3 days, while the normally saprophytic rapid growers are negative. Occasionally a 2-week arylfulfatase tests proves to be a helpful backup procedure for identification of other species of mycobacteria[15]; however, because of the relatively infrequent need for the 2-week test, it will not be further discussed. Two methods for performing the 3-day test are the Center for Disease Control (CDC) procedure and the Wayne modification.

Arylsulfatase—CDC method[15]

Reagents and materials
1. Prepare stock solution of substrate by dissolving 2.6 g phenolphthalein disulfate (tripotassium salt)

in 50 ml distilled water. Sterilize by membrane filtration and store in refrigerator.
2. Liquid medium for preceding substrate, available commercially, may be either Dubos Tween-albumin broth (with ADC enrichment) or Middlebrook 7H-9 broth (with ADC enrichment). Basal medium may be prepared in 180 ml amounts, and after autoclave sterilization, 20 ml enrichment is aseptically added to provide a total volume of 200 ml.
3. Aseptically add 2.5 ml stock substrate (see Step 1) to 200 ml complete broth. Dispense in 2 ml amounts into sterile 16 × 125 mm screw-capped test tubes. This represents the 0.001M substrate for the 3-day test. This finished medium may be stored at room temperature or at 5 C until needed.

As a quality control check on final medium, add a few drops of 2N sodium carbonate (10.6 g anhydrous Na_2CO_3 in 100 ml distilled water) to an uninoculated tube of medium; substrate medium should remain colorless. If it turns pink, this indicates that substrate has broken down, and medium must be discarded. In such cases powdered phenolphthalein disulfate salt may need to be purified. Sufficient purification may be effected by dissolving 3-5 g phenolphthalein disulfate in a minimal amount of distilled water and reprecipitating salt by addition of excess ethanol. Filter precipitated salt off on Buchner funnel, wash with fresh ethanol, dry, and bottle for use in preparation of fresh stock solution.

Controls
1. A tube of uninoculated substrate medium serves as a negative control.
2. Another tube inoculated with *M. fortuitum* should provide a positive control.

Procedure
1. Inoculate substrate medium with 0.1 ml of a 7 d liquid culture (Tween albumin **or** Middlebrook 7H-9 broth) of organism to be tested **or** a spadeful of organisms from a freshly grown slant culture. Incubate at 35-37 C.
2. After 3 days' incubation, remove tubes from incubator and add up to 6 drops 2N sodium carbonate solution. A positive reaction is indicated by an immediate color change from pink to red.
3. If desired, a set of color standards may be prepared to determine intensity of color reaction.[15]

Wayne's phenolphthalein sulfatase test[13,73]

Reagents and materials
1. To 100 ml melted Dubos oleic agar base (Difco Laboratories), add 1 ml glycerol and 65 mg phenolphthalein disulfate (tripotassium salt). Dispense 2 ml amounts into 18 × 160 mm flat-botton, screw-capped vials, and sterilize by autoclaving. Allow to harden with tubes in upright position. NOTE: Commercially available Wayne sulfatase agar (BBL), which already contains the substrate salt, may be used.
2. The control tubes and 2N carbonate solution are prepared as described previously in the CDC method.

Procedure
1. Prepare a barely turbid suspension of test organism by triturating a loopful or spadeful of bacilli in sterile water.
2. Inoculate 1 drop this suspension onto substrate agar.
3. Incubate at 35-37 C for 3 d.
4. Remove from incubator and add 1 ml sodium carbonate solution.

5. Observe for formation of a pink to red band on surface of agar.

Catalase

With the possible exception of some isoniazid-resistant mutants of *M. tuberculosis* and *M. gastri*, all mycobacteria possess catalase. Two modifications of the test for this substance—the semiquantitative and the pH 7/68 C tests—provide information of value in the taxonomy of mycobacteria.

Semiquantitative catalase test[13,15,74,75]

The semiquantitative catalase test divides the mycobacteria into 2 groups, those that produce less than 45 mm of bubbles and those that produce more. In general, *M. kansassii, M. simiae,* most scotochromogens, the normally saprophytic nonphotochromogens, and the rapid growers all produce more than 45 mm of bubbles in this crudely quantitative test. In contrast, the tubercle bacilli, *M. marinum, M. avium* complex, *M. xenopi,* and *M. gastri* produce less than 45 mm of bubbles.

Reagents and materials
1. Lowenstein-Jensen or other egg-base medium is dispensed in 5 ml amounts into 20 × 150 mm screw-capped test tubes. Medium is inspissated for 50 min at 85 C with tubes in an upright position. This provides a butt of solid medium rather than customary slant. NOTE: Lowenstein butt tubes are available commercially.
2. A 10% Tween 80 solution is prepared by mixing 10 ml Tween 80 with 90 ml distilled water and autoclaving for 10 min at 121 C. If Tween settles after autoclaving, swirl to resuspend. Store in refrigerator.
3. 30% Hydrogen peroxide (Superoxol). Store in refrigerator.
4. Just before use mix equal quantities of 10% Tween 80 and hydrogen peroxide. Approximately 1.0 ml mixture will be needed for each test.

Controls
1. An uninoculated tube of medium
2. A known low-catalase strain such as *M. gastri* or *M. avium* complex
3. A hyperactive strain, producing more than 45 mm of bubbles, e.g., *M. gordonae* or *M. terrae* complex

Procedure
1. Inoculate the surface of butt medium with 0.1 ml of a 7 d old liquid culture of the test organism or with a loopful of growth from an actively growing slant.
2. Incubate tubes at 35-37 C for **2 weeks** with **caps loosened.**
3. After incubation, add 1.0 ml Tween-peroxide mixture and allow to stand upright at room temperature for 5 min.
4. Measure in millimeters the height of the column of bubbles above the surface of the medium, and divide the test organisms into 2 groups, those yielding **more** and those yielding **less** than 45 mm of bubbles.

pH 7/68 C catalase test[13,15,76]

When suspended in pH 7 buffer and heated to 68 C for 20 minutes, some mycobacteria lose cat-alase activity; included in this group are *M. tuberculosis, M. bovis,* and *M. gastri.* This "hot catalase" test is especially valuable for strains of tubercle bacilli that are niacin negative or only weakly positive. All nonchromogenic slow growers should be subjected to this test.

Procedure
1. Scrape several spadesful of growth from culture slant of test organism and suspend in 0.5 ml pH 7, 0.067M (i.e., $^1/_{15}$M) phosphate buffer contained in a 16 × 125 mm screw-capped tube.
2. Place this suspension in a 68 C water bath or constant temperature block heater for 20 min. **Time and temperature are critical.**
3. Cool suspension to room temperature.
4. Add 0.5 ml Tween-peroxide mixture.
5. Observe tubes for formation of bubbles, and record as − or +.
6. Hold tubes 20 min before discarding as negative. NOTE: Do not shake tubes because Tween 80 alone may form bubbles when shaken, thereby giving a false-positive reaction.
7. Always include a negative control (e.g., *M. tuberculosis* or *M. gastri*) as well as a positive control (*M. gordonae* or *M. terrae* complex).

Growth rate[13,15]

This was alluded to earlier under "reporting culture results." The clinically significant mycobacteria may be roughly grouped into slow and rapid growers, the former taking more than 7 days to appear on culture media, while the latter are fully matured in less than 7 days (see Fig. 78-2 for this subdivision). Because some rapid growers may require several weeks to grow on primary isolation, it is imperative that proper growth rate be determined using subcultures.

Procedure
1. Either a 7-day broth culture or a saline suspension of organisms from a freshly grown slant is diluted sufficiently to yield isolated colonies.
2. Several 10-fold dilutions of the test organism are inoculated onto either an egg-base or agar-base medium (or both) and incubated at 35-37 C (other temperatures may be needed for organisms with more restricted temperature growth range).
3. Observe culture media at 5-7 days and then weekly thereafter for evidence of grossly visible colonies.

Iron uptake[13,15,70]

In this test, *M. fortuitum* is positive and *M. chelonei* commonly negative, while most other rapid growers are positive. Slow growers and most *M. flavescens* are negative.

Reagents and materials
1. Lowenstein-Jensen slants.
2. A 20% aqueous solution of ferric ammonium citrate. Dispense in small amounts (5-8 ml) and autoclave. If the solution becomes cloudy, discard and prepare fresh.

Controls
1. An uninoculated culture slant (negative)
2. A slant seeded with a known *M. fortuitum* (positive)

Procedure

1. Inoculate medium with 1 drop barely turbid suspension of test organism.
2. Incubate until colonies are grossly visible. Incubate uninoculated control tube at the same time.
3. To all tubes add sterile ferric ammonium citrate, using 1 drop citrate for each ml Lowenstein-Jensen medium (i.e., usually 6-8 drops/slant).
4. Reincubate cultures and examine weekly for 3 wk.
5. A positive reaction is recorded as a rusty brown color of the colonies and a tan color in the medium.

An alternative method for the iron uptake test is to add a final concentration of 2.5% ferric ammonium citrate to Lowenstein-Jensen medium before inspissation. The final medium appears "dirty green." Tube and inspissate as usual. To perform the test, inoculate both an iron citrate–containing slant and an iron citrate–free tube of Lowenstein-Jensen medium with 1 drop barely turbid suspension of the test organism, and incubate. With this method, the colonies and the medium will turn rusty brown as the iron uptake–positive cultures grow (i.e., there is no need to open the tube **after** growth has appeared to add the iron citrate solution). Cultures expected to be negative in this test either (1) will not grow or (2) will grow without observable browning of the colonies.

MacConkey agar[15, 76, 78]

The MacConkey agar test distinguishes the potentially pathogenic *M. fortuitum* complex from the normally saprophytic rapid growers, the former revealing growth and sometimes a color change in the medium within 5-11 days.

Reagents and materials

1. MacConkey agar **without** crystal violet, 20 ml per Petri plate
2. A 3 mm bacteriologic loop and a Petri dish turntable

Controls

1. An uninoculated plate of medium
2. A plate inoculated with *M. phlei* (negative)
3. A plate inoculated with *M. fortuitum* (positive)

Procedure

1. Place plate on turntable, spin table, and touch a loopful of test organism to center of spinning plate and gradually move loop to periphery of plate. This produces an inoculum in form of a spiral. (Alternatively, plates may be streaked as for isolated colonies, but results by this method are not as distinctive.)
2. Incubate plates at 35-37 C (plates may be stacked in an open Petri dish cannister).
3. Read at 5 and 11 d.
4. *M. fortuitum* and *M. chelonei* grow along most of length of spiral; a color change in medium may also be evident. When a very heavy inoculum is used, other rapid growers may grow along beginning of spiral.

Niacin test—Runyon modification[13,15,79]

Test all nonchromogenic mycobacteria for niacin production. Cultures should be 3-4 weeks old on egg-base medium and should have at least 50-100 colonies. (NOTE: Middlebrook 7H-10 medium may also be used provided it is supplemented with 0.1% potassium aspartate.[54] *M. tuberculosis* and the more rarely encountered *M. simiae* are niacin positive, while most other mycobacteria are negative.)

Reagents and materials

1. Screw-capped test tubes, 16 × 125 mm.
2. Sterile water or 0.85% saline.
3. Aniline (4% in 95% ethyl alcohol). Add 4.0 ml *colorless* aniline to alcohol; store at 5 C in a brown bottle. If solution turns yellow, discard and prepare a fresh solution.
4. Cyanogen bromide, 10% aqueous. Dissolve 5 g cyanogen bromide in 50 ml distilled water and store at 5 C in a refrigerator. If crystals appear in refrigerated solution, warm to room temperature to dissolve.

CAUTION: **Cyanogen bromide is tear gas and should be handled only in a well-ventilated safety cabinet. In acid solution it hydrolyzes to hydrocyanic acid; therefore niacin test tubes should be discarded into disinfectant made alkaline by the addition of NaOH.**

Controls

1. Reagent control run on uninoculated medium
2. A negative culture such as *M. gastri* or *M. avium* complex
3. A known positive *M. tuberculosis*

Procedure

1. Add 1.0 ml sterile water or saline to culture slant or Middlebrook 7H-10 drug-free control medium containing the test organism. If culture growth is confluent, puncture through it with a spade or pipet tip because niacin is extracted from the medium not from the bacterial colonies.
2. Place tube or plate so that fluid layers over colonies and allow to stand for 15 min.
3. Remove 0.5 ml extract to a screw-capped test tube.
4. Add 0.5 ml aniline, followed by 0.5 ml (i.e., equal volumes) cyanogen bromide.
5. Observe for a positive yellow color that should form immediately.
   NOTE: Instead of preparing aniline and cyanogen bromide solutions, one may place a commercially available niacin test strip into aqueous extract from step 3.[80,81] Follow manufacturer's directions.

Nitrate reduction[13,15,82]

All mycobacteria should be tested for nitrate-reducing ability about 3 to 4 weeks after colonies are grossly visible on the medium. Species that reduce nitrate include *M. tuberculosis*, *M. kansasii*, *M. szulgai*, *M. flavescens*, the *M. terrae* complex, and most rapid growers (an exception in the latter instance is *M. chelonei*).

Reagents and materials

1. Screw-capped tubes, 16 × 125 mm.
2. Water bath or constant temperature block heater at 37 C.
3. Substrate of 0.01M $NaNO_3$ in M/45 phosphate buffer, pH 7.0, prepared as follows:

$NaNO_3$	0.085 g
KH_2PO_4	0.117 g
$Na_2HPO_4 \cdot 12H_2O$	0.485 g
Distilled water	100.0 ml

4. Test-developing solutions are prepared as follows:

a. *HCl solution* (1:2 dil.). A 1:2 dilution of conc HCl. Add 10 ml HCl to 10 ml distilled water.
b. *Sulfanilamide solution.* Dissolve 0.2 g sulfanilamide in 100 ml distilled water.
c. Dissolve 0.1 g n-naphthylethylenediamine dihydrochloride in 100 ml distilled water.

Store all test solutions and substrate in the dark in the refrigerator. If a precipitate forms in solutions b or c or the reagents change color, discard and prepare fresh reagents.
5. If desired, a color standard may be prepared to help read the test.[15]

Controls
1. A reagent control without organisms (negative)
2. A substrate inoculated with *M. tuberculosis* (positive)

Procedure
1. Triturate 1 loopful or spadeful of organisms from a 4-w-old culture into 2 ml nitrate substrate solution contained in a 16 × 125 mm tube.
2. Incubate in a 37 C water bath for 2 h.
3. Remove from water bath.
4. Add 1 drop HCl solution.
5. Add 2 drops sulfanilamide solution and 2 drops naphthylethylenediamine solution.
6. Examine immediately for a pink to red color.

Result. The formation of a pink to deep red color is a positive test. If no color change occurs, confirm the results by adding a small amount of powdered zinc; this causes an immediate reduction of nitrate to nitrite with the formation of a red color (confirmation of a negative reaction). If no color forms following addition of zinc, this means the organisms have reduced nitrate beyond nitrite into colorless salts. In such cases, repeat the test to confirm the reaction.

NOTE: Nitrite test strips, available commercially, may be used to do this test; however, the strips give reliable results only with strongly nitrate-reducing organisms such as *M. tuberculosis*. Follow manufacturer's instructions.

Pigment production[13,15]

Pigment production was mentioned briefly in the section on reporting culture results. It should be studied both on slow growers that are nonpigmented when grown in the dark and on pigmented cultures that have not been incubated continuously in the dark. Cultures to be tested must be young and actively growing and show well-isolated colonies.

Procedure
1. Inoculate 2 tubes of egg-base medium with a suspension of organisms that will yield isolated colonies when grown.
2. Shield 1 tube from light by wrapping with black paper or aluminum foil.
3. Incubate both tubes at 35-37 C until visible growth is observed on unshielded culture.
4. Remove shield from other culture and record any pigment observed. If culture is nonpigmented, cover half tube and expose other half to light from a 60 W lamp at a distance of 20-25 cm for 1 h. Be certain cap of tube is loosened during light exposure.[83]
5. Replace shield and, with cap still loose, reincubate culture 6-12 h or overnight.

6. A change from nonpigmented to lemon yellow indicates a photochromogen.

Recent studies with *M. szulgai* indicate that it is commonly scotochromogenic when grown at 37 C but may be photochromogenic when tested at 25 C. Although this observation is not unique to *M. szulgai*, it is strongly suggestive of this species; therefore all scotochromogens should be tested for photochromogenicity both at 25 and 37 C.

Pyrazinamidase[15,84]

M. marinum is positive in the pyrazinamidase test at 4 days, while *M. kansasii* is negative. *M. bovis* is negative even at 7 days, while *M. tuberculosis* and the *M. avium* complex are positive within 4 days. This test may be valuable in identifying weakly niacin-positive strains or in separating *M. bovis* from the *M. avium* complex.

Reagents and materials
1. Substrate medium is prepared as follows:

Dubos broth base	6.5 g
Distilled water	1000.0 ml
Dissolve and add	
Pyrazinamide	0.1 g
Pyruvic acid, sodium salt	2.0 g
Agar	15.0 g

Heat to melt agar. Dispense in 5 ml amounts in 16 × 125 mm screw-capped tubes. Autoclave at 121 C for 15 min. Allow to harden upright not slanted.
2. Aqueous ferrous ammonium sulfate, 1%. Prepare fresh before each use.

Controls
1. Uninoculated medium (negative)
2. Tube inoculated with *M. avium* (positive)

Procedure
1. Using a loop or spade, place a heavy inoculum (sufficient to be seen with naked eye) onto surface of each of 2 tubes of medium.
2. Incubate at 35-37 C.
3. Remove 1 tube from incubator after 4 d and add 1.0 ml of ferrous ammonium sulfate solution. Place in refrigerator to prevent growth of contaminants.
4. After 4 h examine tubes for a pink band in agar (positive reaction). Examine tubes against a white background using incident room light.
5. After 7 d remove second tube from incubator and test as described in steps 3 and 4.
   NOTE: If the 4 d test is positive, it is not necessary to retain the tube for the 7 d test.

Sodium chloride tolerance[13,15,72,85]

This test confirms the presence of rapid growers and *M. triviale*; *M. flavescens* may also grow on sodium chloride.

Reagents and materials
1. An egg-base medium (e.g., ATS or Lowenstein-Jensen) is supplemented by addition, prior to inspissation, of sodium chloride to a final concentration of 5%.
2. A similar egg-base medium is prepared without added NaCl (control).

Procedure
1. Inoculate 0.1 ml barely turbid suspension of a broth culture (or saline suspension of bacilli from

a fresh slant) onto both a control slant and an NaCl-containing slant.
2. Incubate at 35-37 C.
3. Examine weekly for growth, and discard after 4 wk.
4. A positive reaction is growth on both the control and the NaCl tubes. A negative reaction is growth on the control, but **not** on the NaCl medium.

Tellurite reduction[13,15,86]

M. avium complex organisms normally are positive in the tellurite reduction test while all other nonpotochromogens usually are negative. Inoculate all nonphotochromogenic, slowly growing mycobacteria for the tellurite test just as soon as sufficient growth appears on the isolation medium.

Reagents and materials
1. Prepare Middlebrook 7H-9 liquid medium with ADC enrichment and Tween 80. **Do not use glycerol.** Place only 5 ml medium into 20 × 150 mm screw-capped tubes.
2. Dissolve 0.1 g potassium tellurite in 50 ml distilled water. Dispense in 2 ml amounts into small screw-capped tubes, autoclave at 121 C for 10 min, and store in refrigerator until needed.

Controls
1. Tube of uninoculated Middlebrook 7H-9 broth (negative)
2. Tube inoculated with *M. avium* (positive)

Procedure
1. Inoculate Middlebrook 7H-9 broth with a **spadeful** of test organisms taken from an actively growing culture slant.
2. Incubate at 35-37 C for **7 d only.** Be certain growth is **heavily turbid.** If growth is not heavily turbid and suspected *M. avium* complex strains do not give a positive test, repeat test with a fresh **heavily turbid** broth culture.
3. Using a capillary pipet, add 2 drops potassium tellurite solution to each test culture and to uninoculated control broth.
4. Reincubate at 35-37 C.
5. Examine cultures on third day after reincubation. **Do not shake tubes.**
6. A positive reaction is indicated by formation of a black, metallic precipitate of tellurium in and around sedimented bacterial cells.

Thiophen–2-carboxylic acid hydrazide (TCH) sensitivity[13, 15, 87-89]

This test is a valuable aid in the identification of suspected *M. bovis,* which is one of the few nonpigmented slow growers susceptible to low concentrations of TCH. Isoniazid-resistant strains of *M. bovis* may be resistant to TCH. *M. tuberculosis, M. avium,* and most other mycobacteria are resistant to the inhibitory action of this compound. The concentration of TCH commonly used in this test is 10 μg/ml; however, recent information[2] indicates that some strains of *M. tuberculosis* also are susceptible to this concentration of TCH. In the event a laboratory is faced with the problem of differential identification of *M. tuberculosis* from *M. bovis* and data suggest the TCH concentration of 10 μg/ml is too high, it may be advisable to use media containing only

1-5 μg/ml of TCH, to which *M. bovis* is susceptible and most *M. tuberculosis* organisms are resistant.[87]

Reagents and materials
1. Prepare 2 batches of complete Middlebrook 7H-10 or oleic acid albumin agar.
2. Pour one as the control medium. To the other add sufficient filter-sterilized TCH to make 10 μg/ml medium (or lesser concentration as suggested previously). The medium may be dispensed into sterile screw-capped tubes or plates.

Procedure
1. Dilute a 7-day-old liquid culture of the test organism in sterile saline to 10^{-2} and 10^{-4} (1:100 to 1:10,000).
2. Using a sterile capillary pipet, inoculate 1 control and 1 drug-containing medium with the 10^{-4} dilution; inoculate a second set of plates with the 10^{-2} dilution.
3. Incubate for 3 wk at 35-37 C in 10% CO_2.
4. Record the organism as sensitive if growth on the TCH medium is less than 1% of that observed on the control medium.

Tween 80 hydrolysis[13, 15, 90]

The Tween 80 hydrolysis test separates the potentially pathogenic from the normally saprophytic members of both the scotochromogens and the nonphotochromogens. It provides confirmatory identification of *M. kansasii.* Inoculate all slow-growing mycobacteria into this test medium.

Reagents and materials
1. Substrate medium

M/15 phosphate buffer, ph 7.0	100.0 ml
Tween 80	0.5 ml
0.1% Aqueous neutral red solution (corrected for actual dye content)	2.0 ml

2. Dispense medium in 2.0 ml amounts in 16 × 125 mm screw-capped test tubes.
3. Autoclave at 121 C for 10 min.
4. Final medium should be amber or straw colored.
5. Store in dark, in refrigerator for no more than 2 wk.

Controls
1. Uninoculated tube of substrate is negative control.
2. Tube inoculated with *M. kansasii* serves as a positive control.

Procedure
1. Inoculate substrate with a spadeful (or loopful) of test organism taken from a freshly grown culture slant. Inoculate positive control also.
2. Incubate at 35-37 C.
3. Read tubes at 5 and 10 d. **Do not shake tubes when reading.** A positive reaction is recorded when fluid (not cells) turns pink or red.
   NOTE: A commercially available concentrated TB-Tween hydrolysis reagent is stable for long periods and provides satisfactory test results.[91] Follow manufacturer's directions.

Urease[13, 15, 84, 92]

The urease test may be useful in identifying both scotochromogens and nonphotochromogens. *M. scrofulaceum, M. szulgai, M. flavescens, M. bovis,* and *M. gastri* are positive, while *M.*

Table 78-2. Rapid growers*

| Test | M. fortuitum complex | | | Others† | |
	M. fortuitum	M. chelonei	M. chelonei ssp. abscessus	M. smegmatis M. vaccae	M. phlei M. vaccae
Pigment	−	−	−	−	+
Arylsulfatase, 3 d	+	+	+	−	−
MacConkey	+	+	+	−	−
NaCl Tolerance	+	−	+	+	+
Nitrate reduction	+	−	−	+	+
Fe (iron) uptake	+	−	−	+	+

*For colony types, see Fig. 78-3, *I* and *J*, and Fig. 78-4, *F* and *J*.
†Only 3 species (*M. smegmatis*, *M. phlei*, and *M. vaccae*) are listed as "others." They are included only as examples of commonly saprophytic species; the text lists many others.

avium complex, *M. xenopi*, and *M. gordonae* are negative. *M. kansasii* is also positive.

Reagents and materials
1. Mix aseptically 1 part Difco-Bacto urea agar concentrate with 9 parts sterile distilled water. **Do not add agar.**
2. Dispense in 3 ml amounts in 13 × 100 mm sterile screw-capped tubes.

Controls
1. Uninoculated tube of substrate as negative control
2. Inoculated substrate tube with *M. scrofulaceum*, *M gastri*, or *M. fortuitum* as positive control

Procedure
1. Inoculate substrate with a spadeful of growth from a young, actively growing culture on solid medium.
2. Incubate at 35-37 C.
3. Observe for color change to pink or red (positive test), and discard all tubes after 3 days.

A much simplified version of the urease test recently reported[93] uses commercially available urea-containing disks. Reported data seem to provide even more distinctive results than those achieved with the method here described.

DIFFERENTIAL IDENTIFICATION OF MYCOBACTERIA

Once the unknown organism has been grown in culture, make a smear and stain for acid-fast bacilli. The presence of either contaminating non-acid-fast organisms or mixed cultures of 2 or more acid-fast species may cause erroneous results in the previously described in vitro tests. If either acid-fast smear results or careful examination of individual colony types on the isolation medium suggests a contaminated or mixed culture, it is necessary to go through single colony isolation or purification procedures before proceeding to the tests for definitive identification.

Once the purity of the isolated organism(s) is ascertained, acid-fast bacilli may be subdivided into several groups on the basis of speed of growth and pigment production (Fig. 78-2). While these preliminary subdivisions are in progress, however, it is advisable to perform all the differential in vitro tests on each unknown organism. Experience has shown that, primarily because of the slow growth of most mycobacteria, it is more economical (from the standpoint of

minimizing time delays in precise species identification) to set up all the tests at one time than to await the results of 1 test procedure before proceeding to the next. In this fashion, once the crude subdivisions depicted in Fig. 78-2 are facilitated, then the "unnecessary" tests that were performed may be either disregarded as irrelevant or the results used purely as supportive evidence of the precise identification effected by the more pertinent tests.

Another thing to be borne in mind considering which in vitro tests should be performed is the level of service that the laboratory provides (discussed earlier in this chapter). The level II laboratory, which is expected only to identify *M. tuberculosis* precisely while merely rough grouping all other mycobacteria, would have only a few tests to perform. Rough grouping of mycobacteria is reliably done simply on the basis of speed of growth and pigment production. The exact speciation of *M. tuberculosis* is attained by use of the niacin, nitrate-reduction, and pH 7/68 C catalase tests. On the other hand, the level III or reference laboratory would be expected to have practical experience with all the in vitro test procedures here detailed.

When rough grouping of the isolate has been realized and the more important differential tests have been selected, then these test results are compared to hypothetical median patterns for the more important species in each group (see Tables 78-2 to 78-6). If the results of the unknown organism match exactly one of the tabulated patterns, identification of the unknown may be considered complete. On the other hand, if test results for the unknown do not match those for any listed species, repeat the tests at least once. Variations from expected test patterns may be

Table 78-3. Niacin-positive nonchromogens*

Test	M. tuberculosis	M. simiae
Nitrate reduction	+	−
Catalase, R°	<45	>45
Catalase, 68 C	−	+
Pigment, photo	−	+

*For colony types see Fig. 78-3, *A* and *B*, and Fig. 78-4, *A*.

Table 78-4. Nonphotochromogens*†

Test	M. bovis	M. avium complex	M. xenopi	M. gastri	M. terrae complex	M. triviale	M. kansasii (nonphoto)
Catalase, R°	<45	<45	<45	<45	>45	>45	>45
Catalase, 68 C	−	+	+	−	+	+	+
Tween hydrolysis	−	−	−	+	+	+	+
Tellurite reduction	−	+	−	−	−	−	−
Nitrate reduction	−	−	−	−	+	+	+
TCH susceptibility	+	−	−	−	+	−	−
NaCl tolerance	−	−	−	−	−	+	−
Urease	+	−	−	+	−	−	+
Pyrazinamidase	−	+	+	−/∓	∓/+	∓/+	−/+

*For colony types, see Fig. 78-3, *C* and *H*, and Fig. 78-4, *E*, *H*, and *I*.
†For *M. ulcerans*, see species discussion.

due to contamination, mixed cultures, strain variation, or improper attention to test performance (e.g., inoculum size, medium, test tube size, incubation time or temperature, etc.). If after this the organism still defies precise speciation, refer to another reference laboratory, such as the Veterans Administration or Center for Disease Control, for consultative assistance.

Following are some comments about the definition of organisms within each of the preliminary subgroups.

Rapid growers

Rapid growers are usually easily defined because mature colonies are visible to the naked eye on subculture in less than 7 days. Potential pathogens in this group include *M. fortuitum, M. chelonei,* and *M. chelonei* ssp. *abcessus,*[10] the three commonly lumped together as the *M. fortuitum* complex. Precise speciation within this complex generally is not clinically important; therefore the simple determination that organisms are positive in 3-day arylsulfatase and MacConkey agar tests would be sufficient to characterize many members of the *M. fortuitum* complex. Should more definitive taxonomy be required within this group, the use of NaCl tolerance, nitrate reduction, and iron uptake tests often facilitates the subdivision (Table 78-2).

Conversely, specific definition of members of the commonly saprophytic rapid growers is rarely necessary for the clinical laboratory; in most cases the laboratory could safely report, "Rapid grower, **not** in *M. fortuitum* complex," for an isolate that gave a negative 3-day arylsulfatase and failed to grow on MacConkey agar. There will be occasion when more exact speciation is needed. The tests listed in Table 78-2 are only slightly helpful in this instance, and the reader should consult more detailed literature.[10,13,94]

Niacin-positive nonchromogens

Once regarded as the most specific in vitro test in mycobacteriology, a positive niacin reaction at one time literally confirmed the identification of *M. tuberculosis*. Although production of niacin is still strong circumstantial evidence that an isolate from pulmonary lesions of man is *M. tuber-*

Table 78-5. Photochromogens*

Test	M. kansasii	M. marinum	M. simiae
Tween hydrolysis	+	+	−
Nitrate reduction	+	−	−
Catalase, R° >45	+	∓	+
Niacin	−	−/+	+
Pyrazinamidase, 4 d	−	+	∓
Arylsulfatase, 2 wk	−/+	+	−

*For colony types, see Fig. 78-3, *D* and *E*, and Fig. 78-4, *B* to *D*.

culosis, it is known that other acid-fast bacilli can produce sufficient niacin to give a positive reaction in this test.[13,72] Among these other mycobacteria is *M. simiae*.[95] Although *M. simiae* originally was isolated from monkeys, a recent report[96] of its synonymy with an organism that causes pulmonary disease in man, *M. habana,*[97] makes it almost certain that clinicians will encounter this "new" *Mycobacterium* in the future. It should be emphasized that the report of Meissner and Schröder[96] strongly suggests the synonymy of *M. simiae* and *M. habana;* if this work is corroborated by others, the name of this new taxon, by priority rule, would be *M. simiae,* and this is the name by which it is here called. Table 78-3 lists the major differences between *M. tuberculosis* and *M. simiae*. The property of photochromogenicity of *M. simiae* should be mentioned for 2 reasons: (1) some strains appear to be scotochromogenic rather than photochromogenic[96] and (2) the photoactivated pigment often requires more light exposure (4 hours) than that commonly employed (1 hour) to express the photochromogenicity in *M. kansasii.*[96] It is important, too, that the laboratory remember that not all *M. tuberculosis* organisms are niacin positive.[72,98] This may be especially true of tubercle bacilli exhibiting multiple drug resistance, a feature not uncommonly associated with slower growth and more sluggish metabolic activity.

Nonphotochromogens

Nonphotochromogens are indeed a complex group of mycobacteria. Not only do they contain potential pathogens (*M. bovis, M. avium* com-

Table 78-6. Scotochromogens*

Test	M. scrofulaceum	M. szulgai	M. xenopi	M. gordonae	M. flavescens	M. kansasii (scoto)
Tween hydrolysis	−	+	−	+	+	+
Nitrate reduction	−	+	−	−	+	+
Catalase, R°	>45	>45	<45	>45	>45	>45
NaCl tolerance	−		−	−	±	−
Urease	+	+	−	−	+	+
Photo-pigment, 25°	−	±	−	−	−	−
Arylsulfatase, 3 d	−	∓	±	−	−	−

*For colony types, see Fig. 78-3, F and G, and Fig. 78-4, G.

plex, and *M. xenopi*) but a number of commonly saprophytic species as well (*M. gastri*, *M. terrae* complex, and *M. triviale*). Mature colonies, as observed on subculture, require more than 7 days to be seen without magnification. Pigmentation is commonly absent, although pale, pastel pigments may be observed. Prolonged exposure to light does not result in pigment intensification. Nonphotochromogenic mutants of *M. kansasii* are extremely rare, but they are included in Table 78-4 to demonstrate the ease with which they may be confused with the *M. terrae* complex; the urease test offers some differential aid in this case. The observation of a negative Tween hydrolysis test (10-day reading recommended here) would quickly identify the potential pathogens (other than the niacin-positive *M. tuberculosis*) in this large group of nonphotochromogens. In this case, however, futher speciation is mandatory because some of these organisms (*M. bovis* especially) respond well to antituberculosis drugs. In contrast, organisms that are Tween hydrolysis–positive (often within 5 days), reduce nitrate, and produce more than 45 mm of bubbles in the catalase test may be lumped together as *M. terrae* complex without need for more precise recognition. *M. bovis* is commonly identified by its lack of reactivity in the tests listed in Table 78-4 (it possesses urease and is susceptible to TCH). *M. gastri* is likewise nonreactive but differs from *M. bovis* in TCH susceptibility and ability to hydrolyze Tween 80. *M. xenopi* is positive in the 68 C catalase test and differs from *M. avium* in that it fails to reduce tellurite.

Not included in Table 78-4, but discussed under individual species names, is *M. ulcerans*, an organism rarely, if ever, seen in temperate climates.

Photochromogens

The unique feature of the photochromogens group is its possession of a photoactivated carotenoid pigment. When grown in the dark, colonies are nonpigmented, but after exposure to light for 1 hour, followed by reincubation for 6-24 hours, they form a lemon yellow pigment. The delayed photochromogenicity observed in *M. simiae* has already been mentioned. The

following require emphasis. (1) Studies on pigment production in the light must be **very carefully** performed, because reactions of some potentially pathogenic photochromogens are similar to those of commonly saprophytic nonphotochromogens (see Table 78-4). (2) Cultures must be well aerated (caps left loose) during exposure to light and subsequent postexposure incubation. (3) If growth is confluent or colonies too old, the characteristic pigment may fail to form following light exposure (be certain to use young, actively growing cultures with isolated colonies). Continuous exposure to light for 2 weeks during incubation may produce orange crystals of β-carotene within colonies of some photochromogens.[99, 100]

All slow-growing photochromogens, *M. kansasii*, *M. marinum*, and *M. simiae*, are potentially pathogenic. It has been reported,[74] however, that strains of *M. kansasii* that produce <45 mm of bubbles in the semiquantitative catalase test are less frequently associated with disease than are the catalase hyperactive strains. *M. marinum* is isolated from superficial lesions, grows best at 30-32 C, and is never to be expected from sputum.

Other differential features of the photochromogens are documented in Table 78-5.

Scotochromogens

The scotochromogen group of organisms, pigmented both in darkness and light, generally produces mature colonies only after 7 days of incubation (*M. flavescens* is intermediate between slow and rapid growers in growth rate and may mature within 7 days on some media). If exposed to light continuously for 2 weeks, many strains reveal intensification of pigment from yellow to orange or brick red. If care has not been observed to protect colonies from light exposure during growth or routine weekly examination, then all scotochromogens should be subcultured to check on production of photoactivated pigment (this is to ensure that an *M. kansasii* organism has not been misdiagnosed). The potential pathogens *M. scrofulaceum* and *M. szulgai* should be identified (because of its pale yellow pigment, another potential pathogen, *M. xenopi*, is included in both Tables 78-4 and 78-6). Both *M. scrofulaceum* and *M. szulgai* are negative in the 5-day Tween hydrolysis test, but the latter often is positive after 10 days. In contrast, most other scotochromogens are positive in 5 days. *M. szulgai* is almost unique among scotochromogens in producing very strong reactions in the nitrate-reduction test (comparable in intensity to *M. kansasii* and some *M. tuberculosis*). The urease test, especially when disks are used,[93] is of great help in separating *M. scrofulaceum* from *M. xenopi, M. gordonae,* and pigmented *M. avium* strains. See Table 78-6 for a summary of the characteristic properties of most commonly encountered scotochromogens; although the scotochromogenic mutant of *M. kansasii* is in-

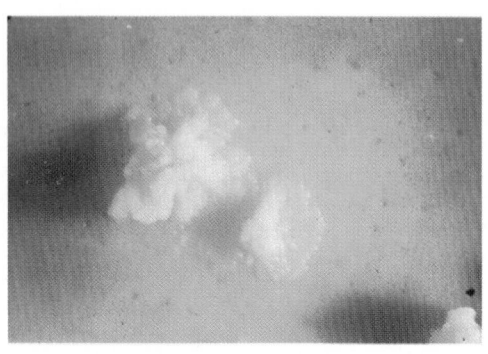

A, *M. tuberculosis.*

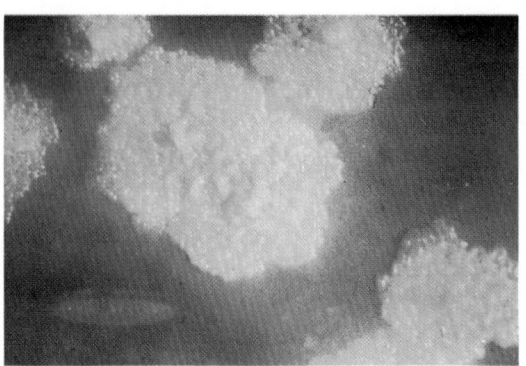

B, *M. tuberculosis.*

C, *M. bovis.*

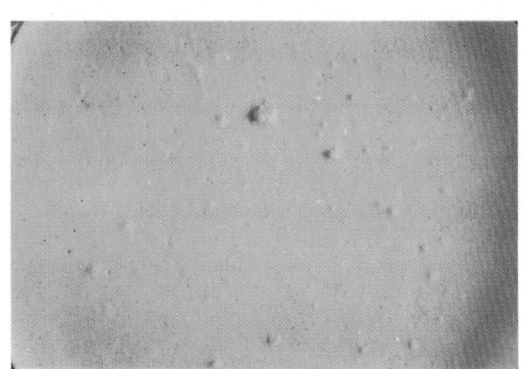

D, Rough *M. kansasii* grown in dark.

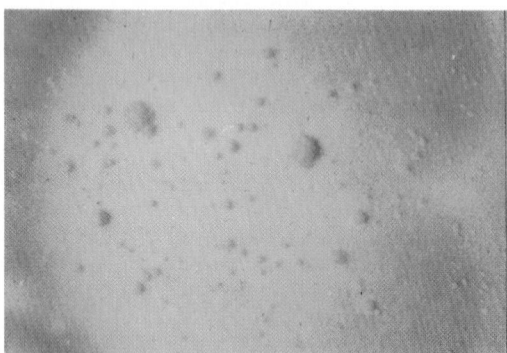

E, Rough *M. kansasii* exposed to light.

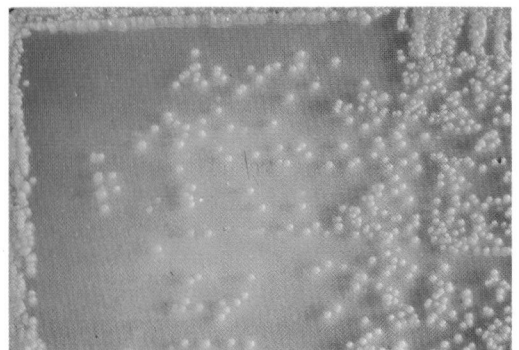

F, Yellow pigmented scotochromogens.

Fig. 78-3. Colonies of mycobacteria grown on egg-base media (close-ups).

cluded in this table, it should be noted that such a mutant has been encountered only as a laboratory variant and not as a patient isolate.

SPECIFIC CHARACTERISTICS OF MYCOBACTERIAL SPECIES

The differential features of many mycobacteria recovered from suspected tuberculosis-like disease in man have been summarized in Tables 78-2 to 78-6. In this section, each species will be discussed individually, not only to summarize its distinctive features but also to permit mention of other species that, for one reason or another, have not yet been dealt with in the text (e.g., *M. leprae* and *M. ulcerans*).

For ease of reference, the names of legitimate or commonly accepted species are recorded alphabetically. Commonly used synonyms, which currently are improper to use, are presented for some species purely as a point of reference for the reader. (Some of these are also presented in Table 78-1.) Because the taxonomy of the mycobacteria is in such a dynamic state, one cannot expect the following list to be completely accurate. Selected examples of some of the different colony types and pigments referred to in

the individual species descriptions following may be seen in Figs. 78-3 and 78-4.

Mycobacterium africanum[101]
Source and habitat

Currently *M. africanum* is limited to central and western Africa where it causes tuberculosis in man; however, global travel could lead to wider dissemination of this species. Suspect strains of *M. africanum* have been isolated from a few African monkeys brought into the United States. Experimentally, *M. africanum* produces little evidence of progressive disease when injected into calves or rabbits (similar to *M. tuberculosis*), severe, progressive, sometimes fatal disease in goats (similar to *M. bovis*), and moderately progressive disease in guinea pigs (personnal communication, H. H. Kleeberg).

Morphology and staining

Staining shows acid-fast rods averaging approximately 3 μm in length.

Growth

M. africanum grows very slowly, often requiring more than 42 days before growth may be de-

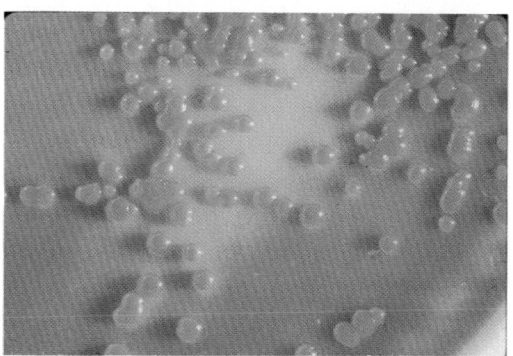

G, Orange pigmented scotochromogens.

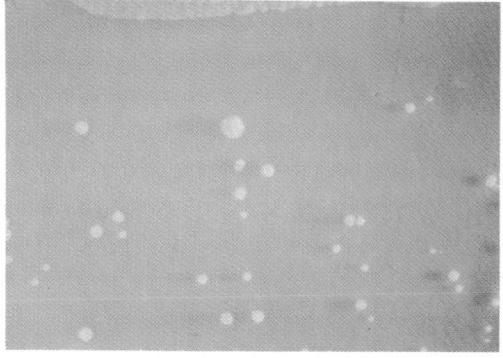

H, Smooth *M. avium* complex.

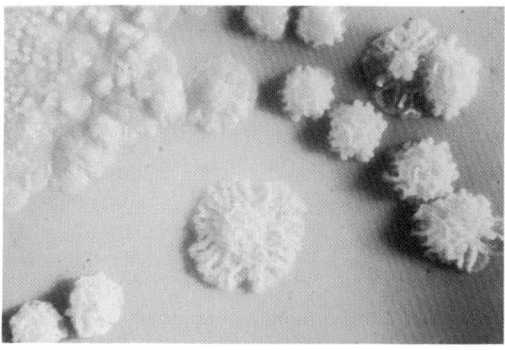

I, Rough *M. smegmatis.*

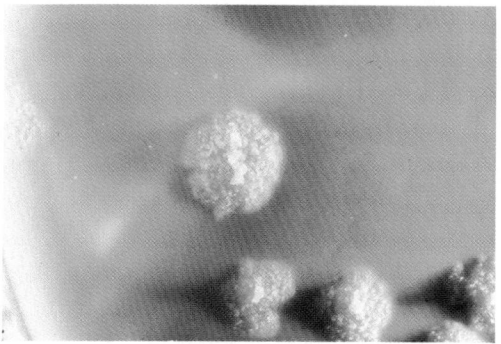

J, Rough *M. fortuitum.*

tected. Colonies usually are dysgonic (like *M. bovis*), sometimes growing down into the medium. Growth is enhanced by the addition of 0.2% pyruvate to the isolation medium.

Differential characteristics

M. africanum exhibits taxonomic variability intermediate between *M. tuberculosis* and *M.*

bovis, suggesting either that these variations may be geographically related or that distinct subspecies of this taxon exist. Niacin test results vary; most strains are negative, but positive reactors are not uncommon. Nitrate reduction is commonly negative; however, positive reactors have been reported. Although commonly susceptible to TCH and pyrazinamide, the organism has

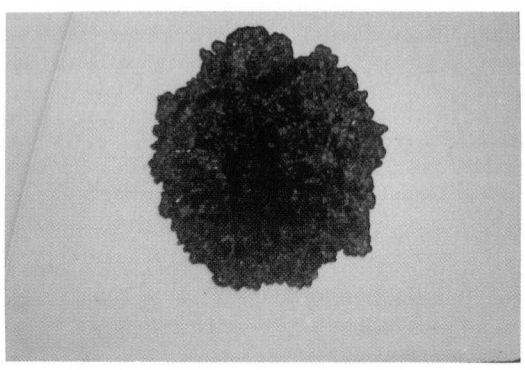

A, *M. tuberculosis;* transmitted light.

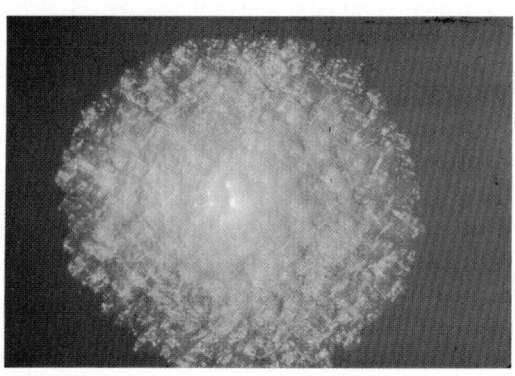

B, Rough *M. kansasii* grown in dark; epi-illumination.

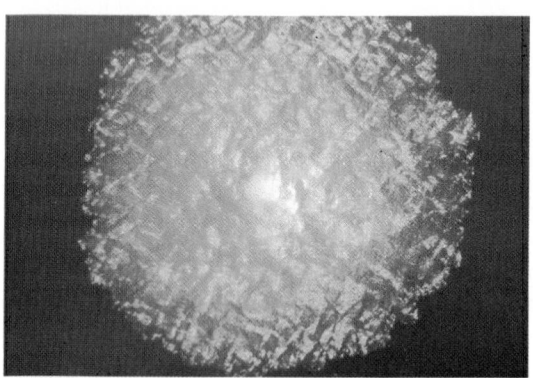

C, Rough *M. kansasii* exposed to light; epi-illumination.

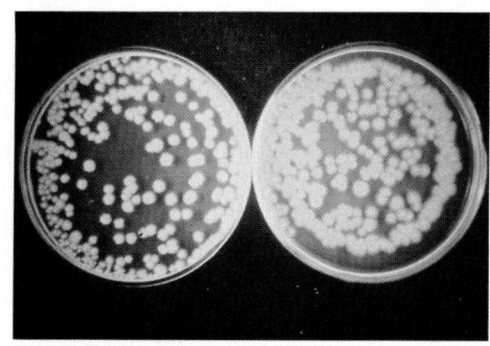

D, Smooth *M. kansasii;* plate on left grown in dark and plate on right exposed to light.

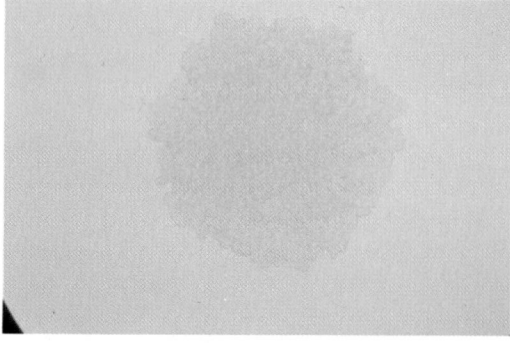

E, *M. triviale:* transmitted light.

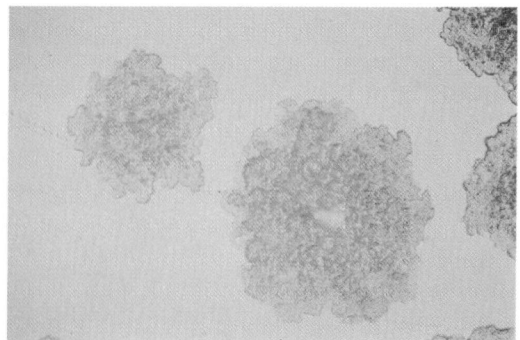

F, Rough *M. fortuitum;* combined transmitted and epi-illumination.

Fig. 78-4. Colonies of mycobacteria on Middlebrook 7H-10 agar (close-ups).

variable susceptibility to amithiozone that appears to be related to geographic areas. Although *M. africanum* appears to be a readily recognized species in Africa, the relatively few strains seen in the United States make it a taxonomic puzzle.

Mycobacterium aurum

See *Mycobacterium parafortuitum.*

Mycobacterium avium[102]
Source and habitat

Precise definition of source and habitat depends on the breadth of one's definition of *M. avium.* The *M. avium* of a decade ago was found to be the causative agent of tuberculosis in fowl and less frequently to be the causative agent of disease in swine, cattle, other lower animals, and rarely man. The majority of contributors to a recent international, cooperative study[11] agreed that *M. intracellulare* should be a synonym of *M. avium.* This, then, broadens the source or habitat range of the *M. avium* complex to include man and soil[103]; also relegated to synonymy with this group is *M. brunense.*[104] Experimentally the disease produced by organisms once referred to as *M. intracellulare* is both less extensive and less severe than that due to *M. avium;* however, in properly administered dosage, the *M. avium* complex can be transmitted to most fowl, swine, rabbits, hamsters, and mice (in the latter 3 cases often causing a Yersin reaction).

Morphology and staining

Bacilli are very pleomorphic, ranging from short, coccoid elements to long rods, with long filamentous forms even observed at some stages of growth on certain media. They are usually strongly acid fast and, like most mycobacteria, usually considered gram positive, although the bacilli do stain with some difficulty.

Growth

The bacilli usually produce smooth, dome-shaped colonies on egg-base media, but growth on oleic acid–albumin agars may be smooth, transparent, and pyramid shaped or hemispherical. Occasionally, rough colonies are seen on both kinds of media. More than one colony type may be seen in the same culture. Appearance of mature colonies commonly requires 10 days or more at 37 C; the temperature of growth ranges from 25-45 C. Although commonly nonpig-

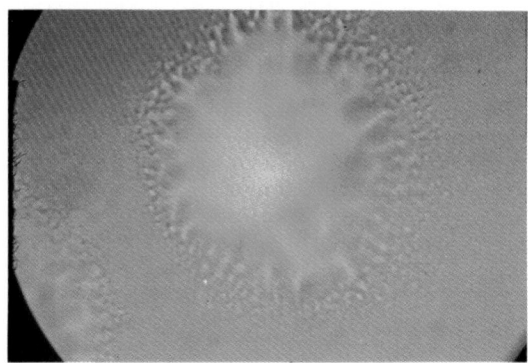

G, Smooth yellow pyramidal scotochromogen; epi-illumination.

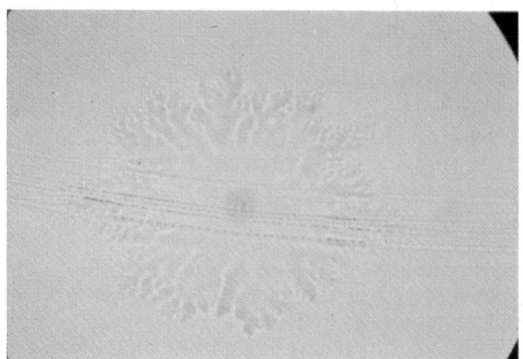

H, Smooth transparent *M. avium* complex; transmitted light.

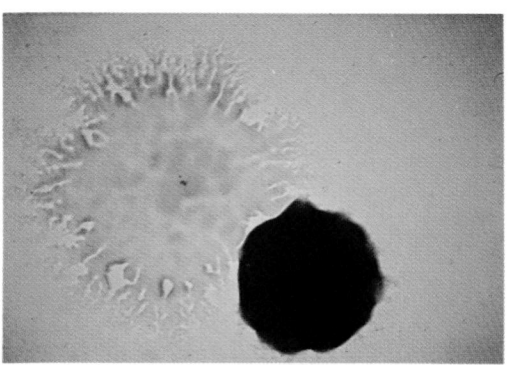

I, *M. avium* complex; transmitted light; smooth transparent and smooth domed colonies.

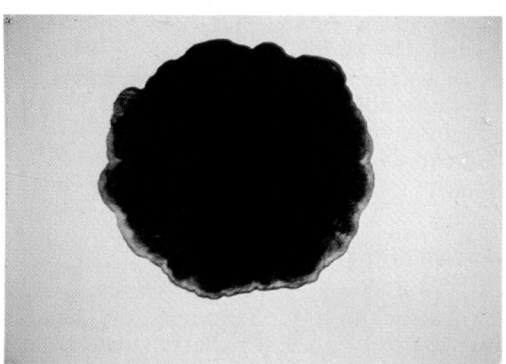

J, Smooth domed colony of *M. fortuitum;* transmitted light.

mented, colonies may reveal pale to deep pigments as they grow older. Those with a yellowish hue may be confused with *M. scrofulaceum*.

Differential characteristics

The 2 most valuable test reactions in diagnosis of *M. avium* are a negative 10-day Tween hydrolysis and a positive tellurite reduction test in 3-4 days. Additionally *M. avium* complex organisms are niacin negative (if only smooth colonies are observed on oleic acid agars, the niacin test need not be performed), fail to reduce nitrate, are urease negative (an aid when confused with *M. scrofulaceum*), and are pyrazinamidase positive (valuable if confusion with *M. bovis* must be resolved).

Mycobacterium bovis[105]
Source and habitat

Commonly referred to as the bovine tubercle bacillus, *M. bovis* is isolated from tuberculous lesions of cattle but will also produce disease in other domestic and wild ruminants, man (though rarely in the United States) and other primates, dogs, cats, swine, parrots, and perhaps birds of prey. Experimentally more pathogenic for animals than *M. tuberculosis*, *M. bovis* produces disease in rabbits, guinea pigs, mice, calves, and goats but not in fowl.

Morphology and staining

Organisms are both gram positive and acid fast. The bacilli are usually shorter (1-2 μm long) than *M. tuberculosis*, although moderately long rods may be observed.

Growth

On primary isolation, *M. bovis* grows very poorly on glycerol-containing medium[57, 58]; in fact, poor or no growth on glycerol-supplemented medium in the presence of growth on the same or other media without glycerol is strongly suggestive of *M. bovis* on primary culture. Media enriched with 0.2% pyruvate are more favorable to growth of *M. bovis*.[55, 56] On egg-base medium, colonies are usually translucent, somewhat smooth, low, small, pyramid shaped, and nonpigmented. On Middlebrook 7H-10 or other agar media, colonies are thin, flat, rough, and usually corded; cording is more pronounced on pyruvate-supplemented media. Growth is commonly dysgonic, often requiring at least 3 weeks for visible colonies to be seen. Temperature range is about 33-39 C.

Differential characteristics

M. bovis is one of the least reactive of the mycobacteria in the in vitro tests, the only consistently positive reactions being in urease activity and production of <45 mm of bubbles in the semiquantitative catalase test. INH-resistant strains may lose catalase activity. On occasion a weakly positive niacin test may be observed; in such cases, differentiation from *M. tuberculosis*

is made by use of nitrate reduction, pyrazinamidase activity (*M. tuberculosis* is positive in 4 days), and TCH susceptibility (*M. bovis* is susceptible). The latter 2 tests and the 68 C catalase test facilitate distinction of *M. bovis* from occasionally troublesome strains of *M. avium*. Rarely is it necessary to resort to animal inoculation to identify *M. bovis*.

Mycobacterium chelonei[3, 10]
Source and habitat

One of the potentially pathogenic rapid growers, *M. chelonei* now includes organisms once referred to as *M. borstelense*, *M. runyonii*, and *M. abscessus*. It has been isolated from soil, sputum from man (with and without associated disease), and abscesses at the site of earlier injections. Experimentally, the organism usually causes only transient lesions in guinea pigs, rabbits, hamsters, and mice, although some reports of grossly visible lesions in organs of mice infected intravenously have been made.

Morphology and staining

The bacilli are quite pleomorphic, varying from short, coccoid to long, narrow forms (0.2-0.5 × 1.0-6.0 μm). Young, actively replicating cells are usually acid fast, while older cultures (>5 days) may exhibit nonacid-fast forms.

Growth

Mature colonies, visible in less than 7 days, are commonly smooth, moist, hemispherical, and nonpigmented both on egg-base and clear agar-base media. Rough colonies are occasionally observed, more often as a result of prolonged incubation of cultures for 3-4 weeks. On corn meal agar, *M. chelonei* does not exhibit the extensive network of filaments commonly associated with *M. fortuitum*. Temperature of growth ranges from 22-40 C.

Differential characteristics

Clinically there seems to be little need to differentiate this organism from *M. fortuitum;* both are potentially pathogenic and commonly give positive reactions in the 3-day arylsulfatase and MacConkey agar tests. When there is a need to segregate this organism from *M. fortuitum*, Table 78-2 suggests that tolerance to 5% NaCl, nitrate reduction, and iron uptake may facilitate the distinction. Additionally, Stanford et al.[106] suggest there may be different in vitro characteristics associated with *M. chelonei* from different geographic areas of the world.

Mycobacterium diernhoferi

See *Mycobacterium parafortuitum*.

Mycobacterium flavescens[10, 94, 107, 108]
Source and habitat

Although *M. flavescens* was originally isolated from drug-treated tuberculous guinea pigs, its occurrence in clinical specimens suggests that it may be a common environmental saprophyte. *M. acapulcense* is suggested to be a synonym of *M. flavescens.*[109]

Morphology and staining

Staining shows rod-shaped acid-fast organisms.

Growth

M. flavescens is capable of growth from 25-42 C, and its intermediate growth rate (6-10 days) results in its placement sometimes with slow growers and sometimes with rapid growers. Growth produces soft, butyrous colonies that exhibit yellow to orange pigmentation and are difficult to remove from the medium.

Differential characteristics

Table 78-6 indicates those tests of value in separating *M. flavescens* from slow-growing scotochromogens, although clinically, its relegation to a gordonae complex (based only on positive Tween hydrolysis) would present no great problem because both species are normally saprophytic. When *M. flavescens* is included with rapid growers, it is grouped with the pigmented *M. phlei–M. vaccae* group, and again, further differentiation seems unwarranted, although the frequent negative reaction of *M. flavescens* in iron uptake may be one way of achieving the separation.

Mycobacterium fortuitum[10, 110]
Source and habitat

One of the potentially pathogenic rapid growers, *M. fortuitum* was originally isolated from a cold abscess of man; however, it has also been isolated from pulmonary disease and injection abscesses of man, lymph nodes of cattle, systemic, nodular disease in frogs, and soil, the latter probably being the normal habitat. Species now considered to be synonymous with *M. fortuitum* include *M. peregrinum*, *M. minetti*, *M. giae*, *M. ranae*, and *M. salmoniphilum*. Experimentally *M. fortuitum* may produce local lesions in kidneys of mice, guinea pigs, rabbits, and monkeys; lesions of the middle ear cause characteristic "spining disease" in mice.[111] These bacilli are rarely associated with generalized or progressive disease in any laboratory animal.

Morphology and staining

Rods are 1-3 μm long, although variations from coccoid to long, branching, filamentous forms have been reported. Young cultures (<5 days) are usually acid-fast, but older growth may exhibit as little as 10% acid-fast cells.

Growth

Most strains will grow from 22-40 C, mature colonies being visible in less than 5 days. On egg-base media, colonies may be soft, butyrous, and hemispherical and multilobate or rosette clustered; rough colonies with heaped centers also are common. Colonies usually are nonpigmented; however, when grown on malachite green–containing media, the colonies may absorb the dye, giving them a green color.[112] On Middlebrook 7H-10 medium, rough colonies are dense with some cording, while smooth forms show hemispherical colonies with entire edges and dark centers. If grown on corn meal agar, the smooth colonies exhibit extensive filament formation, a feature not as evident in the rough colony types.[61,100]

Differential characteristics

Positive reactions in the 3-day arylsulfatase and MacConkey agar tests are usually adequate to identify *M. fortuitum–M. chelonei*. If more precise speciation is needed (such occasions are rare), the tests in Table 78-2 are most valuable.

Mycobacterium gastri[113]
Source and habitat

M. gastri is isolated from human gastric lavage. It may be found in gastric washings or sputa but is not thought to be related to disease; it also is found in soil.[103] *M. gastri* will not produce disease in guinea pigs.

Morphology and staining

Bacilli may be moderately long to long. Cultures are acid fast, but individual cells frequently exhibit cross-barred staining.

Growth

Cultures grow at temperatures from 25-40 C, yielding smooth or rough nonpigmented colonies after more than 7 day's incubation on egg-base media. On oleic acid–albumin agar, colonies are commonly smooth and flat with a granular surface, a regular edge, and occasionally a more dense central spot.

Differential characteristics

A relatively nonreactive organism, *M. gastri* readily hydrolyzes Tween 80, is urease positive, is nitrate negative, and loses catalase activity when heated to 68 C (see Table 78-4).

Mycobacterium gordonae[9, 107, 114]
Source and habitat

M. gordonae is often recovered as a casual isolate from human sputum and gastric washing, but rarely, if ever, is implicated as a pathogen. It may be found in tap water, soil, and other environmental sources.[103] The illegitimate term *M. aquae* has been associated with this organism.

Morphology and staining

Moderate to long acid-fast rods are commonly seen on smear. On occasion these rods may exhibit barred or banded staining.

Growth

On egg-base media *M. gordonae* usually produces smooth yellow to orange colonies that take more than 7 days to be fully mature. On oleic acid–albumin agars the colonies also are commonly smooth, yellow to orange, and hemispherical with entire edge. (Occasionally a more flattened colony with undulating periphery is shown.) On both media, rough colonies may be seen. Growth may occur from 22-39 C but appears optimal at 35 C.

Differential characteristics

M. gordonae exhibits strong catalase activity (>45 mm of bubbles), usually hydrolyzes Tween 80 in less than 10 days, and generally is negative in urease activity (the latter 2 features distinguish it from the potentially pathogenic *M. scrofulaceum*).

Mycobacterium kansasii[3]
Source and habitat

Originally isolated from a pulmonary, tuberculosis-like lesion of man, *M. kansasii* is associated with human, pulmonary disease; it is more rarely recovered from lungs or lymph nodes of cattle and swine. Its source in nature is uncertain; soil surveys have been unproductive,[103] although some strains have been isolated from tap water.[115] Experimentally, *M. kansasii* may prove fatal for hamsters and occasionally for mice. In other animals, however, even very large inocula may prove to be innocuous (chickens) or to cause only self-limiting disease (guinea pigs, rabbits, rats, and monkeys); fatal outcomes are rare. Former synonyms of this species include *M. luciflavum* and the vernacular "yellow bacillus."

Morphology and staining

Acid-fast stains reveal moderately long to long rods that may exhibit extensive acid-fast cross barring, especially if organisms are grown in the presence of fatty acids.

Growth

On egg-base media, *M. kansasii* may produce either smooth or rough colonies that mature in more than 7 days. On oleic acid-albumin agars, colonies likewise are either smooth and flat, with entire edge and dark central spot, or granular to rough, with irregular margin and dense central spot. On both media, colonies are nonpigmented in the dark, but if young, actively growing cultures are exposed briefly (1 hour) to light, they become lemon yellow in the next 6-24 hours. On rare occasions nonpigmented and scotochromogenic mutants of *M. kansasii* are encountered. Continued exposure to light may lead to formation of dark red crystals of β-carotene visible on the surface of colonies. *M. kansasii* will grow at temperatures from 22-40 C.

Differential characteristics

Two other photochromogens, *M. marinum* and *M. simiae* must be distinguished from *M. kansasii* (Table 78-5). The latter rapidly hydrolyzes Tween 80, is niacin negative, reduces nitrate, and is negative in the 4-day pyrazinamidase test.

Mycobacterium leprae

Leprosy, or Hansen's disease, is caused by *M. leprae*, which is second only to the tubercle bacilli as a causative agent of mycobacterial disease in man. In contrast to the other organisms presented in this chapter, *M. leprae* does not grow on artificial media; therefore the diagnosis of leprosy is only presumptive and depends on the correlation of clinically recognizable lesions in which noncultivable acid-fast bacilli may be demonstrated by microscopic examination. The disease commonly occurs in 2 forms, the lepromatous and the tuberculoid types, and it is the former in which the bacilli are most readily demonstrated. The stained bacilli may be observed in tissue sections, skin scrapings, or nasal washings. Shepard has noted[116] 7 conditions that serve to confirm *M. leprae* as the disease agent: (1) there are large numbers of bacilli associated with lepromatous leprosy and rarely with other forms of the disease, (2) the numbers of bacilli observed are rougly proportional to the severity of the disease; (3) the bacilli are most readily found in patients with nasal symptoms and lesions, (4) smears from nasal ulcers are commonly loaded with bacilli, (5) the bacilli are arranged in packets or globi, (6) the bacterial numbers are reduced after successful treatment, as with sulfones, and (7) the bacilli fail to grow on artificial media. With the procedure of Shepard,[116] bacilli may be demonstrated from 2 sources. Most productive of positive smears are scrapings from "involved skin" of lepromatous cases. After cleansing and disinfecting the skin, pinch the involed area between the thumb and forefinger so that the skin blanches (exclusion of blood). Using a sterile scalpel make an incision approximately 5 mm long and 2 mm deep; with the knife blade at right angles to the cut surface, scrape the tissue quickly before blood infiltrates the cut, and smear the scrapings onto a microscope slide. Fix the smear in formalin vapors, cover the smear with gelatin-phenol solution,[117] and again fix in formalin vapors (avoid heat fixing of smears). Although less productive, scrapings from the nasal mucosa or nasal washings may also demonstrate bacilli. Wash nasal mucosa with 500 ml balanced salt solution and concentrate by centrifugation. If the samples are to be cultured (to ensure that bacilli will not grow on routine tuberculosis media), decontaminate sediment with an equal volume of 1N NaOH, neutralize with 1N HCl, recentrifuge, and pour off the supernatant fluid. Suspend sediment in formol milk, smear, and cover with gelatin-phenol to fix.[117]

Staining

Smears should be stained without heat. The usual Ziehl-Neelsen carbolfuchsin is placed on the smear for 20 min at room temperature, rinsed in water, and decolorized with 1% HCl in 70% ethanol. For organisms in tissue sections, use a modified Fite-Faraco stain[118] in which hematoxylin rather than methylene blue is used as a counterstain or employ the method used by the

United States Public Health Service Hospital, Carville, Louisiana, as follows.

Materials
1. Deparaffinizing reagent
   Xylene   2 parts
   Peanut or mineral oil   1 part
2. Acid alcohol, 1%
   Hydrochloric acid, conc   1 ml
   Alcohol, 70%   99 ml
3. Carbolfuchsin solution
   Acid, carbolic,
      melted crystals   2.5 ml
   Alcohol, absolute   5 ml
   Basic fuchsin   0.5 g
   Add distilled water to make 50 ml before use.
   Keeps well at room temperature.
4. Working methylene blue solution
   Methylene blue   0.5 g
   Glacial acetic acid   0.5 ml
   Tap water   100 ml

Procedure
1. Deparaffinize sections with xylene–peanut oil or xylene–mineral oil solution—2 changes, 6 min each.
2. Rinse with running tap water for 1 min. Then drain slides for some 45 s. Do not remove all the oil. There should be a thin film of oil on the slide at all times during the procedure. The oil hastens acid-fast staining without the use of heat.
3. Stain with carbolfuchsin for 20 min at room temperature.
4. Wash in running tap water for 3 min.
5. Decolorize in 1% acid alcohol until the slide is faint pink. This takes approximately 1 min for most slides and slightly longer for larger sections. The acid-alcohol should be changed regularly and never used when it is more than a pink color.
6. Wash in tap water for 5 min.
7. Counterstain with methylene blue for 1-2 min according to desired background.
8. Wash in tap water for 20 s.
9. Allow to air dry. After the slide has air dried thoroughly, wipe excess stain and oil off the slide with a clean cloth dampened with water.
10. Mount in Permount. The slide should be mounted in Permount as soon as possible and never allowed to remain open to the air overnight.

M. leprae rods normally are large and thin (0.2-0.5 × 1.5-9 μm), and the viable cells stain a uniform red color with carbolfuchsin.

• • •

M. leprae, an obligate parasite in man, is communicable from man to man. Experimental transmission to humans and lower animals has been unsuccessful, although Shepard[116,119] has described a procedure that permits successive passages of the organism in the footpads of mice.

Mycobacterium marinum[3, 120]
Source and habitat

Originally isolated from diseased fish and aquariums, *M. marinum* has been the cause of epidemics of "swimming pool granuloma" in man, with lesions commonly observed on the elbow, knee, and digital appendages.[120,121] Synonyms of *M. marinum* are *M. balnei* and *M. platypoecilus*. Attempts to produce disease by intravenous or intraperitoneal injections in chickens, guinea pigs, rabbits, or rats has been unsuccessful, except for occasional scrotal lesions in male animals. Application of bacilli to abraded areas on rabbit skin may cause local granulomas. Large intravenous or intraperitoneal inoculations in mice can cause ulcerations on tail, paws, and scrotum, while footpad inoculation results in local swelling and some ulceration that ordinarily appears faster than the same type lesions caused by *M. ulcerans*.[122] In contrast many poikilothermic species are susceptible to fatal systemic disease if maintained at 30 C following infection.[123]

Morphology and staining

Long acid-fast rods with cross-barred staining are commonly observed.

Growth

On inspissated egg-base media, smooth or rough colonies usually appear after 7 days. Colonies on oleic acid–albumin agars commonly are smooth, having domed centers with either an entire margin or a flat apron with irregular edge. On both media, colonies are nonpigmented in the dark but become lemon yellow if young, actively growing cultures are exposed to light. Capable of growth from 22-35 C, *M. marinum* adapts readily to growth at 37 C.

Differential characteristics

Specimens from superficial body areas should be cultured at 32 C; *M. marinum* should not be expected from sputum or gastric washings. Like *M. kansasii*, *M. marinum* hydrolyzes Tween 80 but differs from the former in being nitrate-reductase negative, positive in the 4-day pyrazinamidase test, and strongly positive in the 2-week arylsulfatase test (sometimes even positive in 3 days).[124]

Mycobacterium neoaurum
See *Mycobacterium parafortuitum.*

Mycobacterium nonchromogenicum
See *Mycobacterium terrae.*

Mycobacterium parafortuitum complex[94]
Source and habitat

Included in the *M. parafortuitum* complex are a number of closely related environmental isolates or species, none of which appears to be related to disease: *M. parafortuitum*, *M. diernhoferi*, *M. aurum*, and *M. neoaurum*.

Morphology and staining

Young cultures are commonly acid-fast, but older cultures (>5 days) begin to lose this feature. Rods are often short and plump (0.5-0.8 × 1-3 μm).

Growth

Dilute inocula reveal mature colonies in less than 5 days. Colonies commonly are smooth and hemispherical and are rarely rough. In the entire complex, pigment ranges from none to yellow or even gray, with light sometimes intensifying the color, especially if exposure is prolonged; gray colonies may become dark brown or gray-black in light. Temperature range may be 20-40 C.

Differential characteristics

All species are positive in iron uptake and Tween 80 hydrolysis, most reduce nitrate, and, like other rapidly growing saprophytes (Table 78-2), all are negative in 3-day arylsulfatase and fail to grow on MacConkey agar. If more precise species definition is needed, consult Saito et al.[94] or the original manuscripts that they reference.

Mycobacterium phlei[3, 10]
Source and habitat

Originally isolated from timothy hay, *M. phlei* is thought to be a common saprophyte; however, recent environmental surveys suggest it is now quite rare.[103] It fails to produce progressive disease in experimental animals.

Morphology and staining

Smears show short (1-2 μm) rods that stain acid fast when young but may become non-acid-fast with age (>7 days).

Growth

Mature colonies that appear on egg-base media in less than 5 days are usually rough, wrinkled, and deep yellow in color. Smooth colonies are sometimes seen. Growth on oleic acid–albumin media is usually restricted, but may be smooth and domed, with flat irregular edges and dark, central granules or rough, flat, and granular with irregular edges. The organism grows at temperatures from 22-52 C.

Differential characteristics

As with *M. parafortuitum* complex, precise speciation of this saprophyte and *M. smegmatis* rarely is necessary. Negative 3-day arylsulfatase and failure to grow on MacConkey agar usually relegate such strains to the category of "rapid grower, saprophyte." If exact identification is needed, consult other papers.[3,10,94]

Mycobacterium scrofulaceum[3, 9, 125]
Source and habitat

M. scrofulaceum was first isolated from a child with cervical lymphadenitis; it is commonly found in patients (notably children) complaining of this type of infection. It is occasionally found in sputum and gastric washing without associated pathology and rarely is associated with pulmonary disease. Commonly regarded as a soil organism,[85,103] *M. scrofulaceum* does not cause extensive disease in experimental animals (rats, hamsters, chickens, and guinea pigs), but intradermal or subcutaneous injection of guinea pigs may cause local abscess and regional lymphadenitis. Exact species name of the taxon was

reviewed,[125] and the name *M. scrofulaceum* was retained over the earlier name *M. marianum* because of possible confusion with *M. marinum*[126]; it is also closely related to *M. paraffinicum*.

Morphology and staining

M. scrofulaceum may be seen as short or long rods, sometimes even as filaments. The cells stain well with acid-fast stains.

Growth

On egg-base medium, mature colonies, which appear after 7 days, are usually smooth and yellow to orange in color. On oleic acid agar media, colonies are usually smooth, hemispherical, and yellow to orange with either entire edge or pyramid-shaped with irregular trailing edge. Rough colonies are only rarely seen on both media. The organism is capable of growth from 22-39 C. The pigment may intensify to brick red if cultures are exposed to light continuously for 2 weeks.

Differential characteristics

Because of cultural similarity to slow-growing saprophytic species, the potentially pathogenic *M. scrofulaceum* should be identified. It is nitrate negative and fails to hydrolyze Tween 80 but gives a positive urease test.[84, 93]

Mycobacterium simiae[95, 97]
Source and habitat

This organism was originally isolated from monkeys,[95] but recent work[96] suggests its identity with *M. habana*,[97] an organism that produces pulmonary pathologic conditions in man. Although it is rarely seen in the United States, a recent report of 1 case[127] suggests that as the result of international travel and immigration more strains may be encountered in North America.

Morphology and staining

Acid-fast rods are seen.

Growth

The bacilli are capable of growth from 22-41 C; mature colonies formed after 7 days of incubation may be either eugonic or dysgonic. Although most strains tend to be slowly photochromogenic (require 4-8 hours of light exposure and longer post-light exposure incubation), some are scotochromogenic.

Differential characteristics

Because they are niacin positive and photochromogenic, *M. simiae* strains must be distinguished from both *M. tuberculosis* and *M. kansasii* (see Tables 78-3 and 78-5). *M. simiae* fails to reduce nitrate, is 68 C catalase positive, and is negative in Tween hydrolysis. Poorly photochromogenic strains of *M. simiae* may be easily confused with *M. avium* complex. If close attention to tests for niacin and photochromogenicity do not facilitate the separation, the culture may have to be subjected to seroagglutination studies.[96,127]

Mycobacterium smegmatis[3]
Source and habitat

As the species name *smegmatis* implies, the organism was first isolated from smegma and later was found in soil and water, although recent surveys suggest its isolation in the natural environment is rare.[103] Experimentally, it fails to produce disease in chickens, mice, hamsters, or guinea pigs.

Morphology and staining

The acid-fast–stained rods are usually thin and range from 3-5 μm in length. Pleomorphic and non-acid-fast forms are more commonly observed in older cultures (>7 days).

Growth

Isolated colonies on egg-base media are fully matured in less than 5 days. Although colonies are commonly rough, heaped-up, and nonpigmented, smooth butyrous colonies also are observed. On oleic acid–albumin media, colonies tend to exhibit a smooth surface over a coarsely folded underlying structure that appears granular on microscopic examination. *M. smegmatis* will grow from 22-45 C.

Differential characteristics

Precise definition of *M. smegmatis* is not possible with tests listed in Table 78-2, and indeed, for clinical purposes exact speciation is not needed. As is the case for all saprophytic rapid growers, inability to grow on MacConkey agar and a negative 3-day arylsulfatase reaction will mark its lack of clinical significance. If more exact identification is necessary, consult detailed papers.[3,10]

Mycobacterium szulgai[128]
Source and habitat

All isolates of the new taxon *M. szulgai* thus far examined have been recovered under conditions indicating complicity in human disease: pulmonary disease, cervical adenitis, and olecranon bursitis.[128,129] At this time nothing is known of the saprophytic nature of *M. szulgai*, but an organism that can grow at temperatures of from 25-40 C has a strong possibility of survival outside the human host. To date little has been done relative to virulence studies in experimental animals.

Morphology and staining

Acid-fast stains reveal rods 1-4 μm long that may exhibit the cross-barred staining often seen in *M. kansasii*.

Growth

On both egg-base and oleic acid–albumin agar media, *M. szulgai* forms either (or both) smooth or rough, somewhat pyramid-shaped colonies that taper to a fine edge that is more commonly irregular. When grown at 37 C, cultures are scotochromogenic, and continuous exposure to light may result in the formation of red crystals in and on the colonies (as noted in *M. kansasii*). When grown in the dark at 25 C, *M. szulgai* is reported[129] to be nonpigmented, but it is reported to acquire yellow pigment following light exposure. This phenomenon of photochromogenicity is less obvious at 30 C than at 25 C, and indeed, others report some difficulty in detecting the photochromogenicity even at 25 C.[130]

Differential characteristics

Because of its potential pathogenicity for man, every effort should be made to identify *M. szulgai*. The unique photochromogenicity at 25 C (when it is manifest) and scotochromogenicity at 37 C should immediately suggest this species. The Tween hydrolysis test is usually positive in 10-14 days, nitrates are reduced, and the 2-week arylsulfatase test is moderately strong[130] (E. A. Selva-Sutter, doctoral dissertation).

Mycobacterium terrae complex[11]
Source and habitat

Included in this complex are a number of closely related, commonly saprophytic species of slow-growing nonphotochromogens that, for clinical purposes, need not be further segregated (even though occasionally seen as casual isolates from sputum or gastric washings): *M. terrae* Wayne, *M. novum*, *M. nonchromogenicum*, *M. terrae* Tsukamura, and sometimes even *M. triviale*. Only on rare occasions have representatives of this complex been associated with human disease; when such instances arise, the culture may be precisely identified as described in the literature.* Limited studies thus far performed indicate this complex to have no pathogenicity for laboratory animals and to be common soil organisms.[3,103,132]

Morphology and staining

Acid-fast rods, usually moderately long to long, are seen.

Growth

Colonies are fully matured after 7 days of growth on either egg-base or agar media. Considering all members of the complex, colonies may be completely smooth, hemispherical to totally rough, and even corded. Usually nonpigmented, occasional isolates exhibit pale pastel pigments. Most species grow well from 22-39 C.

Differential characteristics

The *M. terrae* complex, as a group, are strong catalase producers (>45 mm of bubbles) and are positive in 68 C catalase, in Tween 80 hydrolysis, and usually in nitrate reduction but negative in tellurite reduction.

———
*References 11, 113, 131-133.

Mycobacterium thermoresistible[94, 134]

Like *M. phlei*, *M. thermoresistible* is a thermophilic, pigmented, saprophytic rapid grower whose precise definition for clinical reasons is not usually warranted. Like *M. phlei* and others in this saprophytic group, it is negative on Mac-Conkey agar and in the 3-day arylsulfatase test.

Mycobacterium triviale[133]
Source and habitat

Originally recovered from the sputum of a former tuberculous patient, *M. triviale* is not regarded as a pathogen but probably as an environmental saprophyte.

Morphology and staining

Moderately long acid-fast rods are seen.

Growth

Mature colonies on both egg-base and oleic acid–albumin agar media require more than 7 days to appear. Commonly rough, nonpigmented, and corded, the colonies may be confused with *M. tuberculosis*, especially since a number of isolates came from former tuberculous patients. It is for this reason that so much attention is directed to this one species of the *M. terrae* complex. It is capable of growth from 25-39 C.

Differential characteristics

Distinction from most other members of the *M. terrae* complex is possible because of the ability of *M. triviale* to grow on 5% NaCl. Differentiation from *M. tuberculosis* is achieved because *M. triviale* is niacin negative and positive in 68 C catalase.

Mycobacterium tuberculosis[135]
Source and habitat

Isolated from tuberculous lesions of virtually any organ of man, *M. tuberculosis* is most commonly of pulmonary origin and is an obligatory parasite; it also infects other primates, dogs, parrots, and other animals associated with man. This is the species most commonly recovered from suspected tuberculosis of man. Experimentally, this species produces progressive disease in guinea pigs, mice, and hamsters but is relatively nonpathogenic for rabbits and fowl. Virulence for experimental animals may be lost by routine subculture on artificial media, but maintenance of pathogenicity is facilitated either by passage in well-buffered synthetic media of alkaline pH[136] or by preservation at −70 C.[135,137]

Morphology and staining

Strongly acid-fast rods, measuring 0.3-0.6 × 1-4 μm in size, tubercle bacilli may be straight or slightly curved and often reveal beaded forms when stained. The bacilli have a tendency to aggregate, so that smears of pure cultures often reveal serpentine cord formations very characteristic of *M. tuberculosis* and other tubercle bacilli.

Growth

M. tuberculosis is limited to growth at 33-39 C, with mature colonies taking 10-14 days or more to appear both on egg-base and oleic acid–albumin agar medium. On most media, colonies are rough and heaped (cauliflower-like) with irregular margins and nonpigmented. On oleic acid–albumin agar, colonies always are flat, rough, and corded. The growth is dry, friable, and difficult to emulsify in water or saline.

Differential characteristics

Although a positive niacin test is considered by many to provide unequivocal proof of *M. tuberculosis*, it is well known[72, 96] that other mycobacteria may be positive in this test, that some strains of *M. tuberculosis* may be negative, and that certain non-acid-fast contaminants may give positive niacin tests. For these reasons, the niacin test alone should not be relied on for specific identification of *M. tuberculosis*. Perhaps the two most valuable supportive tests for this taxon are a strong positive reaction in nitrate reduction and a loss of catalase activity at 68 C.

Mycobacterium ulcerans[3, 13]

A causative agent of ulcerative cutaneous or subcutaneous lesions in tropical areas and subtropical areas, *M. ulcerans* has never been isolated from sputum or gastric washings. The ulcers, which have a characteristic undermined edge, increase in size by direct extension to involve large areas. The organism has a limited growth temperature range (30-33 C) and grows extremely slowly, often taking 6-9 weeks or more for growth to be visible. Colonies may begin as tiny, smooth, transparent growth but become low, flat, and rough, with irregular edge after further incubation. Pigment may be none to pale yellow. *M. buruli* is believe to be synonymous with *M. ulcerans*.

Rats and mice may be infected experimentally, but most other species are resistant. Lesions characteristically develop on cooler, exposed, peripheral parts of the body: paws, tail, and scrotum. Inoculation of mouse footpad results in localized ulcerating lesions.[122]

Biochemically, *M. ulcerans* has negative reactions in niacin, nitrate reduction, and Tween 80 hydrolysis tests; catalase activity is >45 mm of bubbles and positive after heating at 68 C. Pattyn and Portaels[71] report *M. ulcerans* to be low in catalase activity and to lose this enzyme on heating at 68 C; reasons for this discrepancy are not apparent and must be resolved. Further characteristics of *M. ulcerans* are documented elsewhere.[71,138]

Mycobacterium vaccae[94]

Another one of the saprophytic rapid growers, *M. vaccae*, may be lumped together with these organisms on the basis of negative reactions in the 3-day arylsulfatase and the MacConkey agar tests.

Mycobacterium xenopi [3, 139, 140]
Source and habitat

First isolated from skin granulomas in toads, M. xenopi is sometimes assoicated with chronic pulmonary disease in man or with disease in the genitourinary tract. Its more frequent isolation as a casual resident in man would support its recent finding in tap water.[141] Experimentally, M. xenopi is rather innocuous for most laboratory animals unless extremely large inocula are used.[140] M. littorale is an illegitimate synonym for M. xenopi.

Morphology and staining

Acid-fast rods are commonly very large and sometimes even filamentous.

Growth

Isolated colonies on egg-base medium are mature in 2 weeks or more, yielding smooth (sometimes rough), initially nonpigmented colonies that become yellow on aging. On oleic acid–albumin agar the colonies are small, compact, and commonly exhibit branching filaments[100,139] that are evident on microscopic examination. The organism is capable of growth from 35-45 C; optimum is 42-45 C.

Differential characteristics

Depending on pigment intensity, M. xenopi may be classed as a scotochromogen (Table 78-6) or a nonphotochromogen (Table 78-4). Recognition is made by observation of small, compact colonies with peripheral filaments observed on oleic acid–albumin agar coupled with positive reactions in 68 C catalase and pyrazinamidase tests and susceptibility to 1 μg/ml INH, together with negative reactions in Tween hydrolysis, urease, nitrate reduction, and tellurite reduction.

Other mycobacteria

A number of other legitimate species of Mycobacterium exist that are not mentioned here. Reasons for this are that (1) they are infrequently isolated in clinical laboratories, (2) they are rarely, if ever, isolated from or shown to cause disease in man (but may be pathogenic for other hosts), (3) they are relatively new species not yet studied, and (4) only 1 or 2 strains are extant. Such a list includes, but is not limited to, the following species: M. asiaticum, M. chitae, M. cuneatum, M. duvalii, M. engbaekii, M. farcinogenes, M. gadium, M. gallinarum, M. lepraemurium, M. microti, M. obuense, M. paratuberculosis, M. petroleophilum and M. (?) thamnopheos.

• • •

From the foregoing it is obvious that through the cooperative efforts of international investigators and the wonders of computer technology the taxonomy of mycobacteria has made great strides since the first designation of the Runyon groups.[5,7,8] Not only has it been possible to de-velop precise, taxonomic criteria to enable exact speciation of the many acid-fast bacilli, but through cooperative efforts of clinicians and bacteriologists, it has proved feasible to lump together into "complexes" those mycobacteria of common clinical significance and similar physical characteristics (speed of growth, pigment). The practicality of the clinical laboratory dealing with mycobacterial complexes rather than numerous, often closely related, species should be obvious. Doubtless to say more new species will be found in the future, but it should be relatively easy to incorporate these into the clinically oriented taxonomy that has evolved over the past 10 years.

DRUG SUSCEPTIBILITY TESTS

Soon after the discovery of streptomycin it became clear that optimal treatment of tuberculosis required the determination of the susceptibility of the infecting organisms to the chemotherapeutic agents. Indeed, in 1947, Pyle[142] demonstrated that there was a time-related increase in the ratio of streptomycin-resistant to streptomycin-sensitive bacteria in strains of tubercle bacilli isolated during the course of therapy. As the proportion of resistant bacteria increased, the disease became refractory to treatment. Similar observations were made in relation to isoniazid, i.e., 64% of the cultures isolated from patients treated for 3 months and 93% of those treated for 9 months were found resistant to this drug.[143] This increase in the proportion of resistant bacteria was caused by the interplay of spontaneous mutations and the selection of drug-resistant mutants directed by the chemotherapeutic agent. Extensive clinical and laboratory investigations demonstrated that the numbers of resistant mutants could be eliminated or at least minimized if antituberculosis treatment was pursued with 2 or more drugs. Furthermore, it also was demonstrated that poor response to chemotherapy was apparent before the selective process was completed; in other words, unresponsiveness to treatment was observed before the bacterial population reached 100% resistance.[144] This observation underlines the difficulty in defining a drug-resistant population for medical purposes. However, current understanding of the factors that affect drug susceptibility testing in the laboratory together with a better understanding of host-parasite relationships in tuberculosis under therapy led to the development of 2 fundamental concepts: the **critical concentration** of the drugs in the medium and the **critical proportion** of mutants in the bacillary population.

The **critical concentration** of the drug is that amount that inhibits the growth of most cells in wild strains of tubercle bacilli without appreciably affecting the growth of the few spontaneously occurring drug-resistant mutants present in these bacillary populations. The critical concentration is usually obtained by finding the minimal quantity of drug that will inhibit the growth of

Table 78-7. Critical concentration of drugs and critical proportion of mutants*

| Drug | Critical concentration (μg) | | Critical proportion (%) |
	Lowen-stein-Jensen	Middle-brook 7H-10	
Isoniazid	0.2	0.2	1.0
Streptomycin	4.0	2.0	10.0
p-Aminosalicylic acid	0.5	2.0	1.0
Kanamycin	20.0	5.0	10.0
Ethionamide	20.0	5.0	10.0
Viomycin	30.0	5.0	10.0
D-Cycloserine	30.0	20.0	10.0
Pyrazinamide†	100.0	50.0	10.0
Rifampin	40.0	1.0	1.0
Ethambutol	2.0	2.0‡	1.0

*From David, H. L.: The bacteriology of the mycobacterioses, United States Public Health Service, Atlanta, 1975, Center for Disease Control.
†Must be performed in media of pH 5.5.[149]
‡6.0 μg is commonly used as the single, clinically significant concentration in Middlebrook 7H-10 medium.

most wild strains of tubercle bacilli isolated from patients before treatment[145]; results depend largely on the medium and testing conditions adopted.

The **critical proportion** of mutants reflects that proportion of drug-resistant bacteria in a microbial population that is still compatible with therapeutic success.[145] It is generally accepted that the critical proportion is independent of the testing conditions. The critical concentration of drugs and the critical proportion of mutants, as determined for different agents on different media, are shown in Table 78-7. In general, when the proportion of mutants reaches or exceeds 1% for any drug, very little benefit may be expected by continuing treatment with that same drug.

Laboratory methods (general principles)

There are 3 general methods for determining drug susceptibility: the absolute concentration method, the resistance ratio method, and the proportion method. In the first 2 methods, best results are obtained when the size of the inoculum does not exceed 100,000 bacilli; in the third method, the size of the inoculum is determined in every test, thereby enabling precise quantitation of the proportion of mutants. These methods are described by Canetti et al.,[145] and their publication should be consulted for details and technics. In the United States the method most generally recommended and used is a modification[15] of the method of proportions as used by Canetti[144] and Middlebrook.[147] The details of the procedure are described later.

Laboratory prerequisites

Drug susceptibility tests are one of the most difficult procedures in mycobacteriology to stan-

dardize. In order to maintain a satisfactory level of performance, the volume of work must be reasonably large (more than 10 susceptibility test patterns per week). Two important procedures must be followed to ensure proficiency and reliability in testing: (1) perform replicate surface plate counts regularly and determine whether the results conform with the Poisson law, or follow recommendations for surface plate counting as outlined by Fenner[148] and (2) run control tests with a standard strain, such as the H37Rv strain of *M. tuberculosis*, every time susceptibility tests are done. To ensure reproducible counts for the standard strain, bacterial suspensions of known titer may be prepared in large volume from which aliquots may be dispensed into Wheaton vials and frozen at -70 C for later use[150,151]; 1.0 ml suspension in 5.0 ml Wheaton vials is a convenient volume.

Primary drug resistance
Indicator for drug susceptibility testing

Primary drug resistance is an epidemiologic concept. It refers to the demonstration of drug resistance in strains of tubercle bacilli isolated from patients who were never before treated. According to Canetti et al.,[145] these are individuals who were initially infected with drug-resistant bacteria excreted by a source case in whom resistance had developed as a consequence of treatment. Surveys of primary drug resistance are important in planning large-scale treatment programs.

In countries like the United States where a continuing primary drug-resistance surveillance program has shown the majority of new patients with tuberculosis (92-95%) to be infected with sensitive bacteria, treatment is initiated once tuberculosis is proved. Although the specific diagnosis of tuberculosis requires the isolation and characterization of the causative agent, the prerequisite of drug susceptibility testing is rarely needed to initiate treatment.

Where continuing drug resistance surveys indicate little primary resistance, there is no need to perform susceptibility tests in all initial treatment cases. Because the number of bacilli decreases rapidly during the initial stages of treatment, drug susceptibility tests should not be performed during this phase. As the number of colonies recovered on isolation media decreases, the chances increase that these represent only a few drug-resistant bacteria and, therefore, that the test will be inconsequential. If, however, the number of bacilli in the secretions begins to increase after an initial fall, then drug susceptibility testing must be performed in order to readjust the therapeutic regimen.

Technical procedures

Although susceptibility tests may be done on either egg- or agar-base media using the single, critical concentrations shown in Table 78-7, it has been our experience that fewer problems are

Table 78-8. Percent of active drug remaining after autoclaving, filtering, and freezing*

Drug at 10,000 µg/ml	Method of sterilization				Stored at −20 C		
	Autoclave	Seitz	Glass	Millipore	3 mo	5 mo	6 mo
Isoniazid	90	92	100	98	98	98	97
Streptomycin	90	88	95	95	95	92	90
p-Aminosalicylic acid	100	90	100	100	85	80	75
Kanamycin	98	90	96	98	98	98	98
Ethionamide	90	80	90	90	95	88	85
Viomycin	94	95	98	95	98	95	94
Ethambutol	98	80	88	90	90	90	90
Cycloserine	0	98	98	98	85	75	65
Pyrazinamide	100	100	100	100	100	100	100
Rifampin	Not tested			100	91	86	

*CDC data.

encountered when studies are conducted on Middlebrook 7H-10 agar contained in plastic quadrant dishes. More complete details for preparation of drug solutions and final media may be found elsewhere.[15]

Direct method

Procedure

1. Stain and read smears of digested, concentrated clinical specimens using Ziehl-Neelsen stain.
2. Count number of bacilli observed in 20-25 oil immersion fields and calculate average number of organisms per field. Select appropriate dilutions of concentrated specimen for inocula as follows:

Microscopy	Dilutions to inoculate
< 1 acid-fast bacillus/field	Undiluted and 10^{-2}
1-10 acid-fast bacilli/field	10^{-1} and 10^{-3}
> 10 acid-fast bacilli/field	10^{-2} and 10^{-4}

3. Using a capillary pipet inoculate 3 drops onto each quadrant of control and drug-containing medium. For patients who have been on treatment it is advisable to inoculate 1 set of media with undiluted inoculum (regardless of smear results) because many observed organisms may represent dead or noncultivable bacilli.
4. Incubate plates in polyethylene bags at 35-37 C in an atmosphere of 5-10% CO_2.
5. Report drug susceptibility test results after 3 wk (sooner if definite drug resistance is observed). Do not discard plates as negative without first examining under 30-60× magnification with a dissecting microscope.
6. Countable colonies should be observed on at least one of control plates. Calculate percentage of resistant colonies that may appear on any of the drug-containing media. If more than 1% of colonies that grow on the control medium also grow on one or more of drug media, then clinical resistance to that drug exists or is rapidly emerging.

Indirect method

The direct test should be done whenever possible because the inoculum is more representative of the bacillary population in the lesions of the host. The indirect test, performed from growth on a primary culture, is necessary in the following instances: (1) primary culture is positive but initial smear examination was negative, (2) reference culture is submitted for drug susceptibility test, and (3) inadequate growth (i.e., less than 50-100 colonies) is observed on the control quadrant of a direct test, necessitating repetition of the test.

Procedure

1. From surface of solid medium, transfer a representative sample of growth (ideally a portion of each colony) to a sterile test tube containing 6-8 glass or plastic beads and 3.0 ml Tween-albumin or Middlebrook 7H-9 broth.
2. Disperse cells on a test tube mixer (5 to 10 min).
3. Allow larger particles to settle. Withdraw supernatant and adjust cell suspension to approximate a MacFarland no. 1 standard using sterile distilled water or 0.85% sodium chloride solution as diluent. (MacFarland no. 1 standard is prepared by adding 0.1 ml 1% $BaCl_2$ to 9.9 ml 1% H_2SO_4.)
4. Dilute to 10^{-2} and 10^{-4}, and use both dilutions to inoculate drug media and controls.

Alternative procedure

1. Use 7 d old cultures of test organism grown in Middlebrook and Cohn's 7H-9 liquid medium.
2. Dilute to 10^{-3}, 10^{-4}, and 10^{-6} in sterile water.
3. Inoculate drug media and controls with each dilution.
4. Incubate, read, and report indirect test exactly as described for direct test.

Sterilization of drugs

The procedure used to sterilize the drugs to be added to the medium must be considered, because the amount of drug that is lost varies with each procedure. Table 78-8 shows the percent of active drug remaining after sterilization by 4 different methods. As a routine procedure, we prefer to use membrane filtration (0.22 µm porosity) to prepare sterile stock solutions of the drugs (unless the drug is received sterile and requires only sterile diluent to solubilize).

Use of drug-impregnated paper disks

In 1966 Wayne and Krasnow[152] proposed the use of drug-impregnated paper disks for susceptibility testing of tubercle bacilli, an approach that could lead to increased standardization of this test procedure. Paper disks containing standardized amounts of drug are available com-

Table 78-9. Drug-containing disks for susceptibility tests

Drug	Amount of drug in disk (μg)	Final drug in medium (μg/ml)
Isoniazid	1	0.2
	5	1.0
Streptomycin	10	2.0
	50	10.0
Ethambutol	25	5.0
Rifampin	5	1.0
p-Aminosalicylic acid	10	2.0
	50	10.0
Kanamycin	25	5.0
Ethionamide	25	5.0

mercially. In the usual drug disk test the disks are placed on the surface of already solidified and inoculated media. In susceptibility testing of tubercle bacilli, however, the disks are aseptically placed in the sectioned quadrants of sterile plastic dishes and measured amounts (5.0 ml) of sterile, complete Middlebrook 7H-10 medium are pipetted over the disks. Dishes are incubated at 25 C overnight to permit the drug to diffuse from the submerged disk into the medium. Because the drug must diffuse throughout 5 ml of medium, it is necessary to use disks containing 5 times the desired quantity of drug. Table 78-9 lists the disks currently available, indicating the quantity of drug per disk and the final concentration of drug in medium (in μg/ml). Since each disk is coded to identify the drug and its concentration, there is no chance for labeling errors. The fact that only 1 batch of plain Middlebrook 7H-10 medium is needed for the disks (as opposed to multiple drug-containing batches when using powdered drugs), and that only in the volume actually needed for the strains to be tested, should prove to be economical of time, media, and drugs. Once the medium has been prepared, it may be inoculated, incubated, read, and reported exactly as described for the other tests. The use of submerged disks has been shown[152-154] to provide as reliable results as routinely performed drug tests.

ASSAY OF ANTITUBERCULOSIS DRUGS IN BODY FLUIDS

The assay of antituberculosis drugs in body fluids, especially in the blood serum, was recommended in the not too distant past as useful in the management of the individual case.[147] At present, however, these assays are of value only when there is reason to believe that the drugs may not be absorbed properly (for example, following surgery of the intestinal tract) or that the drugs may accumulate to toxic levels (for example, in cases of kidney insufficiency). These assays should not be attempted by the average clinical laboratory and must be referred to laboratories specialized in this capacity (level III laboratories). In these laboratories, various chemical or biologic methods of assay are adopted; personnel in such laboratories must be contacted regarding the schedule for drawing the blood, the volume of blood necessary, and the test done for each drug being assayed. Because of the variety of methods used and their distinct prerequisites, no attempt is made to describe them; however, the reader may refer to other sources[147,155,156] for examples of the types of assays that may be performed.

REFERENCES

1. Hawkins, J. E., Karlson, A. G., Wayne, L. G., et al.: Am. Rev. Respir. Dis. **110:**376, 1974.
2. Kubica, G. P., Gross, W. M., Hawkins, J. E., et al.: Am. Rev. Respir. Dis. **112:**773, 1975.
3. Buchanan, R. E., and Gibbons, N. E.: Bergey's manual of determinative bacteriology, ed. 8, Baltimore, 1974, The Williams & Wilkins Co.
4. Buhler, V. B., and Pollak, A.: Am. J. Clin. Pathol. **23:**363, 1953.
5. Timpe, A., and Runyon, E. H.: J. Lab. Clin. Med. **44:**202, 1954.
6. Crow, H. E., King, C. T., Smith, C. E., et al.: Am. Rev. Tuberc. **75:**199, 1957.
7. Runyon, E. H.: Med. Clin. North Am. **43:**273, 1959.
8. Runyon, E. H.: Adv. Tuberc. Res. **14:**235, 1965.
9. Wayne, L. G., et al.: J. Gen. Microbiol. **66:**255, 1971.
10. Kubica, G. P., et al.: J. Gen. Microbiol. **73:**55, 1972.
11. Meissner, G., et al.: J. Gen. Microbiol. **83:**207, 1974.
12. Reznikov, M., and Dawson, D. J.: Appl. Microbiol. **26:**470, 1973.
13. Runyon, E. H., Karlson, A. G., Kubica, G. P., et al: In Lennette, E. H., Spaulding, E. H., and Truant, J. P., editors: Manual of clinical microbiology, ed. 2, Washington D.C., 1974, American Society for Microbiology, p. 150.
14. Runyon, E. H.: Tubercle **55:**235, 1974.
15. Vestal, A. L.: Procedures for the isolation and identification of mycobacteria, Atlanta, 1975, Center for Disease Control.
16. Kestle, D. G., and Kubica, G. P.: Am. J. Clin. Pathol. **48:**347, 1967.
17. Engbaek, H. C., and Weis-Bentzon, M.: Acta Tuberc. Scand. **45:**89, 1964.
18. Engbaek, H. C., and Weis-Bentzon, M.: Acta Tuberc. Scand. **45:**97, 1964.
19. Krasnow, I., and Wayne, L. G.: Appl. Microbiol. **18:**915, 1969.
20. Jones, F. L., Jr.: Dis. Ches. **50:**403, 1966.
21. Vandiviere, H. M., Smith, C. E., and Sunkes, E. J.: Am. Rev. Tuberc. **65:**617, 1952.
22. Carr, D. T., Karlson, A. G., and Stilwell, G. G.: Mayo Clin. Proc. **42:**23, 1967.
23. Kenney, M., Loechel, A. B., and Lovelock, F. J.: Am. Rev. Respir. Dis. **82:**564, 1960.
24. Shaw, J. B., and Wynn-Williams, N.: Am. Rev. Tuberc. **69:**724, 1954.
25. Louden, R. G., Williamson, J., and Johnson, J. M.: Am. Rev. Tuberc. **77:**623, 1958.
26. Geiger, F. L., and Kuemmerer, J. M.: Public Health. Rep. **78:**663, 1963.

27. Gunnels, J. J., Bates, J. H., and Swindoll, H.: Am. Rev. Respir. Dis. **109**:323, 1974.
28. Reagan, W. P.: Clin. Notes Respir. Dis. **11**:3, 1973.
29. Bates, J. H.: Am. Rev. Respir. Dis. **109**:317, 1974.
30. Cashman, H. H., D'Esopo, N. D., Dickinson, W., Jr., et al.: Am. Rev. Respir. Dis. **102**:470, 1970.
31. Sweaney, H. C.: Am. Rev. Tuberc. **45**:103, 1942.
32. Lind, H. E., and Shaughnessy, H. J.: J. Lab. Clin. Med. **27**:531-536, 1942.
33. Oliver, J., and Reusser, T. R.: Am. Rev. Tuberc. **45**:450, 1942.
34. Amercian Lung Association: Diagnostic standards and classification of tuberculosis and other mycobacterial diseases, New York, 1974, The Association.
35. Kubica, G. P., Dye, W. E., Cohn, M. L. et al.: Am. Rev. Respir. Dis. **87**:775, 1963.
36. Kubica, G. P., Kaufmann, A. J., and Dye, W. E.: Am. Rev. Respir. Dis. **89**:284, 1964.
37. Wayne, L. G., Krasnow, I., and Kidd, G. C.: Am. Rev. Respir. Dis. **86**:537, 1962.
38. Petroff, S. A.: J. Exp. Med. **21**:38, 1915.
39. Corper, H. J., and Uyei, N.: J. Lab. Clin. Med. **15**:348, 1930.
40. Warren, N. G., and Lambert, F. W., Jr.: Public Health Lab. **32**:8, 1974.
41. Smithwick, R. W., Stratigos, C. B., and David, H. L.: J. Clin. Microbiol. **1**:411, 1975.
42. Woodruff, C. D., Crombie, D., Medlar, E., et al.: Am. Rev. Tuberc. **54**:428, 1946.
43. Cohn, M. L. Waggoner, R. F., and McClatchy, J. K.: Am. Rev. Respir. Dis. **98**:295, 1968.
44. Cohn, M. L., and Middlebrook, G.: Am. Rev. Respir. Dis. **87**:292, 1963.
45. Kubica, G. P., Kaufmann, A. J., and Beam, R. E.: Am. J. Clin. Pathol. **41**:452, 1964.
46. Novy, F. G., and Soule, M. H.: J. Infect. Dis. **36**:168, 1925.
47. Ebina, T., Nakamura, T., and Inomata, D.: Tohoku J. Exp. Med. **32**:1, 1938.
48. Davies, R.: Br. J. Exp. Pathol. **21**:243, 1940.
49. Schaefer, W. B., Cohn, M. L., and Middlebrook, G.: J. Bacteriol. **69**:706, 1955.
50. Cohn, M. L., Russell, W. F., Jr., and Middlebrook, G.: Am. Rev. Respir. Dis. **82**:579, 1960.
51. Beam, R. E., and Kubica, G. P.: Am. J. Clin. Pathol. **50**:395, 1968.
52. Whitcomb, F. C., Foster, M. C., and Dukes, C. D.: Am. Rev. Respir. Dis. **86**:584, 1962.
53. Miliner, R. A., Stottmeier, K. D., and Kubica, G. P.: Am. Rev. Respir. Dis. **99**:603, 1969.
54. Kilburn, J. O., Stottmeier, K. D., and Kubica, G. P.: Am. J. Clin. Pathol. **50**:582, 1968.
55. Stonebrink, B.: Acta Tuberc. Scand. **35**:Fasc. 1, 1958.
56. Dixon, J. M. S., and Cuthbert, E. H.: Am. Rev. Respir. Dis. **96**:119, 1967.
57. Smith, T.: J. Med. Res. **23**:185, 1910.
58. Weber, A.: Zbl. Bakt. I. Abt. Orig. **64**:243, 1912.
59. Fregnan, G. B., and Smith, D. W.: J. Bacteriol. **83**:819, 1962.
60. Kubica, G. P., and Jones, W. D., Jr.: Zbl. Bakt. (Orig.) **196**:53, 1965.
61. Jones, W. D., Jr., and Kubica, G. P.: Zbl. Bakt. (Orig.) **196**:68, 1965.
62. Vestal, A. L., and Kubica, G. P.: Am. Rev. Respir. Dis. **94**:247, 1966.
63. Feldman, W. H., and Magath, T. B.: Am. Rev. Tuberc. **24**:312, 1931.
64. Weed, L. A.: Am. J. Clin. Pathol. **21**:691, 1951.

65. Goodfellow, M., et al.: J. Gen. Microbiol. **85**:291, 1974.
66. Wayne, L. G., et al.: Int. J. Syst. Bacteriol. **24**:412, 1974.
67. Wayne, L. G., et al.: Int. J. Syst. Bacteriol. **26**:311, 1976.
68. Tsukamura, M.: Tubercle **48**:311, 1967.
69. Käppler, W.: Z. Tuberk. **129**:311, 321, 1968.
70. Wayne, L. G., and Doubek, J. R.: Appl. Microbiol. **16**:925, 1968.
71. Pattyn, S. R., and Portaels, F.: Zbl. Bakt. **A219**:114, 1972.
72. Kubica, G. P.: Am. Rev. Respir. Dis. **107**:9, 1973.
73. Wayne, L. G.: Am. J. Clin. Pathol. **36**:185, 1961.
74. Wayne, L. G.: Am. Rev. Respir. Dis. **86**:651, 1962.
75. Kubica, G. P., et al.: Am. Rev. Respir. Dis. **94**:400, 1966.
76. Kubica, G. P., and Pool, G. L.: Am. Rev. Respir. Dis. **81**:387, 1960.
77. Jones, W. D., Jr., and Kubica, G. P.: Am. J. Med. Technol. **30**:187, 1964.
78. Kubica, G. P., and Vitvitsky, J.: Appl. Microbiol. **27**:917, 1974.
79. Runyon, E. H., Selin, M. J., and Harris, H. W.: Am. Rev. Tuberc. **79**:663, 1959.
80. Kilburn, J. O., and Kubica, G. P.: Am. J. Clin. Pathol. **50**:530, 1968.
81. Young, W. D., Jr., Maslansky, A., Lefar, M. S., et al.: Appl. Microbiol. **20**:939, 1970.
82. Virtanen, S.: Acta Tuberc. Scand. (suppl.) **48**:1, 1960.
83. Wayne, L. G., and Doubek, J. R.: Am. J. Clin. Pathol. **42**:431, 1964.
84. Wayne, L. G.: Am. Rev. Respir. Dis. **109**:147, 1974.
85. Kestle, D. G., Abbott, V. D., and Kubica, G. P.: Am. Rev. Respir. Dis. **95**:1041, 1967.
86. Kilburn, J. O., Silcox, V. A., and Kubica, G. P.: Am. Rev. Respir. Dis. **99**:94, 1969.
87. Bönicke, R.: Naturwissenschaften **45**:392, 1958.
88. Harrington, R., and Karlson, A. G.: Am. J. Vet. Res. **27**:1193, 1966.
89. Vestal, A. L., and Kubica, G. P.: Scand. J. Respir. Dis. **48**:142, 1967.
90. Wayne, L. G., Doubek, J. R., and Russell, R. L.: Am. Rev. Respir. Dis. **90**:588, 1964.
91. Kilburn, J. O., et al.: Appl. Microbiol. **26**:826, 1973.
92. Toda, T., Hagihara, Y., and Takeya, K.: Am. Rev. Respir. Dis. **83**:757, 1970.
93. Murphy, D. B., and Hawkins, J. E.: J. Clin. Microbiol. **1**:465, 1975.
94. Saito, H., et al.: Int. J. Syst. Bacteriol. **27**:75, 1977.
95. Weiszfeiler, J. G.: Die Biologie und Variabilität des Tuberkelbakteriums und die atypischen Mycobakterien, Budapest, 1969, Akademik Verlag, p. 237.
96. Meissner, G., and Schröder, K. H.: Am. Rev. Respir. Dis. **111**:196, 1975.
97. Valdivia-Alvarez, J., Suarez-Mendez, R., and Echemendia Font, M.: Bol. Hig. Epid. **9**:65, 1971.
98. Tsukamura, M.: Am. Rev. Respir. Dis. **110**:101, 1974.
99. Runyon, E. H.: Am. J. Clin. Pathol. **54**:578, 1970.
100. Runyon, E. H.: Identification of acid fast pathogens, ed. 3, Salt Lake City, Utah, 1972, Veterans Administration Hospital.
101. Castets, M., Rist, N., and Boisvert, H.: Méd. d'Afrique Noire No. **4**:321, 1969.
102. Engbaek, H. C., Runyon, E. H., and Karlson, A. G.: Int. J. Syst. Bacteriol. **21**:192, 1971.

103. Wolinsky, E., and Rynearson, T.: Am. Rev. Respir. Dis. **97**:1032, 1968.
104. Kazda, J.: Zbl. Bakt. Abt. I. Orig. **203**:199, 1967.
105. Karlson, A. G., and Lessel, E. F.: Int. J. Syst. Bacteriol. **20**:273, 1970.
106. Stanford, J. L., et al.: J. Med. Microbiol. **5**:171, 1972.
107. Bojalil, L. F., Cerbon, J., and Trujillo, A.: J. Gen. Microbiol. **28**:333, 1962.
108. Wayne, L. G., and Diaz, G. A.: Am. Rev. Respir. Dis. **96**:88, 1967.
109. Stanford, J. L., and Gunthorpe, W. J.: Br. J. Exp. Pathol. **52**:627, 1971.
110. Runyon, E. H.: Int. J. Syst. Bacteriol. **22**:50, 1972.
111. Penso, G., et al.: Rendic. Ist. super. san. **15**:491, 1952.
112. Hartwig, E. C., Cacciatore, R., and Dunbar, F. P.: Am. Rev. Respir. Dis. **85**:84, 1962.
113. Wayne, L. G.: Am. Rev. Respir. Dis. **93**:919, 1966.
114. Wayne, L. G.: Int. J. Syst. Bacteriol. **20**:149, 1970.
115. Bailey, R. K., et al.: Am. Rev. Respir. Dis. **101**:430, 1970.
116. Shepard, C. C.: Amer. J. Hyg. **71**:147, 1960.
117. Hilson, G. R., and Elek, S. D.: Int. J. Lepr. **25**:380, 1957.
118. Armed Forces Institute of Pathology: Manual of histologic and special staining techniques, Washington, D.C., 1957, The Institute.
119. Shepard, C. C.: J. Exp. Med. **112**:445, 1960.
120. Linell, L., and Norden, A.: Acta Tuberc. Pneumol. Scand. suppl. **33**:1, 1954.
121. Schaefer, W. B., and Davis, C. L.: Am. Rev. Respir. Dis. **84**:837, 1961.
122. Fenner, F.: Am. Rev. Tuberc. **73**:650, 1956.
123. Clark, H. F., and Shepard, C. C.: J. Bacteriol. **86**:1057, 1963.
124. Silcox, V. A., and David, H. L.: Appl. Microbiol. **21**:327, 1971.
125. Wayne, L. G.: Int. J. Syst. Bacteriol. **25**:230, 1975.
126. Opinion 53, Judicial Commission, ICSB, Int. J. Syst. Bacteriol. **28**:334, 1978.
127. Krasnow, I., and Gross, W.: Am. Rev. Respir. Dis. **111**:357, 1975.
128. Marks, J., Jenkins, P. A., and Tsukamura, M.: Tubercle **53**:210, 1972.
129. Schaefer, W. B., et al.: Am. Rev. Respir. Dis. **108**:1320, 1973.
130. Selva-Sutter, E. A., et al.: J. Clin. Microbiol. **3**:414, 1976.

131. Tsukamura, M.: Med. Biol. **71**:110, 1965.
132. Tsukamura, M.: Jpn. J. Microbiol. **11**:163, 1967.
133. Kubica, G. P., et al.: Int. J. Syst. Bacteriol. **20**:161, 1970.
134. Tsukamura, M.: Med. Biol. **72**:187, 1966.
135. Kubica, G. P., Kim, T. H., and Dunbar, F. P.: Int. J. Syst. Bacteriol. **22**:99, 1972.
136. Steenken, W., Jr., and Gardner, L. U.: Yale J. Biol. Med. **15**:393, 1943.
137. Kim, T. H., and Kubica, G. P.: Appl. Microbiol. **24**:311, 1972.
138. Pattyn, S. R., et al.: Acad. Roy. Soc. Outre-Mer, Bull. des séances, 1964-1966, pp. 1576-1599.
139. Runyon, E. H.: J. Bacteriol. **95**:734, 1968.
140. Engbaek, H. C., et al.: Acta Pathol. Microbiol. Scand. **69**:576, 1967.
141. McSwiggan, D. A., and Collins, C. H.: Tubercle **55**:291, 1974.
142. Pyle, M.: Proc. Mayo Clin. **22**:465, 1947.
143. Medical Research Council (England): Isoniazid trial, report no. 4, Lancet **2**:217, 1953.
144. Canetti, G., Rist, N., and Grosset, J.: Rev. Tuberc. **72**:218, 1963.
145. Canetti, G., et al.: Bull. W.H.O. **29**:565, 1968.
146. David, H. L.: The bacteriology of the mycobacterioses, United States Public Health Service, Atlanta, 1975, Center for Disease Control.
147. Russell, W. F., Jr., and Middlebrook, G.: The chemotherapy of tuberculosis, Springfield, Ill., 1961, Charles C Thomas, Publisher.
148. Fenner, F.: Am. Rev. Tuberc. **64**:353, 1951.
149. Stottmeier, K. D., Beam, R. E., and Kubica, G. P.: Am. Rev. Respir. Dis. **96**:1072, 1967.
150. Grover, A. A., et al.: J. Bacteriol. **94**:832, 1967.
151. Kim, T. H., and Kubica, G. P.: Appl. Microbiol. **24**:311, 1972.
152. Wayne, L. G., and Krasnow, I.: Am. J. Clin. Pathol. **45**:769, 1966.
153. Griffith, M., et al.: Am. J. Clin. Pathol. **47**:812, 1967.
154. Griffith, M. E., et al.: Am. Rev. Respir. Dis. **103**:423, 1971.
155. Stottmeier, K. D., et al.: Bull. W.H.O. **37**:961, 1967.
156. Lorian, V.: Antibiotics and chemotherapeutic agents in clinical and laboratory practice, Springfield, Ill., 1966, Charles C Thomas, Publisher.

79

GRAM-NEGATIVE BACILLI, VIBRIOS, AND SPIRILLA

Alex C. Sonnenwirth

In this chapter are included the aerobic and facultatively anaerobic gram-negative rods, vibrios, and spirilla.* This group consists of a very large variety of organisms ranging from large rods, which are easily cultivated, to many smaller, coccoid- to coccobacillary-shaped ones, many of which can be cultivated only on enriched media or by special technics.

The terms "enteric bacilli," "enterics," or "enterobacteria" are often indiscriminately applied to various such superficially similar organisms with quite different metabolism, antigenic structure, pathogenicity, ecology, and evolutionary relations. These vernacular terms, in fact, should be applied only to members of the family *Enterobacteriaceae*.

Initial division

A most significant distinction in the initial division of these organisms is between those that can **ferment** sugars and those that utilize sugars **oxidatively** or **not at all** (Table 71-1). Bacteria produce acid from carbohydrates by 2 methods. One is an anaerobic process called **fermentation;** the second, designated **oxidation**, is an aerobic process. Since gram-negative bacteria that attack carbohydrates usually do so exclusively by either fermentation or oxidation, the determination of the type of carbohydrate metabolism carried out by an organism is of taxonomic significance.

The distinction is based on growth in an aerobic (open) tube and in an anaerobic tube (sealed with sterile mineral oil) of Hugh and Leifson's **OF medium** (Chapter 72). Fermenters produce acid in both tubes, oxidizers only in the open tube, and nonutilizers of glucose in neither (glucose can ordinarily be utilized if any sugar can).

Triple sugar iron agar (TSI) can initially be used to differentiate fermentative from oxidative bacteria. A TSI reaction of acid butt with or without an acid slant is indicative of a fermenter. No change of the butt and slant of a TSI or slight alkalinization of the slant is indicative of an oxidizer **or** nonutilizer of sugars. Occasionally an oxidizer will show slight acidity on the slant of a TSI. (In cases where the TSI reaction is doubtful, an oxidation-fermentation test should be carried out using OF base medium with 1% glucose.)

The **fermenters** include both the many genera ordinarily harmless when present in the gut as well as the pathogenic genera of *Enterobacteriaceae* (with *Yersinia* included in the family), *Vibrio, Aeromonas,* and some other more fastidious or rarer genera (*Chromobacterium, Pasteurella, Actinobacillus, Haemophilus, Cardiobacterium*).

Many **nonfermenters** are glucose oxidizers (*Pseudomonas* and many other genera); others cannot utilize glucose or other carbohydrates (*Acinetobacter, Alcaligenes,* etc., Table 79-1). The nonfermenters are found primarily free in nature. However, with the advent of antibiotics and the survival of patients with reduced immune responses, both nonfermenters and the "nonpathogenic" fermenters are encountered with increasing frequency as agents of **opportunistic** (but often very serious) **infection.**

Within the 2 major groups (fermenters and nonfermenters), genera can be differentiated on the basis of various additional characteristics.

The **oxidase** reaction tests for the ability of the electron transport chain to convert certain aromatic amines into colored products: this test clearly distinguishes several genera (Table 79-1).

In the clinical laboratory the oxidase test offers the fastest and most important distinction between these organisms: All gram-negative, aerobic, or facultatively anaerobic rods should be oxidase tested before any further workup is undertaken (for technic of the test, see Chapter 75).

The **flagella** are peritrichous (or absent) in the *Enterobacteriaceae* (see Chapter 68), *Flavobacterium,* and *Alcaligenes,* but polar in *Vibrio, Aeromonas,* and *Pseudomonas.* Other differential characters include sensitivity to bile salts or citrate (used in MacConkey agar and SS agar), in

---

*The **anaerobic,** nonsporeforming gram-negative rods are discussed in Chapter 86.

Table 79-1. Selected differential characteristics of *Enterobacteriaceae* and other gram-negative bacteria*

Family, genus, or species	Glucose metabolism	Oxidase	Growth on Mac	SS	Motility	Nitrate to Nitrite	Gas	Lysine†	Argi-nine‡	Orni-thine†
Enterobacteriaceae, incl. *Yersinia*	F	−	+	+	+, −§	+	−	d‖	d‖	d‖
Vibrio	F	+	+	−¶	+	+	−	+	−	+
Aeromonas	F	+	+	+	+	+	−	−	+	−
Pasteurella	F	+	−¶	−	−	+	−	−	−	d
Pseudomonas	Ox	+#	+	+	+	−	+ or −	− (NC	(NC	(NC)
Achromobacter	Ox	−	d	d	+ (−)	+ or −	−	−	+, −	−
Acinetobacter (anitratum [*Herellea*])	Ox	−	+	−¶	−	−	−	NC	NC	NC
A. (lwofii [*Mima*])	In	−	+	−¶	−	−	−	NC	NC	NC
Moraxella	In	+	− or +	−	−	− or +	−	NC	NC	NC
Flavobacterium	Ox or In	+ (−)	+ (−)	−	+ (−)	−	+ or −	NC	NC	NC
Alcaligenes	In	+	+	(+) −	+	−	+ or −	NC	NC	NC

*F, Fermentative; Ox, oxidative; In, inactive (in OF medium; see text); Mac, MacConkey agar; SS, Salmonella-Shigella agar; +, positive reaction or growth; −, no reaction or growth; (+), delayed positive reaction or poor growth; d, different reactions—+, (+), or −; NC, no change; + (−), majority positive, occasional strain negative.
†Decarboxylases.
‡Dihydrolase.
§In *Yersinia*, motility when present is demonstrable at 20-25 C but usually not at 37 C.
‖Various patterns of reactions.
¶Some strains grow.
#Except *P. maltophilia*.

ability to reduce nitrate to nitrite or gas, and various decarboxylase reactions (Table 79-1).

A multitude of keys and schemes have been constructed for the preliminary recognition and definitive identification of these organisms; Table 79-2, based originally on the widely used schema of Elizabeth King,[1] and more recently extensively revised by Weaver at the U. S. Center for Disease Control,[2,2a] is recommended for the **preliminary recognition** of these bacteria, since it is based on practical criteria such as (1) nature of attack on carbohydrates (fermentative, oxidative, or none), (2) growth on MacConkey agar, (3) oxidase reaction, and (4) nature of flagellation (number, position). The key is intended **only** as a guideline; the groups listed must be identified by the use of a number of differential reactions. (See also Table 79-1).

In general the classification is based on the system used in the 8th edition of *Bergey's Manual*.[3] However, because of the considerable information acquired in the past decade regarding the taxonomic position of many organisms and the general acceptance of certain newer nomenclatural and taxonomic schemes (such as Edwards' and Ewing's system for *Enterobacteriaceae*), a number of newly named (or renamed) genera and species and their differential reactions are listed together with rearrangement and reclassification of certain existing genera and species.

The differences between *Bergey's Manual* and Ewing's classification of *Enterobacteriaceae* are discussed below in detail (Table 79-8), as well as the changes instituted by the (U.S.) Center for Disease Control in the period 1977-1978 (Table 79-9).

Clinical importance[4]

It should be noted that organisms once thought to have little virulence or to be completely nonpathogenic (including members of the normal flora of humans and saprophytes) have been increasingly associated with disease in the developed countries (see, for example, Gale and Sonnenwirth[5]). **Endogenous** infections (due to indigenous organisms) and **nosocomial** (hospital-acquired) infections now represent a large proportion of serious bacterial infections in the United States and other Western countries. On the other hand, typhoid fever (*Salmonella typhi*), bacillary dysentery (*Shigella*), and cholera (*Vibrio cholerae*) are now largely controlled in the Western world (through public health measures), but they still represent serious and periodically recurring problems throughout the rest of the world. Since the mid-1960s the frequency of staphylococcal, pneumococcal, and streptococcal infections has diminished considerably, while the incidence of infections due to enteric bacteria and other gram-negative rods of low virulence has increased strikingly (e.g., *E. coli*, *Klebsiella*, *Enterobacter*, *Serratia*, *Proteus*, *Pseudomonas*). Enteric organisms have always been the most common agents of urinary tract infections, but they are now also the predominant agents in various endogenous and nosocomial infections (surgical wound infections, hospital-acquired pneumonias, etc.). Treatment of such infections is often made difficult by resis-

Table 79-2. Key for presumptive identification of aerobic gram-negative rods*†

Gram-negative fermenters

MacConkey positive
    Oxidase negative
        Enterobacteriaceae, Yersinia pestis, Y. pseudotuberculosis, Y. enterocolitica, Chromobacterium violaceum
           (oxidase variable), HB-5 (oxidase and MacConkey variable)
    Oxidase positive
        Aeromonas hydrophila, A. (Plesiomonas) shigelloides, Vibrio cholerae, noncholera *Vibrio, V. parahaemoly-*
           ticus, V. alginolyticus, Lac + *Vibrio* (halophilic), *Chromobacterium violaceum,* EF-4, HB-5, *Pasteurella*
           haemolytica, Actinobacillus lignieresii, A equuli, Haemophilus aphrophilus
MacConkey negative
    Oxidase negative
        Haemophilus aphrophilus (majority of strains), *H. vaginalis, Actinobacillus actinomycetemcomitans*
           (majority of strains), DF-1, HB-5
    Oxidase positive
        Pasteurella multocida, P. pneumotropica, P. ureae, P. gallinarum, P. "gas," Cardiobacterium hominis,
           EF-4, HB-5, DF-2, *Haemophilus aphrophilus, Actinobacillus actinomycetemcomitans, A. equuli,*
           A. lignieresii, P. haemolytica, Kingella kingae, K. denitrificans (TM-1)

Gram-negative glucose oxidizers

MacConkey positive
    Oxidase negative
        Acinetobacter calcoaceticus (Herellea, anitratus), Pseudomonas cepacia, P. mallei, P. maltophilia,
           P. paucimobilis (IIK-1), Ve-1, Ve-2
    Oxidase positive
        Pseudomonas aeruginosa, P. fluorescens, P. putida, P. cepacia, P. pseudomallei, P. diminuta, P. mallei,
           P. mendocina, P. pickettii, P. "thomasii," P. putrefaciens, P. stutzeri, P. vesicularis, P. paucimobilis
           (IIK-1), IIK-2, *Achromobacter xylosoxidans, Agrobacterium radiobacter, Brucella,* EO-2, *Vibrio*
           extorquens, IIb, *Flavobacterium meningosepticum,* Va-1, Vb-3, Vd-1, Vd-2
McConkey negative
    Oxidase negative
        Brucella, IIe, *Pseudomonas paucimobilis* (IIk-1), *P. mallei*
    Oxidase positive
        Brucella, Flavobacterium meningosepticum, EO-2, *Pseudomonas vesicularis, Vibrio extorquens,* IIb, IIe,
           IIh, IIi-1, *P. paucimobilis,* IIK-2, *Neisseria*

Gram-negative glucose nonoxidizers

MacConkey positive
    Oxidase negative
        Bordetella parapertussis, Acinetobacter (Mima, lwoffi). Pseudomonas maltophilia
    Oxidase positive
        Alcaligenes faecalis, A. odorans, A. denitrificans, Bordetella bronchiseptica, Brucella, Campylobacter
           fetus, IV-f, *Moraxella, Comamonas (Pseudomonas acidovorans, P. testosteroni), P. alcaligenes, P. diminuta,*
           P. pseudoalcaligenes, P. putrefaciens, Vibrio extorquens, IVc-2, IVe
MacConkey negative
    Oxidase negative
        None
    Oxidase positive
        Eikenella corrodens, Brucella, Campylobacter fetus, Moraxella, Vibrio extorquens, IIf, IIj

*From Weaver, R. E.: Gram-negative organisms: an approach to identification (guide to **presumptive** identifications), Atlanta, 1979, Center for Disease Control.

†Key is based on (1) nature of attack on carbohydrates (fermenters, oxidizers, or neither—OF test), (2) growth on MacConkey agar, and (3) oxidase reaction.

tance of the organisms to many antimicrobial agents and by the presence of other serious diseases in the patients.

Thus accurate identification of the organisms described here is imperative. They differ markedly in virulence, which is important for prognosis and for recognizing potential danger to contacts, and in susceptibility to various antimicrobial agents. In addition, identification is essential for epidemiologic investigation of the sources of infection. A typical example of the need for identification is furnished by the

epidemic of hospital-acquired septicemia (at least 400 cases including 40 or more deaths) that was traced to the production of contaminated intravenous solutions (in the early 1970s); the key was a sharp rise in the isolation of 2 relatively unusual organisms, *Enterobacter cloacae* and *Erwinia* (now *Enterobacter agglomerans*), in geographically widely dispersed institutions. Had the clinical microbiology laboratory not carried the identification to the species level, the organisms might have easily been confused with common *Klebsiella* and *Enterobacter* strains, and detection of the source of the epidemic might have been delayed for a long time.

Presumptive and final identifications

As mentioned above, an initial **oxidase test** and determination of the manner of **glucose utiliza-** tion (either by triple sugar iron [TSI] slant or by oxidation-fermentation [OF] medium) serve to distinguish the major group (family or genus) to which the unknown organism likely belongs.

Further identification of the organisms is generally accomplished by inoculation of a portion of a single, isolated colony from an agar plate in

Table 79-3. Presumptive identification I: Gram-negative fermenters, MacConkey positive (growth); oxidase negative*†

	Gas from glucose	Urea	Lysine decar-boxylase	Arginine dihydro-lase	Ornithine decar-boxylase	Lactose	Sucrose	Rhamnose	Motility (C) 35	25	5	Indole
Enterobacteriaceae	Var may be large vol	Var	Var	Var	Var	Var	Var	Var	Var			Var
Yersinia entero-colitica	+ or −, not large vol	+	−	−	+	−(d)	+	−	−	+	+	Var
Yersinia pseudo-tuberculosis	−	+	−	−	−	−	+	−	−	+	+ or −	−
Yersinia pestis	−	−	−	−	−	−	−	−	−	−	−	−
Chromobacterium violaceum	−	−(d)	−	+	−	−	Var	−	+			−‡ (? +)
HB-5	+ or −, not large vol	−	−	−	−	−	−	−				+, w

*From Weaver, R. E: Gram-negative organisms: an approach to identification (guide to **presumptive** identifications), Atlanta, 1979, Center for Disease Control.

†*var*, Variable; *vol*, volume; *d*, variable; *w*, weak +; +, 90% or more +, 1-2 d; + or −, 50-90% +, 1-2 d; −, 90% or more −; − or +, 50-90% − (+), delayed +, 3 or more d.

‡Nonpigmented variants may be positive.

Table 79-4. Presumptive identification II: Gram-negative fermenters, MacConkey positive (growth); oxidase positive*†

	Glu-cose, gas	Mannitol acid	Lactose, acid	Sucrose, acid	Lysine decar-boxylase	Arginine dihydro-lase	Ornithine decar-boxylase	NaCl required	Urea	Indole	Motil-ity
Aeromonas hydrophila	+ or −	+	− or +	+ or −	− or +	+	−	−	− or +	+ or −	+
A. (Plesiomonas) shigelloides	−	−	+ or (+)	−	+	+	+ or −	−	−	+	+
Vibrio cholerae and NCV	−	+	(+)	+ or −	+	−	+	−	−	+	+
Vibrio parahaemo-lyticus	−	+	−	−	+	−	+	+	− or +	+	+
Vibrio alginoly-ticus	−	+	−	+	+	−	+	+	−	+ or −	+
Lac + Vibrio, halophilic	−	+ or −	+ or (+)	−	+	−	+	+	−	+	+
Chromobacterium violaceum	−	−	−	+ or −	−	+	−	−	− or (+)	−‡	+
EF-4	−	−	−	−	−	+ or −	−	−	−	−	−
HB-5	+ or w	−	−	−	−	−	−	−	−	+	−
Pasteurella haemolytica	−	+	+ or −	+				−	−	−	−
Actinobacillus lignieresii and equuli	−	+	+ or (+)	+				−	+	−	−
Haemophilus aphrophilus	w or −	−	+	+				−	−	−	−

*From Weaver, R. E.: Gram-negative organisms: an approach to identification (guide to **presumptive** identifications), Atlanta, 1979, Center for Disease Control.

†+, 90% or more +, 1-2 d; + or −, 50-90% +, 1-2 d; −, 90% or more −; − or +, 50-90% −; (+), delayed +, 3 or more d; *w*, weak +.

‡Nonpigmented variants may be positive.

each of a series of tests established for diagnostic specificity, reproducibility, and high constancy.[6]

Weaver[7] has presented a **guide** to **presumptive identification** of gram-negative aerobic organisms, which is based on his key for initial distinction of these organisms (Table 79-2). The guide for **fermentative organisms** is shown in Tables 79-3 through 79-6; it is highly useful and helpful. For **nonfermenters,** refer to Tables 79-46 through 79-52.

Conventional tests. Several systems (Ewing, Gilardi, etc.) are described in this chapter, concerning both fermenters and nonfermenters, which include well-established series of biochemical and physiologic tests useful for both presumptive and final identification.

Multiple (miniaturized) test kits. As discussed in considerable detail in Chapters 74 and 75 (stool examination), several miniaturized multiple test systems have become available recently

that greatly simplify the identification of the fermenters (*Enterobacteriaceae*, etc.) and are helpful in identifying the nonfermenters (*Pseudomonas*, etc.).

These kits (Micro-ID, General Diagnostics, Morris Plains, N.J.; API 20-E, Analytab Products, Inc., Plain View, N.Y.; Enterotube, Roche Diagnostics, Nutley, N.J.; r/b Enteric, Diagnostic Research, Long Island, N.Y.; Minitek, Bioquest (BBL), Div. of Becton-Dickinson and Co., Cockeysville, Md.) have a long shelf life, are easy to use, and are most convenient especially in smaller, low-volume laboratories.

Automated instruments for identification. The **AMS system** (Vitek, St. Louis), in addition to its ability to enumerate, detect, and identify various organisms in a specimen, now has the capability of identifying *Enterobacteriaceae* grown on agar plates, using a specific biochemical card for this purpose. (See Chapter 74.)

Table 79-5. Presumptive identification III: Gram-negative fermenters; MacConkey negative (no growth); oxidase negative*†

Organism	Catalase	Nitrate reduction	Indole	Lactose, acid	Maltose, acid	
Haemophilus aphrophilus	− or w	+	−	+	+	Esculin not hydrolyzed; coccoid to short rods
DF-1	−	+	−	+	+	Esculin hydrolyzed; long to filamentous rods
Haemophilus vaginalis	−	−	−	−	+	
Actinobacillus actinomycetem-comitans	+	+	−	−	+	
HB-5	−	+	w	−	−	

*From Weaver, R. E: Gram-negative organisms: an approach to identification (guide to **presumptive** identifications), Atlanta, 1979, Center for Disease Control.

†+, 90% or more +, 1-2 d; + or −, 50-90% +, 1-2 d; −, 90% or more −; − or +, 50-90% − (+), delayed +, 3 or more d; w, weak +.

Table 79-6. Presumptive identification IV: Gram-negative fermenters, MacConkey negative (no growth); oxidase positive*†

	Nitrate reduction	Indole	Urea	Xylose	Catalase	Lactose, acid
Pasteurella multocida	+	+	−	+ or−	+	− or +
Pasteurella pneumotropica	+	+	+	+	+	+ or −
Pasteurella ureae	+	−	+	−	w or −	−
Pasteurella gallinarum	+	−	−	− or +	+	−
Pasteurella "gas"	+	+	+	−	+	−
Cardiobacterium hominis	−	+	−	−	−	−
EF-4	+ or +, gas	−	−	−	+	−
HB-5	+	w	−	−	−	−
Kingella denitrificans (TM-1)	+ or +, gas	−	−	−	−	−
Haemophilus aphrophilus	+	−	−	−	− or w	+
Actinobacillus actinomycetem-comitans	+	−	−	− or +	+	−
Actinobacillus lignieresii and *equuli*	+	−	+	+	+	+
Pasteurella haemolytica	+	−	−	+	+	+
Kingella kingae	−	−	−	−	−	−
DF-2	−	−	−	−	+	+

*From Weaver, R. E.: Gram-negative organisms: an approach to identification (guide to **presumptive** identifications), Atlanta, 1979, Center for Disease Control.

†+, 90% or more +, 1-2 d; + or −, 50-90% +, 1-2 d; −, 90% or more −; − or +, 50-90% − (+), delayed +, 3 or more d; w, weak +.

Similar capabilities are also being developed for the **Autobac** (Pfizer, New York) and the **MS-2** (Abbott, Dallas) systems.

Current nomenclature and synonyms

Table 79-7 lists the current nomenclature and the synonyms and earlier usage of a variety of gram-negative fermentative bacteria. See also Table 79-9.

Endotoxins

Endotoxins, complex macromolecules containing lipopolysaccharide, and making up an integral part of the bacterial cell wall, are produced primarily by gram-negative bacteria (e.g., *Salmonella typhi*, *Shigella dysenteriae*, *Vibrio cholerae*, *Brucella melitensis*, *Neisseria gonorrhoeae*, and *Neisseria meningitidis;* also by relatively avirulent gram-negative species like *Escherichia coli*). The toxicity of endotoxins

Table 79-7. Current nomenclature of some fermentative gram-negative rods*

Current usage	Synonyms
Arizona-S. arizonae	Arizona hinshawii
	Salmonella subgenus III
C. freundii (certain bio-types)	Levinea amalonatica
Citrobacter amalonaticus	Levinea amalonatica,
	Citrobacter freundii
	(malonate negative)
Klebsiella pneumoniae	Klebsiella aerogenes
	Klebsiella edwardsii var.
	atlantiae
	Klebsiella edwardsii var.
	edwardsii
Klebsiella oxytoca	Klebsiella pneumoniae
	Ind + or Ind and Gel +
Enterobacter agglomerans	Bacterium typhiflavum
	Erwinia lathyri
	Erwinia herbicola
Hafnia alvei	Enterobacter hafniae
	Enterobacter alvei
Enterobacter sakazakii	Enterobacter cloacae;
	yellow pigment
Morganella morganii	Proteus morganii
Providencia stuartii Ure +	Proteus rettgeri
	biogroup 5
Providencia rettgeri	Proteus rettgeri
	biogroup 1-4
Yersinia enterocolitica	Pasteurella "X"
	Pasteurella enterocolitica
Yersinia pseudo-tuberculosis	Pasteurella pseudo-tuberculosis
Yersinia pestis	Pasteurella pestis
Cardiobacterium hominis	CDC IId
Haemophilus vaginalis	Corynebacterium
	vaginale
DF-1 (CDC)	None
DF-2 (CDC)	None
EF-4 (CDC)	Pasteurella-like organism
HB-5 (CDC)	Haemophilus-like
Kingella denitrificans	CDC TM-1

*Ind, Indole; Gel-gelatin; CDC, Center for Disease Control designation.

seems to reside in the lipid fraction, whereas their specific antigenic determinants reside in polysaccharide (see antigens of *Enterobacteriaceae*). Bacterial endotoxins leave various biological effects (e.g., pyrogenicity, ability to cause shock).

A recently introduced in vitro test, based on the gelation of extracts of blood cells of the horseshoe crab, *Limulus polyphemus* (Limulus assay), can detect very small quantities (pg/ml) of a purified lipopolysaccharide (LPS). The test is also useful for detection of gram-negative bacterial meningitis, gram-negative bacteriuria, and for pyrogen screening of short-lived radiopharmaceuticals and parenteral solutions; its value for the detection of endotoxemia (in gram-negative bacteremia) is controversial at this time. For details of the test, see "Spinal fluid," Chapter 75.

Colicins

Some enteric organisms release highly specific proteins called colicins (type of bacteriocin): molecules that attach to specific receptors on susceptible bacilli, as do bacteriophages, but do not cause lysis of the bacterial cell. Various colicins kill sensitive bacteria by different mechanisms.

The production of colicins (colicinogeny) is controlled by plasmids, which may be transmitted to other enteric bacilli.

Colicins can be used for subdividing strains of organisms for epidemiologic purposes. In such **colicin typing,** enterobacteria are grouped according to the colicins they produce and those to which they are sensitive. Thus *Shigella sonnei* (homogeneous according to phage typing and antigenic analysis) has been divided into 15 types by colicin typing.

Transferable (infectious) drug resistance

The emergence of an organism resistant to a given antibiotic drug in a sensitive bacterial population has been explained as the result of chromosomal mutation and of natural selection. Another type of resistance was demonstrated in 1959 by Japanese workers, who proved that resistance is transmissible from a resistant bacterial cell to a sensitive one by contact (conjugation). This is now known as transferable or infectious drug resistance and occurs both in vivo and in vitro between strains of the same species as well as between organisms of different species (e.g., between *E. coli* and *Shigella*).

This type of resistance is often multiple; e.g., resistance to a number of antibiotics is transferred. The factor responsible is known as RTF (resistance transfer factor), associated with an extrachromosomal element (episome).

Multiple resistance transfer seems to occur mostly among the *Enterobacteriaceae* and some other gram-negative aerobic organisms present in the intestinal tract. The emergence of enterobacterial strains carrying RTF factors is attributed, in part at least, to the continual use of antibiotics in both human and veterinary medicine. Multiple-resistant forms are easily transferred from livestock to humans.

Multiple-resistant strains of *Shigella, Salmonella,* and *E. coli* have been recovered from human epidemics, and transferable drug resistance has been demonstrated also in *S. aureus, Proteus, Pseudomonas,* and *Klebsiella.*

It is not possible to further discuss here this important problem; however, it should be kept in mind that infectious drug resistance poses considerable epidemiologic and clinical problems and emphasizes the need for constant surveillance of the antibiotic snesitivity patterns of organisms in a given locality and also in the patient receiving antibiotic treatment.

For further details the reader is referred to Watanabe,[8] Lebek,[9] Blattner,[10] and Anderson.[11]

Fermenters

ENTEROBACTERIACEAE*
Classification and nomenclature

The classification of the *Enterobacteriaceae* has been a controversial problem in systematic bacteriology and, indeed, constant changes have taken place in the last decade with regard to their nomenclature and identification.

The changes in the nomenclature of the family can be traced, among others, through the various editions of *Bergey's Manual* and the works of Kauffmann.[12] The **taxonomic system** of Ewing and Edwards,[13, 14] eminently practical and useful, has been widely accepted and served as the basis for a **nomenclatural system** proposed by Ewing.[15] The latter was approved by the Subcommittee on *Enterobacteriaceae* of the American Society for Microbiology in 1964,[16] and in amended form, again in 1967.[17]

In the **taxonomic system** for the family *Enterobacteriaceae* (Ewing and Edwards[14]) the types of bacteria that give similar biochemical reactions were placed into **groups.** Some of the groups or genera are related to each other through the similarity in their biochemical reactions and in many cases by close antigenic relationships; such groups were placed into a **division.** The basic criterion for placement of groups in the same principal division is the possession of a **number** of common biochemical characteristics by members of these groups instead of reliance on a **single** characteristic (such as failure to ferment lactose).

*Grateful acknowledgment is made to Dr. W. H. Ewing for permission to use material from his many publications (some with co-workers), 1962-1978 (see references), and for making available much of his unpublished data prior to publication. Parts of this section are based on material from Edwards, P. R., and Ewing, W. H.: Identification of *Enterobacteriaceae,* Minneapolis, 1962 (ed. 2) and 1973 (ed. 3), Burgess Publishing Co.

Ewing has further expanded (1967) and revised his system[18]; his 1973 modification[19, 20] (**eliminating divisions and groups**) is shown in Table 79-8, where it is compared with the taxonomic system for *Enterobacteriaceae* in the eighth edition of *Bergey's Manual.*[3]

Changes

1. Differences between the *Bergey's Manual,* ed. 8,[3] classification and system of nomenclature and Ewing's system[19, 20] pertain to the following:
    a. Bergey's *Citrobacter intermedius* is named *Citrobacter diversus* by Ewing.
    b. *Salmonella arizonae* (subgroup III of *Salmonella*) is *Arizona hinshawii* in Ewing's nomenclature.
    c. *Erwinia herbicola* is *Enterobacter agglomerans* in Ewing's system.
    d. *Hafnia alvei* (new genus VIII in *Bergey's,* ed. 8) is *Enterobacter hafniae* in Ewing.
    e. *Proteus inconstans* (subgroups A and B) in Bergey's now includes *Providencia stuartii* and *Providencia alcalifaciens* of Ewing.
    f. *Serratia marcescens* is the only species of *Serratia* described in *Bergey's Manual,* ed. 8,[3] while Ewing recognizes 3 species, i.e., *S. marcescens, S. liquefaciens* (formerly *Enterobacter liquefaciens*), and *S. rubidaea.*

2. Attention is called to further changes as compared to earlier schemas and *Bergey's Manual,* ed. 7[21]:

a. *Enterobacter.* This is the correct name for organisms formerly listed as *Aerobacter.*

b. "*Paracolon group.*" The term "paracolon" has been used for many years to denote organisms that did not ferment lactose promptly and could not be unequivocally identified as members of recognized genera. Each group of bacteria that ferments lactose promptly also includes counterparts that do not attack this substrate or do so only after prolonged incubation. Failure to ferment lactose does not exclude a culture from a group of which it is otherwise a typical member. An *Escherichia* strain and a culture of *Enterobacter* should not be placed together in a "paracolon group" because each produces acid from lactose after some dealy. Instead each is to be **classified in its appropriate group** regardless of its reluctance to utilize lactose, particularly since the rate of lactose fermentation is not a stable characteristic. Accordingly, this "wastebasket" category has been deleted both by Kauffmann[12] and by Edwards and Ewing[22] and is not recognized by the International Enterobacteriaceae Subcommittee.[23] Neither the generic term *Paracolobactrum* nor the vernacular term "paracolon group" should be used. For a bacteriologic and clinical reappraisal of the "paracolon bacteria" see Fields et al.[24]

c. *Escherichia freundii.* Organisms formerly designated by this epithet are now included in the genus *Citrobacter.*

d. *Edwardsiella* (new tribe and genus) in-

Table 79-8. Classification and nomenclature of *Enterobacteriaceae*

Bergey's Manual, ed. 8 (1974)[3]	*Ewing (1973)*[19,20]
Gram-negative facultatively anaerobic rods	

Family I. *Enterobacteriaceae*	Family *Enterobacteriaceae*
Tribe I. *Escherichieae*	Tribe I. *Escherichieae*
Genus I. *Escherichia*	Genus I. *Escherichia*
Genus II. *Edwardsiella*	*E. coli*
Genus III. *Citrobacter*	Genus II. *Shigella*
C. freundii	Shigella dysenteriae
C. intermedius	Shigella flexneri
Genus IV. *Salmonella*	Shigella boydii
Subgenus I. (most salmonellae)	Shigella sonnei
Subgenus II. (*S. salamae*)	Tribe II. *Edwardsielleae*
Subgenus III. (*S. arizonae*)	Genus I. *E. tarda*
Subgenus IV. (*S. houtenae*)	Tribe III. *Salmonelleae*
Genus V. *Shigella*	Genus I. *Salmonella*
Tribe II. *Klebsielleae*	S. cholerae-suis
Genus VI. *Klebsiella*	S. typhi
K. pneumoniae	S. enteritidis
K. ozaenae	Genus II. *Arizona*
K. rhinoscleromatis	A. hinshawii
Genus VII. *Enterobacter*	Genus III. *Citrobacter*
E. cloacae	C. freundii
E. aerogenes	C. diversus
Genus VIII. *Hafnia*	Tribe IV. *Klebsielleae*
Hafnia alvei	Genus I. *Klebsiella*
Genus IX. *Serratia*	K. pneumoniae
S. marcescens	K. ozaenae
Tribe III. *Proteeae*	K. rhinoschleromatis
Genus X. *Proteus*	Genus II. *Enterobacter*
P. vulgaris	E. cloacae
P. mirabilis	E. aerogenes
P. morganii	E. hafniae
P. rettgeri	E. agglomerans
P. inconstans	Genus III. *Serratia*
Tribe IV. *Yersinieae*	S. marcescens
Genus XI. *Yersinia*	S. liquefaciens
Y. pestis	S. rubidaea
Y. pseudotuberculosis	Tribe V. *Proteeae*
Y. enterocolitica	Genus I. *Proteus*
Tribe V. *Erwinieae*	P. vulgaris
Genus XII. *Erwinia*	P. mirabilis
Amylovora group	P. morganii
Herbicola group	P. rettgeri
Carotovora group	Genus II. *Providencia*
	P. alcalifaciens
	P. stuartii
	Tribe VI. *Yersinieae**
	Genus I. *Yersinia*
	Y. pestis
	Y. pseudotuberculosis
	Y. enterocolitica
	Tribe VII. *Erwinieae*
	Genus I. *Erwinia*
	Genus II. *Pectobacterium*

*Later addition.

cludes the single species *E. tarda* and is included both in *Bergey's Manual*, ed. 8,[3] and in Ewing's schema.[18-20,25]

3. Taxonomic and nomenclatural changes in *Enterobacteriaceae*—Center for Disease Control (CDC) usage (1977-1978).[26] The Enteric Section of the Center for Disease Control has utilized a polyphasic approach to the identification of *Enterobacteriaceae* since about 1975. This approach consists of combining results obtained by utilization of many new biochemical tests, antibiotic susceptibility patterns, species or group specific bacteriophages, deoxyribonucleic acid (DNA) relatedness tests, and computerized identification programs.

This approach has led to proposals for new

Table 79-9. Changes in *Enterobacteriaceae* taxonomy and nomenclature adopted by Center for Disease Control, Enteric Section*†

New designation	Previous designation
Klebsiella oxytoca	*Klebsiella pneumoniae*, indole positive or indole positive and gelatin positive
Enterobacter sakazakii	*Enterobacter cloacae*, yellow pigment
Enterobacter gergoviae	
Hafnia alvei	*Enterobacter hafniae*
Citrobacter amalonaticus	*Citrobacter freundii*, malonate negative, H_2S negative, KCN negative, indole positive, adonitol negative; or *Levinea amalonatica*
Providencia stuartii, urea positive	*Proteus rettgeri*, biogroup 5
Providencia stuartii, biogroup 4	*Providencia alcalifaciens*, biogroup 4
Providencia rettgeri	*Proteus rettgeri*, biogroups 1-4
Morganella morganii	*Proteus morganii*
Yersinia enterocolitica (typical)	*Y. enterocolitica*
Y. enterocolitica, sucrose negative	*Y. enterocolitica*
Y. enterocolitica, rhamnose positive	*Y. enterocolitica*
Y. enterocolitica, rhamnose and raffinose positive	*Y. enterocolitica*
Yersinia ruckeri	Red mouth bacterium

*From Brenner, D. J., Farmer, J. J., III, Hickman, F. W., et al.: Taxonomic and nomenclature changes in *Enterobacteriaceae*, DHEW publ. no (CDC) 78-8356, Atlanta, Oct. 1977, Center for Disease Control.
†Effective date of changes October 1, 1977.

species and also to nonmenclatural changes in existing species. The first of these changes are listed in Table 79-9.

The changes, concerning a new *Klebsiella* species name, two new *Enterobacter* species, acceptance of *Hafnia alvei* over *Enterobacter hafniae*, a new *Citrobacter* species, and changes in *Proteus, Morganella, Providencia,* and *Yersinia* nomenclature, are discussed in detail in the respective sections of the genera involved (below). Those laboratories involved in proficiency testing programs need to be cognizant of these changes in usage.

The family Enterobacteriaceae

The family *Enterobacteriaceae*, according to Ewing,[19] consists of gram-negative, facultatively anaerobic nonsporeforming rods that grow well on artificial media in air. Some species are motile (peritrichous flagella), with nonmotile variants of motile species occurring; some species are nonmotile (atrichous). Glucose (dextrose) is utilized **fermentatively** with the formation of acid or of acid and gas. Nitrates are reduced to nitrites. The indophenol (cytochrome) **oxidase test** is negative and alginate is not liquefied. Pectate is liquefied by members of only one genus (*Pectobacterium*).

Many species are found in the intestines of humans and other animals; some cause intestinal disturbances. Others are parasitic on plants, whereas still others are saprophytes, causing decomposition of dead organic materials.

Table 79-10 lists the essential and principal tests for differentiation of the tribes of *Enterobacteriaceae* in Ewing's system.

Note: The reactions listed in Table 79-10 are only a guide. They are not to be considered sufficient for final identification of Enterobacteriaceae.

The system of classification, nomenclature, and identification procedures described in this section are based mostly on the system of Ewing described above. **It has proved practical in the clinical laboratory and is in general use in the United States.** The changes proposed by the Center for Disease Control (Table 79-9) are also incorporated in the various sections.

The symbols (results) in Tables 79-10 and 79-14 through 79-44 are based on the following grading system used by Ewing:

+: 90% or more positive in 1 or 2 days.
−: 90% or more no reaction.
(+): positive reaction in 3 or more days.
d: different biochemical reactions, +, (+), −.
+ or −: majority of strains +, some cultures negative.
− or +: majority of cultures negative, some strains positive.

Some of these tables are condensed for reasons of space; others contain actual percentage data obtained in various reactions.

Occurrence and pathogenicity in humans

Among the many "enteric" (*Enterobacteriaceae*) organisms, the major pathogens causing various types of gastrointestinal diseases (typhoid, other enteric fevers, gastroenteritis) are *Salmonella* (and *Arizona*), the causative agent of bacillary dysentery, *Shigella*, the agent of

Table 79-10. Differentiation of *Enterobacteriaceae* by biochemical methods*†

	Tribes						
Test or substrate	Escheri-chieae	Edwardsiel-leae	Salmonel-leae‡	Klebsiel-leae§	Prote-eae‖	Yersin-ieae¶	Erwinieae#
Hydrogen sulfide (TSI)	−	+	+	−	+ or −	− or +	d
Urease	−	−	−	− or (+)	+ or −	d	−
Indole	+ or −	+	−	−	+ or −	− or +	d
Methyl red	+	+	+	−	+	+	d
Voges-Proskauer	−	−	−	+	−	−	d
Citrate (Simmons')	−	−	+	+	d	−	d
KCN	−	−	− or +	+	+	d	d
Phenylalanine deaminase	−	−	−	−	+	−	d
Mucate	d	−	d	+ or −	−	n	n
Mannitol	+ or −	−	+	+	− or +	+	d

*Based on data from Ewing[19] and *Bergey's Manual*, ed. 8.[3]

†+, 90% or more positive within 1-2 d; −, 90% or more, no reactions; (+), delayed positive, 3 or more d; d, different biochemical reactions—+, (+), −; + or −, most cultures positive, some negative; − or +, most strains negative, some positive; − or (+), most cultures negative, some positive delayed; n, not known.

‡*S. typhi, S. enteritidis* bioserotype paratyphi-A, and some rare bioserotypes fail to utilize citrate. Cultures of *S. enteritidis* bioserotype paratyphi-A, and some rare bioserotypes may fail to produce hydrogen sulfide; an occasional strain of almost any serotype of salmonellae may be hydrogen sulfide negative.

§Some strains of *E. agglomerans* deaminate phenylalanine.

‖Some cultures of *P. mirabilis* may yield positive Voges-Proskauer tests.

¶Optimal temperature for growth is 30-37 C.

#Optimal temperature, 27-30 C.

yersiniosis, *Yersinia enterocolitica*, and enterotoxigenic and enteropathogenic *Escherichia coli*.

• • •

Other agents of gastrointestinal disease, members of other genera and families, are *Vibrio cholerae, Vibrio parahaemolyticus, Campylobacter fetus*, and *Clostridium difficile* (in pseudomembraneous colitis), as well as certain viruses; rarely, large numbers of *Staphylococcus aureus* or *Clostridium perfringens* (in "food poisoning"). See discussion on "stool examination" (Chapter 75).

• • •

Yersinia, E. coli, some of the *Salmonella, Arizona* can invade the bloodstream and can be found in the blood, urine, and other body fluids, in addition to their occurrence in feces in the course of the disease. The shigellae invade the blood rarely and are present in large numbers in the feces during the acute phase of the disease.

E. coli is a normal inhabitant of the large intestine, being the most common aerobic organism in the human intestine. Certain serologic types of *E. coli* are known to cause severe diarrhea, especially in young infants ("enteropathogenic *E. coli*"); other *E. coli* produce toxins and are involved in severe enteritis (see *E. coli*, below).

E. coli commonly cause urinary tract infections and are found in infections of other organs (meningitis, gallbladder, peritonitis, endocarditis). They are often involved in peritonitis, septicemia following abdominal or genito-urinary tract operations or premature rupture of membranes in pregnancy, and following induced abortions.

Enterobacter, Klebsiella, Citrobacter, Proteus, and *Providencia* strains are found irregularly and in smaller numbers in the normal intestine, but each is capable of causing infections in any part of the human body outside the intestinal canal. Some of these organisms have also been suspected of being involved in intestinal disturbances and diarrheas of varying severity. They are common in urinary tract infections and are frequently isolated from pus or blood. *Serratia* strains have also been isolated from many human infections.[5, 27]

Yersinia enterocolitica (and more rarely *Yersinia pseudotuberculosis*) is involved often in mesenteric lymphadenitis, enteritis, and other syndromes.[28–32]

Antigens of Enterobacteriaceae

Members of the family *Enterobacteriaceae* possess a variety of antigens that can be grouped into 3 major categories—O, H, and K antigens.

The O or somatic antigens. These are antigens of the cell body (soma). They are heat stable, resist heating at 100 C, and are not destroyed by alcohol or dilute acid. They are polysaccharide in nature and determine the somatic subgroups to which the organisms belong. The term **O** (German **Ohne**—without), first applied to non-swarming (i.e., nonflagellated) forms of *Proteus* organisms, is now used as generic term for the lipopolysaccharide somatic antigens of all enteric bacilli and more specifically for their antigenically active polysaccharide components.[4]

The H or flagellar antigens. These are antigens located in the flagella (of motile organisms). They are protein in nature and are inactivated by temperatures over 60 C and by alcohol and acids. The flagellar antigens determine the serotype of a particular strain within the somatic groups of *Salmonella* and some other flagellated organisms.

The designation **H** (German *Hauch*—breath) was originally used to describe the growth of *Proteus* on the surfaces of moist agar plates: the film produced by the swarming of this highly motile organism resembles the light mist caused by breathing on glass.[4]

The K, envelope, or capsular antigens. These are thought of as occurring in sheaths, envelopes, or capsules surrounding the cell. They usually interfere with agglutination by specific O antisera by "masking" the O antigens. The **Vi** antigen of *S. typhi* and certain other *Salmonella*, the various **K** antigens of *E. coli*, and the **K** antigens of the capsular types of *Klebsiella* belong in this category. Most of the K antigens are destroyed by heat (100 C).

The genera of *Enterobacteriaceae* are subdivided generally on the basis of their **O** antigens (*Salmonella, Arizona, Citrobacter, Escherichia, Providencia, Serratia, Yersinia*). The O groups are further subdivided into serotypes characterized by possession of certain O antigen fractions, K antigens, and H antigens. *Shigella* organisms are differentiated on the basis of major somatic (**O**) antigens characteristic of each serotype, not being flagellated, they have no **H** antigens. Although the principal varieties of enteric bacilli can be identified by fermentation and other metabolic reactions in differential media, final identification of many individual species is usually based on antigenic structure. Strains with the same antigenic activity may nevertheless exhibit different metabolic reactions (**fermentative variants** or **biotypes**).

For a more detailed discussion of antigens in the genus *Salmonella*, see "Kauffmann-White scheme" in *Salmonella*, below.

Isolation, media, and growth characteristics

Media for the isolation of *Enterobacteriaceae* and colony characteristics are described under *"stool examination"* (Chapter 75).

All *Enterobacteriaceae* grow well on blood agar. Colonial morphology on blood agar is **not** a differential criterion for these organisms. Most of them grow as rather large, grayish colonies; some are hemolytic.

Preliminary examination of cultures

Fermentation of lactose is a time-honored differential characteristic in the preliminary examination of cultures suspected to belong to *Enterobacteriaceae*. Edwards and Ewing[20] point out that rapid **lactose fermentation** became a major criterion in the early days of bacteriology

Table 79-11. Triple sugar iron agar (TSI) reactions*

Reactions	Possible groups (genera)
Glucose fermented; lactose and/or sucrose fermented	
(1a)	
Acid butt	*Escherichia*
Acid slant	*Klebsiella*
Gas in butt	*Enterobacter*
No H₂S (no blackening)	*Proteus-Providencia*
	Serratia (often scant or no gas)
(1b) Same as (1a) but no gas	*Yersinia enterocolitica*†
	Y. pseudotuberculosis (occasional)
(2)	
Acid butt	*Citrobacter*
Acid slant	*Arizona* (some strains)
Gas in butt	
H₂S produced	
Glucose fermented; lactose and sucrose not fermented	
(3)	
Acid butt	*Salmonella*‡
Alkaline slant	*Proteus*
Gas in butt	Many *Arizona* and some *Citrobacter*
H₂S produced	*Edwardsiella*
(4)	
Acid butt	*Salmonella*§
Alkaline slant	*Shigella*
No gas	*Proteus, Providencia*
No H₂S	*Escherichia* (late or non-fermenters)
	Serratia
	Y. pseudotuberculosis
	Y. pestis
	Y. enterocolitica (2 bio-groups)
No fermentation	
(5)	
Alkaline or neutral butt	*Alcaligenes*‖
Alkaline slant	*Pseudomonas*‖
No H₂S	*Flavobacterium*‖

*Attention is called to certain gram-negative rods that do not belong to *Enterobacteriaceae* but may give confusing reactions on TSI. Refer to cytochrome oxidase reaction for differentiation.

†Some *Yersinia* ferment sucrose and yield acid slant/acid butt, no gas, and no H₂S reaction. *Enterobacter hafniae* produce gas. *Providencia* may or may not produce gas.

‡Majority of *Salmonella* produce gas and H₂S; some produce gas but no H₂S. *S. typhi* produces little H₂S and no gas.

§*S. typhi* and *S. gallinarum* produce no gas. Some *S. typhi* strains produce small amounts of H₂S.

‖These organisms do not belong to *Enterobacteriaceae*. However, since they are lactose negative, they are sometimes inoculated into TSI from isolation plates.

simply because the major enteric pathogens *(Salmonella* and *Shigella)* failed to ferment lactose. At the same time, however, there are a number of other organisms *(Proteus,* certain types of *Escherichia, Enterobacter,* and *Serratia)* that are also lactose negative (or delayed). As pointed out earlier ("paracolon organisms"), failure to ferment lactose does not automatically place an organism into the *Salmonella, Shigella,* or *Yersinia.* Organisms that fail to ferment lactose or do so with delay should be characterized by a combination of tests, not by a single property. Conversely, it is true that **prompt** lactose fermentation does serve well in delineating the "coliform" organisms (most *Escherichia, Citrobacter, Klebsiella,* and *Enterobacter* organisms); but some *Arizona* strains, responsible for diseases similar to those caused by salmonellae, are also rapid lactose fermenters. Here, again, identification of the organism depends on a combination of tests.

In addition, the time-honored lactose fermentation method (for differentiation of pathogenic from nonpathogenic enteric bacilli) proves unreliable when a **lactose-fermenting** *S. typhi,* produced earlier in the laboratory by introduction of a lactose-carrying episome from *E. coli* to *S. typhi,* is involved in typhoid fever. In fact, up to 1% of salmonellae isolated in the United States (1960s) were lactose fermenters. Many lactose-fermenting strains of *Salmonella typhimurium* and *S. oranienburg* have now been isolated from acute diarrheal epidemics in Brazil (1974-75).

Table 79-12. Lysine iron agar reactions*

Lysine iron agar (LIA)	Slant	Butt	Gas	H_2S
Escherichia	K	K or N	− or +	−
Shigella; Y. pseudotuberculosis, Y. pestis	K	A	−	−
Salmonella	K	K or N	−	+(−)
typhi	K	K	−	− or +
paratyphi A	K	A	+ or −	+ or −
Arizona	K	K or N	−	+(−)
Citrobacter	K	A	− or +	+ or −
Edwardsiella	K	K	− or +	+
Klebsiella	K or N	K or N	+ or −	−
Enterobacter				
cloacae	K or N	A	+ or −	−
aerogenes	K	K or N	+(−)	−
hafniae	K	K or N	− or +	−
Serratia	K or N	K or N	−	−
Proteus				
vulgaris	R	A	−	−
mirabilis	R	A	−	−
morganii	K or R	A	−	−
rettgeri	R	A	−	−
Providencia	R	A	−	−

*K, Alkaline; N, neutral; A, acid; R, red (oxidative deamination).

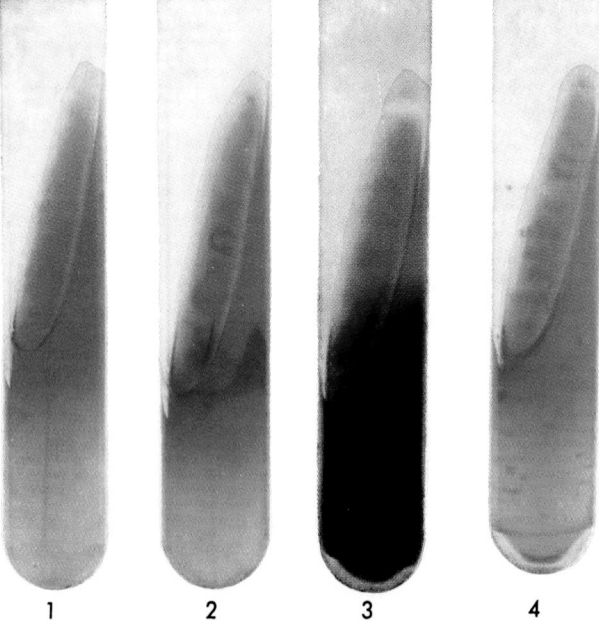

Fig. 79-1. Triple sugar iron agar medium (Hajna). Some typical reactions: **1,** *Shigella:* acid butt, alkaline slant, no gas, no H_2S. **2,** *Salmonella typhi:* acid butt, alkaline slant, no gas, very small amount of H_2S. **3,** Typical *Salmonella:* alkaline slant, acid butt (obscured by large amount of H_2S, gas—see bottom). **4,** Other *Salmonella:* acid butt, alkaline slant, gas, no H_2S. See text for details.

Laboratories relying solely on MacConkey agar and deoxycholate citrate agar for *Salmonella* isolation will not recognize such strains as a *Salmonella*, and therefore the use of bismuth sulphite agar is recommended.

Screening by use of differential and selective media

As described under **stool examination** (Chapter 75), with the use of EMB, MacConkey, deoxycholate, deoxycholate citrate, SS, and other media, it is possible to detect lactose-fermenting and lactose-nonfermenting (or delayed) colonies on the primary plates. The frank coliforms (lactose fermenters) are usually not further examined if a **stool culture** is involved unless enteropathoenic *E. coli* are suspected or specifically searched for. **If the specimen is from any other part of the body, further identification is carried out.**

Caution: Some *Arizona* strains ferment lactose rapidly and can be missed if the colonies are not examined in more detail. The lactose nonfermenters must be screened with the use of **TSI** and **Christensen urea agar,** and, if possible, also with **lysine iron agar** (LIA) and motility medium (see Fig. 75-13). The phenylalanine deaminase test is also very helpful.

Those giving a **rapid** urease reaction (2-6 hours) are *Proteus* organisms. A delayed urease reaction is given by some *Klebsiella, Enterobacter, Serratia,* and *Yersinia. Salmonella, Arizona,* and *Shigella* are urease negative.

TSI reactions. Triple sugar iron agar, designed by Hajna,[33] is an extremely useful medium for the differentiation of gram-negative enteric organisms by means of their ability to ferment dextrose, lactose, and sucrose and to liberate sulfides. The formula contains phenol red indica-

Table 79-13. Schema for differentiation of oxidase-negative, fermentative, catalase-positive, gram-negative bacilli*†

		\multicolumn{7}{c}{*Reactions observed in TSI slants*}						
		K/A H$_2$S +	*K/Ⓐ H$_2$S +*	*K/Ⓐ*	*K/A*	*A/Ⓐ H$_2$S +*	*A/Ⓐ*	*A/A*
Reactions observed in LiA slants	R/A		*P. vulgaris* (rare) *P. mirabilis*	*P. morganii* (rare) *Providencia*	*P. morganii* (rare) *P. rettgeri Providencia*	*P. vulgaris P. mirabilis* (rare)		*P. rettgeri* (rare)
	K/K or N H$_2$S+	*S. typhi* (H$_2$S 1+) *Salmonella* (rare) *Arizona* (rare) *Edwardsiella* (rare)	*Salmonella Arizona Edwardsiella*	*Salmonella* (rare) *Arizona* (rare)	*S. typhi* (rare)	*Arizona Salmonella* (rare)		
	K/K or N	*Salmonella* (rare)		*Enterobacter hafniae Klebsiella Serratia* (occ.)	*Serratia S. typhi* (rare) *Klebsiella* (rare) *Enterobacter hafniae* (rare)		*Klebsiella Enterobacter aerogenes liquefaciens E. coli*	*Serratia*
	K/A H$_2$S+		*Citrobacter*			*Citrobacter*		
	K/A			*E. agglomerans E. coli P. morganii* Paratyphi A *S. flexneri* 6-some biotypes (uncommon) *C. diversus*	*E. coli* (A-D) *Shigella P. morganii E. agglomerans Y. pseudotuberculosis Y. pestis; Y. enterocolitica* (occ.) *A. actinomycetemcomitans C. violaceum*		*E. coli* (rare) *Citrobacter* (rare) *E. cloacae E. agglomerans H. aphrophilus*	*E. coli E. agglomerans C. diversus* (rare) *H. aphrophilus Y. enterocolitica C. violaceum Y. pseudotuberculosis* (occ.)

*From Hall, C. T.: Bacteriology I, January 1973 summary analysis, proficiency survey, Atlanta, 1973, Center for Disease Control.
†*R*, Red, oxidative deamination of lysine; *K*, alkaline slant; *A*, acid slant; *K*, alkaline butt; */A*, acid butt; *Ⓐ*, acid + gas in butt; *H$_2$S +*, hydrogen sulfide production.

Table 79-14. Biochemical reactions of *Enterobacteriaceae* (incl. *Yersinia*), *Aeromonas,* and *Vibrio**†

| | *Escherichieae* | | *Edwardsielleae* | *Salmonelleae* | | | | *Klebsielleae* | | | | |
| | | | | | | *Citrobacter* | | *Klebsiella* | *Enterobacter* | | | |
	Escherichia	*Shigella*	*Edwardsiella*	*Salmonella*	*Arizona*	*freundii*	*diversus*	*pneumoniae*	*cloacae*	*aerogenes*	*hafniae*	*agglomerans*
1. Oxidase test	−	−	−	−	−	−	−	−	−	−	−	−
2. Indole	+	− or +	+	−	−	−	+	−	−	−	−	− or +
3. Methyl red	+	+	+	+	+	+	+	− or +	−	−	− or +	− or +
4. Voges-Proskauer	−	−	−	−	−	−	−	+	+	+	+ or −	+ or −
5. Simmons' citrate	−	−	−	d	+	+	+	+	+	+	d	d
6. Hydrogen sulfide (TSI)	−	−	+	+	+	+ or −	−	−	−	−	−	−
7. Urease	−	−	−	−	−	d^w	d^w	+	+ or −	−	−	d^w
8. KCN	−	−	−	−	−	+	−	+	+	+	+	− or +
9. Motility	+ or −	−	+	+	+	+	+	−	+	+	+	+ or −
10. Gelatin (22 C)	−	−	−	−	(+)	−	−	−	(+) or −	− or (+)	−	d
11. Lysine decarboxylase	d	−	+	+	+	−	−	+	−	+	+	−
12. Arginine dihydrolase	d	d	−	+ or (+)	+ or (+)	d	+ or (+)	−	+	−	d	−
13. Ornithine decarboxylase	d	d‡	+	+	+	d	+	−	+	+	+	−
14. Phenylalanine deaminase	−	−	−	−	−	−	−	−	−	−	−	− or +
15. Malonate	−	−	−	−	+	− or +	− or +	+	+ or −	+ or −	+ or −	+ or −
16. Gas from glucose	+	−‡	+	+	+	+	+	+	+	+	+	− or +
17. Lactose	+	−‡	−	−	d	(+) or +	d	+	+ or (+)	+	d	d
18. Sucrose	d	−‡	−	−	−	d	− or +	+	+	+	d	d
19. Mannitol	+	+ or −	−	+	+	+	+	+	+	+	+	+
20. Dulcitol	d	d	−	d‖	−	d	+ or −	− or +	− or +	−	−	− or +
21. Salicin	d	−	−	−	−	d	(+) or +	+	+ or (+)	+	d	d
22. Adonitol	−	−	−	−	−	−	+	+ or −	− or +	+	−	−
23. Inositol	−	−	−	d	−	−	−	+	d	+	−	d
24. Sorbitol	d	d	−	+	+	+	+	+	+	+	−	d
25. Arabinose	+	d	− or +	+‖	+	+	+	+	+	+	+	+
26. Raffinose	d	d	−	−	−	d	−	+	+	+	−	d
27. Rhamnose	d	d	−	+	+	+	+	+	+	+	+	+ or (+)

*Compiled by A. C. Sonnenwirth, November 1973. Data on *Enterobacteriaceae* from "Differentiation of *Enterobacteriaceae* by biochemical
†+, 90% or more positive in 1 or 2 d; −, 90% or more negative; d, different biochemical types—+, (+), delayed positive (decarboxylase
‡Certain biotypes of *S. flexneri* produce gas; cultures of *S. sonnei* ferment lactose and sucrose slowly and decarboxylate ornithine.
§Gas volumes produced by cultures of *Serratia, Proteus,* and *Providencia* are small.
‖*S. typhi, S. cholerae-suis, S. enteritidis* bioser, paratyphi-A and Pullorum, and a few other ordinarily do not ferment dulcitol promptly.

	Enterobacteriaceae												Aeromonas	Vibrio
	Klebsielleae			Proteeae						Yersinia				
	Serratia			Proteus				Providencia						
	marcescens	*liquefaciens*	*rubidnea*	*vulgaris*	*mirabilis*	*morganii*	*rettgeri*	*alcalifaciens*	*stuartii*	*Y. entero-colitica*	*Y. pseudo-tuberculosis*	*Y. pestis*	*A. hydrophila* (other sp. vary)	*V. cholerae*
1.	–	–	–	–	–	–	–	–	–	–	–	–	+	+
2.	–	–	–	+	–	+	+	+	+	– or +	–	–	+	+
3.	– or +	+ or –	– or +	+	+	+	+	+	+	+	+	+	+	+w
4.	+	– or +	+	–	– or +	–	–	–	–	–, d	–	–	– or +	– or +
5.	+	+	+ or (+)	d	+ or (+)	–	+	+	+	–	–, d	–	+ or –	(+) or –
6.	–	–	–	+	+	–	–	–	–				–	–
7.	dw	dw	dw	+	+	+	+	–	–	+	+	–, d	–	–
8.	+	+	– or +	+	+	+	+	+	+				– or +	
9.	+	+	+ or –	+	+	+ or –	+	+	+	–37 C +22 C	–37 C +22 C	–37 C +22 C	+	+
10.	+ or (+)	+	+ or (+)	+	+	–	–	–	–	–	–	–	+	+
11.	+	+ or (+)	+ or (+)	–	–	–	–	–	–	–	–	–	–	+
12.	–	–	–	–	–	–	–	–	–	–	–	–	+	–
13.	+	+	–	–	+	+	–	–	–	+	–	–	–	+
14.	–	–	–	+	+	+	+	+	+	–	–	–	–	–
15.	–	–	+ or –	–	–	–	–	–	–	–	–	–	–	–
16.	+ or –§	+ or –	d	+ or –	+	+ or –	– or +	+ or –		–	–	–	+ or –	–
17.	–	d	+	–	–	–	–	–	–	–	–	–	– or +	(+)
18.	+	+	+	+	d	–	d	d	(+) or +	+	–	–	+	+
19.	+	+	+	–	–	+ or –	–		d	+	+	+	+	+
20.	–	–	–	–	–	–	–	–	–	–	–	–	–	–
21.	+	+	+ or (+)	d	d	–	d	–	–	–d	+	+	+	–
22.	d	d	+ or (+)	–	–	–	d	+	– or +	–	–, d	–	–	–
23.	d	+ or (+)	d	–	–	–	+	–	+	d	–	–	–	–
24.	+	+	–	–	–	–	d	–	d	+	–	d	d	–
25.	–	+	+	–	–	–	–	–	–	+	+	+	+ or –	–
26.	–	+	+	–	–	–	–	–	–	–	–	–	–	–
27.	–	d	–	–	–	+ or –	–		±	+	–	–		

tests," Enteric Bacteriology Laboratories Chart, DHEW-PHS-CDC, Atlanta, July, 1973.
reactions, 3 or 4 d); + or –, majority of cultures positive; – or +, majority negative; *w*, weakly positive reaction.

S. cholerae-suis does not ferment arabinose.

tor, ferrous sulfate, 1% lactose, 1% sucrose, and 0.1% dextrose. In the case of an organism that ferments dextrose only, the small amount of acid produced by the utilization of dextrose (visible as a yellow slant in the first few hours of incubation) will be oxidized under aerobic conditions in the slant, which then reverts to an alkaline (red) condition. In the butt, under anaerobic conditions, the reaction is not reversed, and the acid reaction (yellow) is maintained. Those organisms producing H_2S will show a blackening of the agar. Lactose- and/or sucrose-fermenting organisms show acid slant and acid butt. Gas formation is shown by bubbles in the butt; the medium is sometimes split.

Table 79-11 lists the various reactions and the possible groups indicated by them on TSI agar; Fig. 79-1 illustrates some typical reactions.

Christensen urea agar. The medium and performance of the test are described in Chapter 72.

Lysine iron agar (LIA) reactions. For details see "Stool examination," Chapter 75. The reactions on LIA slants are shown in Table 79-12.

A summary scheme based on TSI and LIA agar reactions is shown in Table 79-13.

Identification of Enterobacteriaceae

As discussed before, the primary isolation plates and screening by TSI and urea agar (also LIA and phenylalanine deaminase) will allow tentative grouping of the organisms.

1. In the case of **lactose nonfermenters** (as shown by colony appearance on primary plates) or of **lactose and sucrose nonfermenters** (as shown by alkaline slant and acid butt in TSI agar), many workers use growth from the primary plates or the TSI slants for slide agglutination tests with *Salmonella* and *Shigella* polyvalent antisera. This is acceptable when rapid reporting is necessary. See the outline and summary for "screening" of *Salmonella* and *Shigella* organisms for tentative identification of such organisms (Chapter 75, "Stool"); also refer to sections describing the 2 groups below.

Note that by using TSI and LIA slants and the schema in Table 79-13, *Yersinia enterocolitica* and *Y. pseudotuberculosis* can be recognized as a possibility.

Vi antiserum should be used with *Salmonella*-like cultures that are not agglutinated by the polyvalent *Salmonella* antisera (for *S. typhi* and a few other types where the Vi antigen may block the O antigens).

Shigella-like cultures (based on their reactions in TSI agar) that do not agglutinate in polyvalent *Shigella* antisera should be suspended in saline, heated for 30 min at 100 C, cooled, and then retested with the antisera. *Shigella* contains heat-labile antigens that often may block agglutination by the antisera.

If positive agglutination is obtained, a "presumptive" report may be sent out. Further biochemical tests must then be carried out along with additional serologic testing before a "con-

firmed" report for *Salmonella* or *Shigella* is made.

It should be remembered that the term lactose or sucrose nonfermenter is used here to denote organisms that do not utilize these substances promptly (in 24 hours or less); organisms with alkaline slant and acid butt reaction on TSI agar may be slow lactose or sucrose fermenters. For final identification the tests listed in Table 79-14 should be carried out and reference should be made to the description of the various groups in this chapter.

2. For identification of organisms showing **alkaline butt** and **alkaline slant,** refer to "Nonfermenters," below.

3. For identification of **prompt lactose fermenters** (as shown by colony appearance on plates or TSI reaction) **after negative oxidase test,** refer to Table 79-14 and to the sections on *Escherichia, Enterobacter (Aerobacter),* and *Klebsiella.* It should also be remembered that acid slant on TSI agar may indicate sucrose fermentation, not necessarily that of lactose. *Serratia* colonies are lactose nonfermenters on primary plates; when inoculated into TSI, acid slant will be shown due to sucrose fermentation.

Tests for group differentiation of *Enterobacteriaceae* are shown in Table 79-14. These reactions are shown by typical cultures; atypical or aberrant cultures will not necessarily give the exact reactions shown. Final group differentiation can be made with the aid of these reactions and whenever necessary, as outlined under the description of the various groups, by the use of antisera. Species differentiation or serotype determination depends on specific biochemical tests or the use of specific antisera described further in this chapter.

A detailed description on the isolation and **preliminary** identification of *Yersinia enterocolitica* from fecal specimens is given in Chapter 75 (stool examination). Most strains of *Y. enterocolitica* are **urea positive** in 3-24 hours, and most strains are **motile at 25 C,** but very few are motile at **35 C.**

Differentiation of members of the family Enterobacteriaceae from certain other gram-negative organisms

Cytochrome (indophenol) oxidase test. Occasionally gram-negative rods will give reactions similar to those of *Enterobacteriaceae* without fulfilling the criteria for identification in Table 79-14 or by serologic methods. These may be atypical *Enterobacteriaceae* cultures; on the other hand, they may belong to another family, and the tests listed will be misleading for their identification.

An important and very useful test for detecting whether a gram-negative rod resembling *Enterobacteriaceae* is in effect a member of this family or of another is the **(cytochrome) oxidase test.** Ewing and Johnson[34] reported that out of 1222 *Enterobacteriaceae* cultures, including every group listed in Table 79-14, none showed the presence of cytochrome oxidase. On the other hand, every *Aeromonas, Vibrio, Pseudomonas, Pasteurella,* and *Alcaligenes* species (a total of 231 cultures) was cytochrome oxidase positive. None of these organisms belong to *Enterobacteriaceae.* The test is recommended for differentiation of *Aeromonas, Vibrio, Pseudomonas,* and *Alcaligenes* cultures from members of the family *Enterobacteriaceae. (See Chapter 72.)*

Nitrate reduction. With extremely rare exceptions, members of the family *Enterobacteriaceae* reduce nitrate to nitrite, whereas many confusingly similar gram-negative organisms, not members of the family, do not. A negative result, if the test was properly carried out and confirmed (zinc dust!), is of value in the exclusion of otherwise doubtful strains (Table 79-14).

Oxidation vs. fermentation. All *Enterobacteriaceae* attack sugars fermentatively. The OF test is very useful in differentiating organisms that break down carbohydrates oxidatively from the *Enterobacteriaceae* (see Tables 79-1 and 79-2).

Growth on MacConkey, SS, and cetrimide agar. See Table 79-1 for reactions of several genera that may be mistaken for *Enterobacteriaceae.*

Biochemical tests and methods used for differentiation of Enterobacteriaceae

Minimal or essential tests.[35] Indole, methyl red, Voges-Proskauer, Simmons citrate, H_2S (in TSI agar), urease (Christensen urea), motility (at 2 temperatures or room temperature), gas from glucose.

Important additional tests. Lactose, sucrose, salicin, mannitol, adonitol, lysine and ornithine decarboxylase, arginine dihydrolase, phenylalanine agar, KCN.

Other tests of value. Sodium malonate, β-galactosidase (ONPG) organic acid media of Kauffman and Petersen, sodium acetate, sodium mucate, DNase medium, other carbohydrates, e.g., dulcitol, inositol, sorbitol, etc., gelatin liquefaction.

Most of these media and tests are described and interpreted in Chapter 72. They are based mainly on the technics described by Ewing,[36] Edwards and Ewing,[37] and Ewing and Davis.[38] A few are discussed in detail below.

Motility test. A semisolid medium in a test tube is recommended. Stab into top of column to depth of about 5 mm. Incubate at 20-25 C (some workers prefer to use 2 tubes and incubate 1 at 20-25 C and other at 37 C). Examine tube(s) at 4 and 8 hours and after overnight incubation.

Carbohydrate fermentation tests. Commercially available media usually employ phenol red as an indicator. These media are satisfactory for members of the *Enterobacteriaceae.* Ewing[36] recommends Andrade indicator because of easier observance of early fermentation and more clearcut reactions when this indicator is used in fermentation broths. Although semisolid media containing fermentable substances are usable, gas

production can be observed much better in inverted insert tubes in broths.

Decarboxylase tests. The ability or inability of various organisms to decarboxylate certain amino acids can be used for purposes of differentiation. Ewing et al.[39] investigated the decarboxylase activity of a very large number of *Enterobacteriaceae* on lysine, arginine, and ornithine. They employed, in addition to various basal media, an inoculated control without added amino acids for comparison and found the decarboxylase reactions valuable adjuncts for the differentiation of *Enterobacteriaceae* and related organisms. (See Table 79-15.)

KCN broth. Edwards et al.[40, 41] found that ability or inability of an organism to grow in Moeller potassium cyanide medium is another very valuable, differential criterion, in particular for the differentiation of *Salmonella* and *Shigella* organisms, which do not grow, from many other

Table 79-15. Decarboxylase reactions of *Enterobacteriaceae** (Moeller medium)

Genera and species	Lysine	Arginine	Ornithine
Escherichia coli	d†	d	d‡
Shigella			
dysenteriae	–	d	–
flexneri	–	d	–
boydii	–	d	–
sonnei	–	d	+
Salmonella	+	+ or (+)	+
typhi	+	– or (+)	–
paratyphi A	–	– or (+)	+
Arizona	+	(+) or +	+
Citrobacter	–	d	d
Edwardsiella	+	–	+
Klebsiella			
pneumoniae	+	–	–
ozaenae	d	–	–
rhinoschleromatis	–	–	–
Enterobacter			
cloacae	–	+	+
aerogenes	+	–	+
hafniae	+	d	+
liquefaciens	d	–	+
Serratia	+	–	+
Proteus			
vulgaris	–	–	–
mirabilis	–	–	+
morganii	–	–	+
rettgeri	–	–	–
Providencia	–	–	–
Yersinia			
pestis	–	–	–
pseudotuberculosis	–	–	–
enterocolitica	–	–	+

*+, positive within 24 h; (÷), positive after 2-4 d; –, no reaction; + or (÷), majority of strains positive, some late; – or (÷), majority negative, some strains late positive; (+) or +, majority late positive, some positive in 24 h; d, different reactions: +, (+), –.
†87% +.
‡63% +.

Enterobacteriaceae, which grow in KCN broth. The use of KCN broth is recommended.

Phenylalanine deaminase. The formation of phenylpyruvic acid from phenylalanine in the special medium (by deaminase) is a highly specific differential test for the separation of *Proteus* and *Providencia* organisms from other *Enterobacteriaceae.*

Christensen citrate agar. This is a medium for testing citrate utilization in the presence of organic nitrogen. *Shigella* do not utilize citrate, whereas many anaerogenic, nonmotile *E. coli* strains do.

Sodium malonate broth. This is useful in differentiating *Arizona* strains. They utilize malonate, whereas *Salmonella* organisms fail to do so.

Organic acid utilization. The medium, the organic acids used, and the performance of the test are described in Chapter 72. The test is useful for the differentiation of organisms in the *Salmonella-Arizona-Citrobacter* division.

IMViC formula. The mnemonic formula IMViC was used for many years to denote the results of the indole, methyl red, Voges-Proskauer, and citrate test (the i was added for easier pronunciation). Although typical (but not all) *E. coli* cultures give a + + − − formula, and typical *Klebsiella* and some *Enterobacter* species give a + + − − formula, its use if not very helpful if additional tests are not performed, since *Edwardsiella* and some *Shigella* strains also give + + − −, and *Serratia* yields − − + + IMViC formula. Other organisms give intermediate reactions (e.g., + − + −, − + − +, etc.).

Remarks concerning test media and reagents

The reactions shown in Table 79-14 are based on the use of certain specified media and reagents listed in Chapter 72. Adherence to the recommended methods, media, and reagents is important in order to obtain satisfactory tests. It is realized that for many laboratories with restricted facilities the multitude of media listed in Table 79-16 may present some difficulty. However, since the antisera and all of the media listed are available commercially in dehydrated form or as ready-made tubes, even small laboratories should experience no trouble in correctly identifying most of the organisms in the family *Enterobacteriaceae.*

In addition to the media and reagents listed, *Salmonella* polyvalent and group antisera, *Shigella* group antisera, and *E. coli* OB sera should be available, as a minimum, to allow for identification of various members of *Enterobacteriaceae.*

ESCHERICHIEAE (SHIGELLA AND ESCHERICHIA)

Ewing and Edwards[14, 15] placed the *Shigella* and *Escherichia* into a single division (tribe *Escherichieae*), since they are more closely related to each other both biochemically and serologically than either is to any other group.

Major characteristics differentiating the division from others in *Enterobacteriaceae* are shown in Table 79-10. **Typical cultures** belonging to this division are negative in the following tests: Voges-Proskauer, phenylalanine deaminase, and urease; they do not grow in KCN broth or utilize citrate (Simmons citrate agar), and H_2S is not produced in TSI agar. The methyl red test is usually positive, whereas the indole test is variable.

The major biochemical characteristics for the differentiation of genera in the division are listed in Table 79-16. These include **formation of gas from glucose** by the great majority of escherichiae but **not** by shigellae (except for certain biotypes of *S. flexneri* 6, which form gas) and **fermentation of lactose** by most of the *Escherichia* strains but not by most *Shigella* strains (except for *S. sonnei,* which ferments lactose slowly). Shigellae do not ferment salicin, whereas about 50% of escherichiae do. **Shigellae are always nonmotile,** whereas most escherichiae (60-70%) are motile. Lysine decarboxylase is a useful differentiating test: Shigellae are unable to decarboxylate lysine (negative test), whereas most escherichiae give a positive test. Most *Escherichia* strains grow on sodium acetate whereas shigellae do not.

In practice, *Shigella* organisms are identified by **biochemical reactions** and **specific antisera;** since there are close antigenic relationships between members of the 2 groups, it is imperative that both biochemical and serologic methods should be used. Typical *E. coli* cultures present no difficulties in identification, but some anaerogenic (nongasforming), nonmotile varieties of *E. coli* are often mistaken for shigellae. Details for differentiation are found below.

Differentiation is of considerable importance, since shigellae are the causative agents of bacillary dysentery.

Detailed biochemical characteristics for identification of the 2 groups are listed in Table 79-14 and in the section on *Shigella* and *Escherichia.*

SHIGELLA

Shigellae grow well on some differential and selective media employed for *Enterobacteriaceae,* e.g., eosin-methylene blue, deoxycholate, SS, XLD, and MacConkey agar. Some strains grow poorly on SS and deoxycholate citrate agar. Selenite can be used for isolation of shigellae; GN broth was found by some workers to be better. Bismuth sulfite and brilliant green agar are inhibitory for shigellae.

Shigellae are **nonmotile,** gram-negative rods that do not form gas from fermentable carbohydrates (except for certain biotypes of *Shigella flexneri* 6). Salicin, adonitol, and inositol are not fermented. Lactose is fermented only by *S. sonnei* after prolonged incubation. Lysine is not decarboxylated. For details see Tables 79-14, 79-17, and 79-18.

Shigellae show an alkaline slant and acid

Table 79-16. Differentiation within tribe *Escherichieae**†

Test or substrate	Escherichia			Shigella		
	Sign	%+	(%+)‡	Sign	%+	(%+)‡
Indole	+	96.3		− or +	37.8	
Lysine decarboxylase	d	80.6	(1.5)	−	0	
Arginine dihydrolase	d	16.3	(39.1)	d	7.6	(5.6)
Ornithine decarboxylase	d	57.8	(8)	− or +	20§	
Mucate	+	91.6		−	0§	
Sodium acetate	+ or (+)	83.8	(9.7)	−	0	
Christensen's citrate	d	18.1	(22.6)	−	0	
Gas from glucose	+	92		−	2.1‖	
Lactose	+	91.6	(4.2)	d	0.3	(11.4)§
Sucrose	d	53.7	(5.5)	d	0.9	(31.1)§
Salicin	d	36	(12.3)	−	0	
Esculin	d	30.9	(19.7)	−	0	
Motility	+ or −	62.1		−	0	

*From Ewing, W. H.: Differentiation of *Enterobacteriaceae* by biochemical reactions, Atlanta, 1973, (rev.), Center for Disease Control.

†+, 90% or more positive within 1 or 2 d; (+), positive reaction after 3 or more d (decarboxylase tests: 3 or 4 d); −, no reaction (90% or more); + or −, most cultures positive, some strains negative; − or +, most strains negative, some cultures positive; + or (+), most reactions occur within 1 or 2 d, some are delayed; d, different reactions—+, (+), −; w, weakly positive reaction.

‡Figures in parentheses indicate percentages of delayed positive reactions (3 d or more).

§Cultures of S. sonnei usually ferment lactose and sucrose slowly, and strains of this species decarboxylate ornithine. Some isolates of S. sonnei utilize mucate weakly and slowly.

‖Certain biotypes of S. flexneri 6 form gas.

NOTE: Obviously there is no difficulty in differentiation of typical cultures of *E. coli* and shigellae. However, anaerogenic nonmotile forms of *E. coli*, **some** of which often are referred to as Alkalescens-Dispar bioserotypes, may require closer examination before they can be classified as *E. coli*. In attempting to classify a particular strain as *E. coli* or as a member of the genus *Shigella*, biochemical reactivities of the culture should be considered as a whole. Shigellae are much less reactive than *E. coli*, and a culture that produces acid promptly (i.e., within 24 h) from all or most of a wide variety of carbohydrates, such as maltose, rhamnose, xylose, sorbitol, and dulcitol, undoubtedly is not a *Shigella*.

Table 79-17. Biochemical reactions of Shigellae*†

Test or substrate	Sign	%+	(%+)‡	Test or substrate	Sign	%+	(%+)‡
Hydrogen sulfide	−	0		Rhamnose	d	16.6	(6.1)
Urease	−	0		Malonate	−	0	
Indole	− or +	37.8		Mucate	−	3.5	(6.5)§
Methyl red (37 C)	+	100		Christensen's citrate	−	0	
Voges-Proskauer (37 C)	−	0		Jordan's tartrate	+ or +	29.4	
Citrate (Simmons')	−	0		Sodium pectate	−	0	
KCN	−	0		Sodium acetate	−	0	
Motility	−	0		Sodium alginate	−	0	
Gelatin (22 C)	−	0		Lipases			
Lysine decarboxylase	−	0		Corn oil	−	0	
Arginine dihydrolase	d	7.6	(5.6)	Triacetin	−	0	
Ornithine decarboxylase	d	20	(0.3)	Tributyrin	−	0	
Phenylalanine deaminase	−	0		Maltose	d	26.6	(57)
Glucose acid	+	100		Xylose	d	4.3	(11.1)
Glucose gas	−	2.1		Trehalose	d	76.4	(19.3)
Lactose	d	0.3	(11.4)§	Cellobiose	−	2.9	(0.4)
Sucrose	d	0.9	(31.1)§	Glycerol	d	13.8	(39.6)
Mannitol	+ or −	80.5		α-methyl glucoside	−	0	
Dulcitol	d	5.4	(12.7)	Erythritol	−	0	
Salicin	−	0		Esculin	−	0	
Adonitol	−	0		Beta galactosidase	− or +	13.7	
Inositol	−	0		Nitrate to nitrite	+	99.8	
Sorbitol	d	29.1	(21.9)	Oxidation-fermentation	F	100	
Arabinose	d	67.8	(11.2)	Oxidase	−	0	
Raffinose	d	20.7	(19.1)				

*From Ewing, W. H.: DHEW publ. no. (CDC) 75-8098, Atlanta, 1974, Center for Disease Control. Based on examination of 5,166 cultures representative of all 4 species (Ewing, 1971).

†+, 90% or more positive within 1-2 d incubation; (+), positive reaction after 3 or more d (decarboxylase tests, 3 or 4 d); −, no reaction (90% or more); + or −, majority of strains positive, some cultures negative; majority of reactions delayed, some occur within 1-2 d; d, different reactions—+, (+), −; F, fermentation.

‡Figures in parentheses indicate percentages of delayed reactions (3 or more d).

§See text.

Table 79-18. Differentiation of species of Shigella*†

Test or substrate	Subgroup A S. dysenteriae 1-10			Subgroup B S. flexneri 1-5			Subgroup B S. flexneri 6			Subgroup C S. boydii 1-15			Subgroup D S. sonnei		
	Sign	%+	(%+)‡	Sign	%+	(%+)‡	Sign	%+	(%+)‡	Sign	%+	(%+)‡	Sign	%+	(%+)‡
Indole	− or +	43.7	(11.3)	+ or −	61.5			0	(10.3)	− or +	28.8	(31.9)	−	0	(5)
Arginine dihydrolase	d	1.5		−	0§		d	48.9		d	18.1		−	0.5	
Ornithine decarboxylase	−	0		−	0		−	0		−	2.5¶		+	99.4	
Mucate	−	0		−	0		−	0		−	0		− or +	16.4	
Jordan's tartrate	+ or −	78		−	0		−	18.1		− or +	13		+	100	
Gas from glucose	−	0		−	0		− or +	0		−	0		−	0	
Lactose	−	0	(1.6)¶	−	0	(<0.1)	−	0		−	1		d	1.8	(88.1)
Sucrose	−	0	(4.2)	d	1.5	(41.9)	−	0		−	0		d	0.1	(85.4)
Mannitol	−	0		+	93.7		+ or −	82.5		+	97.6		+	98.9	
Dulcitol	−	4.5	(0.5)	−	0		d	9.4	(72.2)	d	6.7	(10.4)	−	0	(1)
Sorbitol	d	29.2	(29.5)	d	30.6	(1.5)	(+) or +	30.2	(59.8)	d	41.8	(36.3)	−	1	(1)
Arabinose	d	43.6	(7.2)	d	65	(8.7)	+ or (+)	54.6	(39.3)	+	94.1		d	94.2	(2.9)
Raffinose	−	0		d	52.8	(28.4)	−	0		−	0.2		−	2.5	(81.5)
Rhamnose	d	32.4	(5.5)	d	6	(6.2)	−	1.6	(3.7)	d	16.6	(1.6)	+ or (+)	77.1	(21)
Maltose	d	12	(77)	d	28.4	(45.3)	(+) or +	16	(74.4)	d	11.2	(66)	+ or (+)	86.4	(6.8)
Xylose	d	3.9	(7.6)	−	1.8	(0.4)#	d	0.5	(18.2)	d	85.2	(57.2)	−	1	
Trehalose	+ or (+)	89.8	(7.5)	+ or (+)	77.8	(12.2)	(+) or +	7.4	(92.6)	+ or (+)	0	(11.2)	+	100	
Cellobiose	−	0		−	0		−	0		−	55.5		d	10.6	(1.8)
Glycerol	d	12.3	(72.5)	−	0		+ or (+)	60	(31.1)	+ or (+)	11.1	(34.8)	d	13	(32.7)
Beta galactosidase (ONPG)	− or +	49.9‖		−	0.8		−	0		− or +			+	95	(32.7)

*From Ewing, W. H.: Differentiation of *Enterobacteriaceae* by biochemical reactions, DHEW publ. no. (CDC) 75-8098, Atlanta, 1974, Center for Disease Control.

†+, 90% positive within 1 or 2 d incubation; (+), positive reaction after 3 or more d (decarboxylase tests: 3 or 3 d); −, no reaction (90% or more); + or −, majority of strains positive, some cultures negative; − or +, majority of cultures negative, some strains positive; (+) or +, majority of reactions delayed, some occur within 1 or 2 d; d, different reactions—+, (+), −.

‡Figures in parentheses indicate percentages of delayed reactions (3 or more d).

§A few doubtful reactions occurred, but these were regarded as negative.

‖Only cultures of S. boydii 13 are positive.

¶Some strains of S. dysenteriae 1 ferment lactose slowly; all are ONPG positive.

#Xylose was fermented by some cultures of the mannitol negative bioserotypes of S. flexneri 4 but not by other strains of serotypes 1 to 5.

butt, no H_2S, and no gas in TSI agar (except for certain biotypes of *S. flexneri* 6, which may form detectable gas).

Disease in humans, distribution and mode of spread

Shigellae are the causative agents of bacillary dysentery. Their habitat is almost exclusively in humans (*S. flexneri* and *S. dysenteriae* have been isolated from dogs and *S. flexneri* also from captive monkeys). Shigellae may cause (1) an inapparent infection, (2) a mild infection showing some abdominal discomfort with few diarrheal stools, or (3) an infection with severe prostration, nausea, extreme pain, and diarrhea in which the discharge contains mostly blood, pus, and mucus. *S. dysenteriae* infections are usually more severe than those caused by the other types.

The organisms are, as a rule, restricted to the gastrointestinal tract, and they rarely, if ever, invade the bloodstream. Diagnosis is made by culturing the organism from the stool.

The most widely distributed types are *S. flexneri* and *S. sonnei*. *S. dysenteriae* 1 seems to occur most frequently in the Far East. Contamination of fingers with fecal material, of toilet seats, and glassware and the consumption of foods or water contaminated with fecal material (by food handlers or flies) are the usual routes of transmission of the infection.

A large percentage (60-70%) of isolations of shigellae from humans are made from children under 10 years of age and, again, a large percentage of the isolates are *S. sonnei;* this organism accounts for about 85% of all *Shigella* isolates in the United States.[42]

For a detailed review of bacillary dysentery see Christie,[43] and for its pathogenesis, Keusch et al.[44]

Nomenclature

The schema originally proposed by Ewing[45] and modified by the *Shigella* Commission of the *Enterobacteriaceae* Subcommittee is based partly on biochemical characteristics and partly on antigenic relationships. Capital letters are used to designate the subgroups and Arabic numerals for the serotypes. It should be remembered that shigellae possess O and K antigens but not H antigens (they are nonmotile).

S. dysenteriae (**subgroup A**) contains those shigellae that characteristically do not utilize mannitol and do not bear significant serologic relationships to members of the other *Shigella* subgroups. There are 10 serotypes: *S. dysenteriae* 1 (Shiga), *S. dysenteriae* 2 (formerly *S. schmitzii),* and serotypes 3-10.

Members of the Providence group sometimes are confused with shigellae because they often fail to utilize mannitol and may be anaerogenic. *Providencia* organisms may be excluded from the genus *Shigella* on the basis of the phenylalanine deaminase reaction, motility,

sodium citrate utilization, and adonitol or inositol fermentation.

Yersinia enterocolitica is motile at 20-25 C, is urease positive, and usually gives an A(cid)/A(cid) reaction on TSI slant.

S. flexneri (**subgroup B**) organisms usually ferment mannitol; there are 6 serotypes and 9 subtypes (1a, 1b, 2a, 2b, 3a, 3b, 3c, 4a, 4b, 5, 6). Members of this subgroup are related to each other through the possession of common group antigens, but each serotype contains a type or main antigen. Note the biochemical differences between serotypes 1-5 on the one hand and serotype 6 on the other (Table 79-18).

S. boydii (**subgroup C**) is composed of 15 serotypes (1-15). They resemble group B organisms biochemically but are antigenically distinct.

S. sonnei (**subgroup D**) ferments mannitol, is indole negative, decarboxylates ornithine, and ferments lactose upon prolonged incubation. Only 1 serotype is known that can occur in the rough (R) or smooth (S) form.

The microorganisms previously known as *S. dispar* and *S. alkalescens* (Alkalescens-Dispar group) are now placed in the *Escherichia* group.

Antigens of Shigella and preparation of antisera

The methods used for **typing** *Shigella* cultures are based on the fact that each serologic type contains a specific or major somatic (O) antigen that is characteristic of the serotype. Certain shigellae also contain group or minor antigens, which in many cases are shared by other serotypes. For example, *S. flexneri* serotypes contain common group antigens, and consequently, each type of this species reacts to some extent in antisera prepared against other serotypes of the species. Such relationships make the use of absorbed antisera a necessity when dealing with *S. flexneri* and certain other types.[17]

The antigenic pattern is rather complex. In addition to the overlapping between the different serotypes, certain of the *Shigella* serotypes are related to members of other groups within the family *Enterobacteriaceae*. The O antigens of 15 *Shigella* serotypes are identical with those of *E. coli* O antigen groups, and there are strong reciprocal O antigenic relationships known between 19 *Shigella* serotypes and *E. coli* O antigen groups.

The **K** antigens of *Shigella* are responsible for the fact that some *Shigella* strains may be made agglutinable by boiling; the envelope antigens are heat labile, and their destruction makes the organism agglutinable by the O antiserum.

It is not necessary to produce one's own grouping sera since they are commercially available.* These

---

*BBL, Div. of BioQuest, Cockeysville, Md.; Difco Laboratories, Detroit; Lee Laboratories, Chicago; Lederle Laboratories, Pearl River, N.Y.; Burroughs Wellcome & Co., Inc., Research Triangle, N.C.

sera must be used, however, in strict adherence to the manufacturer's instructions. If sera are produced in the laboratory, smooth strains are selected and grown on infusion agar slants.

The technic advised for preparation of polyvalent grouping sera by Edwards and Ewing[17] is as follows:

Test culture, after incubation overnight, for smoothness in 1:500 acriflavine and in 1:10 or 1:20 dilution of homologous antiserum for agglutination. Inoculate a meat infusion broth flask, incubate 6-8 h, and heat at 100 C for 2 h. Centrifuge and resuspend organisms in 0.5% formalin-containing saline. Inject animal IV at 4-5 d intervals. Amounts injected are 0.5, 1.0, 2.0, 4.0, and 4.0 ml. Bleed animals after 5-7 d; test serum. If it is satisfactory, exsanguinate animals. Preserve antiserum by adding an equal volume of glycerin.

Polyvalent subgroup A antiserum. Prepared by injecting equal amounts of antigen (S. dysenteriae types 1-7). Absorb* serum with Alkalescens-Dispar organisms (A-D 01) and S. boydii 15.

Polyvalent A-1 antiserum.† Prepare by using S. dysenteriae types 8-10 as antigen. Absorb serum with S. dysenteriae 2 and S. boydii 15.

Polyvalent B antiserum. Use S. flexneri types 1-6. Absorb with A-D 01, A-D 03, and A-D 04 organisms.

Polyvalent C antiserum. Use S. boydii 1-7. Absorb with A-D 01, A-D 03, A-D 04, and S. sonnei R (II).

Polyvalent C-1.† Inject S. boydii 8-11. Absorb with S. boydii 1, S. Boydii 4, A-D 01, and A-D 02.

Polyvalent C-2.† Use S. boydii 12-15. Absorb with S. dysenteriae 2, A-D 01, A-D 02, and A-D 07 organisms.

Sonnei antiserum. Inject cultures of S. sonnei form I(S) and form II(R), variants of single serotype of S. sonnei.

Some type-specific sera are now commercially available. For details of preparation of typing sera refer to Edwards and Ewing.[5,20]

Identification

Organisms from TSI slants selected on the basis of their reactions (or, if urgent reports are needed, from lactose-negative colonies on primary plates) are tested in **polyvalent grouping antisera.** Usually antisera for subgroups A, B, C, and D of Shigella and a serum for the Alkalescens-Dispar group is used.

Slide agglutinations are performed, and only **prompt, complete agglutinations** are taken as positive. Suspensions in saline (or in mercuric iodide solution), **rather thick,** should be employed. For these tests 2 × 3 inch glass slides are convenient. Divide into a number of sections with wax pencil. Place droplet of suspension on slide and then place similar droplet of antiserum below antigen suspension. Mix droplets of antiserum and antigen with loop in such a way as to make a narrow track of mixture (about 5 mm wide and 15 mm long). Mixing may then be continued by tilting slide back and forth. When using commercially prepared antisera, always follow manufacturer's instructions.

Cultures that appear to be shigellae in TSI agar medium but that do **not** react in the grouping antisera should be suspended in plain physiologic saline

solution and heated at 100 C for ½ hr, then cooled, and retested.

Cultures that appear to be shigellae according to their reactions in polyvalent or grouping antisera must be subjected to biochemical tests in order to confirm them as members of the Shigella group.[5] Since Shigella cultures are **nonmotile,** a simple test in semisolid motility medium will eliminate many extraneous cultures. Motile cultures are not Shigella. If sera are not available, biochemical tests should be used for primary differentiation, and suspicious colonies should be submitted to a reference laboratory for serologic typing.

Tables 79-14, 79-17, and 79-18 list the biochemical reactions of Shigella. The cytochrome oxidase reaction is very helpful in differentiating Pseudomonas and Alcaligenes strains from Shigella, if there is some confusion in the interpretation of TSI reactions. Fermentation of lactose and sucrose in 24 hours usually means that the culture is not Shigella. **Any culture that utilizes Simmons citrate, grows in KCN broth, ferments salicin or adonitol, produces H_2S in TSI, and produces urease or that is motile can be excluded from consideration as Shigella.**[46]

Some difficulty may be experienced with anaerogenic (non-gas-producing), nonmotile varieties of E. coli, some of which are often referred to as Alkalescens-Dispar types. The biochemical reactivities of the culture should be considered as a whole. Shigellae are much less reactive than E. coli strains, and a culture that produces acid promptly (i.e., within 24 hours) from all or most of a wide variety of carbohydrates, such as maltose, rhamnose, xylose, sorbitol, and dulcitol, is not a Shigella.[13]

The reactions in Table 79-18 allow differentiation of the **subgroups,** and those in Table 79-19 are the biochemical reactions of **serotypes** of Shigella.

Note: An H_2S-positive strain of Shigella sonnei and an aerogenic (gas-forming) strain of S. boydii type 13 have been encountered.

Subgroup A (S. dysenteriae) is mannitol negative; the other groups, with few exceptions, are mannitol positive. Lactose and sucrose are fermented slowly by S. sonnei only. A positive ornithine decarboxylase test allows rapid confirmation of S. sonnei.

The mannitol-negative S. dysenteriae can be differentiated by performing the indole test (using peptone water, incubated for 2 days): types 1, 3, 4, 5, 6, 9, and 10 are indole negative; types 2, 7, and 8 are indole positive. The existence of some mannitol-negative S. flexneri 6 strains should be kept in mind.

Mannitol-positive shigellae may be subgroup B (S. flexneri), C (S, boydii), or D (S. sonnei). A number of S. flexneri (1, 2, 3, 4, 5) and S. boydii (5, 7, 9) types are indole positive. Mannitol-positive, indole-negative shigellae may be S. sonnei; they give a positive ornithine decarboxylase test and ferment lactose slowly. Other indole-negative strains in this group are S. flexneri 6 and S. boydii 1, 2, 3, 4, 6, 8, and 10.

---

*Antisera should be tested and absorbed as required.
†These antisera are not absolutely necessary.

Table 79-19. Biochemical reactions of serotypes of *Shigella**†

Species and serotype	Mannitol Sign	Mannitol %+	Dulcitol Sign	Dulcitol %+	Xylose Sign	Xylose %+	Rhamnose Sign	Rhamnose %+	Raffinose Sign	Raffinose %+	Glycerol Sign	Glycerol %+	Indole Sign	Indole %+	Ornithine decarboxylase Sign	Ornithine decarboxylase %+
Subgroup A																
S. dysenteriae 1	−	0	−	0	−	0	−	0	−	0	+ or (+)	100	−	0	−	0
2	−	0	−	0	−	0	+	98	−	0	(+) or +	98	+	100	−	0
3	−	0	−	0	−	0	−	0	−	0	(+) or +	100	−	0	−	0
4	−	0	+ or (+)	100	−	0	−	0	−	0	(+) or +	100	−	0	−	0
5	−	0	−	0	−	0	−	0	−	0	+ or (+)	100	−	0	−	0
6	−	0	−	0	−	0	−	0	−	0	− or (+)	38	+	100	−	0
7	−	0	−	0	−	0	(+) or +	90	−	0	−	0	+	100	−	0
8	−	0	−	0	+ or (+)	96	−	8	−	0	+ or (+)	100	−	0	−	0
9	−	0	−	0	−	0	−	0	−	0	+ or (+)	100	−	0	−	0
10	−	0	−	0	+	100	−	0	−	0	−	0	−	0	−	0
Subgroup B																
S. flexneri 1	+	95	−	0	−	0	−	0	d	89	−	0	− or +	35	−	0
2	+	99	−	0	−	0	−	0	d	77	−	0	− or +	44	−	0
3	+	98	−	0	−	0	d	12	d	88	−	0	+ or −	88	−	0
4	+	99	−	0	−	0	d	23	d	82	−	0	+ or −	55	−	0
4	−	0	−	0	d	71	− or +	48	−	3	−	0	+	98	−	0
5	+	99	−	0	−	0	−	5	d	72	d	88	+	95	−	0
6‡	+	>99	d	80	d	4	−	6	−	0	+ or (+)	100	−	0	−	0
6‡	+	100	d	86	d	75	−	0	−	0	(+)	100	−	0	−	0
Subgroup C																
S. boydii 1	+	100	−	1	+ or (+)	97	−	0	−	0	(+) or +	96	−	0	−	0
2	+	100	−	1	−	0	−	0	−	0	+ or (+)	100	−	0	−	0
3	+	100	d	75	d	86	−	0	−	0	+ or (+)	91	−	0	−	0
4	+	99	+ or (+)	28	−	0	−	0	−	0	+ or (+)	100	−	0	−	0
5	+	100	−	0	(+)	94	−	0	−	0	d	61	−	0	−	0
6	+ or (+)	100	(+) or +	100	+	100	−	0	−	0	(+) or +	100	+	100	−	0
7	+	100	−	0	+	98	−	0	−	0	+ or (+)	98	−	0	−	0
8	+	100	−	0	+	94	−	0	−	0	(+) or +	100	+	100	−	0
9	+	95	−	0	−	0	d	80	−	0	(+) or +	82	−	0	−	0
10	+	94	+	100	d	84	−	0	−	0	(+) or +	100	+	100	−	0
11	+	100	− or (+)	34	+ or (+)	100	−	0	−	0	(+) or +	100	−	0	−	0
12	+	100	− or (+)	14	−	0	−	0	−	0	− or +	14	+	100	−	0
13	+	100	−	0	(+) or +	100	−	0	−	0	(+) or −	63	−	0	−	100
14	− or +	29	−	0	−	0	−	0	−	0	+ or (+)	100	+	100	−	0
15	+	90	−	0	−	0	−	0	−	0	(+) or −	64	+	100	−	0
Subgroup D																
S. sonnei	+	99	−	1	−	1	+ or (+)	98	d	84	d	46	−	0	+	>99

*From Ewing, W. H.: Isolation and identification of *Salmonella* and *Shigella*, DHEW publ. no. (CDC) 75-8098, Atlanta, 1974, Center for Disease Control.

†+, 90% or more positive within 1 or 2 d incubation; (+), positive reaction after 3 or more d (decarboxylase tests: 3 or 4 d); −, no reaction (90% or more); + or −, majority of strains positive, some cultures negative; − or +, majority of cultures negative, some strains positive; + or (+), majority of reactions delayed, some occur within 1 or 2 d; d, different reactions—+, (+), −.

‡Some cultures of *S. flexneri* 6 (Newcastle and Manchester biotypes produce gas from fermentable carbohydrates; other shigellae are anaerogenic.

NOTE: In this table percentages of + and (+) reactions are combined.

Cultures of *S. sonnei* occur in two forms, I(S) and II(R), and it is necessary to employ antiserum that contains agglutinins for both forms for identification. *S. sonnei* form I(S) is the smooth form of the micro-organism and form II(R) represents a stage in the degradation of the smooth toward the rough form. Transitional forms between I and II exist and colonies of these transitional forms, as well as of *S. sonnei* I or II, may be encountered on primary isolation plates. Experience has indicated that in acute infections caused by *S. sonnei* one may expect to find I(S) colonies to be predominant whereas in carriers form II(R) colonies of transitional forms predominate (Branham et al., 1952). By careful selection of colony forms I and II for antiserum production and by appropriate absorption of the antisera, it is possible to prepare antisera for differentiation of the two forms of *S. sonnei*. The rough antigens of *S. boydii* 6 are identical with those of *S. sonnei* II, and antisera for the former generally must be absorbed by the latter.[46]

Colicin typing. *S. sonnei* strains can be classified (typed) by the use of colicins. Colicins are antibiotic-like agents and are produced by various gram-negative enteric organisms; they may inhibit the growth of other organisms and a series of indicator organisms with known colicin sensitivities. By growing shigellae on blood agar, colicin production can be detected and *S. sonnei* strains can be typed, a valuable epidemiologic tool for proving or disproving the relatedness of *Shigella* strains obtained in an outbreak. At least 15 colicin types of *S. sonnei* are known; some *S. sonnei* strains do not produce colicins and are considered untypable.

Bacteriophage typing of Shigella sonnei.[42] Recently, about 40% of *S. sonnei* isolates in the United States have been "untypeable" by colicin. A pleage-typing schema was developed by Pruneda and Farmer,[42] which allows differentiation of *S. sonnei* strains highly useful for epidemiologic tracing of strains.

Antibody formation in bacillary dysentery

Agglutinins do appear in the course of the disease, but they develop irregularly. Because of the large number of types capable of causing the disease, the agglutination test would have to be set up against a large number of antigens. In practice, no agglutination tests are used in the diagnosis of *Shigella* infections. Indirect bacterial hemagglutination tests (see Chapter 108) have been employed mainly in epidemiologic studies.

Antimicrobial susceptibility

Since the infection, especially that due to *S. sonnei*, is essentially self-limiting, mild cases often are not treated with antimicrobials, since drug therapy often results in the emergence of multiply drug-resistant strains. (Severely ill patients, young children, and debilitated adults usually are treated with fluids and antibiotics.) While shigellae are usually sensitive to ampicillin, tetracyclines, sulfonamides, kanamycin, chloramphenicol, and colistin, resistance develops quickly and it is necessary to determine the sensitivity pattern of the organism isolated from the patient. Ampicillin has been considered the drug of choice, but this is not true any more in all areas of the United States; trimethoprim-sulfamethoxazole and chloramphenicol are alternative drugs for ampicillin-resistant strains.

ESCHERICHIA
Escherichia coli

E. coli, the "colon bacillus," is so named because it is the predominant **facultative** species in the colon. *E. coli* is normally a bowel organism as are likely some of the *Klebsiella*, whereas *Enterobacter*, *Serratia*, and *Citrobacter* occur infrequently in the normal intestine and are usually free-living saprophytes. These organisms illustrate the difficulty of determining pathogenicity in absolute terms; they are usually harmless in their normal habitat, but they often cause illness when reaching tissues outside the intestinal tract. The "coliforms," mentioned above (together with *Proteus-Providence* organisms), are now the predominant etiologic agents in various **endogenous** (infections due to indigenous organisms) and **nosocomial** (hospital-acquired) infections.

E. coli, the only species of the genus, consists of short rods, motile by means of peritrichous flagella or occasionally nonmotile; they are usually nonencapsulated. The organisms grow well on ordinary media. Growth takes place at 10 and 45 C, with optimum temperature being 30-37 C.

Typical *E. coli* colonies are usually easy to recognize by their characteristic appearance on differential media; they are lactose fermenters, and on EMB (and Endo) medium they have a peculiar metallic sheen. On infusion agar plates the colonies are usually white, entire to undulate, and moist. On blood agar some strains produce β-hemolysis. Smooth and rough variation does occur. Freshly isolated strains are smooth.

The majority of strains are inhibited by enrichment broths and some highly selective media, as described earlier. They produce **acid** and **gas** from a large variety of carbohydrates; some anaerogenic (non-gas-forming) strains do occur (the Alkalescens-Dispar group, formerly in *Shigella*, is now included with *E. coli*). **Lactose** is fermented by the majority of strains but some strains ferment it slowly and some do not ferment it at all. Sodium acetate is utilized as a sole source of carbon; lysine, arginine, and ornithine are decarboxylated by the majority of strains. Indole and methyl red are positive, whereas the Voges-Proskauer reaction and Simmons citrate are negative. The urease test is negative, gelatin is not liquefied, and H_2S is not produced. *E. coli* does not grow in KCN medium. Sucrose is fermented

Table 79-20. Biochemical reactions of *Escherichia coli**†

Test or substrate	Sign	%+	(%+)‡	Test or substrate	Sign	%+	(%+)‡
Indole	+	96.3		Malonate	−	0	
Methyl red	+	99.9		Gas from glucose	+	92	
Voges-Proskauer	−	0		Lactose	+	91.6	(4.2)
Citrate (Simmons')	−	0.2	(0.3)	Sucrose	d	53.7	(5.5)
Hydrogen sulfide (TSI)	−	0§		Mannitol	+	97.5	
Urease	−	0		Dulcitol	d	49.3	(18)
KCN	−	2.6		Salicin	d	36	(12.3)
Motility	+ or −	62.1		Adonitol	−	5.2	(0.4)
Gelatin (22 C)	−	0		Inositol	−	0.9	(0.2)
Lysine decarboxylase	d	80.6	(1.5)	Sorbitol	d	80.3	(1)
Arginine dihydrolase	d	16.3	(39.1)	Arabinose	+	99.3	(0.5)
Ornithine decarboxylase	d	57.8	(8)	Raffinose	d	49.4	(2.1)
Phenylalanine deaminase	−	0		Rhamnose	d	83.5	(3.4)

*From Biochemical reactions given by *Enterobacteriaceae* in commonly used tests (rev.), Atlanta, Sept. 1973, Center for Disease Control.

†+, 90% or of cultures more positive within 1 or 2 d; (+), positive reaction after 3 or more d (decarboxylase tests: 3 or 4 d); −, no reaction (90% or more); + or −, most cultures positive, some strains negative; − or +, most strains negative, some cultures positive; (+) or +, most reactions occur within 1 or 2 d, some are delayed; *d*, different reactions: +, (+), −; *w*, weakly positive reaction.

‡Figures in parentheses indicate delayed reactions (3 d or more).

§An occasional strain may produce hydrogen sulfide.

by about 60% and salicin by about 50% of *Escherichia* strains.

Tables 79-14, 79-16, and 79-20 list reactions of typical *E. coli* and allow differentiation from *Shigella*.

Lactose-negative or late-fermenting E. coli

As pointed out earlier, some *Escherichia* strains ferment lactose late, irregularly, or not at all. Such organisms should be studied carefully. Fermentation of lactose, sucrose, and salicin may be delayed, and tests should be incubated for 7 days before being discarded. With the aid of the reactions in Table 79-20 and, if necessary, serologic methods, such cultures usually can be identified as *Escherichia*.

Slow lactose fermenters should be differentiated from *Shigella sonnei* (always nonmotile and identifiable by agglutination with specific antiserum), *Serratia*, *Arizona*, and *Citrobacter* organisms. Anaerogenic (non-gas-forming) strains may be Alkalescens-Dispar types. Christensen citrate agar and mucate medium are helpful in differentiating *Shigella* and anaerogenic, nomotile *E. coli*.

Alkalescens-Dispar organisms, formerly classified with *Shigella*, are now included in *Escherichia* on the basis of strong relationships of their O antigens with *E. coli* O groups. The organisms are nonmotile, lactose is usually late or it is not fermented; glucose, mannitol, arabinose, maltose, and xylose are fermented with **acid but no gas** production. Salicin usually is not fermented, whereas fermentation of sucrose and dulcitol is variable.

Both O and K antigens are present in the Alkalescens-Dispar group.[17] A grouping serum is available, which can be used to identify types 01 and 02 (formerly *Shigella alkalescens*) and types 03 and 04 (*Shigella dispar*). Their role in enteric infections is not clear; attacks of dysentery have been attributed to these organisms.

Infections in humans
Extraintestinal disease[4]

The most common extraintestinal diseases of humans caused by *E. coli* are those of the urinary tract. In the bladder (cystitis) the infection can be controlled by (appropriate) antimicrobial therapy. In the kidneys (pyelonephritis), lesions may progress despite treatment and may eventually lead to scarring and to destruction.

E. coli is often found in peritonitis, appendicitis, infections of the gallbladder and biliary tract, ureuingitis, and septicemia, along with other enteric bacteria. It frequently infects wounds that become contaminated with urine or feces.

E. coli is now the most frequently encountered species in gram-negative sepsis resulting in bacteremia and in severe shock. This disease is occurring with increased frequency in the very young, in those over age 60, and in debilitated patients (e.g., those on corticosteroid therapy or immunosuppressive agents, or suffering from leukemia); surgery or instrumentation of the intestinal, biliary, or genitourinary tract may also precipitate such sepsis.

The pathogenesis of extraintestinal *E. coli* infections and the factors that determine its invasiveness are not fully understood. However, it seems that the presence of capsular K(1) antigen in certain *E. coli* strains seems to be associated with increased virulence.

Diarrheal disease

It has been known for over 50 years that certain strains of *E. coli* can cause acute **diarrheal disease** in humans, especially in infants.[42,47-50] Some 15 distinct antigenic types were eventually identified as causes of severe diarrhea in small children, especially in nursery outbreaks, and named "**enteropathogenic** *E. coli* (**EEC**)." The mechanism responsible for the development of diarrhea, however, remained unknown and **enteropathogenicity** became synonymous with **serotype.**

More recently, additional *E. coli* strains (**toxigenic strains, ETEC**)[51–56a] previously not considered enteropathogenic (i.e., **not** belonging to the **EEC** serotypes) have been implicated in acute watery **diarrhea.** These strains produce one or both of two **enterotoxins:** (1) a heat-labile enterotoxin (LT) that is closely related to that of *Vibrio cholerae* (below), and (2) a heat-stable (ST) apparently nonantigenic enterotoxin. Heat-labile enterotoxin (LT) is antigenic and highly active in inducing experimental diarrhea. Purified ST is resistant to heating at 100 C for 15 min; it is also capable of causing diarrhea. Injection of the cell-free (LT or LT + ST) enterotoxin into an isolated **loop of rabbit ileum** (for detection of LT) causes massive accumulation of fluid; the toxin effects the secretion of water and electrolytes into the gut lumen,* similar to the action of cholera toxin. For the detection of ST, the material is injected directly into the stomach of the **infant mouse.** Other assays for LT detection are tissue culture systems, i.e., the **mouse Y-1 adrenal cell** (also sensitive to cholera toxin) and the **Chinese hamster ovarian cell test.** These are expensive and laborious tests and are presently not routinely available; when simpler immunologic in vivo tests become available, detection of toxin-producing *E. coli* strains will be practicable in many clinical laboratories. The "enteropathogenic serotyping" practiced in sporadic cases of infantile diarrhea is not useful and has been discouraged, since serotypes and toxin production are not synonymous; serotyping is to be used in investigation of outbreaks[50] (see discussion on "enteropathogenic *E. coli* serotypes and serotyping," below).

Toxigenic strains (ETEC) of *E. coli* are now recognized as worldwide etiologic agents in diarrheal disease of both children and adults, i.e., severe **cholera-like disease, infantile diarrhea,** "**traveler's diarrhea**" ("Montezuma's revenge," "tourist trots"), and **foodborne** and **waterborne outbreaks.** The diseases range from cholera-like "rice-water" diarrhea leading to salt depletion, shock and death, to self-limited mild diarrheas. Diarrhea due to **ETEC** is nonbloody, and there are **no** pus cells (inflammatory exudate) in the feces.

Another enteropathogenic mechanism responsible for **dysentery** has been identified in certain *E. coli* strains. These can penetrate the intestinal epithelium (they are invasive) and cause a bacillary dysentery-like syndrome (colitis) with severe abdominal cramps and pus and blood in the stool. The strains can be assayed by their ability to produce keratoconjunctivitis in the guinea pig's eye (**Serény test**) or their capacity to penetrate cells (HEP-2, Hela) in tissue culture. These **enteroinvasive** *E. coli* (**EIEC**) strains have now been documented in dysentery of both infants and adults.

Some of the in vivo tests for virulence are discussed in detail below ("in vivo tests for *E. coli* virulence properties").

In vivo tests for E. coli virulence properties (toxins, invasiveness)*

Y-1 Mouse adrenal cell test for heat-labile toxin (LT)[57]

LT has been shown to stimulate the enzyme adenylate cyclase with the production of cyclic adenosine monophosphate. This toxin is closely related to *V. cholerae* enterotoxin with regard to both molecular structure and mode of action. In this assay system, LT promotes the conversion of elongated fibroblast-like cells into round, refractile cells.

Equipment
1. Microtiter tissue culture plates, 96 flat-bottom wells, sterile, plastic, with lid
2. Tissue culture roller tube apparatus with 16 × 125 mm tube holder
3. Swinnex filter holder, 25 mm, with 0.45 μm membrane filter
4. Microtiter pipet, 0.025 ml, sterile
5. Syringe, disposable, 5 ml, to accommodate Swinnex filter; 1 ml
6. Vertical laminar flow hood (biological contaminant hood equipped with HEPA filters) (Bellco Glass, Vineland, N.J.)
7. Freezer, −70 or −20 C

Media[38]
1. Ham's F-10 medium (with glutamine and $NaHCO_3$)
2. Y-1 adrenal cell growth medium (Mix 90 ml Ham's F-10, 10 ml FBS (HeLa cell test for invasive potential [see below], and 1 ml AC.)
3. Trypticase soy-yeast extract (TS-YE) broth
4. Trypticase soy agar
5. Casamino acids-yeast extract (CA-YE) broth

Diagnostic reagents
1. Mouse adrenal cell (Y-1) culture, American Type Culture Collection.
2. Phosphate saline solution (for Y-1 assay).
3. Cholera enterotoxin. (Available commercially from Schwarz-Mann, Rockville, MD.) Dilute before use 1:1000 in 0.01M phosphate buffered saline.
4. Strains of *E. coli* producing heat-labile and heat-stable enterotoxins. Available from laboratories actively engaged in research on enteric illness.

Procedure
1. Preparation of Y-1 cell culture: Using standard cell culture technics, grow Y-1 cells on inner surface of 75 sq cm plastic cell culture flasks, using 20 ml Y-1 cell growth medium for 7 d at 35 C in CO_2 incubator. Replace medium on third or fourth day. Examine flasks

---

*Toxin stimulates adenylcyclase, resulting in an increase of adenosine-3¹, 5¹-monophosphate (cyclic AMP, cAMP).

*From Mehlman, I. J., Aulisio, C. C. J., Lovett, J., and Sanders, A.: Enteropathogenic *Escherichia coli*. In FDA Bacteriological analytical manual, ed. 5, Food and Drug Administration, Bureau of Foods, Dir. of Microbiology, 1978, Association of Official Analytical Chemists, Publisher and Distributor.

†Media and reagents are described in detail at the end of this section, following the Serény test.

daily with regard to color of medium and appearance of cells in monolayer. Before preparation of fresh flasks or of monolayers in wells of microtiter culture plates, wash monolayer with 20 ml phosphate saline solution. Add 2 ml 0.25% trypsin. Hold at room temperature until cell sheet has detached. Add 10 ml Y-1 cell growth medium and gently agitate to suspend cells. Centrifuge cells 10 min at 1000 rpm. Discard supernate. Suspend cells in 50 ml Y-1 cell growth medium. Transfer 20 ml aliquots to sterile 75 sq cm flasks for new culture. With slight agitation to maintain cells in suspension, transfer 0.2 ml aliquots to wells of microtiter culture plate. Incubate plates at 37 C in a CO_2 incubator until monolayer in each well is nearly confluent. Examine every 24 h. If cells are rough, discard.

2. Preparation of test filtrates: It is suggested that the investigator inoculate TS-YE broth (5 ml in a 16 × 125 mm screwcap tube) and a slant of trypticase soy agar from each suspected *E. coli* colony on L-EMB agar. It is recommended that 5 colonies from each subsample be examined. Alternatively, TS-YE broth may be inoculated from agar slant. Incubate TS-YE cultures with agitation in roller tube drum 25 h at 37 C. Transfer 0.1 ml of each TS-YE culture to 5 ml CA-YE broth (in a 16 × 125 mm tube). Incubate CA-YE and TS-YE cultures 24 h at 37 C in roller tube drum. If growth occurs in CA-YE, centrifuge culture 30 min at 1200 × g. If growth is poor, substitute TS-YE culture. Filter supernate through 0.45 μm filter. Heat 1 ml aliquot of each supernate 30 min at 80 C. Store filtrates at 4 C until use.

3. Assay: Add 0.025 ml of each heated and unheated filtrate to well of microtiter culture plate. Add 0.025 ml cholera enterotoxin preparation to control well. Simultaneously, examine heated and unheated filtrates of known positive and negative LT-producing strains in adjacent wells. Incubate plates 18 h at 37 C in CO_2 incubator.

Interpretation. A positive test, i.e., the presence of heat-labile enterotoxin in an unheated filtrate and its absence after heat treatment, is shown by a comparison of the wells containing heated and unheated filtrate. Examine preparations of 20× magnification, using inverted stage phase microscope. Criterion for positive response is presence of 50% or more rounded cells in monolayers subjected to unheated LT-containing filtrate or cholera enterotoxin preparation, and 10% or less rounded cells in monolayer subjected to heated filtrate or to filtrate of LT-negative strain. Because of the possibility of nonspecific interfering substances, confirmation is essential. This step, however, is feasible only in research centers where resources are available. A test for diarrhegenic potential in the rabbit ligated loop is usually performed. A second control for both Y-1 and ligated loop tests is suppression of the rounding phenomenon or fluid secretion by treatment of filtrate with anticholera enterotoxin serum. Confirm identity of LT-producing cultures as *E. coli.*

Infant mouse test for heat-stable toxin (ST)

Equipment. Syringe, disposable, 1 ml tuberculin, with 27-gauge needle.

Media. See Y-1 mouse adrenal cell test for heat-labile toxin (LT) above.

Diagnostic reagents
1. Swiss albino mice
2. Evans blue, 2%

Procedure
1. Preparation of hosts: Mice 1-3 d of age must be used. (Available commercially from suppliers such as Charles River Breeding Laboratories, Wilmington, Mass.)

2. Preparation of bacterial filtrates: See Y-1 mouse adrenal cell test for heat-labile toxin (LT) described above. Add 2 drops of 2% Evans blue to 1 ml sterile CA-YE or TS-YE filtrate.

3. Assay: Inject 0.1 ml filtrate percutaneously through translucent mouse skin into milk-enlarged stomach. Use 4 mice for each filtrate. Include known positive and negative controls. Hold mice 3 h at room temperature in filter paper-lined glass Petri dish. Reject all mice not showing blue dye in stomach or showing dye in peritoneal cavity. Sacrifice mice by adding chloroform to chamber. Open each abdomen and remove intestinal tract with exception of stomach and liver. Pool intestines (treated with same filtrate) in tared weighing vessel. Pool remainder of carcasses in another tared weighing vessel. Weigh both vessels on balance (accurate to 0.01 g). Compute ratio of intestinal weight to remaining body weight.

Interpretation. A ratio of 0.082 or greater is considered positive; a ratio of 0.074 or less is considered negative. Filtrates giving ratios of 0.075-0.082 must be reexamined. At present, no independent confirmatory test is available. LT of *E. coli* and cholera enterotoxin give a negative response in infant mouse system. Confirm identity of ST-producing cultures as *E. coli.*

HeLa cell test for invasive potential

Equipment
1. Culture containers, glass prescription bottles, or plastic tissue culture flasks, sterile, 2 oz (57 ml), 3 oz (85 ml), and 6 oz (171 ml) (Costar, Cambridge, Mass.).
2. Carbon dioxide incubator, 95% air—5% CO_2— moisture-saturated atmosphere, maintained at 35 C (Lab-Line Instruments, Inc., Melrose Park, Ill.).
3. CO_2, compressed.
4. Carbon dioxide gas analytical kit. The Fyrite analyzer is satisfactory (Arthur H. Thomas).
5. Cell-counting chamber, Spencer Bright Line or Fuchs-Rosenthal (Preiser Scientific, Charleston, W.Va.).
6. Tissue culture chamber slides, 4 compartments per slide (Lab-Tek units are satisfactory [Miles laboratories, Inc., Naperville, Ill.]).
7. Petri dishes, sterile, 15 × 150 mm or 20 × 150 mm.
8. Pipets, Pasteur; 25 ml, 0.2 ml serologic.
9. Pipet filler, Pro-pipet Spectroline (Arthur H. Thomas Co., Philadelphia).
10. Refrigerated centrifuge, with adapter, to accommodate 13 × 100 mm tubes and covered centrifuge cups to prevent aerosolization of pathogens.
11. Single-edged razor blade.
12. Coplin staining dishes or trays, 100-250 ml (Fisher Scientific Co.).
13. Glass coverslips, 2.5 × 5.1 cm.
14. Microscopes, standard, 900× magnification; inverted stage, 100× magnification (Preiser Scientific, Charleston, W.Va.); and microscope illuminator.
15. Water bath, maintained at 55 ± 1 C and 35 ± 1 C.

Media[58]*
1. Eagle's minimal essential medium, containing glutamine and Earle's salts (MEME).
2. Fetal bovine serum (FBS), sterile, virus-screened, mycoplasma-free, obtained aseptically during slaughter (Flow Laboratories, Rockville, Md.).

---

*Media and reagents are described in detail at the end of this section, after the Serény test.

3. Antibiotic concentrate (AC).
4. Routine HeLa Mammalian cell growth medium (MEME-FBS-AC). Mix 90 ml MEME, 10 ml FBS (2, above), and 1 ml AC.
5. Antibiotic-free medium for cultivation of HeLa cells before infection (MEME-FBS). Mix 90 ml MEME and 10 ml FBS.
6. Dulbecco's phosphate-buffered saline (DPBS).
7. Calcium- and magnesium-free Dulbecco's phosphate-buffered saline.
8. Calcium- and magnesium-free Hanks' phosphate-buffered saline.
9. Trypsin, 0.25%. Suspend 2.5 g 1:250 trypsin (Difco Laboratories, Detroit) in 100 ml calcium- and magnesium-free Hanks' phosphate-buffered saline and let particles settle. Sterilize by filtration. Dilute 10 ml of this solution in 90 ml sterile calcium- and magnesium-free DPBS to prepare 0.25% trypsin.
10. Earle's balanced salts solution (phenol red-free) (**ES**).
11. Heat-inactivated FBS. Heat FBS (2, above) 2 h at 55 ± 1 C.
12. Brain-heart infusion (for HeLa technic), 1.25% in **ES**. Dissolve 12.5 g brain-heart infusion (powder) in 1 L ES. Sterilize by filtration. Final pH should be 7.2 ± 0.2.
13. Bile salts, no. 3, 1% in **ES**. Dissolve 10 g bile salts no. 3 formulation in 1 L ES. Sterilize by filtration.
14. Infection medium (**IM**). Mix 20 ml heat-inactivated FBS (11, above), 10 ml 1.25% brain-heart infusion (12, above), 10 ml bile salts (13, above), and 60 ml ES.
15. Gentamicin in DPBS, 50 μg/ml. Dissolve 50 mg gentamicin (Schering Corp., Kenilworth, N.J.) in 100 ml DPBS to give solution containing 500 μg/ml. Dilute this solution $1 + 9$ in DPBS to give solution containing 50 μg/ml.
16. Lysozyme solution. Weigh 0.3 g lysozyme ($3\times$ crystalline, salt-free, approximately 18,000 IU/mg) (Schwarz-Mann Division of Becton, Dickinson & Co., Rockville, Md.) into 100 ml DPBS and stir to dissolve. Sterilize by filtration.
17. Intracellular growth phase medium (IGP). Mix 80 ml MEME-FBS (5, above), 10 ml gentamicin in DPBS (15, above), and 10 ml lysozyme solution (16, above).
18. Antibiotics currently used in therapy, available as disks.

Diagnostic reagents and stains[58]
1. Human cervical epithelial cell culture. HeLa culture[58] (American Type Culture Collection, Rockville, Md.). Other cultures, including Henle 407 human intestine and human laryngeal carcinoma, gave comparable data; however, HeLa cell culture was more suitable than the aforementioned cultures with regard to culture characteristics.
2. Methanol.
3. Standard invasive and noninvasive control strains of *E. coli*, based on Serény test. (Available from laboratories actively engaged in research on enteric illness).
4. May-Grunwald stain.
5. Giemsa stain.
6. Decolorizing and dehydrating reagents: acetone-xylene $(50 + 50)$ and $(33 + 67)$; xylene.
7. Mounting medium. Dilute mounting medium with xylene to give easily dispensed colloidal suspension; 20 ml Permount (Fisher Scientific

Co., Fairlawn, N.J.) diluted with 5 ml xylene is satisfactory.
8. Vaseline-paraffin, $50 + 50$, wt/wt. Gently heat to melt and to mix. Apply to slides mounted with coverslip to seal. *Caution:* Mixture is flammable.
9. Immersion oil, nondrying, type B (150 centistokes viscosity).
10. Trypan blue, 0.01%. Dissolve 10 mg stain (Allied Chemical and Dye Corp., New York) in 100 ml 0.85% saline.

Procedure[58,61]
1. Preparation of HeLa cell culture: Using standard cell culture technics, grow host cell on inner surface of 3 oz glass prescription bottles or plastic flasks, using 5 ml MEME-FBS-AC medium, for 7 d at 35 C in CO_2 incubator. Replace with fresh medium on fourth day to prevent accumulation of toxic metabolites. In preparing inoculum for pathogenicity testing, wash monolayer once with 5 ml DPBS prewarmed at 35 C. Add 5 ml prewarmed 0.25% trypsin and hold 2 min at room temperature. Aseptically remove approximately 4.5 ml trypsin. Incubate flask at 35 C with occasional agitation. After monolayer has detached and cells are fairly uniformly distributed in residual trypsin, add 25 ml prewarmed MEME-FBS antibiotic-free medium. Estimate cell density using counting chamber. Add sufficient MEME-FBS to dilute suspension to density of 5×10^5 to 1×10^6 cells/ml. With occasional agitation, rapidly transfer 1 ml aliquots to each compartment of chamber slide. Place chamber slides in large Petri dish or other suitable container. Incubate 20-24 h at 35 C in CO_2 incubator. Before infection, aseptically remove medium from each chamber with Pasteur pipet and wash successively with 1 ml aliquots of prewarmed ES and IM.
2. Preparation of bacteria: With needle, inoculate 5 ml veal infusion broth, using growth from veal infusion agar slant. Incubate broth cultures 18-24 h at 35 C. Centrifuge suspension 20 min at $1200 \times g$ at 18 C. Resuspend cells in 5 ml ES. Recentrifuge 20 min at $1200 \times g$. Resuspend in ES to McFarland density standard 2. Dilute latter suspension 1:10 in prewarmed IM.
3. Infection: Transfer 0.2 ml bacterial suspension in IM to compartment of chamber slide. Use 0.2 ml uninoculated IM for negative control. Simultaneously, examine known invasive and known noninvasive strain of *E. coli*, using identical conditions. Incubate 3 h at 35 C in CO_2 incubator.
4. Intracellular growth stage: Remove contents of chamber slides aseptically, using individual Pasteur pipet for each compartment. Wash each compartment twice with 1 ml aliquots of prewarmed ES. Subsequently, wash each compartment with 1 ml IGP. Add 0.8 ml IGP to each chamber. Incubate 2.5 h at 35 C in CO_2 incubator. Examine for change in color of phenol red indicator from red to yellow, indicating production of acid and extracellular growth of bacteria. If there is no change in color between inoculated chambers and negative control, incubate additional 2.5 h. If change in color has occurred, repeat washing procedure above and reincubate. It is suggested that antibiotic sensitivity pattern of culture be determined before pathogenicity testing for optimal use of antibiotics to curtail extracellular growth.
5. Fixation and staining: Remove contents of chamber slides. Wash monolayers 3 times with 1 ml aliquots of DPBS. Add 1 ml absolute methanol. Hold 5 min at room temperature. Remove methanol and side walls of chamber slide. Insert razor blade between gasket and slide and pry gasket gently from slide. Before beginning

staining, do not allow specimen to dry. If necessary, cautiously remove remnants of gasket from slide with razor blade. Immerse slides 10 min in May-Grunwald dye. Withdraw slides, remove excess stain, and immerse 20 min in Giemsa dye. Withdraw slides, remove excess stain, and immerse 10-20 s in water. Rinse twice briefly in acetone. Immerse slides briefly in following sequence of solvents: (1) acetone-xylene (50 + 50), (2) acetone-xylene (33 + 67), and (3) xylene. Examine slide again for remnants of gasket and remove if present. Add drop of mounting medium to each monolayer. Place coverslip on preparation. Remove excess mounting medium by gently blotting. Allow specimens to harden overnight. If necessary to examine preparation immediately, seal it by application of melted Vaseline-paraffin mixture to edges of coverslip.

Microscopic examination and interpretation of data. Examine specimen with oil immersion objective (900× magnification). The criterion for intracellular location of bacteria is parfocality of cytoplasmic ground substance and bacteria. If invasive, *E. coli* and *Shigella* species will be present in cytoplasm, but not in nucleus. On occasion, intracellular bacteria may be located along nuclear membrane. Intracellular bacteria tend to be more elongated than extracellular bacteria. In general, they appear encapsulated, possibly in remnants of phagolysosome. At least one difference between invasive and noninvasive strains is minimal phagocytosis of the latter. In general, the latter tend to be found in less than 1% of the mammalian cells and the number per cell is less than 5. Invasive strains are phagocytized to a greater extent and their number per cell is greater than 5. Frequently, the host cell may appear as a bag of bacteria. Two or more sites of infection may be observed. Tentatively, the following criterion for invasiveness is offered. At least 0.5% of the HeLa cells should contain at least 5 bacteria. For implementation of this criterion, examine 10 fields, randomly distributed, containing 15-30 mammalian cells. It is suggested that each culture be initially tested twice on different slides. A positive response in both compartments would suggest confirmation by the Sereny test. If both are negative, consider the culture noninvasive. If only 1 compartment is positive, perform a third trial, and on the basis of this reaction submit the culture, if positive, to the Sereny reaction.

Sereny test for confirmation of invasive potential[62]

Equipment
1. Instruments for dissecting animals
2. Animal cages

Media
1. Veal infusion broth
2. Veal infusion agar
3. Dulbecco's phosphate-buffered saline (DPBS)

Diagnostic reagents
1. Guinea pigs (less than 6 mo old)
2. May-Grunwald stain*
3. Giemsa stain*

Procedure
1. Preparation of bacteria: With needle, inoculate 30 ml veal infusion broth, using growth from a veal infusion agar slant. Incubate 18-24 h at 35 C. Centrifuge and wash bacteria as described in HeLa cell test for invasive potential above. After last centrifugation, suspend total growth from 30 ml medium in 0.3 ml DPBS.

---

*Described at end of section, following media and reagents.

2. Performance of test: For each culture, use 3 guinea pigs, 1-6 mo of age. Examine eyes for irritation or infection before use. With Pasteur pipet, transfer drop of bacterial suspension to left eye of each animal. Apply drop of uninoculated DPBS to right eye of each animal. Gently open and close eye to spread fluid evenly over conjunctiva. Return animals to individual cages.

Interpretation of data. Examine animals daily for 5-day period. Positive reaction is development of conjunctivitis, ulceration, and opacity in eye treated with bacteria, but not in control eye. Observation by veterinarian is advisable for differentiation of keratoconjunctivitis from conjunctivitis. Confirmation by (1) demonstration of intracellular location of bacteria in corneal epithelial cells, using May-Grunwald and Giemsa stains, and (2) recovery of same culture from lesion on veal infusion agar is essential because of interference from viruses, fungi, chlamydiae, mycoplasmas, and other bacteria. Invasiveness is determined by positivity in at least 2 of 3 trials.

Media. reagents, and stains for E. coli virulence tests

Antibiotic concentrate (AC)

Penicillin G	500,000 IU
Streptomycin	500,000 μg
Distilled water	100 ml

Dissolve antibiotics in water and sterilize by filtration. Antibiotics are available from Flow Laboratories, Rockville, Md.

Casamino acids–yeast extract–salts (CA-YE) broth (Gorbach)

Casamino acids	20 g
Yeast extract	6 g
NaCl	2.5 g
K_2HPO_4	8.71 g
Trace salts solution (below)	1 ml
Distilled water	1000 ml

Mix ingredients with water. Adjust pH with 0.1N NaOH so that value after autoclaving (15 min at 121 C) is 8.5. This medium is not available commercially.

Trace salts solution

$MgSO_4$	50 g
$MnCl_2$	5 g
$FeCl_2$	5 g
Distilled water	1000 ml

Mix ingredients, adding enough 0.1N N_2SO_4 to dissolve salts.

Earle's salts (phenol red-free)

NaCl	6.8 g
KCl	400 mg
$CaCl_2 \cdot 2H_2O$	265 mg
$MgSO_4 \cdot 7H_2O$	200 mg
$NaH_2PO_4 \cdot H_2O$	140 mg
Glucose	1.0 g
$NaHCO_3$	2.2 g
Distilled water	1000 ml

Dissolve ingredients in water. Sterilize by filtration. Final pH should be 7.2 ± 0.2.

Ham's F-10 medium

L-Alanine	8.91 mg
L-Arginine HCl	211.00 mg
L-Asparagine · H_2O	15.00 mg
L-Aspartic acid	13.30 mg
L-Cysteine HCl	35.12 mg
L-Glutamine	146.20 mg
L-Glutamic acid	14.70 mg
Glycine	7.51 mg
L-Histidine HCl · H_2O	21.00 mg
L-Isoleucine	2.60 mg

L-Leucine	13.10 mg
L-Lysine HCl	29.30 mg
L-Methionine	4.48 mg
L-Phenylalanine	4.96 mg
L-Proline	11.50 mg
L-Serine	10.50 mg
L-Threonine	3.57 mg
L-Tryptophan	0.60 mg
L-Tyrosine	1.81 mg
L-Valine	3.50 mg
Glucose	1100.0 mg
Hypoxanthine	4.08 mg
Lipoic acid	0.2 mg
Phenol red	1.2 mg
Sodium pyruvate	110 mg
Thymidine	0.727 mg
Biotin	0.024 mg
Choline chloride	0.698 mg
Folic acid	1.320 mg
Isoinositol	0.541 mg
Niacinamide	0.615 mg
D-Calcium pantothenate	0.715 mg
Pyridoxine HCl	0.206 mg
Riboflavin	0.376 mg
Thiamine HCl	1.010 mg
Vitamin B_{12}	1.360 mg
$CaCl_2 \cdot 2H_2O$	44.10 mg
$CuSO_4 \cdot 5H_2O$	0.0025 mg
$FeSO_4 \cdot 7H_2O$	0.83 mg
KCl	285.00 mg
KH_2PO_4	83.00 mg
$MgSO_4 \cdot 7H_2O$	152.80 mg
NaCl	7400.00 mg
$NaHCO_3$	1200.00 mg
$Na_2HPO_4 \cdot 7H_2O$	290.00 mg
$ZnSO_4 \cdot 7H_2O$	0.028 mg
Distilled water	1000 ml

Dissolve ingredients in water. Sterilize by filtration. Final pH should be 7.0 ± 0.2. Check sterility before use. Also available commercially.

Minimal essential medium (MEME) (Eagle-type with Earle's salts)

L-Arginine HCl	126.4 mg
L-Cystine	24 mg
L-Glutamine	292 mg
L-Histidine HCl·H_2O	41.9 mg
L-Isoleucine	52.5 mg
L-Leucine	52.4 mg
L-Lysine HCl	73.1 mg
L-Methionine	14.9 mg
L-Phenylalanine	33.0 mg
L-Threonine	47.6 mg
L-Tryptophan	10.2 mg
L-Tyrosine	36.2 mg
L-Valine	46.8 mg
D-Calcium pantothenate	1 mg
Choline chloride	1 mg
Folic acid	1 mg
Isoinositol	2 mg
Nicotinamide	1 mg
Riboflavin	0.1 mg
Thiamine HCl	1 mg
Glucose	1 g
$CaCl_2 \cdot 2H_2O$	265 mg
KCl	400 mg
$MgSO_4 \cdot 7H_2O$	200 mg
NaCl	6.8 g
$NaHCO_3$	2.2 g
$NaH_2PO_4 \cdot H_2O$	140 mg
Phenol red	10 mg
Distilled water	1000 ml

Dissolve ingredients in water. Sterilize by filtration. Final pH should be 7.2 ± 0.2.

Trypticase soy-yeast extract (TS-YE) broth

Trypticase soy broth	30 g
Yeast extract	6 g
Distilled water	1000 ml

Dissolve ingredients in water. Autoclave 15 min at 121 C. This medium is not available commercially.

Dulbecco's phosphate-buffered saline (DPBS)

NaCl	8.0 g
KCl	200 mg
Na_2HPO_4	1.15 g
KH_2PO_4	200 mg
$CaCl_2$	100 mg
$MgCl_2 \cdot 6H_2O$	100 mg
Distilled water	1000 ml

Dissolve ingredients in water. Sterilize by filtration.

Calcium- and magnesium-free Dulbecco's phosphate-buffered saline

NaCl	8.0 g
KCl	200 mg
Na_2HPO_4	1.15 g
KH_2PO_4	200 mg
Distilled water	1000 ml

Dissolve ingredients in water. Sterilize by filtration.

Hanks' phosphate-buffered saline (calcium- and magnesium-free)

NaCl	8.0 g
KCl	400 mg
$Na_2HPO_4 \cdot 7H_2O$	90 mg
KH_2PO_4	60 mg
Glucose	1.0 g
$NaHCO_3$	350 mg
Distilled water	1000 ml

Dissolve ingredients in water. Sterilize by filtration.

Phosphate saline solution (for Y-1 LT assay)

Na_2HPO_4	1.07 g
NaH_2PO_4	0.24 g
NaCl	8.9 g
Distilled water	1000 ml

Dissolve ingredients in water. Adjust pH to 7.5.

Giemsa stain

Giemsa stain (Matheson, Coleman & Bell, Norwood, Ohio)	1 g
Glycerol	66 ml
Methanol (absolute)	66 ml

Dissolve stain in glycerol by heating 1.5-2.0 h at 55-60 C. Add methanol. Store stain in tightly stoppered bottle at 22 C for at least 2 weeks. Dilute stock solution with distilled water (1 + 9) before use.

May-Grunwald stain

May-Grunwald stain (Matheson, Coleman & Bell)	2.5 g
Methanol (absolute)	1000 ml

Weigh stain into 50 ml methanol, dissolve by grinding, and dilute to 1 L with methanol. Stir 16 h at 37 C. Hold stain 1 mo at 22 C (room temperature). Filter before use.

Antigens of E. coli

E. coli organisms possess **O** (somatic), **K** (sheath, envelope, or capsular), and **H** (flagellar) antigens. **Groups** are based on **O** antigens (about 160 groups). In addition, there are some 50 **H** antigens and over 90 different capsular **K** antigens. **Serotypes** are based on **K** and **H** antigens.[63]

The **K** antigens, which inhibit the agglutination of living *E. coli* cultures by **O** antisera, are divisible into 3 varieties, **L, A,** and **B,** based on their physical behavior and properties. The serotypes are designated by the **O** antigen and the **B** variety of **K** antigen (i.e., 0125:B15). **O** antisera will not agglutinate live cells, but these will be readily agglutinated by **OB** sera (prepared by using unheated cells containing **O** and **B** antigens). By heating the cell suspension the **B** antigen can be destroyed and the cells become agglutinable by **O** antisera.

Preparation of antisera*

Generally, smooth (S) colony forms are used. O antigens for antiserum production in rabbits are prepared in a number of ways, depending on the presence of the L, B, or A variety. If L or B are present, 6-8 h old infusion broth cultures are heated at 100 C for 2½ h. the L, B, and H antigens are inactivated by this procedure. If A antigen is present or suspected, smooth, translucent O ("K minus") forms are selected from platings. Broth cultures are heat treated as above.

For K antiserum production, nonmotile strains should be used, plated on blood agar base (Difco). For cultures containing B (K) antigens the organisms are alcohol and acetone extracted, and the resulting dried powder is injected into rabbits. H antisera are prepared using motile cultures, the motility of which is enhanced by passage through semisolid medium. For details refer to Edwards and Ewing[22]; for composition of polyvalent antisera see Ewing.[64]

Enteropathogenic E. coli serotypes, infantile diarrhea, and serotyping

As mentioned earlier ("E. coli—disease in humans"), certain serologic types (**serotypes**) of E. coli were believed for many years to be the cause of diarrhea, and such strains were designated "**enteropathogenic E. coli (EEC)**." In the late 1960s the concept of enteropathogenic E. coli changed slowly until it was discovered that **enterotoxin**-producing strains were most often responsible for E. coli-associated diarrheal disease. Further studies found that serologic identification of the organism and its ability to produce enterotoxin were dissociated, i.e., an organism that typed in 1 of the 16 classic enteropathogenic serotypes may or may not actually produce an enterotoxin. Of the possible thousands of combinations of all the **O, K,** and **V** antigens, probably any one of these E. coli serotypes may be enteropathogenic.

By the late 1970s the controversy[50,65,66] on the merits of serogrouping E. coli isolates from sporadic cases of infant diarrhea has been resolved (apparently temporarily) to the extent that the U.S. Center for Disease Control has urged that serotyping for E. coli should only be done on **isolates from nursery outbreaks.**

In addition, a detailed set of instructions has been published by Farmer and colleagues,[65] pointing out that the "abbreviated" typing done earlier by many laboratories (testing with A, B, or C pools of antisera only) is misleading, useless, and should not be done.

*Antisera are available from various biological houses.

The **4 steps required for serotyping** E. coli **are as follows:**[65]

"**Step 1.** Positive agglutination in pools A or B (or C, if used).

"*Report that can be issued:* NONE.

"*Reason:* Many serotypes of E. coli which are not enteropathogenic serotypes agglutinate in these reagents. Some strains agglutinate in pools, but do not agglutinate in the individual antisera. Other strains agglutinate becaus they have strong cross-reactions with members of the pool. These include O antigen groups 4, 11, 13, 19, 23, 25, 35, 43, 48, 62, 66, 68, 73, 75, 80, 86, 90, 102, 116, and 117, and K antigen groups 18, 21, and 38. If the antisera are made from living or formalin-treated cultures, antibodies to flagella that can cause additional unwanted agglutinations will also be present. Many "nonenteropathogenic serotypes" of E coli found in the human gut have these cross-reacting O and K (and H) antigens and can agglutinate in pools A or B (or C). For this reason steps 2 to 4 must be done.

"**Steps 2 and 3.** *Presumptive* identification of O *and* K antigens based on agglutination of living and heated antigen in the individual typing sera.

"*Report that can be issued:* NONE.

"*Reason:* Many strains (given under reason 1) cross-react with the individual reagents. As cited previously, E. coli O75 (a common gut strain) agglutinates strongly in antiserum O126. Thus, step 4 must be done to avoid reporting these cross-reacting gut strains as "enteropathogenic O-K groups."

"**Step 4.** Titration of O antiserum with the presumptive strain.

"This titration will tell if the strain is an "enteropathogenic O group" or a serologically related O group that has not been associated with disease. This step is *essential*, but, unfortunately, most laboratories omit it.

"When all four of these steps have been done and the O and K antigens are known, a report can be issued. This report should warn the physician about "false-positive" strains.

"*Typical report:* This specimen contains E. coli O126:K71 (K71 was formerly called B16). This O-K group has been associated with nursery outbreaks of diarrhea. This particular strain may or may not be the cause of diarrhea."[65]

They also urge that **reports of "no enteropathogenic E. coli isolated"** be discontinued. When a stool specimen does not yield one of the O-K (H) groups of E. coli associated with infantile diarrhea, a more conservative report is required.

"*Typical report:* This specimen was negative for the following O-K serogroups of E. coli: O26:K60, O55:K59, O111:K58, etc. The absence of the above groups does **not** rule out E. coli as the causative agent of this patient's diarrhea."

Gangarosa and Merson[50] also stated that **routine** serogrouping of E. coli in **sporadic** cases of diarrhea using commercial antiserums currently

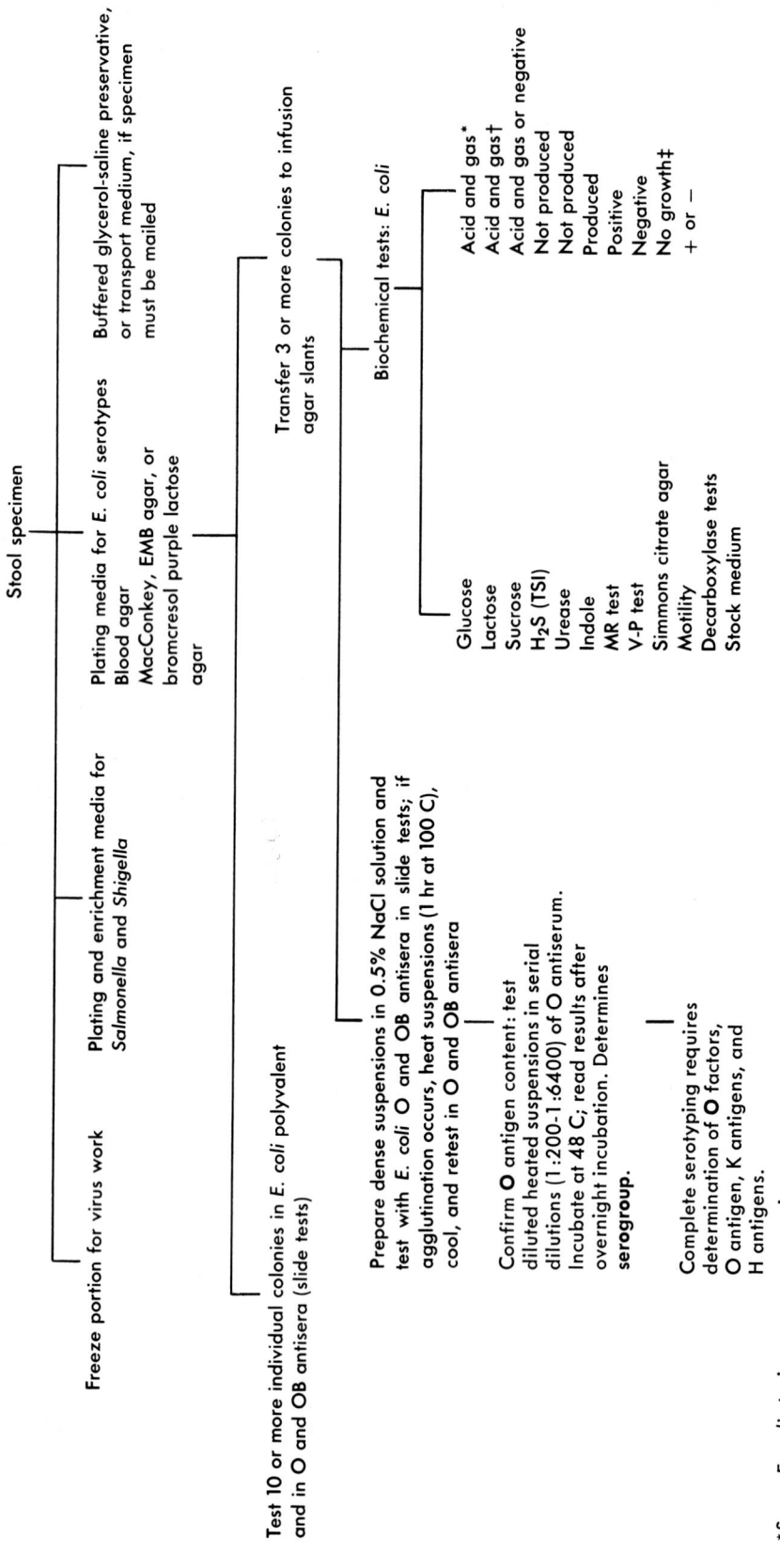

Fig. 79-2. Outline of methods for examination of stool specimens in cases of infantile diarrhea. (Data from Edwards, P. R., and Ewing, W. H.: Identification of *Enterobacteriaceae*, Minneapolis, 1955 [ed. 1] and 1962 [ed. 2], Burgess Publishing Co.; and Ewing, W. H.: Public Health Lab. **27**:19, 1969.)

Stool specimen

Freeze portion for virus work

Plating and enrichment media for *Salmonella* and *Shigella*

Plating media for *E. coli* serotypes
Blood agar
MacConkey, EMB agar, or bromcresol purple lactose agar

Buffered glycerol-saline preservative, or transport medium, if specimen must be mailed

Test 10 or more individual colonies in *E. coli* polyvalent and in O and OB antisera (slide tests)

Prepare dense suspensions in 0.5% NaCl solution and test with *E. coli* O and OB antisera in slide tests; if agglutination occurs, heat suspensions (1 hr at 100 C), cool, and retest in O and OB antisera

Confirm **O** antigen content: test diluted heated suspensions in serial dilutions (1:200-1:6400) of O antiserum. Incubate at 48 C; read results after overnight incubation. Determines **serogroup.**

Complete serotyping requires determination of **O** factors, **O** antigen, **K** antigens, and **H** antigens.

Transfer 3 or more colonies to infusion agar slants

Biochemical tests: *E. coli*

Glucose	Acid and gas*
Lactose	Acid and gas†
Sucrose	Acid and gas or negative
H₂S (TSI)	Not produced
Urease	Not produced
Indole	Produced
MR test	Positive
V-P test	Negative
Simmons citrate agar	No growth‡
Motility	+ or −
Decarboxylase tests	
Stock medium	

*Some *E. coli* strains are anaerogenic.
†Certain *E. coli* strains may require more than 24 h to produce acid from lactose.
‡Occasional strains, otherwise typical, may grow on citrate agar; usually such reactions delayed.

available in the United States is for practical purposes useless. Maybe replacement of the current antisera with newer pools of antisera prepared against selected enteropathogenic, enterotoxigenic, and enteroinvasive strains may be useful for routine laboratory identification of *E. coli.*[50]

The most commonly occurring serotypes previously reported as being involved in "enteropathogenic" *E. coli* diarrhea are as follows:

O26:B6	O112:B11	O126:B16
O44:K74(L)	O119:B14	O127:B8
O55:B5	O124:B17	O128:B12
O86:B7	O125:B15	O136:B22
O111:B4		

An **outline** of methods for examination of stool specimens in cases of infantile diarrhea are outlined in Fig. 79-2. For details, see Edwards and Ewing.[20]

Fluorescent antibody technic in diagnosis of enteropathogenic E. coli serotypes

See Chapter 70.

Antibody response in E. coli infections

See discussion of indirect bacterial hemagglutination, Chapter 108.

EDWARDSIELLA

In 1959 Ewing and associates at the U.S. Communicable Disease Center recognized a group of indole- and hydrogen sulfide-positive, mannitol-negative, gram-negative rods, mostly isolated from humans, as a previously undescribed entity, which they labeled "biotype 1483-59."[67] Sakazaki and Murata (1962)[68] isolated a large number of similar strains from snakes in Japan and proposed the vernacular term "Asakusa group" for these organisms. King and Adler (1964)[69] recovered a previously undescribed strain from an acute case of human gastroenteritis, which they labeled "Bartholomew group."

Ewing et al. in 1965[67] proposed the species name *E. tarda* (tribe Edwardsielleae, genus *Edwardsiella*) for these organisms, after finding that the "Asakusa," "Bartholomew," and "biotype 1483-59" strains were all similar and quite unlike the other genera of Enterobacteriaceae.

Ewing's isolates[70] are mostly of human origin (feces, with or without history of diarrhea, wounds, blood, urine), with a smaller number isolated from warm- and cold-blooded animals and water, whereas Sakazaki's isolates,[71] recovered in Japan, are overwhelming from snakes. In addition to humans and snakes, the organism has also been recovered from cows, alligators, and a sea lion.[72]

Sonnenwirth and Kallus[73,74] reported the first case of meningitis due to *E. tarda,* which proved fatal to a 31-year-old woman who suffered from systemic lupus erythematosus and was on prolonged steroid therapy. The organism was cultured before death from cerebrospinal fluid and after death from brain swabs and heart blood; the second case of (neonatal) meningitis was reported shortly thereafter from Nigeria.[75]

The role of *E. tarda* as a primary etiologic agent (pathogen) remains somewhat uncertain. However, there appears to be little doubt that under certain circumstances (as described above) *E. tarda* may cause severe and occasionally fatal disease. It is believed that more instances of human infections may be uncovered as clinical laboratories become more familiar with this genus and species. In fact, Jordan and Hadley in 1969[76] reported 1 case of liver abscess and septicemia, 3 cases of diarrhea, 3 wound infections, and 1 perirectal abscess, caused by *E. tarda,* and stated that the organism is capable of producing disease patterns similar to those caused by salmonellae.

Definition and identification

E. tarda is a motile, gram-negative rod. H_2S is produced, the indole and methyl red tests are positive. It is Voges-Proskauer, urease, phenylalanine deaminase, and gelatin negative. No growth occurs on Simmons citrate, on sodium acetate medium, or in KCN-containing medium. Ornithine and lysine are decarboxylated. **Glucose** and **maltose** are fermented promptly with gas formation; a very large number of other carbohydrates, including lactose, are not fermented (see Table 79-14 and 79-21). Hence the application of the specific epithet *tarda* (Latin, meaning "slow"), implying inactivity, is fitting. It conforms to the definition of Enterobacteriaceae in that it reduces nitrate, is oxidase negative, and utilizes glucose fermentatively.

The organism grows well on ordinary media, including MacConkey and SS agar, but not on cetrimide agar. According to Sakazaki,[77] it grows on brilliant green and bismuth sulfite agar.

E. tarda gives an IMViC pattern similar to *E. coli:* however, it produces abundant H_2S.

It can be readily differentiated from *E. coli* by additional criteria: *E. coli* ferments mannitol, sorbitol, trehalose, and xylose (about 90% of strains) and is positive in regard to mucate, Jordan's tartrate, and sodium acetate, whereas *E. tarda* is negative in all of the above listed tests.

It is similar to *Salmonella* in regard to H_2S production, ornithine and lysine decarboxylation, and failure to ferment lactose, sucrose, salicin, and adonitol. However, it produces indole and does not ferment mannitol (which is fermented by *E. coli, Salmonella, Citrobacter,* and *Arizona*). See Table 79-21 for a summary of biochemical reactions.

The organism recovered by Sonnenwirth and Kallus[73] was sensitive to chloramphenicol, tetracycline, colistin, ampicillin, and kanamycin. Of the 3 isolates tested by Jordan and Hadley,[76] all

Table 79-21. Differentiation of *Escherichia* and *Edwardsiella**†

Test or substrate	Escherichia			Edwardsiella		
	Sign	*%+*	*(%+)‡*	*Sign*	*%+*	*(%+)‡*
Hydrogen sulfide (TSI)	−	0§		+	99.6	(0.2)
Arginine dihydrolase	d	16.3	(39.1)	−	0	(0.2)
Ornithine decarboxylase	d	57.8	(8)	+	99	(0.2)
Lactose	+	91.6	(4.2)	−	0	
Sucrose	d	53.7	(5.5)	−	0.2	
Mannitol	+	97.5		−	0	
Dulcitol	d	49.3	(18)	−	0	
Salicin	d	36	(12.3)	−	0	(0.2)
Sorbitol	d	80.3	(1)	−	0.2	
Arabinose	+	99.3	(0.5)	d	10.7	(0.2)
Raffinose	d	49.4	(2.1)	−	0	
Rhamnose	d	83.5	(3.4)	−	0	
Xylose	d	82.8	(6.6)	−	0	
Trehalose	+	98.2	(1.8)	−	0.3	
Esculin	d	30.9	(19.7)	−	0	
Mucate	+	91.6		−	0	
Jordan's tartrate	+	97.6		−	0	
Sodium acetate	+ or (+)	83.8	(9.7)	−	0	

*From Ewing, W. H.: Differentiation of *Enterobacteriaceae* by biochemical reactions, Atlanta, 1973 (rev.), Center for Disease Control.

†+, 90% or more positive within 1 or 2 d; (+), positive reaction after 3 or more (decarboxylase tests: 3 or 4 d); −, no reaction (90% or more); + or −, most cultures positive, some strains negative; − or +, most strains negative, some cultures positive; + or (+), most reactions occur within 1 or 2 d, some are delayed; d, different reactions—+, (+), −; w, weakly positive reaction.

‡Figures in parentheses indicate percentages of reactions delayed 3 or more d.

§Some strains produce hydrogen sulfide, but an exact percentage cannot be calculated at present (see text).

were sensitive to chloramphenicol, tetracycline, and kanamycin, 2 were sensitive to ampicillin, but all were resistant to colistin.

Antigenic structure

At least 49 **O** (somatic) and 37 **H** (flagellar) antigens of *E. tarda* have been characterized.

SALMONELLEAE
Salmonella-Arizona-Citrobacter

The 3 genera in this major tribe (see Table 79-8, Ewing's taxonomy) include *Arizona* (formerly *Paracolobactrum arizonae*) and *Citrobacter*, formerly *Escherichia freundii*, with the Bethesda-Ballerup group of organisms.

According to *Bergey's Manual*, ed. 8,[3] the genus *Salmonella* includes the subgenus *S. arizonae*, and *Citrobacter* is a genus; both belong in the tribe *Escherichieae*.

Differentiation of the tribe is based on the biochemical reactions listed in Table 79-10. **Typical** cultures are indole, Voges-Proskauer, urease, and phenylalanine negative. The methyl red test is usually positive, citrate is utilized (Simmons citrate) with few exceptions, and H$_2$S is usually produced. Growth in KCN is variable.

The genera within the tribe are differentiated on the basis of reactions listed in Table 79-22. These include prompt **fermentation of lactose** by the majority of *Citrobacter* strains and usually, but not always, delayed fermentation by *Arizona* organisms, but not by salmonellae; about 1% *of Salmonella* strains ferment lactose in 1-2 days.

Laboratories relying solely on MacConkey agar

and deoxycholate citrate agar for *Salmonella* isolation will not recognize lactose-fermenting salmonellae, and the use of **bismuth sulfite agar is recommended.**

Sucrose is not fermented by salmonellae and arizonae.

The tests considered most useful in the differentiation of *Salmonella* and *Arizona*[78] are indicated in Table 79-22. Martin et al.[79] list lactose, β-galactosidase, dulcitol, malonate, and Jordan tartrate for differentiation of *Salmonella* and *Arizona;* for the differentiation of *Salmonella* and *Citrobacter* the primary tests recommended are KCN and lysine.

Salmonellae and most *Arizona* fail to grow in KCN broth, whereas *Citrobacter* strains grow. Both salmonellae and *Arizona* are lysine positive, whereas *Citrobacter* is negative. *Arizona* and some *Citrobacter* strains are positive in malonate; *Arizona* strains slowly liquefy gelatin. *Salmonella* and *Citrobacter* produce acid in Jordan's tartrate medium. Most but not all organisms in this tribe are **motile**. For identification of organisms in this division refer to Tables 79-14 and 79-22, and to the detailed descriptions of the genera.

On differential media, *Salmonella,* most but not all *Arizona*, and some slow lactose-fermenting *Citrobacter* strains show colorless colonies. Typical *Citrobacter* strains show lactose-fermenting colonies. *Salmonella* and *Arizona* strains grow well on the highly inhibitory media. For TSI and LIA reactions refer to Tables 79-11 and 79-12.

Salmonellae are closely related antigenically

Table 79-22. Differentiation of genera within tribe *Salmonelleae**†

Test or substrate	Salmonella			Arizona			Citrobacter‡		
	Sign	%+	(%+)	Sign	%+	(z+)	Sign	%+	(%+)
Urease	−	0		−	0		d§	70.8	(7.5)
Indole	−	1.1		−	5.1		− or +	21.9	
KCN‖	−	0.3		−	5.7		+ or −	80.6	
Gelatin (Kohn's)	−	0	(1.1)	+ or (+)	12.1	(84.8)	−	0	(1)
Lysine decarboxylase‖	+	94.6¶		+	99.4	(0.3)	−	0	
Ornithine decarboxylase	+	92.7¶		+	100		d	30.7	(0.1)
Lactose	−	0.8#		d**	69.8	(15.6)	d	38.3	(50.9)
Sucrose	−	0.5		−	2.9		d	15.5	(7.9)
Dulcitol††‡‡	d‡‡	86.5	(2.7)	−‡‡	0		d‡‡	58.7	(0.6)
Adonitol	−	0		−	0		− or +	16.3	
Inositol††	d	34.5	(0.8)	−	0		−	2.7	(1.6)
Cellobiose	d	6.5	(76.4)	d	0.5	(69.4)	+ or (+)	66.3	(32.2)
Malonate††	−	0.5		+	94.6		− or +	32.7	
Jordan's tartrate††	+ or −	84.6		−	6		+ or −	83.6	
Beta galactosidase††	−	2.1		+	97.8*d*		+	>90	
Organic acid media									
Citrate	+ or (+)	87	(4.6)	+ or (+)	76.6	(21.3)	(+) or +	49.2	(49.5)
D-tartrate	+ or (+)	84.3	(5.7)	(+) or −	0	(80.3)	(+)	0	(90.9)

*Modified from Ewing, W. H.: Differentiation of *Enterobacteriaceae* by biochemical reactions (rev.), Atlanta, 1973, Center for Disease Control.

†+, 90% or more positive within 1-2 d; (+), positive reactions after 3 or more d (decarboxylase tests: 3-4 d); −, no reaction (90% or more); + or −, most cultures positive, some strains negative; − or +, most strains negative, some cultures positive; + or (+), most reactions occur within 1-2 d, some are delayed; d, different reactions—+, (+), −; w, weakly positive reaction.

‡See "Center for Disease Control Changes, *Citrobacter*"; also Table 79-10.

§Approximately 70% of strains yield positive urease reaction in 1 d.

‖Primary tests for differentiation of *Salmonella* and *Citrobacter*.

¶*S. paratyphi* A is lysine negative; *S. typhi* is ornithine negative.

#Close to 1% of strains ferment lactose in 1-2 d.

**About 70% of strains ferment lactose in 1-2 d; an additional 15% ferment in 3 or more d.

††These tests and substrates are of particular value in differentiation of *Salmonella* and *Arizona*.

‡‡Majority of salmonellae ferment dulcitol promptly, but *S. typhi*, *S. cholerae-suis*, and *S. enteritidis* bioserotypes paratyphi A and pullorum do not. Members of genus *Arizona* are uniformly negative on this substrate.

and have characteristic O and H antigens, and serologic methods (known antisera) must be used for their final identification. There is considerable antigenic overlap between *Salmonella* and *Arizona*. Nevertheless, the commercially available *Salmonella* antisera usually do not agglutinate most *Arizona* strains. When an organism is not agglutinated by *Salmonella* antisera but cannot be excluded from the genus on biochemical grounds, the culture should be submitted to state or federal laboratories that are equipped to perform serologic identification of *Arizona* strains.

Salmonellae and arizonae are major enteric pathogens. Certain *Citrobacter* strains have been associated with cases of enteritis but are not considered true intestinal pathogens. Members of all 3 groups are capable of causing infections in various organs of the body and have been recovered from bacteremias, meningitis, and other serious infections.

SALMONELLA

The salmonellae are among the most widely distributed pathogenic bacteria in nature. They are encountered most commonly in poultry (at least in the United States), also in rodents and livestock, domestic animals, wild animals, arthropods, birds, and reptiles. The usual habitat of the genus is the gastrointestinal tract of animal and human hosts. Salmonellae of animal origin can produce essentially the same clinical diseases in humans as those of human origin; the same serotypes can occur in infections of both humans and animals. Persons contracting *Salmonella* infections react in different fashions, depending on several factors, among which the age and the general health of the patients are, and, to a lesser extent, the strain of the organism are most important. Thus septic infections and meningitis are more frequent in infants and in young animals, due to the lesser resistance of this age group. Similarly, higher mortality is observed in elderly persons, mainly among those suffering from other diseases or confined to institutions.

Within the genus *Salmonella* there exist types that are host-adapted either to humans or to certain lower species and, with some exceptions, these forms occur only in some specific hosts (such as *S. typhi*, *S. paratyphi* A and C, and *S. sendai*, more or less strictly adapted to humans).[80] A few others, e.g., *S. pullorum*, *S. gallinarum*, *S. cholerae-suis*, *S. typhisuis*, and some others are adapted to particular nonhuman hosts but occur in humans also. The far larger number of types, now more than 1500 in number, however, exhibit no host specificity and on occasion might produce disease in any warm-blooded animal.

The ubiquitousness of *Salmonella* poses a major public health problem in the United States and other countries. The literature is replete with *Salmonella* outbreaks traced to foodborne routes (powdered milk, cream cakes, a large variety of meat products, fresh eggs, powdered eggs, coconut meat, whitefish) and contact with pet turtles, dogs, ducks, baby chicks, garden fertilizers containing bone meal, etc. Hospital-acquired epidemics were traced in 1966 to the use of carmine dye capsules used in patients as a fecal dye marker. The dye, manufactured from dried and ground female scale insects and larvae indigenous to Central America, was found to contain *S. cubana*. It is also well documented that feeds for domestic animals very often are contaminated with salmonellae.

Nomenclature

Originally salmonellae were named according to the disease they caused (*S. typhisuis, S. enteritidis,* etc.; the so-called classical species) or after the animals from which they were first isolated. By 1934 the White-Kauffmann terminology was adopted rather generally; this accords specific rank to each antigenically distinguishable *Salmonella* type and each new type ("species") was named after the geographic place at which it was first isolated. By 1978 close to 2000 types had been listed in this schema.

This situation has brought about numerous proposals, ranging from Kauffmann's division of the Salmonella group into 2 subgenera (the third being the *Arizona* group) and subdivided serologically into species, designated **either** by names **or** by antigenic formula (Kauffmann[81] preservation of the "serotype" ("species") designation (subcommittee, 1963[82]), and division of the genus into 3 species (Ewing and Ball,[83]): *S. choleraesuis, S. typhi,* and *S. enteritidis.* The last includes **all** serotypes of salmonellae other than the preceding 2 species. Accordingly, United States usage now recognizes only 3 species (*S. choleraesuis, S. typhi,* and *S. enteriditis*): the first two do not contain subtypes (serotypes), but *S. enteriditis* contains over 1500 serotypes, each written in a nonitalicized form (e.g., *S. enteriditis* serotype paratyphi A, instead of *S. paratyphi* A). In this section both classical names and serotypes ("species") will be employed.

Infections in humans

Salmonellae live in the tissues of reptiles, birds, mammals, and humans; these are the sources of all *Salmonella* infections. Infection is caused by ingestion of food, water, or milk contaminated with the organisms or consumption of animal tissues containing salmonellae (such as uncooked meat, but also processed sausage, eggs, powdered egg, dressed poultry, etc.). Contamination can occur by excreta of humans or animals, by flies carrying excreta or organisms, or by accidental contamination of water systems with sewage or of a well by seepage of surface water.

Oysters and shellfish can cause salmonellosis when taken from waters polluted with sewage.

Important in the spread of infection are the convalescent carriers, who may excrete the organisms for 1-4 months after recovery, and the subclinical, unrecognized cases. Chronic carriers, mainly those of *S. typhi,* are a public health menace and are the main problem in the eradication of typhoid fever.

The clinical manifestations of salmonellosis have been divided into (1) **gastroenteritis,** (2) **bacteremia** or **septicemia** with or without focal (extraintestinal) lesions, (3) **enteric fever,** the classical example of which is typhoid fever, and (4) the **carrier** state. It is important to remember that practically every *Salmonella* strain can produce any of the 4 types of clinical infection, with certain types tending to cause a particular type of clinical manifestation more often than others; also, in some instances a single patient may experience progression from gastroenteritis to enteric fever and possibly to the septicemic form, all due to the same ogranism.

The reader's attention is called to the excellent reviews on salmonellae and salmonellosis, with emphasis on epidemiologic problems and animal sources of *Salmonella,* by Edwards[85] and Bowmer,[86] and the comprehensive volume, *An Evaluation of the Salmonella Problem.*[80] Certain unusual, but increasingly encountered manifestations of salmonellosis were reviewed by Black et al.[87] who describe osteomyelitis, aneurysms, meningitis, and postgastrectomy enteritis due to salmonellae, as well as salmonellosis following surgery and the use of cortisone. For bone and joint *Salmonella* infections, see Ortiz-Neu et al.[88]; infections by salmonellae occurring in the nursery and the hospital are described by Edwards[85] and Williams et al.[89] For salmonellosis in children see Deutch and Sonnenwirth.[90]

The rise in incidence of salmonellosis (excluding typhoid fever) in the United States is reflected by the increase in reported cases from 723 in 1946 to 23,500 in 1975. In contrast, the incidence of typhoid fever in the United States has been declining steadily (from 5590 cases in 1942 to less than 500 in 1967). It is generally accepted that the **reported** number of cases represents only a small fraction of the total cases. Precise diagnosis is possible only when cultures are performed.

For a discussion of the growing problem of salmonellosis in modern society, the reader is referred to Bauer's[84] review.

Gastroenteritis

With symptoms ranging from mild diarrhea to a fulminent form with sudden and violent onset ("food poisoning"), gastroenteritis is the most common clinical manifestation of *Salmonella* infection.

Nausea, vomiting, and diarrhea are common manifestations, followed by fever and prostration lasting 1-4 d. Blood cultures are usually negative, but the organisms can be found in the **stool.** Gastroenteritis is due to consumption of contaminated food, most likely with large numbers of organisms being ingested.

Septicemias

The septicemic type of *Salmonella* infection is characterized by high fever, showing a spiked curve, positive blood cultures, and early focal manifestations. These localizing infections may occur in practically any part of the body, producing abscesses in the pelvic and perineal regions, spleen, and lung, and can cause osteomyelitis, pneumonia, meningitis, peritonitis, endocarditis, etc. *S. cholerae-suis* occupies a special place among the organisms involved in septicemic infections, being apparently extremely invasive.

Typhoid fever and other enteric fevers

Typhoid fever, caused by *S. typhi*, is the classic example of enteric fevers. It is characterized by the stepwise, steady rise of temperature, reaching 104 F, and the appearance of rose spots (rash) and various central nervous system disturbances. Constipation is common in the first week, with accompanying abdominal tenderness. Diarrhea is not a frequent finding in the early stages of the disease, but later the abdominal symptoms may become severe. Intestinal hemorrhage is a frequent occurrence in typhoid fever; intestinal perforation occurs in a small number of cases. Leukopenia and anemia are commonly observed. Respiratory tract involvement may range from mild cough and bronchitis to pneumonia and lung abscess. The fever begins to subside usually after the third week.

Bacteremia occurs in the first 7-10 d, and **blood cultures** are often positive during this period. **Stool cultures** are rarely positive in the first few days of typhoid fever but are positive after the first week, and the organism can often be isolated until convalescence is completed. **Urine cultures** are positive in 25-30% of the cases, beginning after the first 7-10 d of the disease. *S. typhi* has been isolated from bone marrow and spleen, and the gallbladder is invariably infected. Rarely, it has been isolated from the spinal fluid in patients with signs of meningitis.

Enteric fevers caused by salmonellae other than *S. typhi* are usually milder and show few, if any, characteristic symptoms. They usually present fever and general malaise, lasting 1-3 wks. **Blood cultures** are often positive early in the disease; **stool cultures** may be negative in the first week, usually becoming positive afterward.

The carrier state

The carrier state is most often seen with *S. typhi*. About 3% of the patients continue to excrete the organisms for over a year after recovery from typhoid fever (chronic carriers); some continue to do so for many years. *S. paratyphi* B carriers usually excrete the organisms for a much shorter period. In permanent *Salmonella* carriers the organisms usually multiply in the gallbladder. The temporary or chronic typhoid carrier and the convalescent and temporary carrier of other salmonellae present a serious public health problem (food handlers contaminating food, etc.); together with the animal reservoirs of infection, they constitute the 2 principal aspects of *Salmonella* epidemiology.

Antigenic structure

In 1903 Smith and Reagh reported on differences they found in the behavior of the flagellar and somatic antigens of salmonellae, but their work was not appreciated. It was not until

White[91] and Kauffmann[92] studied the antigenic structure of *Salmonella* in great detail that the characteristics of the group became known.

The **Kauffmann-White schema** contains the antigenic classification of the *Salmonella*. The schema is being constantly enlarged as new serotypes are found.

Salmonellae are divided into **groups** on the basis of their major **O** (somatic) antigens. The groups are denoted by the use of capital Roman letters (A, B, C, etc.) and are subdivided (**serotypes**) on the basis of differences in the **H** (flagellar) antigens. The **O** antigens are denoted by Arabic numerals and the **H** antigens by small Roman letters (phase 1) and Arabic numerals (phase 2). All members of the genus possess antigens that fit into the Kauffmann-White schema.

Antigenic variation

In order to elucidate the serologic structure of these organisms it must be taken into consideration that salmonellae show different types of variation that affect their antigenic structure. The following is a brief review of these variations.

H-O variation. The designations "H" and "O" originate from the observation of the spreading (H) and nonspreading (O) colonies of *Proteus*. Subsequently these observations led to the study of the somatic and flagellar antigens of these and other organisms. It was established that O antigens are complex lipopolysaccharide somatic antigens, resistant to heat and alcohol and giving a granular agglutination that develops best when the mixture of antiserum-antigen is incubated at higher, e.g., 50-56 C, temperature for several hours. The H antigens are (protein) flagellar antigens and thus are present only in mobile organisms; they are resistant to formol but not to heat or alcohol and give fluffy clumps in the agglutination test that takes place at lower temperatures, e.g., 37 C, and develops rapidly, usually within 2 h.

Thus motile organisms contain 2 types of antigens (O and H), each of which stimulates its own antibody, with which it reacts exclusively. The nonmotile organisms contain only the somatic (O) antigens. Loss of H antigen (change from flagellated HO form to O form) is rare.

Phase variation. The H antigens are flagellar antigens and therefore are present only in motile cultures. When strains of motil *Salmonella* are plated, 2 types of colonies are observed in most cases. One group of colonies possesses antigens originally considered specific for the type, whereas the other group of colonies shows antigens that are common to many *Salmonella* and were therefore considered nonspecific. Thus the antigens characterizing the "phases" were called "specific" and "nonspecific," antigens of the first group being designated by small Latin letters and those of the second by Arabic numerals.

When the specific H antigens became so numerous that all the letters of the alphabet

Table 79-23. Antigenic formulas of some more common salmonellae (Kauffmann-White schema)

Group	Type	Somatic (O) antigen	Flagellar (H) antigen Phase 1	Phase 2
A	S. paratyphi A	1, **2**, 12	a	−
B	S. paratyphi B	1, **4**, 5, 12	b	1, 2
	S. typhimurium	1, **4**, 5, 12	i	1, 2
	S. abortus bovis	1, **4**, 12, 27	b	e, n, x
	S. san diego	**4**, 5, 12	e, h	e, n, z_{15}
C	S. paratyphi C	**6**, 7, Vi	c	1, 5
	S. montevideo	**6**, 7	g, m, s	−
	S. cholerae-suis	**6**, 7	c	1, 5
D	S. typhi	**9**, 12, Vi	d	−
	S. enteritidis	1, **9**, 12	g, m	−
E	S. anatum	**3**, 10	e, h	1, 6

*All serotypes (species in a particular group possess a number of O antigens and all have at least 1 O antigen (determinant) in common within the group. The boldface number indicates the major O antigen of the group.

had been employed, later investigators found it necessary to designate newly discovered antigens by using index numbers attached to the letter "z"—"z_1," "z_2," etc.

It has become an established custom to call the "specific" phase the "first" phase and the "nonspecific" the "second" phase. Kauffmann and Mitsui proved that certain antigens present in the first phase may also occur in the second phase. They introduced the terminology "alpha" and "beta" phases; the antigens in phase 2 are not related to the nonspecific phase 2 antigens and are peculiar to themselves. The beta phases are denoted by small Roman letters even though they represent phase 2 antigens. This is because the beta phases (e, n) are antigenically related to certain antigens in phase 1 (e, h). The e, n phases are now known to be subject to phase variation. An example of the use of symbols is shown in Table 79-23.

Not all salmonellae are diphasic. Some are monophasic, and in these every colony contains identical H antigens. The monophasic state is characteristic of practically all recognized types containing antigen **g** or **m**. Certain other types are also monophasic. Occasionally 1 of the phases may be weak, and it is necessary to enhance it by using cultural and serologic aids.

Edwards and Bruner recommend the addition of agglutinating serum to semisolid agar, thereby suppressing 1 phase and permitting the spread of organisms containing the other phase. Hajna described a simple modification of this technic. He uses U-shaped culture tubes that are filled with a mixture of Edwards-Bruner semisolid agar with the addition of a small amoung of agglutinating serum of the phase to be suppressed. The medium is inoculated with the culture by barely penetrating the surface of the agar in one branch of the tube. The phase that was not suppressed by the serum may be isolated from the growth in the uninoculated branch of the U tube after incubation.

S-R variation. When this phenomenon was first described, it applied to the colony form and to the stability of the growth in broth cultures. As the original smooth (S) growth on solid media becomes rough (R), the colonies appear to have a rough surface and irregular borders, and the broth cultures form a granular sediment. Slight grades of roughness may be discovered according to the method of Pampana by mixing a drop of a heavy suspension of the organism with a drop of 1:500 acriflavine or Trypaflavine. When the culture is rough, agglutination occurs.

The R form differs from the S form not only in colony morphology but also in its loss of other characteristics, including specific O and Vi agglutinability, ability to absorb and to produce antibodies, toxicity for mice, biochemical activity, and other properties. In practical laboratory work the greatest difficulties are encountered while "typing" strains that do not as yet reveal morphologic roughness but have become serologically rough. Such organisms are frequently encountered among colonies fished from strongly selective media or among strains that have been maintained for a considerable period of time on carbohydrate media before antigenic analysis. A certain number of these strains can be serologically evaluated by using the technic of White, which consists of suspending the growth from the surface of an agar slant in absolute alcohol, heating this mixture for 1 hour at 60 C, and then draining and resuspending it in saline.

The R cultures contain a nonspecific somatic antigen(s) that seems to be common to all salmonellae. Thus roughness of the culture renders it serologically nonspecific. Rough cultures are often isolated from chronic carriers.

V-W variation. The **Vi antigen** was originally discovered in inagglutinable cultures of S. typhi and was thought to be connected with virulence. It also is found in several other salmonellae. It is a surface antigen and is less resistant to heat than are other somatic antigens. It may be preserved by dehydration at a temperature of 60-70 C when its suspension in absolute alcohol is treated *in vacuo*. Colonies of organisms containing Vi antigen are slightly more opaque than the W colonies and have a ground-glass appearance in reflected light. The loss of the Vi antigen is connected with the colony change from V to W form. Although V colonies are susceptible to phage action, W colonies are not. The phage susceptibility of V forms is utilized in the typing of S. typhi strains. Whereas the susceptibility to phage action decreases during the V-W variation, the susceptibility of the strain to phagocytosis increases. An organism gradually losing its Vi antigen first shows a decrease in its ability to absorb Vi antibodies from anti-Vi sera; then a tendency toward reduction in agglutinability with Vi antiserum is demonstrable. Finally the strain shows the typical O structure of the organism.

The serologic properties of Vi antigen and its O agglutination inhibitory power are lost gradually in saline suspension. This change is accelerated in phenolized saline: A Vi culture of S. typhi suspended in phenolized saline ceases to agglutinate in Vi serum and becomes agglutinable in O serum after standing a few hours at room temperature. Therefore a culture suspected of being S. typhi should be suspended in physiologic saline solution and examined immediately by slide agglutination.[93]

Form variation. Certain minor O antigens overlap in the genus; they occur in more than 1 of the O groups (A, B, C, etc.). Certain colonies contain more antigen **12** than others from the same strain. Antigens **6** and **1** are also involved. This is a quantitative difference that is important in the preparation of antisera.

• • •

For a detailed review of the nature and immunochemistry of the O and R antigens of Salmonella and related Enterobacteriaceae, the reader is referred to Lüderitz et al.[94]

Antigenic analysis

The antigenic properties and their variations are utilized in the serodiagnosis of salmonellae. In this section a brief description is given of the principles utilized and of the methods used for preparation of antisera. The methods outlined here are based on those described by Edwards and Ewing.[22, 93] A simplified procedure for serologic identification is described later.

The first step in determining the antigenic structure of salmonellae is the identification of the O antigens. This is accomplished by using pure **O antisera.** To prepare **O** antisera the H antigens must be inactivated. Broth cultures of the organisms are boiled in a water bath 2 h. They may be preserved with 0.3% formalin. Rabbits are given 4 injections at 4 d intervals with the boiled suspension (0.5, 1, 2, and 3 ml). They are bled on the sixth day after the last injection. The serum is preserved with the addition of an equal volume of glycerol.

In a different method (Roschka) the organisms are cultivated on the surface of nutrient agar slants 24 h; then the growth is washed off with saline and kept in the boiling water bath 2 h to destroy H antigens. The

suspension is centrifuged and the sediment is suspended in 95% alcohol and then incubated at 37 C for 4 h. The suspension is again centrifuged and the sediment is washed twice with acetone and then dried overnight at 37 C. The dry powder is suspended in sterile saline for injection.

Vi antiserum is prepared with cultures in the V form. To ensure a pure V culture the culture is plated repeatedly, and V colonies are selected until no W colonies appear on the plates. Edwards and Ewing[93] prepare antigen for Vi serum by scraping the growth of a pure V culture from agar plates, suspending it in absolute alcohol, and dehydrating the bacilli in vacuo. This treatment largely inactivates the H antigens. The dried bacilli are ground to a powder, which is stored in a stoppered tube. Under these conditions the Vi antigen is stable and the powder can be stored without deterioration. It is suspended in physiologic saline just before injection and is administered intravenously without further treatment. The rabbits withstand the injections well, and fairly large amounts can be given. Four injections of this material usually result in the production of a potent Vi serum.

The antisera obtained contain O and H antibodies also; if S. tyhpi is used as antigen, the antibodies must be removed by absorption with the W form of S. typhi. However, if an organism originally named S. ballerup is used as antigen, the serum does not require absorption.

H antisera are prepared with the use of actively motile broth cultures of organisms diluted with an equal amount of saline containing 0.6% formalin. If a particular culture is not sufficiently motile, it may be passed through semisolid agar to enhance motility. A tube of the medium is inoculated on top with the organism. Upon overnight incubation the organisms spread through the medium. The upper part of the medium is heated and poured out of the tube. In the bottom part extremely motile organisms are present. Broth cultures are prepared with these actively motile organisms for antigen production.

Craigie's method employs a tube of semisolid medium with an inner tube that is open at both ends and 1 end extends above the surface of the medium. After inoculation of the small tube (through the extended upper end) the motile organisms descend to the bottom and from there to the surface of the medium in the outer tube.

In case diphasic cultures are used, colony selection may be necessary to obtain colonies that are in phase 1 or 2. Instead of this laborious process, agglutinating serum is added to semisolid agar to immobilize the phase to be suppressed. If a serum with an H titer of 1:1000 is available, 0.1 ml is added to 25 ml of melted agar, and the mixture is poured into a Petri dish. This is inoculated at 1 spot; the unsuppressed phase will swarm across the plate, whereas the suppressed phase (serum against which is in the agar) is immobilized. The organisms are picked from the side of the plate opposite the site of inoculation and used as antigens.

Use of antisera. The O antisera are used in slide agglutination tests. Saline suspension of cultures grown on agar serve as antigens. The glycerolated sera are used in 1:5 or 1:10 dilutions. The test is performed on a slide: A drop of the serum is mixed with a drop of the antigen, the slide tilted about 1 min, and the results read for agglutination (+) or lack of agglutination (−).

The sera are prepared in rabbits by using specific types of Salmonella as antigens. The resulting antisera contain antibodies to a number of O antigens. Marked cross-agglutination occurs between types that have related O antigens. For instance, a strain that has the antigens 4, 5, and 12 will be agglutinated not only by serum derived from an organism with identical O antigens but also by a serum that contains agglutinins for the antigens 4, 12, and 27, since the antigens 4 and 12 are common to both types. Therefore it is necessary to resort to the use of absorbed serum to determine whether an unknown culture contains certain antigens.

Absorbed, single factor sera are prepared from the above sera as needed. Approximately 60 O antigens are presently recognized, and antisera can be prepared for their detection.

For identification of H antigens, Edwards and Ewing use 53 H antisera. These include both multiple and single factor sera. Kauffmann originally recommended the performance of slide agglutination tests for the determination of both O and H antigens. Experience has demonstrated that test tube agglutinations are more reliable because cross-reactions that frequently occur among H factors are more easily eliminated. The titer of the sera for typing of H antigens must be higher than 1:1000, so that O antigens do not interfere with the reaction. For this reason the sera are used in dilutions near their final titer. Equal amounts of diluted serum (usually 1:1000) and formolized antigens are used in single tube tests.

The unknown organism is grown in nutrient broth, and after 24 h 1 or 2 drops concentrated formalin is added. The tests can be carried out after 3 h or more. The reactions are read after a few minutes and again after 1 h incubation at 50-52 C in a water bath.

When the unknown *Salmonella* shows the reactions of only 1 phase, attempts should be made to enhance the other phase, except in cases in which a group of H antigens are found, which occurs exclusively in monophasic types.

The large numbers of antisera described are used in reference laboratories and *Salmonella* centers; for diagnostic laboratory purposes a much smaller number suffices (see discussion on simplified *Salmonella* typing).

For the list of organisms used in preparation of the above O and H antisera, the reader is referred to Edwards and Ewing[20] and Kauffmann.[12]

Agglutinin absorption. For absorbing antisera (to remove agglutinins), organisms grown on agar are used. They are taken up in phenolized saline, washed, and then suspended in 1-2 ml phenol-saline. The serum to be absorbed is added to the cells, mixed, and incubated at 48-50 C for 2 h.

The absorbed H antisera should be titrated against the absorbing strain and the homologous strain in order to ascertain if the absorption is complete and to determine the titer against the homologous strain. Absorbed O antisera should be tested by slide agglutination to make certain that it no longer agglutinates the absorbing strain.

For example, **a single factor O antiserum is prepared as follows:** Serum containing 3 and 10 agglutinins is obtained by injecting rabbits with *S. anatum*, which contains the O antigens 3 and 10. In order to obtain single factor 10 serum, the 3 and 10 serum must be absorbed with *S. newington* organisms, which contain antigens 3 and **15.** In this manner antibody 3 and antigen 3 combine; after centrifugation of the mixture, if absorption is adequate, the serum contains only agglutinin **10,** the agglutinin 3 having been removed. This serum now can be used to determine the presence of a single O antigen, **10,** in an unknown culture.

Certain H antisera (representing antigens a, b, c, d, i, k, r, y, z, z_{10}, z_{27}, z_{29}, z_{36}, z_{37}, and z_{38}) can be used without absorption; others must be absorbed to detect single antigenic components. For detailed procedures regarding absorptions and absorbing strains see Edwards and Ewing.[20]

Isolation of Salmonella

Salmonellae grow well on the usual laboratory media. Differential and selective media and their use are described under "Stool examination" (Chapter 75). Isolation from blood, urine, and other materials is described under the respective headings.

Definition and colonial and biochemical characteristics

The salmonellae are gram-negative, motile, facultative, anaerobic rods that grow well on ordinary laboratory media. The colonies are usually somewhat smaller and more transparent than those of coliform organisms; generally they cannot be distinguished from the latter on the basis of colonial morphology, unless grown on differential media.

On EMB, MacConkey, deoxycholate, and SS agar media they show colorless colonies. On bismuth sulfite agar the well-isolated *S. typhi* colonies are black, surrounded by a black or brownish black zone. Other salmonellae show similar colonies (*S. schottmuelleri, S. enteritidis*), whereas *S. paratyphi* A and certain other types yield flat or slightly raised green colonies. On brilliant green agar they appear as pinkwhite opaque colonies surrounded by a brilliant red medium (*S. typhi* usually does not grow on brilliant green agar).

By definition, salmonellae **do not ferment lactose, sucrose, salicin, raffinose, or adonitol, do not produce indole, and do not show urease activity on Christensen urea agar.** In addition, they are methyl red positive and Voges-Proskauer negative. Most are motile, utilize citrate, and grow on sodium acetate medium; lysine, arginine, and ornithine are decarboxylated and they produce acid in Jordan's tartrate medium. They fail to utilize sodium malonate, do not grow in KCN medium, do not liquefy gelatin or deaminate phenylalanine. With few exceptions, they form gas from glucose, ferment dulcitol, and produce abundant H_2S.

Table 79-24 summarizes the reactions of *Salmonella*. See also Tables 79-14 and 79-22 for differentiation of the genus.

For differential characteristics **within** the genus *Salmonella* see Table 79-25.

NOTE: Approximately 1% of *Salmonella* strains **ferment lactose.** These give a typical *Salmonella* reaction when plated on bismuth sulfite agar, but when plated on MacConkey or SS agar, they show only lactose-fermenting colonies. Lysine decarboxylation (positive in *Salmonella;* use lysine iron agar or decarboxylase tube test) and

Table 79-24. Biochemical reactions of *Salmonella**†

Test or substrate	Sign	%+	(%+)	Test or substrate	Sign	%+	(%+)
Hydrogen sulfide (TSI agar)	+	91.6		Rhamnose	+	90.3	(1.1)
Urease	–	0		Malonate	–	0.5	
Indole	–	1.1		Mucate	d	73.6	
Methyl red (37 C)	+	100		Jordan's tartrate	+ or –	89.3	
Voges-Proskauer	–	0		Stern's glycerol	+ or –	81	
Citrate (Simmons')	d	80.1	(7)	Sodium acetate	d	80	(2.7)
KCN	–	0.3		Sodium alginate	–	0	
Motility	+	94.6		Sodium pectate	–	0	
Gelatin (22 C)	–	0	(1.1)	Lipase	–	0	
Lysine decarboxylase	+	94.6		Maltose	+	96	(1.3)
Arginine dihydrolase	+ or (+)	58.5	(34)	Xylose	+	94	(0.6)
Ornithine decarboxylase	+	92.7		Trehalose	+	93.5	(1.1)
Phenylalanine deaminase	–	0		Cellobiose	d	6.5	(76.4)
Glucose acid	+	100		Glycerol	d	4.5	(17)
gas	+	91.9		α-methyl glucoside	–	3.1	
Lactose	–	0.8		Erythritol	–	3.1	
Sucrose	–	0.5		Esculin	–	0	
Mannitol	+	99.7		Nitrate	+	100	
Dulcitol	d	86.5	(2.7)	Oxidation-fermentation	F	100	
Salicin	–	0	(0.8)	Oxidase	–	0	
Adonitol	–	0		Organic acids			
Inositol	d	34.5	(0.8)	Citrate	+ or (+)	87	(4.6)
Sorbitol	+	94.1	(4)	D-Tartrate	+ or (+)	84.3	(5.7)
Arabinose	+ or (+)	89.2	(0.8)	i-Tartrate	d	3.8	(51.2)
Raffinose	–	3	(0.3)	l-Tartrate	d	9.3	(66.7)

*From Ewing, W. H.: Isolation and identification of *Salmonella* and *Shigella*, Atlanta, 1974, Center for Disease Control.
†+, 90% or more positive within 1-2 d incubation; (+), positive reaction after 3 or more d (decarboxylase tests: 3 or 4 d); –, no reaction (90% or more); + or –, majority of strains positive, some cultures negative; – or +, majority of cultures negative, some strains positive; + or (+), majority of reactions occur within 1-2 d, some are delayed; d, different reaction—+, (+), –; F, fermentation.

Table 79-25. Differentiation of species of *Salmonella**

Test or substrate	S. cholerae-suis			S. typhi			S. enteritidis		
	Sign	%+	(%+)	Sign	%+	(%+)	Sign	%+	(%+)
Hydrogen sulfide (TSI)	+ or –	60		+^{w}	94.4		+	98	
Citrate (Simmons')	(+)	0	(90)	–	0		+	99.3	(0.7)
Ornithine	+	100		–	0		+	99	
Gas from glucose	+	100		–	0		+	97.7	
Dulcitol	d	5	(15)	d	6.2	(31.3)	+	98.3	
Inositol	–	0		–	0		d	42.8	(1)
Trehalose	–	0		+	100		+	100	
Arabinose	–	0		–		(6.3)	+	99.3	
Rhamnose	+	100		–	0		+	95	
Cellobiose	–	0		d	6^w	(31.3)	(+)	5	(92.8)
Erythritol	(+^{w}) or –	0	(85)	–	0		–	0.6	
Sodium acetate	– or (+^{w})	0	(20)	–	0		+	92.4	(2.2)
Mucate	–	0		–	0		+ or –	88.3	
Stern's glycerol fuchsin	–	0		–	0		+	98.2	
Organic acids									
Citrate	– or +	10		– or +	10		+	96	(4)
D-Tartrate	+	95		+ or (+)	87.5	(6.3)	+	91	(5.3)
i-Tartrate	(+) or –	0	(85)	–	0		d	4.7	(57.5)
l-Tartrate	– or (+)	0	(35)	–	0		d	11.8	(75.2)

*From Ewing, W. H.: Isolation and identification of *Salmonella* and *Shigella*, Center for Disease Control, Atlanta, 1974.
†+, 90% or more positive within 1 or 2 d incubation; (+), positive reaction after 3 or more (decarboxylase tests: 3-4 d); –, no reaction (90% or more); + or –, majority of strains positive, some cultures negative; – or +, majority of cultures negative, some strains positive; + or (+), majority of reactions occur within 1-2 d, some are delayed; d, different reactions—+, (+), –; w, weakly positive reaction.

serologic agglutination tests are helpful in the correct identification of such strains. When encountered, they should be submitted to a reference laboratory for confirmation.[83, 95, 96]

Simplified Salmonella typing and identification

Even the small diagnostic laboratory can (and should) carry out a simplified serologic method of *Salmonella* diagnosis. The method of Ewing[97] which is based on the necessity for the identification of certain salmonellae that tend to invade the bloodstream and produce severe enteric fevers, are particularly adapted to humans or tend to become endemic in the population. In institutions (hospitals, etc.) it is particularly important to correctly identify salmonellae so that measures can be taken to prevent or abort any threatening epidemics.

The great majority of *Salmonella* isolated from humans belong to the first 5 somatic O antigen groups, A-E, including the major types that need to be completely identified: *S. typhi* and *S. sendai* (group D), *S. paratyphi* A (group A), *S. paratyphi* B and *S. typhimurium* (group B), and *S. cholerae-suis* and *S. paratyphi* C (group C₁).

Thus the average laboratory can detect the large majority of *Salmonella*, including the types listed above, with the use of somatic **O** antisera for groups A through E, and **H** (flagellar) antisera for antigens a, b, c, d, and i 1, 2, 3, 5, 6, and 7. A **Vi antiserum** and a **polyvalent O *Salmonella* antiserum** containing antibodies to O antigens 1, 2, 3, 4, 5, 6, 7, 8, 9, 10, 12, 15, 19, and **Vi** are also needed; all are available commercially.* By the use of the simplified schema the need for a large number of antisera is obviated; preliminary identification can be carried out even in the small laboratory, with final identification left for *Salmonella* typing centers.

All organisms that cannot be excluded on biochemical grounds from the genus *Salmonella* but are not classifiable by the use of the simplified typing methods should be forwarded to a reference laboratory (usually through state health department laboratories).

Polyvalent antisera. Satisfactory antisera for use in the simplified schema are available from a number of biological houses.† They must be used in strict adherence to the manufacturer's instructions.

• • •

The preparation of antisera is here described for those laboratories which prefer to prepare their own and for illustration of the principles involved.

---

*O antisera for groups F through Z and groups 51-61 as well as a very large number of various H antisera have also become available commercially.

†Difco Laboratories, Detroit; BBL, Div. of BioQuest, Cockeysville, Md.; Burroughs Wellcome & Co., Inc., Tuckahoe, N.Y.; Lederle Laboratories, Pearl River, N.Y.; Sylvana Co., Orange, N.J.; Lee Laboratories.

Edwards and Ewing[22] recommend the use of a **polyvalent serum** that contains agglutinins against the O antigens of the 5 groups, A-E. The polyvalent serum is prepared by injecting rabbits with a mixture (equal amounts) of smooth cultures of the following organisms:

S. paratyphi A	*S. gallinarum*
S. paratyphi B	*S. anatum*
S. thompson	*S. newington*
S. virginia	*S. senftenberg*

The antigens are prepared by method described for preparation of O antisera; injections are given at intervals of 4 d in amounts of 0.5, 1, 2, 4, 5, and 5 ml. A trial bleeding is taken after 4 injections, and titers against each component are determined. If agglutinins against a particular organism are present in low titer, the particular antigen should be doubled in mixture used for next injection. Rabbits are bled 6 d after last injection; serum is preserved with equal amount of glycerol and is standardized. Polyvalent serum should be used in highest dilution in which it will agglutinate all organisms used for injection. Antiserum contains agglutinins for antigens 1, 2, 3, 4, 5, 6, 7, 8, 9, 10, 12, 15, and 19.

Polyvalent serum similar to the one just described is available from a number of biological houses as indicated. (Polyvalent sera containing agglutinins for groups F through Z have become available recently.)

In addition to the polyvalent serum, **serum for each group** is needed. Organisms used to prepare **group O polyvalent antisera** are listed by Edwards and Ewing[22] as follows:

For group A	*S. paratyphi* A
B	*S. paratyphi* B
C¹	*S. thompson*
C²	*S. virginia*
D	*S. gallinarum*
E	*S. anatum* and *S. newington*

Smooth cultures of the indicated organisms are used; 24 h broth cultures are heated at 100 C for 2 h and 0.3% formalin is added. The suspensions are used for injections in rabbits as described under preparation of O antisera. Standardization is performed by preparing different dilutions of each serum and determining the highest dilution at which it will give clear-cut agglutinations in slide tests with the homologous antigen.

A **Vi serum** is also needed. It is prepared, as described earlier, from an organism originally named *S. ballerup*.

Edwards and Ewing[22] use 6 **H sera** prepared as follows:

a	*S. paratyphi* A
b	*S. paratyphi* B, phase 1
c	*S. cholerae-suis*, phase 1
d	*S. typhi*
i	*S. typhimurium*, phase 1
1, 2, 3, 5	*S. thompson*, phase 2, and *S. newport*, phase 2

Preparation of the H antisera has been described. After collection from rabbits, the sera should be titrated by tube tests against the homologous antigens. A titer of 5000 is adequate.

Serologic examination and identification

A "screening" procedure is outlined under "Stool examination" for salmonellae; other reactions and preliminary steps for identification are described earlier in this chapter.

Cultures that produce alkaline slant, acid butt,

H_2S, and gas on TSI agar and do not produce urease on Christensen urea agar are examined.*

1. The growth from TSI slants† should be suspended in saline (use heavy suspensions). The suspension is tested on a **slide with polyvalent O Salmonella serum.**‡ Although the directions of manufacturers vary in some details, in general the test is performed as follows:

1. Using wax pencil, mark off glass plate or microslide into sections about 1 cm².
2. Place 1 drop (about 0.05 ml or 3 mm loopful) polyvalent serum in section of slide.
3. To next square add 1 drop physiologic saline solution. This is control for ensuring that suspension is not autoagglutinable.
4. Add 1 drop or loopful (use sterile loop) of bacterial suspension to saline (step 3). Emulsify thoroughly.
5. Add another loopful of bacterial suspension to serum (step 2) and mix thoroughly.
6. Tilt slide back and forth and observe for agglutination. Positive reactions occur within 30 s to 1 min and are usually clear-cut. Avoid excess evaporation; flakes of dried material might be mistaken for agglutinated bacteria. Saline drop (step 3) should show no agglutination.

2. If positive agglutination occurs, test suspension in a similar manner with individual **O group polyvalent antisera** (A-E). The use of polyvalent sera for groups F, G, H, and others will detect some additional types, but sera A through E are sufficient for the average laboratory.

According to Edwards and Ewing,[22] any culture that is agglutinated in a typical manner by polyvalent serum and by 1 or more of the O grouping sera **may be reported as a presumptive Salmonella,** provided preliminary biochemical examination indicates that it is a member of the genus. **Results should be confirmed by extended biochemical tests,** since many enteric bacteria contain antigens related to the O antigens of *Salmonella.*

Cultures that fail to agglutinate with the polyvalent group antisera should be tested with **Vi** serum. Most freshly isolated S. *typhi* cultures do not agglutinate in O sera but will do so in **Vi** serum. If such is the case, part of the suspension should be boiled for 20 min, and after cooling it should be retested with O group sera and **Vi** serum. S. *typhi* cultures should now react with group D serum and S. *paratyphi* C cultures should react with C₁ serum. **Cultures that continue to agglutinate in Vi serum after boiling but do not agglutinate in the O group sera are most** likely **Citrobacter organisms (Bethesda-Ballerup strains).***

Following positive agglutination with the polyvalent and group antisera, **biochemical tests** must be carried further in order to ascertain that the culture conforms to the characteristics of the genus *Salmonella.* Tables 79-14, 79-24, and 79-25 list the tests to be performed. In small laboratories, because of restrictions on space and labor, not all tests may be available. The following tests are deemed **essential** (minimal) before a **confirmed** report of *Salmonella* isolation may be made:

1. Hydrogen sulfide (TSI)
2. Urease
3. Indole
4. Methyl red
5. Voges-Proskauer
6. Citrate (Simmons)
7. Motility
8. Gas from glucose
9. Lysine
10. Ornithine
11. KCN
12. Lactose

Tests 1, 4, and 6-10 are positive (few exceptions in 6-9); 2, 3, 5, 11, and 12 are negative.

The following additional tests are useful:

13. Sucrose
14. Salicin
15. Dulcitol
16. β-Galactosidase
17. Malonate

Tests 13-17 are all negative.

Cultures that agglutinate in polyvalent *Salmonella* serum and in one or more polyvalent group sera but do not conform to the pattern just described should be submitted to a reference laboratory. Similarly, as stated, cultures that cannot be excluded on biochemical grounds from the genus but are not agglutinated by the polyvalent sera should also be submitted for further identification.

3. Organisms giving positive reactions with the O group sera **should be analyzed further for their H antigens to determine serotype ("species").** Infusion broth tube cultures grown overnight of actively motile cultures are used. The broth culture is inactivated with an equal amount of 0.6% formalinized physiologic saline (6 ml formalin + 8.5 gm NaCl in 1 L distilled water).

Test for H antigens
1. Prepare appropriate dilution of **H antiserum** (directions given by manufacturer).
2. Add 0.5 ml of each serum to be used to separate Kahn tubes (12 × 75 mm), labeled correspondingly. To 1 tube add **only** 0.5 ml saline.

*NOTE: S. *typhi* does not form gas and forms little or no H²S in TSI agar; S. *paratyphi* A produces gas but usually no H_2S.
†Some workers use suggestive colonies from primary plates for testing with polyvalent antisera; this is permissible if rapid reporting is important.
‡Most commercially available polyvalent sera contain Vi antibody. Such sera are preferable to those that do not contain Vi antibody.

*NOTE: Such strains most often show cross-reactions with *Salmonella* somatic (O) group B or C antisera, since they share common O antigens. Refer to *Citrobacter.*

3. Add 0.5 ml culture suspension to each tube.
4. Shake tubes and incubate at 48-50 C for 1 h.
5. Observe for agglutination and record. No agglutination should occur in tube containing saline only.

Edwards and Ewing[22] list the use of H antisera as follows.

Group A cultures. Test with serum a: *S. paratyphi* A produces little or no H_2S, does not utilize citrate, and does not ferment xylose.

Group B cultures. Test with b and i and 1, 2, 3, and 5 H antisera. If agglutination occurs with b or i serum, the culture is mostly likely *S. paratyphi* B or *S. typhimurium*, respectively. If culture is agglutinated only by phase 2 serum (1, 2, 3, 5), phase 1 should be isolated by spot plating cultures on semisolid agar containing 1, 2, 3, and 5 serum (0.1 ml of 1:10,000 titer H serum added to 25 ml melted agar and poured into Petri dish). Phase 1 can be isolated from spreading growth. Or, **inoculate tube of semisolid medium (2-3 ml), to which a loopful of phase 2 serum has been added; this will suppress phase 2 growth and allow phase 1 growth.**

Group C cultures. Test with c and 1, 2, 3, and 5 sera. Those agglutinating with c are either *S. paratyphi* C (trehalose fermented, usually arabinose (also) or *S. cholerae-suis* (trehalose and arabinose not fermented). The majority of *S. cholerae-suis* cultures (Kunzendorf variety) occurs in phase 2; if the group C culture agglutinates in 1, 2, 3, and 5 serum and shows the biochemical characteristics mentioned above, it can be reported as *S. cholerae-suis.*

Group D cultures. Test with a and d and 1, 2, 3, and 5 sera. Cultures that form no gas, give typical biochemical reactions, and agglutinate only in d serum can be reported as *S. typhi.* It should, of course, also agglutinate with Vi serum. *S. sendai*, which occurs mainly in the Orient, should agglutinate both in a and 1, 2, 3, and 5 sera. It is H_2S negative and citrate negative and ferments arabinose immediately, but in xylose and sorbitol it gives delayed reactions.

Group E cultures. These are not examined but are reported as "*Salmonella,* group E."

• • •

Cultures that are not identifiable by the above typing schema should be reported as "*Salmonella,* group —, type undetermined" and sent to a reference laboratory (state, etc.) with identifying information (patient's name, age, sex, source of specimen, clinical diagnosis, and any epidemiologic relationships, if known). Submit cultures on slants of plain infusion agar medium without added carbohydrate; blood agar base medium is a very good choice.

Antimicrobial susceptibility

Chloramphenicol has long been the drug of choice in therapy of typhoid fever and *Salmonella* septicemias; however, chloramphenicol-resistant strains have appeared. Accordingly, antimicrobial sensitivity testing is required, with parenteral ampicillin and trimethoprim-sulfamethoxazole being clinically effective alternatives. Antibiotics are **not** indicated in *Salmonella* gastroenteritis (except in the very young and those over 60), since the disease is brief and limited to the gastrointestinal tract.

Recently, multiply-resistant salmonellae (re-sistant to chloramphenicol, ampicillin, trimethoprim-sulfamethoxazole, and gentamicin) were involved in a hospital epidemic associated with a high mortality among compromised patients.

Salmonella typhi

Although *S. typhi* is not as prevalent in the United States as previously and the number of salmonelloses caused by other members of the genus has increased, the prompt recognition of *S. typhi* is an important laboratory task. Because of its biochemical characteristics, which are at variance with the great majority of salmonellae, the identification of *S. typhi* at times presents a problem to the inexperienced worker.

The organism is anaerogenic (it does not produce gas), and usually only small amounts (or none) of H_2S are seen in TSI agar. The TSI reaction is alkaline over acid (K/A) with a slight blackening at the junction of the butt and slant. It does not utilize citrate (Simmons citrate agar) and fails to ferment dulcitol promptly. As pointed out earlier, some fresh isolates of *S. typhi* do not agglutinate in polyvalent O antisera but give a positive reaction with Vi serum. If such is the case, the suspension should be boiled and retested with O group sera and Vi serum. If the culture is *S. typhi*, it should now react with group D serum. Further studies with H antisera and biochemical tests should be carried out to confirm identity of the culture. (See Table 79-25.)

The organism grows poorly on Hektoen agar and does not grow on brilliant green agar, according to Hickman and Farmer,[98] who studied 2883 strains.

Phage typing

Strains of *S. typhi* can be subdivided on the basis of susceptibility to lysis by specific bacteriophages. At least 72 subtypes carrying the same Vi Ag have been distinguished; the information is useful in investigating epidemics.

Cultures submitted to the Center for Disease Control or regional laboratories for phage typing should be Vi+, sent on egg medium (Pai's medium without glycerin), and accompanied by epidemiologic data.

A phage-typing set for differentiating Salmonellae other than *S. typhi* has been developed by Gershman.[99]

• • •

Antibody formation in salmonelloses and detection of antibodies in patient's serum. See serology, Chapter 106.

ARIZONA

The genus *Arizona* is composed of bacteria related to the members of the genus *Salmonella* but distinguishable from them by biochemical and serologic methods.

Members of the group are gram-negative, motile rods; on differential media the colonies resemble those of salmonellae.* Likewise, the reaction on TSI agar is similar to the latter. Some strains of this group are probably not identified in stool cultures, since they may ferment lactose in 24 hours (approximately 60% of strains); others, however, ferment lactose in 3-10 days.

The organisms were originally isolated from sick lizards and Gila monsters (1939) and were considered *Salmonella* variants. Later they were identified in birds, reptiles, domestic animals, and humans. Kauffmann[100] named the organism *Salmonella arizona*. Largely through the studies of Edwards and co-workers, the status of these organisms has been clarified, and it has become clear that they comprise a group biochemically and serologically distinct from salmonellae.

The single species of the genus is now named *A. hinshawii*.[101] (See Table 79-9.)

Arizona organisms are isolated frequently from fowls, especially turkeys, chicken egg powder, canaries, and various domestic animals such as hogs, dogs, and sheep. The majority of strains from humans have been obtained from stools in diarrheal states, gastroenteritis, and enteric fevers, whereas 30% were isolated from blood and from localized infections (pleural fluid, urine, conjunctivitis, various abscesses, and meningitis). Whether this high degree of invasiveness, more severe than that of non-host-adapted salmonellae, is apparent or real is not known presently. Many strains ferment lactose rapidly, and it is quite possible that such strains are overlooked in stool examinations; thus the high incidence of strains isolated from blood and localized infections may simply be due to the fact that they go unrecognized in cases of diarrhea.

---

*For detailed description of colonies see section on stool cultures, Chapter 75.

Definition[102] and biochemical characteristics

The genus *Arizona* conforms to the definitions of the family Enterobacteriaceae and the tribe Salmonelleae. The biochemical reactions of *Arizona* are similar to those of salmonellae, with the following exceptions: gelatin is liquefied slowly in nutrient medium, sodium malonate is utilized, dulcitol and inositol are not fermented, β-galactosidase is present, and the majority of strains ferment lactose. Table 79-22 lists the reactions useful for differentiation of *Salmonella*, *Citrobacter*, and *Arizona*; Tables 79-14 and 79-26 list the detailed reactions of *Arizona*.

For further details see Edwards and Ewing,[22] and Ewing and Fife.[102]

NOTE:

1. *Arizona* cultures are **lysine decarboxylase positive;** by employing lysine iron agar, in addition to TSI agar, or performing a lysine tube test on suspicious H_2S-positive, lactose-fermenting colonies, these can be distinguished from other lactose-fermenting, H_2S-forming Enterobacteriaceae, which are lysine negative (*Citrobacter*). A positive lysine test also eliminates *Proteus*, *Shigella*, and *S. paratyphi* A (lactose nonfermenters), which give TSI reactions similar to those *Arizona* organisms that do not ferment lactose promptly.

2. Most *Arizona* organisms do not grow in KCN broth, unlike a number of other Enterobacteriaceae.

Antigenic structure

Organisms in the genus *Arizona* have been differentiated into at least 38 O groups with 332 serotypes.[103, 104] Many of the O (and H) antigens are related to *Salmonella* O antigens. The antigen 7a, 7b is identical with *Salmonella* antigen 18, and cross-reactions with *Salmonella* O group K antiserum will occur. When such cross-reactions are found, biochemical characteristics will

Table 79-26. Biochemical reactions of *Arizona**†

Test or substrate	Sign	%+	(%+)‡	Test or substrate	Sign	%+	(%+)‡
Indole	−	5.1		Malonate	+	94.6	
Methyl red	+	100		Gas from glucose	+	99.7	
Voges-Proskauer	−	0		Lactose	d	69.8	(15.6)
Citrate (Simmons')	+	96.8	(2.5)	Sucrose	−	2.9	(0.3)
Hydrogen sulfide (TSI)	+	98.7		Mannitol	+	100	
Urease	−	0		Dulcitol	−	0	
KCN	−	5.7		Salicin	−	2.2	(1.6)
Motility	+	100		Adonitol	−	0	
Gelatin (22 C)	(+) or +	12.1	(84.8)	Inositol	−	0	
Lysine decarboxylase	+	99.4	(0.3)	Sorbitol	+	97.1	(1)
Arginine dihydrolase	(+) or +	25.1	(73.6)	Arabinose	+	99.1	(0.6)
Ornithine decarboxylase	+	100		Raffinose	−	4.1	(0.6)
Phenylalanine deaminase	−	0		Rhamnose	+	95.2	(2.3)

*Based on data from Center for Disease Control (Sep. 1973).[96]

†+, 90% or of cultures more positive within 1-2 d; (+), positive reaction after 3 or more d (decarboxylase tests: 3-4 d); −, no reaction (90% or more); + or −, most cultures positive, some strains negative; − or +, most strains negative, some cultures positive; (+) or +, most reactions occur within 1-2 d, some are delayed; d, different reactions—+, (+), −; w, weakly positive reaction.

‡Figures in parentheses indicate delayed reactions (3 d or more).

Table 79-27. Nomenclature and differential tests for *Citrobacter* species*

Organism	Biochemical characteristics				Synonyms
	H_2S	Indole	Malonate	KCN	
C. freundii	+	−	−	+	
C. diversus	−	+	+	−	L. malonatica, C. intermedius biotype b
C. amalonaticus	−	+	−	+	L. amalonatica, C. intermedius biotype a

*From Brenner, D. J., Farmer, J. J., III, Hickman, F. W., et al.: Taxonomic and nomenclature changes in *Enterobacteriaceae*, DHEW publ. no. (CDC) 78-8356, Atlanta, Oct. 1977, Center for Disease Control.

usually allow differentiation. In any case, identification of *Arizona* strains as salmonellae is not a serious mistake since they produce clinically similar diseases. Polyvalent *Arizona* antisera are commercially available.* *Arizona* strains should be submitted to a reference laboratory for specific serotyping.

CITROBACTER†

The *Citrobacter* genus is composed of members of the family Enterobacteriaceae previously designated as *Escherichia freundii* and certain strains of *Paracolobactrum intermedium* designated as the Bethesda-Ballerup group of "paracolon" organisms. (See also Table 79-9.)

Members of the genus *Citrobacter* are gramnegative, motile rods, the majority of which ferment lactose (frequently delayed) and form H_2S. They are usually negative in the indole and Voges-Proskauer tests, are positive in the methyl red test, and utilize citrate (Simmons citrate agar).

They **do not decarboxylate lysine** and only about ⅕ of the strains decarboxylate ornithine. With few exceptions, they fail to produce indole. The majority of cultures are urease positive, but the reactions are weak (about 70% of the cultures give a positive reaction in 18-24 hours, but not in 1-3 hours as is customary with *Proteus* on urea agar). **They grow in KCN medium,** produce acid in Jordan tartrate medium, and ferment dulcitol and cellobiose.

Citrobacter cultures that hydrolyze urea slowly and ferment lactose or sucrose, slowly or not at all, are frequently confused with salmonellae. The **negative lysine and positive KCN reactions** are of great importance in distinguishing these organisms from salmonellae and arizonae.

Tables 79-27 and 79-28 list the major biochemical characteristics of *Citrobacter*. (See

*Difco Laboratories, Detroit.

†The original Ballerup strain was named *Salmonella ballerup*, since its biochemical properties resemble those of salmonellae and it possesses the **Vi** antigen.

also Tables 79-14 and 79-22.) For further details refer to Davis and Ewing.[105]

Although some strains of the genus have been suspected of producing enteric infections, clear-cut evidence of their role as enteric pathogens is lacking.

The **Bethesda-Ballerup** portion of the group has been extensively studied, and an antigenic schema was established, including 32 O groups and 167 serologic types. Polyvalent sera are commercially available.

Relationships exist between certain O antigens of the *Arizona*, *Salmonella*, and Bethesda-Ballerup groups. Some Bethesda strains show cross-reactions with *Salmonella* B and C_1 group antisera. Some strains possess the **Vi** antigen and thus may agglutinate in polyvalent *Salmonella* antiserum containing Vi antibody. Members of the Bethesda-Ballerup subgroup have been associated with diarrhea in humans, but they are not considered true enteric pathogens. *Citrobacter* strains occur infrequently in the normal stool and have recovered from various pathologic processes.

Citrobacter amalonaticus, C. freundii, and C. diversus[26]

Until 1971 only 1 species of *Citrobacter*, *C. freundii*,[105] was reported by the Enteric Section, Center for Disease Control.

Two groups of H_2S-negative, indole-positive organisms were among the biogroups included in *C. freundii*. One of these was malonate positive and KCN negative; the other, malonate negative and KCN positive. In 1971, Young et al. placed both of these organisms in a new genus, *Levinea*, as *L. malonatica* and *L. amalonatica*.[106] *Bergey's Manual*, ed. 8,[3] calls both of these organisms biotypes of *Citrobacter intermedius*. Since 1971 the Enteric Section has reported the malonate-positive organism as *Citrobacter diversus*,[107] but has continued to report the malonatenegative organism as "biogroup of *C. freundii*."

As of 1978, the malonate-negative organism will be recognized as *Citrobacter amalonaticus*.[26]

Table 79-28. Biochemical reactions of *Citrobacter* species*†

Test	C. freundii	C. diversus	C. amalonaticus
H₂S	+	−	−
Urease	d	d	d
Indole	−	+	+
Methyl red	+	+	+
Voges-Proskauer	−	−	−
Simmons' citrate	+	+	+
KCN	+	−	+
Motility	+	+	+
Gelatin (22 C)	−	−	d
Lysine decarboxylase	−	−	−
Arginine dihydrolase	d	+ or (+)	+
Ornithine decarboxylase	d	+	−
Phenylalanine deaminase	−	−	−
Gas from D-glucose	+	+	+
Acid from:			
Lactose	(+) or +	d	d
Sucrose	d	− or +	d
D-Mannitol	+	+	+
Dulcitol	d	+ or −	−
Salicin	d	(+) or +	(+)
Adonitol	−	+	−
i-Inositol	−	−	−
D-Sorbitol	+	+	+
L-Arabinose	+	+	+
Raffinose	d	−	+
L-Rhamnose	+	+	+
Maltose	+	+	+
D-Xylose	+	+	+
Trehalose	+	+	+
Cellobiose	+ or (+)	+	+
Erythritol	−	−	−
Glycerol	+	+	+
Malonate	d	+	−
Mucate	+	+	+
Jordan's tartrate	+	+ or −	+

*From Brenner, D. J., Farmer, J. J. III, Hickman, F. W., et al.: Taxonomic and nomenclature changes in *Enterobacteriaceae*, DHEW publ. no. (CDC) 78-8356, Atlanta, Oct. 1977, Center for Disease Control.

†+, 90% or more positive within 1-2 d; (+), positive reaction after 3 or more d (decarboxylase tests: 3-4 d); −, no reaction (90% or more); + or −, most cultures positive, some strains negative; − or +, most strains negative, some cultures positive; + or (+), most reactions occur within 1-2 d, some are delayed; d, different reactions—+, (+), or −.

The nomenclatural synonyms are shown in Table 79-27.

DNA hybridization studies[108] showed that *C. diversus* and *L. malonatica* are synonyms. Furthermore, *C. diversus* and *L. amalonatica* are 55-60% related, and *C. freundii* is 50-55% related to each of these species. Additional biochemical studies firmly established that several biochemical tests served to differentiate *C. diversus* and *L. amalonatica* (see Table 79-28).

KLEBSIELLEAE
Klebsiella, Enterobacter, Serratia

The related genera *Klebsiella*, *Enterobacter*, and *Serratia* are members of the tribe *Klebsielleae*. (Recently the species *Enterobacter hafniae* has been renamed *Hafnia alvei* and placed into the newly created genus *Hafnia* [see Table 79-8]). The three genera can be readily identified by biochemical tests including decarboxylase reactions (Table 79-14), and most strains of

Klebsiella and *Serratia* can be typed serologically. These organisms cause serious urinary tract and pulmonary infections in hospitalized patients, and they are second to *E. coli* as causes of gram-negative bacteremia.

Major characteristics differentiating the tribe from others in *Enterobacteriaceae* are shown in Tables 79-14 and 79-29. It can be noted that **typical cultures** in this division are indole, methyl red, phenylalanine deaminase, and H₂S negative. Urease is either not produced or delayed. The organisms grow in KCN broth and Simmons citrate and produce acetylmethylcarbinol (Voges-Proskauer test positive). The majority of strains in this division are inhibited on highly selective media (bismuth sulfite, brilliant green, and deoxycholate citrate agar).

Members of *Klebsiella* and many *Enterobacter* usually **ferment lactose** rapidly, whereas **serratiae usually do not.** They are motile or nonmotile (*Klebsiella*).

Table 79-29. Reactions of members of the tribe *Klebsielleae**†

| | Klebsiella | | | Enterobacter | | | | | | | | |
| | pneumoniae‡ | | | cloacae | | | aerogenes | | | hafniae | | |
Test or substrate	Sign	%+	(%+)§	Sign	%+	(%+)§	Sign	%+	(½+)§	Sign	%+	(%+)
Indole	−	6.8		−	0		−	0.8		−	0	
Methyl red	− or +	11.3		−	3.3		−	1.6		− or +	35	
Voges-Proskauer	+	93.7		+	100		+	100		+ or −	83.6	
Citrate (Simmons')	+	96.8	(0.6)	+	98.9	(0.4)	+	92.6	(2.4)	d	5.6	(63)
Hydrogen sulfide (TSI)	−	0		−	0		−	0		−	0	
Urease	+	95.4	(0.1)	+ or −	74.6ʷ		−	5ʷ		−	6.6ʷ	(2.5)
KCN	+	97.9		+	97.		+	97.5		+	97.3	
Motility	−	0		+	92.4		+	91.7		+	94.1	
Gelatin (22 C)	−	1.9	(0.4)	(+)	0.6	(94.2)	+ or −	0	(61.2)	−	0	
Lysine decarboxylase	+	97.2	(0.1)	−	0		+	97.5		+	99.6	
Arginine dihydrolase	−	0.6		+	92.4	(2)	−	0		d	4.6	(6.6)
Ornithine decarboxylase	−	0		+	93.7	(1.3)	+	95.9	(0.8)	+	98.6	
Phenylalanine deaminase	−	0		−	0		−	0		−	0	
Malonate	+	92.5		+ or −	80.5		+ or −	74.7		+ or −	67.2	
Gas from glucose	+	96		+	99.3		+	95.9	(0.8)	+	98.9	
Lactose	+	98.7	(1)	+ or (+)	76.3	(21.8)	+	92.5	(5)	d	2.8	(11.9)
Sucrose	+	99.3	(0.1)	+	94.1	(0.9)	+	99.2	(0.8)	d	7	(46.5)
Mannitol	+	100		+	99.8		+	100		+	100	
Dulcitol	− or +	33		d	15.2	(0.4)	−	4.1		−	2.4	
Salicin	+	99.7	(0.2)	+ or (+)	69.1	(26.5)	+	99.2	(0.8)	d	11.2	(5.9)
Adonitol	d	89	(0.2)	− or +	22.2		+	97.5		−	0	
Inositol	+	97.2	(0.9)	d	13	(8)	+	96.7		−	0	
Sorbitol	+	99.4	(0.3)	+	90.4		+	98.3		−	0	
Arabinose	+	99.9		+	99.4		+	100		+	99.3	
Raffinose	+	99.7		+	90.7		+	96.7		−	3.8	(1.1)
Rhamnose	+	99.3	(0.4)	d	89.8	(1.2)	+	99.2		+	95.4	(1.1)

*Based on data from Ewing and Edwards,[14] Ewing,[15] and Center for Disease Control.[112a]

†+, 90% or more of cultures positive within 1-2 d; (+), positive reaction after 3 or more d (decarboxylase tests: 3 or 4 d) −; no reaction (90 reactions occur within 1 or 2 d, some are delayed; d, different reactions—+, (+), −; w, weakly positive reaction.

†For *Klebsiella oxytoca*, see text.

§Figure in parentheses indicates delayed reaction (3 d or more).

‖Volumes of gas produced are small (bubble to about 10%).

Biochemical characteristics aiding in the differentiation of the groups (genera) and detailed reactions for identification are shown in Table 79-29. For further details see Fife et al.[109] For the evaluation of the clinical role, antibiotic susceptibilities, and detailed reviews of the group, refer to Weil et al.[110] Edmondson and Sandford,[111] Eickhoff et al.,[112] and Brenner et al.[26]

KLEBSIELLA

The genus *Klebsiella* is composed of members of the family *Enterobacteriaceae* that are **nonmotile, gelatin nonliquefying, lysine decarboxylase positive,** and arginine and ornithine decarboxylase negative. The organisms are indole* and methyl red negative and Voges-

*About 5% of strains are indole positive; see *Klebsiella oxytoca*, **below.**

Proskauer and citrate positive. Lactose, sucrose, sorbitol, and raffinose are usually fermented; gas is produced from inositol, glycerol, and cellobiose. The urease reaction is delayed positive; phenylalanine deaminase and H_2S are negative.[109]

Proper identification of the organism is of concern to the clinician since, traditionally, *K. pneumoniae* (Friedländer's bacillus) was known as the causative agent of severe pneumonia, whereas *Enterobacter* strains were known as occurring in the feces and in urinary tract infections. It is now known that source is not a determining factor, since both *Enterobacter* and *Klebsiella* strains can be isolated from practically any part of the body, and that they have been implicated in septicemias and in diseases of the lung, liver, gastrointestinal tract, and genitourinary tract; still, *Klebsiella* is a

Test or substrate	Enterobacter agglomerans			Serratia marcescens			Serratia liquefaciens			Serratia rubidaea		
	Sign	%+	(%+)‡	Sign	%+	(%+)‡	Sign	%+	(%+)‡	Sign	%+	(%+)‡
Indole	− or +	18.7		−	0.1^w		−	1.8^w		−	2^w	
Methyl red	− or +	44.8		− or +	18.5		+ or −	64.2		− or +	31	
Voges-Proskauer	+ or −	67.9		+	98.7		− or +	49.5		+	92	
Citrate (Simmons')	d	66.6	(19.2)	+	97.6	(1.3)	+	93.6	(6.4)	+ or (+)	88	(2)
Hydrogen sulfide (TSI)	−	0		−	0		−	0		−	0	
Urease	d	27.8^w	(8.4)	d^w	39.7	(22.3)	d^w	3.7	(11)	d^w	4	(16)
KCN	− or +	34.2		+	98.9		+	91.7		− or +	22	
Motility	+ or −	89.4		+	95.5		+	92.7		+ or −	88	
Gelatin (22 C)	d	3	(80.1)	+ or (+)	84.4	(11.3)	+	96.3	(3.7)	+ or (+)	88	(12)
Lysine decarboxylase	−	0		+	99.6		+ or (+)	64.2	(31.2)	+ or (+)	61	(31)
Arginine dihydrolase	−	0		−	0.9^w		−	0		−	0	
Ornithine decarboxylase	−	0		+	99.6		+	100		−	0	
Phenylalanine deaminase	− or +	27.9		−	0		−	0.9		−	0	
Malonate	+ or −	62		−	1.6		−	0.9		+ or −	86	
Gas from glucose	− or +	21.1		+ or −	52.6‖		+ or −	72.5	(0.9)‖	d	35	(4)‖
Lactose	d	40.5	(11)	−	1.3	(4.6)	d	15.6		+	100	
Sucrose	d	77.1	(1.5)	+	99.4		+	98.2		+	96	
Mannitol	+	100		+	100		+	100		+	100	
Dulcitol	d	12.2	(0.6)	−	0		−	0		−	0	
Salicin	d	63.6	(18.8)	+	95	(1.6)	+	96.3		+ or (+)	88	(4)
Adonitol	−	6.7	(0.2)	d	45.6	(13.8)	d	8.3	(5.5)	+ or (+)	88	(2)
Inositol	d	14.2	(4.8)	d	77.3	(6.4)	+ or (+)	64.2	(25.2)	d	35	(16)
Sorbitol	d	23.9	(0.4)	+	99.1	(0.9)	+	97.3		−	8	
Arabinose	+	97.9	(0.4)	−	0		+	97.3		+	100	
Raffinose	d	24.8	(3)	−	1.2	(0.8)	+	90.8	(4.6)	+	96	
Rhamnose	+ or (+)	86.1	(4.3)	−	0		d	16.5	(0.9)	−	4	(2)

or more); + or −, most cultures positive, some strains negative; − or +, most strains negative, some cultures positive; + or (+), most

primary pathogen probably more often than *Enterobacter,* which is considered an opportunist.

Antigens

Typical *Klebsiella* organisms produce large, moist colonies that are due to the formation of large capsules around the organisms (demonstrable by India ink mounts). These capsules contain antigens that are distinct from the somatic (O) antigens. The capsular antigens (K) serve for typing of the organisms. In addition, Kauffmann distinguished a number of antigenic and cultural forms with regard to the O antigens; there are at least 72 capsular types.

"Capsular swelling" reaction for Klebsiella

In their discussion of *Klebsiella* antigens, Ewing and Edwards[22] state that in their opinion no actual swelling of the capsule occurs; rather it is a precipitin reaction occurring on the surface of the capsule. The precipitation of antibody makes the capsule highly refractile and thus easily visible. The loose slime present in the growth also takes place in the reaction. It is recommended for this reason to use a fresh and very dilute suspension for the test; the amount of slime that may interfere with the reaction is greatly reduced.

1. Place on slide 2 drops diluted suspension of the organism (preferably grown on Worfel-Ferguson medium).
2. To 1 drop add India ink and to other add loopful of antiserum. Mix well.
3. Place coverslips over both drops.
4. Examine both mounts: India ink mount is used to ascertain size of capsule. In positive reaction there should be apparent "Quellung" of capsules in drop to which proper antiserum was added.

Identification

Klebsiella grows readily on the usual laboratory media. Characteristically, the typical culture shows large, semifluid, slimy, mucoid, moist colonies. This is due to the formation of capsules. **Most strains ferment lactose** promptly and thus can be recognized on differential media. The growth of the mucoid colonies usually strings out when touched with an inoculating loop. Nonencapsulated strains are also encountered, as are slow lactose-fermenting strains.

For final group identification, perform IMViC reaction, decarboxylase reactions, use TSI (for H_2S), urease test, motility, and gelatin liquefaction (Tables 79-19 and 79-29). It should be remembered that the majority of capsule types 3 and 4 are methyl red negative and Voges-Proskauer positive (IMViC: + − + −). If the organisms are recovered from blood in bacteremia, sputum from pneumonia, or other serious infections, capsular typing should be done.

Klebsiella species

K. pneumoniae (the type species) organisms are short, gram-negative rods that produce large capsules. In infected tissues the rods are usually uniformly ovoid, whereas in cultures longer forms, including filaments, occur. Mucoid colonies, as described above, are usually formed. If subcultured a number of times, the organism may lose its mucoid character and assume the smooth form without capsule. *K. pneumoniae* occurs in a small percentage of normal individuals (respiratory tract, stool). It causes a relatively small number of pneumonias; but the infection is usually severe, due to the destructive action of the organism on the tissues. *K. pneumoniae* lung infections frequently become chronic with the formation of cavities.

K. rhinoscleromatis strains usually form **no gas,** fail to utilize citrate, are methyl red positive,

Voges-Proskauer negative, and citrate negative, and ferment lactose slowly or not at all; they are lysine negative. The organism is implicated in a slowly growing granulomatous tumor in the external nares of the mucosa of the mouth, pharynx, or larynx. In Kauffman's classification the organism has the antigenic formula 2a:3. It is nonpathogenic for mice.

The organism *K. ozaenae* was isolated from "ozena," a type of atopic rhinitis, a condition characterized by an unusually foul odor.

Klebsiella oxytoca (Brenner et al.[26])

In the early 1950s Danish workers found more than 10% of *Klebsiella* isolates to be indole positive. These strains usually liquified gelatin slowly. They were recently shown to be pectinolytic.

The name *Bacterium oxytocum* was revived for the gelatin-liquefying strains, but these strains were not accepted as a new species. They have been considered as an indole-positive, gelatin-positive biogroup of *Klebsiella pneumoniae*.[3,22] A study at the Center for Disease Control (CDC) showed that 6% of some 700 *K. pneumoniae* strains received were indole positive. Slightly more than one-half of the indole-positive strains liquefied gelatin. Only one indole-negative strain liquefied gelatin.[109] Both indole-positive, gelatin-positive and indole-positive, gelatin-negative strains are pectinolytic, while all other klebsiellae are pectate negative.

Deoxyribonucleic acid reassociation is a sensitive method for determining genetic relatedness between organisms. Using this technic Brenner et al. showed that clinical isolates of the 3 recognized species of *Klebsiella*, *K. pneumoniae*, *K. ozaenae*, and *K. rhinoscleromatis*, belong to the same DNA relatedness

Table 79-30. Differentiation within the genus *Klebsiella**†

Test or substrate	K. pneumoniae			K. ozaenae			K. rhinoscleromatis		
	Sign	%+	(%+)‡	*Sign*	%+	(%+)‡	*Sign*	%+	(%+)‡
Urease	+	95.4	(0.1)	d	14.8ʷ	(14.8)		0	
Methyl red	− or +	11.3		+	97.7		+	100	
Voges-Proskauer	+	93.7			0			0	
Citrate (Simmons'*)	+	96.8	(0.6)	d	28.1	(32.4)		0	
Lysine decarboxylase	+	97.2	(0.1)	− or +	35.8	(6.3)		0	
Malonate	+	92.5		−	6		+ or −	50	
Mucate	+	92.8		− or +	25			0	
Sodium alginate (utilization)	+ or (+)	88.5	(9.2)	− or (+)	0	(11)		0	
Gas from glucose	+	96		d	55.5	(9.4)		0	
Lactose	+	98.7	(1)	d	26.2	(61.3)	d	0	(70)
Dulcitol	− or +	33			0			0	
Organic acid media									
Citrate	+ or −	64.4		− or +	18			0	
D-tartrate	+ or −	67.1		− or +	39			0	

*From Ewing, W. H.: Differentiation of *Enterobacteriacea* by biochemical reactions, Atlanta, 1973, Center for Disease Control.
†+, 90% or more positive within 1 or 2 d; (+), positive reaction after 3 or more d (decarboxylase tests: 3 or 4 d); −, no reaction (90% or more); + or −, most cultures positive, some strains negative; − or +, most strains negative, some cultures positive; + or (+), most reactions occur within 1 or 2 d, some are delayed; d, different reactions: +, (+), −; w, weakly positive reaction.
‡Figures in parentheses indicate percentages of positive reactions that were delayed 3 or more d.

group.[113] Indole-positive strains were not included in this study. Jain et al.[114] showed that 4 indole-positive, gelatin-positive strains were in a DNA relatedness group separate from all other *Klebsiella* and *Enterobacter* species. They recommended that these organisms be placed as a new species in a new genus. They did not propose a name.

Brenner, Steigerwalt, and Fife-Asbury at CDC have now studied DNA relatedness in about 30 indole-positive strains that are either delayed gelatin positive or gelatin negative. These strains are clearly different from *K. pneumoniae*, *K. ozaenae*, and *K. rhinoscleromatis*. Most indole-positive strains are 75% or more related regardless of the gelatin reaction. They are 40-60% related to other *Klebsiella* species. In Brenner's group's opinion they should remain in the genus *Klebsiella* and be designated *K. oxytoca*.

K. oxytoca are simple to identify biochemically. Their reactions are typical of *K. pneumoniae* except that they are **indole positive.** They may or may not liquefy gelatin (this reaction may take as long as 30 days). They are pectate positive when tested with von Riesen's method,[115,116] but negative with the pectate test of Martin and Ewing.[22]

Tests of particular usefulness for differentiation of *Klebsiella* species are shown in Table 79-30.

ENTEROBACTER

The genus *Enterobacter* includes **motile** gram-negative rods that are indole and H_2S negative. Gelatin is liquefied slowly by the most common forms (*E. cloacae*). The Voges-Proskauer reaction is positive and lysine decarboxylase is produced (but not by *E. cloacae*). All species produce ornithine decarboxylase. Acid is produced by the majority of species from lactose, sucrose, sorbitol, rhamnose, and arabinose. For differential biochemical characteristics see Tables 79-14 and 79-29.

Enterobacter organisms occur in the intestinal tract of humans and animals and in soil, dairy products, water, and sewage. *Enterobacter* organisms seem to occur often as secondary pathogens, and they have been isolated from sputum, urine, blood, and wounds and have been reported from hospital-acquired infections.[111,117–123]

Enterobacter species

E. aerogenes, E. cloacae, E. hafniae (Hafnia alvei), and *E. agglomerans (Erwinia herbicola)* are listed by Ewing (Tables 79-8 and 79-29) as members of the genus *Enterobacter*. The Center for Disease Control (Brenner et al.[26]) recently has added 2 new species, *E. sakazaki* and *E. gergoviae;* the former *E. liquefaciens* has been moved into the genus *Serratia*, and *E. hafniae* is now known as *Hafnia alvei* (see below). Of these, *E. cloacae* (formerly *Aerobacter* subgroup A) is probably the most commonly occurring form. It differs from the other species in that

it is lysine decarboxylase negative, liquefies gelatin (slowly), and does not form gas from inositol and glycerol.

E. aerogenes (Aerobacter subgroup B) and *E. hafniae* (see Table 79-8 for *Hafnia alvei*, also discussion below) differ mainly in that the former produces acid and gas from adonitol, inositol, sorbitol, and raffinose and is mucate positive. Lactose is attacked by *E. aerogenes* but slowly or not at all by *E. hafniae*.

There also seems to be a rather sharp distinction in the antibiotic susceptibility of these organisms. *Klebsiella* strains seem to be sensitive to cephalothin, whereas *E. cloacae* strains are highly resistant to cephalothin and variably sensitive to ampicillin. Other *Enterobacter* strains seem to be somewhat more susceptible to ampicillin than *E. cloacae*.

A detailed study of bacteriologic and epidemiologic characteristics of *E. hafniae* and *E. liquefaciens* has been reported by Washington et al.[124]

As stated by Brenner et al.,[26] the organisms previously reported by the Center for Disease Control Enteric Section as *Enterobacter hafniae* will henceforth be reported as *Hafnia alvei*. Biochemical reactions for *H. alvei* are unchanged from those reported for *E. hafniae*. The change is purely a nomenclatural one that has been made on the basis of biochemical and DNA studies. Steigerwalt et al.[125] showed that DNA from *H. alvei* was only 15-25% related to DNAs from representative species of all genera in *Enterobacteriaceae*. Relatedness of *H. alvei* to *Enterobacter aerogenes* and *Enterobacter cloacae* was no greater than relatedness of *H. alvei* to strains of *Citrobacter, Edwardsiella,* or *E. coli*. DNA studies between strains of *H. alvei* indicated 2 different relatedness groups with 50-55% relatedness between the 2 groups. Additional, as yet unpublished, biochemical and DNA studies showed 3 separate groups within *H. alvei* (Fanning, Hickman, Cadet, Vaughn, and Brenner, unpublished data). In all probability the species now designated as *H. alvei* will eventually be split into 3 species. These species will form a biochemically and genetically homogeneous genus *Hafnia*.

E. liquefaciens (now moved to *Serratia* as *S. liquefaciens*, see below) is rhamnose negative and liquefies gelatin within 1-2 days. For differentiation see Table 79-29.

Enterobacter agglomerans

This organism is representative of a group of microorganisms called the *Herbicola-Lathyri* bacteria. Ewing and Fife[126] recognized 2 **biogroups** within the species:

1. An aerogenic (gas produced from glucose fermentation) biogroup composed of 4 biotypes
2. An anaerogenic (no gas produced from glucose fermentation) biogroup composed of 7 biotypes

In *Bergey's Manual*, ed. 8,[3] the genus *Erwinia* is divided into 3 groups: the *Amylovora* group, the *Carotovora* group, and the *Herbicola* group. The Herbicola group contains 3 species, one of which has 2 varieties. These *Herbicola* organisms are all contained in *E. agglomerans*. The available data strongly suggest the need to separate these bacteria into more than 1 species.

Of some 300 isolates studied by the CDC Enteric Bacteriology Unit, 180 were from extra-intestinal human sources such as blood, wounds, and the gallbladder; 13 from intestinal human sources; 4 from unknown human anatomic sources; 15 from various species of animals; 5 from foods; 17 from the environment; 23 from unknown sources; and 34 from the collection of D. C. Graham. Furthermore, this organism has been recovered from IV fluids administered to patients who subsequently developed septicemias.

The single most important factor in detecting *E. agglomerans* is the observation of a **yellow pigment.** Unfortunately, numerous strains are unpigmented. As an aid in the early differentiation of *Enterobacter agglomerans,* good use may be made of the characteristics of the organism on triple sugar iron (TSI) and lysine iron agar (LIA) (see Table 79-13). The failure of *E. agglomerans* to decarboxylate or deaminate lysine and the absence of H_2S are important initial observations because these characteristics eliminate large numbers of Enterobacteriaceae from further consideration. The only organisms with common TSI and LIA reactions are *E. coli, Shigella,* some strains of *Proteus morganii,* H_2S-negative strains of *Citrobacter,* and *E. cloacae. E. agglomerans* can be differentiated from most of these biochemically diverse organisms rather easily (see Table 79-29); however, it must be differentiated from some species of *Shigella* by comparing reactivity on a number of tests.

E. agglomerans can usually be differentiated from *Flavobacterium* on the basis of TSI and LIA reactions. The latter organisms yield K/N (alkaline/neutral) or A(cid)/N TSI results and K/N LIA results.

Enterobacter sakazakii[26]

Pigmented strains that biochemically resemble *Enterobacter cloacae* have been isolated in many laboratories. A case report of such a strain first appeared in 1965. A pigmented *Enterobacter* was isolated from an infant with neonatal meningitis in Denmark.[127] DNA relatedness studies showed that the pigmented strains were not closely related to nonpigmented *E. cloacae.*[125] Biochemical differences were not immediately evident between pigmented and nonpigmented strains. Subsequently Farmer showed that the pigmented strains were separable from nonpigmented strains on the basis of DNase and acid production from D-sorbitol reactions. The pigmented strains have been named *Enterobacter sakazakii.* The reactions important in distinguishing *E. sakazakii* from other *Enterobacter* species are shown in Table 79-31; the biochemical profile of *E. sakazakii* is shown in Table 79-32.

The definitive tests for confirming *E. sakazakii* are given below.

1. *Yellow pigment at 25 C.* A single colony is touched and used for inoculating a trypicase soy agar plate or slant. The slant is placed in a 25 C incubator (or at room temperature; 25 ± 3 C) and incubated up to 5 d. After 24-72 h, a bright yellow pigment is visible.

2. *DNase toluidine blue at 36 C.* Commercial DNase medium is made according to manufacturer's instructions, and then 0.1 g/L of toluidine blue dye is added. After dye dissolves, flask is autoclaved at 121 C for 15 min and cooled to 45-50 C. Contents are poured into 100 × 15mm Petri dishes (about 25 ml per dish). Cultures are inoculated in small patch on plate (after medium has dried) and incubated at 36 C for 2-6 d. DNase reaction is considered positive when medium turns pink-red around colony. Nonpigmented *E. cloacae* and most other Enterobacteriaceae are negative, but *Enterobacter sakazakii* gives positive reaction at 2-6 d at 36 C.

3. *Acid production from D-Sorbitol.* D-Sorbitol is added to Andrade's fermentation base or to another good fermentation base (such as commercial phenol red broth base or purple broth base) at a final concentration of 0.5%. Medium is dispensed into tubes and autoclaved at 121 C for 10 min. A single colony is used to inoculate tube, and it is observed for acid production and color change.

Table 79-31. Biochemical reactions to differentiate *Enterobacter sakazakii* from other *Enterobacter* species*

| Species | Biochemical test (% positive)† | | | | | |
| | Yellow pigment | 6-day DNase | D-Sorbitol | Decarboxylases | | |
				Lysine	Arginine	Ornithine
E. sakazakii	100	97	0	0	100	97
E. cloacae	0	0	95	0	97	96
E. aerogenes	0	0	99	99	1	99
Hafnia alvei (E. hafniae)	0	0	0	99	9	99
E. agglomerans	80	A few?	24	0	0	0

*From Brenner, D.J., Farmer, J.J., III, Hickman, F. W., et al.: Taxonomic and nomenclature changes in *Enterobacteriaceae,* DHEW publ. no. (CDC) 78-8356, Atlanta, Oct. 1977, Center for Disease Control.

†Reactions occurred within 48 h at 36 ± 1 C for all tests except yellow pigment (room temperature, 48 h) and DNase toluidine blue (36 C, 3-6 d).

Table 79-32. Biochemical reactions for 32 isolates of (yellow) *Enterobacter sakazakii**

Test	Percent positive within 48 h[†]	Proposed holotype strain (ATCC 29544)	Test	Percent positive within 48 h[†]	Proposed holotype strain (ATCC 29544)
Indole	16	–	L-Rhamnose	100	+
Methyl red	22	–	Maltose	100	+
Voges-Proskauer	97	+	D-Xylose	100	+
Citrate	100	+	Trehalose	100	+
H$_2$S-TSI	0	–	Cellobiose	100	+
Urea	0	–	Glycerol	94	+[2]
Phenylalanine deaminase	Very weak[‡]	Very weak[‡]	αCH$_3$-glucoside	94	+
			Erythritol	0	–
Lysine decarboxylase	0	–	Esculin (black precipitate)	100	+
Arginine dihydrolase	100	+			
Ornithine decarboxylase	97	+	D-Mannose	100	+
			Melibiose	100	+
Motility	94	+	Amygdalin	0	(+[5])
Gelatin (22 C)	0	(+[8])	D-Arabitol	0	–
KCN	94	+	Jordan's tartrate	0	–
Malonate	16	–	Mucate	0	–
D-Glucose acid	100	+	Acetate	94	+
D-Glucose gas	97	+	Lipase (corn oil)	0	–
Acid from:			DNase (36 C)	19[§]	(+[3])
Lactose	100	+	DNase (25 C)	0	(+[6])
Sucrose	100	+	Pectate liquefaction	0	–
D-Mannitol	100	+	H$_2$S PIA	0	–
Dulcitol	6	–	Glucose fermented in OF	100	+
Salicin	100	+			
Adonitol	0	–	Oxidase	0	–
i-Inositol	72	+	NO$_3^-$ → NO$_2^-$	100	+
D-Sorbitol	0	–	Gram-negative rod	100	+
L-Arabinose	100	+	Yellow pigment (25 C)	100	+
Raffinose	100	+	ONPG	100	+

*From Brenner, D. J., Farmer, J. J., III, Hickman, F. W., et al.: Taxonomic and nomenclature changes in *Enterobacteriaceae*, DHEW publ. no. (CDC) 78-8356, Atlanta, Oct. 1977, Center for Disease Control.

†All biochemical reactions are at 36 ± 1 C unless otherwise specified.

‡All isolates produced a slight amount of green when FeCl$_3$ was added to slant (24 h growth). These reactions are much weaker than reactions given by *Proteus* and *Providencia*. We feel that most workers would record these doubtful reactions as "–" or "+ very weak."

§Most of positive DNase reactions were delayed. Cumulative percent positive was as follows (36 C): day 1, 0; day 2, 19%; day 3, 66%; day 4, 78%; day 5, 91%; day 14, 100%. Reactions at 25 C were even slower.

Table 79-33. Biochemical reactions to distinguish *Enterobacter gergoviae* from other species of *Enterobacter* and *Hafnia**[†]

Test	E. gergoviae	E. aerogenes	E. cloacae	E. sakazakii	H. alvei	E. agglomerans
KCN	–	+	+	+	+	d
Urease	+	–	d^w	–	–	d
Lysine decarboxylase	+ or (+)	+	–	–	+	–
Arginine dihydrolase	–	–	+	+	–	–
Ornithine decarboxylase	+	+	+	+	+	–
D-Sorbitol	–	+	+	–	–	d
Sucrose	+	+	+	+	–	d
Raffinose	+	+	(+)	+	–	d
Simmons' citrate	+	+	+	+	d	d
Mucate	–	+	d	–	–	d
Yellow pigment	–	–	–	+	–	d
DNase	–	–	–	(+)	–	–

*From Brenner, D. J., Farmer, J. J., III, Hickman, F. W., et al.: Taxonomic and nomenclature changes in *Enterobacteriaceae*, DHEW publ. no. (CDC) 78-8356, Atlanta, Oct. 1977, Center for Disease Control.

†+, 90% or more; –, 10% or less; d, between 10.1-89.9%; w, weak; (+), positive after 3-7 d.

Table 79-34. Biochemical reactions of *Enterobacter gergoviae**†

Test	Reaction	Percent positive
Indole	−	0
Methyl red	d	36
Voges-Proskauer	+	100
Simmons' citrate	+	97
H₂S	−	0
Urease	+	100
Phenylalanine deaminase	−	0
Lysine decarboxylase	+ or (+)	64 (33)
Arginine dihydrolase	−	0
Ornithine decarboxylase	+	100
Motility	+	97
Gelatin (22 C)	−	0
KCN	−	0
Malonate	+	100
Gas from D-glucose	+	93
Acid from:		
Lactose	d	42 (18)
Sucrose	+	100
D-Mannitol	+	100
Dulcitol	−	0
Salicin	+	94
Adonitol	−	0
i-Inositol	−	0 (30)
D-Sorbitol	−	0
L-Arabinose	+	100
Raffinose	+	100
L-Rhamnose	+	100
Maltose	+	94
D-Xylose	+	97 (3)
Trehalose	+	100
Cellobiose	+	94
α-CH₃-glucoside	−	0
Erythritol	−	0
Esculin	+	94
Melibiose	+	100
Glycerol	+	100
Mucate	−	3
Jordan's tartrate	+	100
Sodium acetate	+	100
Lipase (corn oil)	−	0
DNase (25 C)	−	0
ONPG	+	100
Pigment	−	0
NO₃⁻ → NO₂⁻	+	97

*From Brenner, D. J., Farmer, J. J., III, Hickman, F. W., et al.: Taxonomic and nomenclature changes in *Enterobacteriaceae*, DHEW publ. no. (CDC) 78-8356, Atlanta, Oct. 1977, Center for Disease Control.

†+, 90% or more positive; −, 0-10.0% positive; d 10.1-89.9% positive; ( ), positive reaction in 3-7 d; + or (+), most reactions occur within 1 or 2 d, some are delayed.

Enterobacter gergoviae[26]

Biochemically these organisms are most similar to *E. aerogenes*. Thirty strains were isolated from urine, pus, nasopharynx, and blood from patients in France and Africa. The species was also implicated in a nosocomial outbreak of urinary tract infection.[128] Six strains of *E. gergoviae* isolated from wounds, sputum, and blood were sent to CDC during 1976. They exhibit the following differential biochemical characteristics: urease positive, KCN negative, sorbitol negative, and gelatinase negative.

The biochemical tests used to distinguish *E. gergoviae* from other *Enterobacter* (and *Hafnia*) species are shown in Table 79-33, and a summary of biochemical reactions for *E. gergoviae* is given in Table 79-34.

ERWINIA

The 8th edition of *Bergey's Manual*[3] lists the genus *Erwinia* in the family *Enterobacteriaceae* as plant pathogens or saprophytes; however, it states that one species (*E. herbicola*) has also been isolated from animal and human hosts.

Cooper-Smith and von Graevenitz[129] point out that by 1978, despite the taxonomic confusion (see Edwards and Ewing[20]), *E. herbicola*-like organisms (*E. herbicola-lathyri* group, named *Enterobacter agglomerans;* see *Enterobacter*, above) were known to be significant human pathogens.

A variety of infections with this group in humans have been described,[129–136] including a series of positive blood cultures in 15 patients (in a nonepidemic context).[129]

A detailed description of the organism is given under *Enterobacter agglomerans* (above).

SERRATIA

Cultures of *Serratia marcescens* have been used for many years by bacteriologists for demonstration purposes in the laboratory or for tracer studies because the bright, red pigment (prodigiosin) of some strains is so easily observable. The organisms have always been considered harmless saprophytes, occurring in soil and water, and believed incapable of growing at 35 C.

Since 1960, infections in humans due to *S. marcescens* have been reported with increasing frequency. Gale and Sonnenwirth in 1962[5] recovered 12 cultures of *S. marcescens* from 9 patients in 1 hospital in a period of approximately 6 mo; since then, the organism has been in many (often severe) nosocomial infections.

S. marcescens is usually involved in patients who already have other disorders and who have been on broad-spectrum antibiotic therapy. Indwelling urinary catheters, endotracheal tubes, and tracheostomy tubes put the patient at special risk. *S. marcescens* can cause urinary and respiratory tract infections, septicemia, endocarditis, meningitis, osteomyelitis,[137, 138] and wound infections.[139] Outbreaks of infection have occurred in intensive-care, renal dialysis, and nursery units. The organism has been cultured from irrigating fluids, respirators, nebulizers, liquid soap, and humidifier reservoirs.[139] *Serratia* can be passively transmitted on the hands of hospital personnel.

Most serratiae strains are resistant to 5 or more antibiotics. Gentamicin, tobramycin, kanamycin, chloramphenicol, and carbenicillin are useful, but gentamicin and tobramycin-resistant strains are emerging; amikacin is useful in such cases. Antibiotic therapy should be dictated by the sensitivity pattern of the organism.

Table 79-35. Differentiation of species of *Serratia**†

Test or substrate	S. marcescens			S. liquefaciens			S. rubidaea		
	Sign	%+	(%+)‡	Sign	%+	(%+)‡	Sign	%+	(%+)‡
Voges-Proskauer	+	98.7		− or +	49.5		+	92	
Lysine decarboxylase	+	99.6		+ or (+)	64.2	(31.2)	+ or (+)	61	(31)
Ornithine decarboxylase	+	99.6		+	100		−	0	
Malonate	−	1.6		−	0.9		+ or −	86	
KCN	+	98.9		+	91.7		− or +	22	
Lactose	−	1.3	(4.6)	d	15.6	(21)	+	100	
Adonitol	d	46.5	(13.8)	d	8.3	(5.5)	+ or (+)	88	(2)
Sorbitol									
Acid	+	99.1		+	97.3		−	8	
Gas	−	0		d	57.8	(19.3)	−	0	
Arabinose	−	0		+	97.3		+	100	
Raffinose	−	1.2	(0.8)	+	90.8	(4.6)	+	96	
Xylose	d	7.1	(17.2)	+	99.1	(0.9)	+	98	
Glycerol									
Acid	+	97.2	(1.8)	+	92.2	(6.8)	d	29	(18)
Gas	−	0		d	39.8	(30.1)	−	0	
Melibiose	−	0		d	73.8	(7.5)	+	96	

*From Ewing, W. H.: Differentiation of *Enterobacteriaceae* by biochemical reactions, Atlanta, 1973, Center for Disease Control.
†+, 90% or more positive within 1 or 2 d; (+), positive reaction after 3 or more d (decarboxylase tests: 3 or 4 d); −, no reaction (90% or more); + or −, most cultures positive, some strains negative; − or +, most strains negative, some cultures positive; + or (+), most reactions occur within 1 or 2 d, some are delayed; d, different reactions: +, (+), −; w, weakly positive reaction.
‡Figures in parentheses indicate percentages of delayed reactions (3 or more d).

For a review of *S. marcescens*, a historical perspective, and clinical status, see Yu[27]; the review by Grimont and Grimont[140] includes, in addition, taxonomic and genetic data.

Subdivision of serratiae into 3 species, *S. marcescens* (the most common in clinical practice), *S.* (formerly *Enterobacter*) *liquefaciens*, and *S. rubidaea*, is achieved by biochemical tests[141] (see Tables 79-14, 79-29, and 79-35).

Biochemical characteristics and identification of serratiae

Serratiae are **motile** rods that grow well on the usual laboratory media. Some strains are hemolytic on blood agar. Gelatin is liquefied rapidly,[142] and lysine and ornithine are decarboxylated. All *Serratia* strains produce deoxyribonuclease (DNase). Gas is either not formed from fermentable substances or, if formed, the gas volume is small (10% or less). The pigmented strains constitute only 10% or less of *Serratia* isolates in hospitals. Pigment formation is more pronounced and brighter when the culture is held at room temperature. The pigments, which are water insoluble and diffuse in the agar only when the color is very deep, range from light pink through red to deep purple-red. A characteristic odor of trimethylamine is produced by the cultures.

The Voges-Proskauer reaction is positive in *S. marcescens* and in *S. rubidaea*, but variable in *S. liquefaciens* (Table 79-35). On TSI slants, in which they are often inoculated, since they show lactose-nonfermenting colonies, an alkaline slant/acid butt reaction occurs, with no gas usually formed. Some strains show acid slant/acid butt reaction (depending on rate of sucrose fermentation).

Serratiae are differentiated from enterobacters by their rapid **gelatin** liquefaction, positive reactions in DNase, and failure to produce gas from glycerol acid from arabinose. *Aeromonas* species, which can be sometimes confused with *Serratia* organisms, are cytochrome **oxidase positive** and do not ferment sorbitol but produce acid in arabinose.

At least 15 O and 16 H antigens have been identified; **serotyping**,[143] **bacteriocin** susceptibility **typing**,[144] and **biotyping**[145] are useful for epidemiologic studies.

Selective medium: CT agar.[146] Among the various selective media recommended for *Serratia*, CT agar (Caprylate-Thallous agar) seems to be quite useful in ecologic surveys. For details of the medium, refer to Starr et al.[146]

PROTEEAE
Proteus and Providencia

Ewing[19, 20] lists 2 genera, *Proteus* (4 species) and *Providencia* (2 species), in this tribe, whereas *Bergey's Manual*, ed. 8,[3] recognizes only the genus *Proteus* with 5 species (Table 79-8). Clinical usage in the United States has been based on Ewing's system until recently, when the Center for Disease Control recommended changes in classification, on both genus and species level, as of 1978[26] (see Table 79-9 and below).

PROTEUS*

The organisms in the genus *Proteus* are straight, motile rods. Two species (*P. vulgaris* and *P. mirabilis*) show a **swarming** phenomenon, producing a confluent growth. Swarming

—————
*Ewing.[15, 20]

occurs only in the absence of bile salts. *Proteus* organisms are **lactose negative, urease and phenylalanine deaminase positive.** Two species, *P. vulgaris* and *P. mirabilis*, produce H_2S rapidly and liquefy gelatin. Ornithine decar-boxylase is produced by *P. mirabilis* and *P. morganii.*

The occurrence of the swarming species presents occasional difficulties in the isolation of other organisms present on the same plate.

Table 79-36. Biochemical reactions of species in the tribe *Proteeae*†

Test	Proteus mirabilis	Proteus vulgaris	Providencia alcalifaciens	Providencia stuartii	Providencia rettgeri	Morganella morganii
Indole	− 2‡	+ 98	+ 99	+ 99	+ 100	+ 99.5
Methyl red	+ 99	+ 93	+ 99.9	+ 100	+ 93	+ 97
Voges-Proskauer	v 16	− 0	− 0	− 0	− 0	− 0
Simmons' citrate	v 59	v 11	+ 98	+ 93	+ 96	− 0
H_2S-TSI	+ 94	+ 95	− 0	− 0	− 0	− 0
Urea	v 88	+ 95	− 0	v 15§	+ 99	+ 98
Phenylalanine deaminase	+ 99	+ 100	+ 97	+ 95	+ 98	+ 95
Lysine decarboxylase	− 0	− 0	− 0	− 0	− 0	− 1
Arginine dihydrolase	− 0	− 0	− 0	− 0	− 0	− 0
Ornithine decarboxylase	+ 99	− 0	− 1	− 0	− 0	+ 97
Motility (36 C)	+ 95	+ 95	+ 96	v 86	+ 94	v 88
Gelatin (22 C)	+ 92	+ 91	− 0	− 0	− 0	− 0
KCN	+ 99	+ 100	+ 99	+ 99	+ 97	+ 99
Malonate	− 2	− 0	− 0	− 0	− 1	− 5
D-Glucose-acid	+ 100	+ 100	+ 100	+ 100	+ 100	+ 100
D-Glucose-gas	+ 96	+ 86	v 85	− 0	v 12	v 86
Acid from:						
Lactose	− 2	− 0	− 1	− 4	− 5	− 0
Sucrose	v 19	+ 95	v 13	v 31	v 13	− 1
D-Mannitol	− 0	− 0	− 2	v 13	+ 99	− 0
Dulcitol	− 0	− 0	− 0	− 0	− 0	− 0
Salicin	− 1	v 58	− 1	− 2	v 50	− 0
Adonitol	− 0	− 0	+ 94	− 4	+ 99	− 0
i-Inositol	− 0	− 0	− 1	+ 97	+ 93	− 0
D-Sorbitol	− 0	− 0	− 1	− 3	− 0	− 0
L-Arabinose	− 0	− 0	− 1	− 4	− 0	− 0
Raffinose	− 1	− 0	− 1	− 5	− 9	− 0
L-Rhamnose	− 2	− 9	− 0	− 0	v 75	− 0
Maltose	− 1	+ 96	− 1	− 3	− 2	− 0
D-Xylose	+ 96	v 89	− 1	− 6	v 15	− 0
Trehalose	+ 98	v 30	− 4	+ 99	− 1	v 14
Cellobiose	− 2	− 0	− 1	− 10	− 4	− 0
α-CH_3-glucoside	− 0	v 80	− 0	− 0	− 2	− 0
Erythritol	− 0	− 3	− 0	− 0	v 78	− 0
D-Mannose	− 0	− 0	+	+	+ 100	+ 100
Esculin	− 1	v 59	− 0	− 0	v 30	− 0
Melibiose	−	−	−	−	−	−
D-Arabitol	−	−	−	− 0	+ 99	−
Glycerol	+ 90	v 79	v 12	v 12	v 66	− 5
Mucate	− 0	− 0	− 0	− 0	− 0	− 0
Jordan's tartrate	v 88	+ 93	+ 100	+ 96	+ 96	+ 93
Sodium acetate	v 13	v 23	v 30	v 81	v 59	− 0
Lipase (corn oil)	+ 92	v 87	− 0	− 0	− 0	− 0
DNase (25 C)	v	v	−	−	−	−
$NO_3^- \rightarrow NO_2^-$	+ 94	+ 100	+ 100	+ 100	+ 99	v 89
Oxidase	− 0	− 0	− 0	− 0	− 0	− 0
ONPG	−	−	−	−	−	−
Tyrosine clearing	+	+	+	+	+	+
Pectate	−	−	−	−	−	−

*From Brenner, D. J., Farmer, J. J., III, Hickman, F. W., et al.: Taxonomic and nomenclature changes in *Enterobacteriaceae*, DHEW publ. no (CDC) 78-8356, Atlanta, Oct. 1977, Center for Disease Control.

†+, 90% or greater positive; −, 10% or less positive; v = 10.1-89.9% positive. All reactions are at 36±1 C for 48 h.

‡Number gives percentage positive at 48 h (24 h for phenylalanine, $NO_3^- \rightarrow NO_2^-$, and oxidase). Data were tabulated by W. H. Ewing, B. R. Davis, F. W. Hickman, and J. J. Farmer III from over 1000 cultures submitted to the CDC for identification. Some of data for *Providencia rettgeri* are taken from paper by Penner, J. L., Hinton, N. A., and Hennessy, J. N.: J. Clin. Microbiol. 1:136-142, 1975. When limited data are available no actual percentage is given.

§Estimate based on strains sent to Penner for serotyping.

As described earlier, differential and selective media tend to restrict the swarming of *Proteus* (deoxycholate citrate, SS media). Raising the agar content of medium to 5% or the use of Naylor Lemco agar eliminates swarming and allows the isolation of accompanying organisms.

Since the organisms are **lactose negative,** they sometimes are inoculated into TSI medium from isolation plates. The reactions on this medium and a urease test on Christensen urea agar, where they **usually** give a positive reaction **in 2-4 hours,** allow rapid identification of the organisms.

Biochemical reactions of *Proteus* species are shown in Tables 79-14 and 79-36.

Speciation can be achieved in most instances by the use of 2 tests, namely, H_2S production and ornithine decarboxylase activity, and additionally by indole production, citrate utilization, and mannitol fermentation. The most commonly encountered species, *P. mirabilis*, does not produce indole from tryptophan, while the others do. Clinicians often speak of "indole-positive *Proteus*" (encompassing the other species) and "indole-negative *Proteus*" (*P. mirabilis*). The indole-positive protei are much more resistant to antibiotics than *P. mirabilis*. However, a recently described **indole-negative** *P. rettgeri* strain,[147] involved in nosocomial urinary tract infections, is highly resistant to all antimicrobials in use.

Proteus organisms have an historic interest insofar as Weil and Felix (1917) coined the terms H (*Hauch*, filmy covering) for flagellar, motile organisms and O (*Ohne Hauch*, without filmy covering) for nonmotile organisms while working with *Proteus*. They studied patients with typhus (a rickettsial disease) and found that serum from these patients agglutinated their X19 and X2 *Proteus* strains. Many years later it was found that the cross-reaction is due to a polysaccharide present both in certain *Proteus* strains and in *Rickettsia prowazeki* (see Weil-Felix reaction).

The H and O terminology was later extended to denote somatic antigens (O) and flagellar antigens (H).

For changes in *Proteus* nomenclature see "Changes in *Proteus-Providencia* Taxonomy, CDC Recommendations" in *"Providencia"* below.

Infections in humans

Proteus organisms are commonly found in soil, sewage, and manure. They are found with some frequency in normal human feces, but often in much increased numbers in individuals on antibiotic therapy. The organisms are frequent causes of **urinary tract infection** (both community and hospital-acquired) and are also involved in other, often serious infections, such as septicemia, endocarditis, mastoiditis, or meningitis.

For a review of *Proteus rettgeri* infections, see Arroyo, Sonnenwirth, and Liebhaber.[148]

PROVIDENCIA (PROVIDENCE)

Providence organisms (genus *Providencia*) are motile, phenylalanine deaminase– and indole–positive rods. They do **not** hydrolyze urea, do not produce hydrogen sulfide, and do not liquefy gelatin. Lysine, arginine, and ornithine are not decarboxylated. Lactose and salicin are not fermented.

The designation Providence (originally *Proteus inconstans*) was proposed by Kauffmann.[149] Providence organisms can be mistaken for *Shigella* organisms, but differentiation can be accomplished by demonstrating motility, utilization of citrate, and a positive phenylalanine deaminase test, also positive in the 4 *Proteus* species. The biochemical characteristics of the organisms are listed in Tables 79-14 and 79-36. Ewing recognizes 2 species: *P. alcalifaciens* and *P. stuartii*.[18]

Members of the group occur in urinary tract infections and have been implicated in sporadic cases and outbreaks of diarrhea in humans.

P. stuartii has recently emerged as a major factor in burn infections, displaying marked resistance to many antibiotics,[150] while *P. alcalifaciens* is less frequently encountered and is susceptible to a variety of antibiotics. While gentamicin, kanamycin, carbenicillin, and amikacin are useful for *Providencia*, strains resistant to these antibiotics have already emerged; susceptibility tests are required.

An antigenic schema has been established for the group with 62 O antigen groups and 156 serotypes.

It should be noted here that Ewing's *Providencia* species is named *Proteus inconstans* by *Bergey's Manual*, ed. 8.[3]

Changes in Proteus-Providencia taxonomy— CDC* recommendations[26]

The Enteric Section, CDC, recognizes and reports 7 species of proteae; however, one of these, *Proteus myxofaciens*, is not medically significant and will not be considered further. Biochemical reactions of the other 6 species are given in Table 79-36.

Proteus mirabilis and *Proteus vulgaris* remain unchanged. *P. morganii* has been placed in a new genus, *Morganella*, as *M. morganii*, on genetic grounds (DNA relatedness).

Penner described five **biogroups** of *Proteus rettgeri*.[151] These biogroups are shown and compared with *Providencia stuartii* in Table 79-37; it is clear that, except for the positive urea reaction, biogroup 5 is essentially indistinguishable from *Providencia stuartii*. The O antigens of biogroup 5 are characteristic of *P. stuartii* rather than *P. rettgeri*.[152] By DNA relatedness these strains are indistinguishable from *Providencia*

*Center for Disease Control, Atlanta.

Table 79-37. Comparison of *Proteus rettgeri* biogroups (Penner) with *Providencia stuartii*[*][†]

| Reaction | P. rettgeri biogroup | | | | | | | | | | P. stuartii |
	1a	1b	2a	2b	3a	3b	4a	4b	5a	5b	
Urea	+	+	+	+	+	+	+	+	+	+	−
Trehalose	−	−	−	−	−	−	d	d	+	+	+
D-Mannitol	+	+	+	+	+	+	+	+	+	−	d
Salicin	+	+	+	+	−	−	−	−	−	−	−
L-Rhamnose	−	−	+	+	+	+	−	−	−	−	−
Adonitol	+	+	+	+	+	+	+	+	−	−	−
D-Arabitol	+	+	+	+	+	+	+	+	−	−	−
i-Erythritol	+	−	+	−	+	−	+	−	−	−	−

*From Brenner, D. J., Farmer, J. J., III, Hickman, F. W., et al.: Taxonomic and nomenclature changes in *Enterobacteriaceae*, DHEW publ. no. (CDC) 78-8356, Atlanta, Oct. 1977, Center for Disease Control.
†d, 10.1-89.9% positive; +, 90% or more positive; −, 10% or less positive.

stuartii. They must be viewed as urea positive *P. stuartii* and have been designated as such by Penner[152] and by Brenner et al.[153]

All species of *Proteus* and *Providencia* are **phenylalanine deaminase positive**. The **urea reaction** is relied on to separate urea-positive *Proteus* from *Providencia*.

Urea-negative *Proteus* strains are well documented. In fact, 5% of *P. vulgaris*, 10% of *P. mirabilis*, and 2% of *P. morganii* are urea negative.[20] *Providencia* are listed as 100% urea negative[20]; however, urea-positive strains of *Providencia* are described in several reports in the literature.

In terms of overall biochemical reactions, urea-positive *Providencia stuartii* (or *Proteus rettgeri* biogroup 5) are much more closely related to *P. stuartii* than to *P. rettgeri*.[152] Strains of *P. stuartii* are trehalose positive, adonitol negative, and D-arabitol negative; whereas *P. rettgeri* strains have the opposite reactions. *P. stuartii* strains are easily separated from *P. rettgeri* on the basis of the reactions listed in Table 79-37.

It is clear that the biogroup 5 organisms are **urea-positive** *Providencia stuartii*. The urease gene(s) is probably carried on a plasmid. Both urea-positive and urea-negative organisms have been reported in nosocomial outbreaks,[154] sometimes from the same patient. In the past these were assumed to be caused by both *Proteus rettgeri* and *Providencia stuartii*. We now know that they are due only to *P. stuartii*, some of which are urea positive.

The **true** *Proteus rettgeri* strains (biogroups 1-4) are both biochemically and genetically more closely related to *Providencia* species than to *Proteus* species. For these reasons they have been placed in *Providencia* as *Providencia rettgeri*.

After reviewing biochemical, serologic, and morphologic data on *Proteus* and *Providencia* as well as the DNA hybridization data, the CDC group proposed 3 generic changes: There are 3 related species in *Proteus*, 3 related species in *Providencia*, and a single species in *Morganella*. Additional species will no doubt be added to each of these genera as additional knowledge is accumulated.

YERSINIEAE
Yersinia[28, 29]

In the 7th edition of *Bergey's Manual*,[21] the genus *Pasteurella* was described as consisting of 9 species. Four of these were considered to be important in clinical medicine: *P. pestis*, *P. pseudotuberculosis*, *P. multocida*, and *P. tularensis*. By 1961, in recognition of its fastidiousness and specific growth factor requirements, *P. tularensis* was removed from the pasteurellae and placed in the new genus *Francisella*. It was then proposed that *P. pestis* and *P. pseudotuberculosis* be separated from the *Pasteurella* and placed into a separate genus named *Yersinia* (in honor of the French bacteriologist, A. J. Yersin, who first isolated the plague organism).[155] Other workers[156, 157] demonstrated a clear division of pasteurellae into 2 groups, i.e., those **oxidase positive** (containing cytochrome c in their respiratory electron transport chain) and those **oxidase negative**, and proposed that the oxidase-positive members of the genus be considered the true *Pasteurella* and that the oxidase-negative species should be considered members of the genus *Yersinia*. This was accomplished in the 8th edition of *Bergey's Manual*,[3] where Mollaret and Thal included these organisms in *Yersinia* and placed the genus in the family *Enterobacteriaceae*.

The reasons for placing the *Yersinia* in the family *Enterobacteriaceae* are as follows: (1) both groups are fermenters, i.e., utilize carbohydrates by fermentative pathways; (2) both reduce nitrate to nitrite; (3) 2 of the 3 *Yersinia*, when motile (at 22-25 C but not at 37 C) have peritrichous flagella like the *Enterobacteriaceae*; and (4) both groups are insensitive to bile salts, i.e., they grow on MacConkey agar.[31, 158] In addition, antigenic relationships among the 2 exist,[159] the DNA base composition of *Yersinia* is close to that of several *Enterobacteriaceae*,[160] and DNA/DNA homology studies support the relative closeness of the 2 groups.[161]

The 3 species of *Yersinia* are primarily found in animals (zoonotic bacteria): *Y. pestis* in rodents and insect vectors, and the other 2 species in a wide variety of mammals, and birds, where they may cause extensive epizootic outbreaks or may persist in healthy carriers.

In humans, Y. pestis is the causative agent of plague, while Y. pseudotuberculosis and Y. enterocolitica are responsible for a variety of syndromes (yersiniosis), most commonly enterocolitis and acute mesenteric lymphadenitis (often mimicking acute appendicitis).

Yersinia are relatively large (0.5-1.0 by 1-2 μm) coccobacillary, ovoid- or rod-shaped gram-negative bacteria, nonmotile at 37 C, but Y. pseudotuberculosis and Y. enterocolitica are **motile at 22-25 C**. The organisms are facultative anaerobes with good growth on ordinary media, including MacConkey agar; Y. enterocolitica produces very small translucent colonies on SS agar after 18 hours. All Yersinia ferment glucose, maltose, mannitol, trehalose, glycerol, xylose, and fructose with acid but no gas; they usually do not ferment lactose but produce β-D-galactosidase. They do not ferment dulcitol, inositol, raffinose, and melezitose. On initial isolation, Yersinia (especially Y. enterocolitica) strongly resemble certain other Enterobacteriaceae (especially anaerogenic "atypical coliforms," Proteus morganii, P. rettgeri, shigellae, Providencia) and are easily misdiagnosed.

With the combined use of triple sugar iron (TSI) agar and lysine iron (LIA) agar slants[163] (see Table 79-13), Yersinia can be presumptively differentiated from a large number of other fermentative gram-negative bacilli, with further tests to be undertaken for definitive identification. The TSI reactions are alkaline slant/acid butt, no gas (Y. pestis, Y. pseudotuberculosis); acid slant/acid butt, no gas (Y. enterocolitica, due to fermentation of sucrose; occasional Y. pseudotuberculosis). LIA reactions are alkaline slant/acid butt.

Any lactose-negative gram-negative rod that does not produce H₂S in TSI, is oxidase negative, motile only at room temperature, and is urease positive on Christensen urease agar in 3-24 hours, but is phenylalanine negative, should be suspected of being Y. enterocolitica or Y. pseudotuberculosis, and its further identification pursued.

Yersinia pestis

Y. pestis is a gram-negative rod, 0.5-0.7× 1.5-2 μm, occurring singly; it is **nonmotile.**

It is the causative agent of plague in humans, rats, and ground squirrels; the infected rat flea transmits it from rat to rat and from rat to human. In humans, clinical forms of plague are **bubonic** (most common), **pneumonic,** and **septicemic** plague; rarely, meningitis occurs.[165]

NOTE: **Material suspected of containing Y. pestis must be handled with extreme care; it is hazardous.** Laboratory personnel may become infected via broken skin, mucous membranes, or the respiratory tract through laboratory accidents.

Clinical specimens. The specimens can be aspirates from buboes, pus from the infection site (usually the area of a flea bite), blood (cultivable in routine blood culture bottles), sputum, or throat swabs, to be plated, in addition to blood agar, on MacConkey or deoxycholate agar; autopsy material, such as spleen, liver, lymph nodes, lung, heart blood, or bone marrow, are also used.

Staining. Y. pestis is gram negative and stains bipolarly. The bipolar characteristic is best demonstrated using **Wayson stain** (Chapter 71), the stain of choice for smears made from clinical material or rodent tissues.[21]

Prepare smears and fix with alcohol (preferable) or heat. Add Wayson stain for 7 min, then wash thoroughly with tap water, and allow the slide to air dry.

Bipolar staining ("safety pin" appearance) is not often seen in in vitro preparations (culture) but is very pronounced in tissue impressions, in **bubo** aspirates, and often in pus. **Caution:** Bipolar staining may be shown by other pasteurellae, enteric organisms, and diplococci. Gram stains of broth cultures may show Y. pestis in chains. In older cultures or on media containing 3% NaCl agar or glycerol, involution forms are produced (yeastlike, filamentous, or ring-shaped organisms).

Culture. Primary isolation media are (1) heart infusion agar, (2) blood agar, (3) deoxycholate agar, and (4) MacConkey agar. In laboratories equipped for reference work, antiserum agar and pesticin agar plates are also used. The media may be incubated at 28 C **or** 37 C.[164]

On blood agar base with 5% blood (human, sheep), incubated **at 28 C,** Y. pestis colonies are pinpoint in size. After 48 hours the colonies are 1-2 mm in size, grayish white, and convex. Growth is slower at both 20 C (room temperature) and 37 C. Y. pestis at 28 C produces a flocculent type of growth in broth, adhering to the sides of the tube. If shaken, the growth settles on the bottom. It does not produce a turbid growth.

On deoxycholate agar, growth does **not** appear until the second day when small, reddish, pinpoint colonies are observed.[165]

For a selective medium for Y. pestis, see Knisely et al.[166]

Characteristics. The organism is **nonmotile** at both 37 C and 20 C, an important diagnostic feature. It does not utilize citrate (Simmons), does not grow in KCN, does not produce acid from lactose, sucrose, or dulcitol, but ferments glucose and mannitol (no gas). It is indole, Voges-Proskauer, and urease negative; no H₂S is formed in TSI agar, and it is methyl red positive; lysine and ornithine decarboxylase and arginine dihydrolase are negative, and β-D-galactosidase (ONPG) positive. (See Tables 79-14 and 79-38.) Phenol red broth base (Difco) is a satisfactory medium for carbohydrate tests.

Bacteriophage. Reference laboratories use specific strains of bacteriophage that lyse all known strains of Y. pestis. These phages also

Table 79-38. Differential characteristics of *Yersinia**†

	Y. pestis			*Y. pseudotuberculosis*			*Y. enterocolitica*		
	Sign	%+	(%+)‡	Sign	%+	(%+)‡	Sign	%+	(%+)‡
Motility									
25 C	−	0		(+) or +	50.7	(45)	+	97.5	
37 C	−	0		−	0		−	0	
Urease	−	0		+	100		+	85.6	(10.2)
Phenylalanine deaminase	−	0		−	0		−	0	
Catalase	+			+			+		
Oxidase	−			−	0		−	0	
Simmons' citrate	−			− or (+)	0	(14.5)	−	0§	
H₂S (TSI)	−			−	0		−	0	
Lysine decarboxylase	−			−	0		−	0	
Arginine dihydrolase	−			−	0		−	0	
Ornithine decarboxylase	−			−	0		+	93.2	(4.3)
Esculin hydrolysis	+	100		+	100		d	19.5	(34.7)
β-Galactosidase									
37 C	+			+ or −	91.3		− or +	24.0	
25 C				+ or −	94.2		+	93.3	
Nitrate reduction	+			+	97.0		+	98.7	
Indole	−	0		−	0		− or +‖	40.0	
Methyl red									
37 C	+			+ʷ	100		+	100.0	
25 C				+	97.1		+	97.5	
Voges-Proskauer									
25 C	−			−	0		+ or −	76.3	
37 C	−			−	0		−	0	
Glucose, acid	+			+	100		+	100	
Lactose									
37 C	−			−	0		−	0	(10.2)
25 C				−	0		−	0	(13.6)
Sucrose	−			−	0		+	94.0	
Adonitol	−			+	0		−	0	
Rhamnose	−	0		−	100		−	1.3	
Salicin	− or +	19.0		(+)	1.4	(98.6)	d	22.9	(20.3)
Sorbitol	− or +			−	0		+	98.3	
Cellobiose	−			−	0		+ or (+)	92.4	(7.6)
Xylose				+	100		d	47.4	(10.2)
Mannitol	+			+	100		+	100	
Maltose									
37 C	+			+	90		d	53.4	(41.5)
25 C				+	100		+	94.9	(5.1)
Raffinose	−			− or +	20		−	5.1	
Arabinose	+	30.5		+ or (+)	46.4	(53.6)	+	97.5	(2.5)
Melibiose	d			+	90.0	(10.0)	−	0	
Trehalose	+			+	100		+ or (+)	92.4	(5.9)
Glycerol	−	1.9		+ or (+)	23.2	(76.8)	+ or (+)	61.9	(34.7)

*Percentages from Darland, G., Ewing, W. H., and Davis, B. R.: The biochemical characteristics of *Yersinia enterocolitica* and *Yersinia pseudotuberculosis*, DHEW publ. no. (CDC) 75-8294, Atlanta, 1975, Center for Disease Control; and Ewing, W. H., Tomfohrde, K. M., and Naudo, P.: API Species 1:13, 1977.

†+, 90% or more positive within 1 or 2 d; (+), positive reaction after 3 or more (decarboxylase tests: 3 or 4 d); −, no reaction (90% or more); + or −, most cultures positive, some strains negative; − or +, most strains negative, some cultures positive; + or (+), most reactions occur within 1 or 2 d, some are delayed; *d*, different reactions: +, (+), or −.

‡Delayed reactions (3 d or more).

§At 25 C, 1.7% positive.

‖Many strains isolated in the United States have been indole positive; majority of those isolated in Europe have been indole negative.

lyse *Y. pseudotuberculosis*, but only at 37 C and not at 20 C. For details, see Bahmanyar and Cavanaugh.[164]

Agglutination test. Specific *Y. pestis* antiserum can be used for the agglutination test with ether-methanol-glycerol-formalin–treated cells. The method is used in reference laboratories.

Fluorescent antibody methods. FA methods employing anti-*P. pestis* hyperimmune serum

globulins conjugated with fluorescein isothiocyanate can be used for staining direct smears and tissues, but it is less satisfactory for cultures. Because of the existence of cross-reactions, Goldenberg[167] cautions against uncritical use of the FA method.

Animal inoculations. Guinea pigs or albino mice are used. For details see Goldenberg.[167]

Serologic tests. Precipitin tests with animal

tissue, similar to the Ascoli tests for the diagnosis of anthrax, can be used. For complement-fixation and hemagglutination tests, see Chen and Meyer[168] and Balimanyar and Cavanaugh.[164]

Tests for fraction 1 antigen. These tests are usually conducted in an Ouchterlony gel-diffusion agar plate system. For details, see Bahmanyar and Cavanaugh.[164]

Public health aspects. Suspect and/or confirmed cases should immediately be reported to the local health authority and their instructions for shipment of material should be followed.

Materials suspected of containing plague organisms should be shipped in properly prepated containers with double screw tops. From human cases, material from bubo, skin lesion, excised lymph node, and sputum should be submitted. From autopsies, portions of spleen, liver, and bone marrow can also be included.

In the case of suspected rodents the whole carcass should be submitted, securely packed.

Antimicrobial susceptibility testing. Susceptibility testing of *Y. pestis* is misleading because it usually indicates susceptibility in vitro to penicillin, which is totally ineffective in the treatment of plague. *Y. pestis* is susceptible to streptomycin, tetracyclines, and chloramphenicol. Tetracyclines or chloramphenicol with or without streptomycin are highly effective in the therapy of plague.

• • •

A brief but useful review of the clinical aspects, epidemiology, and diagnosis of plague is that of Butler et al.[169] Serologic responses to *Y. pestis* infection were described by Butler and Hudson[170]; recent experiences with plague in the United States were reviewed by Palmer et al.[171] and Reed et al.[165]

Yersinia enterocolitica and Yersinia pseudotuberculosis[28–32]

The 2 organisms are both relatively large gram-negative coccobacilli and both are capable of producing disease (yersiniosis) in humans.

There is an extensive animal reservoir for *Y. pseudotuberculosis* including mammals (rabbits, cats, sheep, fox, cow, raccoon, various rodents, deer) and birds (turkey, canary, dove, pigeon). *Y. enterocolitica* has been isolated in Europe from both healthy and sick swine, dogs, rabbits, chinchillas, cows, sheep, horses, deer, chinchilla, dogs, frogs, snails, fleas, and laboratory reared primates in the Unites States and, in addition to the above, from swine, cats, beavers, raccoons, various birds, and oysters in Canada. In addition, certain serologic types of *Y. enterocolitica* have been recently recovered from numerous rivers, reservoirs, lakes, and wells both in Europe and North America. The organisms may cause extensive epizootic (animal) outbreaks characterized by diarrhea, lymphadenopathy with necrosis ("pseudotuberculosis"), pneumonia, abortions, liver and spleen abscess, osteomyelitis, and

septicemia. They may also persist latently in healthy carrier animals.[28,32]

It is likely that infection with these animal pathogens mostly occurs through the digestive tract, but no single source has yet been unequivocally identified. The major mode of transmission of *Y. pseudotuberculosis* to humans is probably through food contaminated by animal excreta; other possibilities include direct contact with infected animals and consumption of infected meat. Human-to-human transmission has not yet been reported. In the majority of *Y. enterocolitica* cases, infection undoubtedly occurs through the digestive tract. Occurrence of *Y. enterocolitica* interfamiliar[172] and institutional outbreaks and hospital-acquired infections[173] suggests person-to-person transmission, but foodstuffs and water are likely more important. There is evidence implicating the pig as a major reservoir for human infection in Europe and in Canada; in a recent New York State outbreak affecting 218 school children, foodborne transmission has been unequivocally documented, the infecting organism having been isolated from chocolate milk consumed by the children.[174]

Infection with *Y. pseudotuberculosis* in humans is recognized with moderate frequency in Europe but is relatively rare in the United States. *Y. enterocolitica* infections, recognized first in Europe as affecting animals and then humans, have been increasing and spreading dramatically around the world since 1963; so far 30 countries on 4 continents (except Australia) are known to be affected, with the likelihood that the infection remains unrecognized in several others. The first strains, however, were isolated in New York State (1933-1947) but were misclassified or else labeled as unidentified organisms[31,175]; the isolates, 2 of which are extant, have been identified in retrospect as *Y. enterocolitica*. No other cases of human infection were recognized in the United States for the next 21 years until 1968 when a case of *Y. enterocolitica* meningitis and septicemia was reported from Missouri.[31] By 1976, over 300 cases in humans were known in the United States, some 400 in Canada, and several thousand in Europe. Whether the rapid increase in human *Y. enterocolitica* infections now experienced in the United States and Canada (similar to that seen in the last decade both in Europe and Asia) is due to increased laboratory skill and awareness or represents an actual spread in humans and animals is not known.[30]

Both organisms grow on ordinary media in air or anaerobically, somewhat slower than other enteric bacilli. Both are **motile at 22-28 C but not at 37 C,** which helps distinguish them from *Y. pestis* and other *Enterobacteriaceae.* They produce acid but no gas from glucose, maltose, mannitol, trehalose, glycerol, and xylose; they usually do not ferment lactose, but produce β-D-galactosidase. They are **oxidase negative,** in contrast to species currently charac-

Table 79-39. Biogroups of *Yersinia enterocolitica**†

Reaction	Nilehn[189]					Wauters[188]					Knapp and Thal[187]			
	1	2	3	4	5	1	2	3	4	5	1	2	3	4
Indole	+	+	−	−	+	+	(+)	−	−	−	−	+	+	d
L-Xylose	+	+	+	−	−	+	+	+	−	−	d	+	+	d
Salicin	+	−	−	−	−						−	−	+	d
Esculin	+	−	−	−	−						−	−	+	d
Lactose	+	+	+	−	−	+	+	+	−	−	−	−	−	d
NO₃→NO₂	+	+	+	+	−	+	+	+	+	−				
Trehalose	+	+	+	+	−	+	+	+	+	−				
D-Sorbitol	+	+	+	+	−									
Ornithine decarboxylase	+	+	+	+	−	+	+	+	+	−	+	+	+	d
Voges-Proskauer	+	+	+	+	−									
Beta galactosidase	+	+	+	+	−	+	+	+	+	−				
Sucrose	+	+	+	+	−						+	+	+	d
Sorbose	+	+	+	+	−									
Lecithinase						+	−	−	−	−				
L-Rhamnose											−	−	−	d

*From Brenner, D. J., Farmer, J. J., III, Hickman, F. W., et al.: Taxonomic and nomenclature changes in *Enterobacteriaceae*, DHEW publ. no. (CDC) 78-8356, Atlanta, Oct. 1977, Center for Disease Control.
†+, 90% or more positive in 48 h; −, 10% or less positive; d, 10.1-89.9% positive; (+), delayed, after 48 h.

terized as pasteurellae; both produce urease but not phenylalanine deaminase. On initial isolation, *Yersinia* (especially *Y. enterocolitica*) strongly resemble certain other Enterobacteriaceae (Chapter 29), especially anaerogenic "atypical coliforms," *Proteus, Providencia,* and *Shigella,* and are easily misidentified.

"**Cold enrichment**" (refrigeration of specimens in isotonic saline at 4 C for 1-3 weeks) is useful for selective enrichment and greatly enhances the isolation rate. (See *Yersinia* in "Stool examination," Chapter 75.)

Y. enterocolitica and *Y. pseudotuberculosis* can be distinguished from each other by biochemical tests (Table 79-38), by susceptibility of *Y. pseudotuberculosis* to specific bacteriophages, and by agglutination with specific antisera. The latter 2 procedures are performed in reference laboratories.

Until recently, *Y. enterocolitica* was described as nonpathogenic in the usual laboratory animal (guinea pig, mice, white rabbits) by the intraperitoneal, intravenous, or subcutaneous routes, unlike *Y. pseudotuberculosis,* which is pathogenic in all these animals. However, since 1973 several strains of *Y. enterocolitica* highly pathogenic for mice have been found.[182, 183]

Yersiniosis: clinical manifestations

The most common clinical infections due to these 2 species are **enterocolitis** and **acute mesenteric lymphadenitis** (often mimicking acute appendicitis), the latter affecting predominantly young children; other manifestations are **erythema nodosum** or **polyarthritis, typhoidal syndromes,** and generalized **septicemia.**[32] *Y. enterocolitica* has also been isolated in meningitis, abscesses of the spleen, colon, and neck, local infection at indwelling catheter site, cholecystitis, eye infections, urine, purulent arthritis, and

wounds; occasionally it has been found in feces and lymph nodes of healthy humans.[176-181]

Yersinia enterocolitica

The organism previously described as *Bacterium enterocoliticum, Pasteurella pseudotuberculosis* type B, or *Pasteurella X* was finally named *Y. enterocolitica* in 1964.[183] It is morphologically and culturally related to *Y. pseudotuberculosis,* but differs from it with regard to serology, pathogenicity in animals, bacteriophage sensitivity, and several biochemical reactions.

Isolation. Isolation and recognition of the organism from body areas usually sterile is not difficult, since it does grow well on ordinary media. Isolation from feces, however, requires additional technics and attention.

NOTE: For a detailed description of procedures for isolation and preliminary identification of *Y. enterocolitica* from stool, see *Yersinia* in "Stool examination" in Chapter 75.

The organism grows slower at 37 C than other enteric organisms; for stool culture it is preferable to use MacConkey and *Salmonella-Shigella* (SS) agar plates incubated at room temperature; some atypical strains do not grow on SS agar. Cold enrichment of stool is highly successful in enhancing isolation rate.[184-186] Whenever the organism occurs in epidemic form, it can be recovered from stool in a high percentage of cases, assuming a strong index of suspicion both to grow and recognize it.

Presumptive identification. Little or no bipolarity ("safety pin" appearance) is seen, even when stained with Wayson stain. On triple sugar iron agar (TSI), reactions of typical strains, A/A, are those of anaerogenic (no gas) *E. coli:* both the slant and the butt are acid (due to sucrose fermentation) and no H₂S is produced; however,

Table 79-40. Biochemical characterization of *Yersinia enterocolitica* DNA relatedness groups*†

Reaction	Relatedness group			
	1	*2*	*3*	*4*
L-Rhamnose	–	+	+	–
Raffinose	–	+	–	–
Melibiose	–	+	–	–
α-Methyl glucoside	–	+	–	–
Sucrose	+	+	+	–

*From Brenner, D. J., Farmer, J. J., III, Hickman, F. W., et al.: Taxonomic and nomenclature changes in *Enterobacteriaceae*, DHEW publ. no. (CDC) 78-8356, Atlanta, Oct. 1977, Center for Disease Control; and Hawkins, T. M., and Brenner, D. J.: Isolation and identification of *Yersinia enterocolitica*, Atlanta, 1978, Center for Disease Control.
†+, 90% or more positive; –, 10% or less positive.

there are 2 biogroups that are sucrose negative (see below). Urea agar slants typically turn positive in a 3-24 hours, but phenylalanine is negative.

Definitive identification. Many of the biochemical and physiologic tests used for identification of *Y. enterocolitica* (Table 79-38) show a marked **temperature dependence.** In addition to **motility,** the tests for β-D-galactosidase production, maltose fermentation, and acetoin production (Voges-Proskauer test) are usually positive at 22-25 C but negative at 37 C. Unlike *Y. pseudotuberculosis*, the organism produces ornithine decarboxylase and acetoin, ferments sucrose (typical strains), sorbitol, and cellobiose, but not melibiose or rhamnose (typical strains; for exceptions, see below). Most strains do **not** ferment lactose; many United States isolates are indole positive, in contrast to those in Europe and Canada, which are indole negative.

Biogroups and DNA relatedness groups. *Y. enterocolitica* strains are quite variable biochemically. The 3 schemes used to **biotype** *Y. enterocolitica* are shown in Table 79-39. Most strains of *Y. enterocolitica* are d-methyl glucoside negative, and melibiose negative.[32,187-190]

DNA hybridization data indicate 3 distinct relatedness groups and the possibility of a fourth within strains of *Y. enterocolitica*.[190] The biochemical characteristics of these groups are listed in Table 79-40. Relatedness group 1 contain all of the biochemically typical strains included in biogroups 1-4 of Nilehn and of Wauters, and biogroups 1-3 of Knapp and Thal. There are 2 groups of **sucrose-negative** strains, one of which is typical except for being sucrose negative. These strains are included in biogroup 4 of Knapp and Thal. The second group of sucrose-negative strains is also atypically negative for ornithine decarboxylase, nitrate reduction, Voges-Proskauer, β-galactosidase, sucrose, and sorbose. These strains are in biogroup 5 of Nilehn and presumably in biogroup 5 of Wauters (sucrose was not tested); they are included in biogroup 4 of Knapp and Thal.

Relatedness groups 2 and 3 are both **rhamnose positive.** They are not included in the Nilehn or Wauters schemes but are in Knapp and Thal's atypical biogroup 4. Relatedness group 2 strains are positive for rhamnose, raffinose, melibiose, and α-methyl glucoside. Some of these reactions are often quite delayed at 37 C. This group is substantially more metabolically active at 22 C. Most strains are also citrate positive at 22 C. Relatedness group 3 strains are rhamnose positive, but negative for raffinose, melibiose, α-methyl glucoside and citrate at 22 C and 37 C.

The Center for Disease Control (CDC) Enteric Section (Brenner et al.[26]) restricts the designation on *Yersinia enterocolitica* only to relatedness groups 1 and 4. The CDC will continue to report all rhamnose-negative, sucrose-positive strains as *Y. enterocolitica* (see Table 79-9). Sucrose-negative strains will be reported as a sucrose-negative biogroup of *Y. enterocolitica*. The 2 rhamnose-positive groups will be reported as *Y. enterocolitica*-like rhamnose-positive group and *Y. enterocolitica*-like rhamnose-positive, melibiose-positive group. Both rhamnose-positive groups may be designated as new species in the near future.

Rhamnose-positive groups. The term *Yersinia intermedia* has been proposed for relatedness group 2; the organism causes a wound-type infection but not enteric disease.[190-192] *Yersinia fredericksenii* is proposed for relatedness group 3 (see Table 79-40); these strains do not appear to be enteric pathogens.[190,192]

Serology. There are 34 O antigens and 19 H antigens[193] recognized for *Y. enterocolitica*. Some antigens are shared in common with other bacteria including *Vibrio*, *Salmonella*, and *Brucella*. Most investigators use a tube agglutination test with an O antigen.

Serotype 3 is predominant in Europe, Africa, Japan, and Canada; strains from pigs in various European countries and to some extent in Canada belong to serotype 3, and thus the pig is thought to be a major reservoir for human infection. Serotype 9 is also common in Canada and Europe. In the United States most isolates from humans are serotype 8. Since at this time there are no commercially available *Y. enterocolitica* antisera in the United States, serologic diagnosis has been limited to specific outbreaks, and O antisera prepared against the epidemic strains are used. A number of different O groups have been implicated in the outbreaks, with O groups 5 and 8 being most common.

Diagnosis of *Y. enterocolitica* infection depends on isolation and identification of the organism; serodiagnosis (detection of antibody response in the patient) can be done only where a complete collection of known serotype strains is available.

Clinical manifestations. Clinical manifestations of *Y. enterocolitica* infection are (1) **acute enterocolitis** (most common); (2) **terminal ileitis** with mesenteric adenitis (second most common manifestation); (3) mostly in adults, **erythema nodosum** (predominantly in females) and acute **nonsuppurative polyarthritis,** often preceded by an episode of fever and diarrhea, and **Reiter's syndrome** (arthritis with urethritis and conjunctivitis) (4) **septicemia** is not common and may present as a typhoidlike syndrome (acute septicemic form) or as a subacute localizing form with hepatic or splenic abscesses.

Antimicrobial susceptibility. The organism is usually susceptible in vitro to kanamycin, gentamicin, colistin, chloramphenicol, tetracycline, streptomycin, and the combination sulfamethoxazole-trimethoprim, variably resistant to neomycin and ampicillin, and resistant to cephalothin.

The efficacy of antibiotics in uncomplicated *Y. enterocolitica* gastroenteritis is unknown as is their effect on the carrier state; the infection is usually self-limited. In cases of chronic or fulminating illness, antibiotics are beneficial but therapy should be based, if possible, on susceptibility testing of the isolate.

· · ·

In addition to the references listed above, the reader's attention is called to the review by Morris et al.,[194] Bissett's study on *Y. enterocolitica* isolates in California,[195] the review by Highsmith et al.,[196] and Bercovier's report on the isolation of *Yersinia* strains from a terrestrial ecosystem.[197]

Yersinia pseudotuberculosis

Until about 1960, disease due to *Y. pseudotuberculosis* in humans was thought to occur only as a rare acute **septicemia.** Since then, however, several hundred cases have been recognized in Europe, mostly with **mesenteric lymphadenitis** and some with **enteritis** or **erythema nodosum**[198,199]; the disease has been sporadically seen in the United States since 1938, and its recognition is slowly increasing.[200,201]

Y. pseudotuberculosis can be isolated from blood, mesenteric lymph nodes, effusions from serous cavities, organ specimens, and feces. Wayson's stain reveals the bipolar appearance in most, but not all, isolates.

Cultivation. The organism grows on blood agar and various common media such as MacConkey, EMB, or deoxycholate agar, at both 22 C and 37 C. It grows well in tetrathionate broth. A selective plating medium was recommended by Morris.[202] Colonies on blood agar after 24 hours reach 1 mm, while on EMB or MacConkey agar, they are smaller and lactose negative.

Identification. The organism is motile at 22-25 C and nonmotile at temperatures greater than 28 C, an important diagnostic feature. The TSI overnight reactions are alkaline slant/acid butt, no H_2S, no gas. LIA reactions are alkaline slant/acid butt. Catalase, esculin, methyl red, urease, methyl red, malonate, esculin, and β-D-galactosidase (ONPG) are positive. Phenylalanine

deaminase, oxidase, indole, citrate, lysine, ornithine decarboxylase, and arginine dihydrolase are negative (whereas *Y. enterocolitica* is ornithine positive). Carbohydrates are attacked fermentatively. No gas is produced. Fermentation occurs promptly with glucose, galactose, maltose, mannitol, levulose, mannose, rhamnose, trehalose, and xylose. No fermentation occurs with sucrose, lactose, raffinose, dulcitol, and inositol (see Table 79-38).

Differentiation of Y. pseudotuberculosis and Y. pestis. *Y. pseudotuberculosis* is motile at 20 C, ferments rhamnose, melibiose, and glycerin, and produces urease; in all these respects *Y. pestis* is negative. Antisera containing antibodies against types I-V agglutinate *Y. pseudotuberculosis* and not *Y. pestis*. *Y. pseudotuberculosis* phages lyse all strains but not *Y. pestis*. *Y. pestis* phage does not lyse *Y. pseudotuberculosis* at 20 C (Meyer[203]).

Serology. Six main serotypes, based on 15 somatic (O) antigens, with 8 subtypes have been established.[204] Type I is the most common, occurring in about 90% of cases. Several of the antigens cross-react with some in group B and group D salmonellae, and type VI shows an antigenic relationship with *E. coli* O55. Some degree of cross immunity also exists between *Y. pestis* and *Y. pseudotuberculosis*: killed suspensions of *Y. pseudotuberculosis* protect guinea pigs against infection with *Y. pestis*.

Antibodies have been detected by agglutination or indirect hemagglutination in the sera of acutely ill patients; they rapidly disappear during convalescence (1-4 months).

Animal pathogenicity. The organism is virulent in mice, guinea pigs, gerbils, and white rabbits but not in white rats or hamsters.

Antimicrobial susceptibility. *Y. pseudotuberculosis* is generally sensitive to tetracycline, streptomycin, chloramphenicol, and kanamycin, and is usually resistant to penicillin, ampicillin, carbenicillin, and cephaloglycin. Susceptibility tests are recommended.

Yersinia ruckeri[26]

Yersinia ruckeri was formerly called the red mouth bacterium.[205,206] This organism causes redmouth disease in trout and salmon. No case of human infection caused by this organism has yet been reported. *Y. ruckeri* grows better at 22-25 C than at 35-37 C, and some strains will not grow at the higher temperature.

VIBRIONACEAE

The family *Vibrionaceae*[3] includes, among others, the medically important genera *Vibrio*, *Aeromonas*, and *Plesiomonas*. They are all fermenters.

VIBRIO

The genus *Vibrio* includes gram-negative, nonsporeforming rods with a single rigid curve (or straight rods). They are **motile** by means of a single polar flagellum, are cytochrome (indophenol) **oxidase positive,** and produce acid without gas from dextrose by **fermentation.**[207]

The groups of vibrios associated with human disease are (1) *Vibrio cholerae;* (2) nonagglutinable or noncholera vibrios (known as NAG or NCV, biochemically similar to *V. cholerae* but not agglutinated by *V. cholerae* antiserum); (3) halophilic vibrios, including *V. parahaemolyticus, V. alginolyticus,* and an as yet unnamed lactose-fermenting (L+) vibrio[208]; and (4) the organism previously known as *Vibrio fetus,* now classified as *Campylobacter fetus* and discussed under *Campylobacter* (below).

Some workers consider *V. El Tor* a separate species; others[3,209,210] regard it as a biotype of *V. cholerae.* In any event it is capable of causing epidemic cholera in humans. A number of other *Vibrio* species have been described from various habitats (marine, soil, animal), many of which are similar to *V. cholerae* in morphologic, cultural, and biochemical (but not serologic) characters. For **preliminary** differentiation of *Vibrio* and members of certain other genera see Tables 79-1, 79-2, and 79-4.

Vibrio cholerae*

This organism is found only in the intestine of humans; in nature it is found only in immediate association with cholera cases. *V. cholerae* organisms are slightly curved rods (1-5 μ) that look like commas when freshly isolated and are arranged single or united into C or S forms or in spirals. They are briskly motile, usually by a single polar flagellum. Short comma forms with pointed ends and thickest in the center are characteristic and are seen best in nutrient or bile salt agar culture. Involution forms occur readily.

The organisms are gram negative. The best stain for visualizing the typical comma forms is carbolfuchsin, 1:10, stain for about 5 min.

Provisional, rapid recognition. Examination of liquid cholera stool directly, or after enrichment, by dark-field microscope observation of the characteristic motility of the comma-shaped organisms in a fecal sample helps in rapid recognition (presumptive diagnosis). On addition of group- and type-specific antisera, homologous strains will be clumped and immobilized; however, this test requires diagnostic sera without **any** preservative.[211,212] The World Health Organization[211] does not recommend microscopic stool examination for routine diagnosis.

Identification

As described in Chapter 75 (stool examination), plates inoculated directly with specimen material or from holding media (Cary-Blair fluid medium)

---

*The International Committee on Bacteriological Nomenclature[210] recognized the specific epithet *cholerae* as legitimate. The earlier epithet *comma* will not be used here.

or enrichment (alkaline peptone water) should be examined after 8-10 hours of incubation or after overnight incubation.

Colony characteristics[211]

TCBS agar. In 10-18 hours the vibrios form characteristically **big yellow** slightly convex colonies. These yellow colonies frequenlty become **green** after prolonged incubation, particularly when the organism is an El Tor biotype vibrio.

Pseudomonads and most *Aeromonas* do not grow on this medium. Some *Proteus* (with or without black centers), sporebearing bacilli, and cocci may, however, grow, producing deep yellow colonies of different sizes. TCBS medium may vary in its selective properties according to the producer and the batch.

Gelatin-taurocholate-trypticase-tellurite agar (GTTA agar) (Monsur). Vibrio colonies on this medium are as follows:

1. At 24 hours: small, translucent to transparent with a greyish black center and a turbid halo.

2. At 48 hours: larger colonies 3-4 mm in size with a black center and a well-defined halo.

Frequently, *Proteus* may grow on a plate. The colonies have a greyish center but usually lack the halo.

Nutrient agar. Peculiar, bluish, translucent, glassy, circular, entire, slightly raised colonies, easily distinguishable from opaque coliform colonies. Opaque variant colonies may rarely be seen.

Wilson-Blair modified medium. Translucent colonies with grayish center.

Aronson medium. Transparent, bright red colonies.

D.E.C. medium. Small, clear, colorless colonies.

NOTE: Some strains of *V. cholerae* grow on SS agar and McConkey agar, but many do not.

Serologic examination. The WHO guidelines[211] recommend that suspect colonies should be tested with **polyvalent cholera diagnostic serum** on a slide; this test enables a provisional diagnosis to be made by the following morning. Since agglutinable and nonagglutinable vibrios may coexist and in an enrichment medium the nonagglutinable vibrios may overgrow the agglutinable ones, if one suspicious colony fails to react with the group sera, at least 5 more such colonies should be tested in the same manner before the case is considered negative for agglutinable *V. cholerae.* This is particularly important for the first few suspected cases. If diagnostic serum is not available, the **string test** may be carried out for a presumptive diagnosis (see below) to be confirmed later in the central laboratory.

Slide agglutination test. Use a straight wire rather than a loop to pick up part of a large colony. The agglutination reaction is quicker and better with colonies from BSA (bile salt agar), MEA (meat extract agar), and GA media; colonies grown on a highly selective medium such as

TCBS may agglutinate slowly or weakly, necessitating a re-examination after subculturing on a nutrient agar slant or Kligler iron agar (KIA).

Preliminary biochemical tests

Portions of the agglutinable colonies should be placed on KIA (Kligler iron agar) slants (preferred over TSI slants)[211] to see their characteristics on KIA (red slant and yellow butt without gas in 18 hours), or on TSI slants. If available, LIA slants should also be used[213] because the reactions obtained permit an early presumptive differentiation between most vibrios, *Aeromonas hydrophila*, *Plesiomonas (Aeromonas) shigelloides*, as well as certain other bacteria (see Table 79-13). According to Ewing et al.,[213] the reactions of the majority of strains of certain vibrios and related organisms are as follows:

Microorganism	KIA		TSI		LIA	
	Slant	Butt	Slant	Butt	Slant	Butt
V. cholerae	K*	A	A	A	K	K or N
V. parahaemolyticus	K	A	K	A	K	K or N
V. alginolyticus	K	A	A	A	K	K or N
Vibrio species lac +	A or K	A	A	A	K	K or N
A. hydrophila	K or A	A	K or A	A	K	K or N
P. shigelloides	K or A	A	K or A	A	K	K or N

*K = alkaline, A = acid, N = neutral.

Biochemical and physiologic tests

If one of the miniaturized test kits is used (e.g., API), suspect colonies may be directly inoculated into the kit; LIA and KIA (or TSI) may not be needed. However, Ewing et al.[213] caution that even when kits are used, a nutrient or infusion agar slant be inoculated from suspension used for kit, for serologic work, and reference.

Reactions in conventional testing are as follows: Acid but no gas is produced in glucose, sucrose, mannose, mannitol, maltose, and trehalose within 1-2 days. Acid is produced in lactose after 3 or more days. Indophenol (cytochrome) oxidase, indole, motility, gelatin liquefaction, and lysine and ornithine decarboxylases are positive, whereas arginine is negative, in contrast to *Aeromonas hydrophila*, which gives negative lysine and ornithine but positive arginine tests. (see Table 79-41).

Members of the genus *Aeromonas*, especially *A. hydrophila*, are quite similar in their biochemical reactions to *V. cholerae;* for this reason it is important to include the decarboxylase tests, salicin, esculin (about 60% of *A. hydrophila* strains are positive in the latter 2 tests), and growth test on SS agar (about 85% of *A. hydrophila* strains grow).

Antimicrobial susceptibilities. Some workers recommend testing *Vibrio* strains for their susceptibility to various antimicrobial agents to differentiate *Vibrio* species and *A. hydrophila*. The latter is resistant to penicillin, whereas *V. cholerae* is sensitive or partially sensitive. A vibriostatic pteridine compound, 0/129, seems to be useful in the differentiation of vibrios and aeromonads. With a few exceptions, cultures of *A. hydrophila* are resistant to this substance, whereas *Vibrio* strains are inhibited.

Fluorescent antibody technic. Finkelstein and LaBrec[214] described an FA procedure which, it is claimed, makes a definitive diagnosis possible within 1 hour of taking a sample from the patient. A carrier can be recognized in 7-8 hours. The technic, however, requires costly equipment and a highly trained observer; it is not used routinely.

Tests for distinguishing classical and El Tor vibrios

Hemolysis test[211, 213, 215]

1. Cultivate suspect cultures for 18 h in medium prepared by adding 1.0% casitone to isotonic sodium chloride (0.85%) solution. Dispense in tubes and sterilize at 121 C for 15 min or, grow culture in heart infusion broth (HIB) for 24 h.[211]

2. Add to each 1 ml of culture 1 ml of a 5% suspension of washed sheep erythrocytes in physiologic saline solution.

3. Incubate mixtures at 37 C for 2 h and then place in refrigerator at 4-6 C for 24 h. Hemolysin production is indicated by clearing (lysis) of erythrocytes; read but do not shake tubes.

The El Tor strains isolated currently are usually nonhemolytic in this test, but most of them prove to be hemolytic when tested in the same way after they have been grown in heart infusion broth containing 1% glycerol as a stabilizer.[211]

"String" test.[209] Emulsify, on a slide, a small amount of growth from a 24 h agar slant culture or gelatin agar plate in 1 drop 0.5% saline solution[211] of sodium deoxycholate. Examine the drop for a mucuslike "string" extending from the drop to the loop as it is lifted away from the slide. The following patterns may be observed.

1. + +: A string is observed initially and can still be produced 45-60 s later. All *Vibrio cholerae* and most El Tor biotype cultures give this type of reaction, with the delayed string being even stronger than the initial. Most *Vibrio* species and a few aeromonads give a weaker delayed reaction than that occurring initially.

Table 79-41. Comparison of biochemical reactions of *V. cholerae, V. parahaemolyticus, V. alginolyticus,* and lactose-positive *Vibrio* species*†

Test or substrate‡	V. cholerae			V. parahae-molyticus		V. alginolyticus			Vibrio species (lactose positive, lac +)		
	Sign	%+§	(%+)‖	Sign	%+	Sign	%+	(%+)	Sign	%+	(%+)
Indole	+	100		+	99	+	87		+	97	(3)
Methyl red	+ʷ	95		+	99.5	−	0			NR	
Voges-Proskauer	− or +	47.3		−	0	+	100		−	0	
Citrate (Simmons')	(+ʷ) or −	0	(74ʷ)	+	98	d	20	(47)	d	76	(11)
Lysine decarboxylase	+	100		+	96.5	+	100		+	97	(3)
Arginine dihydrolase	−	0		−	0	−	0		−	0	
Ornithine decarboxylase	+	95.5		+	95.5	− or +	40		+ or (+)	66	(26)
Phenylalanine deaminase	−	0		−	0	−	0		.	NR	
Gelatin (22 C)	+	96		+	100	+	100		+	(1-7 d)	
Gas from glucose	−	0		−	0	−	0		−	0	
Lactose	(+)	0	(100)	−	0	−	0		+ or (+)	81	(16)
Sucrose	+	96		−	5	+	100		−	3	
Arabinose	− or +	10.1		+ or −	81	−	6		−	0	
Mannose	+	99		+	100	+	100		+	100	
Mannitol	+	100		+	100	+	100		+ or −	66	
Salicin	−	0		−	0	d	12.5	(41.7)	+	100	
Esculin	−	0		+	99.5	−	0			NR	
Melibiose	−	0		− or +	15	−	0		d	26	(52)
Motility	+	96		+	99	+	98	(2)	+	97	

*From Ewing, W. H., Tomfohrde, K. M., and Naudo, P. J.: Isolation and identification of *Vibrio cholerae* and certain related vibrios: an outline of methods, API Species **2**:10, 1979.

†+, 90% or more positive within 1 or 2 d; (+), positive reaction after 3 or more d (decarboxylase tests: 3 or 4 d); −, no reaction (90% or more); + or −, most cultures positive, some strains negative; − or +, most strains negative, some cultures positive; + or (+), most reactions occur within 1 or 2 d, some are delayed; d, different reactions: +, (+), or −; w, weakly positive reactions; NR, not recorded.

‡All cultures included oxidase positive, beta galactosidase positive, and reduced nitrate to nitrite. Nitrite not reduced. Detectable hydrogen sulfide not produced in Kligler's iron or triple sugar iron agar. Urease not produced. None ferment dulcitol, inositol, adonitol, xylose, rhamnose, or melezitose.

§Percent positive within 1 or 2 d.

‖Percent positive after 3 or more d (decarboxylase test: 3 or 4 d).

2. +−: A string occurs initially but is absent 45-60 s later. Most *Vibrio* species give this pattern.

3. − −: No string occurs either initially or delayed.

Direct hemagglutination test.[211] Chicken and sheep red blood cells can both be used for this purpose.

1. Make 2.5% suspension of washed (3 times) and properly centrifuged cells in normal saline.

2. Divide clean glass slide into several colonies with glass-marking pencil, and place a 3 mm loopful of suspension in each column.

3. Add small portion of growth from agar slants to red cells with needle or loop and mix well, Clumping of red cells occurs within a few seconds in positive cases.

Known hemagglutinating (El Tor) and nonhemagglutinating (classical) strains should be used as controls for each new suspension of red cells.

Polymyxin B sensitivity test[213, 216]

1. Grow strains to be tested 20-24 h in nutrient broth.

2. Spread inoculum from broth culture over surface of nutrient agar plate, and place 50-unit disk of polymyxin B on plate.

3. After incubation for 24 h at 37 C, observe plates for zones of inhibition.

The classical biotype of *V. cholerae* is sensitive, whereas the El Tor biotype is resistant.

Sensitivity to cholera phage group IV.* This test is performed in reference laboratories. Cholera phage (Mukerjee) group IV used at a routine test concentration lyses cultures of the classical *V. cholerae* but does not lyse the El Tor strains. Cultures to be tested are inoculated in a series of spots on a nutrient agar plate. After the spots are dry, a loopful of phage IV is placed on each spot. After incubation, observe plate for lysis. For details, see Ewing et al.[209]

Serology of V. cholerae

Both somatic **O** antigens and flagellar **H** antigens are present. Burrows has grouped true cholera vibrios according to their O antigens. The A antigen is common to all; all possess, in addition, a second O antigen, either Ogawa (B) or Inaba (C). Thus the formulas for the O forms (sub-O groups) are:

Ogawa	AB
Inaba	AC
Hikojima	ABC

*References 209, 213, 217, 218.

O sera.* Heat cultures (Inaba, Ogawa, and Hikojima separately) for 2½ h at 100 C to inactivate H antigens. Treat with absolute alcohol for 4 h at 37 C, wash with acetone, dry, and grind into fine powder. Resuspend powdered antigen in physiologic saline and give rabbits 4 IV injections, usually at 4 d intervals. First injection consists of 0.5 ml of suspension having density of 24 h broth culture; 1, 2, and 3 ml are given afterward, with density also being increased.

Absorbed antisera.* Use growth from 10 standard Petri dishes per 1 ml undiluted antiserum. Absorb Inaba antiserum with Ogawa and Hikojima strain, respectively, in separate absorptions. Absorb Ogawa antiserum with Inaba strain.

Slide agglutination test.* A loopful of growth (from KIA or fresh nutrient agar slant) is emulsified in about 0.2 ml mercuric iodide solution† in small tubes. A loopful of each such dense suspension is placed on divided slide; then loopful or droplet of antiserum is placed on slide below each droplet of suspension. Suspension and antiserum in each division on slide are then mixed with separate pieces of applicator stick. Mixing should be done in such a way as to form a long narrow band of approximately 5 × 15 mm. Slides may then be tilted back and forth and observed for agglutination. Suitable controls always should be made to assure that agglutination seen is not spontaneous.

Bacteriophage typing

A number of phage lines (Mukerjee, Asheshov) are available to reference laboratories for typing of *V. cholerae*. Bacteriophage also has been used for detection of small numbers of *V. cholerae* in mixtures of materials by placing a spot of phage on the isolation plates after they were inoculated and dried. For details refer to Ewing et al.,[209] and Mukerjee.[219]

Postmortem examination

Cultures from the small intestine, from the gallbladder, and sometimes from the urine may be positive. Macroscopic and histologic appearances of the gut and kidneys: Peyer's patches and solitary follicles stand out prominently as so many small tubercles; there are catarrh, necrosis, and desquamatio of the intestinal epithelium; kidneys are enlarged and pinkish red; glomeruli are swollen; capsular spaces are edematous and tubular epithelium degenerated; and glomerular and intertubular blood capillaries are dilated.

Isolation of V. cholerae from natural sources

Clear water. Pass about 1000 ml water through Millipore filter (Felsenfeld) and drop filter paper from filter into alkaline peptone water or, better still, into

Wilson-Reilly fluid medium* and incubate. Plate few drops from surface and look for vibrio colonies. If any NAG vibrios are found, plating should be done on bile agar medium incorporated with few drops of polyvalent NAG serum.

Turbid and dirty water. Test pH. If it is below 5.0, there is no use in examining it, as all vibrios are killed at this pH. If pH is above 5.0, then proceed as with clear water.

Milk. Enrich by Wilson-Reilly medium or peptone water first and then plate direct or, better, after passing through L3 porcelain candle (Panja). Immerse nonglazed part of candle in alkaline (pH 9)-boric (0.08%)-peptone water and incubate.

Flies, fish, crabs, fruits, vegetables, etc. Same procedure as above.

Halophilic vibrios

V. parahaemolyticus, V. alginolyticus, Vibrio lac+ species

The **halophilic vibrios** are able to grow in seawater and flourish in selective media with high salt content; in fact, they usually do not grow in the absence of salt (at least not on first isolation). The ability of these microorganisms to grow in media, e.g., tryptone broth, that contain various concentrations of sodium chloride[220-222] is as follows[213]:

Organism	NaCl (salt) concentration (%)					
	0	0.5	3	6	8	10
V. parahaemo-lyticus	−	+ or −	+	+	+	−
V. algino-lyticus	−	−	+	+	+	+
Vibrio species Lac+	−	−	+	+	− or +	−
V. cholerae	+ or −	+	+	+ or −	−	−

V. parahaemolyticus

In Chapter 75 (stool examination) procedures for isolation of *V. parahaemolyticus* are detailed, and the organism is briefly described as a marine organism (originally identified by Sakazaki[220]), which is an enteropathogenic, gram-negative rod, facultatively anaerobic, and halophilic (salt-loving).

With a few exceptions, *V. parahaemolyticus* will grow on media used for *V. cholerae* (such as TCBS). However, if the organism is suspected in an outbreak, it is advisable to use media de-

---

*From Ewing et al.[209]

†**Mercuric iodide solution**
1. Stock solution
Mercuric iodine	1 g
Potassium iodide	4 g
Distilled water	100 ml
2. Working solution (1:1000)
Stock solution	10 ml
Physiologic saline solution	90 ml
Formalin	0.05 ml

***Wilson-Reilly medium.** Prepare **solution A** (10 g peptone, 20 g NaCl, and 1 L distilled water; adjust to pH 9.1 with 14% Na carbonate solution and autoclave in 100 ml amounts) and **solution B** (20 g anhydrous sodium sulfite in 100 ml boiling water; then add 0.1 g bismuth ammoniocitrate dissolved in 10 ml boiling water, cool, and add 100 ml 20% glucose solution).

To each 100 ml of **solution A** add 10 ml of **solution B** and 1 ml absolute alcohol before inoculation. It is used in same manner as alkaline peptone water. To make Wilson-Reilly plates, add 2% agar to above medium.

signed for halophilic vibrios.*[222,223] It should be noted, in addition, that it is necessary to add NaCl (0.1 ml of sterile 20% solution per 3.0 ml of medium) to media such as those used for methyl red, Voges-Proskauer, and decarboxylase tests when determining the biochemical reaction of halophilic bacteria using conventional media.

V. parahaemolyticus is a frequent cause of gastroenteritis in Japan, and a number of outbreaks have been reported in the United States.[224,225] Seafood usually is the vehicle of infection. *V. parahaemolyticus* also has been isolated from specimens of extraintestinal origin, including blood (1 of 18 strains described by Hollis et al.[221])

Stool specimen: collection and transport. See Chapter 75, *V. parahaemolyticus*, in "Stool examination." NOTE: Do not refrigerate specimen, since the organism is reported to be sensitive to lower temperatures.

Culture. On TCBS agar, colonies are round, 2-3 mm in diameter, with green or blue centers (lack of a yellow color indicates **no** acid production from sucrose and differentiates this organism from the other cholera organisms. Both *V. parahaemolyticus* and *V. alginolyticus* will grow on commonly used agar media, such as mannitol salt agar (MSA); they grow less well on Hektoen agar,[226] MacConkey agar, and XLD agar.[227] Although distinctive colonies may be observed on these media in 24 hours, the plates should be held for at least 48 hours before they are discarded as having "no growth."

Biochemical tests. Perform tests shown in Table 79-41. Characterizations considered as minimal for typical stool isolates made on TCBS medium include[228]:

1. Reactions on TSI (alkaline slant, acid butt, no gas, delayed or negative H_2S).
2. No growth in 1% trypticase solution with 0% NaCl. Growth in 1% trypticase solution with 3%, 6%, and 8% NaCl.
3. Sucrose not fermented.
4. Oxidase positive.
5. Lysine decarboxylated.
6. Voges-Proskauer negative.
7. Urea usually negative, occasionally rapid positive.

Tilton and Balows[229] state that when minikits (such as API) are used for biochemical testing, the inoculum should be suspended in 0.85%

---

*Bromthymol blue teepol agar[213,222,223]

Yeast extract	3 g
Peptone	10 g
Sodium chloride	40 g
Sucrose	20 g
Bromthymol blue	0.04 g
Thymol blue	0.04 g
Teepol (Shell)	2 ml
Agar	15 g
Distilled water	1000 ml
pH 9	

Sterilize at 121 C for 15 min (if desired). Dispense in Petri dishes.

NaCl, which seems to be sufficient for support of growth.

Antigenic schema. Both **O** antigens and **K** antigens are present; a total of 12 O groups and 52 K types are presently recognized. Antisera are not available at this time commercially in the United States.

Kanagawa phenomenon.[230] The Kanagawa reaction tests for the presence of a specific hemolysin on Wagatsuma agar. A positive reaction has been thought to correlate closely with the pathogenicity of *V. parahaemolyticus* isolates. The isolates that have caused illness in humans are almost always Kanagawa positive, but isolates recovered from seafoods are almost always Kanagawa negative.

Several workers have isolated and purified the thermostable direct hemolysin from culture filtrates of Kanagawa positive cells.[231] The test is performed usually in reference laboratories.

1. To perform Kanagawa test, spot loopful of 18 h culture in trypticase soy 3% NaCl broth onto a well-dried Wagatsuma blood agar* plate. Several spottings may be made in circular pattern on single plate.
2. Incubate at 35 C.
3. Observe results in less than 24 h.
4. Positive test consists of β-hemolysis: zone of transparent clearing of blood cells around colony.
5. It is **very important** to remember that **no observation beyond 24 h is valid in this test.**

Vibrio alginolyticus

V. alginolyticus is not known to be a cause of gastroenteritis. It is important because it must be differentiated from *V. cholerae* and *V. parahaemolyticus* when recovered from stool samples and because it occurs in specimens of extraintestinal origin (ear exudates, wounds, etc.) and as cause of cellulitis in marine wound infections. Its appearance in blood cultures is infrequent. For details of biochemical characteristics, see Table 79-41.

For differentiation of *V. parahaemolyticus* and *V. alginolyticus*, note that *V. alginolyticus* is sucrose and Voges-Proskauer positive, swarms on blood agar, and grows in broth with 10% NaCl added, whereas *V. parahaemolyticus* is negative in all these respects.[229]

---

*Wagatsuma agar[230]

Yeast extract	3 g
Bacto-peptone	10 g
Sodium chloride	70 g
Dipotassium phosphate	5 g
Mannitol	10 g
Crystal violet	0.001 g
Bacto agar	15 g
Distilled water	1000 ml

Adjust to pH 8.0 (do not autoclave). Steam 30 min and temper to 50 C. Add 2 ml suspension of freshly drawn citrated (to give approximately 0.5%) **human** red blood cells that were previously washed 3 times in physiologic saline. Pour plates and allow to harden. Dry plates thoroughly before use. Plates should be used as soon as possible.

Table 79-42. Some characteristics of halophilic
Vibrio species*

	Lac+ Vibrio	*V. parahaemolyticus*	*V. alginolyticus*
Fermentation			
Lactose	+	−	−
Sucrose	−	−	+
Voges-Proskauer	−	−	+
NaCl tolerance	<8%	>8%<10%	>10%

*Personal communication from Dr. R. E. Weaver, 1977.

Lac+ (lactose positive) halophilic Vibrio

In 1976, Hollis et al.[221] reported on the biochemical characterization of strains of halophilic bacteria that were similar to *V. parahaemolyticus* and *V. alginolyticus*, but that were able to ferment lactose; they have been designated lactose positive (L+) *Vibrio*. The L+ *Vibrio* can be differentiated from *V. parahaemolyticus* by a lower salt tolerance and from *V. alginolyticus* by their inability to ferment sucrose. These organisms have been most frequently isolated from blood. Twenty of the 38 strains of *Vibrio* species L+ described by Hollis et al.[221] were isolated from the bloodstream. Skin lesions were present in at least some of the patients who had positive blood cultures. The remaining isolates were from skin lesions, throat, or cornea; none was from feces. This microorganism has not been implicated in diarrheal disease.

By early 1979, Blake et al.[208] reported 2 clinical syndromes distinct from others caused by vibrios: (1) in compromised hosts, after ingestion (raw oysters), the illness began with septicemia (11 of 24 patients died) without gastrointestinal symptoms; (2) in others, i.e., noncompromised hosts, an intense cellulitis was seen following infection of superficial wounds with the L+ *Vibrio*.

Identification. Characteristics of the organism are included in Table 79-41. Distinguishing features of the L+ *Vibrio* and differentiation of the halophilic vibrios are shown in Table 79-42.

AEROMONAS[233–238]

Organisms in the genus *Aeromonas* are gramnegative rods, **motile** by means of polar flagella (occasionally nonmotile), which grow well on various media. The reactions given by these **fermentative** organisms in the biochemical tests used for differentiation of Enterobacteriaceae often resemble the reactions given by the latter, and the differentiation of *Aeromonas* may be somewhat confusing. However, *Aeromonas* strains are **oxidase positive.*** They may be differentiated from *Vibrio, Pseudomonas, Flavobac*

---

*Overman et al.[239] found some oxidase-negative (variable) *Aeromonas* strains; this was due to their being tested on growth on selective and differential media. When grown on sheep blood agar, the organisms were oxidase positive.

terium, and *Alcaligenes* by their lack of pigment formation, positive indole test, and fermentative metabolism (see Tables 79-4, 79-14, and 79-43). See also discussion of *Vibrio cholerae.*

The decarboxylase tests (see Enterobacteriaceae) have been found of value in separating *Aeromonas* cultures from Enterobacteriaceae. The majority of *Aeromonas* cultures are negative in lysine medium, positive in arginine, and negative in ornithine medium, a pattern not given by any of the Enterobacteriaceae (except for *Citrobacter,* where arginine is delayed for 2-3 days).

Several species have been described.[240]

A. hydrophila (*A. punctata, A. liquefaciens*) forms gas from glucose and is Voges-Proskauer positive and hemolytic. These polar flagellated, V-P–positive strains are gelatin, indole, nitrate, and catalase positive and urease negative. They produce acid and gas from glucose, galactose, dextrin, maltose, and mannitol. Lactose fermentation is variable and slow. Raffinose, xylose, dulcitol, and inulin are not fermented.

A. salmonicida (which does not grow at 37 C) and *A. (Plesiomonas) shigelloides* are Voges-Proskauer negative and do not form gas from glucose.

The normal habitat of *Aeromonas* is probably water. The organisms have been isolated from human feces, skin lesions and wounds, blood, gallbladder, and throat and from diverse animals.[241]

PLESIOMONAS[234]

The single species in this genus, *P. shigelloides,* was previously in the genus *Aeromonas.* It is also **oxidase positive** and **fermentative;** differentiating characteristics are given in Table 79-43.

It is Voges-Proskauer negative, often ornithine positive, sucrose negative, mannitol negative, characteristics that differentiate it from *Aeromonas.* It has been isolated from spinal fluid, blood cultures, and feces.[240]

CHROMOBACTERIUM[241–248]

Organisms in this genus are gram-negative, **fermentative, motile** rods, with both 1 polar and usually 1 to 4 subpolar or lateral flagella,[3] that produce violet (or sometimes blue or black) colonies; some strains are nonpigmented.

Two well-defined species are recognized— *C. violaceum* and *C. lividum.* The latter is usually not seen in the clinical laboratory since it does not grow at 37 C ("psychrophil"); however, it does grow at 4-5 C. *C. violaceum* grows abundantly at 35-37 C, but not at 4 C ("mesophil").

The identity of the chromobacteria is usually suspected because of their pigment formation. Some strains, depending on the medium, produce little or no pigment, in which case they may be confused with aeromonads, pseudomonads, or even vibrios. Some violet-pigmented strains occasionally are thought first to be *Serratia.* The optimal pigment formation by chromo-

Table 79-43. Differentiation of *Aeromonas* and *Plesiomonas**†

Test or substrate‡	*A. hydrophila*			*P. shigelloides*		
	Sign	*%+*	*(%+)*	*Sign*	*%+*	*(%+)*
Indole	+ or −	85.5		+	100	
Voges-Proskauer	− or +	44.5		−	0	
Citrate (Simmons')	d	54	(17.5)	−	0	
Lysine decarboxylase	−	18^{vw}	(7.5^{vw})	+	97.7	
Arginine dihydrolase	+ or (+)	80.5	(9.5)	+	95.8	(2.1)
Ornithine decarboxylase	−	0		+ or −	70.2	
Phenylalanine deaminase	− or +^{w}	27^w		− or +^{w}	24.5^w	
Gelatin (22 C) nutrient	+ or (+)	75	(22)	−	0	
Gelatin (charcoal)	+	99		− or (+)	0	(32)
Gas from glucose	+ or −	54.5		−	0	
Lactose	d	12.5	(21.5)	d	59.6	(29.8)
Sucrose	d	80	(2)	−	1.1	(5.3)
Arabinose	d	55	(1.2)	−	0	
Mannose	+	91		d	4	(13)
Mannitol	+	97.5		−	0	
Inositol	−	0		+	95.7	(2.1)
Esculin	+ or −	60		−	0	
Melibiose	d	5.5	(7.9)	d	48	(9)
β-galactosidase	+	100		+	100	

*Modified from Ewing, Tomfohrde, and Naudo.[238a]

†+, 90% or more positive within 1 or 2 d; (+), positive reaction after 3 or more d (decarboxylase tests: 3 or 4 d); −, no reaction (90% or more); + or −, most cultures positive, some strains negative; − or +, most strains negative, some cultures positive; + or (+), most reactions occur within 1 or 2 d, some are delayed; d, different reactions: +, (+), or −; w, weakly positive reactions; vw, very weakly positive reactions.

‡All strains are oxidase positive and reduce nitrate to nitrite. Urease is not produced.

bacteria is achieved at 22 C on media devoid of all meat extracts and containing added mannitol.

The violet pigment, **violacein**, is insoluble in water (e.g., does not diffuse into the medium) and in chloroform. Methods for testing and identification of violacein are given by Sneath.[249]

Chromobacterium violaceum

The organism is facultatively anaerobic and grows well but slowly (1-3 days) in air; it grows on MacConkey agar, with oxidase reaction being variable. For oxidase activity and testing, see Dhar and Johnson.[250] It is usually fermentative, producing acid in fermentation media from a few sugars (not from lactose, adonitol, mannitol, and some strains not even from glucose); see Tables 79-3 and 79-4. In OF medium (use open tube only), acid is produced from 1% trehalose but not from arabinose. The organism grows in KCN, hydrolyzes gelatin, and produces an arginine dihydrolase.

C. violaceum produces hydrogen cyanide, which can be detected in nutrient agar made semisolid by diluting the medium with an equal volume of water.[249] Stab the column of medium; place an indicator paper between the plug and tube. A positive test results in a color change of the paper from yellow to red. Note that some pseudomonads also give a positive test. The indicator paper can be prepared by dipping filter paper strips into saturated aqueous picric acid. After drying the strips, immerse them in a 10% solution of aqueous sodium carbonate. Dry again and keep in an airtight container. They keep for months, even if kept at room temperature.

For cases of human infections, see references 241, 243, 245, and 248.

PASTEURELLA

Organisms in the genus *Pasteurella* are primarily animal pathogens but are also responsible for a variety of syndromes in humans ranging from localized abscesses to septicemias. They are aerobic or facultatively anaerobic, gram-negative, fermentative, nonmotile, ovoid or rod-shaped bacilli (coccobacilli) with bipolar staining common (best demonstrated in Giemsa or methylene blue–stained tissues). They grow best on media containing blood; some grow on MacConkey agar (*P. haemolytica*), but most do not; all species in the genus are **oxidase positive.**

For the evolution of the genera *Pasteurella*, *Yersinia*, and *Frantcisella*, see *Yersinia*, above.

Pasteurella multocida

P. multocida[251-257] is the species most frequently involved in human infections. It is the cause of "hemorrhagic septicemia" in a variety of animals and birds. The organism is frequently carried in the respiratory tract of healthy animals such as sheep, dogs, cats, and rats.

P. multocida, a small, nonmotile, gram-negative coccobacillus, is catalase positive, oxidase positive, **nonmotile** at 37 or 22 C, fermentative, oxidase positive, and **does not grow on MacConkey, EMB, deoxycholate, SS, or centrimide agars.** Small, nonhemolytic, gray colonies are formed on blood agar. They appear either as smooth (iridescent or blue types by oblique transmitted light on dextrose starch agar) or mucoid variants;

Table 79-44. Differential characteristics of *Pasteurella, Actinobacillus, Cardiobacterium, Haemophilus aphrophilus, Eikenella corrodens,* and DF-2*†

	P. multocida	P. pneumotropica	P. haemolytica‡	P. ureae§	A. lignieresii‖	A. equuli¶	A. actinomycetemcomitans	Cardiobacterium hominis	Haemophilus aphrophilus	Eikenella corrodens	DF-2
Glucose	A	A	A	A	A	A	A	A	A	−	A
Xylose	A	A	A	−	A	A	A(−)	−	−	−	ND
Mannitol	A	−	A	A	A	A	A(−)	−	−	−	A
Sucrose	A	A	A	A	A	A	−	+w	+	−	−
Lactose	−	L+(−)	L+(−)	−	A(L)	A	−	−	+	−	A
Maltose	−	A	A	A	A	A	A	+	+	−	A
MacConkey (growth)	−	−	+	−	+	+	−	−	−	−	−
Oxidase	+	+#	+	+	+	+	−	+	−	+	+
Urea	−	+	−	+#	+	+	−	−	−	−	−
Indole	+	+	−	−	−	−	−	+	−	−	−
Lysine decarboxylase	−	−	−	−	−	−	ND				
Ornithine decarboxylase	+	d	d	−	−	−	ND				
Arginine dihydrolase	−	−	−	−	−	−	ND				
Motility	−	−	−	−	−	−	−	−	−	−	−
Melibiose					−	A					

*Based on data from King,[271] Cowan and Steel,[509] Steel and Midgley,[510] Wormser, Bottone, Tudy, and Hirschman,[288] Weaver,[282] and Butler, Mahmoud, and Warren.[511]

†*L*, late; *d*, variable; *ND*, not determined; A, acid; *w*, weak; *v*, variable.

‡Beta hemolytic.

§Hemolysis variable; if present, usually greening.

‖Trehalose, −.

¶Trehalose, A (*A. lignieresii*, no acid). Gelatin, liquefied (*A. lignieresii*, negative).

#May require addition of drop of serum to surface of urea slant.

NOTE: **Common reactions: no gas from glucose; catalase positive; no growth on cetrimide agar; no pigment formed; no H₂S (TSI agar); negative citrate (Simmons'); nitrate reduced. Oxidation-fermentation reaction (OF [Leifson] medium): all fermentative.**

these exhibit marked mouse pathogenicity in contrast to rough variants.

No gas is formed from carbohydrates, the urease reaction is usually negative, nitrate is reduced to nitrite, **indole is produced, and ornithine decarboxylase is produced**; no H_2S is formed in TSI agar, and citrate (Simmons) is not utilized. Glucose, sucrose, and mannose are fermented; most strains also ferment galactose, mannitol, and xylose. (See Tables 79-6 and 79-44; see also reference 258.)

Most strains are sensitive in vitro to penicillin, in addition to other antibiotics usually effective against gram-negative organisms. *P. multocida* is highly pathogenic for mice.

Humans usually are infected by animal bites (cats or dogs) or by inhalation of droplets from the sneeze of an animal. On occasion the organism has been recovered from the throats of healthy humans.

In humans, *P. multocida* may cause systemic infections (septicemia, meningitis),[257] lung abscesses, appendiceal abscesses, and persistent wound infections (after bite).[251, 252, 256] Rarer forms of *P. multocida* infections include epiglottitis, septic arthritis, appendiceal abscess, peritonitis, conjunctivitis, and mouth ulcer.

Based on O antigens, at least 16 serotypes of *P. multocida* are known; each is capable of inducing immunity against the homologous serotype, but instances of cross protection are rare.

Pasteurella pneumotropica

P. pneumotropica causes respiratory infections and abscesses in rabbits, mice, and other laboratory animals, and it also occurs in the mouth and throat of healthy dogs. Following dog or cat bites,[259] it occasionally is involved in human disease with a few fatal cases recorded.[260]

The organism does not grow on MacConkey agar; it is **oxidase positive and urea positive***; it is somewhat sensitive to penicillin, but this is much less marked than in *P. multocida*.

Biochemical and morphologic variants of *P. pneumotropica* have been reported.[261]

Pasteurella haemolytica

P. haemolytica is associated with pneumonia in cattle and sheep; 1 case of human infection in which the organism simulated the ulceroglandular form of tularemia, 1 case in which the organism was isolated from a patient with endocarditis,[262] and a urinary tract isolation have been reported.[263]

P. haemolytica produces β-hemolysis on sheep blood agar, is indole negative, and grows on MacConkey agar. It ferments (no gas produced) glucose, xylose, mannitol, and sucrose; most strains are late or nonlactose fermenters. The oxidase reaction is positive and the urease reaction is negative.[264] (See Tables 79-4 and 79-44.)

---

*It may require addition of a drop of serum to the surface of urea slant.

For biotyping and serotyping of *P. haemolytica*, see Biberstein.[265]

Pasteurella ureae

P. ureae, isolated from the human respiratory tract and from patients with meningitis,[266-268] is regarded as a variety of *P. haemolytica*. It differs from the latter in that it is nonhemolytic, does not ferment xylose, does not grow on MacConkey agar, and is urease positive (usually requires addition of drop of serum to surface of urea slant) (see Table 79-44).

The organism is sensitive in vitro to penicillin and is not pathogenic for mice.

ACTINOBACILLUS

The genus *Actinobacillus* (*A. lignieresii*, *A. equuli*) includes gram-negative bacilli that cause septicemia or granulomatous or suppurative abscesses in horses, cattle, sheep, and pig, and occasionally in humans. An organism of uncertain standing, *A. actinomycetemcomitans*, has been implicated in cases of endocarditis in humans.

The genus includes nonmotile, gram-negative rods that are aerobic and facultatively anaerobic, some requiring increased CO_2 for isolation; they **ferment sugars without gas** production.

Some grow on MacConkey agar and are **oxidase positive** (*A. lignieresii*, *A. equuli*); others do not grow on MacConkey agar and are **oxidase negative** (*A. actinomycetemcomitans*).

For the differential characteristics of *Actinobacillus* sp, see Tables 79-4 and 79-44.

Actinobacillus lignieresii

This organism is usually isolated from "actinobacillosis" of cattle. It is found in lesions of the soft tissues, where abscesses are eventually formed, containing pus with small white granules. Primary cultures are microaerophilic.

The organism is **oxidase positive,** produces small amounts of indole, and ferments (no gas produced) glucose, maltose, sucrose, and mannitol in 48 hours. Nitrate is not reduced. A few cases of isolation from humans have been reported.

See Table 79-44 for differentiation of organism from others in the genus. For further details see Phillips.[269]

Actinobacillus equuli

This organism has been isolated from foals with joint-ill and sleepy disease (Maguire[270]). It is similar to *A. lignieresii*, differing mainly in its prompt fermentation of lactose, liquefaction of gelatin (King[271]), and fermentation of melibiose and trehalose. According to *Bergey's Manual*,[3] it forms H_2S (lead acetate paper test). (See Table 79-44.)

Actinobacillus actinomycetemcomitans

This organism does not grow on MacConkey agar and is **oxidase negative.** The reader is referred to the description of *H. aphrophilus;* the 2 organisms are closely related.

A. actinomycetemcomitans is often isolated concomitantly with *Actinomyces israelii* from patients with actinomycosis; however, the organism has been isolated (often in pure culture) from infections in humans without association with *A. israelii* (see King and Tatum,[272] Page and King,[273] and Sutter and Finegold[274]). In the majority of such reported cases the organism was recovered from blood cultures of patients with endocarditis; see also references 275-281.

A. actinomycetemcomitans does not grow without added CO_2 (**candle jar**); some strains require X factor.

On blood agar, growth is light in 24 hours with colonies punctate to 0.5 mm and nonhemolytic. The colonies increase on continued incubation to 1-2 mm. Colonies vary from strain to strain, from colonies that are convex with a smooth surface to colonies that are domed, have an irregular edge, and a slightly wrinkled surface. After 3-5 days the central area of the colonies may show a 4-6 pointed star formation. When the colony is scraped away, the star formation remains (this is easier to see on clear media than on blood agar).[282]

Differentiation from *H. aphrophilus* is based on the (weak) catalase production and failure to ferment lactose or sucrose of *A. actinomycetemcomitans.* The latter **does** ferment either mannitol or xylose (or both), whereas *H. aphrophilus* does not. Fermentation tests are best performed in media with Andrade's indicator. For a detailed report on the fermentative characteristics of *A. actinomycetemcomitans,* see Pulverer and Ko.[283]

NOTE: The organism produces an acid reaction in both the slant and butt portions of TSI and Kligler slants (even though it does not ferment either lactose or sucrose). This is probably due to the fact that the organism does not grow well enough to produce enough alkaline products to cause a reversion of the slant pH.[282]

CARDIOBACTERIUM

Cardiobacterium hominis[284] is the designation given to a closely related group of bacteria previously designated as group "II D" by the Communicable Disease Center. The original isolates have been obtained from patients with endocarditis,[285] but the organism seems to be part of the normal indigenous respiratory flora.[286] One isolation from spinal fluid was reported[287]; all others to date were cultured from cases of endocarditis.

C. hominis is a small, gram-negative coccobacillus, occasionally pleomorphic, facultatively anaerobic, aerobic growth being dependent on atmospheres with **high humidity ("humidiphile")**; poor or no growth is obtained in the ordinary incubator at 37 C. Increased CO_2 atmosphere and culture in humidors containing filter paper strips saturated with water results in good growth.

C. hominis is a **fastidious** organism requiring rich media (trypticase soy or tryptose blood agar with or without 5% blood, "chocolate" agar, or brain-heart infusion agar and CO_2 incubation); poor growth occurs on nutrient agar; there is **no growth** on MacConkey, Simmons citrate, SS, tellurite, EMB, or Endo agars. On blood agar, punctiform colonies, 1-2 mm in size at 48 hours, are formed at 37 C.

The organism **attacks sugars fermentatively** (see below), **is oxidase positive,** and produces indole (extract with xylene and overlay with Ehrlich reagent); glucose, sucrose, levulose, maltose, mannitol, and sorbitol are fermented, with **no gas production.** Nitrate reduction, urease, catalase, motility, and gelatin liquefaction are negative. H_2S production can be demonstrated with lead acetate paper. In blood cultures (thioglycollate broth), small, discrete, grayish puff balls appear imbedded in the blood-fibrin cloth; in trypticase soy and brain-heart infusion broths, discrete grayish floccules are superimposed on the settled red blood cells.[288]

The organisms require 48-72 hours, under CO_2 (5%), on subculture for developing colonies of about 0.5 mm. Aerobically, in the absence of CO_2, there is no growth of 5% sheep blood, trypticase soy, and chocolate agars.

Fermentation tests and KIA slants should be incubated under CO_2 for 48-72 hours. The organism produces **indole,** unlike *H. aphrophilus,* *A. actinomycetemcomitans,* and *Eikenella corrodens,* all of which are indole negative.

C. hominis is antigenically unrelated to any genera of *Brucellaceae, Streptobacillus, Bacteroides, Corynebacterium,* or *Lactobacillus.*

Fluorescent antibody staining with specific anti–*C. hominis* antiserum can be applied successfully for detecting the organism in nose or throat cultures or for identifying isolates.[284]

The organism is sensitive to penicillin, streptomycin, tetracycline, chloramphenicol, and erythromycin.[285]

For detailed reviews of the organism, see Wormser et al.[288] and Savage et al.[289]

KINGELLA

Henriksen and Bøvre[290] in 1976 proposed the creation of a new genus, *Kingella,* to accommodate the organism originally known as *Moraxella kingii.*[291] *Kingella kingii* is characterized by **β-hemolysis, lack of catalase activity** (different from all other moraxellas), and acid production from glucose and maltose on ascites agar slants with 1% carbohydrate incorporated (like a fermenter), but not in OF (Hugh-Leifson) medium; it is **oxidase positive** (see Table 79-6).

After 1 day small colonies are observed (0.1-0.6 mm) on blood agar plates; after 2-4 days some strains form colonies 1-2 mm in size. A distinct but narrow zone of β-hemolysis is observed on human blood agar; it is more pronounced on rabbit, sheep, ox, or horse blood agar. The organism does not seem to require serum or blood.

It has been isolated from blood, knee joints, bone lesions, and the nose and throat.

Henriksen and Bøvre[292] call attention to the possibility of mistaking this organism for α- or β-hemolytic streptococci or for hemolytic *Haemophilus* species.

The organism does not grow in Leifson's OF medium, but grows well on high-quality nutrient agar and blood agar. There is no need for X and V factors or for added CO_2 in the atmosphere. The organism is highly sensitive to penicillin, erythromycin, oxytetracycline, streptomycin, and chloramphenicol.[290]

HAEMOPHILUS APHROPHILUS AND HAEMOPHILUS VAGINALIS

Haemophilus aphrophilus and *Haemophilus vaginalis* are fermenters and should be described here among other fermenters. However, they are discussed with the other members of the genus *Haemophilus* (below, this chapter) to facilitate the reader's task in finding them.

Nonfermenters

The nonfermenters comprise a heterogeneous group of gram-negative **aerobic** bacilli that do not ferment carbohydrates (see discussion of OF medium, fermentation, and oxidation under "initial division," in the introduction to this chapter). The chaotic nomenclature and classification of many of these organisms have recently been clarified by exhaustive nutritional and genetic studies, and data concerning their ecology, pathogenicity, and antimicrobial susceptibility are gradually becoming available.

The majority of nonfermenters occur variously in the soil, on plants, water, and human skin, while others are found only in the gastrointestinal or genitourinary tract, the oropharynx, and on skin. Of the 30 species and 8 as yet unnamed groups occurring in clinical material,[292] 2 are undoubtedly pathogens (*Pseudomonas mallei* and *P. pseudomallei*), with neither found in nature or among civilians in the United States; 3 other pseudomonads, i.e., *P. aeruginosa*, *P. maltophilia*, and *P. cepacia*, are common in the hospital environment and are etiologically significant in human disease, as are *Acinetobacter*, *Flavobacterium*, and *Moraxella*. Most other nonfermenters are encountered less frequently in the human environment and seem to be of limited (or no) clinical significance.

Nonfermenters comprise about one-fifth (or less) of all gram-negative aerobic or facultatively anaerobic bacilli recovered from extraintestinal specimens in clinical microbiology laboratories, with *P. aeruginosa* being by far the most prevalent (ca. 65%) of all nonfermenters, followed by *Acinetobacter anitratus* (formerly *Herellea*), and *P. maltophilia*.[292]

Many **nonfermenters** are glucose **oxidizers** (*Pseudomonas*, *Acinetobacter*, others); others cannot utilize glucose or other carbohydrates (**nonutilizers**, *Alcaligenes*, *Moraxella*, others; see Table 79-1).

The nonfermenters are found primarily free in nature; with the advent of antibiotics and the survival of patients with reduced immune responses, the nonfermenters (and some fermenters) are encountered with increasing frequency as agents of **opportunistic**, often very serious **infection.**

Presumptive and final identifications

The key originated by King, extensively revised by Weaver,[2, 2a, 7] and shown in Table 79-2, is recommended for the *preliminary* recognition of these organisms. As discussed earlier, the key is based on practical criteria such as (1) nature of attack on carbohydrates (fermentative, oxidative, or none), (2) growth on MacConkey agar, and (3) oxidase reaction. The key is intended **only** as a guideline; the groups listed must be identified by the use of a number of differential reactions (see Tables 79-46 to 79-52 and descriptions of the various genera and groups). Another useful schema is that of Gilardi[293–296]; much highly useful information is found in the works of Pickett et al.,[292, 297–299] CDC publications,[300] and Blazevic.[301]

Conventional tests

It should be emphatically noted here that interpretation of diagnostic data, as given in various tables (in this volume and also in other publications) must be undertaken with the knowledge of the particular **method** on which the data are based.

Pickett[292] sounds a note of warning: a datum generated by a particular **method** regarding a particular **feature** (e.g., **buffered substrate method** for determining **acidification of glucose**) will **not** necessarily be identical with that datum generated for the same feature but by a different method. For example, *P. pseudoalcaligenes* is scored by CDC[2] as "glucose alkaline"; however, Pickett,[292] using different methodology, scores it as "glucose negative." The important point here is not that one method is better than the other, but rather that the bacteriologist should always use a **table** that is applicable to the **method** being used.

NOTE: Weaver's key (Table 79-2) and the criteria in Tables 79-46 to 79-52 are based on the use of conventional media using CDC procedures (see below). The descriptions of the various genera and groups are also based on CDC procedures, unless otherwise noted.

CDC approach to identification of nonfermenters[300]

1. Morphology and preliminary physiologic tests:
   a. Streak unknown culture on blood agar plate for isolated colonies. Incubate 35 C for 18-24 h.
   b. Do **Gram stain** on colonies.
   c. Record cellular and colonial morphology.
   d. Note hemolytic action of colonies.

e. Do **oxidase** test.
f. Pick single colony to:
   (1) Heart infusion agar (HIA) slant
   (2) Heart infusion agar broth (HIB)
   (3) Triple sugar iron (TSI) agar
g. TSI: Use reaction in butt to decide if organism is a fermenter or a nonfermenter.
h. HIA and HIB: Use to inoculate appropriate biochemical sets.

2. Biochemical set used for nonfermentative gram-negative bacteria:

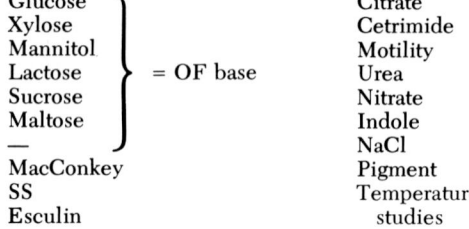

Glucose ⎫
Xylose ⎪
Mannitol ⎪
Lactose ⎬ = OF base
Sucrose ⎪
Maltose ⎪
— ⎭
MacConkey
SS
Esculin

Citrate
Cetrimide
Motility
Urea
Nitrate
Indole
NaCl
Pigment
Temperature studies

3. Inoculation procedure:

Medium	Inoculum	Amount
TSI slant (add lead acetate paper)	HIA slant*	Stab to bottom and streak slant
Sugars: Glucose Xylose Mannitol Lactose Sucrose Maltose Blank		Stab 4 × ½ inch below surface
Motility		Stab once ½ inch below surface
Simmons' citrate		Streak lightly on slant
MacConkey slant SS slant Esculin Nitrate broth Cetrimide Tryptone broth for indole Christensen's urea slant Nutrient broth, 0% NaCl Nutrient broth, 6.0% NaCl Pigment detection: Flo (Medium F) Tech (Medium P) Temperature studies: TGY‡ 25 C TGY 35 C TGY 42 C	HIB†	1 drop

All media are incubated 48 h at 35 C. When necessary, bacteria are stained by Leifson's method for flagellar arrangement.[302]

Gilardi's methodology for identification of nonfermenters[293–296, 303]

1. Morphologic studies[296, 303]:
   a. Prepare smears from 24 h growth on trypti-

*18-24 h heart infusion agar slant.
†18-24 heart infusion broth culture.
‡Tryptone-glucose-yeast extract agar slant.

case soy agar (TSA, BBL). Stain by Gram's method (Hucker's modification).
b. Motility is determined by microscopic examination of a hanging drop preparation of a trypticase soy broth (BBL) culture.
c. To demonstrate flagella, use Gray's method as outlined by Finegold et al.[304]
d. Determine accumulation of poly-β-hydroxybutyrate (PBHB) by Sudan black staining[305] of cultures grown on mineral base medium supplemented with DL-β-hydroxybutyrate used for carbon assimilation studies.[306]
e. Isolated colonies on TSA plates containing 5% (wt/vol) defibrinated sheep blood (TSBA) are examined for morphology and hemolytic activity. Growth characteristics are also observed on Salmonella-Shigella agar (SS agar, BBL), MacConkey agar (BBL), and deoxycholate agar (DC agar, BBL).
f. Fluorescein (pyoverdin) production is detected by exposing cultures on Sellers' differential agar (Difco), Pseudosel agar (BBL), or Pseudomonas agar **F** (Difco) to UV irradiation. Pyocyanin production is determined through the use of Pseudomonas agar **P** (Difco).

2. Physiologic studies[296, 303]:
a. A standard inoculum consisting of one 4 mm loopful of a 24 h TSB culture is used for most tests. Growth from TSA or TSBA culture is used for patch method of inoculation and for inoculating gluconate oxidation and ortho-nitrophenyl-β-D-galactopyranoside (ONPG) tests.
b. *Oxidation of carbohydrates.* Oxidation of 1% (wt/vol) solutions of carbohydrates is tested in OF basal medium (OFBM, Difco) and oxidation of 10% (vol/vol) of lactose is tested in purple agar base (Difco).
c. *Gluconate oxidation.* Production of 2-ketogluconate is detected by adding a loopful of growth and a gluconate substrate tablet (Key Scientific Products) into tube containing 1.5 ml sterile water. After incubation for 24 h, culture is tested for reducing substances by adding Clinitest tablet (Ames Co.) and observing for green or orange color indicative of positive reaction.
d. *ONPG test.* β-D-galactosidase is detected by adding a loopful of growth to β-galactoside test broth (Hyland) and observing for formation of yellow color after overnight incubation.
e. *Nitrate reduction.* Reduction of nitrate to nitrite is determined as outlined by Finegold et al.[304] using trypticase nitrate broth (BBL) plus 1.5% agar. Ability to grow anaerobically in presence of nitrate or nitrite is indicated by development of blue color in butt of Sellers' medium. Nitrogen gas production is ascertained in the 2 former media by production of gas bubbles in condensate as well as in agar butts.
f. *Urease, indole, and hydrogen sulfide production.* Christensen's urea agar (BBL) and Kligler iron agar (KIA, BBL) or triple sugar iron agar (TSI) are used, respectively, for detection of urease and hydrogen sulfide production. Indole production is detected by adding Kovacs' reagent to SIM medium (BBL) cultures after 24 h incubation. With suspicious flavobacteria, indole production is detected by adding Ehrlich's reagent, after xylene extrac-

tion, to tryptone broth (Difco) cultures after 24 h incubation.

g. *Decarboxylase, dihydrolase, and deaminase activity.* Phenylalanine deaminase activity is determined by flooding Phenylalanine Agar (BBL) slant cultures after 24 h incubation with a 1% (wt/vol) ferric chloride solution and observing for development of green color. Arginine dihydrolase and lysine and ornithine decarboxylase activity are detected using Decarboxylase Base Moeller (Difco) overlayed with mineral oil.

h. *Acylamidase activity.* Acylamidase activity is examined using a modified method of the one described by Arai et al.[307] A loopful of growth is inoculated to 1 ml mineral base broth medium used for carbon assimilation studies, supplemented with 0.1% (wt/vol) acetamide. After overnight incubation, 1 drop of Nessler's reagent is added to test medium. A positive reaction is indicated by the immediate appearance of a reddish-brown sediment, demonstrating the presence of ammonia resulting from acylamidase action.

i. *Production of extracellular enzymes.* The patch method of inoculation is used for the following tests with the exception of gelatin liquefaction. **Starch hydrolysis:** Test by flooding TSA plates supplemented with 1% (wt/vol) starch with Lugol's iodine after 24 h incubation and observing for clear zone around patch of growth. **Production of lipase:** Test on agar plate medium supplemented with 1% (wt/vol) polyethylene sorbitan monooleate (Tween 80) described by Sierra,[308] and observing for turbid halo around growth. **Lecithinase production:** Observe for white precipitate around growth on TSA plate supplemented with 10% (vol/vol) egg yolk enrichment (BBL). **Deoxyribonuclease (DNase) activity:** Incorporate 0.01% (wt/vol) toluidine blue into DNase test agar (Difco) and observe for change in indicator to pink around growth. **Esculin hydrolysis:** Observe for black precipitate around growth on TSA plate supplemented with 0.1% (wt/vol) esculin and 0.05% (wt/vol) ferric citrate. **Proteolytic activity:** Determine liquefaction of gelatin in nutrient gelatin.

j. *Indophenol oxidase activity.* Oxidase activity is detected by rubbing growth from TSA or TSBA culture onto oxidase test paper strip (Patho-Tec Co.). Dark blue color appears within 30 s with oxidase-positive strains.

k. *Tolerance to chemical and physical factors.* In the following tests, media are inoculated with broth suspension. **Growth at 42 C** is determined using TSA slant cultures incubated at 42 ± 0.05 C. **Tolerance to 0.03%** (wt/vol) **cetrimide** is tested using Pseudosel Agar plates and to triphenyltetrazolium chloride (TTC) using TSA plates supplemented with 1% (wt/vol) TTC. **Salt tolerance** is determined by adjusting NaCl concentration of TSA plates to 6.5% (vol/vol).

l. *Assimilation of organic compounds as sole source of carbon.* Growth at expense of organic compounds is determined in mineral base medium (MBM) containing (g/L): $MgSO_4$, 0.1; NaCl, 5.0; $NH_4H_2PO_4$, 1.0; K_2HPO_4, 1.0. Respective carbon sources are added to basal medium to give final concentration of 0.03M (pelargonate, DL-norleucine) and 0.015M (acetate). Each medium is adjusted to pH 6.5 ± 0.1. The ingredients, excluding agar, made at double concentration are sterilized by filtration and brought up to working concentration by adding appropriate volume of sterile melted 3.2% agar. Mixture is then dispensed into tubes and slanted.

NOTE: Unless otherwise stated, all cultures are incubated aerobically at **30 C** for 24-48 h.

m. *Antimicrobial susceptibility.* Strains are tested for antibiotic susceptibility according to standardized single-agar disk diffusion (Kirby-Bauer) method (see Chapter 87).

Pickett's methodology for nonfermenters*

Initial subculture of unknown colony is to be made to KIA or TSI (or KIA- or TSI-esculin) to determine if organism is a fermenter or nonfermenter and to obtain massive inoculum needed for **buffered single substrate (BSS) tests.**[297,309,310]

Buffered single substrate tests. Each medium contains single substrate (carbohydrate, alcohol, etc.) that specifically reacts with **preformed** products of **pregrown** organisms in heavy inoculum.

These media are used for determining bulk of secondary characteristics.

Buffered single substrate media.[292] Unless otherwise indicated, all tubed growth media are dispensed in 3 ml amounts into 13 × 100 mm screwcap tubes and steam sterilized (121 C for 15 min).

1. General: All are dispensed into 13 × 100 mm tubes to give final volume of 1.0 ml. Following 5 BSS media are steam sterilized: gluconate, indole, indolepyruvic acid, lysine decarboxylase, and phenylpyruvic acid. Other BSS media (carbohydrates, amides, organic salts, and urea) need not be autoclaved; indeed, some are heat labile and must not be autoclaved.

2. Specific media:
    a. **Indole,** 200 ml single-strength (1×) medium:

L-Tryptophane	1.0 g
NaCl	1.0 g
K_2HPO_4, 0.5M	7.2 ml
KH_2PO_4, 0.5M	0.8 ml
(to give 0.02M, pH 7.6)	
Distilled water	192 ml

    b. **Gluconate,** 200 ml single-strength medium:

Potassium gluconate	4.0 g
KNO_3	0.4 g
KH_2PO_4, 0.5M	16 ml
$NaHCO_3$	0.2 g
(to give 0.04M phosphate, pH 6.5)	
Distilled water	184 ml

    c. **LDC** (lysine decarboxylase), 200 ml single-strength medium:

L-Lysine · HCl	1.0 g
Glucose	1.0 g
KH_2PO_4	1.0 g
(to give pH 4.6)	
Distilled water	200 ml

    d. **PPA** (phenylpyruvic acid), 200 ml single-strength medium:

DL-Phenylalanine	0.8 g
KH_2PO_4, 0.5M	4 ml
K_2HPO_4, 0.5M	4 ml
(to give 0.02M, pH 6.8)	
Distilled water	192 ml

*References 292, 297-299, 309, and 310.

e. **Carbohydrates and alcohols:**
(1) Stock solutions (all are stable for months at room temperature):
(a) 0.5M KH_2PO_4.
(b) 0.5M K_2HPO_4.
(c) A "500×" solution of phenol red and crystal violet (PR-CV) prepared as follows (for 200 ml):

Phenol red	2.0 g
Crystal violet	0.2 g
Distilled water	200 ml

Add concentrated alkali until both ingredients are dissolved.
(d) Substrates: All stock carbohydrates are prepared as "5×" (i.e., 10%) solutions in 20 × 150 mm screwcap tubes. Slight excess of chloroform is added as preservative (filtration for sterilization is unnecessary).
(2) Stock, "10/8×," basal medium. This 10/8× basal is preferable to double-strength (i.e., 2×) medium because it can readily be pipetted cold; a 2× basal contains 0.2 g/100 ml agar and cannot be pipetted satisfactorily without prior heating. For 400 ml:

(a) K_2HPO_4, 0.5M	5	ml
(b) PR-CV, 500×	1	ml
(c) Agar	0.5	g
(d) Distilled water to make	400	ml

(3) Prepare and use:

(a) Basal medium, 10/8× (in 13 mm tube)	0.8	ml
(b) Add closure		
(c) Steam 10 min		
(d) Aseptically add 5× carbohydrate	0.2	ml
(e) Aseptically add inoculum	0.1	ml
(f) Incubate 4-6 d with daily readings		

Note that **all** carbohydrates are added **after** steaming simply to maintain standard procedure for all of these. In fact, one may, if he or she wishes, add heat-stable carbohydrates (e.g., mannitol, sucrose; but **not** labile carbohydrates such as fructose, arabinose, xylose, rhamnose) before steaming.

f. **Amides and organic salts:**
(1) Stock substrates: not all amides and organic salts are used at same final concentration (see Pickett[311] for tabulation of these). Following are 4 of those frequently used:

	Stock g/100 ml	To give g/100 ml
Acetamide, 5×	1.0	0.2
Formate, 5×	1.0	0.2
Nicotinamide, 5×	2.5	0.5
Tartrate, 5×	1.0	0.2

These stocks should be in the range of pH 6.5-7.0. Like carbohydrates, they are stored in 20 mm screwcap tubes over slight excess of chloroform.
(2) Stock, "10/8×," basal medium. For 400 ml:

KH_2PO_4, 0.5M	14	ml
K_2HPO_4, 0.5M	6	ml
PR-CV, 500×	1	ml
Agar	0.5	g
Distilled water to make	400	ml

(3) Prepare and use:

(a) Basal medium, 10/8× (in 13 mm tube)	0.8	ml
(b) Substrate, 5×	0.2	ml
(c) Add closure		
(d) Steam 10 min		
(e) Aseptically add inoculum	0.1	ml
(f) Incubate 4-6 d with daily readings		

g. **Urea,** 200 ml single-strength medium:

Urea	4 g
KH_2PO_4, 0.5M	25 ml
K_2HPO_4, 0.5M	25 ml
PR-CV, 500×	0.4 ml
Distilled water to make	200 ml

Note that formula for urea media differs in respect to concentration of buffer. This urea medium is strongly buffered and hence will give positive tests only with strongly urease-positive organisms.

Some other media of Pickett's

Fluorescence-lactose-denitrification (FLN) medium

Proteose peptone no. 3 (Difco)	1.0	g/100 ml
Lactose	2.0	g/100 ml
Agar	1.5	g/100 ml
Phenol red	0.002	g/100 ml
$MgSO_4 \cdot 7H_2O$	0.15	g/100 ml
K_2HPO_4	0.15	g/100 ml
KNO_3	0.2	g/100 ml
KNO_2	0.05	g/100 ml

If solution of phenol red is used to prepare medium, it must contain no alcohol.
1. Dispense in 4 ml amounts, sterilize, and solidify to give butt and slant of approximately equal length.
2. Inoculate by stabbing and streaking.
3. Read at 24 and 48 h for fluorescence (under UV), acidification of lactose (yellow slant), and denitrification (gas).

Kligler iron agar (or TSI) slants with esculin (KIA-Esc). Use 16-17 ml of commercial medium, supplemented with esculin to give 0.002 g/100 ml (a 1 g/100 ml stock solution of esculin in methanol is convenient for this) per 20 × 150 mm screwcap tube, thus providing butt of about 3 cm and slope of 10 cm extending to constricted neck. Any free fluid on slant medium should be decanted before inoculation.

Motility-nitrate medium

Tryptose (Difco)	1.0	g/100 ml
Infusion agar (Difco)	0.8	g/100 ml
KNO_3	0.1	g/100 ml

1. Dispense in 4 ml amounts, sterilize, and solidify in upright position.
2. Inoculate by stabbing 5-10 mm into medium, incubate, and read at 6 ± 2, 24, and 48 h.
3. Test for nitrite by adding 5 drops reagent and (if nitrite negative) for nitrate by adding few grains of zinc.

Gluconate (double-strength Benedict's solution, modified)

$CuSO_4 \cdot 5H_2O$	17.3	g/100 ml
K_2CO_3	100	g/100 ml
Trisodium citrate dihydrate	173	g/100 ml

1. Incubate inoculated gluconate medium 18-24 h, add 5 drops reagent, mix, heat at 100 C for 2 min, and read.
2. Reduction of blue copper solution to brown color, usually with heavy precipitate, represents positive test.

Nitrate broth. 1 g/100 ml peptone and 0.2 g/100 ml

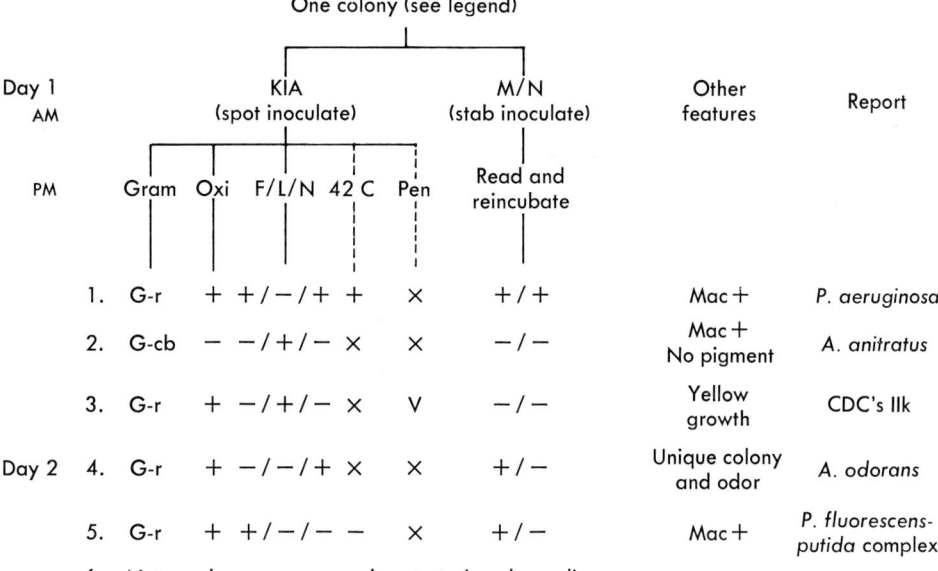

Fig. 79-3. Recommended logistics for processing nonfermentative bacilli. Proceed as follows: (1) During early to midmorning, select a well-isolated colony and "spot" inoculate KIA slant (i.e., a 3-5 mm spot on surface of medium). Stab inoculate (**only** 5-10 mm) M/N medium; incubate both media at 35 C. (2) During mid- to late afternoon, read and reincubate M/N medium; using growth on KIA slant, do Gram stain, do oxidase and catalase tests, and inoculate (stab and streak) a tube of F/L/N medium. If bacterium is oxidase positive and motile, it may be fluorescent pseudomonad; in such instance, lightly inoculate broth medium and incubate this at 42 C. If bacterium is oxidase positive and nonmotile, it may be *Moraxella;* in such instance, check penicillin sensitivity (2-unit disk); this can frequently be done on free area of primary blood agar plate. "Primary" features include colonial morphology, pigmented growth, oxidase, Gram stain, F/L/N medium, motility, growth at 42 C, and penicillin sensitivity. "Secondary" features (**buffered substrate tests, BSS**) include arabinose, glucose or fructose, lactose, acetamide, gluconate, indole, LDC, and urea. *KIA,* Kligler iron agar slant; *M/N,* motility nitrate medium; *Oxi,* oxidase test; *F/L/N,* fluorescence/lactose/denitrification medium; *Mac,* MacConkey agar; *G-r,* gram-negative rod; *G-cb,* gram-negative coccobacillus. (Data from Pickett, J.: Nonfermentative gram-negative bacilli, Current concepts in clinical microbiology course, UCLA Extension Division, Aug. 1976; also syllabus, Am. Soc. Clin. Pathol., Los Angeles Training Institute, 1976; also personal communication, 1977.)

KNO_3. Each tube should receive inverted vial for detection of denitrification.

Reagent for PPA. 10 g/100 ml ferric chloride in 50 vol% HCl (sp. gr. 1.19). Incubate inoculated PPA medium 18-24 h, add 1-2 drops reagent, shake briskly, and read immediately. Green color represents positive test.

For further details on Pickett's methodology and media, see Manclarck et al.,[309] Otto and Pickett,[297] and Pickett.[292, 310] Fig. 79-3 summarizes the steps involved in Pickett's methodology.

• • •

Multiple (miniaturized) test kits. In contrast to the successful application of these kits to the identification of fermenters (especially *Enterobacteriaceae*), the kits have not yet been uniformly successful in the identification of nonfermenters. Several systems are used for this purpose, but they need to be used with caution (see discussion in Chapter 74).

Automated instruments for identification. Similar to the efforts to adapt several automated instruments and systems for the identification of fermenters, developmental work is presently under way for enabling such instruments (AMS system, Vitek, St. Louis; Autobac, Pfizer, New York; MS-2, Abbott, Dallas) to identify nonfermenters.

• • •

Current nomenclature and synonyms of nonfermenters. Table 79-45 lists the current nomenclature, synonyms, and earlier name usage of a variety of gram-negative nonfermentative organisms.

PSEUDOMONADACEAE

The family *Pseudomonadaceae*[3] contains straight or curved gram-negative rods, motile by polar flagella, whose metabolism is respiratory, never fermentative. Of the 4 genera in the family, *Pseudomonas* contains a number of species of medical importance.

PSEUDOMONAS

The organisms in the genus *Pseudomonas* are mostly free-living bacteria widely distributed

Table 79-45. Current nomenclature of some
nonfermentative gram-negative bacilli

Current name	Synonyms; earlier usage
Pseudomonas aeruginosa	Bacillus pyocyaneus
Pseudomonas fluorescens	P. aureofaciens,
	P. chlororaphis,
	P. margialis
Pseudomonas putida	P. ovalis
Pseudomonas cepacia	CDC EO-1, P. multi-
	vorans, P. kingae
Pseudomonas maltophilia	P. melanogena
Pseudomonas putrefaciens	CDC Ib
Pseudomonas stutzeri	P. mendocina, CDC Vb
Pseudomonas paucimobilis	CDC IIK —1
Pseudomonas acidovorans	Comamonas terrigena
Pseudomonas testosteroni	Comamonas terrigena
Pseudomonas pickettii	CDC Va-2, P. pseudo-
	alcaligenes
Acinetobacter	Herellea vaginicola,
calcoaceticus var.	Acinetobacter anitratus,
anitratus	Bacterium anitratum
Acinetobacter	Mima polymorpha,
calcoaceticus var.	Acinetobacter lwoffi,
lwoffi	Achromobacter lwoffi
Flavobacterium odoratum	CDC MIVF
Flavobacterium ssp	CDC II b
Flavobacterium	CDC II a
meningosepticum	
Bordetella bronchiseptica	B. bronchicanis
Achromobacter	CDC III a, III b
xylosoxidans	
Achromobacter spp	CDC Vd —1, Vd-2
Moraxella lacunata	M. liquefaciens
Moraxella osloensis	Mima polymorpha var.
	oxidans
Moraxella phenylpyruvica	Moraxella sp II
Eikenella corrodens	CDC HB-1, Bacteroides
	corrodens
Campylobacter fetus ssp	Vibrio fetus
intestinalis	
Campylobacter fetus ssp	Related Vibrio
jejuni	
Alcaligenes denitrificans	Vc
Achromobacter sp	Vd-1, Vd-2
Agrobacterium radiobacter	Vd-3

in soil and water, while some are parasites (and
pathogens) of plants. Of the many known species,
a small (but growing) number is associated with
disease, often severe, in humans; the most
important of these opportunistic pathogens is P.
aeruginosa. P. (formerly Actinobacillus) pseudomallei, the agent of **melioidosis**, and P. (Actinobacillus) mallei, causing **glanders**, are now
also classified in this genus.

The genus consists of gram-negative rods,
straight or curved but not helical, which are
motile by means of polar flagella (or, with rare
exceptions, nonmotile); they break down sugars
oxidatively without forming gas (usually no acid
in fermentation media; use OF medium to determine sugar reactions), are **oxidase positive**
(except for P. maltophilia and some strains of P.
cepacia), and are strict aerobes,[306,312] except
for those species that can use denitrification as
means of anaerobic respiration.

Diffusible pigments (yellow, green) are produced by many strains and are useful for differentiation. The most common pigments are
pyocyanin ("blue pus")—bluish green, soluble
both in chloroform and water, and **fluorescein**
(pyoverdin)—greenish yellow, fluorescent,
insoluble in chloroform but soluble in water.
Most grow well on ordinary media, including
MacConkey agar and to a lesser extent SS agar.

For major preliminary reactions allowing differentiation of pseudomonads from certain other
gram-negative rods, see Tables 79-46 through
79-52.

P. aeruginosa and many strains of other fluorescent pseudomonads convert gluconate (product of glucose oxidization) to 2-ketogluconate,
which can be detected by appearance of a reducing substance in the medium. The gluconate test
(Chapter 72), especially when performed with
medium made with prepared gluconate substrate* and tested with Clinitest tablets† instead
of Benedict's reagent, is helpful in the identification of P. aeruginosa and some other pseudomonads (however, some strains of Klebsiella,
Enterobacter, and Serratia are also gluconate
positive).[313]

For comprehensive studies on diagnostic criteria and identification procedures of pseudomonads of medical importance see Sutter,[314]
Gilardi,‡ and especially the comprehensive
review by Gilardi[303]; also refer to Stanier et al.[306]
for an exhaustive study of aerobic pseudomonads.

Fluorescein-producing pseudomonads (fluorescent group)
Pseudomonas aeruginosa

P. aeruginosa (known for many years as
Bacillus pyocyaneus) occurs singly, in pairs, or
in short chains of gram-negative rods. It is motile
(monotrichous), grows at 41-43 C but not at 4 C,
and most strains from clinical material are **β-
hemolytic** on blood agar. In addition to other
media, it also grows on **cetrimide agar.** On agar
media the organism forms large, spreading, grayish colonies with irregular edges. The medium
usually has a greenish color due to the pigment
formed. Cultures have a marked odor of trimethylamine (grapelike). In the open tubes of
the OF (Hugh-Leifson) medium, acid is produced from dextrose (glucose) but not from lactose or sucrose (see Table 79-47).

Both **fluorescein** (pyoverdin, yellow-green,
fluorescent) and **pyocyanin** (a blue, water-
soluble, nonfluorescent, phenazine pigment) are
produced by most strains (use Pseudomonas
agar, P and F; see Chapter 72); apyocyanogenic
strains, however, are not uncommon. In TSI
medium no change occurs in the slant or butt
and no H_2S is produced. Both malonate and

---

*Key gluconate substrate tablet, Key Scientific
Products Co., Los Angeles.
†Ames Co., Elkhart, Ind.
‡References 295, 296, 315, and 316.

Table 79-46. Nonfermenters I: gram-negative oxidizers of glucose—MacConkey positive (growth), oxidase negative*†

Species	Growth on MacConkey	Oxidase	Motility	Lysine decarboxylase	Arginine dihydrolase	OF Mannitol	OF Lactose	Nitrate reduction	Notes
Acinetobacter calcoaceticus	+ 99‡ (1)§	− 0	− 0	− 0	− 0	− 2	+ 97 (2)	− 1	
Pseudomonas cepacia	+ 99 (1)	v 87	+ 95	+	− 0	+ 100	+ 99	v 57	Pigment variable
Pseudomonas maltophilia	+ 100	− 10 (?)	+	+ 93	− 0	− 0	v 23	v 39	
Pseudomonas paucimobilis	v 11 (13)	v 75	w	− 0	− 8	− 0	+ 100	− 3	Yellow
Pseudomonas mallei	v 88	v 25	− 0	− 0	+ 100	v 62	v 12	+ 100	
Ve-1	+ 100	− 10	+	− 0	+ 100	v 82	v 6 (28)	v 67	Yellow, esculin +
Ve-2	+ 100	− 9	+	− 0	v 14	+ 100	v 14 (22)	− 6	Yellow, esculin −

*From Weaver, R. E.: Gram-negative organisms: an approach to identification (guide to **presumptive** identifications), Atlanta, 1979, Center for Disease Control.
†+, 90% or more positive in 1-2 d; + or −, 50-90% positive in 1-2 d; −, 90% or more negative; − or +, 50-90% negative; (+), delayed positive reaction (3 or more d; *w*, weakly positive reaction; *v*, variable; *OF*, oxidation-fermentation medium.
‡Percent positive in 1-2 d.
§Percent positive (delayed) in 3 or more d.

Table 79-47. Nonfermenters II: glucose oxidizers—MacConkey positive (growth), oxidase positive*†

Species	Growth on MacConkey	Oxidase	Pyocyanin	Pyoverdin	Indole	H_2S-TSI	Lysine
1. *Pseudomonas aeruginosa*	+ 100‡	+ 100	v 46	v 65	– 0	– 0	– 0
2. *Pseudomonas fluorescens* and putida	+ 100	+ 99	– 0	+ 95	– 0	– 0	– 0
3. *Pseudomonas cepacia*	+ 99 (1)§	v 87	– 0	– 0	– 0	– 0	+
4. *Pseudomonas pseudomallei*	+ 100	+ 100	– 0	– 0	– 0	– 0	– 0
5. *Pseudomonas stutzeri*	+ 100	+ 100	– 0	– 0	– 0	– 0	– 0
6. Vb-3 (*stutzeri*-like)	+ 100	+ 100	– 0	– 0	– 0	– 0	– 0
7. *Pseudomonas mendocina*	+	+	–	–	–	–	–
8. *Pseudomonas "thomasii"*	+ 100	+ 100	– 0	– 0	– 0	– 0	– 0
9. *Pseudomonas vesicularis*	v 89	+ 94	– 0	– 0	– 0	– 0	– 0
10. *Pseudomonas diminuta*	+ 97 (3)	+ 100	– 0	– 0	– 0	– 0	– 0
11. *Pseudomonas pickettii*	+ 100	+ 100	– 0	– 0	– 0	– 0	– 0
12. Va-1 (*Pseudomonas*-like)	+ 99 (1)	+ 100	– 0	– 0	– 0	– 0	– 0
13. *Pseudomonas putrefaciens*	+ 100	+ 100	– 0	– 0	– 0	+ 98	– 0
14. *Pseudomonas paucimobilis* (IIK-1)	v 10 (13)	v 75	– 0	– 0	– 0	– 0	– 0
15. IIK-2	v 81 (17)	+ 98	– 0	– 0	– 0	– 0	– 8
16. *Achromobacter xylosoxidans*	+ 100	+ 100	– 0	– 0	– 0	– 0	v (16)
17. Vd-1 (*Achromobacter*-like)	+ 100	+ 100	– 0	– 0	– 0	v 58	– 0
18. Vd-2 (*Achromobacter*-like)	+ 100	+ 100	– 0	– 0	– 0	v 42	– 0
19. *Agrobacterium radiobacter*	+ 100	+ 100	– 0	– 0	– 0	– 0	– 0
20. EO-2	v 67 (11)	+ 100	– 0	– 0	– 0	– 0	– 0
21. *Brucella*			– 0	– 0	– 0	– 0	NT
22. *Pseudomonas mallei*	v 88	v 25	– 0	– 0	– 0	– 0	– 0
23. *Vibrio extorquens*	v 16	+ 96	– 0	– 0	– 0	– 0	NT
24. *Flavobacterium meningosepticum*	v 89 (3)	+ 99	– 0	– 0	+ 100	– 0	NT
25. IIb, *Flavobacterium spp.*	v 54 (9)	+ 96	– 0	– 0	+ 98	– 0	NT

*From Weaver, R. E.: Gram-negative organisms: an approach to identification (guide to **presumptive** identifications), Atlanta,
†+, 90% or more positive in 1-2 d; + or –, 50-90% positive in 1-2 d; –, 90% or more negative; – or +, 50-90% negative; (+),
‡Percent positive in 1-2 d.
§Percent positive (delayed) in 3 or more d.

	Arginine	Nitrate to gas	Nitrate reduced	Motility	Growth on SS	Urea	OF glucose	OF xylose	OF mannitol	OF lactose	OF sucrose	OF maltose
1.	+ 100	+ 93	+ 98	+ 90	+ 96	v 58	+ 98	+ 92	v 73	− 1	− 0	− 0
2.	+ 99	− 3	v 17	+ 99	v 87	v 20	+ 100	+ 100	v 50	v 25	v 44	v 18
3.	− 0	− 0	v 57	+ 95	− 6	v 60	+ 100	+ 100	+ 99	+ 99	v 86	+ 99
4.	+ 100	+ 98	+ 100	+	v 8 (31)	v 13	+ 100	+ or (+) 86 (14)	+ 99	+ 99	v 66	+ 99
5.	− 0	+ 100	+ 100	+ 100	v 54	v 33	+ 100	+ 100	+ 93	− 0	− 0	+ 100
6.	+ 100	+ 100	+ 100	+ 98	+ 100	v 12	+ 100	+ 97	v 65	− 0	− 0	+ 100
7.	+	+	+	+	+	+	+	+	−	−	−	−
8.	− 0	− 0	v 13	+ 94		+ or (+) 81 (19)	+ 100	+ 100	+ 100	+ 100	− 0	+ 100
9.	− 0	− 0	− 6	v 85	− 6	− (8)	+ 96	v 23	− 0	− 0	− 0	+ 100
10.	− 0	− 0	− 3	+ 98	− 2	v (13)	v 21	− 0	− 0	− 0	− 0	− 0
11.	− 0	v 85	+ 100	v 65	− 0	+ 100	+ 100	+ 100	− 0	− 0	− 0	− 0
12.	− 0	v 86	+ 100	v 81	−' 0	+ 100	+ 100	+ 100	− 0	+ 100	− 0	+ 100
13.	− 0	− 0	+ 100	+ 100	v 48 (6)	v 24	v 24	− 0	− 0	− 0	v 48	v 48
14.	− 8	− 0	− 3	wk	− 0	− 6	+ 100	+ 100	− 0	+ 100	+ 100	+ 100
15.	− 8	− 0	v 13	− 0	− (2)	+ 96	+ 100	+ 100	− 0	+ 100	+ 100	+ 100
16.	v 12 (16)	v 60	+ 100	+ 92	+ 98	− 0	v 78	+ 99	− 1	− 0	− 0	− 1
17.	v 64	+ 97	+ 100	+	+ 97	+ 91	+ 100	+ 100	v 57	− 0	− 0	− 9
18.	v 73	+ 100	+ 100	+	+ 95	+ 92	+ 97	+ 100	+ 100	− 0	+ 100	+ 100
19.	− 3	− 5	v 87	+ 100	v 29	+ or (+) 89 (11)	+ 100	+ 100	+ 100	+ 100	+ 100	+ 100
20.	− 0	− 2	v 85	− 0	− 4	v 74	+ 100	+ 99	v 10	+ 91	− 0	v 20
21.	NT	v 44	+ 100	− 0	− 0	+ 99	v 75	+ 90	− 0	− 0	− 0	− 0
22.	+ 100	− 0	+ 100	− 0	− 0	v 12	+ 100	v 12	v 62	v 12	− 0	v 0 (75)
23.	NT	− 0	v 25	v 23	− 0	v 29	v 40	+ 94	− 2	− 0	− 0	− 2
24.	NT	− 0	− 0	− 0	− 1	+ 8	+ 99	− 3.5	+ 99	v 58	− 0	+ 100
25.	NT	− 0	v 22	− 0	− 0	v 14	+ 92	v 30	− 9	− 0	v 13	+ 92

1979, Center for Disease Control.

delayed positive reaction (3 or more d); *w*, weakly positive reaction; *v*, variable; *OF*, oxidation-fermentation medium.

Table 79-48. Nonfermenters III: gram-negative oxidizers of glucose—MacConkey negative (no growth), oxidase negative*†

Species	Growth on MacConkey	Oxidase	Urea	Indole	OF sucrose	Nitrate reduction	OF xylose	OF maltose	Notes
Brucella	v	v	+	−	−	+	+	−	Tiny; coccoid
			99‡	0	0	100	90	0	
IIe	−	v	−	+	−	−	−	+	
	7	88	0	100	0	0	0	100	
Pseudomonas paucimobilis	v	v	−	−	+	−	+	+	Yellow, nonsoluble pigment
	10 (12)§	75	6 (3)	0	100	3	100	100	
Pseudomonas mallei	v	v	v	−	−	+	v	v	Nonmotile; arginine +
	88	25	12	0	0	100	12	0 (75)	

*From Weaver, R. E.: Gram-negative organisms: an approach to identification (guide to **presumptive** identifications), Atlanta, 1979, Center for Disease Control.

†+, 90% or more positive in 1-2 d; + or −, 50-90% positive in 1-2 d; −, 90% or more negative; − or +, 50-90% negative; (+), delayed positive reaction (3 or more d); w, weakly positive reaction; v, variable; OF, oxidation-fermentation medium.

‡Percent positive in 1-2 d.

§Percent positive (delayed) in 3 or more d.

citrate are utilized; growth occurs in KCN broth and on cetrimide medium; and the catalase test is positive.

Gelatin is liquefied rapidly, and in litmus milk a soft coagulum is formed, with rapid peptonization and reduction of litmus. The reaction is alkaline. Indole is not produced, and nitrates are reduced to nitrites and nitrogen. In liquid media a pellicle is formed.

According to Pickett,[317] *P. aeruginosa* can be identified within 24 hours by determining **fluorescence** and alkalinization of **acetamide** (i.e., acetamide positive). In the context of clinical bacteriology, a fluorescent **and** acetamide-positive nonfermenting gram-negative rod should be reported as *P. aeruginosa*.

Elsewhere, Pickett[292] noted that a fluorescent organism that denitrifies (gas from KNO_3) and grows at 42 C is *P. aeruginosa*. In both instances the media described by Pickett need to be used.

P. aeruginosa occurs infrequently in normal feces and is common in sewage and polluted water. It is found very frequently in pus from lesions and in ear infections, septicemia, genitourinary tract infections, joints, eye infections, and respiratory tract infections. Since the introduction of chemotherapeutic agents and antibiotics, its incidence in wound infections and hospital-acquired infections has been steadily rising, and such incidence equals or in some hospitals surpasses in this respect that of *S. aureus*. It is notorious for the ease with which it colonizes liquids (distilled water with cork bottles, antiseptics such as quaternary ammonium compounds, infusion fluids, eye medications, soap solutions, etc.).

Infection of burns is one of the most common threats of *P. aeruginosa*. Fluorescence of burned surfaces when observed under Wood's light (on a daily basis) was reported to allow early detection of invasive infection. Since the organism is resistant to a great many antibiotics, its identification is important. With hemolytic and pigment-pro-

ducing strains this is not very difficult; but about 10% of the strains do not form pigment and sometimes present a problem in identification.

Such strains can be identified on the basis of acid production from glucose (OF medium), growth on cetrimide and SS agar, oxidation of gluconate, growth at 41-42 C, and positive **oxidase, urease,** and **arginine dihydrolase** tests (see Table 79-47); flagella are monotrichous.

Bacteriophage typing. The identification of individual strains of *P. aeruginosa* with bacteriophages has been accomplished by several workers. There is general agreement that phage typing is useful in the epidemiologic study of *P. aeruginosa* infection. For details, see Sutter et al.[318]

Serologic typing. Verder and Evans[319] classified *Pseudomonas* strains into 10 antigenic groups, and Matsumoto et al.[320] have established 3 more O antigenic groups. Serologic typing may become an important adjunct of *P. aeruginosa* identification, since attempts are made to employ immunotherapy (active and/or passive) in *Pseudomonas* infections. For a review of serologic characterization of *P. aeruginosa*, see Lányi and Bergan.[321]

Pyocin typing. For a review of a system of typing by pyocin production, see Govan.[322]

Encapsulated P. aeruginosa strains. Elston et al.[323] reported an increasing incidence of **mucoid** types of *P. aeruginosa* from clinical material (sputum and urine). When in the mucoid state, they are usually nonmotile; but on successive transfers, when the capsule tends to be lost, motility can be demonstrated. There is a tendency to identify such mucoid organisms as *Klebsiella;* use of the oxidase test, demonstration of oxidation instead of fermentation of glucose, and the Voges-Proskauer test (negative) will readily distinguish such strains from *Klebsiella*. Such mucoid strains are most commonly isolated from the sputum of patients with cystic fibrosis.

Antimicrobial susceptibility. For some years

Table 79-49. Nonfermenters IV: gram-negative oxidizers of glucose—MacConkey negative (no growth), oxidase positive*†

Species	Growth on MacConkey	Oxidase	Indole	Urea	OF glucose	OF xylose	OF mannitol	OF lactose	OF sucrose	OF maltose	Notes
Brucella	v	v	– 0	+‡	v 75	+ 90	– 0	– 0	– 0	– 0	
Flavobacterium meningosepticum	v 89 (3)§	+ 99	+ 100	3 (5)	+ 95 (4)	– 2 (1)	+ 91 (8)	v 43 (15)	– 0	+ 93 (7)	Pale yellow; starch –
EO-2	v 67 (11)	+ 100	– 0	v 74 (3)	+ 100	+ 99 (1)	v 10 (10)	+ 91 (6)	– 0	v 20 (1)	
Pseudomonas vesicularis	v 89	+ 94	– 0	– (8)	+ or (+) 87 (9)	v 21 (2)	– 0	– 0	– 0	+ 98 (2)	
Vibrio extorquens	v 16	+ 96	– 0	v 29 (26)	v 40	+ 94	– 2	– 0	– 0	– 2	
IIb. *Flavobacterium* spp.	v 54 (9)	+ 96	+ 98	14 (28)	+ 92 (6)	v 30 (1)	– 10	– 0	v 13 (10)	+ 92 (6)	Yellow; starch +
IIe	– 7	v 88	+ 100	– 0	+ 100	– 0	– 0	– 0	– 0	+ 100	Esculin –, 0%
IIh	– 0	+ 100	+ 100	– 0	+ or (+) 85 (15)	– 5	– 0	– 0	– 0	+ 95	Esculin +, 100%
IIi-1	– 0	+ 91 (9)	+ 100	v 14 (18)	+ 91 (9)	+ or (+) 87 (13)	– 0	+ 91 (9)	+ 91 (9)	+ 91 (9)	Esculin +, 96%
Pseudomonas paucimobilis	v 10 (13)	v 75	– 0	6 (3)	+ 100	+ 100	– 0	+ 100	+ 100	+ 100	
IIK-2	v 81 (17)	+ 98	– 0	+ 96	+ 100	+ 100	– 0	+ 100	+ 100	+ 100	

*From Weaver, R. E.: Gram-negative organisms: an approach to identification (guide to **presumptive** identifications), Atlanta, 1979, Center for Disease Control.

†+, 90% or more positive in 1-2 d; + or –, 50-90% positive in 1-2 d; –, 90% or more negative; – or +, 50-90% negative; + or (+), most reactions occur within 1 or 2 d; (+), delayed positive reaction (3 or more d); *w*, weakly positive reaction; *v*, variable; *OF*, oxidation-fermentation medium.

‡Percent positive in 1-2 d.

§Percent positive (delayed) in 3 or more d.

the only useful antibiotics were colistin and gentamicin, both of which are more or less toxic. Carbenicillin, much less toxic, is valuable, but highly resistant strains have appeared; carbenicillin is used in life-threatening situations in combination with gentamicin. Recently introduced, tobramycin and amikacin are highly useful against gentamicin-resistant strains; both are relatively toxic. Immunotherapy, both active and passive, has recently been used in burn patients in whom *P. aeruginosa* infection is often fatal; the results have been encouraging. Antimicrobial susceptibility testing should be performed.

Pseudomonas fluorescens

P. fluorescens includes a large number of **fluorescein (pyoverdin)–producing, multitrichous** strains, the characteristics of which are somewhat variable. Stanier et al.[306] distinguish 7 biotypes; generally, strains of this group grow at 5 C but not at 42 C and do not produce pyocyanin pigment. Growth on cetrimide and utilization of sugars in OF medium are variable (see Table 79-47). The gelatin liquefaction test is positive, a characteristic that is valuable in distinguishing *P. fluorescens* from *P. putida* (no liquefaction). *P. fluorescens* strains are common inhabitants of soil and water and have been isolated from clinical material (body fluids) and contaminated blood and blood components.[324] *P. fluorescens* and *P. putida* are susceptible to kanamycin, tetracycline, and gentamicin but are resistant to carbenicillin.

Pseudomonas putida

P. putida does not hydrolyze gelatin and does not denitrify; it produces pyoverdin and thus fluoresces; pyocyanin is not produced. Biotype A strains grow at 4 C, whereas most biotype B strains do not.[314, 325 326] Its occurrence is about the same as that of *P. fluorescens;* both have also been isolated from hospital water sources, ultrasonic nebulizers, and intravenous catheters. Rarely, they have been associated

with emphysema, wound infections, septicemia, and abscesses.

Non-fluorescein-producing pseudomonads Pseudomallei group (P. mallei, P. pseudomallei, P. cepacia)

The pseudomallei group of the genus *Pseudomonas* consists of *P. mallei*, the causative agent of glanders, *P. pseudomallei*, the agent of melioidosis, and *P. cepacia*, widely encountered in the hospital environment.

P. pseudomallei

Melioidosis has long been known as a rare glanderslike disease of humans and other animals in Southeast Asia; it has been observed in Americans who have returned from combat in Vietnam. The causative agent, *P. pseudomallei*, is a common, free-living inhabitant of soil and water in certain tropical and subtropical regions; humans are infected through contamination of skin abrasions and wounds, or by inhalation of dust. Direct transmission from human to human or from animals to humans does not seem to occur. The agent was first isolated in 1910 by Whitmore and Krishnaswami from autopsy lesions of Burmese who died from a glanderslike disease. The first case in the Western Hemisphere was reported by McDowell and Varney (1947).[325]

The clinical symptoms of the disease are highly variable: it is commonly manifested as acute pneumonitis; a pustule or necrotic cutaneous ulcer may be seen sometimes, accompanied by lymphangitis and lymphadenopathy. Septicemia, meningitis, myocarditis, osteomyelitis, arthritis, chronic pneumonia mimicking tuberculosis, splenomegaly, or a fulminant choleralike syndrome may occur. Clinically the disease may mimic a disseminated fungus infection, tuberculosis, plague, typhoid, or viral pneumonia.

The organism is endemic in rodents in Southeast Asia and causes disease in mules, donkeys, sheep, goats, and swine. It has been isolated from soil, vegetables, fruit, and water in the area. Man-to-man transmission has not been shown.

Table 79-50. Nonfermenters V: gram-negative glucose nonoxidizers—MacConkey positive (growth), oxidase negative*†

Species	Growth on MacConkey	Oxidase	OF maltose	Motility	Urea	Beta hemolysis	Notes
Acinetobacter	+	−	−	−	−	v	
(*Mima, lwoffi*)	97‡	0	0	0	5 (4)§	29	
Bordetella	+	−	−	−	+	+	Soluble brown
parapertussis	100	0	0	0	100	100	pigment
Pseudomonas	+	−	+	+	v	−	
maltophilia‖	100	10 (?)	100	95	3 (12)	2	

*From Weaver, R. E.: Gram-negative organisms: an approach to identification (guide to **presumptive** identifications), Atlanta, 1979, Center for Disease Control.

†+, 90% or more positive in 1-2d; + or −, 50-90% positive in 1-2 d; −, 90% or more negative; − or +, 50-90% negative; (+), delayed positive reaction (3 or more d); w, weakly positive reaction; v, variable; OF, oxidation-fermenation medium; NT, not tested.

‡Percent positive in 1-2 d.

§Percent positive (delayed) in 3 or more d.

‖*Pseudomonas maltophilia* oxidizes glucose. However, reaction is frequently weak at 18-24 h and might be interpreted as negative.

The organism shows variable sensitivity to kanamycin, chloramphenicol, tetracycline, novobiocin, and sulfadiazine. It is resistant to ampicillin, streptomycin, cephalosporin, and colistin. In the U.S. Armed Forces, melioidosis was treated with a combination of very large doses of chloramphenicol, kanamycin, and novobiocin for a period of 4 weeks or tetracycline with chloramphenicol. Antibiotic sensitivity testing by the tube dilution technic is highly recommended.[326]

Specimens. Diagnosis is made by isolation of the organism from an abscess, draining sinus tract, blood, urine, sputum, spinal fluid, or visceral biopsy material. Rising antibody titers demonstrated by agglutination or complement-fixation tests are helpful (the antigens are generally not available).

Culture and identification. The organism is a gram-negative, aerobic, motile, filamentous rod; it often shows bipolar staining with Wright, Wayson, or Leishman stain. It grows well on trypticase soy, MacConkey, or blood agar at 35-37 C. **The colonies characteristically demonstrate wrinkling after 48-72 hours of incubation.** In heart infusion broth a heavy pellicle is produced, which shows wrinkling by 48-72 hours. On heart infusion agar, light orange, cream-colored, or bright orange pigment may develop.

The organism is **oxidative**; it attacks glucose, D-xylose, mannitol, lactose, and maltose in OF (Hugh-Leifson) medium (see Table 79-47).

The major reactions useful for the identification of *P. pseudomallei* are described by Weaver[327] as follows:

Positive
  Catalase
  Oxidase
  Simmons citrate
  Nitrate reduction and gas
  Gelatin
  Motility (1-2 polar flagella)
  Acid from:
  10% glucose slant
  10% lactose slant
  Acid produced in OF medium (see above)
  Milk: peptonized
Negative
  Growth on:
    SS agar (few late positive)
    Cetrimide agar
  Indole
  H₂S
  Methyl red
  Voges-Proskauer
Variable
  Sucrose; esculin hydrolysis
  Urease (on Christensen urea medium)

The majority of strains examined by Weaver produced acid slant and neutral or alkaline butts on TSI agar. For data on carbon assimilation patterns see Gilardi.[328]

Identification of the organism is not easy. It has to be differentiated from *P. stutzeri* and *P. mallei*. The former usually develops a yellow pigment and does **not** attack lactose or sucrose; it also reduces **both** nitrate and nitrite with gas

formation. *P. mallei*, on the other hand, is oxidase negative, produces H₂S (using lead acetate paper), does not liquefy gelatin or peptonize milk, and is nonmotile.

In qualified laboratories, guinea pig inoculation and fluorescent antibody tests are used for definitive identification.

All cultures suspected of being *P. pseudomallei* should be submitted to a reference laboratory together with patient's serum samples.

Pseudomonas mallei

Glanders is a severe infectious disease of horses that can be transmitted to humans; it is now extremely rare in the Western world but still occurs in Asia, Africa, and parts of the Middle East. The disease is characterized by nodular, eventually necrotic involvement of the nasal mucous membranes, lymphatics, lymph nodes, and skin, or by an acute or chronic pneumonitis. Fresh isolates of *P. mallei* (previously known as *Actinobacillus, Malleomyces, Loefflerella,* or *Acinetobacter mallei*) may not grow on MacConkey agar (of 7 "stock" cultures examined at the National Communicable Disease Center, Atlanta, 4 strains grew on MacConkey agar)[329]; it is **oxidase negative** and attacks sugars oxidatively (see Tables 79-46 to 79-48).

The organisms are small, slender rods, 0.25-0.4 × 1.5-3 μ, occurring singly, but they may grow into long threads. They are **nonmotile,** gram negative, staining irregularly and often bipolarly.

P. mallei is aerobic; it grows poorly or not at all under strictly anaerobic conditions. Growth is slow, becoming visible in about 2 days. Colonies on Loeffler blood serum are moist, opaque, and slimy, with a yellowish brown tinge. On glycerin veal agar they are whitish and transparent. They acidify and coagulate milk. The medium of choice is glycerin-potato-veal agar formula. **There is growth on blood and heart infusion agar** (it may or may not grow on MacConkey agar). Slimy, tenacious colonies are characteristic.

The principal characteristics of the organism are (1) **no fermentation** of carbohydrates, except occasional slight action on dextrose (perform sugar tests in OF [Hugh-Leifson] medium), and (2) very unevenly staining, granular, gram-negative organisms. Use methylene blue stains.

Specimens are usually from purulent nasal discharges or from pustular eruptions. In chronic cases the material may be from lung lesions or abscesses in various organs. The organism will cross-react with antiserum to *Pseudomonas pseudomallei* and has to be differentiated from other *Pseudomonas* species (*P. pseudomallei* and other pseudomonads are motile).

Animal inoculation—Straus test. Inoculate several male guinea pigs with increasing amounts of the culture. A swollen, red, tender scrotum on second or third day is sign of positive reaction.

Pseudomonas cepacia

P. cepacia (formerly *P. multivorans, P. kingii,* or EO-1 group), a plant pathogen, is genetically

Table 79-51. Nonfermenters VI: Nonoxidizers—MacConkey growth positive, oxidase positive*†

Species	Growth on MacConkey	Oxidase	OF mannitol	OF xylose	Nitrite reduction	Nitrate to gas	Nitrate reduction	H₂S TSI	Urea	Growth on SS	Motility	Flagella	Notes
Alcaligenes faecalis	+ 100‡	+ 100	− 0	− 0	− 0	− 0	v 45	− 0	− (1)	v 78	+ 100	Pe	—
Alcaligenes odorans	+ 100	+ 100	− 0	− 0	+ 100	− 0	− 0	− 0	− 2	+ 100	+ 96	Pe	Fruity odor
Alcaligenes denitrificans	+ 100	+ 100	− 0	− 0	+ 100	+ 100	+ 100	− 0	v 12	v 65	+ 100	Pe	
Bordetella bronchiseptica	+ 100	+ 99	− 0	− 0	NT	− 0	+ 95	− 0	+ 99	+ 99	+ 100	Pe	Strong +
IVc-2	+ 95 (5)§	+ 100	− 0	− 0	NT	− 0	v 11	− 0	+ 100	− 3	+ 100	Pe	Partial +, 24 h
IVe	v 62 (27)	+ 100	− 0	− 0	v 60	v 60	+ 100	− 0	+ 97	− 5	v	Pe	
IVf, Flavobacterium odoratum	+ 96	+ 99	− 0	− 0	v 83	− 0	− 0	− 0	+ 100	v 30	− 0	−	Fruity odor; yellow
Pseudomonas acidovorans	+ 100	+ 100	+ 100	− 0	NT	− 0	− 98	− 0	− 1	v 67	+ 98	P >2	
Pseudomonas testosteroni	+ 96 (4)	+ 100	− 0	− 0	NT	− 0	+ 96	− 0	v 7 (14)	v 22 (11)	+ 100	P >2	
Pseudomonas alcaligenes	+ 96	+ 96	− 0	− 0	NT	− 0	v 54	− 0	− 0	v 38	+ 100	P 1-2	
Pseudomonas pseudoalcaligenes	+ 100	+ 100	− 0	v 32	NT	− 0	+ 90	− 0	− 5	v 84	v 79	P 1-2	Growth at 42 C; fructose+, 82%
Pseudomonas diminuta	+ 97 (3)	+ 100	− 0	− 0	NT	− 0	− 3	− 0	v (13)	− 2	+ 100	P 1-2	Flagella; short wave length and amplitude
Pseudomonas putrefaciens	+ 100	+ 100	− 0	− 0	NT	− 0	+ 100	+ 98	v 24	v 48 (6)	+ 100	P 1-2	
Moraxella	v	+ 100	−	−	v	−	v	−	v	−	−	−	
Brucella	v	+	+ 0	+ 90	v 44	v 44	+ 100	− 0	+ 99	− 0	−	−	
Campylobacter fetus	v	+	−	−	NT	−	+	−	−	−	+	P 1-2	
Vibrio extorquens	v 16	+ 96	− 0	+ 94	NT	− 0	v 25	− 0	v 29	− 0	v 23	P 1-2	Pink pigment

*From Weaver, R. E.: Gram-negative organisms: an approach to identification (guide to **presumptive** identifications, Atlanta, 1979, Center for Disease Control.
† +, 90%, or more positive in 1-2 d; + or −, 50-90% positive in 1-2 d; −, 90% or more negative; − or +, 50-90% negative; (+), delayed positive reaction (3 or more d); w, weakly positive reaction; v, variable; OF, oxidation-fermentation medium; NT, not tested; P, polar; Pe, peritrichous.
‡Percent positive in 1-2 d.

related to *P. pseudomallei* and *P. mallei*.[300] It is frequently recovered from water in the hospital environment, disinfectants, detergents, various medical instruments, and has been isolated from a wide variety of clinical specimens. It is an opportunistic pathogen implicated in a variety of common-source, often hospital-acquired infections.

The organism has polar multitrichous flagella; many strains are **oxidase negative** or produce a very weak oxidase reaction.[303] Some strains grow poorly at 35 C.

For biochemical characteristics, see Tables 79-46 and 79-47; some strains produce a nonfluorescent yellow-green pigment (some strains with purple pigment also exist). The organism oxidizes lactose, maltose, and mannitol, produces lysine decarboxylase, and a positive ONPG reaction.

The organism is resistant to polymyxin and gentamicin and is consistently susceptible only to chloramphenicol and the combination trimethoprim-sulfamethoxazole.

P. cepacia has been isolated from septicemia,[331-333] endocarditis,[333-338] urinary tract infections,[339-342] and wound infections.[343]

Other nonfluorescent pseudomonads

A large number of species of aerobic pseudomonads that do not produce fluorescein have been described. Occasional isolation of such strains from clinical material occurs. They are all oxidase positive (except *P. maltophilia*).

Pseudomonas maltophilia

P. maltophilia, the only consistently **oxidase-negative** pseudomonad, is an occasional opportunistic pathogen. It is widely disseminated in nature and has been associated with bacteremia, endocarditis, pneumonia, urinary tract infections,

and a variety of abscesses and wound infections.[344-347] It is resistant to most antimicrobials except chloramphenicol, colistin, and nalidixic acid.

Biochemical characteristics are shown in Tables 79-46 and 79-50. The organism oxidizes glucose; however, the reaction is frequently weak at 18-24 hours and might be interpreted as negative. It does oxidize maltose (OF medium) and liquefies gelatin. It does not grow on cetrimide or SS agar; lysine is positive. It is unique in that it cannot use nitrate as a principal nitrogen source. Growth at 42 C is absent according to Stanier et al.[306]; Gilardi[315] found growth at this temperature. The organism has multitrichous flagella; some strains produce yellow (intracellular) and brown (diffusible) pigments. See Holmes et al.[347] for a recent review of *P. maltophilia*.

Pickett[317] states that *P. maltophilia* can be identified with a minimum of tests (provided that his methods and media are used): (1) diffuse β hemolysis, (2) negative oxidase test, (3) motile, and (4) lysine decarboxylase positive.

P. alcaligenes and P. pseudoalcaligenes[*]

Strains of this group are nonpigmented and do not liquefy gelatin or produce acid from sugars. They grow at 41 C but not at 4 C and are monotrichous. Glucose is not utilized (OF medium) nor is gluconate oxidized.

For biochemical characteristics, see Table 79-51. *P. pseudoalcaligenes* is nutritionally more active than *P. alcaligenes;* it oxidizes fructose and usually glucose, but not mannitol, and may form acid from several other carbohydrates.[303]

P. alcaligenes and *P. pseudoalcaligenes* have been isolated from inhalation therapy equip-

—————

[*]References 303, 306, 315, and 316.

Table 79-52. Nonfermenters VII: gram-negative glucose nonoxidizers—MacConkey negative (no growth), oxidase positive[*][†]

Species	Growth on MacConkey	Oxidase	Indole	Urea	OF xylose	Nitrate reduction	Notes
Eikenella corrodens	− 0‡	+ 100	− 0	− 0	− 0	+ 100	Ornithine +, 98%; thin, straight rods; nonmotile
Campylobacter fetus	v	+	−	−	−	+	Wavy rods; motile
Brucella	v	+	−	+ 99	+ 90	+ 100	Tiny; coccoid
Moraxella	v	+	−	v	−	v	
Vibrio extorquens	v 16	+ 96	− 0	v 29 (26)	+ 94	v 25	Pink pigment; nonsoluble
IIf	v (11)§	+ 100	+ 100	− 0	− 0	− 0	Moist growth (capsules)
IIj	− 2.4	+ 100	+ 98	+ 100	− 0	− 0	Frequently "sticky" growth

*From Weaver, R. E.: Gram-negative organisms: an approach to identification (guide to **presumptive** identifications), Atlanta, 1979, Center for Disease Control.

†+, 90% or more positive in 1-2 d; + or −, 50-90% positive in 1-2 d; −, 90% or more negative; − or +, 50-90% negative; (+), delayed positive reaction (3 or more d); w, weakly positive reaction; v, variable; *OF*, oxidation-fermentation medium.

‡Percent positive in 1-2 d.

§Percent positive (delayed) in 3 or more d.

ment, raw milk, and various animal and water sources, and in humans from blood, urine, the respiratory tract, and abscesses.[303] They are rarely opportunistic infestious agents. No single antibiotic is uniformly effective against members of these 2 species.[348]

P. acidovorans and P. testosteroni[303, 306, 315]

These organisms do not grow at 41-42 C or at 4 C, do not utilize glucose, lactose, maltose, sucrose, or mannitol (OF medium), and are multitrichous. *P. testosteroni* is distinguished by its ability to grow on testosterone and related steroids.

See Table 79-51 for biochemical characteristics. Generally, negative features are associated with these 2 species. They are relatively easily confused with the alcaligenes group (see above) members.

The 2 organisms have been isolated from human sources including blood, abscess, urine, wound, and respiratory tract, but no clinical significance has been associated with these isolates.[303]

An organism known at one time as *Comamonas*[349] is thought to be the same as *P. acidovorans* and *P. testosteroni*. It was originally named *Vibrio terrigenus*, then *V. percolans*, *Lophomonas alcaligenes*, and finally *Comamonas terrigena*.[350] It is a soil organism, very

rarely found in clinical material. Sonnenwirth[31] isolated it from the blood culture of a patient with pyrexia.

Hugh[351] compared the neotype strain of *C. terrigena* with the type strain of *Pseudomonas testosteroni* and found that they have the same general characteristics, except that *C. terrigena* is urease positive (Christensen urea agar) and citrate negative (both on Simmons and Christensen citrate medium). Accordingly, he proposed that the organism be named *Pseudomonas terrigena*.

The organism is gram negative and rod shaped, with a tuft of polar flagella. It grows at 22 and 37 C. It is a **nonoxidizer** (does not attack dextrose or a number of other carbohydrates in the open tube of the OF medium). It is methyl red, V-P, indole, gluconate, gelatin, H_2S, and phenylalanine deaminase negative. No decarboxylases are demonstrable. It is catalase and oxidase positive and reduces nitrate to nitrite. No water-soluble pigments are formed.

P. stutzeri[303, 306, 328, 352] and P. mendocina[306]

The colonies of freshly isolated strains are light brown after a few days' growth, are rough, dry, wrinkled, and coherent, and can be lifted off as a unit. They resemble craters; on blood agar there is a diffuse lysis after 48 hours (not β). In OF medium, acid is formed oxidatively (in open

Table 79-53. Antimicrobial susceptibility of nonfermenters*†

Organism	Peni-cillin	Novo-biocin	Erythro-mycin	Ampi-cillin	Tetra-cycline	Chloram-phenicol	Strepto-mycin	Cepha-lothin
Pseudomonas aeruginosa								
Pyocyanogenic (110)	0	0	0	0	20	0	15	0
Apyocyanogenic (68)	0	0	4	12	26	15	37	0
P. fluorescens (106)	0	0	4	0	89	40	55	2
P. putida (115)	1	1	11	1	74	27	71	3
P. pseudomallei (7)	0	86	0	71	100	86	0	0
P. capacia (94)	1	45	9	3	13	96	2	1
P. acidovorans (51)	4	45	14	6	90	94	4	8
P. alcaligenss (55)	15	9	55	27	89	62	38	27
P. pickettii (34)	6	0	85	6	100	91	6	74
P. stutzeri (76)	13	1	67	87	95	63	91	1
P. putrefaciens (41)	10	0	93	61	76	98	90	17
P. maltophilia (310)	3	2	8	11	37	88	23	1
P. diminuta (18)	6	100	94	6	100	100	33	78
Xanthomonas (31)	19	42	90	39	90	94	10	3
CDC group VE (27)	7	0	96	93	100	100	96	4
Alcaligenes faecalis (31)	32	23	65	48	87	68	10	45
A. odorans (55)	29	16	40	78	49	45	1	76
A. denitrificans (26)	27	23	54	65	81	58	8	23
B. bronchicanis (23)	17	43	83	26	100	70	13	78
Moraxella (74)	96	91	99	97	100	99	97	100
A. anitratus (644)	1	6	59	23	68	15	81	4
A. haemolyticus (97)	2	11	69	52	72	35	80	11
A. lwoffii (114)	31	24	80	67	82	79	75	39
Flavobacterium (8)	0	99	73	1	22	69	16	0
CDC Group M-4F (8)	13	100	100	13	13	100	0	0
Achromobacter (24)	0	8	8	17	21	42	0	4

*From Gilardi, G. L.: Identification of nonfermentative gram-negative bacteria, New York, 1978, Hospital for Joint Diseases.
†Parenthetical values refer to number of strains examined; other values indicate percentage of strains susceptible. *P. acidovorans* includes closely related CDC group VA-1 strains. *P. diminuta* includes closely related *P. vesicularis* strains. *Moraxella* unnamed flavobacteria. *Achromobacter includes A. xylosoxidans* and unnamed *Achromobacter* species. All strains tested zole), or tobramycin, the percentage being based on the fraction of strains examined. This scheme is not intended for use as an

tube) after 48 hours (Table 79-47). Nitrogen gas bubbles are seen on the surface of nitrate broth. Urease, indole, gelatin, and litmus milk reactions are negative. It does not grow at 42 C. The organism is more sensitive to a variety of antibiotics than *P. aeruginosa*.

P. mendocina, unlike *P. stutzeri*, is arginine dihydrolase positive and maltose negative. The colonies of *P. mendocina* are flat and smooth and contain a carotenoid, pale yellow pigment.[303]

P. stutzeri is differentiated from *P. pseudomallei* by the inability of *P. stutzeri* to oxidize lactose and sucrose, and to produce gelatinase; also, *P. pseudomallei* fails to grow on SS agar.

P. stutzeri has been found in soil and water, animal feces, sewage, stagnant water, baby formula, animals, aerosolization equipment, inanimate surfaces, and eye cosmetics.[303] The organism has been recovered from numerous clinical specimens but has been directly associated with an infectious process only on a few occasions. *P. stutzeri* is relatively antibiotic susceptible and is often susceptible to ampicillin, tetracycline, streptomycin, nalidixic acid, neomycin, kanamycin, polymyxin, gentamicin, and carbenicillin.[303]

P. diminuta (group I-a) and P. vesicularis[303,344]

The organism grows on MacConkey but not on cetrimide agar. Most strains liquefy gelatin and form a soluble brown pigment. Some strains slowly attack glucose in OF medium (open tube) (Table 79-47).

P. vesicularis (Table 79-49)[353] oxidizes glucose, some strains oxidize xylose, and practically all strains oxidize maltose.

P. diminuta has been isolated from water, tissue culture, and inhalation therapy equipment.[344] It has been isolated from human sources but appears to have no etiologic significance. *P. diminuta* is susceptible to chloramphenicol but resistant to polymyxin and gentamicin.

P. putrefaciens[353]

This organism produces H_2S and blackens the butt of KIA (or TSI) slant. It produces ornithine decarboxylase; it does not oxidize glucose (Table 79-51). It rarely has been implicated in human infections[303,353] and is fairly antibiotic susceptible.

Pseudomonas pickettii[296,354,355]

The organism oxidizes glucose and denitrifies and is similar to an unclassified group of clinical isolates designated VA-2. *P. pickettii* is oxidase positive, grows on MacConkey agar at 42 C, and hydrolyzes urea (Table 79-47).

Pseudomonas paucimobilis[356]

This organism was previously referred to as CDC group IIK, biotype 1. It is a yellow-pig-

Nitrofurantoin	Nitrofurazone	Nalidixic acid	Neomycin	Kanamycin	Polymyxin	Gentamicin	Carbenicillin	TMP/SMX	Tobramycin
0	0	0	76	0	100	95	80	0	100
3	6	43	72	56	97	93	66	60	75
4	11	21	94	87	95	97	4	56	88
3	22	43	93	93	98	97	21	20	66
0	43	71	86	100	0	0	0	0	0
0	1	81	53	68	0	13	6	100	0
64	16	98	14	42	80	6	32	89	50
18	45	82	69	75	93	65	71	100	100
0	47	100	26	30	0	21	30	100	35
2	12	92	100	99	100	100	86	80	100
100	100	100	100	100	100	100	83	100	100
0	2	92	32	33	94	46	37	95	27
11	6	6	100	89	56	67	56	71	100
19	29	68	65	39	23	39	68	100	22
4	4	78	100	100	100	100	100	100	48
19	26	68	52	87	87	77	61	100	50
58	44	87	62	20	100	93	96	90	75
4	8	62	31	35	69	15	81	100	0
9	9	96	83	65	91	78	87	100	66
97	99	100	100	100	100	100	95	100	100
2	83	96	99	100	100	99	97	89	100
2	49	97	98	86	100	97	87	91	33
12	74	98	100	100	100	100	96	85	100
26	19	90	47	4	0	30	3	88	4
13	75	100	0	0	0	0	25	100	0
0	0	25	21	8	100	21	88	89	50

includes closely related *P. testosteroni* strains. *P. alcaligenes* includes closely related *P. pseudoalcaligenes* strains *P. pickettii* species include *osloensis, lacunata, nonliquefaciens,* and *phenylpyruvica. Flavobacterium* includes *F. meningosepticum* and were susceptible to lincomycin. Not all strains were tested to gentamicin, carbenicillin, TMP/SMX (trimethoprim-sulfamethoxa-indicator of drug of choice of therapy and is presented only as a diagnostic guide for the identification of nonfermenters.

mented, nonfermentative, gram-negative rod; it has recently been named *Pseudomonas pauci-mobilis.*[356] *P. paucimobilis* is a strict aerobe and produces catalase and polar flagella. The organism tends to appear nonmotile in motility test medium but has a single polar flagellum. It has been isolated from various clinical specimens, especially blood, as well as from sources in the hospital environment.

Most strains (80%) do not grow on MacConkey agar; in addition to glucose, the organism oxidizes xylose, lactose, sucrose, and maltose; about 75% of strains are oxidase positive (Tables 79-47 to 79-49).

Antibiotic susceptibilities of pseudomonads

Gilardi summarized the antimicrobial susceptibilities of nonfermenting, gram-negative aerobic organisms (Table 79-53). **These susceptibilities are not an indicator of drug of choice for therapy.** They are presented only as a diagnostic guide for the identification of these organisms.

ALCALIGENES
Alcaligenes faecalis

A. faecalis (a genus listed in *Bergey's Manual,* ed. 8,[3] as of uncertain affiliation), a short, usually motile, gram-negative rod, is found occasionally in human feces, where it is considered harmless. It has been isolated from blood in septicemia, gallbladder infections, eye infections, meningitis, and pus, and has been implicated in enteritis.

It fails to attack glucose or other carbohydrates in OF medium (inactive, nonfermenter). The organism is frequently mistaken for *Salmonella* in stool cultures, since it is a lactose nonfermenter, and it is mistakenly transferred to TSI slants where it gives a completely alkaline reaction (red butt, red slat). It turns litmus milk alkaline in 2-4 days. It does not produce indole, and is Voges-Proskauer negative (see Tables 79-2 and 79-51).

The organism is strictly aerobic, **oxidase positive,** and grows on MacConkey agar and in KCN broth. Growth on cetrimide agar is variable. The urease and decarboxylase tests are negative. Microscopically it is always rod shaped with peritrichous flagella.

Alcaligenes odorans var. viridans[357]

Alcaligenes odorans var. *viridans* was proposed by Mitchell and Clarke for a number of strains closely resembling *A. faecalis,* except that *A. odorans,* also motile, produces a strongly aromatic, apple like odor on agar media and a green zone of discoloration on blood agar. The organism also grows well on cetrimide agar[315] (see Table 79-51).

Alcaligenes denitrificans (group Vc)

A. denitrificans is similar in most respects to *A. faecalis* except that it reduces nitrate with gas formation (Table 79-51).

ACHROMOBACTER (CDC GROUP Vd AND A. XYLOSOXIDANS)[2, 358–360]

In *Bergey's Manual,* ed. 8,[3] *Achromobacter* is not listed as a genus. Various members of the genus have been reassigned to the genera *Alcaligenes, Arthrobacter, Acinetobacter, Pseudomonas,* etc.

However, a group of bacteria clinically encountered and designated *Achromobacter xylosoxidans*[361] and *Achromobacter* species **(CDC group Vd)** are not included in these reassignments and changes (Chester and Cooper[358]).

The *Achromobacter* strains all grow on MacConkey agar, are **oxidase positive,** and produce no pigment; about one-half of the strains produce H_2S in TSI (4-12 days); they are motile, grow on SS agar, and produce catalase and urease. They reduce nitrate to nitrite and gas, hydrolyze esculin, and deaminate phenylalamine (2-4 days). They oxidize, slowly, glucose and xylose (Table 79-47 and Chester and Cooper[358]).

The organisms produce exceedingly small colonies at 24 hours,[358] but these increase rapidly in size after continued incubation (48 hours) due to elaboration of large amounts of mucoid material. Gram staining reveals gram variability and curved and swollen hooked-end forms.[358]

A. xylosoxidans[361] differs in that it is urease, phenylalamine deaminase, and esculin negative.[358] According to Weaver (Table 49-47), about 78% of *A. xylosoxidans* strains oxidize glucose; however, Chester and Cooper list the organism as a glucose nonoxidizer, but xylose oxidizer.[358]

Yabuuchi et al.[361] described *A. xylosoxidans* as having the following minimal biochemical characteristics: positive reactions for Simmons citrate, indophenol oxidase, and nitrate reduction; peritrichous motility; oxidation of glucose and xylose, but not maltose; and negative reactions for urease, indole production, arginine dihydrolase, and lysine decarboxylase. The species has been divided into 2 Center for Disease Control (CDC) biotypes, IIIa and IIIb: group IIIa reduces nitrate to nitrate only, whereas group IIIb reduces nitrate to gas.[302]

A. xylosoxidans has been isolated from a variety of human body sites (ear drainage in otitis media, spinal fluid, blood, urine, wounds). For details, see Yabuuchi et al.,[361] Pien and Higa,[359] and Holmes et al.[360]

Achromobacter species are resistant to chloramphenicol, nitrofurantoin, cephalothin, and carbenicillin. Most are sensitive to colistin, tetracycline, trimethoprim-sulfamethoxazole combination, and amikacin; only about 50% of strains are sensitive to gentamicin and tobramycin.[358]

A. xylosoxidans strains are mostly resistant to ampicillin (60%), cephalothin, gentamicin, kanamycin, penicillin, and tetracycline (75% resistant), but sensitive to trimethoprim-sulfamethoxazole combination, sulfonamide, carbenicillin, and chloramphemicol (about 72% sensitive, 14% intermediate[359]).

For additional information on *Achromobac-*

ter-like organisms see Baumann et al.[362] Pinter and Bende,[363] DeLey,[364] Gilardi,[296] Brisou and Prévot,[365] Steel and Cowan,[366] and Oberhofer, et al.[367]

ACINETOBACTER

There is a single species, *Acinetobacter calcoaceticus* (temporarily placed in the family Neisseriaceae, *Bergey's Manual*, ed. 8[3]) with 2 recognized varieties, *A. calcoaceticus* var. *anitratus* (formerly *Herellea vaginicola* or *B. anitratus*) and *A. calcoaceticus* var. *lwoffi* (formerly *Mima polymorpha*, oxidase negative).

These are nonfermentative, aerobic, gram-negative rods that are widely dispersed in nature and are commonly part of normal flora (up to 25% of healthy humans may harbor *A. calcoaceticus* on the skin, and it can be occasionally found also in the respiratory tract).[368]

A. calcoaceticus is an opportunistic pathogen; an extensive review of infections involving the organism has been recently published by Glew et al.[369] Nosocomial outbreaks, often with contamination of hospital equipment and hands of personnel, have been reported.[370-372]

The true significance of the finding of *A. calcoaceticus* in clinical specimens is in doubt. Glew et al.[369] felt that only about 2% of isolations in a 2-year period (58 of 3382 isolates) represented clinically significant infection. While noting an unusual seasonal pattern in the occurrence of *A. calcoaceticus* var. *anitratus* in hospital isolations, Retailliau et al.[373] also express some doubt about the role of this organism in nosocomial infection, noting in the meantime that the potential of the organism for causing severe infection is undisputed.

Isolation and identification

The organisms (both varieties) are **oxidase negative, catalase positive, nonmotile,** plump, paired gram-negative rods ("diplobacilli"). In the stationary phase they often appear as diplococci, easily mistaken for neisseriae. *A. calcoaceticus* var. *anitratus* (*Herellea*) grows well on MacConkey agar but poorly or not at all on SS agar. It does not acidify maltose (OF) or produce urease (Table 79-46). It utilizes glucose and lactose oxidatively (OF medium); it also produces acid from 10% (but not from 1%) lactose-containing agar slant.

According to Pickett,[292,317] the organism can be identified rapidly by virtue of its (1) negative oxidase test, (2) lack of motility, (3) coccobacillary appearance on Gram stain, (4) large colonies (> 0.5 mm, 24-hour blood agar plate), and (5) strong lactose positivity (using FLN medium).

A. calcoaceticus var. *lwoffi* (*Mima*) has the same characteristics as var. *anitratus*, except that it is lactose and glucose negative (Table 79-50). Neither of the 2 organisms possess decarboxylases, dihydrolase, or deaminase, and neither grows on cetrimide agar.

Antibiotics of choice are kanamycin, gentamycin, polymyxin B or colistin, the combination trimethoprim-sulfamethoxazole, and carbenicillin. Antibiotic susceptibility tests are required.

For a review of *Acinetobacter*, *Moraxella*, and the *Mimeae*, see Henriksen[374]; for the relationship of *Moraxella*, *Neisseria*, *Branhamella*, and *Acinetobacter*, see Henriksen.[375]

Transformation assay for strains of Acinetobacter and Moraxella osloensis*

There are times when it is virtually impossible to correctly identify some oxidase-negative or oxidase-positive gram-negative coccobacilli with biochemical tests. A more definitive means of speciating the organisms is required. A genetic transformation assay for identification of strains of *Acinetobacter* was described by Juni[376] in 1972. This procedure can also be used for definitive identification of *Moraxella osloensis* strains.[377] Using crude DNA extracts of test strains and auxotrophic mutants of genetically competent *Acinetobacter* or *Moraxella osloensis* strains, transformation assay is carried out on heart infusion agar. Genetically related test strains will convert the auxotroph to prototrophy, and the converted auxotroph will grow on a lactic acid-mineral (LM) agar medium. The unconverted auxotroph will not grow on LM medium.

Preparation of LM medium

1. To prepare 1 L broth medium, add following chemicals to 700 ml distilled water:

KH_2PO_4	1.5 g
Na_2HPO_4	13.5 g
$MgSO_4$	0.1 g

NH_4Cl, 2 g; dissolve in 100 ml distilled water and add slowly while stirring.

$CaCl_2$, 0.1 g; dissolve in 100 ml distilled water and add 10 ml slowly while stirring.

$FeSO_4 \cdot 7H_2O$, 0.1 g; dissolve in 1000 ml of distilled water and add 5 ml slowly while stirring.

Lactic acid (reagent grade) 5 ml
Distilled water. Add to final volume of 1000 ml.
Dispense in 100 ml portions in 8 oz prescription bottles and sterilize at 121 C for 15 min.

2. Prepare 500 ml of 3% agar. Dispense 50 ml portions in 8 oz prescription bottles and sterilize at 121 C for 20 min.

3. To prepare six 30 ml agar plates of LM medium, liquefy 1 bottle 3% agar and mix with 1 bottle broth. After plates have solidified, incubate inverted overnight to dry. Store plates inverted in plastic bags under refrigeration or at room temperature until needed.

Preparation of crude transforming DNA

1. Grow DNA donor culture (test culture) on any suitable medium. Heart infusion agar, blood agar, or nutrient agar are all satisfactory. Age of donor culture is not critical.

2. Suspend loopful of cells into 0.5 ml sterile 0.05% sodium dodecyl sulfate in standard saline citrate (0.15M NaCl, 0.015M sodium citrate). Mix well, immersing all cellular material.

3. Place suspension in 60 C water bath 15-60 min. Check for clearing after 15 minutes.

4. DNA solution may be stored at 3-5 C for months.

---

*From Laboratory methods in special medical bacteriology, Bacteriology Training Branch, Atlanta, 1976, Center for Disease Control.

Transformation assay

1. Spot inoculate portion of heart infusion agar (HIA) plate lightly with 18-24 h culture of auxotrophic (recipient) strain to be transformed. Mix loopful of crude DNA preparation from donor strain into inoculum and spread mixture over area of agar surface about size of dime (18 mm).
2. Inoculate another portion of heart infusion agar plate with recipient strain to serve as non-DNA-treated control.
3. Inoculate third portion of plate with crude DNA preparation **alone** to test its sterility.
4. Incubate HIA plate at 35 C until growth occurs. Incubation times of 4-6 h are usually sufficient for *Acinetobacter. Moraxella* usually require 8-18 h.
5. Examine HIA plate after incubation period. If growth occurs in DNA section for sterility check, heat crude DNA preparation for additional 30 min at 60 C and repeat inoculation of heart infusion agar plate.
6. Inoculate sections of LM plate with cells from each growth area on HIA plate. Incubate LM plate at 35 C for 24 h.
7. Prototrophic transformant colonies should be clearly visible on LM medium. Non-DNA-treated control cells will not grow on this selective medium.
8. If no growth is observed, plate should be incubated additional 24 h. *Moraxella osloensis* may require 48 h incubation period.

MORAXELLA

The moraxella are animal parasites, most commonly present on the mucous membranes, especially in the normal upper respiratory tract. Most moraxella are nutritionally exacting.

The genus *Moraxella* is described in *Bergey's Manual*, ed. 8[3] (in the family *Neisseriaceae*) as nonmotile, small, short, plump, gram-negative, nonpigmented rods approaching coccus shape; there are also some filaments and chains. They are **oxidase positive**, aerobic, and do not utilize carbohydrates. The organisms are also highly **sensitive to penicillin**.

The growth of the 5 species listed (*M. lacunata, M. bovis, M. nonliquefaciens, M. phenylpyruvica,* and *M. osloensis*) is dependent on or improved by the addition of serum or ascitic fluid.

Considerable controversy existed concerning the inclusion of other species and organisms in this genus. At one time oxidase-negative organisms were also placed into the genus (*M. lwoffii* and *M. glucidolytica*).[378,382] Many of the workers investigating the relationships of this genus with the tribes and genera *Achromobacter, Mimeae, Alcaligenes, B. anitratum, Herellea,* and others now agree that the genus *Moraxella* be restricted to oxidase-positive organisms.[378,382]

For the relationship of *Moraxella* with *Branhamella, Neisseria,* and *Acinetobacter,* see the reviews of Henriksen.[374,375]

We define *Moraxella* as nonmotile,* nonspore-forming, nonflagellated, rod- or coccoid-shaped organisms, with a tendency to pleomorphism, that are **oxidase positive,** catalase positive (some exceptions), and obligately aerobic; sugars are not attacked (no acid produced from glucose aerobically or anaerobically). Growth of some strains is improved by addition of blood or serum. They all seem to be sensitive to penicillin, none being able to grow in the presence of 1 unit of penicillin G per milliliter.[361] The organisms are citrate, indole, H_2S, and urease negative (except *M. phenylpyrouvica*) and do **not** form pigment, hemolyze blood agar (except *M. kingii*), or acidify 10% lactose or sucrose slants (see Tables 79-51 and 79-52).

The organisms are variable as to growth on MacConkey agar.

Moraxella nonliquefaciens

M. nonliquefaciens[383] occurs more frequently in the respiratory tract than other *Moraxella*. It usually does not grow on MacConkey agar; it is biochemically inert, except for nitrite positivity. It also requires complex growth factors (most strains require serum or oleic acid).

Moraxella osloensis

The specific name *osloensis* has been assigned by Bøvre and Henriksen[383] to a large group of *Moraxella* organisms characterized by rod-shaped cells and lack of requirement for any specific growth factors (grow on mineral-acetate medium). Almost all strains in the group fail to reduce nitrate to nitrite; gelatin is not liquefied.

This group includes strains designated as *M. duplex,* isolated from the normal human flora (skin, vagina, nose) and from clinical disease (blood, eye, nose, throat, sputum, etc.); also *Mima polymorpha* var. *oxidans,* described as rods (predominating in liquid medium) and coccobacillary (diplococci) on solid medium. The latter organisms are very pleomorphic, do not acidify 10% lactose or 10% sucrose slants, and show good to slight or no growth (+ to −) on EMB and MacConkey agar but none on SS agar. *M. polymorpha* var. *oxidans* has been isolated from patients with septicemia, otitis, pneumonia, meningitis, and urethritis and also from the normal skin, urethra, vagina, etc. It is easily confused with *Neisseria gonorrhoeae,* from which it must be differentiated by (1) sugar utilization (*N. gonorrhoeae* attacks glucose; *Mima* does not) and (2) growth on nutrient agar, EMB, and/or MacConkey agar (*Mima* grows; *Neisseria* does not).

Usually, *M. osloensis* does not grow on MacConkey agar or on SS agar. It is biochemically inert and usually nitrite negative.

• • •

For a transformation assay for strains of *M. osloensis,* see *Acinetobacter,* above.

Moraxella lacunata, M. liquefaciens

M. lacunata (including the biotype *M. liquefaciens*[381]), traditionally known as the **Morax-**

---

*Some gliding (twitching) motility was described by Piéchaud[382] among the true moraxellas. The mechanism of this movement is obscure, and the motility cannot be demonstrated by routine diagnostic technics; for this reason it is not taken into consideration.

Axenfeld bacillus, the type species of the genus, is characterized by requirement for complex growth factors (heart infusion; some strains require serum, oleic acid, or blood). It occurs rarely as a diplobacillus in pus from conjunctivitis and corneal infections. It grows on Loeffler serum slants, which is slowly liquefied, with deep pitting around the colonies. Gelatin is hydrolyzed (add 5% gelatin to appropriate medium; flood with acidic mercuric chloride after 48 hours) and nitrate is reduced to nitrite.

M. phenylpyrouvica

M. phenylpyrouvica was named in 1967 by Bøvre and Henriksen.[384] It is nonhemolytic, grows well on the surface of OF (Hugh-Leifson) medium, is catalase positive, and does not form acid from glucose and maltose. **It is rapidly urease positive on Christensen urea medium; it deaminates phenylalanine.** Pathogenicity is uncertain; it has been isolated from blood, pus, suprapubic ulcers, scalp lesions, and the vulva.

Moraxella bovis

M. bovis requires serum or oleic acid for growth, hydrolyzes gelatin, and does not reduce nitrate to nitrite. It has been isolated from cattle with pink-eye but has not been reported in man.

FLAVOBACTERIUM

Members of the genus *Flavobacterium* (listed as a genus of uncertain affiliation in Part 8 of *Bergey's Manual,* ed. 8[3]) are gram-negative, aerobic, usually **oxidase-positive, nonmotile rods.** Although flavobacteria are fermentative, they are often inactive for several days of incubation (up to 14-21 days) and hence are treated like oxidizers, using unsealed OF media for carbohydrate reactions. Carbohydrates are attacked slowly and with weak acid production (see Tables 79-2, 79-47, and 79-49 for biochemical and physiologic characteristics).

On nutrient gelatin or potato infusion agar they produce yellow, orange, red, or yellow-brown pigmentation; on meat extract or infusion agar these pigments may develop rapidly or in some instances slowly (4-5 days at room temperature).

Approximately 90% of the *F. meningosepticum* strains grow slowly on MacConkey agar,[2] but only about 50% of the IIb group do so.

Four subgroups of *Flavobacterium* are presently recognized: (1) *F. meningosepticum,* (2) unnamed *Flavobacterium* species designated as group IIb, (3) group IIf, and (4) group IVf (*F. odoratum*). They are widely distributed in nature (water, soil, moist areas), including the hospital environment. Members of the group are oxidase positive, form a yellow pigment (hence the name), and are usually nonmotile. Strains isolated from humans are indole positive, but those recovered from the environment often are not.

For an extensive review of the taxonomy of *Flavobacterium,* see McMeekin.[385]

Flavobacterium meningosepticum

Strains obtained from meningitis in infants form a homogeneous group named *Flavobacterium meningosepticum.*[386,387] It has also been reported from septicemia in adults, endocarditis,[388] and outbreak of septicemia in a surgical unit that was traced to contamination of intravenous drugs by the organism,[389] and other hospital-acquired infections.

Short to long, sometimes pleomorphic rods are seen microscopically. Colonies on blood plates grow well in 48 hours; yellow-greenish pigmentation diffuses into agar. The organisms are not hemolytic. They are 1-2 mm in size, smooth, entire, gray-white, and butyrous; on EMB agar clear or blue colonies develop. There is no growth on SS agar. On MacConkey agar no growth may occur on primary isolation, but there is growth after subculture. The organism is catalase and **oxidase positive,** liquefies gelatin, and is urease negative and nonmotile.

For identification, inoculate in TSI agar, citrate slant, nitrate broth, and urea agar. Perform the oxidase test. Those organisms showing a positive oxidase reaction, alkaline TSI throughout, no growth on citrate slant, and no reduction of nitrate should be tested further. Use 10% lactose and 10% glucose slants (the latter is usually positive). For other tests and characteristics, see Tables 79-47 and 79-49.

The organism is indole positive, nonmotile, and glucose and maltose positive (in OF medium; slow and weak); see also Table 79-54.

F. meningosepticum has high virulence for the newborn, especially the premature, in whom it causes epidemics of septicemia and meningitis with a very high fatality rate. While these infections are usually attributed to contaminated hospital equipment and solutions, isolation of *F. meningosepticum* from the female genitals suggests this possible source. The organism also occurs in postoperative bacteremia of adults,

Table 79-54. Biochemical reactions of *Flavobacterium meningosepticum**

Catalase	+		SS	−
Oxidase	+		Motility	−
Gelatin	+		Nitrate	−
Milk†	+		Urea	−
Indole (rare)	+		Methyl red	−
			Voges-Proskauer	−
H₂S‡	+		H₂S, in TSI	−
			Citrate	−
Acid from§:			No acid from:	
Glucose	Mannitol		Adonitol	Raffinose
Lactose	Mannose		Arabinose	Rhamnose
Levulose	Trehalose		Dulcitol	Salicin
			Galactose	Sucrose

*Based on data from King,[271,386] Cabrera and Davis,[387] and Weaver, Tatum, and Hollis.[2]

†Milk is alkaline and is peptonized.

‡Only with lead acetate strip suspended over TSI slant.

§Acid formation is variable and very slow in conventional fermentation media. Acid formation is slow in OF medium with added carbohydrates. There is no change in TSI agar.

in whom the illness is much milder; however, in immunodeficient patients the infection may be fatal.[390]

Infants with fatal flavobacterial meningitis have sometimes had temperatures below normal, whereas adults with flavobacterial septicemia usually have high temperatures and recover rapidly. Since many *F. meningosepticum* strains cannot grow at 38 C, it has been suggested that body temperature is an important factor in the response of infants with flavobacterial meningitis. Six separate serotypes (A-F) of *F. meningosepticum* are known.

The organism has an unusual antimicrobial sensitivity pattern for a gram-negative bacillus: it is susceptible in vitro to erythromycin, novobiocin, rifampicin, and trimethoprim-sulfamethoxazole, to a lesser degree to chloramphenicol and streptomycin, and it is resistant to gentamicin and colistin.

Flavobacterium groups IIb, IIf, and IIj

While *F. meningosepticum* usually produces beige or light yellow pigment, group IIb strains produce markedly orange to yellow pigment. Group IIb does not utilize mannitol or lactose and is starch positive (Table 79-49).

Group IIf colonies are pale yellow-green or gray-green on continued incubation. According to Pickett,[292] his *Flavobacterium* group III may be synonymous with CDC group IIf—these are peritrichously flagellated and feebly motile in hanging drop preparations.

Groups IIb and IIf are only rarely implicated in infections of infants or adults; however, outbreaks of hospital-acquired bacteremia due to group IIb have occurred, while IIf organisms have been isolated from a variety of clinical specimens.

Like the CDC group IIf, IIj is a nonsaccharolytic, gram-negative bacterium that resembles *Flavobacterium*. CDC IIj is generally isolated from lesions that resulted from dog or cat bites or scratches. The organism hydrolyzes urea, liquefies gelatin, and is oxidase positive.

Flavobacterium odoratum

Flavobacterium odoratum was first described by Stutzer and Kwaschnina in 1929.[391] Recently, Holmes et al.[392] compared 9 clinical isolates and 3 cultures of CDC group M IV f with 1 of Stutzer's strains. Biochemical and antimicrobial susceptibility tests and determination of DNA base compositions confirm that both the clinical isolates and CDC group M IVf are *Flavobacterium odoratum*. This organism has been most frequently isolated from urine.

Colonies of this organism are generally lightly yellow pigmented, have strong fruity odor, and have spreading edges. All isolates were found to be nonmotile, nonsaccharolytic, DNase positive, gelatin positive, hydrolyze urea, oxidase positive, and are resistant to carbenicillin, gentamicin, and polymyxin.

Holmes et al.[393] recently examined 24 strains of *F. odoratum* and found them to be resistant to gentamicin, tobramycin, amikacin, carbenicillin, kanamycin, and polymyxin. They were sensitive to erythromycin and (some) to chloramphenicol.

EIKENELLA
Eikenella corrodens

Eikenella corrodens is a facultatively anaerobic, gram-negative, straight, rod-shaped bacterium that stains uniformly and does not demonstrate branching. This organism was formerly known as *Bacteroides corrodens* (also HB-1). In 1972, Jackson and Goodman[394] proposed that the facultatively anaerobic, gram-negative rod be transferred to a new genus and named *Eikenella*, leaving only the strictly anaerobic form to be called *Bacteroides corrodens*. This organism had also been studied by Riley et al.[395] and was designated by them as HB-1. Hill and Goodman suggest that the organism is probably a normal inhabitant of the throat and mouth and may be an opportunistic pathogen. It has been isolated from a number of anatomic sites. From 595 isolates of *Eikenella corrodens* examined at the Center for Disease Control, 43% were recovered from abscesses of the face and the neck, and from fluids of the chest and the lung; 16% from the abdomen, including the peritoneal cavity; and the remaining 40% were isolated from blood culture, brain abscesses, spinal fluids, or miscellaneous anatomic sources.[302] The biochemical characteristics of *Eikenella corrodens* based on

Table 79-55. Reactions of *Eikenella corrodens*[512]

Test	Reaction	Percent positive*
Oxidase	+	100
Catalase	−	9 (weak)
Growth on		
MacConkey	−	0.8
SS agar	−	0
Cetrimide	−	0
Hydrogen sulfide (TSI agar)	−	0
Oxidation-fermentation	Inactive	100
Urease	−	0
Indole	−	0
Methyl red/Voges-Proskauer	−	0
Citrate (Simmons') Alk	−	0
Motility	−	0
Gelatin	−	0
Glucose, xylose	−	0
Mannitol, lactose	−	0
Sucrose, maltose	−	0
Esculin	−	0
Nitrate to nitrite	+	99.7
Pigment (pale yellow)	+	100

*90% or more positive in 1 or 2 d.

the 595 isolates are shown in Table 79-55; see also Table 79-52.

It should be noted that the organism is **oxidase positive**, does **not** utilize carbohydrates, and is lysine and ornithine positive but arginine negative. Colonies of the organism characteristically **pit (corrode) the agar** (blood agar); they are small and are often seen in shallow craters (pits) on the surface of the agar.

Increased CO_2 helps growth of the organism.

E. corrodens is sensitive to penicillin, carbenicillin, ampicillin, tetracycline, but resistant to clindamycin, methicillin, and variably susceptible to cephalothin.

For details of clinical involvement of the organism, see Brooks and White,[396] Brooks et al.,[397] and Goldstein et al.[398]

CAMPYLOBACTER

Campylobacter (family *Spirillaceae*, *Bergey's Manual*, ed. 8[3]) is the generic name proposed in 1963[399] for a group of microaerophilic organisms that clearly differed from *Vibrio* organisms. The type species is *C. fetus* (previously *Vibrio fetus*) which had been known as a cause of abortion in cattle and sheep; other members of the new genus have been associated with diseases of domestic animals, including enteritis of calves and pigs.

The reason for the new genus name and transfer from the genus *Vibrio* for the microaerophilic vibrios was (1) *Campylobacter* strains are microaerophilic to anaerobic (*Vibrio* are facultative anaerobes); (2) they have a respiratory (oxidative) metabolism, whereas *Vibrio* are fermenters; and (3) they have a G + C (guanine and cytosine) content sharply different from that of *Vibrio* (29-36 moles% vs. 40-53 moles%).

Bergey's Manual, ed. 8,[3] lists 3 species: *C. fetus* with 3 subspecies (*C. fetus* ss *fetus*, *C. fetus* ss *intestinalis*, and *C. fetus* ss *jejuni* are considered pathogenic), while *C. sputorum* (ss *bubulus*, ss *mucosalis*, and ss *sputorum*) and *C. fecalis* are nonpathogenic.

C. sputorum ss *sputorum* is a member of the normal flora in the oral cavity of man; the other 2 subspecies of *C. sputorum* are found in swine

(ss *mucosalis*), cattle, and sheep (ss *bubulus*). *C. fecalis* is also present in cattle and sheep.

For an extensive review of the genus *Campylobacter*, see Smibert.[400]

Campylobacter fetus

Campylobacter fetus is a small, slender, and **curved** gram-negative rod, occurring frequently in spiral forms. It is microaerophilic and grows better in an atmosphere of about 10% CO_2 or in thioglycollate broth than in air. Under anaerobic conditions, growth is poor. It is very actively motile (single polar flagellum). Colonies on blood agar are nonhemolytic, round, about 1 mm, smooth, raised, and convex.[3]

C. fetus is **oxidase** and **catalase positive**, reduces nitrate, and is gelatin, indole, and H_2S negative. Carbohydrates are not attacked. There is poor or no growth in methyl red and V-P medium, on Simmons citrate, and on urea agar (for characteristics, see Table 79-52).

C. fetus ss fetus

C. fetus ss *fetus* is the cause of abortion in cattle and has not, to date, been isolated from man. The organism does **not** produce H_2S (lead acetate paper above a culture in broth containing cysteine[401]), does not grow in 1% glycine or at 42 C, and is oxidase positive (see Table 79-56).

C. fetus ss intestinalis

C. fetus ss *intestinalis* causes disease in man (but not gastroenteritis); see Robinson.[402] The organism has been isolated in bacteremia and rarely from spinal fluid.

It can be distinguished from the other subspecies by its growth at 25 C but not at 42 C, growth in 1% glycine, and production of H_2S; it is oxidase positive (Table 79-56). It occurs in cattle, sheep, and humans.

C. fetus ss jejuni

C. fetus ss *jejuni* is now well established as a causative agent of human enteritis.[403, 404] In 1978 there was an outbreak of enteritis in Vermont,[405] involving some 2000 residents, and a

Table 79-56. Characteristics of the subspecies of *Campylobacter fetus*[404a]

Characteristic	Subspecies		
	fetus	*intestinalis*	*jejuni*
H_2S (TSI)	−	−	−
H_2S (lead acetate)	−	+	+
Growth in Brucella broth* + 1% glycine	−	+	+
Growth in Brucella broth + 3.5%NaCl	−	−	−
Growth at 25 C (Brucella broth)	+	+	−
Growth at 42 C (Brucella broth)	−	−	+

*Brucella broth and preparation of various media (glycine, NaCl) is described in detail in Chapter 72, media, under "*Campylobacter* medium."

smaller outbreak in Colorado,[406] in both of which the causative agent was *C. fetus* ss *jejuni;* it also has been reported from other continents.[407, 408]

The organism produces H_2S and grows in 1% glycine and at 42 C but **not** at 25 C; it is oxidase positive (Table 79-56).

C. fetus ss *jejuni* corresponds to the so-called "related vibrios" of King[409]; the organism occurs in cattle, sheep, goats, birds, and man.

Isolation and identification of C. fetus ss jejuni from feces. Detailed instructions are given under stool examination, Chapter 75, for collection and transport, inoculation on selective medium,* incubation, and primary examination of plates. For further details of technics, see Skirrow,[407] Blaser et al.,[408] and Bokkenheuser et al.[404]

Blood culture. Commercial blood culture systems with 10% CO_2 are satisfactory (trypticase soy broth, thioglycollate broth, and supplemented beef-heart infusion broth).[410] Subculture as described below.

Isolation of C. fetus from other clinical specimens. In addition to feces, human specimens from which *C. fetus* ss *jejuni* has been isolated are blood and, rarely, spinal fluid. *C. fetus* ss *intestinalis* has also been isolated from these sources.

For diseases other than enteritis, see Bokkenheuser,[411, 412] and Smibert.[400]

Incubation. Incubate selective plates (Chapter 75) as well as general media (blood agar) at **42-43 C** in anaerobic jar (catalyst removed); evacuate to 15 inches (38.1 cm) Hg twice, and refill each time with either of following gas mixtures: (1) 10% carbon dioxide, 10% hydrogen, and 80% nitrogen; or (2) 5% carbon dioxide, 10% hydrogen, and 85% nitrogen. If facilities for gassing out anaerobic jar are not available, disposable GasPak hydrogen–carbon dioxide generator, **without catalyst,** may be substituted. (Not all strains of *C. fetus* ss *jejuni* grow as well when GasPak generators are used, and some strains may not grow at all.)

Examination of plates and identification. Examine plates after 24, 48, and 72 hours incubation. Colonies of *C. fetus* ss *jejuni* are usually detectable by 24 hours. Colonies vary from pinpoint, glossy-appearing colonies to those that spread over entire surface of agar.

Since *C. fetus* is an **oxidase-positive** organism, the oxidase test is used to screen suspect colonies. This is done by removing a portion of each colony selected and testing it or oxidase on filter paper by Kovacs' technic. (See **oxidase test,** Chapter 72.)

Examine by Gram stain; in wet mounts ob-

****Campylobacter fetus selective medium.**[407] Blood agar base no. 2—Oxoid, with 7% lysed horse blood and 3 antimicrobials, i.e., Vancomycin, 10 $\mu g/ml$. Polymyxin B, 2.5 IU/μl, and Trimethoprim, 5$\mu g/ml$; see media, Chapter 72, and stool examination, Chapter 75. Antimicrobial vial is available from Oxoid.

served by dark-field microscopy, the organism displays a tumbling or darting motility.

Establish the following characteristics:

Test	Result
Oxidase	+
Catalase (done on a slide or blood-free medium)	+
TSI, acid slant or butt	−
H_2S (TSI or SIM)	−
Acid from glucose (broth fermentation or OF medium)	−
Nitrate reduction	+
Motility (wet mount)	+
Growth in Brucella broth*	
at 25 C	−
at 35 C	+
at 42 C	+

Subcultures of initial isolate will usually grow at 42 C in candle jar. If agar media are incubated in room air, there will be no growth or very scant growth.

Differentiation of subspecies of C. fetus

Characteristics that differentiate the subspecies of *C. fetus* are shown in Table 79-56. The ability to grow at 42 C and the failure to grow at 25 C (room temperature may be used if a 25 C incubator is not available) distinguishes *C. fetus* ss *jejuni* from *C. fetus* ss *intestinalis.*

Antimicrobial susceptibility tests

The 3 subspecies of *C. fetus* generally are susceptible to the aminoglycosides, chloramphenicol, erythromycin, clindamycin, furazolidone, and the tetracyclines. The use of these agents in treating uncomplicated diarrheal diseases due to *C. fetus* ss *jejuni* is open to question at the time of writing (1979). Laboratories wishing to perform antibiotic susceptibility tests should recognize that a standardized method for testing *C. fetus* does not exist at this time and that results must be interpreted with great caution.

AGROBACTERIUM

Riley and Weaver[413] (Center for Disease Control) characterized 37 cultures of a gram-negative rod previously designated Vd-3 and found that these organisms are likely identical with *Agrobacterium radiobacter* (family *Rhizobiaceae,* Bergey's Manual, ed. 8[3]).

The organisms rarely occur in clinical specimens; however, microbiologists should be familiar with their characteristics.

Agrobacterium radiobacter and Vd-3 organisms are **glucose oxidizers** (open OF tube), **grow on MacConkey agar,** are oxidase, urease, and phenylalanine deaminase positive, reduce nitrate **and** nitrite, hydrolyze esculin, lack ar-

---

*If Brucella broth is not available, fluid thioglycollate medium may be substituted.

ginine dihydrolase and lysine and ornithine decarboxylase, and produce 3-ketolactose (method of Bernaerts and DeLey[414]) and 2-ketogluconate (method of Moore and Pickett[415]); see also Table 79-47.

Lautrop[416] also isolated a number of *Agrobacterium* strains from clinical specimens.

Miscellaneous, fastidious, or unclassified gram-negative rods

BRUCELLA

Brucella is the smallest of all gram-negative bacteria. It is described as a small, nonmotile, nonsporulating **coccobacillus** or short rod that grows poorly on ordinary media or may require special media. The organisms are **aerobes**, with no growth occurring under strict anaerobic conditions; growth is often improved by CO_2. Brucellae are glucose oxidizers (in appropriate medium), with variable oxidase reactions, that do not grow on MacConkey agar (see Tables 79-48 and 79-49). *Brucella* is described as a genus of uncertain affiliation in Part 7, *Bergey's Manual*, ed. 8.[3]

Brucellae are **obligate parasites** that produce acute, chronic, or inapparent infection in animals and may cause disease in humans; they multiply in phagocytic cells. Localization usually follows the generalized infection (Subcommittee on Taxonomy of Brucellae[417,418]).

The organisms may be coccoid or ovoid rods varying in length from 0.5-2.0 μm and 0.5 μm wide, with no tendency to form characteristic grouping; when observed on smears prepared from solid medium, they appear uniformly distributed. When present in their largest bacillary form, they may show bipolar staining. *B. meli-*

tensis, when recently isolated, is more likely to show coccoid forms, whereas *B. abortus* and *B. suis* are less coccoid and more bacillary. *Brucella* is nonmotile and nonsporeforming, and according to Huddleson[419] is encapsulated.

Three other species, *B. ovis, B. neotomae,* and *B. canis* (from dogs) have been described more recently; of these, only *B. canis* seems to have a role in human disease.[420-426]

Although *Brucella* may grow in media of simple composition and even in synthetic media, these organisms are somewhat difficult to cultivate. Growth is slow, requiring at least 48 hours of incubation at temperatures of 35-37 C. The classic liver infusion, broth or agar, in which best results were obtained in the past, has been supplanted by special preparations, among which tryptose,* Brucella broth and agar,*† and trypticase soy† are quite satisfactory.

In fluid medium the growth is uniform; in old cultures it has a tendency to settle down. In agar media, colonies of freshly isolated *Brucella* organisms appear moist, translucent, and glistening. Older colonies may become opaque. A variety of forms and display of color have been described by Huddleson, making it possible to differentiate a series of changes in colony appearance from the smooth, mucoid to the rough types, which are related to changes in antigenic structure and virulence.[427]

Four main species of *Brucella* are recognized: *B. abortus* (subdivided into 9 biotypes; infects cattle primarily); *B. melitensis* (3 biotypes; mostly infects goats); *B. suis* (4 biotypes; infects swine as well as cattle); and *B. canis* (1 biotype; from dogs).

---

*Difco Laboratories, Detroit.
†BBL, Div. of BioQuest, Cockeysville, Md.

Table 79-57. Differential characteristics of *Brucella* species

| | CO_2 require-ment | H_2S production | Growth in presence of | | | | | Monospecific sera | |
| | | | Thionin* | | | Fuchsin* | | | |
			a	b	c	a	b	B. abortus	B. melitensis
B. melitensis	−	−†	−	+	+	+	+	−‡§	+‡
B. abortus	+‡‖	+‡¶	−	−	−‡#	+**	+**	+‡	−‡
B. suis	−	++‡††	+	+	+	−‡‡	−‡‡	+	−
B. canis	−	−	+	+	+	−	−	−	−

*Data on growth in presence of dyes from Jones[513] and McCullough.[441] Dyes (National Aniline Division, Allied Chemical Corp.) are added to brucella or tryptose agar in the following concentrations: thionin—a, 1:25,000; b, 1:50,000; c, 1:100,000—and basic fuchsin—a, 1:50,000; b, 1:100,000. See text.
†Generally, recently isolated strains of *B. melitensis* fail to produce sufficient amount to blacken the acetate paper. *B. abortus* produces a moderate amount during 4 d, whereas *B. suis* is a strong producer during 4 d. However, strains of *B. suis* isolated in Denmark fail to produce H_2S.
‡Majority of strains.
§Type 2: +, −. Type 3: +, +.
‖Types 1-4, 8, and 9 require CO_2; types 5, 6, and 7 do not.
¶Types 5, 6, and 8 do not produce H_2S.
#Types 1, 2, and 4 give this pattern; type 3: +, +, +; types 5-9: −, +, +.
**Type 2: −, −.
††Types 2, 3, and 4 do not produce H_2S.
‡‡Types 3 and 4: +, +.

Special features

B. melitensis, B. abortus, B. suis, and *B. canis* may be differentiated according to special characteristics in their metabolism and antigenic composition. They differ in their behavior in regard to atmospheric requirements, the formation of H_2S, the effect of dyes on their growth, differences in hydrolysis of urea, susceptibility to lysis by brucellaphage, oxidative metabolic tests,[417] and even differences in resistance to antibiotics.[428] For practical purposes the following procedures are recommended: (1) biochemical tests (CO_2 requirement and H_2S production), (2) bacteriostatic test (Huddleson dye tests), and (3) serologic identification. The tests are summarized in Table 79-57 and are described below.

Serodiagnostic tests

Because of the long incubation period in brucellosis, **antibodies** are frequently demonstrable in the serum by the time the disease is first recognized. **Agglutination** tests are performed with phenolized suspensions of heat-killed smooth (S) bacilli. In fact, because of the increased use of antibiotics administered prior to obtaining cultures, the majority of brucellosis cases are now diagnosed serologically. Of 1644 abattoir-associated cases reported from 1960-1971 in the United States, 85% were diagnosed serologically; confirmation by culture was only obtained in 17% of the cases. For serodiagnostic tests see Chapter 107.

Brucellosis

Bruce, investigating the disease known as Malta fever, Mediterranean fever, or undulant fever, discovered small coccoid organisms in fatal cases of the disease, which he called *Micrococcus melitensis.* Later it was discovered that goats suffered from an infection by this organism and were the source of contagion to humans. The disease was found to be prevalent in Malta and neighboring islands as well as several countries around the Mediterranean Sea. It was reported later in various other parts of the world, including Asia, South Africa, and America. The earliest news concerning human brucellosis in America were the reports of Masser and Garler in 1898[429] and of Craig in 1906.[429] *B. melitensis* may be transmitted to cattle and swine, from which, in turn, humans may be infected.

Bang in 1896-1897 isolated a bacterium responsible for contagious abortion in cattle. It was cultivated for the first time in the United States by MacNeal and Kerr in 1910,[430] but it was not until the work of Evans,[431] published in 1918, that these 2 diseases, one of goats and humans and the other of cattle, were found to be closely related because of the remarkable morphologic, cultural, and serologic resemblances between the 2 organisms.

Traum in 1914 found in fetuses prematurely expelled from sows a bacterium that is related to Bang's disease and Malta fever. This organism

and those discovered by Bruce and Bang constituted the 3 species of the genus *Brucella,* and infection with any of these organisms is termed brucellosis.

Human brucellosis may be manifested in a variety of forms that must be kept in mind in order to avoid confusion. In some individuals the infection has been found to be clinically inapparent; often it is a mild and insidious disease, but not infrequently it is a severe illness and fatal forms may be found. Although the underlying pattern of this illness is generally the same in all cases, there is considerable variation from case to case in regard to associated symptomatology and particularly in the duration of the disease. For this reason it is of practical importance to consider acute, subacute, and chronic forms of brucellosis. Some specialists have found it convenient to add a so-called hyperergic state, which has been found to be associated with an insidious symptomatology for which it has been included in chronic brucellosis.

Because of the peculiar evolution of human brucellosis, one has to be prepared to give proper interpretation to clinical and laboratory findings, since no diagnosis of brucellosis can be sustained without convincing bacteriologic and serologic evidence.

For detailed reviews of brucellosis see Buchanan et al.[432-434] and Martin and Watts.[435]

Brucella canis (isolated originally from dogs[420]) may cause a relatively mild illness in humans.[423] Routine serologic tests for *Brucella* agglutinins do **not** detect antibody to *B. canis.* A total of 18 cases of human *B. canis* infections have been reported in the United States in the period 1967-1977.

Laboratory diagnosis of brucellosis

The battery of tests generally accepted by most experts is as follows: (1) cultivation or isolation of *Brucella* from blood, aseptic fluids, urine, feces, or pathologic material; and (2) detection of antibodies against *Brucella* in the serum of patients (serodiagnostic tests).

For a review of the diagnostic aspects of brucellosis, see Buchanan et al.[433]

Isolation of Brucella. The isolation of *Brucella* from the blood, other aseptic fluids, or pathologic material is the definitive test for the diagnosis of brucellosis. It is necessary to follow good technics for the collection of specimens and the inoculation of reliable media.

Guinea pigs are susceptible to all species and develop an infection after injection of smooth (S) isolates.

Blood culture. Because of the scarcity of *Brucella* in the circulating blood or other body fluids, it has been recognized that liquid media are more adequate than are solid media as a first step in the isolation of these organisms. From liquid cultures, transfers are made to solid media in order to detect growth and identify the isolated bacteria. Media that have acquired wide acceptance are brucella and trypticase soy. Tryptose is also acceptable if previously tested to avoid bacteriostatic batches. When these media are not available, the old liver infusion, beef infusion, and potato infusion are known to be of value for primary isolation.[436]

For laboratories where requests for isolation of brucellae are not frequent, the **classic procedure of blood culture** is as follows. Broth of any of the media mentioned above is distributed in amounts of 75 ml in cotton-stoppered or screw-capped bottles and properly sterilized. The blood or other aseptic body fluids are added to the broth in amounts of 5-10 ml and incubated at 37 C in a closed jar containing CO_2 in a proportion of 10% of the volume. Commercial bottles with 10% CO_2 are satisfactory. **Transfers** from the broth to solid media are performed at regular intervals beginning on the **fourth day** of incubation. The agar slants are incubated in the CO_2 jar and also in ordinary atmosphere. Transfers are made in amounts of 0.2 ml at least for 30 days.

In laboratories where many blood cultures are requested not only for isolation of brucellae but also for general purposes, the **Castañeda technic**[437] has been found to be a practical method. In this procedure both liquid and solid media are placed within the same container. Blood is inoculated into the broth, and without need of entering the bottle for subcultures, transfers are made by the simple procedure of allowing the liquid phase to spread over the agar slant for a short time at regular intervals. This procedure has certain advantages. It reduces manipulation and material as well as chances of contamination during transfers, avoids danger of infection of technicians, and has proved to be as effective as any other method in which the transfer from broth to solid media is required.

Blood cultures for brucellosis should be incubated for a minimum of 3 weeks (preferably for 28 days) before being discarded as being negative. After the acute symptoms have subsided, blood cultures generally are negative; however, antibodies in the patient's serum are usually demonstrable by this time (see Chapter 107).

Preparation of Castañeda's double medium. Glassware may be any 150 ml flat-sided rectangular bottle. Solid media may be prepared with 1 of commercial media mentioned. Original formula is modified to contain 2.5% agar and 0.5% sodium citrate. About 15 ml of this agar medium is placed into each bottle, which is properly protected by means of metal cap or paper cover tied to mouth of bottle. Bottles are autoclaved and medium is allowed to set in 1 of narrow sidewalls. Fluid medium is prepared according to manufacturer's directions but with 2% sodium citrate added. After proper sterilization, broth is distributed in bottles in amounts of 10-15 ml. Sterile rubber stoppers are used to close bottles, and stoppers are protected with sterilized metal caps or paper covers. Bottles are incubated at 37 C for 5-10 d, and those that show no contamination are ready for use.

Considering the difficulty in maintaining the agar

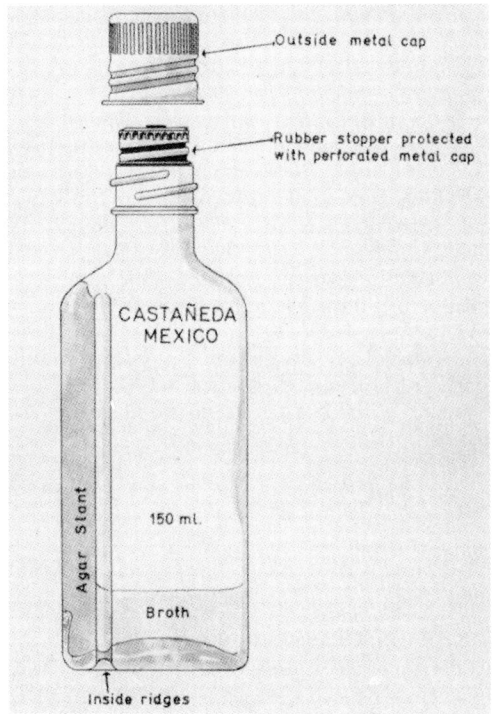

Outside metal cap

Rubber stopper protected with perforated metal cap

CASTAÑEDA
MEXICO

Agar Slant

150 ml.

Broth

Inside ridges

Fig. 79-4. Castañeda bottle for blood culture.

slant in a vertical position, particularly when the outfit has to be sent to another laboratory, Castañeda has developed a **special bottle**[438] that has the following features: The bottle is of rectangular shape with inside ridges that produce a sort of channel along 1 of the narrow sides in which the agar slant is kept and protected against deterioration (Fig. 79-4). The mouth is arranged so that it accommodates 2 stoppers: an inside rubber stopper fixed with a perforated metal cap and a metal exterior protector. When necessary, CO_2 is injected either at the time of inoculation of the blood or at the moment the liquid medium is added. (Castañeda bottles are available commercially.)

Blood must be taken with 20 ml syringe previously sterilized in autoclave. From 5-10 ml blood are injected into bottle through rubber stopper after removing outside protector cap, which may be replaced once operation is finished. Incubate at 37 C, keeping bottle in vertical position. At intervals of 48 h the bottle is tilted to allow fluid mixture to run over slant; bottle is then replaced in incubator. Careful inspection of slant is performed prior to new "transfer." When colonies are detected, bottle is opened, with due precaution, for identification of isolated organism.

Results: When agar layer shows colonies after 24 or 48 h, it is likely that culture has been contaminated. When colonies appear 24-48 h after first transfer, that is to say 72-96 h after inoculation of blood, cultivated organisms have usually been found to be salmonellae, staphylococci, and, less frequently, streptococci, *H. influenzae,* or coliforms. Organisms may be brucellae, but these appear more commonly after third transfer. Salmonellae or other bacteria may also grow after several transfers.

Other specimens. *Brucella* have also been recovered occasionally from bone marrow, biopsied lymph nodes, urine, and spinal fluid.

Selective media for isolation of Brucella from contaminated material. Brucellae are slow-growing and rather delicate organisms that are overgrown by contaminants, particularly gram-positive cocci and *Proteus* organisms. To overcome this difficulty, special media have been recommended. One of the older methods uses any suitable agar medium to which a bacteriostatic dye is added (such as crystal violet in concentration of 1:800,000) and, if necessary, a certain proportion of chloral hydrate to inhibit spread of *Proteus* organisms.

BRUCELLA SELECTIVE MEDIUM—KUZDAS-MORSE[439,440]

Albimi agar	1000 ml
Ethyl violet	1:800,000
Cycloheximide (Actidione*)	100 mg
Polymyxin B	6000 units
Bacitracin	25,000 units

Sterilize stock solutions of Actidione, polymyxin B, and bacitracin by Seitz or Millipore filtration. Keep refrigerated for no longer than 1 week. Add ethyl violet to melted agar before autoclaving. Add other ingredients after agar has cooled to about 50 C. Distribute in Petri dishes.

Even with the most elaborate medium and experience the isolation of *Brucella* from contaminated material is a difficult task.

Identification of Brucella species

For a comprehensive review on the identification of the species and biotypes within the genus *Brucella*, see McCullough.[441]

The cultures suspected of being *Brucella* may be submitted to the tests outlined in Table 79-57. The criteria for an unknown culture are as follows: Smears made from suspected colonies must spread uniformly in saline and, when stained, should show minute coccoid or coccobacillary gram-negative organisms. When suspended in a drop of saline on a slide, the material must agglutinate by the addition of antibrucella serum† and remain uniform with normal serum.

At this point the organism may be sent to a reference laboratory; make certain the organism does not ferment routine glucose medium. The agglutination test must be corroborated by the tube dilution method with a serum of known titer.

CO₂ requirement. Freshly isolated *B. abortus* is CO_2 dependent (5-10%). After a number of subcultures some strains lose this requirement rapidly. The test for CO_2 dependence should be performed as soon as possible after isolation.

Production of hydrogen sulfide. Inoculate surface of brucella agar slants with 24 h agar growth. Place strip

*The Upjohn Co., Kalamazoo, Mich.
†Difco Laboratories, Detroit.

of lead acetate paper* between cotton plug and inside of culture tube, extending ¾-1 inch below plug. Make certain that cotton plug is dry and free from agar. Do not let paper come in contact with inoculated agar surface. Incubate 24 h at 37 C. Remove afterward, label, and tape in record book.

Place new strip in tube. Remove and examine as above after 24 h. Repeat this procedure 4 consecutive days. Record blackening as from − to 4+.[429]

B. melitensis does not produce any change in color or, if so, only a trace of blackening is observed. This is generally true for the majority of recently isolated strains, but there are exceptions to this rule because some strains may produce a definite blackening of the paper. *B. abortus* has a tendency to produce a moderate blackening for 2 or 3 d, whereas *B. suis* commonly produces strongest blackening of all 3 types and for longer periods of time. As previously stated, Danish strains of *B. suis* fail to produce H₂S.

Inhibition by dyes. The most useful procedure for typing *Brucella* is testing the ability of the isolated organism to grow in the presence of certain bacteriostatic dyes. This method was developed by Huddleson.[442]

For species differentiation use Brucella or tryptose agar.† Make up 1% or 0.1% stock solutions (in distilled water) of thionin and basic fuchsin.‡ Add calculated amounts to melted medium to attain concentrations of 1:25,000, 1:500,000, and 1:100,000 of thionin and 1:50,000 and 1:100,000 of basic fuchsin. Distribute dye-containing media into Petri dishes. Several strains, including control strains, should be inoculated onto each plate. Plates should be prepared in duplicate so that 1 can be incubated in ordinary atmosphere and other in CO₂ jar. For inoculum, 48 h cultures grown without dye have been recommended. From these, a loopful is suspended in 0.1 ml saline, and a loopful of this suspension is streaked over test medium.

Other differential characteristics. *B. suis* rapidly hydrolyzes urea; *B. melitensis* and *B. abortus* do so slowly if at all. *B. canis* does not produce H₂S and does not grow in presence of basic fuchsin.[435]

Serologic typing. Serologic differences between *B. melitensis* and *B. abortus* must be detected by means of tests of absorption of agglutinins, but no differentiation is possible between *B. abortus* and *B. suis*. The use of the whole battery of tests summarized in Table 79-5 will help to establish final differentiation.

The monospecific sera used as an aid in typing may be of considerable help, provided that the serum has been properly prepared. One may request monospecific sera from WHO institutions,[436] since it is difficult to prepare reliable material. No specific rules can be followed for the preparation of the sera, and success is attained only with considerable patience and after many trials.

With monospecific sera obtained from the Weybridge Laboratory, Surrey, England, it is possible to differentiate *melitensis* from *abortus-suis* even by a simple slide agglutination. A droplet of saline in which a loop-

*American Indicator Paper Co., Chicago. Strips can be prepared in the laboratory by soaking filter paper in 10% neutral solution of salt. Allow paper to dry and then cut in strips about 15 mm wide and 6-8 cm long.
†Tryptose medium (Difco) and CTA medium (BBL) with incorporated dyes are available ready-made (tubed).
‡National Aniline Division, Allied Chemical Corp., New York.

ful of culture is emulsified on a slide is mixed with a droplet of serum, and after proper movements to the slide, one may notice differences in the effect of each serum. However, a final test is required by which serial dilutions of both sera are mixed with an equal volume of a suspension of the unknown strain. The concentration of this suspension should be close to tube 2 of the McFarland nephelometer.

The serum that produces the higher titers of agglutination after 24-48 h of incubation will indicate the type of the strain under test.

Brucellaphages. The method of determining phage susceptibility is primarily used by reference laboratories. For details see Morgan.[443]

Oxidative metabolic tests. The oxidative uptake rate of a series of amino acids and carbohydrates has been determined for each species. It is a method for use by reference laboratories. For details see Meyer and Cameron.[444]

Fluorescent antibody technics. The direct FA staining procedure for *Brucella* in tissue or in culture is both rapid and sensitive. See Cherry and Moody.[445]

HAEMOPHILUS

The genus *Haemophilus* ("blood loving") includes small, gram-negative, facultatively anaerobic, nonmotile, non-sporeforming bacilli that require certain factors derived from blood for growth on culture media; it is listed as a genus of uncertain affiliation in Part 8 of *Bergey's Manual*, ed. 8.[3]

Some species require **factor V** (replaceable by coenzyme I [diphosphopyridine nucleotide, DPN] or coenzyme II, TPN) or **factor X** (hemin or hematin) **or both.** Whole blood furnishes both factors; growth occurs only if the medium is supplemented with whole blood (or factors X and/or V). Since factor V is easily destroyed by enzymes of unheated red blood cells, heated **(chocolate) agar** is recommended in place of blood agar.

The taxonomic status of 2 organisms, *H. vaginalis* and *H. aphrophilus*, is in doubt at the present time because of uncertainties regarding their need for factors X and/or V; they are discussed below.

The differential characteristics of the *Haemophilus* group are listed in Table 79-58.

Kilian[446] recently developed an identification system that allows the subdivision of *Haemophilus* species into biotypes. The system includes performance of the (1) ALA (porphyrin) test[447]; (2) X and V requirement determinations; (3) indole production; (4) urease production; (5) ornithine decarboxylase activity; (6) production of acids from carbohydrates (phenol red broth base [Difco] with hemin and nicotinamide adenine dinuclueotide added); (7) requirement for increased CO_2 tension; (8) hemolysis of horse blood; (9) hemagglutination test; (10) catalase production; (11) oxidase activity (by Kovacs' method); (12) H_2S production (lead acetate strip in the lid of an inoculated chocolate agar plate and reading after 2 days incubation; (13) ornithine decarboxylase; (14) DNase activity; (15) ONPG (β-galactosidase); (16) PNPG (α-glucosidase); (17) alkaline phosphatase; and (18) nitrate reduction.

Based on this schema, Kilian[446] subdivided *H. influenzae* into 5 biotypes and *H. parainfluenzae* into 3 biotypes. He also recommended that *H. aegyptius*, *H. parahaemolyticus*, and *H. paraphrohaemolyticus* not be accorded specific status. (See other members of *Haemophilus* group, below.)

Goldberg and Washington[448] suggest that **preliminary identification** and **biotyping** of *Haemophilus* can be carried out with a smaller number of tests than those listed by Kilian[446]: In their preliminary scheme they employ (1) the porphy-

Table 79-58. Differential characteristics of some *Haemophilus* species*†

	Growth factors		Iridescence	Capsules	Hemolysis	δ-ALA‡	Indole	Urease	Ornithine decarboxylase
	X	V							
H. influenzae§									
Typable *a-f*	+	+	+	+	0	−	d‖	d‖¶	d‖
Nontypable	+	+	0	0	0	−	d	d	d
H. aegyptius§	+	+	0	0	0	?	−		
H. parainfluenzae§									
Typable	0	+	+	+	0	+	−	d	d
Nontypable	0	+	0	0	0	+	−	d	
H. haemolyticus§	+	+	?	?	+(β)	?	d	+	−
H. parahaemolyti-cus§	0	+	?	?	+	+	−		
H. ducreyi§	+	−		?	±	−	−	−	−
H. aphrophilus§	+(?)	−	?	?	0	+	−	−	−

*Data from Alexander,[456] Buchanan and Gibbons,[3] Kilian,[446] and Goldberg and Washington.[448]

†+, More than 90% of strains positive; −, more than 90% of strains negative; ±, weak or slight; *0*, negative; *d*, 11-89% of strains positive; *?*, not known.

‡δ-Aminolevulinic acid.

§Significant in humans.

‖See text for biotypes of *H. influenzae* and *H. parainfluenzae*.

¶Biotypes 1-4 positive; biotype 5 negative.

rin (ALA, porphyrin biosynthesis from δ-aminolevulinic acid) test; (2) indole; (3) ornithine decarboxylase; (4) urease; (5) oxidase; and (6) catalase tests. They do **not** recommend the determination of X- and V-factor requirements but instead recommend the porphyrin (δ-ALA) test for separating *H. parainfluenzae* and *H. paraphrophilus* from *H. influenzae* and *H. haemolyticus.*

Porphyrin test[449]

The determination of X- and V-factor requirements is notoriously troublesome. Carryover of hemin from the isolation plate may occur; an X- and V-dependent organism may then grow around the V disk or strip, leading to misidentification.

In 1974, Kilian[447] described 2 rapid tests that avoid problems commonly encountered when testing for X-factor requirement.[449] Both tests determine the ability of V-dependent *Haemophilus* to use δ-aminolevulinic acid (ALA) for synthesizing porphyrins and porphobilinogen (heme precursors).

Porphobilinogen can be detected in the medium by using Kovacs' reagent and observing a red color developing. **Porphyrins** can be detected by red fluorescence in the reaction mixture under Wood's light.

The porphyrin test is easier to perform and is more sensitive than the porphobilinogen test. The test yields positive results as early as 2 hours.

Porphyrin test procedure[447,449]
1. Use fresh culture (not more than 24 h old).
2. Use heavy inoculum.
3. Observe fluorescence in darkened room or black box.
4. It is necessary to be sure that *Haemophilus* is tested.

Substrate
1. δ-aminolevulinic acid hydrochloride (ALA),* 2 mM, 31.8 mg/100 ml wt/vol
2. $MgSO_4$, 0.8 mM, 9.62 mg/100 ml wt/vol
3. Phosphate buffer (Sorensen), 0.1M, pH 6.9
Prepare Na_2HPO_4, 14.2 g, in 1 L water and KH_2PO_4, 13.61 g, in 1 L water.
Add 55.4 ml of Na_2HPO_4 solution to 44.6 ml of KH_2PO_4 solution. Add reagent *1* (ALA), 31.8 mg, and reagent *2*, 9.62 mg (mixture can be stored at 4 C for 6 mo).

Test
1. For porphyrin production: make heavy (milky) suspension of organisms in 0.5 ml substrate (in 13 × 100 mm tubes, unsterile) using overnight growth from chocolate agar plate.
2. Incubate tubes in heating block at 35-37 C for 4 h.
3. Observe tubes for red fluorescence (positive test) against white background under Wood's light (dim room lights for reading). Positive test indicates **lack** of requirement of X factor.
4. Tests that are negative (under Wood's light) can be left to incubate for 24 h and then tested with few drops of Kovacs' reagent. Development of red

---

*Sigma Chemical Co., St. Louis.

aqueous layer indicates positive porphobilinogen test (lack of X-factor requirement); no color confirms first negative test (organism **does** require X factor).

Cultivation. It is advisable to use an optimum medium (chocolate, Levinthal, or Fildes' agar) in conjunction with blood agar. Good growth on optimum medium and poor or no growth on blood agar is suggestive of nonhemolytic *Haemophilus* species.[3] Sheep blood agar is not usable for any species of *Haemophilus* that require V factor (rabbit and horse blood agar are suitable).

Staphylococcus streak on sheep blood agar plate can be used for isolation and growth of factor V requiring *Haemophilus*, since staphylococci (like neisseriae and certain yeasts) can synthesize factor V (NAD).

Streak specimen heavily on blood agar plate. With inoculating wire, make single narrow streak of hemolytic staphylococcus (known to produce NAD) through inoculated portion of plate. After 18-24 hours in CO_2 incubation (35 C), very small colonies of *Haemophilus* ("dewdrop" colonies) will be growing in hemolytic zone of staphylococcal colonies ("satellitism"). This phenomenon also can be seen on blood agar plates on which mixed flora is growing (sputum, etc.). *Haemophilus* colonies, quite large, will grow around and next to colonies of staphylococci, pneumococci, neisseriae, and other organisms capable of synthesizing NAD (factor V). *Haemophilus* colonies get smaller as their distance from staphylococcal, etc., colonies increases.

Haemophilus influenzae

H. influenzae, the type species of the genus, produces pyogenic infections frequently in adults[450]; in children it is one of the most frequent causes of meningitis. It may invade the bloodstream, and it may cause empyema, pneumonia, and obstructive infections of the respiratory tract (epiglottitis). It may also cause otitis media, subacute bacterial endocarditis, conjunctivitis, appendicitis, and wound infection.[451]

For an overview of systemic *H. influenzae* disease, see Dajani et al.[452] and Turk and May.[453]

Cultivation

H. influenzae grows poorly on blood agar* but does much better on chocolate agar. Growth is better in media where the contents of the red blood cell are liberated (by heat, Levinthal medium, or by peptic digestion, Fildes medium). Fildes enrichment is available commercially.† CO_2 incubation favors primary isolation. The organism requires both factors X and V when grown aerobically. When grown under anaerobic conditions, it does not require X (involved in the formation of heme-containing enzymes).

---

*Rabbit or guinea pig blood agar is best.
†Difco Laboratories, Detroit.

As mentioned earlier, on blood agar, if the organism grows, it produces tiny colonies. However, if the colonies grow near colonies of staphylococci, neisseriae, or pneumococci (in throat or sputum cultures), they are large and characteristic. This is due to the ability of the organisms mentioned in synthesizing an additional amount of factor V, which diffuses into the medium and stimulates the growth of *H. influenzae*. This is known as the **satellite phenomenon.**

On chocolate agar (containing yeast extract) the colonies appear in about 24 hours; they are small, colorless, and transparent.

In spinal, synovial, or pleural fluids, the organisms are predominantly coccobacillary, **simulating diplococci.** Sometimes short chains are seen, resembling streptococci. Longer bacillary forms also occur along with irregular forms. In cultures, especially when they are at least 24 hours old, the predominant form is the minute, short coccobacillus, which stains rather poorly.

NOTE: In Chapter 75 (spinal fluid), several methods are mentioned for early detection of *Haemophilus*, such as counterimmunoelectrophoresis (CIE, see also Chapter 74) and Quellung test using antiserum.

Identification

The encapsulated varieties of *H. influenzae*, types a, b, c, d, e, and f, produce a specific soluble substance, which is concentrated in the capsule as well. The type of a given strain of *H. influenzae* can be established by capsular swelling, agglutination of the organisms, or precipitation of the soluble substance with diagnostic type-specific serum (available from several commercial sources). When organisms are sufficiently numerous in spinal, pleural, or synovial fluid to be seen on stained smear, species and type may be identified by the **precipitin test or capsular swelling** (see discussion on cerebrospinal fluid, Chapter 75).

For a review of *H. influenzae* serotyping, see Omland[454]; for newer methods (CIE, latex agglutination, etc.) see Ingram et al.[455]

The 2 procedures can also be used with a concentrated suspension of nasopharyngeal mucus from patients with obstructive laryngitis or pneumonia. Alexander[456] recommends collecting the mucus on a small cotton swab passed through the nares to the posterior pharyngeal wall. The swab is placed in a small tube containing 0.2 ml sterile broth.

Encapsulated *H. influenzae* grown from blood cultures or other fluids can be identified usually after 18 hours of growth by demonstration of capsular swelling with type-specific diagnostic antiserum. If the test is negative, inoculate Levinthal agar to test for iridescence of growth. The pathogenic forms produce an iridescent growth on this medium; this can be observed in obliquely transmitted light (on Fildes medium also). If neither iridescence nor capsular swelling can be demonstrated, diagnosis of *H. in-*

fluenzae depends on requirement of both factors X and V for growth. Media for testing the combined and separate action of factors X and V are described in Chapter 72.*

X and V requirement. Disks or strips impregnated with pure compounds (X, V, and X + V)† can also be used to determine requirements of the isolate and allow identification of the organism (especially differentiation of *H. influenzae* and *H. parainfluenzae*). The organism should be picked from the primary plate, preferably diluted in 5 ml sterile trypticase or tryptose broth (to dilute any essential growth factor that may have been carried over from the primary plate), and the inoculum should be spread on a fresh, nonenriched plate (trypticase soy, heart infusion, or tryptic soy agar) using a loop or swab. Aseptically place all 3 strips on the inoculated plate, leaving at least a 20 mm distance between strips. Incubate overnight at 37 C and observe areas of growth **immediately** around the strips. Growth indicates requirement for the adjacent factor. Interpretation should be made by referral to Table 79-58.

The great majority of strains found in meningitis are **type b.** The same type can also be found occasionally in children without signs of infections.

A considerable percentage of the normal population harbors nontypable *H. influenzae* strains in the respiratory tract at some time. Failure to produce iridescence identifies them as nontypable, nonencapsulated varieties.

Biochemical characteristics and biotypes

Sutter and Finegold[457] reported that *H. influenzae* is indole and urease positive, reduces nitrate, and ferments glucose, sucrose, and xylose. More recently, Kilian[446] devised an identification system for the genus *Haemophilus* (see introduction for *Haemophilus*, above); using a variety of biochemical and physiologic characteristics, he was able to subdivide *H. influenzae* into 5 biotypes. Some characteristics of the *H. influenzae* biotypes are shown in Table 79-59.

Both Kilian[446,446a] and Goldberg and Washington[448] found that most of the *Haemophilus* organisms isolated from meningitis (cerebrospinal fluid) belong to biotype I of *H. influenzae* and that practically all of these possessed a capsule of serotype b. In Kilian's study of 130 isolates from meningitis[446] (Norway and Denmark), 93% belonged to biotype I, 4.6% to biotype II, and 2.3% to biotype IV. One strain of biotype I was nonencapsulated (nontypable). All other strains were serotype b.

---

*Blood or chocolate agar contains both factors X and V; yeast extract agar provides factor V only, whereas autoclaved blood agar provides factor X only.

†Taxo X, V, and XV Strips, BBL, Div. of BioQuest, Cockeysville, Md.; Bacto differentiation disks, BV, BX, and BVX (contain bacitracin also), Difco Laboratories, Detroit.

Table 79-59. Some characteristics of *Haemophilus influenzae* and *H. parainfluenzae* biotypes*

	Biotype	δ-ALA (porphyrin)	Indole	Ornithine decarboxylase	Oxidase	Urease
H. influenzae	I	−	+	+	+	+
	II	−	+	−	+	+
	III	−	−	−	+	+
	IV	−	−	+	+	+
	V	−	+, ±	+	+	−
H. parainfluenzae†	I	+	−	+	+	−
	II	+	−	+	+	+
	III	+	−	−	+	+

*Data from Kilian, M.: J. Gen. Microbiol. **93**:9, 1976; Kilian, M., Sorensen, S., and Fredericksen, W. J.: J. Clin. Microbiol. **9**:409, 1979; and Goldberg, R., and Washington, J. A.: Am. J. Clin. Pathol. **70**:899, 1978.
†All V-factor dependent.

Fluorescent antibody technic. Immunofluorescence in conjunction with conventional technics offers a valuable tool for the rapid identification of *H. influenzae* in meningitis.[445,458]

Antimicrobial susceptibility. Since 3-5% of *H. influenzae* isolates are now resistant to ampicillin due to β-**lactamase** production, it is now imperative to determine the susceptibility of strains isolated from blood, spinal fluid, or spaces normally sterile.

A number of β-**lactamase tests,** including rapid iodometric and acidimetric tests, as well as sensitivity testing of *H. influenzae* are described in Chapter 87. Chloramphenicol resistance has also been encountered in *H. influenzae.*[459]

Other members of Haemophilus group

H. haemolyticus. The organism is found frequently in the nasopharynx in the absence of infection. It produces β-hemolysis on blood agar, especially on rabbit blood agar. Sheep blood inhibits its growth. For a survey of hemolytic *Haemophilus* occurence in the throat see Branson.[460]

The organism must be differentiated (by Gram stain) from β-hemolytic streptococci. It is found rarely in subacute bacterial endocarditis. It requires both factors X and V.

H. parainfluenzae. It is found in the normal nasopharynx and occasionally causes subacute bacterial endocarditis. It requires only factor V. The 3 biotypes (Kilian[446]) with some of their characteristics are shown in Table 79-59.

For a review of *H. parainfluenzae* endocarditis, see Jemsek et al.[461]

H. suis. It is not known to be pathogenic in man; it occurs in swine.

H. haemoglobinophilus (H. canis). Isolated from dogs; the organism requires factor X but not factor V.

H. aphrophilus.[457] See below.

H. (C.) vaginalis. Does not really belong in genus; discussed below.

• • •

Kilian[446] has questioned the merit of according specific status to the following:

H. aegyptius (Koch-Weeks bacillus). *H. aegyptius* resembles *H. influenzae* culturally and is related to it serologically. It is associated with conjunctivitis; the organism requires factors X and V. Hemagglutination, according to Kilian,[446] is not a justifiable reason for separating *H. aegyptius* from *H. influenzae.*

H. parahaemolyticus. The organism produces β-hemolysis and is found in cases of subacute bacterial endocarditis. It may cause pharyngitis. It requires only factor V. It is catalase and urease positive, reduces nitrate, and ferments glucose, maltose, and sucrose.[457]

According to Kilian,[446] because the hemolytic properties of the organism are unstable, its differentation from *H. parainfluenzae* is not justified.

H. paraphrohaemolyticus. This organism requires CO$_2$ tension, is urease positive, occurs in the human mouth, and in some pathologic conditions (ulcer of mouth, urethral discharge of adult males,[3] endocarditis[462]).

• • •

H. gallinarum (from fowl), *H. ovis* (from sheep), *H citreus* (from cattle), and *H. piscium* (from fish) are not known to cause disease in humans.

Haemophilus aphrophilus

This organism was isolated from a patient with endocarditis and named by Khairat.[463] Page and King[464] summarized infections due to *H. aphrophilus* in a critical review; see also Bieger et al.[465] Of the 41 patients listed, 17 had positive blood cultures (15 with diagnosis of endocarditis); other isolations were from abscesses (facial and brain), spinal fluid, synovial fluid, wounds, the ear, and pleural fluid. For an extensive clinical and bacteriologic study of *H. aphrophilus* see Sutter and Finegold.[457]

H. aphrophilus is closely related and frequently confused with *Actinobacillus actinomycetemcomitans.* Whereas identification present considerable difficulties, isolation does not seem to be unduly difficult.

Thioglycollate seems to support the growth

Table 79-60. Differential characteristics of *Haemophilus aphrophilus* and *Actinobacillus actinomycetemcomitans**†

	A. actinomy-cetemcomi-tans	H. aphro-philus
Growth in moist air, 24 h‡	–	+
Catalase	+ (weak)	–
Xylose	A (–)	–
Mannitol	A (–)	–
Trehalose	–	+
Absolute CO₂ requirement	+	–
Lactose	–	A
Sucrose	–	A

*Based on data from King,[271] King and Tatum,[272] and Sutter and Finegold.[457]

†A, acid; (–), some strains negative.

‡Many, but not all, strains; on trypticase soy agar.

of the organism when blood is present (blood culture); it grows best in a CO₂-enriched atmosphere (candle jar) or in moist air; most strains do not grow in dry air.[457] Some strains require factor X and therefore media containing factor X (blood or chocolate agar) should be employed for its isolation. After several transfers it seems to lose this requirement.

The organism is small, gram negative, coccoid to coccobacillary, and compares in size with *Brucella*. No capsule seems to be formed.

Growth characteristics and identification. Slight greening occurs on rabbit blood agar in about 48 hours. Colonies (24 hours old) are minute to 0.5 mm in size, usually entire, translucent, and smooth. They attain a size of 2-3 mm after prolonged incubation. Optimal temperature is 37 C. Some strains grow on MacConkey agar; urease, gelatin, catalase, and indole tests are negative.

Fermentation tests[272] in Difco heart infusion broth (with 0.2 ml 1.5% aqueous bromcresol purple per liter of medium, with Seitz filter–sterilized carbohydrates added in 1% concentration) show acid formation in glucose, glycogen, galactose, dextrin, levulose, maltose, mannose, and starch (same as *A. actinomycetemcomitans*). **Acid formation in lactose, raffinose, trehalose, and sucrose and no fermentation of mannitol** and xylose serve to distinguish *H. aphrophilus* from *A. actinomycetemcomitans* (see Tables 79-4, 79-5, and 79-60).

Nitrate is reduced and H₂S is produced (lead acetate paper over TSI). For further details see Sutter and Finegold,[457] King and Tatum,[272] and Young.[466]

Table 79-59 lists some differential characteristics of *H. aphrophilus* and *A. actinomycetemcomitans*.

The organism is uniformly sensitive to streptomycin, chloramphenicol, gentamicin, rifampin, and tetracycline, whereas penicillin, ampicillin,

Table 79-61. Characteristics of *Haemophilus vaginalis**†

Characteristic	Sign	% Positive
Incomplete hemolysis, rabbit blood agar	(+)	(92)
Catalase	–	2
Oxidase	–	6
Nitrate reduction	–	0
Esculin hydrolysis	–	0
Lipase	v	86
Acid from:		
Glucose	+ or (+)	81 (13)
Xylose	v	36 (9)
Mannitol	–	0
Lactose	–	1
Sucrose	v	11 (4)
Maltose	+ or (+)	87 (13)
Fructose	v	60 (23)

*Personal communication from Dr. R.E. Weaver, (Center for Disease Control), 1977.

†+, 90% or more positive within 48 h; ( ), delayed reaction, 3-7 d; –, less than 10% positive; v variable, 10-89% positive. Hemolytic reaction occurs in 2-4 d. Carbohydrate broth is supplemented with 2-3% serum. All strains were not tested for each reaction. Lipase is only characteristic for which less than 50% of strains were tested. Data is based on examination of 126 strains.

methicillin, and erythromycin susceptibility is variable; it is resistant to lincomycin and vancomycin.[457]

For an extensive review of *H. aphrophilus* microbiology and clinical spectrum, see Bieger et al.[465]

Haemophilus ducreyi

H. ducreyi causes chancroid (soft chancre), a venereal disease, in humans. The morphology in the local lesion is characteristic: chains of small gram-negative bacilli occur in strands. Characteristics, diagnosis, and cultivation of the organism are described in detail in Chapter 75 ("Female genital tract").

Haemophilus vaginalis

H. (Corynebacterium) vaginalis is discussed briefly in Chapter 77 (*Corynebacterium*), and in considerable detail (colony appearance, media for isolation, cultivation, role of organism in vaginitis) in Chapter 75 ("Female genital tract").

Biochemical characteristics and salient features of the organism are described here; **the reader is urged to consult the information in Chapter 75.**

The organism is gram variable, rod-shaped, sometimes coccobacillary; it was originally named *H. vaginalis*. Later it was shown that it has no requirement for X and/or V factors; therefore it could not be a member of the genus *Haemophilus*. In 1963 the name *Corynebacterium vaginale* was proposed for it; however, it is **catalase negative** (whereas most corynebacteria are catalase positive) and its cell wall lacks arabinose (which is present in coryne-bacteria), and therefore the organism is likely neither *Haemophilus* nor *Corynebacterium*.

The biochemical and physiologic character-istics of the organism are shown in Table 79-61.

For a recent review of the salient features of *H. vaginalis*, see Greenwood and Pickett.[467] They note fermentation of a variety of carbohy-drates (similar to Weaver's data in Table 79-61) and list a small number of characteristics for the **presumptive** identification of the organism, as follows:

Oxidase*	Negative
Catalase*	Negative
Hemolysis of:	
Human blood†	Positive (96%)
Sheep blood	Negative
Hippurate hydrolysis* (buffered substrate)	Positive (92%)

BORDETELLA
Bordetella pertussis and related species

The genus *Bordetella* consists of 3 species: *B. pertussis*, *B. parapertussis*, and *B. bronchi-septica*. The 3 organisms are associated with whooping cough or infections resembling it.‡

For isolation of Bordetella and the obtaining of specimens and proper media (Jones-Kendrick and Bordet-Gengou media), see discussion on throat and nasopharyngeal specimens, Chapter 75.

Colonies of *B. pertussis* on a Bordet-Gengou plate are small, transparent, entire, convex, and smooth, looking like a small droplet of mercury or a bisected pearl. Colonies appear in not less than 48 hours but usually around 72 hours at 35 C. *B. parapertussis* colonies are larger and duller (in 48 hours) and may show a slight tint of yellow or green. *B. bronchiseptica* colo-nies are usually indistinguishable from *B. pertussis*. All 3 species produce hemolysis on Bordet-Gengou medium in varying degrees.

For staining, the Gram stain is recommended; the counterstain should be left on for 2 minutes. All 3 species are gram negative. On Bordet-Gengou medium, *B. pertussis* shows coccoid

forms, similar to *B. bronchiseptica*, whereas *B. parapertussis* is more rodlike.

NOTE: *B. parapertussis* and *B. bronchisep-tica* grow on ordinary blood agar or plain agar medium, whereas *B. pertussis* does not. The former 2 may grow poorly on blood agar when first isolated; *B. bronchiseptica* eventually grows heavily, whereas *B. parapertussis* grows slowly. *B. bronchiseptica* and *B. parapertussis* also grow on MacConkey agar, utilize citrate, and produce urease (see Tables 79-50, 79-51, and 79-62).

B. pertussis is catalase variable and oxidase positive. It **does not attack** sugars and is non-motile.

B. parapertussis grows on nutrient agar, is urease and citrate positive and oxidase negative, does not reduce nitrate, and is nonmotile.

B. bronchiseptica is catalase, urease, citrate, and oxidase positive, reduces nitrate, and is **motile.**

The identification of *B. pertussis* and *B. parapertussis* is confirmed by agglutination with specific diagnostic antisera* and with fluorescent antibody (FA technic).

For a detailed review of the laboratory diag-nosis of *Bordetella* infections see Lauthrop and Lacey[468]; for an extensive appraisal of pertussis infections see Brooksaler and Nelson.[469]

Fluorescent antibody technics. See Whitaker et al.[470]

FRANCISELLA
Francisella tularensis

F. tularensis is a very small rod coccoidal measuring $0.2 \times 0.3\text{-}0.7$ μ and occurring sin-gly. It is nonmotile and gram negative and usual-ly does not grow on ordinary media. The organ-ism is the causative agent of tularemia ("rabbit fever").

Isolation and cultivation. *F. tularensis* re-quires special enriched media such as cystine-glucose blood agar.† On cystine agar medium, minute, transparent, droplike colonies are formed after 2-5 days of incubation at 37 C; these are mucoid and easily emulsified. The

---

*From subculture on chocolate agar plate.
†"Vaginalis" agar plate (Chapter 75).
‡*Bordetella* is a genus of "uncertain affiliation" in Part 7 of *Bergey's Manual*, eighth edition.[3]

*Commercially available from several manufacturers.
†I encountered a fresh isolate that grew well on sheep blood agar in 4 days.

Table 79-62. Differential characteristics of *Bordetella**†

Characteristic	B. pertussis	B. parapertussis	B. bronchiseptica
Growth on blood-free peptone agar	−	+	+
Browning of peptone agar	−	+	−
Produces urease	−	+	+ (4 h)
Reduces nitrate	−	−	+
Motility	−	−	+

Bordetella is a genus of uncertain affiliation in Part 7 of *Bergey's Manual*, ed. 8.[3]
†−, Negative reaction; +, positive reaction.

optimal growth temperature is 37 C. It is an obligate aerobe. Glucose, maltose, and mannose are utilized (acid produced) without gas production; other carbohydrates are attacked irregularly.

Further identification procedures include **agglutination** by homologous antisera* and the demonstration of virulence by intraperitoneal inoculation of guinea pigs. **The danger of handling infected animals and virulent cultures of F. tularensis cannot be overemphasized.** Masks, gloves, and scrub suits should be worn and material should be handled in a bacteriologic hood.

F. tularensis is not easy to isolate, but the following procedures have been found successful[471]:

1. Inoculate 4 cystine (cystine glucose hemoglobin or blood medium) agar slants and 1 nutrient agar control slant with 0.5 to 1 ml of patient's blood, freshly drawn. Ground tissue material may also be used. Distribute blood over slants before it clots and incubates slants horizontally at 37 C, in air.
2. Observe slants daily for presence of growth. Minute, droplike colonies may appear in 3 to 5 d, but it can take as long as 10 d for them to develop. No growth occurs on nutrient agar slant.
3. Examine stained smear of colony for small, gram-negative coccobacilli. Identify by agglutination with tularemia antiserum.
4. Do not report culture as negative before 3 weeks of incubation.

Guinea pigs can be infected without difficulty, and intraperitoneal injection of a heavy saline suspension of blood or ground-up tissue is the procedure of choice when only small numbers of organisms may be present. **Accidental laboratory infection is an ever-present hazard.** Animal injection, therefore, should not be attempted unless the laboratory worker has been previously immunized against tularemia.

Other specimens for isolation of *F. tularensis* are skin lesions, pleural effusions, conjunctival ulcers, bone marrow, necrotic lesions, liver, spleen, and lungs (autopsy).

Tularemia in animals and humans. Tularemia is an acute, often fatal disease of rodents caused by *F. tularensis.* It is highly infectious and is transmitted to humans from rodents by the bite of a flea or tick or by contamination of the skin or conjunctiva with tissues or body fluids of infected rodents, flies, or ticks. The site of infection in humans is usually marked by a necrotic, punched-out ulcer, which is associated with a regional lymphadenitis. The disease begins with a sudden chill, followed by an irregular fever, lasting 2-3 weeks.

McCoy and Chapin in 1912 found the causative organism in squirrels and named it *Bacterium tularense.* They cultured it, transmitted the infection to various rodents by feeding, nasal inoculation, and injection of blood, and reported positive complement fixation and agglutination

*Commercially available.

for human sera. Francis identified in 1919 the deer-fly fever of Utah with the plaguelike disease of rodents of California, and in 1921 he gave the name of "tularaemia" to the disease because of the bacteremia. He isolated *F. tularensis* from fly-bitten human cases, wild jack rabbits, and 1 ground squirrel, demonstrated agglutinins in human cases, and transmitted infections in laboratory animals with the deer fly, *Chrysops discalis.* Since that time many cases have been described in the United States.

The occurrence of this disease in humans depends on the presence of the disease in wild rodents, especially rabbits, and is often known to be associated with the discovery of sick and dead rabbits in the vicinity. Scratches, abrasions, thorn punctures, etc. have been reported at the site of infection. Infection is acquired from infected tissues or body fluids and may occur in connection with dressing or handling rabbits, woodchucks, or laboratory animals or with the handling of ticks or flies. Infection from person to person has not been reported either by contact, operative procedures, or insects. The disease is found especially in rural districts, among those exposed to ticks and flies and especially those handling wild rabbits, such as hunters, marketmen, housewives, and cooks (Fig. 79-5). **Laboratory infections are frequent.**

Immunity is lasting in humans and may be connected with the long persistence of agglutinins. There is no record of a second attack. Francis described 5 types of this disease: **ulceroglandular tularemia, oculoglandular tularemia, glandular tularemia, typhoidal tularemia, and ingestion tularemia.**

For detecting antibody in suspected patient's serum, a valuable test for establishing a diagnosis, see serology (Chapter 107).

Fluorescent antibody procedures. FA technics are eminently suitable for the detection of the

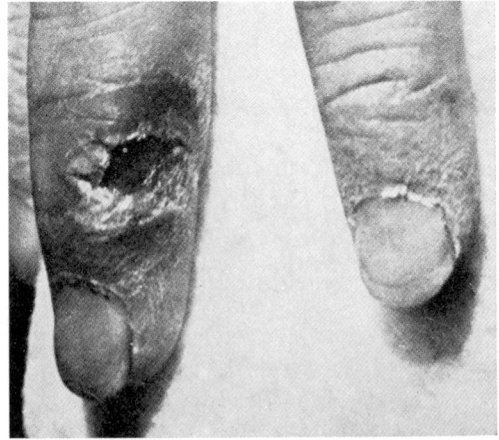

Fig. 79-5. Ulcer of finger 19 days after onset in a marketman who dressed rabbits. (Brown and Hunter.) (From Stitt, E. R.: Diagnosis and treatment of tropical diseases, Philadelphia, P. Blakiston's Son & Co.)

organism in tissues[472] and identification of organisms in cultures.[473]

For a detailed review of the organism, see Eigelsbach[474]; for reviews of epidemics and various clinical manifestations, see Klock et al.,[475] Dienst,[476] and Miller and Bates[477]; for identification, see Karlsson.[478]

STREPTOBACILLUS
Streptobacillus moniliformis

Excellent reviews have been written by Morton[479] and Rogosa.[480]

This organism was also known as *Haverhillia multiformis*, *Streptothrix muris ratti*, and *Actinobacillus murix*. It is a facultatively anaerobic, gram-negative, pleomorphic organism requiring blood, serum, or ascitic fluid for cultivation. The morphology is fairly uniform (bacilli of 2-4 μm in length) in the animal body and in young cultures. In older cultures or in unsatisfactory media the organism is made up of long filaments and chains of bacilli or cocci. The filaments show swelling 2-5 times their own width (Fig. 79-6). Infusion media, properly supplemented, are satisfactory for growth; optimum pH is 7.6. Some strains grow better in an atmosphere of increased carbon dioxide tension. Growth on solid media is better when the medium contains less than the usual 1.5% agar and the atmosphere contains a good deal of moisture. Growth on solid media is relatively slow (2-4 days). Colonies are raised and granular and may reach 5 mm in diameter. The organism does **not** grow on Mac-Conkey agar.

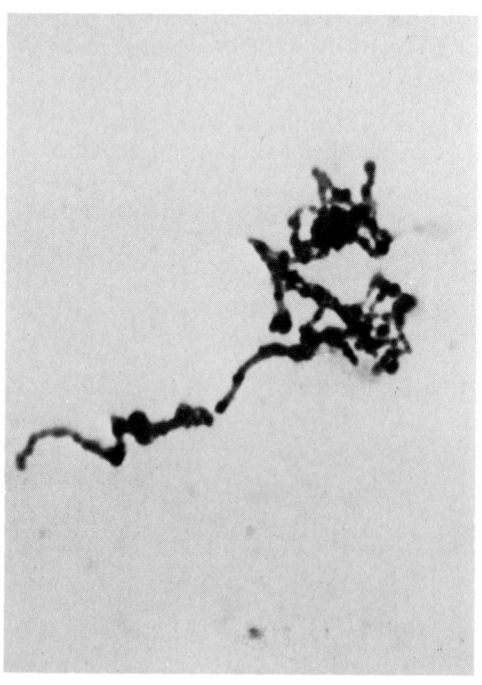

Fig. 79-6. Microscopic morphology—*Streptobacillus moniliformis.* Long filaments in chains, with globular and spindle-shaped swellings. (Giemsa stain.)

S. moniliformis is the cause of one type of rat-bite fever and of Haverhill fever (erythema arthriticum epidemicum) that is characterized by fever, rash, and polyarthritis. Squirrel and weasel bites as well as rat bites and the handling of mice may introduce infection with this organism. Some cases of Haverhill fever may have been foodborne or milkborne. Complications of the disease include endocarditis, pneumonia, arthritis myositis, abscesses, diarrhea, and mastoiditis.[481]

Diagnosis of the infection is best made by culturing the organism from blood (or joint fluid). Blood cultures should be set up so as to yield a final concentration of the patient's blood of nearly 20%. Growth occurs in the form of "bread crumb, fluff balls, or cotton balls" on the surface of the sedimented blood cells or the wall of the culture vessel. An agglutination test is also available.

Penicillin is generally the therapy of choice, and streptomycin is also very active against the organism. One strain highly resistant to penicillin has been encountered.[482] Other drugs that are sometimes effective are tetracycline, erythromycin, chloramphenicol, and bacitracin. The clinical significance of the L phase variant, which is resistant to penicillin, is questionable.

Lambe et al.[483] have reported that in a case of Haverhill fever, sodium polyanethol sulfonate (SPS) incorporated in a blood culture bottle inhibited the growth of *S. moniliformis.*

SPIRILLACEAE
Spirillum

The genus *Spirillum* consists of rigid, helically curved, **crescent-shaped** to **spiral cells**; the cells are described as resembling long screws or portions of a turn. They are usually motile by means of polar flagella, which may occur at 1 or both ends of the cells, and they are gram negative. Several aerobic species have been described and cultured; *S. minor* (*minus*) and *S. volutans* have not been cultivated on artificial media.

A group of curved or helical anaerobic bacteria can be found on the mucous membranes of humans (*S. sputigenum* and others).

Criteria for identification of the cultivable forms are as follows: spirals, 5-10 μm in length, bearing 2-7 coils; motile; litmus milk unchanged; nitrate, V-P, and indole negative; no growth on MacConkey agar; catalase, oxidase and methyl red positive; incapable of fermenting carbohydrates.

For further details consult Williams and Rittenberg.[484]

Spirillum minor (minus)

Spirillum minor (*minus*) causes rat-bite fever. It is motile, showing an extremely rapid darting motion with spinning around the long axis (bipolar tufts of flagella). In blood films, Giemsa and Wright stains are useful for demonstration of the organism. Dark-field examination of a drop of blood from an infected animal is used to demonstrate motility and flagella. The organism is 4-7 μm long and spiral, with 2-5 regular waves, and the body is rigid (the long axis is quite straight).

In rat-bite fever it is important to determine whether *S. minor* (*minus*) or *Streptobacillus moniliformis* is the causative agent. The latter can be grown on enriched media.

Rat-bite fever (sodoku) can be caused, in addition, by mouse, ferret, cat, weasel, and Indian squirrel bites. The bites usually heal rapidly. After 5-15 days the site of the wound swells and becomes purplish. An indurated ulcer usually forms, with a relapsing type fever following. This may go on for months, accompanied by a skin rash.

Miscellaneous Spirillum infections

Species of *Spirillum* other than *S. minor* (*minus*) have been considered nonpathogenic for humans. They have been isolated from stagnant water and putrefying materials. Septicemia[485] and meningitis[486] due to cultivable, aerobic *Spirillum* species were reported. The organism isolated from septicemia grew well on blood and chocolate agar; it did not grow on Endo, phenylethyl alcohol, or milk agar. That isolated from meningitis, classified as *S. serpens,* grew on blood agar and in trypticase soy broth but not on MacConkey agar. Additional cases mentioned by Kowal[485] make it likely that under certain circumstances supposedly nonpathogenic spirilla may be implicated in disease.

BARTONELLACEAE
Bartonella bacilliformis

The family *Bartonellaceae*[487-489] includes *Bartonella bacilliformis,** a small coccobacillus found in or on the blood cells or sometimes in the blood. It also grows in the cytoplasm of tissue cells. The organism shows pleomorphic, coccuslike, ring, oval, rod-shaped (straight or more or less curved), and granular forms. In red blood cells they form a short chain of cocci or a chain of rods, or they may resemble Chinese letters or a circumflex accent. In endothelial cells lining blood and lymph channels of viscera from fatal **Oroya fever** (infectious anemia), they are sometimes discrete and rod shaped but commonly granular or amorphous round masses, distending the cells. In cutaneous nodules (**verruca peruana**) they appear within endothelial cells as rod-shaped organisms or in clusters. They are very slowly motile in fresh preparations of blood in Oroya fever and motile in young cultures. One to 10 unipolar flagella can be demonstrated in culture. *B. bacilliformis* is gram negative; it stains better with Giemsa or Wright stain.

Cultivation can be accomplished in leptospira medium (semisolid nutrient agar containing 10%

fresh rabbit serum and 0.5% hemoglobin; growth appears in about 10 days) or in the yolk sac and chorioallantoic fluid of the chick embryo. Optimum temperature for culture is 28 C.

The organism is the causative agent of Carrión's disease (Oroya fever, verruca peruana).

Distribution. Human bartonellosis occurs only in certain regions of western South America, from approximately 2° north to 13° south latitude. The disease is observed in 2 regions in Peru: one, the Pacific watershed; the other, the Marañon watershed. It is seen near the Peruvian border in Ecuador and in the southwestern part of Colombia.

Transmission. Transmission is by the sandfly *Phlebotomus.* The mechanism of transmission is through feeding.

The only known reservoir in human bartonellosis are humans. Humans and the insect vector are the only living beings known to be naturally infected. The incidence of asymptomatic human carriers in infected areas is 10% or higher.

Diagnosis. The organism must be demonstrated in the peripheral blood. This can be accomplished by examining films, both thin and thick, after staining with Wright or Giemsa stain. When the organisms are not demonstrable in the films, blood cultures must be made. Early in the disease the blood cultures will be positive before the organisms can be found in the blood films.

When the disease is well established, there are irregular fever, rapid and severe anemia, high erythrocytic sedimentation rate, pains in the joints, and enlargement of the lymph nodes, and coupled with history of the environment in which the patient has recently lived, all serve to make the diagnosis.

During the eruptive stage, diagnosis is established by the characteristic appearance of the verrucas, and confirmed by demonstration of the bartonellae in the lesions. Sections should be fixed in Regaud fixative and stained with Giemsa stain.

The verruca may resemble an angioma, an angiofibroma, or a botryomycoma, but these tumors are always single and congenital. The subcutaneous nodules, when they have not eroded the skin, may resemble fatty tumors, fibromas, and similar pathologic conditions. However, the coexistence with typical military verrucas, the localization near the joints, and the course of the disease furnish the diagnosis. In doubtful cases bacteriologic and histologic studies of the lesions should be made. In this period blood cultures are often positive.

The disease is not transmissible to the usual laboratory animals. Even monkeys are difficult to infect.

For further details refer to Weinman.[487,488,490]

CALYMMATOBACTERIUM

C. granulomatis, the causative agent of donovanosis (granuloma inguinale), is discussed in detail in Chapter 75 ("Female genital tract").

---

*The organism is classified in the order Rickettsiales in *Bergey's Manual,* ed. 8.[3]

DF-2 ORGANISM

DF-2 is the designation given by the Center for Disease Control to an unidentified gram-negative rod that has rarely been reported as a human pathogen.[491-493]

The organism has been isolated from the blood of patients with underlying diseases resulting in impaired host defenses. The clinical syndromes involved were cellulitis, septicemia, meningitis, and endocarditis.

In a number of cases (10 of 17 patients[492]) the illness involving DF-2 was preceded by dog bites.

The organism grows slowly on blood or chocolate agar in 10% CO_2, but not on MacConkey agar, is **oxidase** and **catalase-positive**, and is negative for nitrate reduction, indole production, and urease. It produces acid from glucose, lactose, and maltose (not in OF but in broth base with 1% peptone and 3% beef extract).* These features distinguish it from all previously described and classified bacteria.

In TSI (triple sugar iron) agar butt there is either no growth or very poor growth.

The organisms are relatively resistant to aminoglycosides (gentamicin, kanamycin) but are sensitive to the penicillins, erythromycin, and clindamycin.

LEGIONELLA PNEUMOPHILA[494-497] (LEGIONNAIRES' DISEASE BACILLUS, LDB)

An epidemic of pneumonia, involving 183 cases with 29 deaths, occurred among the approximately 5000 persons who attended the American Legion's 1976 summer convention in Philadelphia. The epidemic affected almost wholly those legionnaires who passed through the lobby of, or were accommodated at the Bellevue Stratford Hotel, hence the name of the disease.

Eventually it was found that at least 10 similar outbreaks occurred since 1965 in the United States,[498] and the disease has since been reported in England, Italy, Spain, Canada, Holland, Sweden, Israel, and Australia.

After extensive efforts at the Center for Disease Control, by January 1977 aerobic, gram-negative bacilli had been isolated from lung tissue of several patients by passage through guinea pigs. Suspensions of guinea-pig spleens from animals that became ill were subcultured into chick embryos, which died after 4-6 days. Rods were seen in the yolk sacs, and they finally were grown on enriched Mueller-Hinton agar with 1% hemoglobin and IsoVitaleX[499] (see Media, Chapter 72).

In December 1976 the same organism was successfully isolated directly in vitro from the pleural fluid of a 39-year-old woman in Flint, Michigan, by culturing on commercial enriched chocolate agar (Dumoff).[500]

On the basis of extensive studies involving homology and DNA hybridization, Brenner,

Steigerwalt, and McDade[501] concluded that the organism seems to be a previously unrecognized species that has no known genetic relationship to other bacteria, and proposed the name *Legionella pneumophila*.

Legionnaires' disease (LD) most dramatically presents as a severe pneumonia, but also occurs without pneumonia, i.e., a mild illness characterized by acute self-limited febrile myalgia ("Pontiac fever"[502]), as well as covert subclinical infection. LD is a multisystem disease that, in addition to involving the lungs, often involves the central nervous system, the gastrointestinal tract, and the liver.[496,503,504]

The organism[494]

The etiologic agent of Legionnaires' disease is a fastidious, unusual gram-negative rod that grows only on **specialized media** not generally used when attempting to isolate an unknown bacterial agent. It also requires 3-12 days or more for growth or initial isolation.

The organism does **not** grow on blood agar, infusion agar, or other media without added cysteine. The bacteriologic medium on which the organism was first grown was Mueller-Hinton agar supplemented with 1% hemoglobin and 1% IsoVitaleX. Presently, the charcoal yeast extract agar (CYE) and the Feeley-Gorman (FG) agar are recommended for initial isolation; Mueller-Hinton agar with 1% hemoglobin powder and 2% IsoVitaleX may also be used[494] (see discussion below, laboratory procedures; see also Chapter 72, "Media," and Chapter 75, "Respiratory tract").

L. pneumophila is **not** demonstrable by tissue Gram stain and requires a specialized tissue silver stain (see Dieterle stain, Chapter 71).

Morphology. The bacterium is 0.5-0.7 μm in diameter and 2-3 μm in length. The long forms often are curved; in early passages on agar, the cells are frequently vacuolated. Some of the vacuolated cells are slightly swollen in the region of the vacuoles. The vacuoles can be stained with Sudan black B according to the fat stain procedure.

Fat stain. Fat droplets stain blue-black or blue-gray; the remainder of a cell stains pink.

REAGENTS

1. Sudan black B solution: Add 0.3 Sudan black B to 100 ml 70% ETOH. Agitate to dissolve most of stain and allow to stand overnight.
2. Xylene.
3. Safranin, as used for Gram stain.

PROCEDURE

1. Prepare and heat fix smears.
2. Flood smear with Sudan black B solution and allow to stand 5-15 min.
3. Drain slide and blot dry.
4. Apply xylene to smear several times (either drop by drop or by immersing slide in staining jar containing xylene).
5. Blot smear dry; counterstain with safranin for 30 s. For organisms that stain readily with safranin, di-

---

*Utilization took place in tubes sealed with petrolatum, i.e., the organism behaved as a fermenter.

lute safranin in water and apply for only 5 s. Wash; air dry or blot dry. Examine under oil immersion.

Incubation and temperature. The LDB grows in ambient air but grows better in a candle jar and in 2.5% CO_2. It does **not** grow anaerobically. At 3 days, growth is apparent at 35 C but not at 25 C or 42 C. Cultures will grow at 30 C but not as well as at 35 C.

Length of incubation. On initial isolation, it may take 10 or more days for the organism to grow; on subsequent subcultures marked growth occurs in 3-5 days.

Colonies. Two kinds of colonies are produced: a "dwarf" colony and another, much larger, up to 3 mm in diameter.[496] The colonies of the various strains that have not been transferred more than a few times on the agar are pinpoint in size at 3 days. By 5-7 days, well-isolated colonies may reach a diameter of 3 or 4 mm. The colonies are convex, circular, and have an entire edge. They are gray and glistening. In confluent areas the growth appears to be slightly moist.

Pigment. On **FG** agar (see Media, Chapter 72) there is a distinctive brownish darkening of the colonies and the surrounding agar. Under long-wave (366 nm) ultraviolet light a butter-yellow color is detectable in the 4- to 5-day-old growth.

On CYE agar there is no browning of agar observable. On Mueller-Hinton enriched medium the brown soluble pigment **does** appear.

Carbohydrates. No acid production from carbohydrates has been demonstrated. However, it should be pointed out that the organism does not grow in the commonly used carbohydrate media. Weaver detected no acid from glucose, et al.[505] xylose, mannitol, lactose, sucrose, maltose, or fructose after applying the "rapid sugar" technic (see *Neisseria*, Chapter 76).

Urea. There is no reaction when Christensen's urea slants are inoculated heavily.

Gelatin. The emulsion on photographic film (Kodak, Plus-X) is digested in 48-72 hours when placed in a heavy suspension of the organisms in Mueller-Hinton or heart infusion broth. When the API (Analytab Products, Inc.) gelatin cupule is inoculated with a very turbid saline suspension, a positive reaction occurs in 48-72 hours.

Nitrate. The organism is nitrate negative. Potassium nitrate (0.2%) is incorporated into agar slants in which Fildes' enrichment is substituted for hemoglobin. (Reduction of nitrate by *Pseudomonas aeruginosa* and *Yersinia enterocolitica* can be readily demonstrated with this medium.) The slants are inoculated heavily and are incubated for 7 days.

Oxidase. The LDB is weakly positive by Kovacs' procedure (color change within 10 seconds) with tetramethyl *p*-phenylenediamine dihydrochloride.

Catalase. The organism is catalase positive (72-hour slant cultures). Reaction is very weak

unless growth is "broken up" slightly with a capillary pipet. The "sticky" consistency of the growth apparently reduces contact between the peroxide and the cells.

β-lactamase. The isolates examined produce a β-lactamase on the medium described for detecting penicillinase-producing *Neisseria gonorrhoeae*.[506] The medium does not readily support the growth of LDB and must be inoculated heavily. Both penicillin (2.5 U/ml) and *Sarcina lutea* are incorporated in the medium. The β-lactamase inactivates the penicillin and allows the *S. lutea* to grow.

Starch utilization. LDB is positive for starch utilization on an agar medium that contains starch and is supplemented with iron or Fildes' enrichment rather than hemoglobin. An area of a plate should be heavily inoculated and incubated for 72 hours. The plate should then be flooded with Gram's iodine and observed for a clear zone extending about 4 mm beyond the edge of the bacterial growth.

Branched-chain fatty acid composition. The high content of branched-chain fatty acids in this organism is a striking feature and gives it a unique fatty acid profile, as determined by gas-liquid chomatography (GLC).[505]

Serologic groups of L. pneumophila[507]

Four distinct serologic groups of *L. pneumophila* are recognized at the time of writing:

Serologic group	Antigen (isolate)
1	Knoxville, 1
2	Togus, 1
3	Bloomington, 2
4	LA, 1

Conjugated antisera against serogroup 1 stain some 85% of human strains in the CDC collection.[507]

Laboratory procedures

Indirect fluorescent antibody (IFA) test: See Chapter 107.

Direct fluorescent antibody examination (DFA): See Chapter 70. Specimens to be examined by DFA are fresh or formalin fixed lung tissue obtained at biopsy or autopsy, as well as lower respiratory tract specimens such as transtracheal aspirate, bronchial washing, pleural fluids, sputum, etc. This procedure is most likely to yield the most rapid presumptive diagnosis.

Dieterle silver staining procedure: See Chapter 71. Since this stain is not specific for *L. pneumophila*, it should be confirmed by DFA procedure.

Culture

Media. See Chapter 72, "Media" (*Legionella*, **CYE, FG,** and **chocolate agar** descriptions).

Initial processing, inoculating, incubation, culture examination, and preliminary identification. See Chapter 75, "Respiratory tract"; also "The organism," above.

NOTE: For a recently described procedure allowing cultivation of *L. pneumophila* from blood, see Edelstein et al.[508]

REFERENCES

1. King, E. O.: The identification of unusual pathogenic gram-negative bacteria, Atlanta, 1964, Communicable Disease Center.
2. Weaver, R. E., Tatum, H. W., and Hollis, D. G.: The identification of unusual pathogenic gram-negative bacteria, Atlanta, 1978 (rev.), Center for Disease Control.
2a. Weaver, R. E.: Gram-negative organisms—an approach to identification (guide to presumptive identification), Atlanta, 1979, Center for Disease Control.
3. Buchanan, R. E., and Gibbons, W. E.: Bergey's manual of determinative biology, ed. 8, Baltimore, 1974, The Williams & Wilkins Co.
4. Sonnenwirth, A. In Davis, B., Dulbecco, R., Eisen, H. N., et al., editors: Microbiology, ed. 2, Hagerstown, Md., 1973, Harper & Row, Publishers.
5. Gale, D., and Sonnenwirth, A. C.: Arch. Intern. Med. **109**:414, 1962.
6. Washington, J. A., II: Human Pathol. **7**:151, 1976.
7. Weaver, R. E.: Gram-negative organisms: an approach to identification (Guide to presumptive identifications), Atlanta, 1975 (rev. Nov. 1975), Center for Disease Control.
8. Watanabe, T.: N. Engl. J. Med. **275**:888, 1966.
9. Lebek, G.: Pathol. Microbiol. **30**:1015, 1967.
10. Blattner, R. J.: J. Pediatr. **73**:139, 1968.
11. Anderson, E. S.: Annu. Rev. Microbiol. **22**:131, 1968.
12. Kauffmann, F.: The bacteriology of Enterobacteriaceae, Baltimore, 1966, The Williams & Wilkins Co.
13. Ewing, W. H., and Edwards, P. R.: Int. Bull. Bacteriol. Nomen. Taxon. **10**:1, 1960.
14. Ewing, W. H., and Edwards, P. R.: The principal divisions and groups of Enterobacteriaceae, Atlanta, 1962 (rev.), Communicable Disease Center.
15. Ewing, W. H.: Int. Bull. Bacteriol. Nomen. Taxon. **13**:95, 1963.
16. Subcommittee on Enterobacteriaceae, American Society for Microbiology: ASM News **30**:22, 1964.
17. Subcommittee on Enterobacteriaceae, American Society for Microbiology: ASM News **34**:30, 1968.
18. Ewing, W. H.: Revised definitions for the family *Enterobacteriaceae*, its tribes and genera, Atlanta, 1967, National Communicable Disease Center.
19. Ewing, W. H.: Differentiation of *Enterobacteriaceae*, by biochemical reactions—revised, DHEW publ. no. CDC-74-8270, Atlanta, Aug. 1973, Center for Disease Control.
20. Edwards, P. R., and Ewing, W. H.: Identification of *Enterobacteriaceae*, ed. 3, Minneapolis, 1973, Burgess Publishing Co.
21. Breed, R. S., Murray, E. G. D., and Smith, N. R., editors: Bergey's manual of determinative bacteriology, ed. 7, Baltimore, 1957, The Williams & Wilkins Co.
22. Edwards, P. R., and Ewing, W. H.: Identification of *Enterobacteriaceae*, ed. 2, Minneapolis, 1962, Burgess Publishing Co.
23. International Enterobacteriaceae Subcommittee: Int. Bull. Bacteriol. Nomen. Taxon. **8**:173, 1958.
24. Fields, B. N., Uwaydah, M. M., Kunz, I. J., and Swartz, M. N.: Am. J. Med. **42**:89, 1967.
25. Ewing, W. H., McWhorter, A. C., Ball, M. M., and Bartes, S. F.: The biochemical reactions of *Edwardsiella tarda*, a new genus of *Enterobacteriaceae*, Atlanta, 1967, Communicable Disease Center.
26. Brenner, D. J., Farmer, J. J., III, Hickman, F. W., et al.: Taxonomic and nomenclature changes in *Enterobacteriaceae*, DHEW publ. no. CDC-78-8356, Atlanta, Oct. 1977, Center for Disease Control.
27. Yu, V. L.: N. Engl. J. Med. **300**:887, 1979.
28. Sonnenwirth, A. C.: *Yersinia*. In Lennette, E. H., Spaulding, E. H., and Truant, J. P., editors: Manual of clinical microbiology, ed. 2, Washington, D.C., 1974, American Society of Microbiology.
29. Sonnenwirth, A. C.: Mt. Sinai J. Med. **43**:736, 1976.
30. Sonnenwirth, A. C., and Weaver, R. E.: N. Engl. J. Med. **283**:1468, 1970.
31. Sonnenwirth, A. C.: Ann. N.Y. Acad. Sci. **174** (Art. 2): 488, 1970.
32. Bottone, E. J.: CRC Crit. Rev. Microbiol. **5**(2): 211, 1977.
33. Hajna, A.: J. Bacteriol. **49**:516, 1945.
34. Ewing, W. H., and Johnson, J. G.: Int. Bull. Bacteriol. Nomen. Taxon. **10**:223, 1960.
35. Ewing, W. H.: Differential reactions of *Enterobacteriaceae*, Atlanta, 1966, National Communicable Disease Center.
36. Ewing, W. H.: *Enterobacteriaceae*—biochemical methods for group differentiation, PHS publ. no. 734, Atlanta, 1960, Communicable Disease Center.
37. Edwards, P. R., and Ewing, W. H.: Identification of *Enterobacteriaceae*, ed. 3, Minneapolis, 1973, Burgess Publishing Co.
38. Ewing, W. H., and Davis, B. R.: Media and tests for differentiation of *Enterobacteriaceae*, Atlanta, 1970, Center for Disease Control.
39. Ewing, W. H., Davis, R. B., and Edwards, P. R.: Public Health Lab. **18**:77, 1960.
40. Edwards, P. R., and Fife, M. A.: Appl. Microbiol. **4**:46, 1956.
41. Edwards, P. R., Fife, M. A., and Ewing, W. H.: Am. J. Med. Technol. **22**:28, 1956.
42. Pruneda, R. C., and Farmer, J. J., III: J. Clin. Microbiol. **5**:66, 1977.
43. Christie, A. B.: Br. Med. J. **2**:285, 1968.
44. Keusch, G. T., Jacewicz, M., Levine, M. M., et al.: J. Clin. Invest. **57**:194, 1976.
45. Ewing, W. H.: J. Bacteriol. **57**:633, 1949.
46. Ewing, W. H.: Isolation and identification of *Salmonella-Shigella*, DHEW publ. no. CDC-75-8098, Atlanta, 1974, Center for Disease Control.
47. Bray, J.: J. Pathol. Bacteriol. **57**:239-247, 1945.
48. Ewing, W. H., Tatum, H. W., and Davis, B. R.: Public Health Lab. **15**:118-138, 1957.
49. DuPont, H. L.: Clin. Microbiol. News **1**(11), 1979.
50. Gangarosa, E. J., and Merson, M. H.: N. Engl. J. Med. **296**:1210, 1977.
51. Dorner, F.: *Escherichia coli* enterotoxin: purification and partial characterization. In Schlessinger, D., editor: Microbiology—1975, Washington D.C., 1975, American Society for Microbiology, p. 242.

52. Finkelstein, R. A., Larue, M. K., Johnston, D. W., et al.: J. Infect. Dis. **133**:S120, 1976.
53. Neter, E.: J. Pediatr. **89**:166, 1976.
54. Sack, R. B.: Annu. Rev. Microbiol. **29**:333, 1975.
55. Gorbach, S. L., Kean, B. H., Evans, D. G., et al.: N. Engl. J. Med. **292**:933, 1975.
56. Rudoy, R. C., and Nelson, J. D.: Am. J. Dis. Child. **129**:668, 1975.
56a. Pickering, L. K.: Am. J. Med. Technol. **45**:787, 1979.
57. Sack, D. A., and Sack, R. B.: Infect. Immun. **11**: 334-336, 1975.
58. Scherer, W. F., Syverton, J. T., and Gey, G. O.: J. Exp. Med. **97**:695-710, 1953.
59. Dean, A. G., Ching, Y., Williams, R. G., and Harden, L. B.: J. Infect. Dis. **125**:407-411, 1972.
60. Gianella, R. A.: Infect. Immun. **14**:95-99, 1976.
61. Mehlman, I. J., Eide, E. L., Sanders, A. C., et al.: J. Assoc. Off. Anal. Chem. **60**:546-562, 1977.
62. Sereny, B.: Acta Microbiol. Acad. Sci. Hung. **2**: 293-296, 1955.
63. Ewing, W. H.: Ann. N.Y. Acad. Sci. **66**:61, 1956.
64. Beerens, H., and Castel, M. M.: Ann. Inst. Pasteur Lille **99**:454, 1960.
65. Farmer, J. J., III, Davis, B. R., Cherry, W. B., et al.: J. Pediatr. **90**:1047, 1977.
66. Echeverria, P. D., Chang, C. P., and Smith, D.: J. Pediatr. **89**:8, 1976.
67. Ewing, W. H., McWhorter, A. C., Escobar, M. R., and Lubin, A. H.: Int. Bull. Bacteriol. Nomen. Taxon. **15**:33, 1965.
68. Sakazaki, R., and Murata, Y.: Jpn. J. Bacteriol. **17**:616, 1962.
69. King, B. M., and Adler, D. L.: Am. J. Clin. Pathol. **41**:230, 1964.
70. Ewing, W. H., McWhorter, A. C., Ball, M. M., and Bartes, S. F.: Public Health Lab. **27**:129, 1969.
71. Sakazaki, R.: Jpn. J. Med. Sci. Biol. **20**:205, 1967.
72. Wallace, L. J., White, F. H., and Gore, H. L.: J. Am. Vet. Med. Assoc. **149**:881, 1966.
73. Sonnenwirth, A. C., and Kallus, B.: Am. J. Clin. Pathol. **49**:92, 1968.
74. Sonnenwirth, A. C., and Kallus, B.: Bacteriol. Proc., p. 98, 1967, abst. M221.
75. Okubadejo, O. A., and Alausa, K. O.: Br. Med. J. **3**:357, 1968.
76. Jordan, G. W., and Hadley, W. K.: Ann. Intern. Med. **70**:283, 1969.
77. Sakazaki, R.: Jpn. J. Med. Sci. Biol. **20**:205, 1967.
78. Ewing, W. H.: Differentiation of *Enterobacteriaceae* by biochemical reactions, Atlanta, 1968, National Communicable Disease Center.
79. Martin, W. J., Ewing, W. H., McWhorter, A. C., and Ball, M. M.: Public Health Lab. **27**:61, 1969.
80. Committee on Salmonella, National Research Council: An evaluation of the *Salmonella* problem, publ. no. 1683, Washington, D.C., 1969, National Academy of Sciences—National Research Council.
81. Kauffmann, F.: Int. Bull. Bacteriol. Nomen. Taxon. **13**:187, 1963.
82. Enterobacteriaceae Subcommittee: Int. Bull. Bacteriol. Nomen. Taxon. **13**:69, 1963.
83. Ewing, W. H., and Ball, M. M.: The biochemical reactions of members of the genus *Salmonella*, Atlanta, 1966, National Communicable Disease Center.
84. Bauer, H.: Medicine **52**:323, 1973.
85. Edwards, P. R.: Ann. N.Y. Acad. Sci. **70**:598, 1958.
86. Bowmen, E. J.: Am. J. Med. Sci. **247**:467, 1964.
87. Black, P. H., Kunz, L. J., and Swartz, M. N.: N. Engl. J. Med. **262**:811, 864, 921, 1960.
88. Ortiz-Neu, C., Marr, J. S., Cherubin, C. E., and Neu, H. C.: J. Infect. Dis. **138**:820, 1978.
89. Williams, R. E. O., Blowers, R., Garrod, L. P., and Shooter, R. A.: Hospital infection, London, 1960, Lloyd-Luke.
90. Deutch, M., and Sonnenwirth, A. C.: Clin. Pediatr. **4**:511, 1965.
91. White, P. B.: Medical Research Council, Great Britain, Special Report Series no. 91, 1925.
92. Kauffman, F.: Zbl. Bakt. (Abst. 1) Ref. **95**:519, 1930; **119**:152, 1930; Z. Hyg. **11**:233, 1960.
93. Edwards, P. R., and Ewing, W. H.: Identification of *Enterobacteriaceae*, Minneapolis, 1955, Burgess Publishing Co.
94. Lüderitz, O., Staub, A. M., and Westphal, O.: Bacteriol. Rev. **30**:192, 1966.
95. Porschen, R. K., Hale, D., and Goodman, Z.: Am. J. Clin. Pathol. **68**:416, 1977.
96. Falcao, D. F., Trabulsi, L. R., Hickman, F. R., and Farmer, J. J., III: J. Clin. Microbiol. **2**:349, 1975.
97. Ewing, W. H.: Preliminary serologic examination of *Salmonella* and *Shigella* cultures, Atlanta, 1966, National Communicable Disease Center.
98. Hickman, F. W., and Farmer, J. J.: Am. J. Med. Technol. **44**:1149, 1978.
99. Gershan, M.: J. Clin. Microbiol. **5**:302, 1977.
100. Kauffmann, F.: Acta Pathol. Microbiol. Scand. **18**:351, 1941.
101. Ewing, W. H.: Int. J. Syst. Bacteriol. **19**:1, 1969.
102. Ewing, W. H., and Fife, M. A.: Int. J. Syst. Bacteriol. **16**:427, 1966.
103. Edwards, P. R., Fife, M. A., and Ewing, W. H.: Antigenic schema for the genus *Arizona*, Atlanta, 1965, National Communicable Disease Center (suppl. 1967).
104. Martin, W. J., Fife, M. A., and Ewing, W. H.: The occurrence and distribution of the serotypes of *Arizona*, Atlanta, 1967, National Communicable Disease Center.
105. Davis, B. R., and Ewing, W. H.: The biochemical reactions of *Citrobacter freundii*, Atlanta, 1966, National Communicable Disease Center.
106. Young, V. M., Kenton, D. M., Hobbs, B. J., and Moody, M. R.: Int. J. Syst. Bacteriol. **21**:58-63, 1971.
107. Ewing, W. H., and Davis, B. R.: Biochemical characterization of *Citrobacter freundii* and *Citrobacter diversus*, Atlanta, 1971, Center for Disease Control.
108. Crosa, J. H., Steigerwalt, A. G., Fanning, G. R., and Brenner, D. J.: J. Gen. Microbiol. **83**:271-282, 1974.
109. Fife, M. A., Ewing, W. H., and Davis, B. R.: The biochemical reactions of the tribe *Klebsielleae*, Atlanta, 1965, Communicable Disease Center.
110. Weil, A. J., Benjamin, M. A., and de Guzman, B. C.: Trans. N.Y. Acad. Sci. Ser. II, **27**:65, 1964.
111. Edmondson, E. B., and Sanford, J. P.: Medicine **46**:323, 1967.
112. Eickhoff, T. C., Steinhauer, B. W., and Finland, M.: Ann. Intern. Med. **65**:1163, 1966.
112a. Center for Disease Control: Biochemical reactions given by Enterobacteriaceae in commonly used tests, Atlanta, Sept. 1973 (rev.), The Center.
113. Brenner, D. J., Steigerwalt, A. G., and Fanning, G. R.: Int. J. Syst. Bacteriol. **22**:128-130, 1972.
114. Jain, K., Radsak, K., and Mannheim, W.: Int. J. Syst. Bacteriol. **24**:402-407, 1974.
115. Starr, M. P., Chatterjee, A. K., Starr, P. B., and Buchanan, G. E.: J. Clin. Microbiol. **6**:379, 1977.

116. von Riesen, V. L.: Int. J. Syst. Bacteriol. **26:**143-145, 1976.

117. Edmondson, E. B., and Sanford, J. P.: Medicine **46:**323-340, 1967.

118. Toala, P., Lee, Y. H., Wilcox, C., and Finland, M.: Am. J. Med. Sci. **260:**41-55, 1970.

119. Dans, P. E., Barrett, F. F., Casey, J. I., and Finland, M.: Arch. Intern. Med. **125:**94-101, 1970.

120. Barrett, F. F., Casey, J. I., and Finland, M.: N. Engl. J. Med. **278:**5-9, 1968.

121. Oberhofer, T. R., and Hajkowski, R.: Am. J. Clin. Pathol. **54:**720-725, 1970.

122. Oberhofer, T. R., and Hajkowski, R.: Am. J. Clin. Pathol. **54:**726-732, 1970.

123. Tillotson, J. R., and Finland, M.: J. Infect. Dis. **119:**597-624, 1969.

124. Washington, J. A., II, Birk, R. J., and Ritts, R. E.: J. Infect. Dis. **124:**379, 1971.

125. Steigerwalt, A. G., Fanning, G. R., Fife-Asbury, M. A., and Brenner, D. J.: Can. J. Microbiol. **22:**121-137, 1976.

126. Ewing, W. H., and Fife, M. A.: *Enterobacter agglomerans:* the Herbicola-Lathyri bacteria, Atlanta, 1971, Center for Disease Control.

127. Nissen, R., Nørholm, T., and Siboni, K. E.: Danish Med. Bull. **12:**128-130, 1965.

128. Richard, C., Joly, B., Sirot, J., et al.: Ann. Microbiol. (Inst. Pasteur) **127A:**545-548, 1976.

129. Cooper-Smith, M. E., and von Graevenitz, A.: Curr. Microbiol. **1:**29, 1978.

130. Maki, D. G., Rhame, F. S., Mackel, D. C., and Bennett, J. V.: Am. J. Med. **60:**471-485, 1976.

131. Prats, G., Llobet, J. M., Pericas, R., et al.: Rev. Clin. Española **141:**285-287, 1976.

132. Schneierson, S. S., and Bottone, E. J.: Crit. Rev. Clin. Lab. Sci. **4:**341-355, 1973.

133. Starr, M. P., and Chatterjee, A. K.: Annu. Rev. Microbiol. **26:**389-426, 1972.

134. von Graevenitz, A.: J.A.M.A. **216:**1485, 1971.

135. von Graevenitz, A.: Gram-negative rods as agents of nosocomial disease: some recent developments, with comments on mixed cultures. In Urbaschek, B., Urbaschek, R., and Neter, E., editors: Gram-negative bacterial infections and mode of endotoxin actions, New York, 1975, Springer-Verlag.

136. McHenry, H. C., Gavan, T. L., Hawk, W. A., et al.: Cleve. Clin. Q. **42:**15-32, 1975.

137. Ball, A. P., McGhie, D., and Geddes, A. M.: Q. J. Med. **46:**63, 1977.

138. Tabaqchali, S., Chambers, T. J., and Brooks, H. J. L.: Lancet **1:**306, 1977.

139. Farmer, J. J., III, Davis, B. R., Hickman, F. W., et al.: Lancet **2:**455, 1976.

140. Grimont, P. A. D., and Grimont, F.: Annu. Rev. Microbiol. **32:**221, 1978.

141. Biochemical characterization of *Serratia liquefaciens* and *Serratia rubidaceae,* DHEW publ. no. (HSM)-73-8209, Atlanta, 1972, Center for Disease Control.

142. Ewing, W. H., Davis, R. B., and Reavis, R. W.: Studies on the Serratia group, Atlanta, 1959, Communicable Disease Center.

143. Wilfert, J. N., Barrett, F. F., Ewing, W. H., et al.: Appl. Microbiol. **19:**345, 1970.

144. Sproat, D., and Brown, A.: Am. J. Clin. Pathol. **71:**172, 1979.

145. Grimont, P. A. D., and Grimont, F.: J. Clin. Microbiol. **8:**73, 1978.

146. Starr, M. P., Grimont, P. A. D., Grimont, F., and Starr, P.: J. Clin. Microbiol. **4:**270, 1976.

147. Sonnenwirth, A. C., and Hermann, G. J.: Abstracts of Annual Meeting of the American Society for Microbiology, 1973, abst. no. M190, p. 105.

148. Arroyo, J. C., Sonnenwirth, A. C., and Liebhaber, H.: J. Urol. **117:**115, 1977.

149. Kauffmann, F.: *Enterobacteriaceae,* Copenhagen, 1951, Einar Munksgaarde, Forlag.

150. Overtuft, G. D., Wilkins, J., and Ressler, R.: J. Infect. Dis. **129:**353, 1974.

151. Penner, J. L., Hinton, N. A., and Hennessy, J. N.: J. Clin. Microbiol. **1:**136-142, 1975.

152. Penner, J. L., and Hennessy, J. N.: Int. J. Syst. Bacteriol. **27:**71-74, 1977.

153. Brenner, D. J., Farmer, J. J., III, Fanning, G. R., et al.: Int. J. Syst. Bacteriol. **28:**269, 1978.

154. Penner, J. L., Hinton, N.A., Whiteley, G. R., and Hennessy, J. N.: J. Infect. Dis. **134:**370-376, 1976.

155. Van Loghem, J. J.: Antonie van Leeuwenhoek J. Microbiol. Serol. **10:**15, 1944.

156. Talbot, J. M., and Sneath, P. H. A.: J. Gen. Microbiol. **22:**303, 1960.

157. Smith, J. E., and Thal, E.: Acta Pathol. Microbiol. Scand. **64:**213, 1965.

158. Darland, G., Ewing, W. H., and Davis, B. R.: The biochemical characteristics of *Yersinia enterocolitica* and *Yersinia pseudotuberculosis,* DHEW publ. no. (CDC) -75-8294, Atlanta, 1974, Center for Disease Control.

159. Diaz, R.: Antigenic relationship of *Yersinia enterocolitica* type 9 with other gram-negative species. In Winblad, S., editor: *Yersinia, Pasteurella* and *Francisella,* Proc. Intern. Symp. 1972, vol. 2, Contributions to microbiology and immunology, Basel, Switzerland, 1973, S. Karger, p. 157.

160. Domaradskij, I., Marchenkov, V., and Shimanjuk, N.: New data obtained in comparative studies of plague agent and related organisms. In Winblad, S., editor: *Yersinia, Pasteurella, and Francisella,* Proc. Intern. Symp. 1972, vol. 2, Contributions to microbiology and immunology, Basel, Switzerland, 1973, S. Karger, p. 2.

161. Ritter, D. B., and Gerloff, R. K.: J. Bacteriol. **92:** 1838, 1966.

162. Wetzler, T. F.: Pseudotuberculosis. In Bodily, H. L., Updyke, E. L., and Mason, J. O., editors: Diagnostic procedures for bacterial, mycotic, and parasitic infections, ed. 5, New York, 1970, American Public Health Association, p. 449.

163. Hall, C. T.: Bacteriology. I. Summary analysis, Atlanta, Jan. 1973, Center for Disease Control.

164. Bahmanyar, M., and Cavanaugh, D. C.: Plague manual, Geneva, 1976, World Health Organization.

165. Reed, W. P., Palmer, D. L., Williams, R. C., Jr., and Kisch, A. L.: Medicine **49:**465-486, 1970.

166. Knisley, R. F., Swaney, L. M., and Friedlander, H.: J. Bacteriol. **88:**491, 1964.

167. Goldenberg, M. I.: Health Lab. Sci. **5:**38, 1968.

168. Chen, T. H., and Meyer, K. F.: Bull. WHO **34:**911, 1966.

169. Butler, T., Mahmond, A. A. F., and Warren, K. S.: J. Infect. Dis. **136:**317, 1977.

170. Butler, T., and Hudson, B. W.: Bull. WHO **55:**39, 1977.

171. Palmer, D. L., Kisch, A. L., Williams, R. C., Jr., and Reed, W. P.: J. Infect. Dis. **124:**367, 1971.

172. Gutman, I. T., Otteson, E. A., Quan, T. J., et al.: N. Engl. J. Med. **228:**1372-1377, 1973.

173. Toivanen, P., Toivanen, A., Olkkonen, L., and Aantaa, S.: Lancet **1:**801-803, 1973.

174. *Yersinia enterocolitica* outbreak—New York, Morbid. Mortal. **26**:53, Feb. 18, 1977.
175. Schleifstein, J., and Coleman, M.: *Bacterium enterocoliticum*, Animal Report Division of Laboratories and Research, New York State Dept. of Health, Albany, N.Y., 1943, 56.
176. Jacobs, J. C.: Pediatrics **55**:236-238, 1975.
177. Keet, F. F.: N.Y. State J. Med. **74**:2226-2230, 1974.
178. Delorme, J., and Lafleur, L.: Can. Med. Assoc. J. **110**:281-284, 1974.
179. Nilehn, B., and Sjøstrøm, B.: Acta Pathol. Microbiol. Scand. Suppl. **187**:77-78, 1967.
180. Mollaret, H. H.: Ann. Biol. Clin. **1**:8, 1972.
181. Bottone, E. J., Chester, B., Malowany, M. S., and Allerhand, J.: Appl. Microbiol. **27**:858-861, 1974.
182. Carter, P. B., Varga, C. F., and Keet, F. F.: Appl. Microbiol. **26**:1016-1018, 1973.
183. Frederiksen, W.: A study of some *Yersinia pseudotuberculosis*-like bacteria (*Bacterium enterocoliticum* and *Pasteurella X*), Proc. XIV Scand. Cong. Pathol. Microbiol., Oslo, 1964, pp. 103-104.
184. Eiss, J.: Scand. J. Infect. Dis. **7**:249, 1975.
185. Greenwood, J. R., Flanigan, S. M., Pickett, M. J., and Martin, W. J.: J. Clin. Microbiol. **2**:559-560, 1975.
186. Weissfeld, A. S., and Sonnenwirth, A. C.: Abstracts of Annual Meeting of the American Society for Microbiology, abstr. C(H) 70, 1979, p. 358.
187. Knapp, W., and Thal, E.; Differentiation of *Yersinia enterocolitica* by biochemical reactions. In Winblad, S., editor: Contributions to microbiology and immunology, vol. 2, Basel, Switzerland, 1973, S. Karger, pp. 10-16.
188. Wauters, G.: Contribution a l'étude de *Yersinia enterocolitica*, Ph.D. thesis, Louvain, Belgium, 1970, Vander.
189. Nilehn, B.: Acta Pathol. Microbiol. Scand. **206**:1-48, 1969.
190. Hawkins, T. M., and Brenner, D. J.: Isolation and identification of *Yersinia enterocolitica*, Atlanta, 1978, Center for Disease Control.
191. Bottone, E. J., Chester, B., Malowany, M., and Allerhand, J.: J. Appl. Microbiol. **27**:858-861, 1974.
192. Alonso, J. M., Bejot, J., Bercovier, H., and Mollaret, H. H.: Med. Maladies Infect. **5**:490-492, 1975.
193. Wauters, G., LeMinor, L., Chalon, A. M., and Lassen, J.: Ann. Inst. Pasteur Lille **122**:951-956, 1972.
194. Morris, G. K., Feeley, J. C., Martin, W. T., and Wells, J. G.: Public Health Lab. **35**:217, 1977.
195. Bissett, M. L.: J. Clin. Microbiol. **4**:137, 1976.
196. Highsmith, A. K., Feeley, J. C., and Morris, G. K.: Health Lab. Sci. **14**:253, 1977.
197. Bercovier, H., Brault, J., Barré, N., et al.: Curr. Microbiol. **1**:353, 1978.
198. Mollaret, H. H.: International symposium on pseudotuberculosis, Symp. Ser. Immunobiol. Stand. **9**:45-58, Basel, 1968, S. Karger.
199. Knapp, W.: N. Engl. J. Med. **259**:776-778, 1958.
200. Sonnenwirth, A. C.: Am. J. Clin. Pathol. **56**:546, 1971.
201. Weber, J., Finlayson, N. B., and Mark, J. B. D.: N. Engl. J. Med. **283**:172-174, 1970.
202. Morris, E. J.: J. Gen. Microbiol. **19**:305-311, 1958.
203. Meyer, K. F.: In Dubos, R., and Hirsch, J. G., editors: Bacterial and mycotic infections of man, ed. 4, Philadelphia, 1965, J. B. Lippincott Co.
204. Thal, E., and Knapp, W.: Progr. Immunobiol. Stand. **15**:219-226, Basel, 1971, S. Karger.

205. Ewing, W. H., Ross, A. J., Brenner, D. J., and Fanning, G. P.: Int. J. Syst. Bacteriol. **28**:37, 1978.
206. Ross, A. J., Rucker, R. R., and Ewing, W. H.: Can. J. Microbiol. **12**:763-770, 1966.
207. Subcommittee on Taxonomy of Vibrios Report: Int. J. Syst. Bacteriol. **16**:135, 1966.
208. Blake, P. A., Merson, M. H., Weaver, R. E., et al.: N. Engl. J. Med. **300**:1, 1979.
209. Ewing, W. H., Davis, B. R., and Martin, W. J.: Outline of methods for the isolation and identification of *Vibrio cholerae*, Atlanta, 1966, Communicable Disease Center, Public Health Service.
210. Judicial Commission, International Committee on Bacteriological Nomenclature: Int. Bull. Bacteriol. Nomen. Taxon. **15**:185, 1965.
211. WHO Bacterial Diseases Unit: Guidelines for the laboratory diagnosis of cholera, Geneva, 1974, World Health Organization.
212. Benenson, A. S.: Bull. WHO **30**:827, 1964.
213. Ewing, W. H., Tomfohrde, K. M., and Nando, P. J.: API Species **2**:10, 1979.
214. Finkelstein, R. A., and LaBrec, E. H.: J. Bacteriol. **78**:886, 1959.
215. Hugh, R.: Int. Bull. Bacteriol. Nomen. Taxon. **15**:13, 1965.
216. Han, G. K., and Khee, T. D.: Am. J. Hyg. **77**:184-186, 1963.
217. Ewing, W. H.: *Vibrio cholerae*. In Diagnostic procedures for bacterial, mycotic, and parasitic infections, ed. 5, New York, 1970, American Public Health Association.
218. Feeley, J. C., and Balows, A.: *Vibrio*. In Lennette, E. H., Spaulding, E. H., and Truant, J. F., editors: Manual of clinical microbiology, Bethesda, Md., 1970, American Society for Microbiology.
219. Mukerjee, S.: Bull. WHO **28**:337, 1963.
220. Sakazaki, R., Iwanami, S., and Fukumi, H.: Jpn. J. Med. Sci. Biol. **16**:161-188, 1963.
221. Hollis, D. G., Weaver, R. E., Baker, C. N., and Thornsberry, C.: J. Clin. Microbiol. **3**:425-431, 1976.
222. Sakazaki, R.: *Vibrio parahaemolyticus*: isolation and identification, Tokyo, 1965, Nihon Eiyo Kagky Co. Ltd.
223. Le Clair, R. A., Zen-Yoji, H., and Sakai, S.: Public Health Lab. **28**:82-92, 1973.
224. Center for Disease Control: *Vibrio parahaemolyticus* gastroenteritis—United States, 1969-1972, Morbid. Mortal. **22**:231-232, 1970.
225. Barker, W. H., and Gangarosa, E. J.: Annu. Rev. Med. **25**:75, 1974.
226. Carruthers, M. M., and Kabat, W. J.: J. Clin. Microbiol. **4**:175, 1976.
227. Rubin, S. J., and Tilton, R. C.: J. Clin. Microbiol. **2**:555, 1975.
228. Molenda, J. R.: A review of the clinical bacteriology of *Vibrio parahaemolyticus*, CDC proficiency testing, Bacteriology IV, Atlanta, 1977, Center for Disease Control.
229. Tilton, R. C., and Balows, A.: *Vibrio alginolyticus* and *Vibrio parahaemolyticus*. Check sample no. AMB-19, Washington, D.C., 1977, American Society of Clinical Pathologists, Commission on Continuing Education.
230. Twedt, R. M.: Isolation and identification of *Vibrio parahaemolyticus*. In FDA bacteriological analytical manual, Washington, D.C., 1978, Association of Official Analytical Chemists.
231. Honda, T., Taga, S., Takeda, T., et al.: Infect. Immun. **13**:133-139, 1976.

232. Pien, F., Lee, K., and Higa, H.: J. Clin. Microbiol. **5:**670-672, 1977.
233. Ewing, W. H., Hugh, R., and Johnson, J. G.: Studies on the *Aeromonas* group, Atlanta, 1961, National Communicable Disease Center.
234. Ewing, W. H., and Hugh, R.: *Aeromonas.* In Lennette, E. H., Spaulding, E. H., and Truant, J. F., editors: Manual of clinical microbiology, ed. 2, Washington, D.C., 1974, American Society for Microbiology, pp. 230-237.
235. McCracken, A. W., and Barkley, R.: Clin. Pathol. **25:**970, 1972.
236. Phillips, J. A., Bernhardt, H. E., and Rosenthal, S. G.: Pediatrics **53:**110, 1974.
237. Stephen, S., Achyutha Rao, K. N., Sitaram Kumar, M., and Indurani, R.: Ann. Intern. Med. **83:**368, 1975.
238. Davis, W. A., Kane, J. G., and Garagusi, V. F.: Medicine **57:**267, 1978.
238a. Ewing, W. H., Tomfohrde, K. M., and Naudo, P. J.: API Species **2:**10, 1979.
239. Overman, T. L., D'Amato, R. F., and Tomfohrde, K. M.: J. Clin. Microbiol. **9:**244, 1979.
240. Schubert, R. H. W.: Int. J. Syst. Bacteriol. **17:**23, 273, 1967.
241. von Graevenitz, A., and Mensch, A. H.: N. Engl. J. Med. **278:**245, 1967.
242. Johnson, W. M., DiSalvo, A. F., and Steuer, R. R.: Am. J. Clin. Pathol. **56:**400-406, 1971.
243. Joseph, P. G., Sivendra, R., Anwar, M., and Ong, S. F.: Kajian Vet. (Malaysia-Singapore) **3:**55-66, 1971.
244. Ognibene, A. J., and Thomas, E.: Am. J. Clin. Pathol. **54:**607-610, 1970.
245. Sneath, P. H. A.: Iowa State J. Sci. **34:**243-500, 1960.
246. Victoria, B., Baer, H., and Ayoub, E. M.: J.A.M.A. **230:**578-580, 1974.
247. Sivendra, R., Lo, H. S., and Lim, K. T.: Am. J. Clin. Pathol. **64:**421, 1975.
248. Sivendra, R., and Tan, S. H.: J. Clin. Microbiol. **5:**514, 1977.
249. Sneath, P. H. A., Whelan, J. P. F., Singh, R. B., and Edwards, D.: Lancet **2:**276, 1953.
250. Sneath, P. H. A. In Gibbs, B. M., and Skinner, F. A., editors: Identification methods for microbiologists, pt. A, New York, 1966, Academic Press, p. 15.
251. Dhar, S. K., and Johnson, R.: J. Clin. Pathol. **26:**304, 1973.
252. Hubbert, W. T., and Rosen, M. N.: Am. J. Public Health **60:**1103, 1970.
253. Hubbert, W. T., and Rosen, M. N.: Am. J. Public Health **60:**1109, 1970.
254. Heddleston, K. L., and Wessman, G.: J. Clin. Microbiol. **1:**377, 1975.
255. Jones, F. L., Jr., and Smull, C. E.: Pa. Med. **76:**41, 1973.
256. Tindall, J. P., and Harrison, C. M.: Arch. Dermatol. **105:**412, 1972.
257. Branson, D., and Bunkfeldt, F.: Am. J. Clin. Pathol. **48:**552, 1967.
258. Controni, G., and Jones, R. S.: Am. J. Med. Technol. **33:**379, 1967.
259. Winton, F. W., and Mair, N. S.: Microbios **2:**155, 1969.
260. Miller, J. K.: N.Y. State J. Med. **66:**2527, 1966.
261. Hooper, A., and Sebesteny, A.: J. Med. Microbiol. **7:**137, 1973.
262. Hubbert, W. T.: Bull. Pathol. **6:**67, 1965.
263. Komorowski, R. A., and Farmer, S. G.: J. Urol. **111:**817, 1974.
264. Smith, G. R.: J. Pathol. Bacteriol. **81:**431, 1961.
265. Biberstein, E. L.: Biotyping and serotyping of *Pasteurella haemolytica.* In Bergan, T., and Norris, J. R., editors: Methods in microbiology, vol. 10, New York, 1978, Academic Press.
266. Wang, W. L. L., and Haiby, G.: Am. J. Clin. Pathol. **45:**562, 1966.
267. Starkebaum, G. A., and Plorde, J. J.: J. Clin. Microbiol. **5:**332, 1977.
268. Kolyvas, E., Sorger, R. T., Marks, M. I., and Pai, C. H.: J. Pediatr. **92:**81, 1978.
269. Phillips, J. E.: J. Pathol. Bacteriol. **79:**331, 1960.
270. Maguire, L. C.: Bet. Rec. **70:**989, 1958.
271. King, E. O.: The identification of unusual pathogenic gram-negative bacteria, Atlanta, 1964, Communicable Disease Center (revised, 1967, by R. E. Weaver and H. Tatum).
272. King, E. O., and Tatum, H. W.: J. Infect. Dis. **111:**85, 1962.
273. Page, M. I., and King, E. O.: N. Engl. J. Med. **275:**181, 1966.
274. Sutter, V. L., and Finegold, S. M.: *Haemophilus aphrophilus* infections: clinical and bacteriologic studies. In Kundsin, R., editor: Unusual isolates from clinical material, Ann. N.Y. Acad. Sci. **174(Art. 2):**468, 1970.
275. Goss, J. E., Gutin, R. S., and Dickhaus, D. W.: Am. J. Med. **43:**636-638, 1967.
276. Kayser, F. H., and Bircher, J.: Dtsch. Med. Wochenschr. **1:**21-23, 1967.
277. Mitchell, R. G., and Gillespie, W. A.: J. Clin. Pathol. **17:**511-512, 1964.
278. Overholt, B. F.: Arch. Intern. Med. **117:**99-102, 1966.
279. Sierra, P., and Tonato, M.: Am. J. Med. **47:**809-812, 1969.
280. Thomas, J. R.: South. Med. J. **60:**783-784, 1967.
281. Vogelzang, R. M.: Arch. Intern. Med. **120:**99-101, 1967.
282. Weaver, R. E.: *Actinobacillus actinomycetemcomitans.* In Check sample no. AMB-18, Washington, D.C., 1977, American Society of Clinical Pathologists, Commission on Continuing Education.
283. Pulverer, G., and Ko, H. L.: Appl. Microbiol. **20:**693, 1970.
284. Slotnick, I. J., and Dougherty, M.: Antonie van Leeuwenhoek **30:**261, 1964.
285. Tucker, D. N., Slotnick, I. J., King, E. O., et al.: N. Engl. J. Med. **267:**913, 1962.
286. Slotnick, I. J., Mertz, J. A., and Dougherty, M.: J. Infect. Dis. **114:**503, 1964.
287. Slotnick, I. J.: J. Bacteriol. **95:**1175, 1968.
288. Wormser, G. P., Bottone, E. J., Tudy, J., and Hirschman, S. I.: Am. J. Med. Sci. **276:**117, 1978.
289. Savage, D. D., Kagan, R. L., Young, N. A., and Horvath, A. E.: Microbiology **5:**75, 1977.
290. Henriksen, S. D., and Bøvre, K.: Int. J. Syst. Bacteriol. **26:**447-450, 1976.
291. Henriksen, S. D., and Bøvre, K.: *Moraxella kingii* sp. nov., a hemolytic, saccharolytic species of the genus *Moraxella,* J. Gen. Microbiol. **51:**377-385, 1968.
292. Pickett, J.: Nonfermentative gram-negative bacilli, Current Concepts in Clinical Microbiology Course, UCLA Extension Division, August 1976; also Syllabus, American Society of Clinical Pathologists Training Institute, Los Angeles, 1976 (personal communication, 1977).
293. Gilardi, G. L.: Antonie van Leeuwenhoek **39:**229, 1973.
294. Gilardi, G. L.: J. Appl. Bacteriol. **34:**623, 1971.

295. Gilardi, G. L.: Am. J. Med. Technol. **38**:65-72, 1972.
296. Gilardi, G. L.: Identification of nonfermentative gram-negative bacteria, New York, 1978, Hospital for Joint Diseases.
297. Otto, L. A., and Pickett, M. J.: J. Clin. Microbiol. **3**:566-575, 1976.
298. Pickett, M. J., and Pedersen, M. M.: Am. J. Clin. Pathol. **54**:164 and **54**:178, 1970.
299. Pickett, M. J., and Pedersen, M. M.: Can. J. Microbiol. **16**:351-362, 1970.
300. Jaugstetter, J. E.: The CDC approach to the identification of nonfermentative gram-negative bacteria, Continuing Education Series, Laboratory Training and Consultation Division, Atlanta, 1977, Center for Disease Control.
301. Blazevic, D. J.: Hum. Pathol. **7**:265, 1976.
302. Tatum, H. W., Ewing, W. H., and Weaver, R. E.: Miscellaneous gram-negative bacteria. In Lennette, E. H., Spaulding, E. H., and Truant, J. P.: Manual of clinical microbiology, ed. 2, Washington, D.C., 1974, American Society for Microbiology.
303. Gilardi, G. L.: Mt. Sinai J. Med. **43**:710, 1976.
304. Finegold, S. M., Martin, W. J., and Scott, E. G.: Bailey and Scott's Diagnostic microbiology: a textbook for the isolation and identification of pathogenic microorganisms, ed. 5, St. Louis, 1978, The C. V. Mosby Co.
305. Burdon, K. L.: J. Bacteriol. **52**:665, 1946.
306. Stanier, R. Y., Palleroni, N. J., and Doudoroff, M.: J. Gen. Microbiol. **43**:159, 1966.
307. Arai, T., et al.: Jpn. J. Microbiol. **14**:279, 1970.
308. Sierra, J.: Antonie van Leeuwenhoek **23**:15, 1957.
309. Manclark, C. R., Pickett, M. J., and Moore, H. B.: Laboratory manual for medical bacteriology. ed. 5, New York, 1972, Appleton-Century-Crofts.
310. Pickett, M. J.: Buffered substrates in determinative bacteriology. In Graber, C. D.: Rapid diagnostic methods in medical microbiology, Baltimore, 1970, The Williams & Wilkins Co.
311. Pickett, M. J.: Can. J. Microbiol. **16**:401, 1970.
312. Pseudomonas Subcommittee Report: Int. J. Syst. Bacteriol. **17**:255, 1967.
313. Pease, M., Malcolm, J., Chernaik, M., and Dunlop, S.: Am. J. Med. Technol. **34**:35, 1968.
314. Sutter, V. L.: Appl. Microbiol. **16**:1532, 1968.
315. Gilardi, G. L.: Am. J. Med. Technol. **34**:334, 1968.
316. Gilardi, G. L.: Appl. Microbiol. **16**:1497, 1968.
317. Pickett, J.: The Speciator (Corning Medical) **1**:1, 1978.
318. Sutter, V. L., Hurst, V., and Fennell, J.: Health Lab. Sci. **2**:7, 1965.
319. Verder, E., and Evans, J.: J. Infect. Dis. **109**:183, 1961.
320. Matsumoto, H., Tazaki, T., and Kato, T.: Jpn. J. Microbiol. **12**:111, 1968.
321. Lányi, B., and Bergan, T.: Serological characterization of *Pseudomonas aeruginosa*. In Bergan, T., and Norris, R., editors: Methods in microbiology, vol. 10, New York, 1978, Academic Press.
322. Govan, J. R. W.: Pyocin typing of *Pseudomonas aeruginosa*. In Bergan, T., and Norris, R., editors: Methods in microbiology, vol. 10, New York, 1978, Academic Press.
323. Elston, H. R., and Hoffman, K. C.: Technol. Bull. Reg. Med. Tech. **37**:259, 1967.
324. Gilardi, G. L.: Ann. Intern. Med. **77**:211-215, 1972.
325. McDowell, F., and Varnez, P. L.: J.A.M.A. **134**:361, 1947.
326. National Communicable Disease Center: Morbid. Mortal. Weekly Rep. **16**:127, 1967.
327. Weaver, R. E.: Public Health Lab. **25**:202, 1967.
328. Gilardi, G. L.: Appl. Microbiol. **18**:355, 1969.
329. Weaver, R. E.: Personal communication, 1968.
330. Rogul, M., Brendle, J. J., Haapala, D. K., and Alexander, A. D.: J. Bacteriol. **101**:827, 1970.
331. Yabuuchi, E., Miyajima, N., Hotta, H., and Ohyama, A.: Med. J. Osaka Univ. **21**:1, 1970.
332. Speller, D. C. E., Stephens, M. E., and Viant, A. C.: Lancet **1**:798, 1971.
333. Speller, D. C. E.: Br. Heart J. **35**:47, 1972.
334. Sorrell, W. B., and White, L. V.: Am. J. Clin. Pathol. **23**:134, 1953.
335. Schiff, J., Suter, L. S., Gourley, R. D., and Sutliff, W. D.: Ann. Intern. Med. **55**:499, 1961.
336. Hamilton, J., Burch, W., Grimmett, G., et al.: Antimicrob. Agents Chemother. **4**:551, 1973.
337. Neu, H. C., Garvey, G. J., and Beach, M. P.: J. Infect. Dis. **128**(suppl.):S768, 1973.
338. Rahal, J. J., Simberkoff, M. S., and Hyams, P. J.: J. Infect. Dis. **128**(suppl.):S762, 1973.
339. Ederer, G. M., and Matsen, J. M.: J. Infect. Dis. **125**:613, 1972.
340. Mitchell, R. G., and Hayward, A. C.: Lancet **1**:793, 1966.
341. Hardy, P. C., Ederer, G. M., and Matsen, J. M.: N. Engl. J. Med. **282**:33, 1970.
342. Roberts, J. B. M., and Speller, D. C. E.: Lancet **2**:1099, 1973.
343. Bassett, D. C. J., Stokes, K. J., and Thomas, W. R. G.: Lancet **1**:1188, 1970.
344. von Graevenitz, A.: Clinical microbiology of unusual *Pseudomonas* species. In Stefanini, M., editor: Progress in clinical pathology, vol. 5, New York, 1973, Grune & Stratton.
345. Fischer, J. J.: J. Infect. Dis. **128**(suppl.): S771, 1973.
346. Gilardi, G. L.: Am. J. Clin. Pathol. **51**:58, 1969.
347. Holmes, B., Lapage, S. P., and Easterling, B. G.: J. Clin. Pathol. **32**:66, 1979.
348. Gilardi, G. L.: Appl. Microbiol. **22**:821, 1971.
349. Davis, G. H. G., and Park, R. W. A.: J. Gen. Microbiol. **27**:101, 1962.
350. Hugh, R.: Int. Bull. Bacteriol. Nomen. Taxon. **12**:33, 1962.
351. Hugh, R.: Int. Bull. Bacteriol. Nomen. Taxon. **15**:125, 1965.
352. von Graevenitz, A.: Am. J. Clin. Pathol. **43**:357, 1965.
353. Vandepitte, J., and Debois, J.: J. Clin. Microbiol. **7**:70, 1978.
354. Riley, P. S., and Weaver, R. E.: J. Clin. Microbiol. **1**:1, 1975.
355. Ralston, E. N. J., Palleroni, N. J., and Doudoroff, M.: Int. J. Syst. Bacteriol. **23**:15, 1973.
356. Holmes, B., Owens, R. J., Evans, A., et al.: Int. J. Syst. Bacteriol. **27**:133-146, 1977.
357. Mitchell, R. G., and Clarke, S. K. R.: J. Gen. Microbiol. **40**:343, 1965.
358. Chester, B., and Cooper, L. H.: J. Clin. Microbiol. **9**:425, 1979.
359. Pien, F. D., and Higa, H. Y.: J. Clin. Microbiol. **7**:239, 1978.
360. Holmes, B., Snell, J. S., and Lapage, S. P.: J. Clin. Pathol. **30**:595-601, 1977.
361. Yabuuchi, E., Yano, I., Goto, S., et al.: Int. J. Syst. Bacteriol. **24**:470-477, 1974.
362. Baumann, P., Doudoroff, M., and Stanier, R. Y.: J. Bacteriol. **95**:1520, 1968.
363. Pinter, M., and Bende, I.: Pathol. Microbiol. **31**:41, 1968.

364. DeLey, J.: Antonie van Leeuwenhoek **34**:109, 1968.

365. Brisou, J., and Prévot, N. B.: Ann. Inst. Pasteur Lille **86**:722, 1954.

366. Steel, K. J., and Cowan, S. T.: Ann. Inst. Pasteur Lille **106**:479, 1964.

367. Oberhofer, T. R., Rowen, J. W., and Cunningham, G. F.: J. Clin. Microbiol. **5**:208-220, 1977.

368. Taplin, D., Rebell, G., and Zaiab, N.: J.A.M.A. **186**:166-168, 1963.

369. Glew, R. H., Moellering, R. C., and Kuny, L. J.: Medicine **56**:79-97, 1977.

370. Abrutyn, E. Goodhart, G. L., Roos, K., et al.: Am. J. Epidemiol. **107**:328-335, 1978.

371. Buxton, E. E., Anderson, R. L., Werdegar, D., and Atlas, E.: Am. J. Med. **65**:507-513, 1973.

372. Gilardi, G. L.: Am. J. Med. Technol. **33**:201, 1967.

373. Retailliau, H. F., Hightower, A. W., Dixon, R. E., and Allen, J. R.: J. Infect. Dis. **139**:371, 1979.

374. Henriksen, S. D.: Bacteriol. Rev. **37**:522-561, 1973.

375. Henriksen, S. D.: Annu. Rev. Microbiol. **30**:63, 1976.

376. Juni, E.: J. Bacteriol. **112**:917-931, 1972.

377. Juni, E.: Appl. Microbiol. **27**:16-24, 1974.

378. Henriksen, S. D.: Int. Bull. Bacteriol. Nomen. Taxon. **10**:23, 1960.

379. Henriksen, S. D.: Int. Bull. Bacteriol. Nomen. Taxon. **13**:51, 1963.

380. Baumann, P., Doudoroff, M., and Stanier, R. Y.: J. Bacteriol. **95**:58, 1968.

381. Henriksen, S. D., and Bøvre, K.: J. Gen. Microbiol. **51**:387, 1968.

382. Piéchaud, M.: Ann. Inst. Pasteur Lille **104**:291, 1963.

383. Bøvre, K., and Henriksen, S. D.: Int. J. Syst. Bacteriol. **17**:127, 1967.

384. Bøvre, K., and Henriksen, S. D.: Int. J. Syst. Bacteriol. **17**:343, 1967.

385. McMeekin, T. A.: J. Appl. Bacteriol. **45**:321, 1978.

386. King, E.: Am. J. Clin. Pathol. **31**:241, 1959.

387. Cabrera, H. A., and Davis, G. A.: Am. J. Dis. Child. **101**:289, 1961.

388. Schiff, J., Suter, L. S., Gourley, R. D., and Sutliff, W. D.: Ann. Intern. Med. **55**:499, 1961.

389. Olsen, H.: Danish Med. Bull. **14**:1, 1967.

390. Mani, R. M., Kuruvila, K. C., Batliwala, P. M., et al.: J. Clin. Pathol. **31**:220, 1978.

391. Stutzer, M., and Kwaschnina, A.: Zentralbl. Bakteriol. Parasitenkd. Infectionskr. Hyg. Abt. 1 Orig. **113**:219-225, 1929.

392. Holmes, B., Snell, J. J., and Lapage, S. P.: Int. J. Syst. Bacteriol. **27**:330-336, 1977.

393. Holmes, B., Snell, J. J. S., and Lapage, S. P.: J. Clin. Pathol. **32**:73, 1979.

394. Jackson, F. L., and Goodman, V. E.: Int. J. Syst. Bacteriol. **22**:73-77, 1972.

395. Riley, P. S., Tatum, H. W., and Weaver, R. E.: Int. J. Syst. Bacteriol. **23**:75-76, 1973.

396. Brooks, G. F., and White, A.: South Med. J. **69**:534, 1976.

397. Brooks, G. F., O'Donoghue, J. M., Rissing, P., et al.: Medicine **53**:325, 1974.

398. Goldstein, E. J. C., Kirby, B. D., and Finegold, S. M.: Am. Rev. Respir. **Dis.** 119:55, 1979.

399. Sebald, M., and Vernon, M.: Ann. Inst. Pasteur Lille **105**:897-910, 1963.

400. Smibert, R. M.: Annu. Rev. Microbiol. **32**:673-709, 1978.

401. Blazevic, D. J.: Clin. Microbiol. Newsletter **1**(13): 1, 1979.

402. Robinson, B. L.: Can. Med. Assoc. J. **118**:1087-1088, 1978.

403. Lancet, July 15, 1978, p. 135.

404. Bokkenheuser, V. D., Richardson, N. J., Bryner, J. H., et al.: J. Clin. Microbiol. **9**:227-232, 1979.

404a. Director, Bureau of Laboratories, Identical Memorandum. Center for Disease Control: Diarrheal disease caused by *Campylobacter fetus* subspecies *jejuni*, Atlanta, Aug. 7, 1978, Center for Disease Control.

405. Center for Disease Control: Morbid. Mortal. **27**: 207, 1978.

406. Center for Disease Control: Morbid. Mortal. **2**:226-227, 1978.

407. Skirrow, M. B.: Br. Med. J. **2**:9-11, 1977.

408. Blaser, M., Cravens, J., Powers, B. W., and Wang, W. L.: Lancet **2**:979-981, 1978.

409. King, E. O.: J. Infect. Dis. **101**:119-128, 1957.

410. Guerrant, R. L., Lahita, R. G., Winn, W. C., Jr., and Roberts, R. B.: Am. J. Med. **65**:584-592, 1978.

411. Bokkenheuser, V. D.: Am. J. Epidemiol. **91**:400, 1970.

412. Bokkenheuser, V. D.: Infect. Immun. **5**:222, 1972.

413. Riley, P. S., and Weaver, R. E.: J. Clin. Microbiol. **5**:172, 1977.

414. Bernaerts, M. J., and DeLey, J.: Nature **197**:406, 1963.

415. Moore, H. B., and Pickett, M. J.: Can. J. Microbiol. **6**:35, 1960.

416. Lautrop, H.: Acta Pathol. Microbiol. Scand. Suppl. 187, 1967.

417. Stableforth, A. W., and Jones, L. M.: Int. Bull. Bacterial Nomen. Taxon. **13**:145, 1963.

418. Jones, L. M.: Int. J. Syst. Bacteriol. **17**:371, 1967.

419. Huddleston, I. F.: Mich. Agric. Stat. Technol. Bull. **177**:11, 1941.

420. Blankenship, R. M., and Sanford, J. P.: Am. J. Med. **59**:424, 1975.

421. Carmichael, L. E., and Bruner, D. W.: Cornell Vet. **48**:579-592, 1968.

422. Center for Disease Control: *Brucella* surveillance summary 1972, DHEW publ. no. (CDC)-75-8186, Atlanta, 1974, The Center.

423. Mumford, R. S., Weaver, R. E., Patton, C., et al.: J.A.M.A. **231**:1267, 1975.

424. Carmichael, L. E., and Kenney, R. M.: J. Am. Vet. Med. Assoc. **152**:605, 1968.

425. Spink, W. W., and Morrisset, R.: Trans. Am. Clin. Climatol. Assoc. **81**:43, 1970.

426. Center for Disease Control: Brucellosis annual summary 1977, DHEW publ. no. (CDC)-79-818, Atlanta, 1978.

427. Huddleson, I. F.: Mich. Agric. Stat. Memoir, no. 6, Jan. 1952.

428. Castañeda, M. R., and Carillo-Cardenas, C.: WHO brucellosis report no. 105, 1954.

429. Spink, W. W.: The nature of brucellosis, Minneapolis, 1956, University of Minnesota Press.

430. MacNeal, W. J., and Kerr, J. E.: Infect. Dis. **7**:469, 1910.

431. Evans, A. C.: J. Infect. Dis. **22**:580, 1918.

432. Buchanan, T. M., Faber, L. C., and Feldman, R. A.: Medicine **53**:403, 1974.

433. Buchanan, T. M., Sulzer, C. R., Frix, M. K., and Feldman, R. A.: Medicine **53**:415, 1974.

434. Buchanan, T. M., Hendricks, S. L., Patton, C. M., and Feldman, R. A.: Medicine **53**:427, 1974.

435. Martin, D. W., Jr., and Watts, H. D.: West. J. Med. **122**:232, 1975.

436. Joint FAO/WHO Expert Panel on Brucellosis, first, second, and third reports, FAO Agricultural

Studies no. 14, 1951, no. 67, 1953, and no. 148, World Health Organization, 1958.

437. Castañeda, M. R.: Proc. Soc. Exp. Biol. Med. **64:**114, 1947.

438. Castañeda, M. R.: Bull. Organ. Mond. Santé **14:**795, 1956.

439. Kuzdas, C. D., and Morse, E. V.: J. Bacteriol. **66:**502, 1953.

440. Renoux, G.: Ann. Inst. Pasteur Lille **87:**325, 1954.

441. McCullough, N. B.: Identification of the species and biotypes within the genus *Brucella.* In Bergan, T., and Norris, J. R., editors: Methods in microbiology, vol. 10, New York, 1978, Academic Press.

442. Huddleson, I. F.: Am. J. Public Health **6:**491, 1931.

443. Morgan, W. J. B.: WHO/Bruc./224, 1962, World Health Organization.

444. Meyer, M.E., and Cameron, H. S.: J. Bacteriol. **82:**396, 1961.

445. Cherry, W. B., and Moody, M. D.: Bacteriol. Rev. **29:**222, 1965.

446. Kilian, M.: J. Gen. Microbiol. **93:**9, 1976.

446a. Kilian, M., Sorenson, S., and Fredericksen, W. J.: J. Clin. Microbiol. **9:**409, 1979.

447. Kilian, M.: Acta Pathol. Microbiol. Scand. **82**(B):835, 1974.

448. Goldberg, R., and Washington, J. A.: Am. J. Clin. Pathol. **70:**899, 1978.

449. Lund, M. E., and Blazevic, D. J.: J. Clin. Microbiol. **5:**142, 1977.

450. Snyder, S. N., and Brunjes, S.: Am. J. Med. Sci. **250:**658, 1968.

451. Branson, D.: Am. J. Clin. Pathol. **47:**643, 1967.

452. Dajami, A., Asmar, B. J., and Thirumoorti, M. C.: J. Pediatr. **94:**355, 1979.

453. Turk, D. C., and May, J. R.: *Haemophilus influenzae:* its clinical importance, London, 1967, English Universities Press.

454. Omland, T.: Serotyping of *Haemophilus influenzae.* In Bergan, T., and Norris, J. R., editors: Methods in microbiology, vol. 10, New York, 1978, Academic Press.

455. Ingram, D. L., Collier, A. M., Pendergrass, E., and King, S. H.: J. Clin. Microbiol. **9:**570, 1979.

456. Alexander, H. E.: The *Haemophilus* group. In Dubos, R., editor: Bacterial and mycotic infections of man, ed. 3, Philadelphia, 1958, J. B. Lippincott Co.

457. Sutter, V. L., and Finegold, S. M.: Ann. N.Y. Acad. Sci. **174**(Art. 2):168, 1970.

458. Nahmias, A. J., Brahen, L., and Luce, C.: Antimicrobial agents and chemotherapy—1965, Ann Arbor, Mich., 1966, American Society for Microbiology.

459. Ward, J. I., Tsai, T. F., Filice, S. A., and Fraser, D. W.: J. Infect. Dis. **138:**421, 1978.

460. Branson, D.: Appl. Microbiol. **16:**256, 1968.

461. Jemsek, J.G., Greenberg, S. B., Gentry, L. O., et al.: Am. J. Med. **66:**51, 1979.

462. Geraci, J. E., Wilkowske, C. J., Wilson, W. R., and Washington, J. A., II: Mayo Clin. Proc. **52:**209-215, 1977.

463. Khairat, O.: J. Pathol. Bacteriol. **50:**497, 1940.

464. Page, M. I., and King, E. O.: N. Engl. J. Med. **275:**181, 1966.

465. Bieger, C. R., Brewer, N. S., and Washington, J. A., II: Medicine **57:**345, 1978.

466. Young, V. M.: *Haemophilus.* In Lennette, E. H., Spaulding, E. H., and Truant, J. P., editors: Manual of clinical microbiology, ed. 2, Washing-ton, D.C., 1974, American Society for Microbiology.

467. Greenwood, J. R., and Pickett, M. J.: J. Clin. Microbiol. **9:**200, 1979.

468. Lauthrop, H., and Lacey, B. W.: Bull. WHO **23:**15, 1960.

469. Brooksaler, F., and Nelson, J. D.: Am. J. Dis. Child. **114:**389, 1967.

470. Whitaker, J. A., Donaldson, P., and Nelson, J. D.: N. Engl. J. Med. **263:**850, 1960.

471. Finegold, S. M., Martin, W. J., and Scott, E. G.: Bailey and Scott's diagnostic microbiology: a textbook for the isolation and identification of pathogenic microorganisms, ed. 5, St. Louis, 1978, The C. V. Mosby Co.

472. White, J. D., and McGavran, M. H.: J.A.M.A. **194:**294, 1965.

473. Yager, R. H., Spertzel, R. O., Jaeger, R. F., and Tigertt, W. D.: Proc. Soc. Exp. Biol. Med. **105:**651, 1960.

474. Eigelsbach, H. T.: *Francisella tularensis.* In Lennette, E. H., Spaulding, E. H., and Truant, J. P., editors: Manual of clinical microbiology, ed. 2, Washington, D.C., 1974, American Society for Microbiology, p. 316.

475. Klock, L. E., Olsen, P. F., and Fukushima, T.: J.A.M.A. **226:**149, 1973.

476. Dienst. F. T., Jr.: J. Louisiana State Med. Soc. **115:**114, 1963.

477. Miller, R. P., and Bates, J. H.: Am. Rev. Resp. Dis. **99:**31, 1969.

478. Karlsson, K-A.: Identification of *Francisella tularensis.* In Bergan, T., and Norris, J. R., editors: Methods in microbiology, vol. 10, New York, 1978, Academic Press.

479. Morton, H. E. In Dubos, R. J., and Hirsch, J. G., editors: Bacterial and mycotic infections of man, ed. 4, Philadelphia, 1965, J. B. Lippincott Co.

480. Rogosa, M.: *Streptobacillus moniliformis* and *Spirillum minor.* In Lennette, E. H., Spaulding, E. H., and Truant, J. P., editors: Manual of clinical microbiology, ed. 2, Washington, D.C., 1974, American Society for Microbiology.

481. Pirodda, E.: Otorinolaringol. Ital. **34:**23, 1965.

482. Roughgarden, J. W.: Arch. Intern. Med. **116:**39-54, 1965.

483. Lambe, D. W., McPhedran, J. A. M., Mertz, J. A., and Stewart, P.: Am. J. Clin. Pathol. **60:**854-860, 1973.

484. Williams, M. A., and Rittenberg, S. C.: Int. Bull. Bacteriol. Nomen. Taxon. **7:**49, 1957.

485. Kowal, J.: N. Engl. J. Med. **264:**123, 1961.

486. Edwards, E. E., and Krans, R.: N. Engl. J. Med. **262:**458, 1960.

487. Weinman, D.: *Bartonellaceae.* In Buchanan, R. E., and Gibbons, N. E., editors: Bergey's manual of determinative bacteriology, ed. 8, Baltimore, 1974, The Williams & Wilkins Co., p. 903.

488. Weinman, D.: Bartonellosis. In Infectious blood diseases of man and animals, ed. 2, New York, 1968, Academic Press, vol. 2, p. 3.

489. Schultz, M. G.: Am. J. Trop. Med. Hyg. **17:**503, 1968.

490. Weinman, D. In Dubos, R. J., and Hirsch, J. G., editors: Bacterial and mycotic infections of man, ed. 4, Philadelphia, 1965, J. B. Lippincott Co.

491. Bobo, R. A., and Newton, E. J.: Am. J. Clin. Pathol. **65:**564, 1976.

492. Butler, T., Weaver, R. E., Ramani, T. K. V., et al.: Ann. Intern. Med. **86:**1-5, 1977.

493. Schlossberg, D.: J. Clin. Microbiol. 9:297, 1979.
494. Jones, G. L., and Hebert, G. A., editors: Legionnaires', the disease, the bacterium, and methodology, Atlanta, 1978 (rev.), Center for Disease Control.
495. Sanford, P. J.: N. Engl. J. Med. 300:654, 1979.
496. Vella, E. E.: J. R. Soc. Med. 71:361, 1978.
497. Balows, A. J., and Fraser, D. W., editors: Ann. Intern. Med. 90(4):489-703, 1979.
498. Center for Disease Control: Morbid. Mortal. 27:439, 1978.
499. McDade, J. E., Shepard, C. C., Fraser, D. W., et al.: N. Engl. J. Med. 297:1197-1203, 1977.
500. Dumoff, M.: Ann. Intern. Med. 90(4):694, 1979.
501. Brenner, D. J., Steigerwalt, A. G., and McDade, J. E.: Ann. Intern. Med. 90(4):656, 1979.
502. Glick, T. H., Gregg, M. B., Berman, B., et al.: Am. J. Epidemiol. 107:149-160, 1978.
503. Center for Disease Control: Ann. Intern. Med. 88:363, 1978.
504. Bock, B. V., Kirby, B. D., Edelstein, P. H., et al.: Lancet 1:410-413, 1978.
505. Moss, C. W., Weaver, R. E., Dees, S. B., and Cherry, W. B.: J. Clin. Microbiol. 6:140-143, 1977.
506. Martin, J. E., Jr., and Lewis, J. S.: Lancet 2:605, 1977.
507. Cherry, W. B.: Clin. Microbiol. Newsletter 1(7):1, 1979.
508. Edelstein, P. H., Meyer, R. D., and Finegold, S. M.: Lancet 1:750, 1979.
509. Cowan, S. T., and Steele, K. J.: Manual for the identification of medical bacteria, Cambridge, England, 1965, Cambridge University Press.
510. Steele, K. J., and Midgley, J.: J. Gen. Microbiol. 29:171, 1962.
511. Butler, T., Mahmoud, A. A. F., and Warren, K. S.: J. Infect. Dis. 136:317, 1977.
512. Mehaffey, M. A., and Griffin, C. W., III: Proficiency testing summary analysis, Atlanta, January 1979, Center for Disease Control.

80

THE SPIROCHETES

Alex C. Sonnenwirth

The spirochetes are spiral organisms with slender, flexuous bodies. The smaller forms may have a lower refractile index than true bacteria and can be seen only with the dark-field microscope. The spirochetes are motile. In the eighth edition of *Bergey's Manual*[1] the order *Spirochaetales* includes the family *Spirochaetaceae*, with the genera *Spirochaeta, Cristispira, Treponema, Borrelia,* and *Leptospira. Spirochaeta* are free-living forms (members of the genus are present in H_2S-containing freshwater and seawater mud); *Cristispira* are commensals in the digestive tract of many freshwater and marine mollusks. With few exceptions, members of the genera *Treponema, Borrelia,* and *Leptospira* are parasitic, and some are highly pathogenic. The latter 3 genera are described in detail. For a detailed review of spirochetes, see Johnson.[2]

The type of motility seen under dark-field observation is helpful in distinguishing the members of the 3 genera. Borrelia display a very active rotation around the long axis (corkscrewlike motility) in fresh preparations, with moderate flexion (bending). Sometimes no progression is observed: some translation (movement from place to place) can be seen, and the organisms may move back and forth in the same field. Treponemes show a forward and backward movement (translation), some rotation and slow bending, and twisting or undulation from side to side. Leptospirae progress by undulatory movements and by rapid spinning (rotation) on the long axis; often they dart forward or to and fro, and they may show quick lashing movements of flexion.

Borrelia are larger and longer than the treponemes; the former show shallow, coarse, irregular coils, whereas the latter have tightly wound coils. The leptospirae are described as having extraordinarily fine spirals—so closely wound and so short that they cannot usually be distinguished in stained films and show only as small dots on dark-field examination. Characteristically, 1 or both ends are bent to form a hook.

TREPONEMA

Treponemes are slender spiral organisms that can be distinguished morphologically from the *Borrelia* and the *Leptospira. T. pallidum, T. pertenue,* and *T. carateum* are pathogenic for man, whereas *T. paraluis-cuniculi* causes rabbit syphilis. A group of treponemes, among them *T. dentium (T. macrodentium)* are parasitic in man and occur in the normal mouth, pharynx, lower intestine, and external genitals.

There is general agreement that the pathogenic treponemes have not been cultivated. On the other hand, many of the parasitic or saprophytic treponemes can be cultivated on artificial media.

The term "treponematosis" was first introduced by Butler and Peterson (1927). Hudson[3] stated in his monograph that the disease treponematosis is a universally distributed infection caused by *Treponema,* a genus with 1 species, *pallidum.* Other investigators believe that the various treponemal infections (syphilis, yaws [frambesia], pinta, bejel) are caused by different species of treponemes. Many others agree with Hudson in believing that there is only 1 species of *Treponema* but that different clinical syndromes are produced under the effect of race, diet, climate, and other environmental factors.

As discussed in serology, antibodies can be detected in all the diseases mentioned herein by employing antigens commonly used for syphilis tests (see discussion on serology, Chapter 106).

Treponema pallidum

T. pallidum is a spiral, flexible, thin organism about 0.1-0.2 μm thick and 5-20 μm long. It has 4-14 regular spirals, with the distance between them about 1 μm. The organism exhibits a spinning motion in serum, with slow progression. In more mucoid medium (such as the material from early syphilitic lesions) the motion may be writhing and undulating. It has an axial filament about which the protoplasm is wound.

T. pallidum is the causative agent of syphilis

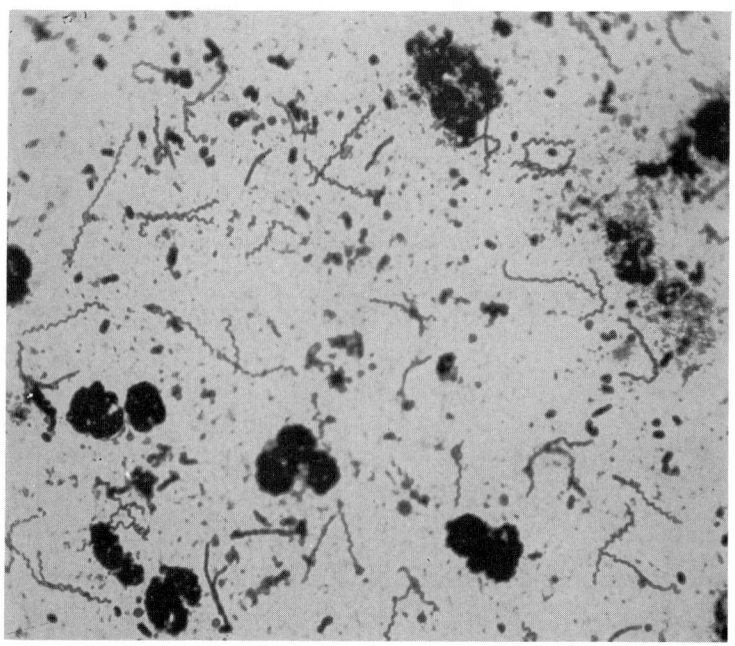

Fig. 80-1. *Treponema pallidum* in biopsy specimen of penile sore. (Stained by Krajian 20 min method.) (From Krajian, A. A., and Gradwohl, R. B. H.: Histopathological technic, St. Louis, The C. V. Mosby Co.)

(For description of disease stages and serologic diagnosis see discussion on serology, Chapter 106). Multiplication is usually by transverse fission.

Since *T. pallidum* **cannot be cultivated in vitro,** diagnosis of syphilis is made (1) by **dark-field demonstration** or **immunofluorescence identification** of *T. pallidum* in primary or secondary lesions, in body fluids, or tissue sections and (2) by **serologic methods.** *T. pallidum* is resistant to staining by bacterial stains; it stains pink with Giemsa stain. Silver impregnation methods, like those of Fontana and Levaditi, Krajian, and Ryu are recommended (Fig. 80-1).

T. pallidum and other pathogenic species of the genus have not been cultivated in vitro. Other treponemes have been cultured on artificial media; they are anaerobes. Such organisms are nonpathogenic. One of these, the Reiter treponeme, has been shown to contain antigens common with *T. pallidum*, and a protein extract of this organism has been used in serologic testing for syphilis. *T. pallidum* is propagated in the testicles of the experimentally infected rabbit.

Dark-field microscopy and detection and identification of Treponema pallidum[4]

A diagnosis of syphilis can be made by the demonstration of *T. pallidum* in suspected and accessible lesions or regional lymph nodes, using dark-field microscopy.* To accomplish this demonstration, proper equipment, adequately

---

*Dark-field examination is also used for demonstrating *Spirillum minus, Leptospira,* and *Borrelia.*

trained personnel, and perseverance are required.

The subject areas to be considered in this presentation are collection and submission of specimens, some elementary principles of dark-field microscopy, adjustment of the microscope, examination of the specimen (including a summary of frequent sources of error), and interpretation of results.

Collection and submission of specimens. The objective in collecting a specimen for dark-field examination is to obtain one as free of red blood cells and tissue debris as practically possible, since these elements will tend to obscure the treponemes.

1. Rubber gloves and other necessary precautions should be used to avoid accidental infection.

2. If lesion is covered with a scab or crust, it should be removed. Cleanse lesion with a gauze sponge wet with tap water or physiological saline. Antiseptics or soap should be avoided because of their potential antitreponemal effects.

3. After drying area, abrade lesion with a dry sponge to provoke slight bleeding and exudation of serum. As oozing occurs, wipe away first few drops, particularly if they contain appreciable amounts of blood, and await appearance of relatively clear serum. It is sometimes necessary to squeeze base of lesion or to apply a suction cup to promote appearance of serum. It is more desirable to obtain serum from depths of lesion rather than from its surface because of greater likelihood of finding motile treponemes.

4. For direct examination, several clean cover slips or slides are applied to oozing lesion, or a capillary pipet may be used to transfer serum from lesion to glass slides. Coverslips and slides are pressed firmly together with exudate between. Coverslip should be evenly depressed or flattened with blunt end of a cotton

swab stick or pencil point in such a manner as to remove air bubbles, etc. Edges of coverglass may be ringed with petrolatum to minimize evaporation, particularly if examination will not be immediate. Drying process has an adverse effect on treponemal motility.

5. If it is not possible to demonstrate organism from lesion after examining several specimens, a sample may be obtained from a **regional lymph node,** particularly if it is palpable. To accomplish this, either wash out or introduce about 0.5 ml physiological saline into a small sterile syringe (2 ml) to which is attached a small hypodermic needle. Disinfect skin overlying node by painting with iodine and alcohol or some other suitable agent. Hold node firmly and insert needle well into node. Ability to manipulate node freely is a good indication that its capsule has been pierced. Inject physiological saline and gently manipulate needle in various directions to macerate tissue, aspirating as much fluid as possible. Discharge aspirated material on slides for immediate examination or into capillary tubes for transmission to laboratory if examination is to be delayed. Delayed examination by use of a capillary tube transport is not as a rule satisfactory.

Lesions of early syphilis that are not manifest but suspected, as well as those observable but relatively less accessible, necessitate special comment and management. **In the male,** the presence of phimosis may make the lesion both inaccessible and nonobservable, although suspected by the examiner. Commonly phimosis can be reduced by persistent traction after application of a clinical lubricant or mineral oil. If this fails, a dorsal slit through the prepuce may be performed; however, this procedure should be used only after specimens obtained by puncture of regional lymph nodes do not reveal treponemes.

In the female, lesions of the cervix and vaginal vault present special problems for the collection of satisfactory material for dark-field microscopy. With visualization by bivalve speculum, all cervical or vaginal discharge of an interfering nature is removed. The lesion is then cleansed with physiologic saline, dried, and abraded as before (in this instance by rubbing with a gauze square held by a Kelly clamp). As bleeding stops and serum exudes, material is obtained, using a pipet equipped with a suction bulb.

In either sex, lesions of the skin in even a fading stage are worthy of multiple small linear incisions or scraping with a sharp scalpel or aspiration of the base of the lesion with a small-caliber hypodermic needle and syringe. This is particularly true of macular lesions and those upon which local medicaments have been used. (Macular lesions are seldom dark-field positive.) Such technics are rarely necessary on papular or moist papular (condylomata lata) lesions that are teeming with *T. pallidum.* Vesicants such as a cantharides patch have been used by some clinicians. Such a patch is retained in place for 24 hours and then serum, aspirated from the resultant blisters, is used for dark-field microscopic examination.

Mucous membrane lesions (patches) usually present little problem except in the mouth, where other treponemes and spirochetes so frequently are a part of the indigenous flora. For this reason, and to avoid contamination of the specimen with these forms, some of which are indistinguishable from *T. pallidum,* the lesion should be cleansed well, then walled off as completely as possible with cotton strips, and again cleansed and dried before being abraded.

If local therapy has been applied to any syphilitic lesion, it may be difficult or impossible to find treponemes. The use of warm compresses of physiologic saline for 24 hours often will facilitate finding the organism. All other treatment of such lesions during this time is absolutely restricted if this procedure is to be fruitful.

Ideally the dark field should be accomplished immediately. Lacking proper facilities to do this, a **capillary tube specimen** should be carefully collected and **promptly** submitted to the nearest laboratory prepared to perform such examinations.

To send a specimen to another laboratory, the capillary tube containing the exudate or aspirate is sealed on both ends with beeswax or a mixture of beeswax and petrolatum. It should be pointed out again that delayed examination by use of a capillary tube transport is not as a rule satisfactory. The tube is then encased in a glass tube of suitable size. Such outfits are generally supplied by state health departments. Measures should be used to facilitate the prompt delivery of specimens to the examining laboratory, since any appreciable delay in transmission may result in questionable findings due to reduced or complete loss of motility of the treponemes.

Principles. The ordinary compound microscope may easily be equipped for dark-field examination by substituting a dark-field condenser for the bright-field or Abbé condenser. In the latter, light rays from the illuminator are concentrated and directed straight upward through the microscope slide and objective lens into the barrel of the microscope (Fig. 80-2, *A*). In the dark-field condenser an opaque stop is arranged to prevent any direct rays of light from entering the objective. All peripheral rays, however, are reflected obliquely to the upper surface of the microscope slide at such an angle that they do not enter the objective lens unless some object is present to reflect them upward (Fig. 80-2, *B*). The field appears dark—hence the term "dark field." When a fluid containing particles, including bacteria or treponemes, is placed on the slide, the oblique rays are reflected from their surfaces upward into the barrel of the microscope, and these particles appear brightly illuminated against a black background.

There are a variety of dark-field condensers, but the paraboloid and cardioid types are most widely used. The **paraboloid condenser,** because of its cost and ease of operation, is satisfactory for use in dark-field microscopy for *T. pallidum.* This condenser contains 1 reflecting surface that because of its configuration does not bring about a sharp focusing of the hollow cone of rays. This

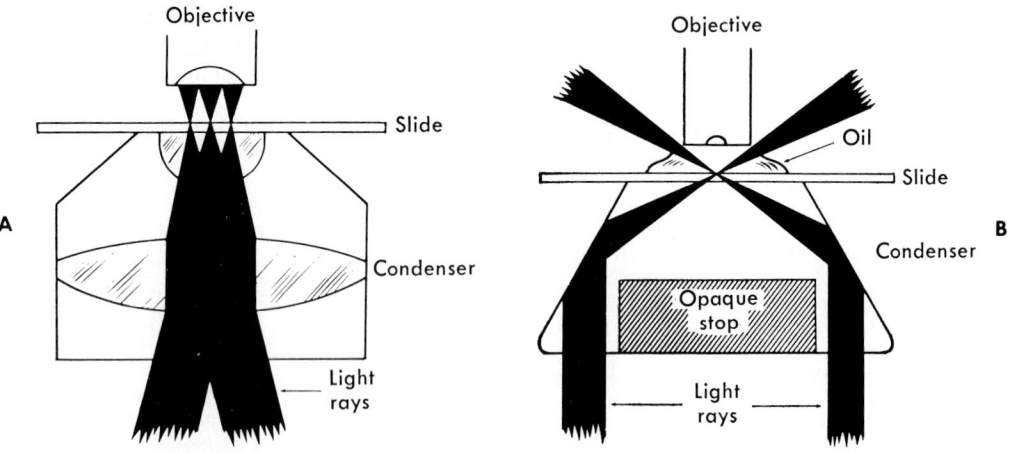

Fig. 80-2. A, Abbé condenser (bright field). **B,** Dark-field condenser. (From Darkfield microscopy for the detection and identification of *Treponema pallidum,* Atlanta, Venereal Disease Branch, Communicable Disease Center.)

characteristic makes it easier to manipulate. An additional advantage is the ability to close down the iris diaphragm of the substage to produce a blacker field. A disadvantage of the paraboloid condenser is that it produces a less intense illumination, making it less desirable when high intensity of illumination is required. However, such intensity of light is not generally needed for visualizing *T. pallidum.*

The **cardioid condenser** possesses 2 reflecting surfaces that produce more intense illumination. Disadvantages of this condenser are the requirement of critical focusing and accurate centering as well as initial high cost due to the use of a quartz lens.

Most dark-field condensers require that the numerical aperture of the oil-immersion objective be reduced below that of the condenser. This is accomplished by inserting a **funnel stop** into the objective.

Adjustment of microscope. There are two general types of microscopes used for dark-field examination: (1) a microscope with a revolving turret or nosepiece containing multiple objectives and an external light source separated from the dark-field condenser and (2) a microscope with a single objective (usually oil immersion) or multiple objectives with the light source attached directly to the underside of the dark-field condenser.

The following steps are necessary for adjustment of the microscope with the **revolving objective turret** and **the external light source:**

1. Replace bright-field or Abbé condenser with a dark-field condenser prescribed for use with microscope model being used. Insert a funnel stop in oil immersion objective. (A funnel stop is not used in a diaphragm objective, but aperture of diaphragm must be reduced for dark-field examinations.)
2. Place external illuminator equipped with an iris

diaphragm in line with and 15-20 cm from plane surface of microscope mirror.
3. Adjust iris diaphragm to a diameter of approximately 20 mm.
4. Using a piece of paper placed across mirror surface, adjust illuminator so that image of filaments of light bulb are shown in sharp focus on center area of plane side of mirror. Remove paper and adjust angle of mirror to direct light through condenser.
5. Adjust height of condenser (raising by rotating top counterclockwise; lowering by rotating top clockwise). Top of condenser should be just slightly below level of fixed stage when substage is raised to its maximum height.
6. Lower substage slightly and place 2-3 drops nondrying immersion oil on top of condenser. Place slide of proper thickness (thickness of slide to be used is engraved on top of most American-made condensers) on fixed stage and raise substage to its maximum height. Oil should make contact with underside of slide and completely cover top of condenser.
7. Focus illuminated specimen with 10 × eyepiece and 10 × (low-power or 16 mm) objective. Light should be centered in field by means of centering screws located on base of condenser. Top of condenser should be rotated up or down until smallest diameter of circular area of intense light is obtained. Following this procedure, adjustments to compensate for slight variations in slide or specimen thickness may be accomplished by racking substage condenser up or down.
8. Objective turret is rotated to bring 45 × (high-dry or 4 mm) objective into place above slide. (It is recommended that microscope be *parfocal.*) Using this combination of 10 × eyepiece and 45 × objective and focusing with fine adjustment, search specimen for suspected treponeme.
9. For identification of suspected organism, turret is rotated so that 1 drop oil can be added to top of coverslip and rotation completed to bring oil immersion lens into contact with oil, giving a continuous optical system. (If a diaphragm lens is used, it should be adjusted by rotating outer collar to

obtain proper opening and passage of light.) Examine suspected organism carefully, all focusing being done with fine adjustment knob only.

The following steps are taken with a microscope containing the **single oil immersion lens and built-in light source** attached to the underside of the condenser:

1. Check built-in light source to be sure that it is connected to rheostat, which is connected to line current. This light should be turned off when not needed for actual observation of specimen; heat generated by this type unit may be sufficient to cause a complete loss in motility of treponeme.
2. Adjust top of condenser by rotation so that it is slightly below fixed stage.
3. Place 2-3 drops oil on top of condenser.
4. Place slide of proper thickness, as engraved on top of condenser, on fixed stage directly over top of condenser. Oil film should completely cover top of condenser when in contact with bottom of slide, and slide should remain flat on stage. Adjustments are made by rotation of top of condenser: raised by rotating counter clockwise, and lowered by rotating clockwise.
5. Add 1 drop oil to no. 1 coverslip.
6. Lower oil immersion objective (equipped with a funnel stop, unless a diaphragm lens is used) until it makes contact with oil. This is observed from side by examiner.
7. Turn on light source.
8. Observed field (adjusting diaphragm lens if necessary) and adjust intensity of light on field by (1) centering mechanism, if available, and (2) rotating top of condenser.
9. Examine specimen carefully, focusing with fine adjustment knob only.

Examination. Verification of the adjustment of the dark-field microscope may be made with a specimen containing nonvirulent spiral organisms prepared from gingival scrapings suspended in a drop of physiological saline on a slide.

Using properly adjusted dark-field equipment, examine the specimens for organisms of characteristic morphology (Fig. 80-3) and motion. A careful and exhaustive search should be made before rendering a negative report. A summary of the more frequent sources of error in the use of this technic may be helpful as a checklist.

1. Preparation error
   a. Inclusion of too many refractive elements (red blood cells, air bubbles, tissue fragments, etc.)
   b. Dirty or defective glassware (fine scratches on slides and coverslips)
   c. Too thick slides and coverslips (1.3-1.5 mm slide thickness with no. 1 coverslip usually satisfactory; however, proper slide thickness usually marked on condenser)
   d. Excessive fluid between glass slide and coverslip, with too rapid flow of liquid across field of vision and too much depth to scan
   e. Too little fluid between glass slide and coverslip, with evaporation effects accentuated
   f. Forgetting to place oil between condenser and slide as well as between objective and coverslip

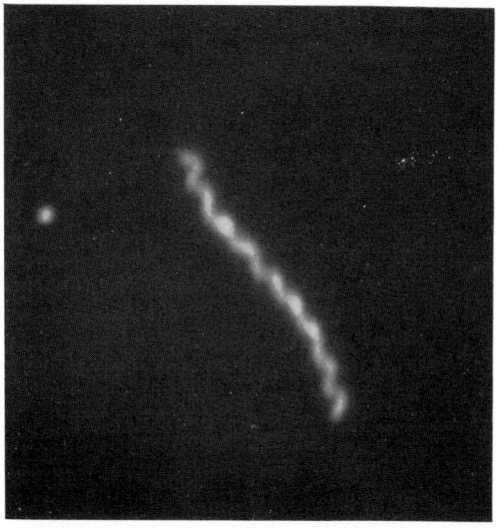

Fig. 80-3. *Treponema pallidum,* ×950 (enlarged ×60). (From *Darkfield microscopy for the detection and identification of Treponema pallidum,* Atlanta, Venereal Disease Branch, Communicable Disease Center.)

2. Condenser error
   a. Not properly centered
   b. Not properly focused
3. Objective error
   a. Too high numerical aperture used
   b. Failure to compensate high numerical aperture with funnel stop or iris diaphragm
4. Inadequate light source

As indicated previously and reemphasized here, definitive differentiation of *T. pallidum* from other treponemes and spirochetes depends not only on size and other morphologic characteristics, but also, and of equal importance, upon characteristic motility. *T. pallidum* appears to be a small spirilliform (corkscrew-shaped) organism with regularly spaced, fairly tightly wound coils. The length is usually 5-15 µm, with an average of 7 µm. This average length is slightly larger than the average red blood cell, and an occasional red blood cell in the preparation can be used as the practical criterion of length. The width seldom varies from 0.25 µm in thickness. The pitch of the spirals appears to be 1 µm. The coiled appearance is maintained despite active motility.

Characteristic movements are forward and backward (translation), rotation about the long axis like a corkscrew, and slow bending, twisting, or undulation from side to side. There is no waving or flattening, as can be noted in large saprophytic spirochetes. The most common bending is in the middle and stiffly executed, as the bending of a coil spring that comes back in place when released. Many other spirochetes have a whiplike lashing movement and rapidly move across the microscopic field, unlike *T. pallidum*.

Interpretation. The demonstration of treponemes of characteristic morphology and motility constitutes a positive diagnosis of syphilis in either primary, secondary, early congenital, or infectious relapse stages, regardless of the outcome of serologic testing. In primary syphilis it may be possible to identify the etiologic agent and to diagnose the disease prior to the appearance of detectable antibodies. Hence, the earliest and empirically most specific means of diagnosing syphilis is by dark-field microscopy.

Every genital lesion should be considered syphilitic until proved otherwise. Those extragenital lesions characterized by indolence, induration, and regional lymphadenopathy should be regarded as probably syphilitic. **Failure to find the organism does not exclude a diagnosis of syphilis.** Negative results obtained in dark-field examination may mean that organisms were not in sufficient numbers in the specimen to be noted, the patient received antitreponemal drugs locally or systemically, the lesion is "fading" or approaching natural resolution or disappearance, the lesion is one of late syphilis, or finally, the lesion is not syphilitic. **The dark-field examination should be repeated at least 3 times, and serologic follow-up should be continued for about 4 months,** at weekly intervals for the first month and biweekly intervals thereafter, before the probability of syphilis is excluded.

In performing an examination of material from suspected lesions, thought should be given to the saprophytic organisms that may normally be present in both **oral** and **genital** lesions. It is again emphasized that a satisfactory cleansing procedure be undertaken. This will tend to eliminate those organisms that reside on surrounding surface areas and may confuse the examiner. The suspected lesion should be dried and isolated as well as possible before taking the serum specimen. In the oral cavity, with care, proper cleansing, drying, and isolation, material may be collected as long as it is not at or near the edge of the gum area. *Treponema microdentium,* which can be confused with treponema pallidum, can normally be found in this area.

Borrelia-like organisms may be found in oral and genital lesions. These may be differentiated from *T. pallidum* by the variability in the length of the organism and number of spirals (3-20), the coarseness of the spirals, the rapid movement back and forth across the field exhibiting a writhing motion, and their extreme flexibility manifested in part by the relaxation of the spirals.

A practical criterion for differentiating *T. pallidum* from nonpathogenic treponemes and spirochetes found commonly in the mouth and not uncommonly upon the genitalia is that when multiple organisms are observed in microscopic fields of the slide, and all are uniform in size, shape, and motility (as described), these will most usually be *T. pallidum.* On the other hand, saprophytic organisms are usually mixed so that any 1 preparation will contain spiral forms of various sizes, shapes, and motility. It must be remembered, of course, that some lesions will contain mixed flora and *T. pallidum.* When in

doubt under such circumstances, the aspirate of the enlarged regional lymph node draining the site of the lesion will contain only *T. pallidum* (if present) and no saprophytic forms.

Caution should be used in interpreting results on slides containing numerous artifacts or refractile objects. The untrained and the unwary may be deceived by miscellaneous pieces of cellular debris, cotton strands, flagellae, cilia, and fine scratches on glass slides. These, and forms (similar to treponemes) made of spiral fibrin filaments can, with brownian movement, be deceptive. Air bubbles, hemoconiae, platelets, epithelial cells, leukocytes, and erythrocytes, with or without rouleaux formation, are other elements that can be readily recognized, but their too-frequent presence make difficult the demonstration of *T. pallidum.*

Immunofluorescent technics for identification of T. pallidum

Fluorescent antibody technics for the demonstration of *T. pallidum* in smears were first reported by Edwards,[5] who employed an **indirect FA** procedure, using serum from a known syphilitic patient (fluorescent treponemal antibody, FTA, reactive). Kellogg and Deacon[6] employed an anti–*T. pallidum* conjugate of human origin in their **direct FA** staining (the "fluorescent antibody dark-field" [FADF] method), sometimes used with a rapid immunofluorescence (RIS) staining procedure.[7] The FADF procedure was said to be as reliable as the conventional dark-field technic for the examination of syphilitic lesions by Jue et al.[8] and was found suitable for the identification of *T. pallidum* in tissues (Yobs et al.[9]; Smith and Israel[10]). (For a general discussion of FA technics see Chapter 70.)

Mothershed[11] produced a fluorescein-conjugated anti–*T. pallidum* serum (absorbed with both tissue powder and nonpathogenic Reiter treponemes, containing group treponemal antigens) from syphilitic rabbits, which is used in a standardized technic (DFATP) by the Venereal Disease Research Laboratory, Center for Disease Control.[12]* The procedure is based partly on the technic of Yobs et al.[9] and is described in detail by Mothershed.[11] It is likely that the direct immunofluorescent identification of *T. pallidum* will be increasingly used since it (1) does not seem to depend on the presence of treponemes with both characteristic motility and morphology, (2) can distinguish *T. pallidum* from saprophytic treponemes (such as those found in the mouth), and (3) also allows mailing of dry, unstained slides to a reference laboratory for confirmation of diagnostic examination. In a recent study[13] the DFATP was found to be as reliable as the dark-field test.

---

*A detailed description of the conjugate and of the technic for its use is available from the CDC, Atlanta, Ga. The conjugate is available commercially from BioQuest Division, Beckton, Dickinson & Co., Cockeysville, Md.

For details the reader is referred to the publications listed above.

Treponema pertenue

The organism is morphologically indistinguishable from *T. pallidum;* it is the causative agent of yaws or frambesia.

The treponemes are present in large numbers in primary and secondary lesions and have been demonstrated in lymph glands, spleen, and bone marrow. They have not been found in the bloodstream, but Castellani successfully infected apes by injecting blood from frambesia patients. Further evidence of their presence in the bloodstream is the dissemination of the secondary lesions over the entire body. Organisms have never been demonstrated in deep organs other than those mentioned, nor in the nodular, ulcerative, scaling, or gummatous lesions of the tertiary stage of the disease. Monkeys and rabbits, as well as apes, can be experimentally infected with frambesia. Hamsters are also susceptible.

Transmission (yaws or frambesia). *Treponema pertenue* is readily transmitted from infected persons to others by direct contact indirect contact (contaminated clothing, bedding, utensils, furniture, soil, and so on) is probably a less important means of spreading the disease. Mechanical transmission by the "gnat" fly, *Hippelates papillipes,* is possible within 7 hours after feeding on open frambesia lesions, by regurgitation of ingested material containing spirochetes. Venereal transmission does occur but is only incidental. Autoinfection may occur during the early course of the disease. Lesions frequently spread locally and to opposing contiguous surfaces, particularly the mouth, anus, and vagina. It is not believed that congenital infection occurs.

Trauma plays an important role in transmission of frambesia. It seems likely that the organisms must come in contact with an abrasion in the skin to initiate successful infection. It is generally accepted that the location of the primary lesion is also the site of infection. Primary lesions occur most frequently on exposed regions of the body that are most likely to be traumatized: the feet and legs. Crowded, unhygienic living conditions foster spread of infection in family groups. Persons of all ages are susceptible to infection with this organism, but the disease occurs most commonly in children.

Immunity. It is believed that 1 attack of yaws confers protection against another in regions where the disease is endemic, the immunity developing slowly and over a period of years. This immunity is not always complete or constant.

Diagnosis. Yaws must be differentiated from syphilis, particularly in the tertiary stages. Little aid can be obtained from the laboratory, since the etiologic agents are indistinguishable, and specific serologic tests are reactive in both diseases. Treponemes can be readily demonstrated by dark-field microscopic examination of serum from primary and secondary frambesia lesions after removal of the crusts. The usual serologic tests for syphilis, complement fixation, flocculation, and other specific tests are reactive in over 99% of patients with early frambesia. The tests become reactive 2-3 weeks after the appearance of the primary lesion. The titer increases rapidly and becomes strongly reactive during the fifth or sixth week. The tests remain reactive for months or years, occasionally becoming nonreactive in the tertiary stage (see discussion on serology, Chapter 106).

Treponema carateum

The organism is morphologically indistinguishable from *T. pallidum;* it is the causative agent of mal del pinto (pinta), a nonvenereal disease of adolescents and young adults in primitive areas of tropical Central and South America who are living under unhygienic conditions.

According to León-Blanco, the distribution of the treponemes in cutaneous lesions in humans varies for the initial lesions of mal del pinto (carate) and pintids and also for lesions of the later phase. In the initial lesions and in the pintids, treponemes are particularly abundant in the epidermis and in the intercellular spaces of the rete mucosum, especially in the acanthotic interpapillary crests, as well as in the epithelial portion of the pilosebaceous follicles. In the dermis they are localized especially in the portion occupied by the inflammatory infiltration, and they are abundant near the blood vessels. It is not exceptional to see them as they traverse the walls of these vessels. In the later phases they have been seen only in the rete mucosum and in the epithelial portion of the pilosebaceous follicles.

Distribution of mal del pinto. Mal del pinto is endemic in rural or suburban areas, stopping at the outskirts of large cities, particularly in countries with a high epidemic index. Where the disease is sporadic, it can be found in large urban centers.

In the intertropical regions of the Americas, the disease is most widely distributed in villages situated in the valleys of large rivers, at an altitude that varies from sea level to 2570 m. In some areas in this zone, incidence reaches 50-90%, whereas in localities a short distance from these zones only 1-2% of the population is affected. Apparently there is no relationship between the disease and geographic conditions. Infection is more frequently seen among inhabitants of villages and small towns situated between mountainous zones and the sea than among residents of towns that lie near the coast. In coastal zones, rural towns and villages show a higher index of infection than less urbanized areas.

In villages with high incidence of the disease it is found in family foci, although intimate contact with pintous patients is not the sole prerequisite for infection. It is frequently observed that in marriages of 1-25 years, 1 marital partner may be ill with the disease whereas the other has remained healthy.

Where the infection is sporadic, pinta is not transmitted to those who live with infected individuals.

Diagnosis. Examination for treponemes in cutaneous lesions and in glands may be carried out by silver impregnation of biopsy material. The dark-field examination may be made of serous matter obtained by puncture of the glands or by erosion and expression of cutaneous lesions. This method is the most rapid and the easiest.

Procedure

1. With a bistoury or curet, make a superficial abrasion in skin of suspected lesion.
2. Apply pressure with a pair of forceps. A few drops of serous matter will be expressed from lesion.
3. If first drops contain many red blood cells, discard until a clear drop is obtained.
4. Mount drop on a slide under a coverglass and examine by means of dark-field microscope.
5. If desired, make a smear and stain by Krajian spirochete method.

Indigenous (oral) treponemes

Oral spirochetes have been divided into 3 groups based on size and number of axial filaments.[2] *T. macrodentium, T. denticola, T. orale, T. scoliodontum,* and *T. vincentii* have been cultivated and well characterized.[1]

T. denticola (dentium, microdentium) is the name designating the small, closely wound *pallidum*-like spirochete most commonly seen in closed fusiospirochetal lesions (lung abscesses) and in the normal mouth (gingival area, tonsillar crypts) of humans. The organism has been cultivated successfully. In addition to its presence in enormous numbers in various processes

(Vincent's angina, etc.), the organism should be taken into account when dark-field examination for *T. pallidum* is carried out from oral lesions, since the inexperienced worker may readily confuse the 2 organisms.

T. denticola shows rapid rotation; when flexion is present the movements are jerky, suggesting that the organism is relatively stiff.

A group of organisms originally named *Borrelia refringens* is now classified[1] into the species *Treponema refrigens, T. vincentii,* and the poorly described *T. buccale.*

T. refringens[1] is not pathogenic; it has been isolated successfully from genital lesions by Hanson and Cannefax[14] and is part of the normal flora of male and female genitalia. *T. vincentii* and *T. buccale* are found in the oral cavity. The organisms, especially *T. vincentii,* are found in profusion in Vincent's angina, ulcerative lesions of the genitals, pulmonary infections, and gingival pyorrhea, often in association with fusobacteria and *Bacteroides* species.

Intestinal spirochaetosis

Harland and Lee[15] described an apparently common form of intestinal spirochaetosis, in which short spirochetes, tentatively classified as *Borrelia* (now *Treponema*) *eurygyrata,* are attached to and penetrate short distances into the surface epithelial cells. Diagnosis can be made on routine histologic preparations. The significance of these findings is unclear at present.

BORRELIA
Relapsing fever

Borreliae are parasitic; some are pathogenic for humans, animals, or birds. *Borrelia recurrentis* is the single species causing **louse-borne** (or

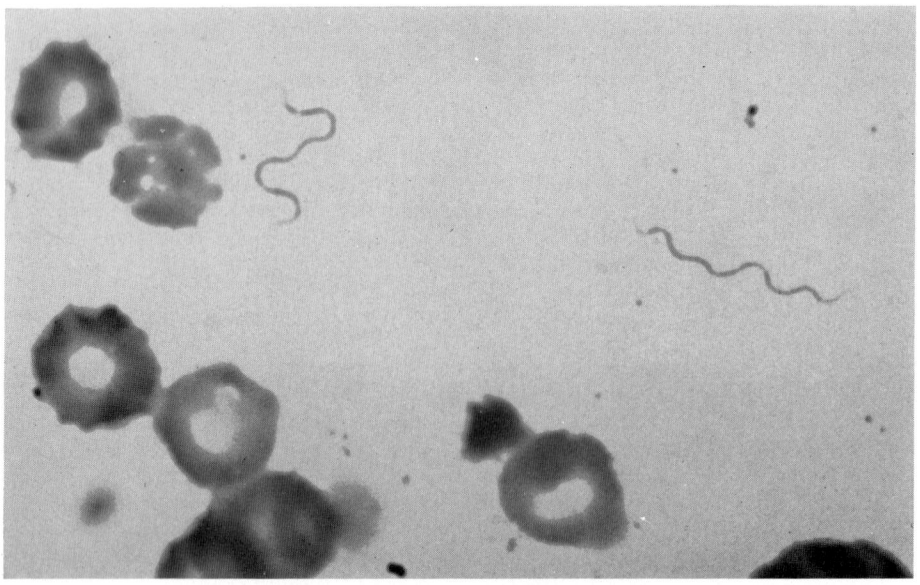

Fig. 80-4. Thin blood film showing spirochetes of relapsing fever. (Wright stain; ×2700.) (From Gradwohl, R. B. H., Benitez Soto, L., and Felsenfeld, O.: Clinical tropical medicine, St. Louis, The C. V. Mosby Co.)

epidemic) **relapsing fever** in humans. The organism is transmitted by the human louse (*Pediculus humanus* ssp. *humanus*).

Other *Borrelia* species are transmitted by soft ticks (*Ornithodoros*) and are responsible for **tickborne** (or **endemic**) **relapsing fever.** Each of these species is named after the tick species transmitting the infection.

The organisms are cylindrical or slightly flattened, with pointed ends, and measure 8-20 μm in length and 0.2-0.3 μm in diameter. Each has about 3-7 large, wavy, irregular, inconstant spirals, each spiral having an amplitude of 1.5 μm. These microorganisms are highly motile and divide by transverse fragmentation. Their spirals are larger, longer, and looser than those of the treponemes.

Borreliae stain readily with Wright, Giemsa, and other bacteriologic stains (Fig. 80-4).

Diagnosis. Tick-borne *Borrelia* species (major agents in the United States are *B. hermsii*, *B. venezuelensis*, and *B. turicatae*) have been grown in Kelly's medium A[16]; more recently, Kelly reported[17] formulations of 2 additional media that support the growth and subculture of *B. recurrentis*. (The organisms grow well in the chick embryo.) Since *Borrelia* isolates cannot presently be speciated by serologic or biochemical methods, dark-field examination, staining by Giemsa or silver stain, or inoculation of animals are the technics utilized in diagnostic work. Serodiagnosis (demonstration of anti–*Borrelia* antibodies) is not generally used; in some cases of relapsing fever, rising *Proteus* OX-K or OX-19 agglutination titers have been described.

Morphologically all the so-called species and strains are identical. Clinically the diseases produced are similar.

During the febrile period the motile spirochetes with lashing movements may be demonstrated in a fresh wet preparation of the patient's blood by dark-field examination, preferably with a high-power, dry objective.

Stained thin or thick blood films are valuable for detection of the microorganisms in the blood.

When the central nervous system is involved, the spirochetes can be demonstrated at times in the cerebrospinal fluids.

Inoculation of laboratory rats with the patient's blood has also been used for diagnosis.

Procedure
1. Place about 5-10 ml patient's blood, taken during febrile period, in a sterile test tube containing a few glass beads and defibrinate by shaking.
2. Inoculate each of 2 rats with 1 or 2 ml defibrinated blood.
3. From second to seventh day examine rat's blood each day for presence of *Borrelia*.
4. Sample of defibrinated blood may be refrigerated for several weeks before inoculation of rats if necessary. Defibrinated blood containing borrelia stored in a refrigerator for 2 or 3 mo still retains its power to infect susceptible test animals.

Laboratory findings. During the febrile period, albuminuria is usually present. The leukocyte count is elevated to about 10,000-20,000 while there is fever. In some cases of louse-borne infections, *Proteus* OX-K agglutinins are present in high titer.

Disease and distribution. Infection with *B. recurrentis* (**louse-borne relapsing fever**) is acquired when a human scratches the area of a louse bite and crushes the *borrelia*-infected louse; the borrelia thus released enter the broken skin. The disease is characterized by recurrent fevers separated by periods of apparent wellbeing. During febrile periods, the borrelia are present in the blood; they are absent during afebrile periods. Since lice prefer 37 C temperature, they leave the febrile patient after feeding on him and becoming infected themselves. Eventually they bite the new host, and if crushed and injured, release borrelia, thus accounting for the spread. Poor personal hygiene, overcrowding, and poverty, usually associated with natural disasters (floods, earthquakes) or wars, favor the multiplication of human lice and the occurrence of louse-borne relapsing fever. Humankind is the reservoir for louse-borne relapsing fever; the borrelia are not transmitted transovarially in the louse.[2] The disease is often found in close association with louse-borne typhus, and in some cases mixed infections of typhus and relapsing fever coexist. Apparently there is no reservoir host other than man in louse-borne relapsing fever, and therefore delousing of people and of their clothing is an effective means of limiting the spread of the disease.

Epidemics have occurred in Asia, Africa, Europe, and America; it is estimated that some 10 million cases occurred during World War II. Most reports of louse-borne relapsing fever now originate in East Afria (Ethiopia, Sudan); the disease is not seen anymore in the United States.

Tick-borne relapsing fever usually occurs sporadically. Infected ticks transmit the spirochetes by biting man. The soft ticks that are known to be naturally infected are *Ornithodorus parkeri*, *O. hermsi*, *O. rudis*, *O. talaje*, *O. moubata*, *O. asperus*, *O. turicata*, *O. tholozani*, *O. erraticus*, and *O. verrucosus*.

The soft tick remains infected for life and passes the infection through its egg; thus *Ornithodoros* is the principal host for the tick-borne borrelia. Man is an accidental host; the borreliae are maintained between the animal hosts and the ticks. Tick-borne relapsing fever exists worldwide with the exception of Oceania, New Zealand, and Australia.

Tick-borne relapsing fever is endemic in the Western part of the United States; recently its presence east of the Mississippi has been reported by Linnemann, et al.[18]

Borrelia refringens. See discussion on Indigenous (oral) treponemes.

Intestinal spirochaetosis. See discussion on *Treponema*.

For an excellent review of *Borrelia* strains, vectors, and human and animal borreliosis, see Felsenfeld's monograph.[9]

LEPTOSPIRA

The genus *Leptospira* belongs to the family *Spirochaetaceae*. The organisms are characterized by a flexible threadlike structure consisting of a large number of fine, regular spiral coils. The amplitude of each coil is approximately 0.5 μm. The length of the entire *Leptospira* usually varies between 6-20 μm. Degenerative forms may reach a length of 40 μm. The width is constant, approximately 0.25 μm. Multiplication is by transverse fission, which may be seen under the microscope.

Leptospirae are visible under the **dark-field microscope**. They look like strings of very closely packed small beads. In liquid media both ends are usually hooked, the center part is rather rigid, and they move slowly through the field, with rapid rotation on the long axis (Fig. 80-5). In viscid media they seem to have some traction and acquire some speed; the middle part appears flexible, the movement becoming snakelike. The ends at times exhibit a whipping motion. They should not be confused with the so-called pseudoleptospirae, which are threadlike fibrin structures expelled from blood cells in blood specimens; these show brownian movement and movement caused by currents in the liquid and are often mistaken for true *Leptospira*.

Leptospira can usually be grown in artificial media; oxygen is required. They are able to pass through the pores of various filters because of their great flexibility, their extreme thinness, and their actively boring movements.

Leptospirae are not stained with simple dyes such as gentian violet. They are stained readily by the **Giemsa** method in blood films and in tissue sections by **silver impregnation** (see below). The primary coils are invisible with the usual fixatives, but good results can be obtained by staining films after drying without preliminary fixation.

Giemsa stain. Use a strong solution with faintly alkaline water.
1. Stain at 37 C for 30 min.
2. Pour off and restain with dilute Giemsa at 37 C for another 30 min.
3. Wash and examine.

Victoria blue may also give good results. Slides should be clean and fat-free. Wash stain off carefully by allowing water to drip on stain-covered glass and rinsing precipitate with water. Leptospirae stain violet, and separate coils can be seen distinctly.

Method of Van Riel.[20] Mix 5 drops *Leptospira* culture with 4 drops May-Grünwald solution and 3 drops distilled water. After 10 min, make smears and examine after drying.

Van Orden Spirochaete Stain.* Because of the capriciousness of staining methods available for

demonstrating spirochetal organisms in **tissue** and the need for a large volume staining technic, the following method has been adapted at the Center for Disease Control, with the Dieterle method as a reference. (This method is similar to the modification used for staining Legionnaire's disease bacillus.)

Materials
1. Rabbit testes were fixed in 10% buffered formalin. Dehydration process (on Technicon [Technicon Instruments, Tarrytown, N.Y.]).
   70% Alcohol, 2 changes (1 h each)
   95% Alcohol, 2 changes (1 h each)
   Absolute alcohol, 2 changes (1 h each)
   Absolute alcohol, chloroform equal parts, 1 change (1 h)
   Chloroform, 2 changes (1 h each)
   Paraffin I, 2 h
   Paraffin II, 2 h
   Paraffin III, for embedding
2. Tissue was embedded and cut 2-4 μm and picked up on albumined slides. Slides were placed in oven at 58-50 C to adhere sections to slide and melt paraffin.
3. Glass staining racks were used, and 10 slides were stained. Hand dipping was eliminated. A known control slide was placed in each rack.

Staining and other solutions
5% Uranium nitrate in 70% alcohol.
10% Fischer gum mastic in absolute alcohol. Allow 2 days to dissolve; filter and stopper well.
1% Silver nitrate. Refrigerate.

Developer solution	$\frac{1}{2}$ original	Other proportions $\frac{1}{2}$ second volume
1. Mix in this order:		
Hydroquinone: 15.0 g	7.5 g	3.75 g
Sodium sulfite: 2.5 g	1.25 g	.625 g
Distilled water: 600 ml*	300 ml	150 ml
Acetone: 100 ml*	50 ml	25 ml
Formalin: 100 ml*	50 ml	25 ml
Pyridine: knocks out bone marrow: 100 ml*	50 ml	25 ml
10% gum mastic in absolute alcohol: 100 ml	50 ml	25 ml

2. Solution turns milky as gum mastic is added, and medium brown on standing.
3. Mix. Store in clear bottle.

Staining and developing procedure
1. Place 1% silver in staining dish in oven to preheat.
2. Xylene I.
3. Xylene II.
4. Absolute alcohol.
5. 95% Alcohol.
6. Distilled water.
7. 5% Alcoholic uranium nitrate in oven at 10 C 3 min. When uranium nitrate precipitates on bottle, make up fresh. Precipitation is due to dirty glassware.
8. Distilled water, 1 dip.
9. 95% Alcohol, 1 dip.
10. 10% Gum mastic, 3 min.
11. 95% Alcohol, 1 dip.
12. Distilled water. Dip for 1 min and drain for 5.

---

*From Sulzer, C. R., and Jones, W. L.[21]

*Shake gently as this solution is added.

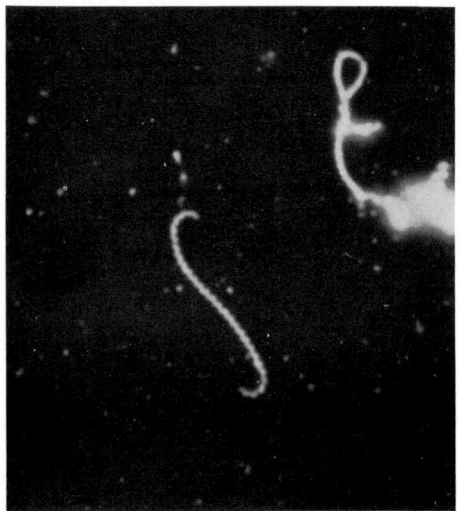

Fig. 80-5. *Leptospira icterohaemorrhagiae.* (Dark field; ×1800.) (Photograph by Prof. T. Y. Kingma Boltjes.)

Turns milky, and gum mastic should adhere to tissue so reticulum will not take silver.
13. 1% Silver nitrate, 55 to 58 C in dark for 4 h.
14. Distilled water, 2 dips.
15. Developer. Dip until pale yellow to golden brown. Cannot overdevelop. After carrying slides through and mounting, leave them under light to make them turn bright yellow. Do not let oven go over 60 C because silver will precipitate out. This step should be done under a hood.
16. Distilled water, 1 dip.
17. 95% Alcohol.
18. Acetone.
19. Xylene I.
20. Xylene II.
21. Mount.

Results. Spirochetes turn black; background turns yellow to light brown. Impression smears for suspected leptospirosis were stained successfully by this method.

Cultivation[21]

Leptospirae have no complicated growth requirements but will grow in rather simple media, a few examples of which follow.

Stuart medium[22]

Asparagine	0.132 g
Ammonium chloride	0.268 g
Magnesium chloride·6H₂O	0.406 g
Sodium chloride	1.808 g
Disodium phosphate	0.666 g
Monopotassium phosphate	0.087 g
Phenol red	0.01 g
Glycerin	5 ml
Distilled water	995 ml

1. Sterilize by autoclaving at 15 psi for 15 min.
2. Cool to less than 50° and **add 8-10% sterile rabbit serum.**
3. Mix well and dispense aseptically.
pH should be 7.4-7.6.
Base is available commercially in dehydrated form (Difco Laboratories, Detroit).

Fletcher medium[23]

Peptone	0.3 g

Beef extract	0.2 g
Sodium chloride	0.5 g
Agar	1.5 g
Distilled water	920 ml

1. Sterilize by autoclaving for 15 min at 15 psi.
2. Cool to 50 C; **add 8-10% sterile rabbit serum.**
3. Mix well. Dispense aseptically and inactivate at 56 C for 1 h on day it is dispensed and 1 h following day. pH should be 7.6-8.
4. Check sterility by incubating for 24 h at 37 **and** for 24 h at 30 C.

Medium is available commercially in dehydrated form (Difco Laboratories; BioQuest).

Vervoort medium, modified by Wolff-Schüffner

Peptone (Witte or Difco proteose no. 3)	1 g
Ringer solution	200 ml
Sørensen phosphate buffer, pH 7.2	100 ml

1. Dissolve in 1000 ml distilled water.
2. Boil until phosphates have been precipitated and filter after cooling. Distribute into small tubes.
3. Sterilize at 100 C. pH is 6.9-7.0.
4. Add 10% sterile rabbit serum and inactivate at 56 C for 30 min. Some rabbit sera agglutinate leptospirae and cannot be used in medium; each rabbit serum must be previously tested.

Noguchi medium

Rabbit serum	1.5 parts
Ringer solution	4.5 parts
Agar, 2%	1 part
Paraffin oil to cover surface	

Noguchi used this medium also in combination with a fluid medium consisting of 1.5 parts rabbit serum and 4.5 parts Ringer's solution poured over solid medium, the whole covered with paraffin oil. A drop of rabbit hemoglobin (1 part defibrinated rabbit blood and 3 parts distilled water) may be added to improve results.

Other media. Various other media such as that of **Cox** (solid medium)[24] and that of Ellinghausen and McCullough, as modified by Johnson and Harris[25] (**EMJH** medium with enrichment), are also used (Difco Laboratories, Detroit).

Other requisites. Leptospirae must be cultivated under aerobic conditions. The optimum temperature for rapid growth in 37 C, but lower temperatures are necessary to keep the cultures alive. **Incubation is usually at 30 C.**

Contaminated cultures can be freed of bacteria by passing them through a membrane filter, by inoculating culture tubes with serial dilutions of the specimen, or by inoculating laboratory animals. The addition of neomycin (final concentrations of 5 μg and 25 μg/ml) to Fletcher's medium is useful in controlling contaminating bacteria.[26]

Viability and resistance

Leptospirae show remarkable viability in cultures. Cultures in Vervoort medium kept in the dark at room temperature without subculturing sometimes remain alive for years. In the semisolid medium of Noguchi a thick layer of leptospirae grows 10-12 mm below the surface, and these organisms may remain fully virulent for years. They do not withstand drying.

Leptospirae are sensitive to acid reaction. They are killed quickly in acid urine. To isolate them from urine, it is advisable to alkalinize the urine by keeping the patient on an appropriate diet for some days before collecting the specimen. They are not sensitive to salts. They may remain alive in seawater for several hours, but they disappear more quickly from salt and brackish water than from fresh water. In undiluted milk they survive only for a short time.

They are killed at 50 C in 10 minute but tolerate low temperatures well. They cannot be preserved by lyophilization, but after quick freezing they can be kept alive at −70 C for several years[27] without losing their virulence.

They have little resistance against the various disinfectants such as iodine and chlorine. Bile kills them quickly. They are not susceptible to sulfonamide drugs.

Classification (species, serotypes) and distribution; leptospirosis

In 1963 the Taxonomic Subcommittee on Leptospira (ICBN) recommended that the genus *Leptospira* be divided into 2 species: *L. interrogans*, representing parasitic strains, and *L. biflexa*, saprophytic strains. Both species were divided into numerous serologic types (**serotypes**). All the pathogenic types seemed to be distinct from the nonpathogenic *L. biflexa* (found in stagnant water, streams, and lakes). In 1967 a World Health Organization expert group[28] recommended that the genus be considered monospecific until it is possible to describe species with confidence. As a result, only one species, *Leptospira interrogans*, was recognized[1,2] as of 1977. Within the genus, however, two "complexes" are recognized: the free-living, saprophytic *Leptospira* are grouped in the **biflexa** complex, while the parasitic (and pathogenic) *Leptospira* are contained in the **interrogans** (or **parasitic**) complex.

The **biflexa** complex organisms are mostly found in surface waters (both fresh and saline). These organisms have also been isolated from bovine urine, horse kidney tissue, frog kidney, and turtles; these isolates do not cause infections in laboratory animals.[2]

The **interrogans** complex includes some 160 **serologic types** (**serovariants**) assembled into 18 **serogroups** on the basis of antigenic relationships. Leptospirosis is worldwide and represents one of the most widespread zoonoses. The pathogenic leptospira occur mostly in domestic animals and rodents, with their habitat being the proximal tubules of the kidneys of the animals and rodents. The leptospira are shed into the urine, and contact with urine containing leptospira (or with contaminated water or soil) results in infection; man is an accidental host. The major source of human leptospirosis in the United States is the dog; recently Feigin et al.[29] demonstrated heavy infection rates among rats in a residential setting as well as human infections transmitted by *immunized* dogs. Thus infection and excretion of leptospira (leptospiruria) can occur even in healthy immunized animals, with subsequent transmission of the infection to humans.

Leptospirosis has been regarded mostly as an occupational disease; however, with increasing time and frequency of recreational pursuits and more frequent contact with wilderness areas and thus wildlife reservoirs, a significant percentage of cases occurs in humans with occupations not usually associated with high risk of leptospirosis.

Human leptospirosis may manifest itself, as an inapparent (subclinical) infection at one end of the spectrum and with meningitis, shock, azotemia, renal involvement, and liver disease at the other extreme. In mild cases a first (septicemic) stage, characterized by presence of leptospira in the blood and spinal fluid, and a second (immune) stage, with development of antibodies, can be distinguished; in severe disease the distinction between the 2 stages is less clear.[29] In a high proportion of patients meningitis develops and leptospiruria occurs. The most common nonspecific symptoms are headache, nausea, vomiting, and mild myalgia. Jaundice occurs frequently in severe forms of the disease.

While the organisms are sensitive in vitro to a number of antibiotics (penicillin G, streptomycin, tetracyclines, erythromycin), the efficacy of antibiotic therapy is limited: It is of questionable value even when given within 48 hours of onset and useless when given later than 48 hours. Large doses of penicillin given within 2-3 days of onset may be of some value.

For a review of human leptospirosis, see Finegold and Meyer,[30] Feigin et al.,[29] and Turner.[31]

Laboratory diagnosis[21]

The diagnosis of leptospirosis can be established by (1) demonstration of the organism and (2) detection of antibody.

Demonstration of organism

Microscopy. Dark-field microscopy is used as screening for leptospira in urine and blood; the procedure is not particularly reliable (see "pseudoleptospirae," above). **Blood** or **spinal fluid** may be examined during the first week of illness; **urine,** on the other hand, should be examined toward the end of the second week, up to 40 days.[30]

Centrifugal method. With this **method,** leptospirae may be demonstrated in the blood in some cases during the first days of the illness.

1. Mix 1 part 1% sodium oxalate solution in phosphate buffer, pH 8.1, with 9 parts blood.
2. Centrifuge 15 min at 1500 rpm.
3. Examine clear plasma under dark-field microscope with low magnification. If no leptospirae are found, centrifuge remainder of the plasma for 20 min at 10,000 rpm. Sediment might show leptospirae.
4. Blood collected in SPS (see discussion on blood culture, Chapter 75) (15-20 ml blood in 4 ml 1% sodium polyanetholsulfonate in saline) can be used for dark-field examination after first centrifu-

gation, and sediment can be obtained from plasma.

This rapid method, which permits an early diagnosis within ½ hour after the sample has been taken, is not absolutely reliable. At times microscopically negative blood yields positive cultures or animal inoculations.

Dark-field microscopy is also used for detecting leptospira in culture media previously inoculated with specimen.

Fluorescent antibody (FA) technic is used in some laboratories for the demonstration of leptospira in the urinary sediment. Urine can be submitted in vials of formalinized, buffered saline solution. The technic has also been used for tissue preparations. For details see Coffin and Maestrone[32] and White et al.[33]

Culture. This is the most reliable method, but often positive results are obtained only after 1½-4 weeks. **Blood** should be cultured as follows.

1. Inoculate 3-5 tubes of a semisolid medium (Stuart, Fletcher, and so on) with 0.03 ml blood (1-2 drops) 5 ml medium.
2. Preferably freshly drawn blood, **drawn between second and tenth day of illness,** should be used, but blood with anticoagulants (see SPS, above) can also be used.
3. Incubate at 30 C for 4 wk. Examine a loopful of culture every 7-10 d by dark-field microscopy (use low- and high-dry magnification).

Culture of blood is rarely successful much beyond the first week of the disease.

Urine should be cultured from the second week on repeatedly, since leptospirae may appear in the **urine** from the beginning of the second week of illness and may be present for another 40-50 days. Direct examination by dark-field microscopy sometimes shows leptospiral in great numbers. If the urine is acid, most of them will be dead and will show the typical rigid appearance. Passage through a susceptible animal (guinea pig, hamster) is necessary to isolate them from urine.

The patient should be given an alkalinizing diet a few days before the specimen is to be collected, to prevent the damage by acid urine. The simplest way to obtain a positive result is to take the second portion of urine of the day and to inoculate the animals intraperitoneally with 1 ml freshly excreted urine at the bedside of the patient. Urine sent to the laboratory seldom contains living leptospirae.

Voided urine can be cultured if the sample is first diluted in buffered saline as follows[34]:

1. Dilute 1840 ml 0.85% physiologic saline solution with 160 ml Sørensen buffer, final pH 7.6
2. With a sterile 2 ml syringe and 20-gauge needle, inoculate 1 drop undiluted urine into a tube of Fletcher medium.
3. With same syringe dilute urine by discharging all but 0.1 ml from syringe and drawing up 0.9 ml buffered saline.
4. Inoculate 1 drop of this 1:10 dilution into 5 ml Fletcher medium.
5. Continue this procedure for 4 additional dilutions.

Alexander[34] states that urine obtained aseptically (e.g., by perforation of bladder) can be cultured directly. Since the undiluted urine may contain growth-inhibiting substances, 1:10 and 1:100 dilutions in saline should also be cultured.

Postmortem material (liver and kidney tissue are preferred) should be examined. The demonstration of leptospirae at autopsy may be possible by dark-field examination of smears from the liver, kidneys, or adrenals. In tissues the silver impregnation method will show leptospirae in these organs. Cultures are useful only immediately after death. In all other cases animal passage is necessary. In chronic animal carriers (rats, dogs, mice, but not rabbits or man) the process in the kidneys is sharply localized to limited parts of the cortical substance; leptospirae will be found in layers on the epithelium of the convoluted tubules. Several organs must be examined before a diagnosis of leptospiral infection can be excluded.

Urine aspirated from the bladder should be cultured (see above).

Kidney tissue should be cultured as follows:

1. Grind with sterile sand.
2. Dilute 1:10 (9 ml Stuart medium or pH 7.2 sterile buffered saline/g tissue) and mix well.
3. Inoculate into Fletcher medium (3 drops into each of 2 tubes).
4. Continue dilutions in syringe as described under urine and inoculate medium.

Cerebrospinal fluid should be cultured in spite of the rarity of isolation of leptospira from spinal fluid. If collected during the first 10 days of illness, the fluid should be cultured by the same method as is blood. Use 0.5 ml fluid for inoculating 5 ml Fletcher medium. Animal inoculations are also indicated.

All leptospiral cultures should be incubated at 30 C. Examine culture tubes with dark-field microscopy at 5- to 7-day intervals[35] as follows.

1. Obtain a small drop a few cm below surface of fluid cultures or from area of linear disk indicating growth of leptospira in semisolid media (1-3 cm below surface; note that absence of disk does not rule out growth of leptospira).
2. Place drop on slide and coverslip.
3. Examine with dark-field microscopy, first with 150 × (low) and then with 450 × (high) dry magnification.

Transfer positive culture to fresh medium; inoculate fresh medium heavily (transfer about 10% original culture). Maintain **stock culture** in Fletcher medium; leptospira will survive for 6-8 wk. They can also be stored, for long-term preservation, by liquid nitrogen refrigeration.[34]

Animal inoculation. Use young guinea pigs, 150-200 g; preferably also weanling hamsters[34] should be used because these animals are sensitive to leptospirae that are only slightly pathogenic for guinea pigs. Gerbils and chinchillas can also be used.

1. Inoculation should be made into peritoneal cavity with 0.5 ml blood.

2. Daily examinations of peritoneal fluid from third day on may show leptospirae even when animal is not ill.
3. If animal develops fever, blood is usually positive, and pure cultures may be obtained by inoculation with blood, obtained by puncture of heart, of suitable media.
4. Guinea pigs dying of leptospirosis show hemorrhages and mostly a severe jaundice. At autopsy liver and kidneys sometimes contain leptospirae in abundance; in other cases very few or none are found. Adrenals are always positive.

White mice are also used; they are susceptible to many strains of leptospirae, but one must bear in mind that white mice may also be spontaneously infected. Ruys et al.[36] found 2 colonies of white mice to be heavily infected with *ballum* serotype organisms that were excreted in large quantities. One must be sure that colony of mice in use is free from spontaneous infection.

Surface water is often the source of infection with parasitic leptospirae, but it is difficult to demonstrate these microorganisms in the water. Microscopically they cannot be distinguished from the nonpathogenic leptospirae, which are often found in water.

A reliable method is that of van Thiel, which brings the warmed water (37 C) into immediate contact with the tissues of susceptible animals either by bathing guinea pigs with an abraded skin in the suspected water or by letting the water flow through the subcutaneous tissue of the animal. By this method even small numbers of pathogenic leptospirae can be isolated.[37]

Detection of antibody: serologic diagnosis

Serologic studies are of great value in diagnosis of leptospirosis. Serum is usually tested, but antibodies can also be found in urine. The antibodies do not usually appear before the seventh to tenth day of the illness. They then increase rapidly and reach the highest titer in the third or fourth week. The reliability of this method depends, however, on the number of strains with which the serum is tested and the method used. (For details see discussion on serology, Chapter 107.)

Antigenic structure and identification of leptospiral serogroups and serotypes

As mentioned earlier, some 160 serotypes (serovariants) of the *interrogans* complex, assembled in 18 serogroups, are known.

The various parasitic strains cause almost the same clinical picture in humans, the differences being unimportant and only in degree. In addition, virulence for animals is not a reliable means of differentiation, even though the pathogenicity of the various types for experimental animals is not the same. Thus far the only reason, but a most important one, for antigenic differentiation is the difference in epidemiology. The serologically different strains often show a quite distinct parasite-host relationship and hence a typical epidemiologic behavior.

The "classification" of leptospirae in serogroups and serotypes is based on various serologic tests (i.e., microagglutination and agglutinin absorption) as discussed by the World Health Organization's expert group on leptospirosis.[28]

Antisera from patients or sera prepared by injection of cultures into rabbits agglutinate cultures of leptospirae often a in high titer.

Because of the faint visibility of the leptospirae in ordinary light, the agglutination is poorly visible macroscopically. Concentrated formalin-killed cultures may show agglutination visible to the naked eye, but unfortunately with these antigens the titers are lower and a much greater quantity of cultures is needed. For rapid **large-scale screening tests** formalin-killed suspensions of leptospirae may be used. The sera are tested **macroscopically** with these antigens on glass slides.[38]

Procedure. In this test leptospirae grown in Stuart medium are killed with formalin (final concentration, 0.5%). After centrifugation, packed leptospirae are resuspended in a solution containing 0.5% formalin, 12% sodium chloride, and 20% glycerin (cells from 40 ml culture). Often pooled antigens are used.

For **serogrouping** (classification as to serogroup; (a group of 2 or more leptospiral serotypes that show close antigenic relationships are considered as a **serogroup**) living cultures are necessary, and the **microscopic agglutination test with live (growing) culture** should be used, as follows:

1. Serial dilutions of standardized rabbit sera (usually a battery of sera against 10-12 serotypes) are prepared with buffered saline (1:25-1:3200). To 0.2 ml serum dilution, 0.2 ml antigen is added.
2. Tubes are shaken and incubated at 30 C for 3 h.
3. A drop from each tube is examined by dark-field microscopy. Degree of agglutination or "lysis" or both is read as negative, 1+ (25% leptospira agglutinated), 2+ (50%), 3+ (75%), or 4+ (75-100%). Endpoint is taken as last dilution showing a 2+ reaction.

In the lower dilutions of a strongly active serum, agglutination is clearly visible; in the higher dilutions, lysis complicates the picture. The conglomerates of agglutinated leptospirae begin to show signs of lysis until at the end only shapeless balls can be found, and finally nothing is seen except a few freely floating single leptospirae. Attention must be called to the fact that sometimes "nests" of leptospirae grow in rich cultures. These may resemble agglutinated leptospirae. In the "nests," however, each leptospira is entire and actively moving; in agglutinated conglomerates the leptospirae have a damaged appearance and the movements finally cease.

Using the above-described test, tentative classification into serogroups can be obtained. For definitive identification the culture should be sent to a leptospira reference laboratory (see agglutinin-absorption procedure below). To

Table 80-1. Important *Leptospira* serogroups and serotypes*

Serogroups and serotypes	Geography	Human disease	Principal animal host	Additional animal host(s)	Note
L. icterohaemorrhagiae	Worldwide	"Weil's disease"	Rattus norvegicus	Other rats, mice, dog, fox, sheep, pig, horse, cattle	Biotypes AB and A and other serotypes
L. canicola	Worldwide	Canicola fever	Dog	Horse, cattle, pig, jackal, hedgehog, golden hamster	
L. pyrogenes	S.E. Asia, U.S.A., Europe	Febrile spirochetosis	Rattus brevicaudatus	Other rodents	Syn. L. salinem
L. ballum	U.S.A., Europe, Canada	(Leptospirosis) Rice-field fever	Mus musculus albus	Other rodents, horse, cow, dog, rabbit, raccoon, fox	
L. pomona	Europe, N. and S. America, Australia, Indonesia, Middle East	Swineherd's disease	Pig	Cattle, horse, rodents, skunk, wildcat	Syn. L. suis, L. australis C
L. hebdomadis	U.S.A., Japan, S.E. Asia, Europe	Seven-day fever	Microtus montebelloi	Cattle, dog, other rodents	L. wolffi and L. medamensis belong to hebdomadis group
L. sejroe†	U.S.A., C.S. Europe, S.E. Asia	Sejroe fever	Mus spicilegus Apodemus sylvaticus	Other rodents, horse, dog, cattle	
L. saxkoebing†	Europe	(Leptospirosis)	Apodemus flavicollis Apodemus sylvaticus	Cattle	
L. grippotyphosa	S. and E. Europe, S.E. Asia, Israel, Africa, U.S.A.	Swamp or mud fever Harvest fever	Microtus arvalis	Other rodents, cattle, raccoon, skunk	L. bovis may be subtype
L. autumnalis	Japan, S.E. Asia, U.S.A.	Autumnalis fever Fort Bragg fever Pretibial fever	Rattus brevicaudatus Apodemus speciosus	M. montebelloi Dog, guinea pig	Serologic biotypes are AB (akiyami A), A (rachmat incomplete), bangkinang
L. bataviae	Africa, Europe, S.E. Asia	Rice-field fever Water fever Indonesian Weil's disease	Rattus norvegicus Micromys minutus soricinus	Other rodents, pig, cat, dog	L. oryzeti identical
L. tarassovi (hyos)†	C.S. Europe, S. America, Australasia	Swineherd's disease	Pig	Horse, cattle, opossum	
L. australis	Widespread	Swamp fever Cane fever	Rattus culmorum Rattus conatus	Other rats, dog, horse, cattle	
L. javanica	S.E. Asia, Europe	(Leptospirosis)	Rattus concolor Rattus brevicaudatus	Other rats, cat	

*Revised from original data of A. C. Ruys, J. W. Wolff, and associates (Schüffner Laboratory) and from Alston, J. M., and Broom, J. C.: Leptospirosis in man and animals, Edinburgh, 1958, E. & S. Livingstone, Ltd.

†Serotype.

avoid the danger of working with living leptospirae and to have a stock of antigen ready at
hand, some laboratories use the **microscopic agglutination test with formalin-killed cultures.**
Use chemically pure formalin; not more than
0.5% impurities may cause nonspecific acid agglutination. When dead cultures are used,
however, the lysis is absent, and agglutination
becomes manifest in much higher dilutions than
with living cultures, in which this phenomenon
has been obscured by the lysis. The titer of the
sera tested with killed antigens is on the whole
somewhat lower than it is when the titer of lysis
is determined with living ones. The incubation
time in this test (killed antigens) is usually at
52 C for 2 hours, then 4 C for 1 hour. Examination
for agglutination under dark field is carried out as
with the live antigens. The results with these
antigens are less specific than with living organisms. The formalin antigens can be kept for a
limited time only (1-2 weeks), because clumping
begins sooner or later, probably caused by formic
acid originating from the formalin under the
influence of light.

Complement-fixation tests are also used, but
their utilization is limited to research laboratories.[39]

**Determination of antigenic structure and
definitive identification.** To determine the antigenic structure of a strain, monovalent rabbit sera
are used, which should have a titer of not less
than 10,000. They agglutinate and lyse strains of
the same serotype to the same titer or sometimes
less, the lowest being $^1/_{10}$ of the titer. Other serotypes may show a strong coreaction, but they do
not reach more than ⅓ of the titer.

Some **serotypes** are serologically closely
related (L. canicola–L. icterohaemorrhagiae);
others are independent (L. bataviae). For an
exact diagnosis, however, **agglutinin-absorption
tests** (usually performed by reference laboratories) are necessary, especially in those cases in
which coreactions are strong.

The **agglutinin-absorption** test first described
by Ruys and Schüffner[40] and improved by
Schüffner and Bohlander[41] is performed as follows:

1. Use a well-grown culture in Vervoort medium,
   killed with 0.5% formalin. Centrifuge 100 ml of
   this culture for 20 min at 10,000 rpm.
2. Pipet off supernatant fluid.
3. Mix remaining 0.45 ml concentrated culture with
   0.05 ml serum diluted to a titer of 1:3000.
4. The antibodies are fixed within 4 h, but mixture
   can be left overnight at room temperature.
5. Centrifuge at 10,000 rpm for 5 min and use supernatant fluid for agglutination tests.

It is difficult to absorb serum with many strains
because a *Liptospira* culture cannot be entirely
deposited at the bottom of a tube, and some fluid
remains in the tube. The serum is diluted with
the remaining culture fluid, and it may become
too greatly diluted if more strains were used. No
absolutely monovalent sera are available. Strains

of the same serotype remove antibodies from a
serum; strains of a related one, only those belonging to the strain itself. The clear-cut results obtained with this method allow exact identification.

Attention is called to the procedure described
by Galton et al.,[34,38] the use of which circumvents
some of the difficulties enumerated above.

Several serotypes are now recognized as serologic and biologic entities in which there is correlation with a distinct epidemiologic behavior.
However, strains considered to be of the same
serotype may show minor serologic differences.
It has been demonstrated, for example, that the
classic Weil strains fall into 2 groups, one complete with the antigens A and B, the other incomplete with only A. Both behave alike pathologi-
cally and epidemiologically so that they may be
considered as 2 biotypes.

A number of other strains have been more or
less exhaustively examined.[42] In Table 80-1 a survey is given of those serotypes that are most
frequently isolated throughout the world. In the
United States, 20 common-source outbreaks of
leptospirosis were reported between 1939 and
1974. The infecting serogroups were *pomona* (10
outbreaks), *autumnalis* (3), *canicola* (3), *icterohaemorrhagiae* (3), and undetermined (1).[43] Between 1965 and 1974 a total of 791 cases of leptospirosis was reported in the United States. The
only states not reporting any cases in the last 70
years are Alaska, North Dakota, and Vermont. It
is generally believed that the disease is underre-
ported, partly because of difficulties in diagnostic
laboratory procedures, but also possibly because
of the low index of suspicion on the part of the
physician.

The most common serogroups (serotypes) responsible for human infections in the first half of
the 1970s in the United States were *icterohaemorrhagiae, canicola, autumnalis, pomona;*
more rarely, *ballum, bataviae, sejroe, grippotyphosa,* and *australis* were involved.

Variability. Until now real variation in serologic behavior has not been observed. No conclusive animal experiments have ever shown a
transition of one type into another. However, exposure of leptospirae to specific antisera led to
the appearance of antigenic variants[44]; results of
such studies suggest that antigenic variability
(instability) may occur in nature.

For further details of diagnostic procedures,
pathogenesis, taxonomy, epidemiology, and therapy see *Current Problems in Leptospirosis Research,*[28] Third report of the Joint FAO/WHO
Expert Committee on Zoonoses,[45] and *Biology of
the Parasitic Spirochetes.*[46]

REFERENCES

1. Buchanan, R. E., and Gibbons, N. E., editors:
   Bergey's manual of determinative bacteriology,
   ed. 8, Baltimore, 1974, The Williams & Wilkins
   Company.
2. Johnson, R. C.: Ann. Rev. Microbiol. **31:**89, 1977.

3. Hudson, E. H.: Treponematosis, New York, 1946, Oxford University Press.
4. Darkfield microscopy for the detection and identification of *Treponema pallidum*, Atlanta, 1962, Center for Disease Control. Reprinted 1974.
5. Edwards, E. A.: Public Health Rep. **77**:427, 1962.
6. Kellogg, D. S., Jr., and Deacon, W. E.: Bacteriol. Proc., p. 60, 1965, abstr. M128.
7. Kellogg, D. S., Jr., and Deacon, W. E.: Proc. Soc. Exp. Biol. Med. **115**:963, 1964.
8. Jue, R., Puffer, J., Wood, R. M., Schochet, G., Smartt, W. H., and Ketterer, W. A.: Am. J. Clin. Pathol. **47**:809, 1967.
9. Yobs, A., Brown, L., and Hunter, E.: Arch. Pathol. **77**:220, 1964.
10. Smith, J. L., and Israel, C. W.: J.A.M.A. **199**:980, 1967.
11. Mothershed, S. M., and Bullard, J. C.: Br. J. Vener. Dis. **44**:201, 1968; Mothershed, S. M.: Appl. Microbiol. **18**:806, 1969.
12. Venereal Disease Research Laboratory: Technique for the direct immunofluorescent identification of *Treponema pallidum* in body fluids and tissue sections (provisional), Atlanta, January 1971, Venereal Disease Research Laboratory, Center for Disease Control.
13. Daniels, K. C., and Ferneyhough, H. S.: Health Lab. Sci. **14**:164, 1976.
14. Hanson, A. W., and Cannefax, G. R.: J. Bacteriol. **88**:111, 1964.
15. Harland, W. A., and Lee, F. D.: Br. Med. J. **3**:718, 1967.
16. Kelly, R.: Science **173**:443, 1971.
17. Kelly, R.: In Johnson, R. C., editor: The biology of the parasitic spirochetes, New York, 1976, Academic Press, pp. 87-94.
18. Linnemann, C. C., Barber, L. C., Dine, M. S., et al.: Am. J. Dis. Child. **132**:40, 1978.
19. Felsenfeld, O.: *Borrelia:* strains, vectors, human and animal borreliosis, St. Louis, 1971, Warren H. Green.
20. Van Riel, J., and Van Riel, M.: Ann. Soc. Belg. Méd. Trop. **38**:1101, 1958.
21. Sulzer, C. R., and Jones, W. L.: Leptospirosis. Methods in laboratory diagnosis, Atlanta, 1978, Center for Disease Control.
22. Stuart, R. D.: J. Pathol. Bacteriol. **58**:343, 1946.
23. Fletcher, W.: Trans. Roy. Soc. Trop. Med. Hyg. **21**:265, 1927-1928.
24. Cox, C. D., and Larson, A. D.: J. Bacteriol. **73**:587, 1957.
25. Johnson, R. C., and Harris, V. G.: J. Bacteriol. **94**:27, 1967.
26. Myers, D. M., and Varela-Diaz, V. M.: Appl. Microbiol. **25**:781, 1973.
27. Annear, D. I.: Aust. J. Exp. Biol. Med. Sci. **36**:1, 1958.
28. WHO Expert Group: Current problems in leptospirosis research, WHO Technical Report Series no. 380, 1967.
29. Feigin, R. D., Lobes, L. A., Anderson, D., et al.: Ann. Intern. Med. **79**:777, 1973.
30. Finegold, S. M., and Meyer, R. D.: In Practice of Medicine, vol. 3, ch 37, New York, 1975, Harper & Row, Publishers.
31. Turner, L. H.: Br. Med. J. **1**:537, 1973.
32. Coffin, D. L., and Maestrone, G.: Am. J. Vet. Res. **23**:159, 1962.
33. White, F. H., Stoliker, H. E., and Galton, M. M.: Am. J. Vet. Res. **22**:650, 1961.
34. Galton, M. M., Menges, R. W., Shotts, E. B., et al.: Leptospirosis, Public Health Service pub. no. 951, Washington, D.C., 1962, U.S. Government Printing Office.
35. Alexander, A. D.: In Lennette, E. H., Spaulding, E. H., and Truant, J. P., editors: Manual of clinical microbiology, ed. 2, Washington, D.C., 1974, American Society for Microbiology.
36. Ruys, A. C., Minkenhof, J. E., and Wolff, J. W.: Proc. Int. Cong. Trop. Med. Malaria **1**:337, 1948.
37. Van Thiel, P. H.: The leptospiroses, Leiden, 1948, Universitaire Pers.
38. Galton, M. M., Powers, D. K., Hall, A. D., et al.: Am. J. Vet. Res. **19**:505, 1958.
39. WHO Technical Report Series no. 113, 1956.
40. Ruys, A. C., and Schüffner, W. A. P.: Nederl. T. Geneesk. **78**:3110, 1934.
41. Schüffner, W. A. P., and Bohlander, L.: Zentralbl. Bakteriol. **144**:434, 1939 (Abt. 1).
42. Wolff, J. W.: The laboratory diagnosis of leptospirosis, Springfield, Ill., 1954, Charles C Thomas, Publisher.
43. Veterinary public health notes, Atlanta, May 1977, Center for Disease Control.
44. Pike, R. M., and Schulze, M. L.: J. Immunol. **81**:172, 1958.
45. FAO/WHO Expert Committee: WHO Technical Report Series no. 378, 1967.
46. Johnson, R. C., editor: The biology of the parasitic spirochetes, New York, 1976, Academic Press.

81

MYCOPLASMA

George E. Kenny

Mycoplasmata are small membrane-bounded organisms without morphologic or chemical evidence of a cell wall. Three genera are recognized among the organisms that parasitize man: *Mycoplasma*,[1] *Ureaplasma*,[2] and *Acholeplasma*[3] (Table 81-1). *Mycoplasma* and *Ureaplasma* are classified in family *Mycoplasmataceae* and *Acholeplasma* is classified in family *Acholeplasmataceae*. *Mycoplasmataceae* are differentiated from *Acholeplasmataceae* in that the former require sterol. These families are classified in order *Mycoplasmatales* in class *Mollicutes*,[1] but the phylogenetic relationships among the genera are not clearly understood. No serologic cross-reactions have been observed between *Acholeplasma* and *Mycoplasma*[4]; this suggests that these organisms are quite distant from each other phylogenetically. Even more interesting is the fact that the organisms now classified in genus *Mycoplasma* can be divided into as many as 6 groups[4] without evidence of serologic cross-reactions between groups when tested by double immunodiffusion, whereby 6 to 10 antigens may be detected. This result suggests that the organisms still classified in genus *Mycoplasma* are strongly heterogeneous and that certain groups of species may be different from each other as *Mycobacterium* is different from *Escherichia*. Clearly, further reclassification of species in genus *Mycoplasma* to new genera will be required to taxonomically reflect their heterogeneity. This will confuse the literature, but it will be necessary in order to view the organisms in their proper perspective. Presently, no common name has been generally accepted for the members of the group, but the terms "mycoplasmas" (the English common name) or "mycoplasmata" (the trivial name) have been used as a common term for members of the order *Mycoplasmatales*. Organisms are defined as members of the *Mycoplasmatales* if they have the following properties:

1. Small size of individual cells (0.3-0.5 μm)
2. Ability to replicate on artificial medium with the formation of typical small colonies (Fig. 81-1) that are imbedded in the agar and frequently show a "fried egg" appearance because of the growth of the organisms in the center of the colony into the agar
3. No ultrastructural evidence of a cell wall
4. Inhibition of growth by specific antisera (Species are separated by the inhibition of growth on agar by specific antiserum.)

Recently, organisms have been recognized from infected tissue cultures that show typical morphology of individual cells ultrastructurally, incorporate uracil,[5] but do not form colonies on known media.[5,6] Thus, it is now clear that organisms exist that are not culturable and that probably belong to the *Mycoplasmatales*. Mycoplasmata also resemble cell wall–defective bacteria both ultrastructurally and by colony morphology. However, no specific relationship has been determined between classic *Mycoplasma* species and bacteria, even though it has long been speculated that mycoplasmata might have arisen from bacteria. Mycoplasmata are differentiated from cell wall–defective bacteria on the basis that the latter usually revert to the parent bacterium on appropriate medium. However, it must be admitted that cell wall–deficient bacteria that do not revert to the parent bacteria would be difficult to distinguish from mycoplasmata. The heterogeneity observed in the *Mycoplasmatales* suggests that if mycoplasmata are derived from bacteria, they could have a number of distinct bacterial parents.

CHARACTERISTICS OF ORGANISMS ISOLATED FROM MAN

Some 9 species are recovered from human sources. A rapidly expanding list of additional species (50+) has been recognized from animal sources; some of these species are related immunologically to species found in humans.[4] The organisms are different metabolically and reflect the differences observed in serologic taxonomy (Table 81-1). The organisms can be divided into 3 groups by physiologic parameters: (1) glucose fermentation, (2) arginine utilization, and (3) urea hydrolysis. The organisms will be discussed separately in terms of their properties.

M. pneumoniae is a slow-growing organism

Supported in part by grants AI 06720, AI 10695, and AI 12005 from the National Institute of Allergy and Infectious Diseases.

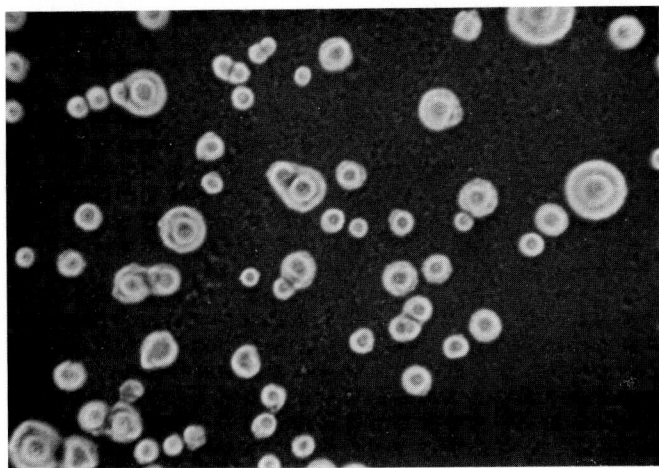

Fig. 81-1. Colonies of *M. pneumoniae* (strain AP-164) on E agar, 10 d incubation. Anoptral phase contrast bar = 100 μm.

Table 81-1. Species of order Mycoplasmatales isolated from humans

Species	Serologic group*	Glucose fermentation	Arginine utilization	Urea hydrolysis	Growth in indicated atmosphere†			Optimum pH
					Air	95% N₂ 5% CO₂	H₂§ CO₂	
M. pneumoniae	5	+	−	−	++++	+	±	7.0-8.0
U. urealyticum	?	−	−	+	+++	+++	+++	5.5-6.5
M. hominis	7	−	+	−	+++	+++	++++	6.5-7.5
M. orale	7	−	+	−	+	+++	++++	6.0-7.0
M. buccale‡	7	−	+	−	+	+++	++++	6.0-7.0
M. faucium‡	7	−	+	−	+	+++	++++	6.0-7.0
M. salivarium	7	−	+	−	+	+++	++++	6.0-7.0
M. fermentans‡	6	+	+	−	++	+++	+++	7.0-8.0
A. laidlawii	2	+	−	−	++++	++++	++++	7.0-8.0

*Serologic groups as defined in Kenny.[4]
†Scores range from ± slight growth to ++++ maximum growth.
‡Only limited data available for wild isolates.
§"GasPak" method.

(generation time 5 hours or greater) that is strongly aerobic and grows very poorly under stringent anaerobiosis. These traits contrast it to all other human species (Table 81-1), which appear to be anaerobic or indifferent to atmosphere. The organisms grow as "spherules" (fluid medium colonies) in broth culture. *M. pneumoniae* is serologically distinct from all other *Mycoplasma* species thus far tested (from both human and animals). Its unique position is also confirmed by its comparative ultrastructure and the 39% guanine plus cytosine (%G + C) in its DNA, a value 5-10% higher than that for all other species in the Mycoplasmatales. Thus, no other species can be used as a reasonable model for study of *M. pneumoniae.*

Ureaplasma contains a unique group in the Mycoplasmataceae that hydrolyzes urea. The human strains are termed *U. urealyticum*, and 8 serotypes (possibly equivalent to species designation in *Mycoplasma* species) are currently recognized.[2] The relationship of *U. urealyt-*

icum to the numerous animal strains is unknown except that those strains tested do not cross react serologically with human strains. *U. urealyticum* organisms are highly unusual in that they require urea for growth[7,8] even in complex biological media. The enzyme behaves like a typical urease with ammonia and CO_2 as products. This behavior produces rapid alkalinity of the medium and has limited growth to fewer than 10^7 colony-forming units per milliliter; this factor has made research on the biochemistry and immunology of these organisms difficult. Recently we found that growth of *U. urealyticum* could be improved by greatly increasing both the buffer and urea content of the medium.[9] The growth of the organism is a function of urea concentration, and titers of nearly 10^8 can be achieved at 32 mM urea. At this concentration of organisms some biochemical studies and studies of the antigens of the organisms have been possible. *Ureaplasma* make very small colonies on agar medium; hence their original name, T-strains (T = tiny). Although the organisms were originally thought to be anaerobic, it is now clear[2] that the apparent anaerobiosis was really a function of CO_2 content of the atmosphere, which served to reduce the pH of the medium to more suitable levels. In adequately buffered medium at pH 6.0, colonies readily appear aerobically even from clinical specimens. Colonies are also larger on buffered medium.

Arginine-utilizing organisms (serologic group 7) possess the arginine dihydrolase pathway and apparently can utilize arginine for energy, but arginine does not appear to be a requirement for growth of all strains. The arginine utilizers show strong serologic relationships between species[4] and are broadly distributed in animals. Some of the species are anaerobic and grow poorly aerobically (e.g., *M. orale* and *M. salivarium*), though this property appears to depend upon the nature of the solid medium. Other species are tolerant of oxygen. Some confusion of terminology is evident for some species: *M. orale* has been termed *M. orale* type 1 and also *M. pharyngis*, *M. buccale* previously was named *M. orale* type 2, and *M. faucium* was called *M. orale* type 3.[10] *M. hominis* type 1 is now *M. hominis* with no serotype designation, since *M. hominis* type 2 has been found to be *M. arthritidis*, a rat species.

A. laidlawii is an organism occasionally recovered from man, but its major habitat appears to be animal feces and sewage. The organism grows rapidly and forms very large colonies. The fact that it ferments glucose may cause confusion with *M. pneumoniae*.

M. fermentans is an unusual organism in that it utilizes both arginine and glucose. This species is related to a large number of animal species that are glycolytic and that have a similar %G + C of 26-28%.[4] The organism appears to be anaerobic, but laboratory strains will grow aerobically. Little information is available on characteristics of wild strains because the organism is seldom isolated.

PATHOGENESIS OF THE MYCOPLASMATALES

On the cellular level the best generalization is that mycoplasmata are surface parasites of nonphagocytic cells.[11] Those strains studied have not been found to be intracellular except in phagocytic cells. Little is understood of the mechanisms by which they produce cellular damage. In animals, mycoplasmata cause primarily respiratory diseases and arthritis. The diseases caused in chickens, pigs, and cattle are of major economic importance. *Spiroplasma* is an interesting group of organisms with properties similar to the *Mycoplasmatales* and causes a variety of "yellow" diseases of plants.[12] One strain of *Spiroplasma* has been found to cause cataracts in infant mice[13]; this finding raises the possibility that these difficult-to-cultivate organisms may be responsible for some animal diseases. The human diseases will be considered in greater detail below.

M. pneumoniae is a major cause of primary atypical pneumonia in humans; it is responsible for as much as 20% of total pneumonia in a civilian population.[14] Although total pneumonia incidence is strongly seasonal, *M. pneumoniae* infections tend to occur throughout the year with occasional epidemics provided that large enough populations are studied.[14] In small populations local epidemics may be recognized. The incubation period is long, about 3 weeks.[15] The highest incidence is found in persons 5-19 years of age, with few cases in persons older than 60 years of age. The organism is not carried as normal flora, but it is clear that a substantial number of subclinical infections occur, with perhaps as many as 5 subclinical infections for every symptomatic case detected.[16] The disease has few complications, but occasional severe cases have been reported in the literature. Treatment with antibiotics such as tetracycline reduces the duration of the illness, but it does not eliminate the organism from throat secretions. Immune mechanisms operate to eliminate the infection since untreated cases recover. However, the length of immunity has been difficult to establish since reinfection with the organism has been documented.[17]

M. salivarium is frequently isolated from the oral cavity and throat. However, the prime habitat of the organism appears to be in the crevice between the teeth and the gingiva. Both an increased frequency of isolation and increased numbers of organisms are found in persons with periodontal disease.[18] The possible role of this species in periodontal disease is difficult to assess because of the great variety of bacterial species also found in the same site.

The role of mycoplasmata in venereal diseases has been difficult to assess because of the high prevalence of these organisms in the genital tract of apparently normal persons. *U. urealyticum* has been isolated from 60% of normal women and 10-40% of male populations.[19,20] The isolation rate of *M. hominis* is more variable, ranging from 10-40% in various male and female populations. The isolation of these organisms is strongly related to sexual activity, with a much higher rate in promiscuous persons. Substantial efforts have been made to relate the isolation of *U. urealyticum* to nonspecific urethritis in males. The results have been highly controversial, and it now appears that the chlamydiae may account for a major portion of these infections.[21] A case can be made for *U. urealyticum* having a role because some groups of patients with high titers of *U. urealyticum* respond clinically to antibiotics toward which chlamydiae are insensitive.[22] A role for *U. urealyticum* in infertility is suspected also. It is clear that *U. urealyticum* and *M. hominis* can be opportunists, particularly in postpartum infections where the organisms have been isolated from the blood stream.

PROCEDURE FOR CULTURE AND IDENTIFICATION
Media

Media for cultivation of mycoplasmata and ureaplasmata contain a peptone, yeast extract,

Table 81-2. Basal media

Ingredient	E agar base	E broth base	Mes agar base
Soy peptone*	20 g	20 g	20 g
NaCl	5 g	5 g	5 g
Glucose	—	10 g	—
Agar†	10 g	—	—
Agarose	—	—	10 g
Mes‡	—	—	4.26 g (20 mM)
2% phenol red (Na salt in H_2O)	—	1 ml	—
Water	1000 ml	1000 ml	1000 ml
Final pH	7.4	7.4	6.0

*"HY-SOY," Humko Sheffield Chemical, 1099 Wall St. West, Lyndhurst, N.J. 07071.
†Difco Noble, Difco Laboratories, Detroit, Mich. 48232.
‡Mes, 2(N-Morpholino) ethane sulfonic acid, Calbiochem, San Diego, Calif. 92112.

Table 81-3. Complete media

	Complete E agar	Complete E broth	Complete Mes agar
E agar base (molten 45-50 C)	65 ml	—	—
E broth base	—	65 ml	—
Mes agar base (molten 45-50 C)	—	—	65 ml
Yeast dialysate	10 ml	10 ml	10 ml
Horse serum	25 ml	25 ml	25 ml
Penicillin (10,000 U/ml)	1 ml	1 ml	1 ml
Thallium acetate (3.3%)	1 ml	1 ml	—

and animal serum. Relatively low agar concentrations are employed for plates to ensure formation of the largest colonies possible because the organisms grow into the agar. Isolation efforts from human specimen materials are directed at 3 organisms: *M. pneumoniae*, *M. hominis*, and *U. urealyticum*. These organisms are all aerobic or aerotolerant, but they have different media requirements. *M. pneumoniae* and *M. hominis* require a medium of pH 7.0-7.5, and *M. pneumoniae* requires fresh yeast extract. In contrast, *U. urealyticum* requires a pH around 6.0,[23] agarose rather than agar, and urea. Accordingly, 2 media are recommended to achieve these objectives; these formulations have been tested in my laboratories for some years and have proven satisfactory. Other successful medium formulations have been described elsewhere.[2,24,25]

Basal agar and broth media. E agar and broth[11,15,26] are used for isolation of *M. pneumoniae* and *M. hominis* and for cultivation of *Mycoplasma* and *Acholeplasma* species in general. Mes agar[9,19] is used for cultivation of *U. urealyticum* and organisms requiring low pH such as *M. salivarium* (Tables 81-2 and 81-3).[18]

Dissolve or suspend ingredients in water, adjust pH with 1N NaOH, and sterilize by autoclaving at 121 C for 15 min (agar medium heated to boiling to solubilize agar before dispensing into smaller aliquots). Basic agar and broth are stored at room temperature until used.

Yeast dialysate[125] is prepared by suspending 450 g Fleischmann's active dried yeast in 1250 ml water. This suspension is heated in an autoclave for 5 min at 121 C (sufficient to heat the yeast suspension to boiling) and permitted to dialyze against 1000 ml of water for 2 d at 4 C. The dialysis casing and contents are discarded and the dialysate is sterilized by autoclaving. The sterile dialysate is stored frozen until used.

Five ml agar is permitted to solidify in each 10 × 35 mm Petri dish. Urea broth for cultivation of *U. urealyticum* is prepared from a soy peptone–fresh yeast dialysate medium[27] supplemented with 25% horse serum, 0.04% urea, 0.004% phenol red, and 100 U penicillin/ml.

Diphasic media. Diphasic E medium is prepared by permitting 3 ml complete E agar medium to solidify in the bottom of a 16 × 125 mm screw-capped test tube. This is then overlaid with 3 ml complete E broth medium.

Isolation of M. pneumoniae

Throat-swab specimens are collected in 3 ml transport medium[15] (0.5% bovine albumin in trypticase soy broth with 100 μg penicillin/ml). Specimens may be stored at 4 C for several days and at −20 C for 1 or 2 weeks. For long-term storage, −70 C has been successful; specimen materials remain viable for years. Plates and diphasic culture tubes are inoculated with 0.1 ml of the specimen in the transport medium. Sputum and other body fluids should be diluted 1:10 and 1:100 before being used for inoculation. The agar plates are incubated aerobically in a tightly sealed container. The agar medium is selective for *M. pneumoniae* under aerobic conditions; under microaerophilic (95% N_2 5% CO_2) conditions or stringent anaerobiosis, *M. orale* and other oral organisms will be recovered. The sealed diphasic cultures are incubated at 37 C and subcultured to agar at 21 and 42 days. Plates should be examined microscopically with a stereoscopic microscope at 20-60× for typical colonies at 2, 5, 10, 15, 20, 25, and 30 days. The agar will be sufficiently clear that the colonies can be observed through the bottom of the plate to avoid cross-contamination. Pseudocolonies[24] are an annoying artifact that can confuse efforts to detect mycoplasmata. Pseudocolonies spontaneously appear as whorls of material on uninoculated plates. Colonies of mycoplasmata transfer poorly with a wire loop, so several methods of propagating colonies are used.

Individual colonies can be excised from a plate with a capillary pipet and inoculated into broth to propagate the agent. Alternatively, a piece of agar with colonies can be excised from a plate with a scalpel or stiff loop and smeared over the plate face down. Diphasic cultures are examined visually for pH shift and microscopically for typical "spherules" (fluid medium colonies) by looking through the side of the tube at the broth with the stereoscopic microscope. Most positive specimens will show typical small colonies, acid production, and spherules by 14 days. However, a significant number of specimens will not show colonies on the primary plate, but will show colonies on the agar subcultures of the diphasic cultures. These 3 factors permit presumptive identification of the organism as *M. pneumoniae;* this is then confirmed by a hemolysis test.[28]

The only other organisms isolated from the respiratory tract under the recommended conditions are *M. hominis,* which grows rapidly and forms large colonies, and *A. laidlawii,* which grows rapidly on subculture, but which also hemolyzes red blood cells. The hemolysis test is carried out by overlaying the colonies with a thin layer of 8% guinea pig red blood cells in saline agar. Incubation is carried out overnight at 37 C; a zone of hemolysis will be observed surrounding the colonies. At this time cultures may be reported as positive for an organism with cultural characteristics of *M. pneumoniae.* Final identification is carried out by inhibition of growth with specific antiserum.[29] One-tenth ml aliquots of serial 10-fold dilutions of the broth culture (1:1, 1:10, 1:100) are spread uniformly over E plates and allowed to absorb; then paper disks (2-3 mm) soaked with antiserum (available commercially) are placed on the plates. Plates are incubated for 4-6 days and read for zones of inhibition of mycoplasmic growth. The test is quite sensitive to excess organisms.[29]

Isolation of other Mycoplasma species and U. urealyticum

Specimens from the genital tract are submitted in the same transport medium as for *M. pneumoniae* and are inoculated on both E agar plates and Mes agar plates. If only 1 atmosphere is to be used, the plates should be incubated in a microaerophilic atmosphere of 95% N_2 5% CO_2, though nearly all strains of *M. hominis* and *U. urealyticum* will grow aerobically on the appropriate medium. However, few data are available on the atmospheric preferences of *M. fermentans.* Urea broth should also be inoculated with 0.1 ml of specimen materials. Since *U. urealyticum* dies rapidly in broth culture after attaining maximum growth, the cultures should be subcultured to agar each day or immediately upon the culture's showing a pH change (the cultures should be observed twice daily). Plates should be examined daily for presence of typical colonies. Colonies of *U. urealyticum* can be differentiated from *M. hominis* by the single-reagent test of Shepard[30] (0.8% $MnCl_2 \cdot 4H_2O$ and 1.0% urea in water). One drop of reagent is added to the agar plate. Colonies of *U. urealyticum* immediately turn brown, whereas *M. hominis* colonies are unaffected. Isolates that produce typical colonies and that prove to be transferable entities are considered to be *U. urealyticum* and are reported as such. Methods for typing *U. urealyticum* strains have not yet advanced sufficiently for general use because of the unavailability of antisera for typing. Isolates of *M.*

hominis are confirmed as such by growth inhibition on agar using specific antiserum (commercially available).

Isolation of *U. urealyticum* and *M. hominis* from blood has been successful. Diphasic culture medium (using Mes agar and urea broth medium) should be prepared with the volume of the fluid phase at least 20 times the sample volume of the blood specimen, and the medium should contain penicillin but not thallium acetate (which inhibits growth of *U. urealyticum,* but not *Mycoplasma* species). Blood should be collected without anticoagulant and directly inoculated into the medium. Cultures should be subcultured to E agar and Mes agar at daily intervals for 1 week and observed for typical colonies.

Controls

It is most important to evaluate the medium used for ability to isolate wild strains of the organisms. Prototype strains may grow well on medium that will not support growth of wild strains. The most common sources of difficulty are the peptone being used (lots of soy peptone vary substantially in ability to isolate *M. pneumoniae*); the lots of serum being used may also give variable results. For isolation of *M. pneumoniae* the isolation rate on agar can be compared to the number of serologic positives obtained when paired sera are tested. In this laboratory the isolation rate was 60% from those who had 4-fold serologic rises when only single throat-swab specimens were tested.[15] Wild strains of organisms can be collected and stored at −70 C in first passage or better, in the original specimen materials, and used to evaluate new lots of serum and medium components.

Isolation of mycoplasmata from tissue cultures

Mycoplasmata are frequent contaminants of animal cell cultures[11]; consequently, requests are frequently made to clinical laboratories for testing of cell cultures. The optimum specimen is cells dispersed in the medium used for cultivation; the organisms both grow in the medium and adhere to the cells. At least 2 plates of E agar medium should be inoculated; one of them should be incubated aerobically (in air or preferably in air with 2.5-5% CO_2) and another plate should be incubated under stringent anaerobiosis (GasPak method or equivalent) to detect organisms such as *M. orale.* Diphasic E agar cultures should be inoculated and 1 culture incubated aerobically and 1 under stringent anaerobiosis. Cultures should be observed daily for a week, and a subculture from the broth should be made on the third or fourth day. The animal cells may resemble mycoplasmata, but they will not be transferable entities and they will not grow on the agar medium, provided that thallium acetate has been included. The morphology of the animal cells can be ascertained by observing the plates immediately after the inoculum has been absorbed. The nonculturable strains will not be recognized by this procedure.[5] It is interesting that *U. urealyticum* has not been recognized as a cell culture contaminant; the organisms die out when inoculated into cell cultures.[11]

• • •

Serology of mycoplasmic infections

For serologic tests used in diagnosis of mycoplasma infections, see Chapter 107.

REFERENCES

1. Edward, D. G., and Freundt, E. A.: Int. J. Syst. Bacteriol. **23:**55, 1973.
2. Shepard, M. C., Lunceford, C. D., Ford, D. K., et al.: Int. J. Syst. Bacteriol. **24:**160, 1974.
3. Edward, D. G., and Freundt, E. A.: J. Gen. Microbiol. **62:**1, 1970.
4. Kenny, G. E.: In Barile, M. F., and Razin, S., editors: The mycoplasmas, vol. 1, New York, 1979, Academic Press.
5. Kenny, G. E.: In Schlessinger, D., editor: Microbiology 1975, Washington, D.C., 1975, American Society for Microbiology.
6. Schneider, E. L., Stanbridge, E. J., and Epstein, C. J.: Exp. Cell. Res. **79:**84, 1974.
7. Shepard, M. C., and Lunceford, C. D.: J. Bacteriol. **93:**1513, 1967.
8. Ford, D. K., and MacDonald, J.: J. Bacteriol. **93:**1509, 1967.
9. Kenny, G. E., and Cartwright, F. D.: J. Bacteriol. **132:**144, 1977.
10. Freundt, E. A., Taylor-Robinson, D., Purcell, R. H., et al.: Int. J. Syst. Bacteriol. **24:**252, 1974.
11. Kenny, G. E.: In Fogh, J., editor: Contamination in tissue culture, New York, 1973, Academic Press.
12. Davis, R. E., and Worley, J. F.: Phytopathology **63:**403, 1972.
13. Tully, J. G., Whitcomb, R. F., Clark, H. F., et al.: Science **195:**892, 1977.
14. Foy, H. M., Kenny, G. E., McMahan, R., et al.: J.A.M.A. **214:**1666, 1970.
15. Grayston, J. T., Foy, H. M., and Kenny, G. E.: In Hayflick, L., editor: The Mycoplasmatales and L-phase of bacteria, New York, 1969, Appleton-Century-Crofts.
16. Chanock, R. M.: N. Engl. J. Med. **273:**1199, 1965.
17. Foy, H. M., Kenny, G. E., Sefi, R., et al.: J. Infect. Dis. **135:**673, 1977.
18. Engel, L. D., and Kenny, G. E.: J. Periodont. Res. **5:**163, 1970.
19. Foy, H. M., Kenny, G. E., Wentworth, B. B., et al.: Am. J. Obstet. Gynecol. **106:**635, 1970.
20. McCormack, W. M., Braun, P., Lee, Y-H, et al.: N. Engl. J. Med. **288:**27, 1973.
21. Holmes, K. K., Handsfield, H. H., Wang, S. P., et al.: N. Engl. J. Med. **292:**1199, 1975.
22. Bowie, W. R., Wang, S. P., Alexander, E. R., et al.: J. Clin. Invest. **59:**735, 1977.
23. Shepard, M. C., and Lunceford, C. D.: J. Bacteriol. **89:**265, 1965.
24. Hayflick, L.: Tex. Rep. Biol. Med. **23**(supp. 1):285, 1965.
25. Kraybill, W. H., and Crawford, Y. E.: Proc. Soc. Exp. Biol. Med. **118:**965, 1965.
26. Kenny, G. E.: J. Bacteriol. **98:**1044, 1969.
27. Kenny, G. E.: Ann. N.Y. Acad. Sci. **143:**676, 1967.
28. Clyde, W. A.: Science **139:**55, 1963.
29. Clyde, W. A.: J. Immunol. **92:**958, 1964.
30. Shepard, M. C.: J. Infect. Dis. **127:**S22, 1973.

82

ANAEROBIC BACTERIA— AN INTRODUCTION

Alex C. Sonnenwirth

GENERAL CONSIDERATIONS*

Anaerobiosis was discovered in 1861 by Louis Pasteur, who introduced the terms *aérobies* and *anaérobies* to designate, respectively, microorganisms that live in the presence and in the absence of oxygen. Within the next 30 years, many diverse types of anaerobic bacteria were isolated and described, and the significant role of several sporeforming, toxin-producing anaerobes in a variety of human diseases (e.g., botulism, gas gangrene, tetanus) was established. The association of non-sporeforming anaerobes (many of endogenous origin) with infections in humans was recognized as early as 1897, but was overlooked and rarely noted for several decades thereafter. Part of this neglect was because of the cumbersome and complex early anaerobic technics, unsuitable for use in clinical laboratories.

A brief survey of the evolution of anaerobic culture technics[1] indicates that until 1916 the methods used were mainly fluid and deep agar shake cultures (Table 82-1). These did not provide for surface cultivation and isolation of single colonies; as a result, many early studies were based on examinations of mixed or anaerobic cultures. In 1916 McIntosh and Fildes introduced an anaerobic jar based on the combustion principle for removal of oxygen, allowing use of agar plates and surface cultivation. It required an electrically heated platinum catalyst and 100% hydrogen, a combination that did not appeal to the self-preservative instincts of many clinical microbiologists. An improved version, the Brewer jar, was introduced in the United States in 1939. The highly reliable roll-tube technic of Hungate[2] described in 1950 made no headway in the clinical laboratory until 1966, when

---

*Modified from Sonnenwirth, A. C.: Anaerobic culture techniques. In Metronidazole: Proceedings of the International Metronidazole Conference (Montreal, 1976), Amsterdam, 1977, Excerpta Medica.

Moore's modifications, known as the VPI (Virginia Polytechnic Institute) method, became available.[3]

Perhaps the greatest single impetus for application of anaerobic technics in the clinical microbiology laboratory has come from Stokes's short 1958 report[4] on the large number of anaerobs isolated from human clinical material with the aid of an anaerobic jar employing a catalyst active at room temperature.

Shortly thereafter a number of major developments occurred in anaerobic methodology: antibiotic-containing media selective for anaerobes were developed,[5] the GasPak (BBL, Cockeysville, Md.), a self-contained combustion jar system with its own gas-generating package,[6] anaerobic chambers,[7,8] and the VPI method[3] were introduced (Table 82-1).

Determination of an optimal system(s) for anaerobic culture requires that different approaches to the nomenclatures, taxonomy, and general methodology of anaerobic bacteriology be emphasized. On the one hand, a busy clinical laboratory must use approaches that are as simple as possible to provide the clinician as rapidly as possible with information needed for proper therapy of an illness. On the other hand, the research laboratory studying the normal flora or attempting to define the role of certain anaerobes in specific disease entities must apply the most detailed and rigorous technics. Anaerobes differ in their sensitivity to oxygen, ranging from those which are just barely anaerobes, such as *Clostridium perfringens*, through moderate anaerobes, capable of growing in the presence of up to 2% to 5% oxygen, to strict anaerobes incapable of growth if there is more than 0.5% oxygen present.[9] For studies of the normal flora, where strict anaerobes are common components, rigorous and sophisticated methods, such as the **anaerobic chamber** (glovebox) or **roll-tube technic**, are imperative. However, the more convenient and simpler anaerobic jar methods are just as reliable. These are suitable for recovery of clinically significant anaerobes from specimens as long as proper collection and anaerobic transport of specimens are carried out, for the

Table 82-1. Brief survey of anaerobic culture technics

Culture technic	Year	Culture technic
Deep shake and fluid cultures	Pre-1915	Reducing agents
	1916	Cooked meat
Surface cultures		
McIntosh-Fildes jar	1916-1921	
Brewer and other jars (heated catalyst)	1939	Thioglycollate broth
	1950	Hungate roll-tube method
Baird-Tatlock ("Torbal") jar (cold catalyst)	1958	
Selective media	1965-1968	VPI modifications
GasPak		of Hungate method
Anaerobic chamber		

Table 82-2. Protocol for anaerobic culture of clinical specimens

Specimens to be cultured routinely for anaerobes

Body fluids normally sterile	Transtracheal aspirates
Blood, bile, synovial, joint, pericardial, peritoneal (ascites), pleural (thoracentesis), transudates; spinal fluid—partial anaerobic culture	Culdoscopy aspirates
	Pus—*aspirated* from deep wound or abscesses— or if "sulfur granules" are present
Abscesses	
Deep aspirates of wounds (identified as "wound aspirate")	Surgical specimens obtained from normally sterile sites (gall bladder, tissue, lymph node)

To be cultured for anaerobes only under special circumstances

Decubitus ulcer	Endometrial aspirate
Wound drainage	Urine (suprapubic aspirate only)

Not to be cultured anaerobically

Bronschoscopic washings	Ileostomy material
Gastric washings	Colostomy material
Sputum	Throat
Urine (voided)	Nose
Vaginal swab	Skin
Feces*	Mouth
Urethra	Episiotomy (swab—no, aspirated abscess—yes)

*For culture of C. difficile, see Chapter 84.

moderate anaerobes include almost all of those known to be pathogenic.[9]

The only acceptable documentation of an anaerobic infection is culture of these organisms from the infected site. This procedure requires the cooperative efforts of the physician and the microbiology laboratory to achieve the requirements of (1) collection of appropriate specimens, (2) expeditious and proper specimen transport, and (3) careful laboratory processing.[10]

Specimen selection

The major consideration here is to avoid contaminating the specimen for anaerobic culture with normal flora, for indigenous anaerobes are often present in such large numbers that even minimal contamination of a specimen with normal flora can give misleading results. Because of this consideration specimens are designated according to acceptability for anaerobic culture (Table 82-2). Specimens that should be cultured anaerobically include (1) normally sterile body fluids; (2) aspirates of abscesses; (3) deep aspirates of wounds; (4) transtracheal and culdoscopy aspirates; and (5) surgical specimens obtained from normally sterile sites. Specimens that should **not** be routinely cultured for anaerobes include those with normal flora, e.g., feces, throat, expectorated sputum, vaginal swabs, etc.[11] (See also Anaerobic infections and anaerobic cultures, Chapter 75).

Collection and transport

Avoidance of contamination with normal flora and protection of specimen from oxygen exposure are imperative. A summary of recommended specimen collection methods is shown in Table 82-3. The optimal methods for lower respiratory tract specimens are transtracheal aspiration or direct lung puncture. In the case of abscesses, the skin or mucosal surface should be decontaminated, and pus should be removed with a syringe. For female genital tract specimens, culdocentesis should be used, if possible, after decontaminating the vagina. For sinus tracts or draining wounds, aspiration by syringe and small plastic catheter should be employed.

Means for proper anaerobic transport include

Table 82-3. Recommended specimen collection methods for anaerobic culture *

Pulmonary	Percutaneous transtracheal aspiration or direct lung puncture
Pleural	Thoracentesis
Abscesses	Needle and syringe aspiration of closed abscess; use of swabs much less desirable
Female genital tract	Culdocentesis to obtain specimens; when possible, after decontaminating the vagina
Uterine	Syringe and small plastic catheter to aspirate through a decontaminated cervical os (contamination from endocervical canal is unavoidable)
Sinus tracts or draining wounds	Aspiration by syringe and small plastic catheter introduced as deeply as possible through decontaminated skin orifice; specimen obtained at surgery from depths of wound or underlying bone lesion always preferable

*Modified from Sutter et al.[11]

(1) syringe technic, i.e., elimination of all air from (specimen-containing) syringe and needle and sticking needle into a sterile rubber stopper; (2) injection of specimen into anaerobic transporter (oxygen-free vial or tube, usually filled with oxygen-free CO_2, commercially available); and (3) if swab must be used, special swab prepared in oxygen-free tube ("anaerobic swab"). After use, swab is placed into second oxygen-free tube, with or without prereduced anaerobically sterilized semisolid transport medium.[11] For details, see Anaerobic culture collection and transport, and Anaerobic infections and anaerobic culture, Chapter 75.

Microscopic examination of clinical materials

Immediately on processing of specimen, a careful Gram stain should be examined. This can provide useful information, such as the cellular characteristics of the material and the relative quantity as well as the morphologic types of bacteria present.

Anaerobic culture systems

In the United States 3 systems are commonly used to culture for anaerobes: roll-tube (VPI) method, anaerobic cabinet (glovebox), and anaerobic jar.

The **roll-tube method** of Hungate, modified by Moore[3,12] and known as the VPI method, is based on the use of prereduced, anaerobically sterilized media (PRAS) stored in sealed tubes, and on the total exclusion of oxygen from the specimen and the media used during inoculation and further manipulations. This is accomplished by continuously passing a stream of oxygen-free gas (CO_2 or nitrogen) through the tubes during manipulation, with the aid of an (commercially available) anaerobic gassing-out apparatus including gas cannula, inoculator, and streaker. In the system each tube becomes its own anaerobic chamber. Advantages include moderate initial cost and space requirements and the fact that growth in the tubes can be inspected at any time without disturbing anaerobic conditions. Disadvantages include requirement for training personnel in technology different from the usual bacteriologic methods, cumbersome steps in

isolating and purifying strains, high cost of media, and inability to use opaque media (see Chapter 70, Anaerobic methods).

The **anaerobic chamber ("glovebox")** comprises vacuum-tight rigid cabinets[8] or flexible plastic bags[7] filled with oxygen-free gas and equipped with an entry lock for introduction of specimens, media, etc., that provide for a large enclosed space, free of oxygen, in which surface cultivation can be used. Its initial cost and space requirement are high, but plates can be inspected at any time under anaerobic conditions, and conventional technics are employed. The Center for Disease Control (CDC) methodology, as described in Chapters 70 and 72, and also in Chapters 83-85, is based on the use of the anaerobic chamber.

There is no doubt that the roll-tube and the anaerobic chamber systems are the most rigorous and efficacious methods in the recovery of the most fastidious and extremely oxygen-sensitive anaerobes, and that the use of one or the other is essential in studies of the anaerobes of the normal flora. Both methods can be useful in clinical laboratories processing large numbers of specimens for anaerobic culture (for further details, see Anaerobic methods, Chapter 70).

The Brewer and Torbal jars (evacuation-replacement types), and especially the GasPak jar,[6] are by far the most commonly used systems now in clinical laboratories. The GasPak jar is a self-contained combustion jar system with its own gas-generating package that eliminates the need for vacuum pumps. It employs a palladinized alumina catalyst active at room temperature; a methylene blue indicator for anaerobiosis is included. It is a simple, convenient system that stimulated the introduction of anaerobic technics into many clinical laboratories. Recent studies[13,14] comparing the efficacy of the GasPak, roll-tube, and anaerobic chamber technics, **employing properly collected and (anaerobically) transported clinical specimens,** indicate that all 3 systems perform equally well in regard to recovery of clinically important anaerobes.

Two special problems are associated with the anaerobic jar system: (1) when plates are inoculated, they are often put into a jar that is left open until more cultures arrive to fill the jar before it is sealed, and thus the plates are exposed to oxygen; (2) sometimes properly and promptly sealed jars are opened to add new plates, again resulting in repeated exposure to oxygen. By using Martin's **holding-flush jar arrangement,**[15] these problems can be easily solved. Inoculated plates are placed into a storage jar covered with an unclamped vented lid through which oxygen-free CO_2 is passing continuously until enough plates accumulate to fill the jar, sealing it and setting up anaerobiosis. The same can be done with media held before inoculation and with plates for subculture. The most economical way to obtain oxygen-free CO_2 is to use a tube filled with copper shavings heated in a thermostatically controlled small electric oven: the CO_2 passes through the hot copper oxidizing it as the O_2 is removed from the CO_2. The copper can be reduced periodically by passing gas containing 3% hydrogen through the heated copper for a few minutes.

The use of **fresh** or **active** catalyst in the anaerobic jar is mandatory; it may become inactivated by moisture or H_2S. Catalysts can easily be reactivated by heating at 160-180 C in a drying oven for 2 hours. **A packet of fresh or reactivated catalyst should be used each time.**

For further details, see Chapter 70, Anaerobic methods.

Blood cultures

Commercially available media, such as tryptic soy broth, thiol broth, Columbia broth (BBL, Cockeysville, Md.), thioglycollate medium 135 C, and trypticase broth, prepared under vacuum with CO_2, usually containing sodium polyanethol sulfonate (SPS), all yield comparable recovery of anaerobes. Since SPS is inhibitory for some gram-positive anaerobic cocci, another anticoagulant, sodium amylosulfate, may be preferable when available. Gram-stained smears and blind aerobic and anaerobic subcultures need to be made.

Media

For jars, freshly prepared or reducible plated media are used (reducible media may contain a chemical reducing agent and palladium chloride and are reduced before use by keeping them in a jar under anaerobic conditions for 1 or 2 days). Recommended media are (1) blood agar with enriched base (Brucella, Columbia, or Schaedler); (2) a liquid medium (PRAS chopped meat–glucose, or supplemented thioglycollate with vitamin K_1, 0.1 $\mu g/ml$, and hemin, 5 $\mu g/ml$); and (3) selective media such as kanamycin-vancomycin laked blood agar.[11] Growth on this latter plate is presumptive evidence for the presence of an obligately anaerobic gram-negative bacillus (about half of all anaerobic isolates from clinical material) and is highly useful for separation of anaerobes from mixed aerobic-anaerobic cultures.

For details, see Media and reagents for anaerobes—CDC, and Media for gram-negative anaerobes—Wadsworth, Chapter 72; see also anaerobic specimens and culture, Chapters 75 and 86.

Incubation

When jars are used, plates should be incubated for 48 hours at 35-37 C. Negative plates should be held for 1 week. If necessary, duplicate plates can be set in 2 jars, so that one set can be examined in 12-24 hours.

Examination and identification

Plates should be examined with a hand lens or with a stereoscopic microscope. All colony types should be quantitated, described, and subcultured for oxygen tolerance, purity, and subsequent identification.

Presumptive identification can be made on the basis of a few observations such as colonial morphology, cellular morphology, Gram stain, and susceptibility to certain antibiotics. A schema for presumptive identification by susceptibility to antibiotics, developed by Sutter et al.,[16] has been used successfully. Other characteristics such as bile and deoxycholate resistance and esculine hydrolysis can also be used. (See Chapters 72, 75, and 86.)

For **definitive speciation,** a large array of biochemical tests is required, details of which are described in the excellent manuals published by the Wadsworth group,[11,17] the VPI group,[12] and the U.S. Center for Disease Control.[18]

Where available, gas chromatography (GLC) for end-product analysis is used for definitive identification of gram-positive cocci, certain clostridia, and some gram-positive non-spore-forming bacilli (for GLC, see Chapter 74).

A **micromethod multitest system** (API-20A) is now available that considerably simplifies performance of biochemical tests and is useful in speciation of certain anaerobes,[19] and another system (Minitek) has been modified and is also useful.[20]

For a brief but useful description of practical anaerobic bacteriology, see Finegold et al.[21]

For further details, see Isolation and identification: various procedures, below.

Susceptibility tests

At present, the majority of clinically significant anaerobes have reasonably predictable susceptibilities to antimicrobial agents. Thus it should be possible for the physician to select an appropriate drug based on presumptive identification of the organism. Therefore, routine susceptibility testing is *not* recommended. However, it may be important in certain circumstances: agar and broth **dilution tests** are used, but they are not feasible in many clinical laboratories. Sutter et al.[11] have developed an **agar disk diffusion** test that can be used in the diagnostic laboratory.

Many laboratories need a method allowing

them to test individual isolates or small numbers at one time. The **microbroth dilution method**[22] and the **broth-disk method**[23] are suitable for such laboratories. The **modified broth-disk** method (Kurzynski et al.),[24] with its aerobic incubation, was evaluated by Rosenblatt, Murray, Sonnenwirth, and Joyce[25] and found to be simple and efficient.

In Kurzynski et al.'s[24] aerobic broth-disk procedure antimicrobial disks are incorporated into 5 ml thioglycollate medium (BBL 11720 or 135 C), each in screwcap tubes, and the tubes are incubated under aerobic conditions (tightened cap in room air). For *Bacteroides melaninogenicus* strains, 0.5 ml supplement of 9 parts rabbit serum and 1 part hemin-menadione stock solution (500 μg hemin, 50 μg menadione) is added.

Number of disks added to each 5 ml thioglycollate medium is as follows:

1 Penicillin 10 μg disk
5 Carbenicillin 100 μg disks
2 Cephalothin 30 μg disks
8 Clindamycin 2 μg disks
2 Chloramphenicol 30 μg disks

Final concentration of antimicrobials (μg/ml) is as follows:

Penicillin   2 μg/ml
Carbenicillin   100 μg/ml
Cephalothin   12.5 μg/ml
Clindamycin   3.2 μg/ml
Chloramphenicol   12.5 μg/ml

Hold tubes 2 h at room temperature, then invert to ensure adequate mixing. Inoculate with 0.1 ml of overnight chopped meat–glucose culture of organism to be tested. Incubate tubes 18-24 h. Susceptibility to drugs is indicated by absence of growth.

For a detailed discussion of antimicrobial sensitivity testing of anaerobes, see Chapter 87.

• • •

The choice of anaerobic system and the extent of identification procedures depends on the size of the laboratory, availability of resources and equipment, workload, and economic considerations. Availability of simplified jar methods, just as effective as the more complex systems, allows practically all clinical laboratories to isolate and characterize clinically significant anaerobes, thereby greatly increasing awareness of the insignificant role and frequency of anaerobes in disease processes.

ANAEROBIC INFECTIONS

Anaerobic bacteria may be involved in any type of infection that can be caused by bacteria. All organs and tissues of the body are susceptible to infection with these organisms. Some infections in which anaerobes of endogenous origin have major etiologic roles are bacteremia, brain abscess, otitis media (chronic), dental infections, aspiration pneumonia, lung abscess, liver abscess, peritonitis, intra-abdominal abscesses, wound infection (following bowel surgery or trauma), puerperal or postabortal sepsis, endo-

Table 82-4. Major habitats of anaerobes commonly found in endogenous infections*

Species	Oral cavity	GI tract	GU orifices	Skin
Actinomyces israelii	+			
Arachnia propionica	+			
Bacteroides fragilis group		+		
B. melaninogenicus group	+	+	+	
Bifidobacterium eriksonii	+	+	+	
Clostridium perfringens		+		
C. septicum		+		
Eubacterium lentum	+	+		
Fusobacterium nucleatum	+			
F. necrophorum	+			
Peptostreptococcus anaerobius	+	+		
Propionibacterium acnes				+

*Modified from Dowell.[27]

metritis, gynecologic infections (e.g., tubo-ovarian abscess), perirectal abscess, and gas-forming cellulitis.[26] Most infections involving anaerobes arise at or near mucosal surfaces, since the major sources of anaerobes in the body are the various mucosal surfaces.

Intra-abdominal infections, most of which arise from the bowel, involve *B. fragilis* commonly; this organism is the dominant member of the normal human colonic flora. Similarly, anaerobic streptococci, prevalent in the mouth, upper respiratory tract, and female genital tract, are often involved in infections of these areas.

Some of the endogenous anaerobes isolated from clinical specimens and their habitats are shown in Table 82-4. Of these, members of the *B. fragilis* group (especially *B. fragilis*, *B. thetaiotaomicron*, and *B. vulgatus*) are by far the most important from the standpoint of human disease.[28-31] They are the most common anaerobes associated with disease in humans and are resistant to a number of antibiotics, e.g., the penicillins and the aminoglycosides (see Chapter 86).

Whereas it is true that most anaerobic infections in humans are **endogenous**, i.e., arising from within and involving indigenous organisms, there are anaerobes, causing diseases in humans, that are of **exogenous** origin (Table 82-5). These include **intoxications** (foodborne illnesses due to preformed toxin, as in botulism, or toxin production at a local wound site, as in tetanus) or **histotoxic infections** (traumatic or nontraumatic), ranging from benign superficial infections to severe uterine infections (following septic abortion) or myonecrosis (gas gangrene).

Table 82-5. Diseases involving anaerobes from exogenous sources[32]

Foodborne illnesses
Botulism
Clostridium perfringens gastroenteritis
Wound infections
Tetanus
Myonecrosis (gas gangrene)
Crepitant cellulitis
Benign superficial infections
Infection following an animal or human bite
Botulism
Septic abortion (contaminated instruments)

Among the factors predisposing to disease involving anaerobes are trauma, ischemia, and necrosis of tissue, and the concomitant multiplication of other bacteria in mixed infections, since these can lower the oxidation-reduction potential of the tissue sufficiently so that multiplication of the obligate anaerobes can occur.

According to Finegold et al.[33] patients with endogenous anaerobic bacterial infections invariably have been compromised in some manner. Some of the predisposing factors include surgical procedures; an underlying illness, such as leukemia, carcinoma, diabetes mellitus, arteriosclerosis, or alcoholism; and the use of antimicrobials or irradiation in therapy.

Clues suggesting infection with gram-negative (or other) anaerobes: clinical and bacteriologic clues. Refer to Chapter 86 (gram-negative anaerobic rods—clues suggesting infection).

ISOLATION AND IDENTIFICATION: VARIOUS PROCEDURES

Wadsworth methodology[11,17]
1. Primary plates should be examined with stereoscopic microscope or good hand lens (5-8x). Colony types should be recorded, Gram stained, and subcultured to:[17]
   a. Blood agar plate (for anaerobic incubation–pure culture)
   b. Chocolate agar (for CO_2 incubation)
   c. Blood agar (for incubation in air)
   d. Egg yolk plate (for lecithinase and lipase)
   Multiple plates can be used, i.e., 4-6 isolates can be inoculated on same plates.
2. Examine primary plates for:[17]
   a. Fluorescence (KVL and blood agar plates)—use Wood's lamp (UV light). Brick red fluorescence is seen with *B. melaninogenicus* or *B. asaccharolyticus*; *Veillonella parvula* also gives red fluorescence, but Gram stain reveals that it is a gram-negative small coccus and not a *Bacteroides*.
   b. Double zones of hemolysis around large colonies of gram-positive rods strongly suggest *Clostridium perfringens*:
   c. If BBE (bile esculin) agar was used, note growth and esculin hydrolysis; if present, this suggests *B. fragilis*.
3. Use of a **holding jar** (see methods, Chapter 70) is strongly recommended if workup of plates is done in air (on bench), since some fresh clinical isolates may die after comparitively short exposure to oxygen.

The Wadsworth group methodology[17] (for details of tests see Chapter 72, Media and methods—Wadsworth methodology) calls at this point for placing the following antibiotic disks on the purity blood agar plate: **kanamycin 1000 μg, colistin 10 μg, and vancomycin 5 μg.** This is a modification[17] of Sutter et al.'s original schema[16] for presumptive identification by susceptibility to antibiotics. The disks are available, on courtesy basis, from Baltimore Biological Laboratory (BBL), Cockeysville, Md.

NOTE: **With the exception of the colistin disk, the disks contain drug concentrations different from those used in the Kirby-Bauer sensitivity test. They should not be used for determining therapeutic susceptibility.**[17]

If the organism examined is a gram-positive coccus, a sodium polyanethol sulfonate (SPS) disk can be placed near the colistin disk for identification of *Peptostreptococcus anaerobius*.

Incubate purity plates (together with primary plates) 48 h.

For identification, it is necessary to carefully determine whether isolates are anaerobic, aerotolerant, or microaerophilic.

Preliminary grouping can be carried out from a pure culture on blood agar plate by observing and recording susceptibility to 3 antimicrobial disks (more than 10 mm zone—sensitive), colony morphology, pigment, hemolysis, fluorescence, pitting, lipase, lecithinase, spot indole test, nitrate reductase, and catalase test.

Subculture to supplemented thioglycollate for inoculation of biochemicals and motility. Inoculate 20% bile if isolate is a gram-negative anaerobic rod.

Several organisms can be identified reliably with these rapid tests:

1. *B. fragilis, B. melaninogenicus* group, *Fusobacterium necrophorum, F. nucleatum, F. mortiferum, F. varium* group (For details, see Chapter 86.)
2. *Peptostreptococcus anaerobius, Veillonella parvula, P. asaccharolyticus* (See Chapter 83.)
3. *Propionibacterium acnes* (See Chapter 85.)
4. *C. perfringens* (See Chapter 84.)

Definitive identification of all isolates should be made whenever possible; however, many laboratories limit their identification procedures to the preliminary grouping tests and, when necessary in important cases, send the isolate to a reference laboratory. For definitive identification, a different set of biochemicals is to be inoculated for each group of organisms (see Sutter et al.[17]). The Wadsworth methodology calls for the use of **PRAS** (prereduced anaerobically sterilized) biochemicals (see Anaerobic methods, Roll-tube VPI technic, Chapter 70; for further details, Holdeman et al.[12]) employing either an open technic with a special (VPI) inoculating apparatus, or inoculating PRAS tubes with a syringe (tubes with a rubber diaphragm are now commercially available from Scott Laboratories, Fiskeville, R.I.). Either way, the use of PRAS tubes is a time-consuming and expensive technic for the average laboratory (Sutter et al.[17]). Resulting pH changes (fermentation) are measured with a pH meter equipped with a thin electrode.

For **GLC** (gas chromatography) procedure, see Chapter 74.

For **micromethods** and **miniaturized kits** used in identification, see below.

• • •

Center for Disease Control (CDC) methodology[34]

The CDC routinely uses an anaerobe glovebox for primary isolation; however, all the procedures used can also be used with an anaerobe jar or a GasPak anaerobe jar.

After incubation:

1. Examine anaerobic and CO_2 plates with hand lens and dissecting microscope.
   a. Observe and record action on blood and egg yolk, and size and shape of colonies.
      (1) Prepare Gram-stained smears for comparison of colonies on different plates. Record shape and location of any spores observed.
      (2) Colonies on egg yolk agar may be used to test for catalase by adding drop of 3% H_2O_2 to suspension of organisms on slide. Expose EYA plates to air for at least 30 min before testing for catalase. Do not use colonies from blood agar plates to test for catalase.
   b. Determine number of different colony types on anaerobe plates.
      (1) For each colony to be transferred, prereduce 1 tube of chopped meat–dextrose medium and 1 tube of thioglycollate medium by heating media in boiling water bath for 10 min. Cool before use.
      (2) Using needle with small loop or heat-sealed 22.5 cm (9 inches) Pasteur capillary pipet, fish each different colony and inoculate tube of chopped meat–dextrose medium and tube of thioglycollate medium. If anaerobes other than clostridia are suspected, add 0.5 ml sterile rabbit serum to thioglycollate medium. Chopped meat medium is best for culturing clostridia, and enriched thioglycollate medium is more suitable for non-sporeforming anaerobes.
   c. Incubate chopped meat and thioglycollate media in anaerobe jar 24-48 h.
2. Be sure to have at least 1 representative colony of each morphologic type seen on original smear. If necessary, restreak plating media to obtain isolated colonies.

Examine plates inoculated with enrichment cultures after incubation. Subculture any colony types not isolated from direct plates to prereduced chopped meat–dextrose and thioglycollate media.

Examine thioglycollate and chopped meat subcultures from isolated colonies. If pure, use these cultures to inoculate appropriate differential media for identification of isolates.

For identification, it is necessary to undertake the following steps:

1. Determine and record cellular morphology and colonial characteristics on blood agar, and Gram stain each colony type; check for purity.
2. Inoculate differential media (thioglycollate base medium with added carbohydrates); see Media, CDC, Chapter 72.
   a. Basic set of differential media includes the following: chopped meat, fermentation base, glucose, mannitol, lactose, sucrose, maltose, salicin, thiogel, iron-milk, indole-nitrite (for indole), indole-nitrite (for nitrite), H_2S medium, motility, esculin, peptone yeast glucose (PYG) agar, and an infusion agar slant. Tube of PYG broth may be added to the basic set to determine metabolic products by gas-liquid chromatography.
   b. Additions to basic set for gram-positive spore-formers: chopped meat–dextrose and urea.
   c. Additions to basic set for gram-negative rodd: xylose, arabinose, rhamnose, trehalose, thioglycollate broth, and 20% bile in thioglycollate broth.
   d. Additions to basic set for gram-positive non-sporeforming rods*: glycerol, xylose, arabinose.
3. Heat all media, except slants and PYG agar, in boiling water bath 10 min. Cool in tap water.
4. Melt PYG agar in boiling bath or autoclave and place in 48 C water bath.
5. Using capillary pipet, inoculate fluid and semi-solid media near bottom of tubes with drop of culture. Expel small amount of inoculum up "line of stab" as pipet is withdrawn. Be sure to expel all air from pipet before placing pipet into into medium. One pipet may be used to inoculate several different media.
6. Mix inoculum and PYG agar by carefully inverting agar tube; allow medium to harden.
7. Inoculate infusion agar slants with drop of culture placed at top of slants. Be sure inoculum runs over surface of slant, not down edge.
8. Inoculate milk last.
9. Include uninoculated tube of Thiogel in each day's run as control for gelatin liquefaction.
10. Incubate infusion agar slants and tubes of PYG broth in anaerobe jar 48 h. Incubate other differential media at 35-37 C in aerobic atmosphere or anaerobically if necessary for fastidious organisms.
11. Streak 2 blood agar plates with 24 h culture. If clostridia are suspected, also streak egg yolk agar plate.
    a. Incubate 1 blood agar plate in candle jar.
    b. With gram-negative rods, add 2-unit penicillin disc in area of heavy inoculum on second blood agar plate. Incubate blood agar plate and EYA plate in anaerobe jar. Anaerobic plates should be incubated at least 48 h before plates are examined.
12. Reading of plates is to be done as follows:
    a. Check plates incubated in candle jar and compare with growth on anaerobic blood agar plates to determine oxygen tolerance of organism. Record as anaerobe (growth only in anaerobe jar), aerotolerant anaerobe (some growth in candle jar but better growth anaerobically), or facultative anaerobe (more or less equal growth).
    b. Check egg yolk agar plates for lecithinase, lipase, and proteolytic enzyme production.
    c. Check anaerobic blood agar plates for hemolysis and colony characteristics. On plates with penicillin disks, any size zone of complete inhibition around disk indicates sensitivity to penicillin. Record as sensitive or resistant.
13. For differential media, biochemical tests are routinely incubated up to 7 d after inoculation, but may be reported as early as 48 h after inoculation if reactions allow identification of isolate. Tubes are inspected daily and results recorded on first, second, and final days of incubation. All tests on fastidious or slow-growing types

---

*To check for spores, inoculate chopped meat agar slants, incubate anaerobically at 30 C for 10-14 d, and perform Gram or spore stains as required.

Table 82-6. List of changes in the nomenclature of anaerobic bacteria[18]

Present designation	Former designations(s)	Present designation	Former designations(s)
Arachnia propionica	*Actinomyces propionicus*	*C. paraperfringens*	*C. barati*
Bacteroides clostridiiformis ssp *girans*	*Fusobacterium girans*	*Eubacterium alactolyticum*	*Ramibacterium alactolyticum, R. pleuriticum*
B. fragilis		*E. lentum*	*Corynebacterium diphtheroides*
ssp *fragilis*	*Bacteroides fragilis*		(CDC Manual),
ssp *distasonis*	*B. fragilis*		*Bifidobacterium*
ssp *vulgatus*	*B. incommunis*		*cornutum,*
ssp *thetaiotaomicron*	*B. variabilis*		*Corynebacterium*
ssp *ovatus*	*B. ovatus*		*group 3*
B. melaninogenicus		*Fusobacterium*	*Sphaerophorus*
ssp *melaninogenicus*	*B. melaninogenicus*	*necrophorum*	*necrophorus*
ssp *asaccharolyticus*	*B. melaninogenicus*	*F. nucleatum*	*Fusobacterium fusiforme*
ssp *intermedius*	*B. melaninogenicus*	*F. mortiferum*	*F. ridiculosum,*
B. oralis			*Sphaerophorus*
ssp *oralis*	*B. oralis*		*ridiculosum*
ssp *elongatus*	*B. oralis*	*Lactobacillus*	*Catenabacterium*
B. pneumosintes	*Dialister pneumosintes*	*catenaforme*	*catenaforme*
Bifidobacterium eriksonii	*Actinomyces eriksonii*	*Propionibacterium acnes*	*Corynebacterium acnes*
Campylobacter sputorum	*Vibrio sputorum*	*P. freudenreichii* ssp *freudenreichii*	*Propionibacterium freudenreichii*
ssp *sputorum*		*P. freudenreichii* ssp *shermanii*	*P. shermanii*
Clostridium cadaveris	*Clostridium capitovale*	*P. granulosum*	*C. granulosum*
C. limosum	*C. species* group P1		
C. ramosum	*Catenabacterium filamentosum, B. trichoides (B. terebrans)*		

may be held up to 3 w. Other exceptions to routine are as follows:

a. Tests for indole and nitrite are made 24 h after good growth is obtained in indole-nitrite medium. This is normally 48 h after inoculation of tubes. In addition, fermentation base medium (control) can be tested for indole after final reading of fermentation test has been made.

b. Tests for catalase on infusion agar and hydrolysis of esculin are normally made at 48 h, and tubes are then discarded.

c. Thiogel may be incubated up to 1 mo before it is reported as negative for liquefaction. Reactions are usually complete in 7 d, however.

d. Occasionally, determination of motility of organism in semisolid motility medium is not possible because of gas production. In this case motility can be checked by microscopic examination of wet mounts prepared from young (6-18 h) broth cultures grown in low-carbohydrate medium such as plain chopped meat medium.

e. Tests for metabolic products are normally made on 48 h PYG broth cultures by gas-liquid chromatography. For method of testing, see Chapter 74, GLC.

For interpretation of reactions in differential media, see Table 72-3, Chapter 72.

Microtechnics and miniaturized kits for identification. The **API-20A** system,[19] containing 16 carbohydrates and tests for indole, catalase, esculin, gelatin, and urea, is used for identification. Whereas it identifies a number of species,

a proportion of clinical isolates is not identified by the system; it is difficult to use with weakly saccharolytic strains, and it is not helpful with asaccharolytic organisms. The **Minitek (BBL)**[20] system, useful with a number of isolates, is also inadequate for identifying asaccharolytic organisms.

Recently, Kilian[35] reported successful use of the API-ZYM system for 20 different preformed enzymes (including phosphatases, esterases, aminopeptidases, and glycosidases) with Actinomycetaceae and related bacteria. The results could be read after 4 h of incubation.

Changes in the nomenclature of anaerobes

A number of changes occurred in the nomenclature of anaerobic bacteria since the last edition (1970) of this work was printed. Some of the changes are shown in Table 82-6.

SEROLOGY OF ANAEROBES

Information regarding human antibodies to anaerobes is limited. Scattered work employing agglutination, gel diffusion, passive hemagglutination, and immunofluorescence demonstrated antibody response to various Bacteroidaceae in patients with *Bacteroides* or *Fusobacterium* infections.

Natural antibodies to Bacteroidaceae are widely distributed in normal adults (Quick et al.[36]); for a review of antibody response to anaerobic bacteria, see Sonnenwirth.[37]

STOCK CULTURES AND SHIPPING OF ANAEROBES

Stock cultures should be prepared from young and actively growing cultures. Sutter et al.[17] recommend supplemented thioglycollate medium for preparation of stock cultures.

1. Add 0.5 ml liquid culture to equal volume of skim milk (20% powdered skim milk in distilled water) in screwcapped 1 dram vial.
2. Freeze and maintain at −70 C.

The Center for Disease Control (CDC)[34] recommends storing non-sporeforming anaerobes, grown on slants, in 0.35-0.4 ml sterile defibrinated rabbit blood, with quick freezing in 95% alcohol–dry ice bath and storing at −42 C in freezer. For sporeformers, use brain storage medium. Inoculate and incubate brain storage medium at 35-37 C. Gram stain daily and look for spores. As soon as spores are noted, store culture at −20 or −42 C, or after 5 d if no spores are noted.

Brain storage medium[34]
1. Add small amount of water to beef or calf brains and mix in blender.
2. Prepare peptone solution, using 20 g peptone in 1000 ml distilled water. Adjust pH to 7.2 − 7.4.
3. Dispense in 13 × 100 mm screwcap tubes. Use 1 part brain and 2 parts peptone solution. Tubes should be over half full.
4. Autoclave at 121 C for 15 min.

Maintenance medium for Actinomyces. See Chapter 85, *Actinomyces*.

Lyophilization of anaerobe cultures[34]
1. Select smooth colony on blood agar, inoculate thioglycollate medium (BBL 135 C or equivalent), and incubate anaerobically at 35-37 C until good growth is obtained.
2. Check purity of culture with Gram-stained smear.
3. If culture is pure, inoculate blood agar slant and incubate anaerobically at 35-37 C for 48 h.
4. Recheck purity of culture with Gram-stained smear.
5. Suspend growth on slant in 0.5-0.75 ml sterile skim milk and dispense approximately 0.25 ml quantities of suspension into sterile 1.0 ml lyophilization ampoules (Virtis). These ampoules have a long tapered stem to allow heat sealing and are prescored for easy opening.
6. Freeze suspensions rapidly by swirling tubes in "slush" mixture of ethanol and dry ice (−70 C) and hold tubes in freezer (−20 C or lower) until lyophilized.
7. Before placing ampoules on freeze dryer, pull vacuum of 5 μ or less (as measured with McLeod gauge) with heavy duty vacuum pump (70-140 L/min) and fill trap with mixture of dry ice and ethanol. Vacuum of 1.2 mm or less must be maintained throughout lyophilization procedure, otherwise suspensions will thaw.
8. After 5-6 h on lyophilization unit, seal ampoules under vacuum using torch fueled with mixture of illuminating gas and air.
9. Check vacuum in ampoules with high-frequency induction coil to ensure proper sealing.
10. Store lyophilized cultures at ambient temperature or under refrigeration.

Shipment of anaerobic cultures.[34] Anaerobic cultures can be shipped to a reference laboratory for identification in tubes of liquid or semisolid media. Plates or slants are not satisfactory. Cultures should be purified before shipment.

Culture can best be shipped in a carbohydrate-free medium containing 0.3% to 1% agar such as motility medium. The medium should be freshly prepared and tubed 5.0-7.5 cm (2 to 3 inches) deep in screwcap tubes. *Clostridium* cultures in plain chopped meat media or cultures of the non-sporeformers in thioglycollate media can also be used for shipment.

Before shipment, a 1.8-2.5 cm (¾ to 1 inch) overlay of melted paraffin or 5% agar should be added to actively growing cultures in either semisolid or liquid media. Screwcaps should be tightened and sealed with waterproof tape.

REFERENCES

1. Sonnenwirth, A. C.: Am J. Clin. Nutr. **25**:1295-1298, 1972.
2. Hungate, R. E.: Bacteriol. Rev. **14**:1-49, 1950.
3. Moore, W. E. C.: Int. J. Syst. Bacteriol. **16**:173-190, 1966.
4. Stokes, E. J.: Lancet **1**:668-672, 1958.
5. Finegold, S. M., Miller, A. B., and Posnick, D. J.: Ernaehrungsforschung **10**:517-528, 1965.
6. Brewer, J. H., and Allgeier, D. L.: Appl. Microbiol. **14**:985-988, 1966.
7. Aranki, A., Syed, S. A., Kenny, E. B. and Freter, R.: Appl. Microbiol. **17**:568-576, 1969.
8. Rosebury, T., and Reynold, J. B.: Proc. Soc. Exp. Biol. Med. **117**:813-816, 1964.
9. Loesche, W. J.: Appl. Microbiol. **18**:723-727, 1969.
10. Gorbach, S. L., and Bartlett, J. G.: N. Engl. J. Med. **290**:1289-1294, 1974.
11. Sutter, V. L., Vargo, V. L., and Finegold, S. M.: Wadsworth anaerobic bacteriology manual, ed. 2, Los Angeles, 1975, Department of Continuing Education in Health Sciences University Extension, and the School of Medicine, UCLA.
12. Holdeman, L. V., Cato, E. P., and Moore, W. E. C., editors: Anaerobe laboratory manual, ed. 4, Blacksburg, Va., 1977, Virginia Polytechnic Institute and State University Anaerobe Laboratory.
13. Killgore, G. E., Starr, S. E., Del Bene, V. E., et al: Am. J. Clin. Pathol. **59**:552-559, 1973.
14. Rosenblatt, J. E., Fallon, A., and Finegold, S. M.: Appl. Microbiol. **25**:77-85, 1973.
15. Martin, J. W.: Appl. Microbiol. **22**:1168-1171, 1971.
16. Sutter, V. L., and Finegold, S. M.: Appl. Microbiol. **21**:13-20, 1971.
17. Sutter, V. L., Vargo, V. L., and Finegold, S. M.: Wadsworth anaerobic bacteriology manual, ed. 3, St. Louis, The C. V. Mosby Co. (In press.)
18. Dowell, V. R., Jr., and Hawkins, T. M.: Laboratory methods in anaerobic bacteriology—CDC laboratory manual, DHEW publ. no. (CDC) 78-8272, Atlanta, 1977, Center for Disease Control.
19. Moore, H. B., Sutter, V. L., and Finegold, S. M.: J. Clin. Microbiol. **1**:15-24, 1975.
20. Stargel, M. D., Thompson, F. S., Phillips, S. E., et al.: J. Clin. Microbiol. **3**:291-301, 1976.
21. Finegold, S. M., Shepherd, W. E., and Spaulding, E. H.: Practical anaerobic bacteriology (Shepherd, W. E., coordinating editor), Cumitech no. 5, Washington, D.C., 1977, American Society for Microbiology.
22. Rotilie, C. A., Fass, R. J., Prior, R. B., and Perkins, R. L.: Antimicrob. Agents Chemother. **7**:311-315, 1975.
23. Wilkins, T. D., and Thiel, T.: Antimicrob. Agents Chemother. **3**:350-356, 1973.
24. Kurzynski, T. A., Yrios, J. W., Helstad, A. G., and

Field, C. R.: Antimicrob. Agents Chemother. **10:**727-732, 1976.
25. Rosenblatt, J. E., Murray, P. R., Sonnenwirth, A. C., and Joyce, J. L.: Antimicrob. Agents Chemother. **15:**351, 1979.
26. Finegold, S. M.: Mt. Sinai J. Med. **43:**776, 1976.
27. Dowell, V. R., Jr.: Am. J. Med. Technol. **41:**32, 1975.
28. Dowell, V. R., Jr.: Wound and abscess specimens. In Balows, A., editor: How to start and when to stop, Springfield, Ill., 1975, Charles C Thomas, Publisher.
29. Finegold, S. M.: Anaerobic bacteria in human disease, New York, 1977, Academic Press.
30. Gorbach, S. L., and Bartlett, J. G.: N. Engl. J. Med. **290:**1177-1184, 1974.
31. Gorbach, S. L., and Bartlett, J. G.: N. Engl. J. Med. **290:**1237-1245, 1974.
32. Jones, G., and Dowell, V. R.: Anaerobic bacteriology in the clinical laboratory, Atlanta, 1976, Laboratory Training and Consultation Div., Center for Disease Control.
33. Finegold, S. M., Marsh, V. H., and Bartlett, J. G.: Anaerobic infections in the compromised host. In Brachman, P., and Eickhoff, T. C., editors: Proceedings of the international conference on hospital infections, Chicago, 1971, American Hospital Association.
34. Dowell, V. R., Jr., and Hawkins, T. M.: Laboratory methods in anaerobic bacteriology, CDC Laboratory manual publ. no. (CDC) 78-8272, Atlanta, 1977, Center for Disease Control.
35. Kilian, M.: J. Clin. Microbiol. **8:**127, 1978.
36. Quick, J. D., Goldberg, H. S., and Sonnenwirth, A. C.: Am. J. Clin. Nutr. **25:**1351, 1972.
37. Sonnenwirth, A. C.: Rev. Infect. Dis. **1:**337, 1979.

83

ANAEROBIC COCCI

V. R. Dowell, Jr.
Alex C. Sonnenwirth

Anaerobic cocci are commonly encountered in clinical materials from a variety of human infections.[1-6] Essentially any region or organ of the body can be involved. With few exceptions these are endogenous infections in which the cocci are derived from the oral cavity, gastrointestinal tract, genitourinary system, or skin of the patient, where they may reside in large numbers. Although there is little doubt that some of the anaerobic cocci isolated from clinical materials are responsible for disease, the pathogenicity of others has not been established with certainty. Mixed infections involving anaerobic cocci are common, and it is difficult to ascribe pathogenicity to any one of the microorganisms involved. On the other hand, serious synergistic infections such as crepitus cellulitis[7] and synergistic gas gangrene as described by Meleney[8] have been well documented.

The gram-positive anaerobic cocci are seen in female genital tract infections, relatively frequently in respiratory tract infections, but less often in intra-abdominal abscesses and infections than are gram-negative anaerobic rods.[6,9,10]

The gram-negative anaerobic cocci, on the other hand, are more often seen in mixed infections but rarely in monoinfections.[11,12] A list of diseases that may involve anaerobic cocci is given in Table 83-1.

The classification of obligately anaerobic cocci of clinical interest is presently in some dispute,[36] despite the detailed classification by Holdeman et al.,[37] which is in some disagreement with *Bergey's Manual* (ed. 8) systematics.[38] Watt and Jack[36] have recently studied a number of anaerobic cocci and have offered a definition for delineating the nature of anaerobic cocci: "cocci that grow well under anaerobiosis and do not grow in 10% CO_2 in air even after incubation for 7 days at 37 C." In addition, they demonstrated that all anaerobic cocci were metronidazole sensitive, whereas microaerophilic, not truly anaerobic cocci are resistant to metronidazole.

Taxonomy

Gram-positive non-sporeforming anaerobic cocci are classified in the eighth edition of *Bergey's Manual of Determinative Bacteriology*[38] as follows:

PART 14 GRAM-POSITIVE COCCI
Family III. *Peptococcaceae*
  Genus I. *Peptococcus* (6 species)
  Genus II. *Peptostreptococcus* (5 species)
  Genus III. *Ruminococcus* (2 species)
  Genus IV. *Sarcina* (2 species)

Recently, Holdeman and Moore[39] proposed a new genus *Coprococcus* to be included in the family *Peptococcaceae*, 2 new *Ruminococcus* species, a new *Streptococcus* species, and recommended that certain species of *Peptostreptococcus* as classified in the seventh edition of *Bergey's Manual of Determinative Bacteriology*[40] be transferred to the genus *Streptococcus*. The characteristics of the genera of the family *Peptococcaceae* (Rogosa) as proposed by Holdeman and Moore[39] are listed in Table 83-2.

The "microaerophilic" streptococci have been a problem in nomenclature and identification. However, these organisms seem to be actually members of the genus *Streptococcus* based on metabolic end-product analysis,[9] and often can

Table 83-1. Diseases that may involve anaerobic cocci and pertinent references to each

1. Central nervous system—brain abscess, meningitis, subdural empyema[6,14,15]
2. Oral and dental—gingival infections,[6] periodontal disease[16]
3. Ear, nose, and throat—otitis media,[14] sinusitis,[17] tonsillar abscess[13]
4. Pleuropulmonary—aspiration pneumonia, lung abscess, pleural empyema[6,18,19]
5. Intra-abdominal—appendicitis,[20-22] liver abscess,[23] pelvic abscess[20-22]
6. Female genital tract—post partum infections,[24,25] tubo-ovarian abscess,[6,14-25] postoperative gynecological infections[6]
7. Cardiovascular—bacteremia,[26] endocarditis[27,28]
8. Bone and joints—osteomyelitis,[6,29] purulent arthritis[27,30]
9. Soft tissues—cellulitis,[20-22,31-34] chronic undermining ulcer[6,35]

Table 83-2. Characteristics of genera in *Peptococcaceae**

Genus	Cell arrangement	Peptone major energy source	Carbohydrate fermented	Lactic acid sole major acid product	Butyric or other 3+ carbon volatile acids produced	Mole % G + C (Tm)
Peptococcus	Diplococci, short chains	+†	−⁺	−	V	36-37‡
Peptostreptococcus	Chains	+	+⁻	−	V	33-35
Coprococcus	Diplococci, chains	−	sr	−	+	39-42
Ruminococcus	Diplococci, chains	−	r	−	−	40-45
Sarcina	Packets	−	r	−	V	29-31

*From Holdeman and Moore.[39]

†−, negative reactions; +, positive reaction; r, required; sr, stimulatory or required; V, variable; where 2 reactions are given (e.g., +⁻), the first is the more usual, and the second is observed less frequently.

‡As reported by Rogosa.[38]

be identified as *S. salivarius, S. mutans, S. anginosus,* or *S. mitis.*

It should be noted that 2 organisms, previously known as *Peptococcus morbillorum* and *Peptostreptococcus intermedius,* are not included here, since they become aerotolerant after one or more subcultures and produce lactic acid without significant amounts of other acids or gas. Therefore, they should be identified as *Streptococcus* species. For definitive identification, gas-liquid chromatography (GLC) is needed.

Major characteristics for differentiation of the anaerobic gram-positive cocci are shown in Fig. 83-1 and Tables 83-2 and 83-3. See also Tables 83-5 to 83-7.

The anaerobic gram-negative cocci are classified in the eighth edition of *Bergey's Manual of Determinative Bacteriology*[38] as follows:

PART 11 GRAM-NEGATIVE ANAEROBIC COCCI
Family I. *Veillonellaceae*
  Genus I. *Veillonella* (2 species)
  Genus II. *Acidaminococcus* (1 species)
  Genus III. *Megasphaera* (1 species)

Identification of anaerobic cocci

Anaerobic cocci include members of the following genera:

Gram-positive	Gram-negative
Peptococcus	*Veillonella*
Peptostreptococcus	*Acidaminococcus*
Streptococcus	*Megasphaera*
Coprococcus	
Ruminococcus	
Sarcina	

Only members of the genera *Peptococcus, Peptostreptococcus, Streptococcus, Sarcina,* and *Veillonella* are commonly isolated from human infections if specimens are collected properly. The others are found in the normal flora of the gastrointestinal tract but seldom if ever are involved in disease. Characteristics of anaerobic cocci are shown in Table 83-3. There is considerable disagreement between the eighth edition of *Bergey's Manual,* ed. 8,[38] and Holdeman and Moore[37, 45] for differentiation of the species in the genera *Peptococcus* and *Peptostreptococcus.* For

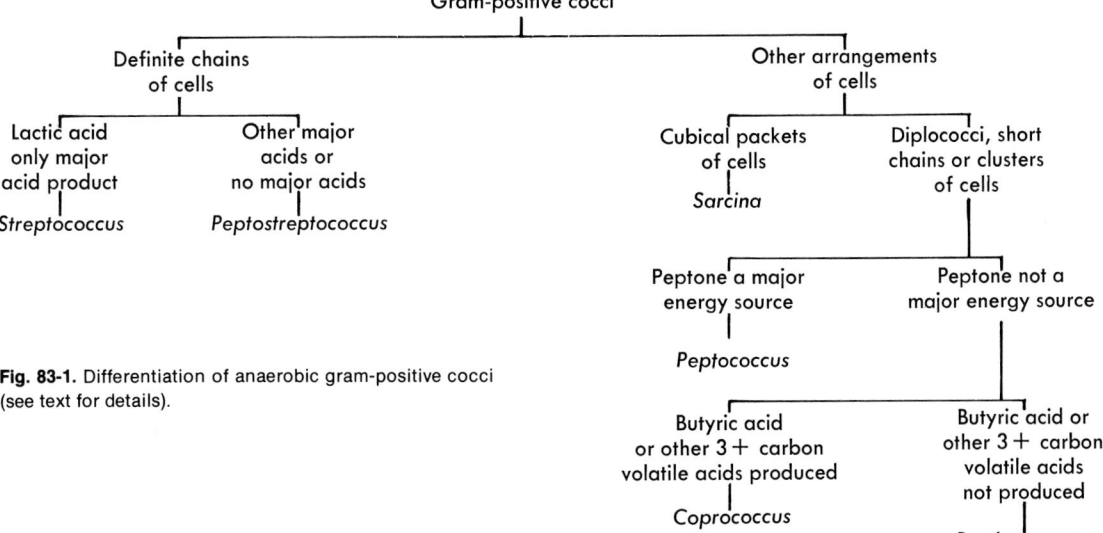

Fig. 83-1. Differentiation of anaerobic gram-positive cocci (see text for details).

Table 83-3. Characteristics of some anaerobic cocci*

Group	Cells in chains	Gram reaction	Catalase	Glucose fermentation	Esculin	Indole	Nitrate reduction	Gelatin liquefaction	Fermentation of						Metabolic products in PYG
									Cellobiose	Glucose	Lactose	Levulose	Maltose	Sucrose	
Peptococcus asaccharolyticus†	−	+	−	−	−	+	−	−	−	−	−	−	−	−	A, B (F, L)
P. saccharolyticus	−	+	+	+	−	−	+⁻	+	−	+	−	+	−	−	A
P. prevotii‡	−	+	−	+	−	−	−	−	−	+	−	+	−	−	A, B (P, F, L)
Peptostreptococcus anaerobius†§	+	+	−	+	−	−	−⁺	−	−	+	−	+	−	−	A, B, IV, IC (P, IB, B, L)
P. micros	+	+	−	−	−	−	−	−	−	−	−	−	−	−	A (F)
P. parvulus	−	+	−	+	−	−	−	+	−	+	+	−	−	−	A, L
Acidaminococcus fermentans	−	−	−	−	−	−	−	−	−	+	−	−	−	−	A, B (PL)
Megasphaera elsdenii	−	−	−	+	−	−	−	−	−	+	−	+	+	−	A, IB, B, IV, VH (PF)
Veillonella parvula	−	−	−	−	−	−	+	−	−	−	−	−	−	−	A, P

*Data from Dowell and Hawkins[41] and Sutter et al.[42] +, Positive reaction; −, negative reaction; A, acetic acid; P, propionic acid; IV, isovaleric acid; IB, isobutyric acid; B, butyric acid; IC, isocaproic acid; and L, lactic acid.

†When tested with 5 μg vancomycin, 10 μg colistin, and 1000 μg kanamycin disks, both *Peptococcus* spp and *Peptostreptococcus* spp are sensitive to vancomycin, resistant to colistin, but variable to kanamycin.

‡*P. prevotii* is not recognized in *Bergey's Manual* (ed. 8) and may be a variant of *P. asaccharolyticus*.

§*P. anaerobius* is markedly inhibited by the anticoagulant sodium polyanethol sulfonate (SPS), and an SPS disk has been used for presumptive identification of the microorganism.[43,44]

Table 83-4. Differential characteristics of anaerobic-to-aerotolerant streptococci*

Characteristic	S. constellatus	S. intermedius	S. morbillorum
Esculin hydrolysis	+	+	−
Glucose fermented	+	+	v
Lactose fermented	−	+	−
Salicin fermented	+[(+)]	+[−]	−
Milk coagulated	−	+	−
Lactic acid sole major product PYG	+	+	+
Growth enhanced by Tween 80	−	v	+ (Tween 80 added)
Aerotolerant after serial transfer	4/5	5/18	1/9

*+, Positive reaction; −, negative reaction; v, variable reaction.

this reason, CDC workers identify the anaerobic cocci as listed in Dowell and Hawkins,[41,46] with the exception that gram-positive cocci producing lactic acid as a sole major product are considered *Streptococcus* species, until the results of more definitive studies have been published. Some differential characteristics of anaerobic-to-aerotolerant streptococci are shown in Table 83-4 (see also Table 83-7).

• • •

Dowell and colleagues[47] have recently developed information related to identification of anaerobic cocci, described below.

Following are characteristics used in the CDC Anaerobe Reference Laboratory for **definitive identification** of anaerobic cocci received from public health laboratories: microscopic features, colony characteristics and hemolysis on anaerobic blood agar, relationship to oxygen (obligate aerobe, facultative anaerobe, microaerophile, aerotolerant anaerobe, obligate anaerobe), growth in enriched thioglycollate broth, various fermentation and biochemical reactions, and acid products produced in PYG medium.[47]

Differential characteristics of the 7 species of anaerobic cocci from human clinical specimens most commonly received by the CDC Anaerobe Reference Laboratory are given in Tables 83-5 and 83-6. These data show that some of the key characteristics for differentiation of these microorganisms are fermentation of glucose, glycerol, and mannose; hydrolysis of esculin; coagulation of milk; indole; catalase; reduction of nitrate to nitrite; and metabolic products (especially butyric, propionic, isocaproic, and lactic acids) in PYG medium.

Practical identification of anaerobic cocci

It is recognized that it is neither practical nor economically feasible in many cases to use a large number of differential media and biochemical determinations for the identification of bacterial isolates in a clinical microbiology laboratory. For this reason, Elliott[48] and Armfield et al. (unpublished data, 1979; also see abstract C198 in Abstracts of the Annual Meeting of the American Society for Microbiology, 1979) have

worked toward development of practical technics suitable for use by clinical laboratories in identification of isolated anaerobic cocci. In these studies, well-characterized reference strains and clinical isolates of various obligately anaerobic and facultatively anaerobic cocci were examined with a large battery of differential tests that included the conventional technics used routinely in the CDC Anaerobe Reference Laboratory and a number of special tests such as inhibition by sodium polyanethol sulfonate (SPS),[49] bacitracin, optochin, and penicillin; decarboxylation of amino acids; effect of Tween 80, formate-fumarate, dithiothreitol, and other additives on growth and reactions on a **presumpto quadrant plate I** containing LD, LD esculin, LD bile, and LD egg yolk media[50] and a **presumpto quadrant plate II,** which contained LD starch, LD glucose, LD milk, and LD DNA media[51] and a disk test for reduction of nitrate[52]; see "Media for anaerobes, CDC usage," Chapter 72.

On the basis of these studies it was concluded that, after pure cultures have been obtained and their relationship to oxygen determined, the common anaerobic cocci can be differentiated with 2 plates and 2 tubes of media:

1. A tube of enriched thioglycollate broth (Thio) to demonstrate chaining of some gram-positive cocci, peptostreptococci, and streptococci.

2. An anaerobe blood agar (AnBA) plate to allow tests for inhibition by SPS and reduction of nitrate.

3. A presumpto quadrant plate I to test for indole, catalase, esculin hydrolysis, H₂S, growth on bile agar, and reactions (lecithinase, lipase, proteolysis) on egg yolk agar.

4. A tube of peptone–yeast extract–glucose (PYG) broth to test for fermentation of glucose and acid metabolic products.

Differentiation of the 7 commonly encountered anaerobic cocci using these characteristics is shown in Table 83-7.

PEPTOCOCCUS

Peptococcus organisms are usually found as members of the normal flora in the respiratory and genital tracts and on the skin. They do occur

Table 83-5. Differential characteristics of common anaerobic cocci received by CDC Anaerobe Reference Laboratory from public health laboratories in United States*

	Peptococcus								Pepto-streptococcus anaerobius		Streptococcus intermedius		Veillonella parvula	
	asaccharolyticus		magnus		prevotii		saccharolyticus							
No. strains	40		31		37		13		25		12		26	
Reaction	Sign	%+	Sign	%+	Sign	%+	Sign	%+	Sign	%+	Sign	%+	Sign	%+
Gram reaction	+	100	+	100	+	100	+	100	+	100	+	100	−	0
Relation to O$_2$	OA	100	OA	100	OA	100	OA	100	OA	100	F/OA	60/40	OA	100
Motility	−	0	−	0	−	0	−	0	−	0	−	0	−	0
Hemolysis (sheep BA)	−	0	−	0	−	0	V	50	−	0	−	0	−	0
Fermentation of:														
Glucose	−	0	−	0	−	0	+	100	V	50	+	100	−	0
Mannitol	−	0	−	0	−	0	−	0	−	0	−	8	−	0
Lactose	−	0	−	0	−	0	−	0	−	0	+	100	−	0
Sucrose	−	0	−	0	−	0	−	0	−	0	+	100	−	0
Maltose	−	0	−	0	−	0	−	0	V	28	+	100	−	0
Salicin	−	0	−	0	−	0	−	0	−	0	+	100	−	0
Glycerol	+	0	−	0	−	0	+	93	−	0	−	0	−	0
Xylose	−	0	−	0	−	0	−	0	−	0	−	0	−	0
Arabinose	−	0	−	0	−	0	−	0	−	0	−	0	−	0
Mannose	−	0	−	0	−	0	+	100	−	0	+	100	−	0
Rhamnose	−	0	−	0	−	0	−	0	−	0	−	0	−	0
Trehalose	−	0	−	0	−	0	−	0	−	0	V	65	−	0
Hydrolysis of:														
Esculin	−	0	−	0	−	0	−	0	−	0	+	100	−	0
Gelatin	−	0	−	0	−	0	−	0	−	0	−	0	−	0
Starch	−	0	−	0	−	0	−	0	−	0	V	50	−	0
Milk coagulation	−	0	−	0	−	0	−	0	−	0	+	100	−	0
Milk digestion	−	0	−	0	−	0	−	0	−	0	−	0	−	0
Indole	+	100	−	0	−	0	−	0	−	0	−	0	−	0
H$_2$S	V	43	V	39	V	37	−	0	−	0	−	0	V	66
Catalase	−	0	−	0	−	0	+	100	−	0	−	0	V	77
Urease	−	0	−	0	−	0	V	33	−	0	−	0	−	0
Nitrate reduction	−	0	−	0	−	0	+	100	V	44	−	0	+	100

*+, Positive reaction exhibited by 90% or more of strains tested; −, negative reaction exhibited by 90% or more of strains tested; V, variable reaction (reaction exhibited by 26-75% of strains tested); OA, obligate anaerobe; F, facultative anaerobe.

Table 83-6. Volatile and nonvolatile acids produced in 48 h peptone–yeast extract–glucose broth cultures of common anaerobic cocci*†

	Peptococcus								Peptostreptococcus anaerobius		Streptococcus intermedius		Veillonella parvula	
	asaccharolyticus		magnus		prevotii		saccharolyticus							
No. strains	40		31		37		13		25		12		26	
Metabolic products	Sign	%+	Sign	%+	Sign	%+	Sign	%+	Sign	%+	Sign	%+	Sign	%+
Volatile:														
Acetic	+	100	+	100	+	100	+	100	+	100	V	65	+	100
Propionic	−$^+$	10	−	0	V	30	−	0	−	0	−	0	+	100
Isobutyric	−	0	−	0	−	0	−	0	V	50	−	0	−	0
Butyric	+	100	−	0	+	100	−	0	V	50	−	0	−	0
Isovaleric	−	0	−	0	−	0	−	0	V	50	−	0	−	0
Valeric	−	0	−	0	−	0	−	0	−	0	−	0	−	0
Isocaproic	−	0	−	0	−	0	−	0	+	100	−	0	−	0
Caproic	−	0	−	0	−	0	−	0	−	0	−	0	−	0
Nonvolatile:														
Lactic	−	0	−	0	−	0	−	0	−	0	+	100	−	0
Succinic	−	0	−	0	−	0	−	0	−	0	−	0	−	0

*+, Positive (acid produced by 90% or more of strains tested); −, negative (acid produced by less than 10% of strains tested); V, variable (acid produced by 26-75% of strains tested); Superscript (−$^+$), acid produced by 10-25% of strains tested.
†Volatile and nonvolatile acids in PYG cultures were identified by gas-liquid chromatography as described by Dowell and Hawkins.[47] We now use 15% SP-1220/1% H$_3$PO$_4$ on 100/120 chromasorb W/AW for volatile acids and 10% SP-1000/1% H$_3$PO$_4$ on 100/200 chromasorb W/AW for nonvolatile acids, both in 6 ft × ¼ inch stainless steel columns.

Table 83-7. Differentiation of common anaerobic cocci*

	Peptococcus				Peptostrep-tococcus anaerobius	Streptococcus intermedius	Veillonella parvula
	asaccharo-lyticus	magnus	prevotii	saccharo-lyticus			
Gram reaction	+	+	+	+	+	+	−
Chains in Thio†	−	−	−	−	+	+	−
Relation to O₂	OA	OA	OA	OA	OA	F or OA	OA
SPS inhibition	−	−	−	−	+	−	−
NO₃ reduction	−	−	−⁺	+	V	−	+
Indole	+	−	−	−	−	−	−
Catalase	−	−	−	+	−	−	V
Esculin hydrolysis	−	−	−	−	−	+	−
H₂S, esculin agar	−	−	−	−	−	−	−
Bile agar, growth	−	−	V	−	−	+	−
Lecithinase, EYA	−	−	−	−	−	−	−
Lipase, EYA	−	−	−	−	−	−	−
Proteolysis, EYA	−	−	−	−	−	−	−
Glucose fermented	−	−	−	+	V	+	−
Acid products	A, B	A	A, (P), B	A	A, (IB), (B), (IV), IC	(A), L	A, P

*+, Positive reaction exhibited by 90% or more of strains tested; −, negative reaction exhibited by 90% or more of strains tested; −⁺, usually negative but positive reaction exhibited by 10-25% of strains tested; V, variable (reaction exhibited by 25-75% of strains tested); A, acetic acid; B, butyric acid; P, propionic acid; IB, isobutyric acid; IV, isovaleric acid; IC, isocaproic acid; L, lactic acid; OA, obligate anaerobe; F, facultative anaerobe; ( ) = variable.
†Chains of 10 or more cells in length.

sometimes in abscesses and other infections; some resemble *Staphylococcus aureus* on Gram stains. Willis[53] actually calls them the anaerobic equivalent of *Staphylococcus*.

P. prevotii is similar to, if not identical with, *P. asaccharolyticus* (see Table 83-3), and *P. magnus* is probably the same as *P. anaerobius*. The species designations of Holdeman et al.[37] do not conform to *Bergey's Manual*, ed. 8.[38]

The organisms are nonhemolytic on blood agar, and their growth is enhanced by Tween 80.

P. asaccharolyticus produces indole but is nonsaccharolytic and nonproteolytic.

The peptococci are sensitive to penicillin, tetracycline, erythromycin, chloramphenicol, clindamycin, lincomycin, and metronidazole.[53]

PEPTOSTREPTOCOCCUS

Peptostreptococci appear microscopically arranged in short or long chains or in pairs. Their colonies are smooth, shiny, circular, and small.

P. anaerobius and *P. intermedius* occur in clinical material more frequently than the other species.

Cultures of *P. anaerobius* develop a foul odor; the organism is sensitive to SPS (sodium polyanethol sulfonate), which serves as a rapid test for its presumptive identification (see Table 83-3).

P. intermedius is nonproteolytic, and most strains ferment glucose, maltose, lactose, sucrose, and fructose.[53]

The antimicrobial susceptibility of peptostreptococci is similar to that of peptococci.

VEILLONELLA

These organisms are small gram-negative cocci that occur in pairs, irregular clumps, and short chains. They occur in the respiratory, genitourinary, and intestinal tracts. Their pathogenicity is in doubt, however; rarely *V. parvula* is found as a single infecting organism.[12]

Willis[53] and Chow et al.[54] state that *Veillonella* strains fluoresce red under UV light (immediately after removal from the anaerobic jar; fluorescence is rapidly lost on exposure of colonies to air[53]).

Veillonellae are sensitive to penicillin, tetracycline, erythromycin, chloramphenicol, clindamycin, and metronidazole, but are resistant to vancomycin and the aminoglycosides.[53]

ACIDAMINOCOCCUS AND MEGASPHAERA [55, 56]

These gram-negative anaerobic cocci were originally isolated from animals. Sugihara et al.[57] have conclusively shown that the 2 organisms (*A. fermentans* and *M. elsdenii*) occur in the feces of normal humans.

They have also isolated *A. fermentans* from a closed abdominal abscess and *M. elsdenii* from a putrid lung abscess.[57]

A case of *M. elsdenii* endocarditis has been recently described.[11]

Acidaminococcus and *Megasphaera* are nitrate negative (*Veillonella* is nitrate positive); *Megasphaera* is fermentative, whereas *Acidaminococcus* is not (see Table 83-3).

REFERENCES

1. Bornstein, D. L., Weinberg, A. N., Swartz, M. N., and Kunz, L. J.: Medicine **43**:207-232, 1964.
2. Bartlett, J. G., and Finegold, S. M.: Medicine **51**:413-450, 1972.
3. Wilson, W. R., Martin, W. J., Wilkouski, C. J., and Washington J. A., II: Mayo Clin. Proc. **47**:639-646, 1972.
4. Weinberg, A. N. In Balows, A., DeHann, R. M., Dowell, V. R., Jr., and Guze, L. B., editors: Anaerobic bacteria: role in disease, Springfield, Ill., 1974, Charles C Thomas, Publisher, pp. 257-265.
5. Martin, W. J.: Anaerobic cocci. In Lenette, E. H., Spaulding, E. H., and Truant, J. P., editors: Manual of clinical microbiology, ed. 2, Washington, D.C., 1974, American Society for Microbiology.
6. Finegold, S.M.: Anaerobic bacteria in human disease, New York, 1977, Academic Press.
7. Altemeier, W. A., and Culbertson, W. R.: Surg. Gynecol. Obstet. **87**:206, 1948.
8. Meleney, F. L.: Ann. Surg. **94**:961, 1931.
9. Finegold, S. M., Martin, W. J., and Scott, E. G.: Bailey and Scott's diagnostic microbiology, ed. 5, St. Louis, 1978, The C. V. Mosby Co.
10. Thomas, C. G. A., and Hare, R.: J. Clin. Pathol. **7**:300-304, 1954.
11. Brancaccio, M. and Legendre, G. G.: J. Clin. Microbiol. **10**:72, 1979.
12. Borchardt, K. A., Baker, M., and Gelber, R.: Ann. Intern. Med. **86**:64, 1977.
13. Sutter, V. L., Vargo, V. L., and Finegold, S. M.: Wadsworth anaerobic bacteriology manual, ed. 2, Los Angeles, 1975, Dept. of Continuing Education in Health Sciences University Extension, and the School of Medicine, UCLA.
14. Heineman, H. S., and Braude, A. J.: Am. J. Med. **35**:682-697, 1963.
15. Swartz, M. N., and Karchmer, A. W.: Infections of the central nervous system. In Balows, A., DeHaan, R. M., Dowell, V. R., Jr., and Guze, L. B., editors: Anaerobic bacteria: role in disease, Springfield, Ill., 1974, Charles C Thomas, Publishers, pp. 309-325.
16. Loesche, W. J.: Dental infections. Anaerobic Bacteria: Role in disease In Ballows, A., DeHaan, R. M., Dowell, V. R., Jr., and Guze, L. B., editors: Springfield, Ill., 1974, Charles C Thomas, Publisher, pp. 409-434.
17. Frederick, J., and Braude, A. J.: N. Engl. J. Med. **290**:135-137, 1974.
18. Bartlett, J. G., Gorbach, S. L., Thadepalli, H., and Finegold, S. M.: Lancet **1**:338-340, 1974.
19. Bartlett, J. G., Gorbach, S. L., Tally, F. P., and Finegold, S. M.: Am. Rev. Respir. Dis. **109**:510-518, 1974.
20. Gorbach, S. L., and Bartlett, J. G.: N. Engl. J. Med. **290**:1117-1184, 1974.
21. Gorbach, S. L., and Bartlett, J. G.: N. Engl. J. Med. **290**:1237-1245, 1974.
22. Gorbach, S. L., and Bartlett, J. G.: N. Engl. J. Med. **290**:1289-1294, 1974.
23. Altemeier, W. A.: Liver abscess. In Ballows, A., DeHaan, R. M., Dowell, V. R., Jr., and Guze, L. B., editors: Anaerobic bacteria: role in disease, Springfield, Ill., 1974, Charles C Thomas, Publisher, pp. 387-398.
24. Swenson, R. M., Michaelson, T. C., Daly, M. J., and Spaulding, E. H.: Obstet. Gynecol. **42**:538-541, 1973.
25. Thadepalli, H., Gorbach, S. L., and Keith, L.: Am. J. Obstet. Gynecol. **117**:1034-1040, 1973.
26. Washington, J. A., II: Bacteremia due to anaerobic unusual and fastidious bacteria. In Sonnenwirth, A. C., editor: Bacteremia: laboratory and clinical aspects, Springfield, Ill., 1973, Charles C Thomas, Publisher, pp. 47-60.
27. Felner, J. M.: Infective endocarditis caused by anaerobic bacteria. In Balows, A., DeHaan, R. M., Dowell, V. R., Jr., and Guze, L. B., editors: Anaerobic bacteria: role in disease, Springfield, Ill., 1974, Charles C Thomas, Publisher, pp. 345-352.
28. Felner, J. M., and Dowell, V. R., Jr.: N. Engl. J. Med. **283**:1188-1192, 1970.
29. Ziment, I., Miller, L. H., and Finegold, S. M.: Antimicrob. Agents Chemother. 1967, pp. 77-85.
30. Ziment, I., Davis, A., and Finegold, S. M.: Arthritis Rheumat. **12**:627-634, 1969.
31. Altemeier, W. A., and Culbertson, W. R.: Surg. Gynecol. Obstet. **87**:206, 1948.
32. Altemeier, W. A., and Culbertson, W. R.: J. A. M. A. **145**:449-457, 1951.
33. Bartlett, J. G., Sutter, V. L., and Finegold, S. M.: N. Engl. J. Med. **287**:1006-1010, 1972.
34. Meleney, F. L.: Ann. Surg. **94**:961-981, 1931.
35. Sandusky, W. R., Pulaski, E. J., Johnson, B. A., and Meleney, F. L.: Surg. Gynecol. Obstet. **75**:45, 1942.
36. Watt, B., and Jack, E. P.: J. Med. Microbiol. **10**:461, 1977.
37. Holdeman, L. V., Cato, E. P., and Moore, W. E. C.: Anaerobe laboratory manual, ed. 4, Blacksburg, Va., 1977, Virginia Polytechnic Institute and State University.
38. Buchanan, R. E., and Gibbons, N. E., co-editors: Bergey's manual of determinative bacteriology, ed. 8, Baltimore, 1974, The Williams & Wilkins Co.
39. Holdeman, L. V., and Moore, W. E. C.: Int. J. Syst. Bacteriol. **24**:260-277, 1974.
40. Breed, R. S., Murray, E. D. G., and Smith, N. R., editors: Bergey's manual of determinative bacteriology, ed. 7, Baltimore, 1957, The Williams & Wilkins Co.
41. Dowell, V. R., Jr. and Hawkins, T. M.: Laboratory methods in anaerobic bacteriology, CDC laboratory manual, HEW, publ. no. (CDC)-78-8272, Atlanta, 1977, Center for Disease Control.
42. Sutter, V. L., Citron, D. M., and Finegold, S. M.: Wadsworth anaerobic bacteriology manual, ed. 3, St. Louis, The C. V. Mosby Co. (In press.)
43. Finegold, S. M., Shepherd, W. E., and Spaulding, E. H.: Practical anaerobic bacteriology. Cumitech no. 5, Shepherd, W. E., coordinating editor, Washington, D.C., 1977, American Society for Microbiology.
44. Graves, J. H., Morello, J. A., and Kocka, F. E.: Appl. Microbiol. **27**:1131, 1974.
45. Holdeman, L. V., and Moore, W. E. C., editors: Anaerobe laboratory manual ed. 2, Blacksburg, Va., 1973, Virginia Polytechnic and State University.
46. Dowell, V. R., Jr., and Hawkins, T. M.: Laboratory methods in anaerobic bacteriology, CDC laboratory manual, DHEW, publ. no. (CDC)-74-8272, Atlanta, 1974, Center for Disease Control.
47. Dowell, V. R., Jr., Armfield, A. Y., Thompson, F. S., and Lombard, G. L.: Personal communication, 1979.
48. Elliott, L. B.: The development of a practical

procedure for the identification of gram-positive cocci in a clinical microbiology laboratory, Chapel Hill, N.C., 1976, University of North Carolina at Chapel Hill, School of Public Health (doctoral dissertation).

49. Graves, M. H., Morello, J. A., and Kocka, F. E.: Appl. Microbiol. **27:**1131-1133, 1974.

50. Dowell, V. R., Jr., and Lombard, G. L.: Presumptive identification of anaerobic nonsporeforming gram-negative bacilli, Atlanta, 1977, Center for Disease Control.

51. Story, S., and Dowell, V. R., Jr.: Abstracts of Annual Meeting of the American Society of Microbiology, Abstr. C24, 1978, p. 281.

52. Wideman, P. A., Citronbaum, D. M., and Sutter, V. L.: J. Clin. Microbiol. **5:**315-319, 1977.

53. Willis, T. A.: Anaerobic bacteriology, ed. 3, London, 1977, Butterworths.

54. Chow, A. W., Patten, V., and Guze, L. B.: J. Clin. Microbiol. **2:**546-548. 1975.

55. Rogosa, M.: J. Bacteriol. **98:**756, 1969.

56. Rogosa, M.: Int. J. Syst. Bacteriol. **21:**187, 1971.

57. Sugihara, P. T., Sutter, V. L., Attebery, H. R., et al.: Appl. Microbiol. **27:**274, 1979.

84

ANAEROBIC SPOREFORMING RODS: CLOSTRIDIA

Alex C. Sonnenwirth
V. R. Dowell, Jr.

GENERAL CONSIDERATIONS

1. Sporeforming, anaerobic, or aerotolerant bacilli are classified in the genus *Clostridium*.

2. The majority of the clostridia are gram positive, but certain species may appear gram negative, particularly in older cultures. According to Smith,[1] many of the species with terminal spores lose the stain readily and gram-positive cells are rarely seen in overnight cultures. Even some of the species with subterminal spores, such as *C. haemolyticum*, often appear only as large gram-negative rods in overnight cultures.

3. Clostridia are sporeforming bacilli, often showing filamentous and plectridial forms. Some (e.g., *C. perfringens*) produce spores only under special conditions.

4. They are catalase negative; a few strains produce catalase.

5. With the exception of *C. perfringens*, they are usually motile.

6. Except for *C. perfringens*, they are non-encapsulated.

7. With the exception of the aerotolerant (microaerophilic) types, *C. tertium*, *C. carnis*, and *C. histolyticum*, all are anaerobic.

8. Clostridia are predominantly saccharolytic (ferment carbohydrates) or proteolytic, but some are neither. Whereas pathogenicity is not limited to any one of these 3 divisions, it is not excluded from any.

9. Some clostridia produce true **exotoxins** and are pathogenic for humans and animals.

10. To distinguish aerotolerant clostridia from aerobic *Bacillus* species, it should be noted that *Bacillus* strains produce catalase and usually do not sporulate when grown anaerobically, whereas clostridia usually do not form catalase but (with exceptions) form spores in an anaerobic environment.[2]

Table 84-1 lists some changes in the nomenclature of anaerobes since the previous edition of this manual was published.

For information on the systematics and diagnostics of the clostridia, see the publications of Smith (1975, 1977),[1,6] Willis (1977),[2] Buchanan and Gibbons (1974),[7] Holdeman et al. (1977),[3] and Sutter et al.[8,8a]; see also Smith and Dowell (1974),[9] Dowell and Hawkins,[10] and Willis (1969).[11]

For information on clostridial diseases, see Finegold (1977),[12] Gorbach and Thadepalli (1975),[13] Smith (1977),[1] and MacLennan (1962).[14]

Table 84-1. Changes in the nomenclature of anaerobic sporeformers

Present designation	Former designation(s)
Clostridium cadaveris	Clostridium capitovale
Clostridium limosum	Clostridium species group P1
Clostridium ramosum	Catenabacterium filamentosum; Bacteroides trichoides (B. terebrans)
Clostridium paraperfringens	Clostridium barati

Proposed for deletion: *Clostridium plagarum* (synonymous with *Clostridium perfringens*)[3,4]; *Clostridium rubrum* (genetically homologous with *Clostridium beijerinckii*).[3,5]

Clostridium

Members of the genus *Clostridium* may be divided as follows: (1) **toxigenic group** (*C. botulinum* A-G and *C. tetani*); (2) **gas gangrene group** (*C. chauvoei*, *C. histolyticum*, *C. novyi* A-D, *C. perfringens* A-E, *C. septicum*, *C. sordellii*, *C. bifermentans*, and *C. sporogenes*); (3) **miscellaneous pathogenic clostridia** (involved in a variety of infections, i.e., bacteremia, abscesses, etc.); (4) *C. difficile*, involved in antibiotic-induced pseudomembranous colitis[15,16]; and (5) **common nonpathogenic clostridia**.

They can also be classified according to their proteolytic and saccharolytic properties (action on milk on the one hand, and on carbohydrates on the other)[2]:

1. **Proteolytic and saccharolytic:** *C. sporo-*

genes, *C. bifermentans*, *C. sordellii*, *C. botulinum* (types A, B, and F).

2. **Proteolytic but nonsaccharolytic:** *C. histolyticum*, *C. botulinum* (type G).

3. **Saccharolytic but nonproteolytic:** *C. cadaveris*, *C. perfringens*, *C. paraperfringens* (formerly *C. barati*), *C. tertium*, *C. fallax*, *C. butyricum*, *C. chauvoli*, *C. botulinum* (types B-F), *C. novyi* (types A-D), *C. sphenoides*.

4. **Nonsaccharolytic and nonproteolytic:** *C. tetani*, *C. cochlearium*.

According to Holdeman et al., *C. perfringens* usually makes up about one half the isolates of clostridia from clinical material; some of the other clostridia commonly encountered in clinical specimens are *C. innocuum*, *C. sordellii*, *C. bifermentans*, *C. sporogenes*, *C. septicum*, *C. ramosum*, and *C. sphenoides*. Five to ten percent of the clostridial isolates will not belong to recognized species; fortunately they usually are nonpathogenic. Dowell and Hawkins[10] enumerate *C. histolyticum*, *C. novyi* type A, *C. chauvoei*, *C. perfringens*, *C. septicum*, and *C. tetani* as commonly encountered pathogenic clostridia.

CLOSTRIDIAL INFECTIONS, CLINICAL SYNDROMES, SPECIMENS, AND LABORATORY TESTS FOR CONFIRMATION
Intoxications

Clostridial intoxications include botulism (*C. botulinum*) and tetanus (*C. tetani*); *C. perfringens* "**food poisoning**" probably also involves preformed toxin; however, it is likely that actual replication of *C. perfringens* in the gut is also involved (see below).

Botulism[18,19]

Botulism is caused by toxins (preformed) of *C. botulinum*. Types A, B, and E are primarily responsible for human botulism.

Botulism almost always involves ingestion of preformed toxin. Toxin is produced usually during improper home canning, i.e., heating for **less** than 30 minutes at a temperature below 121 C. Heating for 30 minutes at 121 C is needed to kill the spores. When not killed, the spores may germinate in the preparation; the vegetative bacteria produce toxin. The toxin can be destroyed by boiling or heating to 80 C for 10 minutes.[18]

Wound botulism[19-23] arises from toxin produced in wounds contaminated with *C. botulinum*. A finding of *C. botulinum* in a culture of a wound is not pathognomonic unless the appropriate clinical picture is present.

Infant botulism is discussed below, following "Isolation of *C. botulinum*."

Collection, handling, and shipment of specimens for detection of botulinal toxin and C. botulinum[10,19]

Most clinical laboratories are not equipped to work with botulinal toxin. For this reason, instructions for collection and handling of such specimens are described here. Botulinal toxins are extremely poisonous. Therefore all materials suspected of containing botulinal toxin should be handled with maximum precaution, and only experienced personnel, preferably immunized with botulinal toxoid, should perform laboratory tests.

All specimens **except those from wounds** should be refrigerated, preferably not frozen, and examined as quickly as possible after collection. **Wound specimens** should be placed in anaerobic transport devices such as Port-A-Cul tubes of vials (BioQuest Division, Becton, Dickinson & Co., Cockeysville, Md.) and sent to the appropriate laboratory without refrigeration for attempted isolation of *C. botulinum*. The date specimens are collected from patients should be indicated on the labels. **Serum samples** must be taken before antitoxin treatment in order to demonstrate the presence of botulinal toxin. Posttreatment serum specimens are sometimes desirable to verify disappearance of the toxin, to determine the amount of antitoxin in circulating blood of the patient after treatment, and to determine how long antitoxin persists.

Ideally 10-15 ml of **serum** should be obtained for laboratory tests. This quantity permits specific identification of the botulinal toxin involved and repeat tests if necessary. Of course, it is impractical to obtain this much serum from some patients, especially from infants. In such cases the amount of serum available should be submitted to the laboratory.

Ideally 25-50 g of **feces** should be collected, preferably prior to antitoxin treatment. However, confirmatory evidence of botulism has been obtained from much smaller quantities. If an enema must be given because of constipation, a minimal amount of fluid (preferably sterile nonbacteriostatic water) should be used to obtain the specimen so the toxin will not be unnecessarily diluted. If the patient has been on any medication that might interfere with toxin assays or culturing of the stool, the laboratory should be notified. For example, it has been demonstrated that anticholinesterase drugs given orally to patients with a prior diagnosis of myasthenia gravis can interfere with mouse botulinal toxin assays of stool extracts.[19]

Specimens sent to a distant laboratory should be placed in sterile leakproof containers and then in insulated shipping containers with refrigerant; they should be labelled "medical emergency" and shipped by the most rapid means available. Cardboard containers are not suitable for stool specimens. Most of the major airlines have a special package-handling service for expedited shipments. The receiving laboratory should be notified in advance by telephone or telegram as to when and how specimens were shipped, when they will arrive, and the waybill or shipping number. If an unavoidable delay of several days is anticipated, the specimens should be kept frozen and then packed in an insulated container with dry ice and proper cushioning material for shipment. The following are appropriate laboratory consultants to notify at CDC prior to shipment of specimens: (1) Charles L. Hatheway, Ph.D. (404)329-3867; (2) George L. Lombard, Dr. P. H. (404)329-3654; or (3) V. R. Dowell, Jr., Ph.D. (404)329-3333.

Detection of Clostridium botulinum and botulinal toxins [10,19]

The procedures detailed here are designed for those laboratories interested in undertaking detection of botulinum toxin and *C. botulinum*.

Seven toxigenic types of *C. botulinum* are recognized on the basis of seven antigenically distinct toxins produced by different strains of the same organism. Cases of human botulism are usually associated with types A, B, or E. Types C and D are frequently involved in outbreaks of botulism in birds and other animals.[1,24] Two human outbreaks due to type F have occurred, one involving liver paste on the Danish isle of Langeland and another in California from venison jerky. No outbreaks in man or animals have been attributed to type G.[25] The most effective means for laboratory diagnosis of botulism is the identification of the specific botulinal toxin in the patient's blood.[26] An indirect laboratory diagnosis can be made by demonstration of the toxin in extracts of the incriminated food. Isolation of the causative organism from food samples and confirmation of the type by mouse neutralization tests also prove helpful in diagnosis.

To detect botulinal toxin in solid food samples, such as meat, it is necessary to extract the toxin in a suitable diluent. Liquid portions of canned foods, extracts, or culture fluids should be centrifuged prior to testing. Clarified materials are inoculated into mice, and any toxin detected is specifically identified by neutralization with type-specific antitoxin. The toxicity of the toxins of *C. botulinum* type E and of the nonproteolytic strains of *C. botulinum* types B and F may be greatly increased by the addition of trypsin.[27,28] For this reason, toxin testing and mouse neutralization should be performed with trypsinized as well as nontrypsinized material. Trypsinization of serum samples is not necessary to activate the toxins.[26]

Examination of specimens for botulinal toxin [19]
Materials and methods
1. Mice: 20-30 g; white ICR strain mice give satisfactory results.
2. Antitoxins: Monovalent (types A-F) antitoxins distributed by CDC contain approximately 10 IU ml when reconstituted. One unit of the corresponding type of antitoxin neutralizes 10,000 mouse IP LD_{50} of toxin types A-D and F, or 1000 IP LD_{50} of toxin type E.
3. Mouse injection: inject mice intraperitoneally with serum or extracts, alone or mixed with antitoxin, using a syringe with a 25-gauge, ⅝ inch needle.
4. Observation of mice: observe mice at intervals (e.g., 4, 8, 12, 18, and 24 h) and then daily for a period of 4 d for signs of illness or death. Although botulinal intoxication usually kills mice within 6-24 h, delayed deaths are occasionally observed. If toxin is present in sufficient quantity all mice injected with test materials will die except those receiving samples mixed with antitoxin specific for the botulinal toxin involved and those injected with heated (held in boiling water for 10 min) extracts because botulinal toxins are heat labile.

NOTE: Signs of botulism in mice begin with ruffling of fur followed in sequence by labored abdominal breathing, weakness of limbs, and total paralysis. Death is caused by respiratory failure. Time between first sign of distress and death varies with amount of toxin mice receive. Death without clinical signs is not adequate evidence that botulinal toxin was present in material injected.[19]

Food samples [10]
Laboratory testing includes extraction and identification of botulinal toxin and isolation of the causative organism. Suspect foods should be examined as soon as possible after they are collected. Leave unopened containers sealed until ready to be examined in the laboratory. Otherwise, collect food samples in sterile containers. Place specimens to be sent to a distant laboratory in a leakproof container, wrap with a cushioning material, pack with ice in a second leakproof, insulated shipping container, and ship by the most rapid means. Notify the recipient laboratory in advance when and how the specimens are being shipped, when they should arrive, and what the waybill or shipping number is.

Preparation of food extract [10]
1. Record all identifying information.
2. If canned foods are to be tested, wipe top of can with solution of 10% Roccal and 70% isopropanol (1 : 1) and place can in a large plastic bag before opening it to prevent formation of an aerosol.
3. Record condition of food (gassy, dark, putrid, etc.) and remove a small sample for a pH determination.
4. Grind food in a sterile, chilled mortar (preweighed).
   a. Place food in mortar, weigh, and record amount of food used. If sufficient material is available, 50 g samples are a convenient size to work with.
   b. Add 1-2 g sterile sand.
   c. Add a small amount (5 ml) of cold gelatin diluent and grind with a sterile pestle until a homogenous suspension is obtained. In some cases where food is extremely dry, it may be necessary to add additional gelatin diluent in order to grind specimen.
   d. After grinding, add sufficient diluent to give a volume of diluent equal to the grams of food employed (vol/wt).
5. Prepare smear and Gram stain. Note size of rods, approximate number and types of organisms present, and presence and location of spores.

Culture of food sample [10]
1. Alcohol treatment.
   a. Using a safety Pro-Pipette or a "broken tip" capillary pipet, place approximately 0.5 ml food suspension in a 13×1000 mm sterile screwcap tube.
   b. Add an equal volume of absolute alcohol and incubate at room temperature for 1 h; mix at approximately 15 min intervals. Alcohol treatment kills vegetative cells but spores should remain viable.[24]
2. Heat 5 tubes of chopped meat–dextrose–starch

Table 84-2. Method of testing serum for botulinal toxin

Tube no.	Vol. of serum (ml)	Vol. of antitoxin* (ml)	Type of antitoxin	Vol. drawn into syringe (ml)	Vol. injected into each mouse (ml)
1	1.0	0	—	0.8	0.4
2	1.0	0.25	A	1.0	0.5
3	1.0	0.25	B	1.0	0.5
4	1.0	0.25	E	1.0	0.5
5	1.0	0.25	F	1.0	0.5
6	1.0	0.25	A-F	1.0	0.5

*Mix antitoxin with serum and incubate for 30 min at 37 C.

medium in a boiling water bath for 10 min. Transfer 3 tubes to a 70 C water bath, and cool other 2 tubes in cold water.

3. Inoculate one of cooled tubes of chopped meat–dextrose–starch medium with an untreated food suspension and second with alcohol-treated food. Inoculate with 0.5-1.0 ml near bottom of tubes with capillary pipet. Try to avoid introducing air bubbles into medium.

4. After equilibration to temperature, inoculate 3 tubes of chopped meat–dextrose–starch medium in 70 C water bath. Start timing. After 10 min, remove 1 tube to cold water, and transfer other 2 tubes to 80 C water bath. After 10 min at 80 C, cool 1 tube and transfer remaining tube to a boiling water bath for an additional 10 min before cooling.

5. Incubate chopped meat–dextrose–starch medium cultures in an anaerobic jar at 30 C. Some types of *C. botulinum* produce little or no toxin at a temperature above 30 C.[28] Maximum toxin production usually occurs after 3-5 days' incubation.

6. **Isolation and identification.** To obtain pure cultures of *C. botulinum*, subculture from chopped meat–dextrose (glucose)–starch tubes to blood and egg yolk agar plates. Streak to obtain isolated colonies. Incubate plates in an anaerobic jar at 35-37 C for 48 h. Pick isolated colonies to tubes of chopped meat–dextrose–starch medium, and incubate at 30 C. Establish identity of pure cultures by conventional cultural and biochemical procedures and toxin type with mouse toxin neutralization test. For further details, see "Isolation of *C. botulinum*," below.

Testing serum for toxin[19]

1. Place 1 ml serum into each of 6 tubes and add 0.25 ml of appropriate antitoxin to last 5 tubes as indicated in Table 84-2.

2. Mix antitoxin with serum by swirling tubes. Try to prevent foaming, which can inactivate toxin.

3. Incubate serum-antitoxin mixtures in 37 C water bath for 30 min.

4. Inject 2 mice intraperitoneally with 0.4 ml untreated serum and 2 mice each with 0.5 ml serum-antitoxin mixtures.

5. Mark each set of mice with dye in a distinctive pattern for identification.

6. Observe mice for signs of botulism and death. If type A, B, E, or F botulinal toxin is present in sufficient concentration, all mice will die within 96 h, except those receiving serum mixtures containing polyvalent (A-F) antitoxin and ones containing monovalent antitoxin corresponding to toxin type.

7. Toxin test that is negative using 0.4 ml of patient's serum described may show botulinal toxin when 0.8 ml is injected per mouse. Volumes larger than 0.8 ml are not recommended since normal serum will sometimes kill a mouse when 1 ml or more is injected. When deaths occur in mice injected with 0.8 ml quantities of serum, neutralization is carried out by adding ⅛ volume of antitoxin (e.g., 2 ml serum plus 0.25 ml antitoxin), incubating 30 min at 37 C, and injecting 0.9 ml into mice.

8. If sufficient serum is not available for a complete toxin neutralization test, priority should be to demonstrate toxin by observing typical signs of botulism in mice after intraperitoneal injection of untreated serum (0.4 or 0.8 ml). If toxin is demonstrated, toxin type should be determined by use of type-specific antitoxin if possible. Exact antitoxin (anti-A, -B, -E, etc.) to employ in performance of neutralization test will depend on quantity of patient's serum available.

Testing stool specimens for toxin

1. Prepare extract.

   a. Weigh 10-50 g feces into sterile, chilled (4 C) mortar.

   b. Add 1 ml cold (4 C) gelatin diluent for each gram of feces.

   c. Mix with sterile pestle until uniform suspension is obtained.

   d. Hold overnight (6-18 h) in refrigerator (4 C).

   e. Centrifuge at $12,000 \times g$ in refrigerated centrifuge (4 C) for 20 min, recover supernatant (SN), and repeat centrifugation to clarify if necessary. Clarified SN is extract used for testing.

2. Test extract in same manner as serum. In addition, test a sample for heat lability and a sample for trypsin activation. Trypsinization sometimes increases toxicity of botulinal toxins.

   a. For heated sample, place 1 ml of extract in a tube, plug with cotton, and heat for 10 min in boiling water bath.

   b. For trypsinized sample, place 1 ml of extract in a tube, add 0.25 ml 0.5% trypsin (Difco 1:250) solution, and incubate at 37 C for 30 min.

3. Schedule for testing extracts is outlined in Table 84-3.

4. If toxin is demonstrated only in trypsinized sample, repeat neutralization tests using trypsinized extract. Add 1.5 ml 0.5% trypsin to 6 ml extract and incubate 30 min at 37 C. Distribute 1.25 ml of trypsinized extract to each of 5 tubes, add 0.25 ml of appropriate antitoxin (monovalent types A, B, E, or F or polyvalent types A, B, C, D, E, or F) per tube, mix, and incubate again for 30 min at 37 C. Inject 2 mice with each trypsinized extract-antitoxin mixture (0.6 ml/mouse). Table 84-4

Table 84-3. Method of testing extracts and culture fluids for botulinal toxin*

Tube no.	Vol. of test material (ml)	Treatment†	Vol. drawn into syringe (ml)	Vol. injected into each mouse (ml)
1	1.0	None	0.8	0.4
2	1.0	Heat 10 min‡	0.8	0.4
3	1.0	Add 0.25 ml trypsin solution	1.0	0.5
4	1.0	Add 0.25 ml anti-A	1.0	0.5
5	1.0	Add 0.25 ml anti-B	1.0	0.5
6	1.0	Add 0.25 ml anti-E	1.0	0.5
7	1.0	Add 0.25 ml anti-F	1.0	0.5
8	1.0	Add 0.25 ml anti–A-F	1.0	0.5

*Certain cultures of *C. botulinum* may produce more toxin than will be neutralized by quantity of antitoxin used in this procedure (1 unit); therefore tests should also be performed on diluted culture fluid, e.g., 10^{-1}, 10^{-2}, etc., if there is no protection with any of antitoxins.
†Mix tubes 3-8 after adding trypsin or antitoxin and incubate for 30 min at 37 C.
‡Plug tube with cotton to minimize evaporation and heat in boiling water for 10 min.

Table 84-4. Neutralization tests on trypsinized extracts and culture fluids*

Tube no.	Vol. of trypsinized test material (ml)	Vol. of antitoxin (ml)	Type of antitoxin†	Vol. drawn into syringe (ml)	Vol. injected into each mouse (ml)
1	1.25	0.25	A	1.2	0.6
2	1.25	0.25	B	1.2	0.6
3	1.25	0.25	E	1.2	0.6
4	1.25	0.25	F	1.2	0.6
5	1.25	0.25	A-F	1.2	0.6

*Trypsinization: 6 ml test material + 1.5 ml 0.5% trypsin; incubate for 30 min at 37 C.
†Mix trypsinized test material and antitoxin and incubate for 30 min at 37 C.

shows details of tests on trypsinized extracts. Trypsinization is only rarely necessary for detecting botulinal toxin.

5. Toxic substances other than botulinal toxin may be present in stool specimen. Diluting sample in twofold increments, titrating extract, and then repeating neutralization test on extract near the end-point dilution may eliminate interference and permit proper identification of botulinal toxin.

Isolation of C. botulinum from stool and food[19]

1. Suspended **stool** and **food** specimens as described under "Testing Stool Specimens for Toxin" and "Preparation of Food Extract" are used for culturing. Large **tissue** specimens may be ground as described for foods. Small tissue specimens should be divided into 2 or more portions so that at least 2 tubes of culture media may be inoculated.
2. Prepare smears of food or tissue suspensions and gram stain. Observe and record staining reaction, morphologic features, and approximate number of bacteria present. Also record size of rods, if present, and location of spores in sporulated cells.
3. Heat 2 tubes of chopped meat–glucose–starch (CMGS) medium in boiling water bath for 10 min. Place 1 tube in cold water and transfer second tube to 80 C water bath. Allow each to equilibrate to temperature.
4. Inoculate by adding 0.5-1.0 ml of suspension into each tube of medium near bottom of tube with capillary pipet. Try to avoid introducing air bubbles into medium.

5. Leave 80 C tube in water bath for 10 min, then place it in cold water.
6. After inoculation and heat treatment, incubate both tubes anaerobically at **30 C** for 4 d.
7. After incubation, remove a portion of culture, centrifuge, and recover supernatant fluid for toxin testing.
8. Screen for toxicity by testing untreated, heated, and trypsinized culture fluids in mice, as shown for tubes 1-3 in Table 84-3.
9. If untreated and trypsinized samples are toxic, perform neutralization tests according to tubes 4-8 in Table 84-3.
10. If only trypsinized sample is toxic, trypsinize 6 ml culture fluid and repeat neutralization tests as described under "Testing Stool Specimens for Toxin" and Table 84-4.
11. Demonstration of botulinal toxin in enrichment cultures from a nontoxic specimen is presumptive evidence for presence of *C. botulinum* in specimen. However, it is desirable to isolate organism for definitive identification when possible.
12. At time of toxicity testing, or 1 or 2 days earlier, subculture from both unheated and heated CMGS cultures onto modified McClung-Toabe egg yolk agar plates and streak to obtain isolated colonies. Incubate plates anaerobically for 48 h at 35 C.
13. Examine plates with hand lens and stereoscopic microscope and pick typical lipase-positive colonies into CMGS medium. Pick several colonies because some isolates may be non-

toxigenic. Incubate CMGS cultures for 4 d at 30 C.

14. If lipase-positive colonies are seen only in growth on plate from nonheated enrichment culture, it might mean that a strain of *C. botulinum* with heat-sensitive spores is present. However, in such a case where there are large numbers of other bacteria present, it may be impossible to isolate *C. botulinum* from plate. If so, try alcohol treatment for spore selection.[17,55a]

   a. Transfer 1 ml unheated enrichment culture to tube and mix with 1 ml absolute alcohol. Hold for 1 h at room temperature and mix every 15 min.

   b. Inoculate 0.5-1.0 ml of alcohol mixture into CMGS medium and incubate anaerobically for 48 h.

   c. Repeat isolation attempt with egg yolk agar.

15. Perform toxicity and toxin neutralization tests on pure cultures.

16. Confirm identity of isolates by biochemical characteristics as described by Dowell and Hawkins.[10]

NOTE: Sometimes it is difficult to isolate *C. botulinum* type E from mixed cultures because of bacteriocin produced by nontoxigenic organisms similar to *C. botulinum*. This can be overcome by using a medium containing trypsin, which inactivates the bacteriocin. Trypticase–peptone–glucose–yeast extract–trypsin (TPGYT) medium may be used in addition to CMGS when such difficulties are encountered, or when one knows beforehand the strain being sought is type E. Dissolve ingredients, adjust pH to 7.0; dispense in tubes, 15 ml/tube. Autoclave for 8 min at 121 C. Prepare a 1.5% solution of aqueous trypsin (Difco 1:250) and filter-sterilize. Just before using medium, drive off oxygen by heating in boiling water bath for 10 min, cool, and add 1 ml trypsin solution.

Infant botulism[19,29-35]

Botulism is caused in young infants by toxin from the germination of ingested spores of *C. botulinum* in the bowel lumen, in contrast to the adult in whom botulism is caused by preformed toxin in contaminated foods or, in rare instances, by wound infection with *C. botulinum*–producing toxin.

Infant botulism was first recognized in 1976 and by early 1979 some 100 cases in infants under 6 months of age (NOTE: an infant case reported in 1978 was 35 weeks of age at onset[19]) had been identified by the Center for Disease Control.[29,31]

Arnon et al.[32] recently demonstrated *C. botulinum* spores in samples of honey; other sources of spores include soil, house dust, and house plants; the evidence linking feeding of honey to infants who later developed botulism is strong. It has now been recommended that **honey not be fed to infants under 1 year of age.**[31,32]

Laboratory tests in infant botulism[35]

Laboratory confirmation. At present, confirmation of the clinical diagnosis of botulism requires the demonstration of botulinal toxin and/or *C. botulinum* in the feces of the infant. All routine laboratory tests (blood chemistry, hematology, urinalysis, etc.) are normal; the cerebrospinal fluid protein has been slightly elevated in a few cases. Although serum samples are frequently useful for laboratory confirmation of botulism in adults, none of the serum samples from infants with botulism examined to date have been positive for botulinal toxin. However, the possibility that some infants may have circulating toxin in their blood during illness has not been excluded (see treatment section).

Collection and shipment of specimens

FECES. A passed stool specimen is preferred for botulinal toxin detection and for isolation of *C. botulinum*.[36] If available, at least 25 g (walnut size) should be collected in a **sterile** container (botulism spores may be present in dust and the environment). However, since it is frequently difficult to obtain stools from infants with botulism, whatever quantity is available, should be collected for testing. If a passed stool is not available, a specimen obtained after a sterile (nonbacteriostatic) water enema can be used. The volume of water used should be limited so that toxin in the feces is not diluted unnecessarily. A specimen volume of 15-20 ml collected after an enema is sufficient. The physician should be guided by the clinical condition and the weight and size of the infant in administering an enema. Fecel samples should always be collected before administration of therapeutic botulinal antitoxin if it is used. Submission of serial stool specimens (approximately biweekly) during the acute and convalescent stages of illness is encouraged since toxin and *C. botulinum* have persisted in the intestinal tract of some infants for many weeks.

SERUM. If possible, serum samples (2 ml or more) for toxin assay should be collected from suspected cases during the acute and convalescent stages of confirmed cases. Convalescent serum should be accompanied by a corresponding stool specimen so that toxin levels in serum (if any) and stool can be compared.

AUTOPSY SAMPLES. Postmortem samples should include serum samples to test for botulinal toxin and samples of intestinal contents to test for botulinal toxin and *C. botulinum*. Intestinal samples should be taken from different levels (e.g., small bowel, proximal colon, distal colon) of the intestinal tract, if possible.

MISCELLANEOUS SPECIMENS. Other specimens that should be collected during an epidemiologic investigation and considered for laboratory testing include foods ingested by the infant or any other suspected item that would have served as a source of *C. botulinum* for the infant, e.g., open containers of cereal, honey, syrups, house dusts, etc.

LABELING SPECIMENS. All specimen containers should be properly labeled, indicating the specimen identification and date and time of collection. In addition, a properly completed requisition or note describing the specimens should accompany them to the laboratory. Since some medications can interfere with botulinal toxin testing, a list of medications the infant(s) is presently receiving should also be submitted.

REFRIGERATION OF SPECIMENS. Unless examined in the laboratory immediately after collection, all specimens to be examined for botulinal toxin and/or *C. botulinum* should be refrigerated (4 C) until tested.

SHIPMENT OF SPECIMENS. Some state health department laboratories provide services for laboratory diagnosis of botulism while others do not; specimens can be submitted to the Center for Disease Control (CDC), Atlanta, during a botulism investigation with concurrence of the state health department. Any specimen shipped to CDC should be placed in a leakproof container, packed with ice or a suitable refrigerant in a second leakproof insulated shipping container, labeled "medical emergency," and shipped by the most rapid means possible.

The following guidelines should be followed in sending specimens to be tested at CDC.

1. Overnight or express delivery is preferred to maintain a quality specimen.
2. Overnight guaranteed service is provided by the United States Postal Service from major cities to Atlanta. An advantage of this system is that the package arrives directly at CDC.
3. Air express (Eastern Sprint, Delta Dash) or Air Freight can also be used.

When shipping specimens to CDC request that shipper (usually hospital laboratory personnel) notify CDC (days: (404)329-3333 or (404)329-3753; nights and weekends: (404)329-3644) of flight, time of arrival of specimens, and waybill or receipt identification number. Airlines do not accept responsibility for notifying CDC, even when requested to do so on shipping label. It is suggested that hospital laboratory personnel responsible for sending a specimen contact the CDC Anaerobe Section **before** sending specimens to ensure that they will be sending appropriate specimens in an expeditious manner. Packages should be addressed to Charles L. Hatheway, Ph.D., Anaerobe Section, Center for Disease Control, 1600 Clifton Road, N.E., Atlanta, Georgia 30333.

• • •

The organism *C. botulinum* is described in detail, together with a number of other major clostridia, at the end of this chapter.

Tetanus[18,37-40]

Tetanus is an intoxication caused by *Clostridium tetani* toxin, an extraordinarily potent exotoxin.

The diagnosis must be made clinically; isolation of the organism from wounds is often not successful.[40] It should be noted that *C. tetani* spores persist in a particular location until anaerobic conditions develop (tissue necrosis, foreign bodies). Once they proliferate and produce toxin, the organisms themselves do not spread beyond their original location (puncture wound, tissue necrosis); it is the circulating toxin that is responsible for the disease.

The organism *C. tetani* is described in detail at the end of this chapter.

Clostridium perfringens food poisoning[18,41-44]

C. perfringens type A accounts for about 15% of reported outbreaks of foodborne disease in the United States. Foods involved are usually those that contain meat or gravy, inadequately or not at all refrigerated after preparation.[18]

The diagnosis is established by anaerobically culturing the incriminated food and growing large numbers of *C. perfringens*.[43]

Type F strains of *C. perfringens* are involved in a rare type of clostridial food poisoning known as **enteritis necroticans,** a severe, sometimes fatal illness.[43]

Examination of foods and feces for Clostridium perfringens[10]

To show that *C. perfringens* is the causative agent in an outbreak of foodborne disease, examine both suspected foods and the feces of patients if possible. Quantitative *C. perfringens* colony counts should be performed on the food samples.[44] At least 3 colony isolates of *C. perfringens* from the food and 3 colony isolates of *C. perfringens* from the feces of each patient should be examined serologically to establish the serotype involved. In large outbreaks, sets of isolates should include 3 or more strains from the incriminated food when the food is available and 3 or more fecal isolates from each of 10 different patients.

Procedure

1. *Enumeration of C. perfringens in food samples.*
   a. Weigh 50 g food sample in mortar. To prepare an initial 1:10 food dilution, grind and dilute sample in 450 ml buffered dilution water as follows*:
      (1) Add 1-2 g sterile sand to contents of mortar.
      (2) Add a portion (15-20 ml) of buffered dilution water to contents of mortar and grind until homogenous suspension is obtained.
      (3) Transfer ground sample to widemouthed bottle; use remaining buffered dilution water to rinse any adherent food from mortar into bottle.
      (4) Mix contents of bottle by inverting 50 times.
      (5) Prepare smear of food suspension for gram staining.
   b. Prepare 10-fold dilutions (10^{-2} through 10^{-6}) by serial transfer of 1 ml diluted sample in 9 ml buffered dilution water.
   c. Plate 10^{-3}, 10^{-4}, 10^{-5}, and 10^{-8} dilutions in duplicate or triplicate in sulfite-polymixin-sulfadiazine (SPS) agar as follows:
      (1) Pipet 1 ml well-mixed dilution into Petri dish.
      (2) Add 15 ml melted agar medium; mix well, and allow agar to solidify.
      (3) When agar is solid, overlay with an additional 4-5 ml SPS agar.
   d. Incubate plates for 24 h in anaerobe jar at 35-37 C.
   e. After incubation, open anaerobe jar and count black colonies in all plates containing 30-300 black colonies. To facilitate counting, use Quebec colony counter with white tissue paper over counting area.
   f. *C. perfringens confirmation.*
      (1) Subculture at least 10 representative black colonies from each culture to tubes of chopped meat–dextrose medium (or thioglycollate medium).
      (2) Incubate chopped meat medium for 4 h at 46 C or overnight at 35-37 C.
         (a) Prepare Gram stains from each chopped meat medium and look for typical gram-positive bacilli with blunt ends and **absence of spores** (usually).
         (b) Prepare wet mounts and check for motility.
         (c) Using capillary pipet, inoculate tube of lactose-motility medium up the "line of stab" with each chopped meat medium culture. Incubate at 35-37 C.

---

*Food sample can also be homogenized and diluted in 450 ml of buffered dilution water in a blender at low speed (8000 rpm) for 2 min.

(3) Examine lactose-motility medium at 24 and 48 h. Reactions are usually complete within 24 h. *C. perfringens* is nonmotile, rarely produces demonstrable spores in chopped meat or thioglycollate media, and produces acid and gas from lactose medium.

g. *Calculation of number of viable C. perfringens per gram of food sample.*

Average plate count ×
Ratio *C. perfringens* to black colonies ×
Dilution = Total count/gram of food

NOTE: If plate counts with 30-300 black colonies are obtained at 2 dilutions, calculate total count for each dilution and average.

h. Save at least 3 different colony isolates of *C. perfringens* from food in chopped meat medium for serologic typing.

2. *Isolation of C. perfringens from feces.*
   a. Inoculate two 25 ml tubes of thioglycollate broth with approximately 1 g of feces or 5 ml of fecal suspension.
      (1) Heat 1 tube in 80 C water bath for 15 min and cool in tap water.
      (2) Incubate both tubes for 4 h at 46 C or 18-24 h at 35-37 C.
   b. After incubating tubes, subculture each thioglycollate broth culture to blood and egg yolk agar plates. Transfer growth from near bottom of broth tubes using a capillary pipet. Place 1 drop on each plate and streak for isolation. Incubate plates for 24 h in anaerobe jar at 35-37 C.
   c. Remove plates from incubator and allow jar to set at room temperature for 2 h (or in refrigerator at 4 C for 30 min) to allow full development of hemolytic patterns.
   d. Open anaerobe jar and subculture at least 1 colony of every type resembling *C. perfringens* to freshly heated and cooled tubes of chopped meat–dextrose medium (or thioglycollate medium).
   e. Confirm *C. perfringens* isolates morphologically and biochemically as in Step 1f.
   f. Save at least 3 different isolates of *C. perfringens* from each fecal specimen examined for serologic typing.

3. *Serologic identification of Clostridium perfringens.*
   a. Using capillary pipette, inoculate tube of *C. perfringens* antigen medium near bottom with approximately 0.5 ml of an 18-24 h chopped meat–dextrose culture. Try to avoid introduction of meat particles. Incubate antigen medium for 18 h at 35-37 C.
   b. After 18 h incubation, examine antigen medium cultures.
      (1) Prepare Gram stain and check for purity.
      (2) Centrifuge culture in plastic centrifuge tube for 10 min at 12,350 × g and discard supernatant fluid.
      (3) Add sufficient 0.4% formalinized 0.85% saline (0.5-1 ml) to sediment to prepare turbid suspension suitable for slide agglutination.
      NOTE: It may be necessary to filter antigen through nonabsorbent cotton wrapped around tip of capillary pipet to obtain homogenous suspension.
   c. *Slide agglutination test.*
      (1) With wax pencil, mark slide into 5 or 6 equal parts.

(2) Place drop of each *C. perfringens* antiserum (Hobbs types 1-13)[19] near top of 1 area. Include drop of normal rabbit serum as a control.
(3) Add drop of antigen near bottom of each area and mix reagents by tilting slide.
(4) Record reaction in 30 sec as:
   Negative = no agglutination
   1+ = 25% clumping
   2+ = 50% clumping
   3+ = 75% clumping
   4+ = 100% clumping

Detection of clostridial toxins: toxin neutralization tests and pathogenicity tests[10]

Tests for clostridial toxins

Although the conditions for toxin elaboration will vary with individual species, clostridial toxins can generally be detected in chopped meat–dextrose cultures incubated 18 hours at 35-37 C.

If *C. novyi* A is suspected, chopped meat medium without dextrose should be used. Cultures suggestive of *C. botulinum* or *C. sporogenes* should be grown in chopped meat–dextrose–starch medium and incubated at 30 C (see section on detection of *C. botulinum* and botulinal toxins above).

Attention must also be given to the age of the culture. Some clostridia, e.g., *C. perfringens*, *C. histolyticum*, and *C. haemolyticum*, are more toxic in young cultures and others, e.g., *C. botulinum*, *C. novyi*, and *C. tetani*, exhibit maximum toxicity after several days' incubation.

1. Do routine tests for toxin on 18 h chopped meat–dextrose cultures incubated at 35-37 C.
2. Pipet 3.0 ml of culture supernate into 12 ml plastic centrifuge tube.
3. Centrifuge at 10,000 rpm (12,350 × g) for 10 min and decant supernatant fluid in clean test tube.
4. Load 1.0 ml syringe with 0.8 ml centrifuged culture fluid and inoculate two 15-20 g mice IP with 0.4 ml each.
5. Observe mice for 3 d. Toxic clostridial cultures will usually kill mice within 24 h after inoculation.
6. Need for further toxin tests for which special media, cultural conditions, or inoculation procedures are used will depend on overall results of cultural, biochemical, and routine toxicity tests.

Identificaton of specific clostridial toxin

1. When it has been demonstrated that a *Clostridium* culture fluid is toxic for mice, it is often helpful in identification of the organism to perform animal protection tests with specific immune serum. Neutralization of toxic culture fluid is usually accomplished by mixing 1.2 ml centrifuged culture fluid with 0.3 ml specific antitoxin, allowing mixture to stand for 30 min at 37 C and inoculating 2 mice IP with 0.5 ml each of material. Since toxicity of *Clostridium* culture filtrates may vary, it is advisable to test culture filtrates diluted 1:5 in gelatin diluent.
2. Cultural characteristics of *Clostridium septicum* and *Clostridium chauvoei* are essentially identical. Isolates resembling either of these organisms should be tested with both *C. septicum* and *C. chauvoei* antisera as well as normal rabbit serum.
3. The commercially available *Clostridium* antisera include:
   C. perfringens types A-E

C. *novyi* types A and B
C. *chauvoei*
C. *septicum*
C. *tetani*
C. *botulinum* types A-F
C. *sordellii*

Tests for pathogenicity

1. Determination of pathogenic properties of anaerobic bacteria is quite useful in evaluating the role an organism may play in a pathologic process. Type of laboratory animal to use and conditions required for demonstration of pathogenicity vary considerably and will depend on species being tested.
2. *Clostridium* cultures are routinely tested for pathogenicity by inoculating a guinea pig IM in the thigh with 0.5 ml of a mixture containing equal parts of an 18 h chopped meat–dextrose culture and 10% calcium chloride.
3. Pathologic changes in guinea pigs after injection with *Clostridium* cultures are quite varied and may include (1) hemorrhagic or gelatinous edema, (2) pockets of gas in the infected tissue, (3) necrosis, (4) digestion of muscle tissue, (5) rapid toxic death with little detectable pathology, and (6) paralysis and/or toxic muscular spasms. Pathologic changes usually occur within a period of 4-5 d; however, guinea pigs should be held for a period of 2 wk before cultures are reported as nonpathogenic for guinea pigs.

Toxin typing of Clostridium perfringens [10]

Most human *C. perfringens* infections or intoxications are due to type A strains. Types A-E are responsible for a variety of diseases in animals. Type A strains produce a lethal α toxin, and all other types produce at least one other major lethal toxin in addition to α-toxin. Differentiation of types is based on detection and specific neutralization of toxins from culture fluids. Tests for toxicity and serum neutralization for typing are done in mice.

C. perfringens types are characterized by the production of one or more of the following lethal toxins:

Type:	A	B	C	D	E
Toxins:	α	αβε	αβ	αε	αι

The ε- and ι-toxins are activated by trypsin; α- and β-toxins may be inactivated by trypsin.

Preparation of centrifuged culture fluid (CCF)

1. Use a 6-16 h (no older) chopped meat–starch culture.
2. Centrifuge culture fluid in polyethylene centrifuge tubes at 10,000 rpm (preferably in the cold) for 10 min.
3. Pour CCF into a 15 × 125 mm tube.
4. For trypsinization mix 1 part 1% trypsin solution with 9 parts CCF in a 15 × 125 mm tube and incubate mixture for 30 min in a 37 C water bath.

Determination of toxicity

1. Inoculate 2 mice IP with 0.5 ml each of untreated CCF.
2. Inoculate 2 mice IP with 0.5 ml each of trypsinized CCF.
3. Observe mice for 48 h. Type A strains usually kill mice within 18 h after inoculation.

Serum neutralization tests

1. When working with toxic isolates from human specimen material, routine neutralization procedure is to test with type A antiserum and normal rabbit serum control. This includes tubes 1, 2, 5, and 6 in Table 84-5. If no deaths occur in mice inoculated with either trypsinized or untrypsinized toxin neutralized with type A antiserum culture is reported as type A. Where deaths do occur, CCF is tested with antisera against remaining *C. perfringens* types.
2. Mix 1.2 ml CCF or trypsinized CCF in 12 × 75 mm tubes with 0.3 ml of particular *C. perfringens* antisera (type A, B, C, D, or E) or normal rabbit antiserum as outlined in Table 84-5.
3. Incubate CCF-serum mixtures for 30 min in 37 C water bath and inoculate 2 mice IP with each mixture.

Histotoxic infections; gas gangrene

MacLennan[14] emphasizes that clostridia represent real danger in humans only when they invade the bloodstream or the muscles (**except** for *C. botulinum* [botulism] and *C. tetani* [tetanus]; see above).

The term "clostridial gas gangrene" is now generally limited to those invasive anaerobic infections of **muscle** that are characterized by severe toxemia, extensive local edema, gas production, and massive death of tissue.[14]

The clostridia are widely distributed in soil, dust, water, and the gut of humans and most animals. They commonly contaminate many

Table 84-5. Mouse toxin neutralization tests of *C. perfringens* centrifuged culture fluids (CCF)[10]

Tube	Mixture injected	Lethality for mice with C. perfringens type				
		A	B	C	D	E
1	Untreated CCF + normal rabbit serum	+	+	+	+	+
2	Untreated CCF + anti-A (anti-α)	−	+	+	−*	±
3	Untreated CCF + anti-C (anti-β)	−	−*	−	−*	±
4	Untreated CCF + anti-B (anti-α + anti-β + anti-ε)	−	−	−	−	±
5	Trypsinized CCF + normal rabbit serum	±	+	−†	+	+
6	Trypsinized CCF + anti-D (anti-α + anti-ε)	−	+	−†	+	+
7	Trypsinized CCF + anti-B (anti-α + anti-β + anti-ε)	−	−†	−†	−	+
8	Trypsinized CCF + anti-E (anti-α + anti-ι)	−	−	−	−	+
9	Trypsinized CCF + anti-E (anti-α + antiι)	−	+	−†	+	−
	Diagnostic toxin identified	α	β + ε	β	ε	ι

*Usually negative, as ε in protoxin form.
†Usually negative, as β-toxin is destroyed by trypsin.

large wounds; however, only a relatively small number of species are pathogenic, and even a smaller number are capable of causing gas gangrene in humans, namely, *C. perfringens, C. novyi, C. septicum, C. histolyticum, C. bifermentans, C. sordellii,* and *C. fallax,* with *C. perfringens* being the most common isolate.[18]

All are pathogenic because of their production of soluble exotoxins. These exotoxins are capable of destroying various tissue and blood cells.

MacLennan classified the histotoxic infections of humans[14] as follows:

1. *Traumatic infections*
   a. Wound infections, consisting of
      (1) Simple contamination
      (2) Anaerobic cellulitis (a heavy clostridial infection involving necrotic tissue already killed; intact muscle is not invaded)
      (3) Anaerobic clostridial myonecrosis; invasion of healthy living muscle by clostridia
   b. Uterine infections (following abortions performed by untrained or unknowledgeable individuals; occasionally following spontaneous abortions)
2. *Nontraumatic infections*
   a. Idiopathic gas gangrene (few cases of gas gangrene unrelated to trauma)
   b. Infected vascular gas gangrene infection by clostridia of tissue already dead from simple ischemia)

For reviews of gas gangrene, see Weinstein and Barza[45] and Caplan and Kluge.[46]

Clostridial septicemia and other infections

C. perfringens septicemia, appendicitis, peritonitis, and cholecystitis are all well-described clinical entities.

C. septicum bacteremia seems to be associated with malignancy, especially cancer of the colon, and hematologic malignancies (see Alpern and Dowell[47] and Koransky et al.[48]).

Clostridial food poisoning and enteritis necroticans are intestinal infections already discussed above (see "Intoxications").

For extensive reviews of anaerobic infections, including clostridial infections, see Finegold,[12] Meyer and Finegold,[18] and Gorbach and Bartlett.[49]

Pseudomembranous colitis: Clostridium difficile

Toxigenic isolates of *C. difficile* have been shown to be a major cause of antibiotic-associated pseudomembranous colitis (PMC) in humans.[15,16,50] Some individuals harbor *C. difficile* in their colon flora without harmful effects. In the presence of certain antimicrobial agents (especially clindamycin), *C. difficile* grows abundantly and produces a cytotoxin that can be demonstrated in the stools of the majority of patients with antibiotic-associated PMC.[51]

Tissue culture assays for the toxin are described by Larson et al.,[52] Chang et al.,[53] Rifkin et al.,[54] and Bartlett et al.[55]

George et al.[56] described a selective and differential medium for isolation of *C. difficile.* The medium consists of an egg yolk–fructose base to which cycloserine and cefoxitin are added.

Selective and differential medium (CCFA) for isolation of Clostridium difficile[56]

Egg yolk–fructose agar base

Protease peptone no. 2 (Difco Laboratories, Detroit)	40 g
Na_2HPO_4	5 g
KH_2PO_4	1 g
NaCl	2 g
$MgSO_4$, anhydrous	0.1 g
Fructose (ICN Pharmaceuticals, Cleveland)	6 g
Agar (BBL, Cockeysville, Md.)	20 g
1% solution of neutral red in ethanol	3 ml
Water	1000 ml

Dispense base in 100 ml portions, sterilize at 121 C and 15 psi for 15 min, and store aerobically at 4 C. Plates

1. Prepare plates by melting basal medium and then cooling to 50 C.
2. Add:

Cycloserine base (Eli Lilly & Co., Indianapolis)	500 µg/ml final concentration
Cefoxitin base (Merck, Sharp & Dohme, West Point, Pa.)	16 µg/ml final concentration
Egg yolk suspension, 50% in saline	5 ml

3. Swirl container vigorously; pour 17-20 ml into 15 × 100 mm Petri dishes.

Stool specimens

1. Blend liquid specimens in vortex mixer with glass beads in large glass screwcap tube in anaerobic chamber until visible homogeneity is achieved.
2. Mix solid and semisolid specimens in high-speed rotary blender for 3-5 min in anaerobic chamber.

Inoculation and incubation. Specimens (after blending) are diluted in a tenfold series (10^1 to 10^9) in 0.05% yeast extract solution in tubes containing glass beads. Inoculate plates with 0.1 ml of each of the dilutions from 10^3 to 10^7.

Place the plates in Gas-Pak jars in the anaerobic chamber, seal the jars, and then remove from the chamber for incubation (48 h).

After incubation, count plates for total bacteria and colonies that might be *C. difficile.* Counts are expressed as log_{10} number or organisms per gram (wet weight) of stool.

Colonies of *C. difficile* have golden-yellow fluorescence on CCFA medium after 24 h, lasting 5-6 days (use long-wavelength ultraviolet light). After 48 h, on uncrowded plates (less than 10 colonies) *C. difficile* colonies measure about 1.5-9 mm (average = 4 mm) in diameter. On blood agar, they fluoresce yellow-green or chartreuse. Colonies on CCFA are yellow, ground glass like, circular with slight filamentous edge, and **lipase and lecithinase negative.**

C. *difficile* cells have subterminal to terminal spores; however, spores are **not** seen on Gram stains made from CCFA, and cellular elongation is marked.

After isolation and subculture (on blood agar), the organism should be identified using physiologic and biochemical tests described in Holdeman et al.[3] or Sutter et al.[8a]; see also Table 84-9 below.

• • •

Isolation and cultivation of clostridia

To make a diagnostic identification of clostridia, (1) the concomitant aerobic flora must be eliminated, (2) the individual anaerobic species must be separated, and (3) the anaerobic species must be identified.

Initial culture. The procedures described in Chapter 75 ("Anaerobic Infections and Anaerobic Cultures") are applicable to isolation and cultivation of clostridia; see also Chapter 82.

In addition to the media described for anaerobes (enriched thioglycollate broth, tube of chopped meat–glucose medium, blood agar, LKV agar, phenylethyl alcohol blood agar), if clostridia are suspected, inoculate 1 egg yolk agar (EYA) plate for the Nagler test (see below), and if available, 1 neomycin blood agar plate, or Columbia agar base with lactose, egg yolk, milk, neomycin, and azide added.

Plain **blood agar plates** incubated aerobically and anaerobically and thioglycollate broth without selective agents should always be used in parallel with selective media; also inoculate MacConkey agar for isolation of aerobic gram-negative rods.

Inoculate media, using at least minimal culture procedure and selective media. Incubate anaerobically at 35-37 C; incubate parallel plates also aerobically.

If Gas Pak jar is used (or other anaerobic jars), incubate 48 hours; however, if adequate specimen is available, a duplicate culture set should be set up and examined after 12-24 hours. An alternative is the use of the Bio-Bag, which allows for examination of the culture at any time[8a] (see Chapter 86 for description of Bio-Bag).

Direct smear. Prepare Gram stains from specimen (exudate, edema) and also from muscle in case of clostridial myositis (gas gangrene). Gram staining of specimens may be lifesaving by alerting the physician to the presence of clostridia.

NOTE: The presence of large gram-positive bacilli in material from a closed (noncontaminated) site, such as fluid aspirated from an injection site, is diagnostic. However, smears made from wounds or tissues contaminated with feces will commonly show clostridia, and they are sometimes seen in wounds at other sites. The laboratory should report that clostridia are present. At the same time, it should be kept in mind that wounds do become contaminated with clostridia without any infection developing; however, even when infection occurs, gas gangrene is much less common than local cellulitis.

Note gram-positive rods **with** or **without spores** because sporulation in tissue is uncommon with

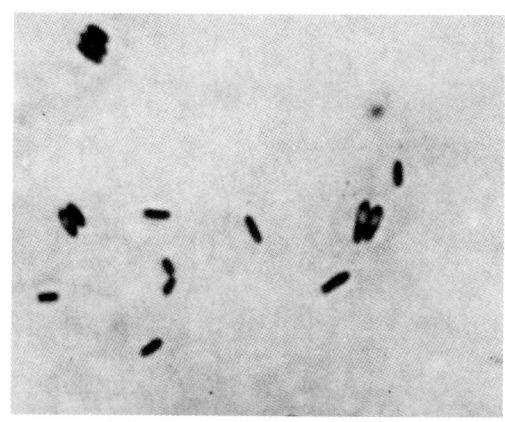

Fig. 84-1. Impression smear from experimental gas gangrene, showing sporulating organism, *Clostridium histolyticum.* (Photomicrograph from slide of Dr. T. F. Wetzler.)

the 2 species frequently encountered, *C. perfringens* and *C. ramosum. C. perfringens* usually appears as large, fat, gram-positive rods, with no spores, in tissue smears; the cells of *C. ramosum* are slender, longer, and often curved, while *C. histolyticum* cells form spores (Fig. 84-1).

Examination of cultures following incubation
1. Make smears from media in tubes and perform Gram stain. Check carefully for gram-positive bacilli, remembering that some clostridia lose gram-staining characteristics fairly early.
2. Examine colonies on anaerobic plates with dissecting microscope or hand lens (8×). Compare anaerobic blood plate with aerobic blood plate. Examine egg yolk half–antitoxin plate for characteristic reactions.
3. Make Gram stains from colonies. All gram-positive bacilli, sporeforming or not, that do not grow well on aerobic plates are suspected of being clostridia.
4. Make Gram stain on minute colonies that appear within 48 h and do not exceed 1 mm in diameter. Gram-positive bacilli with such colony formation probably are microaerophilic clostridia.
5. Microaerophilic clostridia reportedly do not sporulate on aerobic plates.
6. If there are any questionable findings, replate broth culture anaerobically and pick colonies after proper incubation.

Table 84-6 summarizes colonial and microscopic appearance of clostridia.
7. Inspect anaerobic plates. In general, pick the following colonies for transfer:
   a. All colonies exhibiting hemolysis.
   b. All transparent colonies.
   c. All flat, grayish, translucent colonies.
   d. All colonies with emanating, dryish, spreading growth.
      (1) Transfer to an anaerobic blood plate for pure culture; also add kannamycin, 1000 μg disk; colistin, 10 μg disk; and vancomycin, 5 μg disk (as described under "Wadsworth Methodology" in Chapter 82).
      (2) Egg yolk agar plate for lecithinase and lipase determinations.
      (3) Chocolate agar plate for CO_2 incubation.
      (4) Blood agar plate for incubation in air.

Table 84-6. Identification of clostridia; colony form, morphology, and reactions on blood agar*

	Colony form†	He-molysis	Rods‡
C. botulinum A + B	B	+	S to T
C. botulinum C-E	B, E	+	T
C. tetani	FG	+	S
Gas gangrene group			
C. histolyticum	C	+	S
C. novyi A	D	+	S to T
C. novyi B	D, E	+	T
C. perfringens A-E	A	+	TC
C. septicum	DG, F	+	S to T
C. sordellii	DG, A	+	T
Associated species			
C. aerofoetidum	A	+	T
C. bifermentans	DG, A	+	T
C. butyricum	A		T
C. fallax	B	−	S to TC
C. sporogenes	D	+	S to T
C. tertium	C	−	S
Rare species		+	
C. capitovale	C	+	S to T
C. carnis	B	+	T
C. cochlearium	B	+	T
C. difficile	B	−	S to T
C. sphenoides	C	±	T
C. tetanomorphum	E	+	S to T

*Based on data from Sterne and van Heyningen.[57]

†Colony forms on **blood agar:**

A, Large raised colonies, smooth to slightly ridged with entire to undulate margins, 2-4 mm.

B, Smaller, raised colonies, margins like A, 1-3 mm.

C, Minute, raised colonies, smooth to irregular with entire to irregular margins, with short rhizoids.

D, Large colonies, raised, irregular, wide-spreading rhizoids, 3-6 mm.

E, As D, but smaller, finer rhizoids, 1-2 mm.

F, Irregular granular colonies with delicate spreading rhizoids to irregular rhizoidlike structures without a central colony.

G, Tendency to swarm.

‡Rods: S, slender rods; T, thick rods; C, capsulated.

8. After transfers, etc., inspect aerobic plates. Proceed with identification of aerobic organisms. Often wounds, etc., will contain mixture of aerobic and anaerobic organisms.

• • •

One must remember that in working with anaerobic organisms constant checking of an isolated strain for contamination is absolutely necessary. It is rare that a single species of *Clostridium* is isolated from a dirty wound. When only 1 species has been isolated, it is the usual practice to repeat the isolation technic to find other species. When clostridia are recovered from a specimen, at least 5 or preferably 10 colonies should be picked for taxonomic study. When no growth has been observed, a subculture should be made once more from the initial tube to avoid false-negative results.

Identification and differentiation of clostridia

The identification and differentiation of pure culture isolates of clostridia require the determination of cell morphology and colonial charac-

teristics and the performance of a number of physiologic and biologic tests. Additionally, pathogenicity in animals (**toxin production**) is demonstrated, and identification of toxins is performed (the last procedure usually by reference laboratories only).

Antibiotic disk susceptibility. A zone of 10 mm or less is considered resistant. If the **Wadsworth schema** (see Chapter 82) is used, note susceptibility to vancomycin and resistance to colistin: this pattern strongly suggests a gram-positive organism and may be very helpful with some clostridia that stain gram negative and have very few spores.

Nagler reaction (lecithovitellin, LCV, reaction). The Nagler reaction (on egg yolk agar) is very helpful in the presumptive identification of clostridia. Certain clostridia produce opalescence in egg yolk emulsion due to the production by the organism of specific lecithinases. For example, *C. perfringens* secretes a lecithinase (α-toxin); when grown on egg yolk agar, the lecithinase diffuses into the medium, breaking down the lecithin in the egg yolk and producing the **opalescence** (cloudy halo) around the zones of growth. Some clostridia, in addition, also produce a pearly layer (**iridescence**), which is likely due to lipases secreted that break down the free fats in the egg yolk.

Three types of opalescence, namely, (1) a wide zone of opaque precipitate, characteristic of *C. perfringens*, *C. bifermentans*, and *C. sordellii*, (2) a wide zone of precipitation with pearly, iridescent layer, characteristic of *C. novyi* types A and B and *C. botulinum*, and (3) a very narrow zone of precipitate under the colony and a narrow zone of pearly layer characteristic of *C. sporogenes* are helpful in the identification of the clostridia.[58]

NOTE: Aerobic organisms, e.g., some species of *Bacillus* and certain staphylococci, also produce opalescence.

Half-antitoxin plate. The cloudy halo (opalescence) formation by toxin can be specifically inhibited by appropriate antitoxin; diagnosis is greatly facilitated by the use of a half-antitoxin plate.

Dry an egg yolk agar plate for about 15-30 min in incubator. Spread evenly about 5 drops *C. perfringens* antitoxin (polyvalent gas gangrene antitoxin can be used) over one half of egg yolk plate with sterile glass or wire spreader and allow to dry. Inoculate plate with specimen or inoculum prepared from suspected anaerobic growth. Spread inoculum in same pattern over each half of plate. Incubate in anaerobic jar for 24 h or overnight and examine.

On the half of the plate containing no antitoxin, colonies of *C. perfringens* will show a zone of opacity (cloudy halo), but on the antitoxin half of the plate no zones will be seen around the colonies. This is a positive and specific reaction—inhibition of α-toxin by antitoxin—and provided there are no spores and the organism is anaerobic (**no** growth on parallel aerobic plate), the presence of *C. perfringens* can be reported.

Table 84-7. Differentiation of Nagler-positive clostridia[8a]

Species	Indole	Motility	Fermentation of lactose	Gelatin	Urease
C. perfringens	−	−	+	+	
C. paraperfringens	−	−	+	−	
C. bifermentans	+	+	−		−
C. sordellii	+	+	−		+

C. bifermentans and *C. sordellii* give a positive reaction but have abundant spores.

Reactions of various clostridia on egg yolk agar–half-antitoxin plate[59,60]

1. Opalescence produced: *C. perfringens* A-E, *C. botulinum* A-F, *C. sporogenes, C. bifermentans, C. sordellii, C. novyi* A, B, D
2. Pearly layer: *C. botulinum* A-F, *C. novyi* A, *C. sporogenes*
3. Opalescence **inhibited** by *C. perfringens* α-antitoxin: *C. perfringens* A-E, *C. bifermentans, C. sordellii*

The use of an egg yolk–half-antitoxin plate is largely recommended for preliminary differentiation and identification of certain clostridia, especially *C. perfringens.*

The Nagler reaction is recommended by Sutter et al.[8] for the rapid identification of *C. perfringens* and other α-toxin producers. Clostridia that are Nagler positive can be differentiated as shown in Table 84-7.

Presumptive identification. Presumptive identification of commonly encountered clostridia is based by Jones and Dowell[61] on degree of aerotolerance, motility, terminal spores, fermentation of glucose, lecithinase and lipase production, urease production, and toxicity for mice (also gas chromatography, if available). The criteria are given in Table 84-8.

Definitive identification. For definitive identification of clostridia a set of biochemicals is to be inoculated (see Wadsworth methodology and CDC methodology, Chapter 82).

Characteristics of a number of clostridial species are shown in Table 84-9.

Microtechnics and miniaturized kits for clostridial identification. See Chapter 82.

Fluorescent antibody (FA) methods. FA methods for detection and identification of certain clostridia have been devised by English workers[62-65]; however, the technic has had very limited acceptance and is not widely used in the United States.[66]

The fluorescent antibody reagents (*C. septicum, C. chauvoei, C. novyi,* and *C. botulinum* fluorescent sera) are available from Burroughs Wellcome & Co., Research Triangle Park, N.C.

Spore test. A spore test is made to determine the presence of a sporeforming organism in a mixed culture and to isolate it.

1. Inoculate a preboiled, cooled thioglycollate tube or chopped meat medium (preferably containing 0.2% starch) with 0.1 ml of original thioglycollate culture containing unknown gram-positive bacilli.
2. Heat tube at 80 C for 20 min to kill vegetative forms of all bacteria present. This does not kill spores.
3. Incubate for 24-48 h at 37 C.
4. If, after incubation, culture contains grampositive bacilli, transfer to blood agar plates and incubate anaerobically, so that single colonies may be picked.

NOTE: Since *C. perfringens* usually fails to produce spores in certain media, only rarely can it be isolated by the heating procedure.

Tests for pathogenicity and toxin production. See "Clostridial Infections, Clinical Syndromes, Specimens, and Laboratory Tests for Confirmation" above.

Fermentation of carbohydrates, CDC method.[10] Medium used is fermentation base with bromthymol blue added (1 ml of 1% aqueous solution to 1000 ml medium). Some *Clostridium* strains reduce organic indicators to the colorless (leuko) state.

All strains that ferment carbohydrates ferment dextrose (glucose). Use a medium containing dextrose (glucose) as a positive control.

Use as a negative control a tube of sugar-free thioglycollate broth inoculated at the same time as the tubes containing different sugars. This is necessary because some species attack the basal medium, alter the pH, and also produce gas.

Using the positive and negative controls for comparison for reading acid production, read all results in the media containing the carbohydrates as positive, doubtful, or negative.

For interpretation of reactions in various differential media (gelatin, milk, H$_2$S, motility, etc.) see Table 72-3, Chapter 72.

• • •

Clostridium botulinum

Whereas the nonproteolytic strains formerly were designated as *C. botulinum* and the proteolytic ones as *C. parabotulinum,* presently all toxigenic strains are designated as *C. botulinum.* The organism occurs in soils, in vegetable matter of various kinds, in the intestinal tract of animals, but rarely, if ever, in human feces.

C. botulinum, as a group, is divisible into types A, B, C, D, E, and F based on the serologic specificity of the toxins produced (type G is infrequent and not yet known well enough to associate with host species). Types A and E, and less often B, are those found in food poisoning of humans.

Table 84-8. Presumptive identification of commonly encountered clostridia*

Species	Aerotolerant	Motile	Terminal spores	Glucose fermented	Lecithinase (EYA)	Lipase (EYA)	Urease	Toxic for mice†	Volatile metabolic products (GLC) in PYG 48 h. 35 C
C. bifermentans	−	+	−	+	+	−	−	−	A, IC, (P), (IB), (B), (IV)
C. butyricum	−	+	−	+	−	−	−	−	A, B
C. innocuum	−	−	+	+	−	−	−	−	A, B
C. limosum	−	+	−	−	+	−	−	−	A
C. novyi type A	−	+	+	+	+	+	−	+	A, P, B
C. perfringens	−	−	−	+	+	−	−	+⁻	A, B, (P)
C. ramosum	−	−	+	+	−	−	−	−	A
C. septicum	−	+	+	+	−	−	−	+	A, B
C. sordellii	−	+	−	+	+	−	+	+⁻	A, IC, (P), (IB), (IV)
C. sporogenes	−	+	−	+	−⁺	+	−	−	A, P, IB, B, IV, V, IC
C. subterminale	+	+	+	−	+	−	−	−	A, IB, B, IV, (P)
C. tertium	+	+	+	+	−	−	−	−	A, B

*From Jones, G., and Dowell, V. R.: Anaerobic bacteriology in the clinical laboratory, Atlanta, 1976, Center for Disease Control, Laboratory Training and Consultation Division.
+, positive reaction; −, negative reaction; −⁺, majority negative; +⁻, majority positive; may be negative; A, acetic acid; P, propionic acid; IB, isobutyric acid; B, butyric acid; IV, isovaleric acid; V, valeric acid; IC, isocaproic acid; (), variable.
†Toxin neutralization tests aid in identification.

The rods are large, with rounded ends, occurring singly and occasionally in short chains. They are motile by means of peritrichous flagella. Spores are oval and subterminal.

The organism is a strict anaerobe. The colonies are flat, translucent, and granular with a spreading edge.

Types A, B, E, and F ferment glucose, maltose, and sucrose; types C and D ferment glucose and maltose but not sucrose; type G is nonsaccharolytic. All types produce H_2S and are indole negative.

The organism, so far as is known, does not proliferate in the tissue of the host. Botulism is a poisoning (intoxication), not an infectious disease, due to the toxin ingested with the food in which *C. botulinum* has grown. For a review of botulism in the United States see Gangarosa[67] and *Botulism in the United States, 1899-1977*.[19]

Clostridium tetani

The organism *C. tetani* is found in soil and less frequently in the intestinal tract of humans and animals. It is gram positive when young; by 48 hours it may be entirely gram negative. On incubation for 48 hours, **terminal,** spherical spores (in 48 hours they give "drumstick" appearance; see Fig. 84-2) are produced.

Colonies are small and transparent with a tendency to spread as a rhizoid film on solid media. The swarming is a very characteristic feature and can be easily missed because of its delicacy.

C. tetani, one of the strictest anaerobes, is nonsaccharolytic (does not ferment sugars) and nonproteolytic, but does liquefy gelatin in 48 hours and usually produces indole. It produces a very powerful neurotoxin. The rabbit, guinea pig, and especially the mouse are usable for pathogenicity testing. According to Willis,[2] there are at least 10 antigenic types based on flagellar antigens. Toxin is formed by all types and is antigenically identical in all. Variants that are nontoxigenic occur and can occasionally be isolated from wounds in cases of clinical tetanus.

Clostridium perfringens

C. perfringens rods are short and thick (1.5 × 4-8 μm) with rounded ends and occur singly, in pairs, and less frequently in short chains. Spores are found rarely in culture; no spores are seen in smears made from tissue. Capsules are seen on organisms recovered from tissue, but they are usually lost in culture (Figs. 84-3 and 84-4).

C. perfringens is divided into types A, B, C, D, and E, differentiated by the main toxin produced. A type F was distinguished on morphologic grounds and by its heat resistance; this designation is not used anymore because it is very similar to type C. *C. perfringens* grows rapidly, colonies being circular, moist, slightly raised, opaque centered, and entire. No spreading occurs. It is H_2S positive and indole negative

Table 84-9. Characteristics of some Clostridium species*

Species	Aerobic growth	Spores	Motility	Lecithinase	Lipase	Glucose	Mannitol	Lactose	Sucrose	Maltose	Salicin	Glycerol	Xylose	Arabinose	Nitrate reduction	Indole	Esculin hydrolysis	Gelatin hydrolysis	Milk	Toxicity for mice	Organic acids detected by GLC†	Other
C. bifermentans	−	ST	+	+	−	A	−	−	−	A	V	V	−	−	−	+	V	+	CD	−	A, P, IB, (B), IV, IC	Urease negative
C. botulinum																						
A	−	ST	+	−	+	A	−	−	−	A[−]	−[A]	V[−]	−	−	−	−	+[−]	+	CD	+		Toxin neutralization§
B	−	ST	+	−	+	A	−	−	−[A]	A[−]	−[A]	V[−]	−	−	−	−	+[−]	+	(C)(D)	+		Toxin neutralization§
C	−	ST	+	+[−]	+	A	−	−	−[A]	V	−	−[A]	−	−	+[−]	−	−	V	NC(C)	+		Toxin neutralization§
D	−	ST	+	+[−]	+	A	−	−	V	V	A[−]	−	−	−	−	−	V	V	NC	+		Toxin neutralization§
E	−	ST	+	−	+	A	−	−	A	A	−	V[−]	−	−	−	−	−	−	NC	+		Toxin neutralization§
F	−	ST	+	−	+	A	−	−	V	A	A[−]	V[−]	−	−	−	−	+[−]	+[−]	(C)(D)	+		Toxin neutralization§
C. butyricum	−	ST	+	−	−	A	A	A	A	A	A	A[−]	A	A	−	−	+	+	CG	−	A, (P), B	
C. cadaveris ‡	−	T	+	−	−	A	−	−	−	A	−	−	−	−	−	+	−	−	CG	−	A, (IB), B, IV	
C. chauvoei	−	ST	+	−	−	A	A	A	A[−]	A	−	−	−	A	−	−	V	V	(C)	V	A, B	Toxin neutralization§
C. difficile	−	ST	+	−	−	A	A	−	−	−	A[−]	A[−]	−	−	−	−	+	+	NC	V	A, P, IB, B, IV, IC	
C. histolyticum	+	ST	−	−	−	−	−	−	−	−	−	−	−	−	−	−	−	+	CD	V	A, L	Pathogenic for guinea pig
C. innocuum	−	T	−	−	−	A	A	A	A	A	A	−	−	−	−	−	+	−	NC	−	A, B	
C. limosum ‡	−	ST	+[−]	+	−	−	−	−	−	−[A]	−	−	−	−	−	−	−	V	CD	−	A	
C. novyi A	−	ST	+	+	+	A	−	−	−	A	−	A	−	−	−	−	V	+	(C)(G)	+	A, P, B	Toxin neutralization§
C. paraputrificum	−	T	+	−	−	A	A	A	A	A	A	−	A	A	−	−	+	−	(C)(G)	V	A, (P), B, (V)	
C. perfringens	−	ST	−	+	−	A	A	A	A	A	−	A	−	−	V	−	+[−]	+	CG	−	A, (P), B	Spores seldom observed
C. ramosum ‡	−	T	−	−	−	A	A[−]	A	A[−]	A	A	A	−	−	+	−	+	−	(C)(G)	V	A, L, S	Frequently gram negative
C. septicum	−	ST	+	−	−	A	−	A	−[A]	A	−	−	A[−]	−	−	−	+	V	(C)(G)	−	A, B	Toxin neutralization§
C. sordellii	−	ST	+	+[−]	−	A	−	A[−]	A[−]	A	A	A[−]	−	−	+	+	+	+	CD	−	A, (P), (IB), (IV), (IC)	Urease positive
C. sphenoides	−	ST	+	−	−	A	V	A	V	A[−]	A	−[A]	A[−]	A	+	V	+	−	(C)(G)	−	A, L, S	Usually appear gram negative
C. sporogenes	−	ST	+	−	+	A	−	−	−[A]	A	A	A	−	−	−	−	+	+	CD	−	A, (P), (IB), (B), IV, (IC)	
C. subterminale	−	ST	+	−[+]	−	A	−	−	−	A	−	V	A	A[−]	−	−	+[−]	+[−]	CD	−	A, (P), IB, B, IV	
C. tertium	+	T	+	−	−	A	A	A	A	A	V	−	A[−]	−	−	−	+	−	(C)(G)	−	A, B	
C. tetani	−	T	+	−	−	−	−	−	−	−	−	−	−	−	−	V	−	+	NC	+	A, P, B	Toxin neutralization§
C. paraperfringens	−	ST	−	+	−	A	−	A	A	A	A	−	−	−	−	−	−	−	NC	−	A, P, B	
C. cochlearium	−	ST	+	−	−	−	−	−	−	−	−	−	−	−	−	−	−	−	(C)	−		
C. glycolicum	−	ST	+	−	−	A	−	−	−	−	−	−	V	V	+	−	+	+	NC	−	A, P, IB, IV	
C. hemolyticum	−	ST	+	+	−	A	A	−	−	A	−	V	V	−	−	V	−	+	D	V	A, B	Pathogenic for guinea pig
C. malenominatum	−	T	+	−	−	−	−	−	−	−	−	−	−	−	−	+	−	−	NC	−	A, B	
C. perenne	−	T	−	+	−	A	A	A	A	A	A	−	−	−	V	−	A	−	C	−	A, P, B	
C. pseudotetanicum	−	T	−	−	−	A	−	A	−	A	A	−	V	−	V	V	V	V	CG	−	A, P, (IB), (IV)	
C. scatologenes	−	T	+	−	−	A	−	−	−	−	A	−	−	−	−	+	−	+	(C)	−	A, P, B	

*From Dowell, V. R., Jr., and Hawkins, T. M.: Laboratory methods in anaerobic bacteriology: CDC laboratory manual, DHEW Publ. No. (CDC)78-8272, Atlanta, 1977, Center for Disease Control.

+, Positive reaction for 90-100% of strains; −, negative reaction for 90-100% of strains; superscript indicates reaction shown in 11-25% of strains; V, variable reaction; ( ), variable; A, acid reaction (yellow color with bromthymol blue indicator, pH less than 6.0); C, coagulated; D, digested; G, gas; NC, no coagulation; ST, subterminal; T, terminal.

†GLC, gas-liquid chromatography; A, acetic acid; P, propionic acid; IB, isobutyric acid; B, butyric acid; IV, isovaleric acid; V, valeric acid; IC, isocaproic acid; L, lactic acid; S, succinic acid.

‡C. cadaveris was formerly listed as C. capitovale. C. limosum includes organisms formerly listed as C. capitovale. C. limosum includes organisms formerly identified as Clostridium species CDC Group P-1, and C. ramosum includes organisms previously listed as Catenabacterium filamentosum and Bacteroides terebrans.

§Toxin neutralization test is required for species identification.

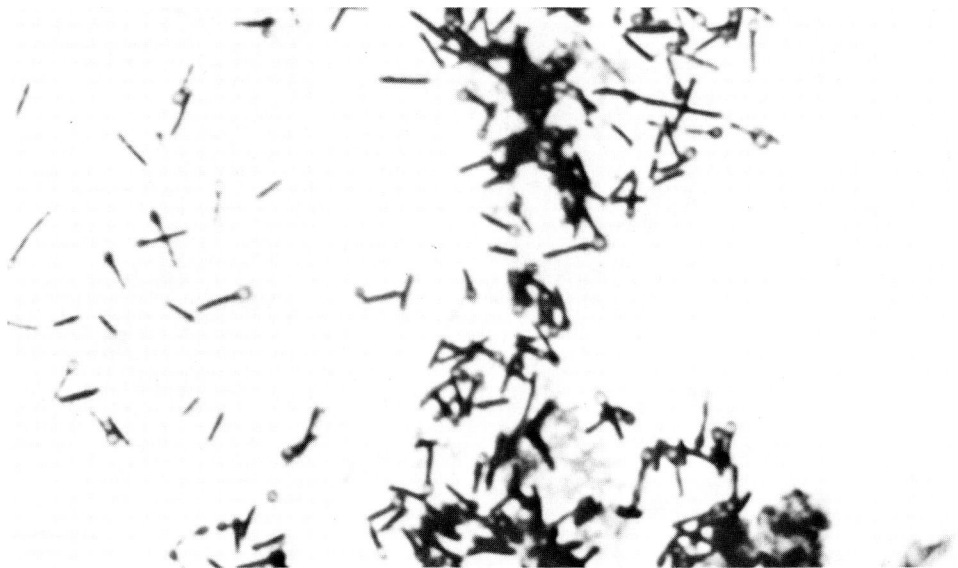

Fig. 84-2. *Clostridium tetani.* Gram-stained preparation of 24 h chopped meat–glucose medium culture. (approx. ×1500.) (From Center for Disease Control Archives.)

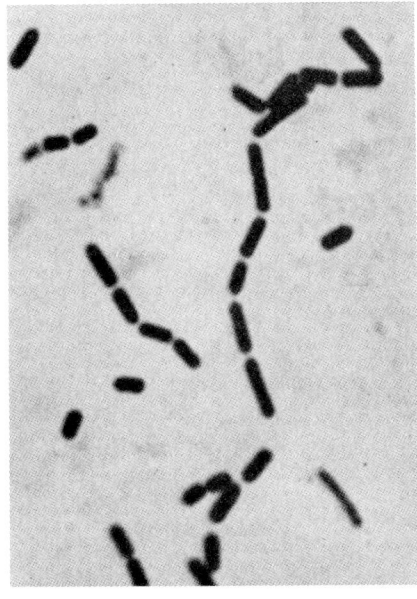

Fig. 84-3. Typical 18 h culture of *Clostridium perfringens*, demonstrating uniform cell size and a tendency to form short chains. (Photomicrograph from slide of Dr. T. F. Wetzler.)

and ferments glucose, maltose, sucrose, and lactose.

As mentioned earlier, spore formation by *C. perfringens* is seldom in evidence on common laboratory media, especially in the presence of fermentable carbohydrate. The organism is non-motile; motility testing should not be performed on hanging drop preparations. Not all strains produce stormy fermentation in milk. The organism is not strictly anaerobic and it grows

rapidly; surface growth can be detected after 4-6 hours' incubation. Most strains of *C. perfringens* produce a **double zone of hemolysis when grown on blood plates.** The inner, narrow zone is usually complete (β-hemolysis), but the outer, wider zone shows incomplete hemolysis.

On egg yolk agar *C. perfringens* produces lecithinase (diffuse opalescence) inhibited by antitoxin; no pearly iridescence is produced. In milk medium rapid fermentation of lactose occurs, with a "stormy clot" reaction. All types ferment sucrose, lactose, maltose, and glucose and produce gelatinase. H_2S is produced but not indole.

A large number of exotoxins are produced (see Willis[2] and Smith[6]). The type to which a particular *C. perfringens* belongs depends on the type and amounts of toxins it produces: type A strains produce mostly α-toxin, type B strains β- and ϵ-toxins, etc.

The α-toxin is lethal, necrotizing, hemolytic, and has lecithinase C activity (the basis for the **Nagler reaction** described above—inhibition of the lecithinase by α-antitoxin).

Some strains of *C. perfringens* produce an enterotoxin that is responsible for *C. perfringens* food poisoning in humans (described above).

C. perfringens is sensitive to penicillin; the cephalosporins are alternatives to it for penicillin-allergic patients. Chloramphenicol and clindamycin are also effective, but not tetracyclines.[68]

Clostridium novyi

The organism *C. novyi* is found in the soil. The rods are large (5-10 × 1 μm) with oval, subterminal spores. It is a strict anaerobe. *C. novyi* is divided into types A-D. There is some spreading of colonies of types A and B.

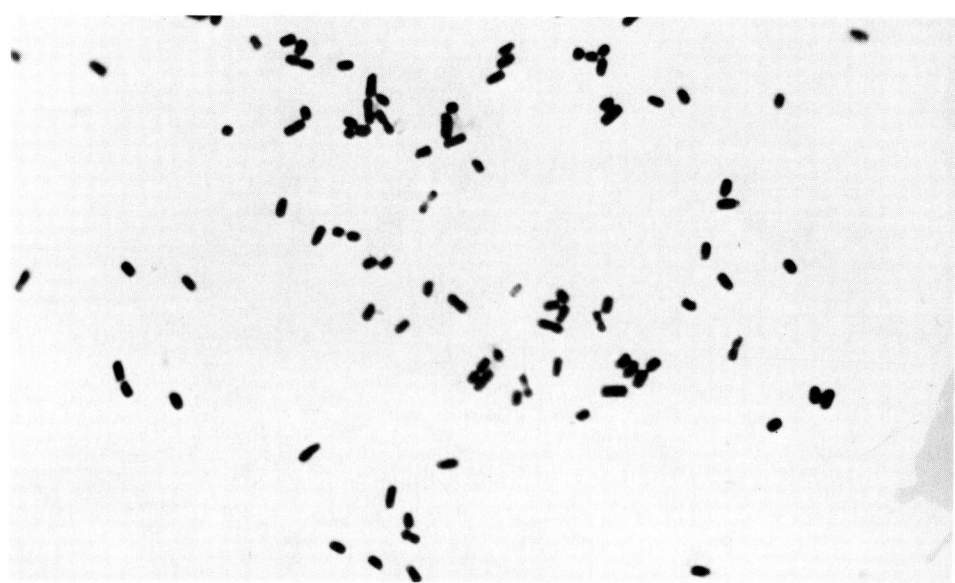

Fig. 84-4. *Clostridium perfringens.* Cells from early log phase culture in chopped meat–glucose medium. (×1200.) (From Center for Disease Control Archives.)

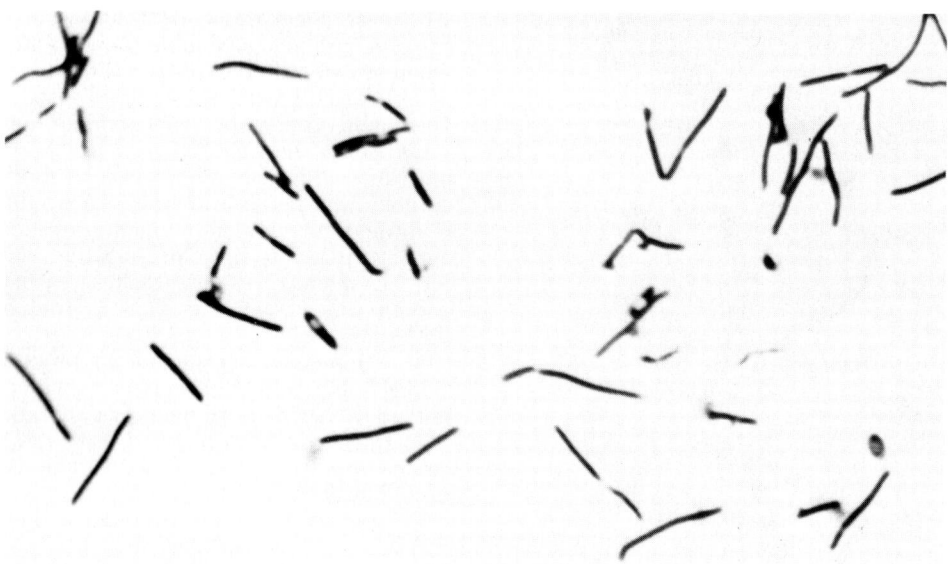

Fig. 84-5. *Clostridium septicum.* Gram-stained preparations of cells from 48 h spreading colonies on CDC anaerobe blood agar. (approx. ×1500.) (From Center for Disease Control Archives.)

Types A-C ferment glucose and maltose; D ferments glucose only. Type A and type B are involved in human gas gangrene. *C. novyi* is relatively difficult to grow, since it is exceedingly sensitive to free oxygen.

Clostridium septicum

The organism *C. septicum* is pathogenic for humans and animals; it is found chiefly in soil. Colonies of *C. septicum* often swarm over the surface of the medium (similar to *C. tetani*) (Fig. 84-5).

C. septicum ferments glucose, maltose, and lactose and produces H_2S but not indole.

Clostridium ramosum

Isolated relatively frequently from a variety of infections, *C. ramosum* is resistant to a number of antimicrobial agents. Several strains are resistant to clindamycin and tetracycline.

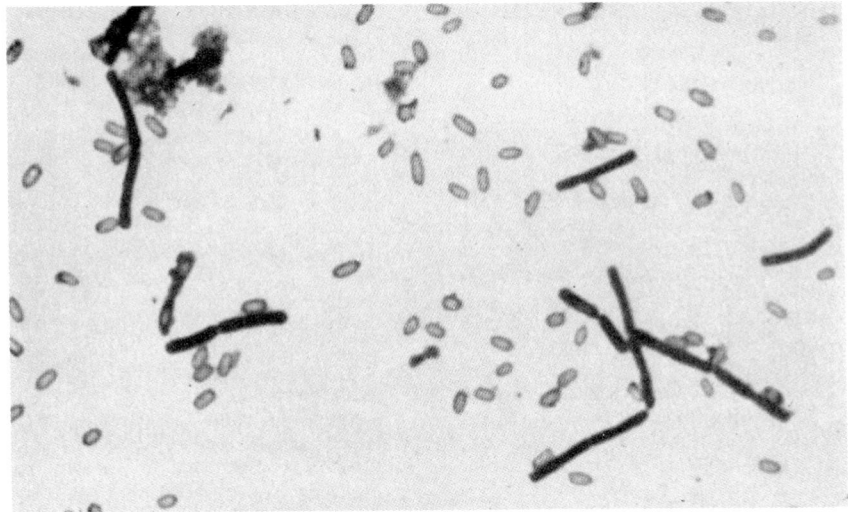

Fig. 84-6. A 48 h culture of sporulating anaerobe *Clostridium bifermentans*. Note relative abundance of extracellular spores. (Photomicrograph from slide of Dr. T. F. Wetzler.)

Table 84-10. Characteristics of commonly encountered *Clostridium* species particularly useful for identification*

Characteristic	Species
Aerotolerant	C. histolyticum, C. tertium
Nonmotile	C. innocuum, C. perfringens, C. ramosum
Terminal spores	C. cadaveris, C. innocuum, C. paraputrificum, C. tertium, C. tetani
Produce lecithinase on egg yolk agar	C. bifermentans, C. limosum, C. novyi, C. perfringens, C. sordellii, C. subterminale
Produce lipase on egg yolk agar	C. botulinum, C. novyi type A, C. sporogenes
Asaccharolytic	C. histolyticum, C. limosum, C. subterminale, C. tetani
Urease positive	C. sordellii
Nonproteolytic (do not hydrolyze gelatin)	C. butyricum, C. innocuum, C. paraputrificum, C. ramosum, C. tertium
Toxic for mice	C. botulinum, C. chauvoei, C. histolyticum, C. novyi type A, C. perfringens,† C. septicum, C. tetani

*From Dowell, V. R., Jr., and Hawkins, T. M.: Laboratory methods in anaerobic bacteriology: CDC laboratory manual, DHEW Publ. No. (CDC)78-8272, Atlanta, 1977, Center for Disease Control.

†The majority of the *C. perfringens* isolates from human sources tested at CDC were nontoxic for mice when tested as described in the section on "Detection of Clostridial Toxins, Toxin Neutralization Tests, and Pathogenicity Tests."

The organism is often much branched, but it also appears in short chains.

Infrequently isolated pathogenic clostridia

Smith[6] lists *C. carnis*, *C. fallax*, *C. colinum*, and *C. limosum* as organisms that seem to be pathogenic but are seldom found in clinical material.

Commonly isolated nonpathogenic clostridia

A large variety of clostridia with no pathogenic propensities are found in soil and in clinical specimens. Among the former (soil) the commonest species are *C. subterminale* and nonpathogenic strains of *C. sordellii*, *C. sporogenes*, *C. mangenoti*, and *C. indolis*. Those most common in clinical specimens are *C. bifermentans* (Fig. 84-6), *C. cadaveris (capitovale)*, *C. innocuum*, *C. subterminale (hastiforme)*.[6]

• • •

Characteristics of commonly encountered clostridia that are useful for identification are shown in Table 84-10.

For a discussion of *C. difficile* and its role in antimicrobial agent–induced pseudomembranous colitis, see "Pseudomembranous colitis," above.

REFERENCES

1. Smith, L. D. S.: Botulism: the organism, its toxins, the disease, Springfield, Ill., 1977, Charles C Thomas, Publisher.
2. Willis, T. A.: Anaerobic bacteriology, ed. 3, London, 1977, Butterworths.
3. Holdeman, L. V., Cato, E. P., and Moore, W. E. C.: Anaerobe laboratory manual, ed. 4, Blacksburg, Va., 1977, Anaerobe Laboratory, Virginia Polytechnic Institute and State University.
4. Nakamura, S., Shimamura, T., Hayashi, H., and Nishida, S.: J. Med. Microbiol. **8**:299, 1975.

5. Cummins, C. S., and Johnson, J. L.: J. Gen. Microbiol. **67**:33, 1971.
6. Smith, L. D. S.: The pathogenic anaerobic bacteria, ed. 2, Springfield, Ill., 1975, Charles C Thomas, Publisher.
7. Buchanan, R. E., and Gibbons, N. E.: Bergey's manual of determinative bacteriology, ed. 18, Baltimore, 1974, The Williams & Wilkins Co.
8. Sutter, V. L., Vargo, V. L., and Finegold, S. M.: Wadsworth anaerobic bacteriology manual, ed. 2, Los Angeles, 1975, Department of Continuing Education in Health Sciences University Extension, and the School of Medicine, UCLA.
8a. Sutter, V. L., Citron, D. M., and Finegold, S. M.: Wadsworth anaerobic bacteriology manual, ed. 3, St. Louis, 1980, The C. V. Mosby Co.
9. Smith, L. D. S., and Dowell, V. R.: Clostridium. In Lennette, E. H., Spaulding, E. H., and Truant, J. P., editors: Manual of clinical microbiology, ed. 2, Washington, D.C., 1974, American Society for Microbiology.
10. Dowell, V. R., Jr., and Hawkins, T. M.: Laboratory methods in anaerobic bacteriology: CDC laboratory manual, DHEW Publ. No. (CDC)78-8272, Atlanta, 1977, Center for Disease Control.
11. Willis, A. T.: Clostridia of wound infection, London, 1969, Butterworths.
12. Finegold, S. M.: Anaerobic bacteria in human disease, New York, 1977, Academic Press.
13. Gorbach, S. L., and Thadepalli, H.: J. Infect. Dis. **131**:S81-S85, 1975.
14. MacLennan, J. D.: Bacteriol. Rev. **26**:177, 1962.
15. Bartlett, J. G., Onderdonk, A. B., Cisneros, R. L., and Kasper, D. L.: J. Infect. Dis. **136**:701-705, 1977.
16. George, W. L., Sutter, V. L., and Finegold, S. M.: J. Infect. Dis. **136**:822-828, 1977.
17. Johnston, R., Harmon, S., and Kautter, D.: J. Bacteriol. **88**:1521, 1964.
18. Meyer, R. D., and Finegold, S. M.: South. Med. J. **69**:1178, 1976.
19. Center for Disease Control: Botulism in the United States, 1899-1977. Handbook for epidemiologists, clinicians, and laboratory workers (Gunn, R. A., coordinating editor), Atlanta, 1979, Center for Disease Control.
20. Gangarosa, E. J., Donadio, J. A., Armstrong, R. W., et al.: Am. J. Epidemiol. **93**:93-101, 1971.
21. Merson, M. H., Hughes, J. M., Dowell, V. R., et al.: J.A.M.A. **229**:1305-1308, 1974.
22. Wapen, B. D., and Gutmann, L.: J.A.M.A. **227**:1416-1417, 1974.
23. Cherrington, M.: Treatment of botulism and wound botulism. In Balows, A., DeHaan, R. M., Dowell, V. R., Jr., and Guze, L. B., editors: Anaerobic bacteria: role in disease, Springfield, Ill., 1974, Charles C Thomas, Publisher, pp. 287-294.
24. Lewis, K. H., and Cassel, K., Jr., editors: Botulism. Proceedings of a symposium, Public Health Service Publ. No. 999-FP-1, Cincinnati, 1964.
25. Gimenez, D. F., and Ciccarelli, A. S.: Zld. Bakt. J. Abt. Orig. **215**:221-224, 1970.
26. Koenig, M. G., Spickard, A., Cardella, M. A., and Rogers, D. E.: Medicine **43**:517-545, 1964.
27. Duff, J. T., Wright, G. G., and Yarinsky, A.: J. Bacteriol. **72**:455-460, 1956.
28. Eklund, M. W., Seiler, D. I., and Poysky, F. T.: J. Bacteriol. **93**:1461-1462, 1967.
29. Brown, L.: J. Pediatr. **94**:337, 1979.
30. Arnon, S. S., Midura, T. F., and Clay, S. A.: J.A.M.A. **237**:1946, 1977.
31. Center for Disease Control: Morbid. Mortal. **27**:249, 1978.
32. Arnon, S. S., Midura, T. F., Damus, K., et al.: J. Pediatr. **94**:331, 1979.
33. Nelson, K.E.: J.A.M.A. **241**:504, 1979.
34. Dowell, V. R.: Hosp. Practice **13**:67, 1978
35. Gunn, R. A., Dowell, V. R., Jr., and Hatheway, C. L.: Infant botulism: clinical and laboratory aspects, Atlanta, Jan. 1978, Center for Disease Control. Bureau of Laboratories, Identical memorandum, Feb. 23, 1978.
36. Dowell, V. R., Jr., McCroskey, L. M., Hatheway, C. L., et al.: J.A.M.A. **238**:1829-1832, 1977.
37. Macrae, J.: Br. Med. J. **1**:730, 1973.
38. Weinstein, L.: N. Engl. J. Med. **289**:1293, 1973.
39. Wessler, S., and Avioli, L. A.: J.A.M.A. **207**:123, 1969.
40. Christensen, N. A. In Eckman, L., editor: Principles on tetanus: Proceedings of the International Conference on Tetanus, Berne, Switzerland, 1967, Hans Huber Publisher.
41. Foodborne outbreaks: annual summary 1970, Atlanta, 1972, Center for Disease Control.
42. Anon.: Lancet **2**:1114, 1977.
43. Nakamura, M., and Schulze, J. A.: Ann. Rev. Microbiol. **24**:359, 1970.
44. Angelotti, R., Hall, H. E., Foter, M. J., and Lewis, K. H.: Appl. Microbiol. **10**:193, 1962.
45. Weinstein, L., and Barza, M. A.: N. Engl. J. Med. **289**:1129, 1973.
46. Caplan, E. S., and Kluge, R. M.: Arch. Intern. Med. **136**:788, 1976.
47. Alpern, R., and Dowell, V. R., Jr.: J.A.M.A. **209**:385, 1969.
48. Koransky, J. R., Stargel, M. D., and Dowell, V. R.: Am. J. Med. **66**:63, 1979.
49. Gorbach, S. L., and Bartlett, J. G.: N. Engl. J. Med. **290**:1289, 1974.
50. Bartlett, J. G., Chang, T. W., Gorbach, S. L., and Ouderdonk, A. B.: N. Engl. J. Med. **298**:531, 1978.
51. Bartlett, J. G.: Rev. Infect. Dis. **1**:530, 1979.
52. Larson, H. E., Parry, J. V., Price, A. B., et al.: Br. Med. J. **1**:1246-1248, 1977.
53. Chang, T. W., Bartlett, J. G., Gorbach, S. L., and Onderdonk, A. B.: Infect. Immunol. **20**:526-529, 1978.
54. Rifkin, G. D., Fekety, F. R., Silva, J., Jr., and Sack, R. B.: Lancet **2**:1103-1106, 1977.
55. Bartlett, J. G., Moon, N., Chang, T. W., et al.: Gastroenterology **75**:778-783, 1978.
55a. Koransky, J. R., Allen, S. D., and Dowell, V. R., Jr.: Appl. Environ. Microbiol. **35**:762, 1978.
56. George, W. L., Sutter, V. L., Citron, D., and Finegold, S. M.: J. Clin. Microbiol. **9**:214, 1979.
57. Sterne, M., and van Heyningen, W. E.: The clostridia. In Dubos, R. J., editor: Bacterial and mycotic infections of man, ed. 3, Philadelphia, 1958, J. B. Lippincott Co.
58. MacLennan, J. D., McClung, L. S., and Smith, L. D. S. In Harris, A. H., and Coleman, M. B., editors: Diagnostic procedures and reagents, New York, 1963, American Public Health Association.
59. Willis, A. T., and Hobbs, G.: J. Pathol. Bacteriol. **75**:299, 1958.
60. Willis, A. T., and Hobbs, G.: J. Pathol. Bacteriol. **77**:511, 1959.
61. Jones, G., and Dowell, V. R.: Anaerobic bacteriology in the clinical laboratory, Atlanta, 1976, Laboratory Training and Consultation Division, Center for Disease Control.
62. Wolf, J., and Barker, A. N. In Gibbs, B. M., and Shapton, D. A., editors: Identification methods for microbiologists. Part B, New York, 1968, Academic Press.

63. Batty, I., and Walker, P. D.: J. Pathol. Bacteriol. **88:**327, 1964.
64. Batty, I., and Walker, P. D.: J. Pathol. Bacteriol. **85:**517, 1963.
65. Batty, I., and Walker, P. D. In Gibbs, B. M., and Skinner, F. A., editors: Identification methods for microbiologists, New York, 1966, Academic Press.
66. Wessler, S., and Avioli, L. A., editors: J.A.M.A. **207:**123, 1969.
67. Gangarosa, E. J.: J. Infect. Dis. **119:**308, 1969.
68. Schwartzman, J. D., Reller, L. B., and Wang, W. L.: Antimicrob. Agents Chemother. **11:**695, 1977.

85

GRAM-POSITIVE, ANAEROBIC, NON-SPOREFORMING BACILLI

V. R. Dowell, Jr.
Alex C. Sonnenwirth

Gram-positive, non-sporeforming, anaerobic bacilli occurring in clinical specimens include members of the following genera: *Actinomyces, Arachnia, Propionibacterium, Bifidobacterium, Lactobacillus,* and *Eubacterium.*[1,2]

Some of these organisms are capnophiles (microaerophilic) or facultative anaerobes; however, most are obligate anaerobes. Practically all are members of the normal flora of humans, either of the mucous membranes or of the skin.

As shown in Table 85-1, there have been a variety of changes in the nomenclature and taxonomy of this group.[3,4] The genus names *Catenabacterium, Cillobacterium,* and *Ramibacterium* are no longer recognized, and species formerly classified as *Corynebacterium* are now included in the genera *Eubacterium* or *Propionibacterium.* The organism earlier listed as *Actinomyces propionicus* is now listed as *Arachnia propionica* in *Bergey's Manual,* ed. 8.[5]

The morphology of these organisms is usually variable and depends often on growth conditions and culture medium. Some show (1) small rods (*A. naeslundii, A. odontolyticus, A. viscosus, B. eriksonii, P. acnes*); (2) large, plump, evenly stained rods (*E. limosum*); (3) club-shaped rods (*A. israelii, B. eriksonii,* other *Actinomyces, E. limosum, Propionibacterium*); (4) rods with bifid (bifurcated) ends (*A. naeslundii, A. odontolyticus, B. eriksonii, E. limosum*); (5) thin filaments, with or without branching (*A. israelii, A. naeslundii, E. alactolyticum, E. lentum*); and (6) "Chinese-letter" configurations (*E. alactolyticum, P. acnes, P. granulosum*). **Branching** is common in *A. israelii* and *A. propionica.*[3]

Because some of these organisms tend to lose their affinity for crystal violet when Gram-stained, they may be misidentified as a (gram-

negative) *Bacteroides* or *Fusobacterium* species. Also it is necessary to search carefully for spores to avoid missing a clostridial species. (*C. ramosum* and *C. perfringens* fail to form spores in ordinary media.)

Culture on egg yolk agar is helpful in differentiating these organisms from clostridia: any lecithinase-producing organism is **not** a non-sporeforming anaerobic bacillus (since none of the latter produce lecithinase).

The definitive identification of this group requires the use of gas-liquid chromatography[2-4] (see Chapter 74) with some exceptions: *P. acnes* and *P. viscosus,* both **catalase positive,** can be recognized without GLC.

Differentiation of gram-positive, anaerobic, non-sporeforming rods to the genus level is shown in Table 85-2. Production of propionic

Table 85-1. Changes in the nomenclature of gram-positive, anaerobic, non-sporeforming bacilli[2]

Present designation	Former designation(s)
Arachnia propionica	*Actinomyces propionicus*
Bifidobacterium eriksonii	*Actinomyces eriksonii*
Eubacterium alactolyticum	*Ramibacterium alactolyticum, Ramibacterium pleuriticum*
Eubacterium lentum	*Corynebacterium diphtheroides, Bifidobacterium cornutum, Corynebacterium group 3*
Lactobacillus catenaforme	*Catenabacterium catenaforme*
Propionibacterium acnes	*Corynebacterium acnes*
Propionibacterium freudenreichii ssp *freudenreichii*	*Propionibacterium freudenreichii*
Propionibacterium freudenreichii ssp *shermanii*	*Propionibacterium shermanii*
Propionibacterium granulosum	*Corynebacterium granulosum*

acid or lack thereof (as determined with GLC) is the major dividing characteristic between *Propionibacterium* and *Arachnia* (propionic acid producers) and the other genera (no production of propionic acid or of catalase).

Clinical significance

Disease involving gram-positive, non-sporeforming, anaerobic bacilli is not as common as that caused by *Bacteroides fragilis* or *Clostridium perfringens*. However, these organisms can cause a variety of human illnesses, either alone or in united infections with other bacteria.[6]

The infections involving these organisms are **endogenous infections**; they involve organisms from the oral cavity, gastrointestinal tract, genitourinary tract, or skin.[6-11]

The infections include actinomycosis, brain abscess, endocarditis, liver abscess, lung abscess, osteomyelitis, peridontal disease, and infections following human or animal bites.[12-16]

Predisposing factors include surgical procedures, dental surgery, tooth extraction, debilitating diseases such as alcoholism, carcinoma, diabetes, or leukemia, aspiration of material from mouth into lungs, and treatment with corticosteroid or immunosuppressant drugs.

Isolation from a single specimen of one of the gram-positive, non-sporeforming, anaerobic bacilli does not necessarily mean that the organism is an etiologic agent of the patient's illness—*Propionibacterium* organisms isolated from bone marrow, blood culture, or spinal fluid always pose a problem. Often *P. acnes* is a contaminant; however, when isolated from properly collected specimens, it may be clinically significant.[14,17,18]

Presumptive identification

Commonly encountered anaerobic, gram-positive, non-sporeforming bacilli can be presumptively identified with aid of a number of characteristics (oxygen tolerance, rate of growth, branding, catalase, indole, esculin, and the antibiotic disk characterization of Sutter et al.[19] [see Chapter 82]), as shown in Table 85-3.

In addition to the characteristics shown in Table 85-3, it should be noted that *A. odontolyticus* develops a pink pigment after incubation at room temperature for 3-4 days, while *A. naeslundii* develops a tan pigment after prolonged incubation.

P. acnes can be identified readily when it is both catalase and indole positive. Indole-negative, catalase-positive bacilli may be *P. acnes*, *A. viscosus*, and other *Actinomyces* species, or *E. lentum*.[19]

For indole determination use the indole spot test (see Chapter 72). Perform the test only on a pure culture plate, since indole can diffuse from an indole-positive colony to an indole-

Table 85-2. Differentiation of gram-positive non-sporeforming anaerobes to the genus level [2]

Rods	
Produce propionic acid	
Catalase usually produced	*Propionibacterium*
Catalase not produced	*Arachnia*
Propionic acid and catalase not produced	
Ratio of lactic to acetic acid produced greater than 1:1	
Lactic acid only major product	*Lactobacillus*
Succinic acid is a major product	*Actinomyces* *
Ratio of lactic to acetic acid produced less than 1:1	
Produce butyric acid plus other acids or no major acids	*Eubacterium* and *Lachnospira*
Butyric acid not produced	*Bifidobacterium*

*A. viscosus is catalase positive. However, this organism is a facultative anaerobe.

Table 85-3. Presumptive identification of commonly encountered anaerobic, gram-positive, non-sporeforming bacilli*

Species	Oxygen tolerance	True branching	Rapidity of growth	Catalase	Esculin	Indole	Vancomycin disks (5 µg)[11]	Colistin disk (10 µg)[11]	Kanamycin disk (1000 µg)
A. israelii	A, M	+	Sl	−	+	−	S	R	S
A. odontolyticus †	A, M	+	Mo	−	V	−	S	R	S
A. naeslundii	M, F	+	Mo	−	+	−	S	R	S
Ar. propionica	A, M	+	Sl	−	+	−			
B. eriksonii	A	−	Ra	−	+	−	S	R	S[R]
E. alactolyticum	A	−	Sl	−	−	−	S	R	V
E. lentum	A	−	Mo	−	−	−	S	R	V
E. limosum	A	−	Ra	−	+	−	S	R	V
P. acnes	A, M	−	Sl	+	−	+	S	R	S

*Data from Dowell and Hawkins[2]; Sutter, Citron, and Finegold[19]; and Jones and Dowell.[20] A, anaerobic; M, microaerophilic; F, facultative; +, positive reaction; −, negative reaction; V, variable reaction; Sl, slow; Mo, moderate; Ra, rapid; S, sensitive; R, resistant (10 mm or less).
†Colonies become red after 4-5 d incubation at room temperature.

Table 85-4. Characteristics of some anaerobic, non-sporeforming gram-positive bacilli*

Species	Motility	Glucose	Mannitol	Lactose	Sucrose	Maltose	Salicin	Glycerol	Xylose	Arabinose	Erythritol	Inositol	Lactose	Raffinose	Ribose	Sorbitol	Trehalose	Esculin hydrolysis	Gelatin hydrolysis	Nitrate reduction	Indole	Milk†	Catalase	Organic acids detected by GLC‡
A. israelii	−	A	V	A^-	A^-	A^-	V	−	A^-	V	−	V	+	+	+	−	+	$+^-$	−	−	−	(C)	−	A,F,L,S
A. naeslundii	−	A	V	A^-	A^-	A^-	V	V	−	A^-	−	V	+	+	V	−	+	+	−	+	−	(C)	−	A,F,L,S
A. odontolyticus	−	A	−	A^-	A^-	A^-	A^-	A^-	V	V	−	−	+	−	+	−	−	V	−	+	−	(C)	−	A,F,S
A. propionica	−	A	A^-	A	A	A	A^-	A^-	A	A	−	−	V	V	+	−	+	$+^-$	$-^+$	+	−	(C)	−	A,P(L),S
B. eriksonii	−	A	V	A	A	A	A	−	−	−	−	−	+	+	−	−	+	$+^-$	−	−	−	(CG)	+	A,L,P(F)
E. alactolyticum	−	A	A^-	−	−	−	−	−	−	−	−	−	−	−	−	−	−	−	−	−	−	NC	−	A,B,H(CF)
E. lentum	−	−	−	−	−	−	−	−	−	−	−	−	−	−	+	−	−	V	−	V	−	NC	−	(A,L,S,F)
E. limosum	−	A	A^-	−	−	−	−	−	−	−	−	−	−	−	−	−	−	−	−	−	−	NC	−	A,B,L(S)
P. acnes	−	A	V	−	−	−	−	A	−	+	+	−	−	−	−	−	−	−	$+^-$	+	$+^-$	C(G)	+	A,P,(IVFLS)

*Data from Dowell and Hawkins,[2] and Sutter et al.[19] +, positive reaction for 90-100% of strains; −, negative reaction for 90-100% of strains; a superscript indicates reaction shown in 11-25% of strains; V, variable reaction; A, acid reaction (yellow color with bromthymol blue indicator, pH less than 6.0).

†C, coagulated; CG, coagulated, gas; NC, no coagulation; (), sometimes detected.

‡A, acetic; P, propionic; B, butyric; IV, isovaleric; H, hexanoic; C, caprylic; F, formic; L, lactic; S, succinic; (), sometimes detected.

negative colony and result in a false-positive reaction.[19, 19a]

Definitive identification

As noted earlier, gas-liquid chromatography and a number of biochemical tests are needed for definitive identification. Those laboratories not equipped to do definitive tests should be capable of maintaining and isolating an anaerobe in pure culture so that it can be sent to a reference laboratory if necessary.

Some definitive characteristics including organic acids detected by GLC are shown in Table 85-4.

Direct examination

Actinomycosis is a chronic disease characterized by the formation of draining sinuses and the presence of so-called "sulfur granules" that are made up of filamentous, branching microorganisms. The granules are white or yellowish grains up to 5 mm in diameter and are usually rather firm. All exudates, sputum, and pleural fluid should be inspected for the presence of granules. Examine gauze dressings that have been in contact with purulent material from draining lesions for granules in the gauze fibers. However, granules are not always present in actinomycosis. (For handling of granules, see discussion on *Actinomyces.*) Gram stains of all specimens should be performed.

Culture

Similar to all other anaerobic cultures, clinical specimens (except blood) should be inoculated at least to the following: (1) thioglycollate medium, enriched; (2) chopped meat, glucose medium; and (3) 2 plates of anaerobic blood-agar plates or one LKV and PEA (phenethyl-alcohol) blood-agar plate.

One plate of blood agar, LKV, and PEA medium should be incubated anaerobically at 35-37 C for a minimum of 2 but preferably for 5 days; other plates should be incubated in candle jar or CO_2 incubator.

Before inoculation, heat liquid media for 10 minutes in a boiling water bath and cool, unless prereduced anaerobically sterilized medium (PRAS) is used.

When actinomycosis is strongly suspected, inoculate 2 sets of primary isolation media (include one brain-heart infusion agar (BHIA) plate in each set) and incubate them in separate anaerobic jars. Handle one set as ordinary anaerobic culture and incubate second set for 5-7 days **before** inspection. Hold liquid cultures (with screwcaps loosened) in anaerobic jar for 2 weeks to detect slow-growing organisms (*A. israelii,* etc.)

Isolation and identification

To determine some of the key characteristics shown in Tables 85-2 and 85-3, inoculate 3 BHIA slants, 1 tube of enriched thioglycollate, and 1 tube of peptone-yeast extract-glucose (PYG) broth. Incubate one BHIA slant in air, one in CO_2, and all others anaerobically, for 24-48 hours. Perform catalase test on (anaerobic) BHIA slant and check pH of PYG broth (for glucose fermentation). For definitive identification, refer to Table 85-4 and to Holdeman et al.,[21] Smith,[22] Willis,[23] and Sutter et al.[19]

ACTINOMYCES

The organisms are anaerobic or microaerophilic, catalase-negative, nonmotile, non-acid-fast, gram-positive rods and filaments; no spores are formed.

The filamentous growth leads to mycelial colonies, and some actinomycetes cause chronic subcutaneous granulomatous abscesses.

For these reasons the actinomycetes were regarded as fungi for many years. As discussed in Chapter 77 (Aerobic actinomycetes), consideration of the fundamental biologic properties of these organisms leaves little doubt about classification of the actinomycetes as bacteria.

1. They lack a nuclear membrane (they are prokaryotic).

2. They are all of bacterial size; their filaments readily segment into bacillary and twig-like forms, with typical dimensions of bacteria.

3. They are all sensitive to antibacterial antibiotics but are resistant to antifungal antibiotics (griseofulvin, nystatin, amphotericin B, and candicidin).

4. Their cell walls contain muramic acid and diaminopimelic acid (lysine in some species), which are characteristic of bacterial walls; they lack chitin and glucans, characteristic of molds and yeasts.

A. israelii, A. naeslundii, A. propionica, A. viscosus, and *A. odontolyticus* are found in the normal mouth, pharynx, various clinical materials, and lesions of actinomycosis. They appear to be strict parasites of humans and of some animal species. *A. israelii* (mostly rough forms) is usually isolated from human lesions or normal human tissues. *A. bovis* (mostly smooth forms) is usually isolated from bovine sources.

Slack et al.[24] established 4 serologic groups of *Actinomyces* by means of fluorescent antibodies. The organisms include isolates from healthy humans and from patients and animals with actinomycosis. There was no correlation between source of the isolate and the serologic group, nor could they distinguish the various "species" by serologic grouping. In extension of the above work, Slack and Gerencser revised the serologic grouping of *Actinomyces.*[25] By means of fluorescent antibody technics, they proposed the establishment of 4 groups: group A, *A. naeslundii;* group B, *A. bovis;* group C, *A. eriksonii;* and group D, *A. israelii.* Since then Brock and Georg[26] showed that at least 2 serotypes of *A. israelii* exist and can be differentiated by FA technics.

For further details, taxonomic relationships, and methodology the reader is referred to Georg,[10,27] Brock et al.,[12] Coleman et al.,[28] Holdeman et al.,[21] and Ajello et al.[29]

Fluorescent antibody (FA) methods

FA methods are eminently suitable for the detection and identification of *Actinomyces* in clinical material as well as in culture. Fluorescent-antibody conjugates have been used for specific staining of *A. israelii* (serotypes 1 and 2), *A. naeslundii, A. odontolyticus, A. viscosus, A. propionica* (serotypes 1 and 2), *P. acnes* (serotypes 1 and 2), *P. avidum, P. granulosum,* and *P. jensenii* in direct smears of clinical materials and in cultures.[6,8,10,12,30]

Simple methods for anaerobic cultivation and CO_2 enrichment[31]

Single tube cultures with anaerobic seals. Cultures may be grown as test tube cultures with **pyrogallol-carbonate seals,** prepared as follows:
1. Clip off cotton plug at end of tube.
2. With rotary motion, push remainder of cotton plug down into tube, leaving a space of about ½-¾ in at top of tube.
3. Insert small wad of absorbent cotton into space.
4. Add 5 drops pyrogallol solution (100 g pyrogallic acid in 150 ml water) and 5 drops 10% sodium carbonate (Na_2CO_3).
5. Plug with a rubber stopper.

After growth has been obtained, usually in 4-8 d, tubes may be placed in a freezer (at or below −20 C) for storage.

NOTE: Whenever available, use of anaerobic jars is preferred to the pyrogallol-carbonate–sealed tubes.

Single tube cultures with CO_2 seals. "Candle jar" conditions may be obtained in test tube cultures by using a seal that gives off CO_2. Prepare as in steps 1, 2, and 3. Then proceed as below:
4. Add 5 drops each Na_2CO_3 (10%) and KH_2PO_4 (1M or 136 g + 1000 ml H_2O).

Media for Actinomyces

Several improved media for the isolation, identification, and maintenance of *Actinomyces* are available.

Actinomyces broth. This is a basic medium modified from Pine and Watson.[32] It may be used as liquid maintenance broth. It is available in dehydrated form (Actinomyces Maintenance Broth) from BBL, Div. of BioQuest, Cockeysville, Md.

Potassium phosphate	15 g
Ammonium sulfate	1 g
Magnesium sulfate	0.2 g
Calcium chloride	0.01 g
Infusion broth	25 g
Dextrose	5 g
Cysteine	1 g
Trypticase	4 g
Yeast extract	5 g
Soluble starch	1 g

Suspend dry material in 1000 ml distilled water. Heat slightly to obtain solution. Dispense and autoclave at 118-121 C for 10 min.

This medium is recommended for fastidious strains, which do not grow well in thioglycollate broth.

Actinomyces, solid medium. Same as *Actinomyces*

broth, with 20 g agar added. Usable for cultivation or maintenance medium.

Actinomyces, semisolid medium. Same as *Actinomyces* broth, with 7 g agar added. Usable as semisolid maintenance medium.

Actinomyces fermentation broth.[29] (Available in dehydrated form from BBL, Division of BioQuest, Cockeysville, Md.)

Potassium phosphate	15 g
Ammonium sulfate	1 g
Magnesium sulfate	0.2 g
Calcium chloride	0.01 g
Infusion broth	25 g
Cysteine	1 g
Trypticase	4 g
Yeast extract	5 g
Bromcresol purple	0.01 g
Distilled water	1000 ml

For fermentation tests add sterile sugar solutions (glucose, xylose, mannitol, raffinose, starch, and glycerol) to give final concentration of 0.5%.

Distribute 5 ml/tube, with inverted Durham tube in place. Use cotton plugs. Autoclave at 15 psi for 15 min. Inoculate tubes of medium containing sugar with 1-3 drops sugar-free, growing culture (heart infusion broth, Difco). Seal tubes with pyrogallol-carbonate seals; incubate at 37 C for 4 wk. Read weekly for acid, gas, or both.

Phenethyl alcohol (PEA) broth.[33] Add phenethyl alcohol (Eastman Organic Chemical no. 313) to *Actinomyces* broth in a concentration of 0.25%. The medium is used as a selective isolation medium; it inhibits *Corynebacterium* species.

Thioglycollate broth, enriched (TST)[33] (BBL, Division of BioQuest, Cockeysville, Md.)

Thioglycollate broth with indicator and glucose	29.5 g
Trypticase soy broth	1.5 g
Tryptose (Difco)	1.3 g
Distilled water	1000 ml

Autoclave at 12 psi for 10 min.

The medium is used for the isolation of individual colonies picked from brain-heart infusion agar plates and also as an isolation medium.

Brain-heart infusion agar. See media, Chapter 72.

Liquid nitrate medium[29]

Heart infusion broth	25 g
Casitone (Difco)	4 g
Yeast extract	5 g
KNO$_3$	1 g
Distilled water	1000 ml

Set pH at 7.0. Dispense 8 ml/tube. Autoclave at 15 psi for 15 min.

Starch medium, Casitone[29]

Heart infusion broth	25 g
Casitone (Difco)	4 g
Yeast extract	5 g
Soluble starch	5 g
Agar	15 g
Distilled water	1000 ml

Autoclave at 15 psi for 15 min in tubes, 8 ml/tube. Slant.

Gelatin medium for Actinomyces[29]

Heart infusion broth (Difco)	25 g
Casitone (Difco)	4 g
Dextrose	5 g
Yeast extract	5 g
Gelatin	100 g
Distilled water	1000 ml

Set pH at 7.0. Autoclave at 15 psi for 15 min, 8 ml/tube.

Reinforced litmus milk[29]

Skim milk powder	100 g
Yeast extract	5 g
Dextrose	3 g
Litmus	750 μg
Distilled water	1000 ml

Set pH at 7.0. Autoclave at 10 psi for 10 min.

Shipment of cultures suspected of being Actinomyces species[31]

1. Liquid media:
   a. Inoculate culture into freshly boiled **thioglycollate broth, enriched (TST)**. Incubate at 37 C for 3-4 d. If growth is apparent at that time, seal by pouring over surface of medium about 3 ml of a sterile melted mixture of equal amounts of paraffin and petrolatum (Vaseline, paraffin jelly). A stock petrolatum-paraffin mixture may be prepared by melting together equal amounts of each. After being mixed well, it may be distributed in 3 ml amounts in plugged tubes for sterilization. These may be stored for use as needed. Seal top of tube with sterile rubber stopper or use a screw cap sealed with masking tape.
   b. If *Actinomyces* broth is used, inoculate tube of broth and incubate under **pyrogallol-carbonate seal** for 3-4 days. If growth is apparent, transfer liquid with culture to a clean sterile tube and seal with petrolatum-paraffin mixture as above.
2. Important points to remember:
   a. *Actinomyces* cultures should not be more than 3-4 days old before shipment. Send airmail if possible.
   b. If liquid or semisolid (0.35% agar) cultures are sent, they should be sealed with petrolatum-paraffin mixture before shipment.

Actinomyces israelii

A. israelii produces a subacute or chronic progressive disease, **actinomycosis,** which occurs in man, cattle, and other animals. The disease is characterized (1) by development of indurated granulating swellings, mainly in connective tissue, (2) by some suppuration, and (3) by the finding of *A. israelii* in the pus or lesions. It develops over a few weeks to a year or more and may spread widely by contiguity. It sometimes points toward the skin and forms fistulae that tend to heal and re-form elsewhere; it is rare that it points toward mucous or serous membranes. The organisms may be disseminated through the blood or in the lungs through the bronchi, with the lymphatic system only rarely involved. In humans, bone lesions are uncommon.

Actinomycosis in man can be **cervicofacial,** with lesions on cheek or submaxillary skin as indurated edematous swellings; **thoracic,** mainly in the lungs, with abscesses and cavities (pleurisy, empyema, involvement of the heart and periocardium also occur occasionally); and **abdominal,** with involvement of practically any organ but most commonly in the region of the cecum and appendix. Recently, actinomycosis associated with intrauterine contraceptive devices (IUD) has been reported.[34]

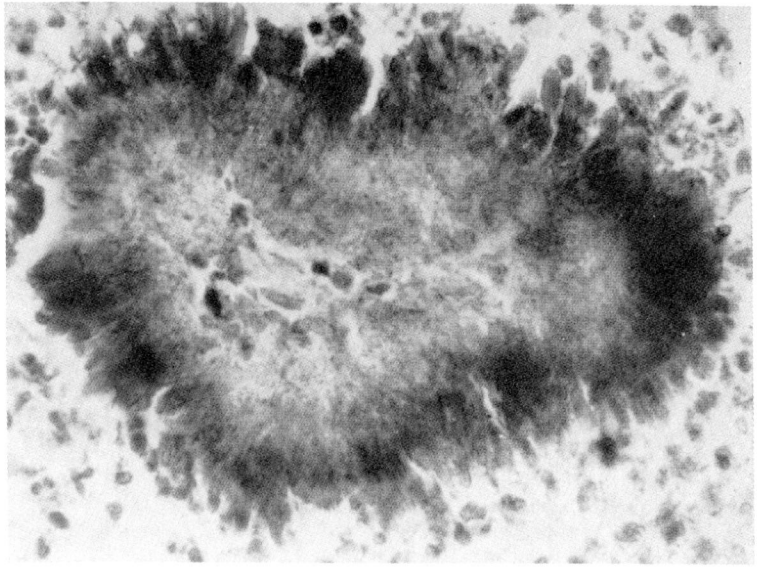

Fig. 85-1. Section of "sulfur granule" from actinomycosis. (×500.) (Courtesy Dr. W. C. Emmons.)

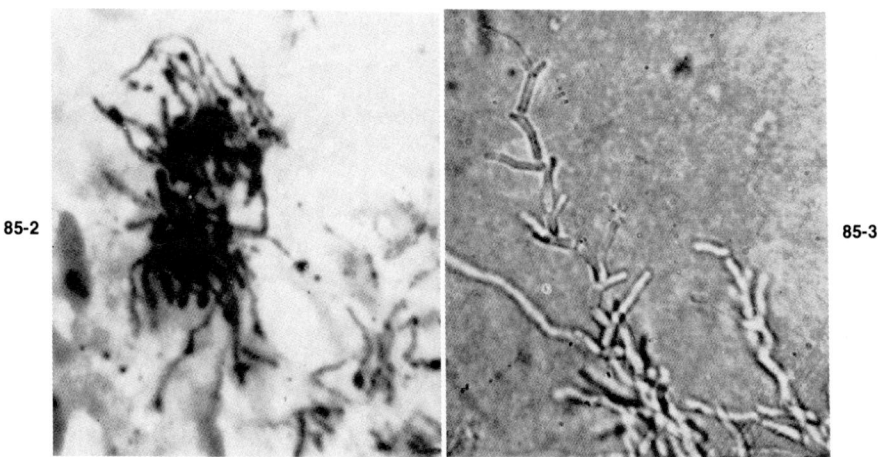

85-2

85-3

Fig. 85-2. Gram stain of *Actinomyces israelii* from crushed granule. (×900.)
Fig. 85-3. Fragile branching mycelium of *Actinomyces israelii* from young culture. (×900.) (Courtesy Dr. W. C. Emmons.)

Material from lesions often contains small gritty flecks known as "sulfur granules." Details of the typical granule are best seen under magnifications of 400 diameters or more (high-dry or oil immersion) (Figs. 85-1 to 85-3). The granule may be circular or irregular in outline or may consist of several colonies of different size and shape that have coalesced. It is composed of a dense reticulum of fibrils that stain gram positive. The ends of the individual filaments may project around the periphery, with or without radially arranged hyaline clubs. The clubs are several times larger than the filaments, the ends of which they enclose.

The finding of microscopically typical "sulfur granules" is considered presumptively diagnostic of actinomycosis in humans; however, the diagnosis cannot be considered as established unless A. *israelii* is isolated from the lesions or is detected and identified by FA procedures in clinical material.

Specimens, culture, isolation, and identification

The usual specimen submitted is pus or sputum. Pus should be examined for presence of granules; the walls of sinuses may be curetted, and the material obtained should be examined. Granules may be found on sterile gauze pads applied over the sinus opening.

Table 85-5. Morphologic characteristics of *Actinomyces israelii, A. bovis, A. naeslundii,* and *Propionibacterium**

Morphology	A. israelii	A. bovis	A. naeslunlii	Propioni-bacterium
A. Gross morphology on BHIA with anaerobic incubation at 37 C 1. Colonies examined after 48 hr under microscope (100×)	Colonies usually only seen microscopically. They appear as a loose mass of long branching filaments on agar surface ("spider" colonies). Or, appear as small whitish granules with a rough surface and a fringed "lacelike" border. Smooth surfaced pinhead-sized colonies with slightly fuzzy edges may occur in some strains—"S" forms	Colonies are usually pinhead-sized, transparent, and look like dew drops. They appear smooth, slightly convex with entire edge. Microscopically they show a smooth but granular surface with a granular or denticulate edge. Some strains are more opaque, rough surfaced and have an irregular or fuzzy border. Rare strains are microscopic in size and appear as mycelial "spider" colonies as seen in "R" A. israelii strains	Colonies similar to those of A. bovis or A. israelii "S" forms most common	Pinhead-size smooth transparent glistening colonies with smooth edge
2. Colonies examined after 7-10 d	Raised irregular to lobulated colonies with white glistening surfaces ("molar tooth" colonies). They tend to indent the agar and are easily moved as a whole. Smooth-surfaced colonies, slightly convex with smooth edges, may occur in some strains—"S" forms	Colonies smooth convex, cream to white, and shining with entire border. Some strains show conical or irregular lumpy surface and scalloped borders (may look like an inverted raspberry). Rare strains produce typical molar tooth colony seen in "R" A. israelii strains	Colonies similar to those of A. bovis or A. israelii "S" forms most common	Smooth colonies that may show granular surface and entire, slightly granular, edge
B. Growth in thioglycollate broth at 37 C	Distinct colonies, rough and lobulated or showing fuzzy edges. Colonies do not break up when tube is shaken. Broth is clear. Smooth strains may appear more diffuse	Most strains produce a soft, diffuse growth. Other strains produce large lobulated bread-crumb colonies, which are easily broken up. Flaky or mucoid growth is seen in some strains. Rare strains produce granular discrete colonies as seen in "R" A. israelii strains	Rapid growth; usually more diffuse than A. bovis. Granular or floccose colonies may be present. Broth somewhat cloudy	Rapid growth; diffuse and often pink. Tend to concentrate along side of tube. Colonies easily broken up. Broth cloudy

*From Ajello, L., Georg, L. K., Kaplan, W., and Kaufman, L.: Laboratory manual for medical mycology, Public Health Service publ. no. 994, Atlanta, 1963, Communicable Disease Center.

Table 85-5. Morphologic characteristics of *Actinomyces israelii, A. bovis, A. naeslundii,* and *Propionibacterium*—cont'd

Morphology	A. israelii	A. bovis	A. naeslundii	Propioni-bacterium
C. Microscopic morphology	Gram-positive rods and branched forms, 1 μm or less in diameter. Variations in diameter and clubbed ends are common. Long mycelial filaments occasionally seen. Nonbranching diphtheroid-like rods may be formed only by "S" forms	Gram-positive diphtheroid forms most common. Difficult to find branching. Some strains somewhat more filamentous. Rare "R" strains show long branching filaments	Similar to *A. Bovis* or *A. israelii* but more irregular forms. Gram-positive short mycelial forms with many branches. Some thick, very irregular forms, and few long mycelial elements varying in thickness throughout. Some diphtheroid-like forms	Gram-positive bacillar or slightly branched organisms, X-, or Y-shaped forms commonly occur

The granules are white or yellowish and range from very small specks to ones 2-5 mm in diameter. They are found more often in pus than in sputum. If granules are found, they should be removed with a sterile capillary pipet or loop into a sterile tube containing a small amount of sterile saline. **Examine under a coverslip; afterward crush and smear on slide; do Gram stain.** Gram-positive branched mycelium will be seen under the microscope.

The granules should be washed in several changes of sterile saline and ground before used as inoculum.

Culture granules, pus, or sputum on brain-heart infusion agar; streak 2 plates and incubate in an anaerobic jar at 37 C (always add about 5% CO_2 to N_2 or H_2 used). Streak duplicate sets of plates for incubation in air **and** under CO_2 (candle jar) at the same time. Examine plates at 48 hour; then return plates to anaerobic jar. Hold under anaerobic conditions for 7-10 days before final examination.

Fluid media are best used if specimen comes from closed, uncontaminated lesion.

Among the several liquid media for selective isolation of *Actinomyces,* the phenethyl alcohol (PEA) broth seems to be useful. Thioglycollate broth, enriched (TST), is also useful as an isolation medium.

Colonies suggestive of *Actinomyces* should be picked from streaked plates and inoculated in thioglycollate broth (or thioglycollate broth, enriched). After growth, plate out again and then pick colonies for biochemical tests.

Appearance of colonies on brain-heart infusion agar.[29] At 48 hours the rough (R) colonies, charac-

teristic of most *A. israelii* strains, can be detected only with a microscope (10× objective). They appear as delicate, branched mycelial filaments on the surface of the agar.

At 7-10 days the R colonies are heaped-up and glistening white with irregular to lobulated surfaces. They are dry and crumbly.

In liquid thioglycollate broth, the colonies grow as "bread-crumb" types, usually 1 cm or more below the surface of the broth.

Smooth colonies (S), characteristic of most *A. bovis* strains, are pinhead-size at 48 hours and usually can be seen with the naked eye. They appear flat and granular when examined with the 10× objective. Seven- to 10-day-old colonies are convex, smooth-edged, cream to white, and circular. They are soft and easily broken. Some strains show irregular or lumpy surface.

Identification

Morphologic characteristics of *Actinomyces* are described in Table 85-5. Physiologic and biochemical characteristics are given in Tables 85-3 and 85-4.

Actinomyces naeslundii

A. naeslundii[35,36] is a facultative anaerobe. The organism is nonhemolytic on blood agar; on BHIA microcolonies appear in approximately 48 hours (about 0.5 mm in diameter). The organism ferments a variety of substrates, but does not attack starch (see Tables 85-3 and 85-4).

Actinomyces odontolyticus

A. odontolyticus is a facultative anaerobe; for a detailed description, see Batty.[37]

Actinomyces viscosus

A. viscosus[38,39] is often overlooked and assumed to be a *Propionibacterium* or *Corynebacterium* species, since it is catalase positive. It hydrolyzes esculin (Table 85-4) and is indole negative.

ARACHNIA

Strains of *Arachnia propionica* and of *Actinomyces* are practically indistinguishable from one another. With gas-liquid chromatography it can be shown that *A. propionica* produces predominantly propionic acid, while *Actinomyces* species produce predominantly acetic acid but not propionic acid.

For further details, see Georg[10,27] and Brock et al.[12]

EUBACTERIUM

Species of *Eubacterium* occur in the mouth or intestinal tract of humans and animals. The organisms are obligately anaerobic.

E. lentum and E. limosum

E. lentum and E. limosum are seen with varying frequency in clinical specimens. Their pathologic significance is in doubt.[17]

E. lentum is nonsaccharolytic and nonproteolytic. It reduces nitrate but does not produce indole.

E. limosum shows some club and swollen forms. It does ferment a number of carbohydrates (Table 85-4).

PROPIONIBACTERIUM

Propionibacterium species[40] are mostly anaerobes, but some strains are microaerophilic. They show typical "diphtheroid" microscopic morphology. *P. acnes*, widely distributed on human skin and hair, the gastrointestinal tract, and the mouth and nose, is catalase positive, produces indole, and reduces nitrate.

BIFIDOBACTERIUM
Bifidobacterium eriksonii

Georg et al. described this organism[41] and originally named it *Actinomyces eriksonii*. It eventually was reclassified as a member of the *Bifidobacterium* genus.[33]

B. eriksonii is an obligate anaerobic organism that produces tiny, glistening colonies on BHIA plates in 48 hours. Seven- to 10-day-old colonies are dull white, soft, and nonadherent to the medium. It is catalase negative, hydrolyzes starch, and produces H_2S; **nitrate is not reduced.** Litmus milk is reduced, and a firm curd is produced. Acid, but no gas, is produced from glucose, mannitol, mannose, raffinose, and glycerol.

As pointed out by Georg et al,[41] the outstanding characteristics of *B. eriksonii* are its morphologic similarity to *A. bovis*, a requirement for strict anaerobiosis, ability to coagulate milk and hydrolyze starch, inability to reduce nitrate, and marked ability to ferment sugars. It seems to cause a form of actinomycosis.[42]

REFERENCES

1. Holdeman, L. V., and Moore, W. E. C., editors: 1972. Anaerobe laboratory manual, Blacksburg, Va., 1972, Anaerobe laboratory, Virginia Polytechnic Institute and State University.
2. Dowell, V. R., Jr., and Hawkins, T. M.: Laboratory methods in anaerobic bacteriology, CDC Laboratory manual. DHEW publ. no. (CDC) 78-8272, Atlanta, 1977, Center for Disease Control.
3. Dowell, V. R., Jr., and Sonnenwirth, A. C.: Gram-positive, non-sporeforming anaerobic bacilli. In Lennette, E. H., Spaulding, E. H., and Truant, J. P., editors: Manual of clinical microbiology, ed. 2, Washington, D.C., 1974, American Society for Microbiology.
4. Moore, W. E. C., and Holdeman, L. V.: Am. J. Clin. Nutr. **25:**1306, 1972.
5. Buchanan, R. E., and Gibbons, N. E., editors: Bergey's manual of determinative bacteriology, ed. 8, Baltimore, 1974, The Williams & Wilkins Co.
6. Dowell, V. R., Jr.: Anaerobic infections. In Bodily, H. L., Updyke, E. L., and Mason, J. O., editors: Diagnostic procedures for bacterial, mycotic and parasitic infections, ed. 5, New York, 1970, American Public Health Association, Inc.
7. Wilson, W. R., Martin, W. J., Wilkowski, C. J., and Washington, J.A.: Mayo Clin. Proc. **47:**639, 1972.
8. Dowell, V. R., Jr.: Laboratory diagnosis of endogenous anaerobic bacterial infections. In Diakos, G. K., editor: Progress in chemotherapy, proceedings of the eighth international congress of chemotherapy, vol. 2, Athens, 1974.
9. Sonnenwirth, A. C.: Incidence of intestinal anaerobes in blood cultures. In Balows, A., DeHaan, R. M., Guze, L. B., and Dowell, V. R., Jr., editors: Anaerobic bacteria—role in disease, Springfield, Ill., 1974, Charles C Thomas, Publisher.
10. Georg, L. K.: The agents of human actinomycosis. In Balows, A., DeHaan, R. M., Guze, L. B., et al.: Anaerobic bacteria—role in disease, Springfield, Ill., 1974, Charles C Thomas, Publisher.
11. Puhvel, S. M., and Reisner, R. M.: Dermatologic anaerobic infections. In Balows, A., DeHaan, R. M., Guze, L. B., and Dowell, V. R., Jr., editors: Anaerobic bacteria—role in disease, Springfield, Ill., 1974, Charles C Thomas, Publisher.
12. Brock, D. W., Georg, L. K., Brown, J. M., and Hicklin, M. W.: Am. J. Clin. Pathol. **59:**66, 1973.
13. Bartlett, J. G., and Finegold, S. M.: Medicine **51:**413, 1972.
14. Felner, J. M., and Dowell, V. R., Jr.: N. Engl. J. Med. **283:**1188, 1970.
15. Finegold, S. M., Rosenblatt, J. E., Sutter, V. L., and Atteberry, H. R.: Scope monograph on anaerobic infections, Kalamazoo, Mich., 1972, The Upjohn Co.
16. Finegold, S. M.: Anaerobic bacteria in human disease, New York, 1977, Academic Press.
17. Sans, M. D., and Crowder, J. G.: Am. J. Clin. Pathol. **59:**576, 1973.
18. Felner, J. M.: Infective endocarditis caused by anaerobic bacteria. In Balows, A., DeHaan, R. M., Guze, L. B., and Dowell, V. R., Jr., editors: Anaerobic bacteria—role in disease, Springfield, Ill., 1974, Charles C Thomas, Publisher.
19. Sutter, V. L., Citron, D. M., and Finegold, S. M.: Wadsworth anaerobic bacteriology manual, ed. 2, Los Angeles, 1975, Dept. of Continuing Education in Health Sciences University Extension, and the School of Medicine, UCLA.
19a. Sutter, V. L., Citron, D. M., and Finegold, S. M.:

Wadsworth anaerobic bacteriology manual, ed. 3, St. Louis, 1980, The C. V. Mosby Co.

20. Jones, G., and Dowell, V. R., Jr.: Anaerobic bacteriology in the clinical laboratory, Laboratory Training and Consultation Div., Atlanta, 1976, Center for Disease Control.

21. Holdeman, L. V., Cato, E. P. and Moore, W. E. C.: Anaerobe laboratory manual, ed. 4, Anaerobe laboratory, Blacksburg, Va., 1977, Virginia Polytechnic Institute and State University.

22. Smith, L. D. S.: The pathogenic anaerobic bacteria, ed. 2, Springfield, Ill., 1975, Charles C Thomas, Publisher.

23. Willis, T. A.: Anaerobic bacteriology, ed. 3, London, 1977, Butterworth & Co.

24. Slack, J. M., Winger, A., and Moore, D. W., Jr.: J. Bacteriol. **82:**54, 1961.

25. Slack, J. M., and Gerencser, M. A.: J. Bacteriol. **91:**2107, 1966.

26. Brock, D. W., and Georg, L. K.: J. Bacteriol. **97:**581, 1969.

27. Georg, L. K.: Diagnostic procedures for the isolation and identification of the etiologic agents of actinomycosis. In Proceedings of the International Symposium on Mycoses, publ. no. 205, Washington, D.C., 1970, Pan American Health Organization.

28. Coleman, R. M., Georg, L. K., and Rozzell, A. R.: Appl. Microbiol. **18:**420, 1969.

29. Ajello, L., Georg, L. K., Kaplan, W., and Kaufman, L.: Laboratory manual for medical mycology, PHS publ. no. 994, Atlanta, 1963, Communicable Disease Center.

30. Lambert, F. W., Jr., Brown, J. M., and Georg, L. K.: J. Bacteriol. **94:**1287, 1967.

31. Georg, L.: Personal communication, 1968.

32. Pine, L., and Watson, S. J.: J. Lab. Clin. Med. **54:** 107, 1959.

33. Blank, C. H., and Georg. L. K.: J. Lab. Clin. Med. **71:**283, 1968.

34. Lomax, C. W., Harbert, G. M., and Thornton, W. N.: Obstet. Gynecol. **48:**341, 1976.

35. Lambert, R. F., Jr., Brown, J. M., and Georg, L. K.: J. Bacteriol. **94:**1287, 1967.

36. Coleman, R. M. and Georg, L. K.: Appl. Microbiol. **18:**427, 1969.

37. Batty, I.: J. Pathol. Bacteriol. **75:**455, 1958.

38. Gerencser, M. A., and Slack, J. M.: Appl. Microbiol. **18:**80, 1969.

39. Radford, B. L., and Ryan, W. J.: J. Clin. Pathol. **30:**518, 1977.

40. Marples, R. R., and McGinley, K. J.: J. Med. Microbiol. **7:**349, 1974.

41. Georg, L. K., Roberstad, G. W., Brinkman, S. A., and Hicklin, M. D.: J. Infect. Dis. **88:**115, 1965.

42. Thomas, A. V., Sodeman, T. H., and Bentz, R. R.: Am. Rev. Resp. Dis. **110:**663, 1974.

86

GRAM-NEGATIVE ANAEROBIC RODS—BACTEROIDACEAE

Sydney M. Finegold

This chapter discusses the obligately anaerobic gram-negative bacilli, with emphasis on organisms occurring in humans and producing disease. These bacteria are important human pathogens. Technics for their cultivation and identification are, for the most part, relatively simple so that even small laboratories can handle them readily. Much information has accumulated on the role of the gram-negative anaerobic rods in infection, and clinicians are now generally aware of their significance. Gram-negative anaerobic bacilli account for 40-45% of all anaerobic isolates from clinical specimens.

CLASSIFICATION

In the eighth edition of *Bergey's Manual* (1974) there are 3 genera in the family *Bacteroidaceae*: *Bacteroides* (22 species), *Fusobacterium* (16 species), and *Leptotrichia* (1 species). This represents a significant simplification from the seventh edition of *Bergey's Manual*, which listed 5 genera and 57 species. Additional species have been proposed since the eighth edition of *Bergey's Manual* was published, but the situation is not too complex considering that some of the *Bacteroidaceae* have not been encountered in humans and others are not medically important. There are several other genera of gram-negative anaerobic bacilli, mostly curved, whose affiliation is uncertain at present. Included are the following genera that have been found in the normal flora of humans and, occasionally, have been isolated from pathologic processes: *Desulfovibrio, Butyrivibrio, Succinivibrio,* and *Selenomonas*.

GRAM-NEGATIVE ANAEROBIC RODS AS NORMAL FLORA

Gram-negative anaerobic bacilli are prevalent on most mucosal surfaces of the body. Knowledge of the presence of specific organisms as normal flora at certain sites is useful in predicting which organisms may be involved in a given

infection since most anaerobic infections arise endogenously in proximity to mucosal surfaces. Thus, *F. nucleatum* and *B. melaninogenicus* would be anticipated, along with anaerobic cocci and *Streptococcus,* in an aspiration pneumonia. In bacteremia of unknown source the presence of a particular organism may suggest the portal of entry (e.g., *B. fragilis* in a male patient would suggest the gastrointestinal tract).

B. melaninogenicus makes up 4-8% of the cultivable flora of the gingival crevice but less than 1% of the coronal tooth surface flora.[1] *F. nucleatum* and *B. oralis* to a lesser extent are also prevalent in the mouth. *Bacteroides* and *Fusobacterium* each account for 4% of the cultivable organisms of dental plaque.[2]

Gram-negative anaerobic rods are not normally found in the stomach or upper small bowel, but *Bacteroides* are encountered in significant numbers in the terminal ileum. In the presence of achlorhydria, obstructive disease, or gastrointestinal hemorrhage, *B. fragilis* may be encountered in the stomach or upper small bowel and thus may be encountered following perforated peptic ulcer or in postoperative infection.[3] In the distal colon (based on studies of feces) the *B. fragilis* group is the dominant organism encountered (mean count 10^{11}/g dry weight feces). *B. vulgatus* is the most prevalent member of this group, with *B. thetaiotaomicron* and *B. fragilis* next in frequency.[4-6]

Bacteroides and *Fusobacterium* are common in the normal vaginal and cervical flora.[7-9] *Bacteroides* (including *B. fragilis, B. oralis,* and *B. melaninogenicus*) and *Fusobacterium* are found in the normal urethral flora,[10,11] and *B. melaninogenicus* and fusiform bacilli are found about the prepuce and elsewhere on the external genitalia.[12-14]

As indicated above, the normal flora may change under abnormal conditions. Hospitalization, serious illness, and antimicrobial therapy may all bring about significant changes.

B. fragilis can synthesize vitamin K; this production in the intestine can be important to the host.[15] Bile acids play an essential role in fat absorption, bile formation, and cholesterol metabolism. Modification of bile acids by intestinal bacteria is important physiologically. The *B. fragilis* group and various species of *Fusobacterium,* as well as certain other anaerobes and certain streptococci, deconjugate bile salts,[16,17] and dehydroxylation is carried out to a limited extent by *B. fragilis.*[17]

The normal bowel flora is also an important defense mechanism. Mice are much more susceptible to experimental *Salmonella* infection after oral streptomycin therapy. This reduces the count of *Bacteroides* in the mouse gut and thus lowers the amount of volatile fatty acids that inhibit *Salmonella.*[18] *Shigella flexneri* and *Pseudomonas aeruginosa* have been shown to be inhibited by similar mechanisms.[19,20]

R factor transfer between donor and recipient strains of *Escherichia coli* in broth culture was completely inhibited by *B. fragilis.*[21]

GRAM-NEGATIVE ANAEROBIC RODS IN PATHOPHYSIOLOGIC STATES

In periodontosis, a rapidly progressive form of peridontal disease seen in younger individuals, recent work implicates 5 different groups of saccharolytic gram-negative anaerobic bacilli, many of which are unclassifiable presently.[22,23] Certain asaccharolytic gram-negative anaerobic rods may contribute to the pathology of relatively rapidly destructive forms of periodontitis.[23]

In various forms of bowel bacterial overgrowth syndrome (blind loop syndrome, gastrocolic fistula, etc.), in which steatorrhea and vitamin B_{12} deficiency are prominent, *Bacteroides* and *Fusobacterium* (as well as other anaerobes and nonanaerobes) may play an important role.[24-30] Bacterial deconjugation of bile acids in the upper small bowel is a major factor in the steatorrhea. Vitamin B_{12} malabsorption is probably related to binding which can be effected by *B. fragilis* as well as *E. coli.*[31]

The syndrome of bypass enteropathy occurs in patients who have undergone ileal bypass for obesity and is manifested by certain intestinal and systemic symptoms resembling those seen in chronic inflammatory bowel diseases. Bacterial overgrowth in the excluded loop accompanies the syndrome and is presumably responsible for it. Various intestinal organisms, including several members of the *B. fragilis* group, have been cultured from such loops.[32]

GRAM-NEGATIVE ANAEROBIC RODS IN INFECTIONS

There are a number of monographs and reviews dealing with anaerobic infections primarily from the clinical standpoint.[33-38] Several others are chiefly bacteriologically oriented but also deal with the role of anaerobes in infection.[39-49] Werner and Pulverer[50] recovered 1244 anaerobic gram-negative bacilli in a period of less than 11 years. Mitchell[51] isolated 1067 strains of gram-negative anaerobic bacilli from clinical material in a 2-year period. Leigh[52] recovered *Bacteroides* from 81% of wound infec-

tions following intestinal surgery. Clark et al.[53] recovered *Bacteroides* from more than 400 patients in a 19-month period.

Anaerobic bacteria may cause any type of infection in which bacteria of any kind may be involved. No organ or tissue is immune to infection with anaerobes. Infections that commonly involve anaerobes include bacteremia, brain abscess, subdural and extradural empyema, chronic otitis media and mastoiditis, chronic sinusitis, dental and oral infections, aspiration pneumonia, lung abscess, necrotizing pneumonia, thoracic empyema, bronchiectasis, intra-abdominal infection of all types, liver abscess, postoperative infections following bowel surgery, vulvovaginal abscess, salpingitis, pelvic peritonitis and abscess, tubo-ovarian abscess, septic abortion, endometritis, infection following gynecologic surgery, anaerobic myonecrosis (gas gangrene), gas-forming cellulitis, perirectal abscess, breast abscess, and osteomyelitis. They may also play a role in certain other serious infections such as endocarditis and meningitis.

Gram-negative anaerobic bacilli are generally recovered in pure culture in up to one-third of infections. It was noted earlier that these organisms account for 40-45% of anaerobic isolates from clinical specimens. The *B. fragilis* group (chiefly *B. fragilis* and *B. thetaiotaomicron*) alone accounts for roughly one-fourth of all anaerobic bacteria isolated from clinical specimens. *B. fragilis* is found in pure culture relatively often. Thus Werner and Pulverer[50] found 22 of 75 isolates of *B. fragilis* and 6 of 19 of *B. thetaiotaomicron* in pure culture. *B. melaninogenicus, B. asaccharolyticus,* and *B. oralis* are also commonly encountered, but seldom in pure culture. Less commonly encountered in clinical specimens are *B. ruminicola* (especially ssp. *brevis*) and *B. corrodens. B. pneumosintes, B. capillosus, B. bivius, B. disiens* (the latter 2 recently proposed as new species[54]), and *B. splanchnicus* (newly described by Werner[55]) are seldom encountered, and other *Bacteroides* species are rare indeed or are never encountered at all in human clinical material. *B. clostridiiformis* is currently felt to be a spore-former, and it is proposed that it be transferred to the genus *Clostridium.*[56,57] As noted earlier it has been proposed that the subspecies of *B. fragilis* be reinstated to species rank.[58] The Subcommittee on Gram-negative Anaerobic Rods of the International Committee on Systematic Bacteriology has proposed species status (as *B. asaccharolyticus*) for *B. melaninogenicus* ssp. *asaccharolyticus. B. multiacidus,* a newly described species from feces of humans and pigs,[59] has not been recovered from infections in humans.

F. necrophorum, encountered much less frequently now than in the preantimicrobial period, is isolated in pure culture a greater percentage of the time than any other anaerobe. The most commonly encountered *Fusobacterium* presently is *F. nucleatum;* it is also found in pure culture

Table 86-1. Frequency of occurrence of gram-negative anaerobic rods in clinical material*

Bacteroides	No. isolates	Fusobacterium	No. isolates
fragilis	57	nucleatum	35
thetaiotaomicron	33	necrophorum	14
distasonis	21	naviforme	6
vulgatus	10	gonidiaformans	5
ovatus	6	mortiferum	5
"fragilis group"	8	varium	2
melaninogenicus		necrogenes	1
ssp. intermedius	35	not speciated	16
ssp. melaninogenicus	19		
ssp. asaccharolyticus	10		
ssp. not determined	24		
oralis	31		
corrodens	16		
ruminicola			
ssp. brevis	14		
ssp. ruminicola	2		
pneumosintes	6		
bivius (group PS)	5		
capillosus	4		
disiens (group I)	3		
splanchnicus	3		
putredinis	2		
praeacutus	1		
furcosus	1		
coagulans	1		
not speciated	43		

*These data are from a total of 728 clinical specimens processed by the Wadsworth Clinical Anaerobic Bacteriology Research Laboratory between August 1972 and December 1975. Subsequently, 3 species not previously encountered (*B. amylophilus, F. glutinosum,* and *F. russii*) have each been recovered once.

with some frequency. Fusobacteria less commonly encountered clinically include *F. naviforme, F. gonidiaformans, F. mortiferum,* and *F. varium.* Other *Fusobacterium* species are rare or not encountered at all in human clinical material.

Table 86-1 presents data on recovery of various gram-negative anaerobic bacilli from unselected specimens received in a clinical bacteriology research laboratory; the data in this table may be skewed by the fact that few female and pediatric patients were studied because of the nature of the hospital where the laboratory is located.

Clues suggesting infection with gram-negative (or other) anaerobes
Clinical clues

1. Location of infection in proximity to a mucosal surface
2. Foul-smelling discharge
3. Necrotic tissue, gangrene
4. Any infection producing gas in tissues or discharges
5. Infection associated with malignancy or other process producing tissue destruction
6. Infection related to the use of aminoglycoside antibiotics (oral, parenteral, or topical)
7. Septic thrombophlebitis
8. Infection following human or other bites
9. *B. melaninogenicus* may produce hematin in tissues, leading to black discoloration of exudate; such discharges may fluoresce red under ultraviolet light
10. Bacterial endocarditis with negative routine blood cultures
11. Clinical setting suggestive of anaerobic infection (e.g., septic abortion, infection related to bowel surgery)
12. Classic clinical picture such as actinomycosis, clostridial myonecrosis (gram-negative anaerobes may also be involved in these conditions)

Bacteriologic clues

1. Gram stain of discharge (or subsequent culture growth) revealing pale, irregularly staining, pleomorphic, slender, gram-negative bacilli or gram-negative rods with tapered ends
2. No growth on routine culture—"sterile pus"; growth in fluid thioglycollate broth or not
3. Failure to grow aerobically; organisms seen on gram stain of original exudate
4. Growth on media containing 75-100 μg/ml kanamycin, neomycin, or paromomycin (particularly if medium also contains 7.5 μg/ml vancomycin)
5. Production of much gas, foul odor in culture
6. Growth in anaerobic zone of fluid thioglycollate broth or of agar deeps
7. Characteristic colonies on agar plates anaerobically

Specimen collection and transport

In collecting specimens for culture in which gram-negative anaerobic rods (or other anaerobes) are considered involved, great care must be taken to avoid "contamination" with normal flora because these organisms are so prevalent on the mucous membrane and other surfaces of the body. For example, voided urine not uncommonly contains anaerobes from the normal urethral flora; obtaining urine by percutaneous suprapubic bladder puncture eliminates this problem. A more common and more difficult problem is the patient with pneumonia or lung abscess in which anaerobes may be involved. Coughed sputum is totally unsatisfactory because of the presence of large numbers of anaerobes from the normal upper respiratory tract flora that contaminate this type of specimen. Bronchoscopically obtained specimens are also not reliable.[60] A recent paper by Wimberley, Faling, and Bartlett[60a] indicates that with the use of a telescoping double catheter plugged at the distal end with polyethylene glycol to protect a bronchial brush it may be possible to get reliable aerobic and anaerobic cultures via a bronchoscope. Transtracheal needle aspiration and direct lung puncture are the only dependable ways to obtain a reliable sample for culture unless material can be obtained from the pleural space in the case of complicating empyema.

Another problem concerns the die-off of anaerobes exposed to oxygen during the interval between obtaining the specimen and the culturing of the specimen in the laboratory. Although anaerobes may survive in thick, purulent specimens of sufficient volume for considerable periods of time,[61] the usual clinical specimen requires special handling. Anaerobic syringe technics or completely filling a small sterile screw-capped tube with specimen (to displace all air) may be useful. Direct placement of a specimen into an ampule or a rubber-stoppered tube that has been gassed out with oxygen-free gas and that contains fluid with reducing substances and an oxidation-reduction indicator such as resazurin[62,63] is excellent. For tissues a miniature anaerobic jar[64] works well. Swabs are the least satisfactory means of transporting specimens for anaerobic culture. When swabs must be used, the miniature anaerobic jar may be employed for transport. Alternatively, the use of prereduced anaerobically sterilized Cary and Blair semisolid transport medium and swabs put up in an anaerobic atmosphere is satisfactory.[63] The Bio-Bag (Marion Scientific Corp.) is an excellent transport setup that can be used for any type of specimen—fluid, tissue, or swab.

Specimen processing and cultivation

It is important to appreciate the usefulness of the direct Gram stain of clinical material. The unique morphology of the gram-negative anaerobes will often alert the microbiologist or clinician to the possibility of infection with these organisms and even to the probable infecting genus or species in some cases. This may be most important in the case of serious infections because these organisms often require 48 hours or longer for growth. Much additional time may be involved to obtain pure cultures in the case of mixed infection and to provide identification. The Gram stain may also suggest the desirability of including special media for inoculation, and it gives information about the relative importance of various organisms in mixed infections and is extremely important for quality control in the laboratory. Dark-field examination is also desirable for detection of motility, spores, and poorly staining forms such as spirochetes.

Certain fastidious anaerobes require technics such as the Hungate roll-tube procedure,[65] modifications of it,[66] or the use of an anaerobic chamber or glovebox.[67] These procedures are necessary for normal flora studies. However, studies to date indicate that such fastidious anaerobes are seldom, if ever, encountered in clinical specimens that have been properly collected and that various anaerobic jar technics are entirely appropriate for clinical bacteriology.[68,69]

Since anaerobic jars are inexpensive, simple to use, widely used in clinical laboratories, and readily allow one to closely examine surface colonies, only the anaerobic jar technic will be described here. Fluid thioglycollate medium, even when supplemented with hemin and other factors, is distinctly inferior to plate culture in anaerobic jars. Anaerobic incubators are effective, but they do not offer enough flexibility for most clinical laboratories. See also discussion of anaerobic methods in Chapter 70.

The various modifications of the Brewer and McIntosh-Fildes jars are all satisfactory. The use of a mercury manometer is preferable to a mechanical gauge unless the latter can be calibrated periodically. When nitrogen or helium is used, 5-7 flushings of the jar are required to displace a sufficent proportion of the oxygen. Whatever gas is chosen, CO_2 and H_2 (5-10% each) should always be included in the final atmosphere because some gram-negative anaerobes require CO_2, and H_2 is necessary to ensure anaerobiosis. Fig. 86-1 shows a good setup for exchanging atmosphere in anaerobic jars. A commercial mixture of 80% nitrogen, 10% hydrogen, and 10% carbon dioxide is very good and is less explosive than pure hydrogen; however, it is somewhat expensive. Furthermore, only cylinders with less than 600 psi should be used, since CO_2 liquefies under higher pressure and the ratio of the gases would therefore not remain constant. One may evacuate and flush 3 or 4 times with nitrogen, as described below, and then, after an additional evacuation, fill the jar for the final time with the nitrogen–hydrogen–carbon dioxide mixture.

A disposable hydrogen generator,[70] which also evolves carbon dioxide, is available commercially (GasPak, BBL) and is easy to use. Both vented

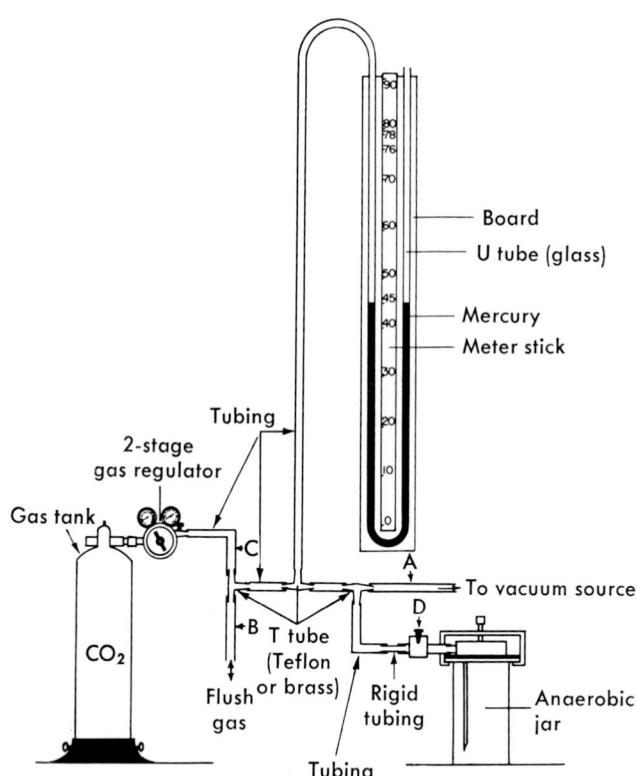

Fig. 86-1. Setup for producing anaerobiosis in jars.

and unvented GasPak jars are available (BBL). This system is the most popular in clinical laboratories today and, because of its simplicity, has done a great deal toward making good anaerobic bacteriology readily available in small hospitals. Considering the time saved, the GasPak system is not noticeably more expensive than others.

Catalysts are readily inactivated by hydrogen sulfide or moisture. They should be regenerated after each use by heating to 160 C in a drying oven for 1½-2 hours; they should then be stored in a desiccator until use.

One may set up a holding jar in which to store inoculated plates until enough specimens are received to set up a full jar with a GasPak envelope.[71] Flowing oxygen-free gas protects the inoculated plates from oxygen.

Various **indicators** of anaerobiosis have been used in media or within (or even on the outside of) anaerobic jars. Methylene blue is widely used, and a convenient sachet is available commercially.[72] Resazurin is preferable. Simple indications that a reaction between the hydrogen and oxygen in a jar is taking place are warmth of the jar lid and accumulation of moisture on the inner surface of the jar soon after it has been set up. Setting up cultures of relatively fastidious anaerobic organisms is an excellent way to determine whether adequate anaerobiosis is achieved in an anaerobic vessel.

Media should be as fresh as possible. Some

workers prefer to store media anaerobically prior to use. The possible advantage of such storage has not been studied formally in the case of clinical anaerobic bacteriology. Many or most commerical media (particularly those that are not prereduced) are inadequate for anaerobic bacteriology. Laboratories wishing to use such media should evaluate them carefully in comparison with laboratory-made media. Liquid media not prepared the same day should be heated in a boiling water bath for 10 minutes before use (discard if not used after such heating).

A good **minimal scheme for processing specimens** is as follows. Inoculate 3 blood agar plates (1 to be cultured anaerobically, 1 under 10% CO_2 in air, and 1 aerobically), a kanamycin-vancomycin–laked blood–agar-vitamin K_1 plate (the latter to be incubated anaerobically), a *Bacteroides* bile esculin (BBE) plate,[63, 72a] and supplemented fluid thioglycollate medium or cooked meat medium. Incubation of the liquid media in anaerobic jars increases their effectiveness but is not practical as a routine procedure. Ordinarily cultures can be examined and subcultured for purity (or processed for identification, if pure) after 48 hours. In the case of seriously ill patients specimens can be set up in duplicate and 1 set examined after 18-24 hours or other appropriate interval. Alternatively, a single-culture setup can be prepared in an anaerobic plastic bag[73] or the

Table 86-2. Instructions for exchanging atmosphere in anaerobic jars (using either nitrogen or helium gas as flush gas) (see Fig. 86-1)

Plates should be incubated right side up so that agar will not accidentally be pulled off Petri dish bottom. Container with calcium chloride should be included to pick up excess water.

Before jar is connected, air should be displaced from gas lines by turning on gases (individually) until flow is obtained at point at which jar is to be connected. When 2-stage gas regulator is used, as for CO_2 in Fig. 86-1, large handle is turned until the gauge reads 2 lb. Small left-hand knob is then opened to obtain flow of gas. Clamp off B and C.

1. Turn vacuum source on. Keep vacuum on until mercury reaches 80 cm on left side of U tube and stabilizes (10 cm on right side). Wait 1 full min. to be sure vacuum is maintained (and therefore that there are no leaks in system). Points of leakage may be detected by applying 1-2% Ivory soap or detergent to all likely places and observing for bubbling. Greater vacuum than this should be avoided, since it causes excessive bubbling of liquid or lifting of agar.
2. Clamp off A and slowly open flush gas B, allowing mercury columns to stabilize near 45 cm.
3. Clamp off B and open vacuum source as in step 1.
4. Repeat this cycle 6-7 times. Each cycle replaces about 90% of the atmosphere.
5. During last cycle, after evacuation, open point C instead of B, and allow CO_2 to enter until left-hand column of mercury is 76 cm (and right 14 cm). This provides 10% CO_2 in the final atmosphere. Close C and open B, as before.
6. When mercury columns stabilize (near 45 cm), close tube clamp at D. Turn off both gas sources. Disconnect and incubate jar. When hydrogen is used as flush gas or during final fill, fewer flushes are required.

Large Kelly hemostats may be used for closing points A, B, and C. These are better than mechanical valves or screw clamps, which may leak, and allow one to cut off and open lines quickly.

Measurements are made by reading the differences between the 2 levels of mercury (80 cm − 10 cm = 70 cm vacuum).

---

commercially available Bio-Bag so that the plates can be examined for growth without disturbing the atmosphere. If possible, original cultures should be reincubated for a total of a total of 2-3 weeks to pick up the rare late-growing anaerobes. It must be remembered that most aerobes found in clinical specimens are facultative. Therefore, all colony types isolated must be subcultured aerobically, under CO_2 in air (the CO_2 culture should be on chocolate agar), and anaerobically to determine which ones are obligate anaerobes. In processing specimens and examining and subculturing anaerobic plates, materials should be exposed to air for as short a time as possible.

The number or relative number of colonies of various types should be noted, since this provides a good indication of the relative importance of each in mixed infections. Colonies should be examined under a stereoscopic microscope for morphologic details.

Common errors in anaerobic bacteriology

Following is a list of common errors in anaerobic bacteriology:

1. Gram stain not prepared directly from clinical specimen. The Gram stain alerts one to the possible presence of organisms requiring special media or conditions of incubation. It also helps one to realize that the technics are defective if organisms seen on the smear fail to grow out.
2. Failure to set up anaerobic cultures promptly from clinical specimens or to keep these under anaerobic conditions pending culture.
3. Use of fluid thioglycollate medium as the only system for growing anaerobes. A number of anaerobes will not grow in this medium, even when it is enriched, and solid media are required to separate the various organisms present in mixed culture. Errors are made at times even when anaerobes have grown in fluid thioglycollate medium. Some workers do not check this medium if growth appears on aerobic plates but assume that the same organism is growing in both. A Gram stain of the broth will often alert one to the additional presence of anaerobes.
4. Use of inadequate commercial media. Failure to use fresh media.
5. Failure to use supplements in media. Vitamin K_1 is required by some strains of *B. melaninogenicus* and often stimulates *B. fragilis*.
6. Failure to use selective media. Some anaerobes may be overgrown by facultative anaerobes and overlooked if selective media are not used.
7. Failure to use a good anaerobic jar. McIntosh-Fildes, Torbal or Baird-Tatlock, and GasPak jars have been found to perform well.
8. Failure to check jars carefully for leaks after they are set up.
9. Catalysts not in good working order when using hydrogen in jars.
10. Using too few flushes when not using hydrogen in jars.
11. Using toxic gas in displacement procedure.
12. Failure to include CO_2 in jars. CO_2 is essential for some anaerobes.
13. Failure to hold cultures for extended periods. Occasionally, fastidious organisms present in small numbers may require 2-3 weeks to grow.
14. Failure to minimize air exposure during processing.
15. Failure to use redox indicator or known fastidious anaerobe in jar.
16. Inaccurate identification and speciation.
17. Use of disk susceptibility technic without standards (or use of Kirby-Bauer aerobic standards).
18. Failure to determine whether organism is a true anaerobe.

Anaerobic blood cultures

There are a number of commercially available media that are satifactory for recovery of anaerobic bacteria.[74] Some contain sodium polyanethol sulfonate (SPS, Liquoid), which may enhance recovery of gram-negative anaerobic rods and other organisms, but which may inhibit *Peptostreptococcus anaerobius*. Some of the media available in unvented bottles (this is important for anaerobic culture) and prepared under vacuum with CO_2 added are tryptic soy broth (Difco), thiol broth (Difco), trypticase soy broth (B-D), thioglycollate medium (B-D), brain-heart infusion broth, and Columbia broth (Difco). A commercially prepared prereduced medium showed no advantage over conventional media.

It is preferable to inoculate the medium directly from the patient via tubing with a needle at both ends (displacing all air from the tubing with blood before inoculating the bottle). Vented bottles must be used for aerobes and fungi.

Daily inspection of bottles and Gram stain and blind anaerobic subculture after 48 hours and before discarding are desirable. Cultures should be held 2-3 weeks, if at all possible.

Identification

The first responsibilities of a clinical laboratory are to recover all anaerobes present, obtain them in pure culture, and keep them alive for study or transmittal to a reference laboratory, if indicated. How much identification is done will necessarily vary from laboratory to laboratory. Certainly the laboratory in a teaching hospital ought to provide reasonably definitive identification. All cases reported in the literature should be accompanied by accurate, detailed description or identification of the organisms recovered. Beyond this the major concern is to provide the clinician with data appropriate to optimum management of the patient's infection. It is of considerable importance to identify the *B. fragilis* group as early as possible, as this group is the most resistant of all anaerobes to antimicrobial agents. Fortunately this is relatively easy to do. Beyond immediate therapeutic considerations, knowledge of the specific identity of an organism may have prog-

nostic implications, serve to identify the likely portal of entry in a bacteremia of uncertain source, etc.

After the organism is isolated in pure culture and established as an obligately anaerobic gram-negative bacillus, a variety of simple tests can be utilized to provide reliable presumptive identification, and then, depending on the laboratory, additional tests may be used to give definitive identification. We have found that it is convenient to place organisms into preliminary groups by means of colonial and microscopic morphology, pigment, hemolysis, pitting of agar, fluorescence under ultraviolet light, motility, susceptibility to bile, indole, and patterns of susceptibility or resistance to special antibiotic-impregnated disks (Table 86-3).

Certain additional tests, none complicated, may then be applied to provide more definitive identification. Table 86-4 shows how the members of the *B. fragilis* group may be identified with the use of the indole test and 3 carbohydrate fermentations. Table 86-5 depicts identification of the members of the *B. melaninogenicus-oralis-ochraceus* group. *B. corrodens* can be verified by observation of nitrite production and hydrolysis of urea. *F. mortiferum* is indole negative and hydrolyzes esculin, whereas *F. varium* typically gives the opposite reactions in these tests. Certain other *Fusobacterium* species may be identified as outlined in Table 86-6. Certain clinical laboratories will find it convenient to use gas chromatographic analysis of end products of metabolism; this can be useful and occasionally is indispensable, even with the gram-negative anaerobic bacilli.[63,75]

Various rapid biochemical methods have been applied successfully with certain anaerobes and may prove useful in the clinical laboratory set-

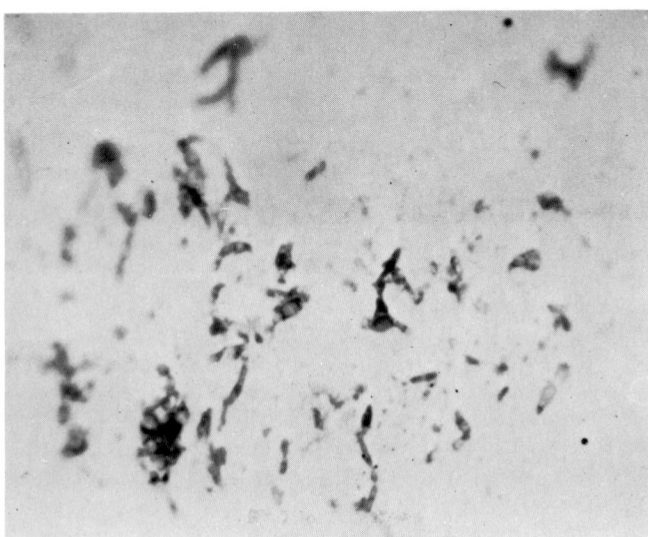

Fig. 86-2. Microscopic morphology—*Bacteroides fragilis.* Note moderate pleomorphism with pseudobranching and irregularity of staining. (From Finegold, S. M.: Med. Times **96:**174, 1968.)

Table 86-3. Preliminary group identification of gram-negative anaerobic rods[*]

Anaerobic rods	Antibiotic disk identification[†] C 10 μg	K 1000 μg	V 5 μg	Lipase	Indole	Cata-lase	Motility	Bile
B. fragilis group	R	R	R	−	V	V	−	No inhibition (or stimulation)
B. melaninogeni-cus-oralis group	V	R	V	V	V	−	−	I
B. corrodens (ureolyticus)	S	S	R	−	−	−[+]	−	I
F. mortiferum-varium group	S	S	R	−	V	−	−	No inhibition (or stimulation)
Certain other Fusobacterium sp.	S	S	R	V	V	−	−	V

[*]− = Negative or absent; −[+] = most strains negative, some positive; V = variable; I = inhibited; S = sensitive, zones ≥ 10 mm; and R = resistant, zones < 10 mm.
[†]C = colistin, K = kanamycin, and V = vancomycin.

Table 86-4. Characteristics of members of B. fragilis group

Characteristics	B. distasonis	B. fragilis	B. vulgatus	B. ovatus	B. theta-iotaomicron
Indole production	−	−	−	+	+
Fermentation of:					
Salicin	+	−	−[+]	+	−[+]
Rhamnose	V*	−	+	+	+
Trehalose	+	−	−	+	+

*V = Variable.

Table 86-5. Characteristics of the B. melaninogenicus-oralis group

Characteristics	B. melaninogenicus ssp. asaccharolyticus	ssp. intermedius	ssp. melaninogenicus	B. oralis
Indole production	+	+	−	−
Nitrate reduction	−	−	−	−
Fermentation of:				
Esculin	−	−	−	−
Glucose	−	+	+	+
Starch	−	+	+	+
Hydrolysis of:				
Esculin	−	−	+[−]	+
Starch	−	+	+	+
Lipase	−	+/−	−	−

Table 86-6. Characteristics of certain Fusobacterium species[*]

Characteristics	F. gonidiaformans	F. naviforme	F. necrophorum	F. nucleatum
Indole production	+	+	+	+
Nitrate reduction	−	−	−	−
Fermentation of:				
Glucose	+	−	−	−
Levulose	−	−	−	+
Mannose	−	−	−	−
Hydrolysis of:				
Esculin	−	−	−	−
Starch	+	−	−	−
Effect of bile on growth	I[†]	I	I	I
Lipase production	−	−	+/−	−

*Organisms whose characteristics do not fit the above species will require additional tests.
[†]I = Inhibition.

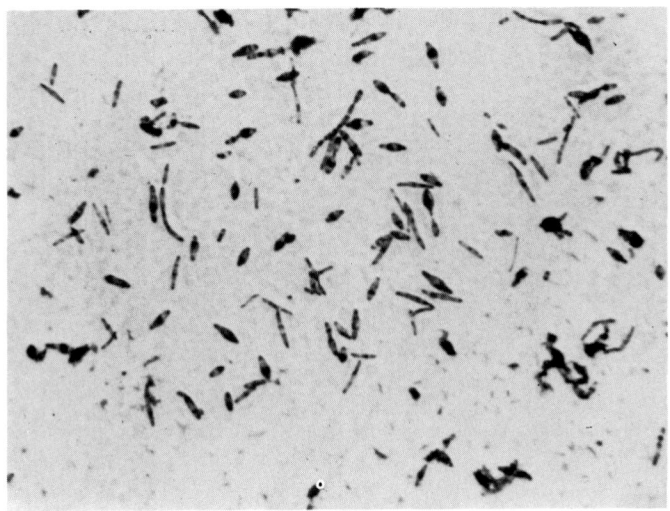

Fig. 86-3. Microscopic morphology—*Bacteroides fragilis.* Pleomorphism and irregular staining are again evident. (From Finegold, S. M.: Med. Times **96:**174, 1968.)

ting.[76-78] It should be pointed out that obligately anaerobic gram-negative bacilli resistant to a 1000 μg disk of kanamycin, with growth stimulated by 20% bile, can be identified as *B. fragilis* group, usually within 24 hours. Commercial miniaturized biochemical systems are also available but presently lack certain important tests or have not had critical, thorough evaluation in the clinical laboratory setting.

L. buccalis is usually a nonpathogen and is normally found in the oral cavity of humans. It stains gram positive in young cultures, and older cells may show gram-positive granules or gram-variable characteristics. Cells often have pointed ends and thus resemble fusobacteria. It is saccharolytic, with lactic acid as the major fermentation product; it does not produce indole.

Typical microscopic and colonial morphology of various *Bacteroidaceae* are shown in Figs. 86-2 to 86-8. Characteristics of motile gram-negative anaerobic bacilli are given in the key below, modified from Holdeman and Moore[75]:

1. Spiral-shaped cells with axial filaments: *Treponema* and *Borrelia*
2. Flagella in tufts on concave side of crescent-shaped cells: *Selenomonas*
3. Polar flagella
   a. Fermentative
      (1) Produce butyric acid: *Butyrivibrio*
      (2) Produce succinic acid
         (a) Spiral-shaped cells: *Succinivibrio*
         (b) Ovoid cells: *Succinimonas*
   b. Nonfermentative: *Campylobacter* (microaerophilic)
4. Peritrichous flagella
   a. Produce butyric acid without much isobutyric and isovaleric acid: *Fusobacterium*
   b. Other than above: *Bacteroides*

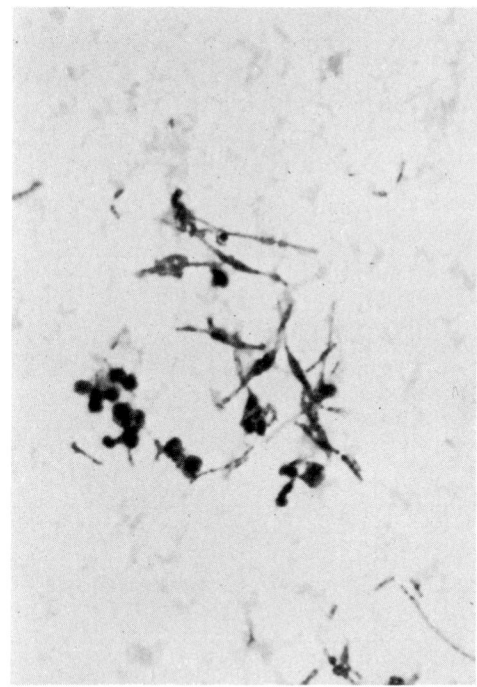

Fig. 86-4. Microscopic morphology—*Fusobacterium mortiferum.* Marked pleomorphism. Note filamentous forms with swellings, large round bodies, and erratic staining. (Gram stain.) (From Finegold, S. M.: Med. Times **96:**174, 1968.)

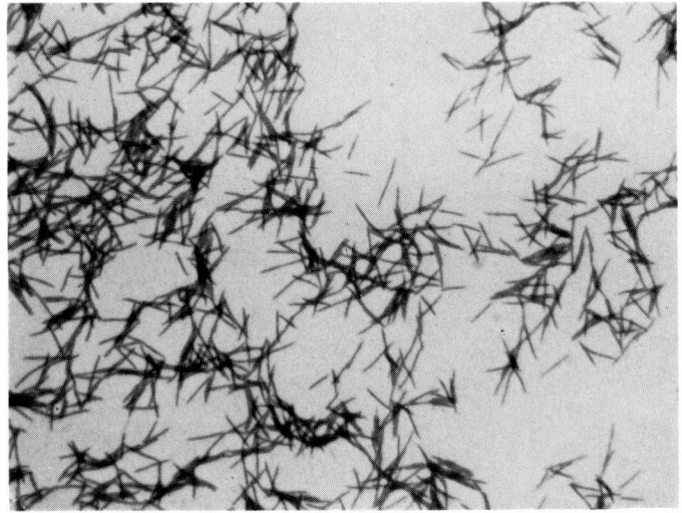

Fig. 86-5. Microscopic morphology—*Fusobacterium nucleatum.* Thin, delicate rods with tapered ends. (From Finegold, S. M.: Med. Times **96**:174, 1968.)

Antibacterial agent susceptibility studies

Patterns of susceptibility of gram-negative anaerobes to antimicrobial agents are relatively constant and predictable. The usual patterns of major organisms in the group are noted in Table 86-7. Aminoglycosides, such as gentamicin and kanamycin, are generally inactive against these organisms (*B. corrodens* [*ureolyticus*] is a notable exception). The activity of erythromycin varies significantly according to the testing procedure, and there are few data on this drug's efficacy clinically. Erythromycin and metronidazole have not been approved by the Food and Drug Administration for use in anaerobic infections, but the latter compound is being studied clinically under FDA authorization. Other penicillins and cephalosporins are frequently less active. Ampicillin, amoxicillin, and carbenicillin are roughly comparable to penicillin G on a weight basis, but the high blood levels achievable (with relative safety) make carbenicillin effective vs. 95% of strains of *B. fragilis*. Methicillin, nafcillin, and

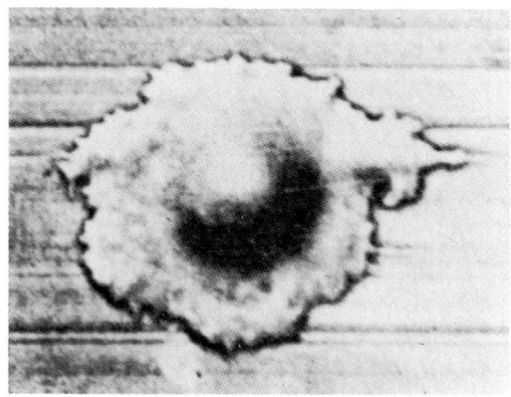

Fig. 86-6. "Fried egg" colony of *Fusobacterium necrophorum.* Note central convexity, relatively flat outer margin, and irregular edge. (From Lahelle, O.: Acta Pathol. Microbiol. Scand. **67**(supp.): 361, 1947.)

Table 86-7. Antimicrobial susceptibility of gram-negative anaerobic bacilli*

	Bacteroides fragilis	*B. melaninogenicus*	*Fusobacterium varium*	Other *Fusobacterium sp.*
Chloramphenicol	+++	+++	+++	+++
Clindamycin	++++	+++	+ to ++	+++
Erythromycin	+ to ++	+++	+	+
Metronidazole	+++	+++	+++	+++
Penicillin G	+	+++†	+++†	++++
Tetracycline	+ to ++	++ to +++	++	+++

*++++ = drug of choice, +++ = good activity, ++ = moderate activity, + = poor or inconsistent activity. There is no difference in activity between drugs rated +++ and those rated ++++; the symbol ++++ indicates a drug with good activity, good pharmacologic characteristics, and low toxicity.
†A few strains are resistant.

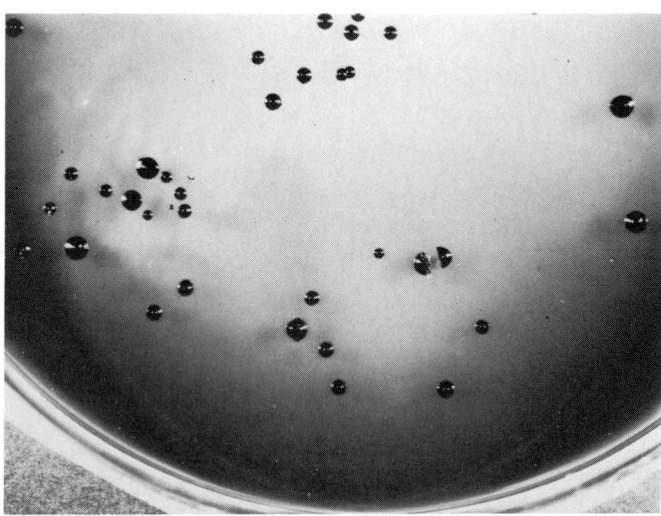

Fig. 86-7. Colony morphology—*Bacteroides melaninogenicus.* Distinctive black color on laked blood agar. One colony has been cut in two; note how half of colony has been moved away from its original site without any disturbance of its integrity. (From Finegold, S. M.: Med, Times **96**:174, 1968.)

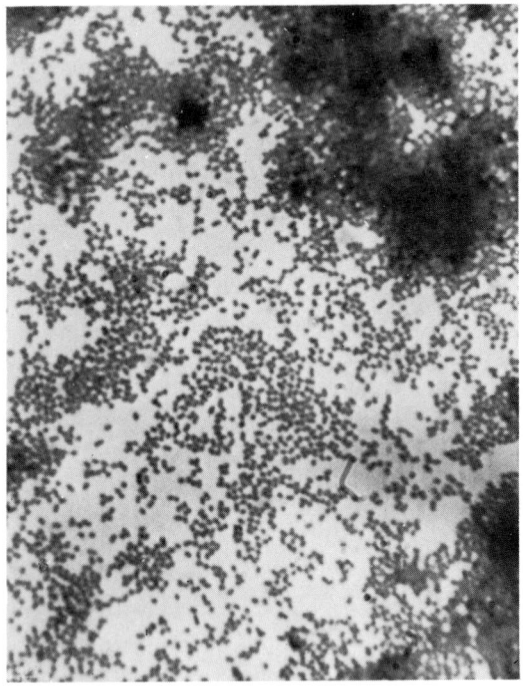

Fig. 86-8. Microscopic morphology—*Bacteroides melanino-genicus.* Organisms are coccobacilli. No pleomorphism or irregularity of staining.

the isoxazolyl penicillins (oxacillin, cloxacillin, and dicloxacillin) are distinctly less active than penicillin G. Cephalothin and cefazolin have relatively poor activity against *B. fragilis* (only 10-30% of strains are susceptible to achievable levels). Cefoxitin, a compound resistant to β-lactamases, is active versus 90% of *B. fragilis*

strains at achievable levels and is effective clinically. Doxycycline and minocycline are more active than other tetracyclines, but susceptibility testing is indicated to ensure activity.

Determination of antimicrobial susceptibility of gram-negative anaerobes may be indicated in serious infections such as bacterial endocarditis, when a patient does not respond to what seems to be an appropriate regimen, and with organisms such as *B. fragilis*, which is often resistant to commonly used agents. β-lactamase is produced by the *B. fragilis* group, *B. oralis*, *B. bivius*, and *B. disiens*, and plasmid-mediated transferable resistance has been demonstrated with *B. fragilis.*

Among the gram-negative anaerobic rods, *B. fragilis* is the most resistant to antimicrobial agents; only chloramphenicol, clindamycin, and metronidazole are consistently active against it. *F. varium*, not commonly encountered, is also relatively resistant; a number of strains are resistant to clindamycin. *B. melaninogenicus* is showing increasing resistance to penicillin G recently. There are no significant differences in susceptibility patterns among the various members of the *B. fragilis* group or the subspecies of *B. melaninogenicus.*

Broth or agar dilution tests—consisting of a series of 2-fold dilutions of drug in a suitable medium, inoculated with the organism to be tested, and incubated anaerobically—are suitable for susceptibility testing of anaerobes. Broth-disk tests (see Chapter 82) are convenient to use for testing small numbers of strains.[79] Agar diffusion (disk) tests may also be utilized. In using any of these types of test, but particularly the disk test, it is important to follow exactly procedures that have been standardized—or to develop one's own standardized procedure. When

Table 86-8. Colonial and microscopic morphology of major gram-negative anaerobic rods

Species	Colony morphology on blood agar	Microscopic morphology
B. fragilis	Convex, white to gray, translucent, glistening	Gram-negative bacilli, rounded ends, may be pleomorphic; may show vacuolation and bipolar staining
B. melaninogenicus	Convex, brick-red fluorescence under ultraviolet light (2 d); brown to black pigment (5-7 d)	Gram-negative, often coccobacillary
B. oralis	Convex, yellowish, translucent, glistening	Gram-negative bacilli, rounded ends
B. corrodens (ureolyticus)	Pinpoint with edges spreading and eroding into agar (5 d or more)	Gram-negative bacilli, rounded ends
F. nucleatum	Convex, glistening with internal iridescent flecking, or raised opaque "bread crumb" colonies	Gram-negative bacilli, slender, spindle shaped with tapered ends, sometimes in pairs end to end; sometimes filamentous
F. necrophorum	Convex, umbonate, opaque center with translucent edge	Gram-negative bacilli with rounded to tapered ends, pleomorphic; sometimes filamentous
F. mortiferum and F. varium	Flat to convex, opaque center with translucent, irregular edge, "fried egg"	Gram-negative bacilli, highly pleomorphic, with round bodies, filaments

this is done, results are entirely reproducible and dependable. Details on specific standardized technics in use at the Wadsworth V. A. Anaerobic Bacteriology Research Laboratory are given elsewhere.[63]

DESCRIPTION OF MAJOR GRAM-NEGATIVE ANAEROBES

The colonial and microscopic morphology of the gram-negative anaerobic bacilli most commonly encountered in clinical specimens are noted in Table 86-8. These morphologic features are often distinctive enough to provide clues to presumptive identification of the organisms. Used together with certain other tests for preliminary grouping (as outlined in the section on Identification), they are valuable in providing the bacteriologist and clinician with early, reliable presumptive identification.

REFERENCES

1. Gibbons, R. J.: Aspects of the pathogenicity and ecology of the indigenous oral flora of man. In Balows, A., DeHaan, R. M., Dowell, V. R., Jr., et al., editors: Anaerobic bacteria: role in disease, Springfield, Ill., 1974, Charles C Thomas, Publisher.
2. Gibbons, R. J., Socransky, S. S., DeAraujo, W. C., et al.: Arch. Oral Biol. 9:365, 1964.
3. Nichols, R. L., Miller, B., and Smith, J. W.: Surg. Clin. North Am. 55:1367, 1975.
4. Finegold, S. M., Attebery, H. R., and Sutter, V. L.: Am. J. Clin. Nutr. 27:1456, 1974.
5. Werner, H.: Arzneim. Forsch. 24:340, 1974.
6. Finegold, S. M., Flora, D. J., Attebery, H. R., et al.: Cancer Res. 35:3407, 1975.
7. Mead, P. B., and Louria, D. B.: Clin. Obstet. Gynecol. 12:219, 1969.
8. Gorbach, S. L., Menda, K. B., Thadepalli, H., et al.: Am. J. Obstet. Gynecol. 117:1053, 1973.
9. Sanders, C. V., Mickal, A., Lewis, A C., et al.: Clin. Res. 23:30A, 1975.
10. Bran, J. L., Levison, M. E., and Kaye, D.: N. Engl. J. Med. 286:626, 1972.
11. Finegold, S. M., Miller, L. G., Merrill, S. L., et al.: Significance of anaerobic and capnophilic bacteria isolated from the urinary tract. In Kass, E. H., editor: Progress in pyelonephritis, Philadelphia, 1965, F. A. Davis Co.
12. Brams, J., Pilot, I., and Davis, D. J.: J. Infect. Dis. 32:159, 1923.
13. Davis, D. J., and Pilot, I.: J.A.M.A. 79:944, 1922.
14. Burdon, K. L.: J. Infect. Dis. 42:161, 1928.
15. Gibbons, R. J., and Engle, L. P.: Science 146:1307, 1964.
16. Shimada, K., Bricknell, K. S., and Finegold, S. M.: J. Infect. Dis. 119:273, 1969.
17. Hill, M. J., and Drasar, B. S.: Gut 9:22, 1968.
18. Bohnhoff, M., Miller, C. P., and Martin, W. R.: J. Exp. Med. 120:805, 1964.
19. Hentges, D. J.: J. Bacteriol. 93:1369, 1967.
20. Levison, M. E.: Infect. Immun. 8:30, 1973.
21. Yale, C. E.: Surg. Clin. North Am. 55:1297, 1975.
22. Newman, M. G., and Socransky, S. S.: J. Periodont. Res. 12:120, 1979.
23. Newman, M. G., Socransky, S. S., Savitt, E. D., et al.: J. Periodont. 47:373, 1976.
24. McKenna, R. D., Beck, I. T., and Epstein, H.: Can. Med. Assoc. J. 83:896, 1960.
25. Lyall, I. G., and Parsons, P. J.: Med. J. Aust. 2:904, 1961.
26. Drasar, B. S., Hill, M. J., and Shiner, M.: Lancet 1:1237, 1966.
27. Tabaqchali, S., Okubadejo, O. A., Neale, G., et al.: Proc. R. Soc. Med. 59:1244, 1966.
28. Polter, D. E., Boyle, J. D., Miller, L. G., et al.: Gastroenterology 54:1148, 1968.
29. Farrar, W. E., Jr., O'Dell, N. M., Achord, J. L., et al.: Am. J. Dig. Dis. 17:1065, 1972.
30. Challacombe, D. N., Richardson, J. M., Edkins, S., et al.: Am. J. Dis. Child. 128:719, 1974.
31. Schjönsby, H., Drasar, B. S., Tabaqchali, S., et al.: Scand. J. Gastroenterol. 8:41, 1973.
32. Drenick, E. J., Ament, M. E., Finegold, S. M., et al.: J.A.M.A. 236:269, 1976.
33. Finegold, S. M.: Anaerobic bacteria in human disease, New York, 1977, Academic Press.

34. Gorbach, S. L., and Bartlett, J. G.: N. Engl. J. Med. **290**:1177, 1237, 1289, 1974.

35. Finegold, S. M., and Rosenblatt, J. E.: Medicine **52**:311, 1973.

36. Balows, A., DeHaan, R. M., Dowell, V. R., Jr., et al.: Anaerobic bacteria: role in disease, Springfield, Ill., 1974, Charles C Thomas, Publisher.

37. Goldsand, G., and Braude, A. I.: Disease-a-month, November 1966.

38. Bornstein, D. L., Weinberg, A. N., Swartz, M. N., et al.: Medicine **43**:207, 1964.

39. Smith, L.DS.: The pathogenic anaerobic bacteria, ed. 2, Springfield, Ill., 1975, Charles C Thomas, Publisher.

40. Werner, H.: Die gramnegativen anaeroben sporenlosen Stäbchen des Menschen, Jena, 1968, Gustav Fischer Verlag.

41. Rosebury, T.: Microorganisms indigenous to man, New York, 1962, McGraw-Hill Book Co.

42. Prévot, A. R.: Biologie des maladies dues aux anaérobies, Paris, 1955, Ernest Flammarion.

43. Prévot, A. R., Turpin, A., and Kaiser, P.: Les bactéries anaérobies, Paris, 1967, Dunod.

44. Beerens, H., and Tahon-Castel, M.: Infections humaines à bactéries anaérobies non toxigènes, Bruxelles, 1965, Presses Académiques Européennes.

45. Weinberg, M., Nativelle, R., and Prévot, A. R.: Les microbes anaérobies, Paris, 1937, Masson et Cie.

46. Dack, G. M.: Bacteriol. Rev. **4**:227, 1940.

47. Lödenkamper, H., and Stienen, G.: German Med. Monthly **1**:233, 1956.

48. Stokes, E. J.: Lancet **1**:668, 1958.

49. Martin, W. J.: Appl. Microbiol. **22**:1168, 1971.

50. Werner, H., and Pulverer, G.: Dtsch. Med. Wochenschr. **96**:1325, 1971.

51. Mitchell, A. A. B.: J. Clin. Pathol. **26**:738, 1973.

52. Leigh, D. A.: Lancet **1**:1081, 1973.

53. Clark, L. P., Marshall, H. A., and Ackerman, N. B.: Surg. Gynecol. Obstet. **138**:562, 1974.

54. Holdeman, L. V.: Personal communication, 1976.

55. Werner, H., Rintelen, G., and Kunstek-Santos, H.: Zentralbl. Bakteriol. [Orig. A] **231**:133, 1975.

56. Kaneuchi, C., Watanabe, K., Terada, A., et al.: Int. J. System. Bacteriol. **26**:195, 1976.

57. Cato, E. P., and Salmon, C. W.: Int. J. System. Bacteriol. **26**:205,1976.

58. Cato, E. P., and Johnson, J. L.: Int. J. System. Bacteriol. **26**:230, 1976.

59. Mitsuoka, T., Terada, A., Watanabe, K., et al.: Int. J. System. Bacteriol. **24**:35, 1974.

60. Bartlett, J. G., Alexander, J., Mayhew, J., et al.: Am. Rev. Respir. Dis. **114**:73, 1976.

60a. Wimberley, N. E., Faling, L. J., and Bartlett, J. G.: Am. Rev. Respir. Dis. **119**:337, 1979.

61. Bartlett, J. G., Sullivan-Sigler, N., Louie, T. J., et al.: J. Clin. Microbiol. **3**:133, 1976.

62. Atteberry, H. R., and Finegold, S. M.: Appl. Microbiol. **18**:558, 1969.

63. Sutter, V. L., Citron, D. M. and Finegold, S. M.: Wadsworth anaerobic bacteriology manual, ed. 3, St. Louis, 1980, The C. V. Mosby Co.

64. Attebery, H. R., and Finegold, S. M.: Am. J. Clin. Pathol. **53**:383, 1970.

65. Hungate, R. E.: Bacteriol. Rev. **14**:1, 1950.

66. Moore, W. E. C.: Int. J. System. Bacteriol. **16**:173, 1966.

67. Aranki, A., Syed, S. A., Kenney, E. B., et al.: Appl. Microbiol. **17**:568, 1969.

68. Rosenblatt, J. E., Fallon, A. M., and Finegold, S. M.: Appl. Microbiol. **25**:77, 1973.

69. Killgore, G. E., Starr, S. E., Del Bene, V. E., et al.: Am. J. Clin. Pathol. **59**:552, 1973.

70. Brewer, J. H., and Allgeier, D. L.: Science **147**:1033, 1965.

71. Martin, W. J.: Appl. Microbiol. **22**:1168, 1971.

72. Brewer, J. H., and Allgeier, D. L.: Appl. Microbiol. **14**:985, 1966.

72a. Livingston, S. J., Kominos, S. D., and Yee, R. B.: J. Clin. Microbiol. **7**:448, 1978.

73. Rosenblatt, J. E., and Stewart, P. R.: J. Clin. Microbiol. **1**:527, 1975.

74. Washington, J. A., II: Anaerobic blood cultures. In Lennette, E. A., Spaulding, E. H., and Truant, J. P., editors: Manual of clinical microbiology, ed. 2, Washington, D.C., 1974, American Society for Microbiology.

75. Holdeman, L. V., Cato, E. P., and Moore, W. E. C., editors: Anaerobe laboratory manual, ed. 4, Blacksburg, Va., 1977, Virginia Polytechnic Institute and State University.

76. Sutter, V. L., and Carter, W. T.: Am. J. Clin. Pathol. **58**:335, 1972.

77. Fay, G. D., and Barry, A. L.: Appl. Microbiol. **27**:603, 1974.

78. Schreckenberger, P. C., and Blazevic, D. J.: Appl. Microbiol. **28**:759, 1974.

79. Rosenblatt, J. E., Murray, P. R., Sonnenwirth, A. C., and Joyce, J. L.: Antimicrob. Agents Chemother. **15**:351, 1979.

87

ANTIMICROBIAL SUSCEPTIBILITY TESTS: LABORATORY TESTING IN SUPPORT OF ANTIMICROBIAL THERAPY

John M. Matsen

Susceptibility tests as generally carried out in the clinical microbiology laboratory are intended to assist the physician in determining appropriate antimicrobial patient therapy. Where specific susceptibility testing data are not available, the physician must rely upon information regarding the likely organisms in the specific disease state and upon the probable susceptibility pattern as predicted from previous laboratory susceptibility summary profiles. Some organisms such as group A *Streptococcus* will provide an almost absolute predictability with respect to susceptibility to penicillin. Other organisms have very little predictability for any of the commonly used antimicrobials. *Proteus rettgeri* is such an organism. The majority of organisms with which the physician must deal in clinical infection settings have a greater or lesser likelihood of susceptibility; this depends upon the specific antimicrobial agent. Factors relating to the antimicrobial, the organism, and the patient's underlying circumstances must be taken into consideration, when susceptibility results are known, in addition to the factors relating to effectiveness and preferred status for a given bacterial organism. Susceptibility data should also provide for the physician some corollary and some understanding of the level of antimicrobial necessary to effectively treat the specific infection.

In those settings where it is desirable to use a combination of antimicrobials, the classic approach to dilution or diffusion susceptibility testing may not provide helpful information regarding the preferred antimicrobial combination. However, special testing can be performed in which organisms are tested together, in varying concentrations, against the organism to be treated. In this specific instance of antimicrobial combination or synergy testing, the laboratory will expend additional personnel time, and for that reason these tests can be costly to perform.

The physician will occasionally need information relating to the behavior of an antimicrobial agent in serum, urine, or other body fluids. The laboratory should be willing to perform these assays or refer them to another laboratory; they can be useful as a predictor of the success of antimicrobial usage and as an indicator in attempting to prevent the toxicity that potentially accompanies the use of a number of therapeutic antimicrobial agents.

Both the estimation of therapeutic success and the prevention of toxicity may be important in the patient with normal excretory function; they are of more frequent concern in the patient who has compromised function. One is much more likely to require assay information when kidney or liver failure or dysfunction is present. Examples of this would include the use of an aminoglycoside antibiotic in a patient in whom the creatinine values were elevated, or the use of chloramphenicol in a newborn infant where the liver conjugating enzymes are immature.

The Schlichter test (serumcidal assay or serum bactericidal titer) has become increasingly important in many clinical microbiology laboratories. This assay is used in assessing therapy for endocarditis, osteomyelitis, or other serious bacterial infections. This test provides a quantitation of the combined effect of serum (or other body fluid) and antibiotic that the patient is receiving. In the absence of foreign body prosthesis or other foreign material, therapy can be anticipated to be successful if bacterial activity has been demonstrated in a dilution of 1:8 or 1:16 or greater. In staphylococcal infections it is preferable to have an activity of 1:32 or greater in endocarditis.

More rapid answers may be desirable both with susceptibility testing and for antimicrobial pharmacology monitoring. Assay information can be provided quickly in many instances. Currently instrumentation and other methodology exist that allow for susceptibility information within 3-6 hours following the isolation of an organism. Studies with urine and other body fluids have also demonstrated that where assessment by Gram stain has indicated the presence of a probable single organism type, susceptibility results can be generated within a short time. Studies I have performed would indicate that there is a substantial increase in the impact that susceptibility information has if it is received simultaneously with preliminary culture information or within a short time after the beginning of therapy in the patient. The longer the result is in arriving, the less the chance that the physician will use those data in altering or modifying therapy.

The pressure for rapid susceptibility and assay testing results has its practical concomitants; if physicians know that rapid answers can be forthcoming, they will learn to expect this service and will plan their therapeutic decisions accordingly.

The clinical laboratory in follow-up to providing rapid answers should also pay attention to the details of result transmission and reporting. The laboratory should call priority susceptibility or assay results in the event of demonstrated susceptibility changes or abnormal assay results or where resistance is demonstrated to the antimicrobial assay agent listed as therapy on the laboratory request slip.

On a routine basis, susceptibility results that do not become available until physicians have made their late afternoon rounds are likely to have a diminishing impact on physician antimicrobial usage. For this reason it is desirable to ensure that results are transmitted as quickly and as timely as possible to be convenient for physician review on the same day that they become available. Another consideration associated with susceptibility testing is that related to the nature of the information required or desired by physicians. Basically the choice relates to the timing of the results and to the consideration of quantitative versus qualitative information.

Until recently clinical laboratories have been limited in their capacity for quantitative susceptibility testing due to the fact that these tests were cumbersome and time consuming. The advent of the Steers[1] replicator and the practical approach, as developed by the Mayo Clinic,[2] have made this a useful quantitative method for those institutions with high susceptibility test volumes. Tube dilution capability, while always available to the routine laboratory, has been prohibitive because of the necessity of performing individual broth dilution sets for each antibiotic. With the advent of microbroth technics the broth dilution technic is now readily available to almost any laboratory choosing to use this form of susceptibility testing as a result of the development of microbroth methods.[3-9] The cost of microbroth testing is comparable to that of the disk diffusion test. Microbroth dilution plates, readily produced or purchased in bulk quantities, provide the appropriate laboratory utility and convenience.[10]

If numerical data are to be provided for physicians, a ready reference for understanding the meaning and interpretation of the numerical values being reported should also be made easily available to physicians. Most commercial firms now producing the bulk microbroth plates or the instrumentation for them will provide tables and reference data sufficient for appropriate physician education.

Disk diffusion testing can also provide a type of quantitative information if one is willing to record zone sizes and extrapolate the range of minimal inhibitory concentrations (MIC) by using previously derived regression plots.[11,12]

TERMINOLOGY

resistance level of susceptibility beyond that normally achieved in the human body by the usual dose given by the usual route of administration.

susceptibility level of antimicrobial at which a given strain or microorganism is inhibited in growth or killed by an antimicrobial compound.

susceptible organism organism inhibited or killed by the concentration of the antimicrobial usually achieved in the serum, other body fluids, and tissues of the patient given the usual dose of the antimicrobial by the usual route of administration.

minimal inhibitory concentration (MIC) (simplest terms) lowest concentration of antimicrobial at which no bacteria growth occurs for a given bacterial strain.

minimum lethal concentration (MLC) or minimum bactericidal concentration (MBC) lowest concentration of antimicrobial at which no viable bacterial cells remain for a given strain.

susceptibility categories the International Collaborative Group[13] proposed 4 susceptibility categories: groups I-IV. Wherever possible the differences between groups should be at least 3-4 full dilution steps in order to give them statistical validity. Each group would not necessarily be employed for each agent.

  group I instances with a high degree of bacterial susceptibility, with a strong likelihood of in vivo response when mild to moderately severe systemic infections were treated with the usual dosage of antibiotic. This would include orally administered antimicrobials where applicable. This group of organisms would be defined as "sensitive" without further qualifications.

  group II level of susceptibility that would conclude that the in vivo response was probable in systemic infections. The antimicrobial should be administered in high dosage or up to the limits of toxicity.

  group III level of susceptibility that would make in vivo response probable in the treatment of localized infections at a site where the antimicrobial would be present in increased concentration by virtue of pharmacokinetic behavior or by direct local application.

  group IV organisms with a degree of resistance that would make the in vivo response improbable. The organisms would be designated "resistant."

  NOTE: The International Collaborative Group further advocates that the application of these categories would be antimicrobial specific, with modifications to fit each agent's unique pharmacokinetic features.

antimicrobial assay determination of the concentration of an antimicrobial present in serum or other body fluid.

serum bactericidal assay   determination of the titer of serum that will, in combination with the antibiotic present in the serum, kill 99.9% of the organisms present as the best inoculum in the serum sample.

GUIDELINES FOR ORGANISM-ANTIMICROBIAL TESTING

The recommendations of the National Committee for Clinical Laboratory Standards and the Center for Disease Control[14,15] suggest the grouping of antimicrobials for susceptibility testing into those used for gram-positive organisms and those used for gram-negative organisms. The gram-negative organism panel may be further subdivided into a panel for gram-negative infections and urinary tract isolates and a separate panel for the pseudomonads and nonfermenter group of organisms as outlined in Table 87-1. Susceptibility testing should be performed only for potential pathogens or for those that are likely pathogens in unusual situations, such as in the compromised patient. Susceptibility testing should not be performed for organisms with predictable susceptibility patterns, as the potential for a laboratory error is greater than the likelihood of the presence of a resistant organism among some species. This point is illustrated by group A streptococci susceptibility testing with penicillin.

Any potential pathogen with a significant proportion of resistant strains will require suscepti-

Table 87-1. Proposed antimicrobials for routine testing

Gram-positive organisms	Enterobac-teriaceae	Other gram-negative organisms
Amikacin	Amikacin	Amikacin
Ampicillin	Ampicillin	Carbenicillin
Cephalothin	Carbenicillin	Colistin (or
	Cefamandole	polymyxin
	Cefoxitin	B)
Chloramphenicol	Cephalothin	Gentamicin
Clindamycin	Chloramphenicol	Tobramycin
Erythromycin	Colistin (or polymyxin B)	
Gentamicin	Gentamicin	Chloramphenicol*
Methicillin, nafcillin, or oxacillin	Tetracycline	Kanamycin*
Penicillin	Tobramycin	Sulfonamide* Tetracycline*
Tetracycline	Nitrofurantoin†	
Vancomycin	Sulfonamide†	
	Trimethoprim-sulfamethoxazole†‡	
	Kanamycin§	
	Nalidixic acid§	

*Reported for nonfermentative bacilli other than *Pseudomonas aeruginosa.*
†Reported for urinary tract isolates only.
‡Trimethoprim-sulfamethoxazole may be efficacious for organisms isolated from other sites.
§May be substituted for other agents, depending upon physician use and preference.

bility testing. Similarly, organisms known to develop resistance rapidly on exposure to antimicrobial agents should be tested again if isolated during therapy; likewise, certain antimicrobial agents such as nalidixic acid and streptomycin, are also known to possess a propensity for the development of organism resistance during their clinical use, organisms not generally considered pathogenic in association with infections in patients with immune deficiencies, etc. And in that context, isolates in those clinical circumstances may well require susceptibility testing that would not otherwise be necessary. Susceptibility testing on normal flora not acting as a pathogen in the clinical setting should be avoided, as should testing on mixed organism cultures.[16] In the latter instance, susceptibility testing should be delayed until the organisms have been separated on isolation plates.

The following organism groups represent those for which susceptibility testing is usually performed: *Bacteroides fragilis,* the *Enterobacteriaceae, Haemophilus influenzae* (ampicillin), *Neisseria gonorrhoeae* (in treatment-failure situations or where resistant organisms are endemic), *Pseudomonas* species and other gram-negative nonfermenter bacilli, *Staphylococcus aureus, S. epidermidis* (when associated with clinical disease), and other unpredictable and infrequently isolated organisms.

Physicians should be aware that most susceptibility data are provided as an inhibitory level. This is of potential concern in infections such as staphylococcal infections where organisms may have a pronounced difference between the inhibitory and bactericidal level for a variety of antibiotics, including those antimicrobials considered bactericidal. For most infections the inhibitory level is adequate information.

Susceptibility data may not provide answers with information that correlate with anticipated urinary tract antimicrobial concentrations. It is generally conceded that urinary tract infections respond to the level of antimicrobial present in the urine and not to the significantly lower level generally present in the serum.[17,18] The disk diffusion methodology may not provide the physician with sufficient information regarding achievable urine antimicrobial levels. Both quantitative inhibitory and bactericidal information can be of considerable assistance in staphylococcal infections, where it is proposed that up to 40% of the strains isolated from clinically significant infections may be termed "tolerant," with a considerable variation and spread between the inhibitory and bactericidal concentrations. Broth dilution testing also allows for the "second-step" determinations necessary for obtaining bactericidal end points.

Testing media

Presently there exists considerable variation in the different testing formulations. There may be significant lot-to-lot and manufacturer-to-manufacturer variations with specific media.

Whereas Mueller-Hinton medium has been chosen because of its growth-potentiating properties for *Neisseria* and for other fastidious organisms, it is vulnerable to lot-to-lot and manufacturer-to-manufacturer variations. There have been continued problems in susceptibility testing media performance. Antibiotics may be outside the limits of quality control as established by regulating agencies and advisory committees.[15] This may relate to cation differences or to the digestion process necessary for the production of the protein components of the media. Much remains to be done in terms of providing a stoichiometrically precise medium, and in terms of the uniform manufacturing processes that will be necessary for a more consistent end product.

The performance of media to be used by a laboratory should be regularly assessed by appropriate quality control means. Media manufacturers should be urged to abide by the constraints of adhering to media performance standards so as to assure a more uniform end result in clinical laboratories.

GENERAL QUALITY ASSURANCE CONSIDERATIONS

All parameters of susceptibility testing should be regularly evaluated in order to ensure confidence in the performance of the test. This section will outline general quality control considerations. Specific methodology quality assurance suggestions will be grouped together after the method description section.

Stock organisms

A collection of all organisms needed to check media, the actual tests themselves, and any needed reagents should be carefully maintained by each laboratory. Cultures may be maintained for the *Enterobacteriaceae* on sealed agar deeps; these may be set at 25 C in the dark or may be maintained at −70 C or in a lyophilized state. Stock cultures of those organisms listed below with ATCC designation may be obtained from the American Type Culture Collection (ATCC) (12301 Parklawn Drive, Rockville, Md. 20852).

1. Disk diffusion susceptibility test: *S. aureus* ATCC 25923, *Escherichia coli* ATCC 25922, *Pseudomonas aeruginosa* ATCC 27853.
2. Broth dilution testing: *S. aureus* ATCC 29213, *Streptococcus faecalis* ATCC 29212.
3. Autobac I: *S. aureus* ATCC 25923, *P. aeruginosa* ATCC 27853, *E. coli* ATCC 29194.
4. Antimicrobial assays: *Bacillus subtilis* ATCC 6633, *Klebsiella pneumoniae* ATCC 27799, *Clostridium perfringens* UUMC 9758.

Stock organism storage

Enterics. Enterics can be stored on small soybean-casein digest agar slants at room temperature in the dark; if not sealed with paraffin, these should be transferred weekly or twice monthly to new slants, or as needed. Reference strains of these organisms are kept in a lyophilized state in the event that the performance of the organisms should change. Both the *E. coli* (ATCC 25922) and the *K. pneumoniae* (ATCC 27799) have proven to be extremely stable over many years. The *P. aeruginosa* control strain, if subcultured daily, has a tendency to develop colonies resistant to carbenicillin. It is suggested[19] that this subculturing be limited to once per week and that a fresh subculture be activated from lyophilized, frozen, or otherwise maintained storage means.

Gram-positive cocci. The *S. aureus* (ATCC 25923) and *S. faecalis* (ATCC 29212) are maintained on sheep blood at room temperature or transferred weekly or when new sheep blood plates are tested. Reference specimens are maintained in a lyophilized or frozen state in the event of question about organism performance.

C. perfringens. *C. perfringens* can be maintained at room temperature in chopped meat media and needs to be transferred to new chopped meat media only once every 3 months.

Media sterility

A portion of each lot of plate media prepared in the clinical laboratory should be incubated to evaluate sterility. Plating media purchased from commercial sources also requires sterility checking. Contamination is a not infrequent problem with the large Mueller-Hinton plates used for disk diffusion susceptibility testing.

Medium performance

Mueller-Hinton plates are tested with both *E. coli* (ATCC 25922) and *S. aureus* (ATCC 25923). These are incubated in an aerobic environment for 24 hours at 35 C. Other parameters to be assessed relate to a pH of 7.2-7.4 at 25 C and an agar depth of 4-5 ml. The surface of these plates should be even and the depth of the agar uniform. Mueller-Hinton broth is tested with the same control organisms as the Mueller-Hinton plates.

It should be noted here that media performance is also tested through the use of antimicrobials in solution, in the agar itself, or as delivered through the vehicle of paper disks. This will be discussed with each method description.

Antimicrobial stock solutions

1. Stock antimicrobials are frozen in readily usable aliquots. Once thawed they are not to be reused.
2. Control organisms should be tested each time a new lot of antimicrobial is prepared or each time a new vial of antimicrobial disks is to be used. The vial of disks should be tested the day previous to its actual insertion into the laboratory usage rotation.
3. Carefully label all antimicrobial material as to the date of expiration, the date received in the laboratory, and the date opened.

4. Discard unused lots of stock solutions after the expiration date. Stocks can be held at −20 C or below for 6 months with the exception of the penicillins and nitrofurantoin.

5. All antimicrobial disks should be frozen at −20 C in desiccated containers. After removal from the freezer these disks should be allowed to equilibrate to room temperature before the containers are opened.

Proficiency testing

Proficiency testing for clinical laboratories becomes an integral part of the monitoring of actual performance. In this context the program conducted by the College of American Pathologists seems to be the one most readily available to laboratories in the United States. The College of American Pathologists will send out proficiency testing for susceptibility disk diffusion testing on a regular quarterly basis. The Center for Disease Control also has a proficiency testing program available to a limited number of clinical laboratories.

DISK DIFFUSION SUSCEPTIBILITY TESTING
Principles

The disk diffusion susceptibility test method involves the addition of a known amount of an antimicrobial agent to a small, absorbent paper disk measuring 6 mm in diameter. The placement of this disk on an agar surface previously streaked with the organism to be tested will result in a concentric zone of inhibited growth for susceptible organisms. The concentric zone of inhibition that results when the test organism is streaked on the agar plate surface, prior to the application of the disk, has been shown to relate linearly to the MIC for most antimicrobials as measured by dilution susceptibility testing.[11,13] Through this relationship the measurement of these zones can be used to predict the in vivo response of the organism.

This correlation is of great significance, and an understanding of this principle is pertinent if one is to truly comprehend the interpretive basis of the test. The histogram that results when one plots these 2 values for each of the test organisms allows for regression analysis.

Fig. 87-1 represents such a regression analysis. A collection of organisms, usually more than 100-150 strains representing the common species of bacteria for which the antimicrobial agent might be used, is tested by both disk diffusion and agar or broth 2-fold dilution methods. Organisms are ideally chosen to provide MIC values evenly spread over the range of achievable body fluid concentrations and to represent all the species for whom use of the antibiotic might be anticipated. Organisms for whom no zone of inhibition occurs are excluded from the calculations of the regression lines. In Fig. 87-1 the ordinate (y axis) denotes the 2-fold MIC susceptibility test results, whereas the abscissa (x axis) is a non-log scale of the disk inhibition zone. The scatter of values for most antimicrobials is linear, and the formula of least squares will provide a mathematical computation of the "regression line" (line of best fit) shown in the figure. This principle does not apply in those situations where the relationship is not linear. In the 2-fold dilution test, as used in this graph, the average "true" value of the MIC is one-half of a 2-fold dilution lower than the observed value. Organism values will be distributed on either side of the regression line, and the organism pattern is a consideration in the derivation of susceptibility category breakpoints.

By defining the achievable serum levels of the antibiotic using the commonly employed dosage given by the usual routes of administration, and by allowing for appropriate organism effect, one arrives at the susceptible MIC value. The zone size corresponding to the MIC value that represents the microgram per milliliter level associated in vivo with organism eradication becomes the susceptibility breakpoint. The intermediate and resistant breakpoints are derived by taking into account factors relating to the toxicity and pharmacokinetics of the individual compounds in addition to the information provided in the regression analysis. The intermediate zone—in addition to providing guidelines indicating the need for maximum dosage requirement if that particular antimicrobial is to be used—also serves as a zone to minimize the misinterpretation of sensitive or resistant values due to the phenomenon of organism scatter.

Pertinent considerations

Indications for disk diffusion susceptibility testing are similar to the indications for susceptibility testing in general. Testing is carried out for those organisms for which there is not a predictable response for a given antibiotic. It follows, then, that one tests organisms such as the *Staphylococcus*, the *Enterobacteriaceae*, *H. influenzae*, *Pseudomonas* species, and other unusual organisms. One does not test, for example, *Streptococcus pyogenes* (group A β-hemolytic) against penicillin, erythromycin, etc. because of the predictable susceptibility. There would be a far greater chance of a laboratory error than of finding a resistant strain in this instance.

In addition to the above recommendations it is also important to understand that the standardized disk diffusion method as now recommended should be used only for rapidly growing organisms for which an end point can be determined within an 18- to 24-hour period. Prolonged incubation beyond that time may result in antimicrobial alteration sufficient for erroneous end-point determinations to result.

There are organisms and antimicrobials that require special test conditions. *H. influenzae*, for example, requires the addition of special nutrients. Streptococci[20] are notoriously poor-growing organisms on Mueller-Hinton medium and

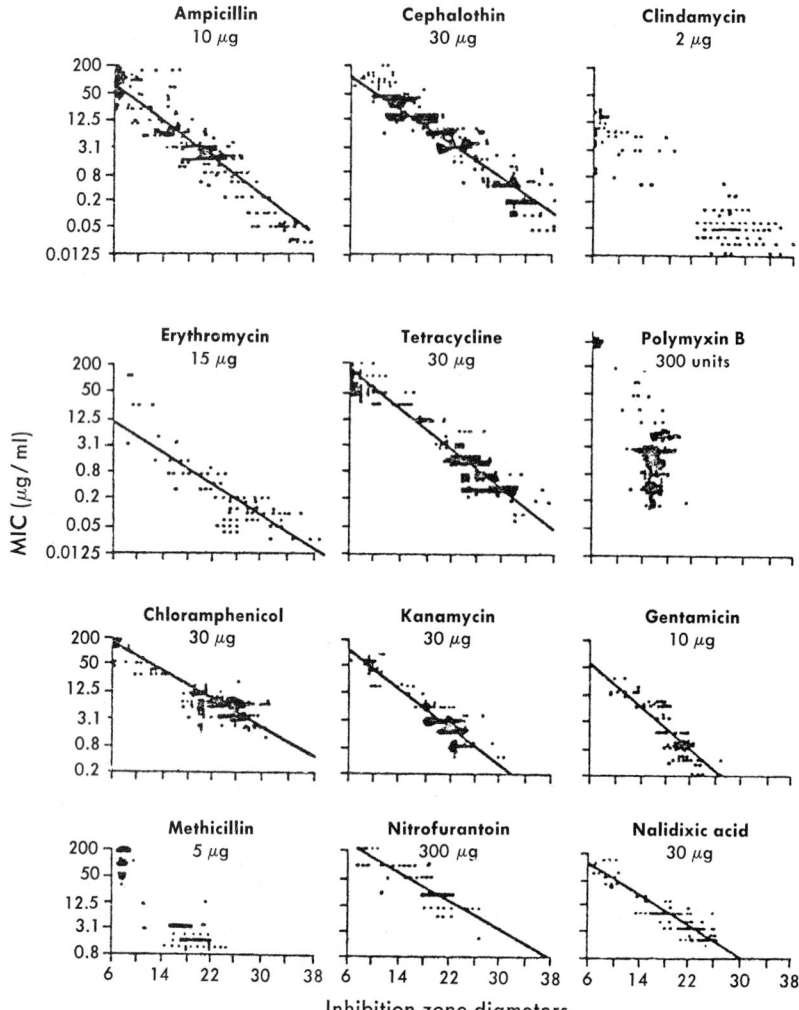

Fig. 87-1. Relationship of zone diameter to agar dilution MIC with some commonly used antimicrobics. **Note:** All except polymyxin and gentamicin show combined data from clinical laboratories of the Universities of Minnesota and Washington; disc content shown below each antimicrobic; polymyxin MICs in U/ml. (Work supported in part by grant RR267 from the Biotechnology Research Branch of the National Institutes of Health. We acknowledge the assistance of Dr. Donald Connelly. For calculation of regression lines see text.)

require the addition of 5% sheep blood. For the testing of sulfonamides or the combination of trimethoprim-sulfamethoxazole, blood additives should be used due to the antagonistic effect of the para-aminobenzoic acid present in blood. When testing is to be carried out with *N. meningitidis* and sulfonamides, special parameters also apply. Agar dilution testing should be employed for *N. meningitidis* as the penicillin disk diffusion susceptibility testing is not yet standardized for this antibiotic-organism combination. Susceptibility testing should not be done with either of the methenamine salts due to the lack of correlation between in vivo and in vitro conditions.

The disk-diffusion method can be used for anaerobic organism susceptibility testing. Special considerations apply for interpretive zone diameters and standardized test conditions when testing anaerobic isolates (see anaerobic susceptibility).

It is recommended at present that only 1 agent from each group of closely related antimicrobials be tested, and due to the Food and Drug Administration action, usually only 1 agent is available. In general this is sufficient for most testing situations, although there are specific instances in which the values derived from 1 agent do not apply to the other related antimicrobials. Dilution testing is indicated in those circumstances where this lack of reciprocity is clinically important.

Table 87-1 outlines general guidelines for the selection of antimicrobials to be tested routinely against rapidly growing aerobic and facultatively anaerobic bacteria.

Recommended methods for disk diffusion testing
Agar diffusion surface-streak method

The high-content disk susceptibility method as proposed by Bauer et al.[21] has now been modified in the recommendations of the FDA[22,23] and the National Committee for Clinical Laboratory Standards.[15] The method recommended here is essentially that of the latter group and varies little from the FDA method. If accurate, reproducible results are to be anticipated, the method must be followed closely.

Media. Although Mueller-Hinton, the recommended medium,[13] supports the growth of most organisms for which susceptibility testing will be done, 5% defibrinated sheep, horse, or other animal blood should be used to provide for appropriate growth of streptococci and other fastidious organisms; 5% laked horse blood–Mueller-Hinton agar, or Mueller-Hinton agar supplemented by Fildes digest or other similar nutrient additive should be employed for testing *Haemophilus* strains.

Plate preparation. It is recommended that 150 mm Petri plates be used, although current recommendations do provide that 100 mm plates can be substituted. Agar depth should be between 4 and 6 mm[24] (20-25 ml agar is required for the 100 mm plates and 70-80 ml for the 150 mm plates). Prepared plates should be stored at 4 C in cellophane wrapping and should be used within a 2-week period. Immediately prior to use plates should be "dried" in an incubator for 30 minutes to facilitate removal of excess surface moisture.

Inoculum preparation. An inoculating needle or loop is touched to 4 or 5 colonies of the organism and inoculated into 4-5 ml of a suitable broth medium (soybean-casein digest or tryptose phosphate broths are recommended). The broth is allowed to incubate at 35 C until the turbidity of the culture compares to that of the recommended turbidity standard prepared by adding 0.5 ml 0.048M $BaCl_2$ (1.175% wt/vol $BaCl_2 \cdot 2H_2O$) to 99.5 ml 0.36N H_2SO_4 (1% vol/vol). The standard should be agitated on a vortex mixer immediately prior to use. Unless the standard is contained in heat-sealed glass tubes it should probably be replaced every 6 months. If appropriately sealed, the standard may last indefinitely.[25] The turbidity of the culture may be adjusted by the addition of sterile saline or broth (if excessive), or additional colonies (if inadequate), providing they are well isolated and are morphologically indistinguishable from those originally selected. The use of a white background and contrasting black lines in combination with an adequate light source greatly facilitates the adjustment of culture turbidity. The modified laboratory view box[25] facilitates the handling of the culture tubes and the standard during the turbidity adjustment. The standard inoculum suspension should be inoculated within 15-20 minutes.

Medium inoculation and disk placement. A sterile cotton swab on a wooden applicator stick is immersed into the standardized inoculum suspension. Excess broth is expressed by pressing and rotating the swab against the inside of the suspension tube. The swab is then streaked evenly in 3 directions on the surface of the agar plate. A final circular motion is made around the agar rim with the cotton swab. This inoculum is allowed to dry for 3-5 minutes, and disks are then applied, either by a mechanical dispenser or by hand using sterile forceps. After placement the disks are pressed firmly and gently to the agar surface. The spatial arrangement of the disks should be such as to obviate the development of overlapping zones of inhibition. This limits the number of disks that can be placed, and the generally recommended limit is 12-13 disks (9 in the outer ring) for a 150 mm plate.

Quality control. Quality control should include all facets of the testing procedure. The Mueller-Hinton medium in the plates should be of appropriate depth (4-6 mm), and excessive drying should be prevented. Plates should be regularly checked for appropriate pH. Disks should be stored frozen (−12-20 C) and should be removed from the freezer as individual cartridges, and the cartridge in use should be kept in a dessicated conatiner at 4 C and allowed to equilibrate to room temperature prior to use each day. Disks should be purchased through a local distributor where storage conditions (4 C) are known or should be purchased directly from the manufacturer. The practice of receiving disks from pharmaceutical representatives is to be avoided because of the unknown storage conditions prior to receipt. A representative disk from each cartridge should be tested with control bacterial strains (*S. aureus* ATCC 25923 for antimicrobials used against gram-positive organisms, *E. coli* ATCC 25922, and *P. aeruginosa* ATCC 27853 for agents to be tested against *Pseudomonas* and related organisms) prior to the use of other disks from that cartridge for routine testing. Control bacterial strains should be tested on a frequent basis, ideally each time a set of susceptibility tests is performed. An easily accessible, easily readable chart is recommended to facilitate recording and interpretation of quality assurance testing. Limits of zone variation for the control of *S. aureus*, *E. coli*, and *P. aeruginosa* are given in Table 87-2; however, it should be emphasized that these excursion limits are rather broad. It is recommended that each laboratory establish its own narrower limits of control.

A separate sheep blood—agar plate should be streaked in quadrants; i.e., 4 or 5 organisms can be put on 1 plate, with the swab used for streaking the surface of each Mueller-Hinton plate. This is done in order to check for inoculum purity.

Interpretation. Zone diameters are measured with a ruler or calipers on the undersurface of the Petri dish under reflected light. If blood has been

Table 87-2. Susceptibility of control strains

Antibiotic	Disk potency	Zone diameter of inhibition (mm)		
		S. aureus (ATCC 25923)	*E. coli* (ATCC 25922)	*P. aeruginosa* (ATCC 27853)
Amikacin	10 μg	18-24	18-24	15-20
Ampicillin	10 μg	24-35	15-20	—
Bacitracin	10 U	17-22	—	—
Carbenicillin	100 μg	—	24-29	20-24
Cephalothin	30 μg	25-37	18-23	—
Chloramphenicol	30 μg	19-26	21-27	6
Clindamycin	2 μg	23-29	—	—
Colistin	10 μg	—	11-15	12-16
Erythromycin	15 μg	23-30	8-14	—
Gentamicin	10 μg	19-27	19-26	16-21
Kanamycin	30 μg	19-26	17-25	6
Methicillin	5 μg	17-22	—	—
Nalidixic acid	30 μg	—	21-25	—
Neomycin	30 μg	18-26	17-23	—
Nitrofurantoin	300 μg	—	20-24	—
Penicillin G	10 U	26-37	—	—
Polymyxin B	300 U	7-13	12-16	—
Streptomycin	10 μg	14-22	12-20	—
Sulfisoxazole	250 or 300 μg	23-27	22-26	6
Tetracycline	30 μg	19-28	18-25	9-14
Trimethoprim-sulfamethoxazole	1.25 μg 23.75 μg	24-32	24-32	—
Tobramycin	10 μg	19-29	18-26	19-25
Vancomycin	30 μg	15-19	—	—

From Thornsberry, C., and Hawkings, T. M.: Agar disc dilution susceptibility testing procedure, PHS, Atlanta, 1977, Center for Disease Control.

added to the Mueller-Hinton agar, the zones are measured from the surface of the agar after removing the cover. The end point is complete inhibition of growth as determined visually, except in the case of sulfonamides where organisms may grow through several generations before inhibition occurs. In this instance slight growth (80% or greater inhibition) is disregarded and the margin of heavy growth is measured. The swarming of *Proteus* is also disregarded, and the margin of heavy growth that is usually clearly apparent is also measured under these circumstances.

Whereas preliminary readings may be obtained as soon as growth patterns become apparent (usually 6-8 hours), readings made at this time should be confirmed at 18-24 hours. Measurement of zones should include the entire diameter of the zone, including the disk. Should colonies be seen within the zone of inhibition, the purity check plate should be analyzed. If it is obvious that more than 1 organism is present, the test should be repeated. If the culture is pure, the colonies are regarded as significant and included in zone size measurement.

Table 87-3 contains the interpretive zone size information along with the MIC correlates for the zone size breakpoints.

Should a physician desire quantitative information, these MIC correlates can be referred to, as can the regression line plots included as Fig. 87-1. One may give a range of MIC values for any given zone size based upon these regression line plots if one strictly adheres to the recommended method.

Agar overlay diffusion method

An alternative method of inoculating disk diffusion test plates is the agar overlay method.[26] This method is also applicable only to tests with commonly isolated, rapidly growing bacterial pathogens such as *S. aureus, Enterobacteriaceae, P. aeruginosa,* and other nonfermentative gram-negative bacilli.

Plate preparation. Mueller-Hinton agar is prepared in 150 × 15 mm plastic Petri plates and poured to a depth of 4 mm.

Inoculum preparation. Four to 5 isolated colonies of the same morphologic type are selected from a primary isolation culture plate. A turbid suspension is prepared in 0.5 ml of brain-heart infusion broth in a 13 × 100 mm tube, which is then incubated at 35-37 C in a water bath or heating block for 4-8 hours. This suspension is mixed well, after incubation, and a 0.001 loopful is transferred to a 9 ml aqueous solution of agar that has been held no longer than 8 hours in a 45-50 C heating block (16 × 125 mm screw-capped tubes are routinely used). Tubes not used within this time are discarded. The melted agar, now inoculated with the test organism, is mixed by being inverted several times before being poured over the surface of the 150 × 15 mm plastic Petri plate containing Mueller-Hinton agar at a depth of 4 mm. The thin layer of melted agar will solidify too quickly on the previously prepared Mueller-Hinton plate unless the plate is first brought to room temperature. The completed plates should be left for 3-5 minutes on a flat surface in order to harden properly before the disks to be placed on the surface are applied as described above.

Incubation. After the disks are placed on the agar surface and pressed to set them, the plates are inverted and within 15 minutes are placed in a 35 C incubator. The plates are incubated for 16-18 hours.

Interpretation. The plates are read in a manner similar to that employed with the surface-streak disk diffusion method, by employing the interpretive criteria contained in Table 87-3.

Included in the rationale in the establishment of sensitive, intermediate, and resistant values is the understanding that they apply for systemic infections (except for nitrofurantoin, sulfonamides, and nalidixic acid). In situations where an antibiotic dose may be safely increased, concentrations far in excess of the levels considered in the establishment of these interpretive values

Table 87-3. Kirby-Bauer zone diameter interpretive standards[15,21-23]

Antimicrobial agent	Disk potency	Inhibition zone diameter (mm)			Approximate MIC correlates	
		Resistant	Intermediate	Sensitive	Resistant	Susceptible
Amikacin[27,]*	30 µg	≤14	15-16	≥17	≥16 µg/ml	≤8 µg/ml
Ampicillin†:						
Enterobacteriaceae and enterococci	10 µg	≤11	12-13	≥14	≥32 µg/ml	≤8 µg/ml
Staphylococcus and penicillin-sensitive organisms	10 µg	≤20	21-28	≥29	≥2.0 µg/ml penicillinase‡	≤0.2 µg/ml
Haemophilus	10 µg	≤19	—	≥20	—	≤2.0 µg/ml
Carbenicillin:						
Proteus and *E. coli*	100 µg	≤17	18-22	≥23	≥32 µg/ml	≤16 µg/ml
P. aeruginosa§	100 µg	≤11	12-14	≥15	≥250 µg/ml	≤125 µg/ml
Cefamandole	30 µg	≤14	15-17	≥18	>32 µg/ml	≤18 µg/ml
Cefoxitin	30 µg	≤14	15-17	≥18	>32 µg/ml	≤18 µg/ml
Cephalothin‖	30 µg	≤14	15-17	≥18	≥32 µg/ml	≤10 µg/ml
Chloramphenicol	30 µg	≤12	13-17	≥18	≥25 µg/ml	≤12.5 µg/ml
Clindamycin¶	2 µg	≤14	15-16	≥17	≥2 µg/ml	≤1 µg/ml
Colistin✗	10 µg	≤8	9-10	≥11	—	—
Erythromycin	15 µg	≤13	14-17	≥18	≥8 µg/ml	≤2 µg/ml
Gentamicin	10 µg	≤12	13-14	≥15	≥6 µg/ml	≤6 µg/ml
Kanamycin	30 µg	≤13	14-17	≥18	≥25 µg/ml	≤6 µg/ml
Methicillin**	5 µg	≤9	10-13	≥14	—	≤3 µg/ml
Nafcillin	1 µg	≤10	11-12	≥13	—	≤3 µg/ml
Nalidixic acid††	30 µg	≤13	14-18	≥19	≥32 µg/ml	≤12 µg/ml
Neomycin	30 µg	≤12	13-16	≥17	—	≤10 µg/ml
Nitrofurantoin††	300 µg	≤14	15-16	≥17	≥100 µg/ml	≤25 µg/ml
Penicillin G: ‡‡						
Staphylococci	10 U	≤20	21-28	≥29	Penicillinase‡	≤0.1 µg/ml
Other organisms	10 U	≤11	12-21	≥22	≥32 µg/ml	≤1.5 µg/ml
Polymyxin B#	300 U	≤8	9-11	≥12	≥50 U/ml	
Streptomycin	10 µg	≤11	12-14	≥15	≥15 µg/ml	≤6 µg/ml
Sulfonamides:						
N. meningitidis only	250/300 µg			≥40		
Other organisms††	250/300 µg	≤12	13-16	≥17	≥350 µg/ml	≤100 µg/ml
Tetracycline	30 µg	≤14	15-18	≥19	≥12 µg/ml	≤4 µg/ml
Tobramycin	10 µg	≤11	12-13	≥14	≥11 µg/ml	≤14 µg/ml
Trimethoprim-sulfamethoxazole[15]	1.25 µg/ 23.75 µg	≤10	11-15	≥17=S/ ≥23=SS	≥200 µg/ml	≤35 µg/ml
Vancomycin	30 µg	≤9	10-11	≥12	—	≤5 µg/ml

*Tentative standard from Bristol Laboratories, Syracuse, N.Y.

†Class disk for ampicillin, hetacillin, and amoxicillin.

‡Resistant strains of *S. aureus* produce penicillinase. There are significant reports of ampicillin-resistant *Haemophilus* strains that produce penicillinase.

§Tentative standards.

‖Class disks for cephalothin, cephaloridine, cephalexin, cefazolin, cephacetrile, cephradine, and cephapirin.

¶The clindamycin disk is used to test susceptibility to both clindamycin and lincomycin. Due to the greater activity of clindamycin, separate interpretative categories of zone diameters are recommended when reporting susceptibility to lincomycin as follows: ≤16=R, 17-20=I, ≥21=S.

✗Colistin and polymyxin B diffuse poorly in agar, and thus the accuracy of diffusion tests is less than that found with other antimicrobics; MIC correlates cannot be calculated reliably from regression analysis.

**Class disk for penicillinase-resistant penicillins (i.e., methicillin, cloxacillin, dicloxacillin, oxacillin, and nafcillin). Nafcillin and oxacillin disks are also available.

††Urinary tract infections only.

‡‡Class disk for penicillin G, phenoxymethylpenicillin, and phenethicillin.

may be reached. Similarly, the concentration of certain antibiotics in the urine may result in urinary levels manyfold higher than the level considered as the resistant value breakpoint in systemic infection. Information is available elsewhere, and space will not allow this chapter to detail the variety of pharmacologic features necessary to outline the approaches that can be made with each group of antibiotics. Suffice it to say that the interpretive values presented in Table 87-3 are rough guidelines that include, in most situations, certain "safety" factors to cover the biologic differences encountered in the organism and in the human host response to the organism and to the antibiotic. Furthermore, the disk producing the greatest zone of inhibition does not necessarily indicate that that particular agent is the agent of choice for a given pathogen. Regression histograms can be used as described elsewhere in this chapter, and the applicability of these curves can be checked by using quality control organism plots to verify that these results are reproducible in one's own laboratory. For further information on regression plots the reader is referred to more detailed sources of information.[11,12,28]

Potential method mistakes

Mistakes can occur with the disk method that may compromise accuracy and reliability, and 1 error may obviously compound another. Some of the more common mistakes are outlined below:

1. Failure to use Mueller-Hinton medium
2. Use of outdated medium or plates
3. Failure to pH test Mueller-Hinton medium and other media-preparation mistakes
4. Use of overnight culture growth without standardization of inoculum or use of improper density-standardization procedures
5. Inaccurate turbidity reference standard (most often due to incorrect preparation, leakage, or evaporation)
6. Failure to express excess fluid from swab used for plate inoculation
7. Excessive time lapse between culture standardization and plate inoculation
8. Outdated or improperly stored disks[29]
9. Prolonged time lapse in applying disks after plates have been inoculated
10. Delays in incubation following inoculation and disk placement that allow antibiotic "prediffusion" prior to optimal organism growth conditions
11. Failure to use quality control strains or use of improper quality control strains
12. Testing of mixed cultures
13. Transcription errors
14. Testing of organisms that require anaerobic incubation or that are so slow in their growth as to preclude a zone reading within an 18- to 24-hour time frame

These problems can be avoided by close adherence to the recommended methodology.

DIRECT SUSCEPTIBILITY TESTING ON CLINICAL MATERIALS

Routine direct application of clinical material is to be avoided, except in emergency situations such as cerebrospinal fluid or other body fluid specimens that result in gram smears indicating that a pure culture may be expected. Mixtures of organisms, common in many specimens, may produce inaccurate interpretations.[16,30] It may be difficult to standardize the inoculum from direct clinical material.[16,31,32] The use of a "purity check" plate will be of great assistance in these emergency situations, as will an assessment of the nature of the "lawn" of inoculum on the susceptibility test plate. Results reported from such emergency tests should, unless a pure culture results and appropriate inoculum has been achieved, be reported as preliminary or tentative and should be repeated and confirmed using one of the recommended methods.[33]

DILUTION TESTING
General considerations
Stock solutions

The preparation of stock solutions requires obtaining standard preparation from either the manufacturer or from laboratory supply firms (also available from United States Pharmacopeia Convention, 12601 Twinbrook Parkway, Rockville, Md. 20852) prepared to provide these testing materials. Antimicrobial preparations meant for human administration are, for the most part, not acceptable as laboratory testing reagents as they may be chemically impure and inaccurate as to stated activity. Laboratory testing materials should:

1. Have a date of expiration clearly visible on the container.
2. Have a readily apparent statement of activity in micrograms or international units per milligram or milliliter of preparation.
3. Be dated on arrival in the laboratory.
4. Be dated when opened.
5. Be stored in a desiccator after opening.
6. Be carefully weighed in an analytical balance or measured with pipets of appropriate volumetric capacity.
7. Be sterilized by membrane filtration when necessary.
8. Be maintained at −20 C or colder.
9. Be dissolved or diluted in the appropriate solvent and diluent (Table 87-4 indicates solvents and diluents to be used in preparation of stock antibiotic solutions from antibiotic powder.)

Inoculum standardization

The use of a barium sulfate standard for standardization is vulnerable to inefficient time expenditure, errors in formation, and, therefore, turbidity inaccuracies, and to visual aberrations due to improper mixing. To ensure the highest likelihood of appropriate efficiency and accuracy, the following steps should be followed:

Table 87-4. Preparation and storage of antimicrobial agents*†

Antimicrobial	Solvent	Dilution
Amikacin	Water‡	Water
Amphotericin B	Dimethyl sulfoxide	Water, adjust to pH 9.0 with NaOH
Ampicillin	Phosphate buffer, pH 8.0, 0.1M§	Phosphate buffer, pH 6.0, 0.1M
Carbenicillin	Water	Water
Cephalothin	Phosphate buffer, pH 6.0, 0.1M	Water
Chloramphenicol	Ethanol	Water
Clindamycin	Water	Water
Cycloserine	Water	Water
Erythromycin	Ethanol	Water
Ethambutol	Water	Water
5-Fluorocytosine	Saline, 0.85%	Saline, 0.85%
Gentamicin	Water‡	Water
Isoniazid	Water	Water
Kanamycin	Water‡	Water
Nalidixic acid	1N NaOH	Water
Nitrofurantoin	Dimethylformamide	Water
Oxacillin	Water	Water
Penicillin‖	Water	Water
Polymyxin B	Water	Water
Rifampin	Dimethyl sulfoxide	Phosphate buffer, pH 7.0
Streptomycin	Water	Water
Sulfonamides	10% NaOH + Hot water	Water
Tetracyclines	Water	Water
Tobramycin	Water	Water
Vancomycin	Water	Water

*Modified from Washington, J. A., II, Warren, E., and Karlson, A. G.: Appl. Microbiol. **24**:1013, 1973.
†Stock solutions are stored in freezer at −35 C. At this temperature, stock solutions of most antibiotics (except penicillins) are stable for approximately 6 mo.
‡Aminoglycoside antibiotics may also be dissolved in phosphate buffer pH 8.0, 0.1M.
§Phosphate buffers should be kept in refrigerator for use as diluents.
‖Penicillins should be replaced monthly.

1. Turbidity standard is prepared by adding 0.5 ml 0.048M $BaCl_2$ (1.175%, wt/vol, $BaCl_2 \cdot 2H_2O$) to 99.5 ml 0.36N H_2SO_4 (1%, vol/vol). This is then equivalent to one-half density of MacFarland no. 1 standard.
2. This should be placed in sealed tube to avoid evaporation fluid loss.[25]
3. Standard should be mixed with vortex mixer prior to each use.
4. Actual process of inoculum standardization can be enhanced and time conserved by utilizing the modified Rh view box apparatus described by Stemper and Matsen[34]; this reference provides both a narrative description of use and a blueprint of the design.
5. Use of a black-on-white background, either as a feature of the apparatus referred to above or separately, will also facilitate turbidity comparison.

Agar dilution

The agar dilution method, as described by the International Collaborative Study Group,[13] has been used on a routine clinical basis primarily for research purposes and in larger clinical laboratories. It probably requires 20 tests out of the 32-36 possible per plate series to make this particular method economical on a day-to-day use basis. If the laboratory is performing more than 20 tests per day, this method has the potential of being the most economical of all the susceptibility test methodologies.

Instrumentation. This method requires the agar-replicating device of Steers et al.[1] in order to achieve the economical advantage described above. Adaptations of the instrumentation are possible using a spring-loaded device that allows for a more rapid and potentially more uniform application of the inoculum to the individual plates. In addition the device as initially described has been modified to use a larger, square plate that provides for 36 inoculum implants[35] (Melrose Machine Shop, Woodlyn, Pa.). The seed plate and inoculating prongs can be made out of either aluminum or stainless steel. It has been my experience that the aluminum construction is much more vulnerable to erosion and pitting. The care of the instrumentation is important. Washington et al.[35] advocate soaking the seed plate and inoculating prongs overnight in 70% ethyl alcohol after scrubbing each section clean with a brush. The sections are then wrapped in a cloth towel and placed in a large glass Petri dish and autoclaved prior to use. Glass rings, sometimes called "Raschig" rings (12 mm × 12 mm, Scientific Glass Apparatus, Bloomfield, N.J.) can be placed around the inoculum of spreading *Proteus* strains in order to inhibit their dispersion across the agar test plate. These rings can be serviced by boiling in water for 20 minutes and then soaking in 70% ethyl alcohol prior to use.

Media. Mueller-Hinton agar (MHA), trypticase-soy agar (TSA), or other agar media may be used for this method. One may also add chocolatized, lysed, or peptic digest of blood for those organisms that require this enrichment. Blood thus modified is usually added in a 5% vol/vol amount. Brain-heart infusion with 5% sheep blood or the medium of Wilkins and Chalgren[36] can be used for testing anaerobic organisms.

Performance standards should be established for each of the several antimicrobials to be used. Cation differences among the 3 media mentioned above may be substantial; in this context, performance—especially with the aminoglycoside antibiotics—can vary from lot to lot, manufacturer to manufacturer, and medium to medium.[37,38]

Antimicrobial preparations. Individual antimicrobials are prepared in sterile distilled water for later addition to the melted agar medium. The simplest approach to this task is to follow a systematized guide such as that presented in Table

Table 87-5. Modified agar dilution—antimicrobial dilution guide[13]*

Antimicrobial solution (µg or IU/ml)	Stock volume (ml)	Volume sterile water to be added (ml)	Concentration as added to melted agar 1:9, etc. (µg or IU/ml)	Final concentration in agar (µg or IU/ml)	Log_2
2000	6.4	3.6	1280	128	7
1280	2	2	640	64	6
1280	1	3	320	32	5
1280	1	7	160	16	4
160	2	2	80	8	3
160	1	3	40	4	2
160	1	7	20	2	1
20	2	2	10	1	0
20	1	3	5	0.5	−1
20	1	7	2.5	0.25	−2

*Can be extended farther.

87-5, as modified from Ericsson and Sherris.[13] Preparing concentrations in this manner allows for a straightforward scheme of the addition of 1.5 ml antimicrobic solution to 13.5 ml agar suspension or of 2 ml antimicrobic to 18 ml suspension for pouring into 100 mm plates.

The use of Table 87-5 is also practical in that only 1 pipet need be used for each series of 3 dilutions. Furthermore, the method as proposed here is not as vulnerable to the same type of cumulative error that may pose a serious problem in fixed and repetitive serial dilution methods.

An abbreviated scheme has been developed for arriving at what may be considered meaningful and pertinent concentrations to be used for agar dilution susceptibility testing. In most instances this relates to 3 or 4 predetermined concentrations.[35] The level of antimicrobial to be tested is determined by an assessment of very susceptible, likely susceptibility in the treatment of systemic infection with the usual dose by the usual route of administration, and levels relating to expected urinary tract concentrations. This abbreviated scheme has obvious economic advantages over a 10- or 12-level 2-fold dilution approach.

Plate preparation. Once the medium has been prepared as per the instructions of the manufacturer of the dry powder, it is allowed to cool to approximately 50 C. The medium is usually prepared in screw-cap bottles as these allow for ease of mixing. These can be held in a temperature range of 45-50 C in an appropriately adjusted water bath.

Considerations in the preparation of plates include the ability to produce a plate that is level and uniform in consistency. In addition the antimicrobials should be evenly distributed throughout the agar medium. Care should be taken to add the antibiotic quickly in order that the agar medium not cool below 45 C, as this temperature lowering could result in partial coalescence of the agar, resulting not only in uneven plates, but in a nonuniform distribution of antibiotic. The addition of an antimicrobial prior to cooling to 50 C can also be detrimental since the increased temperature may have an adverse effect on the activity of certain antibiotics. In the mixing of the antibiotic and agar, one should take care not to introduce bubbles by being too vigorous in the mixing process. Bubbles may cause an uneven surface, and the usual method of handling these bubbles—flaming the surface of the plate—may also have an adverse effect on some antimicrobials. A separate Mueller-Hinton agar plate, without added antibiotics, should also be prepared for each dilution series in order to provide an appropriate growth control.

Plates that have been allowed to harden should be carefully marked as to the type and concentration of antimicrobial agent present. These plates can then be used within a short period of time or can be packaged in plastic bags and stored at 4 C. Studies by Ryan et al.[39] have shown that most antimicrobial agents are stable when stored for 4 weeks in this manner. The exceptions are the penicillins and nitrofurantoin. These should not be stored longer than 1 week. For reference work and other investigational studies, plates should be used within 24 hours of preparation.

Because of the need for uniformity and to obviate the possibility of inoculum spot coalescence, plates should be dried sufficiently to remove agar surface moisture before use.

Blood products are usually added to the agar mixture after the antimicrobial has been added and thoroughly mixed. Once the blood has been added, the plates should be poured immediately in order to avoid the possibility of prepouring agar coalescence. Inoculum is obtained as with other susceptibility test methodologies. Between 4 and 6 morphologically identical colonies are touched with an inoculating loop or needle and suspended in 2 ml of an appropriate sterile medium. Either soybean-casein digest broth (SCDB) or Mueller-Hinton broth (MHB) are routinely used. Streptococci do not generally grow well in MHB, and at least for these organisms the SCDB should routinely be used. There are several approaches to the standardization of the inoculum concentration.[13,35] After the inoculum of 2 ml sterile broth, the organisms are allowed to grow for 2-4 hours at 35 C or are allowed to incubate overnight at the same temperature. The turbidity of the broth culture is then equilibrated to match that of a 0.5 MacFarland standard. This is usually done by diluting the organism suspension with similar broth. A 1:200 dilution is made of the standardized organism suspension using a sterile pipet. This will provide organism numbers in the range of 5×10^6 CFU/ml (colony-forming units). An alternative approach to achieving this concentration is to complete a 1:200 dilution of either an overnight broth culture or a 0.5 broth aliquot that has been heavily inoculated and allowed to incubate for 4 hours.

The inoculum should be transferred without delay in order to obviate organism replication after standardization.

The process of inoculum preparation is facilitated by preparing a rack into which the inoculated broth tubes can be placed in the order determined for transfer to the replicator seed plate. This will also enhance the recording of specimen numbers onto a grid sheet marked such that the location of inoculum in the seed plate can be easily noted.

Inoculum transfer. One well of the seed plate, usually in a corner, is first filled with a suspension of India ink. This will clearly define the orientation of specimen distribution. From the standardized broth tubes an amount of inoculum approximately equivalent to one-half to two-thirds the potential volume of the seed plate well is transferred to that well. In this step individual pipets must be used; since the amount to be transferred is not absolute but approximate, unmarked—and therefore less expensive—Pasteur pipets can be used. The head of the replicating device, containing the individual inoculation prongs, is then placed into the seed plate with the individual prongs resting in the wells. These prongs are constructed so as to deliver approximately 0.001-0.003 ml, which equates to approximately 1×10^4 CFU. The size of the inoculum spot as it eventuates on the agar surface is approximately 5-8 mm.

In the transfer of the inoculum from a seed plate to the agar surface, care should be taken in the hand movements necessary, either in the hand transfer of the inoculating head or in the pressure on the spring-loaded holder used by many laboratories. Pressure on the agar surface with the inoculating head should be avoided. The inoculating head should remain on the agar surface for 3-5 seconds prior to returning it to the seed plate. It has always been my contention that one should move from the least-concentrated antimicrobial plate toward the most concentrated in the series in order to avoid any potential for picking up and carrying undue antimicrobial either to the seed plate or to subsequent plates in the dilution series.

In the section on instrumentation at the beginning of this procedure, it was mentioned that Raschig rings could be used for spreading *Proteus.* Once the inoculation has taken place these rings should be set on the agar. Once the transfer of inoculum has been completed and the cover is replaced, the plate is allowed to stand until the inoculum droplets are absorbed into the agar. The surface of the agar should be carefully visualized immediately after inoculum transfer in order to ensure that there is an inoculum droplet at each location where this transfer should have occurred. On a single-specimen basis a 0.001 urine quantitation loop may be used for the transfer of inoculum from the appropriate seed plate well to the location on the agar surface where any droplets were not transferred.

Incubation. The plates are incubated at 35 C in an inverted position for 16-20 hours. The atmosphere of incubation is usually ambient air. For those organisms requiring increased CO_2, incubation in CO_2 is possible as long as one maintains appropriate control organism comparisons in the same environment. In the event of anaerobic organism testing these plates can be incubated in an anaerobic environment.

Interpretation. The International Collaborative Study, as reported by Ericsson and Sherris, advocated: "In reading end-points, a barely visible haze of growth or single colony is disregarded. If several colonies are found extending more than one dilution beyond an obvious end-point, the purity of this strain is checked and the test repeated."[13] The results are recorded on the grid that has been used to define the geographic location—both in the seed plate and on the agar surface—of the several specimens being tested.

Haemophilus influenzae agar dilution susceptibilities

With the discovery of ampicillin-resistant *H. influenzae* the need has arisen for the routine testing of *H. influenzae* by MIC means, disk diffusion, or β-lactamase production. When several strains of *Haemophilus* are to be tested simultaneously, the agar dilution methodology enhances this evaluation.

A stock antibiotic solution (2500 mg/ml ampicillin) is prepared according to the procedure previously described. This stock solution can be stored at -20 C or lower in aliquots appropriate for the preparation of an agar dilution series. A dilution of this stock ampicillin solution is prepared by adding 0.5 ml stock solution to 3.5 ml sterile distilled water in a sterile tube, thereby giving a working concentration of 320 mg/ml. The less concentrated working solutions are readied by performing doubling dilutions of the 320 mg/ml working solution (2 ml antibiotic solution + 2 ml sterile distilled water in a sterile tube).

Five tubes of Mueller-Hinton agar (18 ml/tube) are then melted, and these are cooled to 50 C and held in a heating block or water bath. To each tube is added 1 ml sterile horse blood or 1% hemoglobin and 0.2 ml IsoVitaleX (BioQuest, Cockeysville, Md.). One ml of the working ampicillin concentrations is then added to each of the tubes of melted Mueller-Hinton agar to provide final agar suspension concentrations of ampicillin in the range of 0.25-32 mg/ml. One tube of melted Mueller-Hinton with added supplements is also prepared. Each of the tubes with the antibiotic and supplement mixture is poured in a sterile 15 × 100 mm plastic plate and allowed to harden. When the plates have hardened, the surface is allowed to dry and the plates are inoculated. The growth from a pure culture (on chocolate or other suitable agar plates) of the *Haemophilus* can be scraped from the agar surface with a sterile platinum loop and can be suspended in 4 ml TSB in order to match the 0.5 MacFarland turbidity standard of approximately 10^8 CFU/ml. This standardized suspension is then diluted 1:100. This can be done by adding 0.04 ml to a 4 ml tube of SCDB. A standardized suspension of *E. coli* 25922 can be prepared from a 2- to 4-hour SCDB culture. The standardized *E. coli* suspension can be diluted 1:100 as described above for *Haemophilus*. If sufficient organisms are present one can use the regular inoculation apparatus of Steers et al.[1] However, for fewer organism numbers it is possible to use a sterile 0.001 ml calibrated inoculating loop and to spot (not streak) 0.001 ml each of these standardized broth solutions into each of the freshly prepared agar dilution plates. It is suggested that a CO_2

atmosphere should not be used unless it is required for the growth of the specific strain.

Interpretation. The interpretation is the same as that described above for the agar dilution method. This MIC testing procedure can be helpful in those situations where there is equivocation with regard to *H. influenzae* disk susceptibility testing. This is clearly one of the areas where MIC testing can be of great value to the physician. This testing can also be of value in those situations where resistance of *H. influenzae* is suspected with ampicillin, in spite of the absence of β-lactamase production. It should be stressed that some strains of *H. influenzae*, resistant to ampicillin, are not β-lactamase producers.

Macrobroth dilution testing

Equipment and testing supplies. This method usually uses 13 × 100 mm tubes and employs either cotton or foam rubber plugs or metal and plastic caps. One can also use 12 × 75 mm tubes with the same kind of coverings. This method is described in detail by Ericsson and Sherris,[13] Washington et al.,[35] and Barry.[40]

Medium. Mueller-Hinton medium is usually used, although historically this testing procedure has employed a wide variety of media, including soy digests, tryptose phosphate, nutrient, Eugon, brain-heart infusion, etc. MIC and MBC values for test organisms can vary widely depending upon the type of media used, the pH of the media, the osmolality, and the electrical conductivity of the medium. It has been my experience that I can vary the MIC values more than 10-fold by varying the medium employed for MIC broth determinations for certain antimicrobials. For the present, media other than Mueller-Hinton

Table 87-6. Modified broth dilution–antimicrobial dilution guide[13]*

Antimicrobial solution (μg or IU/ml)	Stock volume (ml)	Volume of broth diluent to be added	Concentration as added to culture inoculum at 1:2, etc. (μg or IU/ml)	Final concentration in broth (μg or IU/ml)	Log_2
2000	2	13.62 ml	256	128	7
256	2	2 vol	128	64	6
256	1	3	64	32	5
256	1	7	32	16	4
32	2	2 vol	16	8	3
32	1	3	8	4	2
32	1	7	4	2	1
4	2	2 vol	2	1	0
4	1	3	1	0.5	-1
4	1	7	0.5	0.25	-2
0.5	2	2	0.25	0.125	-3
0.5	1	3	0.125	0.063	-4
0.5	1	7	0.063	0.031	-5

*Can be extended farther.

should be used only when organisms fail to grow well in Mueller-Hinton media, as can be the case with some streptococci, for example.

Antimicrobial preparations. The method of preparing stock solutions has been previously described in this section. For the macrobroth method one is again advised to use a systematic table of dilutions. As in the agar dilution discussion, a table modified from the International Collaborative Study Report by Ericsson and Sherris[13] is included (Table 87-6) for perusal and use in the preparation of these dilutions.

Test tubes are labeled for the predetermined dilutions in the test set. These dilutions may be either 2-fold, with a wide or narrow range, or may be established at various predetermined levels in order to derive an appropriate analysis of high- and low-susceptibility information. It has been my experience that when macrobroth dilution testing is done in the laboratory, it is usually done for single-organism determinations. In that context it is still necessary to test appropriate control organisms whenever such determinations are performed. Therefore, in the provisions for this analysis appropriate control organisms must be included and should meet the criteria for dilution susceptibility testing.

Inoculum. In the macrobroth method the aim is for a final concentration of 10^5-10^6 CFU/ml. A 1:1000 or 1:2000 dilution of either an overnight culture or a 4- to 6-hour 0.5 ml broth culture may be used; alternatively, a 1:200 dilution of a broth culture may be standardized to equilibrate to a MacFarland 0.5 standard. One ml antibiotic solution and 1 ml standardized organism suspension are added to each tube.

Incubation. The tubes are incubated at 35 C. Caps or plugs are used in order to preclude evaporation and contamination.

Interpretation. Mueller-Hinton broth is well known for developing a slight turbidity with broth dilution testing. Care must be exercised to ensure comparison with an uninoculated control. The determination of the result is usually made visually and involves judging the least amount of antibiotic that results in complete inhibition of growth. The uninoculated control tube can be helpful in interpreting this visually determined end point.

Macrobroth susceptibility testing also allows for the transfer of aliquots from those tubes that demonstrate no visible growth to agar plate surfaces in order to determine minimal bactericidal concentrations.

Microbroth dilution testing

The development over the past few years of the microbroth dilution method has been favorably received. Microdilution trays made of molded plastic have been available for serologic determinations for several years and have gained great acceptance due to their practicality. However, it is only in recent years that this technic has found wide usage for antimicrobial susceptibility test-ing. Advantages of the method include the availability of commercially prepared trays containing prefrozen antimicrobial dilutions and, for the larger clinical laboratories, the opportunity for the purchase of instrumentation that will allow for the production of plates within an individual clinical laboratory setting.[10]

The description as provided in this section will relate to the entire methodology as if one were beginning at the initial step of preparing the plates. It should be recognized, in the context of the above narrative, that one can begin this process at any procedural step appropriate for the individual laboratory circumstances.

Equipment and instrumentation. The central element of the microbroth dilution system is the molded plastic tray or plate that contains 8 rows of 12 small flat-bottomed or V-shaped cups to which can be delivered a small volume (usually 0.1 ml) of testing suspension. A small device that allows for the dispensing of transparent tape to seal the plates after inoculation will facilitate the performance of this procedure. It is most helpful to use a rack upon which the plate is placed in order to read test results by means of a mirror mounted in the bottom of the rack.

Other items of equipment that may be considered are the specially calibrated loops that can be used for the dilution of antimicrobial solutions and the specially constructed pipets that can be used for the delivery of inoculum. Various levels of mechanization are available, including plates with inoculating heads much like those used for the agar dilution testing. These can be used either manually or in a mechanized frame for the delivery of inoculum for the antimicrobial-containing plates.

Media. The microbroth dilution test can be performed with Mueller-Hinton medium. However, because of the traditional deficiency of important cations in formulations of Mueller-Hinton broth, it is suggested that this medium be supplemented in order to assure appropriate susceptibility results.[19] Studies by Reller et al.[37] indicate that a final concentration of 50 mg Ca and 25 mg Mg/L Mueller-Hinton medium will help to obviate this problem. This can be accomplished by preparing dehydrated Mueller-Hinton broth, as per manufacturer's directions, autoclaving, and then cooling the broth to 4-6 C by overnight placement in a refrigerator. The appropriate concentrations of calcium and magnesium can be derived with $CaCl_2$ and $MgCl_2$. **Presently,** as noted previously, the concentration of these divalent cations is so small in Mueller-Hinton broth as to allow one to disregard any potential presence and add these cations as though there were originally none present.

Antimicrobials. Prefrozen or lyophilized antimicrobial-containing trays are now available from commercial sources for use in the individual clinical laboratory settings. The FDA has developed careful criteria for the quality control of these commercially prepared dilution sets, and the individual clinical laboratory can have reasonable reliance that these trays will perform appropriately. The trays are available individually or multiply packaged.

If preparation of antimicrobial dilutions is to take place in one's own laboratory, it can be done by using a systematized dilution schedule as contained in Table 87-6, or the specially calibrated microdilution loops can be used for serially diluting these trays. If the fully instrumented approach to the preparation of trays is used, then the manufacturer's directions should be closely followed.

Of consideration in the local preparation of the microbroth trays is the matter of using frozen stock solutions. Barry[40] suggests that allowing a stock solution to freeze, preparing the dilutions, transferring those dilutions to the microbroth trays, and then refreezing them for storage —although creating 2 freeze-thaw cycles—may be acceptable.

Indications are that these trays, once prepared, may be frozen in plastic bags for at least 2 weeks. Plates purchased commercially should be used according to the manufacturer's outdate suggestions.

Inoculation. The recommended organism concentration is 5000 CFU/0.1 ml final volume in the tray wells. The inoculators will deliver approximately 5-10 μl/prong or loop or 1-2 μl/pin. The original concentration of the inoculum will be dependent upon the type of inoculating device(s) used. The desired final organism density in the well should be 10^5 CFU/ml. Since certain models of the instrumentation available for preparing antimicrobial suspensions for delivery to the plastic trays have the capacity for altering the volume setting of delivery, one must also take into consideration the volume being delivered to the individual tray wells. Each step should be carefully considered with respect to concentration, volume, and colony-forming units per milliliter. After the inoculum has been delivered to the tray containing the antimicrobials, the tray is sealed with transparent tape and incubated for 16-20 hours at 35 C.

Interpretation. The MIC is taken as the lowest concentration without visible turbidity or a button of cells at the bottom of the well. Gerlach[41] reports 95% reproducibility in end-point determinations, a result consistent with the precision of other susceptibility methods.

Acceleration of result availability. Bartlett[42] has reported that the addition of tetrazolium can accelerate the interpretation of microbroth dilution testing. The reproducibility of this procedure remains to be clearly defined for all antimicrobic substances, and Colvin and Sherris[43] suggest that for appropriate reproducibility an inoculum adjustment must be made. Further investigations are necessary in order to provide a complete understanding of the implications of these more rapid method modifications. Until this is accomplished the broth dilution method should probably be considered a 16- to 20-hour incubation method.

Special considerations. Stacking trays may well preclude appropriate air circulation and may prevent trays from arriving at the appropriate temperature within an expected incubation time period. The longer the incubation time, the less impact this would have on the end result. However, this should be considered in the manner in which trays are placed in the incubator.

Thornsberry et al.[19] suggest that some β-lactamase-producing S. aureus may give low penicillin or ampicillin MICs despite the production of the β-lactamase and probable clinical resistance to penicillin in severe infections. They suggest that all S. aureus tested by the microbroth method be evaluated for the production of β-lactamase in order to obviate a disparate test interpretation.

Automated broth dilution adaptations
Special considerations in automation

It is likely that certain performance guidelines will need to be redefined in order to appropriately utilize the potential of instrumentation. Historically, all new susceptibility methodology has been compared to the agar dilution method, as standardized by the International Collaborative Study.[13] However, it may be more meaningful if the automated methodology procedurally compares more to broth dilution testing, to equate performance to standard or reference broth methodologies.

Any instrumented or automated approach should be expected to perform with the same degree of precision or reproducibility required from other noninstrumented methods. From prior experience with method evaluations it should be hoped that these new technics would approach 95% reproducibility.

The cost should be considered in the overall evaluation of practicality and use of instrumentation. Increased cost may be justified if gains can be documented. In this context the potential advantages of automation might ideally include enhanced precision, objectivity of result interpretations, convenience, uniformity, economy of time, the speeding of results, and potential interface with the computer for both quality control and data processing facilitation.

Quality control considerations, as they apply to automated procedures, create new parameters that must be evaluated with respect to instrument function, maintenance, and performance criteria. Instrumentation for instrumentation's sake is difficult to justify. It should be anticipated that the automated, semiautomated, and instrumented procedures will be critically evaluated; conclusions will be made available to provide information necessary in judging the role instrumentation may play in relationship to the circumstances of an individual clinical laboratory.

Autobac I

Autobac I (Pfizer, Groton, Conn.) is a semiautomated system for measuring antimicrobial susceptibilities of bacteria within a 3- to 5-hour period. The basic overall system is adaptable to several of the chores inherent in clinical microbiology, but the discussion in this chapter will be confined to its use in susceptibility testing.[44-46]

Instrumentation

The system is comprised of 4 separate components—each designed to perform a specific function leading to the end result of susceptibility evaluation. The central component of the system is a light-scattering photometer with associated additional electronic capability allowing it to alter the evaluation mode; this permits it to be umbilicized to a freestanding computer unit that will become more important in future innovations with this instrument. This photometer is important in the standardization of the broth inoculum and in the determination and calculation of susceptibility results.

The second component is a cuvette, comprised of 12 individual test chambers and a thirteenth chamber for growth control. This cuvette is molded such that it can accept and firmly seat a broth inoculum tube. It has a removable thick plastic manifold allowing access to the individual control chambers for the delivery of individual paper disks containing the antimicrobial substances.

The third component is a dispenser that delivers antimicrobial-containing disks to the individual chambers of the cuvette. The specific order of placement of the disks is predetermined and cannot be easily changed, as it must correlate with the printer in the photometer housing.

The fourth component is a combination incubator and shaker. Racks within this incubator-shaker are constructed so as to accept and securely hold in an orderly manner a number of cuvettes. This incubator-shaker has a capacity for variability in temperature control but is in general fixed for a rotation at the rate of 220 rpm. An additional and essential device is a calibration wedge, by which the photometer can be checked and adjusted.

Another noninstrumentation portion of this system is the paper report. This is a multicopy report form that is fed into the photometer housing and onto which the results of the individual cuvette chamber determinations are printed.

Susceptibility testing procedure

The method involves selecting an organism from an initial isolation plate—or transferring an aliquot from what appears to be a pure isolate body fluid specimen—and inoculating it into a saline tube. The saline tube is then placed in the light-scatter photometer housing and either more organism or more saline is added, if necessary, to standardize the inoculum. The photometer has a meter, and the newer models of the Autobac have the capacity for varying the meter reading in order that different inoculum levels may be used. When the meter needle rests in the center portion of the calibrated gauge, standardization has occurred. Two ml of the standardized inoculum are then pipetted into a tube of Eugon broth. While the cuvette is held vertically, the Eugon broth tube is screwed into the cuvette and seated firmly. The cuvette is then inverted on a level surface so that all the broth is distributed to a holding chamber situated at one end of the cuvette. Further manipulations of the cuvette are made to distribute the broth evenly along the length of the cuvette and to deliver 1.5 ml aliquots of the broth into the individual chambers of the cuvette; these have been previously armed with the antimicrobic disks as delivered from the disk dispenser.

The cuvette is then placed in the incubator shaker and rotated at 220 rpm at 36 C for approximately 3 hours; after this the cuvette is seated upon a carriage bar in the light-scatter photometer housing, and the housing lid is closed. A report form is inserted to record the result, and this triggers the machine to begin its computation and to print the results. Sufficient growth must have occurred in the control chamber or the photometer will automatically reject the report slip. If this occurs the cuvette must be incubated for an additional time period. If sufficient growth has occurred in the control chamber, a light-scatter index (LSI) is calculated by means of a minicomputer within the photometer housing. This LSI is a numerical value between 0 and 1 with 0.01 subdivisions. Based upon it, an interpretation of susceptible, intermediate, or resistant is calculated for each antimicrobial agent by using as the reference point the growth index as derived from the growth control chamber in comparison with the events that have transpired in each individual test chamber.

The procedure described above is the basic procedure for use of the Autobac. The variations in test categories require modifications of the antimicrobic disks that are placed into the cuvette. MIC testing can be performed using 2 or 3 concentrations of each antimicrobic at predetermined levels with the end result of susceptibility testing formulated from either the absolute values derived from each growth chamber (formulation will indicate the degree of susceptibility) or by using a mathematical calculation from the high- and low-antibiotic-content disks used in the series. The LSI derivation allows for the mathematical assumption of an MIC value for the test organism based upon a computer-assisted program much akin to the principle of the standard curve or regression analysis.

Problem areas

In the 7-laboratory collaborative study evaluating the Autobac instrument and comparing it to disk diffusion and the International Collaborative Study agar dilution methods, there was an overall agreement of about 90% between the automated results and those of the other 2 methods. In the report of this study by Thornsberry et al.[47] the primary difficulties were encountered with ampicillin and caphalothin testing with certain strains of *Enterobacter*, and with *P. aeruginosa* results obtained with gentamicin, chloramphenicol, and tetracycline. It is now apparent that the Autobac instrument is unlikely to pick up methicillin- or nafcillin-resistant strains of *Staphylococcus*. When strains of staphylococci demonstrate resistance to other antimicrobials in the test battery, it has been shown they should be considered potentially resistant to the penicillinase-resistant semisynthetic penicillins.[48] It is of note in this context that the strains that are methicillin resistant will generally demonstrate resistance to other compounds in the Autobac test battery.

Experience also demonstrates that ampicillin-resistant enterococci should be rechecked for susceptibility by a dilution or diffusion method.

As has been standard practice with the disk diffusion methodology for years, one should also run a purity check on any specimen being tested in the Autobac. This can be accomplished by inoculating individual sections of a blood agar plate to assess purity in growth. Though the Autobac has the potential for doing MIC testing, the primary approach to susceptibility testing at present with this instrument is that of a single-tube broth dilution test, with the report indicating susceptible, intermediate, or resistant based upon light-scatter values previously described.

Other instrumentation

Other forms of susceptibility instrumentation currently marketed are limited to the microbroth dilution methodologies. However, under current test are Automicrobic System or AMS (Vitek, St. Louis, Mo.), MS-2 (Abbott Laboratories, Dallas, Tex.), and Repliscan (Cathra, Minneapolis, Minn.). In addition developmental and clinical testing have been done using radiometric means, laser–light scatter means, and electrical impedance. None of the latter 3 systems is currently projected for marketing within the near future.

It is likely that within the next 2-year time frame susceptibility testing will be available within the clinical laboratories with the Automicrobic, the MS-2, or the Repliscan methodologies. Since these have not been evaluated in routine clinical usage, it seems premature to review their operation or instrumentation in this chapter.

SPECIAL ORGANISM TESTING CONSIDERATIONS
Anaerobes

The susceptibility testing of anaerobic organisms poses special problems for the clinical microbiology laboratory. This is due to the requirements for special atmospheric environment, wide variations in replication times, and other organism-unique features. As a result the methods previously described each require modification for use with anaerobic organisms. Anaerobic susceptibility testing may be carried out with a variety of methods. Special conditions are required, and problems relate to the polymicrobic nature of anaerobic infections— wherein multiple organisms are associated with disease—and to delays in reporting anaerobic susceptibilities that have led to a less than optimal application of these results for patient therapy. As most anaerobic organisms are susceptible to penicillin (*B. fragilis* and some *B. melaninogenicus* are exceptions), these organisms are responsive to therapy by the penicillin class of compounds and also by antimicrobial agents such as chloramphenical, clindamycin, and, variably, the tetracyclines and erythromycin.

Anaerobic susceptibility testing is often of limited physician and clinical usefulness. I specifically inquire of the physician, with any non-body-fluid anaerobic isolate, whether the physician desires susceptibility testing. In almost all instances the physician elects to forgo the susceptibility testing. This area, therefore, represents one of the most selective areas in all of clinical microbiology with respect to the need and clinical usefulness of susceptibility testing. It should be stressed that in the same way that anaerobic infections can develop insidiously, they may be slow in demonstrating clinical and diagnostic test response to therapy.

Anaerobic broth-disk method

The broth-disk method of Wilkins and Thiel[49] is useful. Blazevic[50] has carefully evaluated this method and found it to be reproducible and comparable to standard methodology. For this reason, because of the ease and simplicity of its use, and because of its peripheral association—due to the similar disk usage—with the disk diffusion methodology, it also has potential applicability for a wide spectrum of clinical laboratories. The principle involved in the delivery of antimicrobial to the test environment is the same as previously described for Autobac I, that is, disk elution. The disks, however, are not specially prepared for this method, but rather are multiples of the disks used in the regular disk diffusion methodology. Therefore, the disks are widely available, and the quality assurance of the disks can be associated with the quality control of the Kirby-Bauer methodology.

Medium. The medium employed in this procedure is prereduced brain-heart infusion–supplemented (BHI-S) broth. The supplements are 0.005% hemin, 0.002% menadione, and 0.05% yeast extract. There should be a careful delineation of the amount of medium present, as one is dealing with a quantitative application of antimicrobial agents.

Table 87-7. Broth-disk method for anaerobic susceptibility testing

Antimicrobic	Disk content	No. disks/ tube	Final concentration/ ml
Ampicillin	10 μg	2	4 μg
Carbenicillin	100 μg	5	100 μg
Cephalothin	30 μg	1	6 μg
Chloramphenicol	30 μg	2	12 μg
Clindamycin	2 μg	4	1.6 μg
Clindamycin	2 μg	8	3.2 μg
Doxycycline	5 μg	3	3 μg
Erythromycin	15 μg	1	3 μg
Gentamicin	10 μg	3	6 μg
Penicillin G	10 U	1	2 U
Tetracycline	30 μg	1	6 μg

Inoculum preparation. The inoculum is 1 drop of a turbid 18- to 24-hour culture grown in pre-reduced chopped meat broth, chopped meat–glucose broth, or peptone–yeast extract–glucose broth.

Testing conditions. The test is conducted in an anaerobic environment, either in a glovebox or with the Virginia Polytechnic Institute cannula apparatus. The appropriate number of antibiotic disks is added to the separate tubes of BHI-S for each antimicrobial to be tested (Table 87-7). Each organism is usually tested with all antibiotics, and a tube without disks is inoculated as a growth control. One drop of the turbid overnight culture is added to each tube of the test series, and each tube is then sealed with a rubber stopper and incubated for 18-24 hours at 35 C. After incubation the Gram stain is made of the growth control to assess the purity of the test suspension.

Interpretation. The interpretation of this particular susceptibility test differs from that used for aerobic broth dilution testing. In this particular test one reads and evaluates the susceptibility end point based upon a comparison of the growth in each individual antibiotic tube with that in the growth control tube. Turbidity less than 50% of the turbidity found in the growth control is interpreted as susceptibility. Resistance is the presence of turbidity greater than 50% of the growth control.

Kurzynski et al.[51] have described a modification of this method (**modified "Aerobic" broth-disk method**) in which, using the same basic principle, a susceptibility test is performed in thioglycollate broth incubated in ambient air instead of being incubated anaerobically. The indicated number of disks is added to tubes of broth and the tubes are then kept at room temperature for 2-3 hours in order to allow for the complete elution of the antimicrobial agent into the broth. Diffusion may occur more slowly with this method because of the 0.05% agar present in thioglycollate. The incubation and end points are similar to the methodology described above, although with the more fastidious organisms, 48 hours growth may be necessary. Again a 50% decrease in visible growth is used as an end-point determination.

Rosenblatt et al.[70] found the modified method simple and efficient (except for testing with tetracycline). See "Susceptibility tests," Chapter 82, for details of modification.

Anaerobic agar dilution testing

The protocol for this test is similar to that described for routine agar dilution testing. Several modifications are necessary due to the unique nature of the anaerobic organisms.

Medium. *Brucella* agar (Pfizer, New York, N.Y.) or brain-heart infusion agar can be used. The medium should contain vitamin K_1 (10 mg/ml) and 5% sheep blood or 5% vol/vol (laked defibrinated sheep blood) that has been lysed by repeated freeze-thaw cycles. This is the basic medium to which the antimicrobials are added in the same manner as that described previously for the regular agar dilution method. A subcommittee of the National Committee for Clinical Laboratory Standards has recently recommended that Wilkins-Chalgren medium become the standard medium.[36]

One other consideration should be defined here and that relates to the broth in which the organisms are grown prior to inoculation onto the plates. It seems advisable to suggest that thioglycollate 135 C (BBL, Cockeysville, Md.) without an indicator be used in order to allow for appropriate turbidity comparison. This medium can be enriched with hemin (0.0005%), menadione (0.002%), and $NaHCO_3$ (1 mg/ml).

Inoculum preparation. The inoculum is placed in the wells of the seed plate for use with the replicator device of Steers et al.,[1] or it may be placed using a 0.001 calibrated loop. The thioglycollate broth described above, in which the organism has been grown for 24-48 hours, is equilibrated to a MacFarland 0.5 or MacFarland 1 standard prior to use. There is no further dilution of the broth suspension, and the seed wells are filled one-half to two-thirds as described previously.

Once the organisms have been placed in the seed plate, the test procedure is carried out as described for the International Collaborative Study agar dilution methodology.[13]

Antimicrobials. As noted above the antimicrobials are prepared using the same technic as described for the agar dilution method. The antimicrobials tested are those listed in Table 87-7 for the broth-disk elution method. The plates should be prepared within 18-24 hours of use; they are stored at room temperature to delay absorption of oxygen, which occurs more rapidly at lower temperatures. These plates should be incubated promptly in an anaerobic incubator environment. Susceptibility end points may be readable in 18-24 hours, but may require 48 hours for clear definition.

Whenever this test is performed, a plate containing no antibiotics should be inoculated and incubated simultaneously with the test plates in the same environment. This method is principally used whenever large numbers of anaerobic organisms are to be tested. Its practicality is lessened when only a few organisms are to be tested.

Anaerobic microbroth dilution

The basic methodology for testing anaerobes with the microbroth method is also similar to that employed for regular anaerobic organisms. However, the limitations of this method relate to the fact that the work should be performed, ideally, in an anaerobic glovebox environment. This limits the ability of many laboratories to appropriately perform these tests.

Medium. The medium for this particular procedure is modified, much in the same way that the medium modifications have been previously described. *Brucella* broth or brain-heart infusion broth may be used, and each is best supplemented with menadione (0.005%) and hemin (0.001%). These same media can be used for both inoculum preparation and for antimicrobic dilution.

Disk diffusion susceptibility testing for anaerobic organisms

Sutter et al.[52] have provided guidelines for disk diffusion testing for anaerobes. They advocate the use of *Brucella* agar containing 5% defibrinated sheep blood and 0.5 μg/ml menadione. Rather than using the large plates (150 mm) as generally used for disk diffusion testing, they advocate the use of 90 × 15 mm Petri dishes. The agar is poured to a depth of 5-6 mm and not more than 4 antibiotic disks are applied to each plate. These authors advocate that a few colonies, or a 3 mm loopful from a broth culture, of each strain to be tested are inoculated into a tube containing thioglycollate medium without indicator (thioglycollate 135 C [BBL]) to which is added 5 mg/ml hemin prior to autoclaving and 1 mg/ml NaHCO$_3$ plus 0.5 mg/ml filter-sterilized menadione after autoclaving. These tubes are incubated for 4-6 hours and then diluted to the density of a 0.5 MacFarland standard.

The authors are careful to define the source of cotton swabs to be used (Acme Cotton Co., Valley Stream, Long Valley, N.Y.) and advocate the use of freshly made *Brucella* agar plates. The streaking is done according to the method of Bauer et al.,[21] and the plates are incubated at 37 C in anaerobic incubators. Results are read after approximately 24 hours by measuring the zone of inhibition around the antibiotic disks. The interpretation is made by the zone diameter interpretive chart according to the criteria of Sutter et al.[52] An anaerobic control strain, picked for susceptibility to penicillin, should be tested simultaneously with the test bacteria in order to demonstrate appropriate function of the test.

Category method for anaerobic bacteria

The category test of Stalons and Thornsberry[19] is reported to be simple and reproducible. Anaerobes are tested with 2 or 3 selected concentrations of commonly used antimicrobials. These concentrations conform generally to the categories previously discussed whereby the International Collaborative Study[13] advocates interpretation that defines 4 degrees of susceptibility.

Medium. Thornsberry et al.[19] advocate the use of Schaedler broth (BBL or Difco, Detroit, Mich.) supplemented with menadione (5 mg/ml) and hemin (0.1 mg/ml). They dispense 2.7 ml of this broth into screw-cap 13 × 100 mm tubes. The medium is prereduced prior to use by leaving it in an anaerobic environment for 3 hours or more with the screw cap loosened. An alternative approach is boiling the broth and supplementing it after cooling with the supplements noted above. Following are the concentrations of antimicrobial agents to be used in this test:

Antimicrobial agent	Concentration to test (μg/ml)
Penicillin G	0.25, 16, 128
Tetracycline	2, 8, 32
Clindamycin	2, 8, 64
Erythromycin	2, 4, 64
Chloramphenicol	1, 8

These are prepared in stock solutions containing 1280 μg/ml and may be stored at −70 C. Prior to use in a test the stocks are thawed and diluted to a value 10 times the final desired concentration as there is a further 1:10 dilution during the test.

As with the broth dilution method of Wilkins and Thiel,[49] the antimicrobial agents may also be added by means of paper disks. The authors are careful to point out, however, that it is impractical to use commercial disks, and they suggest that disks of the proper concentrations can be easily prepared in the laboratory by adding the proper amount of antimicrobial to blank disks, drying them, and storing them with a desiccant at −70 C.

Inoculum preparation. The inoculum is prepared by removing an amount of overnight growth from a Shaedler agar plate and suspending it in Shaedler broth in order to adjust the turbidity to that of a 0.5 MacFarland standard. Alternatively, an overnight broth culture can be adjusted to the same turbidity value.

Procedure. Antimicrobial solutions (0.3 ml) are added to provide a concentration 10 times that of the final dilution value to a tube containing 2.7 ml Shaedler broth. Alternatively, if disks are used, one adds the appropriate disks to 3 ml of the broth. A 0.25 ml aliquot of the adjusted inoculum is added by means of a calibrated dropper to each tube containing the antimicrobic and to a tube containing broth but no antimicrobial. The caps are replaced, but not tightened, and the tubes are incubated in a GasPak jar or other anaerobic environment for 18-24 hours at 35 C.

The end point is interpreted as the absence of macroscopic growth. Care should be taken to assure that there is adequate growth in the control broth. The results can be reported as MICs or as categories of susceptibility. For all but chloramphenicol 3 concentrations are tested, permitting interpretations as follows:

Category	Control	Low	Medium	High
I	+	−	−	−
II	+	+	−	−
III	+	+	+	−
IV	+	+	+	+

Susceptibility tests for Neisseria gonorrhoeae

There are 2 types of resistance that exist with *N. gonorrhoeae*. One is a relative resistance that has been recognized for many years. This resistance seems to have reached a peak and has been somewhat constant in recent years. It is because of this type of resistance that 4.8 mil U penicillin is used therapeutically, as contrasted to the much lower levels that at one time were uniformly efficacious in treating this organism. More recently a resistance mediated by penicillinase testing has been recognized. These resistance mechanisms require special understanding and testing considerations. An absolute susceptibility value can be derived, and this is usually done by agar dilution means. Alternatively, one can test for the production of β-lactamase. A disk diffusion test was at one time described by Ronald et al.[53] in which a zone size of 20 mm was equilibrated to a susceptibility of less than 1 U penicillin. This method did not gain wide acceptance. More recently a modified disk diffusion test, using the same breakpoint, has been shown to correlate with β-lactamase production.[19] GC base agar is supplemented with 1% IsoVitaleX. The inoculum is equilibrated to a 0.5 MacFarland standard and applied as with the regular disk method. The method utilizes a single 10 U penicillin disk placed on the plate surface. Strains that produce β-lactamase consistently produce zone sizes less than 19 mm. This method allows most laboratories to test for gonococcal susceptibility patterns and extrapolate the likelihood of β-lactamase production.

It would be unusual for information other than the production of penicillinase to be required for *N. gonorrhoeae*, except in situations of treatment failure or with epidemiologic or in vitro antibiotic activity investigations. In these latter instances agar dilution studies can be performed. The growth from 4 or 5 colonies of the test organism, grown on a chocolate agar or modified Thayer-Martin plate, can be suspended in CSDB and adjusted to the appropriate inoculum level by comparison to a MacFarland 0.5 standard. A 1:20 dilution is made in broth, and this is placed directly onto the surface of antimicrobial plates that have been prepared in the same fashion as the plates described previously. The only modifications required are that dilutions are added to GC medium that has been supplemented with 1 g hemoglobin/100 ml medium and 1 ml IsoVitaleX or Supplement C (Difco); these plates should be used within 48 hours of preparation. The plates are handled as would be other plates in an agar dilution testing situation, with the exception that they should be incubated in an environment of increased CO_2. These tests are read at 24 hours if sufficient growth has occurred, and if not, can be read at 36-48 hours with equal reliability.

A control strain of *N. gonorrhoeae* with a known susceptibility should also be tested. It is recommended that a *Sarcina lutea* strain also be included in order to provide additional technical control. Barry[40] alludes to the fact that the density of the inoculum is an important variable and suggests that this can be assessed by further diluting the adjusted cell suspension by a factor of 50 and streaking it to a chocolate agar plate with a 0.001 ml calibrated loop. An accurate inoculum should result in from 10 to 100 colonies on the plate surface, thus verifying the correctness of the inoculum density.

Susceptibility testing of Neisseria meningitidis

Susceptibility testing of *N. meningitidis* does not have the same implications as the testing of *N. gonorrhoeae* and *H. influenzae*. The reason is that this organism has as yet not demonstrated penicillinase production. However, with the advent of penicillinase production in the somewhat related organisms just discussed, it seems as if it is only a matter of time until the same phenomenon manifests itself in *N. meningitidis*.

It is unusual for *N. meningitidis* to require testing, and when testing is carried out it is primarily in a research setting with penicillin, ampicillin, or chloramphenicol, or for epidemiologic studies. However, due to the facility with which sulfonamides can prevent the acquisition of meningitis by *N. meningitidis*, it is at times desired to carry out susceptibility testing for sulfonamides. In this context a slight modification of the disk diffusion methodology as described by Bennett et al.[54] is used, and the zone of interpretation of 40 mm is used to define susceptibility. Susceptibility testing by the agar dilution method can be carried out as described for *N. gonorrhoeae*.

Susceptibility testing of Staphylococcus aureus with the penicillinase-resistant semisynthetic penicillins

The assessment of resistance of the semisynthetic penicillinase-resistant penicillins to *S. aureus* requires that the incubator temperature be held to 35 C or below to ensure that these organisms will be routinely detected. The detection of resistance can be facilitated also by employing a heavy inoculum, extending the incubation time to 48 hours, and adding 5% NaCl to the testing medium. For all practical purposes unless there is a specific epidemiologic problem requiring added surveillance, these precautions, other than keeping the temperature at 35 C or below, are not necessary.

At present it is best not to use cloxacillin or dicloxacillin as a testing medium for determining susceptibility for *S. aureus*. Drew et al.[55] have shown that these 2 compounds will not reliably detect methicillin resistance. Susceptibility testing, with the disk diffusion method, should be performed with methicillin, nafcillin, or oxacillin disks. Of these, methicillin is the least stable of the 3 compounds. Resistance to the semisynthetic, penicillinase-resistant penicillins is still infrequent in the United States; the finding of a resistant strain should warrant the careful reevaluation of the organism to reaffirm its identity as *S. aureus* and should require retesting with the disk to ensure appropriate disk potency.

It has recently been demonstrated[56] that staphylococci and the semisynthetic penicillinase-resistant penicillins may exhibit a large discrepancy between the MIC values and the MBC level. This phenomenon has been termed "tolerance" and has resulted in a significant increase in the number of laboratory requests for both MBC and MIC determinations. It is thought that as many as 40% of the *S. aureus* strains isolated from clinically significant infections in hospital settings may demonstrate this phenomenon, which is akin to that known for years to occur with the *Enterococcus*. *S. aureus* and enterococci may both appear to be fully sensitive to a penicillin by testing that measures the inhibitory level. However, both may demonstrate at the same time a high bactericidal concentration for the compound being tested. In the same way that additional incubation will at times demonstrate resistance to the semisynthetic penicillins, additional incubation will often more clearly define the phenomenon of tolerance with these strains.

As tolerance may have distinct implications in selected patients, this should be considered by the physician in the approach to the therapy of staphylococcal disease. There are also implications of this phenomenon with respect to laboratory testing, not only in terms of additional requests for MBC values, but also in the potential usage of combined antibiotics (i.e., an aminoglycoside plus a semisynthetic penicillinase-resistant penicillin) and the association that this trend has with the monitoring of therapy with combination-use antibiotics.

It should be noted at this point that *S. epidermidis* is often resistant to the methicillin-nafcillin-oxacillin group of compounds, and the determination of such resistance in the laboratory setting is not unexpected. As many as 25-30% of strains will demonstrate methicillin resistance.

Susceptibility tests for Haemophilus influenzae

Susceptibility testing with *H. influenzae* has acquired increased significance as this organism has recently demonstrated the capacity to produce penicillinase and manifest absolute resistance to the penicillin and other related semisynthetic penicillin compounds that for years have been used without qualm as to therapeutic efficacy. In this context one is likely to test for absolute MIC values, as is desirable in situations such as meningitis. β-Lactamase production can be readily determined, and in most circumstances this information is sufficient. Recently it has been shown that there are strains of *H. influenzae* that demonstrate resistance to penicillin by means other than penicillinase production. For this reason actual susceptibility testing may assume increased significance with this particular organism.

Haemophilus susceptibility testing by agar dilution has been previously described in this chapter.

Broth dilution testing for Haemophilus influenzae

Thornsberry et al.[19] have shown that broth dilution testing will result in better growth of the *Haemophilus* organism if Shaedler's broth supplemented with 5% Fildes reagent is used. Mueller-Hinton broth can also be used but does not provide the same optimum growth as with Shaedler's. The testing procedure used is essentially one of adhering to the protocols of either the microbroth or macrobroth methodologies as previously described, except for the medium employed. The inoculum can be prepared by suspending organisms taken from a chocolate agar plate in Shaedler's broth to equal the density of a 0.5 MacFarland standard.

Interpretation. Susceptible strains of *H. influenzae* almost all have MICs of 1 μg/ml or less. Thornsberry et al.[19] report that ampicillin-resistant strains generally have MICs of 8 μg/ml or higher although occasional strains may have an MIC value of 4 μg/ml. Meningitis-associated strains with MICs of 2 μg/ml or greater should be considered ampicillin resistant.

Disk diffusion testing with Haemophilus influenzae

Mueller-Hinton agar should be supplemented with 1% IsoVitaleX (BBL) and 1% hemoglobin. The pH should be adjusted to 7.2. This preparation surpasses the performance of chocolatized sheep blood because the zones with chocolatized blood are difficult to interpret. Once the special plate contents are prepared, the disk diffusion test is carried out exactly as originally described by Bauer et al.[21]

H. influenzae represents a third test interpretation category for ampicillin testing, and a zone size of 20 mm is used as the breakpoint between resistant and susceptible. Some ampicillin-resistant strains produce zones that approach 19 mm. When this occurs there will almost always be colonies within the zone if the zone created by a resistant strain is as large as 19 mm. Thornsberry et al.[19] indicate that a 10 U penicillin disk can also be applied, as it discriminates the ampicillin-resistant from ampicillin-susceptible strains well using the same interpretive criteria as described for *Haemophilus* with the ampicillin disk.

The resistance of *H. influenzae* to other antimicrobial agents will be perceived using the regular criteria (Table 87-2) for the disk diffusion susceptibility test.

β-LACTAMASE TEST METHODS

The determination of β-lactamase production is rarely carried out except with *H. influenzae, N. gonorrhoeae,* and *S. aureus.* The tests that are described in this section are applicable for any of the 3 organisms, and the testing procedure would be, in essence, similar with each of the 3 with the exception of the growth requirements, which may be different for the former 2 as contrasted to staphylococci. In addition, whereas the production of β-lactamase is usually rapidly demonstrated with *Haemophilus* and *Neisseria,* it can take longer to manifest itself with staphylococci. The test should be allowed to incubate for at least 1 hour. A further difference between *Staphylococcus* and the other 2 is that the β-lactamases produced by staphylococci may be inducible, whereas the β-lactamases of *H. influenzae* and *N. gonorrhoeae* are not.

Four tests will be described for the production of β-lactamase. Each has its advantages and disadvantages,[57] and the applicability varies with regard to the individual laboratory setting and, in the case of the chromogenic cephalosporin test, is dependent upon the availability of the testing material. The advantages and disadvantages of the methods are presented as summarized by Thornsberry.[57]

Advantages and disadvantages

1. Rapid iodometric test
   a. Advantages
      (1) Rapid results available on same day pure culture is available to test
      (2) Reagents readily available and inexpensive
      (3) Easy to perform
      (4) Original culture plate can be used if well-isolated colonies present (grossly contaminated plates not suitable)
      (5) Well-defined, easy-to-read end point
   b. Disadvantages
      (1) Multistep test
      (2) Reagents less stable than the chromogenic cephalosporin
2. Acidometric test
   a. Advantages
      (1) Rapid results available on same day culture is available to test
      (2) Reagents readily available and inexpensive
      (3) Easy to perform
      (4) 1-step test
      (5) Original culture plate can be used if well-isolated colonies present (grossly contaminated plates not suitable)
   b. Disadvantages
      (1) Requires correct pH adjustments
      (2) Reagents less stable than chromogenic cephalosporin

3. Chromogenic cephalosporin test
   a. Advantages
      (1) Can be used easily in the field; simple, easy to perform
      (2) Reagents stable
      (3) Rapid results on same day culture is ready to test
      (4) Original culture plate can be used if well-isolated colonies present (grossly contaminated plates are suitable)
   b. Disadvantages
      (1) Chromogenic cephalosporin may not be readily available; must be obtained from 1 English company (Glaxo, Ltd., Greenford, Middlesex UB6 OHE, England)

Chromogenic cephalosporin test for β-lactamase production in bacteria[57, 58]

Materials. Dissolve 10 mg cephalosporin 87/312 in 1 ml dimethyl sulfoxide (DMSO). Dilute with pH 7.0 phosphate buffer to a concentration of 500 μg/ml. The solution is yellow when viewed in a microdilution plate but may appear more orange in larger volumes. However, the red of a positive test is easily discerned. This solution is stable at 4-10 C for many weeks.

To prepare pH 7.0 phosphate buffer, mix 39.2 ml solution A (0.06M monopotassium phosphate) to 60.8 ml solution B (0.06M disodium phosphate). Solution A contains 9.07 g KH_2PO_4 in 1000 ml distilled water. Solution B contains 9.46 g Na_2HPO_4 in 1000 ml distilled water. This buffer is stable for several weeks at room temperature.

Procedure

Microdilution plate or small tube. Add 0.05 ml cephalosporin substrate to a well of a microdilution plate (or to a small tube). With a loop remove the growth from several colonies of the test organism. Make a heavy turbid suspension in the cephalosporin solution. Mix for 1 min. Observe for color change immediately, after 10 min, and after 1 h. If the culture produces β-lactamase, the substrate will change from yellow to red. β-Lactamase-producing *H. influenzae* or *N. gonorrhoeae* usually turn the solution red in less than 10 min, but staphylococci may take an hour. Run the test with a known β-lactamase- and a non-β-lactamase-producing strain of *N. gonorrhoeae, H. influenzae,* or *S. aureus.*

Agar plate modification. The agar plate should contain the organism in pure culture. Place a drop (approximately 0.05 ml) of the cephalosporin reagent on an area of bacterial growth. Tilt the plate slightly to permit the drop to spread across the plate. If the organism produced β-lactamase the reagent along the streak will turn red, but if it is β-lactamase negative, the reagent along the streak will be yellow. Although the red is not as easily seen as in the test done in the microdilution well, it is generally easy to see. If on rare occasions there is uncertainty, repeat the test in a microdilution well or small tube. Usually the positive test can be read immediately, but the plate should be reexamined after 10 min. However, experience with staphylococci is very limited.

PRECAUTIONS: (1) Primary isolation medium (e.g., modified Thayer-Martin medium) may grow β-lactamase-producing bacteria in addition to the bacteria of interest (e.g., *N. gonorrhoeae*) and may result in a false-positive test; (2) clinical specimens (e.g., urethral discharge, vaginal secretion) cannot be tested directly in the chromogenic cephalosporin test.

Rapid iodometric test for β-lactamase production in bacteria[57,59]

Materials

Sodium or potassium penicillin G. Add sodium or potassium penicillin G powder (most readily available as sodium or potassium penicillin G for intravenous human use) to freshly prepared pH 6.0 phosphate buffer to obtain a solution with a concentration of 6.000 μg/ml. Small aliquots of the penicillin solution can be dispensed into vials that can be tightly sealed and frozen in non-frost-free freezers. Frost-free freezers are unsuitable because repeated thawing cycles destroy the penicillin. Properly stored aliquots can be thawed and used for up to 1 wk or as long as correct results are obtained with control cultures of known reactivity.

1. To prepare pH 6.0 phosphate buffer, mix 87.7 ml solution A (0.06M monopotassium phosphate) to 12.3 ml solution B (0.06M disodium phosphate). Solution A contains 9.07 g KH_2PO_4 in 1000 ml distilled water. Solution B contains 9.46 g Na_2HPO_4 or 11.88 g $Na_2HPO_4 \cdot 2H_2O$ in 1000 ml distilled water. This buffer is stable for several weeks at room temperature.
2. To prepare the penicillin solution weigh small amount of penicillin powder, e.g., 0.5 g (500,000 μg). Divide 500,000 by 6,000 to get number of milliliters buffer needed to dilute penicillin to obtain 6,000 μg/ml (0.6 μg—1.0 U penicillin). In the example, add 0.5 g penicillin G to 83.3 ml pH 6.0 phosphate buffer.
3. Some laboratories prefer to sterilize penicillin solution by filtering it through 0.22 or 0.45 μm membrane filter before using it in assay.

Starch solution. Add 1.0 g soluble starch to 100 ml distilled water. Place in boiling water bath until starch goes into solution. Prepare fresh or store in refrigerator for no more than 1 wk. Smaller volumes of this 1% solution can be made because 10 ml is enough for over 100 tests. Starch designated for use in iodometric tests is commercially available.

Iodine. Dissolve 2.03 g I and 53.2 g KI in 100 ml distilled water. Store at room temperature in brown glass bottle. Prepare fresh when the solution develops excessive precipitate (usually several months). Run the test with known β-lactamase-positive and β-lactamase-negative strains of *N. gonorrhoeae, H. influenzae,* or *S. aureus.*

Procedure. Dispense 0.1 ml penicillin solution into well of microdilution plate or small test tube.

Remove the growth from several colonies of an 18-24 h pure culture with a loop and make a **heavy** turbid suspension in the penicillin solution in the well. An adequate amount of inoculum should produce a cloudy suspension. Stir for 30 s and **let the mixture stand for 1 h at room temperature to allow time for the β-lactamase to break down the penicillin to penicilloic acid.** *H. influenzae* and *N. gonorrhoeae* usually do not require an hour of incubation, but staphylococci may. Add 2 drops starch solution to the suspension of bacteria and penicillin. **Mix.** Add 1 drop iodine reagent with a Pasteur pipet. The solution will immediately turn blue because of the reaction of the iodine and the starch. If the iodine is added prematurely, the enzymatic reaction may stop and a false-negative test may result. Stir the mixture for 1 min. Rapid decolorization indicates the production of β-lactamase. If the solution remains blue for longer than 10 min, the culture did not produce the enzyme.

PRECAUTIONS: (1) Primary isolation medium (e.g., modified Thayer-Martin medium) may grow β-lactamase-producing bacteria in addition to the bacteria of interest (e.g., *N. gonorrhoeae*) and may result in a false-positive test; (2) clinical specimens (e.g., urethral discharge, vaginal secretions) cannot be tested directly in the iodometric test.

Rapid acidometric test for β-lactamase production in bacteria[57,60]

Materials. Two ml 0.5% phenol red solution is added to 16.6 ml sterile distilled water. This solution is then added to a vial containing 20 mil U potassium penicillin G (Pfizer, New York, N.Y.). Sodium hydroxide (1M) is added drop by drop until the test solution turns violet (pH 8.5). The test solution is either used immediately or divided into portions in screw-capped tubes and frozen at −60 C for as long as 1 wk.

Procedure. Dip a capillary tube (0.7-1.0 mm OD) into test solution and allow liquid to flow by capillary action for a distance of 1-2 cm into the tube. The tip of the capillary tube is scraped lightly across several *H. influenzae* colonies from an agar plate (chocolate agar plus 1% IsoVitaleX) that has been incubated 24 h, so that a plug of bacteria fills the bottom of the tube. Allow no air to be trapped between the test solution and the bacteria, since the 2 must be in contact. The filled capillary tubes are incubated at room temperature in vertical position. This is achieved by sticking the empty end of the capillary tube into clay and letting it hang straight down. If the organism produces β-lactamase, the test solution turns a bright yellow in 5-15 min. In the tests with organisms that do not produce β-lactamase, the test solution either does not change color at all or changes to no more than a pale pink. Include a penicillin-resistant *S. aureus* as a positive control and a penicillin-sensitive *S. aureus* as a negative control with each *Haemophilus* tested.

Rapid slide test for penicillinase reagents[61]

Materials. Sterile water (1 ml) is added to penicillin (penicillin G, potassium, for injection [buffered], USP, 1 mil U) vial, and 0.15 ml vol penicillin is removed and frozen at −20 C in 1-dram vials. (Frozen vials may be used for as long as 30 d and once thawed should be discarded after use.)

Procedure. Dissolve 1.5 g KI and 0.3 g I in 100 ml 0.1M phosphate buffer at pH 6.4. This buffer is prepared by the addition of 60 ml pH 6.0 buffer to 40 ml pH 7.0 buffer. The iodine solution is stored in a brown bottle at 4 C. A starch solution (0.4%) is prepared by dissolving 0.4 g solution starch (Difco) in 100 ml distilled water. The solution is then autoclaved and stored at 4 C.

A penicillin-iodine mixture is prepared by adding 1.1 ml iodine solution to a vial containing 0.5 ml thawed penicillin G. Once this mixture has been prepared it should be used within 1 h. A loopful of test organisms is removed from colonial growth on the surface of an agar plate and emulsified in 1 drop of the penicillin-iodine mixture on an ordinary glass microscope slide. Immediately, 1 drop of starch solution is added. A negative test for penicillinase is indicated by the development of purple or lavender that remains for 5 min.

White developing within 5 min indicates a positive test. Most reactions will be complete by 30 s, with a final reading taken at 5 min for the detection of small amounts of penicillinase.

SPECIAL ANTIMICROBIAL TESTING CONDITIONS
Bactericidal activity testing

Since most bacterial susceptibility testing is inhibitory in nature, the answers or results provided may be inadequate, and a lethal concentration may provide more precise and specific information. Such a situation may arise in the patient whose body defense mechanisms are compromised. Since in this circumstance the antimicrobial may lack for the synergism of the host-defense effect, the assessment of the bactericidal activity may become important. It is precisely in this circumstance that an adjustment of antimicrobial therapy may well be warranted based upon the bactericidal test result.

More recently a terminology has developed in which the designation minimal lethal concentration (MLC) has been proposed for the effect previously known as the bactericidal effect. The reader should be aware of the analogy with these terms.

Bactericidal testing is begun by performing a broth dilution test, as if for regular susceptibility testing. An additional step is added, that of making a 1:10 and 1:100 dilution of the control tube or well for purposes of determining the inoculum density. One then takes a 0.01 ml quantitative loop and subcultures from each of the 2 dilutions to one-half of a carefully marked blood agar plate, and, after incubation, calculates the inoculum concentration at the test inception. This plate is then incubated overnight, or in the same time frame as the regular broth susceptibility test. The MIC is recorded in micrograms per milliliter as the concentration in the highest dilution showing no visible growth; by using the same 0.01 quan-

titative loop, all the tubes or wells that have shown no visible growth turbidity are subcultured to a blood or chocolate agar plate. These samples can, by use of this quantitative loop, be taken to one-quarter of a blood agar plate. Again, the plate should be clearly marked as to the tube or well whence the inoculum for that quadrant has been derived.

The plates are incubated overnight at 35 C, and one then records the MBC or MLC in micrograms per milliliter as the concentration and the highest dilution that results in a calculated 99.9% kill of the original inoculum.

The methodology described above is geared for highest efficiency in a clinical laboratory setting; for practical purposes in a routine clinical laboratory setting, the procedure works well. Were one to perform bactericidal testing for reference or investigational purposes, a more carefully defined and volumetrically determined procedure should be performed.

Combination of synergy testing

The rational use of antibiotics—especially in serious infections, in the compromised host, and in unusual and difficult-to-treat circumstances—may require combination therapy for the most advantageous result. In that setting the justification for and effectiveness of such a regimen may require laboratory testing. Such testing can be carried out even when 3 or more compounds are used.[62] Due to the complexity of the

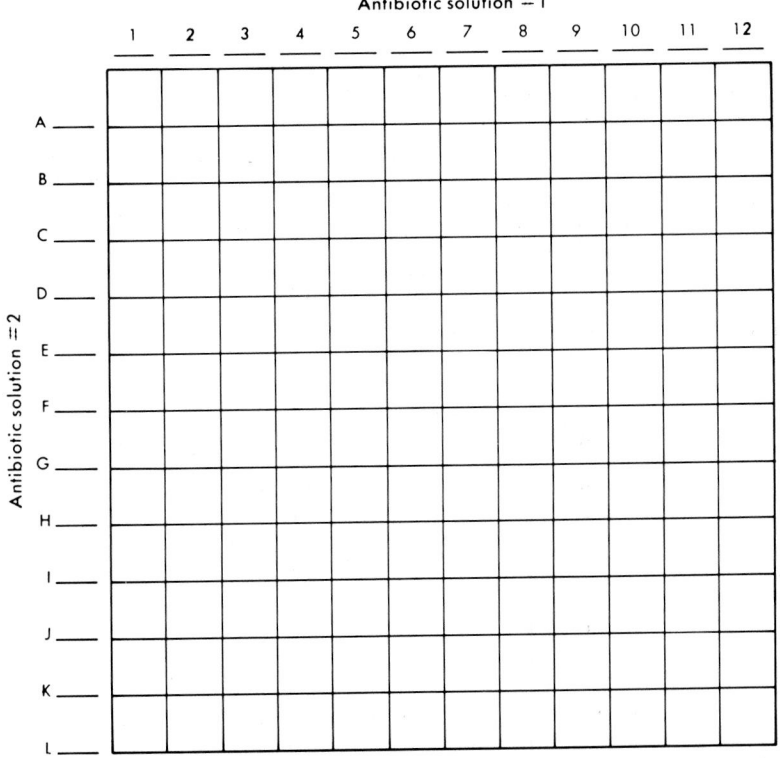

Fig. 87-2. Combination of synergy testing: the use of 2 microtiter plates (see text).

challenge presented by this testing, the method presented here is geared for efficiency and economy of performance.

Materials. The test procedure outlined here requires 2 microtiter plates and a set of 50 μl pipet droppers and 50 μl diluters. Mueller-Hinton broth is used and the antimicrobials to be tested are made up in solutions such that they can be utilized alone or in various combinations. The organisms to be tested should be standardized against 0.5 MacFarland standard and then diluted 1:100 in Mueller-Hinton broth.

Procedure. Two microtiter plates are placed side by side and the second plate is relabeled with the letters I instead of A, J instead of B, K instead of C, and L instead of D. Only 4 rows are used in this second plate (Fig. 87-2). Fifty μl Mueller-Hinton broth is dispensed to all wells except A-1 with a 50 μl pipet dropper. The antibiotic solutions are labeled 1 and 2 and are diluted to contain amounts equivalent to 4 times the final desired concentration. One hundred μl antibiotic solution 1 is added to well A-1, and 50 μl to the rest of the wells in column 1 (B-1) with the pipet dropper. Each well is then serially diluted in column 1 (A-1) across the plates through the wells in column 11 (do not dilute into the wells in column 12). Using the 50 μl pipet dropper, dispense 50 μl of antibiotic solution 2 into each well in row A (1-12). Again using the 50 μl diluters, dilute serially down from each well in row A (1-12) through wells in row K (do not dilute into wells in row L). Add 50 μl of the standardized organism suspension to each of the 144 wells using a 50 μl pipet dropper. Cover the plate with a plastic tape and incubate. The MIC for solution 1 can be obtained from wells 1-11 in row L and the MIC for solution 2 can be obtained from wells A-K in column 12. Well L-12 is the growth

control for the inoculated organism. It is important to have available a synergy-combination studies result chart (Fig. 87-2); this can be easily typed and maintained as a Xerox supply. These sheets should have the letters A-L on the vertical column to the left of the page and the numbers 1-12 across the top of the page in the horizontal column. This will allow for ease of recording, as it will fit nicely with the number and letter scheme on the microbroth tray. Using this form one should list the antimicrobial concentrations, the date, the organisms to be tested, and the results. This sheet also serves as a laboratory worksheet for use in calculating an isobologram. One begins at a point on the left-hand side of the work paper and records sequentially, on a non-log scale, the numbers up to the point of organism susceptibility for that antibiotic. For antibiotic 2, one begins at the same point in the lower corner and works to the right horizontally across the page, again recording the sequential numbers up to the point of organism susceptibility for that antimicrobic. The point of susceptibility for both is marked, and the line is drawn between the two. One then calculates the MIC of the combinations of the 2 organisms and joins those points with the line. If that line falls inside the line that has been drawn to join the 2 MIC values, then an additive or synergistic effect has been demonstrated. If the line joining the plots of the MICs of the combination is outside the line joining the 2 points on the parameters, then antagonism has been demonstrated.

QUALITY ASSURANCE OF SUSCEPTIBILITY PROCEDURES

Each susceptibility test procedure has its own quality control considerations. These specific considerations are presented by testing category.

Table 87-8. Control limits for monitoring precision and accuracy of inhibitory zone diameters obtained in groups of 5 separate observations with *E. coli* ATCC 25922

Antimicrobial agent	Disk content	Individual test control zone diameter (mm)	Accuracy control zone diameter (mm)*	Precision control (range of 5 values†)	
				Maximum	Average‡
Ampicillin	10 μg	15-20	15.8-19.2	6	2.9
Carbenicillin	100 μg	24-29	25.0-28.0	7	3.5
Cephalothin	30 μg	18-23	18.8-22.2	6	2.9
Chloramphenicol	30 μg	21-27	22.0-26.0	7	3.5
Colistin	10 μg	11-15	11.7-14.3	4	2.3
Erythromycin	15 μg	8-14	9.0-13.0	7	3.5
Gentamicin	10 μg	19-26	20.2-24.8	8	4.1
Kanamycin	30 μg	17-25	18.3-23.7	9	4.7
Neomycin	30 μg	17-23	18.0-22.0	6	3.5
Polymyxin B	300 U	12-16	12.7-15.3	4	2.3
Streptomycin	10 μg	12-20	13.3-18.7	9	4.7
Tetracycline	30 μg	18-25	19.2-23.8	8	4.1
Tobramycin	10 μg	18-26			
Trimethoprim-sulfamethoxazole	1.25 μg 23.75 μg	24-32	25.3-30.7	9	4.7

*Mean of 5 values.

†Maximum value minus minimum value obtained in series of 5 consecutive tests should not exceed listed maximum limits, and mean should fall within range listed under accuracy control.

‡In a continuing series of ranges from consecutive groups of 5 tests each, average range should approximate listed value.

Table 87-9. Control limits for monitoring precision and accuracy of inhibitory zone diameters obtained in groups of 5 separate observations with *S. aureus* ATCC 25923

Antimicrobial agent	Disk content	Individual test control zone diameter (mm)	Accuracy control zone diameter (mm)*	Precision control (range of 5 values†)	
				Maximum	Average‡
Ampicillin	10 μg	24-35	25.8-33.2	13	6.4
Cephalothin	30 μg	25-37	27.0-35.0	14	7.0
Chloramphenicol	30 μg	19-26	20.2-24.8	8	4.1
Clindamycin	2 μg	23-29	24.0-28.0	7	3.5
Erythromycin	15 μg	23-30	23.3-28.7	9	4.7
Gentamicin	10 μg	19-27	20.3-25.7	9	4.7
Kanamycin	30 μg	19-26	20.2-24.8	8	4.1
Methicillin	5 μg	17-22	17.8-21.2	6	2.9
Neomycin	30 μg	18-26	19.3-24.7	9	4.7
Penicillin G	10 U	26-37	27.8-35.2	13	6.4
Polymyxin B	300 U	7-13			
Streptomycin	10 μg	14-22	15.3-20.7	9	4.7
Tetracycline	30 μg	19-28	20.5-26.5	11	5.2
Tobramycin	10 μg	19-29			
Vancomycin	30 μg	15-19	15.7-18.3	4	2.3
Trimethoprim-sulfamethoxazole	1.25 μg 23.75 μg	24-32	25.0-31.0	7	3.5

*Mean of 5 values.
†Maximum value minus minimum value obtained in series of 5 consecutive tests should not exceed listed maximum limits, and mean should fall within range listed under accuracy control.
‡In a continuing series of ranges from consecutive groups of 5 tests each, average range should approximate listed value.

Table 87-10. Suggested quality control limits for inhibitory zone diameters tested with *P. aeruginosa* ATCC 27853

Antimicrobial agent	Disk content	Individual test control zone diameter (mm)
Carbenicillin	100 μg	19-25
Gentamicin	10 μg	16-22
Tobramycin	10 μg	19-25
Polymyxin B	300 U	13-18
Colistin	10 μg	11-15
Tetracycline	30 μg	6-14
Chloramphenicol	30 μg	6-12

Disk diffusion testing

The performance of the 3 ATCC strains used for quality control has been carefully defined. Tables 87-8 to 87-10 provide a tabulation of the values expected with respect to the disk zone sizes of the control stains. These are pertinent tables for those using the disk diffusion method and should be maintained for reference. The individual control strains are tested with the various sets of antimicrobics used for the different groups of bacterial organisms, and, therefore there will be overlapping in the antimicrobials tested for *S. aureus* and *E. coli*, *S. aureus* and *P. aeruginosa*, and *P. aeruginosa* and *E. coli*. This provides a double check on the performance of

antimicrobials and for the overall test situation for those agents for which there is duplicate control organism testing.

The control strains should be tested daily or each time the test is performed, and the zone sizes should be recorded on a quality control chart for easy visualization. Should problems arise with zone sizes falling outside the expected range, an investigation must be conducted to determine the reason for the test aberration.

A new vial of antimicrobial disks should be tested the day before its insertion into the regular disk dispenser in order to detect any potential problems. Over the years a large number of vials have been discarded due to the pretest monitoring of their performance. This step is highly recommended; it will preclude the necessity of having to repeat all the susceptibility tests any time any disk from a new vial performs poorly, and it will obviate at least some instances wherein a decision would be made not to report susceptibility results as performed on that day because the zones for the control organisms were not within accepted limits.

Agar dilution

Each agar dilution series should be inoculated with the control strains listed above for dilution testing. At the Mayo Clinic, where agar dilution testing has been used since the 1940s, they advocate also using the *E. coli* (ATCC 25922) and the *S. aureus* (ATCC 25923). They additionally use a strain of *P. aeruginosa* for the control of those compounds usually tested and reported for *P. aeruginosa*. A copy of their means and ranges of MICs with control organisms has been published.[35] In addition to the regular antibiotic agar dilution series plates, it is also important to inoculate a plate that does not contain antimicrobials in order to verify the viability of the test organism. In addition each well of the seed plate should be sampled with an inoculating loop and transferred to a quadrant of a blood agar plate in order to detect the potential presence of contaminants and to verify the purity of the culture.

Results should be carefully recorded on a chart that allows visual comparison with expected susceptibility values for control strains and that allows ready visibility and detection of any apparent problems.

Broth dilution testing

Dilution testing in general presents some special quality control challenges. With broth dilution testing, wherein the majority of what is performed in this country is done as microbroth dilution testing, it is apparent that each dilution set will contain 8-12 two-fold dilutions. In this context control organisms should provide a means of evaluating the performance of each antimicrobial agent, and the values to be expected should be at least 2 two-fold dilutions from either end of the dilution scale for each antimicrobial evaluated. Whereas control stains have been designated for the disk diffusion methodology by virtue of the FDA recommendations and the National Committee for Clinical Laboratory Standards suggestions, for the broth dilution testing the organisms listed above have only semiofficial status. In this context committees are at work to attempt to define appropriate standard reference strains that will provide the wherewithal to test each antimicrobial routinely used in broth dilution testing with common-use strains. In the interim it is suggested that *S. aureus* (ATCC 29213) and *S. faecalis* (ATCC 29212) be used.[19]

The 2 quality control strains noted above for dilution testing should be run with each set of dilutions performed. Since most laboratories will perform susceptibility tests on a number of organisms each day, it is to be expected that, in order to appropriately control the performance of broth dilution tests, test organisms will be run with each group of organisms tested. It should also be noted here that the broth dilution tests are the most vulnerable to inoculum variations and may provide the most accurate test of the highest potential for resistance.

Since the turbidity standard is used for all antimicrobial susceptibility testing standardizations, it should be carefully maintained as described in the general comments section of the Dilution Testing portion of this chapter. The density of the turbidity standards should be checked regularly to ensure their accuracy.

Autobac I

Because one is dealing with disks as a source of antimicrobic and because of the variety of test conditions—including instrument function—control strains of the organisms listed earlier in this chapter for the Autobac should be run with each group of test determinations or on a daily basis. Quality control for any instrumentation should include careful and complete instrument maintenance as well.

General considerations

The 3 methodologies listed above comprise the majority of susceptibility testing performed in the clinical laboratory. Other susceptibility testing situations are in essence modifications of these procedures, and the quality control features suggested for these tests are modified to allow for appropriate assessment of the alternate test performance. In this context it should be stated that there are a number of steps that can provide potential problems in any of these particular tests. However, it is the actual performance with control strains that allows the best opportunity to monitor the overall procedure. While some errors will be more likely to occur than others, some type of log should be kept as to the nature of problems that have occurred and the steps that have been taken to correct these problems and to obviate their recurrence. If one is to appropriately assess performance, one should carefully and periodically check each step of any procedure performed in the laboratory.

Unusual susceptibility testing

The susceptibility testing for anaerobes and for *N. gonorrhoeae, H. influenzae,* and *N. meningitidis*—with their individual test variations—require that the clinical laboratory maintain the capacity for control assessment. However, there are no clearly defined reference strains for these particular tests at present. Therefore, the laboratory should attempt to maintain appropriate stock organism of each of these particular organisms. The *Neisseria* and *Haemophilus* species are difficult to maintain in a clinical laboratory setting short of freezing at −70 C, and even there, there is a great risk of organism loss of viability, especially due to the actual freezing and thawing processes themselves.

ASSAYS OF ANTIMICROBIAL AGENTS
Indications for assays

The performance of a determination of the level of antimicrobial in the serum or body fluid of the patient is usually requested in order to determine potential therapeutic effect of that agent to assess the risk of toxicity. The circumstances in which antimicrobial assays are ordered, therefore, are those situations wherein a low therapeutic-toxic ratio may exist with an antibiotic, as in the case of aminoglycoside antibiotics or in the case of chloramphenicol in newborn infants. Another indication would be with

Table 87-11. Methods for assaying antibiotic levels in serum and body fluids

Antimicrobial	Bioassay method	Control organism	Other antimicrobials that can be present without affecting test validity
Ampicillin	*Clostridium* assay	*C. perfringens*	Aminoglycosides
Amikacin	*Klebsiella* assay	*Klebsiella* ATCC 27799	Ampicillin, carbenicillin, cephalothin, chloramphenicol, clindamycin, other penicillins
Carbenicillin	*Clostridium* assay	*C. perfringens*	Aminoglycosides
Cephalothin	*Bacillus* assay	*B. subtilis* 6633	
Cefazolin	*Bacillus* assay	*B. subtilis* 6633	
Clindamycin	*Clostridium* assay	*C. perfringens*	Aminoglycosides
Chloramphenicol	*Clostridium* assay	*C. perfringens*	Aminoglycosides
Gentamicin	*Klebsiella* assay	*Klebsiella* ATCC 27799	Ampicillin, carbenicillin, cephalothin, chloramphenicol, clindamycin, other penicillins
Nafcillin	*Bacillus* assay	*B. subtilis* ATCC 6633	
Penicillin	*Bacillus* assay	*B. subtilis* ATCC 6633	
Tobramycin	*Klebsiella* assay	*Klebsiella* ATCC 27799	Ampicillin, carbenicillin, cephalothin, chloramphenicol, clindamycin, other penicillins
Vancomycin	*Clostridium* assay	*C. perfringens*	Aminoglycosides

patients in whom the anticipated clinical effect has not been demonstrated; the therapy failure could well be due to individual variations in the pharmacokinetic behavior of the antimicrobial in the patient or to patient, organism, or antimicrobial effects that might work to thwart the action of the antimicrobial. These factors are worthy of assessment because often something can be done to obviate their potential or actual effect in the patient. Antimicrobial assays may also be important in the treatment of severe local infections—where fluid specimens may be available for assay—or in situations where the underlying disease of the patient is such that it is assumed that the antibiotic must do more than the routine task of eradicating the organism.

The list of assay methods includes chemical, turbidimetric, agar diffusion, pH alteration and inhibition, enzymatic, radioimmunoassay, hemoglobin reduction, chromatograph analysis, etc. It is anticipated that radioimmunoassay and high-pressure liquid chromatography will become more and more available in the future. In the interim, and for those hospitals where the availability of instrumentation is seen as a deterrent, there are several bioassay means that can be used effectively in the clinical laboratory to assess the presence of most antimicrobials. The 3 test organisms with their accompanying procedures listed in Table 87-11 would cover well over 90% of the assay requests at the University of Utah Medical Center. For the high-volume aminoglycoside assay requests we use the radioimmunoassay (RIA) during the daytime hours and resort to the bioassay in the evening and on weekends. For the less frequently used aminoglycosides we continue to do the bioassay for economic reasons. When 3 or more radioimmu-

noassays of a specific compound are performed in 1 day, then the cost savings is sufficient to justify performing those tests by RIA on a regular basis. Table 87-11 lists the bioassay methods that can be used in assaying the antibiotic levels in serum and body fluids.

Bacillus subtilis assay

The *B. subtilis* assay can be used for the individual antimicrobials listed in Table 87-12 when no other antibiotics are present. It can also be used as a general method for testing the aminoglycoside antibiotics in the presence of β-lactam antibiotics if β-lactamase is used to inactivate the cephalosporins and penicillins. It represents a means for the testing of the aminoglycosides and also a method for testing the individual antibiotics not covered by other assay methods. The method as described here is extracted from the description by Sabath and Matsen.[63]

Preparation of assay strain. The assay organism is the spore of *B. subtilis* ATCC 6633. This is purchased (Difco) as a lyophilized preparation. The procedure for preparing spores is defined in Sabath and Matsen.[63]

Preparation and storage of assay plates. The assay plates are prepared by adding 0.1 ml *B. subtilis* spore suspension to each 100 ml molten assay medium (Difco antibiotic assay medium no. 5 or Grove and Randall medium no. 5 at 48-65 C), pouring 5 ml uniformly seeded agar into 100 mm plastic Petri dishes, and permitting them to harden on a level bench (check with spirit level) at room temperature. The plates can be used immediately or stored at 4 C in sealed plastic bags for future use; plates stored for less than 2 wk provide results after 2 hr of incubation, and plates stored 2-6 wk require 4-5 h of incubation before readings can be made.

Setting up test. The assay of a single serum requires 2 assay plates and sixteen 0.6 cm (0.25 in.) paper disks

Table 87-12. Anticipated peak antibiotic serum levels (moderate dose)

Antimicrobial	Serum concentration ($\mu g/ml$)	Urine concentration ($\mu g/ml$)
Amikacin (IM)	10-25	150-250
Amoxacillin (PO)	5-7	1000-1500
Ampicillin		
PO	2-4	100-600
IV	3-7	100-600
Carbenicillin		
PO	5-15	600-1200
IV	100-200	600-1500
Cefazolin (IM)	25-50	1500-3000
Cephalexin (PO)	6-20	800-2000
Cephalothin (IV)	10-60	1000-1500
Chloramphenicol (PO)	4-14	50-120
Clindamycin		
PO	2-5	8-25
IV	10-20	20-45
Colistimethate	4-8	50-250
Erythromycin		
PO	1-4	15-50
IV	5-15	50-200
Gentamicin (IM)	4-7	100-300
Kanamycin (IM)	12-30	150-300
Methicillin (IV)	10-20	50-120
Penicillin G (PO)	0.5	70-100
Polymyxin B (IM)	2-6	15
Tetracyclines		
PO	1-4	1200
IM	4-6	100-300
Tobramycin (IM)	4-7	100-300

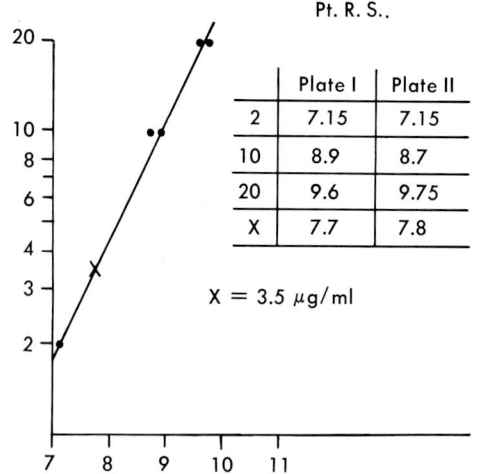

Gentamicin assay

Klebsiella 1296 Date 11/11

Pt. R. S..

	Plate I	Plate II
2	7.15	7.15
10	8.9	8.7
20	9.6	9.75
X	7.7	7.8

X = 3.5 μg/ml

Fig. 87-3. Standard curve used for determining antimicrobial level by bioassay means. *X* represents specimen being tested.

(Schleicher & Schuell Co., Keene, N.H., no. 740-E). The disks are placed in 4 rows of 4 disks in the inverted lid of one of the assay plates, and 0.02 ml (use Land-Levy-type pipet) of the sample is placed on each of the 4 disks in the top row. Three standards are used. Normal human sera (each batch should be checked to be sure it does not contain antimicrobial activity before the "standard" amount of antibiotic is added) containing 12, 6, and 1.5 μg/ml are used for the gentamicin serum assay (suggested standards for other assays are as follows: for streptomycin 25, 12.5, and 3.1 μg/ml; for vancomycin 40, 20, and 10 μg/ml; for kanamycin 27, 9, and 3 μg/ml; and for tobramycin and neomycin 12, 6, and 1.5 μg/ml); 0.02 ml of each standard is placed on each of 4 paper disks. A reference mark should be made on the bottom of each assay plate, and 1 paper disk containing the 12 μg standard should be placed on the surface of the seeded agar near the reference mark, about 1 cm from the edge, and pressed firmly in place with metal forceps. In a similar fashion, samples for assay are placed on the surface of the agar in the sequence going clockwise. Duplicates for each of these 4 disks are placed on the agar surface of the same plate so that pairs containing the same fluid are opposite each other. In an identical fashion the other 8 disks are placed to form a ring on the surface of the seeded agar in the second plate, and the 2 assay plates are placed on a level shelf at 37 C.[63]

Incubation and reading. After about 4 h of incubation, zones of inhibition are visible around the disks containing antibiotic (if gentamicin, at ≥0.37 μg/ml). The zone diameters can be measured with a ruler or, for greater accuracy, with a vernier caliper. The rapidity of result availability will depend upon plate freshness.

Calculation. Results are calculated by forming a standard curve (Fig. 87-3) on semilog paper relating the concentration of antibiotic in the standard sera (log scale) to the diameter (in millimeters) of the zone of inhibition produced. A separate curve is made for each of the 2 plates (each point the mean of the duplicate standards) and diameters of the zones around the 2 sample disks on each plate. The final result of the assay is the mean of the values obtained from each plate. Thus, if plate A gave a value of 5.8 μg/ml and plate B a value of 6.2 μg/ml, the value to be recorded for the sample would be 6.0 μg/ml.

Assay of samples containing more than 1 antibiotic

This agar diffusion assay described can conveniently be used to measure gentamicin or other aminoglycosides in the presence of any other penicillin or cephalosporin currently in use in the United States by simply adding 0.02 ml β-lactamase II–containing fluid (obtainable from Whatman Biochemicals, Maidenhead, Surrey, England) to 0.1 ml serum for assay a few minutes before loading the disks (in calculating results, allow for dilution of sample by enzyme fluid by increasing "apparent" gentamicin value by 20%). Alternatively, an appropriate β-lactamase II–containing fluid may be prepared by simply growing *B. cereus* 569 (obtainable from the American Type Culture Collection, Rockville, Md. ATCC 27348) in Difco brain-heart infusion broth containing 20 μg cephalothin/ml, at 37 C for 18 hours, and using the supernatant fluid as crude β-lactamase II. Should a non-β-lactamase antibiotic (such as tetracycline or clindamycin) be present, the assay should be performed with an assay organism highly resistant to the accompanying antibiotic. The *Klebsiella* bioassay was developed by Lund, Blazevic, and Matsen[64] for the rapid determination of gentamicin of blood

Table 87-13. Susceptibility of *Klebsiella* ATCC 27799 to 18 antibiotics

Antibiotic	MIC*	Zone size† (mm)
Ampicillin	>1000	6
Amikacin	0.8	
Carbenicillin	>2000	6
Cephalothin	300	6
Chloramphenicol	>2000	6
Clindamycin	500	6
Colistin	3.1	14
Erythromycin	800	8
Gentamicin	1.5	20
Kanamycin	>1000	6
Methicillin	>1000	6
Naladixic acid	12.5	16
Nitrofurantoin	500	7
Penicillin G	>2000	6
Polymyxin B	1.5	15
Streptomycin	>1000	6
Tetracycline	>2000	6
Tobramycin	0.2	
Vancomycin		6

*Minimum inhibitory concentration in μg/ml (U/ml for penicillin G and polymyxin B).
†Inhibition zone diameter from disk diffusion method.

and other body fluids, especially for those samples in which there is the presence of other antimicrobial agents (Table 87-13). This assay may also be used for the determination of body fluid and blood levels of tobramycin and amikacin. The basic principles of this test are similar to those previously described for the *B. subtilis* assay. The advantages of this particular approach are that it can be used when other antimicrobials are present, and if one maintains a fresh subculture of this stable organism, one can achieve a reading with almost all test situations within 2½-3 hours of setting up the test. This is especially true if one utilizes the Fisher-Lilly zone reader (Fisher Scientific, Pittsburgh, Pa.).

Media. Antibiotic medium no. 11 (Difco) is employed as follows. Twenty-five ml medium, either fresh or from a single melted agar tube if 15 × 100 mm plates are to be used (or 2 tubes if 15 × 150 mm plates are to be used), is readied. One allows the agar to cool to 50 C and then adds 0.3-0.4 ml of the overnight broth culture of the *Klebsiella,* which had been freshly subcultured the day before. This is mixed well, and 9 ml of this seeded agar is added to each of two 15 × 100 mm sterile Petri dishes. This is to be certain the medium is evenly distributed over the bottom of the plates. It is important that the surface upon which the plates are poured is flat, even to the point of being measured with a spirit level. If several antimicrobial levels are to be done at the same time (up to 5), the contents of the entire tube of seeded agar should be added to each of two 15 × 150 mm sterile Petri plates.

Stock standards of gentamicin, tobramycin, and amikacin are stored at −20 C or lower in concentrations of 5000 μg/ml. The working standards are prepared by diluting the stocks to 200 μg/ml in sterile distilled water (0.2 ml of 5000 μg/ml plus 4.8 ml of sterile water). One ml of this 200 mg/ml stock is added to 9 ml serum diluent. This will provide a 20 mg standard. The 10 mg

standard is prepared by further diluting 5 ml of the 20 mg standard with 5 ml of serum, and the 2 mg/ml standard is prepared by diluting 1 ml of the 10 mg/ml standard with 4 ml of serum.

For the actual test procedure one places 2 sets of disks (3 standards and 1 unknown) in duplicate on the surface of each of 2 assay plates using sterile forceps. One should not place more than 8 disks on a 15 × 100 mm plate. The plate should be labeled underneath each disk with the appropriate designation, and duplicates should be placed opposite each other on the plate. The plates should be incubated singly (do not stack) at 35 C until a clear zone of inhibition appears around the standards. This usually requires 2-3 h.

For patients who have renal failure and are receiving cephalothin, cefaloridine, or cefazolin, it is suggested that one add sterile β-lactamase in order to overcome the potentially high levels of these antimicrobials.

Interpretation. The diameters of the zone of inhibition are measured from the back of the plates using a caliper with a vernier scale and measured to the closest 0.1 mm. A zone reader may also be used. The mean diameter around each pair of standard disks is plotted against the concentration of the standards on 2-cycle semilog graph paper as demonstrated in Fig. 87-3. A line is drawn through the points, and the concentration of antimicrobial in the patient's serum is determined by locating the point of the curve from the appropriate plate for the mean of the diameters of the zone of inhibition around the 2 serum-unknown disks placed on that plate. One averages the result from each plate and reports the result to the nearest 0.1 μg.

Clostridium microassay for the determination of nonaminoglycoside levels

The following antibiotics may be assayed by the *Clostridium* microassay in the presence of gentamicin, tobramycin, or amikacin, since the test organism is resistant to these aminoglycoside antimicrobials: clindamycin, chloramphenicol, vancomycin, carbenicillin, ampicillin, and penicillin; nafcillin cannot be assayed by this method.

Media. Brain-heart infusion (BHI) broth with agarose is used for this procedure.

Test organism. A *C. perfringens* strain is stored in chopped meat–glucose broth and is subcultured as often as a sample is removed from the culture. Two to 3 drops of sheep red blood cells should be added to the new chopped meat glucose and a sheep blood plate should be inoculated as a purity and hemolysis check. Both cultures should be taped to prevent the rubber stoppers from blowing off due to the extreme gas production by the *C. perfringens.*

Standards. The standard concentration is to be used in assaying each of the antibiotics:
  Ampicillin: 2.0, 10.0, and 20.0 μg/ml
  Carbenicillin: 6.3, 12.5, 25.0, and 50.0 μg/ml
  Clindamycin: 0.1, 1.0, 2.0, and 10.0 μg/ml
  Vancomycin: 2.5, 10.0, and 20.0 μg/ml
The standards are to be prepared by diluting the high stock standard to 200 μg/ml in sterile distilled water and then further diluting in sterile human sera to the concentrations noted above.

Procedure. A tube of BHI agar is prepared for each unknown body fluid sample to be tested. This is placed in a 56 C water bath and allowed to cool. One-tenth of the *Clostridium* culture is added to each tube along with 0.9 ml of sheep red blood cells. This is mixed well and pipetted (5 ml) into each of 2 sterile plastic 15 × 100 mm Petri dishes. These plates are allowed to solidify. There is a delivery of 20 μl of each standard solution and unknown to 4 filter paper disks, and these are placed on the surface of the plates, using 2 disks of each standard and 2 disks of unknown on each plate and placing these opposite each other. The plates are sealed in an anaerobe jar. The jar is left at room temperature for 1 h. The jar is then incubated at 37 C for an additional 2 or 3 h. The zone sizes should be read across the total diameter of growth inhibition. Where no growth occurs, no β-hemolysis will be evident, and complete clearing will be evident where the organism has grown. The zone sizes of the standard are plotted on semilog graph paper as shown in Fig. 87-3 and the result extrapolated for the patient unknowns.

As carbenicillin and clindamycin may exceed the standards, it may be necessary to run the serum in dilution, and therefore it is helpful to know what the physician expects the levels to be. Since chloramphenicol is bacteriostatic rather than bactericidal, levels should be allowed to incubate overnight, but should be initially read after 3-4 h incubation.

The BHI-agarose agar for the *Clostridium* antibiotic assay is prepared by taking 18.5 g BHI broth base and adding this to 500 ml water. The BHI broth is heated to almost boiling before adding 5 g agarose. The combination is then reheated to dissolve the agarose. This can then be dispensed in 11 ml amounts in screw-cap test tubes prior to autoclaving at 121 C for 15 min.

Interpretation of assay results

Table 87-12 categorizes anticipated urine and serum concentrations of various antimicrobials following a moderate dose. The pharmacokinetics of the compound, physiologic organ function of the patient, and factors relating to drug administration must all be considered in interpreting the result.

Serum bactericidal testing

The serum bactericidal assay or Schlichter test is used in circumstances of endocarditis and osteomyelitis and for evaluating therapy potential in other serious infections.[65-69] At this time there is considerable discussion as to a standardized method for performing this test. Basically this test employs a process of carefully serially diluting the patient's serum taken while the patient is receiving an antimicrobial agent. The purpose is to determine the titer of the antimicrobial activity of the serum-antibiotic combination against the organism isolated from the infectious process in the patient being studied. There is an actual quantitation of the organisms being used in order to give an indication as to the sensitivity of the test and also to provide a means by which one may assess the reproducibility of precision of the tests; this is desirable should repeat determinations be necessary in the event of switching to oral therapy or to another antimicrobial agent. The interpretation of this test should be generalized to all infections. One may anticipate that the effect achieved in the patient is adequate if a peak bactericidal activity has been demonstrated in a dilution of 1:8 to 1:16 or greater. Some will prefer to measure the trough

level and base a judgment on that response. In the circumstances of staphylococcal infections one usually hopes for an activity of 1:32 or greater in endocarditis. Whereas this test may be extremely helpful in predicting the outcome of osteomyelitis and endocarditis in patients who do not have prosthetic valves or joints, it has been my experience that where prosthetic devices are involved, the outcome is not predictable in the same fashion as it is in the patient with infection with natural heart valves or in the absence of joint prosthesis. This test, in selected infections, is an indicator of therapeutic effect and a predictor of therapeutic success.

Medium. Medium is trypticase–soy broth (TSB) organism. The test organism is the organism isolated from the patient's site of infection. If the patient has endocarditis, then the organism was taken from the blood. If one is testing in circumstance of osteomyelitis, then the organism is either a blood-borne isolate or an isolate aspirated directly from the lesion area. The patient's organism is inoculated into 4 ml of TSB broth. This is incubated aerobically at 35 C for 4 hours or until the broth turbidity matches that of a 0.5 MacFarland standard. It should be noted that endocarditis may be caused by slow-growing organisms such as viridans streptococci that may require the addition of 5% horse serum and overnight incubation. Where serum has been added as a facilitator of growth, it should be used through the entire test in order to enhance the growth of the organism.

Procedure. A sample of blood is obtained from the patient, and one separates the serum aseptically and stores it at −20 C until it is used. If the patient has a positive blood culture, the serum should be filtered prior to use.

Sterile TSB broth (0.5 ml) is pipetted into 7 tubes. The patient's serum is thawed and mixed, and 0.5 ml serum is added to the first tube in the series, which does not have any broth in it. This serves as a nondiluted control tube. One then places the same 0.5 ml serum into the first tube containing TSB broth. One mixes and transfers 0.5 ml from tube 2 to tube 3 and continues to make full serial dilutions through tube 6. Then 0.5 ml is discarded from tube 6, and tube 7 serves as the organism growth control and contains only broth. Therefore, as the set evolves there is 1 tube with 1 serum, 1 tube with only broth, and the other tubes have been serially diluted with the patient's serum in a broth base.

The test organism broth culture is adjusted to a MacFarland standard as noted and a 10^3-10^4 dilution is made. Of the 10^3 dilution 0.5 ml is added to each tube in the series, mixed well, and incubated aerobically at 35 C for 24 h. By using a 0.001 ml quantitative loop, duplicate plates are streaked for counts from the 10^3 and 10^4 dilution tubes and incubated at 35 C for 24 h. After 24 h of incubation the number of organisms present is determined in the 10^3 dilution. The methodology should approximate 10^5 CFU/ml (the actual number will vary from 5×10^4 to 5×10^5 CFU/ml). After 24 h incubation the test organism tubes are shaken and the results recorded as "growth" or "no-growth" on the serum bactericidal assay form. All tubes showing no visible growth are evaluated by inoculating 0.01 ml with a quantitative loop on one-quarter of a sheep blood agar plate. One then incubates overnight at 35 C. The next day the number of colonies from each tube is recorded and the results reported as the highest dilution (least amount of serum) showing no growth or only 1 colony (99.9% killing). A suggested wording for the reporting of these values is as follows: "Organism _____, Source _____, Using a challenge inoculum of _____ organism/ml. The serum bactericidal level is _____. For this method the bacteriologic effects of serum diluted 1:8-1:16 or more are regularly associated with eradication of the organism in patients with bacterial endocarditis. (Exceptions may occur with prosthetic devices or foreign materials.)"

REFERENCES

1. Steers, E., Foltz, E. L., and Graves, B. S.: Antibiot. Chemother. **9**:307, 1959.
2. Washington, J. A., II: Mayo Clin. Proc. **44**:811, 1969.
3. McMaster, P. R., Robertson, E. A., Witebsky, F. C., et al.: Antimicrob. Agents Chemother. **13**:842, 1978.
4. MacLowry, J. D., Jaqua, M. J., and Selepak, S. T.: Appl. Microbiol. **20**:46, 1970.
5. Gavan, T. L., and Butler, D. A.: An automated microdilution method for antimicrobial susceptibility testing. In Balows, A., editor: Current techniques for antibiotic susceptibility testing, Springfield, Ill., 1974, Charles C Thomas, Publisher.
6. Goss, W. A., and Cimijotti, E. B.: Appl. Microbiol. **16**:1414, 1968.
7. Gavan, T. L., and Town, M. A.: Am. J. Clin. Pathol. **53**:880, 1970.
8. MacLowry, J. D., and Marsh, H. H.: J. Lab. Clin. Med. **72**:685, 1968.
9. Gerlach, E. H.: Dilution test procedures for susceptibility testing. In Bondi, A., Bartola, J. T., and Prier, J. E., editors: The clinical laboratory as an aid in chemotherapy of infectious diseases, Baltimore, 1977, University Park Press.
10. Tilton, R. C., Lieberman, L., and Gerlach, E. H.: Appl. Microbiol. **26**:658, 1973.
11. Matsen, J. M., Koepcke, M. J. H., and Quie, P. C.: antimicrobial agents and chemotherapy—1969, Bethesda, Md., 1970, American Society for Microbiology, p. 445.
12. Matsen, J. J., and Barry, A. L.: Susceptibility testing: diffusion test procedures. In Lennette, E. H., Spaulding, E. H., and Truant, J. P., editors: Manual of clinical microbiology, ed. 2, Washington, D.C., 1974, American Society for Microbiology.
13. Ericsson, H. M., and Sherris, J. C.: Acta Pathol. Microbiol. Scand. [B.], suppl. **217**, 1971.
14. Thornsberry, C., and Hawkings, T. M.: Agar disc diffusion susceptibility testing procedure, PHS, Atlanta, 1977, Center for Disease Control.
15. National Committee on Clinical Laboratory Standards: Performance standards for antimicrobial disc susceptibility tests, approved standard ASM-2, Villanova, Pa., 1975, The Committee.
16. Ellner, P. D., and Johnson, E.: Antimicrob. Agents Chemother. **9**:355, 1976.
17. Klastersky, J., Banean, D., Swings, G., et al.: J. Infect. Dis. **129**:187, 1974.
18. Stamey, T. A., et al.: N. Engl. J. Med. **291**:1159, 1974.
19. Thornsberry, C., Gavan, T., and Gerlach, E. H.: New developments in antimicrobial agent susceptibility testing. In Sherris, J. C., editor: Cumitech 6, Washington, D.C., 1977, American Society for Microbiology.
20. Matsen, J. M., and Coghlan, C. R.: Antibiotic testing and susceptibility patterns of streptococci. In Wannamaker, L. W., and Matsen, J. M., editors: Streptococci and streptococcal diseases: recognition, understanding and management, New York, 1972, Academic Press.
21. Bauer, A. W., Kirby, W. M. M., Sherris, J. C., et al.: Am. J. Clin. Pathol. **45**:493, 1966.
22. Federal Register: Rules and regulations **37**:20525, 1972.
23. Federal Register: Rules and regulations **38**:276, 1973.
24. Barry, A. L., and Fay, G. D.: Amer. J. Clin. Pathol. **59**:196, 1973.
25. Washington, J. A., II, Warren, E., and Karlson, A. G.: Appl. Microbiol. **24**:1013, 1973.
26. Barry, A. L., Garcia, F., and Thrupp, L. D.: Am. J. Clin. Pathol. **53**:149, 1970.
27. Kelly, M. T., and Matsen, J. M.: Antimicrob. Agents Chemother. **9**:440, 1975.
28. Chabbert, Y.: Ann. Inst. Pasteur (Paris) **76**:68, 1949.
29. Blazevic, D. J., Koepche, M. H., and Matsen, J. M.: Am. J. Clin. Pathol. **57**:592, 1972.
30. Shahidi, A., and Ellner, P. D.: Appl. Microbiol. **18**:766, 1969.
31. Hollick, G. E., and Washington, J. A., II: Antimicrob. Agents Chemother. **9**:804, 1976.
32. Wegner, D. L., Mathis, C. R., and Neblett, T. R.: Antimicrob. Agents Chemother. **9**:861, 1976.
33. Barry, A. L., Joyce, L. J., Adams, A. P., et al.: Am. J. Clin. Pathol. **59**:693, 1973.
34. Stemper, J. E., and Matsen, J. M.: Appl. Microbiol. **19**:1015, 1970.
35. Washington, J. A., II, Warren, E., Dolan, C. T., et al.: Antimicrobial susceptibility tests of bacteria. In Washington, J. A., II, editor: Laboratory procedures in clinical microbiology, Boston, 1974, Little, Brown and Company.
36. Wilkins, T. D., and Chalgren, S.: Antimicrob. Agents Chemother. **10**:926, 1976.
37. Reller, L. B., Schoenknecht, F. D., Kenny, M. A., et al.: J. Infect. Dis. **130**:454, 1974.
38. Washington, J. A., II, Snyder, R. J., Kohner, P. C., et al.: J. Infect. Dis. **137**:103, 1978.
39. Ryan, K. J., Needham, G. M., Dunsmoor, C. L., et al.: Appl. Microbiol. **20**:447, 1970.
40. Barry, A. L.: The antimicrobial susceptibility test: principles and practices, Philadelphia, 1976, Lea & Febiger.
41. Gerlach, E. H.: Microdilution. I. A comparative study. In Balows, A., editor: Current techniques for antibiotic susceptibility testing, Springfield, Ill., 1974, Charles C Thomas, Publishers.
42. Bartlett, R. C., Mazens, M., and Greenfield, B.: J. Clin. Microbiol. **3**:327, 1976.
43. Colvin, H. J., and Sherris, J. C.: Antimicrob. Agents Chemother. **12**:61, 1977.
44. McKie, J. E., Jr., Borovoy, R. J., Dooley, J. F., et al.: Autobac 1-A 3-hour automated, antimicrobial susceptibility system. II. Microbiological studies. In Heden, C., and Illeni, T., editors: Automation in microbiology and immunology, New York, 1974, John Wiley & Sons.
45. Praglin, J., Curtis, A. C., Longhenry, D. K., et al.: Autobac 1-A 3-hour automated antimicrobial susceptibility system. I. System description. In Heden, C., and Illeni, T., editors: Automation in microbiology and immunology, New York, 1974, John Wiley & Sons.
46. Matsen, J. M., Sielaff, B. H., and Buck, G. E.: Rapid automated bacterial identification with computerized programming of augmented Autobac I results. In Sharpe, A. N., and Clark, D. S., editors:

Mechanizing microbiology, Springfield, Ill., 1977, Charles C Thomas, Publishers.

47. Thornsberry, C., Gavan, T. L., Sherris, J. C., et al.: Antimicrob. Agents Chemother. 7:466, 1975.
48. Cleary, T. J., and Maurer, D.: Antimicrob. Agents Chemother. 13:837, 1978.
49. Wilkins, T. D., and Thiel, T.: Antimicrob. Agents Chemother. 3:350, 1973.
50. Blazevic, D. J.: Antimicrob. Agents Chemother. 7:721, 1975.
51. Kurzynski, T. A., Yrios, J. W., Helstad, A. G., et al.: Antimicrob. Agents Chemother. 10:727, 1976.
52. Sutter, V. L., Kwok, Y., and Finegold, S. M.: In vitro susceptibility testing of anaerobes: standardization of a single disc test. In Balows, A., editor: Anaerobic bacteria role in disease, Springfield, Ill., 1974, Charles C Thomas, Publishers.
53. Ronald, A. R., Eby, J., and Sherris, J. C.: Antimicrob. Agents Chemother. 431:1968, 1967.
54. Bennett, J. V., Camp, H. M., and Eickhoff, T. C.: Appl. Microbiol. 16:1056, 1968.
55. Drew, W. L., Barry, A. L., O'Toole, R. O., et al.: Appl. Microbiol. 24:240, 1972.
56. Sabath, D. L., Wheeler, N., Laverdiere, M., et al.: Lancet 1:443, 1977.
57. Thornsberry, C.: Rapid laboratory tests for β-lactamase production by bacteria, PHS, Atlanta, 1977, Center for Disease Control.

58. O'Callaghan, C. H., Morris, A., Kirby, S. M., et al.: Antimicrob. Agents Chemother. 1:283, 1972.
59. Catlin, B. W.: Antimicrob. Agents Chemother. 7:265, 1975.
60. Thornsberry, C., and Kirven, L. A.: Antimicrob. Agents Chemother. 6:620, 1974.
61. Rosenblatt, J. E., and Neuman, A. M.: Am. J. Clin. Pathol. 69:351, 1978.
62. Berenbaum, M. C.: J. Infect. Dis. 137:122, 1978.
63. Sabath, L. D., and Matsen, J. M.: Assay of antimicrobial agents (antibiotic section). In Lennette, E. H., Spaulding, E. H., and Truant, J. P., editors: Manual of clinical microbiology, ed. 2, Washington, D.C., 1974, American Society for Microbiology.
64. Lund, M. E., Blazevic, D. B., and Matsen, J. M.: Antimicrob. Agents Chemother. 4:569, 1973.
65. Klastersky, J., et al.: J. Infect. Dis. 129:187, 1974.
66. Sabath, L. D., and Taftegaard, I.: Antimicrob. Agents Chemother. 6:54, 1974.
67. Jawetz, E.: Am. J. Dis. Child. 103:113, 1962.
68. Pien, F. D., and Vosti, K. L.: Antimicrob. Agents Chemother. 6:330, 1974.
69. Schlichter, J. G., and MacLean, H. A.: Am. Heart J. 34:209, 1947.
70. Rosenblatt, J. E., Murray, P. R., Sonnenwirth, A. C., et al.: Antimicrob. Agents Chemother. 15:351, 1979.

88

NOSOCOMIAL INFECTIONS AND HOSPITAL EPIDEMIOLOGY

Alice Schauer Weissfeld

The epidemiology and various control measures of nosocomial (hospital-acquired) infections have been the subject of numerous publications beginning in the late 1950s when interest centered largely upon staphylococcal disease.[1-5] Since about 1964 the role of S. aureus in these infections has diminished to some extent, whereas the frequency of infections with gram-negative bacilli has increased appreciably.[6,7] More recently, infections caused by fungi (Candida, Cryptococcus neoformans, Phycomycetes, Aspergillus), viruses (cytomegalovirus, Herpes simplex, Herpes zoster, varicella), and parasites (Pneumocystis carinii, Toxoplasma gondii) have become increasingly common in the severely compromised host.[8]

The average rate of nosocomial infections reported by the Center for Disease Control National Nosocomial Infections Study Report was 356.6 infections/10,000 patients discharged during 1975-1976.[9] According to some estimates the total medical care costs associated with hospital-acquired infections may be up to $1 billion/year.[10]

Among the important consultation references are Hospital Infection (Williams et al., 1966),[11] Infection in Hospitals: Epidemiology and Control (Williams and Shooter, 1963),[12] Control of Infectious Diseases in General Hospitals (1967),[13] Control of Infections in Hospitals (Berlin et al., 1966),[14] Infection Control in the Hospital (American Hospital Association, 1974),[10] Environmental Aspects of the Hospital (U.S. Department of Health, Education, and Welfare, 1967),[15] Control of Communicable Diseases in Man (American Public Health Association, 1970),[16] Isolation Techniques for Use in Hospitals (1973),[17] Infection Control in Health Care Facilities (Cundy and Ball, 1977),[18] Hospital-acquired Infections in Surgery (Polk and Stone, 1977),[19] and the Manual on Control of Infection in Surgical Patients (1976).[20] A concise, basic review of hospital infections is that of LeFrock and Klainer.[8]

Hospitals have followed the recommendation that "every hospital should have an Infection Committee (Hospital Infections Control Committee), charged with the responsibility of investigation, control, and prevention of infections within hospitals"[10] and that through this committee coordination of efforts and cooperation of all hospital departments should be secured,[21] particularly since the accrediting agencies have made the establishment of such a committee mandatory.[22] Hospitals are required to provide, among other measures, "a competent and adequate microbiology service." The membership of the Infections Committee has to include, whenever possible, a bacteriologist or pathologist. The role of the bacteriology laboratory in infection control has been defined as providing (1) diagnostic services, (2) performance of epidemiologic investigations and surveillance, including surveillance of hospital personnel, and (3) environmental control and surveillance (cultures of equipment involved in patient care, periodic checks of sterilizing equipment, and air and surface sampling).[23,24]

The laboratory is also responsible for maintaining and disseminating information on the current status of antibiotic sensitivity patterns of organisms isolated in the hospital (from patients, personnel, and environment). Close cooperation between the laboratory and the infection control nurse and hospital epidemiologist is essential. Recently, for example, our technologists noticed a sharp increase in the number of organisms growing in water cultured from one of the hydrotherapy tanks. Investigations by the hospital epidemiologist revealed that stagnant water in the drain was flowing back into the tank. Flushing the drain for several minutes before filling the tank solved the problem. On another occasion the laboratory noticed a high number of coliform bacteria in dialysate fluid from one hemodialysis bath. The hospital epidemiologist discovered the drain hose for this bath was placed into the commode and then stored inside the bath when the machine was not in use. When this practice was discontinued the number of coliforms returned to zero.

Over the past few years a number of publications have appeared that address the question

Table 88-1. Infection control procedures

Activity	Program	Frequency
Item or area		
Air conditioning		As needed
Anesthesiology	Random items	As needed
Dairy products	Bacterial counts on milk, cream, and ice cream	Monthly
Dietary items	Utensils, glasses, plates, etc. randomly checked	Monthly
Hemodialysis unit	Deionized water and dialysis fluid as sent by unit	Monthly
Ice machines	Bacterial counts on all ice machines in use	Bimonthly
Nursery	Incubator reservoirs	Monthly
	Sink traps and faucets	As needed
	Infant formulas	As needed
Pharmacy	Laminar flow hood	Monthly
	Hyperalimentation fluid	Monthly
Physical therapy	All whirlpools in use cultured by department	Monthly
Respiratory therapy	Culture of swabs sent by department	Monthly
Sterilizers	Spore strips run in all sterilizing equipment	Weekly
Sterilized products	Selected at random from central supply, clinics, operating room, etc. divided between gas and steam	As needed
Surgical soaps	Operating room, emergency room, etc.	As needed
Any area of hospital		As needed
Personnel		
Food handlers	Stool culture, parasite examination	On employment and as needed thereafter
Home care	Nose, throat, and stool culture and parasite examination	On employment (if required by state)
Any personnel	Nose, throat, and stool culture and parasite examination	As needed

of "how far to go" in microbiologic surveillance.[18,25-27] Surveillance of hospital personnel is one area that has undergone modification. Several years ago many hospitals routinely cultured all nursing personnel to determine whether they were carriers of *S. aureus*. Today most hospitals acknowledge that routine culturing of personnel is not justified (with the possible exception of routine stool cultures for new employees in the dietary department)[27]; employee culturing is now limited to investigations of potential cross infections. Similarly, environmental culturing of floors and other surfaces is no longer recommended except in special circumstances.[25,26]

A list of procedures carried out in our laboratory as part of the infection control activities of the microbiology service is shown in Table 88-1. This is intended merely as a guide to the culture of certain areas (at the behest of the infection control committee) for educational and quality control purposes. A number of laboratory procedures employed in prevention and control programs are discussed below. An excellent review of procedures for use in the infection control laboratory is that of Gröschel.[28] Guidelines and procedures have also been published for ice machines,[29,30] large-volume parenteral fluids (including hyperalimentation fluid),[31-34] hemodialysis systems,[35] respiratory therapy equipment,[36] dairy products,[37] and utensils.[38,39]

Sterilizers

Autoclaves and dry-heat ovens should be equipped with recording thermometers. All steam and hot-air sterilizers should be checked at least once each week with *Bacillus stearothermophilus* spores; ethylene oxide gas sterilizers should be checked with each load with *Bacillus subtilis* spores.[27] Heat-sensitive adhesive tape that shows a color change on exposure to moist heat is useful only as an indication that the equipment was placed in the autoclave, but it does not prove that it is sterile. Commercially prepared spore strips (Spordi, American Sterilizer Co., Erie, Pa.) are cultured for 7 days in trypticase soy broth; thioglycollate broth is inhibitory and should not be used. Do not use alcohol-flamed forceps to transfer spore strips to the broth as alcohol may contain viable spores that may not be killed by flaming. A nonsterilized spore strip and an uninoculated tube of broth should be run in parallel. *B. stearothermophilus* strips are incubated at 56 C; *B. subtilis* strips at 37 C. Any tubes showing growth should be Gram stained and subcultured to confirm the presence of *Bacillus* species. Commercial spore ampules (Attest, 3M Co., Minneapolis) are also available. These are incubated in a 56 or 37 C water bath (as indicated) and are observed for growth (indicated by a change of the culture medium to yellow). A nonsterilized ampule should be included as a control.

Sterilized products

Routine sampling of sterilized products is not recommended.[18] However, when it is necessary to test any of these items, culture gauze, dressings, small nontubular instruments, and equipment by placing them in tubes of thioglycollate broth (20 × 150 mm, 30 ml medium) and incubating them at 30-32 C for at least 48 hours. Swab large instruments with a moist swab; then culture swab. Test tubular instruments by rinsing sterile thioglycollate broth through the lumen into a sterile tube; subculture broth to blood agar and thioglycollate broth.

Infant formula[40]

Sampling of commercially prepared formulas is not necessary unless required by state health codes.[27] Several bottles of hospital-prepared infant formula (selected at random from each lot produced) should be tested once a week. Examine the complete, terminally sterilized unit after overnight refrigeration.

Nipple rinse test. Remove nipple with sterile forceps and place in bottle of 50 ml dilution water[37] or neutralizing buffer (Difco, Detroit). Shake 25 times in 10 s. Transfer 1 ml buffer to each of 2 sterile Petri dishes. To one dish add 12 ml melted and cooled violet red bile agar, allow to solidify, and then add 3-4 ml additional medium. To the other dish add same amount of standard methods agar. Invert plates and incubate the first for 24 h and the second for 48 h. Count colonies on Quebec counter, multiply number of coliform colonies (in first plate) by 50, and report coliform plate count per nipple; in second plate count colonies, multiply by 50, and report total bacterial plate count per nipple. There should be no coliform colonies and a total bacterial count per nipple of less than 25.

Formula examination. Transfer 1 ml milk, after mixing, to each of 2 Petri dishes. Add media, incubate, and count as above.

Respiratory therapy[36]

It is unnecessary to sample equipment that has been sterilized. Qualitative sampling of disinfected equipment is recommended. Aerosol sampling is no longer recommended following disinfection since expected levels of contamination would be too low to be detected by this quantitative procedure.

Rinse method (tubing, medication nebulizers, humidifiers, bottles). Pour 40-50 ml (125 ml screw-capped flask) sterile brain heart infusion broth (BHIB) into the tubing or containers and agitate so as to rinse all surfaces. Samples are obtained from inside the tubing by pouring the broth while holding up both ends of the tubing and alternately raising and lowering the ends 50 times. The sampling broth should then be carefully poured or pipetted back into the original flask.

Swab method (exhalation valve, spirometer, mask, mouthpiece, other surfaces). Premoisten a sterile cotton swab in the BHIB (5-6 ml) contained in screw-capped tube. Wring out excess moisture on the side of the tube. Swab the inside surfaces of the item while rotating the swab. Place swab into the broth culture tube and break the stick off below that part that was held.

Incubate the BHIB culture for 18-24 h at 35 C. If turbid, inoculate a loopful of broth onto a blood agar and MacConkey agar plate. Continue to incubate non-turbid broths an additional 24 h before discarding. Identify gram-positive organisms to at least genus and gram-negative organisms to species.

Dairy products[37]

Total count. Mix 1 ml milk or cream or 1 g ice cream, diluted 1:100 through 1:10,000 in sterile saline, with melted and partially cooled sterile plate count agar in a sterile Petri dish. Incubate plates at 35 C when solidified. Count colonies after 48 h incubation. Pasteurized milk and cream should contain no more than 20,000 colonies/ml; pasteurized ice cream should contain no more than 50,000 colonies/g.

Coliform count. Mix 1 ml milk or cream or 1 g ice cream with 10-15 ml melted and partially cooled violet red bile agar. Allow to solidify and overlay with 2-4 ml violet red bile agar. Incubate at 35 C for 18-24 h. The milk or cream should not contain more than 10 coliforms/ml; the ice cream should not contain more than 10 coliforms/g.

Food utensils and food equipment surfaces[38, 39]

Select utensils to be examined at random from shelves or other places where clean utensils are stored; include at least 4 of each type of item. If a direct check of the dishwashing methods is desired, utensils should be selected from those recently washed. Care should be taken to prevent contamination by handling during sampling.

Utensils. Distribute 4.1 ml of neutralizing buffer (Difco no. 0362-15) into 1 screw-cap vial for each group of 4 utensils to be examined. Sterilize at 121 C for 15 min with caps slightly loosened. Use 1 sterile cotton swab on wooden applicator stick for each group of 4 similar utensils. Dip the swab into the neutralizing buffer and squeeze it against the inside of the vial to remove excess buffer, leaving the swab moist but not wet. Rub the swab slowly and firmly 3 times over the significant surfaces of 4 similar utensils, changing the direction each time. After swabbing each utensil, return the swab to the vial of buffer, rotate (whip rinse) the swab in the dilution water, and press out the excess buffer against the inside of the container before swabbing the next of the 4 utensils in the group. Break bud of swab into dilution vial. Make certain that wooden stick snaps just above swab as wood will cause a change in pH of liquid. Use a new swab vial and swab for the next group of utensils.

Utensil	Significant surface
Plates	Three times changing directions—each stroke completely across each of 2 diameters at right angles
Bowls	Three times changing directions—each stroke around the inner surface at a level at which the swab will hug the surface of the bowl. Usually about half way between bottom and rim.
Glasses and cups	Upper 1.25 cm of inner and outer rims
Spoons	Entire inner and outer surface of bowl
Forks	Entire inner and outer surface of tines

Equipment. When swabbing equipment, remove swab from vial and press out excess liquid on the inside wall of vial. Rub cotton portion of swab slowly and thoroughly over approximately 130 cm² of equipment surface. Rub swab slowly and firmly in a path of 1.25 cm width and 40 cm length (to cover approximately 130 cm²), rub swab in reverse direction, and repeat initial stroke (so that same area is covered by the 3 strokes). Return swab to original container of buffered solution, rotate (whip rinse) the swab in the diluent, and press out excess liquid (leaving swab moist but not wet). Using same applicator, swab 4 other 130 cm² areas of the same piece of equipment (including spots that appear difficult to clean and sanitize), rewetting swab and pressing out excess liquid before swabbing successive areas.

After completion of swabbing 5 areas (650 cm²), replace swab in original vial of buffered solution. Break off wooden applicator stick aseptically on rim of container, allowing swab to fall into diluent. Use a new swab container for each piece of equipment examined. Keep the container iced while in transit to the laboratory and until it is plated. Plate the diluent water samples preferably within 4 hours of swabbing, but where this cannot be done, samples must be properly refrigerated and analyzed within 24 h of swabbing.

Laboratory procedure. Shake swab vial containing broken swab 50 times. (Make 50 round trip excursions of 10-15 cm with the container in one hand, striking the palm of the other hand at the end of each cycle, and completing the whole in about 10 s.)

Transfer 1 ml of the dilution water to a sterile Petri dish. Add approximately 10 ml melted Standard Methods (Tryptone glucose yeast extract) agar, mix, incubate for 48 h at 32 or 35 C, and count as in making a Standard Plate Count.

In the case of utensils, report the count as the residual bacterial count per utensil surface examined. For example, if 4 glasses are swabbed, if 1 ml of the 4 ml of the diluent water is plated, and if 56 colonies are counted after incubation, record the count as residual bacterial count/glass (RBC/glass) 56.

Interpretation. The Public Health Service recommends a standard of not more than 100 colonies per surface or utensil swabbed.[38] The *Food Service Manual for Health Care Institutions*[39] says "counts above 100 indicate that dishes and utensils are not clean; bacterial counts in the 30 to 100 range are considered too high for health care institutions. If the count goes above 30, dishwashing and dish-handling should be checked."

For equipment on which 5 areas of approximately 130 cm² each have been swabbed, residual bacterial counts not exceeding 500 are satisfactory, that is, averaging 12.5 colonies/16 cm² of surface or, in the event the 5 areas swabbed are less than 81 cm² each, the counts should not exceed 2 colonies/cm².

Surgical soaps

Routine testing. For routine testing inoculate 40 ml tubes of thioglycollate broth with 0.1 and 1.0 ml of each soap. Smear and stain broth after 48 h; hold tubes for 7 d. If visible contamination (slime, etc.) is apparent, inoculate thioglycollate and, in addition, inoculate duplicate 10 ml tubes of brain heart infusion and trypticase soy broth with inoculating loop. Incubate duplicate tubes at 25 and 37 C.

Hydrotherapy equipment

The Millipore Corporation, Bedford, Mass., manufactures a Total-Count and a Coli-Count Sampler; these are self-contained devices for sampling water. In our hospital these samplers are used for culturing the whirlpool baths. Samples are taken by personnel in the physical therapy department and then brought to the microbiology laboratory for incubation and reading.

Collecting samples. The Sampler consists of a paddle containing a counting grid overlaid with either a nutrient agar (Total-Count Sampler) or a selective agar (Coli-Count Sampler); the paddle fits into a plastic case. Prior to sampling, the paddle is removed and placed on sterile gauze, and 0.2 ml 1% sodium thiosulfate is added to each case to neutralize chlorine in the water. The tank is then filled, the agitators started, and the case is dipped into the tank and filled with water to the top line marked on the case. The paddle is replaced into the case, which is shaken several times and held still for 30 s. The paddle is then removed from the case, the case is emptied, and the paddle is reinserted. The Sampler is incubated, grid side up, at 35 C for 24 h.

Interpretation. Regardless of the sample size introduced into the case, the paddle will only absorb 1 ml of fluid. Therefore the sample volume is always 1 ml.

Total-Count Sampler. All colonies appearing on the surface of the paddle should be counted. Results are reported as colonies/ml. The sample must have less than 200 colonies/ml to be acceptable.

Coli-Count Sampler. Only colonies that are blue or blue-green should be counted. Results are reported as colonies/100 ml. The sample must not contain any coliforms to be acceptable.

Hemodialysis fluid[35]

Millipore's Total-Count and Coli-Count Samplers are used to culture the deionized water used to prepare dialysis fluids as well as the dialysis fluids (see discussion on Hydrotherapy Equipment). Samples are taken by personnel in the hemodialysis unit and brought to the microbiology laboratory for incubation and reading.

Deionized water. It is not necessary to add 1% sodium thiosulfate before sampling as the water is deionized and does not contain any chlorine. Samples are collected at a point where water enters the proportioner, or where it is placed in mixing tanks, depending on the type of system used for preparing dialysis fluids. Total viable counts should not exceed 200 colonies/ml. There should be no coliforms.

Dialysis fluid. It is necessary to dilute the fluid 1:10. This is accomplished by filling the case with dialysate up to the lower line (1:8 ml) and filling the case to the upper line with sterile distilled water (18 ml). Samples should be collected at the termination of the dialysis treatment. In single-pass systems samples should be collected at the point where dialysis fluid leaves the dialyzer. In recirculating systems samples should be collected at the periphery of the recirculating canister containing the coil dialyzer. Total viable counts should not exceed 2,000 colonies/ml. There should be no coliforms.

Ice machines

Millipore samplers should not be used to sample ice machines as they have not been approved at this time (1979) by the Environmental Protection Agency for potable water. Sampling must be done by standard methods.[30] For each 120 ml of sample to be collected, add 0.1 ml 10% sodium thiosulfate to a sampling bottle. Sterilize by autoclaving at 121 C for 15 minutes. Add ice to bottle and allow to melt.

Total count. Add 1 ml of each sample to a Petri dish and mix with standard plate count agar. Incubate plate at 35 C for 48 hours and count. The number of viable bacteria should not exceed 200 colonies/ml.

Coliform count

Presumptive test. Pipet 10.0 ml of melted sample into 5 tubes of 20 ml double strength lactose broth. Incubate at 35 C fo 48 h. Examine each tube at 24 h and again at 48 h. Record gas formation. Note (1) absence of gas formation or (2) formation of gas in the gas vials. If gas is formed within 48 h, this is a positive presumptive test for coliforms. If no gas forms within 48 h incubation, this constitutes a negative test.

Confirmatory test. To confirm the presence of coliforms, inoculate a loopful of broth into 10 ml brilliant green lactose bile broth. Incubate at 35 C for 48 h; examine tube at 24 and 48 h for the formation of gas.

Completed test. If brilliant green lactose broth is positive, inoculate a loopful from each positive tube to a MacConkey plate. There should be no coliforms present for the test to be acceptable.

Laminar flow hoods

Procedure. Place 4 opened blood agar plates inside the hood for 10 min. Space plates evenly throughout hood. Incubate plates at 35 C for 48 h. Identify any organisms grown.

Air sampling

Routine sampling of air is not recommended.[25,26] When indicated, exposure of Petri dishes 30-60 minutes (blood agar or, for staphylococci, mannitol salt agar) to collect bacteria-carrying particles settling from the air is adequate. The procedure is more qualitative than quantitative but can show variations in particle concentrations from place to place. Many more elaborate samplers have been devised for quantitative counts. For a more detailed description of these instruments see Fincher and Mallison.[41]

Surface sampling

Routine surface sampling is not recommended.[25,26] When necessary, examine fabrics by the scrape method of Williams, using Petri dishes containing appropriate selective media. Uncover plate, place the agar surface on the fabric, and sweep the dish back and forth (10 sweeps, 37.5 cm long). Floors may be sampled either by (1) Rodac plates or (2) the swab template method.

Rodac plate

In 1963 Rohde[42] developed a new contact agar culture plate that appeared particularly promising for environmental sampling of hard surfaces. Shortly thereafter Bond et al.[43,44] developed a technic employing the Rodac plate for surveying the microbial contamination of environmental hard surfaces. Subsequently the Rodac plate

sampling technic has become very popular in hospital environmental monitoring programs because of its simplicity in comparison with the older swab template procedure. An abbreviated version of the method appears below. (Sterile Rodac plates and complete details for employing this technic are available from the Falcon Labware Division of Becton-Dickinson, Oxnard, Calif.)

Preparation of plates. BBL trypticase soy agar with lecithin and Tween 80 or BBL standard methods agar with lecithin and Tween 80 are considered media of choice for environmental sampling. Dispense 16.5-17.5 ml of selected media at 48-50 C into each Rodac plate on a level surface. Take care to prevent formation of air bubbles and to keep medium from overflowing. After plates have solidified, several samples are incubated at 37 C for 24 h as a sterility check. Remaining plates should be stored in a refrigerator at 5 C. When sterility is assured, plates can be used for environmental sampling.

Sampling procedure. Holding edges of plate between thumb and middle finger with index finger applied to middle of bottom, remove cover and apply agar surface of plate to sampling site exerting moderate vertical pressure. Do not allow plate to move sideways or smearing will result and plate will be ruined. Replace cover and incubate all plates for 48 h at 37 C. When incubation is completed count colonies on a Quebec Colony Counter.

• • •

A minimum of 15 Rodac plate samples must be obtained from a given environmental surface to be assayed to achieve statistical significance. Based on the studies of Bond et al.[43,44] mentioned above, 60 Rodac plates should be used on a given environmental surface to achieve reliable results.

The Committee on Microbial Contamination of Surfaces of the American Public Health Association[45] suggested that 25 or fewer colonies per plate is considered good, 26 to 50 colonies is considered fair, and more than 50 colonies is considered poor.

Swab template method

Procedure. Use a sterile 10 cm² template; swab floor with swab moistened in neutralizing buffer containing an inactivator for neutralization of residual germicides as necessary. Replace applicator in buffer, shake, and plate out buffer in duplicate 1 ml aliquots. Desirable criteria for floor cleanliness are operating rooms, 0-5 organisms/cm²; wards, 5-10 organisms/cm².[46]

Large-volume parenteral fluids

In-hospital sterility testing of unopened commerical IV products is not recommended.[27,32] When there is a possibility of a contaminated IV fluid, the system should be discontinued entirely, including the removal of cannulas or needles. Two blood cultures should be drawn from 2 independent sites. A sterile closure should be placed on the end of the delivery set tubing, and the suspect IV system should be wrapped in a clean plastic bag and sent to the laboratory for immediate culture. The nature of the solution and the exact lot number should be recorded on the patient's chart and in the permanent laboratory logbook.

Procedure. In the laboratory, all procedures should be performed under a laminar flow hood.
1. Disinfect tubing near clamp release mechanism and let dry.
2. Cut cleaned tubing and drain most of IV fluid into a large flask containing 250 ml double strength BHIB.
3. Disinfect top of bottle, let dry, and draw out 11 ml IV fluid with a sterile syringe.
4. Prepare a Gram stain of material.
5. Place 1 ml into a Petri dish and prepare a pour plate with tryptose blood agar.
6. Inoculate 2 blood culture bottles with 5 ml each of infusion fluid.
7. Refrigerate bottle and save until culture is finished.
8. Place tip of the cannula into tube of heart infusion broth.

Most current recommendations suggest that all cultures be incubated at 35 C for at least 10 days and examined daily for turbidity[27,32]; according to another recent opinion, cultures should be incubated at 20-25 C.[34] Subculture turbid broths to blood and Mac-Conkey agar plates and incubate at 35 C for 18-24 h; reincubate negative plates for an additional 24 h at 35 C, then transfer to room temperature for 5 d before discarding.

If an in-use solution bottle has been opened for at least 6 h, an alternative method, **membrane filtration**, can be used.[32] Aseptically filter the IV solution through a 0.45 μm Millipore field monitor, remove filter from holder, and cut filter in half. Place one-half onto surface of a blood agar plate premoistened with 0.3 ml BHIB; place the other half into a flask containing BHIB. Incubate cultures at 35 C as described above.

Comments. Organisms isolated from IV solutions should be identified to the species level. Antimicrobial sensitivity testing of the gram-negative microorganisms isolated could aid in determining the source of the organisms. Frequently, intrinsic contaminating organisms are multiply sensitive to antibiotics, whereas extrinsic contaminating organisms may be more resistant.[32] Report any positive cultures to the Food and Drug Administration (FDA) immediately.

Hyperalimentation fluid.[32] Aseptically add 50 ml nonturbid solution to an equal volume of double strength BHIB and incubate the remainder at 35 C for evidence of production of turbidity. Turbid in-use solution can be streaked initially to primary isolation media. Incubate plates and broths as indicated for large-volume parenteral fluids.

Carriers

Routine culturing of personnel is not recommended.[27] When necessary, use cotton swabs for nose, throat, anus, and skin; examine stool for enteric pathogens. Moisten nose swabs with sterile saline or water and insert 1-2 cm in the anterior nares. Culture on appropriate selective media.

Nursery incubators

Aspirate some of the water in the incubator wells with a sterile capillary pipet and inoculate it into a tube of thioglycollate broth. Incubate broth at 35 C for 7 days. Subculture broth if turbid and identify any organisms grown.

REFERENCES

1. Center for Disease Control: Selected materials on environmental aspects of staphylococcal diseases, Public Health Service Pub. no. 646, Atlanta, 1959, The Center.
2. Center for Disease Control: Summary of the Conference on Environmental Aspects of Institutional Infections, Atlanta, 1960, The Center.
3. Center for Disease Control: Hospital-acquired staphylococcal disease, Recommendations of the National Conference, Public Health Service and National Academy of Sciences National Research Council, Atlanta, 1958, The Center.
4. Center for Disease Control: Proceedings of the National Conference on Hospital-Acquired Staphylococcal Disease, Atlanta, 1958, The Center.
5. J. Clin. Pathol. **14:**1-99, 1961.
6. Barrett, F. F., Casey, J. I., and Finland, M.: N. Engl. J. Med. **278:**5, 1968.
7. Finland, M.: J. Infect. Dis. **122:**419, 1970.
8. LeFrock, J. L., and Klainer, A. S.: Nosocomial infections, scope monograph series, Kalamazoo, Mich., 1976, The Upjohn Company.
9. Center for Disease Control: National nosocomial infections study report, annual summary 1976, DHEW pub. (CDC) no. 78-8257, Washington, D.C., 1978, U.S. Government Printing Office.
10. American Hospital Association: Infection control in the hospital, ed. 3, Chicago, 1974, The Association.
11. Williams, R. E. O., Blowers, R., Garrod, L. P., et al.: Hospital infection, causes and prevention, ed. 2, Chicago, 1966, Year Book Medical Publishers.
12. Williams, R. E. O., and Shooter, R. A., editors: Infection in hospital, epidemiology and control, a Unesco and WHO symposium, Philadelphia, 1963, F. A. Davis Co.
13. Top, F. H., editor: Control of infectious diseases in general hospitals, New York, 1967, American Public Health Association.
14. Berlin, B. S., and Hilbert, M., editors: Control of infections in hospitals, Ann Arbor, 1966, School of Public Health, University of Michigan.
15. Environmental aspects of the hospital: Infection control (I), supportive departments (II), safety fundamentals (III), administrative aspects (IV). U.S. Department of Health, Education, and Welfare, Division of Hospital and Medical Facilities, Washington, D.C., 1967, U.S. Government Printing Office, no. FS 2.74/3: C-15, C-16, C-17, C-18.
16. Benenson, A. S., editor: Control of communicable diseases in man, ed. 11, New York, 1970, American Public Health Association.
17. U.S. Department of Health, Education, and Welfare: Isolation techniques for use in hospitals, Public Health Service pub. no. 2054, Washington, D.C., 1973, U.S. Government Printing Office.
18. Cundy, K. R., and Ball, W., editors: Infection control in health care facilities: microbiological surveillance, Baltimore, 1977, University Park Press.
19. Polk, H. C., Jr., and Stone, H. H., editors: Hospital-acquired infections in surgery, Baltimore, 1977, University Park Press.
20. American College of Surgeon's Committee on Control of Surgical Infections of the Committee on Pre- and Postoperative Care: Manual on control of

infection in surgical patients, Philadelphia, 1976, J. B. Lippincott Co.

21. Joint Commission on Accreditation of Hospitals, Bull. Joint Comm. Accred. Hosp. vol. 18, 1958; Hospitals 32:49, 1958.

22. Joint Commission on Accreditation of Hospitals: Accreditation manual for hospitals, Chicago, 1973, The Commission.

23. National conference on institutionally acquired infections, Public Health Service pub. no. 1188, Washington, D.C., 1964, U.S. Government Printing Office.

24. Weinstein, R. A., and Mallison, G. F.: Am. J. Clin. Pathol. 69:130, 1978.

25. American Hospital Association Committee on Infections within Hospitals: Microbiologic sampling in the hospital, Chicago, 1975, The Association.

26. American Public Health Association Committee on Microbial Contamination of Surfaces (Favero, M. S., chairman): Health Lab. Sci. 12:234, 1975.

27. Bartlett, R. C., Gröschel, D. H. M., Mackel, D. C., et al.: Control of hospital-associated infections. In Manual of clinical microbiology, ed. 2, Washington, D.C., 1974, American Society for Microbiology.

28. Gröschel, D.: Procedures for infection control laboratory. In CRC handbook series in clinical laboratory science, Cleveland, 1977, CRC Press.

29. Center for Disease Control: Sanitary care and maintenance of ice chests and ice machines, Bacterial Diseases Division, Bureau of Epidemiology, Atlanta, 1975, The Center.

30. Standard methods for the examination of water and wastewater, ed. 14, New York, 1975, American Public Health Association, American Water Works Association, and Water Pollution Control Federation.

31. Center for Disease Control: Infection control in hyperalimentation therapy, Bacterial Diseases Division, Bureau of Epidemiology, Atlanta, 1977, The Center.

32. Mackel, D. C.: Selective growth of microorganisms in parenteral infusion fluids and other solutions: methods of detection. In Infection control in health care facilities, Baltimore, 1977, University Park Press.

33. Phillips, I., Meers, P. D., and D'Arcy, P. F., editors: Microbiological hazards of infusion therapy, Littleton, Mass., 1976, Publishing Sciences Group.

34. National Coordinating Committee on Large Volume Parenterals: Am. J. Hosp. Pharm. 35:678, 1978.

35. American Public Health Association Committee on Microbial Contamination of Surfaces (Favero, M. S., chairman): Health Lab. Sci. 15:174, 1978.

36. American Public Health Association Committee on Microbial Contamination of Surfaces (Favero, M. S., chairman): Health Lab. Sci. 15:177, 1978.

37. American Public Health Association: Standard methods for the examination of dairy products, ed. 13, New York, 1972, The Association.

38. Technical Information Bulletin no. 1, Public Health Service pub. no. 1631, Washington, D.C., 1967, U.S. Government Printing Office.

39. American Hospital Association: Food service manual for health care institutions, Chicago, 1966, The Association.

40. American Academy of Pediatrics: Standards and recommendations for hospital care of newborn infants, ed. 6, Evanston, Ill., 1977, The Academy.

41. Fincher, E. L., and Mallison, G. F.: Intramural sampling of airborne microorganisms. In Air sampling instruments, ed. 4, 1972, American Conference of Government Industrial Hygienists.

42. Rohde, P. A.: Bull. Parenter. Drug Assoc. 17:11, 1963.

43. Bond, R. G., Halbert, M. M., Keenan, K. M., et al.: Development of a method for microbial sampling of surfaces with special reference to reliability, Minneapolis, 1963, University Health Service and School of Public Health, University of Minnesota.

44. Bond, R. G., Halbert, M. M., Putman, H. D., et al.: Survey of microbial contamination in the surgical suites of 23 hospitals, Minneapolis, 1963, University Health Service and School of Public Health, University of Minnesota.

45. American Public Health Association: Committee on microbial contamination of surfaces of laboratory section, Health Lab. Sci. 7:256, 1970.

46. Walter, C. W.: Mod. Hosp. 91:69, 1958.

89

STERILIZATION, DISINFECTION, AND ANTISEPSIS

Dieter H. M. Gröschel

Antimicrobial procedures are necessary to prevent infections in hospitals and clinical laboratories. The laboratory physician and scientist must be familiar with the basic concepts of antimicrobial control measures and agents, not only as they relate to his daily practice, but to his role as a consultant to clinical colleagues and other health care personnel as well. This chapter defines the most important terms, the requirements for and use of antimicrobial procedures and agents, and some test methods to assay or control their effectiveness.

STERILIZATION
Definitions and aims

Sterilization is the physical or chemical process that destroys or eliminates all forms of life; sterility is the condition of being free of microorganisms.[1] This absolute concept causes problems for the hospital and for industry. With the many thousands of items processed daily in an institution or received from industrial sources it is virtually impossible to test each one for sterility. Except for microbiologic media all other objects undergoing a sterility test process are lost for further use; therefore only a representative sample can be tested. The concept of absolute sterility has been replaced by the determination of the statistical probability of the condition of sterility.

Another problem is the limitation of the common test procedure in detecting all living microorganisms. For example, there is no routine testing for infective viruses, psychrophilic and thermophilic bacteria and fungi, and microorganisms having special nutritional requirements. We test only for representative microorganisms and imply that failure to detect them in the sterility test procedure ensures that all microorganisms are killed or eliminated. The United States Pharmacopeia XIX[2] states that the adequacy of a sterilization method must be established by sterility tests. Aside from the use of

biologic indictors, which will be discussed later, culturing methods presented are suitable for revealing the presence of bacteria and fungi in or on pharmaceutical products and devices. The statement is made that in doubtful cases the results obtained by the procedures listed in the USP are conclusive. By this decision a reasonable compromise is reached for both producers and users of sterile products. With this compromise in mind we may accept Bruch's definition of sterilization: it removes or kills living organisms to the extent that they are no longer detectable by an appropriate sampling plan using standard culture media in which they have previously been found to proliferate.[3]

According to Kelsey[4] sterility is a philosophic concept that can never be unequivocally demonstrated in a real world. He proposed to abandon the term "sterility" and use a new term to indicate "the state of having been sufficiently freed from microorganisms to be deemed safe for some special purpose by some competent body." For the laboratory scientist the dilemma can be solved by acquainting himself with and accepting the complex statistical basis of sterility. For commercially sterilized items he should accept the statement that sterilization was conducted and controlled according to USP XIX.[2] For his own institution he should consider making the ideal aim of all sterilization methods the theoretical optimum, freeness of microorganisms, through a responsible program of control. Starkey[5] pointed out that a quality control program must evaluate the challenge to the sterilization process, i.e., the degree and type of microbial contamination before sterilization, the risk of having survivors due to uncontrollable or human error, the complexity of routine controls, and the chance of recontamination before use.

Areas of use

In a hospital environment, sterility often has different connotations for different people. To the bacteriologist a liquid culture medium is sterile if it will not show growth after incubation at 35-37 C for 1-7 days. The pharmacist defines the sterility of intravenous solutions as the result of a sterilization procedure. To the surgeon sterility is a technic practiced in the operating room. The microbiologist's desire for sterility of culture media is dictated by his quality control requirement, i.e., to avoid diagnostic errors in bacteriology or to prevent the destruction of tissue cultures in virology. The pharmacist and the surgeon are interested in sterility in order to prevent hospital-associated infections.

The Spaulding classification of medical and surgical materials[6] is helpful in deciding which items used in patient care need to be sterile. He proposed 3 categories in accordance with freedom from microorganisms: critical, semicritical, and noncritical items. **Critical items** need to be sterile, i.e., free of microbial spores in addition to vegetative bacteria, fungi, and viruses, whereas in the other categories freedom from spores is not required. Critical items are those introduced beneath the surface of the body or attached to other objects so used, such as transfer forceps, scalpel blades, cardiac catheters, components of the heart-lung oxygenator, laparoscopes, and culdoscopes.[7] In addition surgical instruments and linens, syringes and needles, infusion fluids and administration sets, parenteral medications, etc. could be considered critical items. Greene applied the same reasoning to the hospital physical environment[8] to identify critical areas for the care of patients with unnaturally low resistance to infection, for areas where the patient's natural barriers are breached (e.g., surgery), or where hazards of infection transmission are significantly higher than ordinary (e.g., isolation rooms). This can be extended to critical wastes coming from patients with transmissible infections and from clinical and research laboratories.

Methods of sterilization

Sterilization methods used in hospitals and clinical laboratories are determined by the character of the items to be sterilized. The choice of the process requires knowledge of the equipment and of the stability of the material to be sterilized. A sterilization policy demands establishment of objectives, constant supervision of equipment, detailed description of procedure, a monitoring program, and training of all personnel involved.

Physical methods

Steam sterilization. This sterilization method using an autoclave with saturated steam under pressure is the most desirable procedure and is used for glass and certain plastic and metal products as well as for liquids that can tolerate high temperatures and steam. Steam sterilization, according to USP XIX,[2] denotes heating in an autoclave employing saturated steam under pressure at a minimum of 121 C for a minimum of 15 minutes after the material being sterilized has reached 121 C. Autoclaving errors are often due to the fact that the user assumes that the thermometer reading of the autoclave chamber indicates that the critical temperature has also been reached in the center of a pack or in a vessel. Biologic indictors or thermocouples (see discussion on Quality Control in Sterilization) will help to monitor the sterilization process and its efficiency.

The selection of a steam sterilizer will depend on the area of use, desired length of the sterilization cycle (high vaccuum vs. gravity displacement), and funds available. It is advisable to consult with a person experienced in sterilization processes prior to a purchase decision.

The risk of having unsterile products after the steam sterilization process is dependent on equipment problems, which can often be avoided with a good and regular maintenance program, or on human errors such as overloading (failure of steam penetration), underloading (air pockets), inappropriate timing, or selection of the wrong sterilization cycle. Soiled materials must be cleaned prior to steam sterilization and, for the protection of personnel, disinfected prior to cleaning if contamination with infectious microorganisms has occurred or is suspected.

Dry heat sterilization. For the sterilization of heat-stable materials a hot-air oven heated by gas or electricity and usually equipped with a blower or fan is used. At 160-170 C for 2-4 hours materials are not only sterilized, but also rendered nonpyrogenic—an important factor for containers used for injectables or infusion fluids.

The sterilization effect of both dry and wet heat is generally regarded as the result of enzyme inactivation, protein denaturation, or both. Studies with microorganisms have shown that there may be different effects. The time needed to kill spores of *Bacillus subtilis* var. *niger,* one of the bacteria used as a biologic monitor, at 121 C is nearly 2000 times as long in hot air as in steam.[9] Nonaqueous liquids or semisolids such as mineral oil and petrolatum fail to be sterilized by the lack of steam penetration and the low temperature of the steam autoclave. These as well as water vapor–sensitive, heat-stable solids can be sterilized at the higher temperatures of the dry-heat oven.

Detailed discussion of the kinetics of thermal destruction or inactivation of microorganisms may be found in Ernst.[10]

Sterilization by filtration. Heat-sensitive solutions can be sterilized by the physical removal of microorganisms by adsorption and sieving with filters. Most commonly used are membrane filters that yield a relatively particle-free and unaltered sterile product. Both the filter and receptacle are sterilized by a method appropriate to their composition. For injectables and laboratory media it is important to determine the efficiency of the filter, e.g., by testing the retention of very small pseudomonads. The use of pressure on the nonsterile or of suction on the sterile of the filter must be adjusted to the type of filter and filtrate to avoid sterilization failures. Membrane filters may clog, and organisms may grow through the membrane and contaminate the sterile filtrate. Therefore filters should be changed regularly.

Filter elements of porcelain, diatomaceous earth, or sintered material often crack and should best be avoided. For a detailed discussion of sterilization filtration see Fifield.[11]

Sterilization by ionizing radiation. Radiosterilization by γ-rays is used in large scale for the processing of hospital supplies such as syringes and sutures. Radioisotope sources are ^{60}Co and ^{137}Cs with radiation dosages of 2.5-4.5 Mrad. Dosimetry, biologic indictors (*Bacillus pumilus*), and product quality control are required of the manufacturers. The efficiency of the sterilization process depends on the type of material to be sterilized, soil, temperature, and concentration, and radioresistance of the contaminating microorganisms. The use of higher radiation doses (4.5 Mrad) and of the radioresistant *Streptococcus faecium* as a control organism has increased the safety margin. For more details see Boucher,[12] Kelsey,[4] Silverman and Sinskey,[13] and Starkey.[5]

Chemical methods

Sterilization by chemical means became important to the hospital and the clinical laboratories with the introduction of a growing number of heat-sensitive new plastics and delicate instruments. A number of gaseous and liquid sterilizing agents are available but in this chapter only those in common use will be discussed. For information on other chemosterilants see Block[14] and Boucher.[12]

Ethylene oxide. Compared to heat sterilization, ethylene oxide vapor sterilization is slow, complicated, and expensive. However, ethylene oxide damages materials least and can be used for the most sensitive instruments and plastics. Its drawbacks of inhalation toxicity, inflammability, and dependency on humidity and temperature have been overcome by the construction of autoclave-type sterilization chambers and the mixture of the gas with CO_2 or fluorinated hydrocarbons and appropriate safety measures. Nevertheless, the Environmental Protection Agency recently issued a position document together with a rebuttable presumption against registration of pesticide products containing ethylene oxide. There is evidence that ethylene oxide has mutagenic and reproductive effects.[15]

Ethylene oxide sterilizes mainly through its alkylating activity by attachment to sulfhydryl bonds and proteins, thereby interfering with their structure and function. Its effect is most rapid at 30-40% relative humidity but is rather low against dried microorganisms.[12] Gas concentration and temperature are both factors in the rate of killing of microorganisms. The sterilization goods must be thoroughly cleaned before exposure to ethylene oxide to reduce the microbial load and remove protective soil.

The potential toxicity of ethylene oxide–sterilized goods is a special problem. Rubber and certain plastics will absorb ethylene oxide and retain it for varying periods of time. Aeration either at room temperature or in an aeration chamber with filtered, heated airflow is required for the removal of gas residuals. Aeration times will depend on the type of sterilized material, the length of exposure, and the amount of ethylene oxide used. In the presence of chloride atoms in sterilization goods a toxic derivative, ethylene chlorohydrin, is formed. Insufficiently aerated plastic materials in contact with body tissue may also cause the formation of the toxin. It is recommended that surgical devices be left at room temperature for at least 5 days or for 8 hours at 50 C.[16] The Food and Drug Administration recently announced that a proposed rule may be issued that would establish maximum residual limits for ethylene oxide and its reaction products in drugs and medical devices as well as maximum daily exposure levels for drug products.[17]

Despite all drawbacks ethylene oxide gas sterilization is one of the main technics for industrial batch-processing of sterile medical goods and for the sterilization of certain instruments and plastics in hospitals. The selection and use of gas sterilizers should be determined according to the needs of the institution and its financial capabilities. Many hospitals use gas sterilization for applications that could also be handled by a cheaper method of sterilization or by disinfection. For more information on ethylene oxide sterilization see Phillips[18] and Kereluk et al.[19]

Alkaline glutaraldehyde. This dialdehyde is chemically related to formaldehyde but it is claimed to be 2-8 times more sporicidal.[20] In a 2% alkaline aqueous solution it is sporicidal at room temperature and finds wide application in hospitals to disinfect and sterilize plastics, rubber, and delicate lensed instruments. Its disadvantages are the significant loss of activity in the alkaline state (over a 2-week period) due to polymerization, the requirement (for sporicidal activity) to expose items at least for 10 hours, and the need to remove residual glutaraldehyde by rinsing with sterile water. Spaulding et al.[16] reported that simulated in-use tests have shown that for tuberculocidal activity, exposure times of 20-30 minutes are required, and for sporicidal activity, less than 3 to more than 4 hours, depending on species, degree of dryness, and concentration of spores.

It is believed that alkaline glutaraldehyde is active because of its alkylating properties.[12] For additional discussion of glutaraldehyde see Boucher,[12] Spaulding et al.,[6] and Stonehill et al.[21]

Quality control in sterilization

Determinations of the state of sterility are not simple. For the clinical laboratory the microbiologic testing of sterilized objects will bring more problems than benefits. The routine sampling of items that have been properly cleaned, heat-sterilized, and stored is not recommended.[22]

Contamination of commercially sterilized medical items and resulting clinical infection are rare. An ongoing program of infection surveillance is economically more feasible than routine microbiologic sampling. For a discussion of the sampling requirements and their statistical implications see Bruch[3] and Beloian.[23] The problems concerning commercial sterile medical products are summarized in Gaughran and Kereluk.[24]

A realistic **sterilization surveillance program** for hospitals and clinical laboratories includes the combination of systems control of all processes and the use of physical, chemical, and biologic indicators or monitors.

For **wet heat sterilization** pressure gauges and thermometers, preferably temperature-time recorders, should be used. For new steam autoclaves or after repairs a thorough testing of a full load with thermocouples by a qualified service engineer is recommended. In the **hot-air sterilizer** an automated temperature-timer avoids human error. Both heat sterilization procedures may also be monitored by melting-point ampules. One should remember that not all parameters of the sterilization process will be monitored by these means and that certain items may require longer-than-usual sterilization time. Chemical monitors (test tapes and other heat-sensitive color indicators) are usually unsatisfactory, but recently a new chemical indicator was introduced (Thermalog S) that uses a melting-point, steam-penetration, exposure-time combination to monitor steam autoclave performance.[25] Biologic monitoring with a large number of heat-resistant spores is generally accepted as the best substitute for microbial control. The monitors are placed in the center of the load and close to the exhaust valve, since these areas are least likely to be exposed to sterilizing temperatures for an adequate length of time.

Gas sterilization with ethylene oxide is best monitored by testing every load with spore strips. As with heat sterilization, chemical color indicators are not a replacement for biologic monitors. The operator should record temperature, relative humidity, and gas supply during each sterilization cycle.

Liquid chemical sterilization can be monitored by product sampling, but it is probably less time consuming to establish definite policies for the use and the change of sporicidal liquids, the use of sterile rinse water, and appropriate handling and storage of sterile instruments. The effectiveness of chemicals as sporicidal agents is tested by the Association of Official Analytical Chemists (AOAC) sporicidal test.[23, 26]

Spore indicators. For the biologic monitoring of a sterilization process microorganisms are selected that exhibit a high resistance to the respective sterilizing procedure and are more resistant than naturally occurring contaminants. By using a high concentration of these monitor organisms an additional margin of safety is added. For biologic monitoring one can add the test organism directly to a test sample or one can use simulated test samples such as impregnated filter paper strips in paper envelopes. Most hospitals use commercial spore strips to indicate sterility by inference. Spore strips should be purchased only from reputable sources that supply quality control data of their products. Mayernik reporting on a USP collaborative study[27] and Kereluk and Gammon[28] found considerable variations when comparing the label specification of spore strips with their actual performance.

Spores of the thermophile bacillus, *Bacillus stearothermophilus*, are generally used for testing steam autoclaves and spores of *B. subtilis* var. *niger (globigii)* are used for ethylene oxide and dry-heat sterilizers. The Joint Commission on Accreditation of Hospitals recommends testing heat sterilizers **weekly** and gas sterilizers with **each** load.[29] For liquids, ampules containing a spore suspension in culture medium are available.

Culturing spore strips should be the responsibility of the microbiologist. The strips are inoculated with sterile forceps in trypticase soy or a similar broth and incubated at the recommended temperature of 56 C for *B. stearothermophilus* and 37 C for *B. subtilis*. A nonsterilized control of the same lot or batch must be added to ascertain the viability of the spores. Thioglycollate broth is inhibitory and should not be used. Care should be taken that the spore strip cultures are not secondarily infected by unsterile forceps or in a contaminated water bath. The alcohol-flame technic for "sterilizing" forceps should be avoided because alcohol may contain viable spores that may resist the flaming process. The spore strip cultures should be incubated for 7 days to ensure that injured spores have sufficient time for repair of injury and germination. Cultures showing growth on the fifth to seventh day may indicate marginal performance of the sterilizer under the test conditions.[30] All positive cultures and controls must be subcultured to avoid errors due to secondary contamination.

A sterilizer found to perform poorly must be retested immediately while paying strict attention to all parameters. If it fails again, a service engineer should be consulted immediately.

A review of the role of microbiologic indicators in the quality control of sterilization procedures is presented by Kereluk.[30]

DISINFECTION
Definitions and aims

Disinfection is the physical or chemical process that frees from infections; a **disinfectant** is usually a chemical agent that destroys disease or other harmful microorganisms but not ordinarily bacterial spores. It refers to substances applied to inanimate objects.[1] Synonyms of disinfectant are **germicide** and **microbicide**. Specific activity may also be expressed, such as bactericide or virucide. According to Reddish[31] the definition

Table 89-1. Disinfection activity necessary in various hospital areas*

Use areas and risk	Definitions	Microbicidal activity against†					
		Bacteria		Spores	Fungi	Viruses	
		Vegetative	Mycobacteria			Lipid and medium size	Nonlipid and small size
Reused instruments and equipment							
Critical	Introduced beneath surface of body or attached to such object	+	+	+	+	+	+
Semicritical	Contact with internal mucosa	+	+	d	+	+	+
Noncritical	Contact with skin and external mucosa	+	d	−	+	+	d
Hospital environment							
High-risk critical areas	Operating suite, intensive care, incubators, life islands, burn unit, IV preparation	+	+	d	+	+	+
Medium-risk patient areas	Patient areas, therapy and diagnostic rooms, sterile supplies	+	d	−	+	+	d
Low-risk general areas	Administration, cafeteria, waiting rooms	+	−	−	−	−	−
Hospital wastes							
High risk	From infected patients, pathology, laboratories	+	+	d	+	+	+
Medium risk	Regular patient waste	+	d	−	−	d	−
Low risk	Nonpatient areas	d	−	−	−	−	−

*Based on recommendations by Spaulding,[6] Greene,[8] and Fahlberg (see Groschel[34]).
†+, required; −, not required; d, desirable or required in special cases.

includes the purpose and scope of activity of a disinfectant. The American Public Health Association[32] includes physical agents or processes in their definition: disinfection—killing of infectious agents outside the body by chemical or physical means directly applied. Reber[33] offered a scientifically acceptable definition of disinfection: the selective elimination of certain undesired microorganisms in order to prevent their transmission by interfering with their structure or metabolism independently of their functional state. These definitions may be summarized by stating that disinfection is the use of microbicidal agents or processes outside of the body on inanimate objects and aimed at a defined group of microorganisms. As in sterilization, the Spaulding classification[6] of three categories (critical, semicritical, and noncritical) will assist in determining the aims of disinfection for medical and surgical materials. A similar classification may be applied to the hospital environment—critical, patient, or general as defined by Greene[8] or high, medium, and low risk as defined by Fahlberg (as quoted in Gröschel[34]) and to hospital or laboratory wastes (Table 89-1). Noncritical items and areas may be treated with disinfectants of a limited scope of activity that are also known as sanitizers. **A sanitizer** is defined as an agent that reduces the number of bacterial contaminants to safe levels as judged by public health requirements.[1] This term is associated with food and dairy processing and household cleaning. To avoid confusion it should be replaced in the hospital environment by **low-level disinfectant.**[7] As in other antimicrobial measures the effectiveness of disinfectants may be limited by the presence of soil. Therefore disinfection must be combined with or preceded by cleaning. In a **detergent-germicide** a disinfectant is combined with a wetting agent that allows the penetration of organic debris, more exposure of microorganisms, and more rapid antimicrobial activity on inanimate objects. **A germicidal detergent** is primarily a heavy-duty cleaner, especially for housekeeping purposes, with germicidal properties.[35]

Areas of use

Disinfectants are used in hospitals and clinical laboratories for 3 main purposes:

1. To render contaminated objects safe for further use
2. To reduce the microbial contamination of the inanimate environment
3. To prevent spread of microorganisms by contaminated wastes

In the **hospital** many instruments and most equipment used with patients must be sterilized or disinfected before reuse. Semicritical items such as endotracheal tubes, bronchoscopes, cystoscopes, thermometers, and respiratory therapy and anesthesia equipment frequently are disinfected, not sterilized, and noncritical items such as face masks, ECG electrodes, and x-ray equipment usually are subjected to treatment with an intermediate-level chemical disinfectant.[7] Soiled objects must be cleaned before disinfection. Water jets or ultrasound baths with detergents are helpful but should be used in closed containers to avoid environmental contamination with microbial aerosols. If heavily soiled materials are suspected to be contaminated with communicable disease organisms, disinfection with a detergent-germicide should precede the cleaning process and be followed by final disinfection.

In the **clinical laboratory** disinfection is used mainly for environmental cleaning, for discard jars and pans, and for cleaning spills of infectious patient or laboratory materials. The use of disposable supplies has eliminated the need of disinfection prior to cleaning of test tubes, pipets, etc. in many institutions. If one needs to chemically disinfect discarded equipment containing agar or liquids, the concentration of the disinfectant must be adjusted to the soil load and dilution. Microbial contamination of automated equipment such as blood gas machines and waste lines of chemistry equipment poses a special problem. Most companies will instruct laboratory personnel about appropriate decontamination procedures and the disinfectants to be used.

Traditionally a clean hospital is considered to be a safe hospital. This has been interpreted by many that disinfectant must be used for all cleaning procedures in the hospital environment. There is no convincing evidence that the use of disinfectants for cleaning hospital floors and walls has contributed to a safer environment. Finegold et al.[36] and Vesley and Michaelsen[37] could not demonstrate an effect of disinfectants on the reduction of bacteria immediately after cleaning or on the rate of subsequent buildup of bacterial counts on hospital floors. On the other hand, disinfectants are necessary to treat grossly contaminated floors, walls, and furniture. Also the environmental surfaces in high-risk areas such as operating rooms, nurseries, and intensive care units should be disinfected. For infection control purposes, toilets, baths, and hydrotherapy tubs should be treated with disinfectant-cleaners. In laboratories a routine disinfection program is necessary for surfaces that may be contaminated by patient material or during laboratory procedures. Special attention must be paid to the potential hepatitis virus contamination.

With the extensive use of disposable items both in hospitals and in clinical laboratories, the problem of microbial growth in waste materials must be discussed. Previously most hospital wastes including disposable items were incinerated, but clean-air regulations forbid this effective sterilization procedure in most parts of the country. Infectious laboratory waste materials coming from infected patients are usually sterilized prior to discarding but on occasion waste products must be disinfected by chemical or physical means, for example, treatment of hospital sewage by heating before discharge into a public sewage system. Table 89-1 presents some guidelines about the disinfection activity needed for various use areas and various microorganisms.

Requirements on disinfection and disinfectants

Before selecting a disinfectant or a disinfection procedure the user should prepare a list of requirements that must be fulfilled. A disinfectant must be active against microorganisms independently of their functional state and retain its effectiveness under the conditions of use. The process must be compatible with the materials to be disinfected and harmless for the user and the environment. The scope of the activity of the disinfectant is determined by the process or procedure involved, by the types of microorganisms to be eliminated, by the degree of disinfection desired (high, intermediate; or low level) and by the desired rapidity of the decontamination procedure.

Factors that relate to the effectiveness of the disinfectant are (1) the type, physical characteristics, and condition of the material to be disinfected, (2) the stability of the disinfectant before and during use, (3) the compatibility between the disinfectant, the additives, and the diluent, (4) the methods of employment (by hand or machine, as liquid spray or gas, or as a part of a complex procedure), and (5) the disinfectant's cleaning potential.[34] If the user selects a chemical disinfectant he should be aware of the governmental regulations regarding the labeling of such "poisons." Both the Environmental Protection Agency and the Federal Trade Commission review label claims of disinfectants sold in interstate commerce. Thus, certain minimum requirements of activity need to be fulfilled (see discussion on Control of efficacy of disinfectants and disinfection procedures). Other agencies have issued specifications that refer to additional requirements such as toxicity, carcinogenesis, and so on. Information is available from the research departments of disinfectant manufacturers and should be reviewed prior to selection of a product.

Common disinfection procedures and agents
Physical disinfection

Hot water or steam. Boiling in water or exposure of objects to flowing steam is an effective method of destroying pathogens with the exception of certain spores and, possibly, hepatitis virus. Materials that cannot tolerate exposure to 100 C may be treated with hot water of lower temperature, e.g., 30 minutes at 70 C. This hot water disinfection, also called **pasteurization,** is used mainly for respiratory therapy and anesthesia equipment.[38,39]

Ultraviolet light. UV radiation is used in many institutions to reduce the microbial count on surfaces and in air, particularly in biologic safety cabinets and in tissue culture cubicles. The effectiveness of ultraviolet light is dependent on the intensity of the radiation source, its distance to the point of activity, and in the case of air disinfection the speed of airflow. Dust and other soil greatly diminish the effectiveness of ultraviolet radiation. Thus disinfection by UV radiation requires controlled environmental conditions and an experienced user. For detailed discussion see Shechmeister.[40]

Disinfection by mechanical means. Filtration is used mainly for producing clean air with Hepa filters. One may also consider the use of filters for sterilization filtration of liquids as disinfection if certain microorganisms are not retained.

Mechanical removal of microorganisms from objects by processes such as ultrasonic or surfactant cleaning may be considered disinfection if all microorganisms are eliminated, but usually these procedures are used in combination with chemical disinfectants.

Chemical disinfection

High-level chemical disinfectants such as ethylene oxide gas or alkaline glutaraldehyde were previously mentioned in the discussion on Methods of Sterilization.

Dewar[35] reported that the numerous types of disinfectants available in the United States are almost completely based on 6 classes of antimicrobial agents: organometallic compounds, pine oil, quaternary ammonium compounds, iodophors, chlorine compounds, and phenolic compounds.

Organometallic compounds. These agents are considered as bacteriostats and are readily neutralized or inactivated. Thus they are not germicides and should not be used for disinfection in a hospital or laboratory.

Pine oil. Pure pine oil, a natural distillation product of the pine tree, was shown to be inactive against *Staphylococcus aureus* and therefore is used today only in combination with a quaternary ammonium or phenolic germicide, mainly for household purposes.

Quaternary ammonium compounds. At concentrations of 1:1000 to 1:750 they were found to be inadequate for general hospital disinfection because of their limited spectrum of antimicrobial effectiveness (low activity against fungi and pseudomonads, lack of activity against tubercle bacilli) and easy inactivation by anionic matter. Lately they have returned to the hospital in newer preparations that seem to have overcome some of the inadequacies with higher concentrations of the active ingredient and better activity against gram-negative bacteria and fungi. They are quite useful as housekeeping disinfectants in low-risk areas such as hospital floors and nonpatient and food service areas.

Iodophors. As disinfectants the iodophors rank among the 3 most employed agents in hospitals. They consist of iodine bound to a nonionic detergent. They possess broad spectrum activity, are more stable and less corrosive than chlorine compounds, and have low or intermediate germicidal action depending on the concentration of available iodine (0.01-0.05%) and the soil load. Like quaternary ammonium compounds they are used to disinfect clean surfaces and utensils in the food service area of the hospital (at concentrations of 0.01% or less available iodine). At higher concentrations (0.05% or more available iodine) in a detergent-germicide preparation iodophors often are applied for surface disinfection and in discard pans in virus laboratories.

Chlorine compounds. These are powerful germicides with a wide spectrum of activity, lack of poisonous residuals, and a low price. Like other halogens they are highly reactive with organic matter and must be used either on clean surfaces or in high concentration. Both inorganic and organic chlorine compounds are sold, especially for low-level disinfection in food service areas (available chlorine levels of about 0.01%). More concentrated preparations (about 0.5% available chlorine) are used, often in combination with polishing or scouring powders, for bathrooms and toilets. Due to its lack of toxic residuals household bleach (sodium hypochlorite) is an excellent laboratory disinfectant for incubators, tabletops, and spills. For general use it is diluted 1:10 (equals 0.5% available chlorine) and should be prepared daily. For surfaces soiled with hepatitis-virus–containing material the use of full-strength (5%) or 1:5 diluted household bleach is recommended.[41]

Phenolic compounds. Phenolic germicides are by far the most common of all hospital disinfectants. Their use is based on Lister's introduction of carbolic acid over 100 years ago. Since that time synthetic phenolics have been developed to increase the antimicrobial effectiveness against a wider spectrum of microorganisms and to reduce the strong phenolic odor. The majority of presently marketed phenolic germicides contain one or more of the following substituted phenols: o-phenylphenol, o-phenyl-p-chlorophenol, o-phenyl-o-chlorphenol, o-benzyl-p-chlorophenol, and p-tert-amylphenol. The commercially available preparations possess a wide spectrum of germicidal activity, are insensitive to anionic matter, and are superior to other disinfectants in retaining their germicidal activity in the presence of organic soil. At the recommended use dilution (1-4%) phenolic detergent-germicides are excellent disinfectants for use in critical patient care areas and in laboratories. They leave a residual film that is claimed to be bacteriostatic. Therefore **they should not be used in incubators, water baths, and anaerobic or candle jars.** Phenolics are corrosive and irritate the skin. The components p-tert-amylphenol and p-tert-butylphenol may cause permanent depigmentation of the skin.[42] This side effect prompted many hospital housekeepers to switch to quaternary ammonium detergent-germicides for noncritical

areas of the hospital and for floors in patient and treatment rooms.

Alcohols. In concentrations of 70-90% alcohols are an excellent but quite expensive disinfectant of intermediate germicidal activity. Isopropyl alcohol is used widely as an antiseptic and is available in hospitals for rapid decontamination of small objects. It is not lethal for picornaviruses.[43] For emergency disinfection of certain items in the semicritical or noncritical category Spaulding[44] recommends immersion in 75-90% ethyl alcohol for 15 minutes.

Control of efficacy of disinfectants and disinfection procedures

The effectiveness of disinfectants and disinfection processes must be ensured by both **the manufacturer** of a product and by **the user.** Early in this chapter several requirements on disinfectants were listed. Both in vitro and in-use tests have been designed to evaluate disinfectants and disinfection procedures. In the United States a series of official laboratory tests to determine the in vitro activity of disinfectants is known as the AOAC tests. The basic test determines the phenol coefficient of a disinfectant by comparing its activity with that of phenol against standard strains of *Salmonella typhi* as well as *Staphylococcus aureus* and *Pseudomonas aeruginosa.* This test is useful to screen new disinfectants for their antibacterial action but says little about their efficacy in use-conditions. Therefore a **use-dilution test** is added in which stainless steel cylinders are contaminated with test bacteria and exposed to varying dilutions of the test germicide. The maximum dilution of the disinfectant that kills the test organisms on 10 cylinders within 10 minutes of exposure represents the maximum safe use-dilution for practical disinfection. Other AOAC tests were designed for **chlorine compounds** and **germicidal sprays** as well as **tuberculocidal** and **sporicidal disinfectants.** A summary description of the use-dilution test may be found in the previous edition of this book,[35] and detailed methods for all tests may be found in the AOAC publication, *Official Methods of Analysis,*[26] and in Bass.[45]

The use-dilution test has been critized for not accounting for inactivation of disinfectants under use-conditions. In 1969 Kelsey and Sykes described a capacity test with hospital application.[46] Increments of "organic soil" (yeasts) are added to the suspension of test bacteria in 3 concentrations of disinfectant around the recommended use-dilution.

Borneff and Werner,[47] as part of an international effort to standardize testing of disinfectants, proposed a new method for surface disinfection procedures using ceramic tiles and agar impression (Rodac) plates for recovery. Carson et al.[48] warned that laboratory-adapted, subcultured bacteria may not represent the naturally occurring populations in the hospital environment. Therefore in vitro or simulated in-use testing may result in erroneous assumptions about the efficacy of a disinfectant.

The various test methods mentioned above may be used in a well-equipped laboraory to evaluate new disinfectants. Other laboratory methods for controlling the in-use efficacy of disinfectants, including detergent-germicides used for housekeeping purposes, are the measurement of the microbial contamination of disinfectants during actual use by the membrane filter method and the determination of the concentration of disinfectants by a colorimetric procedure.[49]

For the control of disinfection efficacy in hospitals a number of technics have been described. For a low level of expected contamination on smooth surfaces the agar contact method, especially the use of Rodac plates, is most widely accepted and fairly precise. The Committee on Microbial Contamination of Surfaces of the American Public Health Association published arbitrary guidelines for achievable levels of microbial cleanliness of floors in patient rooms by considering up to 25 colony-forming units (CFU) per plate as good, 26-50 as fair, and over 50 as poor performance.[50]

The swab method allows for higher recovery, even from rough and porous surfaces with a high level of contamination, but the precision is only moderate.[51]

The rinse method can be used for hollow items; immersion can be used for small objects. The use of agitation, either manually or mechanically, helps to detach microorganisms. The recovery rate is very high, especially if surface active additives or ultrasound is used for detachment and dispersal of contaminants. For detailed review of technics see Favero et al.[52]

For the monitoring of anesthesia and respiratory therapy equipment several methods have been described.[53] The assembled machine is activated, and the effluent from the patient end of the tubing is collected by an air sampler,[54] through a funnel in a broth tube,[55] or directly onto an agar plate.[56] Mackel of the Center for Disease Control recommends sampling by rinsing of tubings, nebulizers, and humidifiers with sterile broth and by swabbing the exhalation valve. Quantitative assays are performed by the plate dilution method, qualitative by culturing and subculturing on differential media.

The laboratory technician interested in disinfectant testing should always remember that **neutralizers** must be used for all recovery cultures for testing antimicrobial chemicals. Lecithin to neutralize quaternary ammonium compounds and polysorbate (Tween 80) to neutralize phenolics is required in AOAC and other testing, including Rodac plate assays. For halogens, sodium thiosulfate serves as a neutralizer. The addition of blood or serum to the recovery medium also assists in overcoming continued disinfectant activity. A universal neutralizing medium was described by Engley and Dey[57] but the neutralizer effectiveness should always be tested for each compound under investigation. For methodology see Shaffer.[58]

Selection and use of disinfectants in hospitals and laboratories

The selection of a disinfectant for use in a hospital or clinical laboratory is based on 4 parameters: desired effect, class of disinfectant, procedure to be applied, and specific product.

The desired effect of a disinfection procedure is determined by the risk of infection associated with the objects to be disinfected, the degree and type of contamination, and the time available to achieve the desired effect. The type of disinfectant or disinfection procedure will depend on the condition and size of the object to be disinfected, the stability of the disinfectant used, undersirable side effects, the materials to be treated, and level of toxicity for the disinfector and the user of the disinfected object.

The selection of a specific product should be based on (1) its registration by a regulatory agency (e.g., EPA registration number) to ensure minimum effectiveness according to AOAC test procedures, (2) review of label claims and the manufacturer's research and development literature (not the promotional fliers), (3) comparison of the unknown with a known product (either by a comparative in-use test in the user's laboratory or through literature review), and (4) comparison of the price schedules of different producers of similar products.

Phenolic germicide-detergents are most commonly employed in hospitals for the disinfection of surfaces, contaminated objects, and laboratory discard jars and pans. For bathrooms, toilets, and so on hypochlorite compounds are often combined with cleansers and polishers. In virology laboratories and areas with a high risk of hepatitis such as hemodialysis units the use of halogen-releasing disinfectants, especially hypochlorites, is recommended. In low-risk areas new detergent-germicides on a quaternary ammonium basis are used with increasing frequency because of the skin toxicity of phenolics. In food preparation and service areas mainly hypochlorite compounds, iodophor disinfectants, and "quats" in low concentration ("sanitizers") are selected.

For the disinfection of surfaces or equipment soiled with hepatitis virus–containing or suspicious materials the following procedure is recommended[41]:

1. Hands are protected with surgical gloves.
2. The spill is covered with disposable towels to absorb liquid.
3. On nonmetals the entire area is liberally covered with undiluted household bleach (e.g., Clorox, 5% sodium hypochlorite) and allowed to air dry.
4. On metals 2% alkalinized glutaraldehyde is used and left on for 30 minutes. After thorough rinsing with water the surface is dried with paper towels.

5. Towels and gloves are disposed of in autoclavable plastic bags, autoclaved, and discarded.

Broken microbiologic culture tubes and other biohazardous spills are also covered with disposable towels and liberally soaked with either 0.5% sodium hypochlorite (1:10 diluted Clorox) or with a phenolic detergent-germicide at recommended use-dilution. Wetting is important to avoid airborne spread of organisms.

For additional information about the use of hospital disinfectants see Gröschel.[34]

ANTISEPSIS
Definition and aims

Antisepsis is the use of a substance that prevents or arrests the growth or action of microorganisms either by inhibiting their activity or by destroying them. The term "antiseptic" is used especially for preparations applied to living tissue.[1] A legal definition for the United States is contained in the Federal Food, Drug, and Cosmetic Act[59]: "The representation of a drug, in its labeling, as an antiseptic shall be considered to be a representation that it is a germicide, except in the case of a drug purporting to be, or represented, as an antiseptic for inhibitory use as a wet dressing, ointment, dusting powder, or such other use as involves prolonged contact with the body." Mouthwashes, douches, and gargles with a short contact with tissue can be labeled as antiseptic only if they destroy organisms. In the United States there is a clear separation between antiseptics as drugs used on living tissue and disinfectants as pesticides used on nonliving matter due to regulatory legislation assigning the control of the former to the Food and Drug Administration and of the latter to the Environmental Protection Agency. In Europe such strict separation is not known. One speaks about hygienic and surgical hand disinfection if bactericidal agents are applied and defines antiseptics as mainly microbistatic, usually moderately or little soluble in water to be applied to the body surfaces of man and animals.[60]

Areas of use

The aim of antisepsis is the reduction or destruction of undesirable microorganisms on skin and mucosal surfaces while preserving the normal, resident flora. It is obvious that this aim is an ideal one and cannot be achieved by the presently used antiseptics. Depending on their activity and concentrations the present hospital products are used for handwashing, in deodorant preparations, for surgical scrub and preoperative skin preparation, as wound cleansers and prophylactics against infection, for prevention of skin colonization with bacteria and fungi, in athlete's foot control, and as gargles, mouthwashes, vaginal douches, and so on. The definitions of product categories for over-the-counter topical antimicrobials were recently published by the FDA[61]; see Table 89-2.

Table 89-2. Definition of product categories for topical antimicrobials[61]

Category	Definition
Skin antiseptic	A safe, nonirritating antimicrobial-containing preparation that prevents overt skin infection; claims stating or implying an effect against microorganisms must be supported by controlled human studies that demonstrate prevention of infection
Patient preoperative skin preparation	A safe, fast-acting, broad-spectrum antimicrobial-containing preparation that significantly reduces number of microorganisms on intact skin
Surgical hand scrub	A safe, nonirritating, antimicrobial-containing preparation that significantly reduces number of microorganisms on intact skin; a surgical hand scrub should be broad spectrum, fast acting, and persistent
Health-care personnel handwash	A safe, nonirritating preparation designed for frequent use that reduces number of transient microorganisms on intact skin to an initial baseline level after adequate washing, rinsing, and drying; if preparation contains an antimicrobial agent it should be broad spectrum, fast acting, and if possible persistent
Skin wound cleanser	A safe, nonirritating liquid preparation (or product to be used with water) that assists in removal of foreign material from small superficial wounds and does not delay wound healing
Skin wound protectant	A safe, nonirritating preparation applied to small cleansed wounds that provides a protective (physical or chemical) barrier and neither delays healing nor favors growth of microorganisms
Antimicrobial soap	A soap containing an active ingredient with in vitro and in vivo activity against skin microorganisms

Requirements on antisepsis and antiseptics

Concern about hospital-associated infections has stimulated an increasing interest in antisepsis as one of the important control measures. Closer scrutiny of time-honored antiseptics showed that the in vitro tests required by the regulatory agencies have not always reflected their efficacy in practice. The primary requirements of an antiseptic are safety and effectiveness under the conditions of use. This includes the lack of skin or mucosal irritancy, systematic toxicity (usually measured as oral toxicity), and teratogenic, mutagenic, and carcinogenic effects. Absorption blood levels in man must be far below the toxic levels for both long- and short-term exposure, and information is required about tissue distribution, metabolism, and routes of excretion.

Other requirements are stability in both concentrated and use-dilution form, and microbistatic or microbicidal activity against selected test organisms including recent clinical isolates and support of label claims as shown in tests with adult humans. Residual antimicrobial effect is often desired. A major problem with antiseptics of limited antimicrobial spectrum is their possible contamination with resistant microorganisms, a common finding with dispensers refilled from bulk containers. It is a special responsibility of a hospital's infection control service to prevent the spread of nosocomial microorganisms by use of antiseptics and disinfectants that don't work.[62,63]

Commonly used antiseptics

Nonmedicated bar and liquid soaps or detergents are not antiseptics in the sense of the definition, although they may reduce the microbial count temporarily by removing gross dirt, fats, oils, and skin debris.

Heavy metals. Traditionally mercurials were used as mild antiseptics because of their stability and lack of skin and mucosal irritation. Unfortunately they are inactivated by serum, and there is considerable mercury resistance among pathogenic microorganisms. Thus the role of mercurials as antiseptics has diminished. Silver nitrate has been used successfully for almost a century for the prophylaxis of gonococcal infection in the newborn. In recent years silver nitrate and silver sulfadiazene-containing cream were introduced for the treatment of burns. For a detailed discussion of these classes of antiseptics see Block.[14]

Bisphenols. Of the bisphenols, hexachlorophene was the most widely used antiseptic for almost 30 years. It is compatible with soap and detergents, reduces the transient and permanent skin flora, and with continuous use accumulates on the skin surface and has residual antimicrobial effect. It has been used as a 3% soap for surgical scrubs, preparation of operative sites, bathing of newborns, treatment of skin infections, etc. With the shift of hospital-associated infections from gram-positive to gram-negative bacteria the limited effectiveness of this antiseptic came under criticism. The discovery that hexachlorophene can be absorbed through the intact skin of newborns and through damaged skin (e.g., burns) and can cause brain damage has led to considerable curtailment of its hospital use by government regulation.[64]

Chlorohexidine. The recently marketed chlorohexidine gluconate (4%) has replaced hexachlorophene in many hospitals as a surgical scrub, for handwashing, and as a skin wound cleanser. Chlorohexidine, a biguanide, has a long record as an antiseptic in Great Britain.[65] It is the first antiseptic tested and approved by the Food and Drug Administration in accordance with the new guidelines.[61] It has a wider antimicrobial spectrum than hexachlorophene and is active against most microorganisms encountered in the hospital. It is too early to evaluate its impact on the American market.

Alcohols. Ethanol at a concentration of 70-90% (by weight) is a time-honored skin antiseptic and is widely used, especially in Central Europe, as a surgical "hand disinfectant," often in combination with other antimicrobial agents. For routine use 70% by weight is recommened. Alcohol spreads evenly, wets efficiently, and drys slowly.[66] It is stable, little inactivated during use, and rapidly microbicidal. Since alcohol is not sporicidal it may contain bacterial spores if not filter sterilized. Denaturing substances may irritate the skin. Drying can be overcome by the addition of cetyl alcohol or skin care additives. Isopropyl alcohol is equally or more effective and also cheaper.[67] Sterile absorbent pads commonly found in hospitals are excellent for rapid antiseptic treatment of skin.

Iodine and iodophors. Iodine has been used in hospitals for many decades either as an aqueous solution or as a tincture for skin preparation and as a wound antiseptic. Iodine solutions are rapidly microbicidal and stable in closed containers if protected against light. Side effects are due to hypersensitivity to iodine or direct skin damage (iodine burn). For these reasons the concentration of iodine in aqueous solution as well as in tincture has been reduced to 1% and 0.5-1%, respectively. Iodophors have largely replaced the iodine solutions.

Iodophors are bactericidal preparations with a broad spectrum of antimicrobial activity. Iodine is complexed or combined with carriers such as surfactant compounds (e.g., polaxomer-iodine complex) or nondetergent compounds (e.g., polyvinylpyrrolidone-iodine). The antimicrobial activity is dependent on the release of elemental iodine. The rate of iodine release will determine an iodophor's effectiveness, its stability, and its potential for skin irritation. Iodophors are widely used for preoperative skin preparation, surgical hand scrub, and also in the treatment of open wounds and burns. The OTC Antimicrobial 1 Panel expressed concern about the lack of stability of several iodophor preparations and possible interference in wound healing of certain carriers.[61]

Quaternary ammonium compounds. The cationic surface active "quats" have been widely used as antiseptics but there has been much controversy about their limited (mainly gram-positive) antimicrobial spectrum, inactivation with incompatible materials (e.g., serum, soap), adsorption on surfaces of containers and on cotton, and the hazard of contamination with gram-negative bacteria, especially pseudomonads. The OTC Antimicrobial 1 Panel considers quaternary ammonium compounds to be safe and effective in skin wound cleansers but not for other use categories.[61]

Phenols. Phenols and phenolics are rarely used in hospital antiseptics anymore but they may be contained in various over-the-counter preparations. Their safety and effectiveness has not been clearly established. Several European alcoholic antiseptics contain small amounts of phenol derivatives and presumably do not cause any allergic or toxic side effects.

Halogenated salicylanilides and carbanilides. These compounds are used mainly as additives to antimicrobial soaps, especially for the prevention of body odor. The halogenated salicylanilides, tribromsalan and fluorosalan, are not considered safe and effective by the OTC Antimicrobial 1 Panel because of potential toxicity, photosensitization, and limited antimicrobial spectrum. Halogenated carbanilides are still being used in bar soap but additional toxicity studies are required to establish their safety. Their value in preventing skin infections was disputed by the panel.[61]

Control of effectiveness of antiseptics

The Food and Drug Administration requires that antiseptics have certain properties that make them safe and effective. The following in vitro tests are performed for registration[68]:
1. Modified phenol coefficient of Reddish for soluble and liquid antiseptics
2. Serum agar plate method for antiseptic ointments
3. Serum agar cup-plate method for liquid antiseptics in wet dressings, dyes, powders, etc.

The OTC Antimicrobial 1 Panel added to these requirements for topical antimicrobials the inclusion of recent clinical isolates in all in vitro tests and the proof of clinical effectiveness. For surgical scrub testing the glove-juice test is required.[61, p. 33137]

For hospital evaluation of antiseptics the scrub-rinse technics of Price[69] and Cade[70] and the glove-juice test are rather cumbersome. The wipe-rinse test of Peterson et al.[71] is useful for a well-equipped laboratory. For a rapid and simple demonstration of the effects of antiseptic treatment, especially in educational situations, 3 methods have been applied: (1) swabbing of skin or skin stripping with adhesive tape before and after treatment and inoculation on neutralizer agar plates, (2) placing fingertips on the surface of neutralizer agar plates before and after use of the antiseptic, and (3) using contact agar (Rodac) plates to sample skin areas.[72] Since the methods are not standardized they should not be used for investigative work.

REFERENCES

1. Block, S. S.: Definition of terms. In Block, S. S., editor: Disinfection, sterilization, and preservation, ed. 2, Philadephia, 1977, Lea & Febiger.
2. United States Pharmacopoeia, ed. 19, Rockville, Md., 1975, U.S. Pharmacopoeia Convention.
3. Bruch, W. W.: Sterility or microbial control of commercially supplied items. In Brachman, P. S., and Eickhoff, T. C., editors: Proceedings of the International Conference on Nosocomial Infections, Center for Disease Control, August 3-6, 1970, Chicago, 1971, American Hospital Association.
4. Kelsey, J. C.: Lancet **2:**1301, 1972.
5. Starkey, D. H.: Concepts of sterility and degrees of quality control. In Brachman, P. S., and Eickhoff, T. C., editors: Proceedings of the International Conference on Nosocomial Infections, Center for Disease Control, August 3-6, 1970, Chicago, 1971, American Hospital Association.
6. Spaulding, E. H., Cundy, K. R., and Turner, F. J.: Chemical disinfection of medical and surgical materials. In Block, S. S., editor: Disinfection, sterilization, and preservation, ed. 2, Philadelphia, 1977, Lea & Febiger.
7. Spaulding, E. H., and Gröschel, D. H. M.: Hospital disinfectants and antiseptics. In Lennette, E. H., Spaulding, E. H., and Truant, J. P., editors: Manual of clinical microbiology, ed. 2, Washington, D.C., 1974, American Society for Microbiology.
8. Greene, V. W.: Disinfection and sterilization practices in American hospitals. In Bernarde, M. E., editor: Disinfection, New York, 1970, Marcel Dekker.
9. Doyle, J. E., and Ernst, R. R.: Appl. Microbiol. **15:**726, 1967.
10. Ernst, R. R.: Sterilization by heat. In Block, S. S., editor: Disinfection, sterilization, and preservation, ed. 2, Philadelphia, 1977, Lea & Febiger.
11. Fifield, C. W.: Sterilization filtration. In Block, S. S., editor: Disinfection, sterilization, and preservation, ed. 2, Philadelphia, 1977, Lea & Febiger.
12. Boucher, R. M. G.: Am. J. Hosp. Pharm. **29:**661, 1972.
13. Silverman, G. J., and Sinskey, A. J.: Sterilization by ionizing irradiation. In Block, S. S., editor: Disinfection, sterilization, and preservation, ed. 2, Philadelphia, 1977, Lea & Febiger.
14. Block, S. S., editor: Disinfection, sterilization, and preservation, ed. 2, Philadelphia, 1977, Lea & Febiger.
15. Environmental Protection Agency: Fed. Register **43:**3801, 1978.
16. Roberts, R. B., and Rendell-Baker, L.: Anesthesia **27:**278, 1972.
17. Department of Health, Education, and Welfare, Food and Drug Administration: Fed. Register **43:**3800, 1978.
18. Phillips, C. R.: Gaseous sterilization. In Block, S. S., editor: Disinfection, sterilization, and preservation, ed. 2, Philadelphia, 1977, Lea & Febiger.
19. Kereluk, K., Gammon, R. A., and Lloyd, R. S.: Appl. Microbiol. **19:**146, 152, 157, 163, 1970.
20. Borick, P. M.: Adv. Appl. Microbiol. **110:**291, 1968.
21. Stonehill, A. A., Krop, S., and Borick, P. M.: Am. J. Hosp. Pharm. **20:**458, 1963.
22. Bartlett, R. C., Gröschel, D. H. M., Mackel, D. C., et al.: Microbiological surveillance. In Lennette, E. H., Spaulding, E. H., and Truant, J. P., editors: Manual of clinical microbiology, ed. 2, Washington, D.C., 1974, American Society of Microbiologists.

23. Beloian, A.: Methods for testing for sterility and efficacy of sterilizers, sporicides and sterilizing processes. In Block, S. S., editor: Disinfection, sterilization, and preservation, ed. 2, Philadelphia, 1977, Lea & Febiger.

24. Gaughran, E. R. L., and Kereluk, K., editors: Sterilization of medical products, New Brunswick, N.J., 1977, Johnson & Johnson.

25. Witonski, R. J.: Bull. Parenter. Drug. Assoc. 31:274, 1977.

26. Association of Official Analytical Chemists: Official methods of analysis, ed. 10, Washington, D.C., 1970, The Association.

27. Mayernik, J. J.: Bull. Parenter. Drug. Assoc. 26:206, 1972.

28. Kereluk, K., and Gammon, R. A.: Dev. Ind. Microbiol. 15:411, 1974.

29. Joint Commission on Accreditation of Hospitals: Accreditation manual for hospitals, Chicago, 1976, The Commission.

30. Kereluk, K.: Quality control in sterilization procedures: Biological indicators. In Prier, J. E., Bartola, J. T., and Friedman, H., editors: Quality control in microbiology, Baltimore, 1975, University Park Press.

31. Reddish, G. F., editor: Antiseptics, disinfectants, fungicides, and chemical and physical sterilization, Philadephia, 1957, Lea & Febiger.

32. Benenson, A. S., editor: Control of communicable diseases in man, ed. 11, New York, 1970, American Public Health Association.

33. Reber, H.: Zentralbl. Bakteriol. (Orig. B) 157:421, 1973.

34. Gröschel, D.: In von Graevenitz, A., editor: Handbook series in clinical laboratory science; section E, Clinical microbiology, vol. 2, Cleveland, 1977, CRC Press.

35. Dewar, N. E.: Disinfectants, sanitizers, and antiseptics. In Gradwohl's clinical laboratory methods and diagnosis, ed. 7, St. Louis, 1970, The C. V. Mosby Co.

36. Finegold, S. M., Sweeney, E. E., Gaylor, D. W., et al.: Antimicrob. Agents Chemother. 9:250, 1962.

37. Vesley, D., and Michaelsen, G. S.: Health Lab. Sci. 1:107, 1964.

38. Roberts, F. J., Cockcroft, W. H., and Johnston, H. E.: Can. Med. Assoc. J. 101:30, 1969.

39. Nelson, E. J., and Ryan, K. J.: Resp. Care 16:97, 1971.

40. Shechmeister, I. L.: Sterilization by ultraviolet radiation. In Block, S. S., editor: Disinfection, sterilization, and preservation, ed. 2, Philadelphia, 1977, Lea & Febiger.

41. Bond, W. W., and Pattison, C. P.: J.A.M.A. 231:700, 1975.

42. Kahn, G.: Arch. Dermatol. 102:177, 1970.

43. Klein, M., and Deforest, A.: Soap Chem. Spec. 39:70, 95, 1963.

44. Spaulding, E. H.: Assoc. Op. Room Nurs. J. 2:67, 1964.

45. Bass, K. G.: Methods of testing disinfectants. In Block, S. S., editor: Disinfection, sterilization, and preservation, ed. 2, Philadelphia, 1977, Lea & Febiger.

46. Kelsey, J. C., and Sykes, G.: Pharm. J. 101:607, 1969.

47. Borneff, J., and Werner, H. P.: Zentralbl. Bakteriol. (Orig. B) 165:97, 1977.

48. Carson, L. A., Favero, M. S., Bond, W. W., et al.: Appl. Microbiol. 23:863, 1972.

49. Prince, J., and Ayliffe, G. A. J.: J. Clin. Pathol. 25:586, 1972.

50. Vesley, D., Pryor, A. K., Walter, W. G., et al.: Health. Lab. Sci. 7:256, 1970.

51. Angelotti, R., Foter, M. J., Busch, K. A., et al.: Food Res. 23:175, 1958.

52. Favero, M. S., McDade, J. J., Robertsen, J. A., et al.: J. Appl. Bacteriol. 31:336, 1968.

53. Gröschel, D.: In Cundy, K. R., and Ball, W., editors: Infection control in health care facilities, Baltimore, 1977, University Park Press.

54. Reinarz, J. A., Pierce, A. K., Mays, B. B., et al.: Clin. Invest. 44:831, 1965.

55. Edmonson, E. B., and Sanford, J. P.: Am. Rev. Respir. Dis. 94:450, 1966.

56. Nazemi, M. M., Musher, D. M., and Martin, R. R.: Am. Rev. Respir. Dis. 106:920, 1972.

57. Engley, F. B., and Dey, B. P.: CSMA proceedings, fifty-sixth midyear meeting, 1970.

58. Shaffer, H.: Methods of testing sanitizers and bacteriostatic substances. In Block, S. S., editor: Disinfection, sterilization, and preservation, ed. 2, Philadelphia, 1977, Lea & Febiger.

59. Department of Health, Education and Welfare, Food and Drug Administration: Federal Food, Drug, and Cosmetic Act as amended October 1976, Washington, 1976, Ch. II, 201(o).

60. Weuffen, W.: Zentralbl. Bakteriol. (Orig. B) 157:524, 1973.

61. Department of Health, Education and Welfare, Food and Drug Administration: Fed. Register 39:33103, 1974.

62. Sanford, J. P.: Ann. Intern. Med. 72:282, 1970.

63. Frank, M. J., and Schaffner, W.: J.A.M.A. 236:2418, 1976.

64. Department of Health, Education, and Welfare, Food and Drug Administration: Fed. Register 37:20160, 1972.

65. Lowbury, E. J. L., and Lilly, H. A.: Br. Med. J. 1:510, 1973.

66. Price, P. B.: Arch. Surg. 61:23, 1950.

67. Altemeier, W. A.: Surgical antiseptics. In Block, S. S., editor: Disinfection, sterilization, and preservation, ed. 2, Philadelphia, 1977, Lea & Febiger.

68. Roessler, W. G.: Methods of testing antiseptics. In Block, S. S., editor: Disinfection, sterilization, and preservation, ed. 2, Philadelphia, 1977, Lea & Febiger.

69. Price, P. R.: J. Infect. Dis. 63:301, 1938.

70. Cade, A. R.: J. Soc. Cosmet. Chem. 2:281, 1951.

71. Petersen, N. J., Collins, D. E., and Marshall, J. H.: Health Lab. Sci. 10:18, 1973.

72. Ulrich, J.: Health Lab. Sci. 1:133, 1964.

PART VIII

VIRAL AND RICKETTSIAL*
DIAGNOSTIC PROCEDURES

* For taxonomic position of rickettsiae see Chapter 68.

90

VIRUSES: CLASSIFICATION AND GENERAL CONSIDERATIONS

J. Mehsen Joseph

CLASSIFICATION

Earlier classifications of viruses were based on such variable properties as tissue affinities, clinical symptomatology, and distribution in nature. These criteria are insufficient because they are dependent in large measure on the host and other external factors and not on the physicochemical properties of the virus. Since it has been demonstrated that viral genetic material is composed of either RNA or DNA, they can be divided into 2 major groups designated as riboviruses and deoxyriboviruses. Viral nucleic acid (nucleoid) is protected by a shell of protein called a capsid. The capsid is composed of repeating protein subunits or capsomers, which are packed around the nucleic acid core to form particles of either helical or cubic symmetry. Some virus capsids are enclosed in a lipoprotein envelope, which is usually furnished by the host cell. Protein projections or spikes (peplomers) on the envelope are hemagglutinating units. Viruses with helical symmetry are commonly enclosed in an envelope, while those with cubic symmetry are only rarely so enclosed. Enveloped viruses are labile to ether and other lipid solvents because they solubilize the envelope, which is essential for infectivity. The complete infectious particle is referred to as a virion. A classification based on these criteria was approved by the International Committee on the Taxonomy of Viruses in 1963.[1] The animal viruses are placed in 11 major groups based on their nucleic acid composition; there are 6 RNA virus groups and 5 DNA virus groups (Table 90-1). Each group is further characterized on the basis of such properties as size, ether sensitivity, presence of lipid envelope, number of capsomers, and architectural symmetry.

Members of the major groups of animal viruses that have been officially accepted are listed on p. 1994.[2]*

*This list is based on Green, M.: In Horsfall, F. L., and Tamm, E., editors: Viral and rickettsial infections of man, ed. 4, Philadelphia, 1965, J. B. Lippincott Co., with additions and modification.

Table 90-1. Basic properties of viruses*†

Nucleic acid type	Groups	Size (nm)	Presence of envelope	Ether sensitivity	Capsid symmetry	Number of capsomers
RNA	1. Picornaviruses	17-30	−	Resistant	Cubic	—
	2. Reoviruses	70	−	Resistant	Cubic	92 or 180
	3. Togaviruses	20-100	+	Sensitive	Cubic	—
	4. Orthomyxoviruses	80-200	+	Sensitive	Helical	—
	5. Paramyxoviruses	100-300	+	Sensitive	Helical	—
	6. Rhabdoviruses	60-225	+	Sensitive	Helical	—
DNA	1. Papovaviruses	40-45	−	Resistant	Cubic	42 or 72
	2. Adenoviruses	60-70	−	Resistant	Cubic	252
	3. Herpesviruses	120-180	+	Sensitive	Cubic	162
	4. Poxviruses	150-300	+	Some sensitive	Helical	—
	5. Picodnaviruses	15-30	−	Sensitive	Cubic	12

*From International Subcommittee on Virus Nomenclature: Int. Bull. Bact. Nomen. Taxon. **13**:217, 1963; and Horsfall, F. L., and Tamm, E., editors: Viral and rickettsial infections of man, ed. 4, Philadelphia, 1965, J. B. Lippincott Co.

†**Editor's note:** For taxonomic position of **chlamydiae (bedsoniae)** see Chapter 95. The **psittacosis-LGV-trachoma** group contains **both** RNA and DNA, metabolic enzymes, and muramic acid, properties that separate it from the viruses. Members of this group are in the 250-400 nm size range, possess an envelope, are ether sensitive, and have no capsid symmetry.[3]

Picornaviruses
1. Enteroviruses
   a. Polioviruses (3 serotypes)
   b. Coxsackie viruses A (23 serotypes)
   c. Coxsackie viruses B (6 serotypes)
   d. Echoviruses (32 serotypes)
2. Rhinoviruses (120+ serotypes)
3. Unclassified—Mengo virus, Columbian SK virus, encephalomyocarditis, etc.

Reoviruses
1. Reovirus types 1, 2, and 3
2. Colorado tick fever virus

Myxoviruses
1. Orthomyxoviruses
   a. Influenza A, B, and C
   b. Swine influenza
2. Paramyxoviruses
   a. Newcastle disease
   b. Mumps
   c. Parainfluenza types 1-4
   d. Respiratory syncytial virus
   e. Rubeola

Togaviruses
1. Alphaviruses (group A arboviruses)—western encephalitis, eastern encephalitis, Semliki Forest, Sindbis, and 16 other members
2. Flavoviruses (group B arboviruses)—St. Louis encephalitis, Powassan, dengue fever, yellow fever, bat salivary, West Nile, Murray Valley, Japanese B encephalitis, Russian spring-summer complex, and 22 other members
3. Group C aboviruses—Marituba, Caraparu, Oriboca, and 6 other viruses
4. Complexes—California, Bunyamwera, Tacaribe, and 14 other groups
5. Rubella
6. Ungrouped—Rift Valley fever, sandfly fever, epidemic hemorrhagic fever, and over 50 other members

Rhabdoviruses
1. Rabies virus
2. Vesicular stomatitis virus
3. Marburg virus

Coronaviruses
1. Human repiratory viruses
2. Avian infectious bronchitis virus
3. Mouse hepatitis virus

Oncornaviruses
1. Avian leukosis complex
2. Rous sarcoma
3. Murine leukemia
4. Mouse sarcoma
5. Feline leukemia
6. Feline sarcoma

Arenaviruses
1. Lymphocytic choriomeningitis
2. Lassa virus
3. Tacaribe complex

Orbiviruses

Rotaviruses (duoviruses)

Adenoviruses
1. Human adenoviruses (28 serotypes)
2. Simian adenoviruses (12 serotypes)
3. Canine adenoviruses (canine hepatitis)
4. Bovine adenoviruses
5. Murine adenoviruses
6. Avian adenoviruses

Papovaviruses
1. Human papilloma virus (wart)
2. Polyoma virus
3. Simian vacuolating virus (SV-40)

4. Toolan H-1 virus
5. Shope rabbit papilloma

Herpesviruses
1. Herpes simplex, types 1 and 2
2. Herpes B
3. Herpes pseudorabies
4. Varicella zoster
5. Cytomegaloviruses
6. EB virus

Poxviruses
1. Variola
2. Vaccinia
3. Paravaccinia
4. Cowpox
5. Molluscum contagiosum
6. Ectromelia
7. Monkeypox
8. Myxoma
9. Fibroma

Basophilic agents*
1. Chlamydia
   a. Trachoma
   b. Inclusion blennorrhea
2. Miyagawanella
   a. Psittacosis
   b. Ornithosis
   c. Pneumonitis
   d. Lymphogranuloma venereum (LGV)

LABORATORY DIAGNOSIS

Improved and expanded laboratory methods have provided evidence that viruses may be responsible for a wider range of clinical and pathologic conditions than had been previously suspected. For example, it has been show that acute myocarditis and pericarditis may be due to certain Coxsackie group B viruses. It has been suggested that laboratory investigation be employed more extensively to clarify the role of viruses in certain forms of acute and chronic illnesses involving the central nervous system, lungs, liver, gastrointestinal tract, heart, and vessels. It has been demonstrated by laboratory isolation and antigenic experience that occasional cases of paralytic disease resembling poliomyelitis may be due to certain echoviruses and Coxsackie A viruses.

Aseptic meningitis without paralysis, clinically indistinguishable from nonparalytic poliomylitis, may be due to several different viruses such as Coxsackie, echoviruses, mumps, herpes simplex, herpes zoster, lymphocytic choriomeningitis, and equine encephalomyelitis.

To establish a laboratory confirmation of viral infections, direct and indirect methods are employed. Direct examinations are represented by (1) microscopic examination for inclusion bodies as found in rabies and (2) isolation of infective agents in animals, tissue cultures, and chick embryos. Wherever possible, direct isolation of the infective agent is the principal means of laboratory confirmation.

Indirect tests are those in which the level of antibody in the patient's serum for a particular

---

*Editor's note: For taxonomic position of this group see p. 1320.

virus is determined. The tests most frequently employed for this purpose are the neutralization test, complement fixation test, and hemagglutination-inhibition test. In all cases of serologic diagnosis every attempt should be made to obtain paired sera, i.e., an acute phase specimen taken as early in the course of the disease as possible and a convalescent phase specimen taken 14-21 days later, for demonstrating a rise in antibody titer. Both sera must be tested simultaneously for the results to be meaningful. A 4-fold rise in the antibody titer usually indicates recent infection with the virus in question.

Success of laboratory studies of viral disease requires that 3 cardinal rules be observed[4]: (1) freeze the specimens immediately to preserve potency of the virus if the specimen cannot be inoculated immediately into a susceptible host system; (2) obtain paired sera for demonstrating 4-fold rise in antibody titer; and (3) obtain a summary of the case history, which serves as a guide in planning virologic studies.

NEWER VIRUSES

Coxsackie viruses. The initial isolation of the Coxsackie virus was accomplished by Dalldorf and Sickles in 1948.[5] Coxsackie viruses readily infect suckling mice but not adult mice, and 2 groups (A and B) have been established on the basis of the histopathology produced. Group A viruses produce extensive myositis of the skeletal muscles with flaccid paralysis; group B viruses produce focal muscle lesions, necrosis of fat pads, and spastic paralysis.[6]

At the present time there are 23 types of Coxsackie A and 6 types of Coxsackie B viruses. These viruses resemble poliovirus in seasonal incidence and resistance to physical and chemical agents.

Group A virus infections in man are associated with headache, neck stiffness, muscle soreness, and blisters on the pharynx (herpangina). Coxsackie viruses A-7 and A-14 have been associated with paralytic disease indistinguishable from poliomyelitis and A-7, A-9, and A-1 to A-4 with aseptic meningitis.[7]

Coxsackie B viruses are responsible for outbreaks of pleurodynia (stabbing chest pain), or Bornholm disease, and aseptic meningitis. Myocarditis and pericarditis in infants have been associated primarily with B-2, 3, and 4. It is doubtful when they cause paralysis.[8]

Coxsackie viruses may be isolated from throat washings and feces or from spinal fluid in aseptic meningitis. Feces and fluid from blisters are the best sources of the virus.

Coxsackie A viruses are isolated in suckling mice, since most of them do not grow in tissue culture (exceptions are A-9, 11, 13, 15, 16, and 18). Coxsackie B viruses are isolated in monkey kidney tissue culture. Coxsackie B-1, 3, and 5 can also be isolated in HeLa cells.

Echoviruses (ECHO, Enteric Cytopathogenic Human Orphan viruses). Echoviruses were first isolated by Robbins et al.[9] by application of tissue culture for the isolation of viruses from feces in polio-like illnesses.[9] These agents are nonpathogenic for suckling mice, and they grow and produce a cytopathogenic effect (CPE) in human and monkey kidney tissue culture but not in HeLa cells. They are antigenically heterogeneous and do not produce a common complement fixation (CF) antigen. At the present time 32 antigenically distinct types are recognized.

In view of the similarities in physical, biologic, and epidemiologic properties of echoviruses, Coxsackie viruses, and poliomyelitis viruses, they are considered as members of a single group, the **enterovirus group**.[10]

Clinical illness due to echoviruses is characterized by fever, headache, stiff neck and back, and vomiting, without encephalitic disturbance. Echoviruses have been associated with aseptic meningitis, febrile illness with or without rash, and epidemic diarrhea in infants. Paralytic disease is uncommon and without residual paralysis.[11]

Echoviruses types 4, 6, 9, and 16 have been associated with outbreaks of aseptic meningitis, and sporadic cases have been due to most other types. Paralytic disease has been associated with type 6 and sporadic cases with types 2, 4, 9, and 16. Epidemics of febrile illness with rubella-like rash have been associated with echoviruses types 4, 9, 16. Outbreaks of summer diarrhea in infants in hospital nurseries have been due to echovirus type 18. Echoviruses types 8, 10, and 20 have been associated with respiratory-enteric infections.[12]

Echoviruses are most frequently isolated from the throat and stool but rarely from spinal fluid. Monkey kidney epithelial cells are most commonly used for isolation. Suckling and adult mice are not susceptible, except for certain strains of echovirus 9 that produce disease in suckling mice after initial isolation in tissue culture.

Adenoviruses. Rowe et al.[13] in 1953 isolated an agent from tissue cultures of human adenoids that had undergone spontaneous degeneration. Similar agents were isolated by Hilleman and Wenner[14] in 1954 from military recruits with acute respiratory illness. They proposed the term **adenovirus** for these agents.

There are 28 recognized types of adenoviruses of human origin and 12 of simian origin. Adenoviruses have been associated with acute febrile pharyngitis (types 1, 2, 3, and 5), severe infantile pneumonia (7a; rarely types 1 and 3), acute respiratory disease and pneumonia in adults (types 3, 4, 7, and 14), acute follicular conjunctivitis (types 3 and 7a; rarely types 2, 6, 9, and 10), and acute epidemic keratoconjunctivitis (type 8 in severe cases; types 3 and 7a in mild cases).[15] Outbreaks among military recruits have been associated with types 4, 7, 7a, and 14, but in the civilian population they have been mostly type 3.

The principle characteristics are ether resistance, ability to grow and produce CPE in human epithelial cell cultures, nonpathogenicity for animals, and the presence of a soluble CF antigen common to the group.

Adenoids and throat washings are the best sources of these viruses. Frequently they are found in the stool, but they are not definitely associated with enteric infection. HeLa cells are susceptible to all adenoviruses and are recommended for their isolation.

Hemadsorption viruses. In 1956 Chanock[16] isolated a virus from the throats of children suffering from croup and a related agent from children with febrile respiratory illness. These viruses grew in monkey kidney renal cell cultures, and their presence was recognized by the hemadsorption of guinea pig red cells to the tissue culture sheet. Hence they were named **Hemadsorption viruses** types 1 and 2 (parainfluenza 3 and 1).

Sendai virus. The Sendai virus (hemagglutinating virus of Japan or influenza D) was originally isolated by Japanese workers in 1953 from cases of pneumonitis in the newborn.[17] The virus can be grown in the amniotic and allantoic cavities of the chick embryo and is detected by its ability to agglutinate chick red cells (see Parainfluenza, Viruses).

Croup-associated virus. Chanock[16] in 1956 isolated an agent from infants with symptoms of croup, which he named **croup-associated virus (CA virus).** The CA virus produces CPE in monkey kidney and HeLa tissue cultures and agglutinates erythrocytes (see Parainfluenza Viruses).

Parainfluenza viruses. Hemadsorption viruses types 1 and 2, Sendai virus, and croup-associated virus have been placed in a group referred to as **parainfluenza viruses.**[18] Hemadsorption virus type 2 and the Sendai virus have been renamed parainfluenza type 1, the CA virus as parainfluenza type 2, and the hemadsorption virus type 1 as parainfluenza type 3. There are 2 subtypes of parainfluenza type 4.

Because of their affinity for certain mucins and the disease syndrome produced, they are considered as members of the large **myxovirus group.**[19]

Influenza viruses. Influenza viruses[20] are grouped as types A, B, and C on the basis of the type-specific nucleoprotein (NP) antigen contained in the virus core. The CF test using antibody to soluble NP antigen is employed to identify the type of influenza. Subtypes or specific strains are based on the presence of variable surface hemagglutinin and neuraminidase components. Hemagglutination-inhibition (HI) and neuraminidase-inhibition (NI) tests with specific antibody against these antigens are used for strain identification.

Influenza viruses possess 2 antigenically stable internal antigens, the matrix protein (MP) and the nucleoprotein, and 2 antigenically variable surface antigens, the hemagglutinin (HA) and the neuraminidase (NA). Specific antisera have been prepared against all these antigens, and they can be used for characterization of a new viral isolate by CF, HI, NI, and immunodiffusion tests.

The system of nomenclature recommended by WHO[21] is based on characterization of these antigens. Strain designation includes information as to antigenic types of nucleoprotein (type A, B, or C), host origin, geographic origin, strain number, year of isolation, and for influenza A the antigenic character of HA and NA, in that order. A full designation of a given isolate might be expressed as the following: A/Hong Kong/1/68 (H3N2).

Influenza viruses can be isolated in embryonated hen's eggs and in primary kidney cell culture from a variety of mammalian species. For maximum isolation of influenza A and B both systems are recommended. Influenza type C will replicate only in embryonated eggs.

Coronaviruses. With the use of human embryonic tracheal organ culture, a group of previously unidentified viruses has been recovered from patients with acute respiratory disease. These agents bear a close morphologic resemblance to avian infectious bronchitis virus (IBV). When homotypic cultured virus is reacted with antiserum and examined by negative staining with the electron microscope, antibody is found attached to the widely spaced, club-shaped surface projections or spikes on the viral envelope like a cornona or crown, hence the name "coronaviruses." These viruses are extremely difficult to culture by conventional methods. They are recovered by inoculating throat washings from patients onto human embryonic tracheal organ culture. If virus develops in this system, its presence is revealed by the immobilization of cilia on the culture cell walls.[22]

The term "coronavirus" includes the avian infectious bronchitis virus, mouse hepatitis virus, and the human IBV-like viruses. Human coronaviruses are spherical, pleomorphic viruses, measuring 120-160 nm in diameter and containing a core of RNA and an outer lipid envelope with club-shaped peplomers. They are ether and chloroform labile.[23]

These viruses are widespread, occur in cycles, and are associated with a significant proportion of upper respiratory disease in older children and young adults. Strains 229E and OC-38 are among the most common coronaviruses causing respiratory disease in humans. For serologic diagnosis both CF and neutralization tests are useful.

Respiratory syncytial virus. The CCA virus (chimpanzee coryza agent) was originally isolated in 1956 by Morris et al.[24] from chimpanzees with coryza. A similar agent was isolated from children with bronchopneumonia and croup by Chanock et al.[25] in 1957. This agent produced large syncytial masses in monkey kidney tissue culture; hence it was termed **respiratory syncytial virus.** This virus does not grow in the chick embryo or agglutinate erythrocytes; however, it is tentatively classified as a myxovirus.

JH and 2060 viruses. In 1956 Price isolated the **JH virus** from children and adults with respiratory disease. An antigenically related but not identical agent, the **2060 virus,** was recovered by Mogabgab and Pelon in 1957 from recruits with mild respiratory illness. Both of these viruses, which can be recovered from throat washings, grow in monkey kidney cell culture. These viruses were classified as echovirus 28 but are now grouped with the rhinoviruses.

Coe virus. Lennette et al.[26] in 1958 isolated a virus from 4 patients with mild respiratory disease and named the agent **Coe virus.** This virus produces cytopathology in HeLa cell culture but is not capable of hemagglutinating erythrocytes. It is now classified as Coxsackie A-21.

Reoviruses. Reovirus (Respiratory Enteric Orphans) is a term proposed by Sabin in 1959 for those viruses associated with both enteric and respiratory tract infections and formerly designated as being identical with echovirus type 10. The reoviruses are larger than the echoviruses, they produce a CPE in tissue culture that is distinct from the echoviruses, they possess a common CF antigen, and they agglutinate human group O erythrocytes. For these reasons, echovirus type 10 has been removed from the echovirus group and renamed reovirus type 1. There are 3 types of reoviruses currently recognized.[27]

Hepatitis viruses. On the basis of epidemiologic data, 3 distinct types of viral hepatitis have been recognized: hepatitis A, or infectious hepatitis, contracted by oral exposure and having a short incubation period (15-45 days); hepatitis B, or serum hepatitis, transmitted by parenteral exposure and having a long incubation period (50-180 days);[28] recent studies have shown at least 1 additional cause of viral hepatitis, non-A, non-B (NANB) hepatitis, which accounts for a high percentage of posttransfusion hepatitis and has an incubation period intermediate between those of hepatitis A and B.[29, 29 a] It has also been shown that both hepatitis A and hepatitis B can be transmitted by either the oral or parenteral route. Other agents that produce a disease that may mimic viral hepatitis are EB virus, cytomegalovirus, and toxoplasma.

Hepatitis viruses have never been successfully grown in tissue culture. They have been experimentally transmitted to chimpanzees and marmosets for hepatitis A and chimpanzees for hepatitis B. Demonstration of these agents in cases of hepatitis depends on immunologic procedures or electron microscopy.[30]

Hepatitis A (HA antigen). In 1973 Feinstone et al.[31] identified spherical viruslike particles 27 nm in diameter by immune electron microscopy in the stool of patients with hepatitis A during the acute phase of their disease. These particles have been provisionally designated hepatitis A antigen, or HA Ag. Similar particles were detected in stool specimens from volunteers infected with hepatitis A by both oral and parenteral routes. Moreover, antibody specific to HA Ag was detected in epidemiologically proved type A hepatitis. These data suggest that the particles are associated with hepatitis A. Evidence suggests that the virus belongs to the class of parvoviruses. Provost et al.[32] have developed a specific complement fixation test and an immune adherence test to detect antibody to hepatitis A. An examination of antibodies shows no serologic relationship to hepatitis B antigen.[33]

HA Ag–containing serum of infected individuals can transmit a disease to marmosets that is clinically identical to hepatitis A. The agent is present in the blood during the preicteric stage of illness and usually disappears soon after the onset of jaundice.[34] Preliminary serologic data suggest that hepatitis A is a commonplace infection that only occasionally causes clinical illness. Antibody is detectable in 25-30% of the adult population.[28]

Hepatitis B antigen (Australia antigen). Hepatitis B antigen was initially detected in 1965 by Blumberg et al.[35] while studying precipitating antibodies in the Ouchterlony gel diffusion test against human lipoproteins. They noted a previously undetected antigen in the serum of an Australian aborigine and referred to it as the Australia antigen. Other terms that appeared in the literature to describe this antigen are hepatitis-associated antigen (HAA), serum hepatitis antigen (SH antigen), Au/SH antigen, and hepatitis B surface antigen (HBsAg). Since the test procedure detects only the surface antigen, the term "HBsAg" is preferred. The HBsAg is closely associated with the virus of hepatitis B. It has been found to occur in approximately 30% of institutionalized patients with Down's syndrome, 9.4% of lepromatous leprosy patients, and 14% of patients with acute myelogenous leukemia.[36] By means of radioimmunoassay, about 0.5% of the United States population have been found to be carriers of HBsAg and are probably infectious; and 15-25% of sera from young urban adults contain antibody, indicating previous exposure to the agent. Acquisition of antibody occurs most frequently between 15 and 25 years of age.[28]

HBsAg is readily demonstrated in oral secretions, and high transmission rates in families of carriers strongly suggest close personal contact as the primary mode of transmission.[37] The HBsAg has also been demonstrated in genital secretions, breast milk, feces, and urine.[38,39] Other modes of potential transmission are contaminated shellfish, chimpanzees, mosquitoes, and foods. Transmission of hepatitis B virus by blood transfusion has been reduced significantly by eliminating donors found to carry HBsAg. Presently, only 20% of posttransfusion hepatitis can be attributed to this agent.[28]

Several methods have been used to detect the HBsAg in serum and body secretions, e.g., gel diffusion, complement fixation, counterimmunoelectrophoresis, immune electron microscopy, platelet aggregation reaction, passive hemagglutination, and radioimmunoassay. However, the recommended method is radioimmunoassay or a similar third generation test such as passive hemagglutination.[40]

The most striking property of HBsAg is its morphology, which is sufficiently characteristic to be diagnostic. Three types of particles have been observed in blood of patients and carriers. The most numerous are 20 nm spherical particles; also 20 nm filamentous forms are almost invariably present. Both forms are detected in infectious serum. A third type of particle present in about one-third of positive specimens is a double-shelled or "doughnut" form 42 nm in diameter, which is referred to as the Dane particle.[41] The Dane particle is believed to be the hepatitis B virus. HBsAg coats the core of the Dane particle, but the core antigen is antigenically different from spherical and filamentous particles. Because of its different antigenic specificity, the Dane particle is referred to as HBcAg. In clinical cases of icteric hepatitis B the HBsAg is found in the serum several weeks prior to onset of clinical illness and elevation of transaminase level and usually becomes undetectable 1-6 weeks after onset. A persistent carrier state of HBsAg is more frequent in patients with anicteric hepatitis than in those with clinically apparent illness.[42]

It has been clearly established that the Dane particle consists of a core of nucleic acid and an outer surface component, each having specific antigenic properties. The surface component is antigenically similar to the 20 nm particles and appears to be formed as a result of overproduction of surface components of the Dane particle. In addition, is has been established that this surface antigen manifests a group-specific determinant, a, and subtype-specific determinants, d or y, and w or r.

There are 4 major subtypes of HBsAg. Most subtypes contain a common a antigen and either d or y and w or r. The 4 common subtypes are adr, adw, ayr, and ayw. The d and y determinants occur with equal frequency in acute hepatitis; however, d is more common in carriers and cases of chronic hepatitis, and y is found most frequently in drug users and in renal dialysis units. The subdeterminant w occurs most commonly in America, Europe, and Africa, whereas the r occurs in Asia and the South Pacific.[28]

In view of the growing complexity of the antigens, the Committee on Viral Hepatitis of the National Research Council[43] and the World Health Organization Expert Committee on Viral Hepatitis[29] have recommended the following system of nomenclature.

HBeAg e antigen closely associated with hepatitis B infection.

HBsAg hepatitis B antigen found on surface of virus (Dane particle) and on unattached 20 nm particles.

HBcAg hepatitis B core antigen.

Dane particle 42 nm particle containing HBcAg in its core and HBsAg on its surface; same as HBV.

HBV term reserved for hepatitis B virus; originally known as the Dane particle.

HBsAg/adr hepatitis B surface antigen manifesting group-specific determinant, a, and subtype specific determinants, d and r. All recognized subtypes are to be indicated to right of slash.

anti-HBs antibody to hepatitis B surface antigen.
anti-HBc antibody to hepatitis B core antigen.
anti-HBe antibody to e antigen.

Non-A, non-B hepatitis. See Zuckerman[29] and Alter et al.[29b] At the time of writing (1978), no laboratory tests are as yet available for this agent.

Rhinoviruses. Cytopathic viruses were isolated from persons with the common cold by Tyrrell and Parson in 1960.[44] Some virus strains grew only in human embryonic kidney and were termed H strains; others grew also in monkey kidney cultures and were termed M strains. The general name of **rhinoviruses** has been suggested for all these viruses.

Rhinoviruses are clearly distinguished by the fact that they grow best in human cells at a temperature of 33 C, at pH 7.0, and in cultures that are rolled during incubation. In size and ether stability these viruses resemble enteroviruses, but they differ in that they produce colds in volunteers and cannot be isolated from feces.

A number of new H and M strains have been isolated by Tyrrell and Bynoe.[45] At least 62 antigenically distinct serotypes of rhinoviruses—M strains and H strains—have been characterized by Taylor-Robinson and Tyrell.[46]

Coryzaviruses. In 1961 Hamparian et al.[47] described 17 strains of viruses that they isolated from the common cold of children and adults. Because of their association with coryzal disease in man they were designated **coryzaviruses.**

Diploid human fetal lung and kidney cells are used for the isolation of these viruses; they propagate and produce cytopathology. They fail to grow or to cause detectable change in suckling or adult mice, guinea pigs, or embryonated eggs. Hemagglutinins are not produced, and hemadsorption has not been demonstrated.

The coryzaviruses are about 17-18 nm in size, are resistant to ether, and are composed of RNA. Antigenically they are heterogeneous and serologically distinct from other strains of rhinoviruses. However, they resemble rhinoviruses in clinical, biologic, and biophysical properties and are now grouped together.

Rubella virus. In 1961 Weller and Neva[48] and Parkman et al.,[49] working independently, recovered the virus responsible for rubella from military recruits at Fort Dix who were hospitalized with a rubella-like illness.

Rubella virus can be recovered from throat washings, urine, and blood. It replicates in cell cultures of African green monkey kidney and human embryonic kidney but fails to produce hemadsorption, or significant cytopathology in tissue culture. The virus is recognized by the resistance it confers to superinfection with echovirus type 11. In human amnion culture the virus replicates with the production of a characteristic cytopathology.

Hemagglutinin has been demonstrated in baby hamster kidney tissue culture (BHK-21) that has been inoculated with a high multiplicity of virus.

The hemagglutination-inhibition test is now the most rapid, accurate, and economical method for the serologic diagnosis of rubella.

The virus is heat labile but is stable for several years at −60 C. It is rapidly inactivated by ether, chloroform, and sodium desoxychlate and therefore resembles the myxoviruses.

All strains of rubella appear to be antigenically homogeneous and distinct from respiroviruses. Following infection there is a low but consistent rise in neutralizing antibody. CF antibody appears during the second week of onset and reaches a peak titer in 1 month. Hemagglutination-inhibiting antibody appears on the day of onset of rash and reaches peak titer in approximately 6-12 days. This HAI antibody persists for life and is not only the most useful for diagnosis but also for immunity surveys.

Papovaviruses   (PApilloma-POlyoma-VAcuolating agent). See Chapter 91 for adventitious agents in tissue culture. This group includes the papilloma (Shope) virus from rabbit, human wart papilloma virus, polyoma virus from mouse, and SV40 virus, known as vacuolating agent, derived from monkey cells. A number of other papovaviruses are also known.

TORCH complex. The TORCH complex is an acronym devised to focus attention on a group of microbial agents that cause clinically similar manifestations in newborns. Therefore testing for one would indicate the need to test for all agents.[50] The acronym stands for Toxoplasma, Others, Rubella, Cytomegalovirus, and Herpes simplex types 1 and 2. These agents are among the most frequently encountered infections of the fetus and newborn. There is a pressing need to define candidates for the "O" category in the TORCH complex, e.g., Epstein-Barr virus, hepatitis B, varicella, mumps, measles, and influenza.[51]

Infections in newborns by TORCH agents are usually clinically indistinguishable and may result in central nervous system dysfunction, involvement of the eyes and visceral organs, or abnormal growth and development. Inapparent infection is quite common and may escape detection until months or years later when mental or physical impairment becomes evident. Infections in mothers are usually clinically inapparent. Infections with TORCH agents represent a significant problem, and there is need for continuous search for these agents. Diagnosis depends on special laboratory tests.

EB virus. This virus was originally observed in 1964 in cell cultures derived from Burkitt's lymphoma, a highly malignant tumor of lymphoid tissue common among children in central and East Africa.[52,53] EB virus was named for Epstein and Barr, who made the original observation. This virus also occurs in cancerous white blood cells and in a small percentage of white blood cells of healthy donors.

Implication of this virus in **infectious mononucleosis** was first reported by Henle et al. in 1968.[54] They observed that a laboratory technician with infectious mononucleosis developed antibody to the EB virus and was able to cultivate this agent from her leukocytes. This virus has been repeatedly cultivated from leukocytes of patients with infectious mononucleosis and has been demonstrated by electron microscopy and immunofluorescence. Antibody to the EB virus has developed in all patients thus far studied and is determined by the indirect fluorescent antibody technic.[55] Antibody develops late in the acute phase of illness, persists for several years, and is distinct from heterophile antibody. Antibody surveys indicate that infection with this virus is widespread. Incidence in patients with infectious mononucleosis and Burkitt's lymphoma is 100%, but reproduction of these diseases in human volunteers has not been attempted.[56]

EB virus is similar in structure to human herpesviruses (herpes simplex, herpes zoster, and cytomegaloviruses) but is serologically distinct. It is transmissible only to cultured human cells of the hematopoietic system and cannot be freed from these cells or cultured by conventional technics.

NOTE: Various empirical tests used in the diagnosis of infectious mononucleosis are described in Part III, Hematology.

Eaton agent. See Chapter 81, Mycoplasma.

Norwalk agent. Two major groups of agents have been associated with acute nonbacterial gastroenteritis: (1) parvovirus-like agents and (2) reovirus-like agents. The parvovirus-like group contains the Norwalk agent, MC agent, and Hawaii agents, and it is associated with gastroenteritis primarily in adults. Reovirus-like agents contain the orbiviruses and rotaviruses, or duoviruses; they have been found mainly in infants and young children.[58] Evidence suggests that the rotaviruses (duoviruses) are the most important cause of infantile gastroenteritis throughout the world.[59,60]

In 1972 Kapikian et al.[58] reported the visualization by immune electron microscopy of viruslike acute nonbacterial gastroenteritis. These particles have been termed the "Norwalk agent." It has the size, density, and biologic properties characteristic of parvoviruses. The agent is a 27 nm spherical particle that contains DNA, which is ether and acid resistant, heat stable, and does not replicate in tissue cell or organ cultures commonly used for virus isolation.[61]

Clinical manifestations of the illness, which last 24-48 hours, are diarrhea, vomiting, nausea, abdominal cramps, and low-grade fever. The disease is referred to as winter vomiting disease or acute infectious nonbacterial gastroenteritis. Norwalk particles are not detected in the stool prior to onset of illness, but maximal shedding occurs at onset or 24-36 hours thereafter; particles are rarely detectable beyond 72 hours. Evidence for the viral etiology of this disease is based largely on transmission studies performed in volunteers and on serologic responses.

Rotavirus (duovirus). In 1973 Flewett et al.[62] demonstrated the presence of reovirus-like particles by electron microscopy in fecal extracts of infants and children with acute nonbacterial gastroenteritis. These particles, however, are sufficiently different from the reovirus group that other terms have been put forth such as "rotavirus" (radiating subunits resemble a wheel), "duovirus" (double-shelled capsid), and "orbivirus." There is strong epidemiologic evidence that they are responsible for the disease. In addition, serologic evidence of infection has been obtained by immune electron microscopy and by complement fixation.[63] Virus excretion is greatest 3-4 days after onset of illness and is rarely detectable after the eighth day. Stools may be extremely rich in virus particles with 10^9-10^{10} particles per gram. These agents are antigenically related to the Nebraska calf diarrhea virus, and the latter agent, which can be grown readily in tissue culture, is used as antigen in the CF test on human sera.

Complete virus particles have a double-shelled capsid and double-stranded RNA and are approximately 70 nm in diameter. Preliminary studies suggest that they are resistant to ether, bile salts, and heat. Attempts to cultivate these agents have not been consistently successful; therefore they must be detected by electron microscopy.[64]

Rhabdoviruses. Rhabdoviruses are large bullet-shaped viruses that measure approximately 70 × 175 nm and contain single-stranded RNA associated with a nucleocapsid in a helical configuration. They possess a lipoprotein envelope with HA spikes on their surfaces. Because of this structure, they are readily inactivated by ether and other lipid solvents.[65]

In addition to the rabies virus and Marburg virus, 6 arboviruses (Flanders, coccal, Hart Park, Kern Canyon, Klamath, and vesicular stomatitis) have been transferred to this group. This classification is based mainly on their close structural relationship.

Arenaviruses. Viruses in this group are morphologically identical to the LCM prototype virus. These viruses are round, oval, or pleomorphic, and they mature by budding from plasma membranes. They are enveloped viruses with surface projections and a diameter of 50-300 nm. Dense granules 20-30 nm in diameter are found inside the viral particles, hence the name "arenaviruses."[66]

The arenavirus group includes LCM, Lassa, Tacaribe complex, Amapari, Machupo, Tamiami, Junin, Latino, Pichinde, and Parana.

Arboviruses. This is a heterogeneous group of viruses with over 200 members that have in common only the epidemiologic fact that they are arthropod borne; they multiply in blood-sucking insects and are transmitted by bite to a vertebrate.

Unlike other groups, the 2 main antigenic groups, A and B (renamed alphaviruses and flaviviruses), possess common antigens and have been placed in the togavirus group. Togaviruses are spherical viruses, 40-60 nm in diameter, enveloped, and containing single-stranded RNA enclosed in a core of cubic symmetry. They replicate in the cytoplasm and bud through cytoplasmic membranes.

Some viruses originally classified as arboviruses have been allocated to several other groups such as togaviruses, orbiviruses, arenaviruses, and rhabdoviruses.

For the isolation of arboviruses intracerebral inoculation of suckling mice is the most susceptible system. HI antibody to arboviruses possesses a broad spectrum of group reactivity, and thus this test is used to classify these viruses into antigenic groups and for serologic diagnosis. The CF test is highly strain specific.

REFERENCES

1. International Subcommittee on Virus Nomenclature: Int. Bull. Bact. Nomen. Taxon. **13:**217, 1963.
2. Horsfall, F. L., and Tamm, E., editors: Viral and rickettsial infections of man, ed. 4, Philadelphia, 1965, J. B. Lippincott Co.
3. Moulder, J. W.: Annu. Rev. Microbiol. **20:**107, 1966.
4. Maisel, J., Moscovici, C., and Kempe, C. H.: Rocky M. Med. J. **57:**37, 1960.
5. Kamitsuka, P. S., Sorgel, M. E., and Wenner, H. A.: Am. J. Hyg. **74:**7, 1961.
6. Kibrick, S.: Med. Clin. North Am. **43:**1292, 1959.
7. Hammon, W. M., Wonk, D., Ludwig, E., et al.: J.A.M.A. **167:**727, 1958.
8. Kagan, H., and Bernkopf, H.: Ann. Pediatr. **189:**44, 1957.
9. Robbins, F. C., Enders, J. F., Weller, T. H., and Florentino, G. L.: Am. J. Hyg. **54:**286, 1951.
10. Committee on the Enteroviruses: Am. J. Public Health **47:**1556, 1957.
11. Diagnostic procedures for viral and rickettsial diseases, ed. 2, New York, 1956, American Public Health Association.
12. Kibrick, S.: Med. Clin. North Am. **43:**1301, 1959.
13. Rowe, W. P., et al.: Proc. Soc. Exp. Biol. Med. **84:**570, 1953.
14. Hilleman, M. R., and Wenner, J. H.: Proc. Soc. Exp. Biol. Med. **85:**183, 1954.
15. Huebner, R. J.: Mod. Med., p. 103, July 1, 1958.
16. Chanock, R. M.: J. Exp. Med. **104:**555, 1956.
17. Kuroya, M., Ishida, N., and Shiratori, T.: Tohoku J. Exp. Med. **58:**62, 1953.
18. Andrews, C. H., Bang, F., Chanock, R., and Zhanov, V.: Virology **8:**129, 1959.
19. Andrews, C. H., Bang, F. B., and Burnet, F. M.: Virology **1:**176, 1955.
20. Schulman, J. L., and Kilbourne, E. D.: Proc. Natl. Acad. Sci. U.S.A. **63:**326, 1969.
21. Expert Committee on Influenza: Bull. WHO **45:**119, 1971.
22. McIntosh, K., Dees, J. H., Becker, W. B., et al.: Proc. Natl. Acad. Sci. U.S.A. **57:**933, 1967.
23. Bucknall, R. A., King, L. M., Kapikian, A. Z., and Chanock, R. M.: Proc. Soc. Exp. Biol. Med. **139:**722, 1972.
24. Morris, J. A., Blount, R. E., and Savage, R. E.: Proc. Soc. Exp. Biol. Med· **92:**544, 1956.

25. Chanock, R. M., Roizman, B., and Myers, R.: Am. J. Hyg. **66**:281, 1957.
26. Lennette, E. H., Fox, V., Schmidt, N., and Culver, J.: Am. J. Hyg. **68**:272, 1958.
27. Sabin, A.: Science **130**:1387, 1959.
28. Conrad, M. E., and Knodell, R. G.: J.A.M.A. **233**:1277, 1975.
29. Zuckerman, A. J.: Bull. WHO **56**:1, 1978.
29a. Anonymous: Br. Med. J., April 15, 1978, p. 942.
29b. Alter, H. J., Holland, P. V., Purcell, R. H., et al.: Lancet **1**:459, 1978.
30. Maurin, J., and Courouce-Pauty, A. M.: Am. J. Dis. Child. **123**:314, 1972.
31. Feinstone, S. M., Kapikian, A. Z., and Purcell, R. H.: Science **182**:1028, 1973.
32. Provost, P. J., Ittensohn, O. L., Villarejos, V. M., and Hilleman, M. R.: Proc. Soc. Exp. Biol. Med. **148**:962, 1975.
33. Krugman, S. K., Friedman, H., and Lattimer, C.: N. Engl. J. Med. **292**:1141, 1975.
34. Provost, P., Ittensohn, O., Villarejos, V. M., et al.: Proc. Soc. Exp. Biol. Med. **142**:1257, 1973.
35. Blumberg, B. S., Alter, H. J., and Visnich, S.: J.A.M.A. **191**:541, 1965.
36. Blumberg, B. S., Sutnick, A. I., and London, W. T.: Bull. N. Y. Acad. Sci. **44**:1566, 1968.
37. Wright, R. A.: J.A.M.A. **232**:717, 1975.
38. Villarejos, V. M., Visona, K. A., Gutierrez, A. D., and Rodriguez, A. A.: N. Engl. J. Med. **291**:1375, 1974.
39. Feinman, S. V., Krassnitsky, O., Sinclair, J. C., et al.: J. Lab. Clin. Med. **85**:1042, 1975.
40. Shulman, R. N.: Am. J. Med. Technol. **38**:350, 1972.
41. Cossart, Y. E.: J. Clin. Pathol. **24**:394, 1971.
42. Alter, H. J., Holland, P. V., and Purcell, R. H.: J.A.M.A. **229**:293, 1974.
43. Committee on Viral Hepatitis, NRC/NAS: MNR **23**:29, 1974.
44. Tyrrell, D. A. J., and Parson, R.: Lancet **1**:239, 1960.
45. Tyrrell, D. A. J., and Bynoe, M. L.: Br. Med. J. **1**:393, 1961.
46. Taylor-Robinson, D., and Tyrrell, D. A. J: Lancet **1**:452, 1962.
47. Hamparian, V. V., Kelter, A., and Hilleman, M. R.: Proc. Soc. Exp. Biol. Med. **108**:444, 1961.
48. Weller, T. H., and Neva, F. A.: Proc. Soc. Exp. Biol. Med. **111**:215, 1962.
49. Parkman, P. D., Buescher, E. L., and Arstenstein, M. S.: Proc. Soc. Exp. Biol. Med. **111**:225, 1962.
50. Nahmias, A. J.: Pediatr. Res. **5**:405, 1971.
51. Nahmias, A. J.: Hosp. Pract., p. 65, May 1971.
52. Epstein, M., Achong, B. G., and Barr, Y.: Lancet **1**:702, 1964.
53. Epstein, M., Barr, Y., and Achong, B.: Wistar Inst. Sympos. Monogr. **4**:69, 1965.
54. Henle, G., Henle, W., and Diehl, V.: Proc. Natl. Acad. Sci. U.S.A. **59**:94, 1968.
55. Editorial: J.A.M.A. **203**:24, 1968.
56. Med. World News, p. 23, Feb. 2, 1968.
57. Editorial: Br. Med. J. **1**:591, 1968.
58. Kapikian, A. Z., Wyatt, R. G., Dolin, L., et al.: J. Virol. **10**:1075, 1972.
59. Flewett, T. H., Bryden, A. S., and Davies, H.: Lancet **2**:1497, 1974.
60. Bishop, R. F., Davidson, G. P., Holmes, I. H., and Ruck, B. J.: Lancet **2**:1281, 1973.
61. Dolin, R., Blacklow, N. R., Dupont, H., et al.: Proc. Soc. Exp. Biol. Med. **140**:578, 1972.
62. Flewett, T. H., Bryden, A. S., and Davies, H.: Lancet **2**:1497, 1973.
63. Dienstag, J. L., Kapikian, A. Z., Feinstone, S. M., and Purcell, R. H.: Lancet **1**(7910):765, 1975.
64. Parver, W. K., Caul, E. O., Ashley, C. R., and Clark, S. K. R.: Lancet **1**:237, 1973.
65. Howatson, A. F.: Adv. Virus Res. **5**:405, 1971.
66. Lehmann-Grube, F.: Virology monograph 10, New York, 1970, Springer Verlag.

TISSUE CULTURE AND CHICK EMBRYO TECHNICS

J. Mehsen Joseph

TISSUE CULTURE TECHNIC

Multiplication of viruses in tissue culture was first demonstrated unequivocally in 1925. However, it was not recognized until 1949 that multiplication of some viruses was accompanied by degenerative changes in tissue cell cultures, referred to as cytopathogenic effect (CPE), and that this effect was an adequate criterion for presence of a virus.[1] It was further demonstrated that the addition of specific antiserum to the cell culture along with the virus inoculum prevents the development of the CPE.

To avoid bacterial and fungal contamination, antibiotics were used in growth and maintenance media. Antibiotics added to fecal suspensions and throat washings permitted direct inoculation of tissue cultures without resulting contamination.

Trypsin dispersion of cells was reintroduced in 1952, which permitted the development of monolayer cultures. Monolayers are formed by cells that attach to a surface such as glass and flatten out to form a sheet of single-cell thickness. When the cells become overcrowded on the sheet they usually loosen and detach from the glass.[2]

Tissue cultures are referred to as either **primary lines** or **continuous lines.** Primary tissue culture lines are not propagated serially in vitro and are composed of morphologically and biochemically heterogeneous cells. Primary lines have a broader range of viral susceptibility than do continuous lines. One disadvantage is that latent viruses may be present, especially in primary monkey kidney cells, where simiam myxoviruses and the foamy virus are frequent contaminants.

Continuous tissue culture lines are propagated serially and composed of homogeneous-appearing cells. Examples are L cells (mouse fibroblasts) and HeLa cells (human carcinoma of the cervix). Strain HeLa is quite exceptional in that it has a broad spectrum of viral susceptibility.

Tissue fragments and cell suspensions used for tissue culture can be stored at 3-10 C for weeks and at 25 C for longer periods. They may be suspended in glycerin, quick frozen, and stored at −50 to −70 C to maintain viability.

Although tissue cells remain viable over a wide temperature range, virus multiplication is reduced or suppressed at temperatures above or below the 35-37 C range.

Cytopathogenic changes are also affected by the pH of the medium; certain strains of echoviruses and Coxsackie viruses may be inhibited in an acid medium. For this reason it is necessary to maintain the pH of the tissue culture fluid by the addition of sodium bicarbonate or by reducing the concentration of glucose.[3]

For maximum recovery of human viruses, tissue cultures must be maintained at a pH of approximately 7.4 with adequate glucose present in the maintenance medium, and they must be incubated at 36 ±1 C. Many other factors are operative but have not been clearly defined.

Preparation of glassware

Nothing is more essential to successful cultivation of tissue cells than properly cleaned glassware. Thorough cleaning is important to reduce the toxicity of glass, chiefly due to the leaching action of alkali. Hard borosilicate glass such as Pyrex or Kimax is recommended.

Glassware should be cleaned with a mild detergent (e.g., 7X [Linbro Chemical Co., New Haven, Conn.,] or C & M [Calgon Co., Pittsburgh]) so that the detergent ions can be removed with less rinsing. Detergent solutions are more efficient when warm, and boiling is desirable in most instances. Rinsing is considered the most critical step in the cleaning process, and cellular toxicity is not infrequently traced to this step.

Procedure
Old glassware
1. Clean glassware with mild detergent (1:100 dilution of 7X detergent or 1:10 C & M concentrate).
2. Rinse in at least 6 changes of tap water.
3. Soak for 1 h in distilled water containing approximately 0.05% 1N HCl to neutralize alkalinity resulting from detergent.
4. Follow with 3 rinses in distilled water.

New glassware
1. Soak in 25% 1N H_2SO_4 for 1 h.
2. Rinse in 6 changes of tap water.
3. Boil in detergent for 15 min and follow by 6 changes of tap water.
4. Soak for 1 h in distilled water containing 0.05% 1N HCl.
5. Rinse 3 times with distilled water.
6. Dry in inverted position and wrap for sterilization.

New rubber stoppers
1. Boil in 0.5N NaOH for 15 min and rinse 6 times in tap water and 3 times in distilled water.

Glassware that has been used for tissue culture
1. Place immediately into detergent solution until ready to be washed; this greatly facilitates cleaning.
2. Autoclave contaminated glassware before cleaning.
3. To clean, first scrub glassware with brush to remove cellular material from surfaces and rinse in tap water.
4. Place in fresh solution of 7X detergent and boil for 15 min.
5. Drain off detergent and rinse in 6 changes of tap water.
6. Soak for 1 h in distilled water containing 0.05% 1N HCl and then rinse in 3 changes of distilled water.
7. Drain in inverted position and wrap for sterilization.

Miscellaneous
1. Clean pipets by placing them upright in metal cylinder before boiling and rinsing.
2. Scrub screw caps, rubber inserts, and rubber stoppers in 7X detergent and then rinse in 6 changes of tap water. Soak for 1 h in acid water and then rinse in 3 changes of distilled water.

Preparation of reagents

1. Stock antibiotic concentrate
   a. Prepare sterile solution containing 100,000 U penicillin and 100,000 μg streptomycin/ml, using sterile powders commonly available (injectable form).
   b. Since these antibiotics are unstable in solution, store at −20 C to retard decomposition. When thawing, do not expose to excessive heat.
   c. Add 0.1 ml concentrate to each 100 ml tissue culture fluid.
2. Sodium bicarbonate buffer.
   a. Using reagent grade $NaHCO_3$, prepare 1.4% and 7.5% solution and sterilize by positive pressure Millipore (0.22 μm) filtration. Check sterility by inoculating fluid thioglycollate.
   b. Store at 3-10 C.

Autoclaving converts bicarbonate to Na_2CO_3, which is less effective as buffer. This solution is used to adjust pH of tissue culture fluids and acts also as buffer.

3. Hydrochloric acid solution
   a. Prepare 0.1N HCl solution from concentrated HCl, cp.
   b. Sterilize by autoclaving at 121 C for 15 min.

Use this solution for adjusting pH of tissue culture fluids.

4. Phenol red indicator, 0.2%
   a. Place 0.4 g phenol red in flask and add 0.05N NaOH with mixing until almost dissolved.
   b. Add 0.05N NaOH drop by drop until solution is complete.
   c. Bring to final volume of 200 ml with distilled water and adjust to pH 7.0 with 0.05N NaOH.
   d. Autoclave at 121 C for 15 min.

When properly prepared, the solution has a deep red color. Excessive NaOH imparts a purple color that renders the indicator unsatisfactory.[4] This indicator is used in all balanced salt solutions, growth and maintenance media, trypsin solutions, etc. employed in tissue cultures and is incorporated in a quantity of 10 ml stock indicator solution/L (0.02 g dye/L). However, most tissue culture fluids commercially available contain phenol red indicator.

5. Trypsin 1:250 (Difco Laboratories, Detroit)
   Trypsin is used for dispersing and harvesting tissue cells from organs or cell sheets grown in vitro. It may be obtained in powder or crystalline form; powdered trypsin 1:250 has been found to give excellent results. Store the powder at 3-10 C.
   a. Prepare 1% solution of trypsin in Hanks balanced salt solution (Hanks BSS) containing phenol red.
   b. Allow trypsin to dissolve in refrigerator overnight and then sterilize by Millipore (0.22 μm) filtration.
   c. Adjust to pH 7.4 and store in small quantities at −20 C.

Do not expose the trypsin solution to temperatures above 37 C when thawing, since the enzyme will become inactivated. After freezing and thawing several times, a precipitate may form, and the solution loses its effectiveness.

6. Hanks balanced salt solution (Hanks BSS)[4]

Solution A

NaCl	160 g
KCl	8 g
$MgSO_4 \cdot 7H_2O$	4 g
Distilled water	800 ml

Solution B

$CaCl_2$	2.8 g
Distilled water	100 ml

Solution C. Mix solutions A and B and bring to 1000 ml with distilled water; add 2 ml chloroform as preservative. Store at 3-10 C.

Solution D

$Na_2HPO_4 \cdot 12H_2O$	3.04 g
KH_2PO_4	1 g
Glucose	20 g
Distilled water	800 ml

NOTE: Add 100 ml 0.2% phenol red indicator solution to solution D and make up to 1000 ml with distilled water. Add 2 ml chloroform and store at 3-10 C.

Working solution. Hanks BSS is prepared by mixing 1 part solution C and 1 part solution D with 18 parts distilled water. Autoclave at 115 C for 10 min or filter. Store at 3-10 C. Add 2.5 ml 1.4% sodium bicarbonate solution immediately before use.

7. Earle balanced salt solution

Solution A

NaCl	6.8 g
KCl	0.4 g
$MgCl \cdot 6H_2O$	0.17 g
$NaH_2PO_4 \cdot H_2O$	0.14 g
$NaHCO_3$	2.2 g
Glucose	1 g
Distilled water	600 ml

Solution B

$CaCl_2$	10 g
Distilled water	100 ml

   a. Store solutions at 3-10 C. For use, add 2 ml solution B to solution A and add sufficient distilled water to make up to 1000 ml.
   b. Add 10 ml phenol red indicator stock solution and adjust to pH 7.4 with 7.5% solution sodium bicarbonate.

c. Sterilize by filtration and check for sterility.
d. Refrigerate.

Serum

Calf serum is recommended for growth and maintenance of cell and tissue cultures for 2 important reasons: (1) some cell types have less tendency to detach from growth surfaces than they do with certain lots of horse serum; and (2) when monolayers are used for virus studies, there is no need to wash cells free of serum as with human serum.

If serum is obtained from a local abattoir, it must be Seitz filtered in the refrigerator to remove toxic substances, probably lipids, as well as to remove microorganisms. Check serum for sterility and store at 3-10 C.

Growth media

Fluids used for initial outgrowth of cell and tissue cultures are complex and complete mixtures consisting of vitamins, amino acids, inorganic salts, glucose, and undetermined growth factors of serum. Phenol red indicator, bicarbonate, and antibiotics are usually added. Balanced salt solution is the basic diluent for the components of growth media. These media are adjusted to pH 7.4 and stored in the frozen state. Repeated freezing and thawing results in the formation of an undesirable precipitate with a gradual loss of nutritive qualities. (CAUTION: Thawing must be done at a temperature not exceeding 37 C.) If the complete growth medium is to be used within 2 weeks, it should be stored at 3-10 C to avoid the undesirable effect resulting from repeated freezing and thawing.

Every lot of growth medium must be pretested for sterility before the addition of antibiotics. Also, containers must be tightly sealed to prevent the egress of CO_2, which may render the medium too alkaline; one frequently finds it necessary to readjust the pH.

Because of the complexity of growth media, they are beyond the scope of most laboratories. Therefore it is recommended that commercially available stock solutions be obtained. It is recommended that these solutions be purchased in 10× concentration and restored with BSS.

Many kinds of growth media are available; however, only those most frequently used and basic to cell and tissue culture will be described.

Medium 199 (growth)

Medium 199, single strength (prepared by diluting 10× stock 1:10 in Hanks BSS)	80%
Calf serum	20%
Bicarbonate, 7.5%	0.5 ml/100 ml medium

1. Remove quantity needed for sterility test.

Penicillin	100 U/ml final medium
Streptomycin	100 μg/ml final medium

2. Adjust to pH 7.4.

NOTE: This medium is recommended for the growth of strain HeLa cells. However, it is a general purpose medium for the growth of mammalian cells. The formula for this medium is commonly designated as 199_{80}, C_{20}, $Bi_{0.5/100\ ml}$, $P\&S_{100/ml}$.

Basal medium Eagle–growth (BME-growth)

Hanks BSS	87 ml
Amino acid concentrate (100×)	1 ml
Vitamin concentrate (100×)	1 ml
Glutamine concentrate (200 mM)	1 ml
Calf serum	10 ml

1. Adjust to pH 7.4 with 7.5% bicarbonate solution.
2. Remove portion for sterility test.
3. Add 100 U penicillin and 100 μg streptomycin/ml final solution.

NOTE: Stock concentrates of amino acids, vitamins, and glutamine are commercially available. Because of the instability of glutamine, it should be added to the medium just before use. BME is a general purpose medium and may be used for the growth of most cell types of human origin, e.g., HeLa, KB, and human amnion.

Minimum essential medium Eagle–growth (MEM-growth). This medium is prepared in the same manner as BME, except that MEM concentrates of amino acids, vitamins, and glutamine are used. MEM is recommended as the medium of choice for the growth and maintenance of cell lines of mammalian origin except HeLa and monkey kidney epithelial cells.

Lactalbumin hydrolysate medium (medium A)

Calf serum	2%
Lactalbumin hydrolysate	0.5%
Hanks BSS	97.5%

1. Adjust to pH 7.2 with 7.5% bicarbonate solution.
2. Check for sterility.
3. Add 100 U penicillin and 100 μg streptomycin/ml final medium.

NOTE: This solution is recommended for initial outgrowth of monkey kidney epithelial cells. The formula for this medium is usually indicated as C_{20}, $L.H._{0.5}$, $HBSS_{97.5}$, $P\&S_{100/ml}$.

Lactalbumin hydrolysate medium (medium B). Medium B differs from medium A in that Earle BSS is substituted for Hanks BSS. This medium is recommended as a maintenance medium but is used only for growth of monkey kidney cells.

Maintenance media

The preparation of maintenance media is similar to that of growth media, except that 1% serum is used instead of 10-20%. All other ingredients remain the same. Maintenance media permit cells to metabolize at a level satisfactory for virologic and biochemical studies but do not support cellular proliferation. By frequent replacement of the maintenance solution, cell sheets may be kept for several weeks.

Medium 199–maintenance, BME-maintenance, and MEM-maintenance differ from their respective growth media in that they contain only 1% calf serum. These media are used to replace the growth media after a satisfactory monolayer of cells has been obtained and before the cells are used for virologic studies.

Sterility test

All solutions used for the growth and maintenance of tissue cultures must be carefully pretested for sterility on media that will support the growth of bacteria and fungi. As a routine, 2 tubes of fluid thioglycollate and 2 trypticase soy agar slants are inoculated with 1 ml each, and 1 tube of each is incubated at 37 C and 25 C (room temperature) for 7 days.

Continuous propagation of cells in monolayer cultures

Cell lines for establishing continuous cultures are commercially available* as suspensions containing approximately 1 mil viable cells/ml. To serially propagate these lines, follow the general procedure given below. Remember that when the terms "growth media" and "maintenance media" are used, they refer to those media recommended for a particular tissue cell.

Procedure
Cell count
1. Place 1 drop cell suspension on hemacytometer and allow cells to settle before counting.
2. Examine under 100× magnification and count 5 white cell squares and obtain average. Multiply average by 10,000 to determine count/ml. Count small clumps of cells (less than 5) as 1 and larger clumps as ½ the number per clump. If there is crowding of cells in squares, prepare 1:4 dilution of suspension in Hanks BSS and recharge hemacytometer. This dilution factor must be considered when determining count/ml.

Seeding
1. Dispense 600,000 cells to each 200 ml milk dilution bottle or 200 ml prescription bottle to be seeded. Add 15 ml growth medium to each bottle, mix well, and incubate in horizontal position at 36 C. NOTE: If bottle to be seeded has twice surface area of 200 ml milk dilution bottle (approx. 40 cm²), then twice the number of cells are required for seeding.
2. Once bottles are positioned, they should not be disturbed for at least 18-24 h to permit cells to attach to glass surface in uniform pattern.

Adjustment of pH
1. Observe bottles daily and adjust pH of those that appear too acid or too alkaline. The pH should be 7.4-7.6.
2. Make certain each screw cap contains nontoxic rubber liner to prevent escape of CO_2 and consequent alkalinity. Also keep bottles tightly stoppered to prevent loss of CO_2.

Feeding
1. Replace spent growth medium every 3-4 d. To do this, remove two-thirds of spent medium and replace with equal quantity of fresh growth medium. Allow new growth medium to warm to room temperature and check pH by color before adding to cells. Adjust pH if necessary.
2. If cells appear not to be growing well, it may occasionally be necessary to replace all spent medium with fresh medium.
3. Examine bottles daily, using 100× magnification. When complete or near complete cell monolayer has developed, cells should be harvested and new bottles seeded.

Harvesting
1. Remove all but 2-3 ml growth medium and discard.
2. Add equal volume (2-3 ml) 1% trypsin solution to cells to be harvested. Manipulate bottle so that trypsin flows back and forth over cell sheet until cells loosen from glass. Aseptically aspirate fluid with pipet to break up cell clumps. Close bottle tightly and incubate at 36 C for 15 min.

3. Transfer cell suspension to rubber-stoppered 15 ml graduated centrifuge tube and record volume of fluid. Centrifuge for 5 min at 2000 rpm. Discard supernatant fluid and restore to original volume with new growth medium. Mix suspension thoroughly and transfer drop to hemacytometer for cell count, which represents beginning of that procedure (see above for procedure for cell count).
4. Portion of cell suspension may be used to prepare monolayers in test tubes for virus isolation and virus serologic studies as follows.

Seeding test tubes
1. After cell count has been determined, dilute portion with growth medium so that it contains 70,000-100,000 cells/ml. Mix well.
2. Add 1 ml of this suspension to each test tube and screw caps on tightly. Place tubes in test tube tissue culture rack, shake rack to distribute cells, and place in 36 C incubator.
3. Examine tubes daily, and when good monolayer is produced, tubes are ready for use. In most cases, cells are ready in about 3 d. It is seldom necessary to feed cells.
4. Pour off growth medium from those tubes that have a good monolayer and replace with 1 ml maintenance medium. These tubes are now ready for use in viral studies.

Preparation of monolayers of primary cell lines[5]
1. Kill and exsanguinate animal and aseptically remove desired organs such as kidney or liver to sterile container. Wash 4 times with Hanks BSS.
2. Remove tissue layers to be cultured and cut into 1 mm³ pieces. Wash twice with Hanks BSS and discard washings.
3. Transfer tissue to trypsinizing flask (Bellco Glass, Vineland, N.J.). Add 2 vol 0.25% trypsin and allow to react for 6 h at 36 C. Centrifuge mixture at 2500 rpm for 5 min and discard supernatant fluid. Add fresh trypsin and incubate at 36 C for 18 h.
4. Filter through cheesecloth into sterile container. Centrifuge filtrate at 3000 rpm for 10 min and collect sedimented cells. Wash cells in 4 changes of Hanks BSS. In last washing centrifuge suspension at 3000 rpm for 5 min to separate tissue cells from erythrocytes. Resuspend cells in proper growth medium and mix thoroughly.
5. Count cells in hemacytometer and proceed to seed bottles and tubes as described for continuous cell culture.

Preparation of human amnion cells[6]

Media
1. Growth medium
Eagle basal medium (BME)	79%
Calf serum (inactivated)	20%
L-Glutamine, 2.9%	10%
Penicillin	200 U/ml
Streptomycin	200 µg/ml
2. Maintenance medium
BME	98%
Calf serum	2%
Penicillin	200 U/ml
Streptomycin	200 µg/ml

Procedure
1. Obtain human placenta immediately after delivery under aseptic conditions and place in sterile receptacle containing 200 ml Hanks BSS.
2. Suspend placenta and separate amnion from chorion. Remove blood vessels and clotted blood.
3. Wash amnion fragments with several changes of Hanks BSS containing antibiotics.
4. Cut amnion into 1-2 cm² pieces and trypsinize

---

*Microbiological Associates, Walkersville, Md.; Flow Labs, Rockville, Md.; and Difco Laboratories, Detroit.

with 0.25% trypsin, pH 8.0, in same manner as for monkey kidney.

5. Sediment cells by centrifugation at 1000 rpm for 5 min. Decant supernatant.
6. Wash cells twice with growth medium and sediment cells at 1000 rpm for 5 min for each washing.
7. After second washing, packed amnion cells are resuspended in growth medium to final concentration of 500,000 cells/ml.
8. Test tube cultures are prepared by adding 1 ml of this suspension to each tube and incubating in slanted position.
9. On second day of incubation replace with fresh growth medium to remove nonadherent cells. Replace growth medium every third day until confluent monolayer is formed.
10. Replace growth medium with maintenance medium before using cells for virus isolation.

Preparation of monkey kidney tissue culture[7]

1. Remove kidneys aseptically from monkeys anesthetized with pentobarbital sodium and exsanguinated.
2. Remove capsule with sterile scissors and forceps. Place kidney in Petri dish and, using aseptic technic, remove connective tissue and blood clots from organ.
3. Dissect kidney in half and remove medulla. Transfer remaining cortex to another sterile Petri dish.
4. Cut cortex into small fragments approximately 1 cm².
5. Transfer tissue to trypsinizing flask and add 50 ml prewarmed (37 C) 0.25% trypsin, pH 7.3, and stir with magnetic stirrer for 30 min.
6. Discard first run and add 50 ml fresh prewarmed trypsin and stir for 15 min. Collect cell suspension in sterile 200 ml centrifuge bottle containing 10 ml Melnick medium A. Keep suspension at 4 C or in ice bath.
7. Repeat Step 6 until tissue fragments are exhausted.
8. Centrifuge cell suspension at 600 rpm for 10 min. Remove supernatant fluid by suction and resuspend packed cells in growth medium (Melnick medium B) **immediately**. Use approximately 50 ml/bottle of packed cells; mix thoroughly.
9. Filter cell suspension through 6 layers of sterile gauze and collect filtrate in sterile graduated cylinder.
10. Make vital cell count as follows.
    a. To 0.5 ml above suspension, add 1 ml crystal violet solution. Mix well and charge each side of hemacytometer counting chamber with 1 drop from a 1 ml pipet.
    b. Allow 2 min for dye to react and cells to settle in chamber before counting.
    c. Count intact cells in 10 squares (5 on either side of counting area). Total number of cells/ml suspension is determined as follows:

    Total cells in 10 squares $\times$ 3 $\times$ 1000

    d. Adjust cell concentration to 3 $\times$ 10⁵/ml.
11. Seed test tubes with 0.5-0.8 ml, and 10-12 ml for 100 ml bottles.
12. Incubate cultures at 36 C for 24 h without disturbing. Examine daily and change growth medium every third day until confluent monolayer develops. Cell cultures are then ready to use.

Preparation of chick embryo fibroblast cultures[8]

1. Select 9-10 d embryos. Clean egg shells with 70% alcohol and aseptically remove embryo from egg by opening shell over air sac. Place in sterile Petri dish.
2. Remove head, feet, and wings. Place torsos in sterile container and wash in cold Hanks BSS. Decant fluid and mince tissues with sterile scissors, or press embryos through stainless steel screen fitted inside 20 ml syringe.
3. Wash tissue fragments in 3 changes of cold Hanks BSS to remove blood.
4. Sediment fragments by centrifugation at 1000 rpm for 5 min and transfer to trypsinizing flask containing 0.25% trypsin prewarmed to 37 C; wash thoroughly and discard trypsin.
5. Add 50-100 ml prewarmed trypsin and stir on magnetic stirrer for 45 min at 37 C.
6. Filter through 6 layers of sterile gauze and collect filtrate in sterile centrifuge tube. Centrifuge at 1000 rpm for 15 min. Remove trypsin by suction.
7. Wash cells twice with cold Hanks BSS and recentrifuge at 1000 rpm for 15 min. Discard supernatant.
8. Resuspend packed cells in sufficient growth medium (0.5% lactalbumin hydrolysate and 6% calf serum in Hanks BSS) to make 0.25% suspension of tissue.
9. Seed test tubes with 0.5-1 ml of this suspension. Seed 100 ml prescription bottles with 10 ml.
10. Incubate cultures at 37 C for 48-72 h before use.

Preservation of tissue cell cultures[9-11]

Reagents
1. Medium 199 with glycerol or dimethylsulfoxide

199 (10×)	100 ml
Glycerol (sterile)	150 ml
(or dimethylsulfoxide	100 ml)
Calf serum	100 ml
Sterile distilled water	650 ml

   a. Mix ingredients aseptically.
   b. Add antibiotics and bicarbonate.
2. Medium BME with glycerol or dimethylsulfoxide

BME (10×)	100 ml
Calf serum	100 ml
Glutamine (50 mM)	10 ml
(added just prior to use)	
Dimethylsulfoxide	50 ml
(or glycerol	100 ml)
Hanks BSS	740 ml

   a. Add sterile ingredients aseptically.
   b. Just before use, add antibiotics, bicarbonate, and glutamine.
3. Growth media without glycerol (199 or BME)

Procedure
Freezing cells
1. Wash cell monolayer with Hanks BSS.
2. Harvest cells with trypsin and pipet vigorously to break up clumps.
3. Sediment by centrifugation at 1000 rpm for 10 min.
4. Resuspend packed cells in a small volume of growth medium containing glycerol or dimethylsulfoxide.
5. Count cells with hemacytometer and adjust cell density with growth medium (with glycerol or dimethylsulfoxide) to approximately 5 times concentration normally used for seeding bottles (usually 5-10 $\times$ 10⁶ cells/ml).
6. Mix cell suspension thoroughly and dispense in 3 ml quantities into screw-capped vials and seal

with Gel-Seal or into ampules sealed with oxygen torch.

7. Label each vial with type of tissue, growth medium, cell concentration, and date.

8. Place vials at 4 C (refrigerator) for 2 h and then transfer to −20 C (freezer compartment of refrigerator) for 2 h.

9. Cell suspensions are transferred immediately from −20 C to −65 C (Revco freezer) for prolonged storage. Keep in bottom of Revco.

Reviving frozen cells

1. To recover cells, remove vial from −65 C freezer and thaw quickly by agitating vial in 37 C water bath. This process should not require more than 30 s.

2. Transfer contents to centrifuge tube and sediment cells at 1000 rpm for 10 min.

3. Discard supernatant fluid and resuspend packed cells in 10 ml fresh growth medium **without glycerol.** Sediment cells by centrifugation again; discard supernatant and resuspend cells in fresh growth medium **without glycerol** to yield desired concentration (10^5 cells/ml).

4. Transfer contents to 1 tissue culture bottle. **Do not disturb bottle for at least 48 h** and preferably not for 72 h. Change growth medium after this interval and every 3 days until complete monolayer is obtained.

Detection of mycoplasma (PPLO) contamination in tissue cell culture and its eradication

Mycoplasma (PPLO) contamination of tissue cell cultures is a major problem that can seriously affect the interpretation of laboratory results.[12] Not infrequently viral antigens prepared in tissue culture are found to contain a higher titer of myocoplasma than virus; this may account for certain false-positive serologic reactions or cross-reactions observed among viruses.[13,14] Antibiotics commonly used in culture media, e.g., penicillin and streptomycin, do not prevent the growth of these agents. A few strains of mycoplasma rapidly deplete essential nutrients for tissue cells with resulting cytopathology and cell destruction; however, most strains are insidious and fail to produce any detectable microscopic or macroscopic changes. Therefore to detect mycoplasma contamination it is essential to culture the tissue fluid on a suitable agar medium.

There are several sources of mycoplasma contamination of tissue cultures, but the 2 principal sources are the oropharynx of the technician and the serum used in growth and maintenance media. Thus it is important that mouth pipetting should be avoided in preparing reagents and manipulating tissues. Also, the culture and maintenance of mycoplasma should not be done in the same area as tissue culture.[15]

Mycoplasma agar

Yeast extract, 25%	10%
Horse serum	20%
PPLO agar base	70%

Prepare and sterilize agar base. Aseptically add yeast extract and horse serum.

Procedure[16,17]

1. Check all cell lines monthly for mycoplasma; those found to be contaminated are treated with tetracycline (2.5 μg/ml) for 3 successive passages.

2. Collect tissue cells and growth fluid from each of cell lines. Freeze and thaw suspension twice.

3. Inoculate 0.2 ml onto 4 plates per cell line and streak inoculum across mycoplasma agar with glass rod.

4. Incubate 2 plates aerobically and 2 anaerobically at 36 C in moist atmosphere.

5. Examine plates after 48-72 h incubation using 100× magnification. Colonies usually appear in 48 h; however, maintain plates for at least 10 d before discarding as negative.

6. Mycoplasma can usually be identified microscopically on the basis of colony morphology. Colonies are convex, have finely granular texture, grow just beneath agar surface, and develop a characteristic "fried egg" appearance in most instances.

7. To transfer colonies for further identification, cut agar block containing colonies and rub across agar surface. Leave block on agar because growth sometimes occurs only beneath block.

Dienes staining technic[18]

1. Prepare Dienes stain as follows:

Azure II	1.25 g
Methylene blue	2.5 g
Maltose	10 g
Na_2CO_3	0.25 g
Benzoic acid	0.2 g
Distilled water	100 ml

2. Apply stain to several coverslips, using cotton swab. Allow stain to dry.

3. Cut agar block with mycoplasma colonies and place colony side up on microscopic slide.

4. Place coverslip with stain side down on colony and seal edges with melted Vaspar (paraffin containing 10% petrolatum).

5. Allow 10 min for dye to penetrate colonies.

6. Examine with oil-immersion lens.

7. Mycoplasma colonies stain light blue at periphery and bright deep blue in center. Highly pleomorphic organisms can be seen at periphery of colony.

Treatment[19]

1. *Method A.* If cell line is contaminated with mycoplasma, add 2.5 μg/ml tetracycline to growth medium at time new bottles are seeded and maintain this concentration in both growth and maintenance media for at least 3 successive passages. Some strains can be eliminated by this treatment, especially when antibiotic is present during initial outgrowth of cells.[20]

2. *Method B.* Add 800 μg/ml kanamycin to tissue culture fluid of mycoplasma-contaminated cell line. After 3 days change to fresh growth medium containing 200 μg/ml kanamycin and maintain this concentration for 2 successive passages.[21]

Adventitious agents in tissue culture

In addition to mycoplasma contamination of continuous cell lines, endogenous viral contamination of certain primary cell cultures is a frequent occurrence. The virologist must be aware of this and be able to recognize such agents. Since monkey kidney has been the most widely used tissue for virus isolation and viral studies, our knowledge of latent agents encountered in this type of tissue is extensive. Over 60 different simian viruses have been isolated. Hull has studied these in detail and has classified them

Table 91-1. Hull's classification[22] of simian viruses*

Group I	Adenoviruses	SV1, SV11, SV15, SV17, SV20, SV23, SV25, SV27, SV30, SV32, SV33, SV34, SV36
Group II	Enteroviruses	SV2, SV16, SV18, SV19, SV26, SV29, SV35
Group III	Not specified	SA4, SV4, SV28
Group IV	Reoviruses	SA3, SV4, SV28
Group V	Myxoviruses	SV5, SV5A, SV41 (hemadsorbing agents)
Group VI	Herpesviruses	B virus
Group VII	Papovaviruses	SV40 (vacuolating agent)
Group VIII	Miscellaneous	Foamy agent, SA1, SA6

*SV = simian virus; SA = simian agent.

Table 91-2. Susceptibility of chick embryo to various agents in clinical materials*

	CAM	Amniotic cavity	Allantoic cavity	Yolk sac
Eastern encephalitis	+	+	+	+
Western encephalitis	+	+	+	+
Venezuelan encephalitis	+	+	+	+
Influenza types A and B	±	+	+	+
Influenza type C	−	+	−	−
Sendai	−	+	+	−
Mumps	±	+	±	+
Psittacosis	−	±	−	+
Lymphogranuloma venereum	−	−	−	+
Variola	+	−	−	−
Vaccinia	+	−	−	+
Herpes simples	+	+	+	+
B virus	+	−	−	−
Vesicular stomatitis	+	+	+	+
Rickettsias	−	−	−	+

*From Laboratory methods in diagnosis of viral and rickettsial diseases, Atlanta, 1960, United States Public Health Service, Center for Disease Control.

into 8 groups on the basis of their biologic, biophysical, and serologic properties. A summary of this classification is given in Table 91-1.

Probably the most troublesome simian virus is SV5, which produces hemadsorption of guinea pig red blood cells and is therefore confused with human parainfluenza viruses. Thus to suppress the replication of SV5, it is usually necessary to incorporate SV5 antiserum into the growth and maintenance media of monkey kidney tissue cultures used for isolating parainfluenza viruses from human materials. Another virus, the vacuolating agent or SV40, has further complicated matters by its capacity to hybridize with other viruses.

For a more detailed discussion of the endogenous agents encountered in tissue cultures refer to the publications by Hull and Minner[23] and Cottral.[24]

CHICK EMBRYO TECHNIC

Several viruses and rickettsias multiply in the developing chick embryo and are detected either by pock formation on the chorioallantoic membrane (CAM), death of the embryo, or hemagglutinating property of embryonic fluids. The embryo provides a sterile environment free from latent viral infections (except Newcastle disease virus) and remains immunologically inactive throughout its embryonic development.[25]

Pock formation on the CAM is characteristic of variola, vaccinia, herpes simplex, ectromelia, and fowl pox viruses.

Viral infections of the chick embryo usually lead to death, but in most cases viral activity can be detected long before death insues.

The hemagglutinationg property, which is the result of interaction of viruses with receptor sites on the erythrocytes, is associated with viruses such as influenza (types A, B, C), Sendai, mumps, variola, vaccinia, and Newcastle disease.

The route by which the embryo is inoculated depends on the virus to be isolated; some viruses are capable of infecting by any route, whereas others require specific sites (Table 91-2).

Sources of eggs. Eggs of high fertility and free from infection such as Newcastle disease and avian lymphomatosis can be obtained from most commercial hatcheries. Eggs of white leghorns are apparently more susceptible, especially in the case of influenza.

Incubation of eggs. Eggs are incubated at 38 ± 1 C in a relative humidity of 70-80%. A bacteriologic incubator containing a pan of water is usually satisfactory.

The gestation period of the chick embryo is 21 d. One must remember to count the days the eggs were incubated by the hatchery when figuring the gestation period. Eggs that are not used during this period may be refrigerated to prevent the embryos from hatching, or they may be allowed to hatch so that the chicks may be bled to obtain erythrocytes for use in the hemagglutination test.

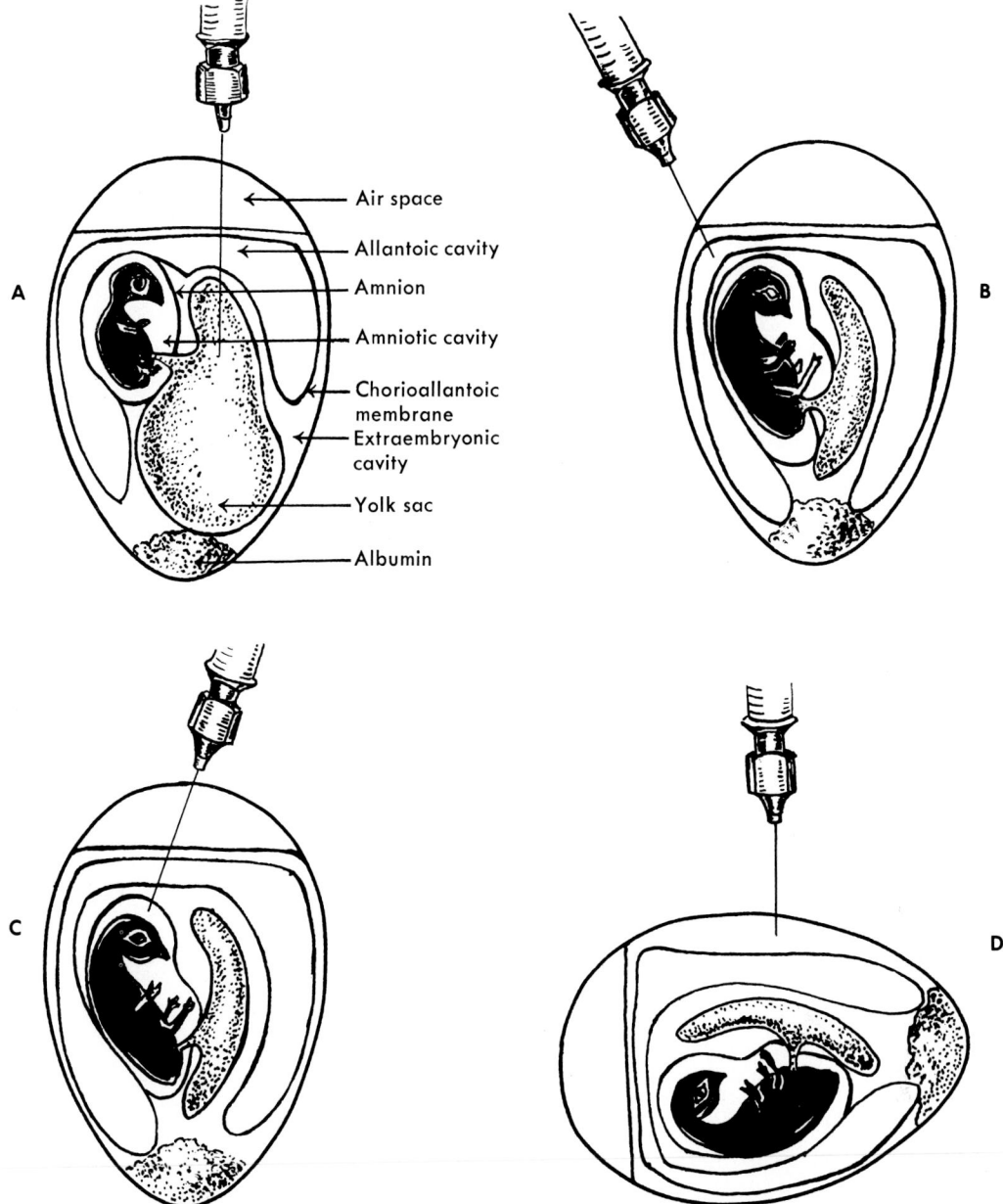

Fig. 91-1. Chick embryo technics. **A,** Yolk sac inoculation. **B,** Allantoic cavity inoculation. **C,** Amniotic cavity inoculation. **D,** Chorioallantoic membrane inoculation. (Drawn by V. Voshell.)

Candling eggs. Candling is necessary to determine whether the embryo is living and to locate the position of the embryo and air space. A simple candling device can be made by placing a 100 W bulb in a box with a small opening at 1 end into which the end of a fertile egg fits snugly. Candle the egg in a dark room.[26]

A live embryo is indicated by spontaneous movement, especially when the egg is warm, and by clearly defined blood vessel shadows. Nonfertile eggs are immediately obvious and should be discarded along with those containing dead embryos.

While the egg is illuminated, mark the position of the embryo and air space on the shell with a pencil.

Inoculation of eggs

Allantoic cavity. Since the allantoic cavity reaches its maximum size in 12 d, use 9-12 d embryos.

1. Disinfect shell over air space with 70% alcohol. Punch small hole in shell over center of air space, using sterile hypodermic needle that has point cut off or egg punch. Traumatic death is less likely if dental-type drill is used. To inoculate, introduce needle (1½ in. length, 23 gauge) into egg at slight angle to long axis of egg and away from embryo.[27] When needle passes just below air space it enters allantoic cavity. Usually 0.2 ml is inoculated by this route.

2. After egg is inoculated, puncture is sealed with petrolatum, cellophane tape, nail polish, or suitable sealer.
3. Inoculated eggs are incubated at 36 C in upright position until allantoic fluid is to be harvested.
4. Before harvesting of allantoic fluid, eggs should be refrigerated for 3 h or placed at −18 C for 30 min to obtain fluid free of red blood cells. Disinfect upper part of shell with 70% alcohol and then cut away shell. Tear away membrane lining air space and cut open transparent allantoic membrane lying underneath. Withdraw fluid with capillary pipet.
5. Portion of fluid is streaked on blood agar to test for sterility.

Amniotic cavity. Amniotic cavity reaches its maximum size at 10-12 d of age, and eggs of this age are used for inoculation.

1. Mark position of air space and embryo by candling. Disinfect shell with 70% alcohol and punch hole in shell at base of air space and just over embryo. Pass needle to point near embryo. When amniotic cavity is entered, embryo will follow movement of needle. If air bubble is introduced with inoculum, it will remain localized in amniotic sac.[28] If sac is missed, bubble will flow to side of shell. Transilluminate egg while making inoculation. Simpler way to inoculate cavity is to cut opening in shell, tear hole in chorioallantois, and pull amniotic membrane up through opening, using pair of forceps. Inoculum is usually 0.2 ml.[29]
2. Seal opening and incubate egg, with opening upright, at 36 C until ready to harvest.
3. To harvest, disinfect shell, cut away shell over air space, tear away membranes, remove allantoic fluid, and then proceed to harvest amniotic fluid. Manipulate cavity with pair of forceps and remove fluid with hypodermic syringe. If cavity is dry, introduce 1 ml Hanks BSS to wash it out.
4. Streak blood agar plate to check fluid for sterility.

Chorioallantoic membrane (CAM). Use 11-14 d old fertile eggs, since viral lesions are more discrete than in younger embryos.

1. Candle egg and mark position of embryo, air space, and area on side of egg free of large blood vessels. Punch hole on side of egg without penetrating membrane and one over air space penetrating membrane. Place drop of sterile saline on side hole and tease membrane apart with needle. With rubber bulb apply negative pressure at air space opening so that chorioallantois drops away from shell. This creates broad flat surface for inoculation.
2. Make inoculations through opening on side of egg by dropping fluid onto membrane. Inoculum up to 0.2 ml is used.
3. After inoculation, seal openings and incubate in horizontal position at 36 C until ready to harvest.
4. To harvest, disinfect shell and cut it away. Cut out portion of CAM and wash it several times in sterile saline. Examine under 10× magnification or by holding it in front of lamp in partially darkened room. Lesions or pocks, if present, are readily visible.

Yolk sac.[26] Use 6-8 d old fertile eggs, since the yolk sac occupies the greater portion of the egg.

1. Candle egg and mark air space and embryo positions on shell. Disinfect shell and puncture hole over the center of air space. Pass 2 in., 22-gauge needle into egg straight downward to depth of 4 cm to enter yolk sac. Inoculum is usually 0.5 ml.

2. Seal opening and incubate in upright position at 36 C until ready to harvest.
3. Yolk is harvested by removing shell, shell membrane, and chorioallantois.
4. Check fluid for sterility by streaking on blood agar.

REFERENCES

1. Enders, J. F., Weller, T. H., and Robbins, F. C.: Science **109:**85, 1949.
2. Merchant, D. J., Kahn, R. H., and Murphy, W. H.: Handbook of cell and organ culture, Minneapolis, 1960, Burgess Publishing Co.
3. Rivers, T. M., and Horsfall, F. L., editors: Viral and rickettsial infections in man, ed. 3, Philadelphia, 1959, J. B. Lippincott Co.
4. Melnick, J. In American Public Health Association: Diagnostic procedures for viral and rickettsial diseases, ed. 2, New York, 1956, The Association.
5. Merchant, D. J., Kahn, R. H., and Murphy, W. H.: Handbook of cell and organ culture, Minneapolis, 1960, Burgess Publishing Co.
6. Dunnebacke, T. H., and Zitcer, E. M.: Cancer Res. **17:**1043, 1957.
7. Younger, J. S.: Proc. Soc. Exp. Biol. Med. **85:**202, 1954.
8. Dulbecco, R.: Proc. Natl. Acad. Sci. U.S.A. **38:**747, 1952.
9. Scherer, W. F.: Exp. Cell. Res. **19:**175, 1960.
10. Swim, H. E., Haff, R. F., and Parker, R. F.: Cancer Res. **18:**711, 1958.
11. Porterfield, J. S., and Ashwood-Smith, M. J.: Nature **193:**548, 1962.
12. Pollock, M. E., and Kenny, G. E.: Proc. Soc. Exp. Biol. Med. **112:**176, 1963.
13. Herdershee, D., Ruys, A. C., and van Rhijn, G. R.: Antonie van Leeuwenhoek **29:**368, 1963.
14. Hayflick, L.: Tex. Rep. Biol. Med. **23:**285, 1965.
15. Lemcke, R. M.: J. Hyg. (Camb.) **62:**351, 1964.
16. Barile, M. F., and Schimke, R. T.: Proc. Soc. Exp. Biol. Med. **114:**676, 1963.
17. Fogh, J., and Fogh, H.: Proc. Soc. Exp. Biol. Med. **117:**899, 1964.
18. Dienes, L.: J. Infect. Dis. **65:**24, 1939.
19. Hearn, H. J., Officer, J. E., Elsner, V., and Brown, A.: J. Bacteriol. **78:**575, 1959.
20. Carski, T. R., and Shepard, C. C.: J. Bacteriol. **81:**629, 1961.
21. Pollock, M. E., Kenny, G. E., and Syverton, J. T.: Proc. Soc. Exp. Biol. Med. **105:**10, 1960.
22. Hull, R. N.: Simian Virus Committee Meeting, National Institutes of Health, Nov. 1961.
23. Hull, R. N., and Minner, J. R.: Ann. N.Y. Acad. Sci. **67:**413, 1957.
24. Cottral, G. E.: Ann. N.Y. Acad. Sci. **55:**221, 1952.
25. Rhodes, A. J., and van Rooyen, C. E.: Textbook of virology, Baltimore, 1953, The William & Wilkins Co.
26. Laboratory methods in diagnosis of viral and rickettsial diseases, Atlanta, 1960, United States Public Health Service, Center for Disease Control.
27. Beveridge, W. B., and Burnet, F. M.: Medical Research Council, Special Reports Series no. 256, 1946.
28. Diagnostic procedures for viral and rickettsial diseases, ed. 2, New York, 1956, American Public Health Association.
29. Burnet, F. M.: Aust. J. Exp. Biol. Med. Sci. **18:**353, 1940.

92

ROUTINE PROCEDURES FOR ISOLATION AND IDENTIFICATION OF VIRUSES

J. Mehsen Joseph

Specimens for isolation should be collected during the phase of the illness when they are most likely to contain the virus in high titer. For example, throat washings for the isolation of the influenza virus should be collected within 48 hours after onset, whereas polio and other enteroviruses may be isolated from feces in high titer as late as 10 days after onset of meningeal symptoms.

In the case of influenza and other acute respiratory diseases, throat washings or throat swabs (infants) are submitted for virus isolation. In the case of enterovirus infections such as poliomyelitis, aseptic meningitis, pleurodynia, and herpangina, stool specimens and throat washings should be submitted. When there is evidence of meningeal involvement, cerebrospinal fluid should be obtained.

Specimens submitted for virus isolation studies are treated as follows:
1. Preparation of suspension from clinical material
2. Decontamination of suspension by antibiotics, high-speed centrifugation, or filtration
3. Low-speed centrifugation to obtain supernatant fluid free of particulate matter
4. Inoculation of supernatant fluid into susceptible host as determined from case history
5. Examination of host for viral effect
6. Typing viral isolates by serologic methods

Acute and convalescent sera are required to complete the laboratory phase of virus diagnosis by providing antigenic confirmation of a virus isolated with respect to the current illness. Isolation of a virus from the brain in encephalitis or the spinal fluid in aseptic meningitis provides direct evidence of an etiologic association. Isolation of an influenza virus from throat washings of a patient with an influenza-like disease strongly suggests that the virus is the causative agent, since this virus is only isolated from throat washings in cases of acute influenza. In contrast, the isolation of an enteric virus from the stool of a patient with aseptic

meningitis does not per se indicate an etiologic relationship, since enteroviruses are occasionally found in the feces of healthy individuals.[1] Additional evidence is obtained by demonstrating a 4-fold rise in antibody titer against the virus isolated.

COLLECTION, TRANSPORT, AND STORAGE OF SPECIMENS

Success in isolating viruses depends on the proper collection, transport, and storage of specimens. Once the viruses are separated from their host cells, they die off rapidly.

Clinical materials to be collected depend on the diagnosis or principal symptoms (Table 92-1).

Respiratory infections—collect throat washings and acute and convalescent sera; postmortem lung, and stool

Aseptic meningitis and paralytic disease—collect at least 3 fecal specimens on different days, throat washings, cerebrospinal fluid and acute and convalescent sera; postmortem brain and spinal cord

Herpangina, pleurodynia, skin rash, undifferentiated febrile illness, infantile diarrhea—collect throat washings, 3 fecal specimens on different days, swab of oral lesions, pleural effusion, and paired sera

Myocarditis and pericarditis—collect specimens as recommended for herpangina and pleurodynia; postmortem heart tissue, swab of oral lesions, pleural effusion, and pericardial fluid

Encephalitis—collect throat washings, acute phase clotted blood, 3 consecutive stool specimens, cerebrospinal fluid, acute and convalescent phase sera; postmortem spinal cord and brain

Chickenpox, vaccinia, and smallpox—collect vesicle fluid, crusts, acute phase clotted blood, and paired sera; postmortem spleen, pancreas, liver, and lung

Cytomegalic inclusion disease—collect urine, saliva, and paired sera

Because of the lability of viruses, specimens should be submitted immediately on collection and introduced promptly into the proper hosts for isolation. Specimens that cannot be processed promptly should be stored at −20 C or perferably at −70 C. Specimens suspected of containing the influenza virus should be stored at 3-10 C or at temperatures below −20 C, since this virus dies off most readily between 0 and −20 C.

If specimens are to be in transit for 24 h or longer,

Table 92-1. Viral and related diseases and clincial materials submitted for laboratory diagnosis*

Illness	Viral or other agent	Specimens to be collected
Respiratory diseases		
Upper respiratory illness	Parainfluenza; adenoviruses; rhinoviruses; respiratory syncytial; echoviruses; coxsackievirus A21; *Mycoplasma pneumoniae*†; reoviruses(?)	Throat washing; stool; paired sera
Exudative tonsillopharyngitis	Adenoviruses; EB virus of infectious mononucleosis	Throat washing; stool; paired sera
Acute lymphonodular pharyngitis	Coxsackievirus (A10)	Throat washing; stool; paired sera
Pharyngoconjunctival fever	Adenoviruses	Throat washing; stool; paired sera
Herpangina; stomatitis; and/or pharyngitis	Coxsackieviruses A; herpes simplex	Throat washing; stool; paired sera; swab of oral lesions
Bronchiolitis	Influenza; parainfluenza; adenoviruses; *Mycoplasma pneumoniae*†; respiratory syncytial	Throat washing; stool; paired sera
Laryngotracheobronchitis (croup)	Parainfluenza; influenza; rhinoviruses; respiratory syncytial; adenoviruses; *Mycoplasma pneumoniae*†	Throat washing; stool; paired sera
Pneumonia	Respiratory syncytial; adenoviruses; influenza; parainfluenza; rubeola; varicella; psittacosis; *Mycoplasma pneumoniae*†	Throat washing; acute phase clotted blood; paired sera
Influenza	Influenza A, A-1, A-2, B, C	Throat washing (must be frozen immediately); paired sera; postmortem lung
Pleurodynia (Bornholm disease)	Coxsackieviruses B	Throat washing; stool; paired sera; pleural effusion
Ophthalmic diseases		
Ocular herpes	Herpes simplex	Eye washing; throat washing; paired sera
Epidemic keratoconjunctivitis	Adenovirus type 8	Eye washing; throat washing; paired sera
Trachoma	Trachoma agent‡	Eye washing; throat washing; paired sera; tarsus scrapings
Inclusion blennorrhea	TRIC agent‡	Eye washing; throat washing; paired sera; tarsus scrapings
Conjunctivitis	Newcastle disease virus	Eye washing; conjunctival scrapings; paired sera
Exanthematous diseases		
Herpangina	Coxsackieviruses A	Throat washing; stool; vesicle fluid; paired sera
Hand-foot-and-mouth disease	Coxsackieviruses A5, A10, A16	Throat washing; stool; vesicle fluid; paired sera
Chickenpox/zoster	Varicella	Throat washing; vesicle fluid; paired sera
Herpes simplex	Herpes simplex	Vesicle fluid; throat washing
Vaccinia smallpox	Vaccinia, variola	Vesicle fluid; throat washing; acute phase clotted blood; paired sera; postmortem liver, spleen, pancreas, and lung

*From Maisel, J., Moscovici, C., and Kempe, C. H.: Rocky Mt. Med. J. **57**:37, 1960; extensively revised by Division of Virology, Maryland State Department of Health, 1969.

†See Chapter 81.

‡**Editor's note:** For taxonomic position of **chlamydiae (bedsoniae)** see Chapter 68. The **psittacosis-LGV-trachoma** group contains **both RNA and DNA**, metabolic enzymes, and muramic acid, properties that separate it from the viruses. Members of this group are in the 250-400 nm size range, possess an envelope, are ether sensitive, and have no capsid symmetry.

Table 92-1. Viral and related diseases and clinical materials submitted for laboratory diagnosis—cont'd

Illness	Viral or other agent	Specimens to be collected
Exanthematous diseases—cont'd		
Dengue fever	Dengue virus types 1-4	Acute phase clotted blood; paired sera
Nonspecific febrile illness with rash	Echoviruses; coxsackieviruses A and B	Throat washing; stool; paired sera
Erythema infectiosum	Unknown	—
Exanthem subitum (roseola infantum)	Unknown	—
Genitourinary tract infections		
Viruria	Echoviruses; coxsackieviruses B; adenoviruses; mumps; cytomegalovirus; rubeola; rubella; vaccinia; herpes simplex	Urine; paired sera
Vulvovaginitis	Coxsackieviruses B; Herpes simplex; lymphogranuloma venereum	Vaginal swab; lesion scraping; paired sera
Central nervous system diseases		
Paralytic disease	Poliovirus types 1, 2, 3; coxsackieviruses A7, A9; echovirus types 2 and 9	Throat washing; stool; cerebrospinal fluid; paired sera; postmortem brain and cord
Aseptic meningitis	Polioviruses; coxsackieviruses A and B; echoviruses; herpes simplex; mumps; lymphocytic choriomeningitis; lymphogranuloma venereum*; psittacosis*	Throat washing; stool; cerebrospinal fluid; paired sera; postmortem brain and cord
Guillain-Barré syndrome	Coxsackieviruses A; echoviruses	Throat washing; stool; cerebrospinal fluid; paired sera; postmortem brain and cord
Meningoencephalitis	Western encephalitis; eastern encephalitis; St. Louis encephalitis; mumps; measles	Throat washing; stool; cerebrospinal fluid; paired sera; postmortem brain and cord; acute phase clotted blood for isolating encephalitis viruses
Subacute sclerosing panencephalitis (Dawson's encephalitis)	Rubeola	Cerebrospinal fluid; blood; postmortem brain
Toxic encephalopathy (Reye's syndrome)	Unknown	Throat swab; stool; blood; postmortem liver, spleen, lung, brain, intestinal contents, blood
Cardiovascular diseases		
Myocarditis and pericarditis	Coxsackieviruses B	Throat washing; stool; paired sera; postmortem heart and pericardial fluid
Miscellaneous diseases		
Cytomegalic inclusion disease	Cytomegalovirus	Saliva; urine; paired sera
Mumps	Mumps	Urine; throat washing; paired sera
Orchitis and epididymitis	Mumps; coxsackieviruses B	Urine; throat washing; stool; paired sera
Intussusception	Adenoviruses	Stool; mesenteric lymph node; paired sera
Lymphogranuloma venereum	LGV agent*	Lesion fluid and pus
Colorado tick fever	CTF virus	Acute phase clotted blood; paired sera
Infantile diarrhea (enteritis)	Echoviruses; coxsackieviruses B	Throat washing; stool; paired sera

*Editor's note: For taxonomic position of **chlamydiae (bedsoniae)** see Chapter 68. The **psittacosis-LGV-trachoma** group contains **both** RNA and DNA, metabolic enzymes, and muranic acid, properties that separate it from the viruses. Members of this group are in the 250-400 nm size range, possess an envelope, are ether sensitive, and have no capsid symmetry.

Continued.

Table 92-1. Viral and related diseases and clinical materials submitted for laboratory diagnosis—cont'd

Illness	Viral or other agent	Specimens to be collected
Miscellaneous diseases—cont'd		
Nonspecific febrile illness	Polioviruses; coxsackieviruses A and B; echoviruses	Throat washing; stool; paired sera
Postperfusion syndrome	Cytomegalovirus; EB virus	Acute phase clotted blood; paired sera
Acute infectious lymphocytosis	Coxsackievirus-like virus; EB virus	Throat washing; paired sera
Gastroenteritis (winter vomiting disease)	Norwalk agent Rotaviruses	Stool; vomitus
Rickettsial diseases		
Rocky Mountain spotted fever	*Rickettsia rickettsii*	Acute phase clotted blood; paired sera; postmortem liver and spleen
Epidemic typhus	*Rickettsia prowazekii;*	Acute phase clotted blood; paired sera; postmortem liver and spleen
Murine typhus	*Rickettsia typhi*	
Q fever	*Coxiella burnetii*	Sputum; urine; cerebrospinal fluid; acute phase clotted blood; postmortem liver and spleen
Rickettsialpox	*Rickettsia akari*	Acute phase clotted blood; paired sera; postmortem liver and spleen

they should be sealed tightly to prevent ingress of CO_2 and should be packed in dry ice.

When the parainfluenza viruses are suspected, the clinical material should be processed promptly, since these viruses are very labile, and a single freezing and thawing greatly reduces the chances of recovering them.

NOTE: When collecting throat washings, the patient should gargle 3 times with 15 ml Hanks BSS, skim milk, or trypticase soy broth or similar broth. Antibiotics (500 U penicillin, 500 μg streptomycin, and 50 Unystatin (Mycostatin)/ml) may be added to the fluid used for gargling, except when contraindicated for the patient. Collect the washings as early in the course of the disease as possible. In the case of influenza this should be not later than 3 d after onset; the virus is rarely recovered 5-7 d after onset.

PREPARATION OF SPECIMENS

Since most clinical materials submitted for virus isolation are grossly contaminated, they must be subjected to methods of decontamination that do not affect the viruses that may be present. The use of antibiotics that are nontoxic to tissue culture cells is the simplest and most practical method. Unfortunately antibiotic treatment is not always successful, and filtration through a Selas or Seitz filter is required. Filtration should be the last resort, since significant amounts of virus adsorb to the filter. Ultracentrifugation may be employed if suitable equipment is available.

Feces
1. Pass cotton swab into center of stool and rotate. Then rotate swab around outside surface. Vigorously agitate swab in 3 ml Hanks BSS contained in Wassermann tube. Express as much fluid from swab as possible.
2. If only a rectal swab is submitted, rotate swab in 1 ml Hanks BSS to prepare suspension.
3. Instead of rotating swab in feces, a 10-20% suspension may be prepared by grinding 1 g feces with 4 ml Hanks BSS in mortar containing small amount of sterile alundum or sterile sand.
4. Centrifuge suspension at 2500 rpm for 20 min. Transfer supernatant fluid to another tube and centrifuge at 3000 rpm for 15 min. Collect supernatant fluid.
5. Add sufficient penicillin, streptomycin, and nystatin (Mycostatin) to supernatant fluid to give final concentration of 500 U, 500 μg, and 50 U/ml, respectively.
6. Incubate at room temperature for 30 min and then inoculate appropriate tissues, as described in following section.

Urine
1. Add antibiotic mixture containing pencillin, streptomycin, and amphotericin B (Fungizone) to specimen and allow to stand at room temperature for 1 h.
2. Centrifuge for 30 min at 3000 rpm at 4 C.

Postmortem tissues
1. Prepare 20% suspension by grinding tissue with Hanks BSS in mortar containing sterile alundum or sterile sand.
2. Transfer suspension to Pyrex test tube. Freeze and thaw suspension 3 times to further disrupt tissue cells, with release of virus.
3. Centrifuge suspension at 3000 rpm for 30 min. Collect supernatant fluid.
4. Add penicillin, streptomycin, and nystatin (Mycostatin) in concentrations recommended for fecal supernatants.
5. Incubate at room temperature for 30 min and then proceed to inoculate tissue cultures, animals, or embryonated eggs.

Throat washings and throat swabs
1. Express material from throat swab in 2 ml Hanks BSS. Add antibiotics to this fluid or to throat wash-

Table 92-2. Viral spectrum of tissue cell cultures*

| Virus | Primary cell cultures | | | | Continuous heteroploid lines | | | | Diploid cell strains | |
	Monkey kidney	Human kidney	Human amnion	Hamster kidney	Monkey kidney	HeLa	KB	HEp no. 2	WI-26 or WI-38	Human embryonic kidney
Eastern equine	0	0	0	+	0	0	0	0	0	0
Western equine	0	0	0	+	0	0	0	0	0	0
St. Louis	0	0	0	+	0	0	0	0	0	0
California	0	0	0	±	0	0	0	0	0	0
Polio 1, 2, 3	+	+	+	0	+	+	+	+	+	+
Coxsackieviruses 1-8, 10-24	0	0	±	0	0	±	±	±	±	±
Coxsackievirus A9	+	+	+	0	+	0	0	0	+	+
Coxsackievirus B	+	+	+	+	+	±	+	+	±	±
Echo 1-20, 22-32	+	+	+	0	+	0	0	0	+	±
Echo 21	−	+	+	0	0	0	0	0	+	0
Influenza A	±	±	0	0	0	0	0	0	±	0
Influenza B	+	+	0	+	0	0	0	0	±	0
Parainfluenza 1-4	+	+	±	0	0	±	±	±	±	0
Adenoviruses 1-32	±	+	+	0	0	+	+	+	±	±
Mumps	+	+	+	+	0	±	±	±	0	0
Respiratory syncytial	±	0	0	0	0	+	+	+	+	0
Reo 1-3	+	±	0	0	0	+	+	+	+	0
Rhino "M" strains	+	+	0	0	0	0	0	0	+	0
Rhino "H" strains	0	+	0	0	0	0	0	0	+	0
IBV-like†	(Human organ tracheal culture)									
Cytomegalovirus	(Human foreskin, human chorion, human embryonic skin and muscle)								+	0
Vaccinia	+	+	+	+	+	+	+	+	+	+
Variola	0	+	0	0	0	0	0	0	0	0
Varicella zoster	±	0	+	0	0	0	0	0	+	+
Herpes simplex types 1, 2	±	+	+	+	0	+	+	+	+	+
Herpes B	+	0	+	0	0	+	+	+	0	0
Molluscum contagiosum	0	0	+	(Also human foreskin)						
Rubeola	+	+	+	±	±	±	±	±	+	±
Rubella	+	±	+	0	0	0	0	0	0	±

*Modified from Laboratory techniques in virology, Atlanta, 1968, Center for Disease Control.

†IBV refers to infectious bovine rhinotracheitis-like viruses that cause respiratory disease in man.

N.B. Rubella virus is most readily isolated in African green monkey kidney; varicella and cytomegalovirus in WI-38.

+ = Virus replicates in tissue; ± = not all strains of virus replicate in the tissue; 0 = virus does not replicate in tissue or has not been adequately determined.

ing to provide concentrations recommended for fecal supernatants.

2. Incubate fluid at room temperature for 30 min to decontaminate. Fluid is then ready for inoculation.

Cerebrospinal fluid and other transudates. Transudates are inoculated without the addition of antibiotics unless there is evidence of contamination.

INOCULATION OF SPECIMEN

Numerous tissue cell lines have become available in recent years, and they vary considerably in their susceptibility to viruses. Certainly it is impractical for the average diagnostic laboratory to use more than a few well chosen lines, and this choice must of necessity depend on the viruses prevalent in the area; animals are likewise selected. Monkey kidney epithelial cells have such a broad host range that they have assumed a role in virology equivalent to that of blood agar in bacteriology. Suckling mice and adult mice are

the animals of choice. Of course, embryonated eggs play a major role in the success of a virus laboratory and are an important part of the routine.

Every virus laboratory should have available at least monkey kidney cells, HeLa cells, WI-38 cells, suckling mice, and embryonated eggs. If funds permit, it is advisable to add human amnion cells (primary line). The viral host range of these other systems is described in Table 92-2, but briefly it is as follows:

Monkey kidney cells—susceptible to polioviruses (1-3), echoviruses (1-20 and 22-38), coxsackieviruses B1-B5, A9, and A14, measles, herpes simplex, adenoviruses, parainfuenza virus type 2, croup-associated virus, and certain strains of influenza

HeLa cells—susceptible to polioviruses (1-3), echoviruses (5, 8, 11, 12, 13), coxsackieviruses B1, B3, B5, A11, A13, A15, and A18, herpes simplex, adenoviruses, and parainfluenza virus type 1

Suckling mice—susceptible to coxsackieviruses A and B, herpes simplex, eastern encephalitis, western encephalitis, St. Louis encephalitis, Venezuelan encephalitis, Japanese B encephalitis, dengue fever, Colorado tick fever, rabies, lymphocytic choriomeningitis, and psittacosis

Embryonated eggs—susceptible to herpes simplex, arthropod-borne encephalitides, psittacosis, lymphogranuloma venereum, mumps, measles, variola, vaccinia, influenza, primary atypical pneumonia, and Newcastle disease

After having selected the most desirable host systems, proceed to inoculate decontaminated clinical materials as follows:

1. Whenever the provisional diagnosis is viral, always inoculate tissue cell cultures. Inoculate 2 tubes of monkey kidney cells with 0.1 ml each and 2 tubes with 0.2 ml each of specimen. Incubate the tubes at 36 C in a stationary tissue culture rack and observe cell sheets daily for 21 d for cytopathology and hemadsorption of red blood cells. Many viruses such as poliomyelitis, echoviruses, coxsackieviruses, and herpes simplex may be detected in cell culture within 2-6 d, whereas some myxoviruses require 1-3 wk.[2]

Specimens that fail to show evidence of viral activity in cell culture within 7 d must be passed at least once before being considered negative. This is done by scraping some cells from the wall of the cell culture tube with a sterile pipet and transferring 0.2 ml to a fresh cell culture and incubating.

All cell cultures showing evidence of viral activity must also be passed to determine whether the effect is transmissible or due to toxicity of the specimen. With experience, toxic effects can be distinguished from viral cytopathology. Cell cultures showing toxic effects are passed on the third day to dilute out this effect.[3]

2. Inject 3 suckling mice intracerebrally with 0.03 ml, 3 intraperitoneally with 0.1 ml, and 3 subcutaneously with 0.1 ml. Disinfect the site of inoculation before and after injection with tincture of iodine. Observe the mice daily for symptoms of flaccid paralysis or spastic paralysis. Death of animals within the first 24 h is usually the result of trauma or toxicity of the specimen. Symptoms caused by viral infection are usually apparent within 3-6 d and death shortly thereafter with such viruses as coxsackieviruses A and B, herpes simplex, psittacosis, Colorado tick fever, and yellow fever. Usually 10-20 d are required for LCM, dengue, the encephalitides, encephalomyocarditis, and rabies. However, since so many factors are operative, involving both the host and the parasite, the final outcome as to whether or not an infection is established may require that the animals be observed for at least 30 d.[4]

Suckling mice that are definitely ill must be removed from the mother's cage; otherwise, on death the mice may be cannibalized by the mother before suitable tissues can be obtained. Using aseptic technic, collect brain and skeletal muscle from mice exhibiting symptoms or that have died. Prepare a 10-20% suspension from pooled tissues in Hanks BSS.[5] Check the suspension for sterility to make certain the animals did not die from a bacterial infection. If this is the case, retreat the original specimen and repeat the inoculations.

If an LCM virus is isolated, it will be necessary to repeat the isolation, using original specimen and a different stock of mice, to make certain that the LCM virus was not latent in the mice and activated by the inoculation.

Suckling mice that have been inoculated and remain healthy must be sacrificed and brain material pooled and passed at least once before being reported as negative.

3. If the provisional diagnosis is mumps, measles, influenza, herpes simplex, vaccinia, variola, molluscum contagiosum, psittacosis, arthropod-borne encephalitides, lymphogranuloma venereum, or vesicular stomatitis, embryonated eggs should be inoculated by the routes recommended for the isolation of specific viruses. Usually it is necessary to inject eggs by 4 routes. In such cases inject the amniotic cavity of 4 fertile eggs with 0.2 ml each, 4 eggs with 0.2 ml each into the allantoic cavity, 4 eggs with 0.5 ml each into the yolk sac, and 4 eggs with 0.2 ml each onto the CAM. Candle eggs daily to detect dead embryos. Harvest the eggs after 72 h for influenza or 5-6 d for other viruses; check the fluids for sterility and for virus by the methods described elsewhere.[6]

Amniotic fluid is viscous and frequently contains debris that may result in false-positive hemagglutination. To avoid this, dilute amniotic fluids 1:10 when testing for hemagglutinating viruses.[7]

Harvested material must be free of blood and microbial contaminants. Bloody fluids are incubated at 37 C for 30 min to dissociate virus from blood cells and then centrifuged at 3000 rpm for 10 min to sediment the red blood cells; the supernatant fluid is examined for viral activity.

If the harvested material is contaminated, retreat the original specimen and repeat the inoculations. Fluids harvested from the same area that are sterile but show no evidence of viral activity are pooled and passed at least one time by the same route before being reported as negative. Never pass negative fluids from dead embryos, except under extenuating circumstances.

Pool positive fluids and pass, if necessary, to increase the titer of the virus and to establish transmissibility of the agent.

DETECTION AND IDENTIFICATION OF VIRAL ACTIVITY IN TISSUE CULTURE

Evidence of viral activity in tissue culture is usually dependent on the production of distinct cytopathogenic effects (CPE) that are visible under low-power ($\times 100$) microscopy and without prior staining. Cytopathology may be represented by a clumping and piling up of rounded cells, by coalescence of contiguous cells to form giant syncytial masses, or by the production of distorted refractile cells with darkened periphery and pyknotic nuclei that progressively degenerate and detach from the glass surface. These cytopathogenic effects begin as small foci of infections and rapidly (e.g. enteroviruses) or slowly (e.g. measles virus) proceed to involve the entire monolayer.[8]

It must be emphasized that the CPE is a criterion of viral activity only and does not enable one to differentiate one virus from another per se, since many viruses produce a similar CPE. Also, the CPE for a particular virus may vary with the tissue cell line in which the virus develops. Nevertheless, certain viruses are sufficiently stable in their CPE that they should come under suspicion when such effects are observed. These cytopathic changes and the viruses usually associated with them are as follows:

1. Formation of rounded and distorted refractile cells with darkened margins and pyknotic nuclei, some cells tend to cluster together; loss of intercellular bridges, progress to complete degenera-

tion of cell sheet quite rapidly: poliovirus, echovirus, coxsackieviruses A and B, herpes simplex, adenoviruses, varicella

2. Fusion of contiguous cells to form multinucleated giant cells (syncytia) that form slowly[9]: measles virus, herpes simplex (strain GC), parainfluenza virus type 1 (Mills strain), respiratory syncytical virus, croup-associated virus

3. Grapelike clustering of rounded cells to form a pock: herpes simplex

Some viruses infect tissue culture cells without producing a visible cytopathogenic effect and must be detected by indirect methods such as the hemadsorption and the hemagglutination tests. Viruses that fall into this category are parainfluenza types 1-3, influenza A and B, and mumps. Recognition must be given to the fact that some strains of parainfluenza and influenza viruses have been found to produce CPE in selected cell lines.[10]

Occasionally infected tissue cell cultures are fixed and stained with polychrome dyes to detect intracytoplasmic and/or intranuclear inclusion bodies. For the most part these inclusion bodies provide only ancillary evidence and are not pathognomonic. Measles and adenovirus inclusions are excellent examples.

Tissue cultures, inoculated as described in the preceding section, are examined daily for at least 21 d for cytopathology and hemadsorption of erythrocytes.[11]

When a distinct CPE is observed, subpass 0.2 ml tissue culture fluid to make certain the agent is transmissible. Also check for bacterial and fungal contaminants, which should be suspected if the maintenance medium is turbid. If the CPE is transmissible and contaminants are ruled out, a virus is suspected. Proceed to identify the virus by the serum neutralization test.

Typing by serum neutralization test

Procedure. Freeze and thaw the tissue culture showing CPE at least once to release adequate virus. Centrifuge at 2500 rpm for 5 min to remove cellular debris. Prepare a 10^{-3} dilution of the supernatant fluid. Add 0.2 ml diluted supernatant fluid to a Wassermann tube containing 0.2 ml 1:10 dilution of known type-specific virus antiserum (1 tube is set up for each virus suspected). The virus antiserum must be heated prior to use at 56 C for 30 min to inactivate nonspecific viral inhibitors that are occasionally encountered in sera. Once a lot of serum has been inactivated the effect is permanent. Most commercial antisera now available are diluted 1:10 prior to use, but this may vary with each lot so that it is necessary to consult the manufacturer's instruction for proper dilution.

Incubate the antiserum-virus mixture at room temperature for 1 h and then transfer 0.2 ml to each of 2 tissue culture tubes. Incubate the tubes at 36 C and examine daily for CPE. Set up a virus control by inoculating 0.1 ml 10^{-3} dilution of culture supernatant into 1 tissue culture tube and incubating with the test. The type-specific antiserum that neutralizes the cytopathogenic effect identifies the virus type. The protective effect should last for at least 4 d beyond the time required for a distinct CPE to show in the control tube.

Identification of echoviruses by intersecting serum schema[12,13]

Preparation of pools
1. Immune sera to be incorporated in pools are inactivated at 56 C for 30 min.
2. Immune serum pools are constructed according to following schema.

Serum pool nos.	6	7	8	9	10
1	E1	E2	E3	E4	E5
2	E6	E7	E8	E9	E10
3	E11	E12	E13	E14	E15
4	E16	E17	E18	E19	E20
5	E21	E22	E23	E24	E25

E = Echovirus immune serum.

Each type-specific immune serum is incorporated into 2 pools. Before constructing pool, it is necessary to determine dilution of immune serum that contains 20 antibody units.

3. Each serum is used in pool at dilution containing 20 antibody units (20 times more concentrated than dilution exhibiting 50% neutralization of 100 TCIDs of virus). For example, if the following were actual titers, pool would be comprised as shown.

Antiserum	50% titer	20 antibody units	Volume in pool (ml)
Echovirus 1	1:2000	1:100	0.1
Echovirus 2	1:1000	1:50	0.2
Echovirus 3	1:500	1:25	0.4
Echovirus 4	1:1000	1:50	0.2
Echovirus 5	1:500	1:25	0.4

Hanks BSS = 10 ml of pool, each serum having 20 antibody units present.

4. After above calculations have been completed for each serum, the 10 pools are composed as illustrated in Step 2.
5. Dispense portions of each pool in volumes convenient for a few tests to avoid reduction in antibody titer due to repeated freezing and thawing of entire pool. Store aliquots at −20 C.

Neutralization test
1. A virus isolate suspected of being an echovirus is arbitrarily diluted 1:100 in Hanks BSS (or 1:10 if agent is weekly cytopathogenic) and tested by intersecting schema.
2. A 0.015 ml vol diluted isolate is added to 0.15 ml of each serum pool.
3. Mix and incubate at room temperature for 1 h or 4 C for 1½ h.
4. Inoculate 0.2 ml of each mixture into single monkey kidney cell culture. Also inoculate 1 tube with 0.1 ml diluted virus isolate as control on viral cytopathic dose. Two uninoculated tissue culture tubes are retained as normal cell controls. Examine each tissue culture tube microscopically before it is used to determine that cells are not undergoing spontaneous degeneration.
5. Inoculated tubes are incubated at 36 C for 7 d and examined microscopically each day during this interval. Earlier readings may detect breakthrough of antigenic relatives.

Interpretation
1. If neutralization of the isolate is observed in 2 pools, its identity is established by the point of intersection in the above schema. To avoid an error in identification, test the isolate against the individual immune serum shared by the 2 pools.

2. If isolate is neutralized by more than 2 serum pools, heterologous activity on the part of one of the immune sera should be suspected.
3. If a mixture of echoviruses is present, neutralization will occur in either one or none of the pools.
4. If complete degeneration of the cell culture is observed during the first 48 h, the virus dose employed is probably too strong, and the test should be repeated with a higher dilution of virus.
5. Neutralization of virus on day 3-4 but with breakthrough of virus by day 7 is suggestive of a "prime" strain of echovirus that does not overlap completely with the prototype strain.

Hemadsorption test

If the provisional diagnosis suggests one of the myxoviruses (influenza, parainfluenza, mumps, etc.), then a hemadsorption test should be performed.

Procedure. Remove the maintenance medium from the tissue culture tube and wash the cell sheet 2 times with Hanks BSS. Add 0.2 ml 0.4% suspension of washed guinea pig erythrocytes to the inoculated tissue cultures that have been incubated for 5 d. After adding the red blood cells, incubate the tubes at 4 C for 30 min and check the cell sheet under 100× magnification for evidence of adsorption of red blood cells to the cell monolayer. If the test is negative, repeat the test at 25 C for 1 h and again check for hemadsorption. If this test is negative, add fresh maintenance medium, reincubate, and test again at 5 d intervals for at least 20 d. Myxoviruses are detected in tissue culture usually within a 5 d incubation period.[14]

It is advisable to wash the tissue culture monolayer with Hanks BSS at least 2 times, since occasionally sufficient virus is contained in the maintenance fluid to block hemadsorption.

Since monkey kidney epithelial cells are frequently contaminated with simian myxoviruses, 0.2% SV5 antiserum must be added to the growth and maintenance media of those tubes used for isolating human myxoviruses.

Typing by hemadsorption-inhibition test. If a positive hemadsorption test is obtained, pass the tissue culture fluid into several tubes and incubate at 36 C for 4 d. After incubation wash each tissue culture twice with Hanks BSS and add 0.6 ml fresh Hanks BSS and 0.2 ml 1:10 dilution of hyperimmune type-specific antiserum (inactivated at 56 C for 30 min) for each virus suspected (usually 1 tube each for influenza types A and B, parainfluenza types 1-3, and mumps). Incubate serum-virus mixtures at room temperature for 30 min; then add 0.2 ml 0.4% suspension of guinea pig red cells and incubate for an additional 30 min at 4 C. Examine the cell monolayer for hemadsorption or hemadsorption-inhibition. A virus control must be included in each test. Identity of the virus is indicated by the type-specific antiserum that inhibits hemadsorption.

Typing adenoviruses by hemagglutination-inhibition (HI) test[15]

Reagents
1. Phosphate-buffered saline, pH 7.2

Na₂HPO₄	1.13 g

(continued)

KH₂PO₄	0.27 g
NaCl	17 g
Distilled water	2000 ml

  a. Store in glass-stoppered bottle at 4 C.
2. Rat erythrocytes, 1% suspension
  a. Collect RBC in 5 vol Alsever's solution and store at 4 C.
  b. Wash 3 times in buffered saline and prepare a 1% suspension in buffer. Mouse RBC may be substituted for rat RBC.
3. African green monkey erythrocytes, 1% suspension
  a. Prepare in same manner as rat erythrocytes. Rhesus RBC may be substituted for African green monkey.
4. Adenovirus isolate
  a. Harvest tissue culture tube showing 3-4+ CPE by freezing and thawing 3 times. Use as antigen in HA test.

Procedure
1. Set up 2 rows of agglutination tubes and label 1 row "rat RBC" and the other "monkey RBC."
2. Prepare duplicate serial 2-fold dilutions of suspected adenovirus culture fluid in 0.4 ml amounts, using buffered saline.
3. Include 0.4 ml 1:2 dilution of normal tissue culture fluid in each row as control.
4. Add 0.2 ml 1% suspension of fresh rat RBC to first row and African green monkey RBC to second row, including cell controls.
5. Mix contents of tubes well and allow to stand 1 h at 37 C or until cells in control tubes have settled to a button.
6. Read and record titer as highest dilution showing 4+ agglutination.
7. Adenoviruses fall into following groups based on species of RBC agglutinated[15]:

	RBC agglutinated		Adenovirus
Groups	Rhesus	Rat	types
I	+	−	3, 7, 11, 14, 16, 20, 21, 25, 28
II-A	−	+	8, 10, 17, 19, 22-24, 26, 27
II-B	+	+	9, 13, 15
III	−	Partial	1, 2, 4-6
IV	−	−	12, 18

8. After determining adenovirus group, identify specific type within group by hemagglutination-inhibition test.

Typing enteroviruses by hemagglutination-inhibition test[16]

Reagents
1. Human O Rh-negative RBC, 0.75% suspension
2. Chicken erythrocytes, 0.5% suspension
3. 0.01M Phosphate-buffered saline, pH 5.8

KH₂PO₄	13.6 g
Normal saline	100 ml

  a. Adjust to pH 5.8.
4. 0.01M Phosphate-buffered saline, pH 7.2

K₂HPO₄	17.4 g
Normal saline	100 ml

Procedure
1. Prepare serial 2-fold dilutions of tissue culture fluid of enterovirus isolate showing 3-4+ CPE, using buffered saline, pH 5.8.
2. Prepare second series of dilutions in buffered saline, pH 7.2. Add 0.4 ml of each dilution to ag-

glutination tubes for pH 5.8 buffer. Repeat for pH 7.2 buffered saline.
3. Add 0.2 ml blood cells suspended in each of buffers.
4. Shake tubes and allow RBC to settle at 4 C for human RBC in each buffer. Repeat at 37 C with human RBC in each buffer. Coxsackievirus A7 agglutinates chicken cells only; echovirus types 3, 6, 7, 11-13, 19-21, 24, and 29, coxsackieviruses A20, A21, A24, B1, B3, and B5 agglutinate human O RBC.
5. Titer is highest dilution at which 1+ agglutination occurs. This dilution is taken as 1 hemagglutinating unit (HAU).
6. If hemagglutination is detected, virus can be identified by HI test. Use 4 HAU in test.
7. Antisera used in HI test must be absorbed with kaolin and human erythrocytes. Sera need not be inactivated.

Detection of virus by cocultivation

Advances in tissue cell culture and development of new methodology have enhanced the detection of some groups of viruses, but the frequency of virus recovery from clinical material is still inadequate for certain agents. It has been established that virus isolation can be enhanced by inoculation of viable tissue cells from the patient, e.g., in varicella zoster. Also, viruses can be demonstrated more readily in cell cultures prepared from organs than from cell cultures inoculated with organ suspensions. In patients with subacute sclerosing panencephalitis (SSPE) the rubeola virus has been successfully recovered only by cultivation of brain cells with HeLa cells, or with BSC-1 cells. Therefore in patients with SSPE this method must be used for isolation of the virus. This technic is called cocultivation and was described by Horta-Barbosa et al.[17] in 1969 for demonstrating the virus in SSPE. In cases of herpesvirus simplex encephalitis, more viral isolations can be made by cocultivation than by inoculating supernatant fluid of tissue homogenates onto cell monolayer. Cocultivation should be used routinely for the laboratory diagnosis of progressive, degenerative neurologic diseases.

Procedure

1. Mince tissue in Hanks BSS into 1 mm³ fragments and trypsinize (Chapter 91).
2. Centrifuge suspension at 600 rpm for 10 min and discard supernatant. Wash cells 3 times in Hanks BSS.
3. Resuspend cells in BME supplemented with 10% heat-inactivated fetal bovine serum to concentration of approx. 8×10^5 viable cells/ml.
4. Plant 2 ml aliquots in tubes and incubate at 36 C. Change growth medium every 2 d until confluent monolayer develops.
5. Trypsinize these cell cultures, wash in Hanks BSS, and perform a viable cell count. Suspend cells in BME to obtain concentration of 3×10^5 viable cells/ml.
6. Prepare mixed cell suspensions of culture patient tissue from Step 5 with cell suspensions of HeLa cells (or other suitable indicator cells) by combining 1 vol 3×10^5 suspension cell/ml patient cells with 2 vol HeLa cells (indicator cells) in BME containing approx. 2×10^5 viable cells/ml.
7. This mixture is seeded in plastic tissue culture bottles and incubated at 36 C.
8. Examine for CPE and change medium every 3 d. Maintain cocultivated cells for 4 wk before considering negative or setting up a second cocultivation.

DETECTION AND IDENTIFICATION OF VIRAL ACTIVITY IN MICE

Suckling mice are the most frequently used animals in the diagnostic virology laboratory, and they are used primarily for the isolation of coxsackieviruses A that, with few exceptions, have not been grown in tissue culture and do not infect adult mice or chick embryos.

Suckling mice infected with coxsackieviruses A develop muscle weakness, tremors, and flaccid paralysis and eventually die; there is diffuse necrosis of skeletal muscle but no involvement of the central nervous system. Symptoms are usually apparent in 3-5 days.

Coxsackieviruses B produce a spastic paralysis with central nervous system involvement and death in suckling mice; there is rarely skeletal muscle necrosis.

Lymphocytic choriomeningitis virus produces symptoms of tremors, convulsions, and generalized rigidity in about 5-12 days, with death 1-3 days after onset of symptoms.

In the case of psittacosis, mice develop tremors, become prostrated, and die within 3-8 days after inoculation.

Adult mice should be inoculated when rabies is suspected; the symptoms in mice are weakness, paralysis, and prostration, with death occurring in 10-14 days with extremes of 3-40 days after intracerebral inoculation.

Mice inoculated intracerebrally with the encephalitis viruses develop symptoms of weakness, tremor, incoordination, convulsions, and paralysis. Mice must be observed for at least 21 days and 1 subpassage made, when results are negative, before reporting is done.[18]

If inoculated mice (suckling or adult) become moribund or die and a subpassage of uncontaminated brain material produces the same result, the causative agent is considered to be a virus and must be identified by the mouse neutralization test (also Negri bodies and FA in rabies) in animals.[19] Make certain the isolate does not grow in tissue cultures available; if it does, then the neutralization test should be performed in tissue culture.

Mouse neutralization test. Prepare a 1:100 dilution of the 20% suspension of positive brain material. Mix 0.2 ml of this dilution with 0.2 ml known type-specific antiserum. Set up a tube for each virus antiserum used. Antisera may be pooled, e.g., coxsackieviruses A, as long as the final dilution of any single antiserum is not greater than 1:10. Incubate the antiserum-virus mixtures at room temperature for 1 h and then inoculate 0.03 ml intracerebrally into each of 5 mice for each antiserum tested. Inoculate 5 mice in the same manner with the 1:100 virus suspension alone to serve as controls.

The antiserum that protects the mice indicates the identity of the viral agent.

DETECTION AND IDENTIFICATION OF VIRAL ACTIVITY IN CHICK EMBRYO

Screen test for viral hemagglutinins. Add 0.5 ml amniotic fluid diluted 1:10 to each of 2 Wassermann tubes. To tube 1 add 0.5 ml 0.5% suspension of chick red cells and to tube 2 add 0.5 ml 0.5% suspension of guinea pig (or human) red cells. Repeat this setup using undiluted allantoic fluid. Add 0.5 ml of each red cell suspension used to 0.5 ml normal saline to serve as a control. Mix and incubate at room temperature for 1 h.[20]

Examine tubes for hemagglutination, which is indicated by a uniform film of agglutinated cells covering the bottom of the tube. Red cells in the control tube settle down to form a compact button that flows when the rack is tilted.

All red cells used in the HA test must be washed 3 times with physiologic saline. Red cells that do not wash with clear supernatant fluid in the third washing should be discarded.

If influenza C is suspected, the test must also be run at 4 C.

Hemagglutination indicates viral activity if bacteria, bacterial toxins, and fungal contamination are ruled out.

Titration of virus by hemagglutination (HA) test. Before the virus can be identified as to type, it is first necessary to establish the concentration of the viral agent in terms of HAU/0.5 ml embryonic fluid (preferably allantoic).

If hemagglutination is detected, prepare serial 2-fold dilutions of allantoic fluid in saline, ranging from 1:2 through 1:1024.

Add 0.5 ml 0.5% suspension of the species of red cells that were agglutinated in the screening test to 0.5 ml of each dilution of allantoic fluid. Mix and incubate at room temperature (25 C) for 1 h. Examine for hemagglutination.[21]

The reciprocal of the highest dilution at which complete hemagglutination occurs is the end point, and 0.5 ml of this dilution contains 1 HAU. Dilute the original allantoic fluid so that it contains 4 HAU/0.25 ml according to the following formula[22]:

$$\frac{\text{Reciprocal of dilution containing 1 HAU/0.5 ml}}{8} = \frac{\text{Dilution of fluid containing 4 HAU/0.25 ml}}{}$$

Proceed to identify (type) the isolate by the hemagglutination-inhibition test.

Virus identification by hemagglutination-inhibition (HI) test.[23] Mix 0.25 ml allantoic fluid containing 4 HAU with 0.25 ml 1:10 dilution of hyperimmune type-specific antiserum (inactivate the antiserum at 56 C for 30 min prior to use). Set up a tube of antiserum for each virus suspected.

Set up a virus control containing 0.25 ml allantoic fluid and 0.25 ml 0.5% suspension of red cells, and a red cell control containing 0.25 ml 0.5% suspension of red cells and 0.25 ml saline.

Incubate all tubes at room temperature (25 C) for 1 h and examine for hemagglutination.

The identity of the virus is indicated by the type of antiserum that inhibits the hemagglutination reaction.

• • •

For a summary of virus isolation procedures see Fig. 92-1.

PLAQUE TECHNIC FOR ISOLATION OF VIRUSES[24]

Reagents
1. Agar 3%
   Agar, Noble   3 g
   Distilled water   100 ml
   a. Autoclave at 118 C for 15 min.

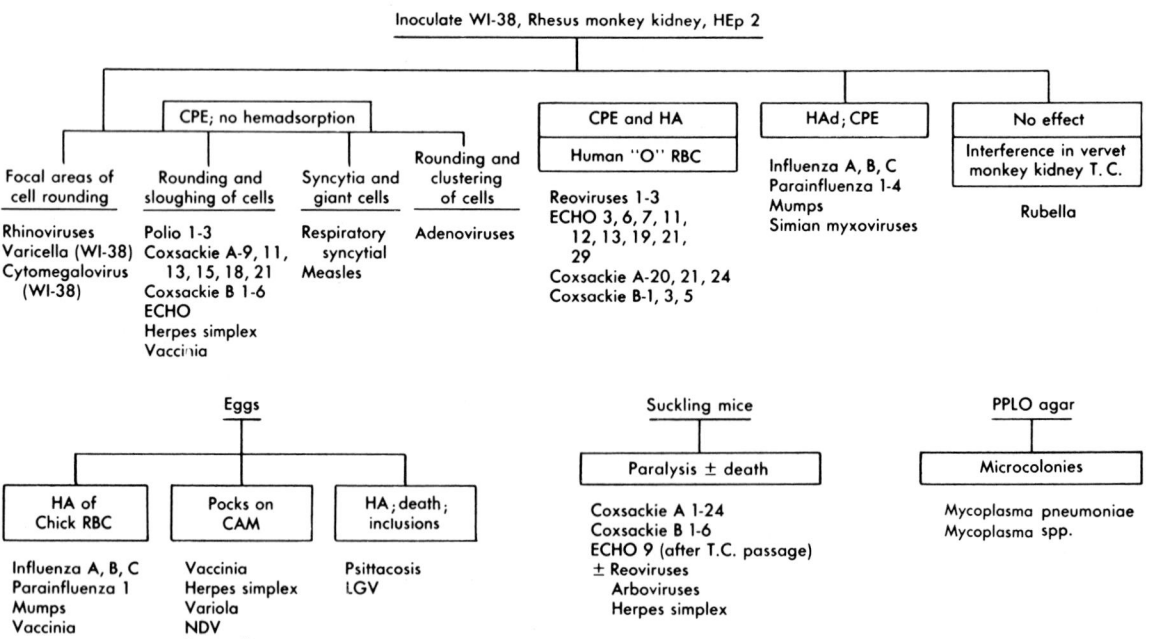

Fig. 92-1. Virus isolation schema. **HA,** hemagglutination; **HAd,** hemadsorption.

2. Glutamine, 3% stock solution

L-Glutamine	3 g
Distilled water	100 ml

   a. Sterilize by filtration at 4 C and store frozen in convenient quantities.

3. BME (2× conc.)

Eagle basal medium (in Earle BSS)	20 ml
Glutamine, 3%	2 ml
Inactivated calf serum	3.6 ml
NaHCO₃, 7.5%	5.6 ml
Neutral red, 1:1000 dilution	3 ml
Penicillin, streptomycin stock	200 U (or μg/ml)
Distilled water, sterile, to	100 ml

Procedure

1. Remove growth medium from monolayer cell cultures and wash 3 times with 5 ml Hanks BSS for 100 ml bottle cultures.
2. Prepare 10-fold dilutions of virus in Hanks BSS and inoculate each 100 ml prescription bottle culture with 0.2 ml. Distribute inoculum evenly over monolayer.
3. Incubate cultures for 2 h at 36 C to permit viral adsorption.
4. Eagle basal medium (2×) is brought to 46-47 C in water bath and mixed with equal vol 3% agar at same temperature. This mixture is held at 46-47 during addition to monolayer cultures with Cornwall syringe.
5. Add 10 ml overlay medium to each bottle and carefully spread over monolayer.
6. Place bottles on flat surface and allow agar to firmly gel for 1 h in the dark. Photodynamic inactivation of some enteroviruses may occur due to neutral red in basal medium.
7. Invert cultures and incubate at 36 C for 2-4 d for polioviruses and 7-10 d for certain echoviruses.
8. Clones of virus can be picked by introducing Pasteur pipet into center of isolated plaque and sucking up portion of agar overlay. Pick portion of each plaque that shows a difference in either size, shape, or plaque periphery and examine separately.
9. By mixing varying dilutions of serum with constant concentration of virus, incubating, and then using a portion of each mixture to produce plaques, serum antibody titer can be established as highest serum dilution that reduces plaque count by 75%.

RAPID DIAGNOSIS BY IMMUNOFLUORESCENCE

Several technics are now available to permit rapid diagnosis of some viral diseases by direct examination of clinical material for the presence of virus. These technics are electron microscopy (see below), counterelectrophoresis (see below), and fluorescent microscopy. Because the direct fluorescent antibody (FA) technic is simple and rapid to perform and the equipment is commonly available in the clinical laboratory, it is being expanded to speed up detection and identification of viruses. The method is, however, complicated by serious problems of nonspecific fluorescence and reagents of low specificity. Usable conjugates are commercially available (Flow Laboratories, Rockville, Md.; Microbiological Associates, Walkersville, Md.) for several commonly encountered agents, e.g., herpesvirus simplex types 1 and 2, cytomegalovirus, and rubella virus. In addition to direct FA on clinical material, the technic can also be used to demonstrate virus in tissue culture inoculated with clinical material before cytopathology is evident.

Immunofluorescent technics are being employed for rapid diagnosis of respiratory virus disease (adenoviruses, influenza, parainfluenza, and respiratory syncytial virus), encephalitis (rubeola, herpesviruses), viral exanthems (rubella, rubeola, herpesviruses), and congenital diseases (CMV and rubella). Applications are continually expanded (Table 92-3).

Cerebrospinal fluid (CSF)

1. Centrifuge CSF at 1500 rpm for 10 min and spot sediment on clean glass slide. Cytocentrifuge may also be used to sediment cells onto slide. Fix in cold acetone (−20 C) for 10 min, air-dry, and rinse in distilled water.
2. Cover smear with unconjugated hyperimmune rabbit antiserum for specific virus and incubate in moist chamber for 30 min at 37 C. Wash once in phosphate-buffered saline (PBS) (pH 7.2) and once in distilled water for 5 min each.
3. Cover smear with fluorescin-conjugated goat antirabbit serum and incubate for 30 min at 37 C. Wash 4 times in PBS for 10 min each and then rinse in distilled water. Blot dry, mount in buffered glycerol saline (pH 8.0), and examine under fluorescent microscope. Include appropriate positive and negative controls each time test is performed.

Biopsy and autopsy specimens

1. Fix cryostat sections of tissues in cold acetone (−20 C) for 1 h, air-dry, and rinse in distilled water.
2. Prepare mixture of conjugated antiserum as follows: 2 parts conjugate, 2 parts PBS (pH 7.2), and 1 part Evans blue (1:200).
3. Flood smear with this mixture and allow to react in moist chamber at room temperature for 30 min.
4. Wash once each in PBS and distilled water for 10 min periods. Mount in buffered glycerol saline and examine. Set up controls as described above.

Vesicular lesions, ulcers, and corneal scrapings

1. Scrape margin of vesicular lesion or ulcer or obtain scrapings from corneal, oral, or genital mucous membranes of infected areas.
2. Air-dry smears and fix in cold acetone (−20 C) for 15 min. Stain with fluorescin-conjugated specific antiserum in moist chamber for 30 min at room temperature. Rinse once each in PBS (pH 7.2) and distilled water for 10 min periods. Mount in buffered glycerol saline (pH 8.0) and examine with fluorescent microscope. Include appropriate controls.

NP aspirates

1. Centrifuge NP fluids or urine specimens at 1500 rpm for 10 min.
2. Prepare 4 smears from sediment of each specimen, fix in cold acetone, and proceed as described for vesicular lesions.

Urine. Process by method described for NP aspirates.

Delayed test

1. Inoculate monolayer tissue culture in tubes with clinical material and incubate 48-72 h (or until CPE is evident).
2. Scrape cells from glass, wash once in PBS, and

Table 92-3. Applications of immunofluorescence to rapid laboratory diagnosis

Disease	Clinical material	Viral conjugates employed
Aseptic meningitis	Cerebrospinal fluid (CSF)	Coxsackieviruses, echoviruses, herpes simplex, mumps, rubeola
Encephalitis	Brain tissue, CSF	Arboviruses, herpes simplex
Subacute sclerosing panencephalitis (SSPE)	Brain tissue, CSF	Rubeola virus
Multiple leukoencephalopathy	Brain tissue	Papovavirus (SV40-like)
Respiratory disease	Throat washings, nasopharyngeal (NP) aspirates	Adenoviruses, influenza, parainfluenza, respiratory syncytial virus
Papilloma (warts)	Cryostat sections of biopsy	Papilloma virus
Burkitt's lymphoma	Lymphocytes	EB virus
Rubella	Throat washings, NP aspirates	Rubella virus
Measles	Urine sediment, NP secretions	Rubeola virus
Skin lesions	Scraping from margin of lesion	Varicella zoster herpes simplex, echoviruses
Acute hemorrhagic cystitis, nephritis	Urine sediment	Adenoviruses, Coxsackie group B
Ocular lesions	Eye scrapings	Adenoviruses, herpes simplex, chlamydia
Cytomegalic inclusion diseases	Urine sediment, NP aspirates	Cytomegalovirus
Colorado tick fever	Peripheral blood RBC	Colorado tick fever virus
Pericarditis, myocarditis, pancarditis	Pericardial fluid, heart tissue	Coxsackie group B

resuspend in PBS to yield approx. 100 cells per field.

3. Add 1 drop 10% bovine serum albumin to each milliliter cell suspension to promote adherence to glass slide.
4. Prepare 4 smears from suspension, air-dry, fix in cold acetone (−20 C), and stain as described for biopsy specimens.

GROUPING OF VIRUSES BASED ON THEIR BIOLOGIC AND BIOCHEMICAL CHARACTERISTICS[25]

Not infrequently viruses are isolated that cannot be identified by the usual serologic procedures, and it becomes necessary to characterize some of their biologic and biochemical properties in order to group them. The most useful properties are nucleic acid type, particle size, sensitivity to ether, and acid lability. All these properties can be readily determined with the basic laboratory equipment commonly found in the clinical laboratory. The technics are described below.

Type of nucleic acid. Several methods are available, but the one most widely used is the inhibition of viral replication in tissue culture by the incorporation of nucleic acid analogs such as 5-fluoro-2-deoxyuridine (FUDR). This chemical antagonist inhibits the multiplication of DNA viruses but not RNA viruses.

1. Dissolve sufficient FUDR in tissue culture maintenance medium to yield final concentration of 10^{-4}M.
2. Two h prior to inoculation of virus, replace fluid in tissue culture tubes with 1.5 ml maintenance containing FUDR.
3. Inoculate 4 tubes with 0.2 ml unidentified virus containing 32-320 TCD_{50}; inoculate 4 tubes with-

out FUDR with 0.2 ml of this virus to compare with tubes containing FUDR.
4. Also inoculate 4 tubes each with poliovirus type I (RNA virus) and adenovirus type 4 (DNA virus) to serve as controls.
5. Incubate all tubes for 2 h, then wash 3 times with Hanks BSS, and refeed with maintenance without FUDR.
6. Incubate tubes at 36 C and observe cultures daily for CPE, hemadsorption, or hemagglutination, depending on which effect the unknown virus exhibits.
7. If virus is of DNA type, its multiplication is suppressed; RNA viruses are unaffected.

Particle size. The size of viruses can be determined by passing a known concentration through Millipore filters with porosities of 50 and 100 nm and then titering the filtrates. Viruses that pass the 50 nm filter without a significant reduction in titer are classified as **small viruses;** viruses that pass the 100 nm but not the 50 nm are classed as **medium viruses;** and those that do not pass through either are considered **large viruses.**

1. Pass 2 ml unidentified virus through Swinny-type adapter attached to syringe and containing a 50 nm Millipore filter. Collect filtrate aseptically. Also pass 2 ml through a 100 nm filter and collect filtrate.
2. Prepare serial dilutions of each filtrate and of original unfiltered viral suspension and determine titer of each after appropriate incubation period, as determined by results of unfiltered viral material.
3. Classify unidentified virus as small, medium, or large virus, as described above.

Ether sensitivity. Some viruses possess an outer envelope of essential lipid that must be present for the virus to be infectious. When these viruses are treated with lipid solvents such as ether or chloroform, their infectivity is considerably reduced or lost. Viruses that lack essential lipids are unaffected.

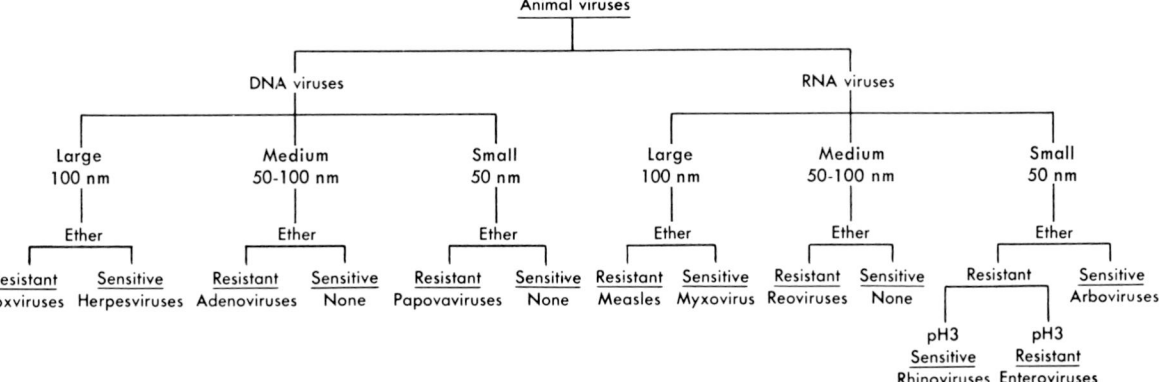

Fig. 92-2. Animal viruses.[26]

1. Mix 1 ml unidentified virus (use undiluted virus) with 1 ml 20% diethyl ether in rubber-stoppered tube. Treat known adenovirus (ether resistant) and myxovirus (ether sensitive) in similar manner.
2. Place tubes in refrigerator (2-10 C) for 18 h.
3. After 18 h treatment, centrifuge tubes at 2500 rpm for 15 min and collect supernatant fluid.
4. Prepare serial 10-fold dilutions of each virus in Hanks BSS.
5. Inoculate 0.2 ml of each dilution in each of 3 tissue culture tubes and label properly.
6. Incubate tissue culture tubes at 36 C for 7 days. Observe tubes daily and record results.
7. Interpret results as follows:
   Ether resistant—no appreciable reduction in infectivity
   Ether sensitive—complete loss in infectivity or a 2-log or greater reduction

Acid lability. Viruses can be grouped on the basis of their acid lability into group I—acid-stable viruses such as adenoviruses, papovaviruses, reoviruses, and picornaviruses; and group II—acid-labile viruses such as myxoviruses, arboviruses, herpesviruses, and poxviruses. Occasionally it is necessary to study this property to differentiate between rhinoviruses and enteroviruses.

1. Prepare 1:10 dilution of unidentified virus in Eagle minimum essential medium free of bicarbonate. Also prepare 1:10 dilutions of known acid-resistant virus (adenovirus) and acid-labile virus (vaccinia).
2. To 2 ml portion of 1:10 dilution of each virus add 0.05 ml 0.1N hydrochloric acid. This should result in pH of 3.0 after adequately mixed. One 2 ml quantity of unidentified virus without addition of acid serves as control.
3. Allow tubes to stand in ice bath for 3 h.
4. Prepare 10-fold dilutions of treated virus and controls in maintenance medium and inoculate 0.2 ml of each into 3 tubes per dilution.
5. Incubate tubes at 36 C and examine daily for viral effect. Calculate $TCID_{50}$ of virus.
6. Interpret results as follows:
   Acid labile—reduction in titer of 2 logs or greater in infectivity
   Acid stable—no apparent reduction in infectivity

• • •

Based on the biologic and biochemical properties described above, Hsuing[26] has devised the schema shown in Fig. 92-2 for tentatively grouping the animal viruses.

DETECTION OF VIRUS PARTICLES BY ELECTRON MICROSCOPY[27]

Electron microscopy has been widely used over the past few years for the study of viral structure and classification of viruses by their distinctive morphology and symmetry. However, the feasibility of using the electron microscope as a diagnostic tool was not accepted due to the belief that the concentration of viral particles in most clinical specimens is too low for detection. This statement is valid because only a minute portion of a specimen can be examined in the field of the electron microscope at one time, and usually 10^9 particles/ml are needed to demonstrate their presence. However, in recent studies of infections such as influenza, parainfluenza, mumps, encephalitis, and respiratory syncytial virus, the nasopharyngeal secretions were found to contain sufficient virus particles to be detected by electron microscopy.[28] By adopting the method of immune electron microscopy one can concentrate the virus particles from larger volumes of clinical specimens, and as little as 10^6 viral particles/ml are sufficient to yield a suitable specimen.

Application of the technic of negative staining to the study of viruses by electron microscopy has permitted identification and grouping of many viruses on a morphologic basis. This method entails the treatment of viral suspensions with a solution of an electron-dense substance such as phosphotungstic acid. One merit of negative staining is that the electron-dense material is capable of penetrating into extremely small regions between the protein subunits of the viral capsid; since the electron beam penetrates sites where the negative stain is not present, the surface configuration of particles is strikingly seen in relief. Negative staining is now commonly employed to detect viruses directly in clinical materials without prior purification.[29]

Immune electron microscopy[30]

Immune electron microscopy was first introduced by Brenner and Horne[31] in 1959. They developed it specifically for visualizing the interaction of antibody molecules with virus particles.

Negative staining provides necessary contrast for visualization of the fine structure of the virus. The dried particles do not change their original structure as they are surrounded and supported by a protein-phosphotungstate complex. That is why the method was adopted by Almeida and Waterson[30] and later by Kapikian et al.[32] to demonstrate and associate viruslike particles (Norwalk agent) in stool from cases of acute infectious nonbacterial gastroenteritis. Immune electron microscopy is the most sensitive method available for establishing the occurrence of an immune reaction, for recognizing the individual antibody molecules of IgG (7S) and IgM (19S), and for detecting viruses in clinical specimens such as throat swabs, throat washings, eye washings, nasopharyngeal secretions, urine feces, or infected tissue cultures.

Materials
1. Specific antiserum or homologous serum from patient
2. 2% Postassium phosphotungstate, pH 6.0
3. Formvar-carbon-coated grids (400 mesh)
4. Hanks BSS with penicillin and streptomycin (100 U/ml)

Procedure
Preparation of specimen
1. Most fluid specimens contain high concentrations of salts, so they are diluted with equal volume of sterile distilled water.
2. Cotton swabs of clinical material can be suspended in 2 ml Hanks BSS.
3. Make 10-20% suspension of stool specimen in Hanks BSS, centrifuge at 3000 rpm for 10 min, collect supernatant, and discard debris.
4. Freeze and thaw infected tissue culture suspension and centrifuge at 3000 rpm for 10 min.

Clarification and concentration
1. Clarify suspension by centrifuging 7000 rpm for 30 min to remove bacteria and debris.
2. Mix 4 parts clarified suspension with 1 part homologous serum (or specific antiserum).
3. Allow to stand at 37 C for 1 h and leave at 4 C overnight.
4. Next morning, centrifuge at 50,000 rpm for 30 min in 5 ml tubes.
5. Decant supernatant and resuspend pellet in 0.1 ml sterile distilled water.

Preparation of grids and staining
1. Mix 0.1 ml resuspended pellet with 0.1 ml 2% potassium phosphotungstate, pH 6.0.
2. Place drop of mixture on 400-mesh Formvar-carbon-coated grid.
3. Withdraw excess fluid with filter paper.
4. Examine under electron microscope.

NOTE: It is important that period between suspending pellet in distilled water and placing grid in microscope should be as short as possible because conditions are nonphysiologic at this time.

Identification. Virus particles are grouped on the basis of 2 characteristics: (1) site of formation of virus within the cell, e.g., cytoplasm or nucleus, and (2) symmetrical property of the virus as seen by negative staining.

From studies on isolated virus particles, it is possible to group them into 3 main symmetry or geometrical categories. These geometrical groups are (1) viruses with icosahedral symmetry, (2) viruses with helical symmetry, and (3) viruses with combined symmetry or complex geometrical patterns. If the nucleocapsid of the virus is surrounded by an envelope, it is termed "compound symmetry" (compound helical or compound icosahedral). If the nucleocapsid lacks an envelope, it is referred to as having "simple symmetry."[33] The grouping of viruses according to their symmetry is given in the outline below.

I. Simple icosahedral symmetry
   A. Adenoviruses
   B. Adeno-associated viruses
   C. Coxsackieviruses
   D. Rotaviruses
   E. Echoviruses
   F. Hepatitis viruses
   G. Norwalk agent
   H. Papovaviruses
   I. Polioviruses
   J. Reoviruses
   K. Rhinoviruses
II. Compound icosahedral symmetry
   A. Cytomegalovirus
   B. Epstein-Barr virus
   C. Herpesvirus simplex
   D. Herpersvirus zoster
III. Simple helical symmetry (no human viruses yet identified with this type)
IV. Compound helical symmetry
   A. Influenza viruses
   B. Mumps virus
   C. Rubeola virus
   D. Parainfluenza viruses
   E. Respiratory syncytial virus
V. Complex or combination symmetry
   A. Arenaviruses (LCM)
   B. Flanders–Hart Park virus
   C. Kern Canyon virus
   D. Molluscum contagiosum
   E. Rabies virus
   F. Smallpox virus
   G. Vaccinia virus
   H. Vesicular stomatitis virus

Diagnostic electron microscopy of fecal extracts for agents of acute nonbacterial gastroenteritis[34]

The technic of electron microscopy is particularly valuable in indentification of viruses recently associated with acute epidemic gastroenteritis (Norwalk agent[32] and rotaviruses, or duoviruses[35]) and the hepatitis A virus[36] in feces. These agents cannot be demonstrated by conventional methods of tissue culture, animal inoculation, etc. The Norwalk agent is associated with gastroenteritis or winter vomiting disease in adults, while rotaviruses, or duoviruses, are found in acute gastroenteritis in infants and children.

Procedure
1. Make a 20-25% (vol/vol) suspension of stool or vomitus specimen in 5 ml Hanks BSS with 1000 U/ml penicillin and streptomycin.
2. Centrifuge suspension at 3000 rpm for 10 min.
3. Remove supernatant and centrifuge at 7000 rpm for 30 min to separate bacteria and debris.
4. Remove supernatant and centrifuge 3-5 ml in ultracentrifuge at 50,000 rpm for 1 h.
5. Resuspend sediment in 0.2 ml distilled water.

6. Touch surface of Formvar-carbon-coated grid (300-400 mesh) to a drop of suspension.
7. Allow to almost dry but not to dry completely.
8. Dip in distilled water 3 times.
9. Dip into 2% potassium phosphotungstate, pH 6.0.
10. Blot dry and examine in electron microscope.

Identification. Refer to electron micrographs in references 32 and 37 for morphology of viruses of gastroenteritis.

Diagnostic electron microscopy of vesicular fluids[38]

Procedure

Preparation of specimen
1. Collect vesicular fluids in capillary tube and seal both ends, or make thick smears on clean glass slides and let them dry.
2. Send specimen in dust-free container to laboratory as soon as possible.
3. In suspected case of smallpox, if pustule is dried up and crust is already formed, send crust in sterile test tube.

Processing of specimen
1. Place drop of sterile distilled water on each smear of microscope slide and rub with inoculating wire to release specimen. Collect material in capillary or Pasteur pipet.
2. If specimen is crust, grind with 0.2 ml sterile distilled water in Griffith's grinder. Collect supernatant in capillary or Pasteur pipet.

Preparation of grid
1. Put drop of specimen from capillary pipet on Formvar-carbon-coated grid (300-400 mesh). Allow to dry.
2. Wash 3 times in distilled water by dipping grid for 10 s each time.
3. Touch surface of grid to drop of 2% potassium phosphotungstate, pH 6.0. Remove excess stain by filter paper.
4. Dry and examine in electron microscope.

Electron microscopic examination of leukocytes (buffy coat) for viruses[39-41]

Procedure

Preparation of leukocytes
1. Mix equal volume of heparinized blood with 2% clinical dextran in physiologic saline.
2. Place tube in slanted (45° angle) position at room temperature for 45 min and allow RBC to sediment.
3. Collect opalescent cell and platelet-rich plasma layer in conical centrifuge tube.
4. Centrifuge for 5 min at $200 \times g$.
   NOTE: Sedimented leukocytes from 1 ml supernatant should yield 5×10^6 cells or 5 mm³ packed cells.
5. Wash 2 times in Hanks BSS using 3 ml/5 mm³ packed cells.

Fixation
1. Mix one part 2.5% glutaraldehyde in 0.1M cacodylate (pH 7.4) with 2 parts 1% osmium tetroxide in 0.1M cacodylate (pH 7.4) within an hour of use and store in ice bath.
   NOTE: Under these conditions, mixture must remain clear and colorless during fixation.
2. Resuspend washed leukocytes in 2 ml cold fixative mixture.
3. After 2 min, transfer to 3 ml conical centrifuge tube and spin at $300 \times g$ for 1 min.

4. Decant superatant with Pasteur pipet and chill pellet briefly on ice.
5. Resuspend in 2 ml fixative mixture and allow to stand on ice 15-30 min.
6. Centrifuge at $300 \times g$ for 1 min.
7. Wash 2 times in cold saline and centrifuge at $300 \times g$ for 1 min.
8. Suspend pellet in uranyl acetate in 0.1M acetate buffer (pH 6.3) and allow to stand at 0 C for 15-30 min.
9. Wash 2 times in normal saline.
10. Warm cell pellet in 50 C water bath for 5 min.
11. Suspend pellet in 3 drops 2% Noble agar (melted and cooled to 50 C). Use warm Pasteur pipet to transfer agar to avoid solidification.
12. Immediately centrifuge suspension in fluid agar at $750 \times g$ for 2 min in carrier half filled with hot tap water.
    NOTE: If solidification is avoided, cells form firm pellet at bottom of tube; if not, cells distribute in fuzzy zone. If latter occurs, remelt agar in steam bath and recentrifuge. Steaming will not affect fixed cells.
13. After centrifugation, solidify agar in ice bath.
14. Add 70% ethyl alcohol and place on ice for 1 h.
15. Remove agar carefully by pipetting.
16. Trim block cell pellet for dehydration and embedding.

Dehydration
1. Wash pellet sections in 3 changes of 70% ethyl alcohol for 5 min each time.
2. Wash with 90% ethyl alcohol for 10 min.
3. Wash with absolute ethyl alcohol for 10 min (2 changes).

Embedding
1. Place pellet section in Epon 812 (Ernest F. Fullman, Inc., Schenectady, N.Y.) (3 changes), 10 min each time.
2. Hold in last change of Epon 812 overnight at 37 C.
3. Next day, place in 3 changes Epon 812 containing 2% accelerator for 5 min each time.
4. Polymerize finally at 60 C for 2 d.

Staining. After cutting sections of 5 μm with ultramicrotome, stain sections with 0.01% lead citrate for 3.5 min. Wash in distilled water and stain with 1% uranyl acetate for 3.5 min. Examine in electron microscope.

DETECTION OF HEPATITIS B SURFACE ANTIGEN (HBsAg OR AUSTRALIA ANTIGEN)

Discovery of the Australia antigen (HBsAg) has provided an important marker for differentiating between the 2 major types of hepatitis, i.e., hepatitis A and B. Because to the significant association between the detection of HBsAg in transfused blood and the transmission of type B hepatitis, blood donors in the United States are required by law to be screened routinely for this antigen. There are a number of other important indications for HBsAg testing: (1) diagnosis of liver disease, (2) management of cases of acute hepatitis and their prognoses, (3) determination of progression from acute to chronic hepatitis in type B hepatitis, (4) detection of carriers in hospital admissions, (5) differentiation between hepatitis types A and B, (6) epidemiologic study of hepatitis outbreaks, (7) surveillance of medical and paramedical personnel who have a high risk of contracting the agent, (8) preoperative testing of patients, (9) screening of obstetrical patients, (10) screening of renal dialysis patients, (11) determination of carrier status of certain groups who might be potential sources of infection, and (12) screening of recipients prior to transfusion.[42]

It is estimated that approximately 90% of patients with type B hepatitis have a positive test for HBsAg, but this varies with the sensitivity of the method employed and with the time and frequency of testing. HBsAg is found most frequently during the incubation period and for 2-3 weeks after acute infection.[43] In acute infections the antigen persists for only 2-3 weeks in most cases and in some cases for only a few days. Persistence of antigen for more than 2-3 months suggests the development of a carrier state or of chronic hepatitis. Studies have shown that a negative test for HBsAg does not necessarily rule out hepatitis due to type B or the carrier state because a negative result may be due to the use of relatively insensitive methods, a delay in collecting specimens for testing, or immune complexes. False-positive reactions are rarely encountered and are due to cross-reactions with guinea pig antibody; the confirmatory neutralization test will detect these reactions.[44]

A variety of methods are available for the detection of HBsAg: (1) agar gel diffusion, (2) counterelectrophoresis, (3) complement fixation, (4) radioimmunoassay, (5) latex agglutination, and (6) reverse passive hemagglutination. The radioimmunoassay (RIA) test is significantly more sensitive than the other methods and detects 40-60% more positive cases than do the others (except reverse passive hemagglutination [RPH]).[45,46] Agar gel diffusion (AGD) is extremely undersensitive and is no longer used for routine testing. It is useful, however, in confirming positive results of other tests by detecting lines of identity by the Ouchterlony modification. As of September 15, 1975, the United States' Food and Drug Administration[47] required that all blood for transfusion must be tested by a third generation test, i.e., RIA or RPHA.

Agar gel diffusion (AGD)[48]

The HBsAg was discovered by using the immunodiffusion (AGD) method of Ouchterlony. AGD is characterized by the diffusion of homologous antigen and antibody toward each other in a semisolid medium where a precipitin reaction occurs at or near a point of optimal proportions. AGD is performed by introducing reactants (antigen and antibody) into separate and opposite wells in an agar gel. Reactants diffuse radially out of their wells, and a visible precipitate forms in a region where there are proper proportions. AGD detects 20-40% of blood donors who are carriers of the antigen. This system is now used primarily for identification or confirmation of precipitin bands by means of so-called "lines of identity."

Several factors affect the formation of percipitin bands and the quantity of precipitate formed.

Excessive concentration of HAA antibody may form soluble antigen-antibody complexes and fail to develop percipitin bands when tested against donor blood containing very low level hepatitis associated antigen. The speed at which the precipitin lines are formed is greater when the temperature is high (37 C), but the quantity of precipitate formed is greater at lower temperatures; therefore it is advisable to keep the agar plates during the diffusion stage at approximately 25 C (room temperature) and in a slightly humid atmosphere.

Other factors that influence the AGD test are pH, electrolyte concentration, and agarose concentration. However, the most important factor is the quantitative ratio of antigen to antibody taking part in the reaction. When optimal concentrations are present, the precipitin lines are sharp.

Reagents
1. 2.0M Sodium chloride solution
2. 0.5M Tris HCl, pH 7.0
3. 0.05M Ethylenediaminotetraacetate (EDTA)
4. Tris buffer

2.0M NaCl	50 ml
0.5M Tris HCl	20 ml
0.05M EDTA	2 ml

   a. Dilute the 1 L with distilled water.
5. 1% Agarose in tris buffer

Agarose	1 g
Tris buffer	100 ml

   a. Dissolve in boiling water bath.
   b. Store at 4-10 C.
   c. Melt in boiling water bath for use.

Procedure
1. Pour 15 ml molten agarose into each Petri dish and allow to harden at room temperaaure. When agarose has hardened, place plates in humidified chamber at 25 c for 24 h and then store at 4-10 C until used.
2. Just prior to use, punch wells 3 mm in diameter and 5 mm from center well according to diagram below.

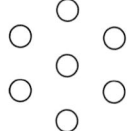

3. Remove agarose from wells with Pasteur pipet attached to vacuum source.
4. As diagrammed below, fill peripheral wells with serum specimens from donors and with control reagents, **using separate** disposable Pasteur capillary pipet for each sample. Be careful not to overfill wells. Positive and negative controls for HBsAg should be run in each rosette.

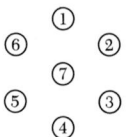

Well 1	Positive HBsAg control serum
Well 2	Donor serum or plasma
Well 3	Donor serum or plasma
Well 4	Negative control serum

Well 5   Donor serum or plasma
Well 6   Donor serum or plasma
Well 7   HBs antibody
5. With disposable Pasteur capillary pipet, fill center with HBs antibody. **Do not overfill wells.**
6. Place immunodiffusion plates in humidified container, place container on level surface, and incubate at 25 C.
7. After 24 h incubation, read plates for immunoprecipitin lines by holding them obliquely under fluorescent desk lamp against black background in darkened room. Approximately 90% of positive serums can be detected after 24 h incubation; however, 48 h incubation may be required to detect serum with low levels of antigen.
8. Plates are kept in humidified chamber for at least 7 d before final reading.
Concentration of serum. Sensitivity of the immunodiffusion test can be increased by concentrating the donor serum with Lyphogel granules as follows:
1. Add 80 mg desiccated acrylamide gel (Lyphogel, Gelman Instrument Co., Ann Arbor, Mich.) to 0.5 ml donor serum.
2. Allow mixture to react for 5 h at 4 C. This concentrates donor serum 5-fold and is used to charge well.
3. Fill well 3 times with serum concentrate in order to achieve a sensitivity similar to that of CEP.

Counterelectrophoresis (CEP)[49]

In 1970 Gocke and Howe[50] reported an electrophoretic procedure, termed "counterelectrophoresis," for the detection of HBsAg. CEP is a modification of the gel diffusion technic; it makes use of the phenomenon of endosmosis to move reactants together in an electric field. In this method the hepatitis antigen and its homologous antibody are placed in opposite wells, parallel to the direction of electric force. An electric current is applied to the test preparation, causing the antigen (HBsAg) to migrate toward the anode and the antibody (anti-HBsAg) toward the cathode by endosmotic flow. Although anti-HBs (γ-globulin) has a net negative charge in the buffer employed in the CEP test, it is unable to move against the endosmotic flow of the buffer; therefore the antibody is carried by buffer flow toward the cathode. The HBsAg also has a net negative charge, but the charge is higher and it migrates toward the anode. When these 2 substances meet in a zone of optimal proportions an immunoprecipitin line forms.

Conditions for performing CEP are critical, and the principles involved must be thoroughly understood to avoid nonspecific reactions. If conditions such as voltage (or amperage), ionic strength of buffer, type of agar, and temperature are not optimal, a reduction in specificity may occur. For this reason, details of CEP must be throughly understood.

CEP offers several practical advantages over AGD for detecting HBsAg: (1) sensitivity is increased; (2) antiserum need not be of extremely high potency; (3) there is a reduction of the time needed for formation of precipitin line; and (4) a large number of specimens can be tested simultaneously. CEP is 10-15 times more sensitive than AGD and will detect most carriers.

Reagents
1. Barbital (Veronal) buffer, pH 8.8, 0.05 μm
   Diethylbarbituric acid   1.84 g
   Sodium diethylbarbiturate   10.30 g
   Distilled water, to   1000.00 ml
   a. Adjust pH to 8.8 with approximately 0.5 ml 50% NaOH.
2. 1% Agarose (Bio-Rad Laboratories, Richmond, Calif.; Seakem [Marine Colloids, Inc., Rockland, Me.]) in barbital (Veronal) buffer, pH 8.8, 0.05 μm
   Agarose   5 g
   Barbital (Veronal) buffer   500 ml
   a. Bring into solution in boiling water bath. Agar gels should not be used freshly poured. Its ideal electrophoretic properties do not become manifest unless stored at least 1 h and preferably 24 h at 4 C after pouring to allow gel particles to equilibrate with contained buffer.
   b. Store unused plates in sealed plastic containers at 4-10 C.
3. Bridge buffer: barbital (Veronal) buffer, 8.8, 0.025 μm
   a. To prepare, dilute buffer in no. 1 above 1:2 with distilled water.
NOTE: For optimal detection of antigen anti-HBs antiserum should have a titer of no less than 1:4 by Ouchterlony immunodiffusion test or 1:8 by CEP when tested against 4 U HBS antigen (i.e., antigen containing serum with titer of 1:4) in test employed.

Precautions
1. Mouth pipetting of specimens and reagents should never be done. Always use disposable capillary pipets with or without hand-pipetting attachment.
2. Disposable plastic gloves should be worn when handling specimens and reagents since positive control antigen is employed in each day's test run.
3. All materials should be autoclaved prior to disposal.
4. Work area should be disinfected daily with solution of dihydrogen chloride (Clorox) or similar disinfectant known to have virucidal activity.
5. Always employ precautions usually taken in handling infectious materials in microbiology laboratory.
6. For optimal detection of antibody, antigen should have a titer of about 1:16 in CEP test. If too strong an antigen is used, low-level antibody will be missed.

Procedure
1. To a thoroughly clean 3¼ × 4 in. lantern slide apply 10 ml 1% agarose (melted in boiling water bath) in barbital (Veronal) buffer, pH 8.8, ionic strength 0.05 μm. Use leveling board for this step and coat to edges of slide. Prior to coating, wipe slides with isopropyl alcohol.
2. Allow agar to harden and then hold in moist chamber in refrigerator for at least 1 h prior to use. Store unused slides at 4-10 C.
3. Cut 3 rows of 12 paired wells 3 mm in diameter and 1 cm apart (i.e., 36 tests per plate). Opposing wells must be exactly parallel to top of plate; otherwise, path of migration will be suboptimal.
4. Thoroughly remove agar plugs from wells with Pasteur pipet attached to vacuum pump.
5. Hold plates in moist chamber in refrigerator until ready for use.

6. Set cold plate of electrophoretic cell to 23 C if equipped with refrigeration.
7. Apply each donor serum or plasma to well (antigen wells) on right (cathodal side) of each pair with Pasteur pipet, filling completely without overflowing. Continue to fill all antigen wells. Include positive and negative controls for hepatitis B agent on each plate.
8. Apply anti-HBs with Pasteur pipet to wells of each pair on anodal (positive) side, again completely filling wells (see diagram).

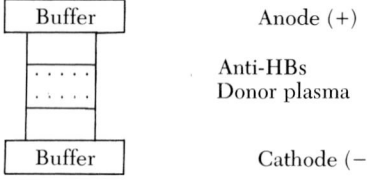

(Input 300 V, 40 mA/1 slide with TEC 400)
(Input 450 V, 40 mA/2 slides with TEC 400)

9. Place lantern slides on Mylar-covered flat plate of electrophoresis cell with donor specimen on negative (cathode) side and anti-HBs on positive (anode) side. Slides should be properly aligned for nondistorted electric flow. Align slides in parallel.
10. When running slides in series connect slides by filling a 1-2 mm separation between each with molten 1% agarose in barbitol (Veronal). Use Whatman 3MM filter paper (Whatman, Clifton, N.J.) to connect plates to buffer troughs. Filter paper wicks should be doubled and well soaked in buffer. Slides may be covered with thin Mylar sheet to retard evaporation during run.
11. Electrophoresis should be done for 1 h at 23 C, 12-15 V/cm (measured between edges of agar plate 30 min after start of run).
12. Read results immediately by holding lantern slide obliquely against fluorescent desk lamp with black background.
13. It is advisable to use fresh buffer for each run.

Reading results
1. Carefully clean bottom of each slide and read immediately.
2. To read slides, place over dark background and read by oblique illumination.
3. Turn lights out to darken room.
4. Read with magnifying lens as well as by unaided eye.

Interpretation
1. If precipitin line is not observed, specimen is reported as "HBsAg not detected by CEP."
2. If precipitin line develops between antiserum well and patient's serum, the specimen is reported as positive for HBsAg. Confirmation can be made by establishing a "line of identity" with a precipitin line from reactants of known HBsAg identity in the Ouchterlony AGD.

Additional comments
1. Serum or reagents contaminated with microorganisms may give nonspecific lines. It is therefore important to employ reasonable aseptic technic in handling these materials.
2. Lipemic serum will give a nonspecific white haze around well, which may mask a positive

reaction. Occasionally they tend to concentrate and precipitate between wells.
3. If CEP is carried out for too long a period, the reaction may be carried into the antigen well and may be missed.
4. Repeated filling of wells may cause many artifacts or multiple precipitin bands to develop as succeeding waves of serum migrate through agar.
5. Drying of agar will cause changes in salt concentration, ionic strength, pH, and porosity of agar. Rapid deterioration in optimal conditions for precipitation quickly occurs.

Complement fixation (CF) test for HBsAg[51]

Among the technics available for detection of HBsAg and antibody, the CF test is most useful for measuring antigen. Although more recent technics such as reverse passive hemagglutination and radioimmunoassay are far superior for measuring anti-BHs, the CF remains one of the most sensitive tests for titering antigen. Sensitivity of the CF test depends on the use of high titer (hyperimmune) antiserum. Because of limited availability of good CF antisera from human sources, attempts have been made to produce antibodies in animals.

Modification of the CF test (Chapter 93) permits the detection of antigen in patients's serum. With a given amount of antibody, CF is proportional to the HBs antigen concentration until an optimum is reached; thereafter, CF decreases with increasing antigen concentration. Because of this phenomenon, a very high titer of HBs antibody must be used to assure adequate antibody for detecting the highest concentration of HBsAg expected in the patient's serum. Antigen excess may give rise to a false-negative reaction; therefore dilutions of the patient's serum are commonly used to avoid this problem.

Procedure
1. For preparation of reagents, standardization of test components, controls, and general test procedures, refer to CF test in Chapter 93.
2. Make serial 2-fold dilutions from 1:4 to 1:2408 of patient's serum (heat activated at 56 C for 30 min) in 0.025 ml amounts in microtiter "μ" plate. Use barbital (Veronal) buffer to dilute serum.
3. Add 0.025 ml anti-HBs serum to each well with diluted patient's serum.
4. Add 0.05 ml complement (containing 5 CH_{50} U) to each well and incubate mixture at 4 C.
5. Next day remove from refrigerator and allow to stand at room temperature for 15 min. Place plate on vibrating platform and add 0.025 ml sensitized sheep RBC. Seal plate and incubate 30 min in 37 C water bath.
6. Centrifuge microtiter plate at 300 × g for 3 min.
7. Read results. Complement fixation is indicated by presence of unlysed red cells, which form button at bottom of well. Positive CF test is indicative of HBsAg. Record dilutions showing 0-30% hemolysis as positive for antigen.

Significance of anticomplementary (AC) activity

It has been noted that AC activity occasionally occurs to high titer in the serum of some patients positive for HBsAg. This activity is due to antigen-antibody complexes, which appear early in the course of hepatitis, disappear during the acute phase of the disease, and reappear in the recovery phase. AC activity at dilution of patient's serum greater than 1:4 is observed in approximately 20% of cases of acute hepatitis.

Radioimmunoassay (RIA)[52]

RIA is a third generation test that is now required for testing of donor blood. RIA is 250-1000 times more sensitive than CEP and slightly more sensitive than CF and RPH. Ausria II-125* is a "sandwich principle" solid phase RIA technic to measure HBsAg levels in serum. Plastic beads coated with anti-HBs (geinea pig) are incubated with patient's serum to detect HBsAg. When antibody tagged with ^{125}I is added, it binds to any HBsAg on the bead to create an antibody-antigen-antibody sandwich. Within limits, the greater the amount of antigen in the patient's serum, the higher the final radioactive count rate.

Procedure†
1. Place 1 bead into well for each patient's serum to be tested.
2. Add 0.2 ml patient's serum to well. Make certain antibody-coated bead is completely surrounded by specimen. Tap reaction tray to release any bubbles that may be trapped in specimen.
3. Set up 7 negative and 3 positive serum controls in similar manner.
4. Apply cover to seal tray and incubate for 2 h in 45 C water bath.
5. Remove tray from water bath and remove sealer. Rinse each well and bead with 10 ml distilled water and aspirate fluid with vacuum aspirator connected to tray containing 2.5% sodium hypochlorite as disinfectant. Washing and aspiration of fluid can be done simultaneously by using disposable pipet or cannula attached to vacuum and Cornwall syringe delivery system. To do this, place pipet attached to vacuum source into bottom of well and simultaneously slowly add 5 ml distilled water with Cornwall syringe. Repeat wash with 5 ml distilled water.
6. After all distilled water has been aspirated from wells, add 0.2 ml ^{125}I-hepatitis B antibody to bottom of each reaction well. Antibody-coated bead must be completely surrounded by antibody. Tap plate to release trapped bubbles.
7. Apply cover sealer to tray and incubate in 45 C water bath for 1 h.
8. Remove tray from water bath. Remove sealer, aspirate antibody solution from wells, and rinse wells and bead with two 5 ml portions of distilled water as in Step 5.
9. Transfer beads to counting tubes and place tubes in suitable well-type γ-scintillation counter to determine counts per minute. Count patient's specimens and controls together.

Results. Presence or absence of HBsAg is determined by relating net counts per minute of patient's serum to net counts per minute of negative control mean times the factor 2%.

If net count rate is higher than mean, cutoff value established with negative control is considered positive for HBsAg.

Mean value of positive controls should be at least 5 times the negative control mean; otherwise, the run should be repeated.

Calculation of cutoff value
1. Calculate negative control mean:

$$\frac{\text{Total count of 7 negative control}}{7} = \text{Net cpm (mean)}$$

2. Discard those individual values in negative control serum that fall outside the range 0.5-1.5 times mean. If more than one negative control value is consistently outside this range, technic should be carefully reviewed.
3. Calculate cutoff value by multiplying net negative control mean by factor 2.1. Unknowns whose net count rate is higher than cutoff value should be considered positive for HBsAg. NOTE: Many γ-counters do not have the capacity for automatically subtracting background. In such a case, one can avoid subtracting background manually and can use uncorrected sample counts per minute by using cutoff value modified as follows:
   (Negative control mean − background) × 2.1 + Background = Cutoff value
4. Calculate positive control: negative control ratio by dividing positive control mean value by negative control mean value after correcting for background. This ratio should be at least 5, or technic may be suspect and run should be repeated.

Interpretation. All HBsAg-positive RIA results must be confirmed by specificity analysis, using the AGD, CEP, CF, RPH, or the RIA neutralization test. If a repeat test shows the sample to be less than 2.1 times the negative control mean, the original result may be classified as a nonrepeatable positive and reported as negative for HBsAg.

Method for specificity confirmation of RIA-positive sera for HBsAg[53]

Several variables in the radioimmunoassay test for HBsAg can give rise to false-positive results and permanent exclusion of donors. One major cause of false-positive results is the presence in the serum of some individuals of antibodies to guinea pig protein, especially among those with allergy to animals. Therefore it is essential to confirm all RIA-positive tests by a special series of specificity-blocking reactions.

Test specimens that are positive by RIA should be confirmed by counterelectrophoresis. If the counterelectrophoresis test is negative, the RIA result must then be confirmed by the specificity verification procedure herein described.

Procedure*
1. Set up 4 Wassermann tubes. Add 0.1 ml patient's

---

*RIA reagents available from Abbott Laboratories, North Chicago, Ill., and Electro-Nucleonics, Bethesda, Md.
†Procedure for Ausria-II, Abbott Laboratories, North Chicago, Ill.

*Reagents for confirmation test are available from Abbott Laboratories, North Chicago, Ill.

Table 92-4. Specificity testing on 3 unknown samples

Inhibiting serum	Patient 1		Patient 2		Patient 3	
	cpm	*Ratio*	*cpm*	*Ratio*	*cpm*	*Patio*
GPS	482	1.2	1970	4.9	1165	2.9
IGPS	521	1.3	482	1.2	2000	5.0
NHS	1405	3.5	2048	5.1	2800	7.0
IHS	1648	4.1	521	1.3	3050	7.6

	Results	*Interpretation*
Patient 1	Inhibited by guinea pig protein	Not an Anti-HB Ag; hence not HB Ag positive
Patient 2	Inhibited by anti-HB Ag serum	True Ag positive
Patient 3	Partially inhibited by guinea pig protein	Possibly too strong an antibody to be inhibited in proportions used; repeat inhibitions with parallel dilutions of positive serum

serum to each tube. Then add to each tube the following reagents:

  Tube 1 0.01 ml normal guinea pig serum (GPS)
  Tube 2 0.01 ml guinea pig anti-HBs (IGPS)
  Tube 3 0.01 ml normal human serum (NHS)
  Tube 4 0.01 ml human anti-HBsAg (IHS)

2. Mix above tubes and incubate for 2 h at room temperature.
3. Transfer 0.1 ml from each inhibition tube to Austria tube.
4. Carry out RIA procedure as described for detection of HBsAg. NOTE: Since small dilution of weakly positive result may give negative results in all tubes, it is advisable to repeat RIA test on untreated serum in parallel with inhibition studies.

Calculation

1. Calculate results as follows: net cpm for test sample divided by mean of net cpm of negative control used in assay.
2. Express results as ratio as illustrated in following example:

$$\frac{\text{Original sample cpm}}{\text{Mean negative control cpm}} = \frac{1300}{400} = 3.25$$

• • •

An example of specificity testing on 3 unknowns is given in Table 92-4.

Neutralization confirmation (alternate method)*

Procedure

1. Add 0.2 ml patient's serum into each of 4 wells of plastic trays containing HBs antibody–coated beads.
2. Add 0.2 ml negative control serum to each of 7 wells containing HBs antibody–coated beads.
3. Add 0.2 ml positive control serum to each of 4 wells containing HBs antibody–coated beads.
4. Tap tray gently to immerse beads completely in liquid. Seal tray and incubate for 2 h in 45 C water bath.
5. Remove seal and completely aspirate fluid from all wells. Wash beads 3 times with 5 ml distilled water for each wash. Aspirate all water from wells.

---
*Reagents available from Abbott Laboratories, North Chicago, Ill.

6. Add 0.2 ml of known HBs antibody–positive serum (confirming antibody serum, Abbott laboratories) diluted 1:5 in saline to 2 of the 4 wells containing beads that were reacted with patient's serum; add 0.2 ml normal control serum to other 2 wells.
7. Add 0.2 ml normal control serum to each of 7 wells containing beads incubated with negative control serum.
8. Add 0.2 ml of known HBs antibody–positive human serum to 2 of the 4 wells used for positive control and 0.2 ml of normal control serum to other 2 wells.
9. Shake tray gently to immerse bead in reagents. Seal plate and incubate 1 h in 45 C water bath.
10. Remove sealer (but not reagents in wells) and add 0.2 ml of ^{125}I-HBs antibody. Shake tray gently to mix reagents.
11. Seal plate and incubate 3 h in 45 C water bath.
12. After incubation, remove sealer and aspirate fluid from all wells. Wash beads 3 times with 5 ml distilled water for each wash.
13. Transfer bead to counting tube and count for 1 min in well-type γ-scintillation counter.

Calculations

1. Calculate average gross cpm of duplicate tests on patient's serum and of 7 negative controls.
2. Calculate percent reduction in counts by using average gross cpm for each of reagents in formula below:

$$\frac{A - B}{A - C} \times 100 = \text{Percent reduction for patient's serum}$$

$$\frac{D - E}{D - C} \times 100 = \text{Percent reduction in positive control serum}$$

where A = average gross cpm (duplicate) for patient's serum reacted with normal control serum; B = average gross cpm (duplicate) for patient's serum reacted with known HBs antibody; C = average gross cpm for 7 negative control sera; D = average gross cpm (duplicate) for positive control serum reacted with normal control serum; E = average gross cpm (duplicate) for positive control serum reacted with known positive HBs antibody.

Interpretation. A specimen is considered as a confirmed positive result if its count rate is reduced by 50% or greater by known positive HBs antibody. However, the positive control count rate must be reduced by 50 or greater by similar antiserum for the test run to be considered valid.

Hemagglutination-inhibition test for detection of hepatitis B antigen[54]

The principle of the hemagglutination-inhibition (HI) test (reagents available form Electro-Nucleonics, Bethesda, Md.) for detecting HBsAg is competitive protein binding of a standard antibody by antigen in the patient's serum and antigen-coated RBC used as an indicator. The procedure is rapid and simple to perform and is highly sensitive and specific for the HBsAg. Concentrations of HBsAg in the range of 1-50 ng can be detected. Reverse passive hemagglutination (RPH; reagents available from Abbott Laboratories, North Chicago, Ill.) is a modification of this procedure in which antibody is used to coat RBC. The HI and RPH tests are considered as "third generation" sensitivity and nearly comparable to RIA. Thus, they are approved by the FDA as substitutes for RIA.

RPH and HI tests for HBsAg can be used also for detection of anti–hepatitis B by slight modification of the test procedure.

Preparation of RBC
1. Collect human group O blood into EDTA and mix with air for 5 min to oxygenate, since this appears to improve subsequent coating. Store at 4 C for 48 h prior to use. Blood can be used for up to 10 d after collection.
2. Wash cells 4 times in 30 vol saline for each wash. Final centrifugation is for 3 min at 3500 rpm.

Storage of coated RBC[55]
1. HBsAg-coated RBC are packed to yield a 55-65% hematocrit. A volume of plasma in EDTA removed from patient's blood from whom cells were collected is added to an equal volume of coated cells and mixed. To this mixture add 1 vol 40% sucrose in distilled water so that final mixture is made up of equal volumes of plasma, coated cells, and 40% sucrose.
2. Mix components and draw into syringe with 21-gauge needle.
3. Add RBC by drops from syringe into wide-mouth thermos flask containing 50 ml liquid nitrogen. As drop of RBC comes in contact with liquid nitrogen it floats for a few seconds before it is frozen and sinks to bottom of flask.
4. Frozen droplets are picked up from bottom of flask and transferred to plastic vial and closed with lid having 3 fine holes to permit liquid or gas to enter or escape while container is tightly closed. Place vials in liquid nitrogen storage tank.
5. When coated cells are needed, remove pellets from liquid nitrogen and put in tube containing at least 10 times their volume of saline at 37 C. Close tube with Parafilm (Fisher Scientific Co., McGraw Park, Ill.) and shake for 10 s. Wash cells twice with 30 times their volume in saline. Centrifuge for 30 s in serofuge. Cells are ready for use.

Coating cells
1. Prepare 1% $CrCl_3$ in distilled water. Store in dark glass bottle at 4 C for up to 7 d. Immediately prior to use, dilute 1:30 in saline.
2. Prepare solution or purified HBsAg protein (Electro-Nucleonics, Bethesda, Md.) in saline having concentration of 0.35 mg/ml. (Absorbance of 1.3 at 280 nm wavelength is equivalent to this concentration).
3. Prepare stock TSP buffer as follows:

Tween 80 (1:20 in saline)	1 ml
Polyvinylpyrrolidone (40,000 mol wt)	25 ml
Difco Hemagglutination Buffer (pH 7.2)	
Sodium azide	1 g
Distilled water	1000 ml

   a. Immediately before use add 3 ml human serum of lipoprotein type Ag (x+ y+), red cell type AB, which is also negative for HBsAg, and anti-HBs to 47 ml stock TSP buffer.
   b. Discard unused portion daily.
4. Determine optimal concentrations of HBsAg and $CrCl_3$ for coating procedure by checkerboard titration of these reagents, i.e., reacting varying concentrations of antigen with varying concentrations of $CrCl_3$.
5. To acid-washed 75 × 12 mm glass tube add 1 vol washed packed cells and an equal vol 0.35 mg/ml isolated purified HBsAg protein. Mix components. Add 1 vol 1:30 dilution 1% $CrCl_3$ and mix for 5 min at room temperature.
6. Wash coated cells in reaction mixture 4 times with saline, centrifuging at 3500 rpm for 30 s after each washing.
7. Suspend coated washed RBC in 10 vol saline. Add 1 vol of this cell suspension to 49 vol TSP buffer to obtain 0.1-0.2% cell suspension.

Standardization of anti-HB
1. Add 0.025 ml TSP buffer to each well of V-shaped microtiter plate.
2. Add 0.025 ml of 1:20 dilution of anti-HB to first well and serially dilute (2-fold dilutions) through twelfth well.
3. To each well add 0.025 ml 0.2% suspension of HBsAg-coated RBC.
4. Cell control consisting of 0.024 ml TSP buffer, 0.025 ml 1:20 dilution anti-HB, and 0.025 ml 2% suspension of uncoated RBC will serve as control for autoagglutination.
5. Seal plates and incubate for 1 h at room temperature.
6. Centrifuge plates in microtiter carrier by accelerating until speed reaches 1200 rpm (requires about 30 s) and then switch off.
7. Remove sealer from plate carefully and incline at 60° angle for 30 min. The unagglutinated cells will run down side of well as smooth stream and agglutinated cells remain at bottom of well as compact button.
8. Read end point of titration as highest dilution of anti-HB showing discrete button of agglutinated cells.
9. Dilution of anti-HB to be used in test for detection of HBs antigen is determined by dividing end point of titration by 4. This gives 4 agglutination units of antibody that is used in the test for antigen.

Procedure for detection of HBsAg
1. Add 0.025 ml TSP buffer to each of 5 wells of V-shaped microtiter plate.
2. Add 0.025 ml patient's serum to first well and make serial 2-fold dilutions through well 5.
3. Add 0.025 ml anti-HB containing 4 units as previously determined.

4. Mix and incubate for 5 min at room temperature.
5. Add 0.025 ml HBsAg-coated RBC.
6. Set up following controls:
   a. Known HBsAg-positive serum.
   b. Known HBsAg-negative serum.
   c. Agglutinator control: 4-well serial 2-fold dilution of 4 units of antibody dilution used in test; serves as back-titration of antibody.
   d. Cell control: 0.025 ml TSP Buffer and 0.025 ml 0.2% cell suspension.
   e. Alloantibody control: 0.025 ml 1:2 dilution of test serum and 0.025 ml 0.2% suspension of uncoated RBC.
7. Seal plates and incubate at room temperature for 1 h.
8. Centrifuge plates and read results of agglutination as described in Step 7 under "Standardization of Anti-HBs." Agglutinated cells form compacted button on bottom of well, while unagglutinated cells tend to stream down side of well when plate is inclined.

Interpretation
1. If HBsAg is present in patient's serum, the anti-HB combines and is unavailable for agglutination of HBsAg-coated RBC. Thus no agglutination indicates presences of HBsAg in patient's serum.
2. If agglutination occurs in all wells containing dilutions of patient's serum, this is interpreted as absence of HBsAg.
3. Positive control serum should inhibit agglutination, and negative control serum should not inhibit. Agglutinator control should show agglutination in the first 2 dilutions only, and cell control should not agglutinate.

DOUBLE IMMUNODIFFUSION TEST FOR INFLUENZA VIRUSES[56,57]

Recently, influenza A viruses have been found to contain a common antigenic matrix protein (MP or membrane protein), which is shared by all strains regardless of the specificity of their HA and NA antigens. Influenza B has a different matrix protein. Therefore it is possible to rapidly identify isolates by the double immunodiffusion test, particularly when the viruses do not react in the HI test with available strain-specific antisera.

By modifying double immunodiffusion (DID) test described for the HBsAg in the manner shown below, it is possible to identify isolates of influenza and other viruses.

Reagents
1. Sodium lauroyl sarcosinate (Sarkosyl NL-97, Geigy Industrial Chemicals, Ardsley, N.Y.), 10%
   a. Add 80 ml distilled water to 100 ml volumeteric flask.
   b. Add 100 g Sarkosyl NL-97.
   c. Mix until dissolved.
   d. Then add distilled water to 100 ml and mix again.
2. Glycine-Sarkosyl NL-97 buffer
   a. Dissolve 0.925 g glycine to 20 ml distilled water in 25 ml volumetric flask.
   b. Adjust to pH 9.0 ± 0.05 with 1N NaOH.
   c. Add 2.5 ml 10% Sarkosyl NL-97 and distilled water to 25 ml.

Preparation of isolate. Acidify culture fluid containing viral isolate (at 4 C) by adding 1N HCl to obtain a final pH of 4.0 ± 0.5. Incubate in ice bath 60 min; then centrifuge at 1000 × g for 10 min at 4 C. Decant supernatant fluid and drain tube upside down on absorbent paper. Resuspend precipitate by adding 0.01 ml glycine-Sarkosyl NL-97 buffer (to disrupt virus) for each milliliter of original culture fluid and mix throughly on Vortex mixer. Use as antigen in DID test.

Performance of test
1. Add 10 μl each reference influenza A and B antiserum to outer wells 1 and 3; add 10 μl of each reference influenza A and B antigen to outer wells 4 and 5 of 6-well agar slide.
2. Allow to stand 15-20 min at room temperature with Petri dish cover to prevent drying of agar.
3. Add 10 μl viral isolate to center well and 10 μg negative control antigen to well 2.
4. Add 5 μl 10% Sarkosyl NL-97 to wells 4 and 5.
5. Incubate slide in moist chamber at 3.7 C for 24 h. Examine slides for precipitin lines of identity. If negative or difficult to read, return slide to Petri dish and flood with 0.85% saline to immerse slide. Allow to soak overnight at room temperature and make final examination of slide.

DIFFERENTIATION OF WILD TYPE AND VACCINE STRAINS OF POLIOVIRUS

With the widespread use of attenuated poliovirus vaccine the use of genetic markers of the virus to differentiate wild type from vaccine strains is common. It is important to characterize all poliovirus isolates from patients with clinical illness. Several markers are available, but the most useful are the "rct" marker and the intratypic serodifferentiation test. The rct marker is a measure of the ability of virulent strains to replicate at 40 C, while vaccine strains show little or no replication at this temperature. This marker test is simple to perform and correlates well with other genetic markers and with pathogenicity for monkeys.

Procedure
1. Prepare serial 10-fold dilutions from 10:1 to 10:6 in sterile serologic tubes (13 × 100 nm) for poliovirus isolate being characterized. Dilutions are made in Hanks BSS, and clean pipet is used for preparing each dilution.
2. Prepare similar dilutions for known attenuated and known unattenuated strain of poliovirus of same type as that isolated from patient.
3. Inoculate 3 tubes of RhMK tissue cell culture with 0.1 ml of each dilution of virus for virus isolate. Repeat process for both attenuated and unattenuated strains. Label properly with type of virus, dilution, temperature of incubation, and date. Place tubes in 36 C incubator.
4. Repeat Step 3 and place tubes **without delay** in 40 C incubator. It is important that tissue culture tubes are equilibrated to 40 C and held at this temperature during inoculation of virus.
5. Tubes at 36 C are read daily after 48 h incubation and CPE recorded.
6. Tubes at 40 C are incubated for 4 d before they are read. It is important that 40 C incubator **not be opened** during this interval. An internal high-low indicator thermometer or continuous recording

thermometer must be used to keep check on temperature.

7. Tissue culture controls to which 0.1 ml Hanks BSS has been added serve as controls for both 36 C and 40 C.

Interpretation

1. Wild, or virulent, strains of poliovirus have comparable titers at 36 C and 40 C.

2. Attenuated, or vaccine, strains of poliovirus have much lower titers at 40 C than at 36 C. Fully attenuated strains usually fail to replicate at 40 C. However, after a single passage in man, this characteristic may be partially or completely lost.

3. Report only those strains that are typically vaccinelike.

REFERENCES

1. McLean, D. M., Rhodes, A. J., Nagler, F. P., et al.: Can. J. Public Health **51**:100, 1960.
2. Syverton, J. T., Scherer, W. F., and Elwood, P.: J. Lab. Clin. Med. **43**:286, 1954.
3. Robbins, F. C., and Enders, J. F.: Am. J. Med. Sci. **220**:316, 1950.
4. Dalldorf, G., Sickles, G. M., Plager, H., and Gifford, R.: J. Exp. Med. **89**:567, 1949.
5. Dalldorf, G.: Ann. N.Y. Acad. Sci. **56**:583, 1953.
6. Kalter, S. S.: Proc. Soc. Exp. Biol. Med. **74**:607, 1950.
7. Diagnostic procedures for viral and rickettsial diseases, ed. 2, New York, 1956, American Public Health Association.
8. Melnick, J. L.: Ann. N.Y. Acad. Sci. **61**:754, 1955.
9. Cheatham, J. W.: Ann. N.Y. Acad. Sci. **81**:6, 1959.
10. Vogel, J., and Shelokov, A.: Science **126**:358, 1957.
11. Chanock, R. M., Parrot, R., Cook, K., et al.: N. Engl. J. Med. **258**:207, 1958.
12. Schmidt, N. J., Guenther, R. W., and Lennett, E. H.: J. Immunol. **87**:623, 1961.
13. Rosen, L.: Virology **17**:335, 1962.
14. Chanock, R. M. Johnson, K. M., Cook, M. K., et al.: Am. Rev. Respir. Dis. **81**:126, 1961.
15. Rosen, L., Am. J. Hyg. **71**:120, 1960.
16. Rosen, L., and Kern, J. K.: Proc. Soc. Exp. Biol Med. **107**:626, 1961.
17. Horta-Barbosa, L., Fucillo, D. A., Zeman, W., and Sever, J. L.: Nature **221**:974, 1969.
18. Howitt, B. F.: Proc. Soc. Exp. Biol. Med. **73**:443, 1950.
19. Beeman, E. A., Huebner, R. J., and Cole, R. M.: Am. J. Hyg. **55**:83, 1952.
20. Lennette, E. H.: Am. Rev. Respir. Dis. **83**:116, 1961.
21. Kalter, S. S., Casey, H., Jensen, K., et al.: Proc. Soc. Exp. Biol. Med. **100**:367, 1959.
22. Jensen, K. E. In American Public Health Association: Diagnostic procedures for viral and rickettsial diseases, ed. 2, New York, 1956, The Association.
23. Committee on standard serologic procedures in influenza studies: J. Immunol. **65**:353, 1950.
24. Lennette, H. E., and Schmidt, N. J. In American Public Health Association: Diagnostic procedures

for viral and rickettsial diseases, ed, 3, New York, 1964, The Association.
25. International Subcommittee on Virus Nomenclature: Int. Bull. Bact. Nomen. Taxon. **13**:217, 1963.
26. Hsuing, G. D.: Bact. Proc., p. 131, 1964.
27. Hayat, M. A.: Principles and Techniques of Electron Microscopy, New York, 1973, Van Nostrand Reinhold co.
28. Doane, F. W., Anderson, N., Zbitnew, A., and Rhodes, A. J.: Can. Med. Assoc. J. **100**:1043, 1969.
29. Almeida, J. D.: Can. Med. Assoc. J. **89**:787, 1963.
30. Almeida, J. D., and Waterson, A. P.: Adv. Virus Res. **15**:307, 1967.
31. Brenner, S., and Horne, R. W.: Biochem. Biophys. Acta **34**:103, 1959.
32. Kapikian, A. Z., Wyatt, R. G., Dolin, L., et al.: J. Virol. **10**:1075, 1972.
33. Horne, R. W.: Virus structure, New York, 1974, Academic Press.
34. Fleisett, T. H., Bryden, A. S., and Davies, H.: J. Clin. Pathol. **27**:603, 1974.
35. Parver, W. K., Caul, E. O., Ashley, C. R., and Clark, S. K. R.: Lancet 1:237, 1973.
36. Feinstone, S. M., Kapikian, A. Z., and Purcell, R. H.: Science **182**:1028, 1973.
37. Flewett, T. H., Bryden, A. S., and Davies, H.: Lancet **2**:1497, 1974.
38. Cruickshank, J. G., Bedson, H. S., and Watson, D. H.: Lancet **2**:527, 1966.
39. Hirsch, J. G., and Fedonko, M. E.: J. Cell Biol. **38**:615, 1968.
40. Harris, T. N., Hummeler, K., and Harris, S.: J. Esp. Med. **123**:161-172, 1966.
41. Hummeler, K., Henle, G., and Henle, W.: J. Bacteriol. **91**:1366, 1966.
42. Kofman, S.: Hepatitis B: a physician's guide to the disease and its associated hepatitis B (Australia) antigen, North Chicago, Ill., 1974, Abbott Laboratories.
43. Sutnick, A. I.: Med. Clin. North Am. **57**:1029, 1973.
44. Feinman, S. V.: Mod. Med. Can. **28**:21, 1973.
45. Lewis, J. H., and Coram, J. E.: Transfusion **12**:301, 1972.
46. Ling, C. M., and Overby, L. R.: J. Immunol. **109**:834, 1972.
47. Federal Register **40**:136 (July 16) 1975.
48. Ridell, N. M.: J. Clin. Invest. **42**:867, 1963.
49. Pesendorfer, F., Krassnitzky, O., and Wewalka, F.: Vox Sang. **19**:200, 1970.
50. Gocke, D. J., and Howe, C.: J. Immunol. **104**:1031, 1970.
51. Purcell, R. H., Holland, P. V., Walsh, J. H., et al.: J. Infect. Dis. **120**:383, 1969.
52. Walsh, J. H., Yallow, R., and Berson, S. J.: J. Infect. Dis. **121**:550, 1970.
53. Overby, L. R., Decker, R. H., and Ling, C. M.: Science 182:1368, 1973.
54. Vyas, G. N., and Shulman, N. R.: Science **170**:332, 1970.
55. Huntsman, I. G., Hurn, B. A., Ikin, E. W., et al.: Br. Med. J. **2**:1508, 1962.
56. Beard, C. W.: Bull. WHO **42**:779, 1970.
57. Dowdle, W. R., Galphin, M. T., Coleman, M. T., and Schild, G. C.: Bull. WHO **51**(3):213-215, 1974.

93

SEROLOGIC DIAGNOSIS OF VIRAL INFECTIONS

J. Mehsen Joseph

Serologic diagnosis is an indirect test in which the level (titer) of antibody in the patient's serum is determined for a specific virus. The tests most frequently used for this purpose are neutralization, hemagglutination-inhibition, and complement fixation. Most of the antigens used in these tests contain live virus, and extreme caution must be exercised. Immunization is recommended for certain neurotropic viruses, particularly poliomyelitis and the encephalitides.

Individuals vary considerably in their antibody response so that an absolute antibody titer cannot be established. Therefore diagnostic significance must be based on a rise in titer between acute and convalescent sera.

In all cases of serologic diagnosis an acute phase serum, taken as early in the course of disease as possible, and a convalescent phase serum, taken 14-21 days later, should be obtained whenever possible. Both sera must be tested simultaneously for the results to be meaningful.

A 4-fold or greater rise in antibody titer is diagnostic. Occasionally an antibody rise to more than 1 virus is observed and may be due to dual infection, antigenic crossing between groups (or types) of viruses, or anamnestic response as a result of previous exposure. Homotypic antibody usually persists longer than heterotypic antibody so that a third serum specimen taken 10-12 weeks after onset may reveal the infecting type.[1]

Diagnostic significance cannot be attached to a single acute phase serum, since antibodies may represent a previous clinical or subclinical infection or previous vaccination; a negative test does not rule out infection.

When only convalescent serum is available, a negative test rules out infection with the virus represented by the antigen used in the test; a positive test is significant only when the titer is as high as or higher than that usually found in persons recently recovered from a similar infection.

Mumps is one instance in which significance can be attached to any titer, in acute or convalescent sera, to the S (soluble) type complement-fixing (CF) antigen, since this antibody disappears shortly after the patient's recovery.

Neutralizing antibody to the enteroviruses usually appears in high titer at the onset of symptoms so that an aucte phase serum must be taken promptly or a rise may not be apparent.

In lymphocytic choriomeningitis, antibody appears late in the course of disease, and a third specimen may need to be taken 2-3 months after onset to demonstrate a rise.

As a general rule CF antibody appears later than neutralizing antibody; its peak titer is lower, and it does not persist as long. Therefore, as in the case of poliomyelitis, CF antibody is usually indicative of recent infection.

Serologic reactions serve 2 important purposes in virology: (1) to confirm that the virus isolated is the etiologic agent and not a latent or carriage strain and (2) to establish an etiology by means of a rising antibody titer in the absence of virus isolation.

Whenever a virus is isolated it should be used as the antigen instead of a stock strain of the same virus, as a more definitive rise in titer is observed.

Quantitation of virus 50% endpoint— Reed-Muench method[2]

Virus used in the neutralization test must be quantitated to determine the tissue culture infective dose ($TCID_{50}$) or the lethal dose (LD_{50}) in the case of animals. The use of a 50% endpoint tends to minimize chance variations that grossly affect a 100% endpoint.

Procedure
1. Prepare serial 10-fold dilutions of virus in Hanks BSS. Inoculate 0.2 ml of each dilution into each of 5 tissue culture tubes or 0.03 ml intracerebrally when mice are used.
2. Incubate tubes at 36 C for 8 d if monkey kidney cells are used and 4 d if cell lines such as HeLa are used.

Mice are observed for 12 d, and all deaths are recorded. Animals dying within 24 h after inoculation are not counted in total deaths, since this effect is due to trauma or toxicity of specimen and not to virus.[3]

Examine each tube for CPE with 100× magnification

Table 93-1. Arrangement of data and calculation of $TCID_{50}$*

Dilution of virus	No. showing CPE or deaths/ no. inoculated	Cumulative CPE or deaths	Cumulative non-CPE or survivals	Cumulative CPE or deaths	
				Fractional	Percent
10^{-4}	6/6	14	0	14/14	100
10^{-5}	4/6	8	2	8/10	80
10^{-6}	3/6	4	5	4/9	44
10^{-7}	1/6	1	10	1/10	10
10^{-8}	0/6	0	16	0/16	0

$$\frac{\%\ \text{Mortality above } 50\% - 50\%}{\%\ \text{Mortality above } 50\% - \text{Mortality below } 50\%} = \text{Proportional distance}$$

$$\frac{88 - 50}{88 - 44} = 0.85\ (\text{or } 0.9)$$

* $TCID_{50}$ endpoint = $10^{-5} + (0.9 \times 1) = 10^{-5.9}$. Antilog of 5.9 = 800,000. Dilution of virus containing 1-$TCID_{50}$/0.1 ml = 1:800,000. If 1:800,000 dilution contains 1-$TCID_{50}$, then 1:80,000 contains 10-$TCID_{50}$ and 1:8000 contains 100 $TCID_{50}$, which is used in the neutralization test.

and determine the 50% endpoint, according to Reed-Muench formula. An example is given in Table 93-1.[1]

Neutralization test in tissue culture

The presence and quantity of neutralizing antibody are measured by the ability of varying dilutions of serum to inhibit specific cytopathology in tissue culture or to protect highly susceptible animals against several lethal doses (LD_{50}) of specific virus. In the chick embryo the inhibition of pock formation on the chorioallantoic membrane (CAM) may be used as an endpoint.

Neutralization tests should be done in tissue culture instead of animals when the specific virus is known to produce a characteristic cytopathogenic effect (CPE) or metabolic change. The tissue culture neutralization test is used primarily for the viruses of poliomyelitis, coxsackievirus B 1-6, coxsackievirus A (types 9, 11, 13, 15, and 18), and echoviruses types 1-32.

In this procedure varying dilutions of the patient's serum are mixed with a constant amount of virus and are then incubated to allow antibody and virus to unite. Portions of each serum-virus mixture are inoculated into a susceptible host system, and after a suitable incubation period the host is examined for inhibition or neutralization of a specific viral effect.[4]

Procedure

1. Inactivate serum specimens at 56 C for 30 min to destroy nonspecific viral inhibitors that may be present.
2. Prepare serial 2-fold serum dilutions from 1:8 to 1:1024 in Hanks BSS. Mix 0.3 ml of each dilution with 0.3 ml test virus containing 100 $TCID_{50}$/0.1 ml. Incubate serum-virus mixtures for 1 h at room temperature and then inoculate 0.2 ml of each mixture into 2 tissue culture tubes.
3. Inoculate 1 tissue culture tube with 0.1 ml lowest dilution of serum used in test to determine its toxicity. Incubate 2 uninoculated tubes with test to serve as tissue culture controls.
4. Set up virus controls by inoculating 2 tissue culture tubes with 0.1 ml test virus dose (100 $TCID_{50}$/0.1 ml). Prepare 1:10, 1:100, and 1:1000 dilutions of test virus dose and inoculate 2 tubes

with 0.1 ml of each for each dilution. Control tubes thus prepared contain 100, 10, 1, and 0.1 $TCID_{50}$, respectively.
5. Incubate all tubes at 36 C and examine controls daily for CPE. When virus controls read 3-4, 2-3, 1-2, ± CPE, respectively, tubes inoculated with serum-virus mixtures should be read.
6. Record titer as reciprocal of highest dilution of patient's serum at which no CPE is detected.

Neutralization test in animals[5]

In this procedure varying concentrations of known virus are mixed with a constant amount of patient's serum and the mixtures are incubated for 1 hour at room temperature or ½ hour at 37 C to allow for interaction of antibody and virus. Then 0.03 ml of each serum-virus mixture is injected intracerebrally or intraperitoneally into susceptible animals that are observed daily for evidence of infection or death.[6]

Inactivation of serum is not recommended, as this destroys certain undetermined heat-labile accessory factors of importance in neutralization.

Set up the test according to the protocol shown in Table 93-2.

Procedure

1. Shake tubes to mix solutions and incubate for 1 h at room temperature or ½ h at 37 C. Inoculate 5 mice with 1 tube intracerebrally or intraperitoneally with 0.03 ml, working backward. Use a different needle and syringe for each row.
2. Observe animals twice daily for 12 d, keeping an accurate record of number that die in each set. Animals dying within 24 h after inoculation are not counted, since their death is usually attributed to trauma.
3. Use Reed-Muench formula to calculate LD_{50} for both acute and convalescent sera. From these results calculate neutralization index by subtracting log LD_{50} for acute serum from that for convalescent serum and taking antilog of difference. For example, if LD_{50} for acute serum is 10^{-4} and convalescent is 10^{-2}, difference $(4 - 2)$ is 2 and antilog of 2 is 100, which is neutralization index. An index of 50 or greater usually indicates infection; an index between 10 and 49 is questionable; an index below 10 is negative.

Table 93-2. Determination of neutralization index

Serum (ml) and virus (in 0.2 ml)	Tube				
	1	2	3	4	5
Row 1—negative serum	0.2	0.2	0.2	0.2	0.2
LD_{50} virus	1000	100	10	1	0.1
Row 2—positive serum	0.2	0.2	0.2	0.2	–
LD_{50} virus	10,000	1000	100	10	–
Row 3—acute serum	0.2	0.2	0.2	0.2	–
LD_{50} virus	1000	100	10	1	–
Row 4—convalescent serum	0.2	0.2	0.2	0.2	–
LD_{50} virus	10,000	1000	100	10	–

Antibody titration by the expensive and time-consuming animal neutralization test should be replaced whenever possible by CF test or tissue culture neutralization test.

Complement fixation (CF) test[1,7,8]

Commercially available CF antigens should be used, since they have been tested for hemolytic, anticomplementary, and antigenic activity.

A decision as to which CF antigens should be tested depends on the diagnosis and reliability of the technic. The following recommendations may be used as a guide:

Clinical diagnosis of infection of the central nervous system: eastern encephalitis, western encephalitis, St. Louis encephalitis, lymphocytic choriomeningitis, mumps (viral and soluble), herpes simplex, herpes zoster, and poliomyelitis
Clinical diagnosis of respiratory infection: influenza A and B, Q fever, psittacosis, adenovirus, respiratory syncytial virus, and parainfluenza (types 1, 2, 3, and 4).

The initial serum dilution recommended for the CF test is 1:4 for poliomyelitis and 1:8 for other viral (and rickettsial) antigens, to avoid nonspecific reactions encountered with more concentrated sera.

To reduce the amount of work involved in performing the CF test and to prevent a tremendous waste of reagents, it is highly recommended that all convalescent sera be screened at only a 1:8 dilution (1:4 for polio) and that those antigens for which the serum is reactive be used for titration. Acute phase sera should not be tested until after the convalescent sera have been screened.

Significant results are obtained only when acute and convalescent sera are tested simultaneously. A 4-fold or higher rise in titer is significant.

In the case of neurotropic viral diseases, serum CF antibody titers usually range from 1:32 to 1:64 and the rickettsial and psittacosis groups, from 1:128 to 1:256.

As a result of the thorough evaluation of the CF test, it has been standardized in every detail, and the new method is referred to as the LBCF test (Laboratory Branch CF test). The LBCF method is useful not only for viruses and rickettsiae, but also for fungi, mycoplasma, and bacteria. The test employs the 50% hemolytic endpoint instead of the previously used, less sensitive 100% endpoint. Commercial antigens and reagents for CF testing are being standardized by the LBCF method. Every effort should be made to adopt this procedure for CF.

Reagents
1. Stock barbital buffer (5 times)

NaCl	83.0 g
Sodium 5,5-Diethylbarbiturate	10.19 g
1N Hydrochloric acid	34.6 g
Stock solution	5.0 ml

   1M $MgCl_2$ and 0.3M $CaCl_2$ (20.33 g $MgCl_2 \cdot 6H_2O$ and 4.4 g $CaCl_2 \cdot 2H_2O$ in 100 ml distilled water)
   a. Transfer first 3 reagents listed above to a 2 L volumetric flask, add 500 ml distilled water, and mix thoroughly.
   b. Add $MgCl_2$-$CaCl_2$ stock solution and mix to dissolve.
   c. Fill to mark with distilled water and mix thoroughly.
   d. Check pH of stock buffer by making a 1:5 dilution with distilled water. pH of diluted stock must be 7.3-7.4. If pH is not in this range, discard and prepare fresh stock buffer. Refrigerate stock buffer.
2. Gelatin-water solution
   a. Add 1.0 g gelatin to 200 ml distilled water.
   b. Bring to boil to ensure solution.
   c. Cool to 25 C and make up to 800 ml with distilled water at room temperature.
   d. Chill in refrigerator.
   Do not hold longer than 1 wk to avoid contamination.
3. Veronal buffered diluent (VBD) containing 0.1% gelatin
   a. Add 4 vol gelatin-water to 1 vol stock buffer.
   b. Store in refrigerator. VBD should not be stored longer than 24 h. **ph of VBD must be 7.3-7.4.** This solution is used throughout test.
4. Alsever solution (modified)

Dextrose	20.5 g
Sodium citrate, $Na_3C_6H_5O_7 \cdot 2H_2O$	8.0 g
Citric acid, C_6H8O7	0.55 g
Sodium chloride	4.2 g
Distilled water to	1.0 L

   a. Sterilize by filtration through Millipore membrane, 0.22 μm pore size. pH should be 6.0-6.2.
   b. Store at 4 C.

Preservation of sheep erythrocytes

Sheep blood should be from a single sheep and collected in Alsever solution (pH 6.1) or 3.8% sodium in 1:1 volumes. Cells must be aged 5 days prior to use in CF test. Erythrocyte suspension is satisfactory for 1 month.

Sheep erythrocytes may be too susceptible or too resistant to action of hemolysin and complement. Reactivity level of a complement fixation technique is greatly influenced by the quality of sheep cells.

Occasionally red blood cells will be found to be very resistant to the hemolytic action of complement and hemolysin. Comparative hemolysin and complement titrations always should be made when new cells are obtained.

The only solution to either of the above situations is to discard the unsatisfactory cells and obtain a new supply.

Standardization of sheep erythrocytes

Target absorbance

Construction of standard cyanmethemoglobin curve. Prepare dilutions of cyanmethemoglobin (cmg) standard in cmg reagent (Hycel, Houston, Tex.) containing 60, 40, and 20 mg/100 ml cmg. Read absorbance of 80% standard, each dilution prepared, and cmg reagent (representing 0 mg/100 ml cmg) in a spectrophotometer at 540 nm wavelength. These readings should fall on a straight line when plotted on regular graph paper against the mg/100 ml cmg of the standards.

Calculation of factor for target absorbance. Factor = Sum of concentrations of standards (80 + 60 + 40 + 20 + 0) divided by the sum of absorbance readings of the standards.

Calculation of target absorbance. Target absorbance = Target mg/100 ml cmg (target mg/100 ml cmg for 2.8% sheep erythrocytes = 35.940) divided by the factor. Factor and target absorbance 540 can be used for all subsequent cell standardizations made with same spectrophotometer, provided the instrument is not moved or unduly jarred.

Preparation of 2.8% erythrocyte suspension. Wash erythrocytes 3 times in 2 vol cold Veronal buffered diluent (VBD), centrifuging at 900x *g* for 10 minutes in a graduated conical centrifuge tube for each wash. Carefully remove supernatant and buffy coat after each wash. After third wash, read packed cell volume and dilute in VBD to 4% cell suspension. If supernatant is not colorless on second washing, cells are too fragile and should not be used. Be certain to prepare enough volume of 4% suspension for a few days. Store at 4 C for no longer than 2 days. Prepare a 2.8% erythrocyte suspension daily as follows:

1. Transfer 1.0 ml 4% suspension to 25 ml volumetric flask. Fill to mark with cmg reagent, mix well, and let stand for 15-45 min at room temperature until cells are lysed.
2. Centrifuge a sample of cell solution at 900x *g* for 10 min and transfer supernatant to a spectrophotometer cuvette.
3. Read absorbance at 540 nm against a reagent blank set at zero. Check a reading of absorbance of a 1:2 dilution of standard cmg (40 mg/100 ml cmg) against standard curve.

4. Calculate dilution necessary to obtain desired 2.8% erythrocyte suspension as follows:

$$\frac{\text{(Absorbance of test suspension)} \times \text{(Volume of 4\% cell suspension)}}{\text{Target absorbance}} =$$

Final volume of 2.8 cell suspension

5. Dilute to 2.8% cell suspension in VBD.

When 2.8% standardized cell suspension shows any degree of lysis after overnight storage in refrigerator, these sheep cells are too fragile for use.

Alternate method

Sheep cell suspension may be standardized by the centrifugation method.

Procedure
1. Prepare 2.8% cell suspension (approx. 670,000 cells/mm³) by adding 34.7 vol VBD to 1 vol packed sheep cells. Shake flask gently to ensure even suspension.
2. To check density of 2.8% suspension, pipet 14.0 ml into graduated centrifuge tube and centrifuge at 600× *g* for 10 min. A 14.0 ml aliquot of properly prepared cell suspension will produce 0.4 ml packed cells. When packed cell volume is under or above 0.4 ml point, cell suspension should be adjusted.

Quantity of VBD that must be added to or removed from cell suspension is determined by following formula:

$$\frac{\text{Actual reading of centrifuge tube}}{\text{Correct reading of centrifuge tube}} \times$$

Volume of cell suspension =

Corrected volume of cell suspension

Example 1 (low density):

Volume of cell suspension	100 ml
Centrifuge tube (15 ml) reading	0.38 ml

$$\frac{0.38 \text{ ml}}{0.40 \text{ ml}} \times 100 \text{ ml} = 95 \text{ ml}$$

Therefore 5 ml VBD should be removed from each 100 ml cell suspension. Centrifuge cell suspension and pipet off desired volume for discard.

Example 2 (high density):

Volume of cell suspension	100 ml
Centrifuge tube (15 ml) reading	0.43 ml

$$\frac{0.43 \text{ ml}}{0.40 \text{ ml}} \times 100 = 107.5$$

Therefore 7.5 ml VBD should be added to each 100 ml cell suspension. Adjusted cell suspension should be rechecked by centrifuging a 14 ml portion.

NOTE: Keep cell suspension in refrigerator when not in use. Always shake flask gently before use to secure an even suspension of erythrocytes.

Preparation of hemoglobin color standards

Color standards are used for reading hemolysin, complement, and antigen titrations. The 30% standard along with adjacent ones for comparison are used for determination of positive

Table 93-3. Labeling in preparation of standards

Percent hemolysis	Hemoglobin solution (ml)	0.28% cells (ml)
0	0.1	1.0
10	0.1	0.9
20	0.2	0.8
30	0.3	0.7
40	0.4	0.6
50	0.5	0.5
60	0.6	0.4
70	0.7	0.3
80	0.8	0.2
90	0.9	0.1
100	1.0	0.0

Table 93-4. Preparation of hemolysin dilutions

Hemolysin dilution (1 ml)		Diluent (ml)		Final dilution of hemolysin
1:100	+	9.0	=	1:1000
1:1000	+	1.0	=	1:2000
1:1000	+	1.5	=	1:2500
1:1000	+	2.0	=	1:3000
1:1000	+	3.0	=	1:4000
1:1000	+	7.0	=	1:8000

and negative results in the diagnositc test. These standards are prepared by combining hemoglobin solution and 0.28% cell suspension as follows:

1. Hemoglobin solution
   a. Pipet 1.0 ml 2.8% cell suspension into 15 × 125 mm test tube.
   b. Add 7.0 ml distilled water and shake mixture until all cells are lysed.
   c. Add 2.0 ml **stock buffer** solution to restore tonicity and mix thoroughly.
2. 0.28% Cell suspension
   a. Pipet 1.0 ml 2.8% cell suspension into 15 × 125 mm test tube, add 9.0 ml VBD, and mix thoroughly.
   b. Label 11 serologic tubes with percentage of hemolysis shown and add hemoglobin solution and 0.28% cell suspension as shown in Table 93-3.
   c. Shake tubes and centrifuge at 600× g for 5 min. Remove from centrifuge without agitation. Store in refrigerator to prevent excessive change in color. Color standards, prepared for reading complement titration, are used next day to read tests.

Hemolysin titration

Procedure

Hemolysin solution (1:100)

VBD	94.0 ml
Phenol, 5%, in 0.85% saline	4.0 ml
Glycerinized hemolysin	2.0 ml

Mix phenol well with VBD before hemolysin is added. Store 1:100 hemolysis solution at refrigerator temperature. Discard if found to contain precipitate. Dilutions of hemolysin of 1:1000 or greater are prepared by making further dilutions of 1:100 solution (Table 93-4).

Determination of hemolysin dilution needed for sensitization of 2.8% sheep cells. Although variation between cells from individual sheep is recognized, a single titration on a particular lot of 1:100 hemolysin solution is generally sufficient.

1. Place 6 tubes, 15 × 125 mm, in rack and label with hemolysin dilutions shown in right column of Table 93-4. Prepare dilutions for titration as shown in Table 93-4. Thoroughly mix each dilution.
2. Label 6 serologic tubes with correct hemolysin dilutions. Add 1.0 ml standardized 2.8% sheep cell suspension to each tube.

3. Add 1.0 ml each hemolysin dilution (1:1000 thru 1:8000) to 1.0 ml portions sheep cell suspension with constant swirling of contents. Incubate 15 min at 25 C. After incubation period, sheep erythrocytes are **sensitized cells** ready for use.
4. Label 6 serologic tubes with hemolysin dilutions. To each tube add 0.4 ml cold VBD and 0.4 ml 1:400 complement dilution (see below). Immediately add 0.2 ml cells sensitized with series of hemolysin dilutions to properly labeled tube. Mix and incubate in 37 C water bath for 1 h. Centrifuge to pack. Read percent hemolysis in each tube by comparison with color standards.
5. Amount of hemolysis obtained with each dilution of hemolysin is plotted on ordinary graph paper as shown in Fig. 93-1. Optimal dilution of hemolysin is determined from graph by inspection. Select a dilution such that further increase in hemolysin does not appreciably change percent lysis. **Optimal hemolysin dilution** is second dilution on "plateau," or 1:2000 (Fig. 93-1). This optimal dilution will ensure a slight excess of hemolysin required for uniform reproducibility.

Sensitized cells for complement and antigen titrations as well as diagnostic tests are prepared by adding 1 vol optimal hemolysin dilution to 1 vol standardized 2.8% cell suspension with rapid swirling. Incubate for 15 min at 25 C before use.

Preparation of 1:400 complement (C') dilution. To make 1:400 dilution of C', draw up undiluted C' in 1.0 ml pipet beyond 0.6 ml mark. Wipe tip of pipet and return excess C' above 0.6 ml mark to stock container. Deliver 0.25 ml of C' (without using last 0.1 ml graduation of pipet) into 99.75 ml cold VBD. **Diluted C' must be kept cold and must be used within 2 h.**

Commercial complement diluted 1:400 generally will yield 30-80% hemolysis for optimally sensitized cells as shown in Fig. 93-1. However, with a less active complement it may be necessary to use a 1:300 dilution for titrations, whereas with a very potent complement it would be necessary to use a 1:500 dilution so that correct percent hemolysis can be obtained for plotting curves.

Complement titration

Complement must be titrated each time tests are run.

Procedure

1. Prepare sensitized cells.
2. Prepare 1:400 dilution of C'.
3. Label 4 serologic tubes and add reagents in order shown in Table 93-5. For greater accuracy, perform titration in duplicate and use average hemolysis for each dilution.
4. Shake tubes and place in 37 C water bath for 30 min. Shake once at 15 min.
5. Centrifuge tubes to pack cells. Determine percent

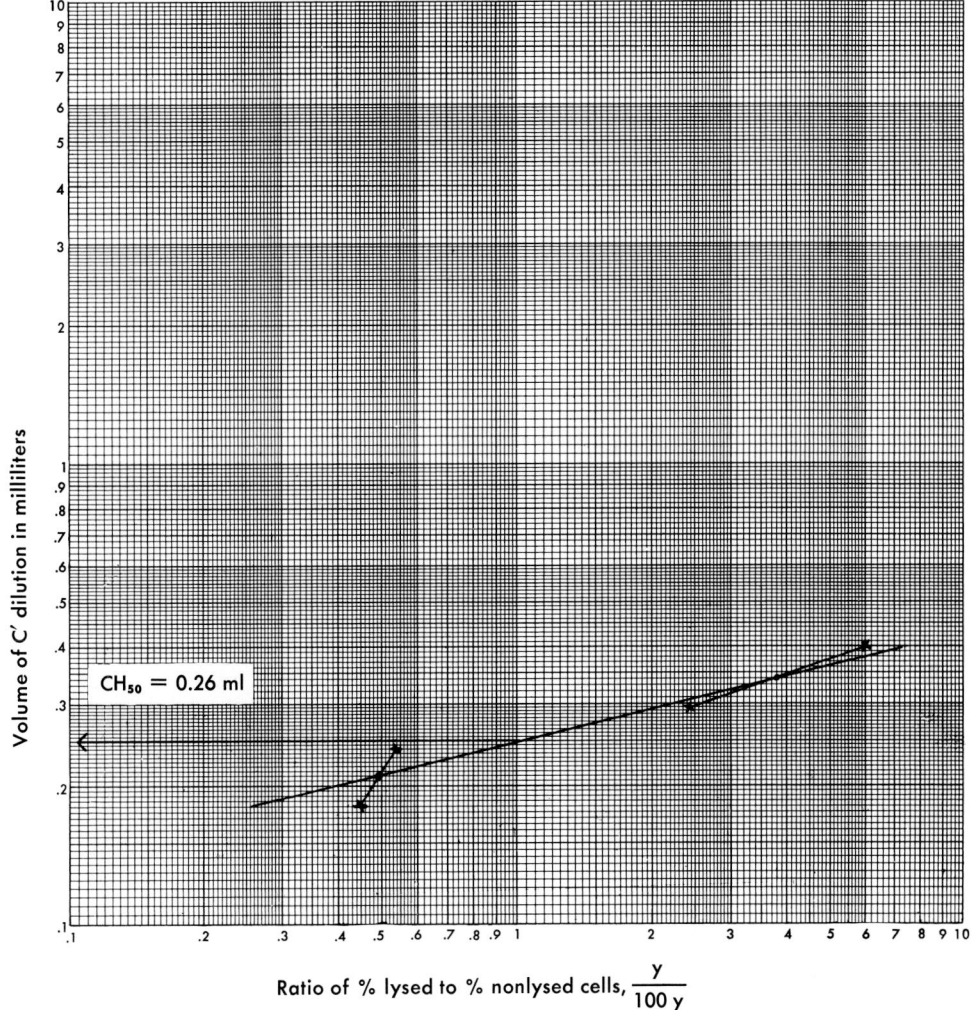

$CH_{50} = 0.26$ ml

Volume of C' dilution in milliliters

Ratio of % lysed to % nonlysed cells, $\dfrac{y}{100\ y}$

Fig. 93-1. Titration of complement.

Table 93-5. Complement titration

	Tube number			
	1	2	3	4
VBD (ml)	0.6	0.55	0.5	0.4
1:400 dilution of C' (ml)	0.2	0.25	0.3	0.4
Sensitized cells (ml)	0.2	0.2	0.2	0.2

hemolysis in each tube by comparing with color standards, interpolating to nearest 5% when a tube does not exactly match one of standards.

6. To determine a 50% unit of complement (1 C'H50) proceed as follows:

Example:

1:400 C' dilution "V" (ml)	Reading in percent hemolysis ("y")	Ratio $\dfrac{"y"}{100\text{-}y}$
0.20	30	0.43
0.25	35	0.54
0.30	70	2.33
0.40	85	5.7

The chart above converts percent hemolysis "y" to the ratio of percent lysed cells to percent nonlysed cells, $\dfrac{"y"}{100\text{-}y}$. For instance, for 35% hemolysis the corresponding value of the ratio $\dfrac{"y"}{100\text{-}y}$ is 0.54. For each of the 4 tubes plot the volume of C' 1:400 in milliliters against ratio found in chart. Join the 2 points plotted for

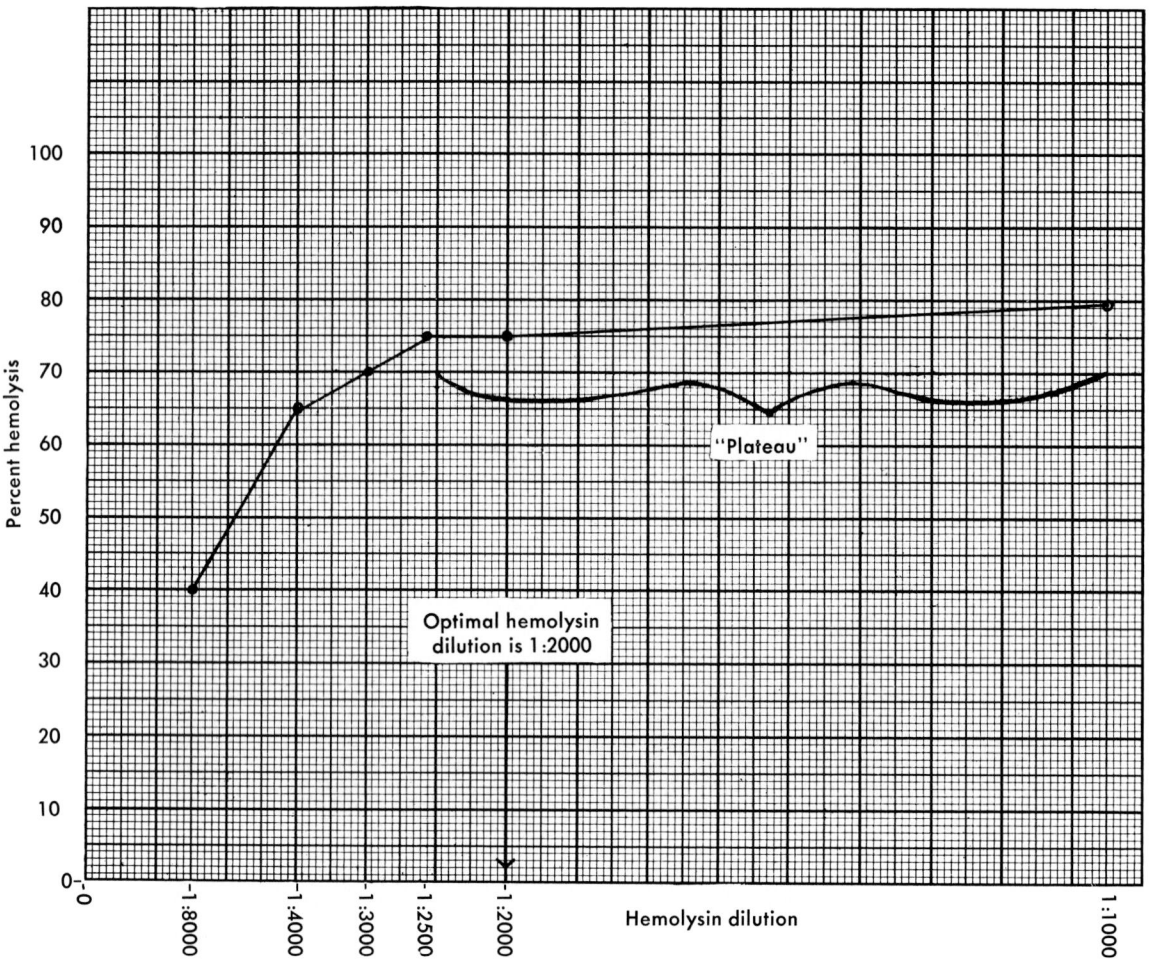

Fig. 93-2. Hemolysin titration.

Table 93-6. Ideal antigen titration (percent hemolysis)

Antigen dilutions* (Use 0.2 ml of each dilution)	Antiserum dilutions (Use 0.2 ml of each dilution)						Complement controls (Number of 50% units)		
	1:8	1:16	1:32	1:64	1:128	1:256	5	2.5	1.25
1:2	0	0	30	90	100	100	100	70	0
1:4	0	0	0	50	70	100	100	90	0
1:8	0	0	0	30	70	100	100	90	0
1:16	0	0	0	40	80	100	100	100	30
1:32	0	0	0	50	80	100	100	100	50
1:64	0	0	30	70	100	100	100	100	50
1:128	50	80	80	100	100	100	100	100	50
1:256	80	100	100	100	100	100	100	100	50
Control antigen	0	0	0	30	70	100	100	90	10
Serum control (1:8)							100	100	50
Tissue control	100	100					100	100	50
VBD							100	100	50

*Optimal antigen dilution in this example is 1:8.

the first 2 tubes and find midpoint (Fig. 93-2). Do the same for the last 2 tubes. Draw a line through the 2 midpoints. Draw a horizontal line through the intersection of this line with the heavy vertical line for a ratio of 1, and read the C'H50 in milliliters of the C' 1:400. **Five C'H50** are required in the test proper.

In the chart the C'H50 is 0.26 ml. Five units are contained in 1.3 ml (5 × 0.26) of the 1:400 dilution. The dilution of C' necessary to obtain 5 C'H50 in 0.4 ml is calculated as follows:

$$\frac{1.3}{400} = \frac{0.4}{x}$$
$$1.3x = 160$$
$$x = 123$$

Hence, 0.4 ml of a 1:123 dilution of complement contains 5 C'H50.

Antigen titration

Dilution of antigen to be used in the test is determined by a checkerboard titration with serial dilutions of a specific "high-titered" antiserum against serial dilutions of antigen as shown in Table 93-6. Total volume in all tubes is 1.0 ml.

1. Prepare 1:8 dilution of antiserum in VBD and inactivate at 56 C for 30 min. Prepare serial dilutions from inactivated serum.
2. Prepare master serial dilutions of antigen, beginning with 1:2 and going beyond expected range of activity.
3. Add 0.2 ml serum dilutions to appropriate tubes as shown in Table 93-6. Add 0.2 ml each antigen dilution to serum dilutions and complement controls. Mix and let stand 10-15 min at room temperature.
4. Add 0.4 ml cold complement containing 5 C'H50 to each tube containing both serum and antigen.
5. Add reagents to complement controls as in Table 93-7.
6. Shake tubes well and place in refrigerator for 15-18 h.
7. Remove tests from refrigerator and allow to stand at room temperature for 15 min while sensitized cells are prepared.

8. Add 0.2 ml sensitized cells to each tube and place in 37 C water bath for 30 min.
9. Centrifuge all tubes not showing **complete** lysis and read by comparison with color standards.

Selection of optimal antigen dilution. "Optimal antigen dilution" is defined as that dilution giving the highest titer with the specific antiserum. Draw a line, known as the **optimal dilution curve,** through the 30% hemolysis endpoints of each antigen dilution, interpolating if necessary. Also examine data for evidence of optimal fixation to the right of this curve, since this will often help in selection of optimal antigen dilutions. In Table 93-6 the 1:8 dilution would be selected as **optimal.** The 1:2 dilution of antigen is anticomplementary (AC) since the 2.5 complement control tube shows less than 85% hemolysis. Acceptable per cent hemolysis in complement control tubes is shown below:

Type of control	Number of 50% units of complement		
	5	2.5	1.25
Antigen	100	85-100	0-75
VBD	100	90-100	40-75
Serum (used for antigen titration)	100	90-100	0-75
Tissue	100	85-100	0-75

Perform a screening test with the 1:8 dilution of patient's serum as follows. If the screen is positive, titer serum. Acute and convalescent sera are tested simultaneously.

1. Prepare a 1:8 dilution of patient's serum in VBD and inactivate for 30 min at 56 C.
2. Cool to room temperature (prepare serial dilution of screen test positives) and transfer 0.2 ml to tubes as shown in Table 93-8. Prepare controls using a known negative serum and appropriate dilutions of a positive serum for each antigen.
3. Add 0.2 ml optimal dilution of antigen (freshly prepared in VBD) to appropriate tubes. Add 0.2 ml normal tissue control antigen at same dilution as test antigen to appropriate tubes.
4. Add 0.2 ml VBD to serum control tubes instead of antigen.
5. Prepare complement dilution to contain 5 C'H50 in 0.4 ml 15-30 min before addition to test by adding C' to cold VBD. Mix gently to avoid foaming. Keep diluted complement cold prior to and during addition to test.
6. Add volumes of cold diluted C' as shown in Table 93-8 and shake to mix. Incubate at 4-6 C for 15-18 h.
7. Remove from refrigerator and leave at room temperature for 15 min.
8. Add 0.2 ml sensitized cells to all tubes. Mix to ensure uniform suspension of cells and place in 37 C water bath for 30 min.
9. Centrifuge tubes not showing complete lysis. Read by comparison with 20%, 30%, and 40% color standards. Provided all controls are satisfactory, record tubes showing 0-30% hemolysis as positive and remainder as negative. Complement control readings are summarized under complement controls. Sera are reported as anticomplementary (AC) if serum control, 1:8 screen

Table 93-7. Addition of reagents (ml) to complement controls

Complement control	Reagents needed	Number of 50% units of complement		
		5	2.5	1.25
Antigen	Antigen	0.2	0.2	0.2
	Complement	0.4	0.2	0.1
	VBD	0.2	0.4	0.5
Serum (1:8)	Serum	0.2	0.2	0.2
	Complement	0.4	0.2	0.1
	VBD	0.2	0.4	0.5
VBD	Complement	0.4	0.2	0.1
	VBD	0.4	0.6	0.7
Tissue	Tissue extract	0.2	0.2	0.2
	Complement	0.4	0.2	0.1
	VBD	0.2	0.4	0.5

Table 93-8. CF test procedure

Tube	Reagents	Serum (ml)	Test antigen (ml)	Tissue antigen (ml)	VBD (ml)	Complement (5 C'H50 in 0.4 ml)*	Sensitized cells (ml)†
1	Test serum	0.2‡	0.2			0.4	0.2
2	Serum control	0.2§			0.2	0.4	0.2
3	Antigen control‖						0.2
a	5U complement		0.2		0.2	0.4	0.2
b	2.5U complement		0.2		0.4	0.2	0.2
c	1.25U complement		0.2		0.5	0.1	0.2
4	Tissue control¶	0.2		0.2		0.4	0.2
5	VBD Control						
a	5U complement				0.4	0.4	0.2
b	2.5U complement				0.6	0.2	0.2
c	1.25U complement				0.7	0.1	0.2
6	Sheep cell control				0.8		0.2

*Leave tubes at room temperature for 15 min before addition of complement.
†Incubate tests for 15-18 h at 4-6 C before addition of sensitized cells.
‡For 1:8 screening dilution and for serial serum dilutions.
§Control for anticomplementary activity of patient's serum.
‖Control for nonspecific fixation of complement.
¶Tissue controls for viral and rickettsial antigens.

dilution without antigen, reads less than 75% hemolysis.

Interpretation. When testing acute and convalescent sera, a four-fold rise in titer is considered significant.

Micromethod for CF test

By use of the micromethod for the LBCF test there is a 10-fold reduction in volume of reagents. For reasons of greater accuracy, complement and hemolysin titrations are performed by the micromethod. Antigen titrations and diagnostic tests are performed in the manner described for the microtest with the following exceptions:

1. Serial dilutions are made in 0.025 ml VBD by transferring 0.025 ml from 0.05 ml master 1:8 dilution dispensed into first well of microdilution plates.
2. Reagents are dispensed with 0.025 ml and 0.05 ml dropping pipets.
3. Volumes of reagents in complement controls are as follows:

VB	5 U (ml)	2.5 U (ml)	1.25 U (ml)
VBD	0.05	0.05	0.05
Antigen or normal tissue	0.025	0.025	0.025
Complement	0.05	0.05 (1:2 dilution of 5 C'H50 dose)	0.05 (1:4 dilution of 5 C'H50 dose)

4. Incubation periods are same as for macrotest, but plates are placed on a vibrating platform shaker after addition of sensitized cells to evenly suspend cells.
5. Plates are sealed with transparent tape before final 37 C incubation period.
6. Unlysed cells are allowed to settle before reading tests.

Hemadsorption-inhibition (HAd-I) test[9]

Viruses of the parainfluenza group are studied by a special modification of the hemagglutination test, termed the "hemadsorption test," which was devised by Vogel and Shelokov in 1957.[10] When these viruses infect tissue cultures they alter the reactivity of the cell sheet so that it characteristically adsorbs guinea pig erythrocytes.

Hemadsorption is not limited, however, to the parainfluenza viruses, since mumps, influenza, and Newcastle disease viruses have been shown to elicit a similar effect.

Inhibition of hemadsorption provides an excellent means for the serologic study of the parainfluenza viruses in particular and the myxoviruses in general.

Titration of virus. Determine quantity of test virus by inoculating 0.1 ml of 10-fold dilutions into each of 4 tubes of monkey kidney cells containing 0.2% simian SV5 antiserum.

After 5 d incubation at 36 C, add 0.2 ml 0.4% washed guinea pig red cells and incubate at 4 C for 30 min. Check cell sheet for hemadsorption using 100× magnification.

The highest dilution at which hemadsorption is detected contains 1-TCID. Employing Reed-Muench formula, determine dilution of virus that contains 100 $TCID_{50}$ and use this dilution in HAd-I test.

Procedure

1. Inactivate patient's serum at 56 C for 30 min and then prepare serial 2-fold dilutions in Hanks BSS.
2. Mix 0.2 ml of each serum dilution with 0.2 ml virus containing 100 $TCID_{50}$/0.1 ml.
3. Incubate serum-virus mixtures for 1 h at room temperature and then inoculate 0.2 ml of each mixture into each of 2 tubes of monkey kidney tissue cells (containing 0.2% SV5 antiserum). Incubate tubes at 36 C.
4. After 5 d add 0.2 ml 0.4% washed guinea pig erythrocytes, incubate at 4 C for 30 min, and then

Table 93-9. Hemagglutinating viruses—species of erythrocytes and temperature requirements

Type of virus	Species of erythrocytes	Temperature (C)
Influenza		
Type A	Chick, human O, guinea pig	4 or 22
Type B	Chick, human O, guinea pig	4 or 22
Type C	Chick	4
Parainfluenza		
Type 1	Chick, human O, guinea pig	4 or 22
Type 2	Chick, human O, guinea pig	4 or 22 (chick at 4 only)
Type 3	Chick, human O, guinea pig	4 or 22
Type 4	Chick, human O, guinea pig	4 or 22 (chick at 4 only)
Mumps	Chick, human O, guinea pig	4 or 22
Newcastle disease	Chick, human O, guinea pig	4 or 22
Rubella	Chick, 1-3 days old	4, 22, 37
Rubeola	Rhesus or vervet monkey	37
Adenoviruses		
Group I	Rhesus or grivet	37
Group II	Rat	37
Group II-A	Rat, rhesus (partial)	37
Group III	Rat (partial)	37
Group IV	No hemagglutination	
Reoviruses		
Types 1 and 2	Human O, rhesus	22 (human), 37 (rhesus)
Type 3	Human O, bovine	22 (human), 4 (bovine)
Echoviruses		
Types 3, 6, 7, 11, 12		
13, 19, 21, 29	Human O	4 or 37
Coxsackieviruses		
Group A-20, 21, 24	Human O	37
Group B-1, 3, 5	Human cord blood	4 or 37
Arboviruses	Goose, day-old chick	37
Variola-vaccinia	Chick	37
Psittacosis	Rat	22

check cell sheets for hemadsorption with 100× magnification.

5. Set up a virus control by inoculating 0.1 ml test virus containing 100 $TCID_{50}$ into each of 2 tubes. Two uninoculated tubes are also included as controls.
6. A positive serum control must be run each time test is set up.

The HAd-I titer of patient's serum is reciprocal of highest dilution that completely inhibits hemadsorption.

Hemagglutination-inhibition (H-I) Test[11]

Strain-specific identification of the influenza virus is an outstanding example of serologic diagnosis by the use of the H-I test. However, this technic is also used for mumps, variola-vaccinia, western encephalitis, St. Louis encephalitis, Japanese B encephalitis, Russian Far East encephalitis, coxsackievirus, echoviruses, dengue, Sendai, and Newcastle disease viruses[1] (Table 93-9).

Titration of virus. Titer virus by hemagglutination test to determine number of HA units/ml. Dilute virus suspension so that 0.25 ml contains 4 HA units that are used in H-I test. Eight HA units/0.25 ml are used for encephalitides.

Red cell suspension. Use 0.5% chicken red cell suspension for myxoviruses, 0.25% suspension of 1-d-old chick red cells for encephalitides, and 0.5% human group O cells for coxsackieviruses and echoviruses.

Suspensions are prepared from red cells washed 3 times in 0.85% saline and sedimented at 2500 rpm for 10 min. Packed cells are suspended in an appropriate quantity of normal saline.

Fresh cells or cells stored in Alsever solution may be used. Cells in Alsever solution stored at 3-10 C are satisfactory for 1 mo.

Treatment of serum.[12] Nonspecific inhibitors of influenza viruses types A and B and some parainfluenza viruses are commonly found in ferret, fowl, and human sera. Before these sera can be tested for H-I antibody, they must be treated to remove these nonantibody substances. Previously trypsin and periodate were employed, but this treatment is not effective for recent isolates of influenza and also destroys some specific antibody. Therefore receptor-destroying enzyme (RDE) treatment has replaced this method. RDE will usually remove serum inhibitors of influenza and most parainfluenza viruses. RDE is prepared from the 4Z strain of *Vibrio cholerae* and contains the neuraminidase enzyme and other proteolytic enzymes. This reagent should be stored at 4 C. (RDE can be obtained from Behring Diagnostics, N. Somerville, N.J.; Burroughs Wellcome Co., Research Triangle, N.C.; Flow Labs, Rockville, Md.; Microbiological Association, Walkersville, Md.)

RDE is titrated using a constant volume of 1% chicken RBC suspension against 4 U/0.5 ml influenza A/PR/8/34(HONI). From this titration a dilution that will contain 100 U/ml RDE is calculated and is the dilution used to treat human, fowl, and ferret sera to remove nonspecific inhibitors. The working dilution in calcium-saline is stable for 1 month at −70 C.

Reagents
1. Calcium-saline solution

CaCl·2H$_2$O	1.0 g
H$_3$BO$_3$	1.203 g
Sodium borate	0.052 g
NaCl	9.0 g
Distilled water to	1000 ml

2. Sodium citrate solution, 2.5%

Sodium citrate	2.5 g
Distilled water to	100.0 ml

3. Receptor-destroying enzyme (RDE) stock
   a. Reconstitute lyophilized RDE with 5 ml sterile distilled water.
   b. Divide into 1 ml aliquots and freeze at −20 C or below.

Titration of RDE
1. Prepare serial 2-fold dilutions (1:8-1:8192) of RDE stock in 0.25 ml calcium-saline diluent.
2. Add 0.25 ml 1% RBC, mix, and incubate at 37 C for 1 h, resuspending RBC every 15 min.
3. Add 0.5 ml PR 8 virus containing 4 HA units, mix thoroughly, and incubate 30-45 min at 25 C.
4. Include cell control that contains 0.25 ml RDE, 0.25 ml RBC, and 0.5 ml normal saline as a check on nonspecific hemagglutination.
5. Read results as soon as cell control has settled to avoid elution of virus from RBC. Highest dilution in which complete hemagglutination does not occur is endpoint dilution. A ring of agglutinated cells (ring positive), which is partial agglutination, is not read as endpoint. Multiply this dilution by 4 to obtain units of RDE/ml.
6. Dilute RDE in calcium-saline diluent so that it contains 100 U/ml. Store in small amounts at −70 C for no longer than 1 mo. Minimal acceptable titer for RDE is 1:256 (representing 1 U/ml). A 1:2.5 dilution of this reagent would contain 100 U/ml. This concentration is usually adequate to inactivate nonspecific inhibitors in most sera, but some may require 200-800 U/ml.
7. To check specificity of RDE, treat normal human and normal fowl sera with 100 U/ml of reagent. Nonantibody inhibitors must not be demonstrated.

Treatment of serum
1. Mix 4 vol RDE (100 U/ml) with 1 vol serum and incubate 12-18 h in 37 C water bath.
2. Add 3 vol 2.5% sodium citrate and heat at 56 C for 30 min to inactivate both RDE and complement.
3. Add 2 vol phosphate-buffered saline (PBS) to give starting dilution of 1:10.

Note. Serum used in the H-I test for the encephalitides must be treated with kaolin to remove nonspecific inhibitors. This treatment consists of mixing 1 vol serum, 4 vol saline, and 5 vol 25% kaolin. Mixture is incubated at room temperature for 20 min with frequent mixing and is then centrifuged at 2500 rpm for 30 min. The supernatant is diluted 1:10 in the process. Hemagglutinating property of encephalitides is pH

sensitive, and saline used as diluent and kaolin suspension must be adjusted to pH 9.0 prior to use.

Procedure
1. Starting with the 1:10 dilution of treated serum, prepare serial 2-fold dilution to 1:1280.
2. Add 0.25 ml of each dilution to 0.25 ml viral antigen containing 4 HA units (8 U for encephalitides) in Wassermann tubes.
3. Shake tubes and incubate at room temperature for 30 min or overnight at 4 C for encephalitides.
4. Add 0.5 ml 0.5% red cell suspension to each tube, mix well, and incubate at room temperature for 45 min or until a distinct button of cells is formed in red cell control tube.
5. Set up a serum control containing 0.25 ml 1:10 serum dilution, 0.25 ml saline, and 0.5 ml cell suspension. If agglutination occurs in this tube, agglutinins must be absorbed from patient's serum before repeating the test. Absorption is accomplished by mixing equal volumes of undiluted patient's serum and packed red cells and incubating at room temperature for 1 h. Include also a red cell control containing 0.5 ml cell suspension and 0.5 ml saline.

The titer of the patient's serum is reciprocal of highest dilution that inhibits hemagglutination.

Rubella hemagglutination-inhibition test (Microtiter)[13]

Reagents
1. Kaolin suspension
   a. Prepare a 25% suspension of acid-washed kaolin in phosphate-buffered saline. Shake suspension vigorously and allow to settle in refrigerator. Decant saline and repeat washing process.
   b. Autoclave kaolin suspension for 60 min at 121 C and then allow to settle overnight at 4 C. Decant saline and replace with an equal volume of dextrose-gelatin-Veronal buffer. Store at 4 C until used.
2. Dextrose-gelatin-barbital (Veronal) buffer (DGV)

Barbital	0.58 g
Gelatin	0.6 g
Sodium barbital (Veronal)	0.38 g
CaCl$_2$	0.02 g
MgSO$_4$·7H$_2$O	0.12 g
NaCl	8.5 g
Dextrose	10 g
Distilled water	1000 ml

   a. Dissolve gelatin and Veronal in 250 ml distilled water with gentle heat.
   b. Dissolve remaining reagents in 750 ml distilled water.
   c. Combine 2 solutions and sterilize by Millipore filtration. Store at 4 C.
3. Erythrocytes
   a. Erythrocytes from 1- to 2-d-old chicks are collected in Alsever solution and stored at 4 C until used (suitable for approximately 1 wk).
   b. On day they are used, wash RBCs 3 times in 10 vol DGV and pack at 1600 rpm for 12 min.
   c. Prepare an 0.16% suspension in phosphate-buffered saline (PBS), pH 6.2, which is used in H-I test.

Treatment of serum
1. Mix 0.2 ml patient's serum with 0.2 ml DGV.
2. Add 0.6 ml 25% kaolin suspension and shake vigorously. Incubate 20 min at room temperature.
3. Resuspend kaolin and centrifuge for 20 min at 2500 rpm. Do not remove supernatant fluid.

4. Add 0.05 ml 50% chick RBC suspension, shake well, and refrigerate at 4 C for 1 h with agitation 2-3 times. Centrifuge at 2500 rpm for 20 min.
5. Collect supernatant fluid and heat-inactivate for 30 min at 56 C. This represents a 1:4 dilution.

Hemagglutination-inhibition test
1. Add 0.05 ml 1:4 dilution of adsorbed serum to 1 well of a Microtiter "V" plate. Add 0.025 ml DGV to 8 other wells.
2. Prepare serial 2-fold dilutions using an 0.025 ml loop by transferring 0.025 ml from first well through ninth well. Dilution range is from 1:4 to 1:1024.
3. Add 0.025 ml rubella antigen diluted in DGV to contain 4 HA units to each well.
4. Prior to incubation of test set up a back titration of antigen, using 8, 4, 2, 1, and 0.5 HA unit/0.05 ml. Also prepare a red cell control, an isoagglutinin serum control, and positive and negative serum controls.
5. Incubate all plates in an ice bath or refrigerator for 2 h.
6. Place each plate on a shaking machine and add 0.05 ml cold 0.16% suspension of chick erythrocytes.
7. Allow red cells to settle for 2 h in an ice bath or overnight in a refrigerator.
8. Check controls; if they read properly, then read hemagglutination patterns of test sera.
9. Antibody titer is considered to be reciprocal of highest serum dilution causing complete inhibition of hemagglutination.

Measles (rubeola) hemagglutination-inhibition test[14]

Reagents
1. Calf serum diluent
   a. Use normal saline containing 0.5% inactivated calf serum as a diluent.
2. Kaolin
   a. Prepare a 25% suspension of acid-washed kaolin in normal saline.
   b. Add phenol red and adjust pH with 1N NaOH to pH 7.0. This eliminates spontaneous agglutination due to acidity of some batches of kaolin.
   c. Centrifuge at 2000 rpm for 10 min and wash sediment once with 5 vol saline.
   d. Restore to 25% suspension with normal saline.
3. Erythrocytes
   a. African green monkey RBCs are preserved in 2 vol Alsever solution.
   b. Wash cells 3 times in normal saline.
   c. Pack RBCs by centrifugation at 2000 rpm for 10 min.
   d. Prepare a 1% suspension in calf serum diluent.
   e. Lyse 0.5 ml in 4.5 ml distilled water and measure absorbance on a BD spectrophotometer at a wavelength of 640 nm.
   f. Adjust concentration of original 1% suspension to 0.45-0.5 absorbance.

Hemagglutination test
1. Prepare 0.4 ml amounts of serial 2-fold dilutions of virus in calf serum diluent.
2. Add 0.2 ml 1% suspension of African green monkey erythrocytes to each tube.
3. Mix and incubate at 37 C for 1 h and read hemagglutination by pattern method.
4. Highest dilution of virus showing definite hemagglutination (1+) contains 1 HA unit.
5. Use 8 HA units/0.4 ml in H-I test.

Treatment of serum
1. Dilute patient's serum 1:5 in calf serum diluent.
2. Mix this with an equal volume of 25% kaolin suspension. Incubate the mixture at room temperature for 20 min.
3. Centrifuge and collect supernatant fluid, which is considered a 1:10 serum dilution.
4. Add 0.1 ml 50% suspension of African green monkey RBC to 1 ml 1:10 serum dilution.
5. Mix and incubate for 1 h at 4 C. Mix suspension every 15 min to increase adsorption of heteroagglutinins.
6. Centrifuge at 2000 rpm for 10 min and collect supernatant fluid.

Hemagglutination-inhibition test
1. Prepare 0.2 ml quantities of serial 2-fold dilutions of patient's serum ranging from 1:10 to 1:1024. Use calf serum diluent for preparing dilution.
2. Add 0.2 ml rubeola virus containing 4 HA units to each serum dilution.
3. Mix and incubate at room temperature for 1 h.
4. Add 0.2 ml erythrocyte suspension to each tube.
5. Mix and incubate at 37 C for 1 h.
6. Include following **controls**
   a. Antigen back titration
   b. Serum control for heteroagglutinins to monkey RBC: 0.2 ml lowest dilution of patient's serum used in test + 0.2 ml diluent + 0.2 ml RBC suspension
   c. RBC control: 0.2 ml RBC suspension + 0.4 ml diluent
   d. Positive serum control
7. Titer of patient's serum is considered to be reciprocal of highest dilution that completely inhibits hemagglutination.

Indirect fluorescent antibody (IFA) technic for titration of rubella antibodies[15]

A procedure for the detection and titration of rubella antibody was developed in 1964 by Brown and co-workers. The source of antigen consists of coverslip cultures of continuous-line LLC-MK2 monkey kidney cells that are chronically infected with the RA strain of rubella virus. This indirect technic is a 2-step reaction using 2 sera—the first one is an unlabeled human serum (patient's serum) and the second is a fluorescein-labeled goat antiserum to human γ-globulin. In the first step the reaction is between antigen and antibody, in the second step antigen and bound antibody of the patient's serum acts as an antigen and combines with fluorescein-conjugated antiglobulin antibody. This is a Coombs-type reaction. (For further discussion of FA technics see Chapter 70).

Procedure
Preparation of chronically infected tissue culture
1. Seed 250 ml milk dilution bottles with 20 ml medium 199 containing 80,000 LLC-MK2 cells/ml chronically infected with RA strain of rubella.
2. Incubate infected cells at 33 C, since higher temperatures usually result in greater loss of rubella virus from tissue cells.
3. Every other day remove 10 ml spent medium and replace with 10 ml fresh medium.
4. If cells show decreasing titer of cell-associated virus, restore by adding rubella virus when seed-

ing new bottles or when Leighton tubes are prepared.

5. Trypsinize bottles of chronically infected LLC-MK2 after 28 d as follows:
   a. Pour off medium.
   b. Wash each bottle with 10 ml warm phosphate-buffered saline, pH 7.4.
   c. Add 5 ml warm 0.25% trypsin (36 C) solution and incubate at 36 C.
   d. When cell sheet begins to crack, pour off trypsin and let bottles stand until cells are released from glass.
   e. Suspend cells in 20 ml medium 199 and pipet vigorously to disperse clumps.
   f. Prepare bottles or Leighton tubes as follows:
      Bottles: Four new bottles can be prepared from 1 bottle of cells. Add 5 ml cell suspension and 15 ml medium 199 to each new bottle.
      Leighton coverslip cultures: Sixty tubes can be prepared from 1 bottle of cells. Dilute 20 ml cell suspension to 120 ml with medium 199 and dispense 2 ml to each tube. **Medium is not changed** on these tubes. Harvest coverslips after fourth day and not later than sixth day. This **time interval** is **critical.**

Staining of chronically infected and normal coverslip cultures

1. Carefully remove coverslips from Leighton tubes and rinse 3 times in PBS, pH 7.4. Allow to drain.
2. Fix in acetone for 10 min at room temperature, wash in PBS, and reimmerse in fresh acetone for another 10 min. Fixed coverslips may be stored at 4 C until needed.
3. Allow coverslips to air dry at least 30 min.
4. Coverslips are stained as follows:
   Unknown serum
   a. Add 1-2 drops each dilution of patient's serum (1:8, 1:16, 1:32, 1:64) made in normal saline to infected coverslip cultures.
   b. Add 1-2 drops lowest dilution of patient's serum (1:8) to a normal uninfected coverslip culture.
   Positive control serum
   a. Add 1-2 drops appropriate dilutions of known rubella-positive human serum to infected coverslip.
   b. Add lowest dilution of this serum to a normal coverslip culture.
   Negative control serum
   a. Add a1:8 dilution of rubella-negative human serum to an infected coverslip.
   b. Add a similar dilution to a normal coverslip culture.
   Tissue control
   a. Add saline to an infected coverslip culture.
   b. Repeat using a normal coverslip culture.
5. Incubate all coverslips in a moist chamber for 1 h at 36 C.
6. Rinse in PBS, pH 7.4, for 10 min in 3 changes of buffer.
7. Drain coverslips to remove excess buffer.
8. Add 2 drops conjugated antihuman globulin to all coverslips and incubate in a humidified atmosphere for 1 h at 36 C.
9. Rinse in PBS for 10 min with 3 changes in buffer.
10. Immerse all coverslips in distilled water for 10 s to remove saline, which may crystallize on coverslip and interfere with results.
11. Air dry coverslips and mount in buffered glycerol-saline, pH 7.6.
12. Examine slides by fluorescence microscopy using a UG-5 exciter filter and an OG-4 and OG-5 barrier filter combination.
13. Reactions are graded according to brilliance of fluorescence, and serum endpoint is reciprocal of highest serum dilution giving a 3+-4+ stain.
14. Specific staining is intracytoplasmic and perinuclear, but not intranuclear.

Interpretation

1. Positive controls
   a. Rubella immune serum + Infected coverslip culture = Specific fluorescence
   b. Rubella immune serum + Normal coverslip culture = No fluorescence
2. Negative controls
   a. Negative serum + Infected coverslip culture = No fluorescence
   b. Negative serum + Normal coverslip culture = No fluorescence
3. Unknown serum
   a. Grade fluorescent reactions from 0 to 4 according to brilliance.
   b. Highest serum dilution exhibiting 3+-4+ staining is taken as titration endpoint.

Detection and titration of Epstein-Barr virus (EBV) antibody by IFA[16]

Because of the association of high levels of antibody to the EB virus with several diseases and a very definite association with infectious mononucleosis, there is growing interest in diagnostic laboratory services for this agent. A number of cell lines have been isolated that are lymphoblastic in character and grow freely in culture media without attachment to the surface of the glass vessel. Several of these cell lines contain the EBV and can be used to detect and quantitate antibody in patients' sera. Two such cell lines are EBV-3 and HR-1.

Infectious mononucleosis can usually be diagnosed by the heterophil antibody test; however, false-positive reactions occur in some cases and remain negative in others.[17] EBV infections, particularly in children, often have a negative heterophil test, and the clinical picture is usually atypical. EB virus antibody studies are helpful in these cases.[18]

Preparation of EBV antigen

1. Seed a 100 ml screw-cap bottle with 1-2 times 10[6] HR-1 cells/ml RPMI-1640 medium* to which 20% inactivated fetal calf serum is added. Approximately 50 ml medium is contained in each bottle. To continuously propagate lymphocyte culture, split each bottle of cells into 2 new bottles every 4 d.
2. Incubate cells 3-4 d at 36 C undisturbed so that cells will settle to bottom.
3. To prepare antigen slides, remove cell culture from incubator, draw off supernatant from cells, and discard.

---

*RPMI-1640 medium can be obtained from Grand Island Biological Company, Grand Island, N.Y.; Microbiological Associates, Walkersville, Md.; and Flow Laboratories, Rockville, Md.

4. Resuspend cells in 25 ml pH 7.2 PBS in a graduated 50 ml centrifuge tube.
5. Mix cells well and do a viable cell count.
6. Centrifuge cells for 10 min at 1500 rpm in a refrigerated centrifuge. Repeat centrifugation and washing procedure with PBS 2 times.
7. Resuspend cells in PBS to make a cell concentration of 10 mil cells/ml.
8. Put 0.05 ml cell suspension (500,000 cells) in each uncoated circular area on an epoxy-coated microscope slide (Cel-Line Associates, Minotola, N.J.) and dry slides at 37 C.
9. Fix cells on slides with acetone for 10 min at room temperature.
10. Dry slides at room temperature. Store slides in air-tight plastic bags at −20 to −50 C.

Indirect FA procedure
1. To titer patient's sera follow steps 4-13 of rubella IFA procedure (see above).
2. Titer of test serum is highest dilution exhibiting fluorescence comparable to positive serum control endpoint, or 2+ fluorescence. No fluorescence should be visible at a 1:10 dilution of negative control serum.

Titration of other viral antibodies by IFA technique

If performed properly the IFA technique (developed by Laboratories of the Maryland State Department of Health and Mental Hygiene) provides and alternative approach to serodiagnosis of a variety of viral infections. It is a simple and rapid method for detection of antibodies. Titers are mostly comparable to those of CF. Specific IgM also can be detected by this method.

Preparation of antigen slides
1. Use heavy inoculum to infect appropriate tissue cell culture tubes (Table 93-10) and incubate at 36 C.
2. When 75% of monolayer shows CPE, cell suspensions are made. For cell-associated viruses (varicella and CMV), trypsinize cells with 0.25% trypsin solution; for others, scrape off tissue growth into cell culture fluid to make suspension.
3. Wash suspension 3 times with phosphate-buffered saline (PBS), pH 7.2, and sediment cells at 500 rpm for 2 min. Resuspend cells in PBS with

1 ml/tube. Use a suspension of uninfected cells made similarly as a negative control.
4. Make smears on prelceaned FA slides (10 circles per slide) and allow to dry in 36 C incubator.
5. Fix smears in acetone for 10 min at room temperature.
6. Store slides at −20 C (good for 6 mo) until used. Slides can be stored at 4-10 C for about 4 wk.

Procedure
1. Prepare serial 2-fold dilutions of test sera and positive and negative control sera in pH 7.2 PBS, starting at 1:8.
2. Remove required number of appropriate slides from stock stored in refrigerator or freezer and allow to attain room temperature.
3. Wash slides in distilled water and allow to dry.
4. Cover a separate smear with a drop of each dilution of test serum.
5. Place slides in moist chamber and incubate at 36 C for 30 min.
6. Immerse slides in pH 7.2 PBS in staining jar and agitate on mechanical rotator at 20 rpm for 20 min.
7. Rinse in distilled water and blot dry.
8. Place slides in moist chamber and cover smears with fluorescin-labeled antihuman globulin diluted to 1:10 in 0.2% Evans blue in pH 7.2 PBS and incubate at 36 C for 30 min.
9. Repeat steps 6 and 7.
10. Mount smears with drop of pH 8.0 buffered glycerol saline and coverslip.
11. Examine slides with FA microscope equipped with BG-12 exciter filter and OG-1 barrier filter.

Detection of IgM antibody

For specific IgM antibody detection, incubate test serum dilutions on antigen slides for 3 hours at 42 C to ensure attachment of immunoglobulin, and use fluorescin-labeled μ-chain-specific antihuman IgM globulin in place of whole antihuman globulin. With the longer incubation period a partial exchange takes place between IgM and IgG molecules, allowing more of the slower diffusing IgM molecules to attach to the antigen.

Interpretation. The IFA titer of patient's serum is the highest dilution at which definite yellow-green fluorescence is observed in the infected cells (uninfected control cells show reddish fluorescence). Absence of specific antibody is indicated by an absence of yellow-green fluorescence in any of the cells.

Cold hemagglutination test[19]

See Chapter 107 for procedure and discussion.

Table 93-10. Source of viral antigens for IFA test

Viruses	Source of antigen	Incubation period to obtain (hours) 75% infection
Herpes types I and II		18-24
Varicella zoster	Infected W138 cells	72
Cytomegalovirus		72
Vaccinia virus		48
Rubeola virus	Infected AGMK cells	48
Mumps virus		48
Influenza virus	Infected RMK cells	72

REFERENCES

1. Laboratory methods in diagnosis of viral and rickettsial diseases, Atlanta, 1960, United States Public Health Service, Communicable Disease Center.
2. Reed, L. J., and Muench, H. A.: Am. J. Hyg. **27:**493, 1938.
3. Contreras, G., Barnett, V. H., and Melnick, J.: J. Immunol. **69:**395, 1952.
4. Lazarus, A. S., Johnston, E. A., and Galbraith, J. E.: Am. J. Public Health **42:**20, 1952.
5. Whitman, L.: J. Immunol. **56:**97, 1947.
6. Olitsky, P. K., and Casals, J.: J.A.M.A. **134:**1224, 1947.

7. United States Public Health Service: Standardized diagnostic complement fixation method and adaptation to microtest, PHS pub. no. 1228 (Public Health Monograph no. 74), Washington, D.C. 1965, U.S. Government Printing Office.

8. Mayer, M. M.: In E. A. Kabat and M. M. Mayer, editors: Experimental immunochemistry, ed. 2, Springfield, Ill., 1961, Charles C Thomas, Publishers.

9. Chanock, R. M., Parrot, R., Cook, K., et al.: N. Engl. J. Med. **258:**207, 1958.

10. Vogel, J., and Shelokov, A.: Science **126:**358, 1957.

11. Rhodes, A. J., and van Rooyen, C. E.: Textbook of virology, Baltimore, 1953, The Williams & Wilkins Co.

12. Ada, G. L., French, E. L. and Lind, P. E.: J. Gen. Microbiol. **24:**409, 1961.

13. Stewart, G. L., Parkman, P. D., Hopps, H. E., et al.: N. Engl. J. Med. **276:**554, 1967.

14. Rosen, L.: Virology **13:**139, 1961.

15. Brown, G. C., Maassab, H. F., Veronelli, J. A., et al.: Science **145:**943, 1964.

16. Henle, G., and Henle, W.: J. Bacteriol. **91:**1248, 1966.

17. Joncas, J. H.: Prog. Med. Virol. **14:**200, 1972.

18. Klemola, E., von Essen, R., Henle, G., et al.: J. Inf. Dis. **121:**608, 1970.

19. Diagnostic procedures for viral and rickettsial diseases, ed. 2, New York, 1956, American Public Health Association.

94

CYTOLOGIC AND CYTOCHEMICAL TECHNICS FOR STUDY OF VIRAL INFECTIONS

J. Mehsen Joseph

Viral infections of host cells are associated with alteration in cell morphology, physiology, or biochemical composition. By selecting the appropriate cytologic staining technic, infection may be demonstrated before any outward evidence is apparent in unstained preparations.[1] Appropriate staining procedures are shown in Table 94-1.

Cytologic methods are employed in the study of inclusion bodies, elementary bodies, and morphologic changes in tissue culture.

By use of the appropriate technics, typical inclusion bodies are demonstrated in the spleen and lung of mice infected with psittacosis or in impression smears of the yolk sac membrane of the infected chick embryo. Elementary bodies are rendered discernible in impression smears made from plaques of epithelial hyperplasia on the chorioallantoic membrane (CAM) of the chick embryo infected with vaccinia or variola viruses; these viruses produce elementary bodies in tissue culture and inclusion bodies called "Guarnieri bodies" in the tissues of man. In tissue culture the measles virus produces large acidophilic intranuclear and intracytoplasmic inclusion bodies and multinuclear giant cells that resemble the Warthin-Finkeldey giant cells observed in the tissues and nasal discharge of man. Herpes simplex produces multinucleated giant cells with intranuclear inclusions only, and parainfluenza type 3 virus produces multinucleated giant cells but no inclusion bodies. Parainfluenza virus type 2 may produce syncytia containing eosinophilic intracytoplasmic inclusions. These morphologic alterations are well revealed by proper cytologic methods.[2]

Intranuclear inclusion-bearing cells in urinary sediment and tissues of man, which are pathognomonic of cytomegalic inclusion disease, are demonstrated by the modified Giemsa technic. Cytomegaloviruses produce similar inclusions in tissue culture.[3]

Rabies is a classic example of a positive diagnosis based on the demonstration of inclusion bodies (Negri bodies) with Seller stain. However, with other virus diseases inclusion bodies provide only ancillary evidence.

Cytologic and cytochemical staining technics may be used to reveal the presence of dual viral infections in tissue culture by demonstrating 2 different types of inclusion bodies or by demonstrating the presence of viral DNA and RNA, since a virus forms one or the other but not both kinds of nucleic acid. A dual infection of measles

Table 94-1. Materials and technics used in demonstrating viral inclusions

Virus	Material	Staining procedure
Adenovirus	Tissue culture	May-Grünwald-Giemsa
Cytomegalovirus	Urinary sediment	Giemsa
Herpes simplex	Tissue culture	May-Grünwald-Giemsa
Lymphogranuloma venereum	Bubo fluid	Giemsa
Measles	Tissue culture	May-Grünwald-Giemsa
Psittacosis	Spleen, air sac, meninges, yolk sac	Macchiavello or Castañeda
Rabies	Brain	Seller; see also rabies FA technic
Trachoma	Conjunctival scrapings	Giemsa
Varicella	Vesicle fluid	Herzberg
Variola-vaccinia	Vesicle fluid	Herzberg
Yellow fever	Liver	Hematoxylin and eosin

and adenovirus may be detected by cytochemical methods since the former contains RNA and the latter contains DNA.

Macchiavello stain[4]

This is an excellent stain for demonstrating extracellular and intracellular rickettsiae and elementary bodies of the psittacosis-LGV group of agents. Rickettsiae appear as red-staining coccoid forms. Psittacosis elementary bodies stain red and are usually found in clusters in macrophages. Early developmental forms of the psittacosis agent appear as large coccoid bodies and stain blue. These are called "initial bodies" and cannot be considered diagnostic. Bacteria stain blue, but a few may stain red. They are readily differentiated by size.

Preparation of stock solutions
1. Basic fuchsin, 0.5%
   a. Dissolve 0.5 g in 100 ml phosphate-buffered saline (pH 7.4) and filter just prior to use.
2. Citric acid, 0.5%
   a. Dissolve 1 g in 200 ml boiled distilled water.
3. Methylene blue, 1%
   a. Dissolve 1 g in 100 ml boiled distilled water.

Procedure
1. Air dry smears or impression slides and fix gently with heat.
2. Stain with basic fuchsin for 45 min and drain off stain.
3. Dip in citric acid for 30 s, then wash thoroughly in tap water for 2-5 min.
4. Stain with methylene blue for 30 s and wash in tap water.
5. Air dry and examine stained smears.

Gimenez stain[5]

Rickettsiae in yolk sacs are not stained well by the Macchiavello stain; therefore the Gimenez stain is now more commonly employed. A special modification of this technic is needed for *R. tsutsugamushi*. Rickettsiae stain a bright red; the cells, greenish blue; and the background, slightly green.

Preparation of solutions
1. Stock solution of carbol basic fuchsin
   a. Mix 100 ml 10% basic fuchsin in 95% ethanol with 250 ml 4% aqueous phenol and 650 ml distilled water.
   b. Store solution 48 h at 37 C before use.
2. Stock solution of 0.1M sodium phosphate buffer, pH 7.45
   a. Mix 3.5 ml 0.2M NaH_2PO_4 with 15.5 ml 0.2M Na_2HPO_4 and 19 ml distilled water.
3. Working solution of carbol basic fuchsin
   a. Mix 4 ml stock solution with 10 ml pH 7.45 phosphate buffer.
   b. Filter solution immediately and again before every staining.
4. Aqueous malachite green oxalate, 0.8%
   a. Dissolve 0.8 g in 100 ml distilled water. Stain is useful for several months.
5. Aqueous $Fe(NO_3)_3 9H_2O$ solution, 4%
   a. Dissolve 4 g $Fe(NO_3)_3 9H_2O$ in 100 ml distilled water.
6. Aqueous fast green FCF, 0.5%

   a. Dissolve 0.5 g fast green FCF in 100 ml distilled water.

Procedure. For all rickettsiae (except *R. tsutsugamushi*) and for psittacosis as follows:
1. Make a very thin smear from yolk sac tissue (from which excess yolk has been drained) on a clean slide.
2. Air dry and fix by passing through a flame.
3. Cover with carbol basic fuchsin (working solution) and stain for 2 min.
4. Wash thoroughly in tap water and stain with malachite green for 6-9 s.
5. Wash with tap water and stain again with malachite green for 6-9 s.
6. Wash in tap water and blot dry.

For *R. tsutsugamushi* the procedure is the same except that smear is covered with carbol basic fuchsin for 2 min and then washed with tap water. Then 4-6 drops 4% ferric nitrate is put on smear, which is then washed immediately and thoroughly with tap water. Red color will nearly disappear. Fast green FCF is applied for 15-30 s. Slide is washed in tap water and dried.

Castañeda stain (Bedson modification)[6]

Rickettsiae and psittacosis-LGV agents grown in the chick embryo or animals are readily stained by this procedure. Elementary bodies stain deep blue.

Preparation of solutions
1. Weiss mordant
   a. Prepare by dissolving 7.5 ml glacial acetic acid in 100 ml neutral formalin.
2. Formol blue solution

0.067M Phosphate buffer (adjusted to pH 7.0)	90 ml
Azure II (1% in methyl alcohol)	10 ml
Formalin	5 ml

3. Counterstain
   a. Dissolve 0.25 g safranin in 100 ml distilled water.

Procedure
1. Fix smears in Weiss mordant solution and wash thoroughly in distilled water.
2. Stain for 10 min in formol blue solution.
3. Wash thoroughly and counterstain with safranin for 5 s.
4. Wash with tap water, dry, and examine.

Herzberg Victoria blue stain[7]

This procedure is recommended for staining elementary bodies of variola, vaccinia, varicella, and herpes simplex.

Stain
1. Dissolve 3 g Victoria blue in 100 ml distilled water and heat to 60 C for 30 min.
2. Age solution in a brown bottle 14 days; filter before using.

Procedure
1. Air dry smear 24 h; wash in distilled water for 10 min.
2. Dry smear at 37 C for 1 h.
3. Stain 5 min for vaccinia, 20 min for varicella, and 30 min for herpes simplex.
4. Rinse in distilled water, dry, and examine.

May-Grünwald-Giemsa stain[8,9]

This is the most commonly used staining technic for tissue culture studies. It is recommended for monolayer cultures and is used to demonstrate ribonucleic acid (RNA) and deoxyribonucleic acid (DNA). RNA proteins stain blue, whereas DNA proteins stain red-purple.

Preparation of solutions
1. May-Grünwald stain
   a. Dissolve 0.25 g dye in 1000 ml absolute methyl alcohol. Age for 1 mo prior to use.
2. Giemsa solution
   a. Dissolve 1 g Giemsa stain in 66 ml glycerol by heating at 55-60 C for 1½ h.
   b. Add 66 ml methyl alcohol.

Procedure
1. Wash tissue culture monolayer for 15 min in 3 changes of Hanks BSS.
2. Fix 5 min is absolute methyl alcohol.
3. Stain 10 min in stock May-Grünwald solution.
4. Stain 20 min in dilute Giemsa solution (stock Giemsa diluted 1:10 with distilled water).
5. Rapidly dehydrate in 2 changes of acetone. Do not allow slide to dry.
6. Clear by rinsing in 3 changes of acetone-xylene (2:1), 3 changes of acetone-xylene (1:2), and 10 min in fresh xylene.
7. Mount in balsam and examine.

Methyl green–pyronin stain[8]

Deoxyribonucleic acid and ribonucleic acid may be differentiated by this technic. Methyl green is specific for DNA, which stains green, and pyronin is specific for RNA, which stains red.

Preparation of solutions
1. Stain
   a. Dissolve reagents in following order:
      Methyl green, 0.5 g, in 50 ml distilled water containing 0.5% phenol
      Pyronin Y, 0.5 g, in 50 ml distilled water containing 0.5% phenol
   b. Mix solutions of methyl green and pyronin Y; then add following reagents:
95% Ethanol	2.5 ml
Glycerin	20 ml
2. FAA fixative
95% Ethyl alcohol	90 ml
Glacial acetic acid	5 ml
Neutral formalin	5 ml

Procedure
1. Fix tissue in cold FAA fixative for 60 min.
2. Rinse in 50% ethanol and then in distilled water.
3. Stain 20-25 min in methyl green-pyronin solution.
4. Wash in distilled water.
5. Dehydrate with acetone for 3 s.
6. Clear in 2 changes of xylene.
7. Mount in Clearite (Hartman-Leddon Co., Philadelphia) or balsam and examine.

Acridine orange stain[10]

Since acridine orange characteristically stains both DNA and RNA, this procedure is recommended as a rapid, simple technic for determining the type of nucleic acid of a virus isolant. DNA virus particles fluoresce yellow-green, and RNA virus particles turn a flaming reddish orange. Mixed viral infections caused by DNA and RNA viruses can be detected by examining acridine orange–stained tissues. Determination of nucleic acid composition is an important first step in virus identification.

Preparation of solutions
1. Carnoy fixative
   a. Mix 75 ml 95% ethyl alcohol and 25 ml glacial acetic acid.
2. McIlvaine buffer, pH 3.8
Disodium phosphate	10.081 g
Citric acid monohydrate	13.554 g
Distilled H_2O	1000 ml
   a. Refrigerate when not in use.
3. Acridine orange stain
   a. Dissolve 0.5 g acridine orange in 100 ml McIlvaine buffer.

Procedure
1. Wash cell monolayer in phosphate buffer, pH 6.8.
2. Fix Leighton coverslip for 20 min in freshly prepared Carnoy fixative solution.
3. Rinse for 2 min in 3 changes of McIlvaine phosphate buffer (pH 3.8).
4. Stain for 30 min with 0.5% acridine orange solution in buffer (pH 3.8).
5. Wash for 30 min in 3 changes of McIlvaine buffer.
6. Mount in buffer pH 3.8 and seal with nail lacquer.

Alternate procedure
1. Fix smears in equal parts of diethyl ether and 95% ethyl alcohol for 1 h.
2. Dip 5 min each in 80%, 70%, and 50% alcohol and 5 min in distilled water.
3. Dip 4 times in 1% acetic acid.
4. Place in distilled water for 2 min.
5. Place in McIlvaine buffer for 3 min.
6. Stain in 0.01% acridine orange for 3 min.
   a. Stock solution is 0.1% acridine orange in distilled water and 2 ml Tween 80/L for better penetration.
   b. Working solution is prepared by diluting 1 part stock with 9 parts McIlvaine buffer, pH 3.8.
   c. Store both solutions at 2-10 C.
7. Place in McIlvaine buffer (pH 3.8) for 4 min for differentiation.
8. Mount with buffer (pH 3.8) beneath coverslip.

RNA material stains bright red; DNA material stains green-yellow.

Hematoxylin and eosin stain[8]

This procedure is recommended for paraffin-embedded and sectioned tissues. Histopathologic changes that are used to differentiate coxsackievirus A from coxsackievirus B are best observed by this technic.

Preparation of solutions
1. Alum hematoxylin solution
   a. Dissolve 0.6 g hematoxylin, 5.0 g ammonium alum, and 0.1 g $NaIO_3$ in 70 ml distilled water.
   b. Add 2 ml glacial acetic acid and 30 ml glycerol.
   c. Filter and dilute 1:20 with distilled water prior to use.
2. Sodium bicarbonate solution
   a. Dissolve 1 g in 100 ml distilled water.
3. Eosin Y solution
   a. Dissolve 0.5 g in 100 ml distilled water.

Procedure
1. Rinse in 3 changes of Hanks BSS.
2. Fix in neutral buffered formalin 30 min.
3. Rinse in distilled water.
4. Stain with a 1:20 dilution of alum hematoxylin solution for 10 min.
5. Rinse in tap water.

6. Treat with 1% bicarbonate solution until cells turn blue.
7. Rinse in distilled water.
8. Dehydrate by rapidly exposing to 2 changes of acetone.
9. Rinse in 3 changes of acetone-xylene (2:1), 3 changes of acetone-xylene (1:2), and finally in xylene.
10. Clear in fresh xylene for 10 min.
11. Mount in Clearite and examine.

Modified Giemsa stain[11]

This procedure is recommended for staining urinary sediment for intranuclear inclusion bodies pathognomonic for cytomegalic inclusion disease.

Preparation of solutions
1. Fixative
    a. Mix equal parts of ethyl ether (USP) and absolute ethyl alcohol.
2. Stain
    a. Prepare a 2% solution of Giemsa in 100 ml Sørensen phosphate buffer (pH 7.2).

Procedure
1. Centrifuge urine at 2500 rpm for 15 min.
2. Spread sediment on a clean glass slide that has been coated with a thin film of 25% bovine albumin in physiological saline.
3. Fix while still moist by immersing in alcohol-ether solution for 10 min.
4. Stain with Giemsa solution for 1 h.
5. Wash in Sørensen buffer (pH 7.2) for 3 min.
6. Examine with or without mounting in Permount (Fisher Scientific Co., St. Louis, Mo.) or balsam.

Seller stain

The **microscopic diagnosis of rabies** is dependent upon the demonstration of intracytoplasmic inclusion bodies in neuronal cells of brain tissue. These inclusions are termed "Negri bodies" and are well-revealed with Seller stain.

Negri bodies are acidophilic inclusions containing 1-20 internal basophilic granules. With Seller stain the matrix stains pink and the internal granules stain blue to deep blue.

Intracytoplasmic inclusions are observed in brain tissue of a variety of animals infected with viruses of distemper, encephalitis, hepatitis, etc., and these must be differentiated from Negri bodies. Nonrabies inclusion bodies may be differentiated from rabies as follows[12]:

Nonrabies inclusion bodies	Negri bodies
Absence of internal granules	1-20 internal basophilic granules
Definite pink matrix	Matrix pink with faint blue tinge
Homogeneous matrix	Heterogeneous matrix
Usually highly refractile	Usually nonrefractile

Preparation of solutions
1. Methylene blue stock solution
    a. Dissolve 1 g methylene blue in 100 ml absolute methyl alcohol (acetone free).
2. Basic fuchsin stock solution
    a. Dissolve 1 g basic fuchsin in 100 ml absolute methyl alcohol (acetone free).
    b. Store in refrigerator (2-10 C).

3. Seller stain
    a. Mix 2 parts methylene blue stock solution with 1 part basic fuchsin stock solution.
    b. Adjust stain to obtain proper color differentiation of brain tissue. Stroma should appear rose-pink in thin areas of smear.
    c. Adjust with methylene blue or basic fuchsin, depending on whether blue or red is dominant in stained brain smear.
    d. Keep solution tightly stoppered to prevent evaporation of alcohol.
    e. Check stain periodically with rabies-positive brain tissue.

Procedure
1. Amputate animal's head, taking it to laboratory as soon as possible before decomposition sets in. In summer it is advisable to pack head in ice during transportation. Operator should wear rubber gloves.
2. Place head upon a board and remove skull cap by sawing. Remove brain from skull.
3. Make an incision straight down on 1 side of hemisphere into lateral ventricle.
4. At posterior part of floor of lateral ventricle, make an incision deep down into cortex. Here is found a structure known as Ammon's horn, where Negri bodies are most likely to be found.
5. Prepare smears by spreading brain tissue between 2 sides or by making impressions. Include smears from right and left Ammon's horns and right and left cortical areas of cerebrum and cerebellum in each examination.
6. While tissue is still moist, dip slides in Seller stain and quickly remove (3 s).
7. Rinse immediately in running tap water.
8. Dry without blotting and examine.

Fluorescent antibody (FA) technic for diagnosis of rabies

The diagnosis of rabies has been traditionally based on the demonstration of Negri bodies in brain tissue of rabid animals. However, these inclusion bodies cannot be demonstrated in approximately 10% of the naturally infected animals, and in rabid bats this may be as high as 25-30%. In 1958 Goldwasser and Kissling[13] adapted the fluorescent antibody technic to the identification of rabies antigen in the brain tissue of animals in which Negri bodies failed to form. By this technic fluorescent "dustlike" material

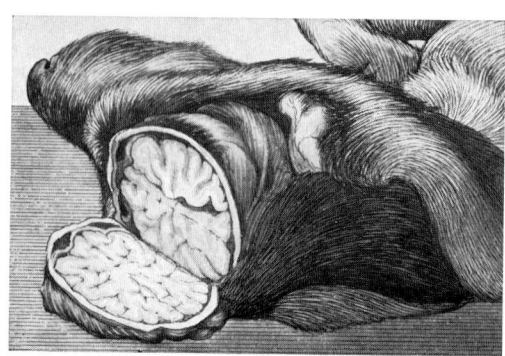

Fig. 94-1. Section through dog's head for Negri bodies examination.

representing viral antigen is characteristically observed in Negri body–negative brain tissue of rabid animals; in Negri body–positive tissue both large fluorescent bodies (Negri bodies) and "dustlike" viral antigen are observed.

This technic has now become an established routine in most laboratories concerned with the diagnosis of rabies to supplement the Seller technic and mouse inoculation. All 3 methods must be used for the maximum number of positive results. A few animals have been found rabies-positive by the FA technic but negative by both the seller technic and mouse inoculation and a few positive by mouse inoculation but negative by FA and Seller technics.

Reagents are commercially available.* Reagents for control and standardization may be obtained from the Center for Disease Control, Atlanta.

A general discussion of the principles and applications of the fluorescent antibody technic are given in Chapter 70.

Reagents

1. Prepare phosphate buffer stock solutions as follows:
    Solution A, 0.1M K_2HPO_4
    Solution B, 0.1M $NaH_2PO_4 \cdot 4H_2O$
2. Prepare a working buffer pH 7.6-7.8 by mixing A and B:

Solution A	91.5 ml
Solution B	8.5 ml
Distilled H_2O to	900 ml

    Sterilize by autoclaving at 121 C for 20 min.
3. Prepare a 10% suspension of egg yolk in phosphate buffer. Use 6- to 7-d embryonated eggs. Store at 4 C.
4. Using aseptic technic, prepare a 20% suspension of CVS strain rabies–infected mouse brain in 10% yolk buffer. Centrifuge at 3000 rpm for 20 min and collect supernatant. Store at −20 C.

---

*Difco Laboratories, Detroit; BBL, Division of Bio-Quest, Cockeysville, Md.

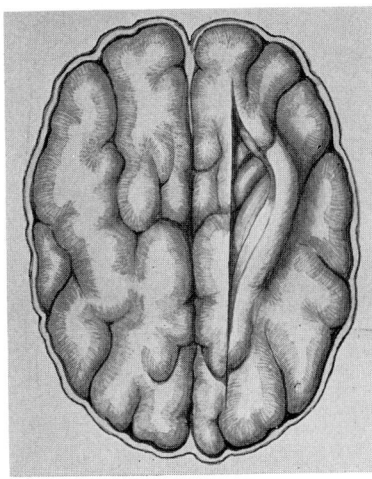

Fig. 94-2. Dog's brain, showing method of locating Ammon's horn.

5. Also prepare a 20% suspension of normal mouse brain in 10% yolk buffer. Centrifuge and collect supernatant. Store at −20 C.
6. Dilute antirabies conjugate with equal volume of normal mouse brain suspension. Store in approximately 1 ml quantities at −20 C.
7. Dilute a second portion of antirabies conjugate with CVS mouse brain suspension. Store in approximately 1 ml quantities at −20 C.
8. Prepare 2 touch impression smears on a FA microslide. Always prepare at least 2 slides from different regions of brain. Whenever possible, make smears from Ammon's horn, cerebrum, and cerebellum.
9. Touch impressions should also be prepared from known positive mouse brain (using CVS strain) and from uninfected mouse brain. These control slides can be stored at −20 C, after fixation in acetone, for at least 1 mo.
10. Air dry touch impressions and immediately fix in acetone at −20 C for 4 h. Remove and air dry slides at −20 C prior to staining.

Procedure[14-16]

1. Remove slides from freezer and warm to room temperature.
2. Ring each smear with a wax pencil to retain conjugate.
3. Cover 1 smear on each slide with antirabies conjugate diluted in normal mouse brain suspension and other smear with conjugate diluted in CVS mouse brain suspension.
4. Place slides in a large Petri dish containing moistened filter paper and incubate at 35 C for 30 min.
5. Drain conjugate and wash slides by dipping in phosphate buffer for 1 min; then place in a second buffer solution for 9 min.
6. Rinse in distilled water by dipping slides 3-4 times.
7. Cover smears with rhodamine B and incubate in moist chamber for 30 min at 35 C.
8. Repeat phosphate buffer and distilled water rinses.
9. Air dry or blot dry and mount in glycerol buffer pH 7.6-7.8. Seal coverslip with nail polish. (To prepare, mix 9 parts neutral glycerin with 1 part buffer.)
10. Examine with 5840 exciter filter and W-2A barrier filter.

REFERENCES

1. Love, R.: Ann. N. Y. Acad. Sci. **81:**1, 1959.
2. Rose, H. M.: Viral infections of infancy and childhood, New York, 1960, Paul B. Hoeber.
3. Bancroft, J., Seybolt, J. F., and Windhager, H. A.: Acta Cytol. **5:**182, 1961.
4. Adams, J. M.: Newer virus diseases, New York, 1960, Macmillan.
5. Gimenez, D. F.: Stain Techn. **39:**135, 1964.
6. Laboratory methods in the diagnosis of viral and rickettsial diseases, Atlanta, 1960, United States Public Health Service, Communicable Disease Center.
7. Rhodes, A. J., and van Rooyen, C. E.: Textbook of virology, Baltimore, 1953, The Williams & Wilkins Co.
8. Merchant, D. J., Kahn, R. H., Murphy, W. H.: Handbook of cell and organ culture, Minneapolis, 1960, Burgess Publishing Co.
9. Staff of Tissue Culture Course: An introduction to

cell and tissue culture, Minneapolis, 1953, Burgess Publishing Co.

10. Bertalanffy, L. V., and Masin, M. F.: Cancer **11**:873, 1958.
11. Hanshaw, J. B., and Weller, T. H.: J. Pediatr. **58**:305, 1961
12. Tierkel, E. S., and Neff, H. O.: Rabies—laboratory methods in diagnosis, Atlanta, 1957, Communicable Disease Center, United States Public Health Service.

13. Goldwasser, R. A., and Kissling, R. E.: Proc. Soc. Exp. Biol. Med. **98**:219, 1958.
14. Goldwasser, R. A., Kissling, R. E., Carski, T. R., and Hosty, T. S.: Bull. WHO **20**:579, 1959.
15. Cherry, W. B., Goldman, M., and Carski, T. R.: Fluorescent antibody techniques, Public Health Service pub. no. 729, 1960.
16. McQueen, J. L., Lewis, A. L., and Schneider, N. J.: Am. J. Public Health **50**:1743, 1960.

95

LABORATORY METHODS IN DIAGNOSIS OF RICKETTSIAL INFECTIONS

J. Mehsen Joseph

The generic name *Rickettsia* was proposed by da Roche-Lima in 1916 to honor Dr. H. T. Ricketts, who died of epidemic typhus fever while studying the etiology of this disease.

Rickettsiae are small, gram-negative, pleomorphic, coccobacillary microorganisms that measure 0.3-0.5 μm. Their size and shape are not reliable criteria for identification. They are nonmotile, nonsporeforming, and nonfiltrable agents that are visible with the light microscope.[1]

Rickettsiae are difficult to stain with the usual aniline dyes and require special staining methods such as Giemsa or Macchiavello. They stain reddish purple with Giemsa stain. With the Macchiavello method they stain bright red, except for scrub typhus, which stains blue. Rickettsiae are difficult to demonstrate in fixed tissues (the stains and staining technics mentioned are described in Chapter 94).

Rickettsiae are obligate intracellular parasites that die quite rapidly when separated from their host tissues. (See also Chapter 68 for a discussion of rickettsiae and their taxonomic position.)

Rickettsiae multiply by transverse fission similar to that of true bacteria. They usually grow intracellularly as clusters or colonies in the cytoplasm of tissue cells, except spotted fever rickettsiae that grow in both the cytoplasm and nucleus. *Rickettsia quintana* of trench fever is the only member of the group that has been grown in vitro on cell-free media.

All members are sensitive to *p*-aminobenzoic acid and broad-spectrum antibiotics such as the tetracyclines and chloramphenicol. These agents have a rickettsiostatic effect and must not be used to decontaminate clinical materials prior to inoculating host systems or incorporated into tissue culture media.

Rickettsiae contain 2 principal antigens: (1) a soluble group-specific antigen that can be removed by repeated washing of the organism and (2) a species-specific antigen that is firmly incorporated in the cell wall and cannot be removed by washing. Both react in the complement fixation (CF) test. The soluble group antigen is the type commercially available and recommended for diagnostic use because of its broad antigenic coverage.

Concentrated suspensions of rickettsiae, except Q fever, are toxic to adult mice, which die within a few hours after intravenous inoculation. Specific antiserum neutralizes this effect.

Each rickettsia has an arthropod vector and an animal reservoir, and human infections occur wherever there is a close association of man with ectoparasites and animal reservoir (Table 95-1).

Infection in man is characterized as an acute febrile illness with sudden onset and skin rash (except Q fever). Rickettsiae multiply in the endothelial cells of the aterioles, venules, and capillaries throughout the body.[2]

Laboratory diagnosis is based on the isolation and identification of the causative agent or on the demonstration of specific and rising antibody in serial serum specimens taken from the patient.

Primary isolation of rickettsiae is attempted by inoculating blood taken from the patient during the febrile phase into adult male guinea pigs and adult albino mice. Rickettsiae are demonstrated in impression smears of the spleen and testicular tissues. Scrotal reactions in guinea pigs may be useful in differentiating among epidemic typhus, murine thyphus, and Rocky Mountain spotted fever.

The principal serologic tests are the **Weil-Felix agglutination test** (see Chapter 107) and the **complement fixation test** (see Chapter 93). For a recently described **microimmunofluorescence test** employing rickettsial antigens, see Philip et al.[12] and Hechemy et al.[13] See also discussion of "Febrile agglutinations," Chapter 107.

Rickettsiae that produce disease in man may be placed in 4 groups: (1) typhus fever, (2) spotted fever, (3) Q fever, and (4) tsutsugamushi fever.

Table 95-1. Rickettsial diseases of man*

Group	Disease	Etiologic agent	Mode of transmission	Natural reservoir	Geographic distribution
Spotted fever	Rocky Mountain spotted fever	R. rickettsii	Wood tick; dog tick	Wild rodents and rabbits, dogs and sheep	United States
	Rickettsialpox	R. akari	Mite	House mouse	North Atlantic seaboard states; Russia
	Boutonneuse fever	R. conori	Tick	Dogs; small rodents	
	South African tick fever	R. conori	Tick	Small wild rodents, dogs	Mediterranean, Africa
Typhus	Epidemic typhus	R. prowazeki	Human body louse	Man, rodents	Worldwide
	Brill-Zinsser disease	R. prowazeki	Recrudescence of latent infection of epidemic typhus		United States, Europe
	Endemic typhus	R. mooseri (R. typhi)	Rat flea	Small rodents	Worldwide
Tsutsuga-mushi	Scrub typhus	R. orientalis (R. tsutsu-gamushi)	Mite	Wild rats and mice	Japan, Malay, Sumatra
Q fever	Q fever	C. burneti	Air-borne usu-ally, also tick and milk	Small mammals, cattle, sheep, goats	Worldwide
	Trench fever	R. quintana	Body louse	Man ?	Europe, Mexico

*From Smadel, J.: Rickettsial disease. In Diagnostic procedures for virus and rickettsial diseases, ed. 2, copyrighted, New York, 1956, American Public Health Association.

Rickettsiae are classified in the eighth edition of *Bergey's Manual* (1974) as follows:

Order I. *Rickettsiales*
  Family I. *Rickettsiaceae*
    Tribe I. *Rickettsieae*
      Genus I. *Rickettsia*
      Genus II. *Rochalimaea*
      Genus III. *Coxiella*
    Tribe II. *Ehrlichieae*
      Genus IV. *Ehrlichia*
      Genus V. *Cowdria*
      Genus VI. *Neorickettsia*
    Tribe III. *Wolbachieae*
      Genus VII. *Wolbachia*
      Genus VIII. *Symbiotes*
      Genus IX. *Blattabacterium*
      Genus X. *Rickettsiella*
  Family II. *Bartonellaceae*
    Genus I. *Bartonella*
    Genus II. *Grahamella*
  Family III. *Anaplasmataceae*
    Genus I. *Anaplasma*
    Genus II. *Paranaplasma*
    Genus III. *Aegyptionella*
    Genus IV. *Haemobartonella*
    Genus V. *Eperythrozoon*
Order II. *Chlamydiales*
  Family I. *Chlamydiaceae*
    Genus I. *Chlamydia*

It is customary to group rickettsiae according to their vectors as follows:

1. **Tick-borne typhus**
   Rocky Mountain spotted fever
   North Queensland tick typhus
   Kenya fever
   Boutonneuse fever
   Siberian typhus
2. **Louse-borne typhus**
   Epidemic typhus
   Relapsing typhus (Brill's disease)
   Trench fever
3. **Flea-borne typhus**
   Endemic typhus
4. **Mite-borne typhus**
   Tsutsugamushi fever
5. **Others**
   Q fever
   Rickettsialpox

TYPHUS FEVER GROUP

Epidemic typhus, murine (endemic) typhus, and Brill-Zinsser disease are the principal diseases of the typhus fever group. The causative agent of epidemic typhus is *R. prowazeki,* and the vector is the human body louse. *R. mooseri* is the agent of endemic typhus, and the vector is the rat flea. Brill-Zinsser disease is a recrudescence of epidemic typhus. Epidemic typhus is characterized clinically by fever, chills, severe aches, and rash spreading out from the back and chest.

Table 95-2. Differentiation between epidemic typhus and murine typhus rickettsiae*

Differential test	R. prowazeki	R. typhi (mooseri)
Guinea pig (intraperitoneal)	Rickettsemia, fever, no scrotal reaction	Fever and scrotal swelling
Albino rat (intraperitoneal)	No persistent brain infection	Persistent infection in brain for at least 1 y
Hamster (intranasal)	Transient lung infection	Rapidly fatal lung infection
Complement fixation test	Differentiate with species-specific antigen	
Toxin neutralization test	Toxin is specific for each species	

*Based on data from Rhodes, A. J., and Van Rooyen, C. E.: Textbook of virology, ed. 4, Baltimore, 1962, The Williams & Wilkins Co.

Similar but milder symptoms are observed in endemic typhus.

Rickettsiae can be isolated from blood obtained during the febrile phase by inoculating the adult male guinea pig. The infected guinea pig responds with fever only in the case of *R. prowazeki* or fever and scrotal swelling in the case of *R. mooseri*. By subpassing peritoneal fluid, tunica vaginalis, and splenic tissue, rickettsiae increase in concentration and can be seen in impression smears made from the surfaces of spleen and scrotal tissue (Table 95-2). Cross immunity and CF antibody tests aid in identification of the isolate.

The Weil-Felix reaction is positive to high titer for *Proteus* OX-19 during the second week of illness and reaches a maximum of about 1:640 to 1:1280 late in the third week. After recovery the titer declines rapidly. A weak response is detected for *Proteus* OX-2 but is negative for *Proteus* OX-K.[3]

The patient responds with CF antibody about 7-9 days after onset of symptoms, and a peak titer is attained on the twelfth to sixteenth day. The CF antibody level declines slowly over a period of 3-6 months and remains at a low level for years.

SPOTTED FEVER GROUP

The principal diseases in the spotted fever groups are Rocky Mountain spotted fever *(R. rickettsii)*, rickettsialpox *(R. akari)*, boutonneuse fever *(R. conori)*, and South African tick fever *(R. conori)*. Clinically they are characterized by malaise, fever, myalgia, and rash that spreads from the extremities to cover the entire body. Rickettsialpox is so named because of the generalized rash that resembles chickenpox.

Ticks serve as vectors, except in the case of rickettsialpox that is transmitted by a mite.

Rickettsiae may be isolated from blood by the intraperitoneal inoculation of adult male guinea pigs (adult albino mouse is the animal of choice for rickettsialpox). Fever develops 2-3 days after inoculation, with scrotal necrosis and usually death. Blood, spleen, and testicular tissue is subpassed to increase the concentration of rickettsiae, which can be demonstrated in smears of spleen and tunica vaginalis.

Rickettsiae are identified by the cross-immunity test, using known viable strains of spotted fever rickettsiae. Also, the neutralization test may be used, which consists of mixing rickettsiae form inoculated guinea pigs with known specific antiserum.

The CF test is the most reliable serologic technic for differentiating the spotted fever group from the epidemic typhus and scrub typhus groups. CF antibody appears during the second week of illness and persists for years. The suppressive effect of broad-spectrum antibiotics on the CF antibody response limits the usefulness of this test.

Q FEVER

Coxiella burneti is the etiologic agent of Q fever and is the most stable and resistant member of the rickettsial group. The disease is characterized by fever, malaise, respiratory symptoms, and patchy pneumonia but no rash.

Rickettsiae can be isolated from blood, sputum, urine, and postmortem tissues by the intraperitoneal inoculation of guinea pigs. Infected guinea pigs develop fever within 7-10 days. Guinea pigs showing symptoms are killed, and a 10% suspension of spleen is subpassed to healthy guinea pigs. Several passages are required before rickettsiae can be seen in impression smears of splenic tissue.[4]

To identify the etiologic agent, serum is obtained from infected guinea pigs 4-6 weeks after infection and examined for specific CF antibody to Q fever. Also animals that recover are challenged with viable Q fever stock strains to demonstrate cross protection.

The hazard of infection with *C. burneti* is quite great, and isolation should not be attempted unless adequate facilities are available.

Serologic diagnosis is much safer and simpler, and the CF test is the method of choice. It is usually advisable to employ both the Italian Henzerling and the American 9-mile strains as CF antigens. CF antibody usually appears during the second week of illness and reaches a peak 4-6 weeks after onset. Agglutinins appear early during the first week of illness and reach a peak during the fourth week. The Luoto capillary agglutination test may be used to detect agglutinins.

Both CF and agglutinating antibodies persist in high titer for several months and then decline to low levels.

It should be remembered that the Q fever CF antigen is highly specific and does not cross-react with other rickettsial agents.

SCRUB TYPHUS GROUP (TSUTSUGAMUSHI GROUP)

Scrub typhus is caused by *R. tsutsugamushi* and is transmitted to man by a mite. Wild rats and mice constitute the natural reservoir of infection. The disease is characterized by an abrupt onset with chills, fever, and a rash on the trunk that spreads to the extremities.

The causative agent can be isolated from febrile phase blood or necropsy tissue by inoculating adult albino mice intraperitoneally. Mice usually die within 8-10 days and show a serofibrinous peritonitis and an enlarged spleen. Not all strains are lethal to mice on primary isolation, and it is therefore necessary to subpass suspensions of spleen from healthy as well as from sick animals. Subpassage of blood, peritoneal fluid, liver, and lung is also advisable.

Rickettsiae may be seen in smears prepared from the spleen and from parietal cells scraped from the peritoneum and stained with Giemsa. Rickettsiae appear as purple-stained intracellular and extracellular diplococci or coccobacilli.

Isolates are identified by challenging survivors with specific virulent stock strains of rickettsiae, and a cross immunity identifies the species involved.

The most useful serologic method is the nonspecific Weil-Felix test. Antibody to the *Proteus* OX-K strain appears during the second week of illness and reaches a maximum titer 7-10 days later. Antibody then begins to decline rapidly and within 5-6 weeks is no longer detectable. Antibodies to *Proteus* OX-19 and OX-2 do not develop.

A 4-fold rise in titer to *Proteus* OX-K is diagnostic, but the titer of a single serum specimen must be 1:160 or greater to be significant.

It must be remembered that the spirochetes of relapsing fever may evoke an antibody response to *Proteus* OX-K.[5]

Soluble antigen used in the CF test is specific for scrub typhus, but only about 50% of the patients develop CF antibody. Therefore a negative test has no significance. Also strains of scrub typhus are antigenically heterogeneous so that a single satisfactory CF antigen is not available.

COLLECTON OF SPECIMENS

Rickettsemia is associated with all rickettsial infections of man, and blood is the principal source of the etiologic agent. During the febrile stage, collect 10 ml heparinized or clotted blood aseptically in sterile Wassermann tubes. If clotted blood is obtained, remove the serum and save for serologic studies. Grind the clot to rupture the cells and add sufficient Hanks BSS (without antibiotics) to prepare a 10% suspension.[4]

In fatal cases postmortem spleen and liver may be used for isolation of rickettsiae.

Sputum and urine are good sources of rickettsiae when Q fever is suspected. They must be treated with 100 units penicillin/ml specimen and incubated 30 min at 36 C prior to animal inoculation. Broad-spectrum antibiotics and streptomycin must not be used because of their rickettsiacidal effect.[4]

All rickettsiae, except Q fever, lose their viability rapidly when separated from their host cells. Specimens should be stored at −18 C and, if possible, at −70 C.

Collect paired serum specimens to demonstrate the presence and rise of specific antibody. Where possible, 3 specimens are desirable. The first specimen should be collected during the first week of illness, the second specimen 1 week later, and the third specimen 4-5 weeks after onset.

ISOLATION OF RICKETTSIAE
Guinea pig inoculation

Inoculate 3 disease-free, adult male guinea pigs intraperitoneally with 5 ml patient's blood. Observe the animals daily and record their rectal temperature and scrotal reactions. A rectal temperature of 40 C or higher indicates fever.

Guinea pigs infected with rickettsiae almost invariably develop fever. Fever is usually detected during the first postinoculation week for Rocky Mountain spotted fever, rickettsialpox, and endemic typhus and early in the second week for Q fever and epidemic typhus.

Scrotal reactions are apparent at the onset of fever or shortly thereafter. Rickettsiae are placed in 3 groups on the basis of scrotal responses.[5]

> Group I: scrotal swelling
>   *R. conorii*
>   *R. mooseri*
>   Some strains of *R. akari* and *R. rickettsii*
> Group II: scrotal necrosis
>   *R. rickettsii*
> Group III: no scrotal response
>   *C. burnetii*
>   *R. prowazekii*
>   Some strains of *R. tsutsugamushi*

In group I the scrotal reactions are characterized by erythema, edema, and swelling. In group II there is erythema, edema, and macular scrotal rash; rash extends to adjacent tissues; macules become purpuric, necrotic, and ulcerate; ulcers heal, leaving scars; animal may die before scrotal response develops to the ulcerative stage.

Kill 1 of the animals that develops fever with or without scrotal reactions and collect blood, peritoneal exudate, spleen, and tunica vaginalis (if scrotal reactions develop). Prepare 10% suspensions of spleen and testicular tissues in Hanks BSS and subpass by injecting 5 ml intraperitoneally into 2 adult male guinea pigs. Blood and peritoneal exudate are injected without dilution. (Table 95-3.)

Blind passage is usually unrewarding when all guinea pigs inoculated remain well. If there is any suspicion, a passage should be made and

Table 95-3. Isolation and passage of rickettsiae from clinical materials and associated serologic response*

Rickettsiae	Animal used for isolation	Response of animal	Passage material 10% suspension	Death on passage	Serologic reactions	
					Weil-Felix	CF
R. prowazekii	Adult male guinea pig	Fever	Spleen, brain	Never	OX-19	Positive with typhus fever group antigen pox antigens
R. mooseri	Adult male guinea pig	Fever and scrotal swelling	Tunica, spleen	Never	OX-19	Positive with typhus fever group antigen
R. rickettsii	Adult male guinea pig	Fever and scrotal necrosis	Spleen, tunica, whole blood	Usual	Indeterminant	Positive with spotted fever and rickettsial-pox antigens
R. conorii	Adult male guinea pig	Fever and scrotal swelling	Tunica	Rare	Indeterminant	Positive with spotted fever and rickettsial-pox antigens
C. burnetii	Adult male guinea pig	Fever	Spleen	Infrequent	—	Positive with specific antigen
R. akari	Adult albino mice	Roughened fur and inactivity	Spleen	Usual	—	Positive with spotted fever and rickettsial-pox antigens
R. tsutsuga-mushi	Adult albino mice	Roughened fur and inactivity	Spleen	Usual	OX-K	Positive in 50% with appropriate antigen

*Adapted from Smadel, J.: Rickettsial diseases. In Diagnostic procedures for virus and rickettsial diseases, ed. 2, copyrighted, New York, 1956, American Public Health Association.

serum collected after 28 days and tested for CF antibody.

Prepare impression smears from the surface of the spleen and tunica vaginalis (if scrotal reactions are observed). Also prepare smears from scrapings of the parietal peritoneum and peritoneal exudate. Fix smears with absolute methyl alcohol and stain with Giemsa or Macchiavello stain (see Chapter 94).

Mouse inoculation

Inoculate 6 adult albino mice intraperitoneally with 0.5 ml patient's blood taken during the febrile period. Observe animals daily for signs of illness.

Mice infected with R. akari (rickettsialpox) usually show signs of illness 10-14 days after inoculation and may die shortly thereafter. Roughened fur, abdominal distention, labored respiration, enlarged lymph nodes, enlarged edematous liver, and dark engorged spleen characterize the infectious process.

Mice infected with R. tsutsugamushi (scrub typhus) become ill within 8-10 days and many die within 10 days after inoculation. On autopsy one may observe enlarged spleen and lymph nodes, congested liver, serofibrinous peritonitis, pleural edema, and hemorrhagic pneumonia.

Not all strains of rickettsiae are lethal for mice on primary isolation. Those of low mouse virulence include newly isolated strains of R. akari and R. tsutsugamushi and practically all strains of C. burnetii and R. mooseri.

If the inoculated mice fail to show any signs of clinical disease, kill and autopsy 1 mouse after 14 days and check for splenomegaly and peritonitis. If pathologic evidence is lacking, kill a mouse 21 days after inoculation and autopsy. Kill and autopsy the remaining mice on the twenty-eighth day, and if no lesions are found, report as negative (Table 95-3).

If minimal peritonitis and splenomegaly are observed, suspect R. akari, R. mooseri, R. tsutsugamushi, and C. burnetii. Subpass peritoneal exudate and splenic tissue through adult mice until rickettsiae are observed in smears prepared from the peritoneal and splenic surfaces.

If illness, subcutaneous ascites, and death of mice ensue, suspect R. akari and R. tsutsugamushi. Subpass until rickettsiae are observed in smears.

If the rickettsiae remain nonlethal for mice and scrotal reactions do not develop in guinea pigs, suspect C. burnetii and R. tsutsugamushi; if scrotal swelling develops in guinea pigs, suspect R. mooseri and R. akari. Subpass to demonstrate rickettsiae in stained smears of peritoneal and splenic surfaces.

Chick embryo

Primary isolation of rickettsiae in the chick embryo is too variable and should not be used for isolation from clinical materials. The exceptions are rickettsialpox and Q fever rickettsiae that are highly infective on primary isolation. After isolation, rickettsiae can be adapted to luxuriant growth in the yolk sac of the embryonated egg, and high titers are obtained.

IDENTIFICATION OF RICKETTSIAE
Neutralization test[6]

This procedure is especially useful for identifying rickettsiae of Rocky Mountain spotted fever (*R. rickettsii*).

Obtain serum from infected guinea pigs during the febrile period and use as test blood rickettsiae.

Mix 0.5 ml specific antiserum with 0.1, 0.25, and 0.5 ml, respectively, of the test blood rickettsiae. Incubate mixtures at room temperature (25 C) for 30 min. Inoculate 2 adult male guinea pigs with each mixture and observe daily for fever and other signs of illness. Inoculate 0.25 ml unneutralized test blood rickettsiae as a control. The specific antiserum that protects the animals for 28 days without any signs of illness while those in the control group become ill or die indicates the infecting rickettsial species.

Rickettsiae from the spleen or peritoneum may be substituted for those in blood.

Cross-immunity test

Animals that become ill following inoculation of clinical material but recover are challenged with known strains of viable rickettsiae to determine their immunity. This is an indirect means of identifying the original infecting strain.

Inoculate convalescent animals with 100 infectious doses (ID_{50}) of known rickettsial strains (American Type Culture Collection, Rockville, Md.) by intraperitoneal inoculation. Observe daily for illness or death. Animals surviving 28 days indicate the original infecting strain of rickettsiae.

Convalescent CF antibody test

Obtain serum from convalescing guinea pigs and titer for complement-fixing antibodies for known specific rickettsial antigens (see Chapter 93 for CF procedure).

The specific antigen that results in the fixation of complement identifies the strain of rickettsiae present in the original clinical material.

SEROLOGIC DIAGNOSIS
Complement fixation test[7]

The complement fixation test is the most practical and most reliable serologic method for differentiating rickettsiae as to Rocky Mountain spotted fever group, typhus fever group, Q fever, and scrub typhus group. Reactions to group-specific rickettsial CF antigens are shown in Table 95-4. Since most commercial CF antigens* represent soluble group-specific antigens, a positive serologic test indicates only a particular group of rickettsiae and not a specific species of rickettsiae. Species-specific antigens can be prepared, but the method is so time consuming and expensive that it is not practical.[4]

Procedure. The CF test is performed according to the technic described for viral antigens (Chapter 93), using 2 full units of complement and 2 units of CF antigen. Fixation is allowed to take place overnight at 4 C.

It may be necessary to use antigens for both the Henzerling and the 9-mile strains of Q fever. Also antigens of several scrub typhus strains should be used as they vary widely in their antigenic composition.

Interpretation. A 4-fold or greater rise in CF titer between acute and convalescent phase serum specimens is considered diagnostic. If an acute phase serum is not available, a specimen taken 4-6 weeks after onset and one taken 12-14 weeks after onset may reveal a decline in titer that has diagnostic significance. When only a single convalescent phase serum is available, significance is given to a titer greater than 1:160. However, it must be remembered that CF antibodies may persist in high titer for many years after rickettsial infection or immunization.

Since group-specific antigens are used, results must not be interpreted as to a specific agent, except in the case of Q fever. Report results as "CF titer of spotted fever group," "CF titer of epidemic murine group," etc.

Broad-spectrum antibiotic therapy may suppress or completely inhibit the CF antibody response so that caution is required in interpreting a negative result.[8]

Weil-Felix agglutination test[9, 10]

This test is described in Chapter 107.

---

*Lederle Laboratories Division, American Cyanamid Co., Pearl River, N.Y.; Parke, Davis & Co., Detroit; Markham Laboratories, Chicago.

Table 95-4. Reactions of rickettsiae to group-specific CF antigens

| | Reaction with rickettsial CF antigens | | | | |
Disease	*RMSF*	*Rickettsialpox*	*Epidemic typhus*	*Murine typhus*	*Q fever*
Rocky Mountain spotted fever (RMSF)	++++	++++	–	–	–
Rickettsialpox	++++	++++	–	–	–
Epidemic typhus	–	–	++++	±	–
Murine typhus	–	–	±	++++	–
Q fever	–	–	–	–	++++
Scrub typhus (tsutsugamushi fever)	–	–	–	–	–

Luoto capillary agglutination test[11]

This test was originally devised for the serologic diagnosis of Q fever in cattle and has been shown to be highly specific and sensitive.

Procedure

1. Prepare 2-fold serum dilutions ranging from 1:10 to 1:640.
2. Using 9 mm capillary tubes, draw each serum dilution into a tube until it is one-third full; then fill remainder with test antigen.
3. Seal both ends of each capillary tube with wax and place upright in a Plasticine block.
4. Incubate for 2 h at 37 C and then read degree of agglutination.

Microimmunofluorescence test

See Philip et al.[12] and Hechemy.[13]

REFERENCES

1. Topping, N., Bengtson, I., Henderson, R., et al.: National Institutes of Health Bull. no. 183, 1945.
2. Simmons, J. S., and Gentzkow, C. J.: Medical and public health laboratory methods, Philadelphia, 1955, Lea & Febiger.
3. Burrows, W.: Textbook of microbiology, ed. 16, Philadelphia, 1954, W. B. Saunders Co.
4. Diagnostic procedures for viral and rickettsial diseases, ed. 2, New York, 1956, American Public Health Association.
5. Rivers, T. M., and Horsfall, F. L.: Viral and rickettsial infections in man, ed. 3, Philadelphia, 1959, J. B. Lippincott Co.
6. Parker, R. R.: J.A.M.A. **110:**273, 1938.
7. Platz, H., Reagan, R. L., and Wertman, K.: Proc. Soc. Exp. Biol. Med. **55:**173, 1944.
8. Lennette, E. H., Clark, W. H., Jensen, F. W., and Toomb, C. J.: J. Immun. **68:**591, 1952.
9. Zarafonetis, C. J. D., Ingraham, H. S., and Berry, J. F.: J. Immunol. **52:**189, 1946.
10. Joseph, J. M.: Laboratory methods, Bureau of Laboratories, Maryland State Department of Health, Baltimore, 1962.
11. Luoto, L. A.: J. Immunol. **71:**226, 1953.
12. Philip, R. N., Casper, R. A., Ormsbee, M. G., et al.: J. Clin. Microbiol. **3:**51, 1976.
13. Hechemy, K. E., Stevens, R. W., Sasowski, S., et al.: J. Clin. Microbiol. **9:**292, 1979.

MEDICAL PARASITOLOGY

96

GENERAL CONSIDERATIONS

Michael H. Ivey

Chapters 96-100 review the fundamentals of medical parasitology and provide useful information about parasitologic problems encountered in the diagnostic laboratory. Emphasis is placed on information relevant to intelligent laboratory diagnosis. The reader should consult other references for detailed information on prevention, control, symptoms, pathology, and treatment.

CLASSIFICATION

Parasitic animals that live in or on humans include a wide variety of forms from several diverse phyla. They vary from single-cell protozoa only a few micrometers in size to tapeworm species that may reach 6 meters in length. Although closely related forms may look similar in shape and size, they usually have distinctive morphologic characteristics. These morphologic characteristics along with the parasite's life history provide the main basis for classification and identification.

The classification of parasitic animals is based on the International Code of Zoological Nomenclature. Each parasite is placed in a **phylum, class, order, family, genus, and species.** In some cases subgroupings such as subphylum, suborder, superfamily, subfamily, and subspecies are used to classify parasites further. Each parasite has been given a scientific name according to laws of priority. The name consists of the genus and species designation assigned to that particular organism. For example, *Enterobius vermicularis* and *Necator americanus* are the genus and species names given pinworms and hookworms, 2 different species. The use of genus and species designation, spoken of as binomial nomenclature, eliminates confusion that might arise from use of common names that vary from country to country. The parasitic animals (other than arthropods) frequently encountered in humans are presented in a classification scheme similar to that used by Faust et al.[1]

  I. Phylum Protozoa; subphylum Mastigophora
    A. Superclass Mastigophorasica
      1. Class Zoomastigophasida

        a. *Enteromonas hominis*
        b. *Embadomonas intestinalis*
        c. *Chilomastix mesnili*
        d. *Giardia lamblia*
        e. *Trichomonas hominis*
        f. *Trichomonas vaginalis*
        g. *Trichomonas tenax*
        h. *Leishmania donovani*
        i. *Leishmania tropica*
        j. *Leishmania braziliensis*
        k. *Trypanosoma cruzi*
        l. *Trypanosoma rhodesiense*
        m. *Trypanosoma gambiense*
        n. *Trypanosoma rangeli*
    B. Superclass Sarcodasica
      1. Class Rhizopodasida
        a. *Entamoeba histolytica*
        b. *Entamoeba hartmanni*
        c. *Entamoeba coli*
        d. *Entamoeba gingivalis*
        e. *Endolimax nana*
        f. *Iodamoeba bütschlii*
        g. *Dientamoeba fragilis*
        h. *Naegleria fowleri*
        i. *Hartmannella* sp.
        j. *Acanthamoeba* sp.
  II. Phylum Protozoa; subphylum Apicomplexa
    A. Class Sporozoasida
      1. Subclass Coccidiasina
        a. *Isospora belli*
        b. *Isospora hominis*
        c. *Toxoplasma gondii*
        d. *Sarcocystis lindemanni*
        e. *Plasmodium falciparum*
        f. *Plasmodium vivax*
        g. *Plasmodium malariae*
        h. *Plasmodium ovale*
  III. Phylum Protozoa; subphylum Ciliophora
    A. Class Ciliasida
      1. *Balantidium coli*
  IV. Protozoan of uncertain status
    A. *Pneumocystis carinii*
  V. Phylum Nematoda
    A. Class Aphasmidia
      1. *Trichinella spiralis*
      2. *Trichuris trichiura*
      3. *Capillaria hepatica*
      4. *Capillaria philippinensis*
    B. Class Phasmidia
      1. *Strongyloides stercoralis*
      2. *Ancylostoma duodenale*
      3. *Ancylostoma braziliense*
      4. *Ancylostoma ceylanicum*
      5. *Necator americanus*
      6. *Trichostrongylus* sp.
      7. *Enterobius vermicularis*

8. *Ascaris lumbricoides*
9. *Angiostrongylus cantonenis*
10. *Toxocara canis*
11. *Wuchereria bancrofti*
12. *Brugia malayi*
13. *Onchocercus volvulus*
14. *Acanthocheilonema perstans*
15. *Mansonella ozzardi*
16. *Loa loa*
17. *Drancunculus medinensis*

VI. Phylum Acanthocephala
    None important
VII. Phylum Platyhelminthes
    A. Class Trematoda
        1. Subclass Digenea
            a. *Schistosoma mansoni*
            b. *Schistosoma haematobium*
            c. *Schistosoma japonicum*
            d. *Fasciola hepatica*
            e. *Fasciolopsis buski*
            f. *Echinostoma ilocanum*
            g. *Opisthorchis felineus*
            h. *Clonorchis sinensis*
            i. *Heterophyes heterophyes*
            j. *Metagonimus yokogawai*
            k. *Paragonimus westermani*
    B. Class Cestoidea
        1. Subclass Cestoda
            a. *Taenia saginata*
            b. *Taenia solium*
            c. *Echinococcus granulosus*
            d. *Echinococcus multilocularis*
            e. *Hymenolepis nana*
            f. *Hymenolepis diminuta*
            g. *Dipylidium caninum*
            h. *Diphyllobothrium latum*
VIII. Phylum Annelida
    A. Class Hirudinea (leeches)
        1. *Liminatis* sp.
        2. *Dinobdella* sp.
        3. *Haemadipea* sp.
IX. Phylum Arthropoda
    The species of medical importance are too numerous to list. The arthropods of medical importance are placed in one of the following groups:
    A. Crustacea, e.g., copepods, crabs, and crayfish (serve as intermediate hosts)
    B. Chilopoda, e.g., centipedes (venomous) and millipedes (venomous)
    C. Arachnida, e.g., scorpions (venomous), spiders (venomous), ticks (venomous and vectors), mites (vectors)
    D. Pentastomida, e.g., tongue worms (endoparasites)
    E. Insecta, e.g., sucking lice, true bugs, beetles, bees, wasps, ants, flies, fleas (depending on species may be venomous, biologic or mechanical vectors, intermediate hosts, or parasitic)

BIOLOGIC CONSIDERATIONS
Definitions and host-parasite interactions

Different species of organisms that live together have a **symbiotic** relationship. This association may manifest itself in several ways. If the relationship is beneficial for both the association is termed **mutualism.** However, if one species benefits significantly while the other is not affected the association is termed **commensalism.** The participants in this relationship are the **host**

and the **commensal.** In another type of symbiotic relationship one species benefits at the expense (implying that harm occurs) of another. This association is recognized as **parasitism,** and the participants are designated **parasite** and **host.**

These definitions present philosophic and semantic difficulties in common usage. For example, the nonpathogenic intestinal organisms such as *Entamoeba coli, Endolimax nana,* and *Iodamoeba bütschlii* probably never injure the host; thus they are true commensals by the above definition. Yet most authorities refer to them as parasites. More confusion arises if the organism can transform from commensal to parasite. For example, *Entamoeba histolytica* probably lives as a commensal in humans most of the time but definitely possesses the potential to cause symptoms and pathology, thus becoming a parasite. Smyth's[2] definition of a parasite (i.e., an organism that lives in intimate contact with another species and is "metabolically dependent" on it to some degree) tends to soften or eliminate the problem associated with definitions that require a judgment concerning whether one organism lives at the "expense" of another. The metabolic dependency may be the need for nutritional components or physiologic stimuli that control the maturation process of the parasite. This definition classifies according to dependency on the host and eliminates the necessity to classify on the basis of injury or noninjury to the host, a status that is often difficult to determine.

The outcome of the host-parasite encounter varies greatly. Some parasites are frequently highly virulent, overcome the host's immune response to a large extent, and cause disease. Others cause little or no discernible harm. Either they lack virulence potential or the host immune response contains or conquers the parasite. In recent years still another facet of host-parasite balance has become apparent. Potentially dangerous parasites may live in humans and cause relatively little harm until steroids, cytotoxic drugs, or other therapeutic measures compromise the host's immune system. Under such circumstances latent infections of *Strongyloides, Toxoplasma, Pneumocystis,* and other parasites may flourish, causing considerable harm to the patient.

How do we become infected with parasitic animals? Much of the answer depends on where the organism lives in our bodies; how and in what form it or its progeny escape from our bodies; how and where the organism lives, develops, and persists outside the body; and what customs and habits we have that may facilitate transmission. Parasitic organisms may infect persons following (1) ingestion of water or food contaminated with feces that contain the organism, (2) ingestion of the infective stage that resides in an animal or plant tissue (having undergone some development in that plant or animal before it became infectious for humans, (3) active penetration of the skin by invasive forms, (4) inoculation by an arthropod vector, or (5) person-to-person spread following close body contact.

Transmission via fecal contamination is the primary means of spread of all intestinal protozoa. Many helminths (e.g., *Enterobius, Hymenolepis, Taenia,* and *Echinococcus*) infect humans in a similar manner, although in some instances the eggs given off by the worms must develop outside the body for a time before becoming infectious. *Ascaris lumbricoides, Trichuris trichiura,* and *Toxocara* species are examples of the latter case.

Transmission of many helminths depends on a person's eating food prepared in a manner that does not kill the infective form residing in the food. In most cases infection results from ingestion of raw or partially cooked food. *Trichinella spiralis* and *Taenia solium* are usually contracted from eating improperly cooked pork. *Diphyllobothrium latum* and *Clonorchis sinensis* are transmitted by ingestion of improperly cooked fish. Other examples of transmission via foods are described in subsequent chapters.

Several helminths infect humans by skin penetration. In most cases, however, improper disposal of feces affords the chance for development of the form that can infect by this route. Examples of parasites that infect via skin penetration are *Necator americanus, Strongyloides stercoralis,* and *Schistosoma mansoni.*

Several protozoan infections and some nematode infections are transmitted by arthropod vectors. Mosquitoes transmit malaria and *Wuchereria bancrofti* infections. Different species of insects transmit trypanosomal, leishmanial, and other filarial infections.

Personal contact may serve as a means of transmission in a few instances. *Trichomonas vaginalis,* for example, is thought to be transmitted primarily by sexual contact or intimate contact with clothing or towels of infected persons. *Entamoeba gingivalis,* a commensal of the mouth, is probably transmitted by kissing. Various arthropods (e.g., *Phthirus pubis, Pediculus humanis,* and *Sarcoptes scabiei*) usually require close body contact for spread from person to person.

The presence or absence of parasites in a community depends largely on the presence of adequate hosts, environmental conditions, and cultural factors that facilitate transmission. Before a parasite can infect another host a set sequence of events must take place. The sequence may be fairly simple, involving only improper disposal of feces containing the infectious stage by one host and ingestion of the infectious stage by another unsuspecting host. This happens in all feces-borne diseases—viral, protozoan, or bacterial. In other cases the sequence of events that must take place before spreading to another host can occur may be complicated, involving economic, biologic, and cultural factors. For example, *Fasciolopsis buski* eggs, after passing from the human intestinal tract in the feces, require a period of development in fresh water. The emerging larval form must penetrate a specific species of snail before developing further. Subsequent larval forms developed from the original leave the snail and encyst on the undersurface of water plants. Humans acquire infection usually by peeling the water plant with their teeth to get at the nut inside the plant. The sequence of events for infection must take place in that order and illustrates how a person's habits are responsible for parasite transmission. Many other examples could be cited where personal habits such as improper disposal of feces or improper cooking of food are the means by which parasites survive and perpetuate themselves.

There are many thousands of animal parasites, but humans are regularly parasitized by only a few dozen. In some cases our customs do not bring us in contact with a parasitic species to which otherwise we are susceptible. This is the case with parasites such as spirurids, Acanthocephala, and most tapeworms that encyst in insects as the intermediate host. People rarely eat insects and are only rarely infected by these types of parasites, although they are susceptible. Fortunately, however, we are not susceptible to the majority of parasites afflicting other animals.

Some parasites may infect a variety of host species, while others may be capable of existing in only one host species. The reasons for this phenomenon are not clear. Apparently in their genesis and evolvement most parasites adapted themselves to the physiology and habits of their host(s). This adaptation increased their ability to infect that host but decreased their ability to infect other hosts with different habits and physiologic makeups.

REFERENCES

1. Faust, E. C., Beaver, P. C., and Jung, R. C.: Animal agents and vectors of human disease, ed. 4, Philadelphia, 1975, Lea & Febiger, p. 479.
2. Smyth, J. D.: Introduction to animal parasitology, Springfield, Ill., 1962, Charles C Thomas, Publisher, p. 470.

97

PHYLUM PROTOZOA

Michael H. Ivey

Protozoa are single-celled organisms belonging to the phylum protozoa. Many authorities classify them as members of the animal kingdom. Protozoans such as amebae and ciliates are phagotrophic, lack cell walls, and thus are easily identified as animals. Other forms, however, are more difficult to categorize. For example, some flagellated protozoa have plantlike cell walls. Others are phagotrophic, some osmotrophic, and still others photosynthetic. Another group, the slime molds, resemble plantlike fungi at 1 stage of their life cycle and animallike amebae in another stage.

The major microbial groups recognized today are probably descendants of ancient evolutionary lines that preceded the emergence of the 2 great lines that eventually gave rise to the more complex plants and animals. The more recent descendants of plants or animals generally have characteristics that make classification relatively simple. Most classification problems occur in those microbial organisms that possess characteristics of both plants and animals. They are probably more representative of organisms found before plant and animal lines emerged.

The problem of classifying microbial organisms has been resolved for the moment by placing them in a kingdom separate from the plant or animal kingdoms. Thus all unicellular, coenocytic, or undifferentiated multicellular organisms are placed in the kingdom *PROTISTA*. The organisms (protists) all have a relatively simple biologic organization. Within the past 20 years electron microscopy studies have revolutionized our knowledge about the way these cells function. There are basically 2 different kinds of protist cells. The less differentiated **procaryotic** cells include the bacteria and bluegreen algae. These cells lack a membrane-lined nucleus and other membrane-bound organelles such as mitochondria, chloroplasts, or Golgi apparatus. The nucleus of procaryotes is naked, consisting of a single chromosome.

The relatively complex **eucaryotic cells** include protozoa, fungi, and most algae. In these organisms nucleus and other organelles (e.g.,

mitochondria, Golgi apparatus, organellular ribosomes) are membrane bound. Eucaryotic organisms are genetically more complex than procaryotic organisms in that the nucleus may contain several chromosomes. In some instances sexual as well as asexual modes of reproduction occur. The only eucaryotic cells lacking mitochondria are certain anaerobic protozoa and fungi that obtain energy exclusively by fermentation of organic compounds. There are many other fundamental differences between procaryotic and eucaryotic cells implicit in the presence or absence of the intracellular organelles mentioned above. For a more complete discussion of these differences consult Stanier et al.[1]

The protozoa of medical importance to humans may be divided into at least 4 groups on the basis of morphology, means of locomotion, or means of reproduction. Flagellates all possess whiplike locomotory structures called flagella at some stage in their life cycle, whereas amebae move by simple extrusions of the protoplasm (pseudopods). Sporozoan parasites possess no special locomotory structures but do have a sexual cycle in addition to the asexual cycle common to other protozoa. Finally, ciliates possess and move by means of cilia.

Many protozoan species are not pathogenic. However, they may be difficult to differentiate from pathogenic species. For this reason the laboratory diagnostician must be familiar with characteristics of nonpathogenic as well as pathogenic species.

The general procedures utilized for diagnosis of the protozoa (see Chapter 100 for details of laboratory procedures) vary according to where the parasite is found in the body. The malarial parasites and blood or tissue flagellates (*Trypanosoma* and *Leishmania*) are usually detected in stained smears of blood or tissue. In the case of the blood or tissue flagellates cultivation procedures and animal inoculation are often useful diagnostic tools. The intestinal and atrial parasites, with a few exceptions, may be found as a motile trophozoite stage or a nonmotile, resistant cyst stage. In some cases, especially the intestinal flagellates, the type of movement of the trophozoites is enough to effect identification.

The fecal specimen containing trophozoites must be examined soon after collection or else the trophozoite degenerates and becomes uni-

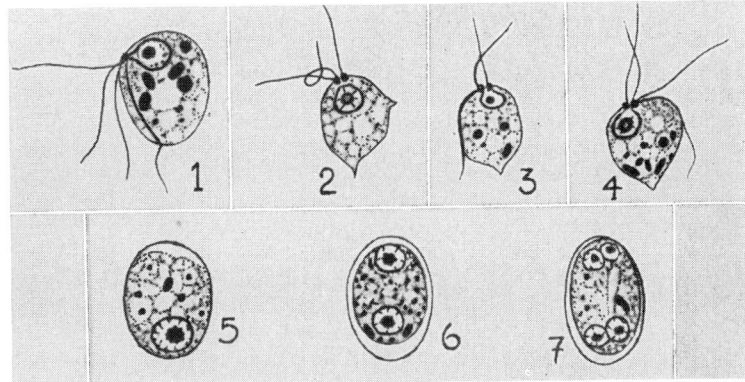

Fig. 97-1. *Enteromonas hominis.* **1,** Typical form of trophozoite with 4 flagella, 3 free and 1 recurrent. **2,** Recurrent flagellum is not clearly visible. **3,** Only 2 anterior flagella are visible. **4,** Typical form showing 2 blepharoplasts. **5-7,** Cysts uninucleate, binucleate, and quadrinucleate (mature) respectively. (From Kourí, P., and Basnuevo, J. G.: Lecciónes de parasitología y medicina tropical, Havana, Editorial Profilaxis S.A.)

dentifiable by any procedure. The cyst stage of the intestinal protozoa usually must be stained with iodine or hematoxylin to be identified, although size and shape often enable one to make a tentative identification without stains. Usually fecal specimens containing the cyst stage can be preserved in the refrigerator for several days without destroying morphologic features necessary for identification. The detailed morphologic structures described under each species are never clearly seen unless hematoxylin or similar permanent stains are used. All the intestinal protozoa possessing a cyst stage can be effectively concentrated by $ZnSO_4$ flotation or formalin ether sedimentation procedures. Trophozoites are not readily concentrated by any procedure.

SUBPHYLUM MASTIGOPHORA; SUPERCLASS MASTIGOPHORSICA
Species of intestinal and atrial flagellates

Enteromonas hominis, Embadomonas intestinalis, Chilomastix mesnili, Giardia lamblia, and *Trichomonas hominis* live in the intestinal tract of humans; *T. tenax* is found in the mouth and *T. vaginalis* in the genitourinary tract. All possess active trophozoite stages, and all except *Trichomonas* species possess cyst stages able to resist adverse conditions for varying lengths of time. Cysts may be readily concentrated by $ZnSO_4$ flotation or by one of the sedimentation procedures.

Enteromonas hominis

E. hominis probably has cosmopolitan distribution but apparently is not found or reported often in humans. The trophozoite is the active stage in humans, whereas the cyst is probably the resistant stage that is transferred from person to person by fecal contamination. The trophozoite lives in the large intestine and multiplies by binary longitudinal fission. Nuclear division in the cyst also results in multiplication. The pres-

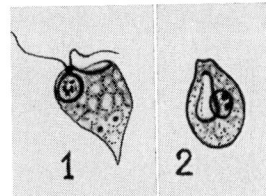

Fig. 97-2. *Embadomonas intestinalis.* **1,** Trophozoite. **2,** Cyst. (Adapted from Dobell and O'Connor; from Kourí, P., and Basnuevo, J. G.: Lecciónes de parasitología y medicina tropical, Havana, Editorial Profilaxis S.A.)

ence of this organism causes no demonstrable symptoms.

The trophozoite (Fig. 97-1) is pear shaped or ovoid, measuring 4-10 × 3-6 μm. In stained specimens a single nucleus with a large karyosome may be seen. In front of the nucleus are 4 flagella arising from a group of dotlike blepharoplasts. One of the flagella adheres closely to 1 side of the body and trails off the posterior end of the organism. In fresh specimens seen under the microscope the trophozoites exhibit jerky movements. The oval cyst (Fig. 97-1) measures 6-8 × 3-4 μm and possesses 2-4 nuclei with equal numbers at each end. Diagnosis of the trophozoite stage is based on demonstration of the organism in saline mounts of feces. Cyst stages may be identified in iodine-stained feces. Morphologic details, however, show up best in hematoxylin-stained preparations.

Embadomonas intestinalis

E. intestinalis, a seldom reported nonpathogenic inhabitant of the intestinal tract, probably has a cosmopolitan distribution. An active trophozoite and resistant cyst stage exist. Transmission occurs through the cyst by fecal contamination. The trophozoite (Fig. 97-2) measures 4-9 × 3-5 μm. In hematoxylin-stained specimens a single nucleus with a centrally located karyosome may be seen. Characteristically a cleftlike cytostome may be seen near the nucleus. The pear-shaped cyst measures 4-7 × 3-4 μm, contains a single nucleus, and appears to have a double-contoured wall. Diagnosis is based on demonstration of the trophozoite in saline or the cyst in iodine smears of feces. The cytostome of the trophozoite or the pear shape of the cyst is characteristic. Morphologic detail shows up best in hematoxylin-stained preparations.

Chilomastix mesnili

C. mesnili, a nonpathogenic inhabitant of the intestinal tract, has a cosmopolitan distribution but probably is more frequent in warm climates. An active trophozoite and resistant cyst stage oc-

cur. The infection is transmitted through the cyst by fecal contamination. The pear-shaped trophozoite (Fig. 97-3) measures 6-20 × 3-10 μm. A large spherical nucleus is present along with a characteristic spiral groove curving across the body. A well-defined oblong cytostome about twice as long as the nucleus may be seen extending below the nucleus. The live trophozoite is propelled by 3 anterior flagella and exhibits a spiral, jerky motion. The lemon- to oval-shaped cyst (Figs. 97-3 and 97-15) measures 6-10 μm in length, averaging 8 μm. Characteristically the cyst protrudes eccentrically at one end, breaking the symmetry of the other pole. A nucleus and cytostome may be seen in well-stained preparations. Diagnosis is based on demonstration of the trophozoite in saline or the cyst in iodine-stained

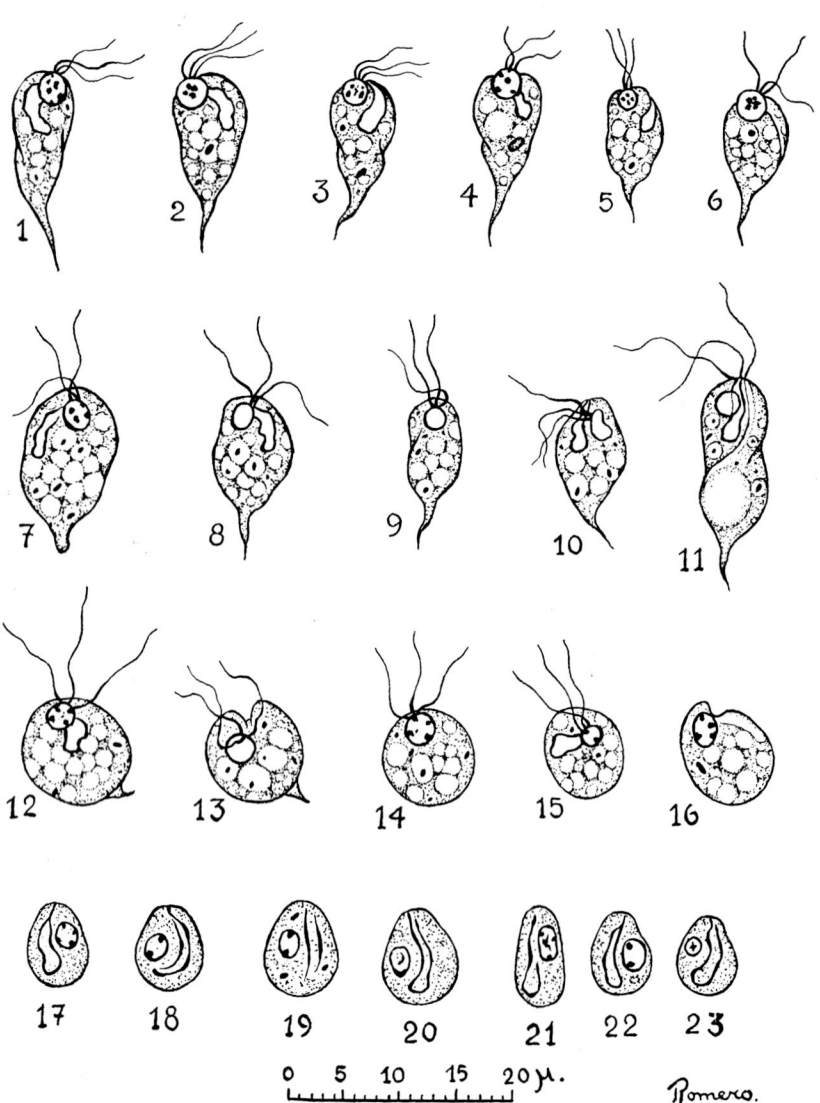

Fig. 97-3. *Chilomastix mesnili.* **1-11,** Trophozoites. **12-16,** Rounded or spherical trophozoites in the process of dying. **17-23,** Cysts. (Iron-hematoxylin stain.) (After Kourí, P., and Basnuevo, J. G.: Lecciónes de parasitología y medicina tropical, Havana, Editorial Profilaxis S.A.)

fecal smears. The spiral movement and spiral grooves are typical of the trophozoite, whereas the size and eccentric protuberance on one end characterize the cyst.

Giardia lamblia

This parasite has a cosmopolitan distribution and lives in the area of the duodenum, upper jejunum, and occasionally the gallbladder. The cyst stage is resistant to external environment and is the stage transmitted from person to person via fecal contamination.

Apparently *Giardia* can persist in the body and cause few if any symptoms. In recent years, however, reports of explosive outbreaks of symptomatic giardiasis have reemphasized the pathogenic potential of this organism.[2-5] Children are more frequently affected than adults. Symptoms most frequently reported are diarrhea, steatorrhea, weight loss up to 4.5 kg, and abdominal pains. Less frequent are complaints of nausea, fever, and intestinal malabsorption. Stool specimens from patients with giardiasis frequently have the consistency of porridge, are light in color, have no blood present, and have a fishy odor.

The mechanism of pathogenicity is not well understood. Intestinal malabsorption has been attributed to the apparent ability of the organism to literally coat or cover the mucosal surface.[6,7] Observed abnormalities in villus structure have been attributed to *Giardia*.[8,9] In other instances where such abnormalities were not apparent malabsorption has been explained as due to "coating" or interference with enzyme activity or microvillar function.[10] Most authorities believe *Giardia* to be strictly a lumen dweller. Recent reports[10-12] presented evidence that *Giardia* actually invades intestinal mucosal cells. At present the relationship of mucosal invasion to pathophysiology is controversial.

The pear-shaped trophozoite (Fig. 97-4) is bilaterally symmetrical with a broad, rounded anterior and a tapering posterior. Size varies from 9-21 μm in length by 5-15 μm in width. At the anterior end 2 nuclei, each with a large karyosome, may be seen lying within a sucking disc. A pair of slender axonemes (some authorities mis-

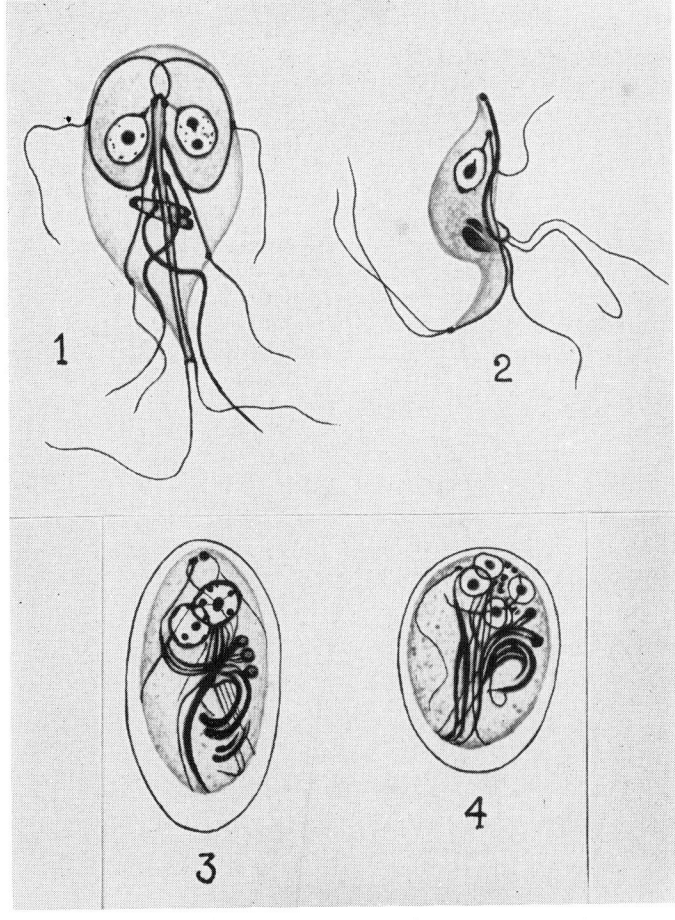

Fig. 97-4. *Giardia lamblia.* **1,** Trophozoite form, front view. **2,** Side view of trophozoite. **3,** Cystic form with 2 nuclei. **4,** Mature quadrinucleate cyst. (Adapted from Dobell and O'Connor; from Kouri, P., and Basnuevo, J. G.: Lecciónes de parasitología y medicina tropical, Havana, Editorial Profilaxis S.A.)

takenly call these structures axostyles), originating from blepharoplast above the nuclei, run the median length of the organism. A pair of dark-staining, short, rodlike median bodies is found approximately in the center of the organism.

The ovoid cyst (Figs. 97-4 and 97-15) measures 8-14 μm in length by 7-10 μm in width. In stained specimens the contents of the cyst may shrink from the cyst wall, leaving a clear space. Four nuclei, the axonemes, and short thick fibrils may be discerned in stained specimens.

Laboratory diagnosis is based on demonstration of the trophozoite or cyst in feces. Fecal examinations are often unproductive.[13] In addition to saline and iodine-stained fecal smears, concentration technics should be used. If these are negative and giardiasis is still suspected, duodenal aspirates should be examined. The live trophozoite exhibits an irregular progression, rotation, and rocking movement. In stained specimens the shape, size, character of nuclei, sucking disc, axonemes, and fibril aid in identification. Detailed morphologic structures are apparent only with hematoxylin or similar stains. However, iodine stain will show enough detail to make identification of the cyst possible.

Trichomonas hominis

This parasite has a cosmopolitan distribution and is a nonpathogenic inhabitant of the large intestines. No cyst stage has been described. Apparently the trophozoite is relatively resistant to adverse conditions and is the stage transmitted from person to person via fecal contamination.

The trophozoite (Fig. 97-5) may assume a variety of shapes. The organism possesses a rather large nucleus with 3-5 flagella seen trailing off from a blepharoplast located near the nucleus. A curved rigid axostyle extends the length of the organism and slightly beyond it. A rather heavy costa forms the base of attachment for the undulating membrane that runs the length of the organism and trails off into a free flagellum.

The nervous, jerky, rotating movements, the undulating membrane, and the axostyle serve to distinguish this organism from others in the feces. In stained specimens the axostyle and prominent costa are characteristic. Diagnosis is made in simple saline smears, since the trophozoite is destroyed or distorted by the usual iodine stains and concentration procedures. The organism is easier to identify in the living state than in stained smears.

Trichomonas vaginalis

T. vaginalis, a cosmopolitan parasite, inhibits the genitourinary tract of humans. The organism divides by binary fission. No cyst stage is known. In view of the limited ability of the organism to survive outside the host, it must be assumed that the primary mode of transmission is by sexual contact and secondarily by contaminated clothing, towels, and so on. The reported prevalence of *T. vaginalis* is much greater in females, but this may be due in part to the fact that males invariably have asymptomatic infections. In females the organism may be associated with varying degrees of vaginitis and vaginal discharge, or the organism may cause no observable symptoms. Thus the organism may be an opportunist, requiring the presence of relatively high host pH, certain other organisms, or other factors not yet known in order to cause symptoms. Also there may be pathogenic and nonpathogenic strains of *T. vaginalis* that account for the variable effects of this organism on the host.

The organism resembles *T. hominis* in general morphology. It differs in that *T. vaginalis* is usually larger that *T. hominis*, measuring 5-15 μm in length. Unlike *T. hominis* the undulating membrane does not extend the entire length of the body. However, the diagnosis of *T. vaginalis* presents no problem, since it is the only trichomonad found in the vagina or urethral tract. Diagnosis may be made by microscopic examination of vaginal exudate, urethral discharge, prostatic secretions, or, occasionally, centrifuged urine. *T. vaginalis* exhibits the typical nervous, jerky trichomonad movement and possesses a characteristic undulating membrane. *T. vaginalis* can

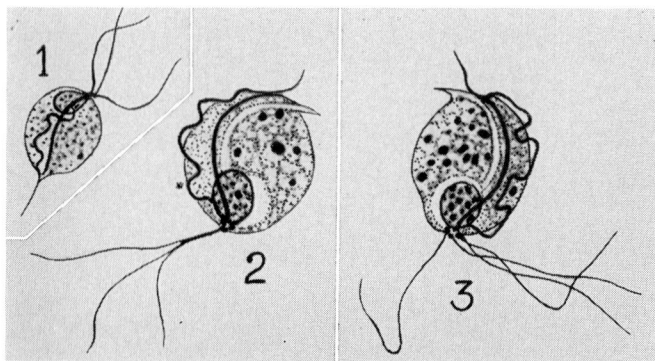

Fig. 97-5. *Trichomonas hominis.* **1,** Small specimen with 3 anterior flagella. **2,** Large specimen with 3 anterior flagella. **3,** Specimen with 4 anterior flagella. (After Dobell and O'Connor; from Kourí, P., and Basnuevo, J. G.: Lecciónes de parasitología y medicina tropical, Havana, Editorial Profilaxis S.A.)

be detected more often by cultivation in one of several media available for the purpose.

Trichomonas tenax

T. tenax is considered a nonpathogenic inhabitant of the mouth, although a higher incidence is reported in unclean or diseased mouths. Apparently transmission is by direct contact such as kissing. The organism resembles the other trichomonads in general morphology and movements. However, it is site specific and is the only species found in the mouth. Diagnosis is made either by examining smears of debris from diseased gums or carious teeth or by cultivation.

Blood and tissue flagellates

Several species of *Leishmania* and *Trypanosoma* are capable of infecting humans. Depending on the species involved, parasites of the genus *Leishmania* can cause cutaneous leishmaniasis, diffuse cutaneous leishmaniasis, visceral leishmaniasis, or post-kala-azar dermal leishmaniasis. *Trypanosoma gambiense* and *T. rhodesiense* are causative agents of African sleeping sickness. *T. cruzi* is the etiologic agent of Chagas' disease. Another trypanosome of South and Central America, *T. rangeli,* can give rise to parasitemia but no apparent symptomatology.

All of these parasites require 2 hosts in their life cycles, a susceptible mammal (including humans) and a blood-sucking insect vector. Sand flies belonging to the genera *Phlebotomus* and *Lutzomyia* transmit leishmanial infections. Various species of *Glossina* (tsetse flies) serve as vectors of *T. rhodesiense* or *T. gambiense.* The Western hemisphere trypanosomes *T. cruzi* and *T. rangeli* are transmitted by triatomid bugs (species of *Triatoma, Rhodnius,* and *Panstrongylus*).

The blood and tissue flagellates undergo morphologic transformation when transferred from the mammalian host to the insect vector. A similar reverse transformation occurs when the vector inoculates the parasite into the mammalian host. The morphologic forms (Fig. 97-6) possess discernible features of diagnostic value. Formerly the 4 known morphologic forms were called leishmanial, leptomonad, crithidial, and trypano-

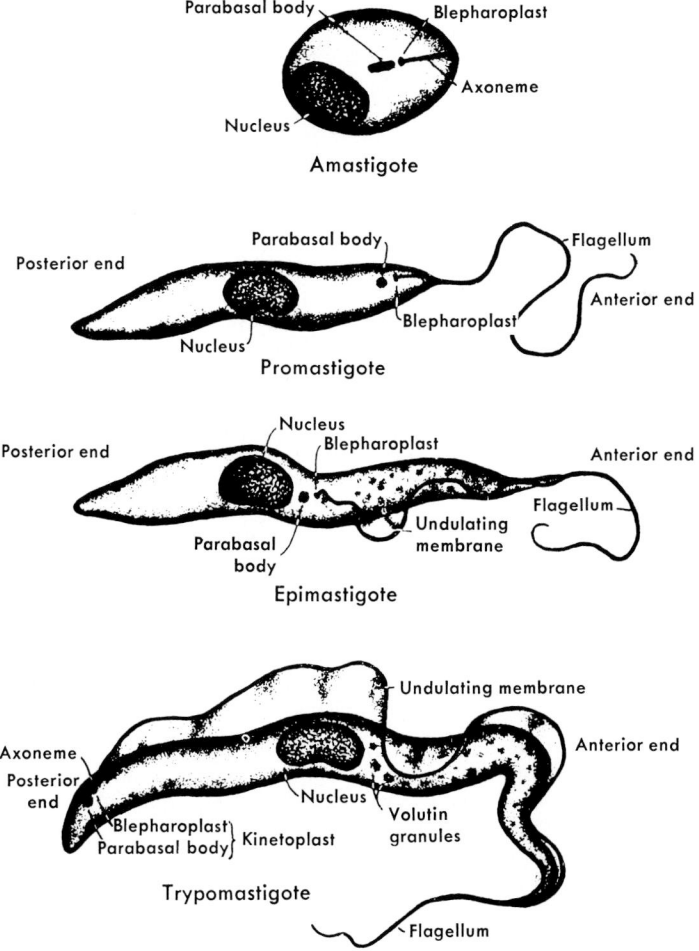

Fig. 97-6. Morphologic forms occurring in genera *Leishmania* and *Trypanosoma.*

Table 97-1. Stages of species of *Leishmania* and *Trypanosoma* in humans and in the insect host*

Species	Stage of parasite			
	Amastigote (leishmanial)	Promastigote (leptomonal)	Epimastigote (crithidial)	Trypomastigote (trypanosomal)
Leishmania tropica	Found in macrophages of skin and sub-cutaneous tissue	In midgut and, later, proboscis of sand fly (vector): transfer stage to humans	Absent	Absent
Leishmania braziliensis	Same as *L. tropica*	Same as *L. tropica*	Absent	Absent
Leishmania donovani	Found in macrophages in liver, spleen, bone marrow, and lymph nodes	Same as *L. tropica*	Absent	Absent
Trypanosoma rhodesiense	Absent	Absent	In salivary glands of tsetse fly (vector)	In proboscis of tsetse fly; transfer stage to humans; present in bloodstream and lymph nodes
Trypanosoma gambiense	Absent	Absent	Same as *T. rhodesiense*	Same as *T. rhodesiense*
Trypanosoma cruzi	Found in macrophages of skin, lymph nodes, liver, spleen, brain, etc.	Transitional stage only	In midgut of triatomid bug	In hindgut and feces of triatomid bug; transfer stage to humans; present in bloodstream during acute episodes

*Adapted from Faust, E. C., Beaver, P. C., and Jung, R. C.: Animal agents and vectors of human disease, ed. 4, Philadelphia, 1975, Lea & Febiger.

somal forms (shown in parentheses in Table 97-1). In a newer terminology, widely accepted by most authorities, the forms are renamed amastigote, promastigote, epimastigote, and trypomastigote (Fig. 97-6) respectively. All 4 forms possess a nucleus, a parabasal body, and a blepharoplast. The latter 2 structures collectively are called the kinetoplast. The undulating membrane if present originates from the blepharoplast. In recent years a great deal of valuable information has accumulated on flagellate ultrastructure and the relationship of structure to function during cyclic changes. The interested reader should consult Vickerman[14] for an authoritative review of this subject.

The amastigote is an intracellular parasite of mammals (including humans), less than 4 μm in size, that multiplies intracellularly in patients with leishmaniasis (all forms) and Chagas' disease. The trypomastigote is an extracellular parasite stage found in various *Trypanosoma* infections of humans and other mammals. The other morphologic stages, promastigotes and epimastigotes, occur primarily in the insect vector or in in vitro culture medium. Promastigotes are part of the life cycle of *Leishmania* species and are found in the intestines of the infected sand fly vector or, if inoculated, in culture medium. Epimastigotes as well as trypomastigotes occur in the insect vectors of African sleeping sickness and Chagas' disease. Table 97-1 summarizes where the various morphologic forms occur in the mammalian host and insect vectors.

Laboratory diagnosis of the blood and tissue flagellates depends on demonstration of the organism and to a lesser extent on in vitro cultivation, animal inoculation, or serologic tests. *Leishmania* infections can be diagnosed by demonstrating the amastigote in stained biopsy material or in many instances by cultivating the organisms in appropriate medium. Complement fixation, slide agglutination, fluorescent antibody, and skin tests also may be useful. *T. gambiense* and *T. rhodesiense* infections are diagnosed by finding trypomastigotes in wet mounts or stained smears of blood, swollen lymph node exudate, or spinal fluid. Inoculation of rats or mice is useful in the rhodesian but not the gambian form of sleeping sickness. Chagas' disease can be diagnosed by finding trypomastigotes in blood smears or amastigotes in biopsy material, by xenodiagnosis, by in vitro cultivation, or by serologic tests. For more detailed information on diagnosis refer to the section on each parasite and to Tables 100-3 to 100-5.

Visceral leishmaniasis

Traditional textbook presentations suggest that *Leishmania donovani* is the only etiologic agent of visceral leishmaniasis. Many recently published texts still adhere to this view. Observed differences in clincial disease or organism characteristics are simply explained away as strain variations within the one recognized species. However, support for this concept has eroded in the past decade. Recent epidemiologic, immuno-

Table 97-2. Geographic and age distribution, laboratory animal susceptibility, and cultural characteristics of *Leishmania* causing visceral leishmaniasis

Parasite species or subspecies	Clinical name and age distribuion	Susceptible animals	Growth in vitro	Geographic distribution
Leishmania donovani (*L. d. donovani*)	Visceral leishmaniasis, kala-azar; all age groups	Hamsters	Usually adequate	Bengal, Assam, Bangladesh, Thailand, Burma, Sumatra, Pakistan, Sudan, Ethiopia, Somalia, Fjibouti, Kenya, Chad, Niger, Dafur, Gabon
Leishmania infantum (*L. d. infantum*)	Infantile visceral leishmaniasis or kala-azar; children especially susceptible; adult asymptomatic	Hamsters and dogs; possibly gerbils, rats, and gerboas	Difficult to isolate	Countries surrounding the Mediterranean Sea, northern China, Near Eastern countries, Nigeria, USSR
Leishmania chagasi (*L. d. chagasi*)	New World visceral leishmaniasis; primarily in infants and children	Hamsters	Very difficult to isolate	Argentina, Paraguay, Bolivia, Columbia, Venezuela, Salvador, Guatamala, Mexico, Guadaloupe, several sections of Brazil

logic, biologic, and clinical data suggest that the *Leishmania* causing visceral leishmaniasis belong to a complex consisting of several species or subspecies. Many authorities believe that adherence to the traditional concept of a single-species etiologic agent promotes confusion as to the true meaning of the observed differences in epidemiology, biology, immunology, and clinical manifestations associated with this disease. Similar speciation problems exist with the *Leishmania* responsible for cutaneous leishmaniasis.

Each member of the *L. donovani* complex has certain characteristics that justify its being considered a separate species or subspecies. For example, each can be differentiated serologically; each has different DNA buoyant densities, and each has special charactertics in conncection with the disease that it causes in humans or the reservoir host. Table 97-2 summarizes certain characteristics of members of the *L. donovani* complex.

Members of the *L. donovani* complex are the causative agents of visceral leishmaniasis or kala-azar. The prototype of this complex, *Leishmania donovani donovani*, causes kala-azar in all age groups. Dogs appear to be the most important animal reservoir, allthough in certain areas, especially India, they appear to be of no importance. Another member of this complex, *L. d. infantum*, is a causative agent of infantile visceral leishmaniasis. The fox and jackal appear to be important wildlife reservoirs, and the dog appears to be the major domestic reservoir. The third member of this complex, *L. d. chagasi*, causes visceral leishmaniasis in the Western Hemisphere. However, some authorities consider that the taxonomic status of *L. d. chagasi* is not well defined and that perhaps it is the same organism as *L. d. infantum*. Dogs and possibly foxes are reservoirs.

Life cycle—epidemiology. In humans the amastigote multiplies by binary fission in the en-

dothelial cells of the reticuloendothelial system. Eventually the parasites destroy the cells and invade new ones. The amastigotes are ingested by various species of *Phlebotomus* or *Lutzomyia* and transform into promastigotes in the insect intestines. Within the sand fly the promastigote multiplies by longitudinal fission. Eventually (1-2 weeks) they migrate to the anterior portion of the buccal cavity, where they can be injected into humans when the fly takes a blood meal. Kala-azar is limited to sharply defined areas due to the inability of the sand fly to travel more than a few hundred yards from its breeding place. Sand flies breed in rubble, cracks in houses, and places near human habitation.

The infection in humans is frequently fatal unless treated. It may follow an acute, subacute, or chronic course over a period of a week, a few weeks, or 2-3 years. The symptoms of infection are related to changes in the reticuloendothelial system, especially the spleen, bone marrow, and liver. Destruction of cells in these organs may give rise to anemia early in the infection and eventually leukopenia, prolonged clotting time, and an increase in blood volume, thiocyanate space, and interstitial fluid. Usually the Coomb's test becomes positive, and cold agglutinins to red blood cells can be detected as well as platelet and leukocyte agglutinins. Characteristically the serum albumin and IgM levels are decreased and the IgG levels are greatly increased. Erythropoiesis is greatly increased; granulopoiesis is decreased.

A cutaneous form of leishmaniasis called postkala-azar dermal leishmaniasis may occur in patients with inadequately treated visceral leishmaniasis. In such instances cutaneous eruptions develop several months after cessation of the treatment. Amastigote forms can be recovered from the cutaneous lesions.

Morphology. The etiologic agent occurs intracellularly in various leukocytes or endothelial

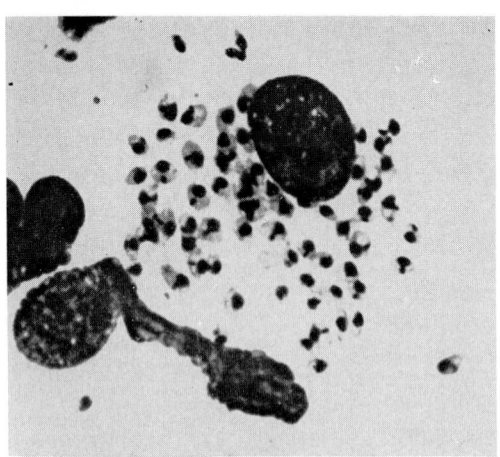

Fig. 97-7. *Leishmania donovani* amastigotes in stained smear from spleen puncture. (From Hunter, G. W., III, Frye, W. W., and Swartzwelder, J. D.: A manual of tropical medicine, Philadelphia, 1960, W. B. Saunders Co.)

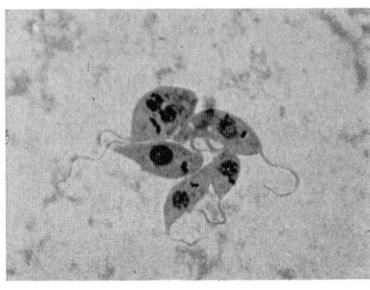

Fig. 97-8. Promastigote stages in culture of *Leishmania braziliensis* in NNN medium. (From Pessôa, S. B. In Gradwohl, R. B. H., Benitez Soto, L., and Felsenfeld, O.: Clinical tropical medicine, St. Louis, The C. V. Mosby Co.)

cells (Fig. 97-7). In Giemsa- or Wright-stained preparations the amastigotes appear as small, nonflagellated oval bodies measuring 2-3 × 1-2 μm. Within the pale blue cytoplasm of the parasite may be seen a relatively large red-staining nucleus. At right angles to the nucleus a dark-staining parabasal body may be evident. During the staining procedure the parasitized host cell often ruptures, releasing the amastigotes. On microscopic examination such organisms will appear outside the host cells.

The promastigotes occur either in the insect vector or in culture and closely resemble the promastigotes of other *Leishmania* species (Fig. 97-8). Their size will usually vary from 15-25 μm in length and 1.5-3.5 μm in width. Short, stumpy forms may occur. All promastigotes typically possess a single flagellum at the anterior and a large centrally located nucleus.

Diagnosis. Laboratory diagnosis depends on demonstration of the parasite either in stained tissue or blood, by culture, animal inoculation, or one of several serologic tests. Fig. 97-7 illustrates

amastigotes seen in a stained smear of spleen tissue. The diagnostic method of choice will vary with the experience of the clinician and the species of *Leishmania* to be isolated. Giemsa- or Wright-stained blood smears have proved of value in diagnosing kala-azar in India but not in other areas. If present the organisms are frequently found in white cells along the edges of the smear. Spleenic puncture probably reveals more positive cases than do any other procedures, but some clinicians object to the inherent hazard of the procedure to the patient. Sternal and liver punctures are safer but reveal fewer positive cases. Gland puncture has proved of value in the Mediterranean and Sudan regions, where glandular involvement is common. In the Sudan, organisms are often recovered from nasal secretions. Skin scrapings of lesions are frequently of value in the Sudan and India, especially in inadequately treated patients that subsequently develop post-kala-azar dermal leishmaniasis. Any of the above tissue material may be inoculated into NNN culture medium in combination with antibiotics. *L. d. donovani* is easier to culture than *L. d. infantum* or *L. D. chagasi*. In positive cases the promastigotes are evident after 7-30 days of cultivation.

Diagnosis via inoculation of laboratory animals is not recommended. Gerbils, gerboas, and rats are susceptible to *L. d. donovani* and *L. d. chagasi*. In past years nonspecific chemical tests were widely used to detect elevated euglobulin and decreased albumin ratios that occur in patients with kala-azar. The addition of chemicals such as antimony, formalin, or distilled water to the serum of patients with elevated euglobulins will cause precipitates or gels to form. Obviously any other conditions that cause an altered euglobulin-albumin ratio will give positive tests also. Such tests are being replaced by more reliable procedures.

Complement fixation and skin tests have long been accepted as useful diagnostic tests (Table 100-5). More recently the hemagglutination and fluorescent antibody technics have been shown to be of diagnostic value. Best results are obtained with antigens prepared from *Leishmania* rather than the antigens prepared from *Mycobacterium* species that have been used in the past. Consult Bray[15] and Dumonde and Preston[16] for recent reviews of this subject. For detailed diagnostic information see Tables 100-3 and 100-4.

Cutaneous leishmaniasis

As previously stated the taxonomic status of all of the *Leishmania* species are undergoing reevaluation. Traditionally cutaneous leishmaniasis has been thought to be caused by either *Leishmania tropica* in the Old World or by *Leishmania braziliensis* in the Western Hemisphere. Lumsden[17] suggested that there are 3 complexes that may be etiologic agents of cutaneous leishmaniasis. The members of each complex with their

Table 97-3. Geographic distribution and laboratory animal susceptibility of *Leishmania* species causing cutaneous leishmaniasis

Parasite complex and species	Clinical name	Known geographic distribution
L. tropica complex		
L. t. tropica (or *L. tropica*)	Cutaneous leishmaniasis, oriental sore	Urban areas in countries surrounding the Mediterranean Sea, Near Eastern Asia
L. t. major (or *L. major*)	Zoonotic cutaneous leishmaniasis	Rural areas of Israel, Jordan, Turkmen, Kazakh, USSR, Iran, Senegal, Mali, Sudan, Niger, Nigeria, Angola, Namibia
L. aethiopica	Diffuse cutaneous leishmaniasis (DCL)	Ethiopian highlands, Mount Elgon, Kenya, possibly southwest Yemen
L. mexicana complex		
L. m. mexicana	Chiclero's ulcer, bay sore	Southern Mexico, Honduras, Guatamala, Panama
L. m. amazonensis	Cutaneous leishmaniasis (DCL)	Northern Brazil, Southern Venezuela
L. m. pifanoi		Venezuela
L. braziliensis complex		
L. b. braziliensis	Cutaneous and mucocutaneous leishmaniasis, expundia	Brazil, Amazonian Peru, Ecuador, Bolivia, Venezuela, Paraguay, Columbia
L. b. guyanensis	Pian bois, bosch yaws, forest yaws	Guyana, Surinam, Brazil, Venezuela
L. b. panamensis	Cutaneous leishmaniasis	Panama, possible elsewhere in Central America
L. peruviana	Uta	Western Andes of Peru

clinical names and geographic distribution are summarized in Table 97-3.

The *Leishmania tropica* complex characteristically gives rise to cutaneous lesions that are confined to the skin and do not tend to visceralize or spread. Hamsters and mice are usually susceptible, and usually the organisms can be cultured without difficulty. The 2 best known members of this complex are *L. t. tropica* and *L. t. major* (some authorities contend that *L. t. major* deserves seperate species status, *L. major*, on the basis of its unique antigenic, nosologic, and epidemiologic characteristics). A third species, *L. aethiopica*, appears to be a member of this complex but possesses characteristics (clinical, antigenic, and laboratory animal susceptibility) that probably warrant classifying it as a separate species within the complex. *L. t. tropica* occurs primarily in urban areas and produces a single dry sore that usually heals spontaneously with scarring within a few months. Usually no animal reservoir hosts are involved in the epidemiology of *L. t. tropica*. In contrast *L. t. major* occurs primarily in rural areas, causes a moist, weeping sore, and reservoir hosts are an important part of the epidemiology. *L. t. major* (or *L. major*) is essentially a zoonotic infection.

A second more recently defined complex, the *Leishmania mexicana* complex, occurs in various areas of the Western Hemisphere (Table 97-3). Members of this complex are characterized as zoonotic parasites, relatively fast-growing organisms in culture and in hamsters. In hamsters metastatic spread occurs, but the inflammatory response is poor and lesions usually contain many amastigotes. Cutaneous lesions in humans are usually mild with no nasopharyngeal involvement. The prototype member of this complex, *L. m. mexicana*, causes a mild infection in humans (i.e., a single cutaneous lesion that is self-healing or a persistent, chronic ear lesion). The second member of this complex, *L. m. amazonensis*, occurs throughout the Amazon Basin. It rarely infects humans but can give rise to mild lesions, usually single or limited. There is no predilection for the ear tissue or the nasopharynx. An occasional disseminated cutaneous leishmaniasis (DCL) has been reported. The third member of this complex, *L. m. pifanoi*, occurs in Venezuela and is only known to cause DCL.

The third complex responsible for cutaneous leishmaniasis is the *Leishmania braziliensis* complex. Members of this complex grow relatively slowly in culture and in hamsters. The importance of wild animals as reservoirs has not been established. In hamsters the host response is marked and lesions have moderate or scanty amastigotes. There is no tendency for metastatic spread. The lesions in humans are single or multiple, often extensive and disfiguring. *L. b. braziliensis* frequently causes destructive cutaneous lesions, frequently large, persistent, and disfiguring, and frequently involving the nasopharyngeal area.

The second member of this complex, *L. b. guyanensis*, causes single lesions or it may spread to form many crateriform ulcers over the body. It also spreads along the lymphatics but probably does not involve the nasopharynx.

A third member of this complex, *L. b. pana-*

mensis, causes single or few shallow crateriform lesions and may metastasize as nodules along the lymphatics. It probably does not spread to the nasopharynx.

The last known member of this complex, perhaps a separate species by itself, *L. peruviana,* occurs along the western slopes of the Peruvian Andes up to a height of 3000 m. It is the only form not associated with forested areas. The disease manifests itself as a single or limited number of self-healing lesions with no nasopharangeal involvement. The clinical designation for this infection is uta.

The life cycle of all species of *Leishmania*

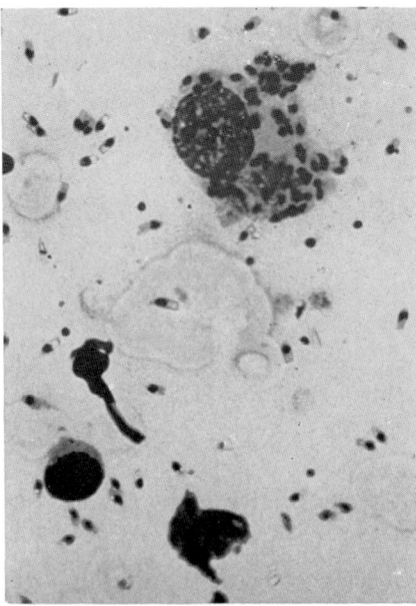

Fig. 97-9. Smear of material obtained from puncture of non-ulcerative lesion of mucocutaneous leishmaniasis; macrophage containing 62 amastigotes may be observed (Giemsa stain). (After Pessôa and Barretto in I. Meeting of Dermat. & Symph., Brazil, 1944; from Gradwohl, R. B. H., Benitez Soto, L., and Felsenfeld, O.: Clinical tropical medicine, St. Louis, The C. V. Mosby Co.)

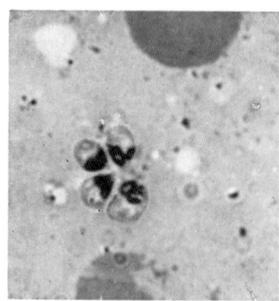

Fig. 97-10. *Leishmania braziliensis.* Parasites in rosette pattern. Smear from ulcer. (From Pessôa, S. B. In Gradwohl, R. B. H., Benitez Soto, L., and Felsenfeld, O.: Clinical tropical medicine, St. Louis, The C. V. Mosby Co.)

causing cutaneous leishmaniasis is essentially the same as that described for *L. donovani.* Different species of sand flies (*Phlebotomus* or *Lutzomyia*) serve as vectors. Various types of animals may serve as reservoirs, the exact type varying from area to area. Dogs, cats, or some rodents are most often involved as reservoirs.

Unlike kala-azar, cutaneous leishmaniasis is a localized infection involving the cutaneous tissues. The presence of the *L. tropica* complex organisms gives rise to a raised crateriform lesion with a depressed ulcerated center. The base of the lesion is granulated. Secondary bacterial infection is common. The lesions eventually heal with scarring. Infection with parasites belonging to members of one of the other complexes causes lesions characteristic for that species. Depending on the species the lesions may be solitary *(L. tropica),* may involve predominantly the mucocutaneous tissues *(L. braziliensis),* may involve the ear *(L. mexicana),* or may give rise to diffuse lepromatous-like lesions or other manifestations.

Morphology. The morphology of the various *Leishmania* species is identical to that described for *L. donovani* (Figs. 97-7 to 97-10).

Diagnosis. Laboratory diagnosis is based on demonstration of the amastigote within leukocytes in Giemsa-stained smears of tissue or aspirates taken from the indurated edge of the lesion. The appearance of *L. tropica* and *L. mexicana* in stained cutaneous lesion smears is identical to that seen for *L. braziliensis* (Figs. 97-9 and 97-10). Smears from the floor of the ulcer are usually negative. The organism may be demonstrated by inoculating lesion material into NNN medium containing antibiotics and incubating at 22-24 C until promastigotes appear. Members of the *L. mexicana* and *L. tropica* complexes grow better in culture media than members of the *L. braziliensis* complex.

The Montenegro skin test is a useful diagnostic tool. Intradermal injections of phenolized promastigotes provoke an erythematous wheal in 48 hours that may last 4-5 days. Routine serologic tests have not proved of value in diagnosis of cutaneous leishmaniasis. For detailed diagnostic information see Tables 100-3 to 100-5.

Trypanosoma cruzi

Geographic distribution. *T. cruzi,* the causative agent of Chagas' disease, occurs throughout South and Central America and Mexico. Although *T. cruzi* has been reported in wild animals and various species of triatomid bugs in the United States, only 2 cases have been reported in humans.

Life cycle—epidemiology. *T. cruzi* multiplies in humans as an amastigote in practically every organ of the body. The reticuloendothelial system, cardiac muscle, and central nervous system are most frequently involved. The amastigotes transform into trypomastigotes and escape from dying infected cells and invade new cells. The transitional, nonmultiplicative trypomastigotes may be detected in the peripheral circulation, especially during febrile episodes. Eventually these forms invade cells and transform into amastigotes and multiply. Thus 2 stages of *T. cruzi* occur in humans. The nonmultiplying trypomastigote is a temporary stage, found only in the bloodstream and intracellularly just prior to escape from the cell. The multiplying amastigote occurs intracellularly and is the essential stage. Amastigotes or trypomastigotes are ingested by triatomid bugs belonging to the genera *Triatoma, Rhodnius, Panstrongylus,* and others. In the midgut of the triatomid bug the organism transforms to the epimastigote stage and multiplies. Eventually the epimastigotes migrate to the hindgut and transform into trypomastigotes in about 1-2 weeks, increasing in numbers by binary fission. As the infected bug feeds on a person, it defecates and the trypomastigotes find their way from the feces into the bite wound or mucous membranes. The organisms are engulfed by nearby macrophages and transform into amastigotes. A characteristic nodular or ulcerated skin lesion (chagoma) often develops at the bite site. The regional lymph nodes may be involved. In a large percentage of cases a unilateral palpebral edema occurs. Eventually the infection spreads through the lymph channels and bloodstream to other tissues. The systemic infection can take an acute or chronic course from the beginning or can transist from the acute to a chronic state. Symptoms depend largely on organs and tissues affected. Children are more acutely affected than are adults.

Chagas' disease is essentially a zoonotic infection. In typical endemic areas people live in primitive mud plaster houses with straw roofs that provide shelter for the bugs during the day and close proximity to the people when the bugs seek a blood meal at night. In areas where houses are reasonably bugproof the disease is virtually nonexistent. Opossums, raccoons, armadillos, dogs, cats, and various others animals are natural reservoirs of infection.

Morphology. In tissue sections typical amastigotes identical to those of *Leishmania dono-*

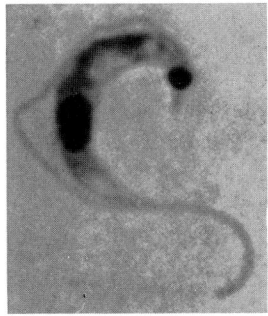

Fig. 97-11. *Trypanosoma cruzi* in human blood. (Giemsa stain; ×2000.) (From Mazza, S. In Gradwohl, R. B. H., Benitez Soto, L., and Felsenfeld, O.: Clinical tropical medicine, St. Louis, The C. V. Mosby Co.)

vani may be seen. They are 1.5-4 μm in length, oval, and when stained with Wright or Giemsa stain show a large deep and red nucleus and a dark-staining parabasal body. The trypomastigotes (Fig. 97-11) appear in the blood as long, thin, crescent-shaped forms about 20 μm in length. The large nucleus stains red or violet. The undulating membrane runs the length of the body, trailing off into a free flagellum. The kinetoplast is relatively large when compared with that of other trypanosome species affecting humans.

Diagnosis. Every effort should be made to demonstrate the organisms. The trypomastigote is seldom seen in blood except during the acute febrile stages. Preferably a thick drop of blood should be stained with Giemsa or a sample of blood should be concentrated by differential centrifugation. Hoff[18] described a promising method of concentrating trypomastigotes by lyzing red cells in 0.87% NH_4Cl followed by examination of centrifuged sediment for motile trypomastigotes.

Probably more infections are discovered by inoculation of blood or tissue into NNN medium or blood agar slants with a saline overlay. Obvious growth usually occurs in the liquid phase within 1 week, and trypomastigote, amastigote, and epimastigote forms may be seen. Blood or tissue may also be inoculated intraperitoneally into laboratory animals such as guinea pigs or young mice, and the infection may be detected in the animal blood 1-4 weeks (average 10 days) after inoculation.

An ingenious and often successful method for diagnosis of Chagas' disease is xenodiagnosis. Noninfected laboratory-bred triatomid bugs are allowed to feed on a patient thought to have the disease. If infected the *T. cruzi* may be detected in the bugs' feces in approximately 10 days.

Serologic tests have proved of values in chronic cases of Chagas' disease. The complement fixation test has been of special value. An antigen recommended by Kelser[19] is widely used, easy to prepare, and sensitive. However, frequent cross-reaction with sera from patients with syphilis and leishmaniasis occurs. A purified antigen described by Fife and Kent[20] reduces or eliminates many of these cross-reactions. The IHA technic[21] and recently a soluble fluorescent antibody technic[22] have proved useful. A latex test[23] and direct agglutination test[24] show considerable promise as screening tests. Consult Segovia[25] for a recent authoritative review of the immunology of Chagas' disease.

For detailed information on diagnosis of Chagas' disease see Tables 100-3 to 100-5.

Trypanosoma rhodesiense and Trypanosoma gambiense

Geographic distribution. *T. rhodesiense* infections occur sporadically in isolated areas of the upland savannahs of east central Africa. *T. gambiense* is more widely distributed over much of central western Africa. Cases may be sporadic or on occasion reach near epidemic proportions. Both species are etiologic agents of clinically different forms of African sleeping sickness known as rhodesian and gambian sleeping sickness.

Life cycle—epidemiology. In humans the trypomastigote of both species inhabits and multiplies in the connective tissue tissue spaces of various organs, the reticular tissue of the lymph nodes and spleen, the intercellular spaces of the brain, and the lymph channels.

African sleeping sickness affects primarily the lymph nodes and central nervous system. *T. gambiense* infections usually begin with glandular involvement and progress to central nervous system involvement over several years. With *T. rhodesiense* there is less glandular involvement and more acute involvement of the central nervous system, causing death within 1 year unless treated. Gambian sleeping sickness depresses the general immune response to other organisms.[26] This might explain the known increased susceptibility of patients with African sleeping sickness to secondary infections.

The principal vectors of *T. gambiense* are *Glossina palpalis* and *G. tachinoides*, whereas *G. morsitans* and *G. swynnertoni* are the major vectors of *T. rhodesiense*. The *Glossina* (tsetse flies) ingest trypomastigotes when taking a blood meal. Within the fly midgut the trypomastigotes multiply, and those that migrate to salivary glands transform into epimastigotes. These forms also multiply and in a few days become infective trypomastigotes. The cycle in the tsetse fly requires 20-30 days before infective trypomastigotes develop.

In general *T. gambiense* infections occur in agricultural communities and *T. rhodesiense* occurs only sporadically, primarily in individuals associated with sparsely populated game animal districts. *T. rhodesiense* exists only in areas where game animals live. Thanks to development of a new serologic tool that allows differentiation of *T. rhodesiense* and *T. gambiense* from other trypanosomes, workers recently found that lions, hyenas, sheep, cattle, goats, and reedbucks serve as reservoirs for *T. rhodesiense*.[27,28] On the other hand *T. gambiense* has no required association with game animals, being found in areas cleared of game. However, many domestic animals as well as wild antelopes can be experimentally infected and probably are important reservoirs or sources of infection for humans.

Morphology. *T. gambiense* and *T. rhodesiense* are morphologically identical. The trypomastigote stage of the 2 species (Figs. 97-12 and 97-13) varies from 8-30 μm. They are polymorphic, and some forms are long and narrow, possessing a long trailing flagellum, whereas others may be short and stumpy, lacking a trailing flagellum. When stained with Giemsa and examined microscopically the nucleus of the trypomastigote is seen as a large reddish purple body located near the center of the organism. An undulating membrane arises posteriorly from a blepharoplast situated just in front of a larger parabasal body and runs the entire length of the body. The blepharoplast and parabasal body, collectively called the kinetoplast, are almost indistinguishable from each other. The cytoplasm of the organism stains pale blue.

Diagnosis. Laboratory diagnosis is based on demonstration of the trypomastigote (Figs. 97-12 and 97-13) in blood, lymph node exudate, bone marrow, or cerebrospinal fluid. Early diagnosis is important clinically, since the late stages of African sleeping sickness are relatively resistant to therapy. Thick and thin blood smears Giemsa or Wright stained frequently are positive during fe-

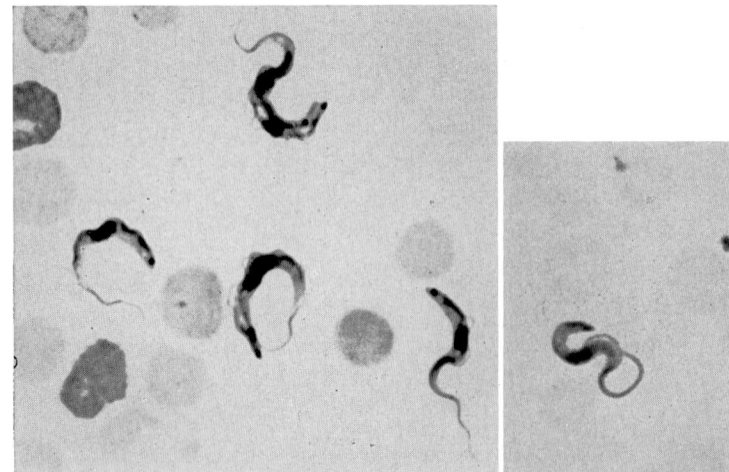

97-12

97-13

Fig. 97-12. *Trypanosoma gambiense* in peripheral blood. (From Felsenfeld, O. In Gradwohl, R. B. H., Benitez Soto, L., and Felsenfeld, O.: Clinical tropical medicine, St. Louis, The C. V. Mosby Co.)
Fig. 97-13. *Trypanosoma rhodesiense* in peripheral blood. (From Felsenfeld, O. In Gradwohl, R. B. H., Benitez Soto, L., and Felsenfeld, O.: Clinical tropical medicine, St. Louis, The C. V. Mosby Co.)

brile stages but seldom in the chronic late stages. Differential centrifugation of blood will concentrate the trypomastigotes and reveal more positive cases. Stained or unstained biopsy material from the posterior cervical lymph nodes or any other swollen lymph node probably reveals more positive cases than any other procedure. Trypomastigotes also can be detected in the centrifuged sediment of the cerebrospinal fluid of patients exhibiting central nervous system symptoms. Indirect evidence of late-stage sleeping sickness is indicated by finding an increase in mononuclear leukocytes in the spinal fluid.

If the above methods are unsuccessful, laboratory animals such as mice, guinea pigs, and young rats can be inoculated intraperitoneally with blood or spinal fluid sediment. Trypomastigotes usually appear in the blood after 1 week.

The organism may be demonstrated by cultivation in Tobie and Weinman media. Weinman[29] believes that cultivation is the most sensitive method.

Serologic tests are not used routinely. Some workers consider precipitin and double-diffusion tests reliable. FA tests have been used successfully to detect antibody. Most patients show elevated IgM levels using standard radial immunodiffusion methods. However, infection should be confirmed by demonstrating the organisms.

For further information of diagnosis see Tables 100-3 to 100-5.

SUBPHYLUM MASTIGOPHORA; SUPERCLASS SARCOVASICA
Amebae

The intestinal amebae that commonly infect humans belong to the genera *Entamoeba, Endolimax, Iodamoeba,* and *Dientamoeba.* Several free-living soil amoeba, *Naegleria, Acantho-*

amoeba, and *Hartmannella,* may be found in the nasopharyngeal cavity and central nervous system of humans. One species, *Naegleria fowleri,* causes a fatal infection (primary amebic meningoencephalitis) in humans. All amebae of humans live in the body as **trophozoites** and multiply by binary fission as long as suitable environmental conditions exist. The trophozoites of most species can secrete a membrane to form a tough wall around themselves and become a **cyst,** a resistant stage that can survive outside the body. A transitional **precyst** stage may also be seen in the feces of humans. The cyst is the stage transmitted from person to person, usually via contaminated food or water.

Five species of the genus *Entamoeba* are seen in humans. *Entamoeba gingivalis* is found in the mouth and is the only *Entamoeba* species in humans that lacks a cyst stage. *Entamoeba coli, E. hartmanni,* and *E. histolytica* are found in the large intestines. *Entamoeba polecki,* a swine ameba, occasionally is reported in the feces of humans. All are nonpathogenic with the exception of *E. histolytica,* which although nonpathogenic most of the time can cause overt disease. Elsdon-Dew[30] presents a lucid discussion and review of the controversy concerning the virulence or nonvirulence of *E. histolytica.* In much of the literature prior to the 1960s *E. hartmanni* was called "small race *E. histolytica*" and was considered nonpathogenic "most" of the time. Presently *E. hartmanni* is considered a valid species with no known virulence potential for humans.

Higher primates and less frequently dogs may harbor the species of amebae found in humans. Another amebae, *Entamoeba moshkovskii,* closely resembles *E. histolytica* and is frequently found in sewage. Apparently it is a free-living species as all attempts to demonstrate that it is an

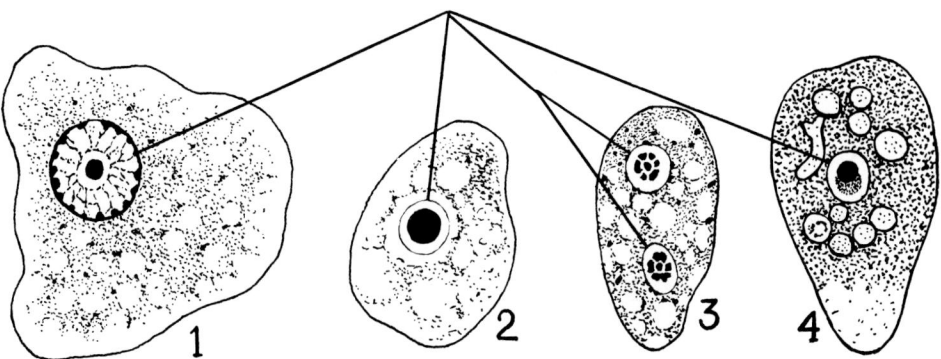

Fig. 97-14. Genera of amebae. Nuclear characteristics (partly according to Brumpt and Dobell). **1,** *Entamoeba:* small central or eccentric karyosome and denticulated layer of peripheral chromatin. **2,** *Endolimax:* voluminous karyosome, delicate nuclear membrane without peripheral chromatin. **3,** *Dientamoeba:* usually 2 nuclei with delicate nuclear membrane without peripheral chromatin, and numerous karyosomes in rosette formation. **4,** *Iodamoeba* (*Pseudolimax*): voluminous central spherical karyosome surrounded by layer of achromatic granules, crescent shaped in cysts, and delicate nuclear membrane without peripheral chromatin. (From Kourí, P., and Basnuevo, J.G.: Lecciónes de parasitología y medicina tropical, Havana, Editorial Profilaxis S.A.)

intestinal parasite have failed. *E. histolytica*-like amebae of humans have been thoroughly reviewed by Goldman.[31]

Many laboratory procedures are available for diagnosis of amebic infections. The trophozoites are usually identified in fecal smears stained with a permanent stain or a vital stain. With either type of stain identification is based primarily on characters of the nucleus (Fig. 97-14). Organisms belonging to the genus *Entamoeba* possess a small centrally or eccentrically located karyosome and a definite lining of chromatin material around the nucleus periphery. *Endolimax* possess a large karyosome and lack the peripheral nuclear chromatin. *Dientamoeba* trophozoites usually have 2 nuclei, each consisting of a cluster of separate chromatin particles; no peripheral nuclear chromatin is present. *Iodamoeba* trophozoites possess a relatively large karyosome and usually an associated cluster of achromatic granules; no peripheral nuclear chromatin is present.

The cysts may be identified in iodine-stained smears (Fig. 97-15) or iron-hematoxylin–stained

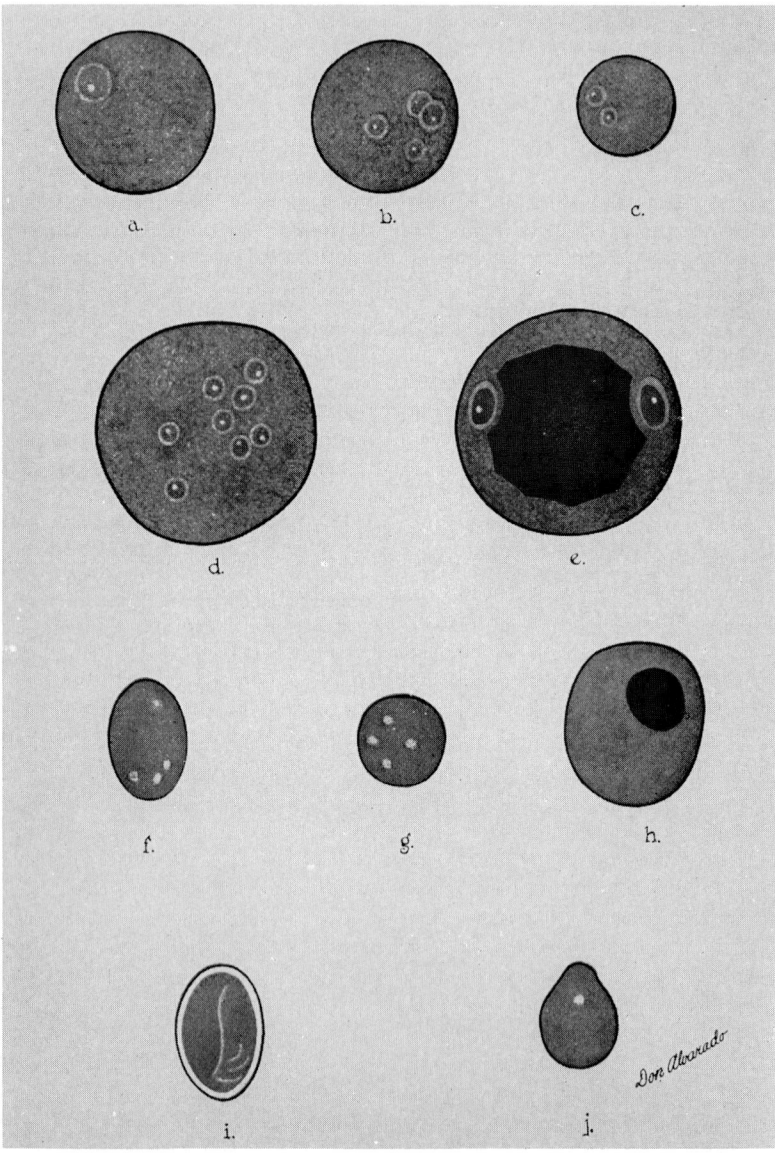

Fig. 97-15. Cysts of some intestinal protozoa in direct fecal smears, fresh, unpreserved, iodine stained. **a,** Uninucleate cyst of *Entamoeba histolytica.* **b,** Quadrinucleate cyst of *E. histolytica.* **c,** *E. hartmanni.* **d,** Mature cyst of *Entamoeba coli.* **e,** Immature cyst of *E. coli.* **f, g,** *Endolimax nana.* **h,** *Iodamoeba bütschlii.* **i,** *Giardia lamblia.* **j,** *Chilomastix mesnili.* (Courtesy Louisiana State University School of Medicine; from Hunter, G. W., III, Frye, W. W., and Swartzwelder, J. C.: Manual of tropical medicine, Phildelphia, 1960, W. B. Saunders Co.)

fecal smears, the cyst size and number of nuclei being important characters in identification. Only the cyst stages can be effectively concentrated. Sedimentation and flotation procedures are used for concentration of the cysts.

A more complete discussion of laboratory diagnosis is presented under diagnosis of *E. histolytica*.

Entamoeba histolytica

Geographic distribution. *E. histolytica*, the causative agent of **amebiasis,** has a cosmopolitan distribution. The prevalence varies from 2% or less in temperate zone countries with good sanitation to 80% in some tropical communities. However, prevalence may reach 50% in closed institutional populations in temperate zone countries.

Life cycle—epidemiology. The active trophozoites live in the large intestine, most frequently in the ileocecal region, the first part of the ascending colon, and in the sigmoid-rectal region. The trophozoites multiply by binary fission. For reasons not understood some of the trophozoites in the intestinal lumen expel their nutritional material and become rounded transitional forms called **precysts.** The precyst secretes a resistant membrane and becomes a cyst. The immature cyst contains only 1 nucleus, but as the cyst matures the nucleus undergoes 2 divisions to produce a quadrinucleate cyst. The cyst stage is relatively resistant and can survive outside the body for relatively long periods in a moist, cool environment. Although trophozoites, precysts, and cysts may pass in the feces, only the cysts are significantly involved in transmission, the other stages quickly perishing outside the host. Once ingested the quadrinucleate ameba escapes from the cyst and soon divides into uninucleate trophozoites.

E. histolytica is usually transmitted directly from person to person by food handlers, housekeepers, and so on, or by food or drink contaminated by excreta of infected persons. The usual source of infection is the carrier, who exhibits few if any symptoms. Persons with diarrhea or dysentery excrete primarily (but not exclusively) the trophozoite stage. Since this stage is not adapted for survival outside the body and probably could not survive the gastric juices if ingested, diarrheic or dysenteric persons are not important sources of infection. Cockroaches and flies may serve as a source of infection by transporting cyst-containing feces to food or water ingested by persons. The cyst may survive, apparently without damage, for 48 hours in the intestinal tract of insects. In some instances insects have been shown to be an important source of infection, especially in military camps, work camps, and similar installations.

The cyst stage is relatively resistant to adverse conditions. Cysts may survive several days or weeks in cool water but are quickly destroyed by temperatures below −5 C or above 40 C. They are also sensitive to desiccation. The effectiveness of disinfectants is variable, decreasing as the associated organic matter increases. The usual level of chlorine present in drinking water is not enough to readily kill cysts. In the past, serious outbreaks of amebiasis have occurred when chlorinated water supplies became rather heavily contaminated with feces containing *E. histolytica* cysts. Modern filtration and chlorination plants probably reduce the chances of infection, but they are not perfect measures, particularly if the water source becomes contaminated **after** leaving the water plant. This occasionally occurs in instances of faulty plumbing design and cross-connections.

Undoubtedly the main sources of infection are carriers who serve as food handlers, either in private homes or public places. Cooked or raw food may be contaminated after it has been prepared. Secondary sources of infection are insects and vegetables customarily eaten raw, contaminated by human feces. Although the old maxim "Do not eat it unless it is cooked or can be peeled" is a wise one, it does not take into consideration those instances in which food is contaminated after cooking, either by food handlers or insects.

As might be expected a large number of cases occur in crowded institutions such as military camps, schools, nurseries, hospitals, and so on, especially if personal hygiene standards are low. Although a number of other animal species have been found infected in nature, they probably do not play a major role in the epidemiology of this disease.

Although some strains of *E. histolytica* may be more pathogenic than others, all strains probably are potentially pathogenic. The so-called nonpathogenic small race *E. histolytica* is now recognized as a separate species, *E. hartmanni*.

At any time the majority of persons harboring *E. histolytica* exhibit few if any noticeable symptoms. They are asymptomatic carriers. Elsdon-Dew,[30] like most authorities, believes that *E. histolytica* lives as a commensal in the lumen of such individuals, causing no damage at all. Certain American authorities, however, believe the ameba causes damage but that the host is able to contain the parasite and repair any damage done to the intestinal mucosa by the parasite. In either case, when host resistance is lowered the parasites invade the deeper layers of the intestinal tissue, overcoming the host's ability to contain or repair tissue damage. A symptomatic case of amebiasis develops. The intestinal lesions vary from slight, superficial erosion of the intestinal mucosa to extensive, deep lesions.

If the trophozoites reach the muscularis mucosae, they may digest the wall of mesenteric venules, enter, and be carried to the liver or less frequently to other parts of the body. The trophozoites filtered out in the liver may be destroyed by host defenses or may establish a colony that eventually causes an amebic hepatic abscess by lytic necrosis of adjacent liver tissue. Most abscesses involve the right lobe of the liver.

Although the most frequent extraintestinal site of ameba localization is the liver, foci may infrequently be found in the lungs, brain, skin, and rarely other areas of the body. These foci may be secondary, resulting from extension of the amebic hepatic abscess, or may arise from the initial invasion of the blood by the trophozoites.

Morphology

Living Entamoeba histolytica in fresh unstained preparations

TROPHOZOITES. The living trophozoite of *E. histolytica*, observed in unstained preparations, appears as a more or less rounded, colorless, refractile organism 15-60 μm in diameter, with an average size of 18-25 μm. The existence of large and small strains, producing large and small cysts respectively, has been long accepted. Recent work by Freeman and Elsdon-Dew[32] indicates that trophozoite size in cultures is dependent on bacterial associates. Perhaps the same is true in the host. The trophozoite shows a hyaline ectoplasm and a finely granular endoplasm, usually well differentiated, especially when the protozoan is moving. As a general rule the nucleus is not observable in a fresh specimen, although at times it can be seen in the form of a ring of small refractive granules within the cytoplasm. In fresh feces the trophozoites contain neither bacteria nor nutritional vacuoles, but these may be present in the endoplasm of dead and degenerated forms. The presence of red blood cells in the endoplasm is almost pathognomonic in the differential diagnosis of this species, since other species rarely show red blood cells in the endoplasm of their trophozoites.

Pseudopodia may be long and narrow (fingerlike) or short and wide. They project rapidly. Locomotion is the result of forward extensions of hyaline ectoplasm, with the granular endoplasm then flowing into the fingerlike extension. This motion is so active in fresh feces that there is no clear differentiation between ectoplasm and endoplasm; the pseudopodia seem to be projections of total cytoplasm. As the feces cool, the movement of the ameba becomes slower, and (1) the projection of the hyaline ectoplasm that forms the pseudopodium and (2) the projection of granular endoplasm into the pseudopodium may be seen. Later the ameba becomes less motile until the protozoan becomes rounded and dies.

PRECYSTS. In the process of becoming a precyst the trophozoite becomes immobilized, rounded, smaller, and expels its nutritional contents. The nucleus, when visible, may appear as a series of yellow refractive granules distributed in a circle or in the form of a rounded mass, yellow and refractive when viewed by artificial light. Oval or rod-shaped bodies are observed in the cytoplasm. These rods have rounded ends and have a hyaline appearance similar to chromatoid bodies frequently observed in the younger cyst forms of this species. A cyst wall is lacking.

CYSTS. Cysts appear as round hyaline bodies with a cyst membrane that is more refractive than the rest of the cytoplasm. The diameter of the cysts varies from 10-20 μm. *E. histolytica*-like cysts with diameters less than 10 μm are identified as *E. hartmanni*.

The nucleus of the cyst has the same appearance as that of the trophozoite. In newly formed cysts only 1 nucleus is seen. After division this nucleus forms 2 and by the second division 4 nuclei. This number is characteristic of mature cysts and predominates in specimens obtained from fecal matter. In fresh specimens the nuclei are barely perceptible; the cytoplasm appears colorless and refractive, free of all nutritional inclusions, and in young or immature cysts glycogen vacuoles may be observed. **When stained with iodine** (Fig. 97-15) cysts are yellow, the cytoplasm loses its refractivity and appears finely granulated, nuclei are discernible, and the glycogen contained in the vacuoles stains a mahogany red color. The glycogen vacuole attains its maximum size in uninucleated cysts. In immature cysts ovoid or rod-shaped chromatoid bodies may be observed. The nature of these bodies has not been definitely determined. They stain a deep black with iron-hematoxylin (Fig. 97-16). They usually disappear in older, mature cysts. If the immature cyst lacks the chromatoid bar it may be difficult to differentiate from immature *E. coli* cysts. If the cyst is small and the 4 nuclei are small and of equal size, it is almost certainly a mature 4-nucleated cyst of *E. histolytica*; if the 4 nuclei are unequal in size and shape it is probably an immature cyst that on maturing will have 8 nuclei and is almost certainly a cyst of *E. coli*.

Entamoeba histolytica stained with iron-hematoxylin

TROPHOZOITES. In well-stained preparations the cytoplasm of the trophozoites stains grayish or violet and is granular in appearance with an alveolar and spongy structure. If the feces are fresh and the amebae have not degenerated, the cytoplasm will not contain bacteria, but red blood cells may be observed. The nuclear elements stain intensely black in contrast to the gray or pale violet color of the cytoplasm. The nuclear elements are the nuclear membrane, chromatin granules on the inner surface of this membrane in the form of a cogged wheel, and the small karyosome, usually central but at times slightly eccentric, all stained an intense black. Sometimes traces of a linin net can be observed in the form of thin fibrils radiating from the center to the periphery.

CYSTS. Iron-hematoxylin or other permanent stains clearly show the structural characteristics of protozoa, even in cases in which these characteristics may not have been observed in examination of the living specimens and in fresh specimens stained with iodine. In preparations stained by iron-hematoxylin the cysts (Fig. 97-16) show characteristic morphology and structure. They are spherical, oval, or rarely irregular. The

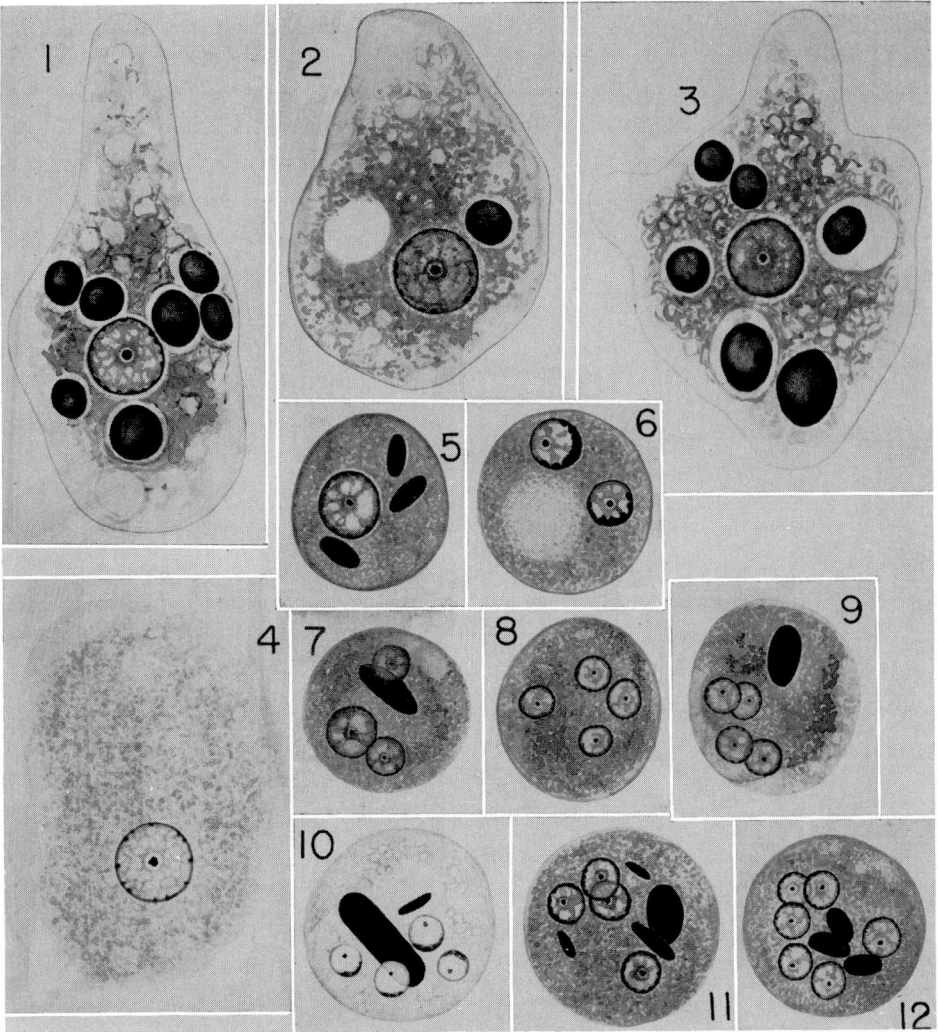

Fig. 97-16. *Entamoeba histolytica.* **1-3,** Trophozoites from single case, showing ingested red blood cells. **4,** Trophozoite from another case, showing delicate cytoplasm and typical nucleus. **5-12,** Various cysts, with and without chromatoid bodies, showing 1, 2, 3, 4, and 6 nuclei of varying character. In exceptional cases 8 nuclei are present. Chromatoid bodies are commonly present in young cysts, absent in older cysts. (Courtesy Winthrop-Stearns, New York.)

wall does not stain with hematoxylin but appears as a colorless halo around the cyst. The cytoplasm stains a grayish blue, whereas the nucleus and the chromatoid bodies are of a contrasting intense black color. The number of nuclei in mature cysts is usually 4. Rarely cysts have been observed with 6 or 8 nuclei.

Diagnosis. The laboratory diagnosis of intestinal amebiasis is based on demonstration of the organism in feces. Serology has developed into an increasingly valuable tool for diagnosis of extraintestinal amebiasis and possibly invasive intestinal amebiasis. A more detailed discussion of this subject is presented at the end of this section on diagnosis. The important morphologic characteristics of the common intestinal amebae, except *E. hartmanni,* are summarized in Table

97-4. The differential characteristics of *E. hartmanni* are summarized later in this chapter. Well-accepted laboratory procedures and their applications are summarized below. For a more detailed discussion of laboratory diagnosis of amebiasis consult references 33 and 34. An older publication[35] covers most of the basic principles plus a valuable review of microscopy technics appropriate for diagnosis of amebiasis. A short, concise authoritative review by Ridley[36] provides useful practical information about the laboratory diagnosis of amebiasis and other tropical diseases.

Collection and preservation of specimens. Stool specimens should be collected in a watertight cardboard container. If possible the stool specimen should be examined immediately after

Table 97-4. Important characters of intestinal amebae

	Entamoeba histolytica	Entamoeba coli	Endolimax nana	Iodamoeba bütschlii	Dientamoeba fragilis
Trophozoite (living)					
Usual size (μm)	10-30	10-50	6-12	9-20	5-20
Intracellular inclusions					
Red blood cells	Sometimes present	Absent or rare	Absent	Absent	Absent
Bacteria debris	Absent in fresh feces	Present	Present	Present	Present
Vacuoles	Scanty	Numerous	Numerous	Numerous	Numerous
Pseudopodia	Formed rapidly, finger shaped, hyaline	Formed slowly, blunt, granular	Like *E. coli*	Like *E. coli*	Like *E. coli*
Motility	Directional progression	No directional progression	—	—	—
Trophozoite (stained with iron-hematoxylin)					
Nuclei number	1	1	1	1	2 (usually)
Karyosome	Single, small, centrally located	Single, larger, eccentrically located	Irregular, large, eccentrically located	Variable shape, large, variable location; achromatic granules around karyosome	4 granules closely grouped together
Chromatin	Thin peripheral layer, minute regular dots	Heavy peripheral layer, coarse irregular dots	Peripheral chromatin absent	Like *E. nana*	Like *E. nana*
Cyst (stained with iodine)					
Size (μm)	6-15	10-30	4-8 × 8-14	5-16	No cyst
Shape	Spherical	Spherical, sometimes oval	Variable, usually oval	Irregular	—
Glycogen	Present in young cyst, diffuse	Present in young cyst	Not obvious	Compact, stains dark brown, diagnostic	—
Cyst (stained with iron-hematoxylin)					
Nuclei number	1-4	1-8	1-4	Usually 1	—
Size of nuclei (μm)	1-2	2-3	1	3-4	—
Chromatoid bodies	Cigar shaped, diagnostic if present	Splinterlike with pointed or square ends	Seldom seen	Seldom seen	—

passage. If this is not possible the specimen should be preserved. Specimens, especially those containing cyst stages, can be stored in the refrigerator for several hours without undue harm. Ideally part of the specimen should be mixed with a chemical preservative until it can be processed. Formalin, 10%, can be used to preserve cysts for subsequent concentration procedures and iodine-stained temporary mounts. Polyvinyl alcohol (PVA) fixative preserves trophozoites as well as cyst stages for subsequent preparation of permanent smears. Preservatives such as merthiolate-iodine-formalin (MIF) and phenol-alcohol-formalin (PAF) can be used effectively to preserve trophozoites and cyst stages for subsequent concentration or temporary mounts. Scholtens[37] described a simple method for preserving all stages of protozoa in Schaudinn's solution that enables the laboratory worker to concentrate the specimen and more easily prepare permanent smears.

The physician or laboratory worker should recommend and obtain stool specimens free of substances likely to interfere with diagnosis, in-

Table 97-5. Important characteristics of fecal specimens from patients with amebiasis or bacillary dysentery

	Amebiasis	*Bacillary dysentery*
Macroscopic	Semisolid or liquid, often streaked with blood or mucus; fecal elements include offensive odor, acidity	Gelatinous mucus, bright red blood; fecal elements decrease with severity and include inoffensive odor, alkalinity
Microscopic	Clumped red cells, white cells scarse and degenerate; numerous motile *Entamoeba histolytica* present	Red cells not clumped, numerous normal white cells; few organisms, usually nonmotile macrophages, present

cluding (1) antidiarrhea preparations such as bismuth and kaolin; (2) radiologic preparations such as barium sulfate; (3) biologically active drugs such as sulfonamides, antibiotics, and antiprotozoal and antihelmintic drugs; and (4) antacids and laxatives such as mineral oil, magnesium hydroxide, and enema solutions such as water, soap, hypertonic salt solutions, and irritants. If such substances were used by the patient, then 1 or preferably 2 weeks should be allowed to elapse after cessation of use before collecting a stool specimen for examination.

In routine populations surveys, examination of 1 stool specimen per person will have to suffice. In a clinical setting, examination of only 1 stool specimen is inadequate because of the well-known erratic discharge of amebae in the feces. For this reason 3 or more specimens should be examined over 1-2 weeks. Although specimens obtained by purgation will frequently contain more organisms, they probably reveal no more positive cases than a series of normally passed stools. In addition trophozoites in a purged stool are often difficult to identify. If purged feces are to be collected, sodium sulfate (Glauber salts) or phosphosoda is preferred to magnesium sulfate (Epsom salts) as a purgative. Yarinsky and Sternberg[38] recommend examination of the first 2 stools passed after purgation. Material collected during sigmoidoscopy should be examined immediately for motile trophozoites in temporary saline wet mounts. Care must be taken not to confuse tissue cells or macrophages with *E. histolytica*. Organisms exhibiting progressive *E. histolytica*-like motility should be sought in the temporary smears. In addition to temporary mounts some of the material should be smeared on a slide with PVA for subsequent permanent staining.

Liver aspirates require special treatments to free the amebae from the coagulum (see Chapter 100). Amebae are more likely to be found in the last portion of the aspirate. Add streptodornase-steptokinase to portions of the entire specimen to achieve 10 U/ml aspirate. Incubate the mixture at 37 C for 30 minutes with repeated shaking before examining for motile *E. histolytica*.

Methods of examination. The procedures generally used for demonstration of *E. histolytica* are as follows. For more detailed information see Chapter 100.

1. *General macroscopic and microscopic examinations of the stool specimens.* Although these types of examinations will not give a definitive diagnosis, they often provide the laboratory worker with valuable clues that may aid in differential diagnosis of amebiasis and bacillary dysentery. Observe and record the consistency of the specimen (e.g., formed, soft, loose, or watery), color, and abnormal elements (e.g., blood or mucus). See Table 100-1 for a more complete listing of gross fecal characteristics. In addition certain microscopic characteristics may give valuable information. Table 97-5 summarizes macroscopic and microscopic characteristics of feces from patients suffering from amebiasis or bacillary dysentery. Remember that cysts are most likely to be found in formed or soft stools, while trophozoites predominate in diarrheic or dysenteric stools.

2. *Temporary wet mounts.* These can be prepared directly from stool specimens, sigmoidoscopic scrapings, or liver aspirates. Stool specimens mounted in physiologic saline are examined for trophozoites and cysts. Those prepared with iodine are examined for stained cyst stages. Less frequently used temporary mounts include vital stains for trophozoites and MIF for cysts. Unless unmistakable features of *E. histolytica* trophozoites are seen (typical motility and presence of red blood cells intracellularly), final identification should be based on permanently stained smears of trophozoites or preferably stained smears of cyst stages.

3. *Concentration procedures.* These are probably the single most efficient method for detecting protozoan cysts. Both the formalin-ether sedimentation and zinc sulfate flotation procedures are effective when performed correctly. Neither technic is suitable for concentrating trophozoites. The formalin-ether sedimentation technic is less subject to technical errors and is the procedure of choice.

4. *Permanently stained fecal slides.* Amebae can be identified with greater certainty in permanently stained fecal smears. Not only will identification be easier, but often this method will reveal organisms, expecially trophozoites, not found by other technics. Smears can be prepared from fresh feces or from feces preserved in PVA or Schaudinn's solution. A variety of stain procedures have been found effective. Variations using iron-hematoxylin, trichrome, or chlorazol black have proved reliable.

5. *Staining of amebae in biopsy or autopsy material.* Routine hematoxylin-and-eosin-stained sections are unsatisfactory for demonstrating amebae. As a screening procedure formalin-fixed sections can be stained with periodic acid–Schiff. The amebae stand out as bright red bodies, but the exact morphology is seldom clear. Follow-up staining of sections with iron-hemotoxylin or trichrome will bring out typical morphology.

6. *Cultivation.* In appropriate media, amebae can be cultured from fresh stool specimens but seldom from older specimens. Specimens that cannot be cultured immediately after passage should be refrigerated. Frequently used media include the modified Boeck and Drbohlav medium and Balamuth's medium. Identification of organisms that flourish in these media requires that permanently stained smears be prepared and examined. Because of the uncertainties of cultivation, the identification by cultivation is not a routine procedure for the average laboratory.

Recommended stool examination protocol. The following is suggested as an adequate examination protocol for hospitals and clinics.

1. Collect a series of normally passed specimens. Since amebae appear in feces at irregular intervals, more positive cases will be discoverd if a minimum of 3 stool specimens collected over 1-2 weeks are examined. Examine for consistency, color, elements (e.g., blood, mucus), and the presence of *E. histolytica* cysts or trophozoites.
2. If prompt delivery of stool specimens to the laboratory is not possible, mix a portion of the feces in PVA or Schaudinn's solution to preserve trophozoite and cysts. Trophozoites are more likely to predominate in liquid stool specimens. Formed stool specimens are more likely to contain cyst stage and can be preserved in 10% formalin for subsequent concentration procedures or staining with iodine.
3. Examine saline mounts of fresh feces for trophozoites and iodine-stained fresh or formalin-preserved feces for cyst stages.
4. Concentrate specimens that are likely to contain cyst stages (formed and soft specimens).
5. Prepare permanently stained slides of fresh or PVA- or Schaudinn-preserved feces of (a) all *E. histolytica*–positive specimens for a permanent record, (b) soft or diarrheic specimens, which are more likely to contain trophozoites, and (c) are specimen that contains amebae unidentifiable by temporary mounts.

Criteria for identification of E. histolytica. Accurate identification of *E. histolytica* requires a microscope equipped with a calibrated ocular micrometer. The microscope should have a low-power objective for searching wet mounts, a high-power dry objective for more careful study of organisms encountered, and an oil-immersion objective for examining permanently stained smears. It is seldom possible to identify *E. histolytica* from observation of one organism or a single morphologic feature. In most instances the identification can be made if one of the following features is seen in several organisms in wet mount preparations:

1. Trophozoites with directional movement in saline mounts, containing red blood cells
2. Trophozoites over $12\mu m$ in diameter in saline mounts, with relatively clear cytoplasm and directional movement
3. Cysts over $10\ \mu m$ in diameter, with 1-4 *Entamoeba*-type nuclei (in iodine stain mount) and distinct rod-shaped chromatoidal bodies
4. Cysts over $10\mu m$ in diameter, most of them containing 4 *Entamoeba*-type nuclei

If findings are positive, prepare permanently stained slides for confirmation and a permanent record whenever possible.

Presumptive interpretation of laboratory findings. Dysenteric stools with gross blood and mucus, hematophagous *E. histolytica*, and very little cellular exudate strongly suggest acute amebic dysentery. A similar interpretation would be given to sigmoidoscopic material containing hematophagous *E. histolytica*, especially if there is a history of dysentery.

Stool specimens that are more or less diarrheic and contain some mucus, with or without gross blood, are more difficult to interpret. The presence of hematophagous *E. histolytica* indicates amebiasis, probably with hemorrhagic ulceration. The presence of nonhematophagous *E. histolytica* indicates amebiasis possibly without significant invasion of bowel mucosa. The presence of *E. histolytica* cysts only indicates amebiasis with possibly no significant intestinal tissue involvement.

Formed or soft stool specimens that contain *E. histolytica* cysts but not necessarily trophozoites indicate amebiasis with possibly no intestinal tissue involvement. The presence of *E. histolytica* cysts in feces of patients without symptoms is of clinical concern. Although the infection may be asymptomatic at that moment, there is always the potential danger of subsequent tissue invasion. In some instances deep local lesions with spread to the liver occur without noticeable intestinal symptoms.

On the other hand, if *E. histolytica* trophozoites are found in the stools of dysenteric patients, they may or may not be the etiologic agent. *Shigella* and *Salmonella* infections may be responsible for the dysenteric symptoms with the presence of *E. histolytica* only an incidental finding. Thus in regions with a prevalence of asymptomatic amebiasis, attention must be given to the characteristics of the fecal specimen (Table 97-5). If a typical bacillary exudate is present, then a role of *E. histolytica* in the symptomatology remains suspect.

In cases of suspect amebic liver abscess organisms may or may not be found in the feces. The mere presence of *E. histolytica* in the feces is not direct proof of amebic liver abscess. The recovery of organisms from liver abscesses is difficult. Fluid obtained by open drainage or closed aspiration from positive cases often has a "typical" anchovy paste or chocolate color. However the color may be white, cream colored, greenish, or yellowish. Amebic liver abscesses are generally bacteriologically sterile. In some instances, especially if aspiration has been attempted earlier, the recovered aspirate may show signs of bacteria (e.g., foul smell and greenish or yellowish color). Visualization of liver abscesses by radiographic and ultrasonic technics[34,40] often provides the clinician useful information for diagnosis and evaluation of subsequent therapy.

Immunodiagnostic methods. In the past few years several immunodiagnostic procedures have been thoroughly evaluated and found suitable for use as routine diagnostic tests. Several studies demonstrated that invasive amebiasis almost always gives rise to detectable antibodies. The newer serologic methodologies and the availability of better antigens have resulted in tests of high sensitivity and specificity. Some serologic tests may detect antibodies for long periods after termination of infection; thus a positive serologic result is not by itself an adequate basis for the diagnosis of active amebic infection. However, a negative serologic test by the more sensitive methods helps the physician rule out invasive amebiasis. Certain of these tests are suitable for epidemiologic studies.

Several of the better known procedures are listed below with comments about their usefulness.

1. *Indirect hemagglutination test.* This method is the most sensitive of the routinely used methods. Titers of 1:128 are considered indicative of past or present infections. Usually 95% or more of amebic abscess cases are positive. A high percentage (over 50%) of invasive and asymptomatic amebiasis cases also are positive by IHA. Antibody titers may remain elevated several years after successful treatment. The high level of sensitivity and long duration of detectable antibody limit the usefulness of the IHA procedure in highly endemic areas. Also the IHA procedure is not well suited for the laboratory that performs the test on only single specimens at sporadic intervals.[41] However, Farshy and Healy[42] described a method for preparing sensitized cells that retained their original sensitivity for a year or more. Such preparations would be extremely useful in the laboratory that performs only a few tests per year. Comparisons of IHA with other methods has been reported by several workers.[41,43-45] The technic has value as a seroepidemiologic tool[46] and as a tool for differential diagnosis of amebiasis and inflammatory bowel disease.[47]

2. *Immunodiffusion tests.* Gel diffusion precipitin tests have proved reliable and specific indicators of antiamebic antibody. The test is almost always positive with sera from patients with amebic liver abscess. It is slightly less sensitive than IHA in detecting antibody in sera from patients with invasive or asymptomatic ame-

biasis. The simplicity of the test is commendable. One potential drawback is the necessity of waiting 48 hours before being certain of negative reactions. A sophisticated variant of this test, the cellulose acetate diffusion test,[41] gives faster results. Recently Krupp[45] evaluated counterimmunoelectrophoresis as a serologic tool and found it reliable, rapid, and more sensitive than IHA.

3. *Complement fixation tests.* These tests are not widely used because of the complexity of the test system. Generally the complement fixation test is less sensitive than IHA or immunodiffusion tests.

4. *Latex agglutination tests.* These tests provide reliable, specific results and are only slightly less sensitive than IHA.[41] They require a minimum of equipment and can give results rapidly. Commercial kits are available (Sermeba, Ames Co., Elkhardt, Ind.). The test is usually negative in noninvasive amebiasis and may serve as a useful indicator of clinical status of the infection.

5. *Fluorescent antibody tests.* These tests appear to be sensitive and reliable but require further evaluation. A soluble-antigen fluorescent antibody test has been used with promising results.[49] Using conventional indirect FA technics Ambroise-Thomas and Kien Truong[50] found the test specific and that it detected 100% of hepatic abscess cases, 59% of amebic dysentery cases, 31% of amebic colitis cases, and 15% of asymptomatic cyst passers. Titers were high in hepatic abscess cases and dropped rapidly within 2 months after successful therapy. If this observation is generally true, IFA should be extremely valuable in evaluating therapy.

6. *Skin tests.* Interest in skin tests has revived since the development of antigens derived from bacteria-free cultures. Skin tests probably will be most valuable as an epidemiologic tool. Skin tests done on individuals with low IHA titers may provoke a rise in IHA titer. Although skin tests do not induce IHA antibody in normal persons, skin test antigen concentrations of 8 μm or higher can sensitize normal persons, giving rise to subsequent "positive" skin reactions.[53]

Primary amebic meningoencephalitis

Recent reports demonstrated that certain free-living water amebae can cause fatal primary meningoencephalitis. Fatal cases have been reported from the United States, Belgium, Australia, England, and Czechoslovakia. All cases, with a few exceptions, have resulted in death in spite of vigorous treatment with combinations of antibiotics, sulfa compounds, and other chemotherapeutic agents. Illness begins with headache, mild fever, and sometimes sore throat and rhinitis. Over the next 3 days headache and fever increase and vomiting and neck rigidity develop. Soon after, the patient becomes disoriented, lapses into a coma, and dies 5-7 days after the onset. At autopsy the base of the brain and cerebellum are covered with exudate such as occurs in other forms of acute meningitis. Primary amebic meningoencephalitis should not be confused with the rarely occurring invasion of the central nervous system by *Entamoeba histolytica*. Such infections arise secondarily following primary infection of the large intestines.

Most cases studied to date occurred following swimming or diving in ponds or indoor pools containing free-living amebae. Apparently these amebae gain entrance to the nervous system via the nasal passages. Evidence strongly suggests that they invade along the olfactory nerves, cause early damage to the olfactory bulbs, then spread widely via the subarachnoid space.

Classification of the free-living soil amebae capable of causing amebic meningoencephalitis is somewhat controversial. Tentatively the chief offender has been identified as *Naegleria fowleri*. (*Naegleria aerobia* is a commonly used synonym, reflecting some of the taxonomic confusion and controversy over which name has priority.) In hematoxylin-and-eosin-stained tissue sections this ameba ranges 5.2-9.1μm (average 7.4μm) in size[54] and exhibits a large nucleolus similar to that seen in *Iodamoeba bütschlii*. *N. fowleri* is an aerobic organism that can be isolated and cultured from spinal fluid or fresh brain tissue containing the amebae. The amebae will develop and destroy cells in the usual tissue culture systems. They can also be cultured on an agar surface in the presence of *Escherichia coli* or recovered from mice inoculated intracerebrally.[55] Growth without bacteria (axenic culture) is possible using heat-killed (60 C for 1 hour) *Escherichia coli* to seed the agar medium.[56] In culture the trophozoite stage is quite active. The nuclear division of *Naegleria* differs from certain closely related amebae (*Hartmannella* or *Achanthamoeba*) discussed below, since the nucleolus does not disappear but divides and the halves migrate to the poles of the mitotic spindle. *Naegleria* is especially unique in that a variable percentage (usually less than 15%) of cultural forms transform into flagellated forms within 2-12 hours after addition of distilled water to the medium that contains the amebae. The actively swimming flagellates possess 2 flagella but revert to amebic form several hours later.

Another species of *Naegleria*, *N. gruberi*, frequently can be isolated from natural bodies of water. Although similar to *N. fowleri*, it is not pathogenic for mice, it will not grow at 45 C as does *N. fowleri*,[57] and the cyst wall has 5 exit pores, while *N. fowleri* has none.[58] Antigenic differences have been demonstrated by agglutination and fluorescent antibody tests.[59-61] Apparently these tests hold great promise as a means of identifying these amebae more conclusively.

Some confusion exists as to whether free-living soil amebae belonging to the *Hartmannella* or *Acanthamoeba* group may cause fatal infections. With the exception of 1 or 2 cases[62] these organisms do not cause fatal infections. However, organisms of this type have been isolated from the nasal passages of healthy persons and the spinal fluid of a patient who survived the infection[63] and are occasionally reported as contaminants in tissue cultures. Furthermore these organisms can cause fatal or chronic meningoencephalitis in experimentally infected mice, rabbits, and monkeys. Further work is needed to clarify their disease potential in humans. Although many reports consider *Hartmannella* and *Acanthamoeba* as synonyms, Page[64,65] suggests that they are separate genera.

In tissue sections *Hartmannella* and *Acanthamoeba* are approximately twice as large as *Naegleria*. Unlike *Naegleria*, the other species form cyst stages in tissue. In culture both organisms are sluggish, exhibit contractile vacuoles, and possess a very large nucleolus that disappears during mitosis. *Acanthamoeba* has spinelike pseudopodia, but *Hartmannella* does not. As mentioned above, neither *Acanthamoeba* or *Hartmannella* produce flagella when exposed to distilled water. *Hartmannella-Acanthamoeba* infections, unlike *Naegleria* infections, do respond to treatment with sulfadiazine.

Consult Carter[66] for a balanced review of most aspects of primary amebic meningoencephalitis and for an introduction to the recent literature.

Procedures for detection and isolation of *Naegleria* are described in Chapter 100.

Nonpathogenic intestinal amebae

The nonpathogenic amebae found in the feces that might be confused with *E. histolytica* are *E. coli*, *E. hartmanni*, *Endolimax nana*, *Iodamoeba bütschlii*, and *Dientamoeba fragilis*. With the exception of *D. fragilis*, their distribution, life cycle, and the methods used in diagnosis are the same. *E. coli* and *E. nana* are probably more prevalent than *E. histolytica* in most areas, but *I. bütschlii* and *D. fragilis* are not common. *D. fragilis* differs only in that the cyst stage is unknown, and consequently those technics applicable to cyst differentation do not apply. Table 97-4 lists the intestinal amebae and the major characteristics of each.

Entamoeba coli

The *E. coli* trophozoite (Fig. 97-17) is somewhat larger than *E. histolytica*, measuring between 18-50μm in diameter. Usually bacteria and cellular debris are obvious in the endoplasm. The living trophozoite is sluggish and does not show the progressive motility seen in *E. histolytica*. The pseudopodia extruded are frequently blunt and granular, not fingerlike and hyaline like *E. histolytica*. In stained trophozoites the peripheral chromatin granules appear coarse and irregular; the karyosome is usually eccentric and slightly larger than that of *E. histolytica*.

The precyst stage measures about 20μm and cannot be differentiated accurately from precysts of *E. histolytica*.

The cysts are spherical and occasionally irregular, especially in preserved specimens. They

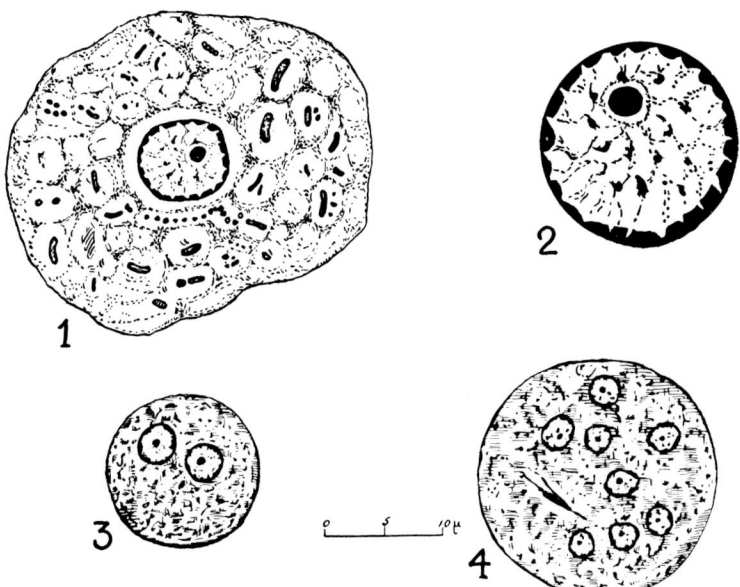

Fig. 97-17. *Entamoeba coli.* **1,** Trophozoite without hyaline ectoplasm, without erythrocytes in endoplasm, but containing bacteria. Nucleus central with eccentric karyosome and thicker than that of *E. histolytica.* **2,** Nucleus greatly enlarged to show its characteristics. Thicker denticulated peripheral chromatin, eccentric karyosome thicker than in *E. histolytica,* and small chromatic granules disposed in spaces between karyosome and nuclear membrane. **3,** Small binucleate cyst. **4,** Normal sized mature cyst with 8 nuclei. (Iron-hematoxylin stain.) (After Langeron and Rondeau du Noyer; from Kourí, P., and Basnuevo, J. G.: Lecciónes de parasitología y medicina tropical, Havana, Editorial Profilaxis S.A.)

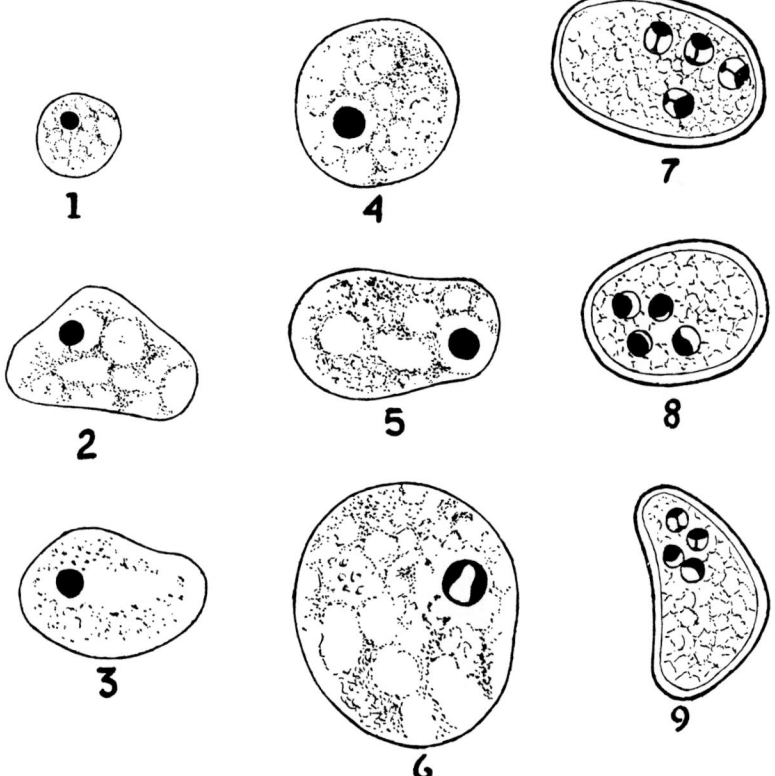

Fig. 97-18. *Endolimax nana.* **1-6,** Trophozoites of different sizes (after Brumpt). **7-9,** Cysts. (After Wenyon and O'Connor; from Kourí, P., and Basnuevo, J. G.: Lecciónes de parasitología y medicina tropical, Havana, Editorial Profilaxis S.A.)

measure 10-30 μm in diameter. Iodine-stained cysts (Fig. 97-15) possess 1-8 ringlike nuclei, depending on the maturity of the cyst. Cysts with less than 5 nuclei may be confused with *E. histolytica*. Usually, however, immature *E. coli* cysts are larger than those of *E. histolytica*, and the nuclei differ in their diameters. In iron-hematoxylin–stained cysts (Fig. 97-17) the splinterlike chromatoid bar if present and the character of the nucleus help differentiate *E. coli* from *E. histolytica*.

Endolimax nana

The trophozoite of *E. nana* (Fig. 97-18), measuring 6-12 μm (average 8 μm) in diameter, is usually smaller than *E. histolytica*. Movement of the living trophozoites is sluggish like *E. coli*. In iron-hematoxylin–stained specimens (Fig. 97-18) the karyosome appears as a large, more or less rounded dot. The nucleus lacks peripheral chromatin.

The iodine-stained cyst (Fig. 97-15) is oval or, less frequently, spherical. It is typically smaller than other cysts, measuring 5-16 μm in diameter. The nuclei appear as holes resembling vacuoles in the endoplasm and lack the ringlike appearance of *E. histolytica* and *E. coli*. In hematoxylin-stained cysts (Fig. 97-18) the large eccentrically located karyosome of each nucleus is characteristic. The peripheral chromatin lining is absent.

Iodamoeba bütschlii

The *I. bütschlii* trophozoite varies from 9-20 μm in diameter. Intracellular inclusions and motility resemble those of *E. coli*. The iron-hematoxylin–stained trophozoite (Fig. 97-19) exhibits a large irregular or rounded karyosome with a cluster of achromatic granules. Peripheral chromatin lining is absent. The nuclear characters of the stained cyst (Fig. 97-19) resemble those of the trophozoite. The most prominent feature of the cyst is the large clear vacuole that represents the area previously occupied by the glycogen mass. In iodine-stained cysts (Fig. 97-15) the glycogen mass is sharply demarcated and stains a characteristic dark mahogany brown.

Dientamoeba fragilis

The *D. fragilis* trophozoite varies from 5-20 μm in size. Intracellular inclusions and motility resemble those of *E. coli*. There is no cyst stage. The iron-hematoxylin–stained trophozoite (Fig. 97-20) exhibits 1 or 2 nuclei; each nucleus appears as several closely grouped granules, usually 4. Peripheral chromatin is lacking.

Occasionally *D. fragilis* infections have been

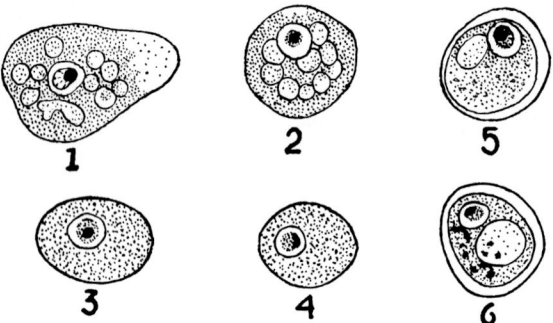

Fig. 97-19. *Iodamoeba bütschlii.* **1, 2,** Trophozoites. **3, 4,** Precystic forms. **5, 6,** Mature cysts with glycogen vacuoles and single nucleus. (Original figure of Brumpt; from Kourí, P., and Basnuevo, J. G.: Lecciónes de parasitología y medicina tropical, Havana, Editorial Profilaxis S.A.)

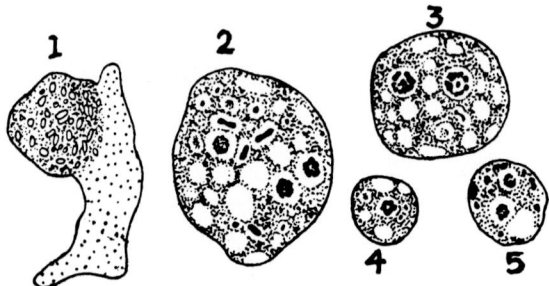

Fig. 97-20. *Dientamoeba fragilis.* **1,** Living trophozoite. **2-5,** Trophozoites, fixed and stained. (After Jepps and Dobell; In Kourí, P., and Basnuevo, J. G.: Lecciónes de parasitología y medicina tropical, Havana, Editorial Profilaxis S.A.)

associated with diarrhea, although this contention is controversial.

Entamoeba gingivalis

E. gingivalis, as its name implies, is an inhabitant of the mouth and not the intestinal tract. It occurs frequently in persons with unhygienic mouths. It is apparently a commensal form, living on the margins of the gums, and thrives best on unhealthy gums. It can be demonstrated in material removed from the gum margins or between the teeth. There is no known cyst stage. The trophozoites measure 5-35 μm in diameter and extrude their pseudopodia much like *E. histolytica*. In stained specimens (Fig. 97-21) the nucleus has a small centrally located karyosome and distinct peripheral chromatin lining not unlike that of *E. histolytica*.

Entamoeba hartmanni

E. hartmanni has long been said to be synonymous with small race *E. histolytica*. Burrows[67]

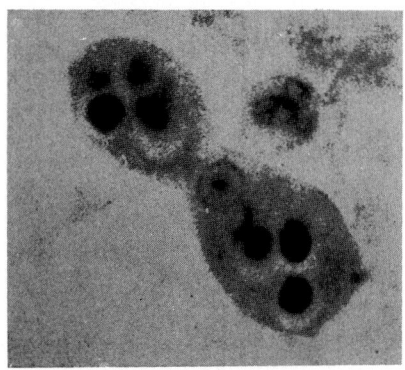

Fig. 97-21. *Entamoeba gingivalis.* Trophozoite. Nucleus is seen in central portion, remnants of ingested leukocytes in food vacuoles. (Iron-hematoxylin stain; ×3000.) (Original photomicrograph of E. Beltrán; from Gradwohl, R. B. H., Benitez Soto, L., and Felsenfeld, O.: Clinical tropical medicine, St. Louis, The C. V. Mosby Co.)

reviewed the subject and presented morphologic evidence as to the validity of separating this species from *E. histolytica*. Differentiation is possible, according to Burrows, in carefully stained iron-hematoxylin smears. Although most authorities agree that *E. hartmanni* is a valid species, they disagree on the usefulness of nuclear characteristics as criteria for speciation. At present their size, antigenic characteristics, and lack of pathogenicity are considered the most reliable features of *E. hartmanni*. The average laboratory should base diagnosis on the size of the organism. *E. histolytica*-like cysts 10 μm or less in diameter and *E. histolytica*-like trophozoites 12 μm or less in diameter are considered to be *E. hartmanni*.

Blastocystis hominis

B. hominis, a yeast, appears in the stool as a spherical body, colorless and refractive, varying in size from 2-15 μm in length (Fig. 97-22). In some specimens only small forms are seen, whereas in others medium forms are found, and in still others, very large forms. The small forms are frequently confused with cysts of amebae.

When stained with iodine, the characteristic structures can be seen well. It has a relatively thick peripheral ring of protoplasm in which may be seen 1 or more nuclei with a dense karyosome and a central or slightly eccentric vacuole. It stains well with Gram stain and iron-hematoxylin. *B. hominis* is usually regarded as nonpathogenic, but occasionally it is seen in large numbers in diarrheal or dysenteric states, alone or associated with spirochetes, and in patients in whom it is otherwise impossible to ascertain any other cause for the disturbance. Many times the disturbance disappears with the successful eradication of the *Blastocystis*.

SUBPHYLUM APICOMPLEXA

The subphylum Apicomplexa (formerly Sporozoa) contains 2 classes of medical importance to humans. The class Piroplasmasida

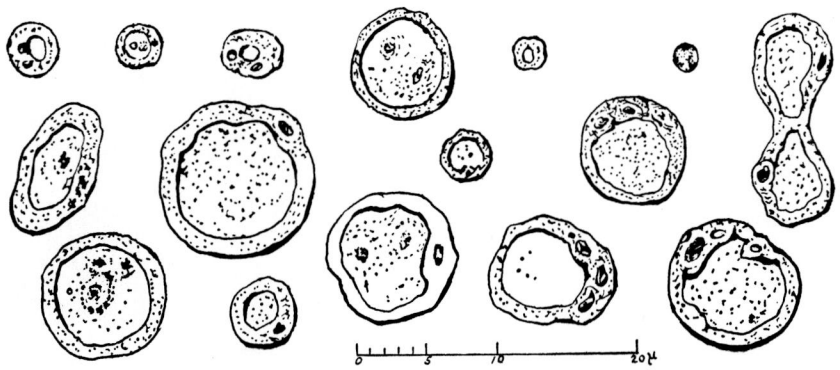

Fig. 97-22. *Blastocystis hominis* (after Langeron and Rondeau du Noyer). This organism is found frequently in human feces. (From Kourí, P., and Basnuevo, J. G.: Lecciónes de parasitología y medicina tropical, Havana, Editorial Profilaxis S.A.)

contains one genus, *Babesia,* of minor medical importance. Although *Babesia* causes an important disease of cattle, babesiosis or red water fever, only a few cases have been described in humans.

The class Sporozoasida contains several parasites of considerable importance to humans. Coccidian parasites belonging to the genus *Isospora* or *Sarcocystis* occur frequently in humans, giving rise to relatively benign infections. *Toxoplasma gondii* occurs even more frequently but is potentially a dangerous infection. The best known parasites in this class are the malarial parasites belonging to the genus *Plasmodium.* An estimated 200 million cases of malaria occur each year with an estimated 2 million deaths attributed to this parasite.

Some authorities place *Pneumocystis carinii* in the class Sporozoasida. Other authorities contend that this organism is a fungus. Although its taxonomic status remains unclear, it is discussed briefly in this chapter because it has long been considered a protozoan by many authorities.

Malarial parasites of humans

Four species of plasmodia affect humans: (1) *Plasmodium vivax,* the causative agent of benign tertian malaria; (2) *P. malariae,* the causative agent of quartan malaria, (3) *P. falciparum,* the causative agent of estivoautumnal, subtertian, or malignant tertian malaria, and (4) *P. ovale,* a relatively rare form causing ovale malaria. The life cycles of all 4 species are similar. The major points of difference involve the species of *Anopheles* serving as a vector and the clinical course of the disease. Refer to standard parasitology texts for details on these points.

The *Plasmodium* parasite requires a vertebrate (human) and an invertebrate host (*Anopheles* mosquito) to complete its life cycle. The parasites undergo an asexual phase (schizogony) in humans. A sexual phase (gametogony and sporogony) takes place in the mosquito.

The phase in humans begins when the female mosquito, while taking blood, injects sporozoites into the person. The sporozoites quickly disappear from the bloodstream, invading the parenchymal cells of the liver. Within these cells the malarial parasites multiply asexually, producing a cluster of nuclear elements (Fig. 97-23). The dividing mass of elements is called a schizont. The schizont may reach 60 μm in size and contain from 1000-40,000 nuclear elements. Eventually the schizont matures, and each nuclear element becomes an independent organism called a merozoite. The merozoites escape and invade more liver cells. There may be 1-4 generations of schizonts before parasites begin to appear in the red blood cells. The prepatent period varies with the species: *P. falciparum* averages about 5 days, *P. vivax* and *P. ovale* 8 days, and *P. malariae* about 14 days. The earliest stage in the red blood cell is called a trophozoite or "ring" stage. Initially the trophozoite consists of a red-staining dotlike nucleus and a connecting ring of bluestaining cytoplasm. As the trophozoite grows the cytoplasm increases and some pigment is produced. After a time nuclear division occurs, giving rise to a multinucleated parasite (schizont or segmenter) within the blood cell. The nuclei continue to divide until a number is reached that is consistent for that species of *Plasmodium.* In the case of *P. vivax* the final number of nuclei produced is 15-20; *P. malariae,* 6:12; *P. ovale,* 8-10; and *P. falciparum,* 8-32. As the schizont matures the nuclei become separate entities surrounded by cytoplasm. Each entity or organism is called a merozoite. The red cell ruptures, releas-

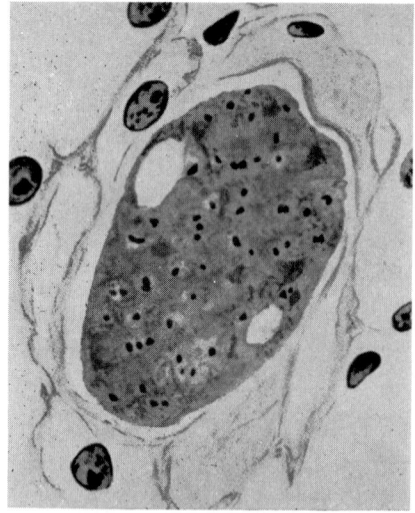
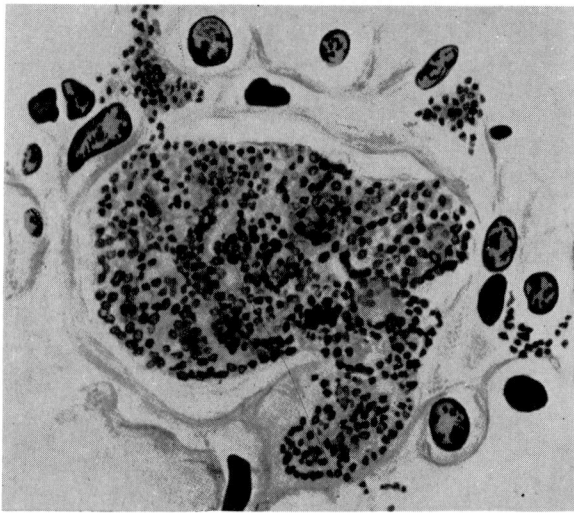

Fig. 97-23. Preerythrocytic phase. Schizonts of *Plasmodium vivax* showing development in human liver on seventh day after experimental sporozoite infection. (From Shortt, H. E., and Garnham, P. C.: Trans. R. Soc. Trop. Med. Hyg. **41**:705, 1948.)

ing the merozoites, which then enter new red blood cells to start the cycle anew as young trophozoites.

After several generations of merozoites have been produced, microgametocytes and macrogametocytes begin to appear in circulating erythrocytes. The gametocytes have their own characteristic morphology and undergo no further development unless ingested by the invertebrate host, the *Anopheles* mosquito. In the mosquito the microgametocyte gives off several motile spermlike gametes. One of these penetrates and fertilizes the macrogamete. The resulting zygote becomes a motile ookinete that penetrates the midgut to the outer limiting membrane, where it becomes a resting body or oocyst. Within the oocyst thousands of sporozoites develop. After 1-3 weeks the oocyst ruptures and the sporozoites that reach the salivary glands may be injected into a human at the mosquito's next blood meal.

The cycle in humans is primarily asexual, involving a cyclic development of the trophozoite into a schizont that releases merozoites to reinitiate the cycle. In recently acquired infections merozoite release occurs sporadically and at irregular intervals. If the infection is allowed to persist long enough the development of parasites and reinvasion of red blood cells become synchronized, and at regular intervals the merozoites escape from the old red cells and invade new ones. In the case of *P. vivax* and *P. ovale* infections the cycle occurs every 48 hours; *P. malariae*, every 72 hours; and *P. falciparum*, irregularly between 37 and 48 hours. The initiation of the classic symptoms of malaria is directly related to the cyclic release of the parasites from red blood cells. A cold stage develops soon after rupture of red cells and release of the merozoites. The patient may experience a frank chill, nausea, and vomiting. These symptoms are probably due to the body's reaction to toxic by-products released when the merozoites escape from the red cells. Also symptoms in part may be due to anaphylactic-like reactions to antigenic components of these by-products. The temperature begins to rise. In less than 1 hour the disease shifts into a hot stage lasting several hours. By this time over 90% of the merozoites have entered red blood cells, and the patient may experience a burning fever, rapid respiration, and a severe headache. Then follows a sweating stage that may last 1-3 hours. By now all the parasites are in red cells and actively growing. The patient sweats profusely and feels exhausted, and the temperature begins to drop. After the temperature returns to normal the patient has no symptoms until the cycle of symptoms is again repeated when the next crop of merozoites escapes from infected red cells. The cyclic occurrence of symptoms continues until the infected individual develops immunity. As stated before, the cycle occurs every 48 hours with *P. vivax* and *P. ovale* and every 72 hours with *P. malariae*. The cycle

and symptoms in *P. falciparum* infections are irregular and not as characteristic. There is usually no chill or sweating stage, and the fever stage is prolonged. For this reason *P. falciparum* infections are more severe. Another reason for the seriousness of *P. falciparum* infection is that the young trophozoites tend to accumulate in the capillaries and cause capillary occlusions with resultant tissue anoxia and necrotic foci. In vital organs this can lead to especially serious consequences.

If blood smears are taken from an infected individual the stage found in the infected cells will be dependent on the age of the infection and the cyclic nature of the parasites. In recently acquired infections the cyclic development of the parasite is unsynchronized and various stages may be found. After synchronization has occurred 1 stage will tend to predominate, although others may be infrequently present. Gametocytes may be present at any time except early in the infection. It must be remembered that in the case of *P. falciparum* infections only young trophozoites and gametocytes are routinely found. The older trophozoites and schizonts accumulate in capillaries and are seldom seen in circulating blood except in terminal cases.

The preerythrocytic stages of *P. vivax* and *P. ovale* may persist in liver cells after the erythrocytic stages have been eliminated by the host's immune response or by chemotherapy effective against the erythrocytic stages. Months or years later, perhaps when the immunity of the host has declined, the preerythrocytic stages may reinvade the red cells and initiate a recurrence of symptoms. Such relapses can be prevented by concurrent or sequential administration of drugs effective against the erythrocytic and preerythrocytic stages. Apparently the preerythrocytic stages of *P. falciparum* and *P. malariae* do not persist, and drugs effective against the erythrocytic stages will produce a complete cure.

Morphology of malarial parasites
Plasmodium vivax

The various stages of *P. vivax* seen in Giemsa-stained thin and thick blood smears are shown in Figs. 97-24 and 97-25; their characteristics are summarized in Table 97-6. The earliest stage in the development of the asexual form, the trophozoite, consists of a red dot of chromatin and a delicate ring-shaped strand of sky blue cytoplasm. The parasite is about one-third the red cell diameter. As growth occurs more sky blue cytoplasm becomes obvious and the chromatin mass enlarges. The cytoplasm assumes a variety of shapes and is usually widely and irregularly scattered across the red cell. The infected cell appears larger than normal cells. Frequently but not always, pink spots (Schüffner's dots) appear throughout the red cell. Granules of greenish brown pigment are present in old trophozoites and subsequent forms. The chromatin undergoes division to form the schizont stage, and succes-

Text continued on p. 2102.

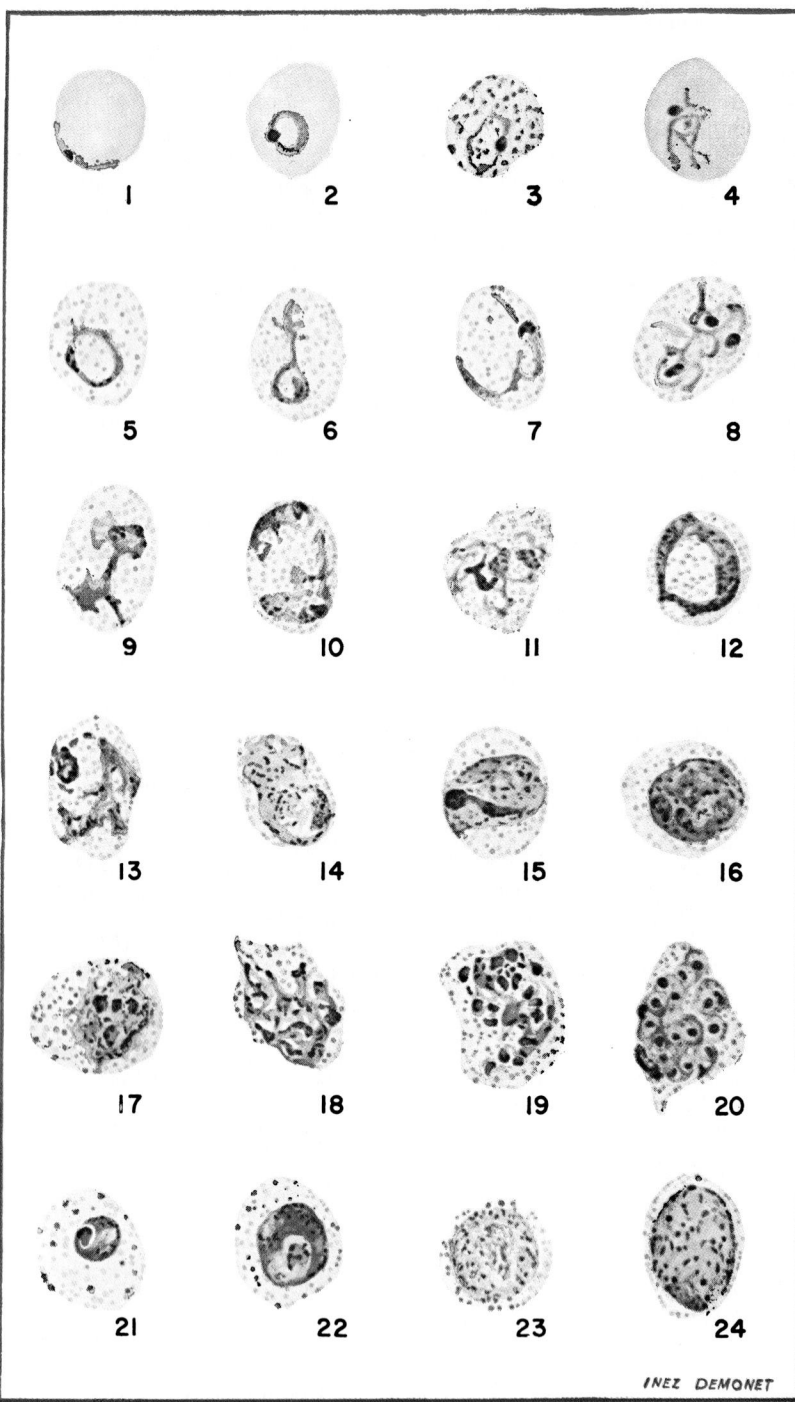

INEZ DEMONET

Fig. 97-24. *Plasmodium vivax.* **1,** Normal sized red cell with marginal ring form trophozoite. **2,** Young signet ring form trophozoite in macrocyte. **3,** Slightly older ring form trophozoite in red cell showing basophilic stippling. **4,** Polychromatophilic red cell containing young tertian parasite with pseudopodia. **5,** Ring form trophozoite showing pigment in cytoplasm, in enlarged cell containing Schüffner's stippling (*dots*). (Schüffner's stippling does not appear in all cells containing growing and older forms of *P. vivax,* as would be indicated by these pictures, but it can be found with any stage from fairly young ring form onward.) **6, 7,** Very tenuous medium trophozoite forms. **8,** Three ameboid trophozoites with fused cytoplasm. **9, 11-13,** Older ameboid trophozoites in process of development. **10,** Two ameboid trophozoites in 1 cell. **14,** Mature trophozoite. **15,** Mature trophozoite with chromatin apparently in process of division. **16-19,** Schizonts showing progressive steps in division (presegmenting schizonts). **20,** Mature schizont. **21, 22,** Developing gametocytes. **23,** Mature microgametocyte. **24,** Mature macrogametocyte. (From Wilcox, A.: Manual for the microscopical diagnosis of malaria in man, Department of Health, Education, and Welfare, Public Health Service, Washington, D. C., 1960, U. S. Government Printing Office.)

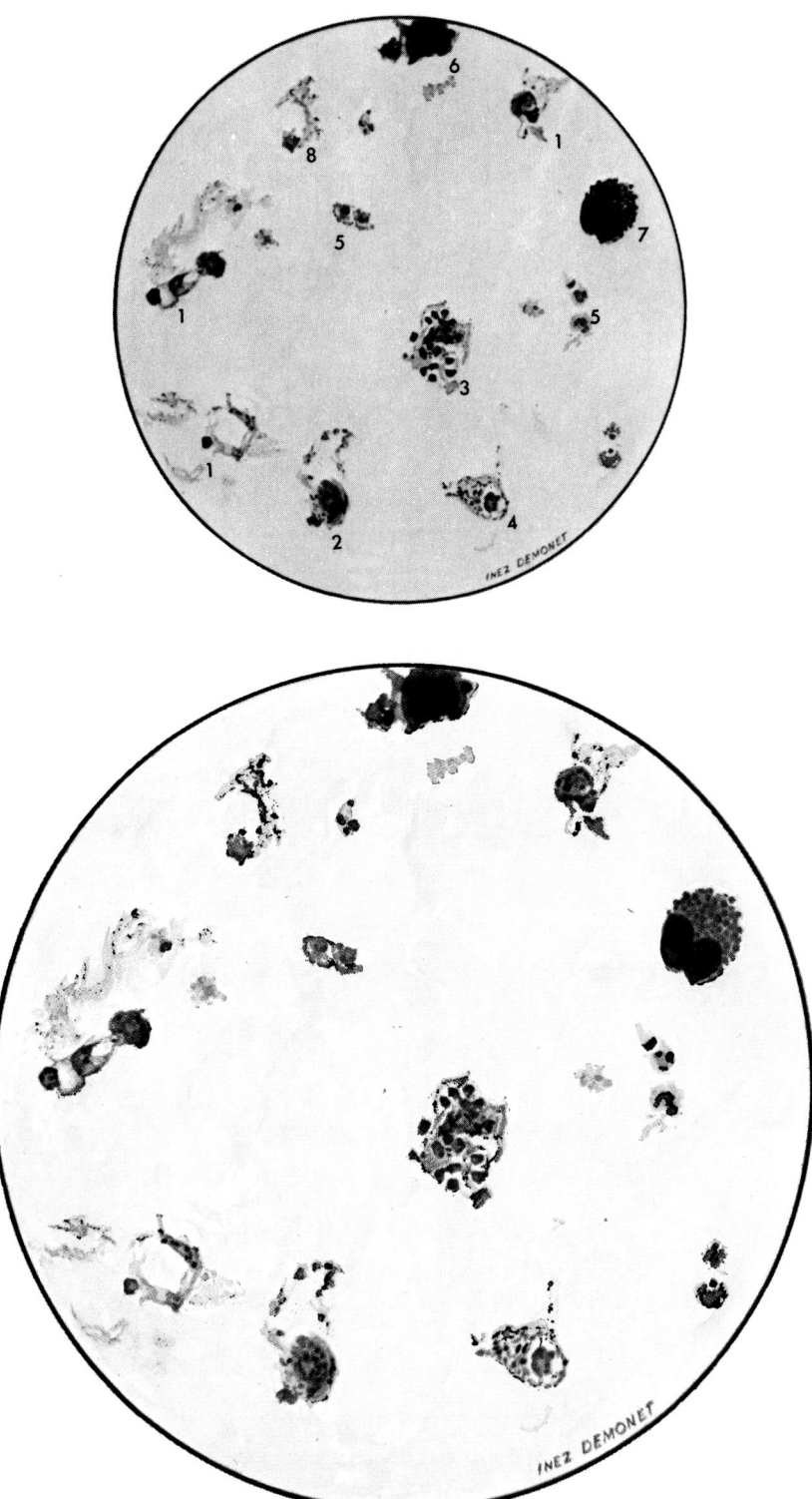

Fig. 97-25. *Plasmodium vivax* in thick smear. **1,** Ameboid trophozoites. **2,** Schizont: 2 divisions of chromatin. **3,** Mature schizont. **4,** Microgametocyte. **5,** Blood platelets. **6,** Nucleus of neutrophil. **7,** Eosinophil. **8,** Blood platelet associated with cellular remains of young erythrocytes. (From Wilcox, A.: Manual for the microscopical diagnosis of malaria in man, Department of Health, Education, and Welfare, Public Health Service, Washington, D. C., 1960, U. S. Government Printing Office.)

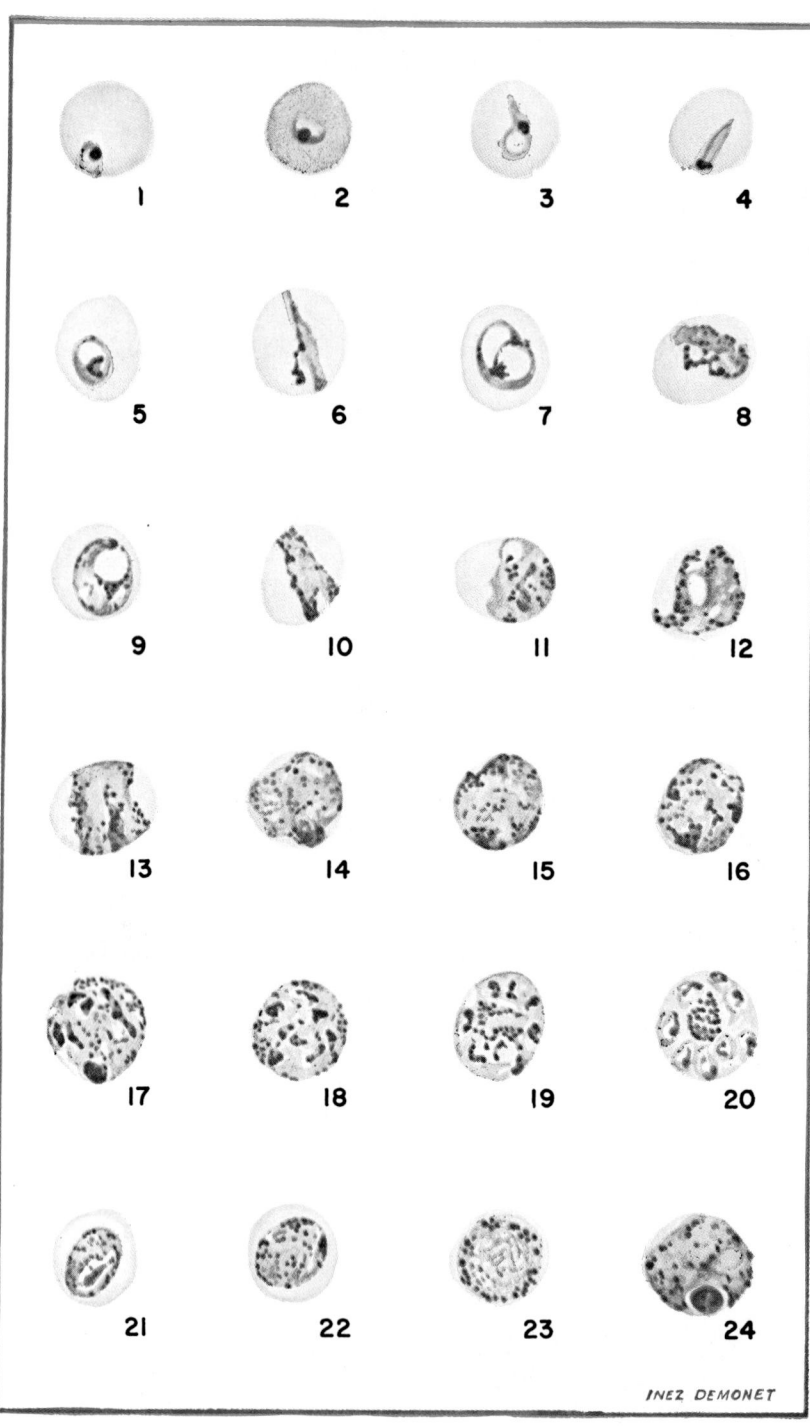

Fig. 97-26. *Plasmodium malariae.* **1,** Young ring form of trophozoite of quartan malaria. **2-4,** Young trophozoite forms of parasite showing gradual increase of chromatin and cytoplasm. **5,** Developing ring form trophozoite showing pigment granule. **6,** Early band form trophozoite: elongated chromatin, some pigment apparent. **7-12,** Some forms that developing trophozoite of quartan may take. **13, 14,** Mature trophozoites, 1 a band form. **15-19,** Phases in development of schizont ("presegmenting schizonts"). **20,** Mature schizont. **21,** Immature microgametocyte. **22,** Immature macrogametocyte. **23,** Mature microgametocyte. **24,** Mature macrogametocyte. (From Wilcox, A.: Manual for the microscopical diagnosis of malaria in man, Department of Health, Education, and Welfare, Public Health Service, Washington, D. C., 1960, U. S. Government Printing Office.)

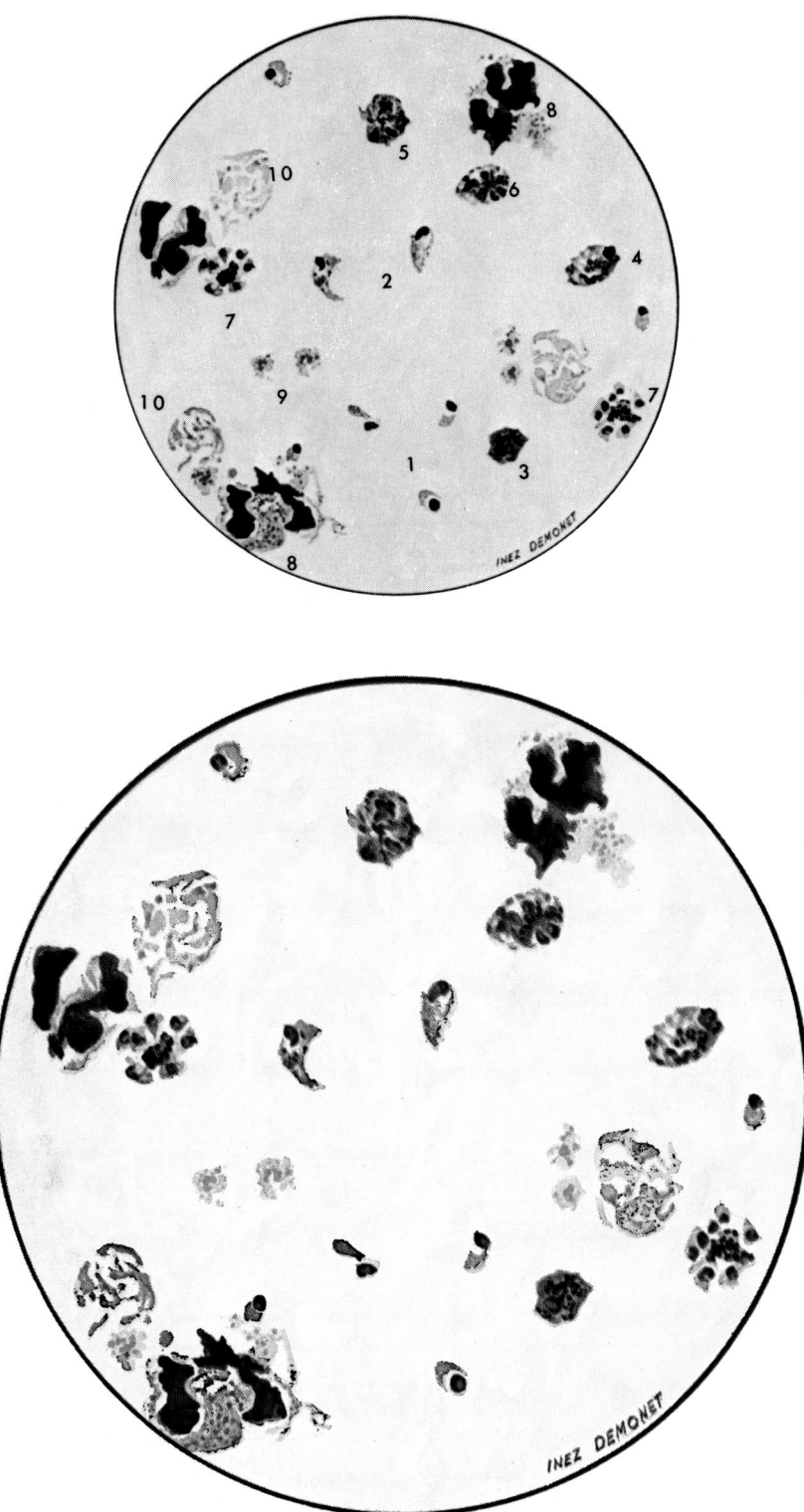

Fig. 97-27. *Plasmodium malariae* in thick smear. **1,** Small trophozoites. **2,** Growing trophozoites. **3,** Mature trophozoites. **4-6,** Schizonts (presegmenting) with varying numbers of divisions of chromatin. **7,** Mature schizonts. **8,** Nucleus of leukocyte. **9,** Blood platelets. **10,** Cellular remains of young erythrocytes. (From Wilcox, A.: Manual for the microscopical diagnosis of malaria in man, Department of Health, Education, and Welfare, Public Health Service, Washington, D. C., 1960, U. S. Government Printing Office.)

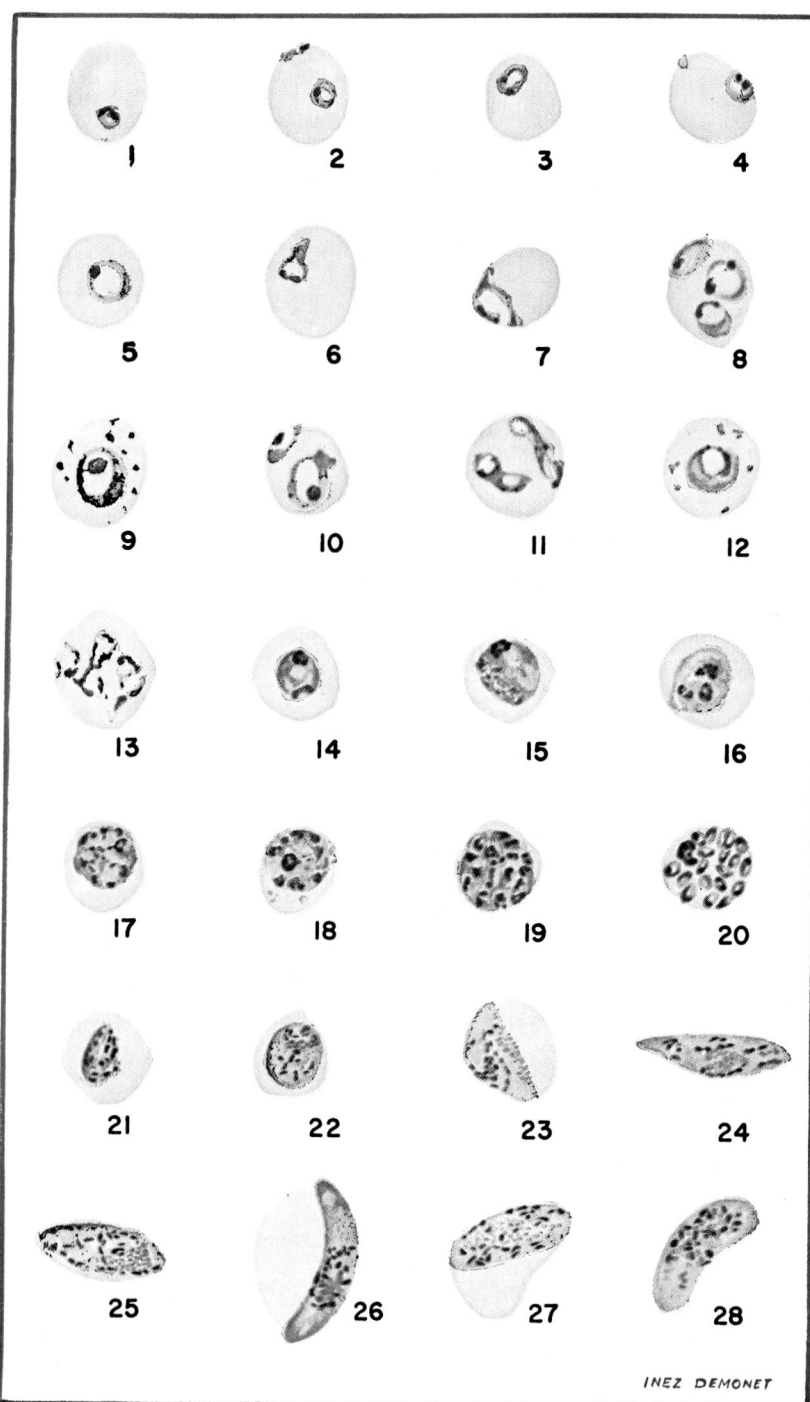

INEZ DEMONET

Fig. 97-28. *Plasmodium falciparum.* **1,** Very young ring form trophozoite. **2,** Double infection of single cell with young trophozoites, one a "marginal form," the other "signet ring" form. **3, 4,** Young trophozoites showing double chromatin dots. **5-7,** Developing trophozoite forms. **8,** Three medium trophozoites in 1 cell. **9,** Trophozoite showing pigment in cell containing Maurer's dots. **10, 11,** Two trophozoites in each of 2 cells, showing variations of forms that parasites may assume. **12,** Almost mature trophozoite showing haze of pigment throughout cytoplasm. Maurer's dots in cell. **13,** Estivoautumnal "slender forms." **14,** Mature trophozoite showing clumped pigment. **15,** Parasite in process of initial chromatin division. **16-19,** Various phases of development of schizont (presegmenting schizonts). **20,** Mature schizont. **21-24,** Successive forms in development of gametocyte, usually not found in peripheral circulation. **25,** Immature macrogametocyte. **26,** Mature macrogametocyte. **27,** Immature microgametocyte. **28,** Mature microgametocyte. (From Wilcox, A.: Manual for the microscopical diagnosis of malaria in man, Department of Health, Education, and Welfare, Public Health Service, Washington, D. C., 1960, U. S. Government Printing Office.)

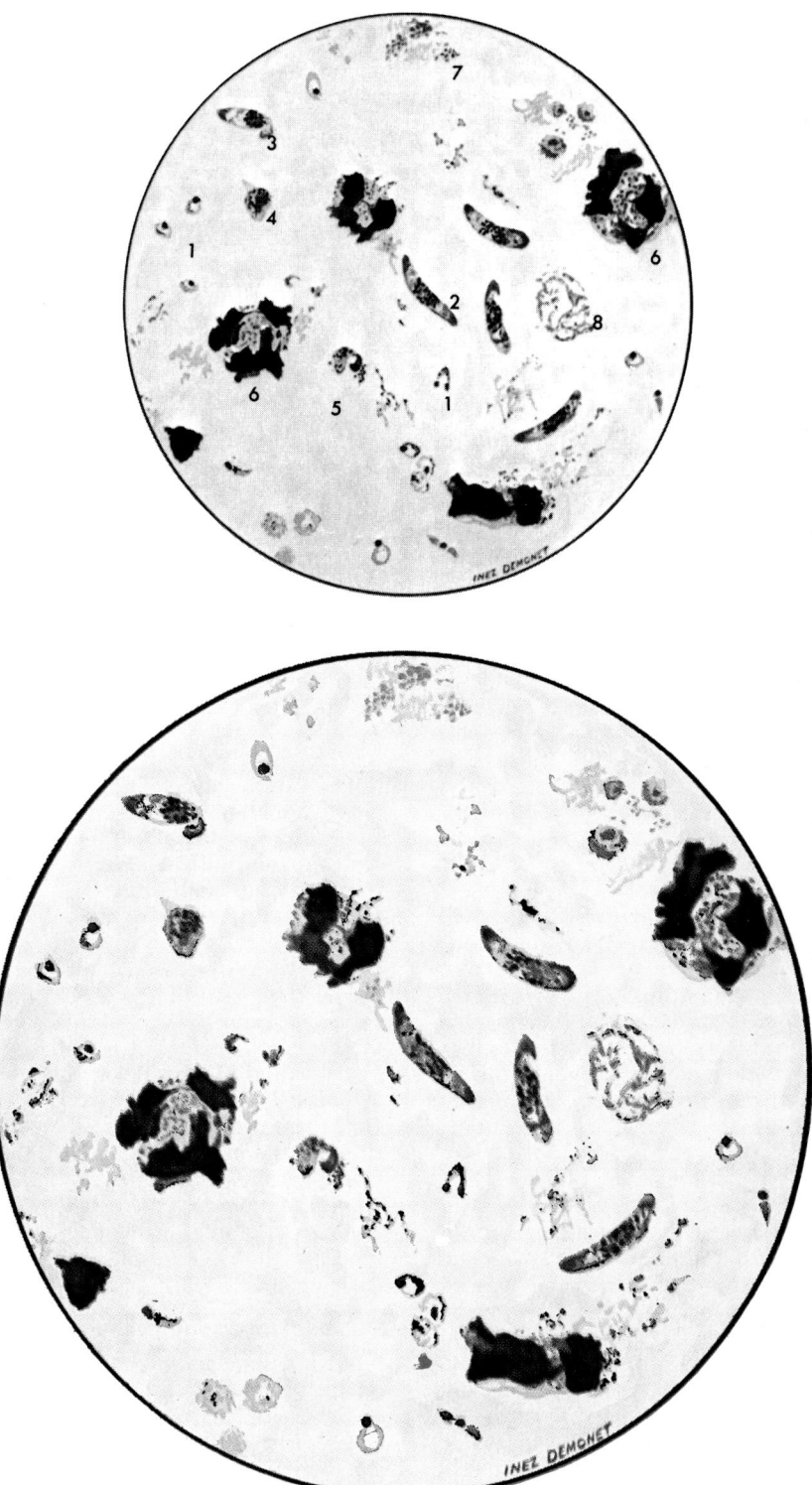

Fig. 97-29. *Plasmodium falciparum* in thick film. **1,** Small trophozoites. **2,** Gametocytes, normal. **3,** Slightly distorted gametocyte. **4,** "Rounded-up" gametocyte. **5,** Disintegrated gametocyte. **6,** Nucleus of leukocyte. **7,** Blood platelets. **8,** Cellular remains of young erythrocyte. (From Wilcox, A.: Manual for the microscopical diagnosis of malaria in man, Department of Health, Education, and Welfare, Public Health Service, Washington, D. C., 1960, U. S. Government Printing Office.)

Table 97-6. Differential points of 3 common malarial parasites of humans

	Plasmodium vivax	Plasmodium malariae	Plasmodium falciparum
Size of infected red cells	Enlarged	Reduced	No change
Color of red cells	Pale	Intensified	No change
Stippling of red blood cell	Schüffner's dots may be observed	None	Maurer's dots rarely may be seen
Size of trophozoite	Large (one-third diameter of blood cell)	One-third diameter of blood cell	Very small (one-fifth diameter of red blood cell)
Number of nuclei in each trophozoite	1, rarely 2	1, sometimes 2	2 or more not uncommon
Nuclei in mature schizont	12-24, average 16	6-12, average 8	8-36 (average 18-24), seldom seen
Shape of asexual forms	Irregular, spread out	Band or compact form	Not seen after early ring stage
Pigment in asexual forms	Greenish brown, fine	Greenish black, coarse	Dark brown
Size of gametocytes	Fills most of red blood cell	Fills most of red blood cell	Diameter about one-half red blood cell; length may appear to be outside blood cell
Shape of gametocytes	Round or oval	Round or oval	Crescent or banana-shaped
Pigment of sexual forms	Scattered, fine greenish brown	Clumped, coarse, greenish black	Centralized
Lenght of asexual development	48 h	72 h	48 h

sive divisions occur until 12-24 (average 16) chromatin fragments are produced. The cytoplasm then undergoes subdivision, enclosing each of the chromatin masses. The mature schizont, containing the merozoites, fills most of the red cell. More pigment granules are present as well as perhaps the characteristic Schüffner's dots.

The mature male gametocyte (microgametocyte) often fills the entire cell. The pale blue or grayish cytoplasm is more regularly distributed. The chromatin material is dispersed and not in a compact mass. The pigment appears darker than that in the schizont and is uniformly distributed. The mature female gametocyte (macrogametocyte), in contrast to the microgametocyte, possesses a darker blue cytoplasm, evenly distributed granules of brownish green pigment, and an eccentrically located compact mass of chromatin.

Plasmodium malariae

The various stages of *P. malariae* as seen in Giemsa-stained thin and thick blood smears are shown in Figs. 97-26 and 97-27; their characteristics are summarized in Table 97-6. The young trophozoite or ring forms of *P. malariae* are about the same size as those of *P. vivax*. The cytoplasm tends to be a darker blue and more compact, and frequently the cytoplasm stretches across the red cell in a band form. Unlike *P. vivax*, *P. malariae*–infected cells are normal sized. The pigment is coarse, greenish black, and more prevalent than in *P. vivax*. Mature schizonts contain 6-12 (average 8) merozoites, frequently in a circular (rosette) arrangement with a centrally located mass of pigment. The gametocytes resemble those of *P. vivax* except that they are

smaller, are in normal sized cells, and the pigment is coarser. No Schüffner's dots are seen in trophozoites, schizonts, or gametocytes.

Plasmodium falciparum

The various stages of *P. falciparum* as seen in Giemsa-stained blood preparations are shown in Figs. 97-28 and 97-29; their characteristics are summarized in Table 97-6. The ring stage of *P. falciparum* is smaller than that of *P. vivax*, occupying about one-fifth of the cell. Multiple infection of red cells is common. The trophozoite in some cells may be located on the extreme periphery of the erythrocyte. These marginal forms, called appliqué or accolé forms, occur frequently in *P. falciparum*. Occasionally red-staining clefts, called Maurer's dots, may be seen in the cytoplasm of infected cells. The older trophozoites and schizonts are seldom seen in the peripheral blood. The gametocytes are characteristically crescent-shaped bodies, although young gametocytes may be shorter and more oblong. The microgametocyte stains a darker blue, and the pigment and chromatin material are more compact.

Plasmodium ovale

Plasmodium ovale resembles *P. vivax* in the length of its asexual cycle and in the presence of Schüffner's dots, but its other morphologic characteristics more closely resemble *P. malariae*. Unlike *P. vivax*, Schüffner's dots may be observed frequently in the young trophozoite. Infected cells are frequently distorted, assuming oval or irregular shapes. The color and compactness of the cytoplasm resemble those of *P. malariae*. The mature schizont has 6-12 (average 8) merozoites. The gametocytes resemble closely

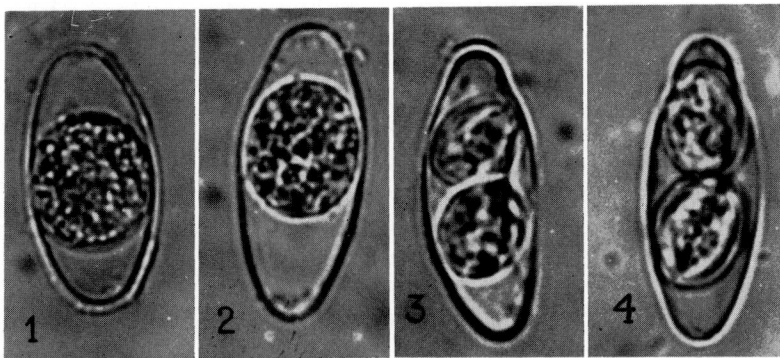

Fig. 97-30. *Isospora belli.* Human coccidia. **1, 2,** Oocysts with 1 sporoblast in concentrated specimen, method of Willis; fresh feces recently passed. **3, 4,** Oocysts with 2 sporocysts, from 48 h culture of fecal material concentrated by method of Willis. Each sporocyst produces 4 sporozoites. Thus 2 sporocysts × 4 sporozoites = 8 sporozoites. (From Kourí, P., and Basnuevo, J. G.: Revista de medicina tropical y parasitología; and Lecciónes de parasitología y medicina tropical, Havana, Editorial Profilaxis S.A.)

those of *P. vivax* but are usually smaller and more spherical.

Diagnosis of malarial infections

Definitive diagnosis of malaria is made by demonstration and identification of the malarial parasite in stained blood smears. Giemsa and Wright stains are frequently used to stain blood. Most authorities prefer Giemsa stain for identification of malaria. Many other staining procedures have been devised but have not been used as widely as these two. Field stain was often used during World War II because of the rapidity with which stained preparations could be made.

Thick or thin blood smears may be examined. Thick smears are preferred by the experienced worker because they allow many more positive cases to be discovered. The concentration of blood in a small space on the slide allows the laboratory worker to examine in 5 minutes the volume of blood that would require 15 minutes or more examination on a thin smear. However, frequently the parasites in thick smears are distorted and difficult for the inexperienced worker to identify. More characteristic parasite morphology is seen in thin blood smears. Thus in some cases it may be necessary to prepare both types of smears to effect identification. The laboratory worker should make every effort to accurately identify the species because if the infection is *P. falciparum* there is cause for grave concern and immediate treatment. If the infection is *P. vivax* or *P. ovale* a different treatment regimen is required because of persisting preerythrocytic stages.

As successful eradication programs eliminate or markedly decrease the malaria incidence, diagnostic acumen or consciousness may decrease. Careful examinations should be done on all persons returning from malarious countries. Although malaria has been eradicated from the United States, recently that country experienced a marked increase in imported malaria, primarily in servicemen returning from Viet Nam. Several persons died unnecessarily of undiagnosed *P. falciparum* infections. Thus special concern and attention must be given to malaria, even in countries where the disease is technically eradicated.[68]

Serodiagnosis of malaria has progressed to the point that it is a useful tool for epidemiologic studies and detection of blood donors responsible for transmission of malaria to recipients. Both IFA and IHA tests have shown at least 95% sensitivity and 99% specificity. For an introduction to literature associated with these tests consult Lennett et al.[69] Neither of these procedures, however, should replace examination of stained blood smears for primary diagnosis of malaria.

Coccidian parasites of humans
Isospora belli and Isospora hominis

These intestinal parasites have been reported most often in the tropics and subtropics. The life cycle is not known, but it is assumed that both an asexual cycle and a sexual cycle take place in the intestines. The asexual cycle probably resembles closely that described for malaria (i.e., trophozoites within intestinal tissue cells become schizonts that liberate merozoites, and so on). At some point gametocytes are formed, fertilization occurs, and zygotes (oocysts) are produced. In the case of *I. belli* the oocysts given off in the feces contain 1 or 2 nuclear bodies called sporoblasts. After development of the 2 sporoblasts into 2 sporocysts, each sporocyst nucleus divides twice, producing 4 nuclei per sporocyst within the oocyst. The nuclei develop into sporozoites. If the mature oocyst is ingested, the sporozoites are released to begin the cycle anew.

The stage observed in the feces is the oocyst (Fig. 97-30). The oocysts of *I. belli* are about 20-33 μm long and 10-19 μm wide. *I. belli* oocysts found in the fresh feces contain 1, rarely 2, sporoblasts. The oocyst matures in 18-36 hours, giving rise to 2 thin-walled sporocysts, each containing

4 sporozoites. *I. hominis* oocysts usually are passed fully developed. Often the oocyst wall is absent, and the relatively thick-walled sporocysts are seen either singly or in pairs, each containing 4 sporozoites. The ovoidal sporocysts measure 10-16 × 7.5-12 μm. Recent evidence strongly suggests that *I. hominis* should be reclassified and placed in the genus *Sarcocystis*.

The parasite has been reported in healthy individuals and in those complaining of diarrhea or colic. Most patients, however, have mild intestinal symptoms. Apparently the infection in humans is self-limiting and lasts only a few days. Diagnosis is based on identification of the oocyst in the feces.

Toxoplasma gondii

Toxoplasmosis is a common infection in most parts of the world. A wide range of warm-blooded animals is susceptible to the parasite. In the human population prevalence rates of 25% or higher are common. Prevalence tends to be lower in dry, cold climates.

Life cycle—epidemiology. Five stages are known to occur in the life cycle of *Toxoplasma*. All 5 stages occur in cats and other members of the cat family Felidae. Only 2 of these stages occur in humans, other mammals, and birds: (1) and extraintestinal intracellular trophozoite (Fig. 97-31) found in a wide range of cell types during the acute stages of infection and (2) a cyst stage found in chronic or latent infection (Fig. 97-31, *A*). The other 3 stages, found only in felines, are intestinal intracellular proliferative (asexual) trophozoites, intestinal gametocytes, and oocysts that pass in the feces.

Cats become infected by ingesting an acutely ill animal containing extraintestinal trophozoites or by ingesting chronically infected animals containing the cyst or by ingesting infective oocysts passed in the feces of another cat. Whichever stage is ingested, schizogonic (asexual) stages develop in the intestinal epithelium. These give rise to gametes that unite. The fertilized macrogamete becomes an oocyst that passes undeveloped in the feces (Fig. 97-31, *A*). Within 3-4 days sporulation occurs, producing an infective oocyst containing 2 sporocysts (Fig. 97-31, *A*). Extraintestinal trophozoites and cysts also develop in the cat just as they do in mammals and birds.

The time required after initial infection for an oocyst to appear in the infected cat's feces depends on the stage of the parasite that the cat ingests. If oocysts are ingested the prepatent period (time required for oocysts to appear in the feces) is 20-24 days; if extraintestinal trophozoites or cysts are ingested the prepatent periods are 5-10 days and 3-5 days respectively. These observations suggest that these stages in the life cycle of *Toxoplasma* occur sequentially and that ingestion of "later" developmental stages shortens the time required for completion of the life cycle in the cat.

Humans may acquire the infection by ingestion of oocysts passed in cat feces or by ingestion of inadequately cooked animal tissue containing the extraintestinal stages (especially the cyst) of this parasite. In most instances the infection in humans is benign or asymptomatic. Those persons who do develop acute disease have symptoms that resemble infectious mononucleosis, spotted fever, or typhus. Fever, rash, and lymphadenopathy are frequently seen in such cases. Although the individual recovers from the acute infection phase, the cysts apparently survive in the tissues for years. Later in life rupture of the cysts in the eye with subsequent multiplication or allergic reactions may cause chorioretinitis. Some authorities estimate that over 30% of retinochoroiditis is due to *Toxoplasma*. In recent years reactivation of latent toxoplasmosis has been reported in patients whose immune response has been compromised by malignant disease or use of cytotoxic or immunosuppressive drugs.

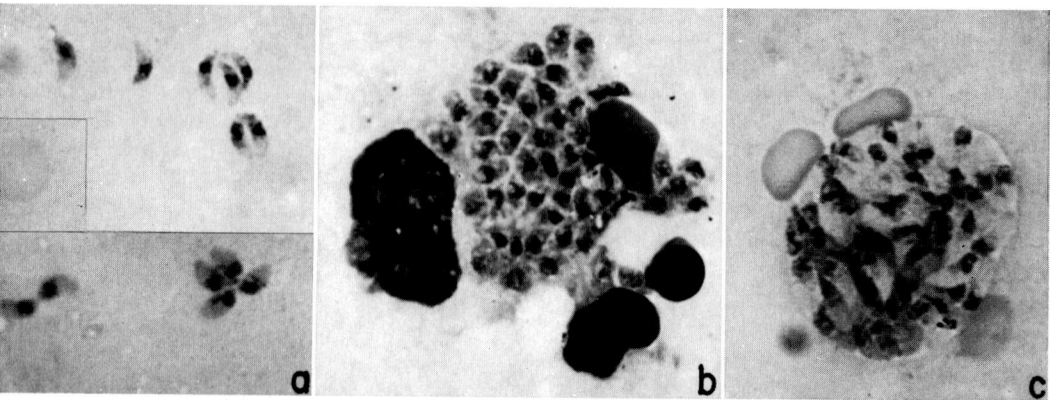

Fig. 97-31. Toxoplasma as seen, **a**, free in stained smears of peritoneal exudate or tissue, **b**, intracellularly, and, **c**, as pseudocyst in film of brain. (Wright stain; × 800; reduced from photomicrograph with magnification of 1000 diameters.) (From Sabin, A. B.: J.A.M.A. **116:**101, 1941.)

The most severe form of toxoplasmosis occurs in the newborn who acquires the infection transplacentally, especially during the last 6 months of gestation. The mother develops a primary case of toxoplasmosis, usually asymptomatic, during pregnancy and passes the infection transplacentally to her unborn child. Epidemiologic evidence suggests that transplacental infection occurs only if the mother becomes infected for the first time during pregnancy. Subsequent children are not endangered by a latent infection. At birth the infected child often shows signs of chorioretinitis, cerebral calcification, and less frequently hydrocephalus or microcephaly. Psychomotor disturbances are common. These symptoms tend to be irreversible, and surviving children often have impaired sight and CNS symptoms and are mentally retarded.

Morphology. The extraintestinal trophozoite is crescent shaped, measuring 4-7 μm long and 2-4 μm wide. The nucleus is nearer the rounded end. In Giemsa- or Wright-stained preparations the cytoplasm (Fig. 97-31) stains blue and the nucleus reddish purple. Intracellular forms may appear singly or in clusters. Within the cell the organism may lose its crescent shape and resemble leishmaniasis, especially within endothelial and mononuclear cells. The pseudocyst (Fig. 97-31) varies from 30-100 μm in diameter. The pseudocyst and cyst stages have been used synonymously by most workers, but Lainson presented experimental evidence that early in the infection a mass of organisms enclosed in a delicate membrane may be present. This structure may be called a pseudocyst. Later in chronic phases of the infection a true cyst state occurs (Fig. 97-32, A), the organisms being enclosed in a tough, thick-walled cyst.

Diagnosis. Indications for laboratory tests for suspected toxoplasmosis are (1) lymphadenopathies resembling glandular fever but giving negative Paul-Bunnell reactions or symptoms resembling Hodgkin's or other malignant diseases, (2) choroidretinitis, and (3) congenital illness manifested by hydrocephalus, meningitis, hepatomegaly, jaundice, or purpura.

Serologic tests play an important role in the diagnosis of toxoplasmosis. Formerly the complement fixation and methylene blue tests were the procedures of choice. A widely used complement fixation test devised by Warren and Sabin becomes positive relatively late in the course of the disease. The methylene blue test devised by Sabin and Feldman proved the most reliable and extensively used serologic test for many years. It is based on the fact that the cytoplasm of *Toxoplasma* organisms, when acted on by specific antibody, lose their affinity for the dye methylene blue. The titer or end point of the test is considered that dilution of serum that prevents methylene blue from staining the cytoplasm of 50% of the organisms under observation. A titer of less than 1:16 is of doubtful significance. Infected individuals as a rule develop titers of 1:256 or higher 10-20 days after infection. The high level may persist for several years. The vast majority of healthy persons have titers of 1:64 or less. The chief disadvantage of the dye test is that it requires living *Toxoplasma*.

The indirect hemagglutination test has gained favor in recent years. It is easier to perform and gives results similar to the dye test.[70] Titers higher than 1:256 reflect experience with *Toxoplasma*. The indirect fluorescent antibody test has also proved specific and reliable.[71] Detection of IgM antibody aids diagnosis of suspected toxo-

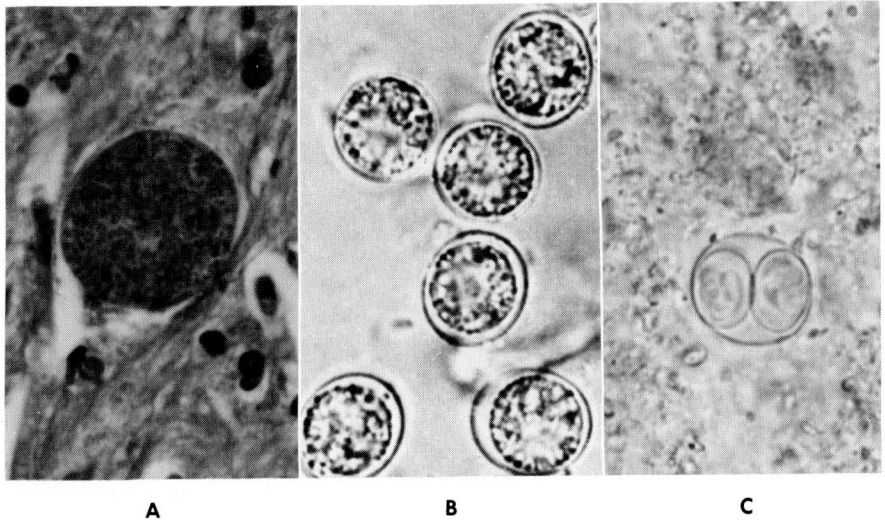

Fig. 97-32. *Toxoplasma gondii.* **A,** Cyst in brain of chronically infected mouse. ($\times$480.) **B,** Oocysts from fresh feces of cat 4 days after ingestion of cysts. Oocysts are approximately 10 $\times$ 12 μm. **C,** Oocyst containing 2 sporocysts, each containing 4 sporozoites after 7 days in vitro cultivation of feces from infected cat. (From Faust, E. C., Beaver, P. C., and Jung, R. C.: Animal agents and vectors of human disease, ed. 4, Philadelphia, 1975, Lea & Febiger.)

plasmosis in newborn infants or early infection in adults.[71] Consult Lunde[72] for review of technical factors and use of various serologic procedures. Consult Anderson and Remington[73] for review of transmission, clinical syndromes, and diagnosis of toxoplasmosis.

Isolation of *T. gondii* from suspected cases can be attempted without much difficulty. Giemsa-stained impression smears of lymph nodes, bone marrow, spleen, brain, and other tissues often reveal the organism (Fig. 97-31). Body fluids or tissues can be inoculated intraperitoneally into young mice. Such mice usually die of a fulminating infection within a few days, and many organisms can be demonstrated in Giemsa-stained ascitic fluid from the peritoneal cavity. Serum from surviving inoculated mice may also be tested for antibody against *Toxoplasma*.

Sarcocystis lindemanni

Until recently the taxonomic affiliations of *Sarcocystis* were unknown, although electron microscopy studies suggested that organisms of this genus were related to the Sporozoasida. In addition the infection in humans was of minor interest, since it has not been associated with any definite symptoms. In humans they appear as whitish streaks grossly visible in muscle fibers. In hematoxylin and eosin stains the whitish streaks appear to be compartmented or septate cysts (Miescher's tubules) that range up to 5 cm in length and are filled with crescent-shaped organisms (Rainey's corpuscles) measuring 5-12 μm in length by 2-4 μm in breadth. The cysts have been found most frequently in muscle fibers of the tongue, larynx; esophagus, diaphragm, chest, abdomen, and myocardium. Similar cysts frequently can be found in the tissues of domestic and other animals. Many have been described as separate species, but their validity remains questionable. The mode of transmission was unknown until recently.

Recent evidence, succinctly summarized by Markus et al.,[74] indicates the coccidian nature of *Sarcocystis*. The general life cycle involves 2 hosts, predator and prey. The predator (dogs, cats, humans, and possibly other primates) becomes infected by eating cyst-containing tissue of the prey. These organisms undergo gametogony below the intestinal epithelium of the predator and give rise to oocysts. Unlike *Isospora felis, I. rivolta, I. belli,* and *T. gondii,* the oocyst wall usually ruptures, and single, fully sporulated sporocysts pass in the feces. When ingested by the prey host (e.g., domestic animals, rodents, birds) the organisms undergo schizogony in tissue and organs, ultimately giving rise to cysts in muscle tissue.

It is now apparent that some if not all of the free sporocysts seen in the feces of cats, dogs, and humans are *Sarcocystis* species rather than *Isospora* species. Thus the coccidian parasites *Isospora, Sarcocystis,* and *Toxoplasma* must be differentiated when seen in the feces of susceptible hosts. *Sarcocystis* oocysts, usually seen as free sporocysts (Fig. 97-33, *A* and *B*) pass fully developed in the feces of dogs, cats, and humans. The average sporocyst size is 12.9 × 8.7 μm (range 11.6-14.9 × 8.2-10.4 μm). Oocysts of *I. hominis* (*Sarcocystis?*) also pass fully developed in the feces of humans; however, usually the oocyst ruptures and the free sporocysts are found in the feces. The sporocysts vary in size from 10-16 × 7.5-12 μm. Oocysts of *I. belli* (Fig. 97-30) also are found in the feces of humans. Characteristically they are intact, undeveloped, and range from 20-33 × 10-19 μm in size. Oocysts (Fig. 97-32, *B*) of *Toxoplasma* also may be found in the feces of cats but not of dogs or humans. They are intact, undeveloped, and measure approximately 12 × 10 μm.

Babeosis

Babesia causes an important hemolytic infection of cattle known as babeosis, piroplasmosis, or red water fever. Other mammals including

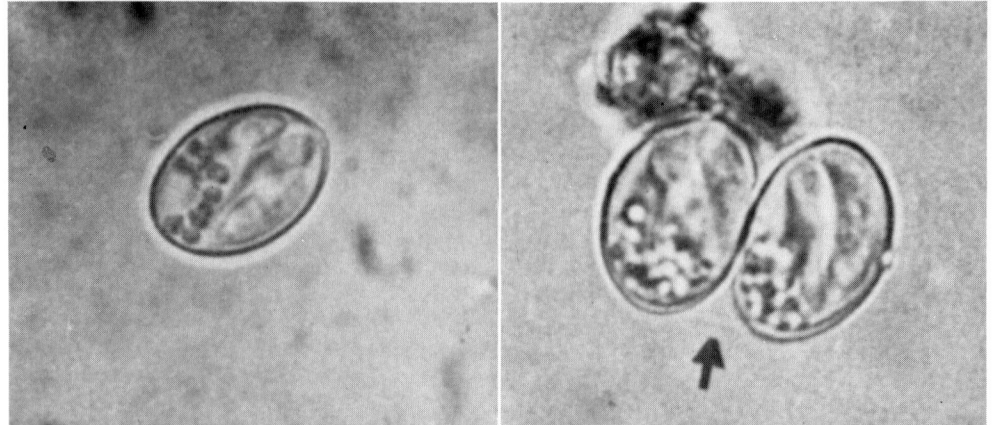

Fig. 97-33. *Sarcocystis fusiformis* from cat feces. (×2000.) Fresh preparations. **A,** Free sporocyst containing sporozoites. **B,** Intact oocyst (thin oocyst wall arrowed). (From Markus, M. B., et al.: J. Trop. Med. Hyg. **77:**250, 1974.)

dogs and cats can be infected with other species of *Babesia*. Ticks serve as the vectors of *Babesia*. In the mammalian host the parasite multiplies asexually as a trophozoite in red blood cells. The organism destroys the erythrocytes and invades other cells. Ticks become infected by ingesting infected red cells. These ticks, however, do not transmit the parasite back to humans or other mammals, as they usually take only 1 blood meal as an adult before laying their eggs and dying. Instead the organisms invade the developing ova within the tick and subsequently invade the salivary glands of the tick's progeny. The organisms continue to multiply and can be transmitted to the mammalian host when the tick takes a blood meal.

The first 3 cases reported in humans occurred in persons whose spleens had been removed, suggesting that alteration of the normal immune response was necessary before a person could be infected. Subsequently several cases have been reported in apparently healthy persons with no history of blood transfusion or parenteral drug use. All these cases occurred on Nantucket Island off Cape Cod, Mass.[75]

The parasites cause an acute hemolytic episode in humans. The parasites are best seen in Giemsa-stained thin blood smears as teardrop-like or ovoid to spherical bodies within erythrocytes. Pairs or tetrads of organisms may be seen. The organisms may be confused with *P. falciparum*, another organism that is seen in erythrocytes primarily as a trophozoite.

Pneumocystis carinii

Although recognized as a distinct disease-causing entity for more than 60 years, the true nature of *Pneumocystis carinii* remains a mys-

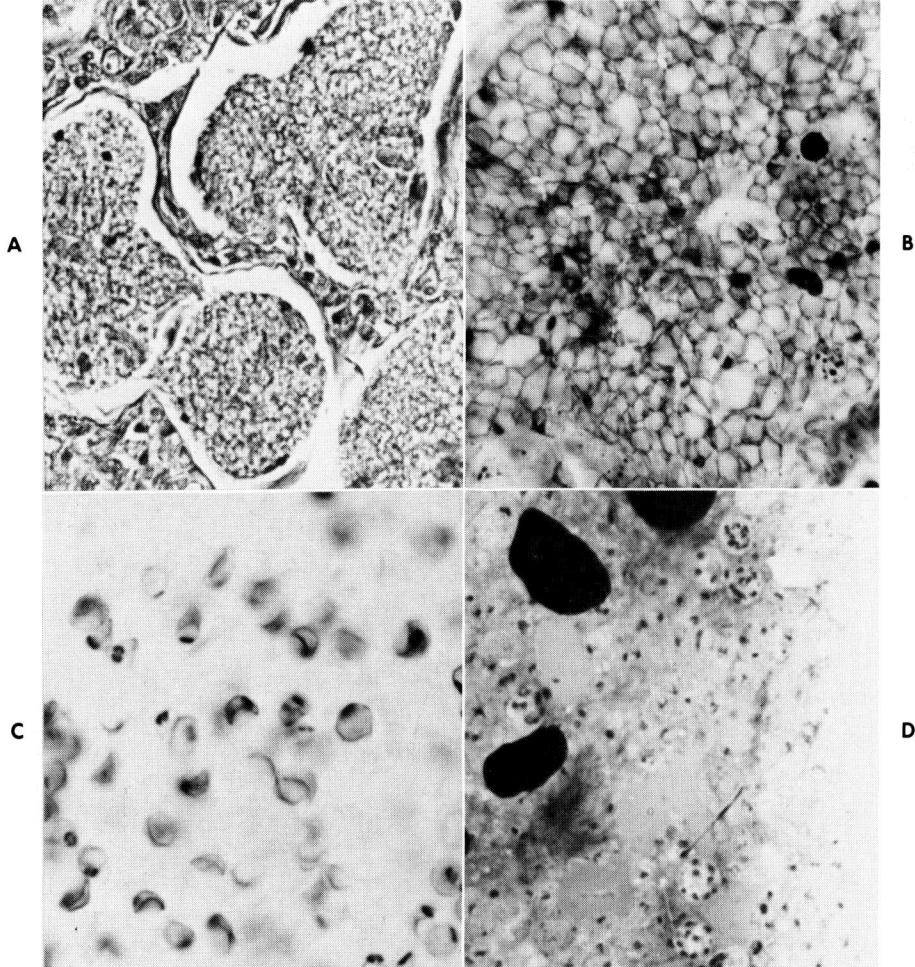

Fig. 97-34. *Pneumocystis carinii* in human lung. **A,** Section showing characteristic honeycomb pattern of alveolar exudate. (H & E stain; about ×400.) **B,** Section prepared with Warthin-Starry stain to emphasize honeycomb pattern of material in alveoli. (×1200.) **C,** Section stained with Gomori's methenamine silver stain to show characteristic comma-shaped thickening in cyst wall of parasite. (×1200.) **D,** Impression smear of lung showing several parasites with 8 nuclei and numerous uninucleate forms. (From Faust, E. C., Beaver, P. C., and Jung, R. C.: Animal agents and vectors of human disease, ed. 4, Philadelphia, 1975, Lea & Febiger.)

tery. Some authorities contend that the organism is a fungus, while others, representing the older view, believe the organism is a protozoan with close affinities to the coccidia.

Pneumocystis carinii afflicts the immunosuppressed host. The early literature described the disease as interstitial plasma cell pneumonia occurring predominantly in premature, malnourished, and debilitated infants. It is now recognized that all age groups are afflicted and that the disease occurs as an opportunistic infection in patients with primary immune deficiency disorders, leukemia, Hodgkin's disease, or other conditions requiring prolonged use of some combination of immunosuppressive drugs, antibiotics, or cytotoxic drugs.

P. carinii apparently occurs frequently in humans and other animals. Although the organism may exist in the healthy host, disease develops only after suppression of immunity via other disease or use of drugs that depress the normal immune response. Symptoms may merge with the underlying disease. Those most frequently associated with *Pneumocystis* pneumonia are dyspnea and nonproductive cough without pleurisy or upper respiratory complaints. Fever is common in adults but frequently absent in infants. X-ray examination typically shows bilateral diffuse or patchy interstitial infiltrate.

Laboratory diagnosis depends on demonstration of the organism in aspirates or tissue. Collection of sputum or tracheal or bronchial aspirates is a safer procedure but reveals fewer positive cases than open or closed lung biopsies or needle aspiration of infected lung. For recent reviews on diagnostic procedures consult Burke and Good,[76] Walzer et al.,[77] and Hughes et al.[78] Aspirates or tissues should be stained with Giemsa or by Gomori's methenamine silver procedure. Scarce organisms are easier to detect with methenamine silver technic, but organism morphology is best shown with Giemsa. Kim and Hughes[79] reported that polychrome methylene blue (Hema-Tek) and Wright stains give results similar to those obtained with Giemsa, while toluidine blue O stain gives similar results of the more complicated methenamine silver stain procedure.

In stained smears at least 2 types of organisms may be seen in the honeycombed exudate (Fig. 97-34, A and B) filling the alveolar spaces. A round or ovoid trophozoite, measuring 1.5-12 μm in diameter with a single nucleus, may be seen with Giemsa stains (Fig. 97-34, D) but not with methenamine silver stains. The "cyst," containing 2-8 smaller forms (trophozoites), measures 7 μm (Fig. 97-34, D), and the pear-shaped, crescentic, or ameboid organisms within the cyst measure 1 μm. In methenamine silver stains the cyst is easy to detect and shows characteristic comma-shaped thickenings in the cyst wall (Fig. 97-34, C). Hematoxylin and eosin and other stains show the characteristic honeycomb pattern of the exudate but do not show the organism.

Complement fixation tests[80] and immunofluorescent technics[81-83] have been used successfully to detect antibody against *Pneumocystis*. Immunofluorescent technics also can detect organisms in tissue.[84] European workers report

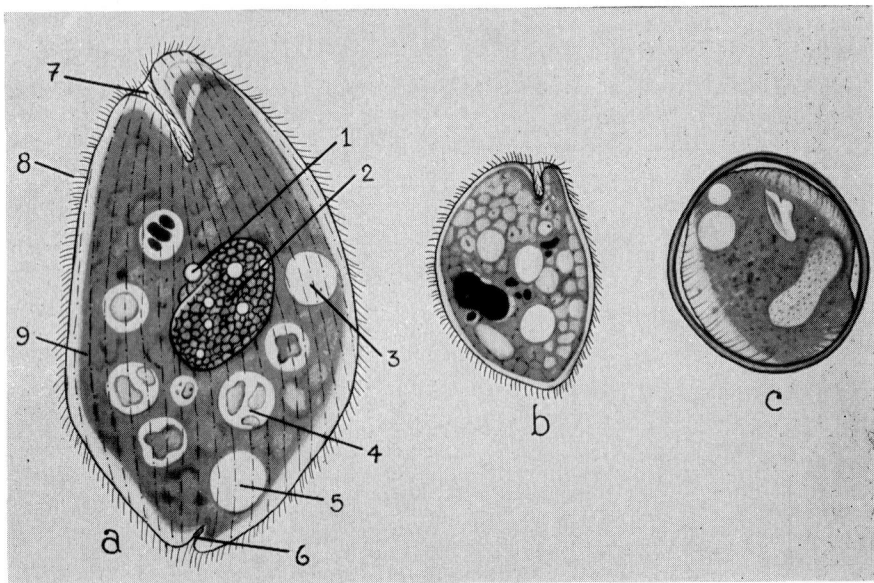

Fig. 97-35. *Balantidium coli.* **A,** Living trophozoite in feces of pig. Left side. **B,** Trophozoite stained with iron-hematoxylin, from human feces; ventral surface, half diameter of **A. C,** Living cyst in feces of pig; same diameter as **B. 1,** Micronucleus. **2,** Macronucleus. **3,** Anterior contractile vacuole. **4,** Nutritional vacuole. **5,** Posterior contractile vacuole. **6,** Anus or cytopyge. **7,** Mouth or cytosome. **8,** Cilia. **9,** Longitudinal stria. (Redrawn from Dobell and O'Connor: In Kourí, P., and Basnuevo, J. G.: Lecciónes de parasitología y medicina tropical, Havana, Editorial Profilaxis S.A.)

greater sensitivity with such tests than workers in the United States (75% vs. <35%). None of the tests have been perfected or evaluated sufficiently to be used routinely.

Balantidium coli

Geographic distribution. This parasite has an extensive distribution in hogs throughout the temperate and tropical areas. It is also found in certain monkeys in the tropics. The infection is relatively rare in humans and is reported most frequently in warm climates.

Life cycle—epidemiology. The trophozoite of *B. coli* is found in the large intestines of humans, monkeys, and pigs. At times the trophozoite secretes a cyst wall, which enables the organism to survive outside the body when passed in the feces. No increase in the number of nuclei occurs, as is the case with most amebae. The mode of transmission is by fecal contamination.

B. coli apparently may live in humans as a commensal, causing no symptoms or damage. In most cases intestinal symptoms resembling those of intestinal amebiasis develop. The organism may actively penetrate into the mucosa, but extraintestinal involvement is rare.

The exact relationship *B. coli* in animals has with *B. coli* in humans remains obscure. About 50% of persons with *B. coli* infection have a history of contact with infected animals, especially pigs. However, the organism has never been successfully transmitted experimentally from animal to person. It is likely that this parasite is poorly adapted to humans, and only an occasional strain is able to infect people readily.

Morphology. The trophozoite is much larger than the average protozoan parasite, varying in size from 50-100 μm in length by 40-70 μm in width. The trophozoite (Fig. 97-35) is ovoid, covered with cilia, and exhibits constant motion in freshly passed feces. The anterior end is slightly narrowed, and on one side an oral opening, the cytostome, can be seen. Less obvious is an opening at the posterior end, the cytopyge. The most obvious characteristic in stained specimens is the large peanut-shaped macronucleus. The cyst (Fig. 97-35) has similar morphologic characteristics and measures 45-65 μm in diameter.

Diagnosis. Laboratory diagnosis is based on demonstration of the trophozoite or cyst in feces. The methods utilized to identify the intestinal amebae are adequate to demonstrate this parasite.

REFERENCES

1. Stanier, R. Y., Doudoroff, M., and Adelberg, E. A.: The microbial world, ed. 3, Englewood Cliffs, N.J., 1970, Prentice-Hall, p. 873.
2. Moore, G. T., et al.: N. Engl. J. Med. **281**:402, 1969.
3. Morbid. Mortal. **19**:455, 1970.
4. Walzer, P. D., Wolfe, M. S., and Schultz, M. G.: J. Infect. Dis. **124**:235, 1970.
5. Thompson, R. G., Karandikar, D. S., and Leek, J.: Lancet **1**:615, 1974.
6. Barbieri, D., DeBrito, T., Hoshino, S., et al.: Arch. Dis. Child **45**:466, 1970.
7. Notes, W. M.: Gastroent. **63**:1085, 1972.
8. Ament, M. E., and Rubin, C. E.: Gastroenterology **62**:216, 1972.
9. Hoskins, L. C., Winaiver, S. J., Broitman, S. A., et al.: Gastroenterology **53**:265, 1967.
10. Morecki, R., and Parker, J. G.: Gastroenterology **52**:151, 1967.
11. Brandborg, L. L., Tankersley, C. G., Gottleib, S., et al.: Gastroenterology **52**:143, 1967.
12. Gupta, R. K., and Mehta, S.: Indian J. Med. Res. **61**:743, 1973.
13. Kamath, K. R., and Murugasi, R.: Gastroenterology **66**:16, 1974.
14. Vickerman, K.: In Fallis, A. M., editor: Ecology and physiology of parasites, Toronto, 1970, University of Toronto Press, p. 258.
15. Bray, R. S.: Rev. Microbiol. **28**:189, 1974.
16. Dumonde, D. C., and Preston, P. M. In Sadun, E. H., and Cohen, S., editors: Immunology of parasitic diseases, Oxford, Blackwell Scientific Publications.
17. Lumsden, W. H. R.: Trypanosomiasis and Leishmaniasis, New York, 1974, Associated Scientific Publishers.
18. Hoff, R. J. Parasitol. **60**:527, 1974.
19. Kelser, L.: Am. J. Trop. Med. Hyg. **16**:405, 1936.
20. Fife, E. H., and Kent, J. F.: Am. J. Trop. Med. Hyg. **9**:512, 1960.
21. Carmargo, M. E., Hoshino, S., and Sequiera, G. R. V.: Rev. Inst. Med. Trop. Sao Paulo **15**:81, 1973.
22. Toussaint, A. J., Tarrant, C. J., and Anderson, R. I.: Proc. Soc. Exp. Biol. Med. **120**:783, 1965.
23. Pelligrino, J., and Katz, N.: J. Parasitol. **57**:771, 1971.
24. Allain, D. S., and Kagan, I. G.: J. Parasitol. **60**:179, 1975.
25. Segovia, S. A.: Bull. WHO **50**:459, 1974.
26. Greenwood, B. M., Whittle, H. C., and Molyneux, D. H.: Trans. R. Soc. Trop. Med. Hyg. **67**:846, 1973.
27. Robson, J., and Rickman, L. R.: Trop. Anim. Health Prod. **5**:187, 1973.
28. Geigy, R., Kauffmann, M., Rogers, D., et al.: Acta Tropica **30**:12, 1973.
29. Weinman, D.: Trans. R. Soc. Trop. Med. Hyg. **54**:180, 1960.
30. Elsdon-Dew, R.: Adv. Parasitol. **6**:1, 1968.
31. Goldman, M.: Bull. WHO **40**:355, 1969.
32. Freedman, L., and Elsdon-Dew, R.: Am. J. Trop. Med. Hyg. **8**:327, 1959.
33. WHO Tech. Rep. Ser. **421**:52, 1969.
34. Healy, G. R.: Bull. N.Y. Acad. Med. **47**:478, 1971.
35. Schwartzwelder, C.: Am. J. Clin. Pathol. **22**:379, 1952.
36. Ridley, D. S.: J. Clin. Pathol. **27**:435, 1974.
37. Scholtens, T.: J. Parasitol. **58**:633, 1972.
38. Yarinsky, A. E., and Sternberg, S. deB.: Am. J. Clin. Pathol. **40**:598, 1963.
39. Mathews, A. W., Gough, K. R., Davies, E. G., et al.: Gut **14**:50, 1973.
40. Bieler, E. V., Meyer, B. J., Jansen, C. R., and Dutoit, D.: S. Afr. Med. J. **48**:308, 1974.
41. Sodeman, W. A., and Dowda, M. C.: Gastroenterology **65**:604, 1973.
42. Frashy, D. C., and Healy, G. R.: Appl. Microbiol. **27**:11, 1974.
43. Krupp, I. M., and Powell, S. J.: Am. J. Trop. Med. Hyg. **20**:414, 1971.
44. Juniper, K., Worrell, C. L., Minshew, M. C., et al.: Am. J. Trop. Med. Hyg. **21**:157, 1972.

45. Krupp, I. M.: Am. J. Trop. Med. Hyg. **23:**27, 1974.
46. Healy, G. R., Kagan, I. G., and Gleason, N. N.: Health Lab. Sci. **7:**109, 1970.
47. Healy, G. R., and Kraft, S. C.: Am. J. Digest. Dis. **17:**97, 1973.
48. Heilblum, M., and Cordero, C. B.: Dis. Colon Rectum **16:**368, 1973.
49. Gore, R. W., and Sadun, E. H.: Exp. Parasitol. **22:**316, 1968.
50. Ambroise-Thomas, P., and Kien Truong, T.: Am. J. Trop. Med. Hyg. **21:**907, 1972.
51. Savanat, T., Bunnag, D., Chongsuphajasiddhi, T., and Viriyanond, P.: Am. J. Trop. Med. Hyg. **22:**168, 1973.
52. Meerovitch, E., and Scott, F.: J. Parasitol. **59:**1134, 1973.
53. Kirkpatrick, C. H., Lunde, M. N., and Diamond, L. S.: Am. J. Trop. Med. Hyg. **21:**18, 1973.
54. Cerva, L., Zimak, V., and Novak, K.: Science **163:**575, 1969.
55. Culbertson, C. G., Ensmninger, P. W., and Overton, W. M.: J. Protozool. **15:**353, 1968.
56. Anderson, K., and Jamieson, A.: Pathology **6:**79, 1974.
57. Griffin, J. L.: Science **178:**869, 1972.
58. Lastovica, A. J.: Int. J. Parasitol. **4:**139, 1974.
59. Anderson, K., and Jamieson, A.: Pathology **4:**273, 1972.
60. Cerva, L., and Kramer, J.: Folia Parasitol. **20:**113, 1973.
61. DeJoncheere, J., Van Dijck, P., and van de Voorde, H.: Appl. Microbiol. **28:**159, 1974.
62. Robert, V. B., and Rorke, L. B.: Ann. Intern. Med. **79:**174, 1973.
63. Callicott, J. H., Nelson, E. C., Jones, M. M., et al.: J.A.M.A. **206:**579, 1968.
64. Page, F. C.: J. Protozool. **14:**499, 1967.
65. Page, F. C.: Protozool. **14:**709, 1967.
66. Carter, R. F.: Trans. R. Soc. Trop. Med. Hyg. **66:**193, 1972.
67. Burrows, R. B.: Am. J. Trop. Med. Hyg. **8:**583, 1959.
68. Sonnenwirth, A. C., Keating, J. P., and Waltman, S.: J.A.M.A. **209:**687, 1969.
69. Lennette, E. H., Spaulding, E. H., and Truant, J. P., editors: Manual of clinical microbiology, ed. 2, Washington, D.C., 1974, American Society for Microbiology.
70. Fairchild, G. A., Greenwald, P., and Decker, H. A.: Am. J. Trop. Med. Hyg. **16:**278, 1967.
71. Sulzer, A. J., and Hall, E. C.: Am. J. Epidemiol. **86:**401, 1967.
72. Lunde, M. N.: Health Lab. Sci. **10:**319, 1973.
73. Anderson, S. E., and Remington, J. S.: South. Med. J. **68:**1433, 1975.
74. Markus, M. B., Killick-Kendrick, R., and Garnham, P. C. C.: J. Trop. Med. Hyg. **77:**248, 1974.
75. Healy, G. R., Spielman, A., and Gleason, N.: Science **192:**479, 1976.
76. Burke, B. A., and Good, R. A.: Medicine **52:**23, 1973.
77. Walzer, P. D., Perl, D. P., Krogstad, D. J., et al.: Ann. Intern. Med. **80:**83, 1974.
78. Hughes, W. T., Price, R. A., Kim, H. K., et al.: J. Pediatr. **82:**404, 1973.
79. Kim, H. K., and Hughes, W. T.: Am. J. Clin. Pathol. **60:**462, 1973.
80. Barta, K., and Lsek, H.: Ann. Intern. Med. **70:**235, 1967.
81. Brozoko, W. J., Madalinski, K., and Nowoslawski, A.: Ann. N.Y. Acad. Sci. **177:**156, 1971.
82. Norman, L., and Kagan, I. G.: Infect. Immunol. **8:**317, 1973.
83. Lim, S. K., Eveland, W. C., and Porter, R. J.: Appl. Microbiol. **26:**666, 1973.
84. Brozoko, W. J., Madalinski, K., Krawczynski, K., and Nowoslawski, A.: Exp. Med. Microbiol. (Poland) **19:**397, 1967.

98

HELMINTHS

Michael H. Ivey

PHYLUM NEMATODA

It has been estimated that there are 500,000 distinct species of nematodes. The great majority of these are free living, existing in varied habitats such as salt water, fresh water, and soil. An estimated 80,000 species are parasitic for 40,000 species of vertebrates. This does not include those nematodes parasitizing invertebrates. Only about 50 species of nematodes have been reported in humans, and only about a dozen of these parasitize humans with regularity. Nevertheless they make their presence felt. Stoll estimated that there were 2000 million human nematode infections among the existing 2200 million people. In many areas certain nematode infections, combined with other diseases and malnutrition, cause severe health problems.

Morphology (general). Nematodes are thread-like and cylindrical in appearance, varying in size from less than 1 mm to 75 cm or more. The sexes are separate. Fig. 98-1 illustrates the relative size and shape of the more important nematode species infecting humans. The body wall consists of a tough impermeable chitinous-like cuticle. But unlike chitin, it cannot be digested in potassium hydroxide. More likely the cuticle is a keratinlike or collagenous substance. It is marked by regularly arranged transverse striations or annulations and is secreted by the hypodermis, a subcuticular epithelium that thickens into 4 cords or lines, 1 dorsal, 1 ventral, and 2 lateral. These cords carry the nerve fibers and in some species the lateral excretory canals.

Fig. 98-2 illustrates the basic structures in the typical nematode. The **digestive system** consists of a **mouth** leading into a **buccal cavity** or **buccal capsule.** There follows an **esophagus** and tube-like **intestine** terminating as a **rectum** and **anus** near the posterior end of the worm. The arrangement or absence of lips and presence of teeth or cutting plates in the mouth are sometimes useful features in identification of adult worms.

The **nervous system** consists of a **nerve ring** around the esophagus just anterior to the excretory pore. From this ring extend longitudinal nerve trunks both anteriorly and posteriorly. The large dorsal nerve trunk and ventral nerve trunk are contained in the dorsal and ventral cords. These trunks unite at various points toward the posterior portion of the worm.

The **excretory system,** illustrated in Fig. 98-2, consists of 2 **lateral excretory canals** or **tubes** that lie in the lateral cords and open to the outside of the body by means of an anteriorly located **excretory pore.** However, many modifications of the excretory system exist among different species. In some species the lateral excretory canal may be lacking.

All the nematodes parasitizing humans have separate sexes. The males are usually smaller and have a curled posterior end or a posterior end that flares into a tentlike structure called the **copulatory bursa.** The **male reproductive organs,** situated in the posterior third of the body, consist of a **testis, vas deferens, seminal vesicle,** and **ejaculatory duct** that opens into the **cloaca.** The cloaca opens to the outside of the worm and serves as a common terminal opening for both the digestive and reproductive systems. Males usually possess a pair of spicules just dorsal to the ejaculatory duct that apparently serve to guide the sperm during copulation. In some nematode forms such as the hookworms the male reproductive organs terminate at the very end of the worm in a tentlike structure called the bursa.

Life cycle (general). The nematodes have relatively simple developmental cycles compared with the trematodes and cestodes. Humans may be infected in 1 of 4 general ways. (1) The simplest way, utilized to perpetuate *Ascaris, Trichuris,* and *Enterobius,* is for humans to ingest the infectious or embryonated egg containing the larva. (2) Humans may also be infected by ingestion of meat containing the infected larvae (*Trichinella*) within its tissues. (3) Humans may be infected by larval forms of parasites (*Necator* and *Strongyloides*) that penetrate the skin. The infectious larval forms, **filariform larvae,** develop from eggs or larvae deposited on the ground in the feces. (4) Humans may be infected by the bite of an appropriate infected insect vector. The filarial worms are dependent on insects to transmit progeny from person to person.

Laboratory diagnosis (general). The specific details regarding methods and technics used in laboratory diagnosis are discussed in Chapter

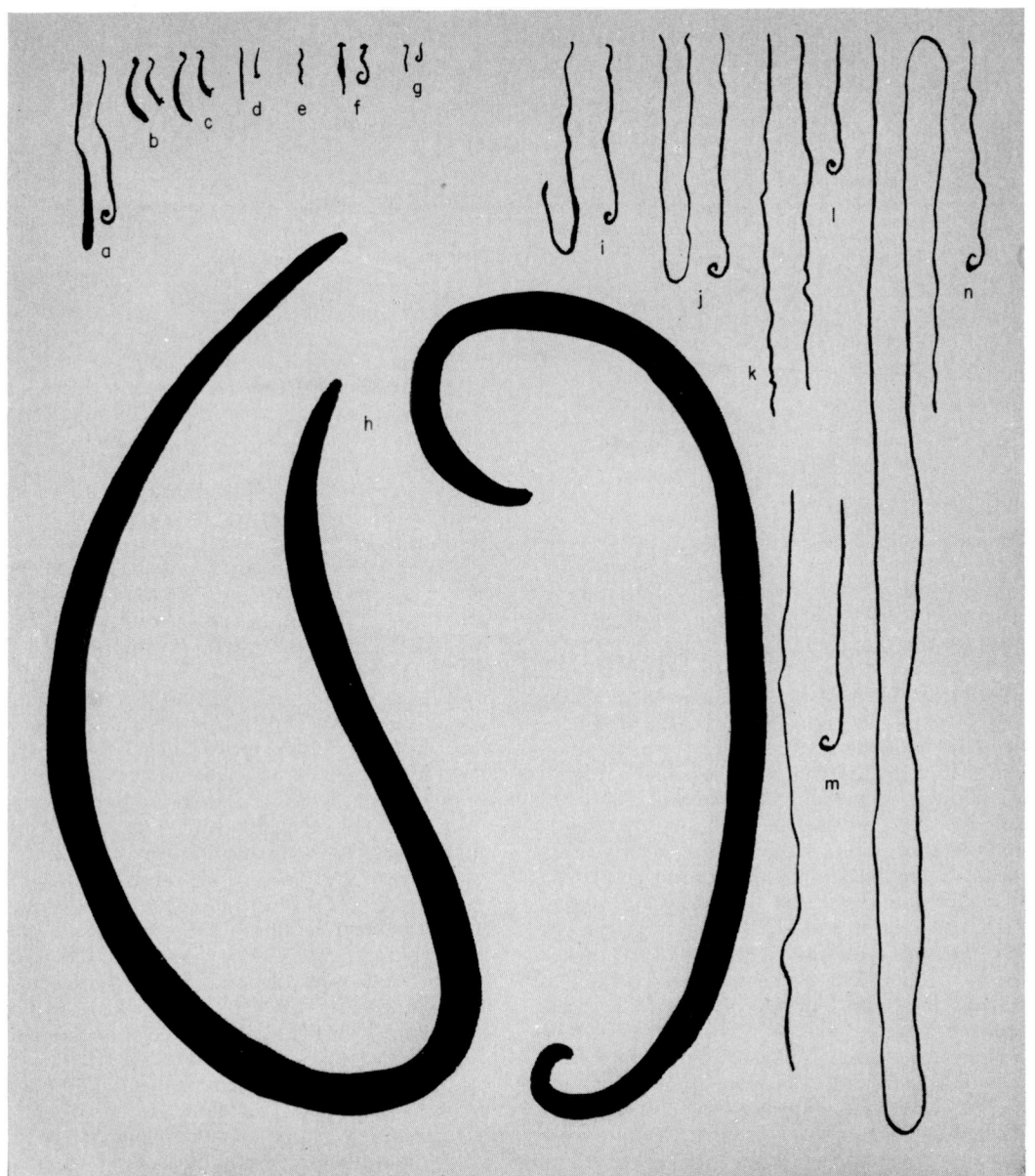

Fig. 98-1. Outline drawings of important nematode parasites of humans, drawn to scale. *a, Trichuris trichiura,* female (left) and male (right). *b, Necator americanus,* female (left) and male (right). *c, Ancylostoma duodenale,* female (left) and male (right). *d, Trichostrongylus orientalis,* female (left) and male (right). *e,* Female parasitic *Strongyloides stercoralis. f, Enterobius vermicularis,* female (left) and male (right). *g, Trichinella spiralis,* female (left) and male (right). *h, Ascaris lumbricoides,* female (left) and male (right). *i, Loa loa,* female (left) and male (right). *j, Acanthocheilonema perstans,* female (left) and male (right). *k,* Female *Mansonella ozzardi. l, Brugia malayi,* female (left) and male (right). *m, Wuchereria bancrofti,* female (left) and male (right). *n, Onchocerca volvulus,* female (left) and male (right). (From Faust, E. C.: Animal agents and vectors of human disease, Philadelphia, 1955, Lea & Febiger.)

100. The principles of laboratory diagnosis of nematode infection are briefly discussed.

In general, laboratory methods that demonstrate the parasite microscopically are preferred to other types of tests. *Ascaris, Trichuris, Strongyloides,* and hookworm infections may be readily diagnosed by the presence of character-istic eggs or larvae in the feces (Fig. 98-3). Microscopic artifacts, pseudoparasites, and so on, frequently confused with helminth eggs, are shown in Fig. 98-21. The number of positive cases discovered is greatly increased when concentration technics such as zinc sulfatre flotation on formalin-ether sedimentation are used.

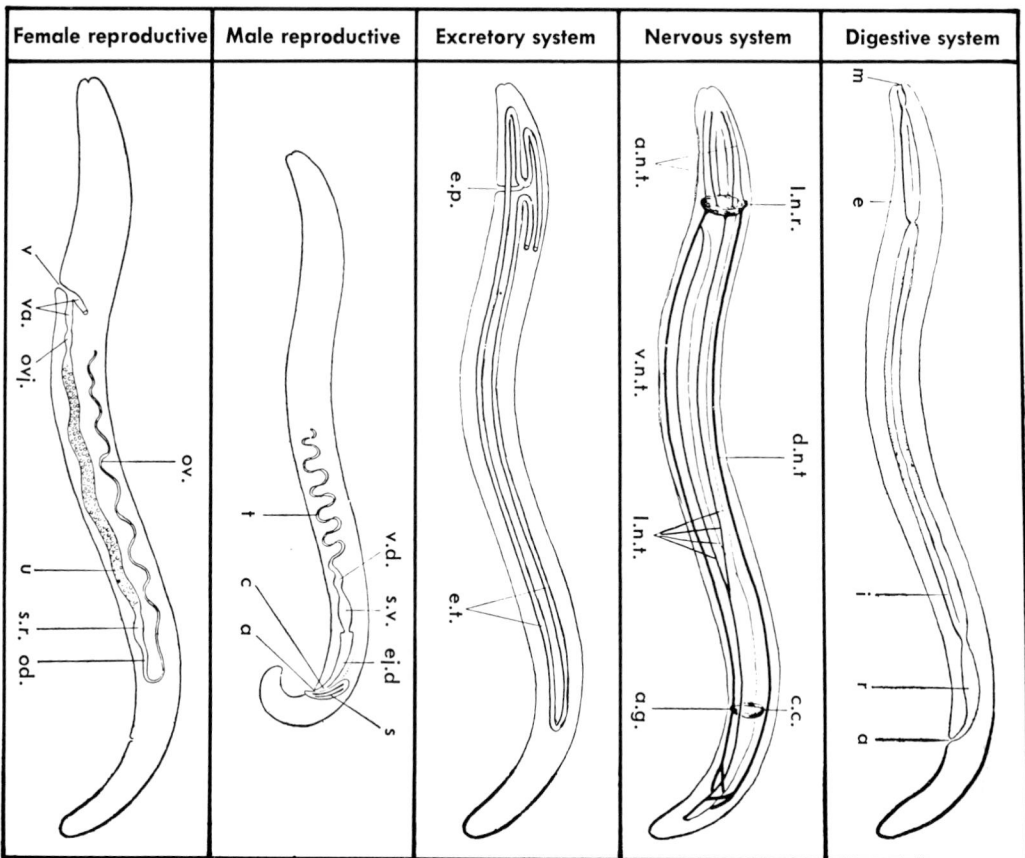

Fig. 98-2. Morphology of typical nematode. **a**, Anus; **a. g.**, anal ganglion; **a. n. t.**, anterior nerve trunks; **c**, cloaca; **c. c.**, circumcloacal commissure (male); **d. n. t.**, dorsal nerve trunk; **e**, esophagus; **e. p.**, excretory pore; **e. t.**, excretory tubules; **e. j. d.**, ejaculatory duct; **i**, intestine; **l. n. r.**, circumesophageal ring; **l. n. t.**, lateral nerve trunks; **m**, mouth; **o. d.**, oviduct; **ov.**, ovary; **ovj.**, ovejector; **r**, rectum; **s**, spicules; **s. r.**, seminal receptacle; **s. v.**, seminal vesicle; **t**, testis; **u**, uterus; **v**, vulva; **va.**, vagina; **v. d.**, vas deferens; **v. n. t.**, ventral nerve trunk. (From Belding, D. L.: Textbook of parasitology, ed. 3, New York, 1965, Appleton-Century-Crofts.)

Several nematodes do not give off larvae or eggs in the fecal stream. Thus methods other than facal examination must be used to detect the parasite's presence. In *Trichinella* infections the adult female worm deposits larvae that migrate to the voluntary muscles or other tissues. No easily detectable phase is ever present in feces or blood circulation. Thus diagnosis depends on either serologic tests or muscle biopsy to demonstrate the larvae. The filarial infections may be detected by examination of blood for larval forms (*Wuchereria, Mansonella, Acanthocheilonema*) or by examination of skin scrapings for larval forms (*Onchocerca*). Blood specimens may be concentrated by the Knott technic or stained with Giemsa stain to facilitate identification.

Adult worms recovered from feces can be identified either by macroscopic or microscopic observation of shape or pertinent structures. Sometimes it may be desirable to clear the worm specimen, either to aid in identification or as a preliminary step in preparation of a permanent slide mount of the worm for future reference and study. Although nematodes may be preserved in 70% alcohol–5% glycerin, specimens should be placed in hot glycerin-formalin or lactophenol solutions or glacial acetic for clearing if permanent slide preparations are desired. See Chapter 100 for details.

Species of Nematoda
Trichinella spiralis

Geographic distribution. *T. spiralis* has a cosmopolitan distribution, probably being found wherever pork is consumed. Its prevalence is undoubtedly higher in the United States and Europe than in the Tropics or Orient.

Life cycle—epidemiology. Humans become infected by ingesting raw or partially cooked meat (usually pork) containing viable encysted infected larvae. In the stomach or intestines the cyst walls surrounding the larvae are digested, freeing the larvae, which then penetrate the mucosa of the small intestine and undergo a series of molts, developing into adults in 2-3 days. After fertilization the female burrows into

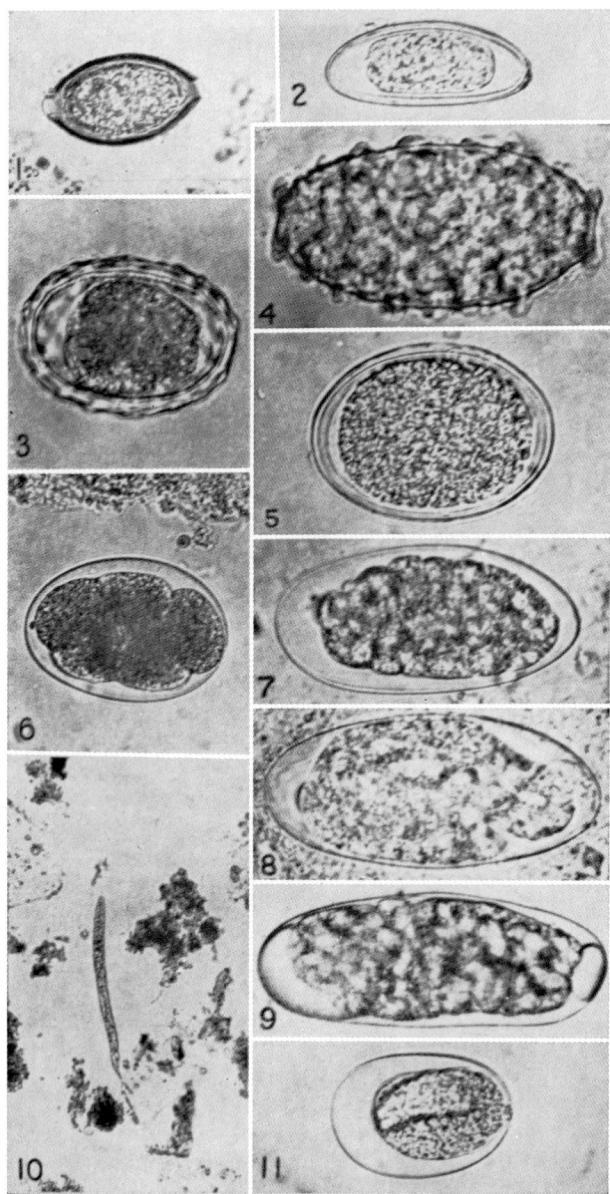

Fig. 98-3. Common nematode eggs. **1,** Whipworm, *Trichuris trichiura.* **2,** Pinworm, *Enterobius vermicularis.* **3,** Large roundworm, *Ascaris lumbricoides,* fertilized egg. **4,** *Ascaris,* unfertilized egg. **5,** *Ascaris,* decorticated egg. **6,** Hookworm egg. **7,** Immature egg of *Trichostrongylus orientalis.* **8,** Embryonated egg of *T. orientalis.* **9,** Egg of *Meloidogne javanica,* a plant nematode, which sometimes is found in stools. **10,** Rhabditiform larva of *Strongyloides stercoralis,* the stage usually found in the stool. **11,** Egg of *S. stercoralis,* rarely seen in the stool. See Fig. 98-21 for objects in feces most often confused with helminth eggs. (**1-9** and **11,** ×500; **10,** ×75.) (From Hunter, G. W., III, Frye, W. W., and Swartzwelder, J. C.: A manual of tropical medicine, Philadelphia, 1960, W. B. Saunders Co.)

the mucosa and begins larvipositing about the fifth to seventh day. Larvipositing may continue for several weeks, 1 female giving off as many as 1500 larvae. The adults are short-lived, usually dying within a few weeks. The larvae find their way into the lymphatics or venules and eventually into the general circulation. The larvae may penetrate practically any tissue or organ, but only those larvae that enter striated or voluntary mus-

cles develop into infected larvae. The muscles most often invaded are diaphragm, larynx, tongue, abdomen, biceps, deltoids, and other active muscles. In the muscles the larvae increase from 0.1 to 1.0 mm in size. A host reaction results in cyst walls forming around the larvae in about 1 month. Calcification may begin about the sixth month. The larvae remain alive in a dormant state within the cyst, perhaps for years, until the host is ingested, freeing the larvae to start the cycle over again.

T. spiralis, unlike many parasites, may infect many different species of animals. In nature the parasite has been found in almost all meat-eating animals. Under experimental conditions non-carnivorous animals such as rabbits, guinea pigs, cattle, and sheep can be readily infected. However, the main source of infection in humans is the pig. The infection is maintained in pigs by the practice of feeding hogs raw garbage containing pork scraps. The rat may play a minor role in maintenance of *Trichinella* in hogs, as conceivably hogs, especially improperly fed hogs, may eat recently dead infected rats. However, rats are not considered an important factor in perpetuation of trichinosis.

In the United States an estimated 16% of the population harbor *T. spiralis* as determined by surveys 20-30 years ago of larvae present in examined human cadavers. Recent surveys indicate a decreasing incidence. However, few cases are diagnosed, probably because most infections are light and subclinical. Clinical cases, sometimes severe or even fatal, usually result from ingestion of pork prepared from a single heavily infected hog. Subclinical cases probably result from ingestion of commercial pork products prepared from the pooled meat of many hogs. Although 1 hog may be infected, the larvae are diluted by pooling with other hogs. Meat products such as wieners, various sandwich meats, and sausages, which may not be cooked or are only partially cooked, probably serve as vehicles for many subclinical infections.

The great majority of infections are light, and consequently symptoms are so mild that the infected individual goes undiagnosed. Heavier infections may cause symptoms resembling many other diseases because the larvae affect so many parts of the body. However, in classic cases symptoms may be attributed to 3 overlapping phases in the life cycle.

The **first phase** is the result of the presence of the excysted larvae developing to adults in the intestines. They may initiate nausea, vomiting, diarrhea, and other gastrointestinal symptoms. A typhoid-type fever, maculopapular eruptions, and profuse sweating also may occur. As long as the adult worms are present, usually about 2-3 months, gastrointestinal symptoms may be present.

The **second phase** of symptoms begins after the female worms larviposit and is the result of the migrating larvae. Beginning about the seventh day after infection, there may be marked edema about the eyes, muscular pains, respiratory difficulties, difficulty in swallowing and speech, myocarditis, encephalitis, meningitis, and ocular disturbances. Other symptoms may occur, depending on the tissue invaded and the extent of damage. An eosinphilia is usually initiated about the fourteenth day, reaching a peak about the twenty-first day. Eosinophil counts usually vary between 15-40%, but in some cases eosinophilia as high as 50-90% may be present.

The **third phase** of symptoms, overlapping with the other phases, begins about 6 weeks after infection as the larvea becoming encysted. Generalized edema, skin eruptions, and various sequelae of tissue damage, caused by larval invasion, may occur. In fatal cases death usually occurs between the fourth and sixth week. Recovery from severe infection may take several weeks or months.

Morphology. The adult worms are small; the male measures about 1.5 mm and the female about 3-4 mm in length. The male is readily recognized by the presence of 2 caudal appendages at the posterior end. The vulva of the female is in the anterior fifth. Both sexes have a characteristic column of cell bodies in the anterior portion of the worms. The adults are rarely seen in the feces and when seen are often degenerated and hardly recognizable. Larvae are seen free only occasionally in blood smears or if muscle containing infective larvae is digested. The larva measures 80-120 μm at birth and possesses the characteristic column arrangement of cell bodies in the anterior of the worm.

Diagnosis. Diagnosis of *Trichinella* infections in the early stages is almost impossible. Symptoms may be suggestive but are not definitive. Examination of feces is usually fruitless, since adults are seldom recovered and there is no diagnostic egg stage produced by the female. Presumptive diagnosis may be made on the basis of (1) suggestive symptoms and history of eating pork and (2) skin tests and serologic tests. However, diagnosis is seldom arrived at in time to prevent the larvae from invading the tissues.

A commercial skin test antigen, originally developed by Bachman, has value as a presumptive diagnostic tool. By the third week infected persons will usually give a specific immediate reaction (within 15 minutes) to intradermal injection of the trichina antigen. Occasionally delayed reactions occur in the first week of infection and at other times, but they are not considered reliable. About 85-90% of infected individuals will react positively. Interpretation of the test must take into consideration that a positive reaction may be due to (1) a recent infection, (2) an old infection, or (3) a biologic false-positive reaction. Thus a negative skin test may be of greater diagnostic significance than a positive test, since the test is negative in only about 10% of infected individuals. The complement fixation test, although still considered reliable, has been largely displaced by other serologic technics. In the United States the bentonite flocculation test has proved relatively sensitive and very specific. It detects antibody in serum from patients by the third week of infection, revealing peak titers several weeks later. Usually the test reverts to negative 2-3 years after infection. The indirect fluorescent antibody test has proved even more sensitive and just as specific. Flocculation tests

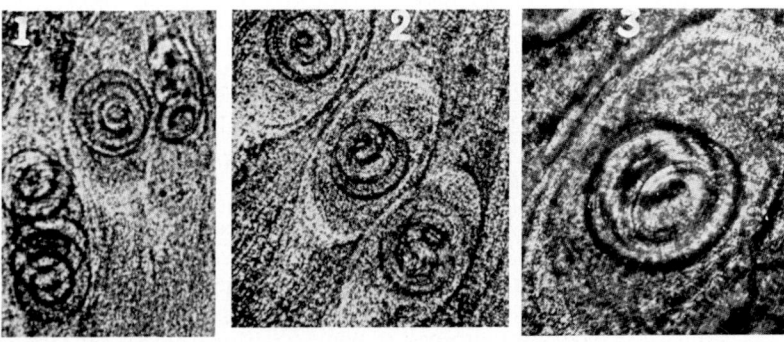

Fig. 98-4. *Trichinella spiralis.* **1-3,** Larvae in diaphragm muscle. Experimental infestation of white rat. (Courtesy Dr. G. Bachman, Puerto Rico.) (Various magnifications.) (Originals of Kourí.)

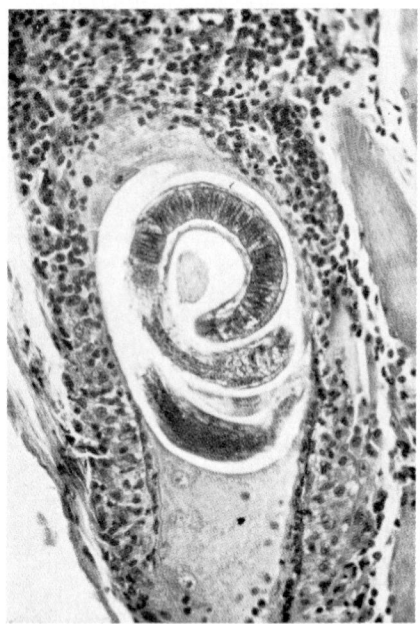

Fig. 98-5. Section of *Trichinella spiralis* in muscle.

using latex or cholesterol-lecithin particles have been evaluated and proved reliable. These latter 2 tests are available commercially, are simple to perform, and are especially suitable for the small laboratory that performs the test only occasionally. Futher details on serologic procedures are given in Chapter 100.

Precipitin tests have been made using sterile living larvae. The larvae, after being placed in contact wih *Trichinella* antibodies, develop precipitates around the oral and anal orifices. Although considered sensitive, the test would require the laboratory to maintain animals infected with *T. spiralis*, a task beyond the average laboratory.

Definitive diagnosis of trichinosis can be made by demonstration of (1) the adult in feces, (2) larvae recovered from blood, and (3) larvae seen in muscle biopsy. Demonstration of the adult is rarely accomplished and is not a profitable diagnostic endeavor, although the adult stage is the one that must be eliminated if the inevitable larviposition and subsequent damaging larval invasion are to be prevented. Occasionally larvae are found in blood smears, representing the circulatory larval phase following larviposition by the female. Larvae may be demonstrated by means of muscle biopsy in patients recovering from trichinosis. Snips of muscle removed after the third week of infection may reveal larvae on microscopic examination. The muscle tissue may be pressed between 2 slides and examined under about 100×. Typical larvae are seen in Fig. 98-4. One must ascertain that the larvae seen in the muscle are not encysted; this would represent an old infection and not one of recent origin. In stained sections of muscle containing *T. spiralis* the inflammatory response will suggest whether the infection is recent (Fig. 98-5). A more sensitive method of revealing larvae is to digest the muscle in 1% pepsin and HCl at 37 C for about 1 hour and then to examine the sediment for motile larvae freed from their encysted states. Although more sensitive, this method does not differentiate between an old and recent infection.

Trichuris trichiura

Geographic distribution. *T. trichiura* has a cosmopolitan distribution but is more abundant in warm, moist climates.

Life cycle—epidemiology. The adult worms of *T. trichiura*, commonly called whipworms, live in the large intestine of humans. Some authorities believe that whipworms found in primates and pigs are the same species that affect humans. The female worms give off undeveloped eggs that pass in the feces. With proper moisture, shade, and temperature the eggs become infectious in 3-6 weeks. Humans become infected by ingesting the egg. Once ingested the eggs hatch, liberating larvae that may invade the intestinal villi for a few days but eventually find their way to the cecum and develop into adults in

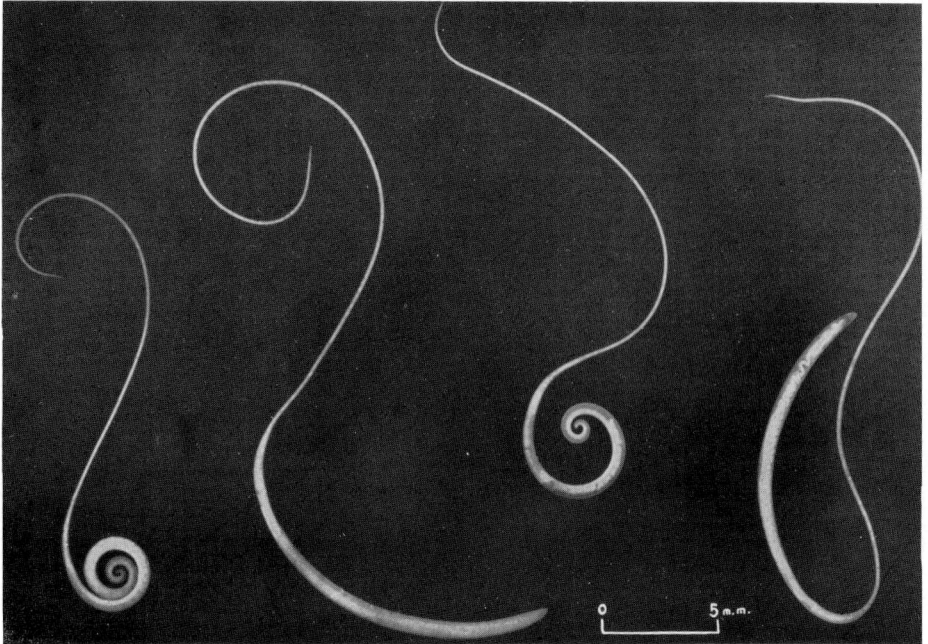

Fig. 98-6. *Trichuris trichiura.* Photograph of male and female. Millimeter scale. (Original of Kourí.)

about 3 months. The adult worm may live several years.

The adult worm embeds its threadlike anterior portion in the mucosa. The extent of damage is usually dependent on the number of worms present. Light infection may cause only vague abdominal pain and gastric disturbances. Heavier infections may result in marked inflammation of the colon, perhaps appendicitis, bloody diarrhea, anemia, loss of weight, and prolapse of the rectum. Jung and Beaver have pointed out that frequently *Trichuris* and *Entamoeba histolytica* are found in the same person, and one must ascertain which, if not both, are responsible for the diarrhea, and other symptoms.

Trichuris infections have been termed "dooryard" infections because in many rural areas infections are maintained by children defecating around the door, under the house, or in the yard. A focus of infection builds up in the area where the children play, and opportunities for infection occur as the children play in the dirt or perhaps contaminate food in the household. However, infection is not restricted to children, since adults may be infected by ingestion of contaminated dirt or food. Although transmitted by the same method, *Ascaris* infections will occur in areas where *Trichuris* is not common. This is probably because the eggs of *Ascaris* are considerably hardier and survive under more adverse conditions. However, in areas especially suitable for *Trichuris* egg development *Trichuris* infections tend to be heavier because *Ascaris* adults live only about 9 months, whereas *Trichuris* adults live for years, thus tending to build up in numbers upon reinfection.

Morphology. Adult worms (Fig. 98-6) are easily recognized by their characteristic whiplike shape. In both sexes the main body of the worm is relatively thick and tapers into a threadlike anterior end. The male is recognized by the characteristic curled posterior end. Various reproductive and digestive structures may be seen within the worms. The brown-stained egg (Fig. 98-3) measures about 22 × 50 μm and is barrel shaped, possessing pluglike elements at the 2 poles.

Diagnosis. Laboratory diagnosis is based on identification of the characteristic egg in the feces (Fig. 98-3). Either simple saline smears or concentration of feces may be done to demonstrate the eggs. Concentration procedures such as zinc sulfate flotation and ether sedimentation may be performed. Usually a heavy infection will be easily picked up by a simple smear examination, whereas light infections may be missed.

Capillaria infections of humans

Capillaria species are closely related to *Trichuris* and exhibit similar morphology in adult and egg stages. *C. hepatica* is a tissue parasite in the liver of rats, other rodents, and occasionally other mammals. Eggs, measuring 51-67 × 30-35 μm, have a velvety outer shell perforated with minute pores. The eggs are deposited and retained in the liver until the infected animal is eaten by a predator or scavenger. The eggs are liberated by host digestion and are passed in the feces. In the soil the eggs develop to the infective stage and are capable of infecting a susceptible host when ingested. Less than a dozen authentic cases have been reported in humans. The clinical picture resembles that of visceral larva migrans. Occasionally a person develops a spurious infection by ingesting cooked liver from infected animals. This results in eggs being passed in the feces but does not result in active infection. Normally diagnosis is made by liver biopsy.

In northern Luzon in the Philippines a newly discovered species of *Capillaria, C. philippinensis*, causes epidemic severe, often fatal, spruelike diarrheal disease. The infection apparently is acquired by eating small uncooked fish. Apparently the infection is intensified via internal autoinfection, which results in large numbers of adults and larvae in the intestinal mucosa. Diagnosis is made by finding eggs (45×21 μm), adult or larval stages, in the feces.

Strongyloides stercoralis

Geographic distribution. The distribution is cosmopolitan but spotty. Heaviest prevalence occurs in tropical and subtropical countries where warmth and moisture favor growth.

Life cycle—epidemiology. *S. stercoralis* is an amazingly versatile parasite. The adult females penetrate deeply into the mucosa at all levels of the intestine, favoring perhaps the mucosa of the duodenum and upper jejunum. Apparently the males are not tissue parasites and are passed in the feces a few weeks after reaching adulthood. In any event the male is not necessary for fertilization as the female is parthogenetic. Within the intestinal tissues the female gives off eggs that hatch in the tissues, releasing rhabditiform larvae that find their way into the lumen and pass in the feces.

The larvae at this point may evolve through an indirect cycle, more common in the tropics where environmental conditions are more likely to be favorable, or the larvae may evolve through a direct cycle, more common in the temperate zones. In the indirect cycle the rhabditiform larvae, after several molts, develop into free-living male and female adults in about 36 hours. They mate, and the female gives off eggs that hatch, releasing rhabditiform larvae. The free-living cycle may continue indefinitely, or at some point, usually after the first free-living generation, the rhabditiform larvae, instead of developing into free-living adults, become infective filariform larvae. The filariform larvae penetrate the skin of humans, find their way into the circulation, and are carried to the lungs, where they break out of the pulmonary capillaries into the alveoli. After several days of development the worms travel up the respiratory tract to the epiglottis and are swallowed. The worms mature into adults in about 28 days.

In the direct cycle of development, more common in the temperate zone, the rhabditiform larvae develop directly into infective filariform larvae, omitting the free-living generation(s).

The parasite can also perpetuate itself by means of autoinfection or hyperinfection. Larvae entrapped in fecal debris at the perianal region develop into filariform larvae and infect the individual without ever technically leaving the host. Apparently it is also possible in some cases for rhabditiform larvae to develop to the filariform stage unusually fast and to penetrate the intestinal wall without ever leaving the host. Also apparently larvae may be trapped in alveoli, where they develop into adults, and produce offspring that may reach the filariform stage. In still another variation rhabditiform larvae may penetrate the intestines of extremely debilitated patients instead of passing with the feces. The ability to autoinfect makes *Strongyloides* potentially a very dangerous parasite in that individuals may acquire heavy, debilitating infections without reexposure to an outside source of infection. Recently a severe, sometimes fatal strongyloidiasis has been described in patients receiving immunosuppressive or cytotoxic drugs. Apparently depression of the immune response triggers autoinfection with potentially disastrous results. All patients scheduled to receive drugs that compromise the immune system should be examined for *Strongyloides* before beginning treatment with immunosuppressives.

Cases of strongyloidiasis occur sporadically in the United States. It may reach epidemic proportions in some closed communities, especially among mentally retarded patients.

Although cats and dogs are infected with an apparently identical species, they are not thought to be important as reservoirs. Apparently the parasite develops best in saturated topsoil in warm subtropic or tropic areas. Environmental conditions combined with improper disposal of feces are responsible for perpetuation of *Strongyloides*. However, once infected an individual may remain infected for years because of the parasite's potential for autoinfection.

Larval penetration may result in erythema, edema, hemorrhagic papules, possible secondary bacterial infection, and in general a condition that resembles "ground itch" caused by hookworms. Urticarial wheals may develop at the site of larval penetration. As the larvae migrate through the lungs, small areas of hemorrhage and inflammation develop. In some cases the host reaction may trap larvae, which then may develop to adults in the lung. Often the adult females in the intestines may cause chronic inflammation with variable gastric symptoms. Light infections frequently cause no intestinal symptoms, whereas moderate infections cause diarrhea alternating with constipation. Heavy infections, probably the result of autoinfection, may cause diarrhea and thin, watery stools containing an excess of mucus. Persistent eosinophilia, usually 8-15% but occasionally 40% or more, and sharp pains in the pit of the stomach often occur in infected individuals.

For a recent review of the clinical manifestations of strongyloidiasis, roentgenographic features, and differential diagnostic problems consult Berkman and Rabinowitz.[1]

Morphology. The eggs of *S. stercoralis* usually hatch before reaching the lumen of the intestine. Occasionally eggs are observed after purgation or severe dysentery or duodenal aspiration. They resemble hookworm eggs but are smaller and contain motile larvae. The adult stages of *Strongyloides* are shown in Fig. 98-7. The parasitic female (Fig. 98-7, *A*) measures about 2 mm in length, is translucent, and possesses a long cylindrical esophagus. The free-living male and female (Fig. 98-7, *B* and *C*) measure about 0.7 mm and 1 mm respectively and resemble typical free-living nematodes. The rhabditiform larva (Fig. 98-7, *D*), usually 200-300 μm long, has a relatively short buccal cavity and a conspicuous genital primordium halfway down the intestines. The filariform larva (Fig. 98-7, *E*). measures about 550 μm in length and possesses a characteristic cleft at the tip of the tail, sometimes referred to as the caudal notch.

Diagnosis. Laboratory diagnosis is usually based on demonstrating the rhabditiform larvae in fecal smears. *Strongyloides* rhabditiform larvae may be recognized by the relatively short buccal cavity (Figs. 98-7, *D*, and 98-8, *A*) and relatively large genital primordium. Occasionally other larval nematodes may be found in fecal specimens. If feces has been held several hours before examination, hookworm and *Trichostrongylus* species eggs (limited primarily to Asia and U.S.S.R.) may hatch, liberating larvae resembling *Strongyloides*. Also occasionally free-living larvae are found in fecal specimens. These forms usually are ingested and pass through the intestinal tract quickly, not causing infection. Fig. 98-8 indicates differential characteristics of larvae found in feces. Hookworm larvae have a relatively long buccal cavity and an inconspicuous genital primordium. *Trichostrongylus* larvae have a noticeable dorsal bend just prior to the anal opening and a minute bulbar swelling at the tip of the posterior end. Free-living *Rhabditis* larvae usually have a characteristic mid-esophageal bulb.

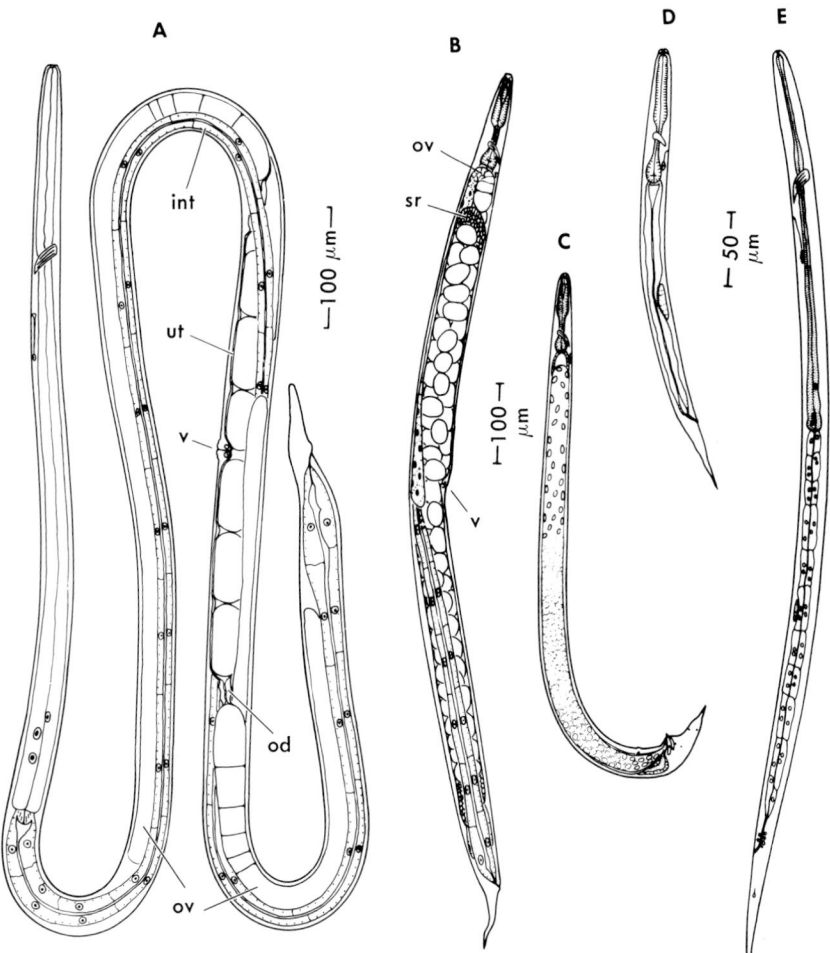

Fig. 98-7. *Strongyloides stercoralis.* **A,** Parasitic female. **B,** Free-living female. **C,** Free-living male. **D,** First-stage (rhabditiform) larva from fresh fecal specimen. **E,** Third-stage (filariform) larva. *Int,* intestine; *od,* oviduct; *ov,* ovary; *sr,* seminal receptacle; *ut,* uterus containing eggs; *v,* vulva. (Camera lucida drawings courtesy Dr. M. D. Little and Journal of Parasitology.)

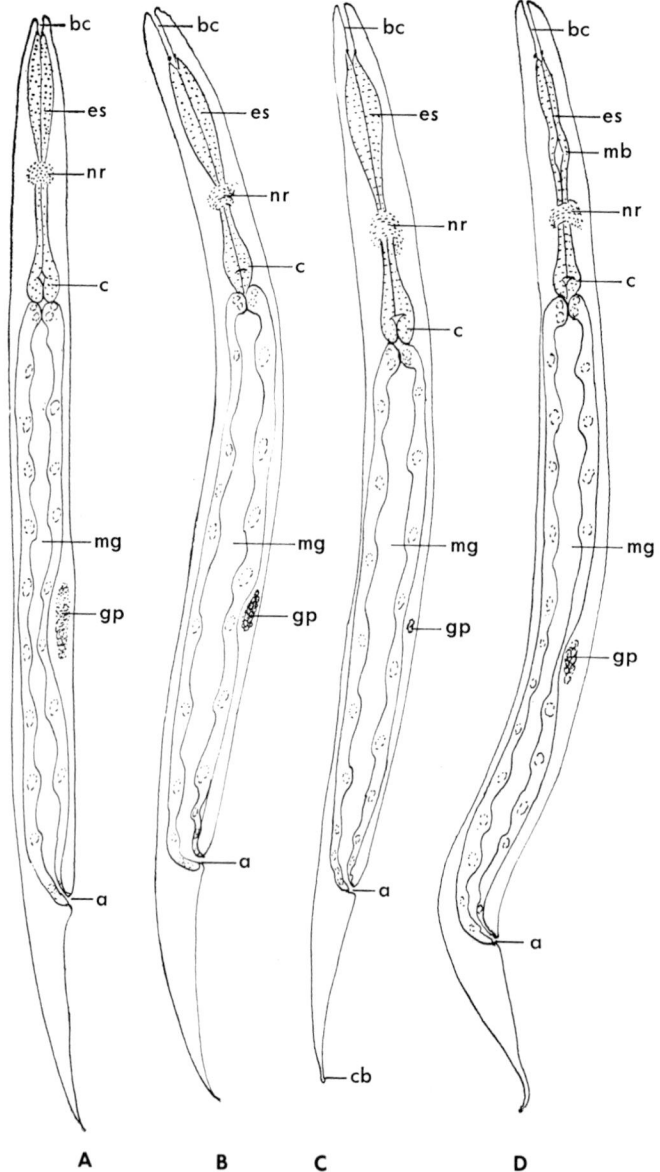

Fig. 98-8. Diagram of rhabditiform larval stages of, **A,** *Strongyloides,* **B,** hookworms, **C,** *Trichostrongylus,* and, **D,** *Rhabditis. a,* Anus; *bc,* buccal chamber; *c,* cardiac bulb; *be,* beadlike swelling of caudal tip; *es,* esophagus; *gp,* germinal primordia; *mb,* midesophageal bulb; *mg,* midgut. (From Faust, E. C., and Russell, P. F.: Craig and Faust's clinical parasitology, Philadelphia, 1957, Lea & Febiger.)

Culture of feces by the Harada-Mori filter-paper technic (Chapter 100) often detects infections missed by simple fecal examinations. Also this technic enables the laboratory worker to better differentiate *Strongyloides* from other nematode larvae found in feces.

Many times larvae can be demonstrated in duodenal aspirates after unsuccessful attempts to demonstrate larvae in the feces. Investigators differ in their opinions of the relative efficiency of the 2 procedures. If strongyloidiasis is suspected, it would be wise to utilize both procedures in attempts to confirm the diagnosis.

Aspirates can be obtained by intubation or by use of duodenal capsule technics (Entero-Test) available commercially.

Ancylostoma duodenale and Necator americanus

Geographic distribution. *A. duodenale* and *N. americanus* are the 2 important species of **hookworms** found in humans. The life cycle and epidemiology of these 2 species are almost identical. *A. duodenale* is found most extensively in southern Europe, the north coast of Africa, northern India, north China, and Japan. Scat-

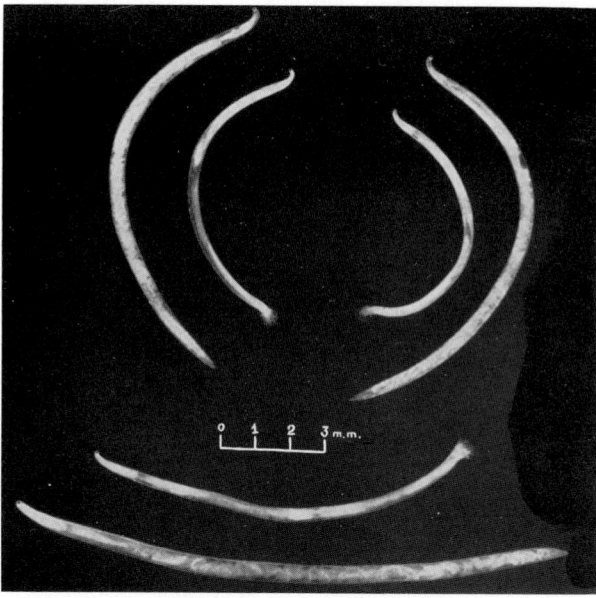

Fig. 98-9. *Necator* and *Ancylostoma.* Top, *Necator americanus,* male and female (2 pairs); bottom, *Ancylostoma duodenale,* male and female (1 pair). Millimeter scale. (Original of Kourí.)

tered foci occur in other countries, probably as a result of migration of infected persons. In the Western Hemisphere the parasite is found in parts of Brazil, Chile, Paraguay, and Peru. *N. americanus* predominates in the Western Hemisphere, central and south Africa, southern Asia, Melanesia, and Polynesia. A third hookworm species, *Ancylostoma ceylanicum,* occurs in humans throughout Southeast Asia. Foci exist in Brazil and India. Morphologic features of adult worms of this species are described by Yoshida.[2]

Life cycle—epidemiology. The adult worms live in the small intestines, attached to the intestinal mucosa. The female gives off eggs in the 2-8 cell stage, which pass in the feces. Under favorable conditions the eggs develop rapidly and hatch in 1-2 days, liberating rhabditiform larvae. The larvae feed on bacteria and organic debris and undergo 2 developmental molts before becoming nonfeeding infective filariform larvae. The filariform larvae usually remain encased in the cuticle following the second molt. The larvae infect humans by penetrating the skin, usually bare feet. The larvae migrate to the bloodstream and are carried to the lungs, where they break out of the capillaries into the air sacs. They then migrate up the respiratory tract to the epiglottis; they are swallowed and undergo 2 additional molts before maturing into adults in the small intestines in about 6 weeks. However, the larvae of *A. duodenale* may be ingested and may develop into adults without migrating from the intestines. The majority of adults live less than 1 year but may live several years in some cases.

The pattern of acquisition of hookworm infection varies considerably. Usually a source of infective filariform larvae is built up in shady moist areas as the result of repeated promiscuous defecation. Persons, usually barefooted, become infected when walking over areas containing the larvae. Infections have also resulted from use of feces as fertilizer, contact with soiled laundry after allowing time for filariform larvae to develop, and many other ways. On occasion domestic animals may ingest human feces and redeposit it in places people are more likely to frequent.

The highest prevalence of hookworm is found in warm tropical areas, primarily because hookworm larvae require a large amount of moisture during development and cannot survive freezing temperatures.

Larval penetration may cause a dermatitis or "ground itch" complicated by secondary bacterial infections. Larval migration through the circulatory system and respiratory tract usually causes little significant host response unless the infection is heavy. Repeated infections may cause a host immune response capable of walling off larvae in various tissues. Eosinophilia and leukocytosis may result form larval entrapment and subsequent destruction.

The severe effects of hookworm infection result from the adults' attachment to the villi and ingestion of blood. The worms may move from one site to another, leaving behind a bleeding lesion. The extent of damage caused by the adults depends on the number of worms and the ability of the host to compensate for the blood loss. One worm may remove 0.5 ml or more of blood per day. Heavy infections plus poor diet can result in marked anemia and physical debilitation.

Morphology. Fig. 98-9 indicates the size and form of *A. duodenale* and *N. americanus.* Fig.

Table 98-1. Characteristics of human adult hookworms

	Necator americanus	*Ancylostoma duodenale*	*Ancylostoma ceylanicum*
Length (mm)			
Female	9-11	10-13	10.5 ± 0.82
Male	7-9	8-11	8.1 ± 0.33
Buccal capsule	1 Pair of ventral cutting plates	2 Pairs of ventrally curved teeth	2 Pairs of ventral teeth
Vulva	Anterior half of body	Posterior half of body	Posterior half of body
Bursa	Broader than long, split dorsal rays, lateral rays unequally distributed	Long and wide, single dorsal ray, lateral rays equally distributed	Small bursa, externodorsal rays short and stout, lateral rays longest toward ventral rays
Shape	Head strongly curved and hooked in appearance	Head lacking, hook appearance	Same as *A. duodenale*

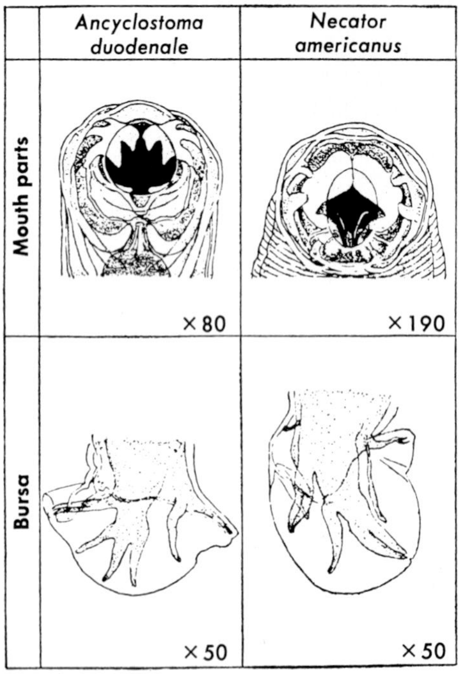

Fig. 98-10. Mouth parts and bursae of hookworms of humans. (Redrawn from Looss, 1911; from Belding, D. L.: Textbook of parasitology, ed. 3, New York, 1965, Appleton-Century-Crofts.)

98-9 presents the salient morphologic features used to identify *A. duodenale* and *N. americanus*. Table 98-1 summarizes differential characteristics of the human hookworms. *A. duodenale* adults are grayish white, slightly curved, and 8-13 mm long, depending on the sex. The mouth or buccal capsule is well developed and contains 2 pairs of ventrally located teeth (Fig. 98-10). The males have a characteristic broad bursa with a single dorsal ray and 3 equal length lateral rays. In the female the vulva is located just posterior to the middle of the worm. *Necator* adults are smaller than *Ancylostoma*, and the heads are curved to form a hooklike silhouette. The buccal capsule is provided with inconspicu-

ous cutting plates instead of teeth (Fig. 98-10). The male bursa is long and wide with a characteristic ray arrangement. In the female the vulva is situated in the anterior portion of the worm.

The rhabditiform larvae have been described and discussed under the section dealing with *Strongyloides*. As shown in Fig. 98-9 the buccal cavity of the hookworm larva is relatively long, and the genital primordium is inconspicuous.

The characteristic egg of the hookworm (Fig. 98-3) measures about 60×38 μm in *Ancylostoma* and 70×38 μm in *Necator*, but they cannot be differentiated. The eggs are in the 4-cell stage when passed and develop no further until exposed to air.

Diagnosis. Laboratory diagnosis is based on finding the characteristic egg (Fig. 98-3) in feces. Species differentiation is not possible by egg characteristics. Differentiation of species may be made by studying adult worms passed in the feces either naturally or after treatment or by identification of larvae from Harada-Mori fecal cultures (see Chapter 100). Differential characteristics of human hookworms are summarized in Table 98-1.

Simple fecal smears will usually uncover hookworm cases of clinical significance. Light infections are often missed by simple fecal smears but can usually be demonstrated by flotation or sedimentation procedures. However, light infections are not usually serious clinical problems.

The number of eggs being passed in a given unit of feces can be quantitatively determined by utilization of the Stoll technic or Beaver technic. These are not diagnostic procedures but technics to determine the number of eggs being passed. With knowledge of the approximate number of eggs given off per female worm per day the worm burden can be approximated. At times this is useful information, since the worm burden is directly related to the severity of hookworm infection.

Ancylostoma braziliense and Ancylostoma caninum

These 2 parasites are normal hookworm parasites of cats and dogs and undergo life cycles in

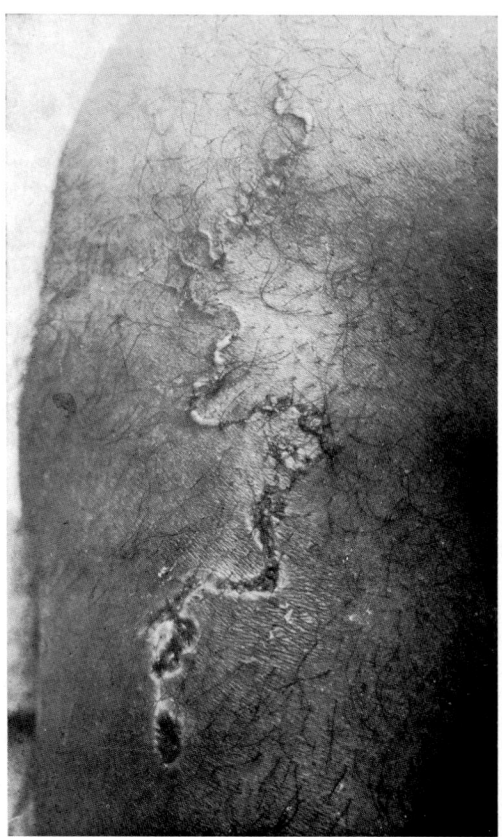

Fig. 98-11. Clinical case of larva migrans studied by Dr. Kouri. Lesions on internal surface of right leg and knee.

these animals similar to that described in humans. However, the filariform larvae of these 2 species, especially *A. braziliense*, will penetrate the skin of humans. Because persons are abnormal hosts, the larvae rarely go further than just beneath the skin. The larvae may tunnel underneath the skin, causing erythematous, raised, and vesicular lesions, often secondarily infected with bacteria (Fig. 98-11). This condition has been clinically termed **creeping eruption** or **cutaneous larval migrans.** The larvae may persist in the skin for weeks, the severity of the infection dependent on the number of larvae present.

Most cases have been reported along the Gulf of Mexico and coastal areas of the United States. However, isolated cases have been reported in the northern United States.

Diagnosis is based on clinical appearance. There are no laboratory diagnostic procedures.

Trichostrongylus species

An estimated 5.5 million people, almost exclusively natives of Asia and the U.S.S.R., harbor *Trichostrongylus* parasites. Several species, *T. colubriformis, T. probolurus, T. vitrinus, T. orientalis,* and others, have been described in humans. The species normally parasitize cattle, sheep, camels, and other animals. The eggs (Fig. 98-3) resemble those of the hookworm but are usually longer (70-90 × 40-50 μm) and have more pointed ends.

Infection is acquired via ingestion of filariform larvae. The larvae attach to the mucosa and develop into adults without any extraintestinal migration. Infection with these species is usually not serious unless large numbers of worms are present. The worms are difficult to remove with standard anthelmintics. Failure to distinguish between *Trichostrongylus* and hookworms has led to conflicting reports on efficiency of therapy.

Angiostrongylus cantonensis

In humans the worm *Angiostrongylus cantonensis* may provoke eosinophilic meningoencephalitis. Humans acquire the infection by eating certain invertebrates (slugs, snails) that contain the infective larvae. Several species of rats serve as normal definitive hosts and harbor the adult worms primarily in the pulmonary arterioles. Eggs are laid, which develop and hatch in small blood vessels. The larvae escape by breaking out of the blood vessels, migrating up the respiratory tract, and passing in the feces. The larvae develop to the infective stage in slugs, land snails, and land planarians. The rat completes the cycle by eating the infected invertebrate host. The larvae mature in the pulmonary arteries and veins and in the blood vessels of the central nervous system. Experimentally infected rats tolerate a small number of worms, but heavy infections often prove fatal.

Humans are abnormal hosts and acquire the infection in those countries where the attraction of raw invertebrates as a delicacy coincides with the zoonotic rat-parasite-slug cycle. In humans the larvae and young adult fail to complete the normal cycle, dying in the brain, meninges, or spinal cord. To date human cases have been reported or suspected in Thailand, Cambodia, Vietnam, Indonesia, Taiwan, Tahiti, Hawaii, Marshall Islands, and possibly other Pacific islands. The disease is characterized by headache, stiffness of back and neck, and CNS symptoms. Pleocytosis with a high eosinophilia count is common. At present there is no method of demonstrating the parasite except at autopsy. Skin tests show some promise as a diagnostic tool. Recently the IHA test was found to be of value.[3]

Another species of *Angiostrongylus, A. costaricenis,* has been described in Central America. The worms have been found in the sections of intestinal walls removed from preschool children with acute abdominal symptoms.

Enterobius vermicularis

Geographic distribution. *E. vermicularis,* commonly called pinworm or seatworm, has a cosmopolitan distribution.

Life cycle—epidemiology. The adult worms live at all levels of the large intestine. The gravid female migrates out of the anus, usually at night, and lays eggs on the perianal and perineal skin.

The female may die at this point or may retreat back into the anus to return another night. The eggs, infectious within a few hours after being deposited, may be transferred back to the host by hand-to-mouth transfer or they may spread to bed clothing and linen and be picked up by other persons. Once ingested the eggs hatch, liberating larvae that eventually reach the large intestine and mature to adults in about 1-2 months. The adults live about 2 months.

Poor personal hygiene is responsible for spread of pinworms, especially among small children. However, spread of eggs to clothing, linen, and even dust will often provide a source of infection for the entire family. Pinworm infection may cause loss of sleep and anal pruritus due to adult migrations. Occasionally adult worms may migrate into the vagina, fallopian tubes, or peritoneal cavity, where they die and become encapsulated.

Morphology. The adult male measures 2-5 mm and the female 8-13 mm. Characteristic size and shape of adults may be seen in Figs. 98-12 and 98-13. The adult worm has a prominent esophageal bulb and anteriorly located cuticular blisters that are characteristic of the species.

The egg (Fig. 98-3) measures about 55 × 25 μm, is flattened on one side, and contains a motile larva.

Diagnosis. Laboratory diagnosis is usually based on finding the characteristic egg (Fig. 98-3) in swabs or scrapings made from the perianal region. This material should be obtained either late at night or on arising in the morning before bathing or defecation. Because of the egg-laying habits of the female, eggs are seldom found in fecal smears made from stool samples.

The cellophane tape technic is considered the best diagnostic procedure. Examination of several perianal impression smears over several days should be done before a negative diagnosis is made. See Chapter 100 for details of the procedure.

Ascaris lumbricoides

Geographic distribution. *A. lumbricoides* has a cosmopolitan distribution.

Life cycle—epidemiology. The adults live in the small intestine. Eggs in the 1-cell stage are passed in the feces and must undergo development in shady, moist soil for about 3 weeks before becoming infectious. The infectious eggs

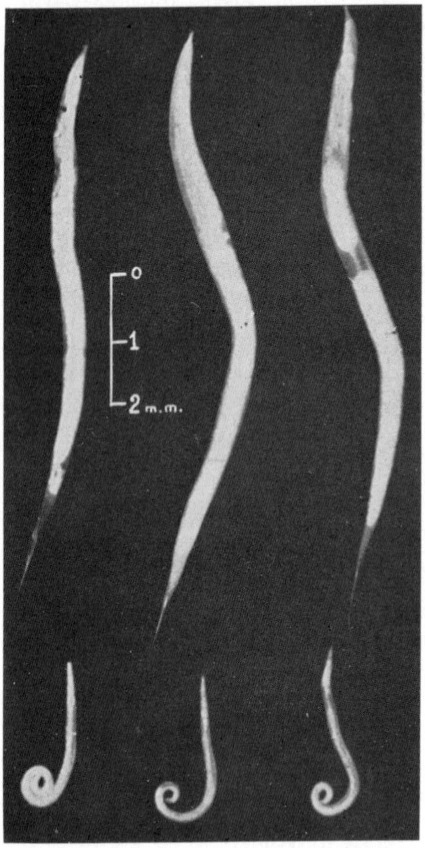

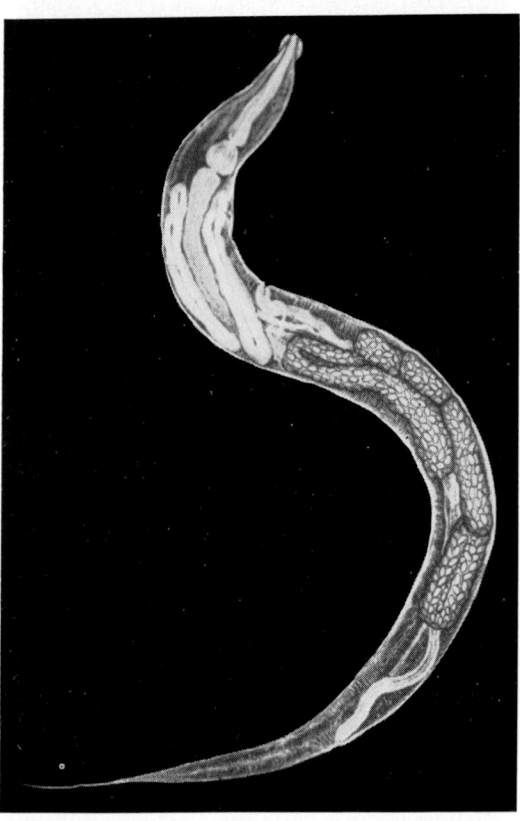

Fig. 98-12. *Enterobius vermicularis.* Top, 3 females, showing characteristic fine, long tail; bottom, 3 males, much smaller, with posterior extremity coiled upward. (Original of Kourí and Basnuevo.)

Fig. 98-13. *Enterobius vermicularis.* Pregravid female parasite. Observe cuticular cervical expansions, muscular esophagus, with its 2 portions, intestine, ovaries, uterus, vulva, and anus. (Original of Kourí and Basnuevo.)

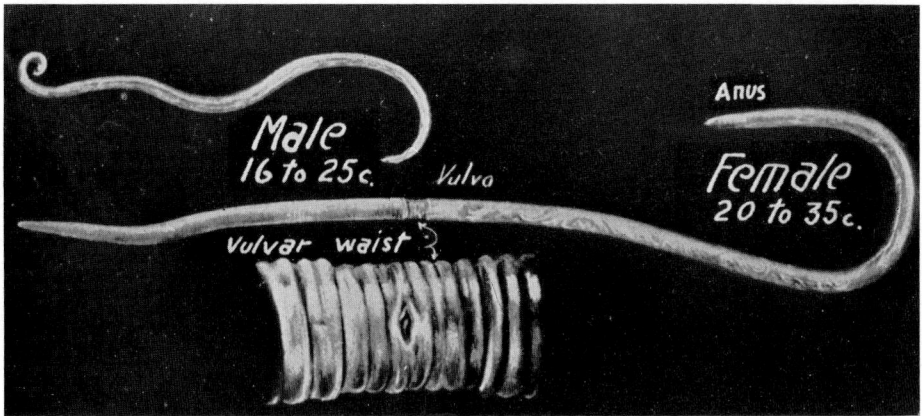

Fig. 98-14. Male and female *Ascaris lumbricoides*, natural size. Vulvar waist magnified. (Original of Kourí.)

are ingested and hatch in the small intestine. The liberated larvae penetrate the intestinal wall, reach the circulatory system, and are carried to the lungs. After about 2 weeks of development in the lungs the larvae break out into the air sacs and travel up the respiratory tree to be swallowed. The larvae mature to adults in about 2 months and have a life span of less than 1 year.

The pattern of infection for *Ascaris* is similar to that described for *Trichuris*. The greatest number of infections occurs in children. The eggs of *Ascaris* are resistant to external conditions and have survived as long as 6 years in experimental patches of ground.

Ascaris infections are usually well tolerated. During migration through the lungs the larvae may provoke inflammatory responses that give rise to *Ascaris* pneumonitis. The cardinal symptoms are dyspnea, cough, rales, transient eosinophilia, and pulmonary infiltration. These symptoms disappear within a week or two as the larvae leave the lungs and migrate to the intestines. The adults may cause vague abdominal pains. Large numbers of adults may cause intestinal obstructions. Occasionally adults will undertake potentially dangerous migration, especially if irritated by some ingested substance or inadequate treatment. Cases of worms migrating up the bile duct, pancreatic duct, or respiratory tract or perforating the intestines have been recorded.

Morphology. The adults are a dull cream color. The females (Fig. 98-14) measure 20-35 cm, whereas males measure 16-25 cm in length. The cuticle is finely striated and to the inexperienced observer may appear to be segmented. The mouth (Fig. 98-15) has 3 lips, 1 dorsal and 2 latero-ventral.

The fertile eggs vary in size from 45-75 × 35-50 μm. As shown in Fig. 98-3, the typical egg is 1 celled and thick shelled. The exterior is rough and mammillated in appearance, although sometimes the rough exterior is missing (Fig. 98-3). Infertile eggs (Fig. 98-3) are usually considerably longer than fertile eggs, lack interior cellular differentiation, and many vary in appearance.

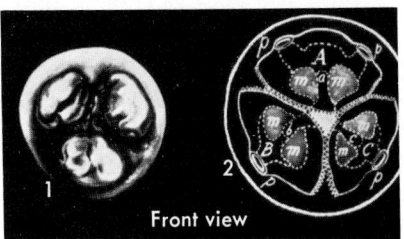

Fig. 98-15. *Ascaris lumbricoides.* Anterior extremity showing mouth with 3 lips. (**2,** Gruart's sketch; other drawing after Kourí.)

Diagnosis. Laboratory diagnosis is based on finding typical eggs (Fig. 98-3) in the feces. Fertile eggs are characteristic, but infertile eggs are often incorrectly identified or missed altogether. Some evidence has been presented that many *Ascaris* infections in urban areas are missed because infections are so light that fertilization does not occur and only hard-to-identify infertile eggs are passed in the feces. Fertile eggs are readily concentrated by flotation technics. The opposite is true of infertile eggs.

Visceral larva migrans

Visceral larva migrans is caused most frequently by nematode larvae migrating through extraintestinal viscera of various animals, causing granulomatous lesions. This condition has been recognized as a distinct disease entity since 1952. Almost all cases have been described in the United States in children.

Visceral larva migrans results when parasites of other animals infect humans and utilize them as a transport (paratenic) host. When the final (predator) host ingests tissues of the transport host that contain larvae, then the larvae develop into adults in the intestines. *Toxocara canis* and *T. cati*, ascarids of dogs and cats, have been definitely implicated. These parasites undergo a life cycle in dogs and cats similar to *Ascaris*, but in humans and other transport hosts the *Toxocara* larvae never complete their migratory pattern. Most often the larvae are found in the liver, but the lungs, kidney, heart, brain, and eye also have been affected. Undoubtedly other animal parasites that have an internal migratory pattern could potentially cause visceral larva migrans. Consult Beaver[4] for a detailed account of larva migrans.

Symptoms vary, depending on the location of the parasite. Characteristically a persistent eosinophilia, enlarged liver, bronchial asthma, and a history of eating dirt are usually present.

There is no reliable laboratory diagnostic procedure other than liver biopsy and identification of the larva in liver section. Nichols[5,6] presented an excellent experimental study of problems and criteria utilized in the identification of larva in tissue sections of animals infected with *Toxocara* larvae and other larval species. See also Chitwood and Lichtenfels[7] for an excellent reference on identification of helminths in tissue sections. Serologic tests are available but are not considered reliable. Recent information on serology is summarized in Table 100-5.

Wuchereria bancrofti

Geographic distribution. W. *bancrofti*, or Bancroft's filariasis, occurs in a large number of subtropical and tropical countries. It is found primarily along coastal areas of countries with a long hot season and high humidity. The most highly endemic areas are the Samoan, Ellice, Tokelau, and Fiji islands. It is found in central Africa, Madagascar, Mediterranean Coast of Africa, Spain, Italy, Yugoslavia, Hungary, Turkey, India, Pakistan, Burma, Malaysia, Thailand, Philippines, Indonesia, China, Korea, Japan, West Indies, Central America, and northern South America.

Life cycle—epidemiology. The adult worms live in the lymph vessels and glands, the females discharging microfilariae that are enclosed in an egg membrane or sheath. The microfilariae remain in the lymph or blood circulation until ingested by certain mosquitoes. W. *bancrofti* microfilariae in most areas exhibit a nocturnal periodicity and are more prevalent in the blood circulation from 10 PM-2 AM. However, in certain South Pacific islands and the Philippines there is no periodicity. Manson-Bahr believes the nonperiodic form possesses sufficiently distinct morphologic characteristics to justify calling it a separate species, W. *pacifica*. However, other observers believe these differences are not great enough to justify such a designation.

Aedes, *Culex*, *Anopheles*, and *Mansonia* mosquitoes may serve as vectors in various geographic locations, with a *Culex* species usually being the most important. After ingestion by the mosquito the microfilaria penetrates the stomach wall and develops into a sausagelike stage. Within about 2 weeks the larva undergoes 2 molts, elongates, and migrates to the proboscis. During the mosquito's blood meal the larva

breaks free from the mosquito labium and crawls across the skin, penetrating at the bite site or other skin abrasions. The larva migrates to the lymphatic vessels, matures to an adult in about 9 months, and may live 12 years or longer.

Perpetuation of endemic wuchereriasis depends on many factors. The environment is important in determining whether larval development in the mosquito will take place. A hot humid climate, temperatures above 80 F and humidity of 90% or higher, is necessary for optimal larval development. Environments providing this temperature and humidity are limited primarily to coastal areas in the tropics and subtropics. The density of the mosquito vector and the density of the microfilariae in the blood determine to a large extent the probability of acquisition of infection.

Wuchereriasis is characterized by lymphangitis and lymphadenitis probably caused by allergic reactions to the presence of the adult worms. The male genital organs, the arms, and the legs are most often involved. Persons exposed to reinfection for many years may develop chronic inflammatory reactions that lead to lymphatic obstruction and to the grotesque cases of elephantiasis. It is erroneously thought by some that all persons with *Wuchereria* develop elephantoid appendages. Elephantiasis develops only following continued exposure to reinfection over a long time, leading to chronic allergic reactions and serious lymph obstruction. However, in many cases, even though exposed to reinfection for long periods of time, individuals never develop inflammatory reactions associated with elephantiasis.

Morphology. The adult worms are creamy white and threadlike. The male worms may measure 40 mm, whereas the female worms are longer, ranging from 80-100 mm. Two rings of small papillae are present on the slightly swollen cephalic region. On the male the ventrally curved tail may possess a maximum of 8 preanal and 4 postanal pairs of papillae. Posterior to these papillae are 2 pairs of larger papillae and 1 pair of smaller ones.

The characteristics that are useful in differentiating W. *bancrofti* microfilariae from other sheathed species are presented in Table 98-2. Fig. 98-16 illustrates the important differences diagrammatically. As seen under the microscope the microfilariae are graceful in appearance with sweeping curves. Other ensheathed species tend to be stiff in appearance with secondary kinks.

Fully developed W. *bancrofti* microfilariae, as seen in thick blood films, measure 230-296 μm in length by 7.5-10 μm in width. The tip of the head bears a spinelike stylet, and the cephalic space between the head and the beginning of the nuclei is as broad as it is long. Microfilariae, adequately stained with Giemsa or preferably hematoxylin, exhibit a nerve ring, excretory pore, excretory cell, g (genital) cells, and an anal pore that are certain percentage distances from the head.

Table 98-2. Characteristics of sheathed microfilariae found in blood

Characteristics	Wuchereria bancrofti	Brugia malayi	Loa loa
Periodicity	Usually nocturnal	Nocturnal, but not absolute	Diurnal
Appearance	Graceful, flowing curves	Irregular curves with secondary kinks	Irregular curves with secondary kinks
Length	230-296 μm, average 260	177-260 μm, average 220	250-300 μm, average 275
Anterior stylets	1	2	1
Cephalic space	As broad as long	Twice as long as broad	As broad as long
Excretory pore	Small (29)*	Large (30)*	Large (32)*
Excretory cell	Small (31)*	Large (37)*	Large (37)*
Genital (g_1) cell	Small; uniform in size; g_1 (70)*	Larger; g_1 (68)*	Larger; g_1 (69)*
Anal pore	(82.5)*	(82.3)*	(82)*
Tail	Terminal nuclei absent; tapers to point	2 terminal nuclei present and elongate	Nuclei all the way to tip

*( ), percentage distance from anterior end.

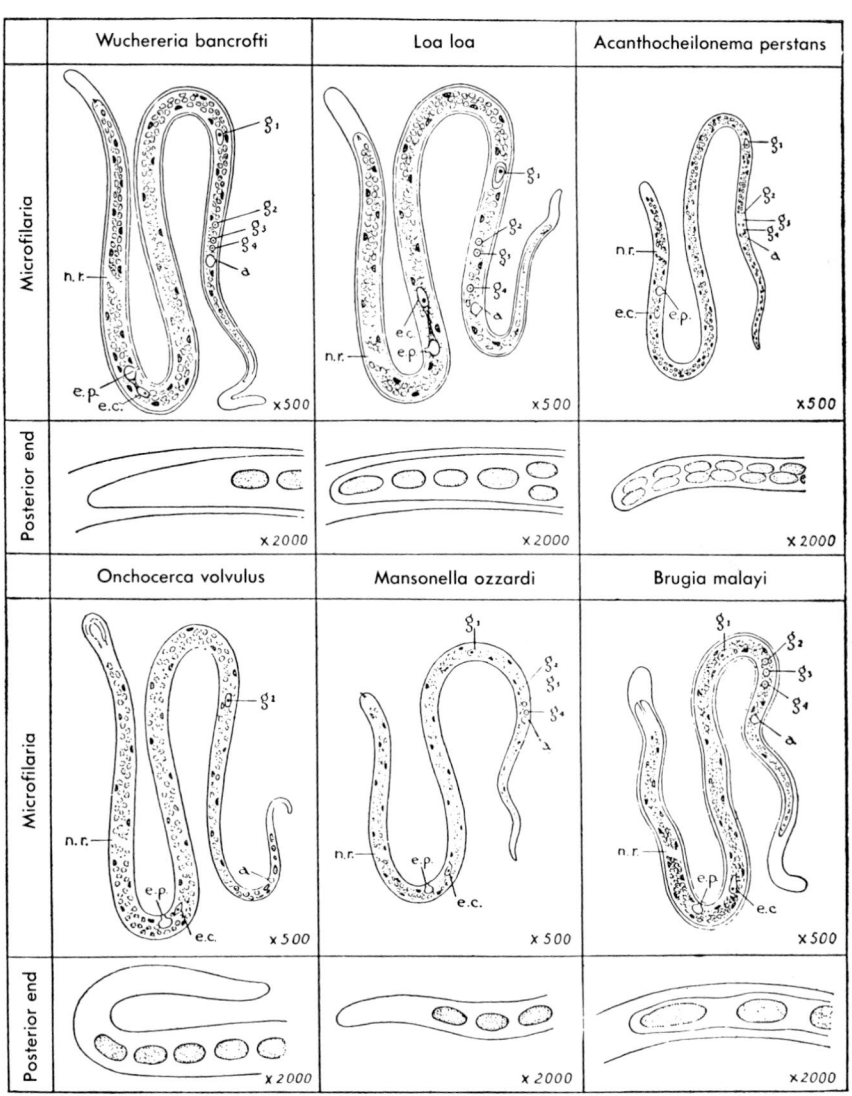

Fig. 98-16. Microfilariae of humans. *a,* Anal pore (tail spot); *e.c.,* excretory cell; *e.p.,* excretory pore; g_1-g_4 first, second, third, and fourth genital cells; *n.r.,* nerve ring. (From Belding, D. L.: Textbook of clinical parasitology, New York, 1952, Appleton-Century-Crofts.)

Table 98-3. Key for identifying the most common microfilariae of humans

		3′. Body nuclei or somatic cells do not extend to tip of tail; cephalic space equal to diameter of head; noctural periodicity (or nonperiodic?)	*Wuchereria bancrofti*
	3. Sheathed	3″. Nuclei extend in broken row to tip of tail; cephalic space twice diameter of head; nocturnal periodicity	*Brugia malayi*
1. Microfilariae in peripheral blood		3‴. Nuclei extend in continuous row to tip of tail; diurnal periodicity	*Loa loa*
		4′. Nuclei extend to tip of tail; frequently in double row	*Acanthocheilonema perstans*
	4. Unsheathed	4″. Nuclei do not extend to tip of tail	*Mansonella ozzardi*
2. Microfilariae of skin and subcutaneous tissues		2′. Nuclei do not extend to tip of tail; head enlarged; curved tail	*Onchocerca volvulus*
		2″. Body nuclei or somatic cells extend to tip of tail; curved tail	*Dipetalonema streptocerca*

These differences, summarized in Table 98-2, are useful in separating the sheathed microfilariae from one another because they are constant for the species. The last 5% of the microfilaria is devoid of nuclei, a point important in distinguishing this species from *B. malayi* and *Loa loa.*

Diagnosis. Definitive diagnosis rests on demonstration of microfilariae in the blood. In early clinical cases microfilariae can usually be demonstrated in peripheral blood from 10 PM-2 AM in the periodic type or all 24 hours in the nonperiodic type. In patients with elephantiasis frequently microfilariae cannot be demonstrated.

Thick blood smears stained with Giemsa or preferably Delafield hematoxylin are recommended for routine demonstration and identification of microfilariae. Occasionally airborne spores of saprophytic fungi such as *Helicosporium lumbricoides* may accidentally contaminate blood films and may be confused with microfilariae.[8] In cases in which microfilariae are few, the Knott[9] concentration procedure or microfilter technic[10] may be utilized to advantage. Table 98-3 presents in key form features useful in identifying microfilariae.

Serologic tests are not as reliable as might be expected because of unavailability of a specific antigen. Antigens used in complement fixation tests and skin tests are prepared from *Dirofilaria immitis*, the dog heart worm. The antigen is group specific and will react with antibodies directed toward other filarial infections. The group-specific nature of the antigen probably accounts for the observed false-positive skin test reactions, since persons in endemic areas are exposed to nonhuman filarial forms as well as to *Wuchereria*. Skin tests may be positive in old cases that are no longer active. Complement fixation tests are useful in differentiating these cases because

usually complement-fixing antibodies are present only in active cases.

Although biopsy of lymph node material to demonstrate adult worms is possible, it is not recommended, since the procedure may precipitate further lymphatic obstruction.

Brugia malayi (formerly Wuchereria)

Geographic distribution. *B. malayi*, or Brug filariasis, is found in the Philippines, Malaysia, India, Vietnam, Sumatra, Celebes, Borneo, New Guinea, Ceylon, China, Korea, Japan, and Indonesia. In some localities its distribution overlaps with that of *W. bancrofti.*

Life cycle—epidemiology. The life cycle of this form is essentially the same as that described for *W. bancrofti.* The primary mosquito vectors are species of *Mansonia* and *Anopheles*, with the former genus the more important. The microfilariae have a nocturnal periodicity, a peak being reached at 4 AM. However, the periodicity is only partial, since microfilariae may be found in the blood most of the day, unlike *W. bancrofti.* The effects of this parasite on the host are similar to those caused by *W. bancrofti.* Characteristically it affects the legs, and there is rarely any genital involvement.

Morphology. The adult worms have an appearance similar to those of *W. bancrofti.* The adult male measures 22-23 mm in length, and the posterior portion undergoes about 3 complete loops, unlike *W. bancrofti.* One large pair of papillae is present just in front of the cloaca and 1 pair behind. Two smaller pairs are nearby. The female measures about 55 mm in length. The vulva is 0.92 mm from the anterior end and the anal pore 0.94 mm from the posterior end. The ensheathed microfilariae of *B. malayi* (Fig. 98-14) measure 177-230 μm in length. They may be distinguished from *W. bancrofti* microfilariae

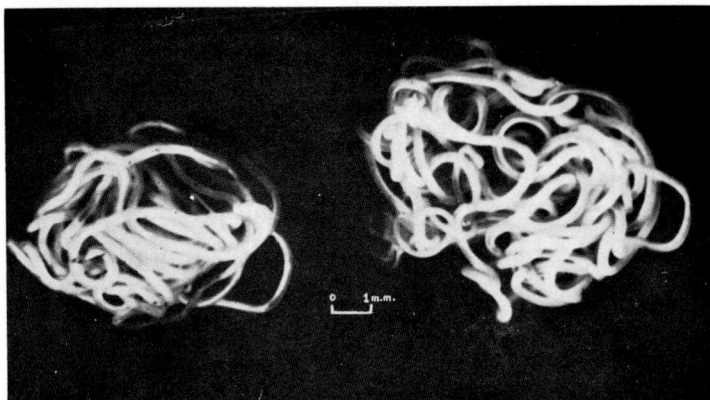

Fig. 98-17. *Onchocerca volvulus.* Enlargement of bundles of *Onchocerca volvulus.* (Original of Kourí.)

by the presence of 2 discrete nuclei at the tip of the tail and a cephalic space twice as long as broad. Usually *B. malayi* microfilariae are stiff appearance with secondary kinks. The location of the excretory cell relative to the excretory pore and the relative location of the genital cells are characters of some value in identification. Table 98-2 indicates characteristics utilized to identify this species. Fig. 98-16 illustrates useful morphologic features.

Diagnosis. Specific diagnosis depends on demonstration of the characteristic microfilariae. A peak microfilaremia usually occurs around 4 AM, but *B. malayi* is less periodic than *W. bancrofti.* Methods for laboratory diagnosis are the same as those described for *W. bancrofti.* Features useful in identifying microfilariae are presented in key form in Table 98-3.

Onchocerca volvulus

Geographic distribution. In the Western Hemisphere onchocerciasis, the blinding filariasis, is confined chiefly to Central America and Mexico in areas having elevations between 70-135 m. Coffee plantations in Guatemala and the southern states of Mexico are the main endemic centers, although cases have been reported in other areas of Latin America. In Africa onchocerciasis has been reported in Sierra Leone, Liberia, Ghana (Gold Coast), Chad, Central African Republic, Congo, and Gabon (these 4 formerly French Equatorial Africa), The Congo, Sudan, eastern Tanzania (Tanganyika), Uganda, Nigeria, Kenya, and other areas.

Life cycle—epidemiology. The adults are usually located in tumorlike nodules in the subcutaneous tissue. The microfilariae given off by the female are usually found in the nodule, in the dermis, and in the tissues of the eye. A fly belonging to the genus *Simulium* ingests the microfilariae while feeding on a human. After ingestion the microfilariae migrate into the thoracic muscles, undergo 2 molts, and then migrate to the labium and are ready to infect a human when the *Simulium* fly (black gnat) takes another blood

meal. The larvae require at least 6 days for development in the fly before becoming infective. The larval forms leave the fly and apparently enter a person through the bite site made by the fly and develop into adults in the subcutaneous tissue. A host reaction eventually walls off the worms in a tumorlike cyst, although some worms may remain free in the tissues.

Infections with *O. volvulus* give rise to painless nodules containing adult worms. The nodules may be found any where on the body, but in the Western Hemisphere head nodules predominate. Various types of dermatitis, rash, and skin involvement also may occur. The most serious consequence of infection, especially in Guatemala, is ocular damage resulting from microfilariae invasion of the eye and the resultant host inflammatory response to their presence. Partial loss of vision or even blindness may result.

Morphology. The adult worms, as seen in excised nodules, are tightly coiled, the males measuring 19-42 mm and the females, 33-50 mm in length. Fig. 98-17 portrays 2 masses of worms freed from the tumor by artificial digestion.

The microfilariae (Fig. 98-16) are 221-350 μm long and 5-9 μm wide. The anterior and posterior ends of the microfilariae contain no nuclei. The tip of the tail is sharply pointed.

Diagnosis. Definitive laboratory diagnosis may be made by microscopic examination of skin biopsy material for microfilariae or by excision of nodules and demonstration of adult worms and microfilariae. Skin biopsies are usually made by scraping epidermis from the shoulder region or the ear and making a saline mount. Under the microscope microfilariae may be seen struggling out of the epidermis mounted in saline. Skin biopsy is the method of choice because of the ease with which it may be performed. The stained microfilaria has no nuclei at the tip of the tail, a pointed tail, and a strong affinity for methylene blue. Although the nodule may be removed and examined for the presence of the adult worm and microfilariae, this procedure is usually associated with treatment and control aspects and less with laboratory diagnosis. Table 98-3 presents in key form characteristics useful in differentiating the microfilariae.

In certain parts of Africa another species of microfilariae, *Dipetalonema streptocerca*, may be found in skin biopsies and must be differentiated from *O. volvulus*. *D. streptocerca* microfilariae measure 180-240 μm in length and have nuclei to the tip of the tail, a blunt tail, and little affinity for methylene blue.

Loa loa

This parasite is restricted to Africa, being especially prevalent in west and central Africa. Its distribution may overlap that of *Wuchereria bancrofti*. The males measure 30-34 mm and the females measure 50-70 mm in length and live in subcutaneous tissues. The microfilariae, found in blood primarily during the day light hours, must be ingested and undergo development in the intermediate host, certain species of flies belonging to the genus *Chrysops*, before becoming infective for humans. In humans the migration of adult worms may provoke temporary inflammation and Calabar swellings. Not infrequently worms may be seen migrating across the eye, causing considerable inflammation in the process. Laboratory diagnosis is based on finding characteristic ensheathed larvae in the blood. The nuclei extend to the tip of the tail. The microfilariae have an affinity for methylene blue (*Wuchereria* does not). Characteristics useful in identification are summarized in Tables 98-2 and 98-3 and are illustrated in Fig. 98-16.

Acanthocheilonema perstans

A. Perstans, or *Dipetalonema perstans*, is distributed throughout tropical Africa, South America, and New Guinea. Its distribution may overlap that of *Wuchereria bancrofti* and requires differentiation from the latter. The adult worms, 45-80 mm in length, live in the peritoneal cavity, pleural cavity, pericardium, mesenteries, or retroperitoneal tissues and usually cause little if any damage to the host. However, recent workers described several patients that were incapacitated while infected with this worm. The nonperiodic microfilariae are found in the blood. The vectors are various species of *Culicoides*. The characteristics useful in identifying *A. perstans* microfilaria are summarized in Table 98-3 and are illustrated in Fig. 98-16. The unsheathed microfilariae measure about 200 μm in length, and the nuclei extend to the tip of the tail.

Mansonella ozzardi

This parasite has been reported only in the Western Hemisphere. The parasite is present in the West Indies, Panama, Yucatan, the Guianas, Colombia, Venezuela, and Argentina. The adult female worm measures 65-81 mm in length. A complete male has never been described. The adults live in the mesenteries and visceral fat and cause little if any host reaction. The unsheathed

microfilariae are found in the blood, measuring about 200 μm in length. Various species of *Culicoides* serve as the vectors. Laboratory diagnosis is based on identification of the unsheathed microfilariae in stained blood films. The tail is pointed and contains no nuclei at the tip. See Table 98-3 and Fig. 98-16 for additional features.

Dracunculus medinensis

Geographic distribution. *D. medinensis*, the guinea worm, serpent worm, or dragon worm, is found in the Nile Valley, central equatorial Africa, and northern and western coasts of Africa. In Asia the worm is reported in Arabia, Persia, Afghanistan, Turkestan, Pakistan, extensive areas of India, U.S.S.R., and New Guinea. In North America *Dracunculus*, possibly a different species, has been found in fur-bearing animals.

Life cycle—epidemiology. The adults develop in the body cavity and connective tissue. When sexually mature, about 9-12 months after infection, the female migrates to the subcutaneous tissues and surfaces of the body that come in contact with water frequently (i.e., the arms and legs). As the worm approaches the skin surface it apparently secretes a toxic substance that causes a blister formation that ulcerates to the outside on contact with water. On contact with water the anterior end of the worm uterus ruptures, releasing motile larvae into the water. The extrusion of larvae may occur over time as the ulcer is reexposed to water until all the larvae are released. The larvae are ingested by a freshwater crustacean, *Cyclops* species, and undergo development for 2 or 3 weeks. Humans are infected by ingesting *Cyclops* containing infective larvae. The larvae after ingestion penetrate the intestines and mature to adults in the body cavity and connective tissue.

Where dracontiasis is endemic, the drinking water of the populace usually contains many *Cyclops*, the intermediate host. Also the water supply is usually designed so that persons actually have contact with the water to obtain a supply, thus affording opportunity for larvae to be liberated from the ulcer.

Infection may cause some allergic reactions, but secondary bacterial infection is probably the most dangerous consequence. Usually the infection is not noticed by the host until the female worm approaches the surface of the skin.

Morphology. The adult female measures 500-1200 mm in length. The seldom-recovered male measures 45 mm or less. The vermiform larva measures 500-750 μm in length and possesses a long, filiform tail with conspicuous striations.

Diagnosis. Diagnosis is based on appearance of the primary blister and subsequent ulcer formation revealing the presence of the female worm.

PHYLUM PLATYHELMINTHES— CLASS CESTOIDEA

The helminths belonging to the class Cestoidea are commonly referred to as cestodes or **tape-**

worms. All the tapeworms of humans require an intermediate host, with the exception of *Hymenolepis nana*. The tapeworms are ribbon shaped, segmented, lack a digestive tract, and are hermaphroditic. Electron microscope studies of the main body of tapeworms have revealed that villi-like structures make up the body surface. It is thought that these structures function somewhat like the villi in the human intestines, especially in absorption of carbohydrates from the host intestinal tract. Restriction of host intake of carbohydrate adversely affects the adult worm, causing a reduction in glycogen content, stunting of growth, or eventually causing the worm to be unable to persist. However, similar restriction of host intake of protein has no effect on the worm. This suggests that the worm absorbs its protein requirements from the intestinal mucosa.

The tapeworms parasitizing humans are classified either in order Pseudophyllidea or order Cyclophyllidea on the basis of distinct morphologic and life cycle differences. The tapeworms of humans may be classified into order and genera as indicated below.

Class **Cestoidea**
Order **Pseudophyllidea**
   Genus *Diphyllobothrium*
Order **Cyclophyllidea**
   Genus *Hymenolepis*
   Genus *Taenia*
   Genus *Echinococcus*
   Genus *Dipylidium*

Morphology (general). The adult tapeworm may vary in size from 3 mm-10 m, depending on the species. However, all tapeworms are composed of 3 fairly distinct regions: (1) the **scolex,** (2) the **neck,** and (3) **strobila** or chain of segments (proglottids). The scolex or head of the tapeworm (Fig. 98-18) is adapted for attaching to the intestinal wall. The scolex of cyclophyllidean tapeworms is somewhat oval, has suckers that aid in attachment, and may or may not have a rostellum armed with hooks. The scolex of pseudophyllid-

ean tapeworms *(D. latum)* has no suckers but is modified into a spoon-shaped structure (Fig. 98-33) with a dorsal and a ventral groove. Immediately behind the scolex is a neck region composed largely of germinal tissue that gives rise to the proglottids. As the proglottids are budded off the posterior end of the neck, they are pushed posteriorly, gradually developing from immature to mature and finally to gravid proglottids. The immature proglottids are sexually undeveloped and possess no definitive structures of note. The sexually mature proglottids possess the organs of both sexes (Fig. 98-18). The arrangement of the sexual organs is characteristic in each species and often is useful in identification. The sexual organs of the gravid proglottids have atrophied, and much of the space within each segment is occupied by the egg-filled uterus. Species of *Diphyllobothrium* possess a uterine pore; eggs are extruded through it and pass in the fecal stream. The uterine pore is lacking in the other tapeworms of humans, and the eggs escape only as the gravid proglottids break off from the strobila or degenerate, releasing the eggs.

There is considerable group variation in morphology of the larval tapeworms. The various stages such as cysticercus larva, cysticercoid larva, hydatid cyst, etc. are illustrated in Fig. 98-19. The ciliated coracidium of pseudophyllidean tapeworms *(D. latum)* breaks out of the egg after a period of development. The coracidium is ingested by the first intermediate host, certain freshwater crustacea, loses its cilia, and evolves into an elongate procercoid larva with a posterior spherical appendage containing embryonal hooklets. The procercoid larva develops into a solid, wormlike plerocercoid larva if ingested by appropriate species of fish.

The egg of the cyclophyllidean tapeworm is fully developed on passage in the feces and contains an oncosphere or hexacanth larva possessing 6 hooklets. The morphologic features of the egg are discussed under each species. The onco-

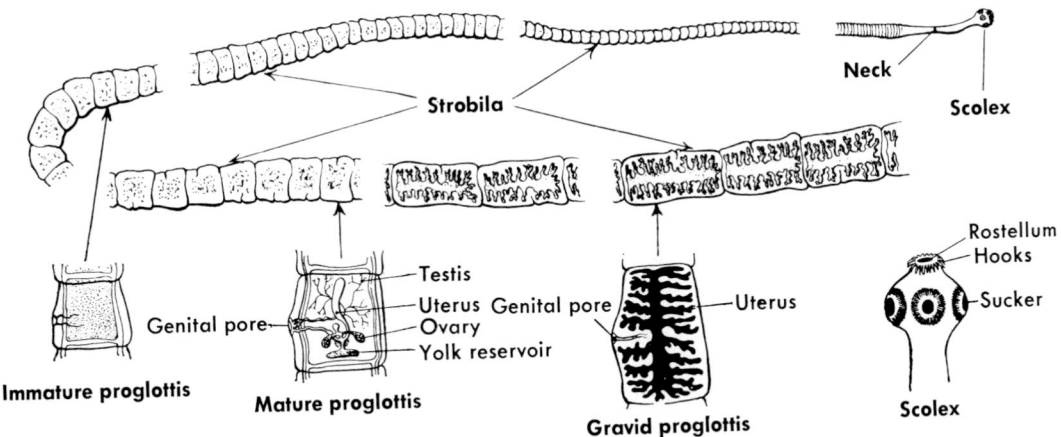

Fig. 98-18. Morphologic features of tapeworm. (From Medical protozoology and helminthology, Bethesda, Md., 1955, United States Naval Medical School, National Naval Medical Center.)

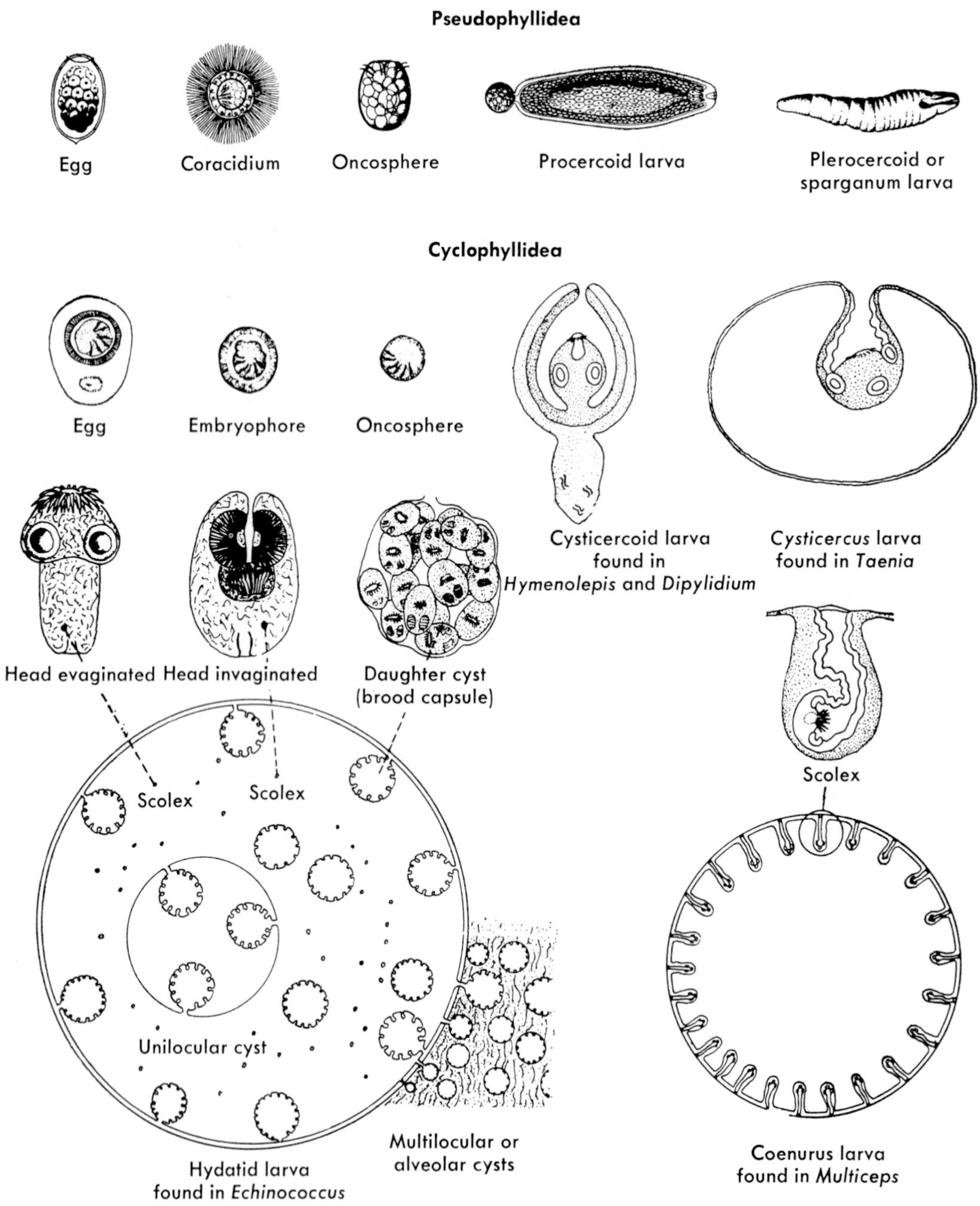

Pseudophyllidea

Egg · Coracidium · Oncosphere · Procercoid larva · Plerocercoid or sparganum larva

Cyclophyllidea

Egg · Embryophore · Oncosphere

Cysticercoid larva found in *Hymenolepis* and *Dipylidium*

Cysticercus larva found in *Taenia*

Head evaginated · Head invaginated · Daughter cyst (brood capsule)

Scolex · Scolex

Scolex

Unilocular cyst

Multilocular or alveolar cysts

Hydatid larva found in *Echinococcus*

Coenurus larva found in *Multiceps*

Fig. 98-19. Immature stages of human tapeworms. (From Medical protozoology and helminthology, Bethesda, Md., 1955, United States Naval Medical School, National Medical Center.)

sphere may develop into 1 of several larval forms, depending on the species. The oncosphere of *Hymenolepis* or *Dipylidium* develops into a cysticercoid larva that possesses an invaginated scolex and a solid tail. The oncospheres of *Taenia* develop into cysticercus larvae, each possessing an inverted scolex enclosed in a relatively spacious fluid-containing bladder. The oncosphere of *Echinococcus* becomes a hollow bladder called a hydatid cyst. The inner layer of the cyst consists of germinal tissue that may give rise

to brood capsules containing many invaginated scolices, each capable of developing into an adult worm in the definitive host. Other variations and structures within the hydatid cyst are discussed in more detail under *Echinococcus*. The *Multiceps* oncosphere may develop into a coenurus larva consisting of a hollow bladder lined with germinal tissue that buds off scolices. The coenurus larva occurs most frequently in sheep, rarely in humans.

Life cycle (general). Humans may be the

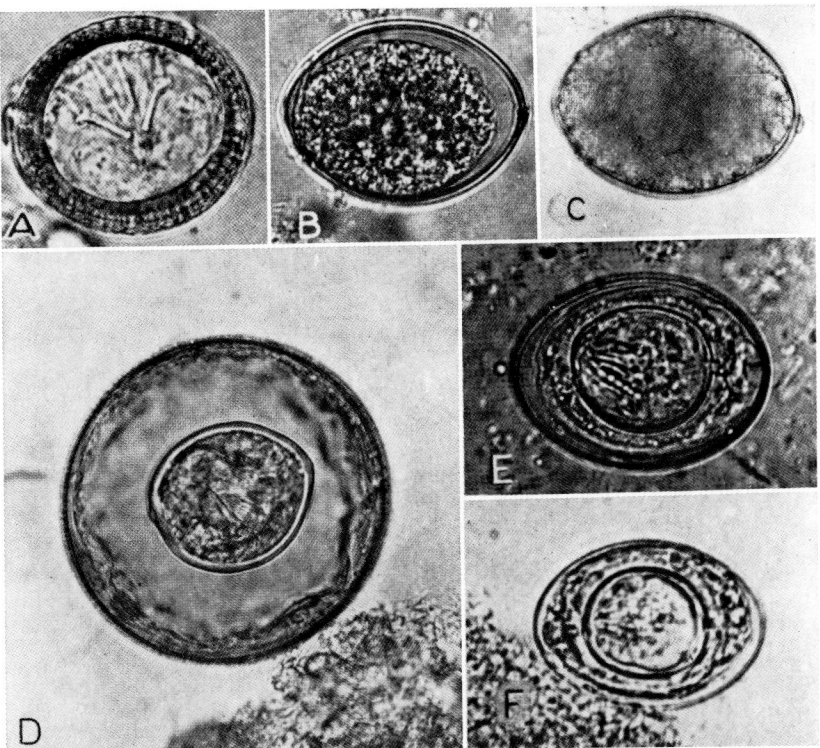

Fig. 98-20. Some cestode eggs. **A,** *Taenia* sp. (×570). **B, C,** *Diphyllobothrium latum* (×500). **D,** *Hymenolepis diminuta* (×650). **E, F,** *Hymenolepis nana* (note polar filaments) (×750). See Fig. 98-21 for objects in feces often confused with helminth eggs. (From Hunter, G. W., III, Frye, W. W., and Swartzwelder, J. C.: Manual of tropical medicine, Philadelphia, 1960, W. B. Saunders Co.)

definitive host and harbor the adult worm of *Diphyllobothrium latum, Taenia* sp., *Hymenolepis* sp., and *Dipylidium caninum.* Humans become infected with *H. nana* by ingesting the egg, whereas *H. diminuta, Taenia* sp., *D. latum,* and *D. caninum* infections are contracted by ingestion of the animal serving as the intermediate host and harboring the infective larval stage. Depending on the species of tapeworm, the intermediate host may be anything from a fish to an insect or domestic animal.

In some cases humans can serve as an intermediate host, harboring the larval stage of the parasite species. Thus humans may harbor larval stages of *Taenia solium* or *Echinococcus* species.

Laboratory diagnosis (general). Infections of *H. nana, H. diminuta,* and *D. latum* are diagnosed by identification of characteristic eggs in the feces (Fig. 98-20). The eggs of species of *Taenia* are characteristic of the genus, and species differentiation must be made on the basis of scolex and proglottid characteristics. Only the eggs of *Hymenolepis* are concentrated adequately by flotation procedures. Other cestode eggs are best concentrated by sedimentation procedures. Microscopic artifacts, pseudoparasites, etc. that might be confused with helminth eggs are shown in Fig. 98-21.

Frequently gravid proglottids are passed in the feces and may be the first overt sign of infection to the patient. Under normal conditions the gravid proglottids of *T. saginata, T. solium,* and *D. caninum* separate from the strobila and pass in the feces. They may or may not rupture or disintegrate in transit, releasing the eggs into the main fecal stream. The proglottids of these species are characteristic, and species identification can be made usually by examining the proglottids between 2 slides under a dissecting microscope. The proglottids of *T. saginata* and *D. caninum* are muscular and may migrate over the surface of the feces. Frequently *T. saginata* proglottids migrate from the anus, leaving a trail of eggs along the way. Often these eggs are detected by cellophane tape impressions of the perianal region, such as is used for *Enterobius vermicularis.* Unlike the *Taenia* species and *Dipylidium,* the gravid proglottids of *D. latum* do not normally break away from the strobila; rather, eggs are extruded periodically from the ventral uterine pore. The terminal proglottids of *D. latum* break off only as they disintegrate beyond recognition. In the case of *Hymenolepis* species the eggs are usually released by disintegration of terminal gravid proglottids. Thus the proglottids of *D. latum* and *Hymenolepis* species are not normally found in the feces unless the worm or its segments are prematurely expelled.

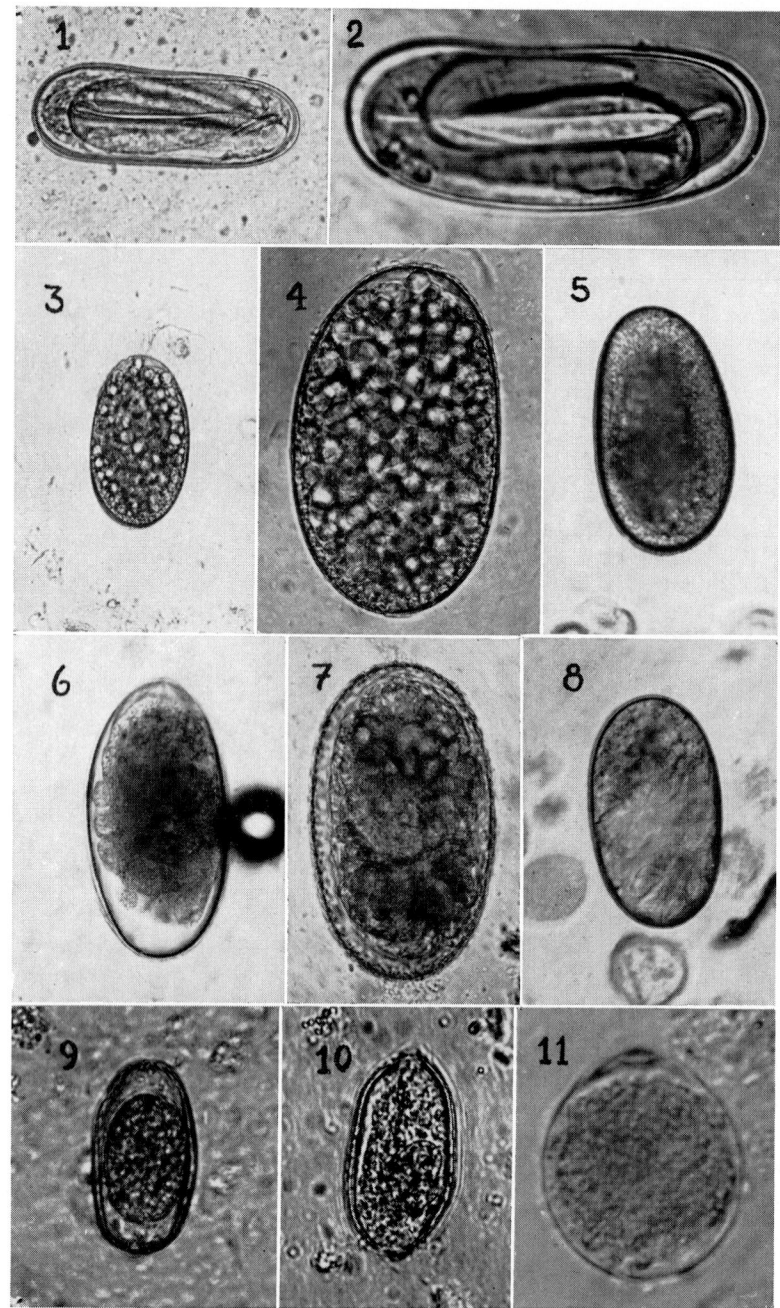

Fig. 98-21. Microscopic pseudoparasites. Eggs in transit and nonparasitic elements found frequently on microscopic examination of human feces. **1, 2,** Egg of *Heterodera radicicola*. **3-8,** Eggs of *Tyroglyphus* sp. in different stages of development. **9, 10,** Vegetable elements sometimes confused with eggs of helminths or with coccidia. **11,** Pine pollen grains, which frequently contaminate the stools. (Originals of Kourí.)

Humans may serve as the intermediate host for *Echinococcus granulosus* or *T. solium* and may harbor a somatic larval stage rather than the in testinal adult stage. In such cases no eggs or pro-glottids are passed in the feces, and diagnosis must be based on clinical, serologic, and roent-genographic evidence. Skin tests and various serologic tests (complement fixation, floccu-lation, and hemagglutination) have been used successfully for presumptive diagnosis of *E. granulosus*. Skin tests, roentgenograms, and biopsy have been used with some success for cysticercosis or larval *T. solium* of humans. See also Chapter 100.

Species of Cestoidea
Taenia saginata

Geographic distribution. *T. saginata*, the beef tapeworm, has a worldwide distribution.

Life cycle—epidemiology. The adult worm lives in the small intestine, attaching to the mucosa with its suckers. The terminal gravid proglottids break off from the main body of the worm and pass in the feces. The eggs may or may not be found in the main fecal stream, depending on whether the proglottids rupture, releasing the eggs into the fecal stream. The eggs, infectious immediately, are ingested by the intermediate host, cattle. Other animals such as buffalos and less frequently giraffes, llamas, and antelopes may serve as intermediate hosts. Sheep and goats have also served as experimental intermediate hosts. Reported cases of humans being the intermediate host are very rare. In the intermediate host the eggshell disintegrates, and the liberated oncosphere penetrates the intestinal wall and reaches the blood or lymph circulation to be filtered out in the striated muscles. Here the larva transforms into the cysticercus larva or bladder worm (Fig. 98-19) *Cysticercus bovis* and requires about 60-75 days to become infective for humans. Individuals acquire *T. saginata* infections by ingesting raw or partially cooked beef containing the cysticercus larvae. In humans the larva evaginates and develops into an adult worm in 2-3 months. The adult may persist for years.

The presence of the adult worm may cause abdominal discomfort, hunger pains, loss of weight, weakness, and infrequently nausea, vomiting, headache, and diarrhea. However, many cases are asymptomatic.

Morphology. The beef tapeworm of humans ordinarily reaches a length of 4.5-6.0 m, but worms up to 15 m have been recorded. The scolex (Fig. 98-22) measures less than 2 mm in diameter and possesses 4 round suckers situated at intervals around the head. The scolex is unarmed, containing no hooks that are typical of *T. solium* (Fig. 98-24). The scolex is followed by a short neck region about one-half as broad as the head and several times as long. The neck is followed by the progressing series of immature, mature, and gravid proglottids. The mature proglottids are broader than long and contain roughly twice the number of testes (300-400) as does *T. solium*. The gravid proglottids (Fig. 98-23) are longer than broad, measuring 5-7 mm in width and about 20 mm in length. There are 15-20 main lateral extensions on each side of a median uterus that runs the length of the proglottid. The typical *Taenia* egg (Fig. 98-20) is spherical or ovoid, measuring 31-43 μm in diameter, and cannot be distinguished from eggs of *T. solium, Multiceps,* or *Echinococcus.* The oncosphere has 6 hooklets. The outer eggshell is thick and heavily marked with radial striations.

The mature cysticerci, seen only in the intermediate host, are oval in shape, opalescent, and measure 7.5-10 mm in breadth to 4-6 mm in

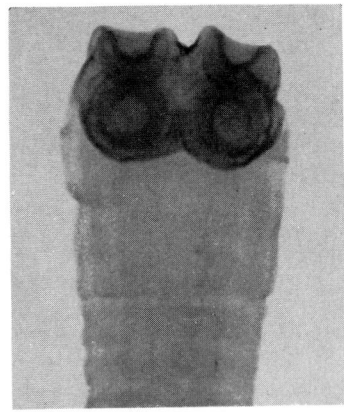

Fig. 98-22. *Taenia saginata* scolex.

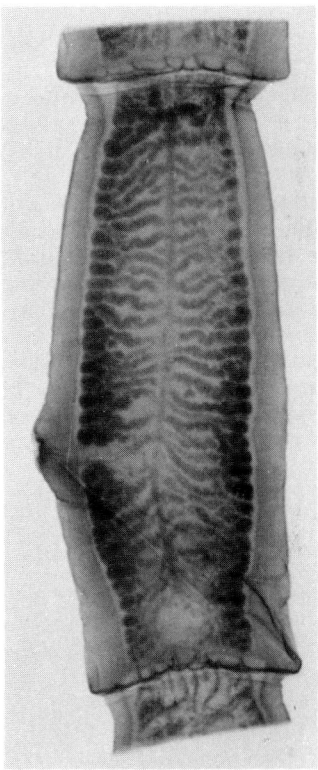

Fig. 98-23. *Taenia saginata* gravid proglottid.

length. Very few cases of infection with *C. bovis* have been reported in humans.

Diagnosis. Definitive diagnosis of *T. saginata* infections can be made on the basis of characteristic scolices or gravid proglottids (Figs. 98-22 and 98-23) in the feces. Definitive diagnosis cannot be made on the basis of eggs seen in the feces, since *T. saginata* and *T. solium* eggs are indistinguishable. However, *Taenia* eggs found on cellophane tape impressions such as used for the diagnosis of *Enterobius vermicularis* would strongly indicate a *T. saginata* infection, as the proglottid of this species is more active and more likely to migrate out the anus, leaving a trail of eggs in the perianal region.

The proglottid usually can be identified by pressing it between 2 slides and counting the number of lateral extensions of the uterus. *T. saginata* has 14-35 extensions, or branches, on each side of the uterus versus 7-16 for *T. solium*. If the number of lateral branches does not clearly indicate *T. saginata*, then the absence of a third lobe of the ovary, a cirrus pouch that does not extend to the longitudinal excretory vessel, and the presence of a vaginal sphincter are diagnostic.[11] The small scolex is difficult to find in feces. Attempts should be made to locate it, especially after treatment. Perhaps the most efficient method of searching for scolices is to emulsify the feces and filter through a sieve of fine enough mesh (30-50 mesh) to prevent passage of the scolex.

Taenia solium

Geographic distribution. *T. solium*, the pork tapeworm, is cosmopolitan to all pork-eating countries. Infection has become relatively rare in the United States.

Life cycle—epidemiology. The adult worm is found in the small intestine. The life cycle is essentially the same as described for *T. saginata*, except that pigs and rarely other mammals serve as intermediate hosts and are the source of infection for humans. One other important difference is that humans may easily serve as the intermediate host and may harbor the larval form *Cysticercus cellulosae*. This may occur if a person ingests the egg or if, as some believe, reverse peristalsis occurs in an individual harboring the adult worm and the eggs are carried back to the stomach or duodenum, affording an opportunity for them to hatch and develop into cysticerci larvae.

The adult worm may cause vague abdominal discomfort, diarrhea, constipation, loss of appetite, and weakness. In cases of cysticercosis the effects on the host depend on the location of the larvae. They are found in order of frequency in the subcutaneous tissues, eye, brain, musculature, liver, and lungs. Symptoms usually begin after the cysticerci die and there is a marked tissue reaction to their distintegration products.

Morphology. The adult pork tapeworm usually measures from 1.8 to over 6 m in length. The scolex (Fig. 98-24) is about 1 mm in diameter and has 4 suckers distributed around the head and a prominent terminal rostellum with 2 circular rows of hooklets. The scolex is followed by a short neck, which gives rise to immature, mature, and gravid proglottids. The mature proglottid is nearly square and has 150-200 testes, compared with 300-400 for *T. saginata*. The gravid proglottid (Fig. 98-25) is similar to *T. saginata* in size. There are between 7-13 (average 9) main branches on each side of the median uterus running the length of the gravid proglottids.

The egg (Fig. 98-20) cannot be distinguished from that of *T. saginata*, *Echinococcus*, or *Multiceps multiceps*. The egg is spherical, measuring 31-43 μm in diameter. The encased oncosphere has 6 hooklets, and the thick outer shell of the egg is heavily marked with radial striations.

Diagnosis. The presence of eggs in the feces denotes the presence of a *Taenia* worm. Species identification must be made on the basis of the gravid proglottid or scolex. The gravid proglottid, when pressed between 2 slides, will reveal a uterus with 7-16 (average 9) main lateral branches on each side. *T. saginata* has between 14-35 lateral branches on each side. If the number of lateral branches does not clearly indicate *T. solium*, then the presence of a third lobe of the ovary, a cirrus pouch that extends to the longitudinal excretory vessel, and the absence of

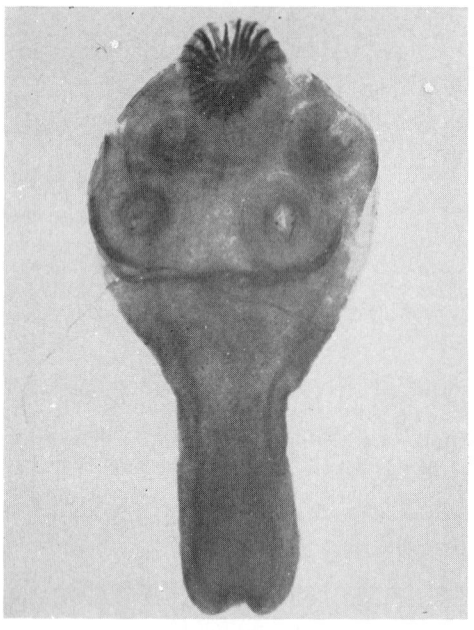

Fig. 98-24. *Taenia solium* scolex.

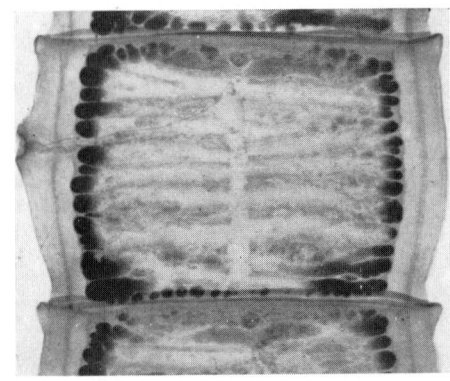

Fig. 98-25. *Taenia solium* gravid proglottid.

a vaginal sphincter are diagnostic.[11] The scolex, usually sought only to determine efficacy of treatment, may be found by passing emulsified feces through 30-50 mesh wire. The scolex will be trapped in the web of the mesh and may be identified on the basis of the armed rostellum (Fig. 98-24).

In cases of cysticercosis the larvae may be located in the musculature and central nervous system by means of roentgenograms if the larvae have calcified. In subcutaneous tissue the cysticerci often are present as characteristic nodules. Identification of the excised cystocercus is made on the basis of 2 rows of hooks. In tissue sections the cysticercus larva (Fig. 98-26) hooks and suckers may be discerned.

Skin tests and serologic tests have proved to be of limited value in the presumptive diagnosis of cysticercosis because the antigen preparations are group specific rather than species specific. The indirect hemagglutination test appears to be the most sensitive and useful test available.[12] Antigen preparations are not generally available.

Echinococcus granulosus

Geographic distribution. *E. granulosus* infection, or hydatid disease, of humans occurs most extensively in sheep-raising countries, mainly in temperate and subtropical zones. Algeria, Cape Colony, Tanzania, Israel, Syria, southern Australia, Tasmania, New Zealand,

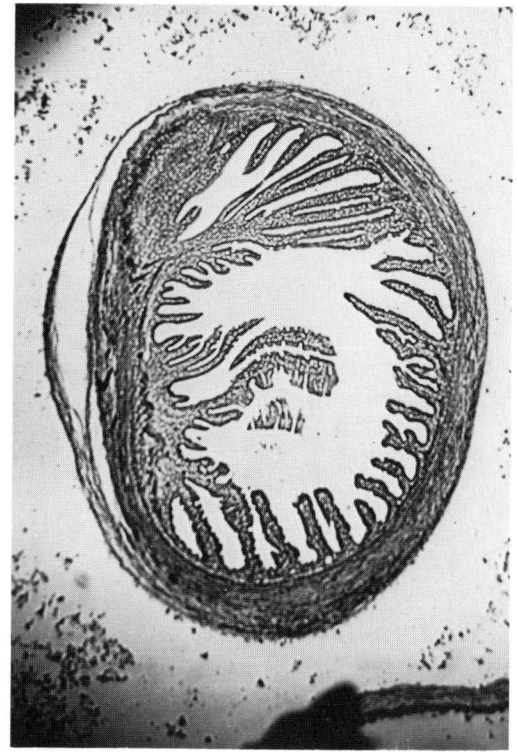

Fig. 98-26. Cross section of *Cysticercus cellulosae*, larval stage of *Taenia solium*.

central Europe, Argentina, Uruguay, and Paraguay are regions of relatively high prevalence in humans. However, the disease has been reported infrequently in persons in other countries. Most cases reported in the United States have been traced to sources outside of the country. Still, a number of cases have been reported in the Mississippi Valley area and in a few other states. Recently important endemic foci have been discovered in California, New Mexico, Arizona, Alaska, and Canada.

Life cycle—epidemiology. The adult worm resides in the small intestine of the dog. Other animals such as wolves, jackals, foxes, and cats may harbor the adult but are not thought to be of epidemiologic importance. The egg, passed in the feces, is infectious immediately and may be ingested by a number of suitable intermediate hosts. The most common are sheep, cattle, and pigs. However, in Alaska and Canada dogs and wolves become infected by eating infected moose carcasses. Humans and a wide variety of other animals may occasionally serve as an accidental intermediate host. In humans the egg hatches, liberating the oncosphere, which penetrates the intestinal wall and reaches the circulation, only to be filtered out either in the liver or lungs and infrequently in other tissues. About 70% of all human infections occur in the liver. After being filtered out, the oncosphere transforms into a hollow bladder or cyst and begins to grow. The ultimate size of the cyst is dependent on location and other not well-understood factors. The cyst, measuring 1 mm in diameter after 1 month, may eventually range from the size of an orange to that of a basketball in 10-20 years. The outside periphery of the cyst consists of a laminated, nonliving cuticle. Lining the inner surface of the cuticle is a nucleated germinal layer that buds off brood capsules, inside which a number of scolices develop. Sometimes because of pressure the mother cyst may form daughter cysts, within which brood capsules develop. During cyst development much fluid may accumulate. Free brood capsules and free scolices, collectively called hydatid sand, may be found in this fluid. Secondary formation of hydatid cysts may occur if the cyst ruptures, allowing the escape of brood capsules and scolices, all of which have the potential to form secondary hydatid cysts.

Another type of development occurs if the oncosphere settles in the bone tissue. Not being limited by a host reaction, the cyst develops along the bone canal in haphazard fashion.

The dog, the main definitive host, becomes infected by eating infected carcasses containing the hydatid cyst. Within the dog the scolices evaginate and develop into adults. Humans are never infected with the adult worm and serve only as an accidental intermediate host, harboring the cyst. Most frequently humans contract the infection from close contact with infected dogs. Many infections probably occur during childhood as a result of transferring eggs from dog fur

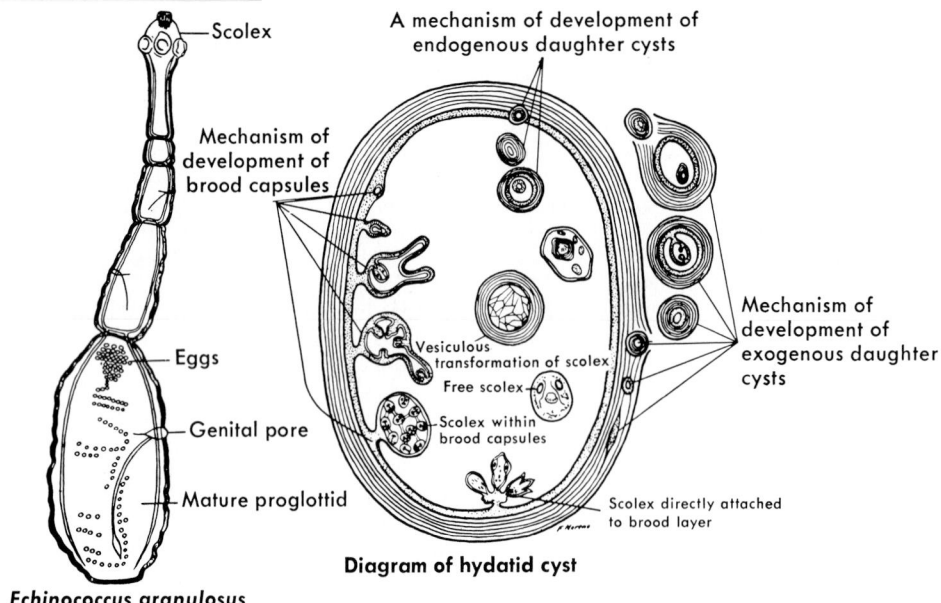

Scolex

A mechanism of development of endogenous daughter cysts

Mechanism of development of brood capsules

Eggs

Vesiculous transformation of scolex

Free scolex

Genital pore

Scolex within brood capsules

Mature proglottid

Mechanism of development of exogenous daughter cysts

Scolex directly attached to brood layer

Diagram of hydatid cyst

Echinococcus granulosus

Fig. 98-27. Schematic drawing of *Echinococcus granulosus*. Adult parasite (left) and larva in hydatid cyst (right). (According to Leuckhart; from Kourí, P., and Basnuevo, J. G.: Lecciónes de parasitología y medicina tropical, Havana, Editorial Profilaxis S.A.)

to the mouth. However, infection may occur from ingestion of food or water contaminated with dog feces containing the eggs. In Alaska and Canada the feces of infected sled dogs or wolves contaminate the snow and ground surface water that are often the only source of drinking water.

The growth of the cyst in humans may cause mechanical trauma to the adjacent tissues. Leakage of the cyst may result in secondary hydatid cysts that cause trauma in other tissues. Also, individuals may become hypersensitive to hydatid antigens, and if subsequent rupture of the cyst occurs anaphylaxis may result.

Morphology. The adult (Fig. 98-27), found primarily in dogs, is a minute worm, measuring 3-6 mm in length. The scolex, about 0.3 mm in length, has 4 suckers and is armed with 28-50 hooklets. There are only 3 proglottids, 1 immature, 1 mature, and 1 gravid. The mature proglottid contains 45-65 testes. The gravid proglottid is about one-half the total length of the worm and possesses a uterus with lateral branches containing relatively few eggs. The genital pore is located on the lateral surface about midway down the gravid segment.

The eggs, about 30-39 μm in diameter, are indistinguishable from *Taenia* eggs. The unilocular hydatid cyst of humans (Fig. 98-27) may be seen in its entirety only on surgical removal. The size varies with the age of the cyst and possible host resistance. Within fertile cysts free scolices or hydatid sand (Fig. 98-28) and brood capsules may be recovered. The scolices are invaginated and typically possess a row of hooklets.

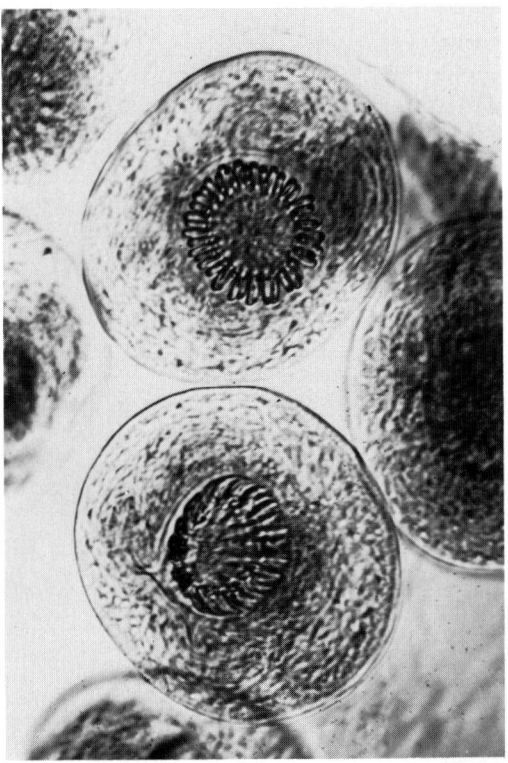

Fig. 98-28. *Echinococcus granulosus*, hydatid sand.

Diagnosis. Hydatid disease usually is not diagnosed until the cyst has reached considerable size. Symptoms may indicate a tumor. Roentgenograms may be useful for diagnosis of pulmonary cysts, osseous cysts, or calcified liver cysts. Persistent eosinophilia may or may not occur. A hydatid thrill may be demonstrable on large abdominal cysts. Although exploratory cyst puncture is possible, it is not recommended because of the danger of secondary echinococcosis and anaphylaxis caused by leakage of material from the punctured cyst.

Serologic tests have proved useful in presumptive diagnosis of hydatid disease. The merits of the skin test (Casoni test) have been reviewed by Magath.[13] The reaction to intradermal injection of the antigen occurs within 5-15 minutes. The skin test remains positive for life and is positive in 65-90% of proved cases. The Kagan et al.[14] hemagglutination test has proved slightly more sensitive than the bentonite flocculation and much more sensitive than the complement fixation test. However, the complement fixation test gave no false-positive reactions, whereas the former tests gave 10-14% false-positive reactions. Similar findings were reported by Garabedian et al.[15] Kagan et al.[16] found hydatid fluid to be a better antigen than scolices or hydatid membrane for the hemagglutination or bentonite flocculation tests. Studies by Kagan et al.[17] on the nonspecificity of serologic tests used in diagnosis of hydatid disease indicated that in slightly over 25% of persons tested cases diagnosed as liver cirrhosis, nephrosis, erythematosus, multiple myeloma, hypogammaglobulinemia, or agammaglobulinemia gave some degree of false-positive serologic reactions with hemagglutination and bentonite flocculation tests used for echinococcosis. Most of these false-positive reactions, however, could be ruled out if HA titers of 1:32 and BF titers of 1:5 or higher were reported as positive results. More recently the use of partially purified antigens has eliminated many nonspecific reactions.

Echinococcus multilocularis

Geographic distribution. *E. multilocularis*, the causative agent of alveolar hydatid disease, occurs most frequently in south central Europe and U.S.S.R. Cases have been reported in Alaska, South America, Australia, New Zealand, and other locations.

Life cycle—epidemiology. The life cycle is essentially the same as that of *E. granulosus*, except that the fox is the most important definitive host and dogs, wolves, and cats are of secondary importance. The natural intermediate hosts are field mice and various other small mammals. Humans are accidentally infected on ingestion of contaminated soil, vegetables, or fruits. In humans the oncosphere does not develop into a typical unilocular hydatid cyst. The larva, usually found in the liver, forms a spongelike slow-growing mass of small cysts that proliferate by budding. The alveolar cyst was at one time thought to be a variant of *E. granulosus*, but recent work has established *E. multilocularis* as a separate species, with the adult worm possessing distinct morphologic characteristics.

Morphology. The adult worm, found in foxes, dogs, and cats, ranges in size from 1.2-3.7 mm. There are usually 4 proglottids, the 2 mature proglottids containing 17-26 testes each. The gravid proglottid is shorter than the rest of the strobila, and the uterus is wide and without lateral branches. The genital opening is located near the middle in the gravid segment. The egg is a typical *Taenia* type and cannot be identified as to species. The alveolar cyst has an ill-defined border, irregular cavities with thin and crumpled membranes. Few brood capsules and scolices are seen, and these are usually seen in the vesicles.

Diagnosis. Frequently diagnosis is not made until autopsy. Diagnosis may be established by histologic examination of liver biopsy material for germinal tissue, scolices, or brood capsules. Serologic tests and skin tests utilized for unilocular hydatid cysts may be done, but their reliability has yet to be ascertained, although work by Kagan et al.[16] indicates potential usefulness.

Hymenolepsis nana

Geographic distribution. *H. nana*, the dwarf tapeworm, has a cosmopolitan distribution. It occurs most frequently in temperate and tropical climates.

Life cycle—epidemiology. The adult worm is attached to the mucosa of the small intestines. Usually the terminal gravid proglottids degenerate while still attached to the worm, releasing the eggs to pass in the feces. The egg, infectious immediately, is ingested by a human host and hatches, releasing an oncosphere that penetrates into an intestinal villus and develops into a cysticercoid larva. After about 4 days the larva returns to the lumen and matures into an adult in 2-3 weeks. The adult worm probably has a life span of only a few months.

There is some evidence that autoinfection may occur (i.e., eggs hatch before leaving the body), especially if the host's resistance is lowered by concurrent infections. Humans may also be infected from strains of *H. nana* parasitizing mice and rats. Under experimental conditions certain species of beetles and fleas may serve as intermediate hosts. On ingestion of the egg by these insects the oncosphere develops into a cysticercoid larva. Rodents and possibly humans could become infected by ingestion of the infected beetle. However, this mode of transmission is probably not important.

Infections in humans are usually mild, but toxic symptoms, abdominal pains, diarrhea, convulsions, and insomnia may occur. Symptoms are more severe in small children and in persons harboring large numbers of worms. Infections are more common in children.

Morphology. The adult worm (Fig. 98-29) is relatively small, measuring 25-45 mm in length. The scolex has 4 suckers and a short rostellum armed with 20-30 hooks. The rostellum may be invaginated into the tip of the scolex. The egg (Fig. 98-20) is ovoid and is 30-47 μm in diameter. The egg contains an oncosphere with 3 pairs of hooklets. The oncosphere is enclosed in an envelope, and threadlike filaments may be seen trailing off the slightly thickened poles.

Diagnosis. Diagnosis is based on finding the characteristic egg (Fig. 98-20) in feces. Unlike other cestode eggs, *Hymenolepis* eggs may be readily concentrated by zinc sulfate flotation methods.

Hymenolepis diminuta

Geographic distribution. *H. diminuta*, the rat tapeworm, has a cosmopolitan distribution among rats and mice but occurs only occasionally in humans.

Life cycle—epidemiology. *H. diminuta* is normally a parasite of mice and rats, humans acquiring the infection accidentally. The adult worm lives in the small intestine and eggs are passed in the feces. Various species of fleas, cockroaches, beetles, moths, and other arthropods may serve as intermediate hosts. The larvae of certain rat fleas and the flour beetle *Tenebrio molitor* are

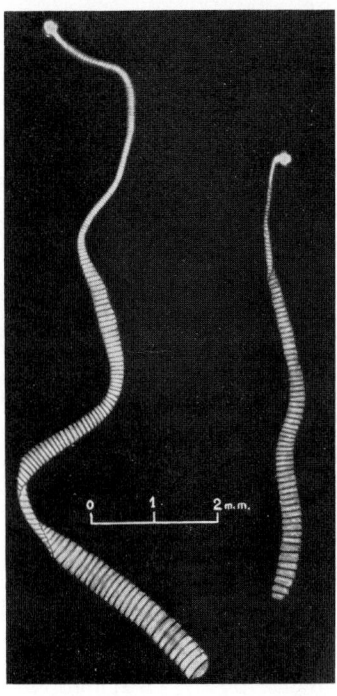

Fig. 98-29. *Hymenolepis nana.* Two specimens. Dark background. Greatly enlarged. Parasites fixed in 10% formalin. (Original of Kourí.) (From Kourí, P., and Basnuevo, J. G.: Lecciónes de parasitologia y medicina tropical, Havana, Editorial Profilaxis S.A.)

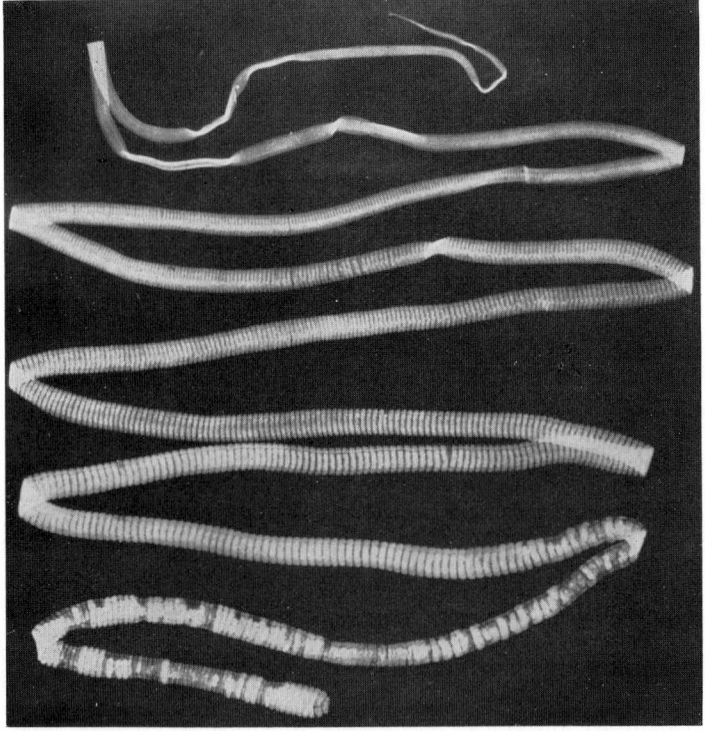

Fig. 98-30. *Hymenolepis diminuta.* Specimen 75 cm long, obtained by autopsy of rat. Scolex is very small. All proglottids, gravid proglottids included, are wider than long. It is difficult to see separation between proglottids with naked eye.This segmentation is clearly noted if parasite is observed with magnifying glass, as in this photograph. (From Kourí, P., and Basnuevo, J. G.: Lecciónes de parasitología y medicina tropical, Havana, Editorial Profilaxis S.A.)

the most important. On ingestion of the egg by the intermediate host the oncosphere escapes and develops into a cysticercoid larva. Humans become infected by accidentally ingesting insects harboring the cysticercoid larva. The infection occurs mostly in children. The symptoms most often attributed to this parasite are vague gastrointestinal complaints, diarrhea, and abdominal pain.

Morphology. The adult worm measures 10-18 cm in length (Fig. 98-30). The scolex has an unarmed rostellum and 4 suckers. Mature proglottids are wider than long, each containing a central ovary flanked by 2 testes on one side and 1 on the other. The almost spherical egg (Fig. 98-20) varies in diameter from 60-86 μm, and the outer egg layer has a yellowish brown color. The inner membrane surrounding the 6-hooked oncosphere is separated from the outer membrane by a layer of gelatinous material.

Diagnosis. Diagnosis is based on finding the characteristic egg (Fig. 98-20) in the feces. Unlike other cestode eggs, *Hymenolepis* eggs may be concentrated by flotation technics.

Dipylidium caninum

Geographic distribution. *D. caninum*, the dog tapeworm, is cosmopolitan among dogs and cats and occurs infrequently in humans.

Life cycle—epidemiology. The adult worm lives in the small intestine. The gravid proglottid either disintegrates, releasing eggs in the feces, or it actively migrates from the anus, leaving behind a trail of eggs. The egg is ingested by the larval stage of certain species of dog fleas or cat fleas. Within the flea an oncosphere escapes from the egg and develops into a cysticercoid larva. Humans are accidentally infected by ingesting the infected flea. The infection is more common among children and is probably the result of affectionate playing with pets, ingesting fleas accidentally in the process. The infection may result in mild gastric disorders.

Morphology. The adult worm is small, measuring 15-70 cm in length. The scolex has an armed rostellum. The mature proglottid is longer than wide and possesses 2 sets of male and female reproductive organs. A genital pore on each lateral margin of the proglottid is found in both mature and gravid proglottids (Fig. 98-31) and is characteristic of the species. The eggs, seen infrequently in the feces, occur in packets of 5-30 and are enclosed by a capsule.

Diagnosis. The first sign of infection is usually the presence of the muscular, actively moving proglottid on the fecal mass. The long slender proglottids (Fig. 98-31) may be identified by the presence of a genital pore on each lateral margin. The eggs are characteristically in packets but are not frequently seen in the feces.

Diphyllobothrium latum

Geographic distribution. *D. latum*, the fish or broad tapeworm, is most prevalent in the Baltic

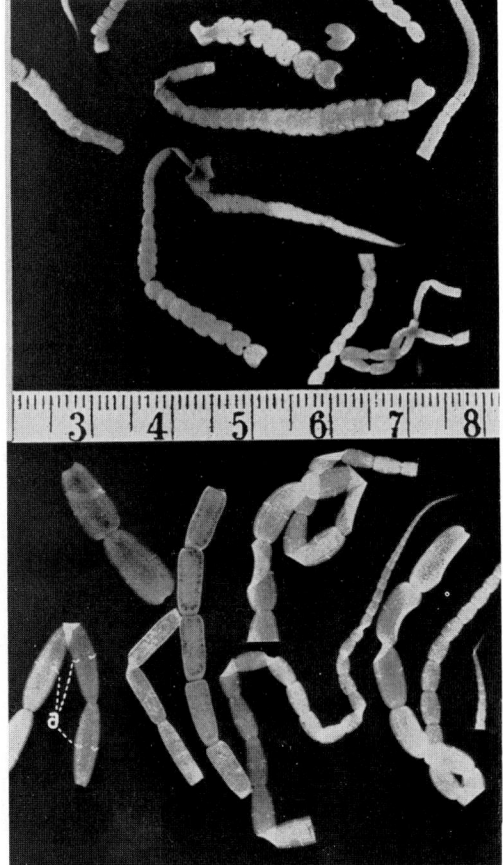

Fig. 98-31. *Dipylidium caninum*. Fragments of strobila of different specimens. Note variability in shape of segments. Some are biconvex, others heart shaped. Some are long, broad, and thin; others are narrow, short, and thick. Some have almost parallel sides. In segments marked *a*, double genital system is clearly visible. Fixed in 10% formalin; dark background, illuminated from above. Millimeter scale. (Originals of Kourí.)

countries, western U.S.S.R., parts of Scandinavia, and parts of the United States and Canada. In the United States cases have been reported in the Great Lakes regions of Wisconsin, Minnesota, and Michigan. A few scattered cases have been reported elsewhere.

Life cycle—epidemiology. The adult worm lives in the small intestine and passes eggs in the feces. After approximately 2 weeks of development in water the egg hatches, releasing a free-swimming ciliated coracidium. The coracidium is ingested by freshwater copepods belonging to the genus *Cyclops* or *Diaptomus*. Within the copepod the coracidium transforms into an elongated procercoid larva (Fig. 98-19) in 10-20 days. Further development occurs only if the infected copepod is ingested by 1 of 20 or more species of freshwater fish. Within the fish the procercoid migrates into the flesh and transforms into a wormlike plerocercoid (Fig. 98-19) in 1-4 weeks. Infected small fish may be ingested by larger fish, and the plerocercoid will reestablish

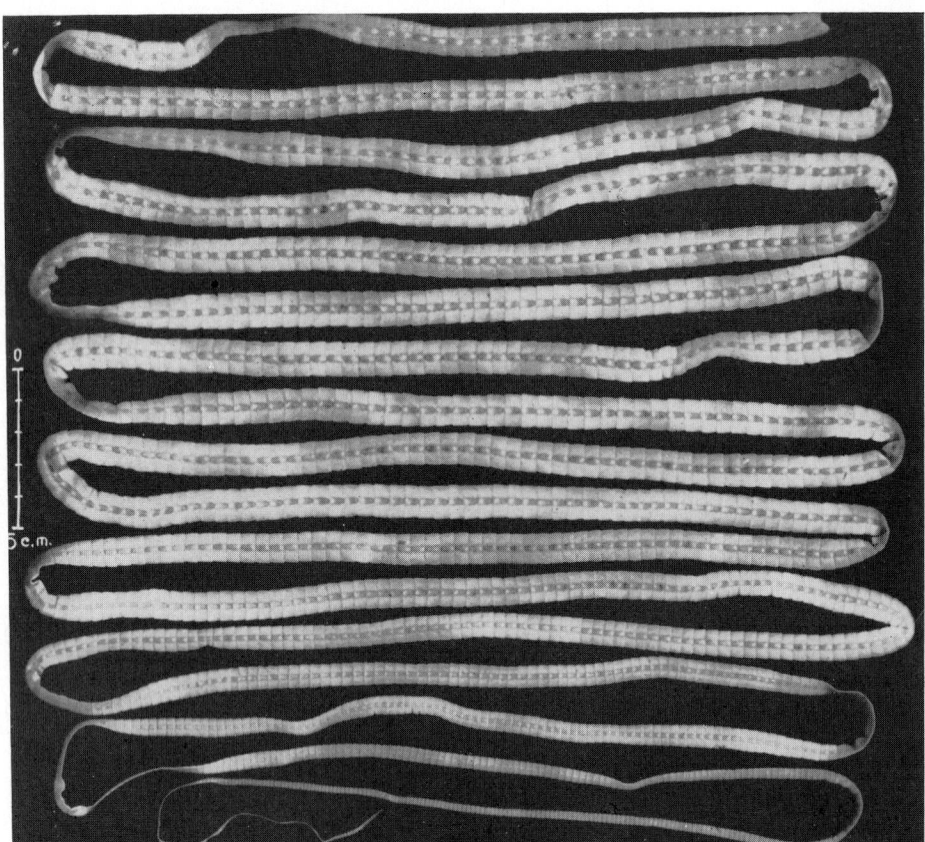

Fig. 98-32. *Diphyllobothrium latum.* Complete adult specimen expelled during treatment. (Kourí; from Kourí, P., and Basnuevo, J. G.: Lecciónes de parasitología y medicina tropical, Havana, Editorial Profilaxis S.A.)

in the larger fish. Different species of pike, trout, and salmon harbor the plerocercoid larva and are sources of infection for humans. In the United States blue pike, sand pike, and burbots are frequently infected. Humans become infected by ingesting raw or partially cooked fish containing the plerocercoid larva. The larva develops into an adult in a few weeks and may live several years.

The majority of infected individuals show few if any symptoms. Occasionally infections of *D. latum* are associated with a condition resembling pernicious anemia, especially if the worm is attached in the area of the jejunum. Studies have indicated that the parasite competes with the host for vitamin B_{12}, which is essential for adequate erythrocyte development.

Dogs, cats, foxes, and many other fish-eating mammals as well as humans may harbor *D. latum* and possibly serve as a reservoir for maintaining the infection in nature. The infection is widespread among fish in many of the small lakes around the Great Lakes. The infection is most prevalent among people of Jewish, Russian, Finnish, and Scandinavian origin, who frequently eat raw or inadequately cooked fish.

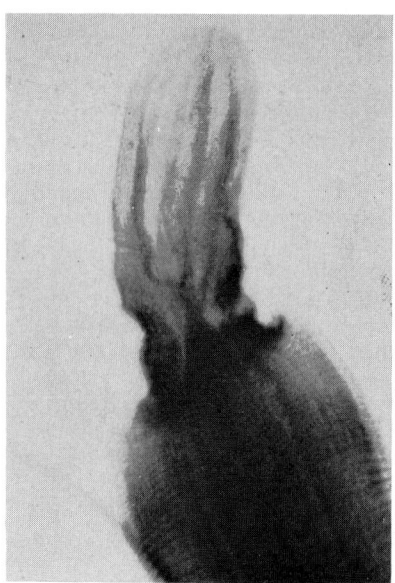

Fig. 98-33. *Diphyllobothrium latum* scolex.

Morphology. The adult tapeworm (Fig. 98-32) may reach 10 m or more in length. The scolex (Fig. 98-33) is elongated, spoon shaped, and possesses 2 longitudinal grooves. The proglottids are broader than long, usually 2-4 mm in length by 10-12 mm in width. Located in the center of each proglottid (Fig. 98-32) is a characteristic coiled uterus that resembles a rosette. A genital pore is present in the flattened surface in the anterior third of the proglottis. The yellowish brown egg, undeveloped when passed in the feces, is ovoid in shape and about 75 × 45 μm in size. At 1 pole of the egg an inconspicuous operculum may be discerned, and at the other a small knoblike projection may or may not be discernible.

Diagnosis. Diagnosis of the *D. latum* infections is based on finding the characteristic egg (Fig. 98-20) in the feces. Proglottids are seldom recognized in the feces unless prematurely expelled by treatment or other means. Diagnosis may be confirmed after treatment by examination of expelled proglottids for characteristic rosette arrangements of uteri.

Sparganosis

Sparganosis has a cosmopolitan distribution but occurs rarely in humans. Most reported cases have occurred in Indochina, Japan, and China. The term sparganum has been used loosely to mean the plerocercoid larva found in the second intermediate host. Humans may serve as the second intermediate host to a number of species of *Diphyllobothrium* that parasitize cats and dogs as adults. Also possibly other genera belonging to the order Pseudophyllidea and normally parasites of birds, as adults, may cause sparganosis in humans.

The mode of infection for humans varies. In the Orient fresh frogs are often split open and used as a plaster over a sore eye or wound. The plerocercoid larva escapes from the flesh of the frog and enters human flesh. Humans may also acquire the infection by ingestion of various amphibians, reptiles, and birds harboring the plerocercoid larvae. These larvae, being in an abnormal host, may migrate anywhere in the body. Experimental evidence indicates that humans may contract sparganosis by ingestion of *Cyclops* species containing the procercoid larva, this stage then transforming into a plerocercoid larva.

In humans the larvae reside primarily in the subcutaneous tissues. Symptoms depend on the number and location of the larvae. The affected tissue becomes edematous and painful to touch. In a few human cases a peculiar budding type of larva known as *Sparganum proliferum* has been reported. Unlike other spargana, this larva produces branches and proliferates, these new entities also being capable of proliferation. In these cases the invaded tissue may become honeycombed and nodular.

Diagnosis of sparganosis is made following surgical removal of the larvae. The sparganum larva is a whitish, wrinkled, ribbon-shaped worm a few millimeters in width and several centimeters in length. The anterior end is structurally suggestive of the sucking grooves of the mature scolex.

PHYLUM PLATYHELMINTHES — CLASS TREMATODA

Within the phylum Platyhelminthes the classes **Cestoidea (tapeworms)** and **Trematoda (flukes)** are of medical interest. The tapeworms are discussed elsewhere. The flukes are further divided into subclasses Monogenea and Digenea. Members of the former subclass are primarily ectoparasites of various aquatic animals and are of no medical concern. The subclass Digenea contains those flukes of importance to humans. Trematode infections of humans are not native to the United States. For this reason trematode infections are looked upon by many in the United States as either rare, exotic, or of no immediate concern. In many countries, however, certain fluke infections are of paramount importance. Various species of schistosomes (blood flukes) cause an estimated 100 million or more infections. The other flukes of humans also parasitize many millions. Unlike many of the nematode and cestode worms, the trematodes, especially the blood flukes, can cause serious medical problems.

Morphology (general). With the exception of the schistosomes, all the adult trematodes of humans are hermaphroditic, possessing both male and female reproductive organs. The size and shape of trematodes vary considerably, as seen in Fig. 98-34. The typical hermaphroditic fluke (Fig. 98-35) is usually flat, elongated, and more or less leaf shaped. Usually at the anterior end an oral sucker may be seen. In most flukes a ventral sucker (acetabulum) is also present. The digestive tract (cecum) usually is forked and ends blindly, there being no anal opening connecting the digestive tract to the outside. Thus to get rid of accumulated waste products the flukes make use of an excretory system consisting of a complicated arrangement of branched tubules. Waste material is funneled into the excretory duct by a fine network of flame cells scattered throughout the body of the worm. The flame cells are united in a characteristic definite arrangement, varying in different trematode groups. The waste material passes from the flame cells into the excretory duct, down to the bladder, and escapes through the posterior excretory pore.

The reproductive system (Fig. 98-35) is rather complex. The male system usually consists of 2 testes, the vas efferens uniting into a vas deferens that leads to the seminal vesicle and retractile copulatory organ, the cirrus. The female system consists of an ovary with its oviduct, which are joined by a vitelline (yolk) duct. At this junction there may be a duct that leads to a seminal receptacle and a side duct called Laurer's canal that ends blindly or opens to the body surface. Sur-

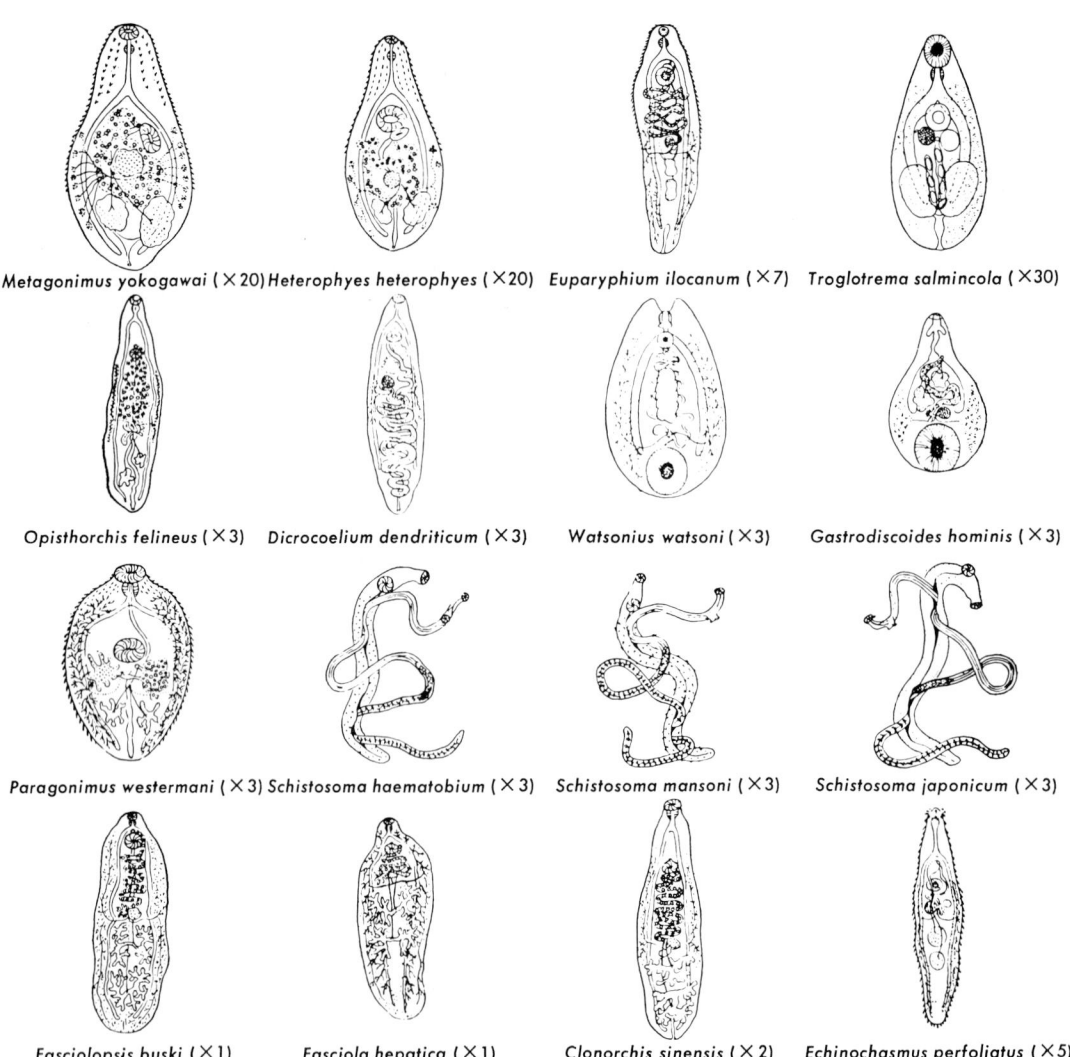

Metagonimus yokogawai (×20) *Heterophyes heterophyes* (×20) *Euparyphium ilocanum* (×7) *Troglotrema salmincola* (×30)

Opisthorchis felineus (×3)   *Dicrocoelium dendriticum* (×3)   *Watsonius watsoni* (×3)   *Gastrodiscoides hominis* (×3)

Paragonimus westermani (×3) *Schistosoma haematobium* (×3)   *Schistosoma mansoni* (×3)   *Schistosoma japonicum* (×3)

Fasciolopsis buski (×1)   *Fasciola hepatica* (×1)   *Clonorchis sinensis* (×2)   *Echinochasmus perfoliatus* (×5)

Fig. 98-34. Trematodes of humans. (From Belding, D. L.: Textbook of clinical parasitology, New York, 1952, Appleton-Century-Crofts.)

rounding the junction of the uterus, oviduct, seminal receptacle, and yolk ducts are a cluster of unicellular glands called Mehlis' gland. The uterus winds its way up the body to the genital pore. The relative positions of the ovary and testes, position of the uterus, arrangement of vitellaria, presence or absence of a seminal receptacle, and other characters are useful in identifying the adult stages of hermaphroditic trematodes. The schistosomes have separate sexes, and other characteristics are used to differentiate the adults. These characteristics are discussed in the section dealing with schistosomes.

The morphology of the larval forms of trematodes is complex and varied. These stages are not found in humans, except for the egg stages. The morphologic features of the eggs are described under each species. In addition to the egg there develop miracidia, sporocysts, rediae, cercariae,

and metacercariae (Fig. 98-36), depending on the species. The miracidium (Fig. 98-36, *A*) hatches from the egg and is a free-living stage, moving by means of cilia. The miracidium possesses a primitive gut, penetration glands, one or more pairs of flame cells, excretory tubules, an excretory pore, and a cluster of germinal cells that subsequently give rise to the next generation of organisms. The free-swimming miracidium must penetrate into an appropriate snail host in order to develop into a sporocyst. In some species (*Clonorchis* and *Dicrocoelium*), however, the trematode egg is ingested, hatches within the snail, and the miracidium then develops into a sporocyst. The sporocyst (Fig. 98-36, *B*) is an irregularly shaped sac, inside which the germ cells give rise to several daughter sporocysts or rediae. Daughter sporocysts are produced by the schistosomes, whereas rediae are produced by most

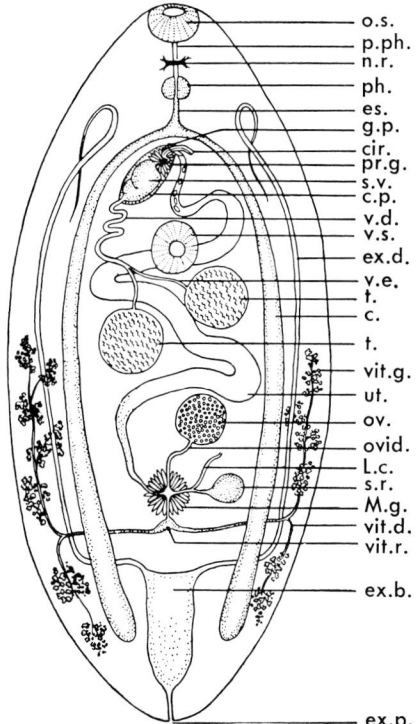

o.s.
p.ph.
n.r.
ph.
es.
g.p.
cir.
pr.g.
s.v.
c.p.
v.d.
v.s.
ex.d.
v.e.
t.
c.
t.
vit.g.
ut.
ov.
ovid.
L.c.
s.r.
M.g.
vit.d.
vit.r.

ex.b.

ex.p.

Fig. 98-35. Diagrammatic fluke to illustrate principal morphologic characteristics. *c.,* Cecum; *cir.,* cirrus; *c.p.,* cirrus pouch; *es.,* esophagus; *ex.b.,* excretory bladder; *ex.d.,* excretory duct; *ex.p.,* excretory pore; *g.p.,* genital pore; *L.c.,* Laurer's canal; *M.g.,* Mehlis' gland; *n.r.,* nerve ring; *o.s.,* oral sucker; *ov.,* ovary; *ovid.,* oviduct; *ph.,* pharynx; *p.ph.,* prepharynx; *pr.g.,* prostate glands; *s.r.,* seminal receptacle; *s.v.,* seminal vesicle; *t.,* testis; *ut.,* uterus; *v.d.,* vas deferens; *v.e.,* vas efferens; *vit.d.,* vitelline duct; *vit.g.,* vitelline glands; *vit.r.,* vitelline reservoir; *v.s.,* ventral sucker. (From Chandler, A.C., and Read, C. P.: Introduction to parasitology, New York, 1961, John Wiley & Sons.)

other species of trematodes. The redia (Fig. 98-36, *C*) possesses an oral sucker, saclike gut, and germinal cells that form germ masses. From the daughter sporocysts or rediae there develop cercariae that escape from the sporocyst or redia and eventually from the snail. Thus 1 miracidium develops into a sporocyst, which gives rise to several daughter sporocysts or rediae, which in turn produce hundreds or thoudands of cercariae. The rate of multiplication among trematodes is tremendous, but it is necessary because of the high mortality of the forms infective for humans.

After leaving the snail the cercariae of schistosomes must penetrate the skin of a human to continue development toward adulthood. The cercariae of other trematodes transform into metacercariae in or on some animal or vegetation before becoming infective for humans. The cercaria (Fig. 98-36, *D*) consists of a main body and a tail that may be single, as illustrated, or forked, as occurs among the schistosomes. The cercaria possesses an oral and ventral sucker, digestive

tract, excretory system, various spines, penetration glands, and cystogenous glands. The metacercaria stage (Fig. 98-36, *E*) occurs after the cercaria penetrates a host or attaches to vegetation. Essentially the metacercaria is an encysted cercaria that has lost certain cercarial features (i.e., tail, spines, and lytic glands).

Life cycle (general). Humans always harbor the adult stage. *Fasciolopsis, Heterophyes, Metagonimus, Echinostoma,* and *Gastrodiscoides* adults parasitize the intestinal tract, whereas adults of *Fasciola, Clonorchis, Opisthorchis,* and *Dicrocoelium* are found in the bile ducts. *Paragonimus* is usually located in the lungs or other tissues. The *Schistosoma* species are found in veins near the intestines or the bladder. Trematode eggs pass in the feces, urine, or sputum, depending on the species. The eggs of some species are fully developed at passage, whereas others require a maturation period. After the eggs reach water and mature, they may hatch, liberating miracidia that seek a specific snail host. In some species the eggs may be ingested by the snail before hatching (*Clonorchis, Opisthorchis,* and others). Within the snail the miracidium transforms into a bladderlike sporocyst that may produce several daughter sporocysts in the case of the schistosomes or several rediae in the case of other trematodes. The daughter sporocysts produce and liberate thousands of cercariae over a period of time. The rediae may do the same or in some species produce a generation of daughter rediae that finally produce and liberate many thousands of cercariae.

The free-living cercariae escape from the snail and must reach a suitable animal or plant host within a few days. The schistosome cercariae penetrate the skin of humans, reach the circulatory system, and eventually must reach the portal circulation before developing into adults. The cercariae of other trematodes penetrate certain fish or crustacea or attach to aquatic vegetation and encyst, becoming the metacercariae after a period of development. The cercariae of *Fasciola hepatica* attach to various grasses, whereas those of *Fasciolopsis buski* encyst on water chestnuts and caltrops. *Clonorchis, Heterophyes, Opisthorchis,* and others develop into metacercariae in various species of fish. *Paragonimus* cercariae become metacercariae in freshwater crabs and crayfish.

Humans become infected with the metacercariae-forming trematodes by ingesting the host harboring the metacercariae. Ingestion of raw or inadequately cooked fish, crayfish, or vegetation accounts for all infections. Within human the metacercariae mature directly to adults.

Laboratory diagnosis (general). In general, laboratory methods utilized for diagnosis are similar to those used for nematodes and cestodes. Fig. 98-38 illustrates most trematode eggs of humans, and Fig. 98-21 illustrates artifacts commonly encountered. The most commonly used technics are (1) saline smear, (2) sedimentation,

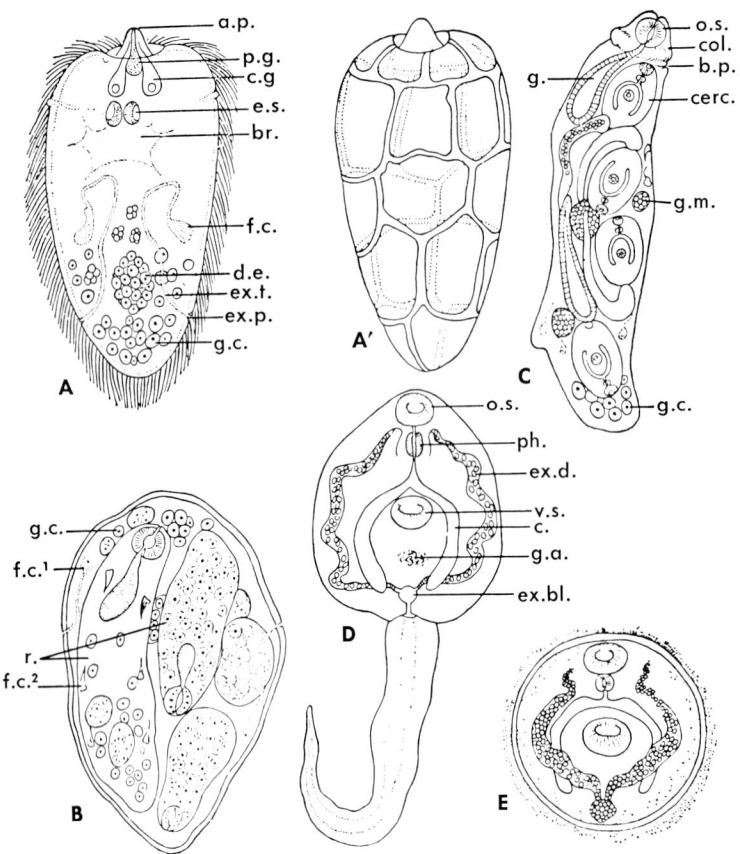

Fig. 98-36. Stages in life cycle of fluke. **A,** Miracidium showing internal organs. **A′,** Ectodermal cells. *a.p.,* apical papilla; *br.,* brain; *c.g.,* cephalic gland; *d.e.,* developing embryo; *e.s.,* eyespot; *ex.p.,* excretory pore; *ex.t.,* excretory tubule; *f.c.,* flame cell; *g.c.,* germ cells; *p.g.,* primitive gut. **B,** Sporocyst. *f.c.¹,* flame cell of sporocyst; *f.c.²,* flame cell of redia; *g.c.,* germ cells; *r.,* developing rediae. **C,** Redia. *b.p.,* birth pore; *cerc.,* developing cercaria; *col.,* collar; *g.,* gut; *g.c.,* germ cells; *o.s.,* oral sucker; *g.m.,* germinal mass. **D,** Cercarcia. *c.,* cecum; *ex.bl.,* excretory bladder; *ex.d.,* excretory duct; *g.a.,* genital anlage; *o.s.,* oral sucker; *ph.,* pharynx; *v.s.,* ventral sucker. **E,** Encysted metacercaria. (From Chandler, A. C., and Read, C. P.: Introduction to parasitology, New York, 1961, John Wiley & Sons.)

(3) centrifugation, (4) acid-ether technic, and (5) hatching for miracidia (schistosomes only). The saline smear is performed in the usual manner. However, if schistosome eggs are being sought, mucus flecks and strands on the outside on the fecal mass should be examined under a cover-slip. Simple sedimentation of feces in 0.5% glycerinated tap water concentrates schistosomes, *Clonorchis, Opisthorchis,* and *Heterophyes* to a degree. The method is simple and inexpensive but requires time. Centrifugation of strained feces has proved of some value in concentrating eggs but is decidedly inferior to the acid-ether technic (AMS III), which is the best method available for trematode egg concentration. As a specialized procedure, viable schistosome eggs may be demonstrated by placing feces in water. The schistosome eggs will hatch in a few hours, and the miracidia may be observed swimming in the water.

In suspected cases of paragonimiasis, sediment of sputum treated with NaOH is examined for eggs. The sedimented urine of suspected cases of *Schistosoma haematobium* is examined for eggs. Rectal or sigmoidoscopic biopsies are of value in schistosome infections.

Serologic tests and skin tests are of limited value in diagnosis of trematode infections. They have been used considerably in cases of schistosomiasis, primarily as a secondary diagnostic tool or to evaluate the effectiveness of therapy. Complement fixation tests, precipitin and agglutination tests, and skin tests have been studied, using adult eggs, cercariae, or sometimes miracidia as antigens. The significance of these tests is discussed in more detail under schistosomiasis.

For further details see Chapter 100.

Species of Trematoda
Schistosoma japonicum

Geographic distribution. *S. japonicum,* the oriental blood fluke, occurs only in the Far East.

The parasite is endemic in parts of Japan, China, Taiwan (Formosa), the Philippines, and Celebes. An estimated 46 million persons harbor the parasite in these areas.

Life cycle—epidemiology. The adult worms live in the superior mesenteric veins draining the small intestine, although the inferior mesenterics and caval system may be invaded. The female deposits many eggs in the small venules. Early in the infection the eggs work their way through the tissue rapidly and find their way to the lumen of the intestine to pass in the feces. Those eggs that reach water hatch, liberating miracidia that seek out a specific amphibious snail host belonging to the genus *Oncomelania*. The miracidium penetrates the snail and develops into a saclike sporocyst. The sporocyst produces several daughter sporocysts that in turn produce thousands of cercariae over a period of months. After leaving the snail the cercariae swim about in the water and must find a suitable host within a day or two or else perish. The cercariae penetrate the skin of humans and via the blood circulatory system find their way to the intrahepatic portal circulation. After a few weeks' development in the portal circulation the worms migrate to the mesenteric veins and mate. Eggs may begin to be deposited as early as 5 weeks after infection.

Transient dermatitis, pulmonary involvement, and hepatitis may occur early in infection due to cercarial penetration and migration, but the main effects of *S. japonicum* infection are caused by the host reaction to the eggs given off by the adult female. Passage of eggs through tissue causes trauma, and the resultant inflammatory response causes polyp formation and fibrosis of the intestines. Frequently eggs are filtered out in the liver, causing inflammation.

Humans become infected by wading through shallow water in irrigation ditches, canals, and rice fields that harbor the infective cercariae. The cercariae arise from amphibious snails, *Oncomelania*, that live in closer proximity to these waters. Opportunities for the snail to become infected are provided by promiscuous defecation, by use of human feces as fertilizer in rice crops, and from the feces of other infected mammals. Control of this parasite has proved especially difficult because of animal reservoir hosts and the time-honored custom of using human feces for fertilizer on crops such as rice.

Morphology. The gross morphologic features of the human schistosomes are illustrated in Fig. 98-37. *S. japonicum* male adults, unlike the other human species, lack the tuberculated cuticle (Fig. 98-34). The males average 12-20 mm in length, possess a characteristic gynecophoric canal, oral sucker, ventral sucker, and 7 testes. The slender female, often found within the gynecophoric canal averages 26 mm in length. The ovary is located in the middle of the body, and the uterus is long, usually containing 50-300 eggs. The egg (Fig. 98-38) is broad, oval, and measures 70-90 × 50-70 μm in size. The egg contains a developed miracidium. Rarely a small knob may be seen on one lateral surface of the egg.

Diagnosis. Definitive diagnosis of schistosomiasis japonica is made by demonstrating the egg (Fig. 98-38) in feces or in rectal biopsy material. Eggs are often difficult to demonstrate by the direct smear technic, especially early light infections and old chronic cases. More positive cases will be detected by concentration technics. The standard formalin-ether sedimentation technic will concentrate eggs. However, the AMS III sedimentation technic gives better results. Sigmoidoscopic examination of early cases may reveal erythematous nodular lesions and submucosal plaques. Chronic cases may exhibit papillomas. Aspiration, scraping, and biopsy of suspect lesions may reveal schistosome eggs.

Rectal biopsies have proved useful in evaluating effectiveness of therapy. If therapy is unsuccessful, viable eggs will continue to be found in biopsy material. Serologic procedures such as the complement fixation test and intradermal test have been utilized effectively by some workers. Apparently the *Schistosoma* antigen preparation currently used is group specific and will react with antibodies against the other schistosomes. The serologic procedures are discussed in more detail under *S. mansoni.*

A simple procedure that has proved of value in light infection involves diluting feces in water, allowing time for the eggs to hatch, and then examining the water surface for motile miracidia. The procedure is a simple, inexpensive, sensitive method of detecting **viable** eggs.

Schistosoma mansoni

Geographic distribution. *S. mansoni* (European workers and the World Health Organization prefer the generic name *Bilharzia*) is important along the Nile Delta, much of the eastern coast of Africa, west Africa, Congo River area, South Africa, and Madagascar. In the Western Hemisphere foci of infection are found in Brazil, Venezuela, Surinam (Dutch Guiana), Puerto Rico, Dominican Republic, Martinique, and other Caribbean islands. An estimated 29 million persons harbor this parasite.

Life cycle—epidemiology. The basic life cycle of *S. mansoni* is the same as that of *S. japonicum*. It differs in that the adult worms reside primarily in the inferior mesenteric venules, with eggs being found primarily in the venules and capillaries of the large intestine and lower small intestine. Eggs may be transported to the liver, whereas eggs and adults may find their way to the lungs via anastomoses between the mesenteric-portal veins. Although *S. mansoni* produces relatively few eggs and thus less damage, the type injury caused by this parasite is similar to that caused by *S. japonicum*. The intermediate snail host is one of various species of *Biomphalaria* on the African continent and pri-

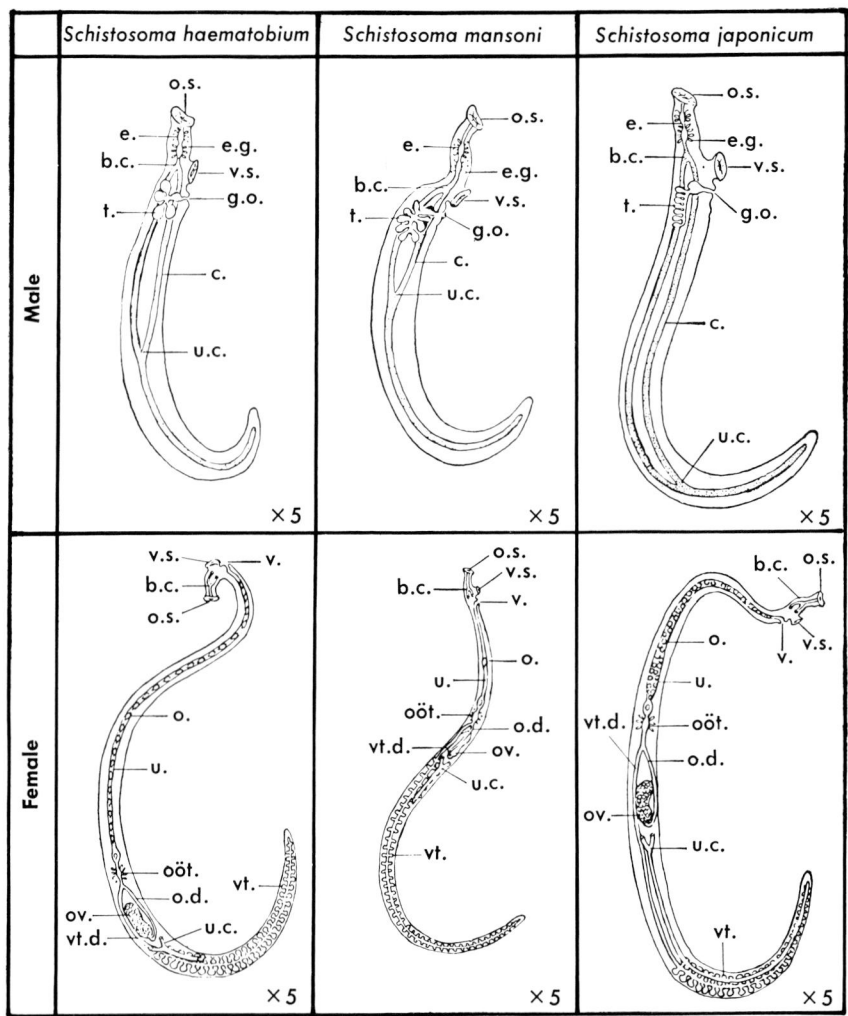

Fig. 98-37. Schematic representation of morphology of important schistosomes of humans. *b.c.,* Bifurcation of ceca; *c,* ceca; *e,* esophagus; *e.g.,* esophageal glands; *g.o.,* genital orifice; *o,* ova; *o.d.,* oviduct; *oöt.,* oötype; *os.,* oral sucker; *ov.,* ovary; *t,* testes; *u,* uterus; *u.c.,* union of ceca; *v,* vulva; *v.s.,* ventral sucker; *vt.,* vitellaria; *vt.d.,* vitelline duct. The breadth of the female worms has been doubled. (From Belding, D. L.: Textbook of clinical parasitology, New York, 1952, Appleton-Century-Crofts.)

marily *Australorbis glabratus* in the Western Hemisphere. Infection results from contact with cercariae. In endemic areas the cercariae are found in canals used in agricultural irrigation or in streams used for washing clothes, bathing, etc.

Morphology. The gross morphologic features of *S. mansoni* are illustrated in Fig. 98-37. *S. mansoni* males (Figs. 98-34 and 98-37) possess prominent cuticular tubercles, 6-9 testes, and average 6-10 mm in length. Like the other schistosomes, an oral sucker, ventral sucker, and a gynecophoric canal are present. The female averages 7-14 mm in length. The ovary is located in the anterior part of the worm, and the uterus is short, usually containing only 1 egg at a time. The characteristic lateral-spined egg (Fig. 98-38) is large, measuring 114-175 μm in length by 45-68 μm in diameter.

Diagnosis. Laboratory diagnosis of *S. mansoni* infections is based primarily on demonstration of the egg in feces or biopsy material. Flecks of mucus from the feces may be examined in a simple smear, or eggs may be concentrated by sedimentation or the AMS III technic. The hatching techinc may also be utilized to demonstrate viable eggs. In chronic cases rectal biopsies or concentration technics reveal more infections. The rectal biopsy can also by utilized to evaluate success of therapy by noting whether viable eggs are in the biopsy specimen.

Much information has accumulated recently on the value of serologic and intradermal tests in *S. mansoni* infection. None of these procedures replace diagnostic efforts to demonstrate the egg; rather, they serve as screening devices. Usually a positive skin reaction occurs in infected per-

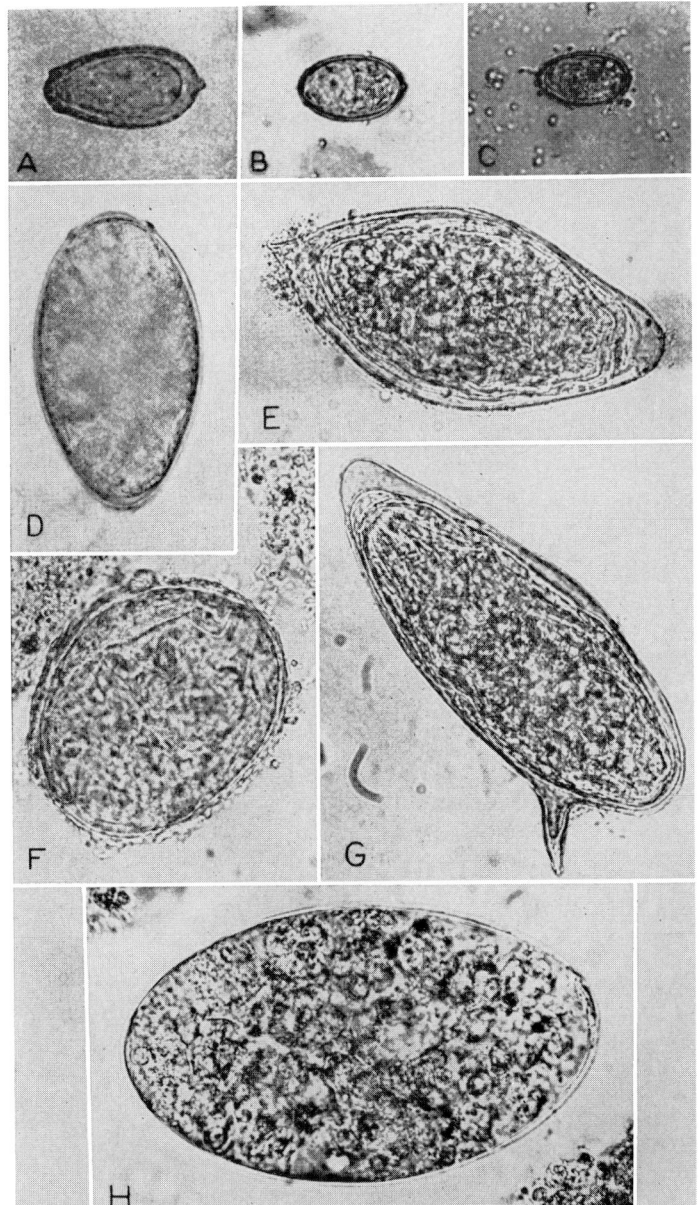

Fig. 98-38. Some trematode eggs. **A,** *Clonorchis sinensis.* **B,** *Heterophyes heterophyes.* **C,** *Metagonimus yokagawai.* **D,** *Paragonimus westermani.* **E,** *Schistosoma haematobium.* **F,** *Schistosoma japonicum.* **G,** *Schistosoma mansoni.* **H,** *Fasciolopsis buski.* See Fig. 98-21 for objects in feces often confused with helminth eggs. **(A,** approx. ×710; **B-H,** approx. ×430.) (From Hunter, G. W., III, Frye, W. W., and Swartzwelder, J. C.: Manual of tropical medicine, Philadelphia, 1960, W. B. Saunders Co.)

sons injected intradermally with either adult or cercarial antigens. Precipitin or agglutinating antibodies are formed against cercariae and eggs (circumoval antibodies). Antibody levels against the cercariae are high early in the infection and low later in the infection. The reverse is true in the case of circumoval antibody. Chaffee and Nieves[18] and Anderson and Naimark[19] found the complement fixation test using adult or cercarial antigens to be quite reliable, although the former workers noted cross-reactions with sera from patients with paragonimiasis. Anderson[20] reported on an interesting flocculation type of test for schistosomiasis that was quite specific within the schistosome group except for cross-reactions with persons infected with *Trichinella spiralis.* Buck and Anderson[21] and Allain et al.[22] reported on use of CF, slide flocculation, and BF tests. All presented problems in sensitivity and specificity but were considered useful diagnostic aids. The indirect fluorescent antibody test using tissue sections of adult worms gives increased sensitivity and specificity.[23]

Schistosoma haematobium

Geographic distribution. *S. haematobium*, or *Bilharzia haematobia*, occurs throughout much of Africa and the Middle East. The parasite is endemic in the Nile Valley and occurs in many parts of Africa, frequently in the same areas as *S. mansoni*. In the Middle East cases have been reported in Israel, northern Syria, Saudi Arabia, Iran, and Iraq. In Europe the parasite is present in Portugal and Cyprus. Recently a foci of infection has been found in the Maharashtra (formerly Bombay) state of India. An estimated 39 million persons harbor *S. haematobium*.

Life cycle—epidemiology. The life cycle of *S. haematobium* is essentially the same as that described for *S. japonicum* except for final location of the adult in the host and the choice of snail intermediate hosts. The adult worms reside in the vesical and pelvic plexuses of the venous circulation and the veins of the lower colon and rectum. The eggs deposited by the female worm work their way through the bladder or intestinal tissue to pass either in urine or feces. The miracidia are liberated from the eggs after they reach water and seek snails belonging to the genus *Physopsis* or *Bulinus*. As with the other species of schistosomes, the major damage results from trauma and host reaction to the eggs. The principal organ affected is the urinary bladder. The genital organs, rectum, lungs, and other organs may be involved. Damage to the liver is seldom as severe as that caused by the other schistosomes of humans. The epidemiology is the same as that described for *S. mansoni*.

Morphology. The adult male (Figs. 98-34 and 98-37) possesses 4 large testes and a cuticle that is finely tuberculate; it measures 10-15 mm in length. The ovary of the adult female (Fig. 98-37) is located in the posterior half of the body, and the uterus is long, usually containing 20-30 eggs. The females measure on the average 20 mm in length. The egg, as seen in the urine (Fig. 98-38), measures 112-170 × 40-70 μm. The egg is identified by a characteristic terminal spine. Other species of schistosomes such as *S. matthei*, *S. intercalatum*, *S. spindale*, and *S. bovis* also produce terminal-spined eggs. These schistosomes are primarily parasites of other animals, although in certain areas of Africa considerable numbers of human beings may be infected with certain of these species.

Diagnosis. The laboratory diagnosis of *S. haematobium* infections is primarily based on demonstration of the typical terminally spinal egg (Fig. 98-38) in urine, feces, or biopsy material from the bladder or rectum. The AMS method, sedimentation method, hatching technic, or water centrifugal sedimentation method may be utilized for fecal examinations as well as the simple fecal smear. In all suspected cases the sediment of the last few drops of passed urine should be examined for eggs, as this is the route by which most viable eggs leave the host. Baldran et al.,[24] however, presented evidence that more positive cases could be uncovered by rectal biopsy than by urine examination alone. Several workers have reported that persons infected with *S. haematobium* often harbor chronic urinary infections of *Salmonella*. Such infections are difficult to eradicate unless the schistosome infection is treated.

Serologic procedures for *S. haematobium* have not been utilized extensively under experimental conditions because of the difficulty of adapting this parasite to laboratory animals. However, since the schistosome group has common antigens and one species cannot be differentiated from another serologically, one may assume that the serologic and intradermal tests discussed under *S. mansoni* are applicable to *S. haematobium* infections.

Schistosomal dermatitis

Schistosomal dermatitis, or swimmer's itch, is caused by the cercariae of other animals penetrating the skin of humans. Cases have been reported most often in the United States along beaches in the Great Lakes region, New England, Oregon, Florida, and California and sporadically in other countries. Bathers, fishermen, and clam diggers are most frequently affected. The cercariae of certain bird trematodes, especially those species of *Trichobilharzia*, are most frequently involved in the United States. These cercariae penetrate human skin and may migrate as far as the lungs but apparently no farther. Eventually the individual becomes sensitized, and on reexposure the cercariae are trapped in the skin and die. Their presence may cause allergic reactions manifested in papular eruptions of varying severity. Diagnosis is based on clinical appearance and history of exposure. No procedures are available to demonstrate the parasite.

Fasciola hepatica

Geographic distribution. *F. hepatica*, the sheep liver fluke, is primarily a parasite of sheep and occurs in most sheep-raising countries. Infections in humans have been reported in Venezuela, Uruguay, Chile, Argentina, Puerto Rico, Cuba, Costa Rica, Lebanon, Syria, China, Russia, France, Italy, Corsica, Spain, Hungary, Romania, Salonika, Algeria, Afars and Issas (French Somaliland), South Africa, Hawaii, and Queensland of Australia.

Life cycle—epidemiology. The adult worm lives in the bile duct and gives off immature eggs that pass in the feces. In water the egg develops and hatches in about 2 weeks, releasing a miracidium that penetrates a *Lymnaea* snail or related species and develops into a sporocyst. The sporocyst gives rise to 2 rediae generations that produce many cercariae. The cercariae leave the snail host and encyst on water vegetation, transforming to metacercariae capable of surviving several months. Various mammals are infected by ingesting vegetation containing the metacercariae. In the host the metacercaria excysts, penetrates the intestinal wall, and bores into the liver parenchyma. Seven to 8 weeks later the metacercaria reaches its final habitat, the bile duct, and develops into an adult. The adult in the bile duct may live as long as 10 years. Some damage may be caused by metacercarial migration through the liver. Within the bile duct constant irritation and inflammation caused by the presence of the worms may eventually cause cirrhosis of the liver. The severity of the infection in humans is related to the number of worms and duration of infection.

Although sheep and cattle are the main hosts, goats, camels, dogs, and some other carnivores may harbor the adult. Several species of snails may serve as intermediate host, enhancing biologic persistence of the parasite. Forage pastures containing small ponds or streams create an ideal environment for maintenance of the parasite.

Morphology. The adult worm (Fig. 98-39) is large, flat, brownish, and leaf shaped, measuring

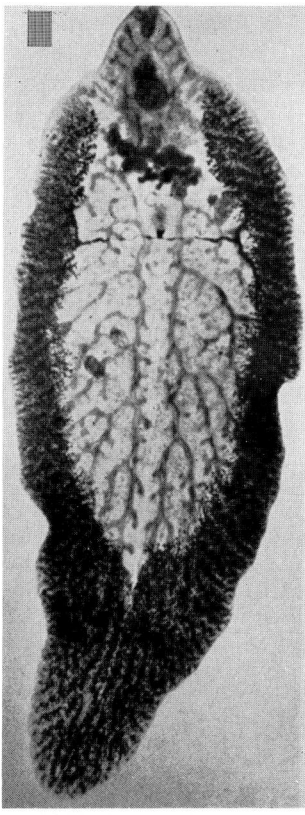

Fig. 98-39. *Fasciola hepatica,* characteristic shape with anterior conical prolongation. White central oval zone is occupied by testes. Dark zone contains vitelline glands. White central zone is crossed by 2 intestinal branches with lateral external ramifications. Trunks and their branches end in blind pouches. (Original of Vigueras and Moreno.)

about 25 mm in length and 13 mm in breadth. The anterior end tapers off to a conelike projection. The anterior portion of the cuticle is covered with scales, but the posterior surface may be smooth. A ventral and oral sucker are present, the ventral sucker being only slightly larger than the oral one. The testes, ovary, and bifurcate ceca are branched and are distributed widely throughout the body of the worm. The egg measures 130-150 μm in length by 63-90 μm and resembles closely the egg of *Fasciolopsis buski* (Fig. 98-38). The egg is immature at passage, possesses an operculum, and is light yellowish brown.

Diagnosis. Laboratory diagnosis is based on demonstration of the egg (Fig. 98-38) in feces or from material obtained by duodenal or biliary drainage. Occasionally, if raw liver containing adult worms is eaten, the eggs will pass on through the intestine, and a false diagnosis may be made. To eliminate this possibility the patient should be placed on a liver-free diet a few days before examination. Eggs may be concentrated by the formalin-ether sedimentation method but not flotation methods. Complement fixation, precipitin, and intradermal tests have been described but are not used routinely.

Fasciolopsis buski

Geographic distribution. *F. buski,* the large intestinal fluke, is widely distributed in pigs and humans in areas of eastern Asia, central and south China, Taiwan, Annam, Tonkin, Pakistan, Thailand, Assam, Malaysia, Sumatra, and Borneo.

Life cycle—epidemiology. The adult worms live in the small intestine of humans or pigs and occasionally dogs. Undeveloped eggs are passed in the feces. In water they mature, hatch, and liberate miracidia that penetrate snails belonging to the genus *Hippeutis* or *Segmentina.* In the snail a sporocyst and 2 generations of rediae develop before finally producing cercariae. The cercariae leave the snail host and encyst on water vegetation such as water caltrops, water chestnuts, or bamboo and transform into metacercariae. As metacercariae the trematodes may survive many months. Humans become infected by ingesting the roots, bulbs, pods, or stems of various water plants containing the metacercariae. Within humans the metacercaria develops directly into an adult in the small intestine.

The damage caused by the parasite is usually directly related to the number present. Worm attachment to the mucosa results in inflammation and possibly ulcer formation. Toxic and allergic reactions to worm secretions may be the most serious consequence of infection. Facial edema, ascites, abdominal pains, and an elevated eosinophilia may be present.

Morphology. The adult worm (Fig. 98-40) measures 20-75 mm in length and 8-20 mm in breadth. It is a large fleshy worm with a spined integument and lacks the anterior cephalic cone characteristic of *Fasciola.* The oral sucker is

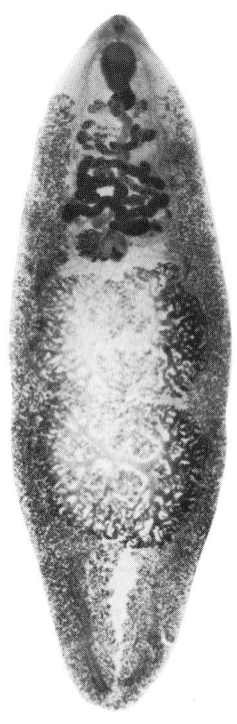

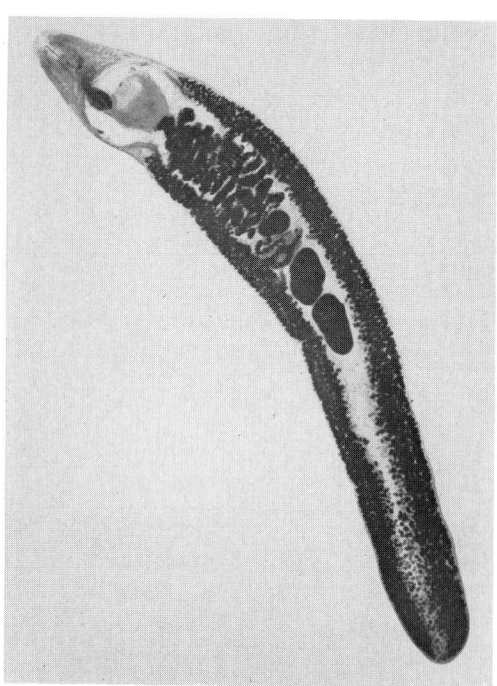

Fig. 98-40. *Fasciolopsis büski.*

Fig. 98-41. *Echinostoma* sp.

much smaller than the ventral sucker. The testes are located in the posterior half of the body; the intestinal ceca are not branched. The egg (Fig. 98-38) measures 130-140 μm in length by 80-85 μm in breadth and is difficult to differentiate from *F. hepatica* eggs.

Diagnosis. Laboratory diagnosis is based on demonstration of the egg (Fig. 98-38) or adult worm (Fig. 98-40) in the feces. The egg is not easily differentiated from that of *F. hepatica.* Another species of *Fasciola*, *F. gigantica*, occurs occasionally in humans, but usually the eggs are longer than *F. büski* eggs, measuring 160-190 μm in length. The usual sedimentation concentration technics may be utilized for diagnosis of *Fasciolopsis* eggs.

Echinostoma species

The echinostomes are parasites of many kinds of vertebrates, especially aquatic birds. The infection in humans is accidental and relatively rare. *E. ilocanum* in the Philippines and Java, *E. lindoensis* in Celebes, and *E. cinetorchis* in Japan are among the more important species. Human cases have been reported in the Philippines, Malaysia, Celebes, Japan, Java, and a few other localities in Asia. Humans acquire the infection by ingestion of the secondary intermediate host, which may be any number of edible freshwater snails containing the encysted metacercariae. For some echinostomes other freshwater mollusks may serve as the second intermediate host. The adult worms attach to the wall of the small intestine and may produce inflam-

mation, ulceration, and diarrhea. The undeveloped eggs seen in the feces vary in size according to species but are often difficult to differentiate from *Fasciolopsis* eggs. Adult worms, seen only after treatment, may be recognized by the circumoral spines seen at high magnification. The adult worms (Fig. 98-41) are relatively slender, but size varies considerably between species.

Dicrocoelium dendriticum

D. dendriticum is a common parasite of the bile passage of many herbivores in many parts of the world but occurs rarely in the bile duct of humans. Fully embryonated eggs are passed in the feces and are ingested by land snails. After the usual developmental cycle the cercariae are liberated from the snail in slime balls. If the slime balls are ingested by ants, the cercariae develop into metacercariae. Humans become infected by accidentally ingesting ants containing the metacercariae. The adult worm (Fig. 98-42) measures 5-15 mm in length; its testes are found in the anterior third of the body. The eggs are dark brown, fully developed, possess a large operculum, and measure 38-48 × 22-30 μm.

Opisthorchis species

O. felineus and *O. viverrini* have been described in humans. The former species is prevalent in central and eastern Europe, Siberia, and parts of the Far East; the latter species is prevalent in Thailand. The adult worms live in the bile ducts of humans, dogs, and cats. Fully developed eggs are passed in the feces and are ingested by

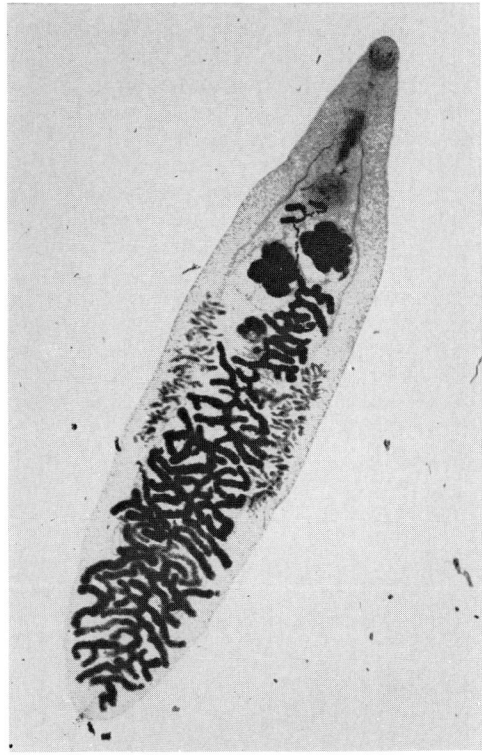

Fig. 98-42. *Dicrocoelium dendriticum.*

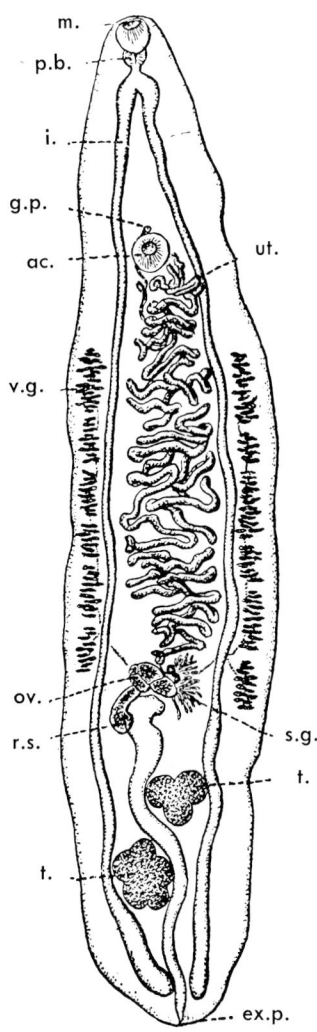

Fig. 98-43. *Opisthorchis felineus* from cat. *m.,* Mouth; *p.b.,* pharynx; *i.,* gut; *g.p.,* genital pore; *ac.,* ventral sucker; *ut.,* uterus; *vg.,* vitellarium; *ov.,* ovary; *s.g.,* shell gland; *r.s.,* receptaculum seminis; *t.,* testes; *ex.p.,* excretory pore. (×15.) (After Stiles and Hassall; from Fantham, H. B., Stephens, J. W. W., and Theobald, F. V.: The animal parasites of man, London, Bale, Sons & Danielsson, Ltd.)

snails. Within the snail the eggs hatch, and the miracidia develop into sporocysts, rediae, and finally cercariae, which leave the snail and penetrate freshwater fish to develop into metacercariae. Humans become infected by ingesting raw or pickled fish containing the metacercariae. The adults residing in the bile duct may cause varying degrees of injury. Generally pathogenicity is of low degree. The adult worm (Fig. 98-43) measures 7-12 mm in length and 2-3 mm in breadth, tapering anteriorly and rounded posteriorly. The oral and ventral (acetabulum) sucker, unlike *Clonorchis*, are of about equal size. The testes are lobate rather than branched in tandem fashion as seen in *Clonorchis*. The egg (Fig. 98-44) measures about 11 × 30 μm and is similar to *Clonorchis* eggs but has a less pronounced shouldering at the margin of the operculum. Laboratory diagnosis is based on demonstration of the egg or adult worm in the feces.

Clonorchis sinensis

Geographic distribution. *C. sinensis,* the Chinese liver fluke, is prevalent in most of China, Taiwan (Formosa), Japan, Korea, and Indochina. Although cases of clonorchiasis are reported in the western world, they occur either in Orientals who have recently migrated from endemic areas or in persons who have eaten frozen, dried, or pickled infected fish shipped from endemic areas.

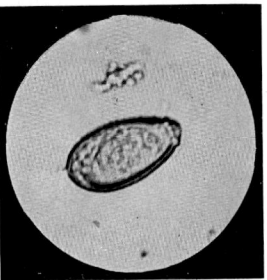

Fig. 98-44. Egg of *Opisthorchis felineus.* (×1000.)

Life cycle—epidemiology. The life cycle of *Clonorchis* is essentially the same as that described for *Opisthorchis*. Several species of snails and fish serve as first and second intermediate hosts respectively.

Morphology. The adult worm (Fig. 98-45) measures 10-25 mm in length and 3-5 mm in breadth. The oral sucker is somewhat larger than the ventral sucker (acetabulum); the latter is located in the posterior part of the anterior third of the body. The characteristic testes are branched and lie one behind the other in the posterior third of the body. The yellowish brown egg (Figs. 98-38 and 98-45) is 27-35 μm in length by 12-20 μm in breadth and is fully embryonated. The egg has a pronounced shouldering at the margin of the operculum. On the end opposite the operculum a small knoblike projection may be seen.

Diagnosis. Laboratory diagnosis is based on demonstration of the egg (Fig. 98-45) in the feces and duodenum or biliary drainage. The egg must be distinguished from that of *Metagonimus yokagawai, Heterophyes heterophyes,* and *Opisthorchis* species. The eggs of *Opisthorchis* (Fig. 98-44) are more elongated, usually 3 times longer than broad. The eggs of *Heterophyes* and *Metagonimus* are hard to differentiate, but both lack the distinct shoulder at the margin of the operculum that is seen in *Clonorchis* eggs. Also the operculum of *Clonorchis* is broader in relation to length. *Clonorchis* eggs also possess a more pronounced knob on the end opposite the operculum. The adult *Clonorchis* resembles *Opisthorchis* but may be differentiated on the basis of characteristics of the testes and relative size and location of the suckers to one another. Serologic

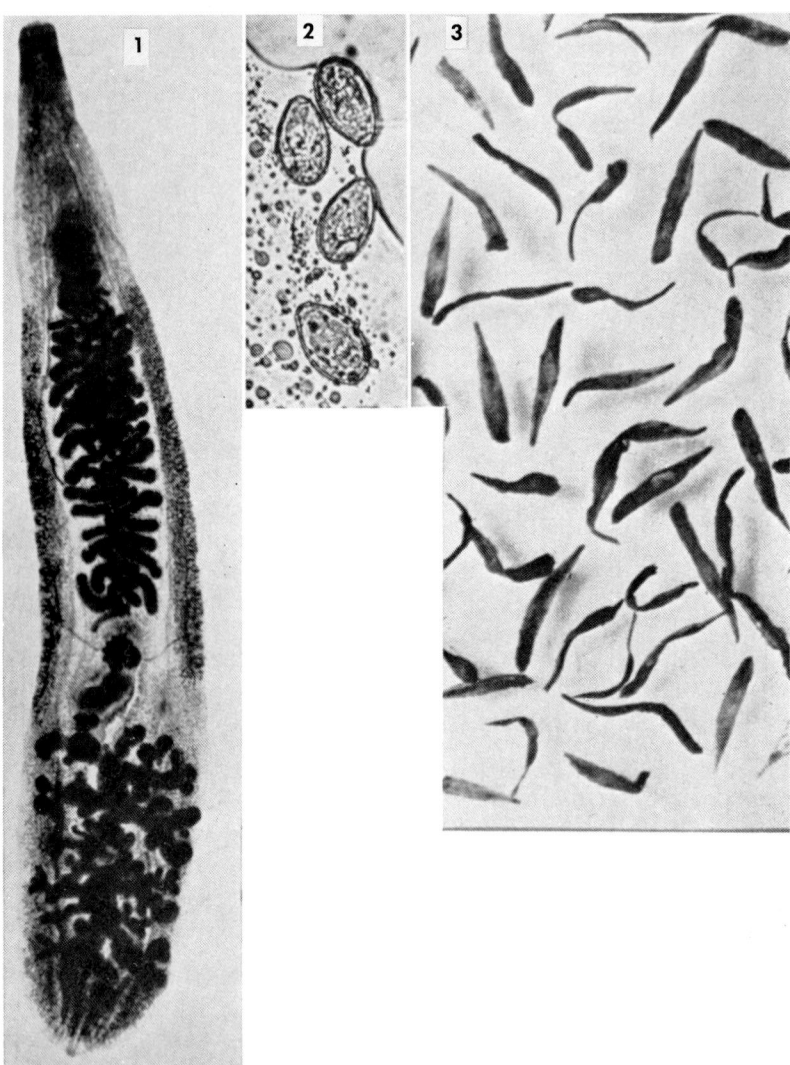

Fig. 98-45. *Clonorchis sinensis.* **1,** Photomicrograph of specimen stained with Meyer acid hemalum. (×12.) **2,** Photomicrograph of eggs in bile obtained by duodenal intubation. **3,** Photograph natural size. (Originals of Kourí.)

tests are not used routinely for diagnosis. The indirect hemagglutination test,[25] complement fixation, and skin tests[26] have been used with some success.

Heterophyes heterophyes

H. heterophyes is common in the Nile Delta, Japan, Korea, Taiwan, central and south China, and the Philippines. The adult worms (Fig. 98-50) live in the intestinal tract; otherwise the life cycle (i.e., choice of intermediate host) is similar to that of the *Clonorchis sinensis*. The presence of worms usually causes mild abdominal upsets. However, some workers have presented evidence that when humans are infected with certain species of *Heterophyes* the eggs may cross the intestinal barrier and lodge in various organs and tissues, causing serious inflammatory foci. The adult worm (Fig. 98-46) measures less than 2 mm in length, is spined, and possesses a large genital sucker adjacent to the ventral sucker. The egg (Fig. 98-38) measures about 29 × 16 μm, is slightly darker yellow-brown than *Metagonimus* eggs, but otherwise is indistinguishable from them. Diagnosis is made by demonstration of the egg in the feces.

Metagonimus yokagawai

M. yokagawai is prevalent in parts of China, Japan, Indonesia, maritime provinces of U.S.S.R., Siberia, Spain, Israel, and the Balkan States. The adult worm (Fig. 98-47) lives in the small intestine and has a life cycle very similar to that of *Clonorchis*. Infections with this parasite are usually mild, but occasionally heavy infection may be serious, especially if eggs cross the intestinal barrier and become lodged in other tissues. The adult worm (Fig. 98-47) measures less than 3 mm in length, is spined, and characteristically has the ventral sucker located off the right of the median line. The egg (Fig. 98-38) measures 28-38 × 15-17 μm and, although slightly darker, is difficult to distinguish from eggs of *Heterophyes*.

Paragonimus westermani

Geographic distribution. *P. westermani*, the oriental lung fluke, has a wide distribution and is especially prevalent in central China, Japan, Korea, Taiwan, and the Philippines. Other foci of lung fluke infection in parts of Africa, Vietnam, Indonesia, New Guinea, Malay Peninsula, parts of India, Brazil, Peru, Ecuador, Venezuela, Costa Rica, and Mexico are probably caused by other species of *Paragonimus*.

Life cycle—epidemiology. Typically the adult worm lives in encapsulated pockets of the lung. Undeveloped eggs are given off by the adult and pass up the respiratory tree to be eliminated either in the sputum or swallowed and passed in

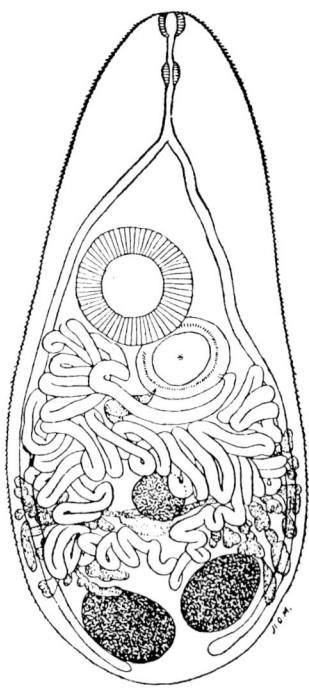

Fig. 98-46. *Heterophyes heterophyes* (after Mönnig); adult, ventral face. Note that posterior extremity is thicker than anterior. Note also large ventral sucker (acetabulum) and immediately behind it characteristic genital sucker. The 2 testes are oval, posterior, and horizontal. (×60.) (Kourí, P., and Basnuevo, J. G.: Lecciónes de parasitología y medicina tropical, Havana, Editorial Profilaxis S.A.)

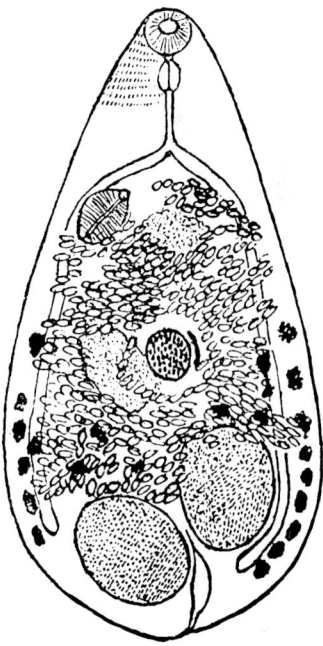

Fig. 98-47. *Metagonimus yokogawai.* Spines are shown only over small part of skin. (×50.) (After Leiper; from Fantham, H. B., Stephens, J. W. W., and Theobald, F. V.: The animal parasites of man, London, Bale, Sons & Danielsson, Ltd.)

feces. In water the egg develops and hatches in about 3 weeks, liberating a miracidium. The miracidium seeks and penetrates various species of snail hosts and produces successive generations of sporocysts, rediae, and cercariae. The cercariae leave the snail host and invade the muscles and viscera of freshwater crabs or crayfish. Humans become infected by ingesting freshwater crabs or crayfish containing the metacercariae. Within humans the metacercariae excyst and migrate through the intestinal wall and the diaphragm to the vicinity of the bronchioles, where they develop to adults within cystlike capsules formed as part of the host reaction to the parasites. Not infrequently the metacercariae never reach the lungs but develop to adults in the pleural cavity, genitourinary system, cerebrum, abdominal cavity, subcutaneous tissues, testes, and other places. In these instances the sites other than the lung are blind alleys in that there is no way for the eggs to escape from the body to perpetuate the life cycle.

Many types of mammals harbor *P. westermani* and serve as a reservoir source for maintaining the parasite in nature. In areas where paragonimiasis is endemic, crayfish and freshwater crabs are often eaten raw or pickled. In the United States a species of *Paragonimus* exists in nature among mammals, but only 1 case has been reported in a human. On the basis of slight morphologic differences some observers call this species *P. kellicotti*, whereas others believe that the separate species differentiation is not justified.

The infection varies from mild to severe, usually depending on the number of worms present and their location. The reader may consult Sadun and Buck[27] and Kim and Walker[28] for a rather complete review of pathogenesis, diagnosis, and treatment. The presence of the worm in the lung usually results in a productive cough of reddish brown sputum. The character of the sputum and radiologic evidence often resemble those found in tuberculosis.

Morphology. The reddish brown adult worm (Fig. 98-48) is ovoid and thick bodied, measuring 8-20 mm in length by 4-8 mm in width. The branched testes are located in the posterior third of the body. In stained specimens a lobate ovary may be seen to 1 side of the ventral sucker, with the uterus located on the opposite side. A long, slender bladder extends most of the length of the worm. The golden brown, operculate, underdeveloped egg (Fig. 98-38) measures 80-115 × 48-60 μm, averaging 85-53 μm. It appears slightly flattened, with slight "shoulder" margins at the operculum end.

Diagnosis. Definitive laboratory diagnosis of paragonimiasis is based on demonstration of the egg (Fig. 98-38) in sputum or feces. The eggs must be differentiated from those of *Diphyllobothrium latum*. Eggs are frequently found in the sputum, although many examinations over a period of weeks may be necessary to demonstrate the egg. Characteristically the egg masses in spu-

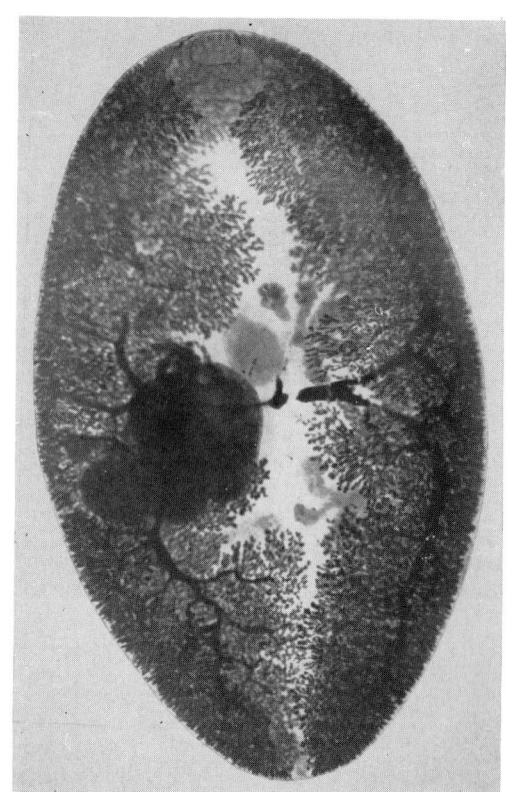

Fig. 98-48. *Paragonimus westermani.* (From Markell, E. K., and Voge, M.: Diagnostic techniques in medical parasitology, Philadelphia, 1958, W. B. Saunders Co.)

tum appear as rusty brown flecks, or the sputum may be tinged with blood. Fecal specimens are more frequently positive in children than in adults, since children have a greater tendency to swallow sputum. Best results on fecal examinations are obtained by use of concentration technics such as the AMS III. Sadun and Buck[27] noted that almost 10% of their patients were diagnosed by means other than sputum or fecal examinations. In these cases eggs were found either in the pus of the empyema, by pleural puncture, or urine examination.

In addition to the examination of various specimens for eggs, a leukocytosis and eosinophilia of 10% or more may be suggestive in the early stages of the disease. Sadun and Buck[27] found intradermal tests valuable in differentiating paragonimiasis from tuberculosis, especially in those under 14 years of age. The authors, using purified antigen, found that cross-reactions occurred between *Paragonimus* and *Clonorchis*, but cases of paragonimiasis always produced a larger wheal with the *Paragonimus* antigens, even if *Clonorchis* and *Paragonimus* were present concurrently.

REFERENCES

1. Berkman, Y. M., and Rabinowitz, J.: Am. J. Roentgenol. Radium Ther. Nucl. Med. **115:**306, 1972.

2. Yoshida, Y.: J. Parasitol. **57**:983, 1971.
3. Suzuki, T., Liu, K. H., Chen, S. N., et al.: Jpn. J. Parasitol. **22**:187, 1973.
4. Beaver, P. C.: J. Parasitol. **55**:3, 1969.
5. Nichols, R. L.: J. Parasitol. **42**:349, 1956.
6. Nichols, R. L.: J. Parasitol. **42**:363, 1956.
7. Chitwood, M., and Lichtenfels, J. R.: Exp. Parasitol. **32**:407, 1972.
8. Norman, L., and Donaldson, A. W.: Am. J. Trop. Med. Hyg. **4**:89, 1955.
9. Knott, J. I.: Trans. R. Soc. Trop. Med. Hyg. **31**:191, 1939.
10. Desowitz, R., and Hitchcock, J. C.: Am. J. Trop. Med. Hyg. **23**:877, 1974.
11. Proctor, E. M.: So. Afr. Med. J. **46**:234, 1972.
12. Proctor, E. M., Powell, S. J., and Elsdon-Dew, R.: Ann. Trop. Med. Parasitol. **60**:146, 1966.
13. Magath, T. B.: Am. J. Clin. Pathol. **31**:1, 1959.
14. Kagan, I. G., Allain, D. S., and Norman, L.: Am. J. Trop. Med. Hyg. **8**:51, 1959.
15. Garabedian, G. A., Matossian, R. M., and Sudian, F. G.: Am. J. Trop. Med. Hyg. **8**:67, 1959.
16. Kagan, I. G., Norman, L., and Allain, D. S.: Am. J. Trop. Med. Hyg. **9**:248, 1960.
17. Kagan, I. G., Norman, L., Allain, D. S., and Goodchild, C. G.: J. Immunol. **84**:635, 1960.
18. Chaffee, E. F., and Nieves, E. E.: Am. J. Trop. Med. Hyg. **67**:727, 1957.
19. Anderson, R. I., and Naimark, D. H.: Am. J. Trop. Med. Hyg. **9**:600, 1960.
20. Anderson, R. I.: Am. J. Trop. Med. Hyg. **9**:299, 1960.
21. Buck, A. A., and Anderson, R. I.: Am. J. Epidemiol. **96**:205, 1972.
22. Allain, D. S., Chisholm, E. S., and Kagan, I. G.: Public Health Rep. **87**:550, 1972.
23. McCarten, W. G., Nzelibe, F. N., Simonton, L. A., and Fife, E. H.: Exp. Parasitol. **37**:239, 1975.
24. Baldran, A., Alfi, D. E., Pfschner, W. C., et al.: Am. J. Trop. Med. Hyg **4**:1068, 1955.
25. Guillermo, P., Wykoff, D. S., and Jung, R. C.: Am. J. Trop. Med. Hyg. **9**:367, 1960.
26. Sadun, E. H., Walton, B. C., Buck, A. A., and Lee, B. K.: J. Parasitol. **45**:129, 1959.
27. Sadun, E. H., and Buck, A. A.: Am. J. Trop. Med. Hyg. **9**:562, 1960.
28. Kim, S. K., and Walker, S. E.: Acta Psychiatr. Neurol. Scand. **36**(suppl. 153):1, 1961.

99

ARTHROPODS

Michael H. Ivey

Arthropods are well known for their beneficial and destructive effects in the field of agriculture. Many species of arthropods also affect human health and well-being. Arthropods may affect the health of humans directly by invading and destroying tissue or by stings and bites and indirectly by transmitting disease agents. It is beyond the scope of this section to consider arthropods as transmitters of human disease. The arthropods and the diseases they transmit are listed in Table 99-2.

Arthropods characteristically are bilaterally symmetric, have a firm exoskeleton, and possess a segmented body with jointed appendages. Arthropods affecting human health belong to one of several classes.

Members of the class Chilopoda (centipedes and millipedes) possess a head and a trunk consisting of a series of similar segments, each with 1 or 2 pairs of legs. Members of the class Crustacea (crabs and copepods) are aquatic animals possessing 5 or more pairs of legs and 2 pairs of antennae. Members of the class Arachnida (ticks, mites, spiders, and scorpions) possess 4 pairs of legs as adults and no antennae. Members of the largest group, the class Insecta, possess 3 pairs of legs as adults, and the body is divided into a head, thorax, and abdomen. Members of the class Pentastomida are tongue shaped or moniliform with external pseudosegments.

ARTHROPODS INFESTING OR INVADING MAN
Sarcoptes scabei

Life cycle—epidemiology. *S. scabei*, the human itch mite, has a cosmopolitan distribution and infest domestic animals as well as humans. The infection in humans is called scabies and in other animals, mange. The adult mites burrow into tender epidermal areas between fingers, toes, shoulder blade, small of back, and genitalia. During its burrowing the female deposits eggs that hatch in a few days, releasing larvae. The larva begins its own burrow, maturing rapidly into a nymph, then into an adult, and then lays more eggs. The entire cycle from egg to egg may take only 1 or 2 weeks. Thus the parasite may spread quite rapidly. Transmission of this mite is usually by contact with an infested person, clothing, or bed linen contaminated with some stage of the mite. The infestation may cause intense irritation and itching. Scratching may cause secondary bacterial infections.

Diagnosis—morphology. Diagnosis is made by obtaining skin scrapings from affected parts containing the adults or immature stages. It is best to examine the affected skin closely, using a hand lens, to find the cutaneous burrows several millimeters to centimeters in length. The eggs may be in any portion of the burrow, but the adult female is at the terminal end of a fresh burrow. The skin should be mounted in 1 or 2 drops of 20% potassium hydroxide to effect clearing and then should be covered with a coverslip and examined microscopically.

The adult female (Figs. 99-1 and 99-2) measures from 330-450 μm in length by 250-350 μm in width. The male is considerably smaller and is rarely seen. The adult possesses 4 pairs of short

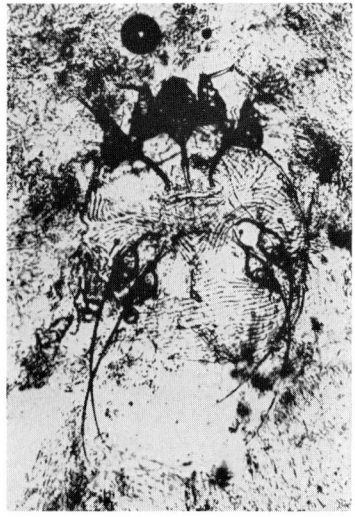

Fig. 99-1. Diagnosis of infestation by *Sarcoptes scabiei* var. *hominis* by slice, scrape, and smear method. Ventral view of female adult. (Official U. S. Navy photograph; photomicrograph by Lt. Comdr. E. A. Hand, (MC) USNR: U. S. Naval Med. Bull. **46**:834, 1946.)

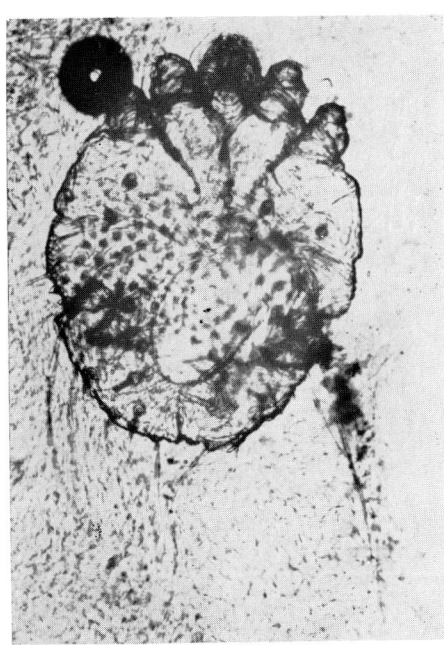

Fig. 99-2. Diagnosis of infestation with *Sarcoptes scabiei* var. *hominis* by slice, scrape, and smear method. High power of adult female showing egg in oviduct. (Official U. S. Navy photograph; photomicrograph by Lt. Comdr. E. A. Hand, (MC) USNR: U. S. Naval Med. Bull. **46:**834, 1946.)

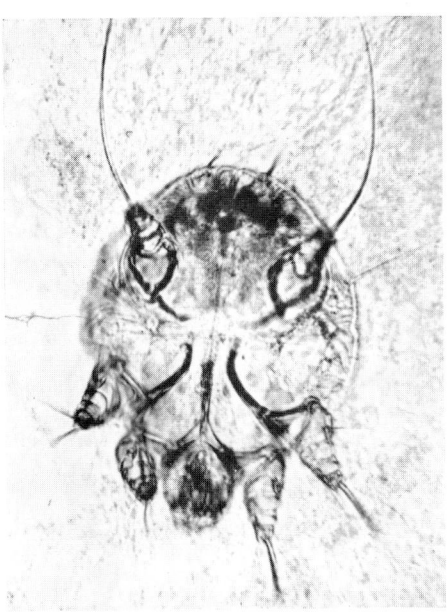

Fig. 99-3. Diagnosis of infestation with *Sarcoptes scabiei* var. *hominis* by slice, scrape, and smear method. Hexapod larva. High power. (Official U. S. Navy photograph; photomicrograph by Lt. Comdr. E. A. Hand, (MC) USNR: U. S. Naval Med. Bull. **46:**834, 1946.)

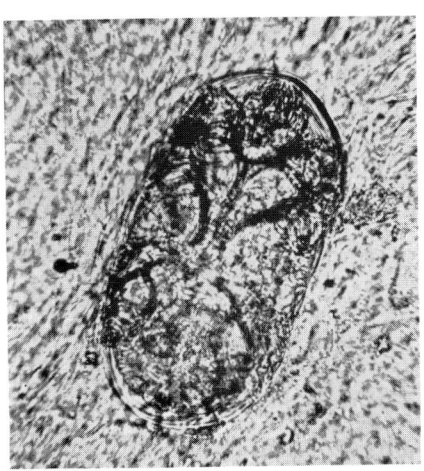

Fig. 99-4. Diagnosis of infestation with *Sarcoptes scabiei* var. *hominis* by slice, scrape, and smear method. Egg with embryo. High power. (Official U. S. Navy photograph; photomicrograph by Lt. Comdr. E. A. Hand, (MC) USNR: U. S. Naval Med. Bull. **46:**834, 1946.)

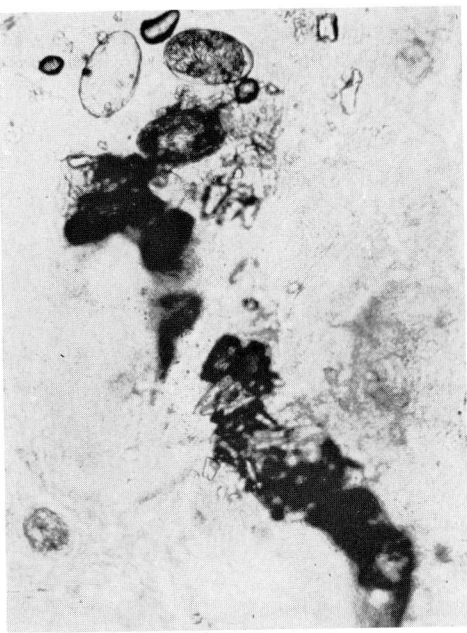

Fig. 99-5. Diagnosis of infestation with *Sarcoptes scabiei* var. *hominis* by slice, scrape, and smear method. Burrow showing eggs and mite feces or scybala. (Official U. S. Navy photograph; photomicrograph by Lt. Comdr. E. A. Hand, (MC) USNR: U. S. Naval Med. Bull. **46:**834, 1946.)

stump legs. One pair of legs may be seen on each side of the mouth parts, whereas the other 2 pairs of legs are located further back on the body and trail off in long hair bristles. The larval form (Fig. 99-3) possesses only 3 pairs of legs, 2 pairs around the mouth parts and 1 pair ventrally located. The eggs (Figs. 99-4 and 99-5) may also be seen in skin scrapings.

Pediculus humanus

Life cycle—epidemiology. *P. humanus,* the human body or head louse, has a cosmopolitan distribution but is associated with poor personal hygiene and environments in which persons are crowded together, especially during wars. Two varieties are recognized, the head louse, *P. humanus* var. *capitis,* and the body louse, *P. humanus* var. *corporis.* The head louse infests the scalp and deposits eggs (nits) onto hairs, where they are firmly attached. The eggs hatch in about 10 days, releasing nymphs that mature into adults in about 2 weeks. The adult and nymph feed on the blood. Outbreaks of epidemic proportions occur occasionally in school-age children.

The body louse has a similar life cycle but resides primarily on the body. The lice usually hide in the seams of clothing during the day and feed at night when the host is asleep. Lice can live about 15 days without a blood meal. The lice are extremely sensitive to temperature and will leave a person with high fever. Lice are transmitted from person to person by contact with clothing, hats, or hair of infected persons.

Heavily infested persons may develop characteristic papules and pruritus that probably are the result of hypersensitivity to the saliva and feces of the insect. Secondary bacterial infection may also occur. However, the most important role of the *P. humanus* is as **transmitter of epidemic typhus, trench fever, and epidemic relapsing fever.**

Diagnosis—morphology. The female body louse (Fig. 99-6) measures 2-4 mm in length and the male, 2-3 mm in length. The head louse is somewhat smaller and lighter. The head is spoon shaped, and the legs are equipped with terminal claws for grasping (Fig. 99-6). The relatively large abdomen is ridged and with obvious segments. The egg (Fig. 99-7) of the head louse measures about 0.8 mm; it is attached to hairs and resembles that of the crab louse. The eggs of the body louse are more frequently found in the clothing.

Diagnosis is based on finding the egg (nit) (Fig. 99-7) or the adult louse (Fig. 99-6).

Phthirius pubis

Life cycle—epidemiology. *P. pubis,* the pubic or crab louse, has a cosmopolitan distribution. It is found on the hairs of the genital region and occasionally on other parts of the body. The fe-

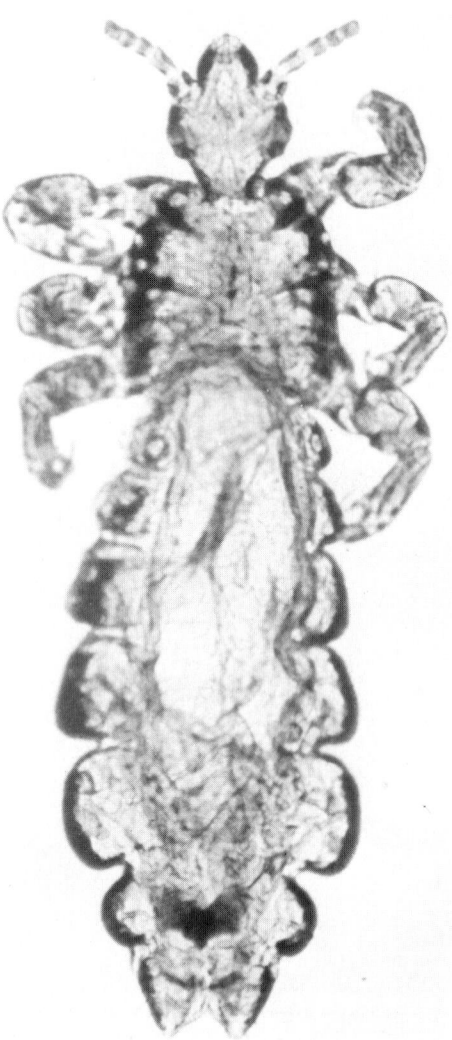

Fig. 99-6. Female body louse (*Pediculus humanus*).

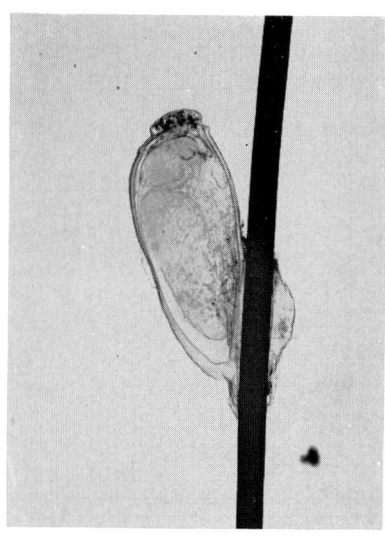

Fig. 99-7. *Pediculus humanus* egg (nit) attached to hair.

Table 99-1. Species of fly larvae most frequently causing myiasis in humans

Species	Tissue(s) invaded	Geographic location
Dermatobia hominis	Skin	Central and South America, Mexico
Hypoderma sp.	Skin, eye	North temperate zone
Gasterophilus sp.	Skin, rarely intestines	North America, Europe
Oestris ovis	Eye, nasopharynx	U.S.S.R., northern Africa, rare in U.S. and Europe
Rhinoestrus purpureus	Eye	Mostly U.S.S.R.
Cordylobia anthropophaga	Skin (usually feet)	Africa
Chrysoma bezziana	Nasal, skin, ear, vagina	Asia, Ethiopian region
Callitroga hominivorax	Skin	Western Hemisphere
Auchmeromyia luteola	Intermittent blood suckers	Africa
Wohlfahrtia magnifica	Skin, nasal, ear, eyes, vagina	Mediterranean region, U.S.S.R.
Wohlfahrtia vigil	Eyes, skin	U.S., Canada
Sarcophaga haemorrhoidalis	Skin, intestines	Tropical and subtropical zones
Calliphora sp.	Skin (lesions)	Tropical and subtropical zones
Fannia canicularis	Urethral tract	Widespread
Musca domestica	Intestine, urethral tract	Cosmopolitan

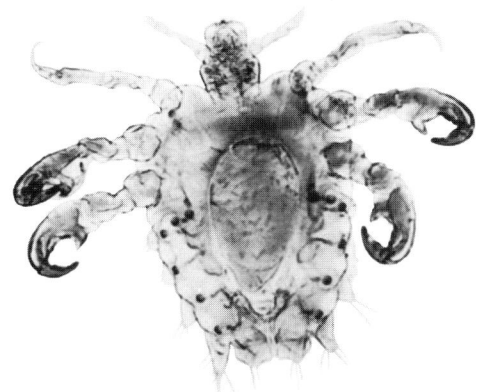

Fig. 99-8. Crab louse of humans, *Phthirius pubis*.

male deposits eggs (nits) on hairs. The developmental cycle is similar to that described for *Pediculus humanus*. Transmission is by close contact with infested individuals, their clothing, towels, etc. The lice do not travel readily, and transmission is dependent on transferral of the adult, nymph, or egg stages from one person to another.

The crab louse transmits no known disease. However, there may be local irritation and hypersensitive reactions to the presence of the insect. Secondary bacterial infection may occur.

Diagnosis—morphology. Diagnosis is made by demonstrating the adult (Fig. 99-8), nymph, or egg on pubic hair. The adult measures 1-1.2 mm in length and is relatively oblong or turtle shaped. It possesses 3 pairs of conspicuous legs, the latter 2 pairs possessing huge terminal claws for grasping onto hairs. The abdominal segments are indistinct.

Myiasis

Myiasis refers to a condition caused by fly larvae that invade living tissue. Invasion of tissue by fly larvae may be a necessary part of the developmental life cycle of the particular species, or it may be more or less accidental. Flies in the latter category usually deposit eggs in decaying organic matter but occasionally deposit eggs in foodstuff or perhaps lesions. All flies must undergo a similar developmental sequence. The adult deposits eggs in a suitable environment. The eggs develop and hatch, releasing larvae. The larvae develop into pupae and finally adults. Myiasis of humans in most instances is caused by deposition of the egg on tissue, and the resultant injury is due to larval development. Fly larvae have been recovered from skin, nasal passages, eyes, ears, urinary tract, and intestinal tract. The species of fly larvae most frequently affecting humans and the tissues invaded are shown in Table 99-1. Hundreds of species of flies have caused myiasis in humans at one time or another, and other sources should be consulted for more detailed accounts of myiasis. The consequences of myiasis vary with the tissue affected. In the skin painful ulcers may be produced. In the eye severe irritation and pain are usually present. Nasal myiasis results in severe irritation and sometimes death. Intestinal myiasis may cause nervous symptoms as well as intestinal irritation.

Definitive diagnosis of myiasis is made by finding the larvae, which are small whitish yellow to light brown, wormlike, and usually consist of 11-12 segments. Usually each segment has a crown of fine hooklets or hairs. The mouth shows 2 deeply stained, sharp hooklets. On the posterior end of the larva are dark spots that are the openings to the respiratory structures. The larval stages are difficult to identify as to species, although they may be classified into groups on the basis of certain patterns on the stigmal plates on the posterior segment. Positive identification as to species is based on adult morphology and requires an expert in fly classification. If live larvae (maggots) are obtained, they should be placed in a cotton-plugged container with raw meat on moist sand 5-10 cm deep at room tem-

Table 99-2. More important arthropod transmitters of disease to humans

Class and genus	Disease	Etiologic agent	Arthropod's role
Class Crustacea			
1. *Cyclops* (copepod)	Dracontiasis	*Dracunculus medinensis*	Copepod ingest larvae from water; humans infected by ingesting infected copepods
2. *Cyclops* (copepod)	Diphyllobothriasis	*Diphyllobothrium latum*	Copepod ingests coracidium; humans infected by ingesting fish that ingested copepod
3. *Diaptomus* (copepod)	Diphyllobothriasis	*Diphyllobothrium latum*	Copepod ingests coracidium; humans infected by ingesting fish that ingested copepod
4. Various crabs, crayfish	Paragonimiasis	*Paragonimus westermani*	Crab infected by cercariae; humans ingests infected crab
Class Arachnida			
1. *Dermacentor* (ticks) *Rhipicephalus* *Amblyomma* *Ornithodorus* and others	Spotted fever Q fever Tularemia	*Rickettsia rickettsi* *Coxiella burneti* *Francisella tularensis*	Tick ingests agent from infected human; human infected at blood meal of tick or inhalation of tick feces (Q fever)
2. *Ornithodorus*	Endemic relapsing fever	*Borrelia duttoni*	Tick ingests agent from infected human; human infected at blood meal of tick
3. *Trombicula* (mite)	Scrub typhus	*Rickettsia tsutsutsugamushi*	Mite ingests agent from infected human; human infected at blood meal of mite
4. *Allodermanyssus* (mite)	Rickettsialpox	*Rickettsia akari*	Mite ingests agent from human or mice; human infected at blood meal of mite
Class Insecta			
1. *Pediculus humanus* (lice)	Epidemic typhus Trench fever Epidemic relapsing fever	*Rickettsia prowazeki* *Rickettsia quintana* *Borrelia recurrentis*	Louse ingests agent from human; human infected by bite, feces, or crushing of louse; agent enters bite site
2. *Xenopsylla* (flea) *Pulex* (flea)	Plague	*Yersinia pestis*	Flea ingests agent from infected human or rat; human infected at blood meal of flea
3. *Xenopsylla*	Murine typhus	*Rickettsia typhi*	Flea ingests agent from infected human or rat; human infected via flea feces
4. *Ctenocephalides* (flea)	Dipylidiasis	*Dipylidium caninum*	Flea larva ingests egg; dog and human infected by ingesting flea
5. *Anopheles* (mosquito)	Malaria	*Plasmodium* sp.	Mosquito ingests sexual stages; progeny injected back into human
6. *Aedes* (mosquito)	Yellow fever	Yellow fever virus, dengue virus	Mosquito ingests agent from infected human; human infected at blood meal of mosquito
7. *Culex, Aedes, Mansonia*	Encephalitis Western equine St. Louis Eastern equine Japanese B	Viruses	Mosquito ingests agent from infected human or animal; human infected at blood meal of mosquito
8. *Culex, Aedes, Anopheles, Mansonia*	Filariasis	*Wuchereria bancrofti* *Brugia malayi*	Mosquito ingests microfilariae from humans; human infected at blood meal of mosquito
9. *Glossina* (tsetse fly)	Sleeping sickness	*Trypanosoma gambiense* *Trypanosoma rhodesiense*	Fly ingests trypanosome from infected human or animals (?); human infected at blood meal
10. *Simulium* (black fly)	Onchocerciasis	*Onchocerca volvulus*	Fly ingests microfilariae from infected human; human infected at blood meal of fly
11. *Chrysops* (deer fly)	Loiasis	*Loa loa*	Fly ingests microfilariae from infected human; human infected at blood meal of fly

Table 99-2. More important arthropod transmitters of disease to humans—cont'd

Class and genus	Disease	Etiologic agent	Arthropod's role
	Tularemia	Francisella tularensis	Fly ingests bacteria from infected human or rodents; human infected at blood meal of fly
12. Phlebotomus (sand fly)	Leishmaniasis (all kinds)	Leishmania donovani, L. tropica, L. braziliensis	Fly ingests Leishmania from infected human; human infected at blood meal of fly
	Bartonellosis	Bartonella bacilliformis	Fly ingests agent from infected human; human infected at blood meal of fly
13. Triatoma, Rhodnius, Panstrongylus (triatomid bug)	Chagas' disease	Trypanosoma cruzi	Bug ingests agent from human or animals; human infected by inoculation of feces as bug ingests blood

perature. The larvae will develop in the meat and enter the sand to pupate before becoming adult flies. Once the adult emerges it may be identified by an entomologist. Care should be taken that maggots seen in urine or feces were not the result of egg deposition **after** the specimen was passed.

Tunga penetrans

T. penetrans, the chigoe flea, is found in humans and other animals in tropical and subtropical climates. The flea life cycle consists of egg, larva, pupa, and adult stages. The fertilized female chigoe flea burrows under the skin, preferably under the toenails, where she feeds on blood. The female enlarges due to blood engorgement and egg development, causing a painful area often secondarily infected with bacteria. If allowed to persist the female eventually expels her eggs onto the soil and then drops off the host.

Diagnosis is made by detecting the dark posterior of the flea protruding from the burrow. The flea may be removed surgically and studied further.

HARMFUL EFFECTS OF ARTHROPODS
Arthropods as transmitters of disease

Arthropods are of major importance as transmitters of disease. It is beyond the scope of this section to consider this subject. Certain arthropods, especially various species of flies and cockroaches, have been incriminated as mechanical carriers of fecal-borne diseases. These insects often feed or breed in fecal debris and later visit human food supplies, carrying the infectious agent with them. Certain flies, *Hippelates* species transmit yaws and conjunctivitis by mechanical transfer of the organism from person to person. Other arthropods serve as biologic carriers and vectors of diseases. The infectious agent is ingested or penetrates into the arthropod and undergoes development or multiplication within its body. The arthropod then transmits the disease back to humans while seeking a blood meal or on being ingested. In rickettsial diseases the infectious agent may be passed congenitally

to the offspring of the vectors, ticks or mites. A summary of the more important arthropods that transmit disease to humans is shown in Table 99-2.

Other harmful effects of arthropods

In addition to transmitting diseases arthropods affect human health by their bites or stings. Well known are the painful effects of bee and wasp stings. Occasionally stings of these insects result in death, especially in hypersensitive individuals. In the southern United States and Latin America fire ants, *Solenopsis saevissima* var. *richteri*, can cause painful pustular eruptions by their stings. The bite of the black widow spider, *Latrodectus mactans*, can cause much pain, abdominal muscle rigidity, respiratory difficulties, and even death. The severity is related to the size of the spider and the victim. Other spiders may cause painful necrotic lesions. The bite of the

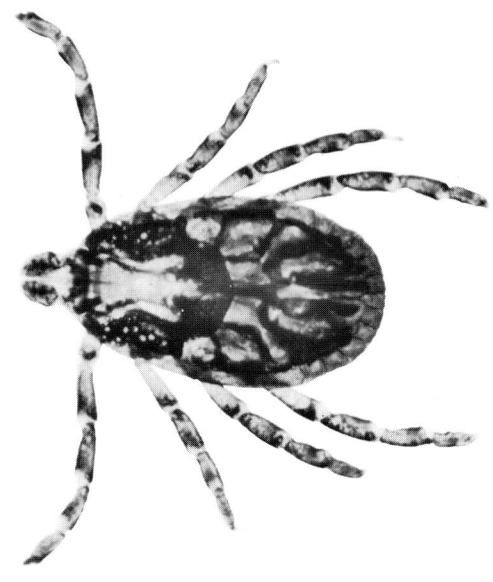

Fig. 99-9. Adult *Dermacentor* tick.

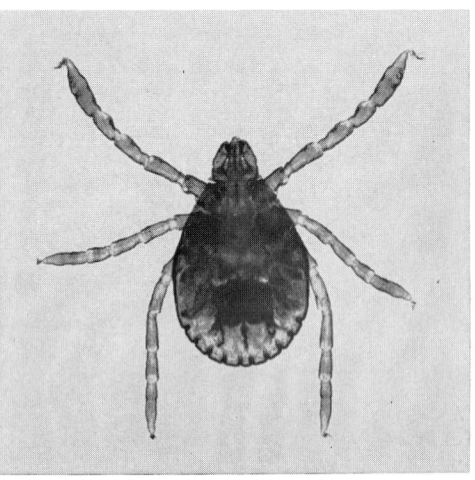

Fig. 99-10. *Dermacentor* larva. Note only 3 pairs of legs; adult has 4 pairs.

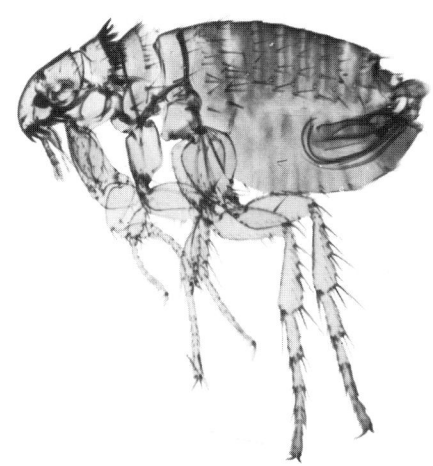

Fig. 99-11. Dog flea, *Ctenocephalides canis.*

brown spider, *Loxosceles reclusus* and other species of this genus, has been shown to cause painful necrotic lesions. Scorpions, belonging to the genus *Centruroides*, may cause painful reactions and may be very dangerous in the southwest United States and Mexico where the scorpions grow quite large.

In addition to transmitting various diseases, certain ticks may cause a condition known as tick paralysis. The tick, attached somewhere on the body but usually along the spinal column, apparently secretes a toxic substance that produces a progressive ascending flaccid motor paralysis. The only cure is the removal of the tick. Adult ticks (Fig. 99-9) may be recognized by their saclike shape and the presence of 4 pairs of legs as adults. Larvae (Fig. 99-10) resemble adults but possess only 3 pairs of legs.

A minor but persistent problem is caused each summer by the larval chigger, *Eutrombicula alfreddugesi*. This larval mite injects lytic fluid that causes irritable spots. Scratching to relieve the intense itch often causes a secondary bacterial infection.

Certain relatively large arthropods may bite or sting humans. The centipede if provoked will inject a toxic substance causing a local reaction. Millipedes may secrete a mildly irritating fluid.

Various species of fleas (Fig. 99-11) may either transmit disease or cause irritating bites.

Occasionally pentastomes (tongue worms) occur in humans. The adults live in the lungs and body cavities of reptiles, birds, and mammals. Eggs escape in the sputum. If ingested by a human the larvae escape from the eggs and migrate to the liver, spleen, lymph nodes, lungs, and other sites. They transform into nymphs and remain encapsulated in the host tissue. In most cases the parasite causes no demonstrable symptoms. Rarely marked inflammation develops in multiple infections. Diagnosis usually occurs postmortem as an incidental finding. Recent epidemiologic evidence suggests that pentastomiasis may predispose to cancer.

100

LABORATORY PROCEDURES IN PARASITOLOGY

Michael H. Ivey

Intestinal or fecal parasites
General considerations

Fecal specimens are best collected in water-tight cardboard containers. The specimen should not contain urine, oils, magnesium, barium, aluminum, bismuth, or iron salts, since they may alter morphologic features of protozoa. If purged stools are to be collected, sodium sulfate (Glauber's salts) should be used as the purgative.

A record should be made of the kind of fecal material examined. The consistency, color, and nature of the feces should be described in some manner. The code in Table 100-1 has been found useful.

Before making a microscopic examination of a fecal specimen, examine the gross specimen for consistency and the presence of blood, mucus, or other elements as suggested above. Occasionally worms or proglottids may be seen in the fecal mass by the naked eye. Tapeworm proglottids and scolices, adult *Enterobius, Ascaris,* and *Trichuris,* and hookworms may be identified if present in the feces. The worms may be picked off the fecal mass. If recovery of worms that may not be visible is desired, the feces may be made into a watery suspension and poured through a series of graduated sieves stacked on each other. Usually 3 sieves—10, 20, and 40 meshes—will suffice. Additional water is then poured through the sieves to remove excess fecal debris. Worms, if present, may be seen either with the naked eye or with the aid of a hand lens. The worms are best seen against a black background.

The consistency of the fecal specimen determines the manner in which it should be processed for examination for protozoa. Loose, diarrheic, or watery stools, containing primarily the trophozoite stage, must be examined **immediately,** or typical trophozoite movement ceases and the organism degenerates beyond recognition. Formed stools contain primarily cyst stages and may be kept in the refrigerator several days without destroying morphologic characteristics. Fecal specimens to be examined for helminth eggs may be stored in the refrigerator for several days without harm. However, if the fecal specimen cannot be examined soon after passage, it is usually best to preserve portions of the specimen by one of the methods considered (see "Preservation of parasites found in feces," pp. 2171-2174).

The laboratory worker has access to numerous diagnostic procedures of proved worth. The choice of tests depends on the condition of the specimen and on the availability of equipment, time, and interest. The following procedures are adequate for the different types of specimens.

1. **Fresh specimen**—direct saline for protozoa, helminth eggs, and larvae; iodine smear for protozoan cysts; vital stain for identification of trophozoites if a hematoxylin- or trichrome-stained smear is not done; concentration by zinc sulfate flotation or formalin-ether sedimentation for protozoan cysts and helminth eggs or larvae; hematoxylin- or trichrome-stained permanent smears of protozoa-positive specimens for confirmation and reference purposes.
2. **Old specimens**—zinc sulfate flotation or formalin-ether sedimentation for protozoan cysts, helminth eggs, or larvae. Protozoan trophozoites are not likely to be identifiable in old specimens.
3. **Preserved specimens**—in formalin: formalin-ether sedimentation for cysts, eggs, and larvae. In Merthiolate-iodine-formalin (MIF): direct wet smears for all forms. In polyvinyl alcohol (PVA): hematoxylin- or trichrome-stained films for protozoan trophozoites and cysts.
4. **Aspirated material from colon**—direct saline smear and hematoxylin- or trichrome-stained smears for trophozoites.

DIRECT FECAL SMEARS (TEMPORARY)
Direct saline fecal smear

Helminth eggs can be detected and usually identified under low-power magnification (100×), but high-power magnification (430×) may aid in identification after finding them under low power. Amebic trophozoites and cysts can be detected, but they must be stained for positive identification (exception, *Entamoeba histolytica* cysts containing chromatoid bars or trophozoites containing red blood cells). The trophozoites or flagellates can be identified by characteristic appearance and locomotion. Vital stains (pp. 2167-2168) are suitable temporary preparations, whereas permanent smears may be stained with hematoxylin (p. 2168) or trichrome (p. 2169). The permanent stains give better results than temporary stain preparations.

Procedure
1. Place 1 or 2 drops physiologic saline on a slide.
2. With applicator stick, select a 1-2 mg fecal sample

Table 100-1. Fecal characteristics

Consistency	Color	Nature
1. Hard (resists puncture)	1. Black	1. Nearly all pulp and fiber
2. Formed (can be punctured)	2. Dark brown	2. Conspicuously fibrous
3. Soft (can be cut)	3. Brown	3. Scanty to moderate fiber
4. Mushy (can be reshaped)	4. Pale brown	4. All colloidal feces
5. Loose (assumes shape of container)	5. Yellow	5. Feces with scanty mucus
6. Diarrheic (flows)	6. Green	6. Feces with much mucus
7. Watery (pours)	7. Clay	7. Mucus with scanty feces
	8. Other	8. Other (blood, barium, etc.)

(1 mg feces is about 1 mm³). Avoid selecting non-fecal elements unless schistosome eggs or amebae are suspected, in which case select flecks of mucus and blood.

3. Stir into saline and make homogeneous suspension. Remove coarse fibers, seeds, sand, etc.

4. Cover with 22 × 22 mm cover slip. If of proper consistency, print of newspaper will be just legible through smear after applying cover glass.

5. Satisfactory smear contains maximum of observable fecal elements without any objects of protozoan size (8-30 μm diameter) being obscured. If preparation is too dilute or too concentrated, discard it and prepare another. For convenience many laboratory workers prepare saline fecal smear on one end of slide and iodine-stained fecal smear on other end of same slide to aid in identification of protozoan cysts.

Examination of smear. The fecal sme   should be examined under low-power magnification. A magnification of 100× is ample for detecting the presence of protozoan cysts or helminth eggs. After detecting suspicious objects, examine closely under 430× for greater morphologic detail. Do **not** look for fecal parasites routinely with 430×. This is a time-consuming procedure that may result in fewer parasites being detected. However, certain very small protozoans may be overlooked unless a portion of the slide is checked at 430×. The fecal smear should be examined systematically. Start at the lower left edge of the smear and examine field by field until you reach the lower right edge. Then move the preparation **up** 1 field and move back toward the left. Examine the entire preparation in this left to right, right to left manner. Obviously this can only be done correctly by using a mechanical stage. Without a mechanical stage you increase your chances of missing parasites as well as chances of contaminating your fingers with fecal material.

Common errors to avoid

1. Making preparations too thick, with the result that parasites are obscured in the dense fecal masses; there should be no large clumps of fecal material under the cover glass.

2. Making preparations too thin, with the result that parasites are not detected unless extremely numerous; the desired density of the fecal emulsion on the slide is often described as one that is **uniform throughout** and through which the print of a newspaper can be discerned after applying the cover slips.

3. Failure to use cover slips, with resultant drying of the smear, fogging and contamination of the lens, and rapid loss of the stain.

4. Employing tap water instead of physiologic saline; tap water destroys or alters trophozoites.

5. Failure to employ both saline- and iodine-stained smears on a fecal slide; both sides of the double fecal smear serve distinct purposes and supplement each other.

6. **Most beginners use too much illumination.** Keep the substage condenser near the stage.

Control light primarily by adjusting the aperture of the substage diaphragm and secondarily by means of ground glass or blue glass filters. With proper lighting, fecal objects will exhibit maximum color contrast and depth when examined.

Direct iodine-stained fecal smear

Special solution required
1. Iodine stain. For preparation see "Reagents," p. 2195.

Procedure
1. Place 1 drop iodine on a slide.
2. Proceed as described under "Direct fecal smear" (p. 2166).

This method stains protzoan cysts for identification but is not suitable for protozoan trophozoites because the stain renders them unidentifiable.

Direct fecal smear—Merthiolate-iodine-formalin (MIF)[1]

This stain may be used as a preservative stain (MF) or as a temporary direct wet smear for identification of all protozoan stages. The trophozoite stains immediately, whereas the cyst stains more slowly.

Special solutions required
1. Lugol's solution. See p. 2194.
2. Merthiolate-formalin (MF) solution. See p. 2194.

Procedure
1. Combine 1.0 ml MF solution and 0.1 ml freshly prepared Lugol's solution in small tube. If Lugol solution is over 1 wk old, increase 0.1 to 0.125 ml; if over 2 wk old, increase to 0.15 ml. Reduce volume of tincture of Merthiolate in MF solution by same volume that Lugol's solution is increased. These stain ingredients should be combined only just prior to use in fecal smear.
2. Place 1 drop MIF stain into 1 drop distilled water on slide and make wet smear as described under "Direct saline fecal smear" (p. 2166).

Direct fecal smear—Quensel vital stain[2]

The Quensel vital stain may be used as a quick, easy way to identify amebic trophozoites in temporary fecal smears. The Quensel-stained nuclei present the same morphologic characteristics seen in permanent hematoxylin preparations. Amebic cysts, ciliates, and flagellates do not stain. *Dientamoeba* nuclei do not stain as well as desired. *Blastocystis hominis* stains nicely and can be easily differentiated from amebae. However, none of the vital stains is considered the equal of hematoxylin- or trichrome-stained smears.

Special solution required
Quensel solution. See p. 2195.

Procedure
1. Emulsify small amount of feces in large drop of Quensel solution and cover with coverslip.
2. After 10-20 min, examine under low- and high-power magnification. After a period of time (1-2 h), organisms overstain and can no longer be identified.

Direct fecal smear—Valet-Weinstein-Otto vital stain[3]

This stain was designed to stain trophozoites of the intestinal amebae in fresh preparations and, in particular, to be used for the differentiation of *Entamoeba histolytica* in routine examinations.

Special solution required
Valet-Weinstein-Otto stain. See p. 2195.
Procedure
Use of stain. Trophozoites may be stained by mixing small quantity of fecal material into 1 or 2 drops of stain on slide. Coverslip is added and preparation examined in usual manner. Trophozoites from culture are stained in similar manner by mixing 1 drop culture with 1 drop stain on slide.

Staining reactions. Critical differential staining of trophozoites is completed in 3-5 min at pH 4.6-4.8 or in 5-15 min at pH 5.2-5.4. With latter range, organisms do not tend to overstain. During the first few minutes trophozoites usually round up and can be located by their refractility while the particulate material stains a light purple against the faintly pink background of the solution. Gradually the nucleus and karyosome stain purple-black and the cytoplasm a light purple. Trophozoites from cultures do not differ in their staining reactions. Mature amebic cysts rarely stain, but occasionally penetration into young cysts occurs. Trophozoites of flagellates usually become immobilized and tend to swell to some extent; however, characteristic structures of the various species often become more easily visible. The chromatin in the nucleus of *Chilomastix mesnili* stains a light purple; the nucleus of *Trichomonas hominis* colors slowly, with many small purplish granules becoming visible; the nuclear membrane, fibrils, and flagella of *Giardia lamblia* stain a purple-black, whereas the cytoplasm stains a light purple-pink color. In *Blastocystis hominis* the cytoplasm and nuclei stain faintly, whereas the vacuole usually disappears. The entire cell becomes dull and graunlar in appearance. Nuclei and cytoplasm of leukocytes, macrophages, and epithelial cells stain similar to amebae.

Perianal fecal debris examination[4]

The fecal material from around the anus is usually examined for diagnosis of *Enterobius* (pinworm) infections. Often *Taenia* eggs, undetected by direct smear examinations, are also found in perianal swabs.

The fecal swab should be collected either late at night or early in the morning before bathing or defecation. Three or 4 samples, collected on alternate nights, should be examined before a negative diagnosis for pinworms is made.

Procedures
1. Cut a 6 in. strip of adhesive cellulose tape and bend over sides of tongue depressor, sticky side out. (Tongue depressors that have been squared on one end are easier to handle.)
2. Holding tape close to sides of applicator with finger and thumb, spread buttocks to expose anus and press sticky tape surface against right and left perianal folds.
3. Place tape, sticky side down, on clean slide containing drop of toluene or xylene. Be sure the section of tape containing fecal debris comes in contact with toluene. Excess tape on either side of slide may be cut and discarded.

4. Search for pinworm eggs under low-power magnification ($100\times$).

PERMANENTLY STAINED FECAL SMEARS
Iron-hematoxylin–stained fecal smears

The iron-hematoxylin–staining procedure utilized for staining intestinal protozoa reveals the best morphologic detail and is recommended for trophozoites or unidentifiable cysts seen in saline or iodine wet preparations. Permanent smears should be prepared as soon as possible after specimens have been passed to prevent trophozoite deterioration. However, such deterioration may be prevented either by refrigeration of the specimen or, better, by preservation in polyvinyl alcohol (PVA). For PVA preservation see p. 2172. Formalin preserved protozoan cannot be stained with hematoxylin or trichrome.

Special solutions required
1. Fixative (Schaudinn solution). See p. 2194.
2. Iodine-alcohol. See p. 2196.
3. Mordant. See p. 2196.
4. Iron-hematoxylin stock stain, diluted. See p. 2195.
5. Destaining solution. See p. 2196.
6. Carbolxylene. See p. 2196.

Procedure. Directions for the procedures appear simple but in reality considerable practice is required before consistently good results are obtained. Using applicator stick, make thin smear of feces on clean 3×1 in. slide. If necessary, dilute feces with physiologic saline. **The smear must not be permitted to dry at any step of the procedure.** If it is necessary to interrupt the staining schedule before or after the mordant stain process, smears may be stored in 70% alcohol indefinitely without subsequently changing the regular procedure. If it is necessary to interrupt between the mordant and stain, store smears in 70% alcohol, but repeat the mordanting step when ready to complete the staining.

1. Fix smears in Schaudinn solution 5 min at 50 C or 1 h at room temperature. (**Omit this step if smears are fixed in PVA.**)
2. Place in iodine-alcohol 5 min (20 min for PVA smear).
3. Place in 50% alcohol 3 min.
4. Wash in tap water 3 min.
5. Place in mordant 10-20 min at 40-50 C or 12-24 h at room temperature. This solution must be prepared fresh daily.
6. Wash in water (distilled or tap), 2 changes for 3 min (total).
7. Place in diluted iron-hematoxylin 5-10 min at 40-50 C or 12-24 h at room temperature.
8. Wash in tap water, 2 changes, 3 min (total).
9. Place in destaining solution; time required is determined by periodic microscopic examination. This is the critical step in this technic. Destaining usually requires 1-3 min or more, depending on smear thickness, organism, and other factors. Before observing under microscope, place coverslip over wet preparation to keep it moist. Examine under low and high power. Organisms may be totally black at first, but as destaining proceeds, nuclear structures become evident. Slide is properly stained (and destained) when structures can be seen within nucleus, but chromatin still stains black. Cytoplasm should stain grayish or blue.
10. Wash in gently running water at least 5 min (30 min preferred).

11. Place in 70% alcohol containing a few drops saturated lithium carbonate solution per Coplin jar for 3 min.
12. Place in 95% alcohol 3 min.
13. Place in carbolxylene 3 min.
14. Place in xylene 3 min.
15. Mount in Permount; use no. 1 coverglass.
16. Examine at least 15 min using oil-immersion objective.

Automatic destaining technic. All steps are same as outlined above except 2 % aqueous solution of phosphotungstic acid or saturated picric acid solution (made up at least 1 day prior to use) is substituted for destaining solution used in step 9. Time required for destaining in phosphotungstic acid solution is not critical—merely 2 min or longer. Destaining in picric acid usually requires 5-10 min and must be monitored to prevent excessive destaining.

Trichrome-stained fecal smear

The trichrome technic is a rapid procedure giving good results for routine identification of intestinal protozoa in fresh fecal specimens. Instructions for preparation and handling of fecal smears to be stained are described above (see Procedure). The trichrome stain is stable and may be used repeatedly. Any volume of stain lost during use may be replaced with additional stock solution. The iodine-alcohol may also be used repeatedly. Other solutions should be discarded after the day's use. Staining of over 14 smears daily tends to weaken the stain. Strength will return if the stain is exposed to air 3-8 h.

Special solutions required
1. Schaudinn fixative. See p. 2194.
2. Iodine-alcohol. See p. 2196.
3. Trichrome stain. See p. 2196.
4. Xylene or toluene.

Procedure
1. Smear feces on slides with sticks or brushes and **immediately** place in Schaudinn fixative for 1 h at room temperature (omit this step if fixed in PVA); overnight fixation is acceptable. Amount of feces spread on slide should be thin enough that newsprint can be read through smear. If stool is hard, it will be necessary to soften with saline before making smears on slide.
2. Place in 70% ethyl alcohol 5 min.*
3. Place in 70% ethyl alcohol plus iodine (portwine color) 2-5 min (10 min for PVA smear).
4. Place successively in 2 changes of 70% ethyl alcohol for 5 min in each solution.*
5. Place in trichrome stain 10 min.
6. Dip briefly (2-3 s) in 90% acidified ethyl alcohol (1 drop glacial acetic acid in 10 ml alcohol).
7. Dip once or twice in 100% ethyl alcohol to remove decolorizing agent.
8. Place in 2 changes of 100% ethyl alcohol for 2-5 min each.*
9. Place in 2 changes of xylene or toluene for 2-5 min each (10 for PVA smear).*
10. Quickly mount in Permount or other mounting medium; use no. 1 thickness coverglass.

Staining reaction. Thoroughly fixed and well-stained *E. histolytica* trophozoites and cysts exhibit blue-green

---

*Slides may be left in this solution several hours or overnight.

tinged with purple cytoplasm. *E. coli* cysts are slightly more purple. Karyosomes of nuclei stain brilliant ruby red. Degenerated organisms stain pale green. Organisms in thick smears stain neutral shades of red and green. Background material usually stains green, resulting in noticeable color contrast with protozoa. If nonstaining cysts or predominantly red-stained cysts are seen in trichrome-stained PVA-preserved specimens, it usually indicates incomplete fixation due to poor emulsification of feces in PVA.

Chlorazol black E–stained fecal smear

Fixation and staining take place in a single solution in this simple procedure. The stain gives good results with fresh fecal smears but is less satisfactory with PVA-fixed material. (PVA-fixed specimens stain better with iron-hematoxylin or trichrome). See p. 2194 for stain preparation.

The optimum staining dilution and time must be determined for each liter of new stock solution. Stock stain remains stable indefinitely, and stain dilutions may be used repeatedly until it "wears out," i.e., when slides appear visibly red rather than greenish black at the end of the staining period. (Approximately 20 slides can be stained adequately in a 50 ml Coplin jar before stain deteriorates.) Stain deterioration is dependent on the number of slide stains and not on time. Slides that are inadequately stained (red appearance) can be restained in fresh stain.

The optimum dilution and staining time must be determined for each stock solution of stain. Trial smears should be stained in varying dilutions of stain as outlined below.

Stock stain	Basic solution	Hours
Undiluted	—	2-3
1	1	2-4 to overnight
2	1	2-4
1	2	2-overnight
1	3	4-overnight

More than one dilution-time combination may give good results. The choice may depend on the laboratory schedule and urgency of diagnosis. The range must frequently satisfactory is a 1:2 dilution for 2 hours or a 1:3 for 4 hours or overnight. A dilution producing good overnight staining does not appear to overstain when left in stain for several days.

Staining technic
Stock stain (use dilution and time predetermined as outlined above)	2 h to overnight
Ethyl alcohol 95%	1-15 s
Ethyl alcohol 100%	5 min
Xylene	5 min

Mount in Permount and cover with no. 1 coverglass

CONCENTRATION TECHNICS FOR PARASITES IN FECES

Many different concentration procedures and modifications of procedures are available for concentrating helminth eggs and larvae and protozoan cysts. With the exception of the Merthiolate-iodine-formaldehyde concentration

(MIFC) procedure, none of the procedures claims to concentrate amebic trophozoites.

Concentration procedures may be divided into 2 general types—**flotation** and **sedimentation.** Flotation procedures concentrate most nonoperculated helminth eggs and all protozoan cysts. Schistosome eggs do not concentrate well by flotation procedures. In flotation procedures the specific gravity of the suspending fluid (usually zinc sulfate at sp gr 1.18) causes the eggs and cysts to float to the top, whereas the heavier debris sinks to the bottom. Sedimentation procedures concentrate all helminth eggs and protozoan cysts, and in a sense they are more versatile than flotation procedures. In sedimentation procedures the parasites concentrate in the sediment at the bottom of the tube, and the mass of the fecal debris collects in a stratified layer above the sediment.

Formalin-ether centrifugal sedimentation technic[5]

The formalin-ether sedimentation technic is excellent for the detection and identification of protozoan cysts and helminth eggs and larvae of most all intestinal parasites. The technic is also very useful for examining stools containing fatty substances that interfere with the performance of the zinc sulfate centrifugal flotation method. It is not satisfactory for trophozoites.

1. Place approximately 10 ml 10% formalin in saline into small beaker or unwaxed paper cup. Add feces (about size of marble) to solution and mix well, using 2 applicator sticks. Let stand minimum of 30 min for adequate fixation.
2. Strain fecal suspension through small funnel or 4 oz cone-shaped paper cup containing 2 layers of wet cheesecloth gauze into 15 ml centrifuge tube. Squeeze excess fluid from feces by pressing cheesecloth with applicator sticks.
3. Centrifuge at 1500 rpm 2 min. Decant supernatant by turning tube upside down. About 0.5-1.0 ml sediment should be present. If too much is present, resuspend sediment in formalin-saline, pour off part of it, and centrifuge again. If too little feces is present, then emulsify and strain additional feces as described in steps 1 and 2, add to tube of feces, mix, and centrifuge again.
4. Fill tube about half full with 10% formalin-saline and mix well with sediment.
5. Add approximately 3 ml ether, plug tube with rubber stopper, and shake vigorously at least 30 s. Hold tube away from body during shaking, since shaking may cause increased pressure in tube. Remove stopper with care.
6. Centrifuge at about 1500 rpm 3 min. Four layers should result as follows: (1) small amount of sediment at bottom containing most of parasites, (2) layer of formalin, (3) plug of fecal debris, and (4) top layer of ether.
7. Carefully ring plug of debris with applicator stick to free it from sides of tube. Pour off supernatant fluid. If necessary, use cotton swab to clean debris from walls of tube.
8. Mix remaining sediment with small amount of fluid that drains back from sides of tube.

9. Use applicator stick to drag drop of sediment to lip of tube. Place drop of sediment on slide and mix with similar amount of iodine stain.

NOTE: If specimen has been previously washed, strained, and fixed in formalin, take 10 ml thoroughly mixed specimen and start at step 5. For unwashed, preserved specimens start at step 2.

Merthiolate-iodine-formaldehyde concentration (MIFC)[1]

Specimens in MIF preservative (p. 2170) can be concentrated by this method. The procedure concentrates all helminth eggs and protozoa. It has the additional advantage of staining all stages of protozoa for identification purposes. The specimen should be processed within 1 week of preservation or the method may lose its efficiency.

Special solutions required
1. MF preservative solution. See p. 2194.
2. Lugol solution. See p. 2194.
Procedure
1. Pour 2.35 MF solution in 0.15 ml Lugol solution and mix immediately. Quickly add feces (approximately the size of a pea) and thoroughly mix. Proportions may be doubled if desirable to examine larger fecal sample.
2. Mix MIF-preserved specimen thoroughly.
3. Strain mixture through 2 layers of wet surgical gauze into cup or beaker and pour into 15 ml centrifuge tube. Ideally, strained specimen should contain about 0.5 ml sediment.
4. Add 4 ml ether to tube, stopper, and shake vigorously. If ether remains on top after shaking, add 1 ml tap water and shake again.
5. Remove stopper and let stand 2 min.
6. Centrifuge 1 min at 1600 rpm. Four layers will appear in tube: (a) ether layer on top, (b) plug of fecal detritus, (c) MIF layer, and (d) bottom layer of sediment containing protozoa and helminth eggs.
7. Loosen fecal detritus plug by ringing with applicator stick.
8. Quickly, but carefully, pour off all but bottom layer of sediment.
9. Mix sediment, pour drop on slide, mount with coverglass, and examine under low-power magnification (100×).

Zinc sulfate flotation concentration[6,7]

The zinc sulfate flotatin method concentrates protozoan cysts and most nonoperculate helminth eggs. The zinc sulfate method is unsuitable for fatty stools. The formalin-ether sedimentation method is better suited for eggs of trematodes and large tapeworms (*Taenia* and *Diphyllobothrium*); otherwise both methods give similar results.

Special solution required
Zinc sulfate solution, sp gr 1.18. See p. 2196.
Procedure
1. Using 2 applicator sticks, transfer about 0.3 ml (½ tsp) feces to small tube (about 13 × 100 mm) and thoroughly mix with 2-3 ml water. After mixing, fill tube within 2-3 mm of top with water.
2. Centrifuge at approximately 1500 rpm for 1 min. Discard **all** supernatant fluid.

3. Add approximately 1-2 ml zinc sulfate solution (sp gr 1.18) and resuspend sediment by tapping tube sharply with 1 finger while holding top of tube with other hand. As an alternative, use applicator to resuspend sediment.
4. Fill tube within 2-3 mm of top with additional zinc sulfate solution. Strain suspension through 2 layers of gauze into paper cup. Discard gauze and return suspension to tube. Add enough zinc sulfate to fill within 2-3 mm of rim.
5. Centrifuge at approximately 1500 rpm for 1 min. Allow centrifuge to come to a stop without interference or vibration.
6. While centrifuge is slowing down, place ⅓-½ of drop of iodine (or water, if not interested in protozoan cyst identification) on slide.
7. Without removing centrifuge tube, take freshly flamed and cooled bacteriology loop (or any 26- to 28-gauge wire with loop diameter of 5-7 mm) and remove 1 or 2 loopfuls from center of surface film. To do this bend loop portion of wire 90° so that loop is parallel with surface of fluid. **Do not** push loop deep into fluid but rather **touch** surface with loop and collect film of fluid within loop for transfer to microscope slide.
8. Add coverglass and examine.

Common sources of error
1. Stool contains oil or other substances that interfere with egg or cyst accumulation on surface.
2. Too heavy a fecal suspension.
3. Failure to pour off all water prior to addition of zinc sulfate.
4. Unbalanced centrifuge or interference with natural slow down of centrifuge.
5. Dipping beneath surface with loop rather than collecting fluid from surface.
6. Failure to collect sample promptly after centrifugation.

Acid–sodium sulfate–triton–ether concentration (AMS III method)

This procedure, commonly called the AMS III method, was described by Hunter et al.[8,9] The method concentrates eggs and larvae of all helminths and is the method of choice for concentration of schistosome eggs.

Special solutions required
1. HCl–sodium sulfate solution. See p. 2196.
2. Triton NE (Triton-30*)

Procedure
1. Emulsify enough feces in 10-12 ml water to yield 0.5-1.0 ml fecal sediment after completion of steps 2 and 3 below.
2. Strain through 2 layers of gauze moistened with hydrochloric acid–sodium sulfate solution into cup or beaker and transfer to 15 ml calibrated centrifuge tube.
3. Wash 3 times by centrifugation (1 min at 2000-2500 rpm), discarding supernatant fluid each time and mixing sediment with fresh acid–sodium sulfate solution.
4. After final wash, discard supernatant fluid and add 5 ml acid–sodium sulfate solution, 3 drops Triton, and 5 ml ether. Stopper and shake vigorously 30 s.
5. Centrifuge 1 min at about 1500 rpm. Four layers should appear: (a) ether at top, (b) plug of fecal

detritus, (c) an acid–sodium sulfate layer, and (d) bottom layer of sediment containing parasite eggs.
6. Ring fecal detritus with applicator stick to break its contact with walls of centrifuge tube. Pour off supernatant fluid.
7. Add tap water to 0.4 mark, mix sediment, and pour drop on slide, cover, and examine under low-power magnification (100×).

Egg hatching for schistosome miracidia

This especially sensitive test demonstrates indirectly the presence of viable schistosome eggs that might go undetected by other technics. It takes advantage of the fact that viable schistosome eggs placed in water will hatch in a few hours, releasing motile, easily seen miracidia. The procedure is best used if other examination procedures have given negative results.

Procedure
1. Place approximately 5 g feces in about 75 ml water. Use chlorine-free tap water throughout entire procedure, since tap water may contain sufficient chlorine to kill miracidia. Chlorine-free water may be prepared by boiling tap water and cooling to room temperature.
2. Mix feces and water thoroughly. Add about 125 ml water, mix again, and strain through 2 layers of moist gauze into graduated cylinder.
3. After 1 h pour off supernatant fluid and resuspend sediment in small amount of water.
4. Pour into 500 ml Erlenmeyer flask and fill flask almost to lip with water. Cover all but neck of flask with aluminum foil or similar material.
5. Allow flask to stand overnight at room temperature. Eggs will hatch, liberating miracidia, which will collect in neck of flask due to positive phototrophic response. Against dark background, miracidia will be seen as minute, white organisms swimming on straight course. Hand lens and adjacent light source are helpful in observing miracidia.
6. **Caution:** If water is cloudy, miracidia will not accumulate in neck of flask. Subsequent washing after step 3 should be done in such cases.
7. Coprozoic, free-living ciliates, e.g., *Colpoda steini*, may appear in fecal-contaminated water but should not be confused with miracidia. To confirm identification, transfer a few organisms to slide and examine. Weak iodine solution or dilute methylene blue will immobilize miracidia.

PRESERVATION OF PARASITES FOUND IN FECES
General considerations

Fecal specimens that cannot be examined soon after passage should be preserved to prevent alteration of characteristic protozoan morphology. Refrigeration at 3-5 C in a closed container will preserve protozoan cysts for several days. For semipermanent preservation formalin, polyvinyl alcohol (PVA), and Merthiolate-iodine-formalin (MIF) are frequently employed. Formalin preserves all helminth stages and protozoan cysts but destroys protozoan trophozoites. PVA preserves protozoan trophozoites and cysts. MIF preserves all stages of helminths and protozoa and also stains protozoa for identification. Perma-

---

*A wetting agent obtainable from Rohm & Haas Co., Philadelphia, Pa.

nent preservation of protozoan cysts and trophozoites is possible in iron-hematoxylin–stained fecal smears (p. 2168) or trichrome-stained smears (p. 2169). Such preparations may be made from fresh fecal specimens or PVA-preserved specimens but not formalin-preserved specimens.

Formalin preservation of feces
Preservation of bulk specimens for reference purposes

1. Mix fecal specimen thoroughly with saline and strain through 2 layers of gauze to remove coarse debris. Pour into graduated cylinder.
2. After allowing at least 1 h for sedimentation, pour off supernatant fluid and replace with about 5 vol of 10% formalin. Use of hot (60 C) formalin is preferable as it will prevent development of helminth eggs. In cold formalin some eggs will continue to develop to the infective stage.
3. Repeat sedimentation again and pour off supernatant fluid.
4. If feces is to be stored for long period of time, it is desirable to change formalin once or twice a year. Protozoan cysts preserve better if the 10% formalin is made up in 0.85% saline.

Preservation for transport to diagnostic center

1. Mix pea-sized portion of feces with about 5 vol 10% formalin in test tube or vial.
2. Plug test tube or vial for transport to laboratory. Cysts and helminth eggs may be preserved in this manner for several days or weeks. Trophozoites are destroyed.
3. Such specimens may be examined by simple saline or iodine smear (pp. 2166-2167) or, preferably, by formalin-ether sedimentation technic (p. 2170).

Polyvinyl alcohol (PVA) preservation of feces

PVA fixative preserves trophozoites well. Although protozoan cysts may be distorted in PVA smears, they are adequately preserved and can usually be identified without undue difficulty. PVA is the fixative of choice for preserving watery or dysenteric stools and material aspirated from sigmoidoscopy. Liquid fecal material or culture material seldom remains on a slide in sufficient quantity to make a good iron-hematoxylin smear. PVA serves as an adhesive as well as a preservative and overcomes this problem. PVA can be used to preserve feces contained in vials or used directly on a slide in preparation of a fecal smear for iron-hematoxylin staining. For preparation of PVA see p. 2194.

Preservation of specimens for future slide preparation

Add 1-2 ml fecal specimen to 8-10 ml PVA fixative and mix **thoroughly.** Trophozoites are preserved indefinitely. Smears for staining may be prepared immediately or later. Formed stools should be diluted in saline before emulsifying in PVA.

PVA smears

1. Place 1 drop of dysenteric stool, diluted feces, or culture sediment in 3 drops of PVA on slide and mix. If prepared from PVA-preserved material from vial, place 1 or 2 drops of mixed material on slide.

2. Smear material over approximately two-thirds of the slide surface. Smear must be relatively thin or else it may peel off during staining process. Place slide in horizontal position and allow to dry thoroughly (preferably overnight in 37 C incubator).
3. Dry PVA smear may be stained by conventional iron-hematoxylin or trichrome staining procedures. Since organisms have already been fixed, immersion in fixative is omitted. PVA film is placed in 70% alcohol-iodine 10-20 min for removal of mercuric chloride crystals. Remaining steps depend on technic employed.
4. For acceptable staining technics for PVA see iron-hematoxylin technic (p. 2168) and trichrome technic (p. 2169). If unsatisfactorily stained organisms are obtained from PVA-preserved specimens, it usually indicates incomplete fixation due to poor emulsification. Thorough emulsification of soft stools (or formed stools diluted with saline) with PVA will yield satisfactorily stained organisms.

Preservation of feces in Schaudinn solution

Scholtens[10] described an improved technic for recovery of intestinal protozoa using Schaudinn solution. After fixing fecal specimen in Schaudinn, material is diluted 1:2 in 0.85% saline, filtered through 1 layer of gauze, and centrifuged 3 min at 2000 rpm. Sediment is added to 1 drop Mayer's albumin (equal parts egg white and glycerine) on slide and smeared thinly over portion of slide. After drying at room temperature 5-10 min, smear is placed in 70% ethyl alcohol plus iodine as part of sequence of iron-hematoxylin or trichrome staining procedures. Procedure concentrates protozoa at least twice, and there is less tendency for organisms to wash off slides.

Merthiolate-iodine-formalin (MIF) preservation of feces

MIF serves as an excellent preservative and stain for protozoan cysts, trophozoites, and helminth eggs and larvae. The MIF direct smear examination technic is decribed on p. 2167. The MIF solution used for preservation differs from that used for immediate examination.

Special solution required
1. MF for preservation purposes. See p. 2194.
2. Lugol solution. See p. 2194.
Procedure
1. Add 9.4 ml MF preservative solution to 0.6 ml Lugol solution and mix immediately.
2. Quickly add approximately ¼ tsp (1g) feces and thoroughly mix. It is important that 2 solutions be combined only just prior to addition of feces. Also, too much feces must not be added or fixation and staining will not be satisfactory. If it is desirable to preserve larger amounts of feces, multiple proportions of solutions and feces may be used.
3. To examine, draw off top of surface layer of sedimented feces and place on slide.
4. Crush large particles; cover and examine. Best staining results occur if only fresh feces are preserved. Initial iodine-staining reaction may change to eosin stain. Iodine phase may be renewed by addition of 1 drop fresh MIF solution to slide preparation.
5. If desired, MIF-preserved fecal specimens may be concentrated by MIFC technic (p. 2170).

Preservation and staining of helminths
Adult helminths—adult trematodes

Most adult trematodes are muscular and will contract to an extreme degree when exposed to fixatives. If specimens are numerous and not especially muscular (*Clonorchis* or *Fasciolopsis*), relax them by chilling in cold saline or by shaking vigorously in saline for several minutes before pouring fixative over them. With many specimens it will be necessary to place cover slips or slides on them to prevent undue contraction when fixative is added. However, such restraints may distort size and arrangement of internal organs of the trematodes.

Procedure for preservation
1. Relax worms in cold saline or by shaking worms vigorously for several minutes in warm saline.
2. Place relaxed worm or worms on slide or glass plate, restrain if necessary, and pour hot (60-63 C) alcohol-formol-acetic fixative (p. 2194) over specimens. A better procedure, if relaxed worms do not contract too vigorously, is to drop worms directly into hot fixative.
3. Leave worms in dish of fixative at room temperature for 3-12 h.
4. Replace fixative with 2 changes of 50% alcohol for 20-60 min each and store in 70% alcohol until ready to stain, using one of the staining technics described below.

Semichon carmine stain technic
1. Cover specimen with Semichon carmine (p. 2196) diluted 1:2 with 70% alcohol for 1-8 h.
2. Remove stain and wash twice with 70% alcohol to remove excess stain.
3. Destain in 0.5% HCl in 70% alcohol until specimens are light pink in color against white background. Internal organs should be colored.
4. Wash specimens in 2 or 3 changes of 70% alcohol to remove acid and to prevent further destaining.
5. Dehydrate by successive treatments with 80% and 95% alcohol (1 h each).
6. Clear specimen by passing through xylene–95% alcohol mixtures with following proportions: (a) 1 part xylene, 3 parts alcohol, (b) 1 part xylene, 1 part alcohol, (c) 3 parts xylene, 1 part alcohol, and (d) undiluted xylene. Leave in each solution about 1 h.
7. Transfer specimens to slide, remove excess xylene, and mount in Clarite or Permount.

Hematein staining technic
1. Return specimens from 70% alcohol storage to water by successively treating with 50%, 30% alcohol, and water for 60 min each.
2. Place in hematein (p. 2195) for 1 h. Then wash in 3 changes of tap water, 5 min each.
3. Destain in 35% acid-alcohol (6 drops conc. HCl to 100 ml 35% alcohol) until blue color changes to pink against white background.
4. Place in ammonia water (2 drops NH$_4$OH in 500 ml) for 20 min. Then wash thoroughly in several changes of tap water.
5. Dehydrate successively with 30%, 50%, 70%, 80%, and 95% alcohol, 20 min to 1 h each. Then clear and mount as directed in steps 6 and 7 of Semichon technic.

Adult cestodes

Tapeworms will contract when placed directly in fixatives. Thus they should be relaxed in saline

prior to fixation. After relaxation in saline, place small specimens on a glass slide or plate and straighten out. Wrap slide in tissue paper and slowly add hot (60-63 C) neutral 10% formalin. (Acid fixatives will destroy characteristic calcarous corpuscles.) Transfer worm into neutral 10% formalin. A large specimen should be relaxed, wound around a beaker or graduate cylinder, and hot fixative poured over it. The worm should be unwound before it hardens, cut into convenient lengths, and fixed further on glass plates under slides flooded with fixative. After 3-24 h replace fixative with 2 changes of 50% alcohol for 20-60 min, then store in 70% alcohol until ready to stain. Cestodes may be stained by either of the methods given for trematodes above or by the more widely used Delafield hematoxylin stain technic given below.

Delafield hematoxylin stain technic
1. Return specimen to water from storage in 70% alcohol by successively treating with 50%, 30% alcohol, and water for 60 min each.
2. Place in Delafield hematoxylin stain (p. 2194), diluted with 9 parts distilled water for 1 to several hours. Then wash in several changes of water.
3. Place successively in 30% and 50% alcohol for 30-60 min each.
4. Destain in 70% acid-alcohol (6 drops conc. HCl/100 ml alcohol) until light reddish purple. Change alcohol if it becomes noticeably colored.
5. Wash in 2-3 changes of 70% alcohol to remove acid and to prevent further destaining.
6. Place in 70% alkaline alcohol (2 drops NH$_4$OH in 500 ml alcohol) until specimen becomes decidedly bluish in color.
7. Dehydrate through 80% and 95% alcohol, preferably several hours in each, changing the latter at least once. Then clear and mount as for adult trematodes.

Adult and larval nematodes

Nematodes can be fixed and preserved indefinitely in 10% formalin. For clearing, the worms can be transferred from formalin to glycerol-alcohol (p. 2194), or the living worms can be fixed and cleared by placing in hot (60-63 C) glycerol-alcohol solution. The vessel containing worms in glycerol-alcohol should be covered with paper that excludes dust but allows the alcohol to evaporate. By the time the alcohol evaporates (several days), the worms have cleared sufficiently for examination. Nematodes stain poorly and there is seldom need to stain them for identification purposes. Below is outlined a suitable method for mounting nematodes.

Procedure
1. Leave worms in glycerol-alcohol (p. 2194) at room temperature in open vial until all alcohol evaporates. Cover vial with paper to exclude dust.
2. Clean circular coverglasses of 2 sizes, differing by at least 3 mm in diameter. Smallest size should cover specimen to be mounted.
3. Place smaller cover glass on cork or vial set in Plasticine. Cork or vial diameter should be less than coverglass diameter.
4. Heat glycerol-jelly (p. 2196) to 60-70 C in water bath. Transfer drop of medium to center of cover-

glass. Correct amount must be determined by experience, since there must be no excess later.

5. Transfer 1 or more worms to medium on coverglass. Those large enough to be seen without difficulty can be picked up on a needle and placed in glycerol-jelly. Smaller species or larvae should be concentrated in as little fluid as possible and transferred to coverglass. It may be best to transfer worms to coverglass and remove excess fluid before adding glycerol-jelly.

6. Pick up larger cover glass with finger and thumb, breathe on it to condense film of moisture, and lower it toward smaller coverglass with 2 coverglasses as nearly parallel and concentric as possible. When coverglasses make contact, immediately lift and invert preparation so that small coverglass is uppermost. Keep level to prevent shifting of coverglass. Glycerol-jelly should not travel far beyond edge of smaller coverglass. If this does occur, coverglasses should be separated and specimens returned to glycerol for remounting.

7. Place properly prepared mount in refrigerator for a few minutes to set gel, then examine microscopically to see whether preparation is satisfactory. Margin of larger coverglass must be free of glycerol-jelly to distance of almost 1 mm to ensure strong seal later.

8. Place mounting medium on slide and lower preparation into mounting medium with larger coverglass uppermost.

Permanent mounts of helminth eggs

The following procedure may be used for preparation of permanent slides of helminth eggs. However, none of the procedures of this type produces slides that last indefinitely. Fecal suspension containing eggs should be strained through several layers of gauze to remove large particles. If eggs are scarce, it may be necessary to concentrate the eggs by formalin-ether sedimentation technics and then suspend the eggs in 10% formalin for slide preparation. The amount of feces and the number of eggs per drop of fluid should be adjusted to provide preparations similar to those seen on direct fecal smear examination.

Procedure

1. Place clean slide on turntable and with camel's hair brush spin a ring of asphaltum–gold size mixture (2 parts asphaltum; 1 part gold size). Outside diameter of ring should be equal to diameter of round coverslip to be used. Ring should be about 2 mm in width. Asphaltum–gold size mixture should be about consistency of glycerin. If it is too thick, thin with xylol.

2. Set slide or series of slides aside to dry for 24 h. If deeper cell is desired, 1 or more additional layers may be applied to ring at 24 h intervals. Large numbers of slides may be prepared and set aside indefinitely for future use.

3. At the time mount is to be completed, an additional fresh ring of shellac–gold size mixture (equal parts shellac and gold size) is spun on top of asphaltum–gold size mixture. Shellac–gold size mixture should be about consistency of glycerin. If too thick, thin with 95% alcohol.

4. With medicine dropper, immediately place 1 drop of formalin-fixed fecal specimen in center of cell.

Experience will aid in judging how much liquid to add, but as a rule add more than enough to fill cell and let it run out over ring when coverslip is pressed on cell.

5. Touch round coverslip to one side of cell and lower it slowly onto cell. Liquid should spread evenly and cover the entire cell without trapping any bubbles.

6. Gently press edges of coverslip down to bring margin in firm contact with shellac.

7. Set slides aside to dry in flat position at room temperature.

8. The following day any slides showing signs of evaporation of fecal suspension should be discarded. Remaining slides should be placed on turntable and additional ring of shellac and gold size spun, overlapping margin of coverslip to seal it to slide.

9. After 24 h or more, spin final ring of asphaltum–gold size mixture. Such preparations should be checked periodically and resealed if flaking of asphaltum occurs.

CULTIVATION OF PARASITES FROM FECES
General considerations

Cultivation of parasite forms in feces is most often attempted for *E. histolytica*. However, occasionally feces are cultured to recover filariform stages of hookworms *Trichostrongylus* or *Strongyloides* for identification purposes.

There are numerous media available for cultivation of *E. histolytica* and other amebae. Diagnosis by this method should not replace microscopic examination procedures. More positive cultures will occur if fresh specimens, likely to contain viable trophozoites, are used to inoculate culture medium. Old or mailed specimens may contain viable cysts, but these stages often fail to excyst and multiply to detectable numbers. However, some laboratories report considerable success even with cultures made from mailed specimens. The **modified Boeck-Drbohlav** medium (below) is the medium of choice in many laboratories. **Balamuth medium** (p. 2175) has proved a good medium for isolation of most intestinal protozoa and is quite stable. Nelson's medium,[11] not described here, also gives good results.

Cultivation of feces for nematode larvae may be carried out by the Harada-Mori method (p. 2175) or by the older method of culturing eggs or larvae in animal charcoal. Cultivation makes it possible to concentrate larvae otherwise undetected in regular fecal examinations because of few numbers. Also, eggs and larvae may not be specifically identifiable in the stages present in a fecal sample. For example, eggs and early larval stages of *Strongyloides*, hookworms, and *Trichostrongylus* are less easily differentiated than the infective larvae. *Necator* and *Ancylostoma* can be differentiated as infective larvae, but eggs or early larval stages cannot.

Modified Boeck-Drbohlav medium

The modified Boeck-Drbohlav medium is used for cultivation of *E. histolytica*. It requires no serum overlay, but preparation procedures are somewhat involved.

Preparation of Locke solution

Sodium chloride	8	g
Calcium chloride	0.2	g
Potassium chloride	0.2	g
Magnesium chloride	0.01	g
Sodium phosphate (Na$_2$HPO$_4$)	2	g
Sodium bicarbonate	0.4	g
Potassium phosphate (KH$_2$PO$_4$)	0.3	g
Distilled H$_2$O	1000	ml

1. Add chemicals to distilled water in order given.
2. Mix until dissolved. Boil 10 min. Some precipitate will form.
3. Cool to room temperature and filter through paper.
4. Sterilize in autoclave 15 min at 121 C.

Preparation of medium. Add Locke solution to 270 ml well-beaten egg and mix well. Filter mixture through surgical gauze and place under vacuum to draw out all small bubbles. Dispense into tubes (15 × 125 mm) in 4.5 ml amounts. Allow pressure in jacket of autoclave to reach 15 psi. Then place tubes in autoclave in slanted position and close exhaust valves and door of chamber. This maneuver will trap enough air in chamber to assure proper inspissation. Allow steam pressure from jacket to enter chamber and allow it to rise to 15 lb/in.^{2} (psi) in chamber. Hold at this pressure for 15 min. Cut off steam supply and allow pressure to drop gradually with all doors and valves tightly closed. Allow slants to cool; then cover with 6 ml Locke solution and autoclave in usual manner.

Inoculation of medium. Add approximately a 5 mm loop of sterile rice powder (Difco Laboratories, Detroit) to each tube just prior to use. (Rice powder is sterilized by dry heat 2½ h at 150 C.) Inoculate about 1.5 ml fluid or semifluid feces into each of 2 tubes. If fecal specimen is formed (not fluid), inoculate pea-sized portion and mix with as little agitation as possible. To one of these tubes add enough penicillin and streptomycin to give final concentration of 200-250 U or μg/ml overlay. Incubate at 37 C for 24 h; then examine a few drops of sediment microscopically. All cultures not showing trophozoites are transferred to fresh medium. Inoculate about half of sediment/transfer, incubate at 37 C for 48 h, and examine again. Sediment may be fixed in PVA (p. 2172) and smears stained permanently (p. 2168) to aid in identification. Organisms may also be identified by Quensel stain smears (p. 2167). To maintain amebae, transfer every 2 or 3 d.

Balamuth medium[12]

Add 36 g dried egg yolks to equal volume of distilled water. Mix well and add 125 ml 0.8% sodium chloride solution. Mix thoroughly, then boil 10 min, stirring constantly. Dilute to original volume with distilled water and press through double layer of muslin. Dilute to 125 ml with 0.8% saline and sterilize in autoclave at 15 psi for 20 min. Cool to temperature below 10 C and filter through Buchner funnel, using medium grade filter paper. Add equal amount of 0.067M phosphate buffer, pH 7.5, to yolk mixture. **To prepare phosphate buffer,** mix 43 ml 1M dipotassium phosphate solution and 7 ml 1M monopotassium phosphate solution; then add 14 parts distilled water to 1 part of this mixture to make 0.067M buffer. Prepare solution of Wilson or Lilly liver concentrate by making 5% suspension, filtering, and autoclaving. Add 1 part liver extract to 9 parts

buffered yolk infusion. Distribute in tubes in 7-10 ml quantities and sterilize in autoclave 20 min at 15 psi. Before use add loopful of sterile rice powder.

Medium can be prepared from fresh egg yolks as follows: Boil 4 eggs 15 min and discard whites. Add 125 ml 0.8% saline to yolks. Proceed as above, except that routine filter paper may be used for filtration through Buchner funnel.

Harada-Mori culture for nematode larvae

The Harada-Mori culture method aids in the differentiation of *Strongyloides. Trichostrongylus, Necator,* and *Ancylostoma.* The technic is simple and requires no special laboratory equipment.

Procedure

1. Add about 7 ml distilled water to test tube. Take strip of filter paper with width about same as that of test tube and length slightly less than that of test tube and smear about 0.5 g feces on filter paper strip, leaving 5 cm at one end free of feces.
2. Insert smeared strip into test tube with unsmeared end reaching bottom of tube. Fecal smear itself should not be immersed in water. Cover top of test tube with cellophane and secure with rubber band.
3. After 8-10 d at room temperature, remove filter paper strip with forceps. **Caution:** Infective larvae may move to top of filter paper strip or to under surface of cellophane. Avoid contact.
4. Place tube containing larvae in water bath at 50 C for 15 min. Then shake and transfer to 15 ml conical centrifuge tube. Centrifuge, remove supernatant fluid, and examine sediment under low-power magnification (100×).

Key for identification of filariform larvae*

1. a. Larva about 500 μm long and without sheath; esophagus nearly half length of body; tail blunt or forked . . . . *Strongyloides stercoralis*
   b. Esophagus about one-fourth length of body of sheathed larvae; longer than 600 μm . . . 2.
2. a. Body length about 750 μm; intestinal lumen not straight but zigzagged; end of tail rounded and knoblike . . . . *Trichostrongylus* spp.
   b. Body length about 590 μm, and sheath length about 660 μm; sheath conspicuously striated, most clearly observed around tail portion of body; mouth "spears" appear dark; anterior end of body (not sheath) rounded, like the small end of a hen's egg; anterior portion of intestine as wide as esophagel bulb; tail end sharply pointed. . . . . *Necator americanus*
   c. Body length about 660 μm, and sheath length about 720 μm; sheath less clearly striated; mouth "spears" less conspicuous; anterior end of body (not sheath) blunt; intestine narrower in diameter than esophageal bulb; tail end blunted . . . . . . *Ancylostoma duodenale*
3. Exceptions:
   a. Occasionally infective larvae will be found exsheathed and sheath striations accordingly unavailable.
   b. It should te recalled that *Strongyloides stercoralis* has free-living generation; male and fe-

---

*From Hsieh, H. C.: WHO Technical Report Series, no. 255, pp. 27-30, 1963.

male adults as well as immature larvae may consequently be encountered.

Barrett-Yarbrough medium for Balantidium

Cultivation of fecal material is not routinely done for diagnosis of *Balantidium coli* infections. However, in instances in which teaching material is desired, the Barrett-Yarbrough medium has proved of value.

Preparation of medium. Prepare mixture of 1 part inactivated human serum and 16 parts 0.5% sodium chloride. Sterilize by filtration and tube in 8 ml amounts. Inoculate tube with 0.1 ml feces and incubate at 37 C for 24 h. Transfer should be made every 1 or 2 d. Growth is better if Locke or Ringer solution with dextrose is substituted for sodium chloride solution.

QUANTITATIVE EGG COUNT

Quantitative egg count procedures are used to determine the intensity of worm burden in an individual. Such information may aid the physician in determining whether the worm infection is incidental or a matter of direct concern. For example, hookworms present in large numbers often cause anemia, although if present in small numbers, they may contribute little or nothing to an existing anemia. Also such information gathered from a community provides an index of the status of a helminth problem in the community. For example, even though the majority of a population is infected with a particular worm, if the worm burden is very low, then control or treatment measures would not be as urgent as in a population with a heavy worm burden. Quantitative egg count procedures are not recommended for diagnosis of infection. The Stoll dilution technic[13] or Beaver direct smear technic[14] may be used to quantitate egg counts. The former procedure is given below.

Stoll procedure[13]
1. Fill Stoll flask* to 56 ml mark (lower) with 0.1N NaOH solution.
2. Carefully add feces to bring contents up to 60 ml mark (upper) without soiling neck of flask.
3. Add 6-8 glass beads, stopper, and shake vigorously. Allow to stand 12-24 h with occasional shaking.
4. Shake vigorously with up-and-down motion (avoid circular motion that might concentrate eggs in small area) and **immediately** withdraw exactly 0.075 ml with Stoll pipet.* Wipe outside of pipet to remove excess fecal suspension.
5. Transfer 0.075 ml sample to slide, cover with 22 × 30 coverglass, and count eggs in entire preparation. This is number of eggs in 0.005 ml sample of feces:

$$\left(\frac{4}{60} \times \frac{0.075}{1} = 0.005\right)$$

6. Multiply count by 200 to convert to eggs/ml.
7. Correct for stool consistency by multiplying egg/ml count as follows: hard-formed (difficult to puncture with applicator), × 1; mushy-formed

---

*Stoll flasks and pipets available from Arthur Thomas Co., Philadelphia, Pa.

Table 100-2. Intensity of hookworm infection

Eggs/ml formed feces	Intensity of infection
100-699	Very light
700-2,499	Light
2600-12,599	Moderate
12,600-25,099	Heavy
25,100 and over	Very heavy

(can be cut with applicator), × 2; mushy-diarrheic (nonliquid but takes shape of container), × 3; and diarrheic (liquid), × 4. Report corrected count as **eggs/ml formed stool.**

Interpretation. Each female *Ascaris* produces an average of about 2000 eggs/ml feces and each female hookworm and whipworm produces about 45 eggs/ml. Thus the approximate number of female worms can be determined by dividing egg count/ml formed feces by the number of eggs produced/ml by the worm in question. Since male worms will make up half the worm burden, multiply the calculated female worm burden by 2 to arrive at the total approximate worm burden.

For hookworms, Table 100-2 serves as a guide to the intensity of the infection.

Tissue, body fluid, and atrial parasites

General considerations

The tissue–body fluid complex may be inhabited by many different helminths or protozoa. Selection of a single type of tissue or fluid specimen usually narrows considerably the spectrum of potential parasite possibilities. However, it is often necessary to examine several types of tissues or fluids to demonstrate a given parasite (see below). Chapters 97 and 98 or standard reference texts should be consulted for information on parasite life cycles and on the course of disease in relation to possible presence of the organism and the stage that would be present.

Parasites found in common tissues and fluids

Table 100-3 summarizes the specimens, parasites, and the frequency of specimen used in diagnosis.

Specific procedures used for diagnosis

Table 100-4 summarizes the specific procedures used for diagnosis of the common tissue parasites. The examination procedures referred to in Table 100-4 are coded from A to G as indicated. The discussion on each parasite form of interest should be consulted for additional information on examination procedures.

Direct blood examination
Fresh smear

Direct blood examination of a fresh smear is done primarily for detection of motile organisms

Table 100-3. Specimen-parasite summary

Specimen	Frequency of specimen use in diagnosis	Parasite
Blood	Frequently used	*Plasmodium vivax, P. malariae, P. falciparum, P. ovale, Trypanosoma gambiense, T. rhodesiense, T. cruzi, T. rangeli, Wuchereria bancrofti, Brugia malayi, Loa loa, Mansonella ozzardi, Acanthocheilonema perstans, Leishmania donovani, especially the Indian form*
	Rarely used	*Toxoplasma gondii, Trichinella spiralis*
Urine	Frequently used	*Dioctophyma renale, Schistosoma haematobium*
	Infrequently used	*Wuchereria* (associated with chyluria)
	Rarely used	*Entamoeba histolytica, Trichomonas vaginalis, Strongyloides stercoralis, Schistosoma mansoni*
Sputum	Frequently used	*Paragonimus westermani*
	Infrequently used	*Echinococcus granulosus*
	Rarely used	*Entamoeba histolytica, Schistosoma* sp.
Spinal fluid	Frequently used	*Toxoplasma gondii, Trypanosoma gambiense, Trypanosoma rhodesiense*
	Infrequently used	*Naegleria, Hartmanella, Acanthamoeba*
	Rarely used	*Trichinella spiralis*
Duodenal contents or bile	Infrequently used	*Giardia lamblia, S. stercoralis, Fasciola hepatica, Clonorchis sinensis, Opisthorchis* sp.
Tissue or tissue fluid		
Proctoscopic aspirate	Frequently used if lesions present	*Entamoeba histolytica*
Proctoscopic biopsy	Frequently used	*Schistosoma mansoni, S. haematobium, S. japonicum*
Liver lesion biopsy or aspirate	Frequently used if lesions present	*E. histolytica, Echinococcus* sp., *Toxocara canis*
Splenic biopsy or aspirate	Frequently used	*Leishmania donovani, T. gondii, Trypanosoma cruzi*
Liver biopsy and aspirate (no lesion visible)	Infrequently used	*L. donovani, Schistosoma* sp.
	Rarely used	*Toxoplasma gondii, Trypanosoma cruzi*
Lymph node biopsy or aspirate	Frequently used	*T. cruzi, T. gambiense, T. rhodesiense*
	Infrequently used	*T. gondii*
	Rarely used	*L. donovani, Wuchereria, Brugia*
Bone marrow	Frequently used	*L. donovani, T. cruzi*
Muscle	Frequently used	*T. cruzi* (heart autopsy), *T. spiralis, Cysticercus cellulosae* (*Taenia solium* larva)
	Incidental	*Sarcocystis lindemanni*
Lung lesions	Frequently used	*Pneumocystis carinii*
	Infrequently or rarely used	*E. histolytica, Strongyloides, Echinococcus granulosus*
Skin lesion or scrapings	Frequently used	*L. tropica, L. braziliensis, L. donovani* (postkala-azar), *Onchocerca* microfilariae, *Acanthocheilonema streptocerca*
	Rarely used	*E. histolytica*
Vaginal smear	Frequently used	*Trichomonas vaginalis*
Eye	Infrequently or rarely used	*Toxoplasma, Loa loa, Onchocerca, Toxocara*

present in the blood such as the trypanosomes or microfilariae. The examination may be done on a drop of fresh blood or on concentrates of several milliliters of fresh blood. Examination of blood for microfilariae must take into account the possible nocturnal or diurnal periodicity of the various species.

Procedure

1. Place small drop of blood on slide and cover with coverglass. Fresh blood from earlobe or fingertip as well as blood from venipuncture with or without anticoagulant may be used.
2. Examine preparation systematically under high-

power (430×) magnification for trypanosomes and low-power (100×) for microfilariae. For best results blood layer should be about thickness of 2 red blood cells.
3. To concentrate fresh blood for trypanosomes, collect about 10 ml blood in citrate solution. Centrifuge at 1000 rpm 3 min. Discard sediment and centrifuge supernatant fluid at approximately 2000 rpm 15 min. Examine sediment under high-power (430×) magnification. If desired, make a smear, air dry, and stain with Giemsa (p. 2179).
4. To concentrate fresh blood for microfilariae, use the Knott method (p. 2179) or membrane filter method (p. 2180).

Table 100-4. Examination procedure summary

Parasites	Specimen	Examination procedure*
Plasmodium sp.	Blood	B
Trypanosoma gambiense	Blood	A, B, D, E
Trypanosoma rhodesiense	Spinal fluid	A, B, D, E
	Lymph node biopsy or aspirate	B, D, E
	Bone marrow	B, D, E
Trypanosoma cruzi	Blood (febrile episode)	A, B, D, E, F, G
	Liver biopsy or aspirate	B, C, D, E
	Splenic biopsy or aspirate	B, C, D, E
	Lymph node biopsy or aspirate	B, C, D, E
	Bone marrow	B, C, D, E
	Heart muscle	C, D, E
Leishmania donovani	Blood	B, D, G
	Liver biopsy or aspirate	B, C, D, E
	Splenic biopsy or aspirate	B, C, D, E
	Lymph node biopsy or aspirate	B, C, D, E
	Bone marrow	B, C, D, E
Leishmania tropica and	Blood	G
Leishmania braziliensis	Ulcer scrapings	B, D, E
Trichomonas vaginalis	Vaginal smear	A, D
Toxoplasma gondii	Blood	G
	Spinal fluid	B, E
	Liver biopsy or aspirate	B, C, E
	Splenic biopsy or aspirate	B, C, E
	Lymph node biopsy or aspirate	B, C, E
	Brain	B, C, E
Entamoeba histolytica†	Proctoscopic aspirate	A, B, C
	Liver lesion aspirate	A, D
	Lung lesion aspirate	A
	Skin lesion	A
	Bloody sputum	A
Naegleria fowleri	Spinal fluid	A, D, E
	Brain	C, D, E
Strongyloides stercoralis†	Duodenal aspirate	A
Trichinella spiralis	Blood	G
	Striated muscle biopsy	A
Toxocara canis (visceral larva migrans)	Blood, liver biopsy	G
Wuchereria, Brugia, Loa, Mansonella, Acanthocheilonema	Blood	A, B, G
Onchocerca, Acanthocheilonema	Skin scrapings	A
Echinococcus granulosus and	Blood	G
Echinococcus multilocularis	Fluid from liver or lung cyst or lesion	A
Cysticercus of *Taenia solium*	Found in all tissues	A, C, G
	Biopsy of subcutaneous tissue most frequent procedure	
Schistosoma mansoni† and	Blood	G
Schistosoma japonicum†	Proctoscopic biopsy	A
Schistosoma haematobium	Proctoscopic biopsy	A
	Urine	A
Paragonimus westermani	Sputum	A
	Blood	G

*Examination procedure code: A, unstained (fresh) smear; B, stained smear; C, histologic section; D, culture; E, animal inoculation; F, xenodiagnosis; and G, serologic or skin test.
†This parasite is usually demonstrated in feces.

Stained smear for blood protozoa and microfilariae

Stained thick or thin blood smears may be examined to demonstrate parasites that circulate in the blood. Although the motile species such as the trypanosomes and the microfilariae can easily be demonstrated in fresh smears, detailed morphology studies are possible only after the organisms are stained. Nonmotile species such as the malarial parasites and *Leishmania donovani* might be missed altogether unless stained.

For diagnosis of malaria, thick smears are preferred over thin smears by experienced workers because they allow many more positive cases with low parasitemia to be discovered. The thick smear concentrates blood in a small space on the slide and enables the laboratory worker to examine the same volume of blood about 3 times faster than possible by thin smear. However, frequently the parasites in thick smears are distorted and difficult for inexperienced workers to identify. More characteristic morphology is seen in thin smears. Therefore, often it is desirable to prepare both thick and thin smears on the same slide for examination.

Stained thin smears are useful for detection of moderate or heavy trypanosome infections, but other diagnostic procedures should be utilized if blood smears are negative. Stained thick smears are recommended in the search for *Leishmania donovani* before attempting to demonstrate the organism in other tissues to avoid unnecessary biopsies of internal organs. *Leishmania* organisms are most often found in endothelial cells, large mononuclear cells, and, rarely, neutrophilic leukocytes. Microfilaria can be identified to species in stained blood smears.

Either Giemsa or Wright stain may be used for staining blood protozoa, but the Giemsa stain is superior. Giemsa stains microfilariae adequately, but hematoxylin (below) gives better results. Giemsa stain may be prepared from powder or purchased as a concentrated stock from commercial sources. Each new lot of stain should be checked, since there may be some variation in staining reactions with different lots. Permanent preparations of blood smears should be mounted with Permount and covered with a cover glass.

Smears to be stained should be stored in a dust-free container to protect fresh smears from flies and cockroaches. Thin smears should be fixed in methyl alcohol and thick films laked in distilled water **before** storage if slides cannot be stained within 48 hours of preparation. Store slides at temperatures below 27 C to prevent undesirable heat-fixation or unlaked thick films. If a large number of thick films are being laked during staining, change the staining solution every 50 slides to prevent accumulation of excess hemoglobin.

Giemsa staining procedure

Special solutions required
1. Giemsa (commercial or prepared). See p. 2194.
2. Buffer solution for Giemsa. See p. 2196.

Procedure
Thin smear
1. Touch alcohol-cleaned slide to small drop of finger or earlobe blood so that drop of blood is near one end of slide. Place slide, blood side up, on table; take second slide, holding it at 30° angle to first slide, and draw it back into drop of blood. Then push forward so that blood spreads out and trails angled slide. Amount of blood should be small enough so that it is used up before spreader slide reaches end of first slide. Allow to air dry.
2. Fix smear by immersing in absolute methyl alcohol 2-3 min.
3. Place in stock Giemsa stain diluted 1:50 with pH 7.0 buffer for 1 h. Staining time can be reduced to 20 min by using 1:20 dilution of Giemsa. **Diluted Giemsa stain should be prepared fresh each day.**
4. Dip slides briefly in buffer. Allow slide to drain and dry. Examine under oil immersion.

Thick smear in vertical position.
1. Touch alcohol-cleansed slide to drop of finger or earlobe blood. Using corner of another slide, spread blood in large enough rectangular pattern so that blood flows slowly and does not immediately form a drop at lower edge when slide is tilted. If desired, thin smear can be prepared on other end. Allow slide to dry in flat position overnight.
2. If for *Plasmodium* spp., place dry smear in Giemsa stain diluted 1:50 with pH 7.0 buffer for 45 min. If for *L. donovani*, flood dried film with aqueous solution of 4 parts 2% glacial acetic acid and 1 part 2% crystalline tartaric acid for 5-10 min. Drain off solution, fix in methyl alcohol, wash thoroughly, and place in 1:50 Giemsa for 45 min.
3. Wash slide gently for 2 min. Dry and examine under oil immersion.
4. Thin and thick smears may be prepared on same slide by allowing thin smear, but not thick smear, to be fixed with methyl alcohol and then staining with Giemsa as described above. Stain with thin smear uppermost.

Concentration by Knott procedure and staining of blood microfilariae with Delafield hematoxylin

Procedure
1. Place 1 or 2 ml venous blood in 10 ml 2% formalin in distilled water. (This procedure ruptures all red cells.)
2. Centrifuge mixture for 5 min at 2000 rpm. Transfer sediment to slide and examine under low power (100×) for microfilariae; if present, allow smear to dry.
3. Fix in equal parts ether and 95% ethyl alcohol for 10 min.
4. Air dry and stain in undiluted Delafield hematoxylin (p. 2194) for 40-60 min.
5. Rinse quickly in 0.05% HCl and wash in running water until blue color appears in film.
6. Air dry and search for parasites under low power (100×). Identify under oil immersion.

NOTE: Thick blood smears containing microfilariae can be stained with Delafield hematoxylin as follows: (1) place air-dried thick smear in distilled water for 10 min; (2) dry and fix in equal parts ether and 95% alcohol for 10 min; (3) stain with undiluted Delafield hematoxylin for 10 min; (4) place in 0.05% HCl for 5-10 min; and (5) wash in tap water for 5 min, dry, mount in Permount, and examine.

Concentration of microfilariae by membrane filter technic[15]

This technic will detect positive cases of microfilaremia missed by counting chamber or thick-blood film examination. It is particularly well suited for epidemiologic studies done under field conditions.

Draw 1 ml venous blood into 10 ml syringe containing suitable anticoagulant (0.1 ml of 5% sodium citrate) and 9 ml of 10% solution of Teepol in physiologic saline. Shake gently 1 min to accomplish complete hemolysis. Replace needle with Swinney filter holder containing 25 mm membrane filter (Millipore Corp.) of 5 µm porosity placed over supporting filter pad paper of same size. Moisten pad before placing membrane over it. Write code number on edge of moist membrane with waterproof-ink marker. With gentle pressure on syringe piston, force hemolyzed blood through filter. Wash membrane 3 times by passing 10 ml physiologic saline through it. Remove membrane from holder and place in hot (60-63 C) Harris hematoxylin (Ortho Diagnostic Co.) for 5 min. Immerse membrane briefly in running tap water until membrane is blued. Allow membrane to dry thoroughly and then place on glass microscope slide. Clear with immersion oil or, if a permanent preparation is required, use mounting medium such as Permount.

CULTIVATION OF BLOOD AND TISSUE PARASITES

The human trypanosomes and leishmanias frequently can be isolated by inoculating suitable media with blood, tissues, or tissue juices from infected patients. Numerous media and modifications of media have been described and used successfully. Only a few of the better known and more reliable media are described here. For more complete information on various media the reader is referred to Burrows[16] or Belding.[17] *Trypanosoma cruzi* and *L. donovani* are relatively easily cultivated on NNN medium. *T. gambiense* and *T. rhodesiense* are more difficult to cultivate and subculture. However, Weinman[18] devised a medium that gave excellent results for primary isolation and subculture.

NNN medium for Leishmania sp. or T. cruzi

Preparation. Add 14 g Bacto-agar and 6 g sodium chloride to 900 ml distilled water and bring to boil. Adjust ph to 7.0 with 1N sodium hydroxide. Dispense in 3 ml amounts to screw-capped or rubber-stoppered tubes and sterilize. Tubed medium may be stored in refrigerator several months without deteriorating. Just before use, melt tubed medium in boiling water bath or in autoclave. Cool to 48-50 C and add 1 ml sterile defibrinated rabbit blood (at 48-50 C) to each tube. Mix blood into medium, then slant and allow to harden. After medium has solidified, place in 37 C incubator overnight to test for bacterial contamination. Discard all medium that is contaminated.

Inoculation
1. *Leishmania donovani* in white cells: Collect 10 ml blood aseptically and mix with 50 ml sterile saline. Centrifuge at 750 rpm for 5 min. Remove supernatant fluid and centrifuge at 1500 rpm for 5 min. Inoculate sediment into tubes of NNN medium.
2. For *T. cruzi* inoculate several tubes with 0.5-1.0 ml blood taken during febrile episode.

3. If tissue is to be inoculated into culture medium, please refer to appropriate section of this chapter dealing with various tissues for information on how to handle tissue.
4. Inoculate each tube with 50 units penicillin and 50 µg streptomycin contained in 0.5 ml saline to inhibit bacterial growth. (Trypanosomes and leishmanias will not grow in presence of bacteria.)
5. Incubate culture at room temperature and examine loopfuls of fluid at weekly intervals for at least 1 mo.

Weinman medium for African trypanosomes[18]

Preparation. An autoclaved base and nonheated blood portion comprise the medium.
1. Add 31 g Difco nutrient agar and 5 g plain agar to 1000 ml distilled water. Heat to boiling to dissolve, cool to 45 C, and adjust pH to 7.3. Autoclave; then store in refrigerator until needed.
2. Centrifuge citrated human blood. Remove plasma and inactivate at 56 C for 30 min. Wash red cells 3 times in sterile saline by suspension and centrifugation.
3. Melt agar base and cool to 45 C. Mix equal volumes of prewarmed inactivated plasma and packed, washed red cells. Add 1 part plasma–red cell mixture to 3 parts base. Mix and dispense in 5 ml amounts and allow to harden in slanted position for several days at room temperature or overnight in refrigerator. Incubate slants at 37 C overnight to test for sterility. Store slants in refrigerator. Medium is stable for at least 6 mo.

Inoculation
1. Either inoculate 0.1 ml blood directly onto slants or add 0.1 ml polyvinyl sulfuric acid (PVSA) to each ml blood and promptly inoculate 2.0 ml PVSA-blood mixture to each tube. PVSA, in addition to being an anticoagulant, inactivates complement and prevents it from inhibiting trypanosome growth.
2. Add dihydrostreptomycin sulfate, 0.5 mg/ml blood, or penicillin, 2000 µ/ml blood, to control contamination.
3. Tilt inoculum over slant and incubate in darkness at room temperature.

Examination
1. Irrigate slant surface of culture with overlay fluid to wash down colonies.
2. Remove drop of fluid and examine under high-power magnification (430×).
3. Cultures rarely become positive before 5 d or after 30 d after inoculation.

Tobie medium for trypanosomes[19]

Preparation. Place 1.5 g Bacto-beef (Difco), 2.5 g Bacto-peptone (Difco), 4.0 g NaCl, and 7.5 g Bacto-agar (Difco) in 500 ml distilled water and dissolve. Adjust pH to 7.2-7.4 with NaOH, then autoclave 20 min at 15 psi (121 C). Cool to 45 C and add heat-inactivated (56 C for 30 min), defibrinated whole rabbit blood to achieve 1 part blood to 3 parts base medium. Dispense in 5 ml amounts, slant, and allow to harden. Overlay hardened slants with 2.0 ml Locke solution (8.0 g NaCl, 0.2 g KCl, 0.2 g CaCl$_2$, 0.3 g KH$_2$PO$_4$, 0.25 dextrose, and 100 ml distilled H$_2$O).

Inoculation. Inoculate tubes with 0.1-0.5 ml amounts blood. Incubate at room temperature. Maximum growth usually occurs between 10-14 d. Antibiotics may be used as in Weinman medium to prevent bacterial growth.

NOTE: Better growth may occur on this medium if

NaCl content per 500 ml is reduced to 2.5 g. A further modification of this medium, reported by Hunter et al. (1966),[20] is as follows: infuse 25.0 g Bacto-beef (Difco) in 500 ml distilled water 1 h. Heat mixture 5 min at 80 C. Filter through ordinary filter paper; then add 10.0 g Neopeptone (Difco), 10.0 g Bacto-agar (Difco), and 2.5 g NaCl. Adjust pH to 7.2-7.4 with NaOH, then autoclave at 15 psi (121 C) for 20 min. Cool to 45 C and add defibrinated rabbit blood to make 10% concentration. Dispense, cool, and overlay as described for original medium above. This medium will support growth of leishmanias as well as human trypanosomes.

Simplified trypticase serum medium for Trichomonas vaginalis

Kupferberg et al.[21] devised a simple medium that is useful for isolation and cultivation of *T. vaginalis*. Cultivation has proved superior to microscopic examination of vaginal exudate in demonstrating this organism. The medium may be prepared in modified form as described below or purchased commercially* in dehydrated form.

Preparation of medium. Add 20 g trypticase (BBL), 1.5 g cysteine HCl, and 1 g maltose to 850 ml distilled water. Adjust pH to 6.0. Add 1 g Difco agar and boil to dissolve agar. Add 0.6 ml 0.5% methylene blue (this step is optional). Readjust volume to 850 ml and tube medium in 8.5 ml amounts. Autoclave at 15 psi for 15 min. Store medium in refrigerator until used. Medium will keep 2 or 3 wk. Just prior to use, add 0.5 ml sterile serum (pH adjusted to 6.0) and 1 ml penicillin-streptomycin mixture containing 500 U/ml to each tube. Human, beef, and sheep serum may be used as serum source. Sterilize serum by filtration.

Inoculation of medium. Inoculate tube of medium with swab containing vaginal exudate from suspected patient. Incubate at 37 C and observe 4 or 5 d. Most tubes are usually positive in 1 or 2 d.

Diamond medium for Trichomonas

Diamond[22] medium is similar to simplified trypticase serum (STS) medium. It is a richer medium and in my hands has proved more satisfactory than STS medium for long-term maintenance of *Trichomonas vaginalis*. For initial isolation, however, both media appear about equal.

Preparation of medium. Add 20 g trypticase (BBL), 10 g yeast extract, 5 g maltose, 1 g cysteine HCl, and 0.2 g ascorbic acid to 900 ml distilled water. Adjust pH to 6.0 and add 0.5 g agar. Boil to dissolve agar and tube in 4.5 ml amounts. Store in refrigerator until used. Medium will keep at least 2-3 wk. Just prior to use, add 0.5 ml sterile human serum (adjusted to pH 6.0) and 0.5 ml penicillin-streptomycin mixture containing 500 U of each antibiotic per milliliter. Serum can be pooled and sterilized by means of a Seitz filter after adjusting pH.

ANIMAL INOCULATION AND XENODIAGNOSIS
Animal inoculation

Blood from infected patients may be injected into susceptible lab animals and the parasite

---

*Difco Laboratories, Detroit, Mich., or BBL, Division of BioQuest, Cockeysville, Md.

demonstrated in the blood or tissues of the animal. However, the procedure should not be relied on to the exclusion of direct microscopic examination and culture technics. Approximately 1 ml blood with an appropriate anticoagulant can be injected intraperitoneally into a 15 g mouse. Correspondingly, larger amounts of blood can be injected into rats, hamsters, guinea pigs, and other animals. The usual procedure for each suspected parasite is outlined below.

Trypanosoma cruzi. Blood is taken from patients, especially during febrile episode, and injected into mice, rats, guinea pigs, hamsters, puppies, or kittens. Young male mice, weighing 12-15 g are usually the most convenient animals. Inoculate each mouse with 0.5-1.0 ml citrated or heparinized blood from patient. Mice can be rendered more susceptible by injecting 5 mg cortisone acetate subcutaneously at the same time. After 4 d check mouse tail blood every day by direct examination (p. 2176) for trypanosomes at 430× magnification. If this blood is negative after 3 wk, sacrifice mice by withdrawing as much heart blood as possible, using 24-gauge needle attached to 1 ml tuberculin syringe. Express blood into tube of NNN medium (p. 2180). Similarly, heart tissue or bone marrow can be collected and macerated aseptically, then inoculated into NNN medium.

Trypanosoma gambiense and Trypanosoma rhodesiense. Inject suspect patient blood into several guinea pigs, rats, or mice. Examine ear or tail blood at 2- or 3-day intervals (p. 2176) at 430× magnification for trypanosomes. If blood is negative after 1 mo, withdraw blood from heart and inoculate into several tubes of Weinman medium (p. 2180).

Leishmania. Aspirates or biopsy material, obtained aseptically from cutaneous ulcers, lymph nodes, spleen, liver, bone marrow, or spinal fluid, may be used. Inoculate 0.25-1.0 ml of material intraperitoneally or intratesticularly into 2- to 4-month-old hamsters. The leishmanias may be demonstrated in liver, spleen, and bone marrow. However, the method is not used frequently because it often requires 2 mo or longer before the animal shows signs of disease.

Toxoplasma gondii. Inject suspensions of glandular tissue or fluid, spinal fluid, blood, bone marrow, or enucleated eye tissue into young white mice. For tissue preparation see Splenic aspirate or biopsy (p. 2183). Inoculate 0.03 ml intracerebrally and 0.1-1.0 ml intraperitoneally into same animal. Each animal should be injected subcutaneously with 5 mg cortisone acetate just prior to tissue inoculation. If any inoculated animals show ascites or other signs of illness, they should be sacrificed, and fresh and Giemsa-stained smears of peritoneal exudate examined microscopically. Giemsa-stained smears of brain and spleen also should be examined microscopically. If animals inoculated with material from patient do not develop any symptoms in 1 wk, they should be sacrificed and blind passage of their tissues made into additional mice. Material from brain and spleen should be aseptically macerated and injected into mice. Three blind passages should be made in attempt to demonstrate organisms.

Xenodiagnosis

This method is used for diagnosis of *Trypanosoma cruzi*. Uninfected laboratory-bred triatomid bug nymphs in a gauze-covered container are placed in contact with the forearm of the patient suspect. After the bugs feed to repletion they are kept at room temperature. Examine bug fecal material for flagellates after 10-14 days and afterward at weekly intervals for 2 mo or longer. Light infection can often be detected by this method.

EXAMINATION OF TISSUES AND BODY FLUIDS
Urine examination

Schistosoma haematobium eggs and the flagellate *Trichomonas vaginalis* are commonly found in the urine of infected individuals. In cases of wuchereriasis with chyluria, microfilariae may be found in the urine. Eggs of *Doctophyma renale*, an exteremely rare nematode parasite of humans, also are found in urine. In those rare cases in which *Entamoeba histolytica* invades the genitalia, trophozoites may be recovered from urine. On rare occasions *Strongyloides stercoralis* larvae are found in urine. If, however, urine is contaminated with feces, *Strongyloides* larvae may be mistakenly reported as "found in urine."

Procedures
Fresh smear
1. Collect urine toward end of micturition.
2. Centrifuge 2-4 min at 2000 rpm and examine sediment under 100× magnification.

Stained smear. Not done.
Culture. Not done although *Trichomonas vaginalis* may be cultured from urine (p. 2182).
Animal inoculation. Not done.

Sputum examination

Few parasites are found in sputum. *Paragonimus westermani* infections are most frequently diagnosed by finding eggs in sputum. Other than cases of suspected paragonimiasis, routine examination of sputum for animal parasites is not done. Rarely, *E. histolytica* trophozoites, *Strongylolides*, or *Ascaris* larvae have been found in coughed-up blood, mucus, and tissue from lung infection foci. *Echinococcus granulosus* cyst material and eggs of schistosomes have been recovered in similar material.

Procedures
Fresh smear
1. For suspected cases of paragonimiasis, mix sputum with 5 vol 5% sodium hydroxide and let stand 2-3 h, with occasional mixing.
2. Centrifuge at 2000 rpm for 2 min. Examine sediment.
3. If eggs are scarce, if may be necessary to process sputum collected over a 24-48 h period.

Stained smear. Not done.
Culture. Not done.
Animal inoculation. Not done.

Spinal fluid examination

The African trypanosomes, *Trypanosoma gambiense* and *rhodesiense,* may be recovered from spinal fluid of late stage cases of sleeping sickness. *Toxoplasma gondii* has been recovered

from cases with central nervous system involvement. In rare instances *Trichinella* larvae and *Trypanosoma cruzi* have been found in spinal fluid.

Recently free-living soil amebae, *Naegleria fowleri* have been isolated from fatal cases of meningoencephalitis. Other soil amebae, *Acanthamoeba,* have also been isolated from spinal fluid of a nonfatal case of meningitis.

Procedures
Fresh smear
1. If only a small amount of fluid is available, place drop on slide, cover with coverglass, and examine under high-dry magnification (430×).
2. If several milliliters are available, centrifuge at 500 rpm for 15 min and examine sediment in similar manner.

Naegleria is best seen by phase microscopy at 100× or 430×. Cover fluid with coverslip, seal with mineral oil, and keep slide at 37 C during examination.
Stained smear
1. For *Trypanosoma* or *Toxoplasma,* spread drop of fluid or sediment on slide and allow to air dry.
2. Stain with Giemsa as described for blood films (p. 2179).
3. Examine under dry (430×) and oil-immersion lens.

Culture
1. For **trypanosomes,** process as described for blood (p. 2180).
2. **Soil amebae** will grow in usual tissue culture systems but may be difficult for beginner to differentiate from neutrophils. Amebae also can be isolated on 1.5% Difco agar containing bacteria as described by Culbertson et al.[23] Prepare 1.5% solution of Difco agar in distilled water. Either add 0.1 ml live *Escherichia coli* suspension just prior to pouring 8 ml agar into sterile Petri dish or streak 4 cm diameter area of center surface with bacteria after agar solidifies in plate. Allow excess moisture to dry from inverted plate. Place small drop (0.05-0.1 ml) of spinal fluid or tissue emulsion in center of plate. If excess fluid is a problem, place inoculum on sterile antibiotic disk. Place inoculated plate in airtight container and incubate at 37 C. Examine 24 h later with 10× lens for signs of globular objects (amebae) migrating from bacterial zone. Cysts will form after several days if amebae are present.

Cerva[24] reported good growth of *Naegleria* for maintenance purposes in 2% Bacto-Casitone and 10% fresh horse, calf, or rabbit serum. Transfers were made every 5 d. See also Duma[25] for other maintenance media.
Animal inoculation
1. For trypanosomes and toxoplasma, process as described for animal inoculation (p. 2181).
2. For *Naegleria* or other soil amebae, inoculate 11-13 g mice intracerebrally with spinal fluid sediment or tissue emulsion. Inject through skull into frontal lobe of brain with ¼ in., 27-gauge needle. Draw each inoculum for each mouse separately. Observe mice 2 wk. If symptoms occur, remove brain aseptically and make microscopic examinations, cultures, and histologic sections. For best results, tissue for histologic sections should be preserved in 10% formalin as soon as possible after death. See Culbertson[26] for greater details on animal inoculation and other aspects of diagnosis.

Duodenal and bile aspirates

Although not done routinely, some investigators claim that more infections of *Giardia lambia* or *Strongyloides stercoralis* are uncovered by examination of duodenal aspirates than by fecal examination. Most investigators, however, rely on fecal examinations to detect these 2 parasites and examine duodenal aspirates only if fecal examinations remain negative despite clinical symptoms suggestive of infection with one of these parasites.

The duodenal contents may be sampled simply and conveniently by the duodenal capsule technic (Entero-Test*). The device consists of a weighted nylon string enclosed within a gelatin capsule. One end of the line protrudes from the capsule and can be taped to the side of the patient's face. The capsule is swallowed and the line is carried into the duodenum by peristalsis following dissolution of the gelatin capsule. The line is retrieved after 4 hours. The bile-stained mucus adhering to the string is removed by pulling the string between glove-encased thumb and finger, and letting the material fall into a Petri dish. Usually 4 or 5 drops of material are recovered.

The specimen should be examined immediately for motile organisms. If examination of the material must be delayed longer than 1 hour after collection, then preserve the material in 5-10% formalin.

Fasciola hepatica, Clonorchis sinensis, and *Opisthorchis* spp. are found in the bile duct. Aspirates of the duodenum or bile duct may reveal eggs of these parasites. Normally such infections are detected by fecal examination. However, *Fasciola hepatica* eggs closely resemble eggs of *Fasciolopsis buski,* an intestinal parasite. A differential laboratory diagnosis of the two can be made if eggs are found in uncontaminated bile fluid. It should be remembered that eggs of any of several intestinal parasites may be recovered if the duodenal aspirates are contaminated with detritus from the small intestine.

Procedures
Fresh smear
1. Mucus from duodenal aspirates should be examined under low-power magnification (100×). In the case of *Strongyloides*, active rhabditiform larva may still be in the egg. (Those found in feces have almost always hatched from the egg.) Such egg-encased larvae will usually hatch in 10-15 min and may then be examined more closely with iodine stain, if necessary.
2. Sediment may be concentrated by centrifugation before examination, if desired.
3. Eggs of parasites of bile duct are most frequently found in darkest bile.
4. Retrieve mucus suspended in bile and examine under low magnification (100×). Dilute with saline if necessary.

Stained smear. Not done.
Culture. Not done.
Animal inoculation. Not done.

Proctoscopic aspirate or biopsy

Proctoscopic aspirates may reveal *Entamoeba histolytica* trophozoites, indicating amebic lesions of the lower sigmoid colon and rectum. However, such material is not recommended for **routine** diagnosis of amebiasis, since the infected individual may have no lesions in the area or he may be a cyst passer. Such examination should be resorted to only **after** fecal examination gives negative results.

Proctoscopic biopsy often detects eggs of *Schistosoma mansoni, S. haematobium,* or *S. japonicum* that have been deposited in the lower mesenteric and rectal venules and have worked their way into the adjacent tissues of the sigmoid colon and rectum. *S. haematobium* may be demonstrated from cystoscopic biopsy material from the bladder.

Entamoeba histolytica
Procedures
Fresh smear
1. Collect material by means of Volkmann spoon or through sigmoidoscope.
2. Place in saline, cover with coverglass, and examine immediately. Since tissue cells often resemble *E. histolytica,* diagnosis of amebiasis is more reliable if material is preserved immediately and then stained with permanent stain.

Stained smear. Preserve material in PVA (p. 2172) and prepare permanently stained smear (p. 2168) when desired. Material can be smeared on a slide, fixed in Schaudinn fixative, and then permanently stained.
Culture. See Cultivation technics (p. 2174).
Animal inoculation. Not done.

Schistosome eggs
Procedures
Fresh smear
1. Obtain by sigmoidoscope a small piece of mucosa from middle valve of Houston about 10 cm from anus.
2. Place specimen in tap water 3-5 min.
3. Flatten between 2 slides and add drop of water and coverglass.
4. Examine under low-power magnification (100×). Live schistosome eggs have normal shape and are golden yellow. Dead eggs are usually black and miracidium structure is distorted.

Stained smear. Not done.
Culture. Not done.
Animal inoculation. Not done.

Splenic aspirate or biopsy

Splenic aspirates and biopsy material are especially suitable for demonstrating *Trypanosoma cruzi, Leishmania donovani,* and *Toxoplasma gondii.* Splenic puncture can be dangerous in inexperienced hands, and for this reason sternal puncture (bone marrow) is often a preferred alternative diagnostic material, especially in young infants or early cases in which the spleen is soft and not greatly enlarged. However,

---

*Obtained from Health Development Corp., 2411 Pulgas Ave., Palo Alto, Calif. 94303.

splenic puncture has not proved unduly hazardous in endemic areas provided a size 20 or
smaller needle is used. Stained smears, cultures,
animal inoculations, and histologic sections can
be made from splenic material.

Procedures
Fresh smear. Not done.
Stained smear
1. Using forceps, touch fresh tissue to glass slide
   several times until 2-3 cm² area is covered with
   thin film of cells. Do not streak tissue along slide.
   As an alternative, tissue can be pressed between 2
   slides and smears made by pulling slides across
   each other until they separate.
2. Allow smear to air dry and stain with Giemsa as for
   blood (p. 2179).
3. Examine under high magnification (430×). If parasites are seen, examine under oil immersion for
   detailed morphology.
Histologic section. Fix, section, and stain tissue by
standard histologic methods.
Culture
1. For *Trypanosoma* and *Leishmania* collect spleen
   tissue aseptically and cut into small pieces under
   aseptic conditions.
2. Aseptically introduce one or more pieces of tissue
   into fluid condensate of each tube of NNN medium.
3. Incubate and examine as described for blood cultures (p. 2180).
Animal inoculation
1. Collect splenic tissue aseptically and grind with
   sterile mortar and pestle with about 9 parts sterile
   saline. Grind until suspension will pass through
   21- or 22-gauge needle. Suspension must be even
   finer if it is to be inoculated intracerebrally as recommended for *Toxoplasma.*
2. Draw suspension into needle and syringe and
   inoculate up to 1.0 ml intraperitoneally into appropriate species of animals (p. 2181).
3. Follow the animals as described on p. 2181.

Liver aspirate, biopsy, and lesions

Liver aspirates and biopsies provide material
for demonstrating *Trypanosoma cruzi, Leishmania donovani,* and *Toxoplasma gondii.* Examination of liver aspirates and tissue for protozoa is
not done routinely except perhaps at autopsy.
More positives are usually found from examination of spleen or bone marrow.

Liver lesions caused by *Echinococcus granulosus, E. multilocularis,* and *Toxocara canis* may
be seen by the naked eye in instances where the
liver is exposed for view. The diagnosis of *Echinococcus granulosus* is usually made on clinical
and serologic grounds. Such a diagnosis can be
confirmed by examination of fluid from the
hydatid cyst for scolices on surgical removal of
the cyst. Diagnosis of *E. multilocularis* is usually
made on clinical and serologic grounds. *E. multilocularis* is seldom discovered until autopsy, at
which time germinal tissue and possibly scolices
will be seen. *Toxocara canis* larvae may be encased in granulomatous lesions visible to the eye
at laparotomy. Such lesions can be biopsied and
sectioned for study.

Entamoeba histolytica may cause abscess formation in the liver. The great bulk of purulent
material in the abscess contains no amebae.
Material scraped from the abscess wall may be
examined microscopically for motile amebae
mixed with PVA on slide (1 drop aspirate with 2-3
drops PVA) and examined as permanently
stained smear or inoculate material into culture
medium (p. 2174). If the amebic abscess is bacteriologically sterile, fecal bacteria must be
added to the culture medium to obtain enough
growth for serial transfer.

Trypanosoma, Leishmania, and Toxoplasma
Procedures
Fresh smear. Not usually done.
Stained smear. For protozoa proceed as described for
splenic aspirate and biopsy (p. 2183).
Culture
1. See Splenic aspirate and biopsy (p. 2183) for tissue
   preparation methods.
2. For *T. cruzi* and *L. donovani* as described earlier
   for blood culture (p. 2180).
Histologic section. Fix, section, and stain according
to standard methods.
Animal inoculation
1. For tissue preparation see Splenic aspirate and
   biopsy, p. 2183.
2. For *T. cruzi, L. donovani,* and *Toxoplasma*
   proceed as described on p. 2181.

Lymph node aspirate or biopsy

Lymph node material is especially useful for
demonstrating *Trypanosoma gambiense* or *T.
rhodesiense.* When the postcervical nodes are
palpable, this is the material of choice for these
trypanosomes. *T. cruzi* is often found in enlarged
cervical and inguinal lymph nodes during the
acute phase of disease. *Leishmania donovani*
may be found in similar material, especially in
the Mediterranean and Sudan cases. *Toxoplasma*
organisms may be found in lymph nodes of acute
cases with lymphadenitis.

Procedures
Fresh smears. Fluid material from lymph node puncture should be examined for motile trypanosomes
under high-power magnification (430×).
Stained smears. As described for splenic aspirate and
biopsy (p. 2183).
Culture. As described for blood culture (p. 2180), but
culture is seldom done for lack of sufficient material.
Animal inoculation. As described for blood inoculation (p. 2181), but inoculation is seldom done for lack of
sufficient material.

Bone marrow

Examination of bone marrow obtained from
the sternum or iliac crest is the diagnostic
method of choice for *Leishmania donovani.* If
blood examination and inoculation fail to demonstrate *T. cruzi,* then bone marrow examinations
should be considered before splenic puncture.

Procedures
Fresh smear. Primarily used for motile trypanosomes. Place material in drop of saline and cover with

coverglass. Examine under high-dry magnification (430×).

Stained smear. Make thin smear and allow to dry. Stain with modified Giemsa procedure as described for *Leishmania* in blood (p. 2179)

Culture. Primarily used for *Leishmania donovani* but may be useful for trypanosome infection. After obtaining specimen, inoculate appropriate media as described for blood culture (p. 2180), except use smaller inoculum.

Animal inoculation. Seldom done for *Leishmania donovani* because it takes several months for animals to become positive. Material is inoculated into animals as described for animal inoculation with blood (p. 2181).

Muscle biopsy

Examination of bits of muscle tissue may make possible a definitive diagnosis of trichinosis or cysticercosis (*Taenia solium* larva infection). *Trichinella* larvae may be found in most voluntary muscle tissue. The pectoralis major muscles and to a lesser extent the deltoid, biceps, and gastrocnemius may be biopsied and examined. However, immunologic tests (p. 2186) are used more often for diagnosis of trichinosis than muscle biopsy. Similarly *Toxocara canis* larvae are found occasionally in muscle, but they are found most frequently in the liver, brain, or other organs.

For *Trichinella spiralis*, obtain a snip of muscle and place on a slide with a drop of saline. Tease muscle fibers into small strands and press material between 2 slides. Examine under low power (100×). Larvae from an infection that may have been acquired in the past will be encased in a cystlike host reaction, whereas larvae from a recently infected host may be smaller and lack the pronounced cystlike reaction. Tissue sections of recent infections will show more or less acute inflammatory changes around the larvae, which will be absent in older infections. Infections are more likely to be detected if the muscle is digested in a 1% HCl and 1% pepsin mixture at 37 C and the sediment examined. However, such a procedure does not differentiate between an old and recent infection.

Taenia solium larvae, causing cystocercosis, may be found in almost any body tissue. In descending order of frequency they have been found in subcutaneous tissue, eye, brain, musculature, heart, liver, lungs, and abdominal cavity. Biopsy material from nodules in subcutaneous tissue is used for diagnosis in most cases. Carefully dissect the larvae out of the nodular tissue and demonstrate the characteristic hooklets and suckers under the microscope by compressing the larvae between a slide and coverglass.

The protozoan, *Sarcocystis lindemanni*, is usually an incidental finding discovered at autopsy. The cysts may be found in muscles, especially in the chest, esophagus, diaphragm, and abdomen. To the eye they appear as minute white streaks within the muscle fiber. Microscopically, a cystlike body containing round- or crescent-shaped spores is seen. Although pathogenic for domestic animals, it causes no known disease in humans. Diagnosis is by microscopic demonstration of the cyst.

Trypanosoma cruzi has a predilection for heart muscle. In tissue taken at autopsy the organism may be demonstrated in tissue sections, by cultivation (p. 2180), and by animal inoculation (p. 2181) technics.

Lung lesions

The hydatid cyst of *Echinococcus granulosus* may be found either in the liver or, less frequently, in the lung, particularly at the base. Diagnosis is usually made from the case history, symptoms, x-ray films, and immunologic tests. The diagnosis may be confirmed by examination of hydatid cyst fluid on surgical removal of the cyst. Such fluid may reveal scolices and germinal tissue.

Adults of *Paragonimus westermani* may be found in the deeper layers of the lungs near the bronchioles. They typically provoke a granulomatous reaction progressing to fibrous encapsulation. In addition to the lungs, the worms may reside in the liver, intestinal wall, mesenteric lymph nodes, muscles, testes, brain, peritoneum, or pleura. Diagnosis is made on clinical grounds and by demonstration of eggs in sputum. Adults are seldom recovered, except at autopsy.

Amebic abscesses of the lung caused by *Entamoeba histolytica* are most frequently, but not always, extensions of a hepatic abscess through the diaphragm. If the abscess involves a bronchus, pinkish yellow or anchovy-colored material may be coughed up that contains trophozoites. The presence of amebic lung abscess is usually diagnosed on clinical grounds, hepatic involvement, and the presence of trophozoites in sputum.

Pneumocystis carinii may be found in lung tissues, usually at autopsy. Although not common, it may give rise to an interstitial plasma cell pneumonia in premature or debilitated babies in the first 3 mo after birth. Adults receiving immunosuppressive or cytotoxic drugs may develop *Pneumocystis* pneumonia. In hematoxylin-eosin–stained tissue, parasites appear as lightly stained foamy masses. Better differentiation of cyst stages occurs with the use of the methenamine silver stain procedure.

Skin scrapings and lesions

Leishmania tropica and *L. braziliensis* typically cause ulcerlike lesions on various parts of the body. Following inadequate therapy, *L. donovani* may cause postkala-azar dermal leishmanoid as evidenced by appearance of nodules and depigmented areas that may contain the organism. *Onchocerca volvulus* and *Acanthocheilonema streptocerca* microfilariae may be found in skin scrapings of normal tissue. Rarely *Entamoebia histolytica* may spread from an intestinal or extraintestinal site and cause lesions of the perianal region or abdominal wall. Even rarer are reports of amebic lesions of the vagina and penis.

Leishmania tropica-braziliensis

Procedures

Fresh smear. Not done.

Stained smear. Make small incision through skin at edge of ulcer and insert glass capillary tube. Force tube into tissue **below ulcer bed** and collect tissue fluid by capillary attraction. Avoid collecting blood. As alternative method, puncture tissue just back of and near edge of ulcer with 25-gauge hypodermic needle and inject few drops of sterile saline solution. Aspirate gently until material is just visible in syringe. Express material on slide, make smear, and allow to air dry. Stain with Giemsa as described for thin blood smear (p. 2179). Examine under high-dry (430×) and oil-immersion (960×) magnifications.

Culture. After obtaining specimen, inoculate NNN medium as described for blood culture (p. 2180). Antibiotics must be added to prevent bacterial overgrowth.

Animal inoculation. Possible, but not usually done. Subcutaneous inoculation of material into hamsters will give rise to cutaneous lesions.

Leishmania donovani and postkala-azar dermal leishmanoid

Use the same procedures applied to *Leishmania tropica-braziliensis* above. Excise small nodule and cut into pieces for smears and cultures. Parasites seldom are seen in macular or erythematous lesions.

Onchocerca volvulus and Acanthocheilonema streptocerca

Remove a small piece of epidermis from any part of the body (shoulder or earlobe is used by many) by means of a sharp razor blade. The skin sample may be so superficial that no bleeding occurs. Mount specimen in saline and separate tissues slightly with dissecting needles. Observe under low-power magnification (100×) for active microfilariae. Adult worms of *Onchocerca* may be recovered from nodules in subcutaneous tissues. However, this procedure is done primarily for treatment and not diagnosis.

Entamoeba histolytica

Amebae may be recovered from the necrotic base of the irregular ulcer and examined under low-power (100×) and high-dry magnification (430×). Make the diagnosis on the basis of motile trophozoites.

Vaginal smears

Trichomonas vaginalis is associated with or may cause vaginitis. Diagnosis of acute cases is routinely accomplished by examination of exudate from vaginal smears. More positives are uncovered by culture technics. Males may harbor the organism in the urethral tract with no symptoms and serve as carriers of the infection.

Procedures

Fresh smear

1. Take vaginal smear and place small amount of exudate in a drop of saline.

2. Examine under low-power magnification (100×) for motile flagellates.

Stained smear. Not done.

Culture. Several types of media are available,* although medium by Diamond is probably superior (p. 2181).

Serologic and immunologic procedures

General considerations

Serologic and immunologic procedures used in diagnosis of parasitic diseases are of secondary importance to those procedures that demonstrate the parasite. However, in those diseases in which demonstration of the parasite is difficult, immunologic tests assume an important diagnositc role. In the case of trichinosis, echinococcosis, amebiasis, kala-azar, Chagas' disease, and toxoplasmosis, immunologic tests are important. Occasionally tests are used to aid in the diagnosis of other parasitic diseases such as filariasis, schistosomiasis, paragonimiasis, malaria, and cutaneous leishmaniasis. Kagan and Norman[26] summarized current information about serologic testing for parasitic diseases. Most antigens used in serologic tests for parasitic infections are relatively crude. In highly sensitive tests (passive hemagglutination, immunofluorescent technics, and other sandwich technics) lack of specificity often presents problems. Tests with lower sensitivity (flocculation, agglutination, precipitin, and complement-fixation tests) show greater specificity at the expense of sensitivity. Consequently it is desirable to test suspect sera simultaneously with an appropriate low sensitivity–high specificity test and a high sensitivity test. Many new tests are reported in the literature as serologic technology continues to expand. Enzyme-linked immunoabsorbent assays show great promise in detecting small amounts of antibody and may prove extremely valuable if they are specific. Table 100-5 summarizes the current status of immunodiagnositc tests for parasitic infections. Table 100-6 gives information on commercial sources of various antigens, reagents, and kits.

Trichinosis

Many different types of serologic tests have been utilized for diagnosis of trichinosis. The bentonite flocculation (BF)[28-30] test is the test of choice because of specificity, ease, and speed of performance and stability of reagents. The test becomes positive after the third week of infection. Generally peak titers occur several weeks later and then gradually return to negative within 2-3 years. This makes the BF test useful in differentiating recent infection from one that might have been acquired several years earlier. Titers of 1:5 or higher are considered significant. If possible, rising titers should be demonstrated.

*Commercially available from Difco Laboratories, Detroit, Mich., and BBL, Division of BioQuest, Cockeysville, Md.

Table 100-5. Summary of immunodiagnostic tests for parasitic infections

Disease	Test*	Status	Reference
Trichinosis	BF	Test of choice	27, 28, 30
	CF	Accepted as useful	32
	HA	Useful, needs further evaluating	40
	LA	Accepted as useful	32-34
	CL	Accepted as useful	35
	FA	Accepted as useful	31
	ST	Accepted as useful	27
Filariasis	BF	Useful, needs further evaluating	43, 44
	HA	Useful, needs further evaluating	43, 44
	CF	Useful, needs further evaluating	45
	ST	Experimental	45
Echinococcosis	BF	Test of choice	53, 56
	HA	Test of choice	53, 56
	CF	Accepted as useful	52
	LA	Useful, needs further evaluating	55, 56
	ST	Accepted as useful	52, 56
Cysticercosis	HA	Accepted as useful	32, 60, 61, 104
	CF	Accepted as useful	61
Schistosomiasis	CF	Test of choice	62-64, 105
	CL	Accepted as useful	32, 65, 66
	FA	Accepted as useful	69, 106
	BF	Accepted as useful	67, 68, 105
Clonorchis	CF	Test of choice	74
	HA	Accepted as useful	74, 107
	ST	Useful, screening test	74
Paragonimiasis	CF	Useful, needs further evaluating	76, 77
	ST	Useful, needs further evaluating	78
Visceral larva migrans	HA	Useful, but not reliable	49, 53
	BF	Useful, but not reliable	53
	ST	Experimental	50
	FA	Experimental	51
Amebiasis	HA	Test of choice	108-111
	GD	Test of choice	108-111
	FA	Accepted as useful	112, 113
Leishmaniasis (visceral)	CF	Test of choice	82
	FA	Accepted as useful	80, 82
	GD	Experimental	83
	ST	Accepted as useful	81
Chagas'	CF	Test of choice	32
	HA	Acceptable for epidemiology	87
Toxoplasmosis	Dye test	Test of choice	95
	HA	Accepted as useful	91, 92, 114
	FA	Accepted as useful	93
	ST	Accepted as useful for screening	90
Malaria	FA	Useful for epidemiology	97-99
	HA	Experimental	98, 114, 115

*BF = Bentonite flocculation, CF = complement fixation, HA = hemagglutination, LA = Latex, CL = cholesterol-lecithin, FA = fluorescent antibody, ST = skin test, GD = gel diffusion.

The immunofluorescence test is the test of choice for maximum sensitivity.[31]

Other tests such as the latex agglutination (LA) test[32-34] and cholesterol-lecithin (CL) flocculation test[35] are good simple diagnostic tests for small laboratories. These commercially available antigen preparations should appeal to laboratories that desire a rapid, reliable serologic test

that requires no preparation of antigen (see Table 100-6).

Below are presented procedures for preparation of 2 different antigen extracts of *Trichinella spiralis* larvae. The crude extract is easier to prepare than the acid-soluble protein antigen. However, the latter is considered a slightly superior antigen.

Table 100-6. Listing of commercially available parasitic antigens

Company	Disease	Type of reagent
Italdiagnostic, Rome, Italy	Echinococcosis	Latex test kit
	Toxoplasmosis	Latex test kit
	Toxoplasmosis	CF test antigen
ICN Chemical & Radioisotope Division, Irvine, Calif.	Toxoplasmosis	IF test kit
	Amebiasis	Agar gel test
Hyland Laboratories, Los Angeles	Amebiasis	Countercurrent electrophoresis kit
	Chagas' disease	Countercurrent electrophoresis kit
	Trichinosis	Latex test kit
Behringwerke, Marburg, Germany	Chagas' disease	Latex test kit, CF
	Schistosomiasis	Skin test antigen
	Echinococcosis	Skin test antigen
	Toxoplasmosis	CF and latex test antigen and sera
Wellcome Reagents Ltd, Beckenham, Kent, England	Amebiasis	IF antigen
	Chagas' disease	IF antigen
	Echinococcosis	IF antigen
	Leishmaniasis	IF antigen
	Schistosomiasis	IF antigen
	Toxoplasmosis	IF antigen
	Trichinosis	IF antigen
	African trypano-somiasis (3 antigens)	IF antigen
Cooke Laboratory Products, Alexandria, Va.	Toxoplasmosis	IF test kit
Ames Co., Elkhart, Ind.	Amebiasis	Latex test kit
Electro-Nucleonics Laboratory, Inc., Bethesda, Md.	Toxoplasmosis	IF test kit
Canalco, Inc., Rockville, Md.	Toxoplasmosis	IHA, microhemagglutination kit
Difco Laboratories, Detroit	Trichinosis	Bentonite flocculation test reagents
ICL Scientific, Fountain Valley, Calif.	Trichinosis	Slide agglutination test
Cordis Laboratories, Miami	Amebiasis	Countercurrent electrophoresis kit
Natural Veterinary Assay Laboratory, Tokyo, Japan	Toxoplasmosis	IHA sensitized cells

Crude antigen extract

The technic of larval collection is a University of North Carolina Department of Parasitology method modified by Moore.[36] The procedure markedly reduces host protein and bone particles from the antigen preparation.

Procedure. Infect 10 mice with 500-600 *Trichinella* larvae each (see Larsh and Kent[37] for technical details of larvae collection and standardization). Thirty days later sacrifice, skin, and eviscerate mice. Place 5 carcasses in Waring blender with about 250 ml digestion fluid (0.7% pepsin and 1% HCl). Blend for approximately 15 s. Repeat blending procedure with other 5 carcasses. Place all homogenized carcasses in bucket with a total 6 L warm digestion fluid. Digest mixture for 90 min at 37.5 C, stirring constantly with magnetic stirrer. Filter digested mixture through 4 layers of cheese cloth into three 2 L flasks. Fill each flask within ½ in. of brim. Stretch piece of wet gauze (36 × 44 squares/in.) tightly over mouth of each flask and secure with rubber band. Place 250 ml beaker over mouth of each flask and invert, with bottom of beaker in contact with gauze-covered flask opening. Stabilize upside-down flask with aid of ring stand. Add saline to level of about ½ in. above gauze-covered opening. Larvae will migrate through gauze and into saline. Gently agitate flask after 30 min. At end of 1 h lift flask out of beaker. Pool larvae present in beaker and wash larvae several times by allowing them to settle through several changes of saline. At end of fourth washing perform biuret test on supernatant fluid, and, if test is negative, larvae are ready for further processing. Either lyophilize larvae and then grind them up by mortar and pestle, followed by overnight extraction in cold saline (20 ml/ml larvae), or, preferably, break up larvae by sonic vibration, followed by overnight extraction in cold saline. Next day centrifuge extract at 10,000 × g for 30 min and discard sediment. Add Merthiolate to extract to final concentration of 1:10,000 and store at −20 C or lower. Antigen remains stable for many months.

Melcher antigen[38]

Extract 2 g lyophilized powdered larvae (yield of approximately 10 infected rats) with petroleum ether in Soxhlet apparatus for 7 d. Adjust temperature of Soxhlet so that apparatus empties once every 15 min. After removing larvae from ether, extract them in borate buffer (pH 8.3) at 4 C overnight. During extraction procedure agitate contents gently at intervals. Next day centrifuge extract at 10,000 × g for 30 min and discard sediment. Cool supernatant fluid to 4 C and lower pH to 4.8 with 0.2N HCl. Remove precipitate that forms by centrifugation again. Clear supernatant is Melcher antigen and should be kept frozen until use.

Bentonite flocculation test[30]

Preparation of "stock bentonite" particles. The objective of the following procedure is to prepare a stock suspension of bentonite particles of uniform size (approximately 3-5 μm) by fractional centrifugation. Homogenize 0.5 g no. 200 Standard Volclay (Wyoming bentonite) in 100 ml glass-distilled water in Waring blendor for 1 min. When particles are to be used without lyophilization, ordinary distilled or demineralized water may be used.

Transfer suspension to glass-stoppered 500 ml graduated cylinder and add glass-distilled water to 500 ml. Shake and allow to stand 1 h.

Transfer supernatant suspension to 50 ml centrifuge tubes and centrifuge at 500 × g for 15 min. Decant supernatant fluid and recentrifuge at 750 × g for 15 min. At this speed all but very small particles are sedimented. Supernatant fluid is discarded, and sediment resuspended in 100 ml glass-distilled water by blending in Waring blendor for 1 min. This is "stock bentonite suspension." It has been stored in refrigerator 6 mo without loss of activity. In event of contamination with molds, suspension is discarded. If bentonite particles are to be preserved by lyophilization, sedimented particles are blended with 20 min (and not 100 ml) glass-distilled water. Two 10 ml aliquots are lyophilized, and when needed, each vial is reconstituted in 50 ml distilled water.

Preparation of "stock antigen." Shake thoroughly stock bentonite suspension and transfer 20 ml to flask containing 10 ml trichina antigen. Mix and store at 4 C overnight. Antigen is adsorbed onto the particles in this step.

On following day add 5 ml 0.1% thionin or thionin blue O solution in water and allow to stand 1 h to ensure complete adsorption of dye to coated particles. This is "stock antigen" and may be used at least 3 mo after preparation if kept at 4 C.

Preparation of "test antigen." Shake thoroughly stock antigen suspension and transfer 8 ml to 50 ml round-bottomed centrifuge tube. Wash twice with 10 ml 0.85% saline by centrifugation at 1000 × g for 5 min. This removes nonadsorbed antigen from suspension.

Resuspend sedimented particles in 4 ml saline. Since saline causes flocculation of coated bentonite particles, small amounts of Tween 80, a nonionic surface-active reagent, are added to suppress this nonspecific flocculation. Prepare fresh solution of Tween 80 by dissolving 0.5 ml in 99.5 ml distilled water. Add 0.1 ml Tween 80 solution to antigen. Shake well.

Test with saline and normal serum (1:100) as described under performance of flocculation test. If particles are agglutinated, additional 0.1 ml amounts of Tween 80 are added until flocculation has entirely disappeared in negative serum and less than 50% of particles in saline are flocculated. Usually about 0.2 ml Tween 80 will be sufficient for 4 ml antigen.

At this point 2 positive control sera, 1 of high titer and 1 of low titer, should be tested, since excess Tween 80 may have been added, causing antigen to become insensitive. If titer of positive control serum is more than 1 tube lower than expected, excess Tween 80 has been added. Antigen may be washed once in 10 ml saline, centrifuged, and sediment resuspended in 4 ml saline. Readjust as before, using smaller amount of Tween 80. This standardized, adjusted antigen (test antigen) has been used from 4-6 wk when stored at 4 C.

Technic of performing test. Sera to be tested should be inactivated 30 min at 56 C. Each serum is diluted with 0.85% saline 1:5, 1:10, and 1:20. Positive sera are further diluted until flocculation is read as negative.

1. Pipet 0.1 ml serum onto wax-ringed slide and add drop of standardized test antigen with pipet that delivers 60-80 drops/ml.
2. Agitate slide on rotating shaker 15 min at 100-120 rotations/min.
3. Examine under dissecting microscope for presence of agglutination or flocculation.

Reading the test. 4+ reaction—all particles are agglutinated; 3+ reaction—75% of particles are agglutinated; 2+ reaction—50% of particles are agglutinated; 1+ reaction—25% of particles are agglutinated. A 3+ or 4+ agglutination is considered positive. A 2+ or 1+ reaction is negative. For each series of tests, saline control and negative and positive serum controls should be made.

Complement-fixation test

Many reliable complement-fixation tests have been devised for trichinosis serology.

Several complement fixation schemes are described elsewhere in this text. The variety of tests makes comparisons between laboratories difficult. The U.S. Public Health Service published a monograph, *Standardized Diagnostic Complement Fixation Method and Adaptation to Micro Test,** which recommends and describes in detail a standardized complement-fixation test and a micro adaptation suitable for large-scale testing or experimental tests when reagents are in short supply. Adoption of such a test by most laboratories would allow more accurate evaluation of results in different laboratories. The test described above uses the 50% hemolytic complement-fixation technic, adheres to the theoretical principles used by previous workers, and can be used as a practical day-to-day test with all antigens, including parasite antigens.

An enzyme-linked immunoabsorbent assay, using horseradish, has been used successfully to detect antibody against *Trichinella* 3 days after experimental infection of pig.[39]

Skin tests

Kagan[27] presented a review of past experience with the skin test. A commercial skin test antigen, similar to the crude saline extract of Bozicevich,[28] is available. Results with this and other antigen preparations have been variable. Apparently cross reactions with other helminth infections do occur. There is need for a sys-

---

*Available from U.S. Government Printing Office, Washington, D.C., by requesting Public Health Service pub. no. 1228 (Public Health Monograph no. 74) at $0.30 a copy.

tematic evaluation of the skin test. Because of cross reactions, probably more significance should be placed on a negative test than on a positive test. In positive tests an immediate reaction is apparent and reaches its zenith in 10 min and then begins to fail. Although delayed reactions have been reported, they are not diagnostically reliable.

Filariasis

Serologic tests are not used routinely to aid in diagnosis of filarial diseases because procedures that demonstrate the microfilariae have proven satisfactory in most instances. Also, it is difficult to procure satisfactory antigens to perform serologic tests. The most commonly used antigen for skin-testing suspected cases of wuchereriasis has been extracts of *Dirofilaria immitis,* the heartworm of dogs. The antigen is group-specific and reacts with other filarial infections. Bozicevich and Hutter[41] described a satisfactory skin test antigen prepared from *D. immitis.* Bozicevich et al.[42] described an antigen prepared from adults of *Onchocerca volvulus* that was satisfactory for skin tests and complement-fixation tests against cases of onchocerciasis.

Kagan et al.[43,44] evaluated the bentonite flocculation and indirect hemagglutination (HA) tests for serologic diagnosis of filariasis. Cross reactions with *Trichinella, Ascaris,* and schistosomiasis antisera were observed. They recommended that both tests be used and that (1) a 1:200 HA titer and negative bentonite test be viewed with caution; (2) a 1:200 HA test and a positive bentonite test be considered positive; and (3) a 1:400 or higher HA test be considered positive. The literature on immunologic diagnosis of filariasis is a large one. The interested reader should refer to Kagan,[45] Kagan,[32] and Jachowski[46] for reviews on this subject.

Increasing interest in the filarial etiology of tropical eosinophilia has led to serologic investigations in this area. Many workers believe humans are constantly sensitized, if not infected, with filarial species of lower animals. Serologic diagnosis and differentiation presents formidable problems. Pacheco and Danaraj[47] will introduce the reader to the literature on this subject.

Visceral larva migrans

Although the term "visceral larva migrans" (VLM) may refer to any immature helminth that migrates in the body, current usage makes the term primarily applicable to *Toxocara canis.* Specific immunologic tests for VLM are not available. Cross reactions are common with sera from patients with *Ascaris.* Similar cross reactions have been observed with antibody against a wide spectrum of other parasites (helminth, protozoan, and bacterial). Thus positive serology for VLM must be viewed with caution.

Hemagglutination and bentonite flocculation tests with crude somatic antigens of *Ascaris* and *Toxocara* adults are used routinely by the National Communicable Disease Center in the United States. Kagan[32] reported that antiserum will usually show a higher titer with the antigen of the species of larvae invading the body. Experimental work has suggested that larval somatic antigens and larval metabolic antigens are superior to adult antigens.[48,49] Wiseman and Woodruff[50] reported promising results with a skin test using an adult *Toxocara* antigen. FA using frozen sections of *Toxocara* larvae has shown promise.[51] A recently developed enzyme-linked immunoabsorbent assay using *Toxocara* larval antigen shows great promise.

Echinococcosis

Serologic tests have proved extremely useful as a diagnostic aid in cases of echinococcosis. Magath[52] reviewed his experiences with the complement-fixation test and intradermal test. Using hydatid fluid as the antigen, 93% of 41 proved cases of hydatid disease gave a positive complement-fixation test and 87% of 42 cases gave a positive immediate type skin test within 5-15 min after injection of 0.05 ml antigen diluted 1:50,000. The complement-fixation test became negative 2-6 mo after successful cyst removal, whereas the skin test remained positive for life.

Bentonite flocculation (BF) and hemagglutination (HA) tests have been developed for routine use and have proved more sensitive than the complement-fixation test. Titers of over 1:400 in the HA test and 1:5 or higher in the BF test are considered positive and specific diagnostic tests. Directions for the test are given in earlier publications.[53,54] A latex agglutination suitable for a screening test has been found 100% sensitive and 97% specific when compared with the HA and BF tests (Szyfres and Kagan[55]). These tests and the skin test were evaluated (Kagan et al.[56]). The sensitivity varied from 82% for serum from persons with liver cysts to 33-50% for serum from persons with lung cysts.

In some cases nonspecific serologic reactions of hydatid fluid antigen occur with serum of patients ill with other diseases. It has been found that patients ill with liver cirrhosis, nephrosis, lupus erythematosus, multiple myeloma, hypogammaglobulinemia, and agammaglobulinemia showed some degree of serologic reactivity in 28% of 129 patients tested with the bentonite flocculation and hemagglutination tests. However, if doubtful reactions were excluded and repeat tests were run, only about 7% of these patients were positive by the hemagglutination test and 8.5% by the bentonite flocculation test. Analysis of *Echinococcus granulosus* antigens from pigs and *E. multlocularis* antigens from cotton rats revealed the presence of host protein in these antigens and evidence that these parasites have common antigens with host liver. It was suggested that production of autoantibodies by the host may account for the nonspecific reactions, since the *Echinococcus* antigens, especially *E. multilocularis,* do contain host material. Differences in albumin-globulin ratio did not appear to affect serologic nonspecificity.

Crude hydatid fluid antigens are complex mixtures of host and parasite proteins. Immunoelectrophoretic analysis revealed at least 19 antigenic components with only 10 of these of parasite origin.[57] Studies indicate that hydatid antigens can be partially purified by column chromatography technics.[58] Similar success has been achieved with *E. multilocularis* antigens from experimentally infected gerbils.[59] This antigen may prove superior to hydatid fluid antigen because it can be collected from animals infected under controlled conditions and is readily available.

Immunofluorescent and immunoelectrophoretic technics give good results and are under evaluation in many parts of the world.

Cysticercosis

Serologic tests have not been utilized extensively for diagnosis of cysticercosis (larval *Taenia solium* infections), primarily because of the presence of cross reactions.

IHA, double diffusion precipitin (DD), and CF tests have been used most frequently. Of these, IHA appears to give the best results. In South Africa the test was 85% positive in proven cases of cysticercosis and 5% positive with unrelated hospital patients.[60] Spinal fluid gave higher titers than serum. Biagi et al.[61] found the IHA superior to other tests. Both studies reported cross reactions in cases with *T. saginata* or *Coenurus*.

Schistosomiasis

Serologic tests have been utilized by many workers to aid in the diagnosis of schistosomiasis. Most of the reported work has been done with *Schistosoma mansoni*, but since there are common antigens among the human species of schistosomes, the general principles elucidated with one species probably hold for all. Although many of the serologic tests utilized are the standard types, in general, they are performed only in endemic areas or in laboratories with the experimental facilities to provide a source of antigens.

The complement-fixation test is probably the most reliable test available. The reader is referred to the work of Anderson and Naimark,[62] Sleeman,[63] and Chaffee and Nieves[64] for analysis of this test with fractionated antigens and comparison with other serologic procedures.

Other tests such as the cholesterol-lecithin (CL),[32,65,66] BF,[67,68] and FA[69] tests have also proven of value. The CL and BF tests use a delipidized cercarial antigen. The FA uses cryostat sections of adult worms. These tests detect 70-80% of positive cases. Positive trichinosis cases give positive reactions in most schistosome serologic tests.

The intradermal skin test has considerable value because of the ease of performance. Most workers agree that antigens prepared from the adult worms give the best results. Kagan et al.[70] rightly emphasized the necessity of standardizing the nitrogen content of such antigens. The skin test appears better suited for epidemiologic studies rather than for clinical diagnosis.

Much work of experimental nature has been performed with egg, miracidial, and cercarial antigens, using a variety of fluorescent, precipitin, and agglutination type tests. Most of these tests are not suitable for diagnostic work.

Several excellent review papers (Jachowski,[71] Jachowski,[72] Kagan,[32] Jachowski and Anderson,[66] and Kagan and Pelligrino[73] are available that critically review the vast literature associated with immunologic diagnosis of schistosomiasis.

Clonorchiasis

Most serologic studies dealing with *Clonorchis sinensis* have produced equivocal or unsatisfactory results. Sadun et al.,[74] working with a purified antigen, found the intradermal and complement-fixation tests fairly reliable. Moderate cross reactions occurred, using the intradermal test, in persons with paragonimiasis and schistosomiasis, but this was not thought to be a serious obstacle, since this type of patient presents different clinical symptoms. With the complement-fixation test some cross reactions occurred in individuals infected with paragonimiasis, schistosomiasis, tuberculosis, and leptospirosis. In these studies the antigen was adult *Clonorchis* obtained from infected rabbits. The lipid-free borate-extracted antigen used in complement-fixation tests and the acid-soluble protein antigen used in intradermal tests were prepared by the method of Melcher.[38] For a brief review of the literature on immunodiagnosis of clonorchiasis, the reader is referred to Jachowski.[75]

Paragonimiasis

Sadun et al.[76] and Sadun and Buck[77] reported on rather extensive tests on patients with paragonimiasis, using the intradermal and complement-fixation tests. These workers obtained their adult antigen material from experimentally infected dogs and cats. The methods of Melcher[38] were used to prepare the antigens. The acid-soluble protein fraction was found superior for the intradermal test and the acid-insoluble (alkaline soluble) fraction best for complement-fixation tests. Cross reactions in cases of schistosomiasis and clonorchiasis were observed. However, in the case of the intradermal test, the wheal produced was always larger with the homologous antigen. Thus, by using both *Clonorchis* and *Paragonimus* antigens in endemic areas in which these infections overlap, one may tentatively differentiate the infections on the basis of relative wheal size. Toshisada et al.[78] isolated a skin test *Paragonimus* antigen by column chromatography that did not cross react when used on *Clonorchis* patients.

Amebiasis

The development of technics to cultivate *Entamoeba histolytica* axenically[79] provided reliable soluble antigens, and more reproducible, standardized tests were developed. At present the IHA, DD, and FA methods appear to be the best tests available at the moment. For a detailed discussion of these tests and others consult Chapter 98.

Visceral leishmaniasis (kala-azar)

The complement-fixation test has proved reliable in the hands of various workers. An antigen containing BCG or promastigotes gives the best results. The test is considered "specific" and is recommended in conjunction with other laboratory procedures done to demonstrate the organism. IHA and IF also give good results using promastigotes or amastigotes as antigens.[80]

The skin test has proved a useful screening device in diagnosis and in surveys[82] The fluorescent antibody[82] and gel diffusion technics[83] have shown some promise.

Several other tests, nonantibody-antigen reactions, may be performed on the serum of suspected cases of kala-azar. These tests take advantage of an altered albumin-globulin ratio and are nonspecific in that positive reactions occur in other diseases affecting the albumin-globulin ratio.

Formol-gel test (aldehyde reaction)

Place 1 ml of patient's serum, free from erythrocytes, in 9 mm test tube. Add 1 drop 40% (commercial) formaldehyde.

Positive result is indicated by complete coagulation of serum. Coagulation is complete if serum does not move when tube is inverted or shaken. One hour is allowed for coagulation process.

It has been noted that serum of a patient with kala-azar becomes coagulated in a few seconds and not in a few hours.

The test, like other serologic tests, is not absolutely specific. Although it is always negative in normal individuals, solidification of the serum takes place in other diseases besides kala-azar, e.g., malaria, leprosy, bouba, and alastrim, although the process takes a long time. In American visceral leishmaniasis the reaction is slow in the early stages but increases in rapidity with the degree of infection. It is useful in the diagnosis of American visceral leishmaniasis in the early stages and also can be used for evaluating the results of therapy.

Brahmachari test (reaction of Ray)

The Brahmachari test consists of formation of a turbid ring at the point of contact between serum and distilled water. Allow 2 or 3 ml distilled water to flow slowly down walls of test tube containing 1 ml of serum. Turbid ring forms at point of contact in positive cases; the stronger the reaction, the more definite the ring.

Cutaneous leishmaniasis

An intradermal test (**Montenegro test**) has proved of value in cases of cutaneous leishmaniasis in which the organisms are difficult to demonstrate. The antigen, prepared from cultures of the organism, is suspended in phenolized saline and is injected underneath the skin. Positive reactions show the formation of a specific papule, which reaches a peak in about 48 hours, remains 4 or 5 days, and then regresses and disappears. The test is positive in about 95% of proved cases.

FA tests using amastigotes have given good results.[84] Most other serologic tests do not detect antibody in sera from cases of cutaneous leishmaniasis.

Chagas' disease

The complement-fixation test has proved of value in the diagnosis of *Trypanosoma cruzi* infections, especially in chronic cases in which the organism is difficult to demonstrate. The major objections to the test have been the cross reactions with syphilis and *Leishmania* infections. Chaffee et al.[85] markedly reduced cross reactions with syphilitic sera by utilizing an antigen that had been lyophilized and extracted with ether and alkaline saline. Their antigen proved stable for at least 2 years. Further work by Fife and Kent[86] produced a lipid-free protein fraction that gave no reactions with syphilitic sera and few reactions with cases of cutaneous leishmaniasis. The antigen has remained stable in a lyophilized state for at least 5 years.

The HA test[87] also gives good results but is not as specific as the CF test. It is well suited to epidemiologic studies.

Toxoplasmosis

Serologic procedures play an important part in the diagnosis of toxoplasmosis. The **dye test**[88] has proved the most reliable and sensitive procedure. The test takes advantage of the fact that the cytoplasm of *Toxoplasma* organisms, once exposed to specific antibody, lose their ability to absorb methylene blue. The dye test titer is that dilution of anti-serum capable of preventing the cytoplasm of 50% of the *Toxoplasma* from being stained with methylene blue. The dye test becomes positive early in the infection and remains positive for years. The chief drawback of the dye test is that it requires living organisms.

The **complement-fixation test** has as its main advantage the fact that stable extracts of *Toxoplasma*-infected chorioallantoic membranes of chick embryos[89] may be used as antigens. However, the complement-fixing antibody appears later in the course of infection and disappears sooner. Used in conjunction with the dye test, it can give valuable information, especially if the complement-fixation test becomes positive in the face of persisting positive dye tests.

The **intradermal skin test**[90] becomes positive during infection and remains positive for years. Its greatest drawbacks have been the occurrence of negative reactions in infected persons and the presence of many reactors in the general population. Like the tuberculin test, the skin test for *Toxoplasma* gives information on the past experience of the individual but not the present status.

Several new serologic procedures have been developed in recent years. Jacobs and Lunde[91] and Fairchild et al.[92] have reported on a **hemag-**

glutination test (**HA**) for toxoplasmosis. In addition to not requiring a live antigen source the test proved quite sensitive. HA titers higher than 1:256 indicate recent experience with *Toxoplasma*. Another test, the **FA (fluorescent antibody)** test, is becoming increasingly more valuable as it is reliable and does not require living antigen as the dye test does. Indirect fluorescent antibody titers of 1:64 or higher are considered significant. Use of class-specific conjugates of IgM provides a powerful tool for diagnosing active toxoplasmosis in newborn.[93] Carver and Goldman[94] devised a method of staining paraffin and frozen tissue sections with fluorescein-labeled antibody, which should prove a useful tool for the pathologist searching for *Toxoplasma* in tissue sections. It also should enable differentiation of *Toxoplasma* from *Leishmania* and *Histoplasma* infections, all morphologically very similar in tissue sections.

Methylene blue dye test—Sabin-Feldman

The procedure for the Sabin-Feldman (methylene blue dye) test is presented in part as recommended by Brooke and Sulzer.[95] The original should be consulted for full details.

Materials
1. Antigen. Viable *Toxoplasma* organisms are obtained from peritoneal exudate of mice inoculated 72 h previously. Exudate should contain at least 50 mil organisms/ml and be free of bacterial contamination.
2. Accessory factor serum. Human serum containing no antibodies to *Toxoplasma* is required. It must not modify staining of cytoplasm with methylene blue in more than 10% of tested organisms.
3. Methylene blue–buffer solution. Prepared daily by mixing 1 part saturated medicinal methylene blue solution in 95% ethanol with 9 parts pH 11 buffer (97.3 ml 0.53% Na_2CO_3 and 2.7 ml 1.91% $Na_2B_4O_7 \cdot 10H_2O$). Buffer tablets are available commercially.

Procedure
1. Dilute serum in 0.9 % sodium chloride to 1:16, 1:64, and 1:256. Also include in series as controls a tube containing known positive serum, one containing saline, and another containing accessory factor.
2. Prepare *Toxoplasma* antigen by mixing 0.2 ml peritoneal exudate, 0.02 ml 1% heparin, and 0.8 ml accessory factor. **Keep refrigerated and use within 1 h of preparation.**
3. Add 0.1 ml *Toxoplasma*–heparin–accessory factor mixture to all tubes except saline control, which should receive 0.02 ml undiluted exudate.
4. After incubating 1 h at 37 C, 0.1 ml methylene blue–buffer solution is added to each tube and shaken.
5. A drop from each tube is placed on slide and number of stained and unstained parasites counted. Highest dilution is that dilution in which 50% or more of organisms have unstained cytoplasm.

Titers of 1:16 or less are of doubtful significance. In some areas 50% or more of the population may have positive dye tests. Serologic results are best interpreted in cases of suspected congenital toxoplasmosis. If both the mother and over 4-month-old infant have titers of 1:256 or more, it is highly suggestive, especially if symptoms compatible with toxoplasmosis are present.

Fluorescent antibody staining of tissue sections

Below are presented directions for staining paraffin sections with fluorescein-labeled antibody as described in part by Carver and Goldman.[94] The original article should be consulted for full details.

Procedure
1. Globulin is separated from pools of human sera, revealing high dye test titers, and conjugated with fluorescein isocyanate according to method of Coons and Kaplan[96] and treated with liver powder twice to reduce nonspecific staining of tissue elements.
2. Conjugates are diluted just prior to use with 2.5% crystalline bovine serum albumin in pH 7.5 Veronal HCl saline buffer. Degree of dilution must be determined for each conjugate pool and each series of tissues. Optimal dilution is that giving maximum specific organism staining and minimum nonspecific tissue staining.
3. Tissues are suitable for labeling **only** if they have been fixed in Wolman-Behar fixative (1 part glacial acetic acid to 19 parts absolute ethanol). Fixation for several hours to several days should be allowed.
4. After fixation, tissues are embedded in paraffin and cut at 4 μm on rotary microtome. Sections are floated on slides moistened with commercial detergent.*
5. Before staining, paraffin is removed and section partially dehydrated by passing through usual series of xylol and alcohols (to 70%).
6. After allowing sections to air dry, approximately 0.05 ml conjugate is placed on section and staining is allowed to proceed for 1 h at 37 C in moist chamber.
7. Shake off conjugate and wash slide in saline and then tap water 30 and 10 min, respectively.
8. Air dry preparation, mount in alkaline-buffered glycerol, and examine under fluorescent microscope.
9. After fluorochroming procedure, sections may be washed free of mounting medium and restained with celestine blue B and phloxine, followed by usual dehydration and mounting procedures.

Malaria

Primary diagnosis of malaria depends on demonstration of the parasite in stained blood smears. However, the FA and HA procedures are of value in epidemiologic surveys. The FA test is especially useful for investigating suspect blood donors who may have infected a recipient via blood transfusion or outbreaks due to common usage of contaminated needles. Tobie et al.[97] and Collins et al.[98] contributed greatly to the evaluation of FA tests. Using a thick smear preparation,

---

*Aerosal, Eimer & Amend, New York, N.Y.

the FA technic detects 95% of known positive cases[99] with a low (1%) false-positive rate.

The HA test is especially suited for mass survey work.[100] Modifications using lyophilized red cells make the test more useful and reproducible.[101] Malaria-infected children under 5 years of age may give negative reactions with the HA test[102] whereas they give positive reactions with the FA test.

Reagents

Fixatives and preservatives

Alcohol-formol-acetic fixative (AFA). AFA is a widely used fixative for fixing cestodes and trematodes. Worms must be transferred from this fixative to 70% alcohol within 24 h for best results.

Formalin, commercial	10 ml
Ethyl alcohol, 95%	50 ml
Glacial acetic acid	2 ml
Distilled water	40 ml

Bouin fixative for pathologic tissue. Tissue suspected of containing parsites may be fixed in this fluid.

Picric acid, saturated aqueous	75 ml
Formalin, commercial	25 ml
Glacial acetic acid	5 ml

Formalin. Some workers confuse formalin and formaldehyde. Commercial formalin contains approximately 37% formaldehyde by weight. This solution should be thought of as a 100% formalin solution and dilutions made accordingly. Thus 10% formalin is commercial formalin diluted 1 part in 9 parts water (and in essence contains 3.7% formaldehyde). Five percent formalin is a good preservative for protozoan cysts, helminth larvae, and *Hymenolepis* eggs. Ten percent formalin is a good preservative and fixative for other helminth eggs and nematode adults.

Glycerol-alcohol fixative. Glycerol-alcohol fixative is frequently used to kill, clear, and preserve nematodes.

Ethyl alcohol, 95%	90 ml
Glycerol	10 ml

Merthiolate-formalin (MF) preservative. MF preservative is used in combination with Lugol solution (below) to preserve and stain protozoa.

Formalin, commercial	25 ml
Tincture of Merthiolate (no. 99 Lilly 1:1000)	200 ml
Glycerol	5 ml
Distilled water	250 ml

Lugol solution

Iodine crystals (powdered)	5 g
Potassium iodide	10 g
Distilled water	100 ml

1. Dissolve potassium iodide in distilled water.
2. Add iodine crystals slowly and shake until in solution.
3. Filter and store in brown bottle. Make fresh solution every 3 wk.

Polyvinyl alcohol (PVA) fixative.* PVA is a widely used preservative for protoxoan trophozoites, especially amebae. The solution prepared as described below uses PVA powder.*

---

*Commercially available as PVA Medical Fixative Solution (500 ml bottles) and PVA powder (Elvanol 71.30) from Delkote, Inc., Wilmington, Del.; PVA powder (Gelvatol, grade 3-60) available from Shawingan Resins, Inc., Springfield, Mass.

Ethyl alcohol, 95%	156 ml
Mercuric chloride, saturated aqueous	312 ml
Glacial acetic acid	25 ml
Glycerol	7.5 ml
PVA powder	20 g

Add PVA powder to alcohol slowly, with stirring. Break up clumps with stirring rod. Heat solution to 75 C and stir continuously until solution becomes clear. This may take several hours if lumps are not dispersed. After clearing, add other components. When solution clears, allow it to cool. Slight clouding may be present but will not affect quality of solution. Keep PVA solution in closed container at room temperature until needed, then decant desired amount without disturbing sediment.

Schaudinn fixative. Schaudinn fixative is used to fix and preserve fecal smears prior to staining for identification of intestinal protozoa. Mercuric chloride–ethyl alcohol mixture will keep indefinitely. Once glacial acetic acid is added, solution should be utilized and discarded same day.

Mercuric chloride, saturated aqueous	200 ml
Ethyl alcohol, 95%	100 ml
Glacial acetic acid	12 ml

Stains for helminths and protozoa

Chlorazol black E stain.[103] Used for fixing and staining intestinal protozoa in fecal smears or tissue sections.

Basic solution

Ethyl alcohol, 90%	170 ml
Methyl alcohol	160 ml
Glacial acetic acid	20 ml
Liquid phenol	20 ml
Phosphotungstic acid, 1%	12 ml
Distilled water	618 ml

Stock stain

Chlorazol black E dye	5 g
Basic solution	1000 ml

1. Grind dye at least 3 min with mortar and pestle.
2. Add small amount of basic solution and grind until smooth paste is obtained.
3. Add more solution and continue grinding 5 min.
4. Allow particulate matter to settle a few minutes and pour supernatant into clean, dry container.
5. Add more solution and continue grinding and decanting solution and store stain in bottle for 4-6 wk.
6. Filter black cherry–colored liquid through Whatman no 12 filter paper before use. Keep filtered stain in closed bottle.

Delafield hematoxylin. Delafield hematoxylin is widely used for staining cestodes, trematodes, and microfilariae. Dissolve 1 g hematoxylin crystals in 10 ml absolute ethyl alcohol and add, dropwise, to 100 ml saturated aluminum ammonium sulfate (ammonia alum). Leave open and exposed to light for several weeks until hematoxylin is oxidized to hematein. Filter and add 25 ml glycerol and 25 ml methyl alcohol (for use, see p. 2179).

Giemsa stain. Giemsa stain is the most widely used stain for blood protozoa. Microfilariae stain well with Giemsa, although perhaps they stain better with Delafield hematoxylin. Giemsa stain may be purchased from commercial sources as a concentrated stock, but each new lot should be tested because there may be variation in staining reactions produced by different lots. Some workers prefer to prepare their own stock solution. Directions for preparing stock solutions are given below.

Powdered Giemsa	1 g
Glycerol	66 ml
Methyl alcohol, absolute	66 ml

Grind stain in mortar with little glycerol. Add remainder, mix thoroughly, and pour into flask. Heat in 55 C water bath until stain dissolves. Cool and add methyl alcohol. Allow to stand 2-3 wk. Filter and store in brown bottles away from light. Dilute with buffer (p. 2196) before use (for staining procedure see p. 2179).

Hematein. Hematein is used for staining trematodes or cestodes (p. 2173). Dissolve 25 g aluminum potassium sulfate (potassium alum) in 500 ml distilled water. Grind 0.5 g hematein (Forbes-MacAndrews, color index no. 1246) in mortar with 10 ml 90% ethyl alcohol. Add ground hematein slowly to alum solution with stirring. Wash out mortar with alum solution and add to remainder. Stir several minutes. Allow to stand 30 min; then filter. Stain keeps 2 mo or longer in refrigerator.

Iodine stain for protozoa. Iodine stain is used for staining protozoan cysts in temporary wet mounts. Dissolve potassium iodide in distilled water. Add iodine crystals and shake thoroughly. Since solution will be saturated, some excess of crystals will remain. Store stock solution in brown, glass-stoppered bottles away from light. For use, decant or filter into brown glass dropping bottles. When solution lightens (usually several days), discard and replace with fresh stain. If stock solution fades or fails to stain protozoan cysts properly, add a few iodine crystals to again create excess of iodine crystals.

Potassium iodide	1 g
Powdered iodine crystals	1.5 g
Distilled water	100 ml

Iron-hematoxylin stock stain. Iron-hematoxylin stock stain is used for permanently staining protozoa in fecal smears.

Hematoxylin powder	10 g
Ethyl alcohol, 95% 100 ml	100 ml

Keep stock stain in stoppered bottle 6-8 wk before using. **To make hematoxylin stain for fecal smears, dilute stock stain by mixing 5 ml stain with 95 ml distilled water before use. Diluted stain will be a delicate violet.**

Lugol solution. Lugol solution is used as part of Merthiolate-iodine-formol (MIF) stain for protozoa. Prepare fresh solution every 3 wk.

Potassium iodide	10 gm
Powdered iodine	5 gm
Distilled water	100 ml

Merthiolate-formalin (MF) solution. This MF solution is used for staining protozoa for direct examination (p. 2167) or MIFC concentration (p. 2170). A slightly different MF preservative (p. 2184) is used for long-term preservation of protozoa. The 2 solutions should not be confused.

Formalin	0.125 ml
Tincture of Methiolate (no. 99	
Lilly 1:1000)	0.775 ml

Multiple proportions of this solution may be prepared, since the solution is reasonably stable if stored in a stoppered brown bottle.

Quensel solution[2]
1. Decant 20 ml saturated solution of Sudan III in 80% alcohol.
2. Mix with 30 ml saturated and filtered aqueous solution of methylene blue (medicinal).
3. Filter mixture into 50 ml 10% aqueous solution of cadmium chloride (cp for scientific purposes).
4. Gently shake occasionally 15-20 min (a voluminous flocculent precipitate develops and fluid becomes almost colorless).

5. Filter and remove all excess liquid from precipitate by placing filter paper with precipitate on another filter paper. Leave overnight.
6. Transfer precipitate to fresh filter and rapidly pass through 25-30 ml distilled water.
7. Dissolve washed precipitate in 250 ml distilled water.
8. Filter within a few days if fine crystals of cadmium chloride precipitate.

Valet-Weinstein-Otto vital stain[3]
This stain is used as a vital stain for protozoan trophozoites.
1. Prepare 2.5% soution of crystal violet by dissolving stain in warm distilled water.
2. Make 1% hematoxylin solution by adding powder to slowly boiling distilled water.
NOTE: Stains certified by the Biological Stain Commission are suggested. Both should be powdered.
3. Add 0.4 ml triethanolamine to 100 ml boiling hematoxylin in solution. Allow to boil additional 2-3 min. Cool to approximately 50 C. Cooling is important.
4. Slowly add entire volume of hematoxylin-triethanolamine solution to 20 ml 2.5% crystal violet, combining with constant stirring, resulting in immediate formation of precipitate. Mixing procedure must not be reversed.
5. Filter through medium-grade paper. As filtrate is collected, it is poured back into filtering stain, mixing thoroughly each time. Filtrate is repoured 4-5 times. Total final filtrate is discarded.
6. Using approximately 10 ml portions distilled water, slowly wash down precipitate adhering to sides of filter paper so that it collects on bottom of cone. Do not use more than a total of 50 ml wash water. This removes uncombined crystal violet and excess triethanolamine.
7. Allow precipitate to remain in funnel to dry. This may be speeded up in incubator at 37 C. When thoroughly dried, stain is removed from filter paper and stored in dry, stoppered container. In this form it is stable indefinitely.
8. Buffered solvent for dried stain is prepared as follows:
   a. Acetic acid solution: Bring 16.82 ml glacial acetic acid up to volume of 1 L, using distilled water.
   b. Sodium acetate solution: Dissolve 19.72 g salt ($NaC_2H_3O_2 \cdot 3H_2O$) in distilled water to make 1 L solution. Most critical staining will be obtained using buffered solutions falling within pH range of 4.5-5.5. The following mixtures, using above solutions, are isotonic with physiologic saline.

Acetic acid solution	Sodium acetate solution	pH
102 ml	98 ml	4.6
80 ml	120 ml	4.8
42 ml	158 ml	5.2
29 ml	171 ml	5.4

9. Prepare 0.05% solution of dried stain in acetate buffer. Stain will dissolve slowly but not completely within period of 2-3 wk. Occasional shaking will aid in dissolving. At end of this time, solution should be filtered and undissolved stain discarded. If allowed to stand for a longer period, solution may stain too deeply; however, this may be corrected by diluting with buffer. Filtered stains may develop sediment after several weeks,

but this does not modify staining reaction. Solution should be filtered periodically. (See p. 2168 for procedure.)

Semichon carmine stain. Semichon carmine stains is used for staining trematodes (p. 2173).

1. Slowly add 1 vol glacial acetic acid to 1 vol distilled water.
2. Add carmine powder slightly in excess of that which dissolves immediately.
3. Heat to 95-100 C for 15 min; then cool and filter.
4. Before use, dilute with equal volume of 70% ethyl alcohol.

Trichrome stain. Trichrome stain is used in a rapid staining technic for intestinal protozoa.

Chromotrope 2 R or fast fuchsin G	0.6 g
Light green SF	0.15 g
Fast green FCF	0.15 g
Phosphotungstic acid	0.7 g
Glacial acetic acid	1 ml
Distilled water	100 ml

Add glacial acetic acid to dry components of stain, mix, and allow to stand 15-30 min. Then add distilled water. Stain should be purple (for use, see p. 2169).

Solutions for concentration technics

HCl−sodium sulfate solution. HCl−sodium sulfate is used exclusively in acid−sodium sulfate technic (p. 2171) for concentration of schistosome eggs. Prepare HCl of specific gravity of 1.018 by adding 45 ml concentrated HCl to 55 ml distilled water. Prepare sodium sulfate solution of gravity of 1.08 by dissolving 9.6 g dry anhydrous sodium sulfate in 100 ml distilled water. Combine equal parts of HCL and sodium sulfate solutions. Final mixture should have specific gravity of 1.08.

Zinc sulfate solution. Zinc sulfate solution is used for concentration of protozoan cysts and helminth eggs and larvae. Dissolve 331 g in 1000 ml distilled water. This gives only an approximation of desired specific gravity. Check with hydrometer and add zinc sulfate or water accordingly until specific gravity is 1.18. Keep solution in stoppered bottle and check specific gravity at intervals.

Miscellaneous solutions

Buffer solution for use with Giemsa stain (p. 2194): Prepare 2 stock 0.067M buffer solutions:

1. 0.067M Na_2HPO_4 9.5 g/1000 ml (disodium phosphate)
2. 0.067M $NaH_2PO_4 \cdot H_2O$ 9.2 g/1000 ml (sodium acid phosphate)

Prepare buffer solution used in staining procedure by combining stock solutions in amounts indicated below to obtain desired pH. Filter buffer before use, prepare fresh weekly, and check pH occasionally.

pH	0.067M Na_2HPO_4	0.067M $NaH_2PO_4 \cdot H_2O$	Distilled water
6.8	49.6 ml	50.4 ml	900 ml
7.0	61.1 ml	38.9 ml	900 ml
7.2	72.0 ml	28.0 ml	900 ml
7.4	80.3 ml	19.7 ml	900 ml

Carbolxylene. Carbolxylene is used in iron-hematoxylin staining procedure for protozoa in fecal smears.

Xylene	3 parts
Melted phenol crystals	1 part

Glycerol-jelly. Glycerol-jelly is used for preparing permanent mounts of nematode adults and larvae.

Place 6 g gelatin in 40 ml distilled water 15 min. Then heat in 65-75 C water bath to melt gelatin. Dissolve 1 g phenol in 50 ml glycerol and add gradually to gelatin while stirring. Store in stoppered bottle away from light to prevent darkening.

Iodine-alcohol solution. Iodine-alcohol solution is used in iron-hematoxylin–staining procedure for intestinal protozoa. Prepare **stock solution** by adding iodine crystals to 70% alcohol to make dark, concentrated solution. **For use,** add drop by drop to 70% alcohol until urine-colored solution is obtained. Exact concentration of this solution is not critical.

Mordant solution. Mordant solution is used in iron-hematoxylin–staining procedure for intestinal protozoa. To distilled water add purple crystals of ferric ammonium sulfate to make about 4% solution. Stir until color is that of dark urine; then either remove crystals or pour off supernatant fluid. Fresh mordant solution should be made each day.

Destaining solution. Destaining solution is used in iron-hematoxylin–staining procedure for intestinal protozoa. Dilute above mordant solution 1:4. Destaining solution should have color of pale urine.

REFERENCES

1. Sapero, J. J., and Lawless, D. K.: Am. J. Trop. Med. Hyg. **2**:613, 1953.
2. Svensson, R.: Acta Med. Scand. **70** (suppl.):15-16, 1935.
3. Valet, C. A., Weinstein, P. P., and Otto, G. F.: Am. J. Trop. Med. Hyg. **30**:43, 1950.
4. Beaver, P. C.: Am. J. Trop. Med. Hyg. **29**:577, 1949.
5. Ritchie, L. S.: Bull. U.S. Army Med. Dept. **8**:326, 1948.
6. Faust, E. C., D'Antoni, J. S., Odom, V., et al.: Am. J. Trop. Med. Hyg. **18**:169, 1938.
7. Faust, E. C., Sawitz, W., Tobie, J., et al.: J. Parasitol. **25**:241, 1939.
8. Hunter, G. W., III, Ingalls, J. W., and Cohen, M. G.: Am. J. Clin. Pathol. **16**:721, 1946.
9. Hunter, G. W., III, Hodges, E. P., Jahnes, W. G., et al.: Bull. U.S. Army Med. Dept. **8**:128, 1948.
10. Scholtens, T.: J. Parasitol. **58**:633, 1972.
11. Nelson, E. C.: Am. J. Trop. Med. Hyg. **27**:545, 1947.
12. Balamuth, W.: Am. J. Clin. Pathol. **16**:380, 1946.
13. Stoll, N. R.: Am. J. Hyg. **3**:59, 1923.
14. Beaver, P. C.: J. Parasitol. **36**:451, 1950.
15. Desowitz, R. S., and Southgate, B. A.: S.E. Asian J. Trop. Med. Public Health **4**:179, 1973.
16. Burrows, R. B.: Microscopic diagnosis of the parasites of man, New Haven, Conn., 1965, Yale University Press.
17. Belding, D. L.: Textbook of parasitology, ed. 3, New York, 1965, Appleton-Century-Crofts.
18. Weinman, D.: Proc. Soc. Exp. Biol. Med. **63**:456, 1946.
19. Tobie, E. J., von Brand, T., and Menland, B.: J. Parasitol. **36**:48, 1950.
20. Hunter, G. W., Frye, W. W., and Schwartzwelder, J. C.: A manual of tropical medicine, ed. 4, Philadelphia, 1966, W. B. Saunders Co.
21. Kupferberg, A. B., Johnson, G., and Sprince, H.: Proc. Soc. Exp. Biol. Med. **67**:304, 1948.
22. Diamond, L. S.: J. Parasitol. **43**:488, 1957.
23. Culbertson, C. G., Ensminger, P. W., and Overton, W. M.: J. Protozool. **15**:353, 1968.
24. Cerva, L.: Science **163**:576, 1969.
25. Duma, R. J.: Clin. Lab. Sci. **3**:163, 1972.
26. Culbertson, C. G. In Manual of clinical microbiol-

ogy, ed 2, American Society of Microbiologists, 1974.
27. Kagan, I. G., and Norman, L. In *Manual of Clinical Microbiology*, ed. 2, American Society of Microbiologists, 1974.
28. Bozicevich, J., Tobie, E. J., Thomas, E. H., et al.: Public Health Rep. **66:**806, 1951.
29. Sadun, E. H., and Norman, L.: J. Parasitol. **41:**476, 1955.
30. Kagan, I. B.: J. Infect. Dis. **107:**69, 1960.
31. Sulzer, A. J., and Chisholm, E. S.: Public Health Rep. **81:**729, 1966.
32. Kagan, I. G.: Am. J. Public Health **55:**1820, 1965.
33. Bloomfield, N., and Snook, G. W.: Cornell Vet. **52:**569, 1962.
34. Maraschi, T. F., Bloomfield, N., and Newman, R. B.: Am. J. Clin. Pathol. **37:**227, 1962.
35. Anderson, R. I., Sadun, E. H., and Schoenbechler, M. J.: J. Parasitol. **49:**642, 1962.
36. Moore, L. L. A.: J. Elisha Mitchell Sci. Soc. **81:**137, 1965.
37. Larsh, J. E., Jr., and Kent, D. E.: J. Parasitol. **35:**45, 1949.
38. Melcher, L. R.: J. Infect. Dis. **73:**31, 1943.
39. Ruitenberg, E. J., Steerenberg, P. A., Brosi, B. J. M., and Buys, T.: Bull. W.H.O. **51:**108, 1974.
40. Kagan, I. G., and Bargai, V.: J. Parasitol. **42:**237, 1956.
41. Bozicevich, J., and Hutter, A. M.: Public Health Rep. **53:**2130, 1944.
42. Bozicevich, J., Donovan, D., Mazzotti, L., et al.: Am. J. Trop. Med. Hyg. **27:**51, 1947.
43. Kagan, I. G., Norman, L., and Allain, D. S.: Am. J. Trop. Med. Hyg. **12:**548, 1963.
44. McQuay, R. M.: Am. J. Trop. Med. Hyg. **16:**161, 1967.
45. Kagan, I. G.: J. Parasitol. **49:**733, 1963.
46. Jachowski, L. A., editor: Am. J. Hyg. monograph series no. 22, pp. 72-74, 1963.
47. Pacheco, G., and Danaraj, T.: Am. J. Trop. Med. Hyg. **15:**355, 1966.
48. Collins, R. F., and Ivey, M. H.: Am. J. Trop. Med. Hyg. **24:**460, 1975.
49. Krupp, I. M.: Am. J. Trop. Med. Hyg. **23:**378, 1974.
50. Wiseman, R. A., and Woodruff, A. R.: Trans. R. Soc. Trop. Med. Hyg. **64:**239, 1970.
51. Annen, J. M., Eckert, J., and Hess, V.: Acta Trop. **32:**37, 1975.
52. Magath, T. B.: Am. J. Clin. Pathol. **31:**1, 1959.
53. Kagan, I. G., Norman, L., and Allain, D. S.: Am. J. Trop. Med. Hyg. **9:**248, 1960.
54. Kagan, I. G., Allain, D. S., and Norman, L.: Am. J. Trop. Med. Hyg. **8:**51, 1959.
55. Szyfres, B., and Kagan, I. G.: J. Parasitol. **49:**69, 1963.
56. Kagan, I. G., Osimani, J. J., Varela, J. C., and Allain, D. S.: Am. J. Trop. Med. Hyg. **15:**172, 1966.
57. Chordi, A., and Kagan, I. G.: J. Parasitol. **51:**63, 1965.
58. Norman, L., and Kagan, I. G.: J. Immunol. **96:**814, 1966.
59. Norman, L., Kagan, I. G., and Allain, D. S.: J. Immunol. **96:**822, 1966.
60. Proctor, E. M., and Elsdon-Dew, R.: S. Afr. J. Sci. **62:**264, 1966.
61. Biagi, F., Navarrette, F., Pina, A., et al.: Rev. Med. Hosp. Gen. Mexico City **24:**501, 1961.
62. Anderson, R. I., and Naimark, D. H.: Am. J. Trop. Med. Hyg. **9:**600, 1960.
63. Sleeman, K. H.: Am. J. Trop. Med. Hyg. **9:**1, 1960.
64. Chaffee, E. F., and Nieves, E. E.: Am. J. Trop. Med. Hyg. **6:**727, 1957.
65. Anderson, R. I.: Am. J. Trop. Med. Hyg. **9:**299, 1960.
66. Jachowski, L. A., and Anderson, R. I.: Bull. W.H.O. **25:**675, 1961.
67. Kagan, I. G.: Bull. N.Y. Acad. Med. **44:**262, 1968.
68. Allain, D. S., Chisholm, E. S., and Kagan, I. G.: Public Health Rep. **87:**550, 1972.
69. Kagan, I. G., Sulzer, A. J., and Carver, K.: Am. J. Epidemiol. **8:**63, 1965.
70. Kagan, I. G., Pellegrino, J., and Memoria, J. M. P.: Am. J. Trop. Med. Hyg. **10:**200, 1961.
71. Jachowski, L. A., editor: Am. J. Hyg. Mono. series no. 22, pp. 82-83, 1963.
72. Jachowski, L. A., editor: Am J. Hyg. Monograph Series, no. 22, pp. 97-104, 1963.
73. Kagan, I. G., and Pellegrino, J.: Bull. W.H.O. **25:**611, 1961.
74. Sadun, E. H., Walton, B. C., Buck, A. A., and Lee, B. K.: J. Parasitol. **45:**129, 1959.
75. Jachowski, L. A., editor: Am. J. Hyg. Monograph Series, no. 22, pp. 79-80, 1963.
76. Sadun, E. H., Buck, A. A., and Walton, B. C.: Milit. Med. **127:**187, 1959.
77. Sadun, E. H., and Buck, A. A.: Am. J. Trop. Med. Hyg. **9:**562, 1960.
78. Toshisada, S., Takei, K., and Yoneyama, K.: J. Infect. Dis. **114:**315, 1964.
79. Diamond, L. S.: J. Parasitol. **54:**1047, 1968.
80. Kien Truong, T., Ambroise-Thomas, P., Ouilici, M., et al.: Bull. Soc, Pathol. Exot. **62:**1077, 1969.
81. Shaw, J. J., and Lainson, R.: Trans. R. Soc. Trop. Med. Hyg. **69:**323, 1975.
82. La Placa, M., Pampiglione, S., Borgatti, M., and Zerbini, M.: Trans. R. Soc, Trop. Med. Hyg. **69:**396, 1975.
83. Bray, R. S., and Lainson, R.: Trans. R. Soc, Trop. Med. Hyg. **60:**605, 1966.
84. Walton, B. C., Brooks, W. H., and Arjona, I.: Am. J. Trop. Med. Hyg. **21:**296, 1972.
85. Chaffee, E. F., Fife, E. H., and Kent, J. F.: Am. J. Trop. Med. Hyg. **5:**763, 1956.
86. Fife, E. H., and Kent, J. F.: Am. J. Trop. Med. Hyg. **9:**512, 1960.
87. Cuadrado, R. R., and Kagan, I. G.: Am. J. Epidemiol. **86:**330, 1967.
88. Sabin, A. B., and Feldman, H. A.: Science **108:**660, 1948.
89. Warren, J., and Russ, S. B.: Proc. Soc. Exp. Biol. Med. **67:**85, 1948.
90. Frenkel, J. K.: Proc. Soc. Exp. Biol. Med. **68:**634, 1948.
91. Jacobs, L., and Lunde, M. N.: J. Parasitol. **43:**308, 1957.
92. Fairchild, G. A., Greenwald, P., and Decker, H. A.: Am. J. Trop. Med. Hyg. **16:**278, 1967.
93. Anderson, S. E., and Remington, J. S.: S. Med. J. **68:**1433, 1975.
94. Carver, R. K., and Goldman, M.: Am. J. Clin. Pathol. **32:**159, 1959.
95. Brooke, M. M., and Sulzer, A. J.: Public Health Lab. **13:**136, 1955.
96. Coons, A. H., and Kaplan, M. H.: J. Exp. Med. **91:**1, 1950.
97. Tobie, J. E., Abele, D. C., Hill, G. J., et al.: Am. J. Trop. Med. Hyg. **15:**676, 1966.
98. Collins, W. E., Jeffery, G. M., Guinn, E., and Skinner, J. C.: Am. J. Trop. med. Hyg. **15:**11, 1966.
99. Sulzer, A. J., Wilson, M., and Hall, E. C.: Am. J. Trop. Med. Hyg. **18:**199, 1969.

100. Desowitz, R. S., and Saave, J. J.: Bull. W.H.O. **32:**149, 1965.
101. Meuwissen, J. H. E. T., and Leenwenberg, A. D. E. M.: Trans. R. Soc. Trop. Med. Hyg. **66:**666, 1972.
102. Voller, A., Meuwissen, J. H. E. T., and Goosen, T.: Bull. W.H.O. **51:**662, 1975.
103. Gleason, N. N., and Healy, G. R.: Am. J. Clin. Pathol. **43:**494, 1965.
104. Proctor, E. M., Powell, S. J., and Elsdon-Dew, R.: Ann. Trop. Med. Parasitol. **60:**146, 1966.
105. Buck, A. A., and Anderson, R. I.: Am. J. Epidemiol. **96:**205, 1972.
106. McCarten, W. G., Nzelibe, F. N., Simonton, L. A., and Fife, E. H.: Exp. Parasitol. **37:**239, 1975.
107. Guillermo, P., Wykoff, D. S., and Jung, R. C.: Am. J. Trop. Med. Hyg. **9:**367, 1960.
108. Sodeman, W. A., and Dowda, M. C.: Gastroenterology **65:**604, 1973.
109. Krupp, I. M., and Powell, S. J.: Am. J. Trop. Med. Hyg. **20:**414, 1971.
110. Juniper, K., Worrell, C. L., Minshew, M. C., et al.: Am. J. Trop. Med. Hyg. **21:**157, 1972.
111. Krupp, I. M.: Am. J. Trop. Med. Hyg. **23:**27, 1974.
112. Gore, R. W., and Sadun, E. H.: Exp. Parasitol. **22:**316, 1968.
113. Ambroise-Thomas, P., and Kien Truong, T.: Am. J. Trop. Med. Hyg. **21:**907, 1972.
114. Lunde, M. N.: Health Lab. Sci. **10:**319, 1973.
115. Sulzer, A. J., and Hall, E. C.: Am. J. Epidemiol. **86:**401, 1967.

MEDICAL MYCOLOGY

101

GENERAL CONSIDERATIONS

George S. Kobayashi
Demosthenes Pappagianis

Included among the vast number of organisms capable of producing pathologic processes in human beings and animals are the fungi.[1-4] Although historically, and for reasons of convenience, the fungi have been placed in the plant kingdom (phylum Eumycotina), differing views exist on the evolutionary development of these organisms.[5-6a] Several hypotheses have been put forward on their origin and these are based, in part, on the morphologic, cytologic, and chemical similarities exhibited by fungi when compared to various other forms of life, e.g., bacteria, protozoa, and algae. A currently popular theory on this interesting and highly speculative question postulates a polyphyletic origin in the systematic development of fungi.[6a] This view presupposes points of phylogenetic divergence from the protozoa and the autotrophic algae.

The fungi exhibit a large array of morphologic forms. They may exist on the one extreme as unicellular structures or on the other as multicellular filamentous colonies with a tendency toward cellular differentiation. Some species of fungi are dimorphic in that they possess the ability to grow and multiply in either a unicellular or a filamentous form, depending upon the environment. Germination and subsequent multiplication of a single haploid cell may yield yeast cells, multicellular molds, specialized sexual organs, fruiting structures, a variety of spore forms, or other specialized cells.

All fungi are **heterotrophic** and, with a few exceptions, **obligately aerobic.** They do not possess a photosynthetic or an autotrophic chemical mechanism for the production of energy or the synthesis of protoplasmic constituents. The absence in fungi of the photodynamic pigment chlorophyll is 1 criterion that distinguishes these organisms from algae and plants. For this reason fungi require organic nutrients to live. They obtain these nutrients by parasitizing or living in symbiosis with other forms of life and with decaying organic matter (meat, wood, and leather). The metabolic capabilities of fungi are diverse. In nature they are responsible for much organic degradation, which results in a myriad of new and frequently unusual organic compounds. Several economically important processes take advantage of the unique metabolic pathways of fungi, e.g., the production of vitamins, antibiotics,[7,8] enzymes, organic acids, alcohols, and esters.

Fungi cause many of the known plant diseases, account for damage to agricultural products estimated in the millions of dollars, and also cause disease in man and animals. Of the estimated 50,000-200,000 species, only about 50 are recognized to be pathogens of man. Some saprobic* fungi may also invade tissues and cause lesions under certain unusual circumstances.[9-11] The circumstances that predispose a small number of individuals to infection by these fungi are unknown. In some instances these organisms are found as part of the indigenous flora of man and may obfuscate the etiology of certain disease conditions. Fungus spores are ubiquitous,[12,13] produced in large numbers, easily disseminated in air currents, and frequently encountered as laboratory contaminants. For these reasons it is important that accurate evaluations and identifications be made of all fungi isolated from clinical specimens. The diseases with fungus etiology are called the **mycoses** and, with few exceptions, they may be categorized into 4 groups, depending upon the tissue level at which the infection is primarily localized. These categories are: the **superficial mycoses** (the outermost layers of epidermis and hair); the **dermatomycoses** (the epidermis, hair, and nails); the **subcutaneous mycoses** (subcutaneous tissue, fascia, and occasionally bones); and **systemic mycoses** (internal organs).

The microscopic morphology of fungi is extremely important in identification, and for this reason numerous illustrations have been provided in the text of this section. We are indebted to Dr. Malcolm McGavran, formerly of the Washington University School of Medicine, St. Louis, who assisted us in the photomicrographic work.

---

*Throughout this section the terms "saprobic" and "saprobe" are used in preference to "saprophytic" and "saprophyte" to emphasize the distinction between fungi and plants.

REFERENCES

1. Conant, N. F., Smith, D. T., Baker, R. D., et al.: Manual of clinical mycology, ed. 3, Philadelphia, 1971, W. B. Saunders Co.
2. Emmons, C. W., Binford, C. H., and Utz, J. P.: Medical mycology, ed. 2, Philadelphia, 1970, Lea & Febiger.
3. Rippon, J. W.: Medical mycology: the pathogenic fungi and the pathogenic actinomycetes, Philadelphia, 1974, W. B. Saunders Co.
4. Wilson, J. W., and Plunkett, O. A.: The fungous diseases of man, Berkeley, Calif., 1965, University of California Press.
5. Alexopoulos, C. J.: Introductory mycology, ed. 2, New York, 1964, John Wiley & Sons.
6. Bessey, E. A.: Morphology and taxonomy of fungi, Philadelphia, 1950, Blakiston Co.
6a. Webster, J.: Introduction to fungi, London, 1970, Cambridge University Press.
7. Brian, P. W., Curtis, P. J., and Hemming, H. G.: Trans. Br. Mycol. Soc. **29:**173, 1946.
8. Oxford, A. E., Raistrick, H., and Simonart, P.: Biochem. J. **33:**240, 1939.
9. Brown, C., Jr., Propp, S., Guest, C. M., et al.: J.A.M.A. **152:**206, 1953.
10. Henrici, A. T.: J. Bacteriol. **39:**113, 1940.
11. Torack, R. M.: Am. J. Med. **22:**872, 1957.
12. Conant, N. F.: Mycologia **29:**597, 1937.
13. Emmons, C. W.: Trans. N.Y. Acad. Sci. **17:**157, 1954.

102

CHARACTERISTICS OF FUNGI

George S. Kobayashi
Demosthenes Pappagianis

The wide spectrum of morphologic forms exhibited by fungi include single cells, the yeasts, and multicellular filamentous colonies, the molds, and mushrooms.

COLONIAL MORPHOLOGY

In general, yeast colonies are soft, pasty, and resemble those produced by bacteria, but in a few instances they may be mucoid, friable, or waxy in consistency. These colonies are composed of oval or spherical cells that reproduce asexually by budding (**blastospore** formation) or by cell division (**fission**). In some species of yeasts there is a pronounced elongation of the daughter cells that are formed. These cells have a tendency to remain attached in a "sausagelike" arrangement and resemble the principal vegetative tubular element (**hypha**) (**-ae**) of the molds. The "sausagelike" arrangement of cells is termed **pseudohypha** (**-ae**).

Molds are composed of branching hyphae that intertwine, anastomose, and grow by apical extension. These tubular filaments may be separated by cross walls (**septa**) or the cross walls may be absent (**cenocytic**). Collectively, the mass of intermingled hyphae is called **mycelium.** On the surface of solid or liquid media, young mold colonies have a characteristic cottony or velvety appearance that usually darkens with age and may become powdery or granular. This appearance is due to the aerial mycelium that projects above the surface of the colony and usually bears the reproductive cells of the organisms.

MICROSCOPIC MORPHOLOGY

Cytologically, the fungi are complex in that they possess a true nucleus with a well-defined nuclear membrane, mitochondria, and an endoplasmic reticulum. It is not uncommon to find many nuclei within 1 given cell. They also possess a rigid cell wall that contains, among other constituents, either chitin or cellulose.

Budding, fission, and apical growth are all examples of **asexual reproduction.** In addition many fungi have the ability to produce, asexually, other specialized cells called **spores.** The general process of asexual reproduction results in the formation of new haploid cells without involvement of nuclear fusion. Spores that develop on specialized hyphae are called **conidia** and those that result from fragmentation of hyphal cells, **oidia** or **arthrospores.** Certain fungi produce a thick-walled cell that behaves much like a resting cell and is termed a **chlamydospore.** Some species of fungi (e.g., in the class Phycomycetes) produce, endogenously, spores within a round, terminal structure. The large structure is called a **sporangium** and the spores, **sporangiospores.** The asexual spores that are produced may vary in

Table 102-1. General characteristics of classes in the division Eumycotina*

Class Phycomycetes

Cenocytic mycelium, although septa may be formed by some species; asexual spores (**sporangiospores**) produced usually within a sac (**sporangium**); unicellular motile sporangiospores formed by some aquatic genera; sexual reproduction involves conjugation of compatible haploid gametes, gametangia, or morphologically differentiated hyphal branches and results in the formation of diploid zygotes; includes *Rhizopus, Mucor,* and watermolds

Class Ascomycetes

Septate mycelium; variety of asexual spores produced; sexual reproduction results in the formation of spores (**ascospores**) that are produced within a sac (**ascus**); includes the perfect yeasts, *Penicillium, Aspergillus,* and ergot

Class Basidiomycetes

Septate mycelium; variety of asexual spores produced; clamp connections may be present between cells; sexual spores (**basidiospores**) produced externally on specialized structure (**basidium**); includes mushrooms

Form class—Fungi Imperfecti

Septate mycelium; sexual stage not observed; shape, size, color, and mode of production of asexual spores are the basis for identification of the genus and species of fungi in this form class; includes most of the fungi pathogenic to man

*True fungi.

color, shape, and size, but they are relatively constant for any given species. The morphology of the spores and the method by which they are produced constitutes the basis for identifying most of the species in which a sexual cycle has not been observed.

In fungi that possess a **sexual cycle** (perfect stage) the process involves the fusion of 2 compatible nuclei to form a diploid nucleus, followed by reduction division to yield progeny with haploid nuclei. The conjugation process is accomplished in a variety of ways, but it is a constant feature of any given class of fungus. Classification of the fungi is based on the mode of reproduction and the cytology of the hyphal elements.[1] A simplified scheme and some of these criteria are presented in Table 102-1.

Most of the fungi pathogenic for man and animals fall into the form class **Fungi Imperfecti** (Deuteromycetes), but pathogenic species of fungi that belong to the classes **Ascomycetes** and **Phycomycetes** are known. With 1 exception,[2] the class Basidiomycetes does not contain any known pathogens for man but is of interest medically because of the allergies induced by the spores and the toxic and hallucinogenic properties of some mushrooms.[3]

MORPHOLOGIC VARIATION

After long continuous cultivation of some species of fungi or incubation under suboptimal conditions, morphologic changes may occur, and these may be manifested in many ways. In colonies of yeast there may be smooth to rough variation similar to that exhibited by some bacteria. Sectoring may also occur, and this appears as wedge-shaped areas that may be different in color or texture from the main body of the colony.

Any mutation characterized by rapidly growing, thin hyphae and partial or complete loss of sporulation has been termed **pleomorphism**.* Some of these changes are temporary or reversible; others appear to be permanent.

DIMORPHISM

Several species of fungi are capable of growing either in a multicellular form (mold) or in a unicellular form (yeastlike or spherule), depending on environmental conditions. This phenomenon has been termed **dimorphism** and is not unique to fungi alone. Some of the nutritional, biochemical, and environmental factors that regulate this phenomenon in fungi are known. While changes in macromolecular synthesis during phase transition have been described,[5] much still remains unknown. Most of the systemic mycoses are caused by fungi that have the capacity to grow in either form. In general they reproduce in a unicellular form in tissue and a multicellular filamentous form in culture at room temperature.

---

*The original definition of pleomorphism, as defined by the eminent mycologist DeBary, designated the morphologic changes observed in the rust fungi as they appear on their different host plants and is quite different from the term as it is used here.

REFERENCES

1. Cummins, C. S., and Harris, H.: J. Gen. Microbiol. **18**:173, 1958.
2. Kwon-Chung, K. J.: Mycologia **67**:1197, 1975.
3. Paaso, B., and Harrison, D. C.: Am. J. Med. **98**:505, 1975.
4. Gilardi, G. L.: Bact. Rev. **29**:406, 1965.
5. Cheung, S. C., Kobayashi, G. S., Schlessinger, D., et al.: J. Gen. Microbiol. **82**:505, 1975.

103

METHODS FOR STUDY OF MEDICALLY IMPORTANT FUNGI

George S. Kobayashi
Demosthenes Pappagianis

In general the methods and technics employed in the laboratory study of fungi are similar to those used to study bacteria. However, certain procedures differ and these have been developed to apply especially to mycology.

COLLECTION AND HANDLING OF CLINICAL SPECIMENS

The methods employed in the collecting and handling of clinical specimens are of considerable importance to the isolation and identification of fungi. The sampling procedures vary according to the area and type of tissue involved. Although selective media are currently employed in the isolation and culture of most pathogenic fungi, it is important to use sterile technics wherever possible. This is especially applicable to skin surfaces that may be heavily contaminated with bacteria, dirt, and epithelial debris. Seventy percent alcohol is swabbed onto the affected area and allowed to air-dry prior to sampling. In some instances, such as superficial and cutaneous infections of the skin and nails, scrapings may be taken with a dulled scalpel or the edge of a glass slide, examined microscopically, and cultured on a suitable medium at room temperature (about 25 C); or they may be placed into a clean container, such as an envelope, and mailed to the diagnostic laboratory. In mycotic infection involving the hair of the scalp or beard, the hairs may be plucked or clipped and handled in the same manner as that described for skin and nail scrapings.

On the other hand, biopsies and specimens from subcutaneous tissues, fluids, and other organs (liver, lung, lymph nodes, bone marrow, spinal fluid, and blood) must be handled much differently. It is imperative that these tissues be examined microscopically and cultured as soon as possible before autolytic processes and bacterial growth make the specimen unsuitable for diagnostic procedures. Cultures taken in this manner are incubated at **room temperature** and at **37 C.** Clinical materials of this type should not be mailed, since they are frequently decomposed or overgrown with bacteria and of no value when they reach the diagnostic laboratory.

The most suitable vehicle for transport of fungus cultures is an agar slant medium in an 18 × 150 mm culture tube. The tubes should be stoppered with a plug of cotton rather than plastic screw caps or snap caps, since the latter types of closures can produce a tight seal and inhibit growth of fungi. If the culture is to be incubated before transport, the screw-capped tube is suitable, provided that the stopper is loosened to allow growth of fungi, then tightened prior to dispatching.

Pertinent data (patient's name, physician's name, site from which specimen was taken, date, and the presumptive diagnosis) should accompany all clinical specimens submitted to the diagnostic laboratory.

DIRECT EXAMINATION OF CLINICAL SPECIMENS

A rapid presumptive diagnosis of mycotic infection can be made by microscopic examination of clinical specimens. This procedure can be performed whenever a light microscope is available. The materials from suspected lesions are placed on a clean slide and covered with a glass coverslip. Epithelial debris and tissue cells that are present can be hydrolyzed by alkali without altering the structure of the fungus elements that are present. Ten percent potassium hydroxide is routinely used as a clearing solution, although lower concentrations of alkali containing an anionic wetting agent, e.g., Tergitol, and dye may be used.[1] The alkaline solution is carefully placed at the edge of the coverslip and allowed to flow under it. The slide is heated gently to hasten hydrolysis. After cooling, the coverslip is pressed firmly with the aid of a rubber eraser until only a thin layer of material is left. The slide is then examined for fungus elements, using low-power (10×) and high-dry (45×) magnification only. Because of the relatively large size of fungus cells, microscopic examination using oil immersion (100×) is unnecessary.

Exudates from abscesses and draining sinus tracts should be examined in wet-mount preparation as described above for skin scrapings. Exudates should also be smeared directly on clean slides, air-dried, and heat fixed. These can be Gram stained and then examined.

When spinal fluid is submitted for mycologic examination, the fluid should be centrifuged, the supernatant fluid removed, and the sediment examined microscopically for yeastlike cells. If an encapsulated organism is suspected, a small drop of **India ink*** emulsified with the sediment will aid in demonstrating the presence of the capsule.

Biopsy specimens and other large tissue fragments should be reduced in size prior to microscopic examination and culture. This can be done by mincing the tissue with a sterile scalpel blade or grinding in a sterile mortar. In certain situations use of an abrasive, such as sterile sand, will facilitate the grinding procedure. The ground specimen is then emulsified in sterile saline, and portions of this material can be examined and cultured accordingly.

CULTURE MEDIA

Fungi grow on a variety of laboratory media under various environmental conditions. For selective isolation of pathogenic fungi from clinical materials, advantage is taken of metabolic characteristics of the fungi.

A classic example is **Sabouraud glucose agar** (40 g glucose, 10 g peptone, 20 g agar in 1 L distilled water) in which a high sugar concentration and simple adjustment of the hydrogen ion concentration to pH 5.6 results in a complete medium selective for growth of fungi. Most fungi tolerate this acidic environment, whereas bacterial growth is inhibited or delayed. Unfortunately, saprobic fungi grow as well as, or better than, the pathogens, and they frequently overgrow the plate. A greater degree of selectivity for isolation of pathogenic fungi can be attained by incorporation of antibiotics in a modification of the basic Sabouraud dextrose agar formula. One such **selective medium** contains 0.005% chloramphenicol and 0.04% cycloheximide (Actidione) and is commercially available in dehydrated form.†

Chloramphenicol inhibits bacterial growth and cycloheximide inhibits growth of most saprobic fungi. A few fungi that have been implicated in

disease processes will not grow on this medium. These are *Cryptococcus neoformans, Aspergillus fumigatus, Allescheria boydii, Trichosporon cutaneum,* and some species of *Candida.* Therefore, for **primary isolation** of fungi from clinical specimens, cultures should be prepared in duplicate on **media with and without added antibiotics.** As an alternative procedure, media containing antibacterial antibiotics such as chloramphenicol are useful to reduce bacterial growth yet allow growth of saprobic fungi that have been implicated in disease processes of debilitated patients. One set of cultures should be incubated at **room temperature** and the other set at **37 C.** After the isolation of fungi from clinical specimens on selective antibiotic media, the organism should be transferred and maintained on a medium without antibiotics. It is important to remember that the yeast phase of systemic fungi is sensitive to cycloheximide when incubated at 37 C. Cultures should be held for 4 weeks before they are discarded as negative for fungi.

Occasionally some fungi cannot be identified on the basis of their growth characteristics on selective isolation media; these must be grown on special media. **Potato dextrose agar** stimulates the formation of spores and is prepared from an infusion of potatoes (200 g), glucose (20 g), and agar (20 g). Another medium that also stimulates spore formation is **neutral wort agar.** Both media are available commercially (see media for fungi, Chapter 72).

When the situation calls for consideration of a specific fungus or group of fungi, special media may be required to aid in the identification of the organism. These media are described in the text under the special circumstances in which they should be employed (e.g., see *Cryptococcus neoformans* for Christensen urea agar).

STAINING TECHNICS FOR HISTOPATHOLOGIC STUDIES

Although study by histologic technics is one of the most valuable means of diagnosis in pathology, dermatology, and other medical specialties, it has its limitations. One important reason for this is the similarity in the histologic picture of many infectious diseases so that if the causative organism cannot be demonstrated, a specific diagnosis cannot be made. Nevertheless, these observations frequently contribute to a working diagnosis of the disease process. Routine tissue sections stained with hematoxylin and eosin will demonstrate fungus elements; unfortunately, they stain poorly and frequently cannot be distinguished with ease from tissue elements. However, several other staining methods are available; although they are not specific for fungi, fungus cells stain much more intensely than surrounding tissue elements. The basis for many of these staining procedures is the chemical nature of the cell walls of fungi. The cell walls are rich in polysaccharide materials that can be hydro-

---

*A useful preparation is the following: India ink, 15 ml; aqueous Merthiolate 1:1000, 15 ml; aqueous Tween 80 1:100, 0.1 ml; filter through paper before use.[2]

†Mycosel (BBL), Mycobiotic agar (Difco Labs.), and Mycology agar (Case Labs.).

lyzed by periodic or chromic acid to release free aldehyde radicals. The numbers and types of free aldehyde groups made available by this hydrolytic procedure determine the intensity of staining of the fungus elements present. These can react with other substances, e.g., Schiff base, to give a color.

Periodic acid–Schiff staining technic (Gridley)[3]
Principle

Leucofuchsin (colorless Schiff reagent), formed by the reaction of basic fuchsin with sulfurous acid, is converted to a colored aldehyde addition product by cell walls of fungi that have been hydrolyzed with chromic or periodic acid. The cell walls of fungi stain an intense red after this reaction because of the large number of free aldehydes that are present. These aldehydes are produced by the periodate or chromate oxidation of the glucan and mannan polysaccharides that are present in the walls of fungi.

Gridley fungus stain[3]

Reagents
1. 4% Chromic acid solution (freshly prepared)
Chromium trioxide (CrO_3)	4 g
Distilled water	100 ml
2. Coleman feulgen reagent
Basic fuchsin	1 g
Distilled water	200 ml
Potassium metabisulfite ($K_2S_2O_5$)	10 ml
Activated carbon (Norit)	0.5 g
   a. Dissolve basic fuchsin in boiling distilled water, cool, and filter.
   b. To filtrate add 2 g potassium metabisulfite and 10 ml 1N hydrochloric acid.
   c. Keep solution in dark for 24 h, and then add 0.5 g activated carbon (Norit).
   d. Filter solution. Resulting filtrate should be colorless.
   e. Store at 4 C.
3. Sulfurous acid solution
Sodium metabisulfite ($Na_2S_2O_5$), 10%	6 ml
1N hydrochloric acid (HCl)	5 ml
Distilled water	100 ml
4. Aldehyde-fuchsin solution
Basic fuchsin	1 g
Ethyl alcohol, 70%	200 ml
Paraldehyde [($CH_3CHO)_3$]	2 ml
Hydrochloric acid (concentrated (HCl)	2 ml

   This solution is mixed and kept at room temperature for 3 d. Resulting deep blue solution is filtered and stored at 4 C.
5. Metanil yellow solution
Metanil yellow	0.25 g
Distilled water	100 ml
Glacial acetic acid (CH_3COOH)	0.25 ml

Procedure
1. Paraffin sections (6 μm thickness) of well-fixed tissues are deparaffinized to distilled water.
2. Place into 4% chromic acid solution for 1 h.
3. Wash in running tap water (5 min).
4. Place in Coleman reagent (15 min).
5. Rinse in sulfurous acid (3 changes).
6. Wash in running tap water (5 min).
7. Place into aldehyde-fuchsin solution for 15-20 min.
8. Rinse off excess stain with 96% ethyl alcohol.

9. Counterstain with metanil yellow solution.
10. Wash well in running water.
11. Dehydrate to absolute ethyl alcohol.
12. Clear with xylene and mount stained sections.

Microscopic observations
1. Hyphal filaments stain deep rose.
2. Conidia stain deep rose to purple.
3. Elastic tissue and mucin stain deep rose.
4. Background stains yellow.

Gomori methenamine–silver nitrate technic[4]
Principle

The chemical basis for the reaction depends upon the availability of free aldehyde groups for he reduction of an alkaline methenamine–silver nitrate complex to metallic silver. The free aldehydes are liberated from the chromic acid treatment of fungus cell wall polysaccharides.

Reagents
1. Chromic acid solution, 5%
Chromium trioxide (CrO_3)	5 g
Distilled water	100 ml
2. Methenamine–silver nitrate solution (stock)
Silver nitrate (5% $AgNO_3$)	5 ml
Methenamine (3% $[CH_2]_6N_4$)	100 ml

   Shake to dissolve white precipitate. Resulting clear solution is stable at 4 C.
3. Sodium bisulfite, 1%
Sodium bisulfite ($NaHSO_3$)	1 g
Distilled water	100 ml
4. Borax, 5%
Sodium borate ($Na_2B_4O_7$ $10H_2O$)	5 g
Distilled water	100 ml
5. Gold chloride, 0.1%
Gold chloride ($AuCl_3 \cdot HCl \cdot 3H_2O$)	0.1 g
Distilled water	100 ml

   This solution may be used repeatedly.
6. Sodium thiosulfate, 2%
Sodium thiosulfate ($Na_2S_2O_3 \cdot 5H_2O$)	2 g
Distilled water	100 ml
7. Light green stock solution
Light green, S. F. (yellow)	0.2 g
Distilled water	100 ml
Glacial acetic acid (CH_3COOH)	0.1 ml

   One part of light green stock solution to 5 parts distilled water is used as the counterstain.

Procedure
1. Paraffin sections (ca. 6 μm thickness) of well-fixed tissues are deparaffinized to distilled water.
2. Place into 5% chromic acid solution for 1 h.
3. Wash in running tap water (10 min).
4. Place into 1% sodium metabisulfite for 1 min.
5. Wash in running tap water (5 min), then rinse further in 3 changes of distilled water.
6. Place into methenamine–silver nitrate solution and incubate at 45-50 C for 1 h. Methenamine–silver nitrate solution is prepared by adding 25 ml stock methenamine–silver nitrate solution to equal portion of distilled water that contains 1-2 ml 5% borax.
7. Rinse in 2-3 changes of distilled water.
8. Tone in 0.1% gold chloride for 5 min.
9. Place in 2% sodium thiosulfate solution for 1 or 2 min.
10. Wash thoroughly in running tap water.
11. Counterstain with diluted light green solution.

Microscopic observations
1. Fungi stain black.

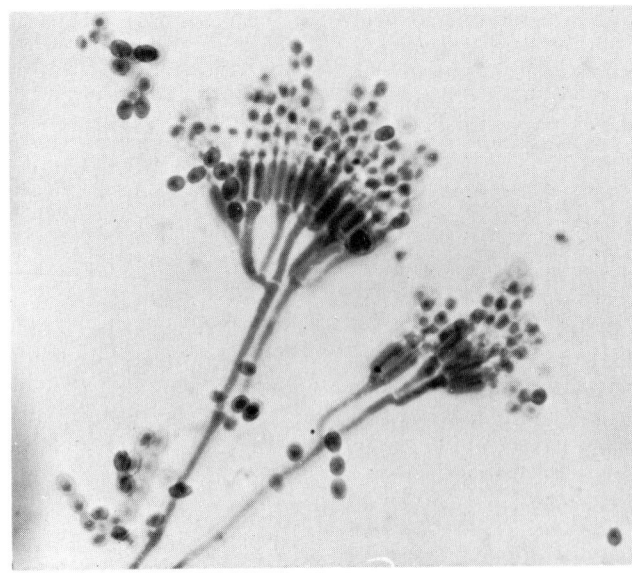

Fig. 103-1. Conidiophores and conidiospores of *Penicillium* sp. (×680.)

2. Mucin stains taupe to dark gray.
3. Background stains pale green.

SPECIAL MYCOLOGIC TECHNICS

Macroscopic characteristics of the colony such as rate of growth, texture, and pigmentation of obverse and reverse surfaces should be noted and recorded. It is necessary, however, to observe the **microscopic morphology** of the organisms to identify them properly.[5] A small portion of the colony is removed with a stiff wire needle. The material is placed into a drop of fluid (e.g., lactophenol cotton blue*) and teased apart with sterile, stiff dissecting needles. A glass cover slip is carefully placed over the specimen, and the preparation is examined with 10× or 45× objective. This practice may be unsatisfactory, however, in that the hyphae are broken, the spores are disrupted, and the physical relationships between spores and hyphae cannot be determined.

The **slide culture method** will obviate these criticisms and in addition will allow continuous microscopic observations of the growing colony (Figs. 103-1 and 103-2). There are several ways to prepare these slides; one of them is summarized as follows:

1. Microscope slide and cover slip, supported on bent glass rod, are sterilized in Petri dish containing circle of filter paper or blotter.

---

*Lactophenol–cotton blue mounting fluid[6]

Phenol	20 g
Lactic acid	20 g
Glycerin	40 g
Distilled water	20 ml

Mix together and dissolve by gently heating, then add 0.5 g Poirrier blue (cotton blue).

2. Several blocks of supporting growth medium (Sabouraud dextrose agar) 1 cm² and 2-3 mm deep are cut from sterile agar plate that has been previously prepared.
3. Sterile block of medium is carefully placed on slide in Petri dish.
4. Fungus to be studied is inoculated on all 4 sides of agar block, using a stiff wire inoculating needle.
5. Sterile cover slip is gently placed on top of agar block, using pair of forceps.
6. About 5 ml water is placed on filter paper in Petri dish to minimize drying of culture.
7. Cultures prepared in this manner are incubated at room temperature and examined periodically or until sporulation occurs.
8. At a suitable time, i.e., when spores are abundant, cover slip is gently lifted off and mounted onto clean microscope slide.
9. Agar block is removed and discarded. Clean cover slip is mounted on slide that supported block of agar.
10. Edges of cover slip may be sealed with petroleum jelly, fingernail polish, Harleco mounting fluid, or asphalt tar varnish.

ANIMAL STUDIES

Laboratory animals, inoculated with clinical materials, are occasionally employed for primary isolation of fungi. This technic is also useful for studies with pure cultures and for confirmation of the diagnosis of certain mycotic infections, especially where dimorphic fungi are involved.

These procedures are simple and are summarized as follows:

Laboratory animals (mice, guinea pigs, rats, hamsters) are housed in cages at room temperature (25-27 C) and fed and watered ad libitum. Inoculum will vary, depending upon the specimen. Portions of **clinical specimens** (sputum, bronchial washings, pus) are emulsified with antibiotics (10,000 U penicillin and 1000 μg

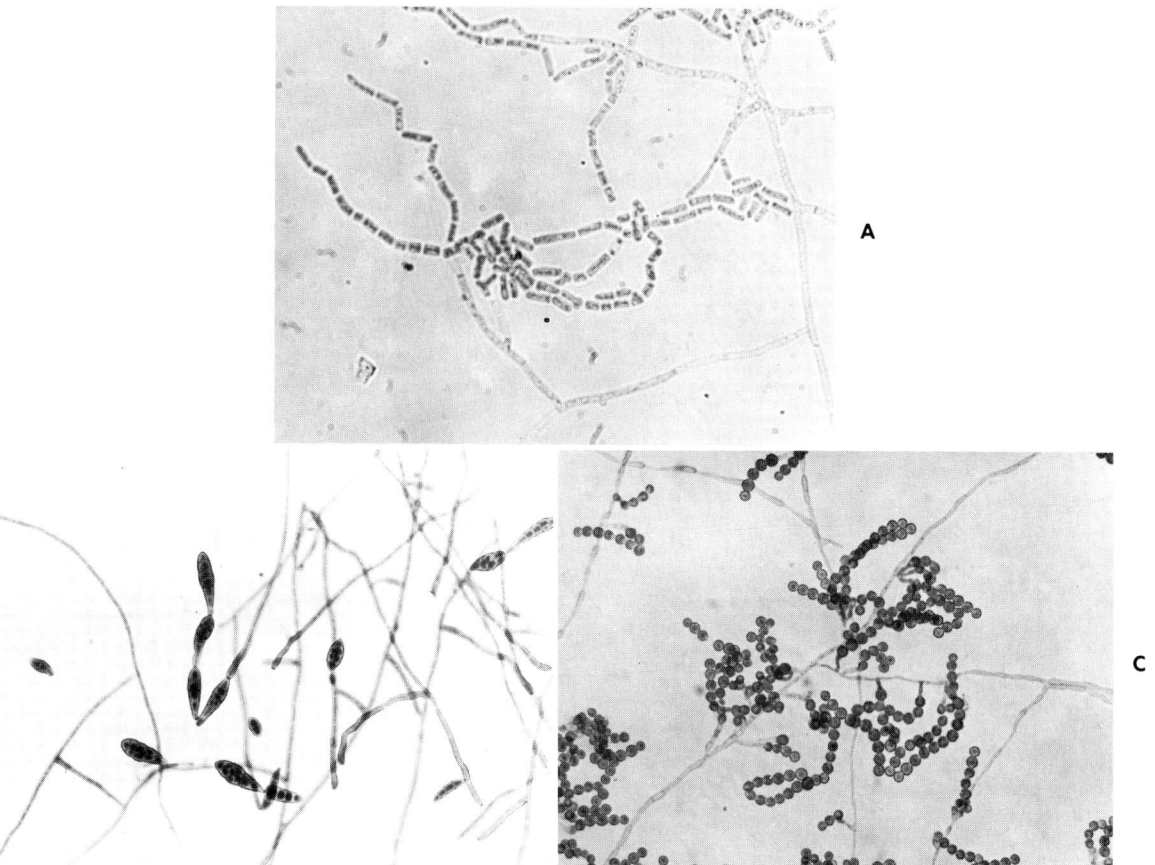

Fig. 103-2. Slide culture preparations. **A,** *Oospora* sp. (×680.) **B,** *Alternaria* sp. (×272.) **C,** *Scopulariopsis* sp. (×400.)

streptomycin/ml sample). For inoculation of pure cultures a saline suspension of spores and hyphal fragments is prepared from the organism. The technic for preparing suspensions of pure cultures will vary with the fungus that is under investigation.

Several **routes of inoculation** are employed (intraperitoneal, intratesticular, intravenous, and intracerebral) Each route may have certain advantages, depending upon the organism under investigation. These will be covered in detail under the specific fungus.

Necropsy studies must be performed on each animal that succumbs. Similarly, those animals that survive for 4 weeks should be sacrificed and necropsied. Cultures should be made from the liver, spleen, lungs, diaphragm, and nodes. These are seeded onto cycloheximide agar and Sabouraud dextrose agar and incubated at room temperature.

Obvious lesions should be examined under the microscope (10× and 45×) in the manner previously described (see Direct examination of clinical specimen). Tissues may also be placed in 10% formalin (4% for formaldehyde) for histopathologic studies.

STOCK CULTURE COLLECTION AND MAINTENANCE

It is beyond the scope of these chapters to describe all of the saprobic fungi, a task that would require several volumes. However, it is useful to study a selected group, especially those that are commonly encountered in the laboratory. These organisms are often found in clinical materials as contaminants or as part of the indigenous flora of man and animals. These organisms are considered to be the bane of bacteriologists when they are found growing in their cultures. To the mycologist, on the other hand, the repeated isolation of the same saprobic organism from several consecutive specimens of a patient may be of clinical significance. This is especially true when morphologic structures suggestive of fungi are observed in the lesion, and no other recognized pathogens have been isolated.

There has been a wealth of literature concerning the role of saprobic fungi in disease processes. In such cases they may act either as the primary source of the lesion or as a secondary invader. These fungi are frequently found in individuals with underlying diseases such as diabetes mellitus, leukemia, lymphoma, and aplastic anemia, or in patients receiving steroids, antibiotic drugs, antimetabolite drugs, or radiation therapy.

To determine which species of fungi are most populous in the laboratory environment, several Petri plates of Sabouraud dextrose agar may be exposed in critical areas and then incubated. It has been estimated that only a dozen or so organisms will be repeatedly isolated. Several taxonomic keys and well-illustrated reference books on mycology should be consulted for the identification of these organisms. In some cases, however, it may be necessary to consult an experienced mycologist or to send a particular isolate to a person who has specialized in the study of the particular genus under consideration.

Cultures that have been properly identified and are representative of various genera and species of pathogenic and saprobic fungi frequently become part of the stock collection of the diagnostic laboratory. The preservation and propagation of these cultures will, at times, prove to be a problem. Various storage methods have been suggested, each of which has its shortcomings.

Room-temperature maintenance. This method is usually unsatisfactory because the medium tends to dry out rapidly, necessitating frequent, time-consuming subculture to fresh medium. However, **cultures can be stored at room temperature if they are covered with a layer of sterile mineral oil.** The oil must completely cover the agar surface to prevent desiccation of the medium. Fungi remain viable for several years in this condition. When cultures are transferred from oil, the inoculating needles must be carefully heated to prevent spattering. Heavy mineral oil (Soybolt viscosity 330 at 212 C) can be sterilized at 120 C for 45 minutes.

Low-temperature maintenance. The problem of desiccation can be reduced by placing the stock cultures at refrigerator temperatures (4 C). Newer "frost-free" refrigerators have low relative humidity, and cultures may dry out rapidly unless tightly stoppered. The lower temperature will obviate the problem of frequent subculture, but some fungi do not survive well in this environment. Cultures may be stored at freezing temperatures (−20 C) for extended periods of time, usually 1-3 years. Many organisms remain viable without morphologic changes at this temperature.

Mite control. Another problem in the maintenance of stock cultures is mite control. These arthropods (class Arachnida) may inadvertently be introduced into the laboratory by mite-infested animals or cultures received from outside sources. Once mites establish residence, they contaminate other cultures by crawling from 1 tube to another. Mites may be exterminated by fumigation with 1,4-dichlorobenzene (p-dichlorobenzene), without damage to the cultures. Cultures are placed into a wide-mouthed jar or desiccator that has been seeded with crystals of 1,4-dichlorobenzene. The container is sealed, and the cultures are left in this environment for about 4 hours. This treatment should be repeated within 1 week. The incubator or room-temperature storage area should be cleaned with an insecticide, such as O,O-dimethyl dithiophosphate of diethyl mercaptosuccinate (malathion), to destroy all the mites and eggs that may be present. Other methods for the control of mites in fungus cultures are available.[7]

SAFETY PRECAUTIONS

Emphasis should always be placed on the use of sterile technic whenever mycologic studies are performed, to protect laboratory personnel, to obtain pure cultures, and to minimize contamination of the laboratory environment with airborne spores of ubiquitous fungi. A bacteriologic hood, ventilated and with effluent air filters, provides additional safety and should be used especially for work with cultures on solid media.

A towel, either cotton or absorbent paper, well-moistened with 2% Amphyl or 5% cresol should be placed on the work bench. All procedures should be performed over this area. A stiff wire needle (Nichrome, 22-gauge), hammered flat and bent at about 90°, should be flamed to redness before and after use. When moist specimens or stock cultures in mineral oil have been transferred with the needle, the needle should be heated gradually to redness. Gradual heating prevents spattering and dissemination of viable, pathogenic organisms.

All clinical specimens, culture tubes, slides, Petri plates, and instruments should be placed in a metal container and autoclaved (15 psi for 20 minutes) prior to discarding. Pipets should be submerged in disinfectant overnight. Infected animals and tissues should be placed in a waterproof container and incinerated. At the end of each work period, all cultures should be placed in suitable containers, preferably a wire basket or rack, and placed in the incubator or room-temperature holding area. The laboratory work area must be cleaned and wiped with disinfectant. Proper caution in handling cultures minimizes laboratory accidents. In the event that cultures are dropped or spilled, the debris should be flooded with disinfectant and disposed of carefully. Hands, face, and personal effects should be washed with soap and water.

REFERENCES

1. Swartz, J. H., and Lamkin, B.: Arch. Dermatol. **89:**89, 1964.
2. Littman, M. L.: J. Infect. Dis. **101-**51, 1957.
3. Gridley, M. F.: Am. J. Clin. Pathol. **23:**303, 1953.
4. Grocott, R. G.: Am. J. Clin. Pathol. **25:**975, 1955.
5. Emmons, C. W.: Arch. Dermatol. **30:**337, 1934.
6. Linder, D. H.: Science **70:**430, 1929.
7. Nibley, C., and Newton, A.: J. Invest. Dermatol. **28:**373, 1957.

104

THE MYCOSES

George S. Kobayashi
Demosthenes Pappagianis

SUPERFICIAL MYCOSES
Pityriasis versicolor (tinea versicolor)

Pityrosporum orbiculare has been conclusively demonstrated to be the etiologic agent (formerly *Malassezia furfur*)[1] of pityriasis versicolor (tinea versicolor), a chronic superficial infection of the skin most frequently affecting the chest and back but sometimes involving the neck, face, shoulders, and arms. The lesions are variable in size and are characterized by branny, scaling patches that appear dry. They are yellow to brown, depending on the normal pigmentation of the patient, and may fluoresce under Wood's ultraviolet light. The disease is worldwide in distribution and prevalent in both tropical and temperate climates.

Laboratory methods

P. orbiculare can be demonstrated with ease in skin scrapings treated with 10% potassium hydroxide (Fig. 104-1) or in biopsy specimens stained with periodic acid–Schiff stain. The organisms appear in considerable numbers as short, rather thick, pleomorphic, hyphal elements and as clusters of spherical cells. Routine cultures of clinical material are not normally taken since direct microscopic examination shows cells that are pathognomonic. The lipophilic yeastlike organism, however, grows well at 37 C on Sabouraud's agar containing antibiotics and layered with sterile lanolin or olive oil.

Tinea nigra

Although various members of the genus *Cladosporium* are ubiquitous and frequently encountered as laboratory contaminants, *C. wernecki* is the causative organism of tinea nigra, which is a superficial fungus infection of the palms of the hands but which may on rare occasions involve the soles of the feet. It is most commonly seen in tropical climates but has been reported to occur in the temperate zones. Clinically the disease presents itself as macular patches that appear as brown to black discolorations of the involved skin surfaces.

Laboratory methods

Microscopic examination of alkali-treated scrapings reveal dark-colored septate hyphae and budding cells. The organism can be isolated from clinical specimens on media containing cycloheximide. Microscopic examination of young cultures reveals 1- or 2-celled yeastlike structures (Fig. 104-2). On aging, the culture becomes dark olive to black, and mycelial growth predominates.

Black piedra

The fungus *Piedraia hortai* is an ascomycete responsible for black piedra, an infection of hairs of the scalp. The disease is characterized by the development of firmly adherent, hard, black nodules located predominantly on distal portions of the hairs (Fig. 104-3). These nodules are masses of dark hyphae firmly cemented together to form concretions in which asci develop. The asci contain 8 fusiform (spindle-shaped) ascospores.

Laboratory methods

P. hortai can be isolated on media containing cycloheximide. Smooth, black, raised colonies are produced. Hyphae and many intercalated chlamydospores are seen on microscopic examination. The sexual stage of this fungus can occasionally develop on routine culture media.

White piedra

White piedra, caused by *Trichosporon cutaneum*, is a fungus infection of the hairs of the beard and mustache. The infection occurs most commonly in the tropical zones but has been reported in the United States on rare occasions.[2] Soft, white to light brown nodules composed of a dense network of mycelium form along infected hairs.

Laboratory methods

The fungus is sensitive to cycloheximide and must therefore be isolated on an antibiotic-free medium. Cream-colored yeastlike colonies

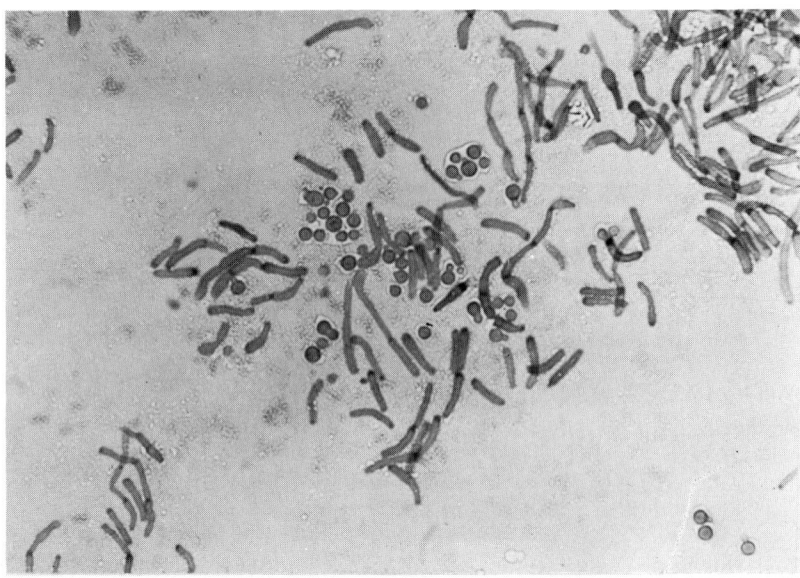

Fig. 104-1. Hyphae and spherical cells of *Malassezia furfur* from scrapings of skin. (×440.)

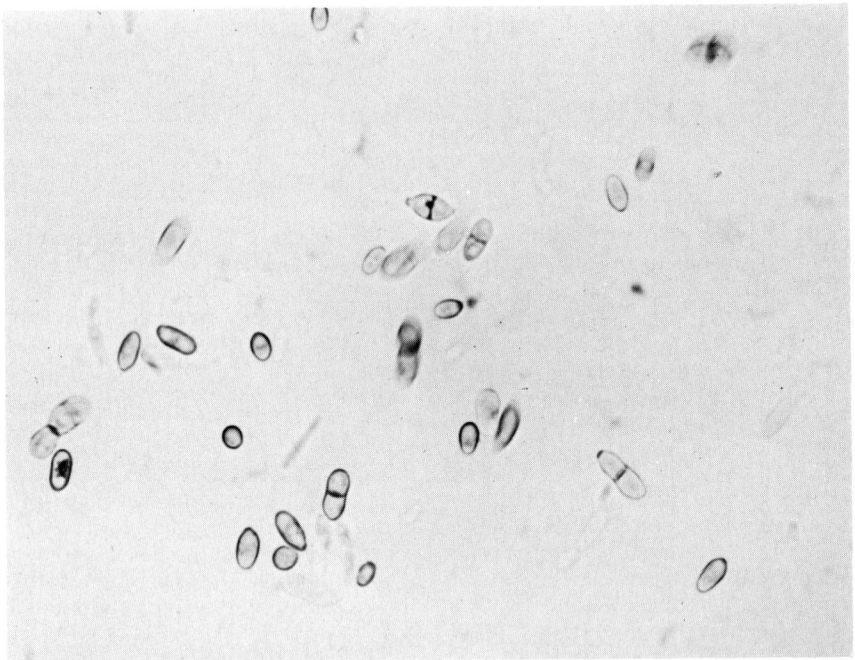

Fig. 104-2. Yeastlike cells of *Cladosporium wernecki* from culture at room temperature. (×680.)

develop rapidly, and with age they become wrinkled and yellowish gray. Microscopically the fungus appears as septate hyphae that readily fragment into arthrospores or blastospores (Fig. 104-4). *T. cutaneum* is a nonfermenting fungus but will assimilate glucose, sucrose, maltose, galactose, and lactose. Nitrate is not utilized; the glycoside, arbutin, is hydrolyzed.

DERMATOMYCOSES (CUTANEOUS MYCOSES, DERMATOPHYTOSES, RINGWORMS, TINEAS)

The tissue levels of infection caused by the fungi responsible for the dermatomycoses are limited almost entirely to the epidermis, hair, and nails. Occasionally they invade deeper into the dermis; but involvement of internal organs,

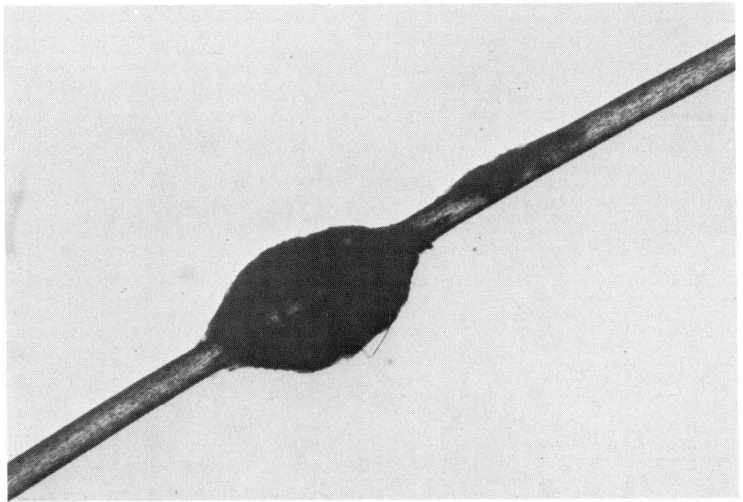

Fig. 104-3. Hair infected with *Piedraia hortai.*(×69.3.)

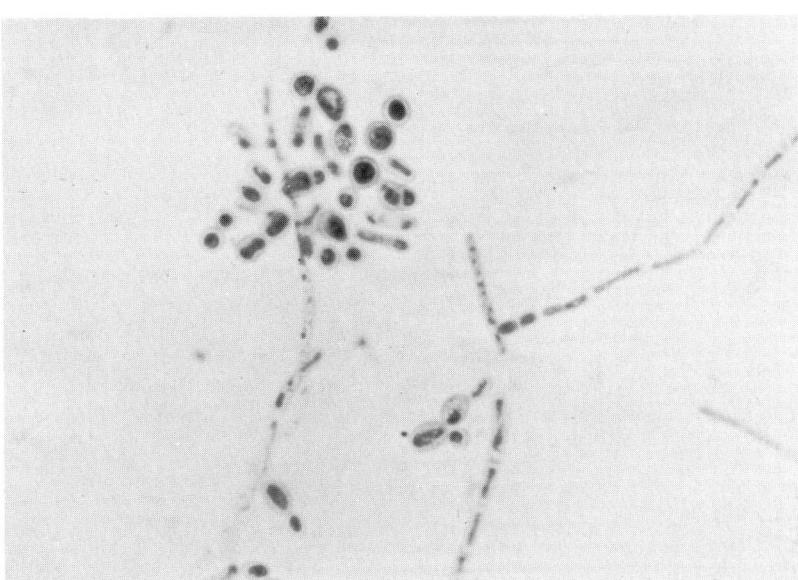

Fig. 104-4. Dimorphic characteristic growth in vitro of *Trichosporon cutaneum* at room temperature. (×680.)

as occurs in disseminated mycotic infection, is rare. These fungi have also been described as the "keratinophilic" fungi because of their ability to utilize keratin, a protein found in skin and its appendages.[3-5] Keratin, however, is not an essential metabolite for these organisms. The reason for the high degree of selectivity of epidermal tissue for the growth of these fungi is unknown.

The descriptive clinical terms for these cutaneous infections are "ringworms" or "tineas" (Latin, worm). The infections are categorized clinically according to the areas of the body involved, e.g., **tinea capitis** (scalp),[6,7] **tinea barbae** (beard), **tinea corporis** (body), **tinea cruris** (groin), **tinea pedis** (foot), **tinea manus** (hand), and **tinea unguium** (nails).

One notable advance in the study of this group of fungi is in the area of their taxonomy. As a result of the careful studies of several workers, especially Emmons (1934)[8] and Georg (1957),[9,10] the cumbersome number of species described, estimated in the hundreds, has been reduced to a practical working group.

Microsporum, Trichophyton, and Epidermophyton

The etiologic agents of the dermatomycoses fall into 3 genera of the form class Fungi Imperfecti: *Microsporum, Trichophyton,* and *Epider-*

mophyton. The ascigerous stage ("perfect form") of a number of dermatophytes has been observed in mating studies with several species, and these fungi have been appropriately placed into the class Ascomycetes (Table 104-1). The nomenclature of these fungi most frequently used in the United States is that of the Communicable Disease Center of the U.S. Public Health Service. Epidemiologic studies reveal that there are geographic differences in the distribution of these fungi.[13-15] Furthermore, the various species of each genus may be grouped according to host preferences (Table 104-2).[13] Some species found almost solely in association with man are classified as **anthropophilic** species; others in association with animals, **zoophilic;** and still others most frequently as soil saprobes, **geophilic.** The zoophilic and geophilic species can occasionally infect man.[16-19]

In general the mycelia produced by this group of fungi are undifferentiated, and species identification is based primarily on the conidia produced (Table 104-3 and Figs. 104-5 to 104-8). These conidia may be large and multicellular (**macroconidia**) or small and unicellular (**microconidia**). In addition to the production of macroconidia and microconidia, some of these organisms produce other morphologic structures such as chlamydospores, spiral hyphae, nodular bodies, chandeliers, and racquet hyphae. These structures will be produced commonly by some species and infrequently by others.

Pleomorphic changes (see morphologic variation, in Chapter 102) are frequently associated with this group of fungi. When such changes occur, it may be impossible to identify the fungus. The tendency toward pleomorphic change can

Table 104-1. Ascigerous stage of various dermatophytes*

Imperfect form	Perfect form
Microsporum gypseum	*Nannizzia incurvata*
	N. gypsea
M. fulvum	*N. fulva*
M. nanum	*N. obstusa*
M. Cookei	*N. cajetani*
M. vanbreuseghemii	*N. grubyia*
Trichophyton ajelloi	*Arthroderma uncinatum*
T. terrestre	*A. quadrifidum*

*For a detailed listing see reference 12.

Table 104-2. Classification of the dermatophytes according to habitat*[13]

Anthropophilic species	Zoophilic species	Geophilic species
Microsporum audouini	*Microsporum canis*	*Microsporum gypseum*
M. nanum	*M. distortum*	*Trichophyton ajelloi*
M. distortum	*M. vanbreuseghemii*	
M. vanbreuseghemii	*Trichophyton gallinae*	
Trichophyton tonsurans	*T. mentagrophytes*	
T. mentagrophytes	*T. verrucosum*	
T. rubrum	*T. equinum*	
T. schoenleini		
T. violaceum		
T. ferrugineum		
T. gourvilii		
T. megninii		
T. soudanense		
T. yaoundei		
Epidermophyton floccosum		

*Based on data from Ajello, L.: Ann. N.Y. Acad. Sci. **89**:30, 1960.

Table 104-3. Generic characteristics of dermatophyte macroconidia*

Genus	Frequency	Size (μm)	No. of septa	Thickness of wall	Surface of wall	Manner of attachment
Microsporum	Very numerous (Exception: *M. audouini*)	5-100 × 3-8	3-15	Thick (Exception: *M. gypseum M. nanum*)	Rough	Singly
Trichophyton	Usually rare	20-50 × 4-6	2-8	Thin	Smooth	Singly
Epidermophyton	Numerous	20-40 × 6-8	2-4	Intermediate	Smooth	In groups of 2-3

*From Ajello, L., Georg, L. K., Kaplan, W., et al.: CDC Laboratory manual for medical mycology, PHS pub. no. 994, Washington, D.C., 1963, U.S. Government Printing Office, p. D-8.

be minimized by frequent transfer of such fungi to sporulating media (see culture media, in Chapter 103) or by storage at freezing temperatures (see stock culture collection, in Chapter 103). Cultures that do not produce morphologic structures characteristic for any species may be identified on the basis of their biochemical behavior on various substrates.

These fungi tolerate a wide range of pH, but the optimal range is about pH 6.8. They grow best at 25-35 C. Several keratinophilic fungi can be grown on hair, and it has been assumed that the enzymatic activity that allows them to decompose the protein is derived from a keratinase. However, this enzyme has not been clearly demonstrated in these species.[3,4,20] Nutritionally some species have specific vitamin requirements.[21,22] This characteristic is a rather stable one and is useful in their identification.

Laboratory methods

The diagnosis of dermatomycosis is usually based on such clinical findings as alopecia, scaling lesions, eroded nails, and broken hairs. Definitive diagnosis, however, must be confirmed by the observation of fungus elements in clinical specimens or isolation of the agent by culture. In general, clinical specimens taken from suspected areas may be placed into a clean envelope and sent or mailed to the diagnostic laboratory. A portion of these specimens must be examined by direct microscopy and the remainder seeded onto a suitable agar medium (see culture media, in Chapter 103). For microscopic examination, skin scales and nail clippings should be treated with alkali to hydrolyze and clear the epidermal proteins and epithelial debris present. Fungus elements are resistant to such treatment and will be seen as highly re-

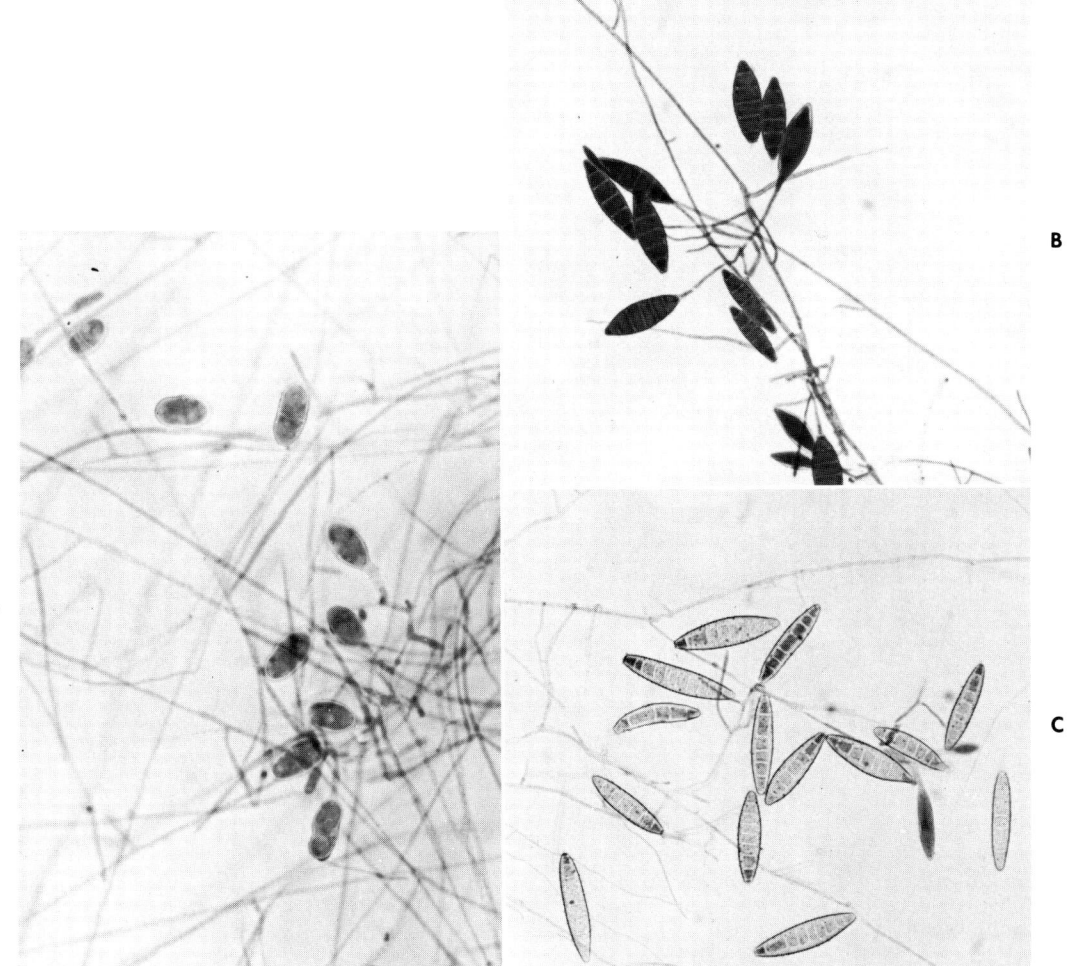

Fig. 104-5. A, Macroconidia of *Microsporum nanum.* (×440.) **B,** Macroconidia of *M. gypseum.* (×272.)
C, Macroconidia of *M. canis.* (×272.)

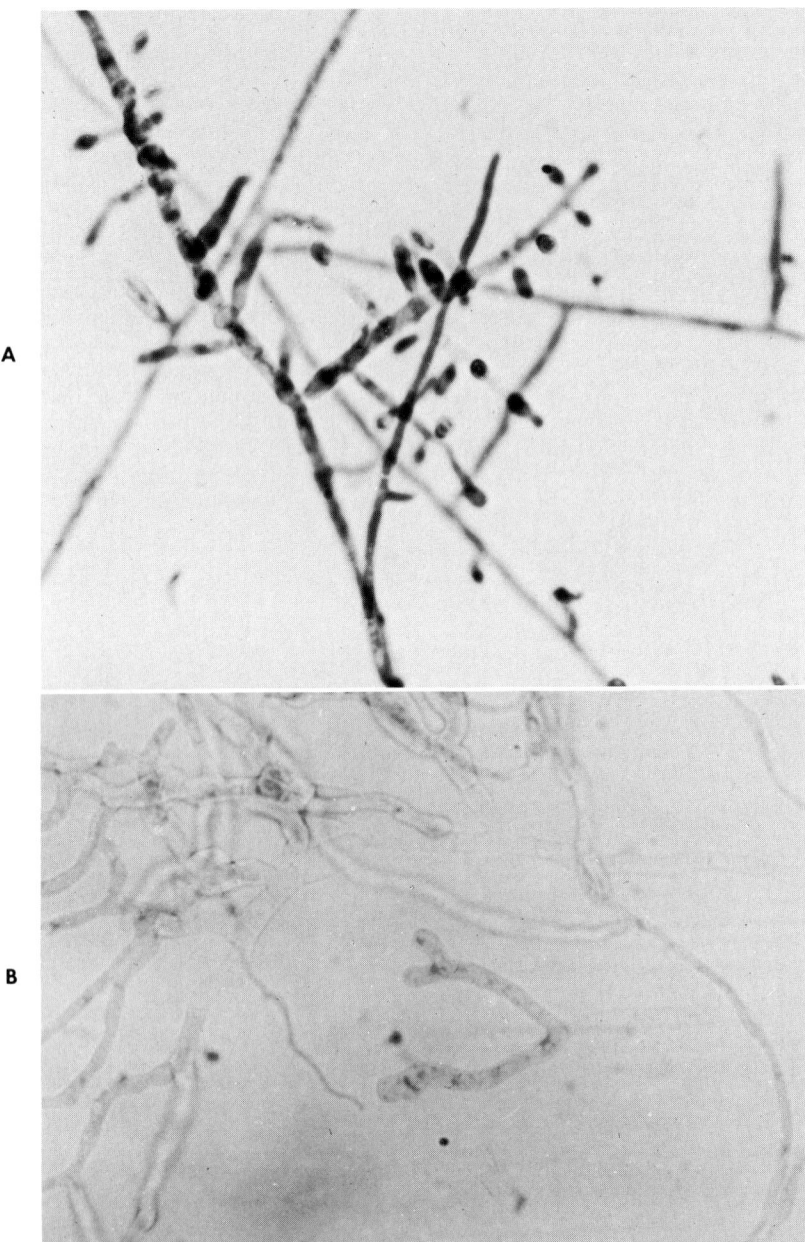

Fig. 104-6. A, Microconidia of *Trichophyton mentagrophytes.* (×680.) **B,** Favic chandelier of *T. schoenleini.*
(×680.)

fractile, branching filamentous structures (Fig. 104-9).

Fragments of hair may be mounted in lactophenol–cotton blue and examined under high dry magnification (45×). Hair infections may be endothrix or ectothrix, depending on where the spores are formed (Figs. 104-10 and 104-11). In some cases invasion of the hair is characterized by the presence of hyphae only within the hair shaft proper. This type of hair infection is referred to as **favic** and is commonly seen in the

clinical entity of **favus** *(Trichophyton schoenleini).* A useful aid in the clinical diagnosis of tinea capitis is **Wood's light** (366 nm).[23-25] Hair stubs infected by some species of *Microsporum* *(M. audouini, M. canis, M. distortum,* and *M. ferrugineum)* usually fluoresce bright yellow-green when examined in the dark under this ultraviolet light. Hairs infected with *T. schoenleini* may appear bluish white under these conditions. Examination of the lesions of tinea capitis in this manner further serves as an aid in preferentially

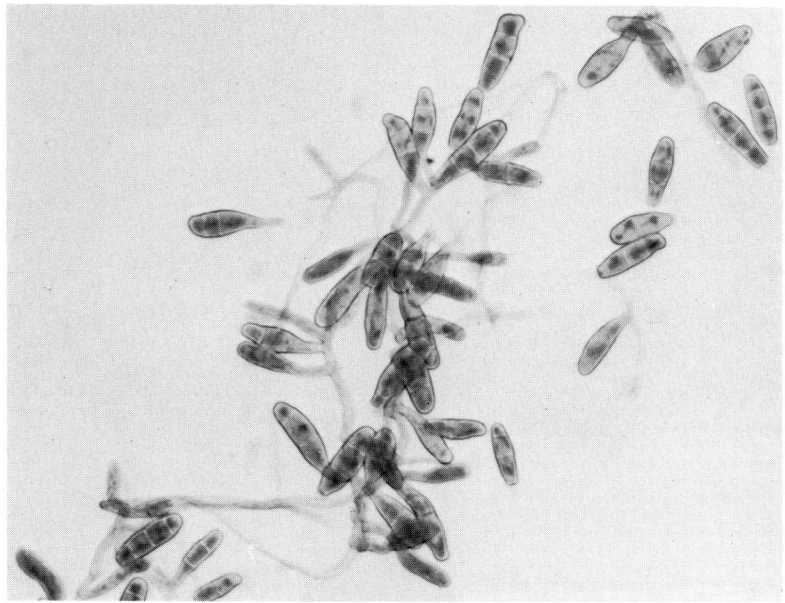

Fig. 104-7. Macroconidia of *Epidermophyton floccosum.* (×272.)

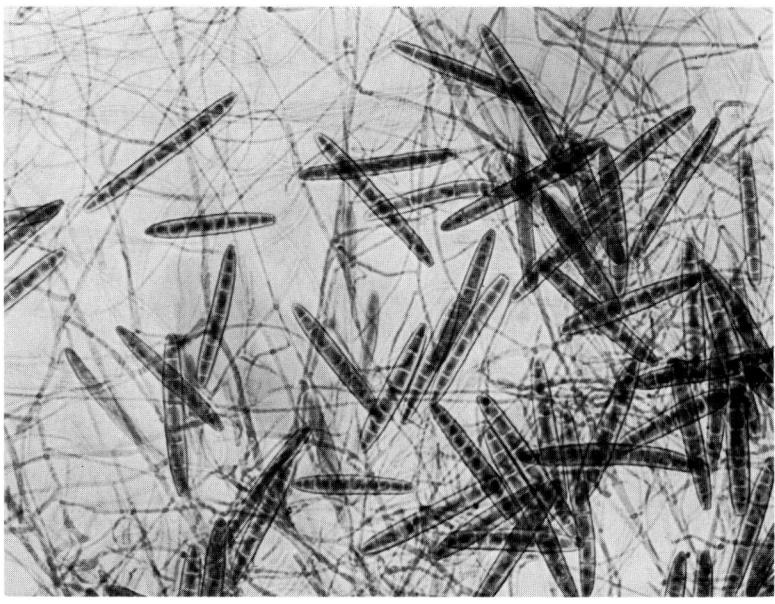

Fig. 104-8. Macroconidia of *Trichophyton ajelloi.* (×272.)

plucking infected hairs for microscopic and cultural examination.

It is beyond the scope of this section to describe all of the growth requirements that are employed in taxonomic studies. These are especially useful in the genus *Trichophyton*. Reference should be made to Georg and Camp (1957),[10] Georg (1952),[9] and to the *Laboratory Manual for Medical Mycology* (Ajello, Georg, et al., 1963).[26] Some general characteristics of se-

lected dermatophytes are presented in Table 104-4.

Two basal media employed in nutritional tests for the identification of various species of the genus *Trichophyton* are **casein agar** and **ammonium nitrate agar.** *M. canis* and *M. gypseum* grow and sporulate well on **rice medium,** whereas *M. audouini* does not. For description of these media see Chapter 103, Methods for Study of Medically Important Fungi.

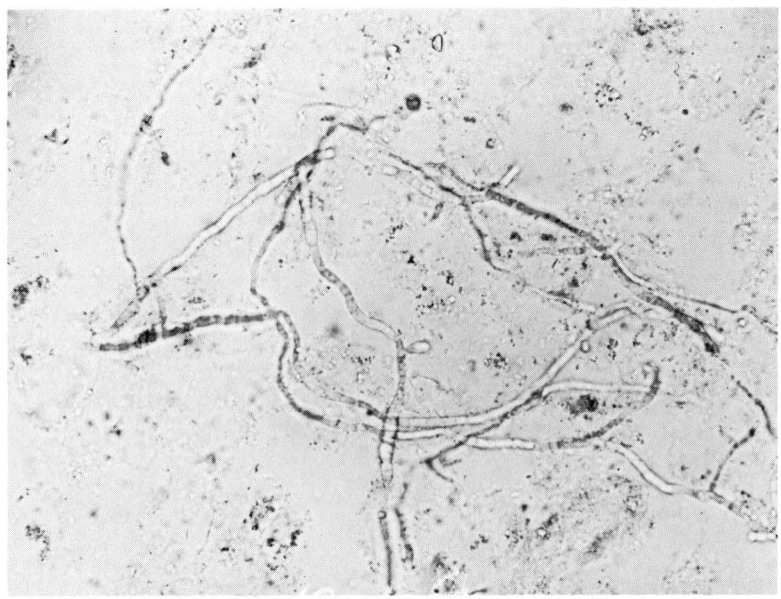

Fig. 104-9. Branching filaments of dermatophyte in scrapings of skin. (×400.)

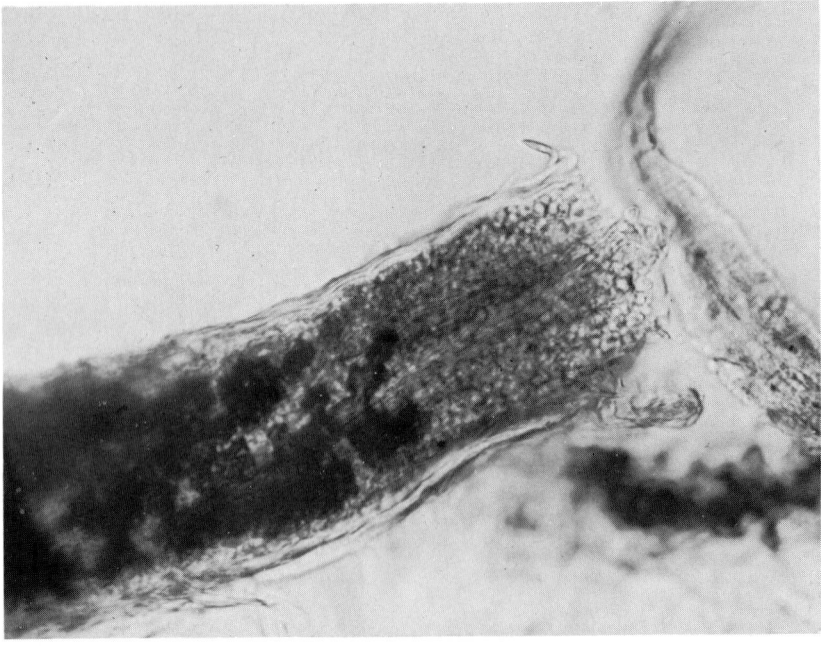

Fig. 104-10. Endothrix hair infection from which *Trichophyton tonsurans* was cultured. (×272.)

SUBCUTANEOUS MYCOSES
Sporotrichosis
Sporothrix schenkii (Sporotrichum schenkii)

Sporothrix schenkii is a dimorphic fungus that lives saprobically on various forms of living or decaying vegetation.[27,28] The disease, sporotrichosis, is worldwide in distribution and has occurred in epidemic form. This organism causes a subacute or chronic infection usually limited to the skin and subcutaneous tissues but sometimes involving fascia and bones. On rare occasions this organism may be the cause of systemic disease.[29] The clinical manifestations of primary cutaneous and lymphatic sporotrichosis are

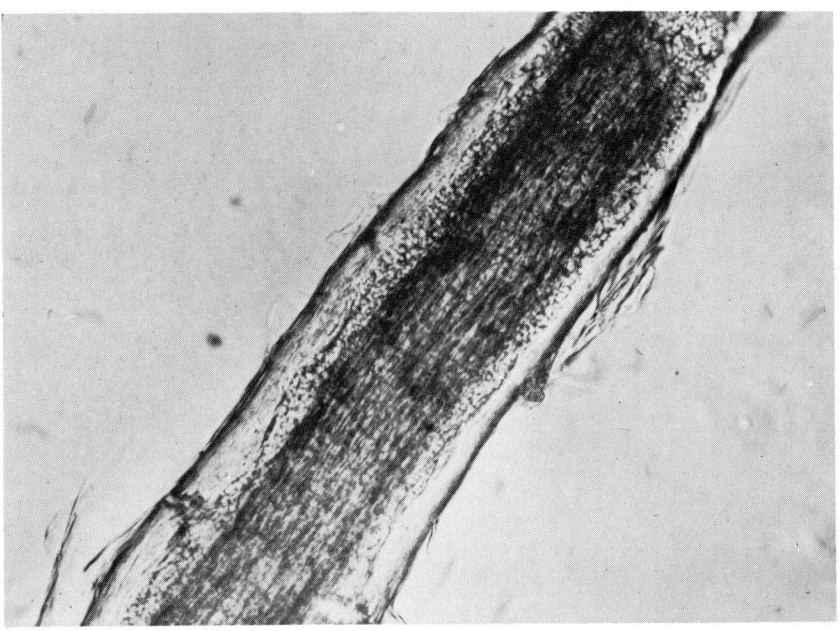

Fig. 104-11. Ectothrix hair infection from which *Microsporum audouini* was cultured. (×272.)

Table 104-4. Macroscopic, microscopic, and nutritional characteristics of selected dermatophytes*

Genus	Species	Gross colonial morphology	Microscopic features	Special nutritional studies
Tricho-phyton	rubrum	Cottony to granular; red to yellow	Delicate hyphae with tear-shaped microconidia produced laterally along filaments	None; on potato dextrose agar red pigment produced
T.	mentagro-phytes	Cottony to granular; buff to red	Club-shaped macroconidia sometimes produced; clusters of small, round, microconidia, which in some strains may be tear-shaped; spiral hyphae may be seen	None
T.	verrucosum	Moist, glabrous, heaped; dull yellow	Tear-shaped microconidia, ant-lerlike branched hyphae	Thiamine required
T.	violaceum	Heaped, waxy, irregular; violet	No conidia as a rule; hyphae tortuous and tangled	Grows better in thiamine-containing medium
T.	tonsurans	Velvety to granular; yellowish to brown	Abundant microconidia produced; large, teardrop to club-shaped, in clusters	Grows well on media with thiamine added
T.	ajelloi	Cottony to powdery; cream to orange-tan, may produce reddish pigment	Smooth-walled, large, elongated macroconidia; microconidia produced by some strains	None
Micro-sporum	audouini	Velvety, moist; tan to peach	Macroconidia rarely produced; terminal chlamydospores formed; no distinguishing features	Grows poorly on polished rice
M.	canis	Cottony; yellow to orange	Rough, thick-walled macro-conidia, spindle-shaped	Grows profusely on polished rice
M.	gypseum	Matted, granular to cottony; cinnamon color	Rough, thin-walled macroconidia, spindle-shaped	Grows well on polished rice
Epider-mophy-ton	floccosum	Velvety to powdery; greenish yellow	Broad, calvate, smooth-walled, multicelled macroconidia produced terminally; no microconidia	None

*Based on data from Ajello, L., Georg, L. K., Kaplan, W., et al.: CDC Laboratory manual for medical mycology, PHS pub. no. 994, Washington, D.C., 1963, U.S. Government Printing Office.

characterized by painless, chancriform papules, which slowly enlarge, break down, and ulcerate. These enlarged papules and ulcers usually appear along the lymphatics that drain the primary inoculation site. Small, oval to "cigar-shaped," yeastlike cells develop in tissues. These cells are difficult to detect in tissue stained with hematoxylin-eosin, but periodic acid–Schiff and methenamine silver stains will delineate them from other tissue elements.

Laboratory methods

The organism can be isolated in the mycelial phase at room temperature on selective media containing antibiotics. Within 7 days moist, white, leathery colonies appear. Radiating furrows develop, and with age the colony takes on a wrinkled appearance. The white growth darkens and may become brown to black. The mycelial phase is composed of delicate hyphae about 1.5-2 μm in diameter. Numerous pyriform (flame-

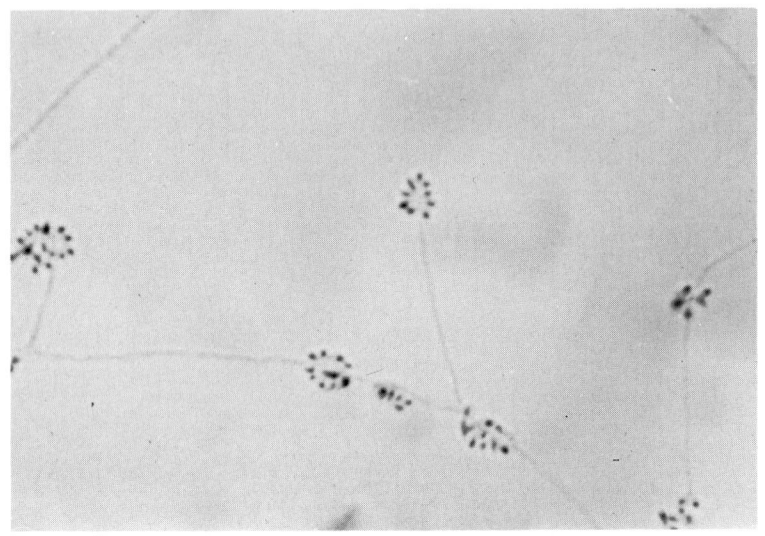

Fig. 104-12. Slide culture preparation of *Sporothrix schenkii* incubated at room temperature. (×450.)

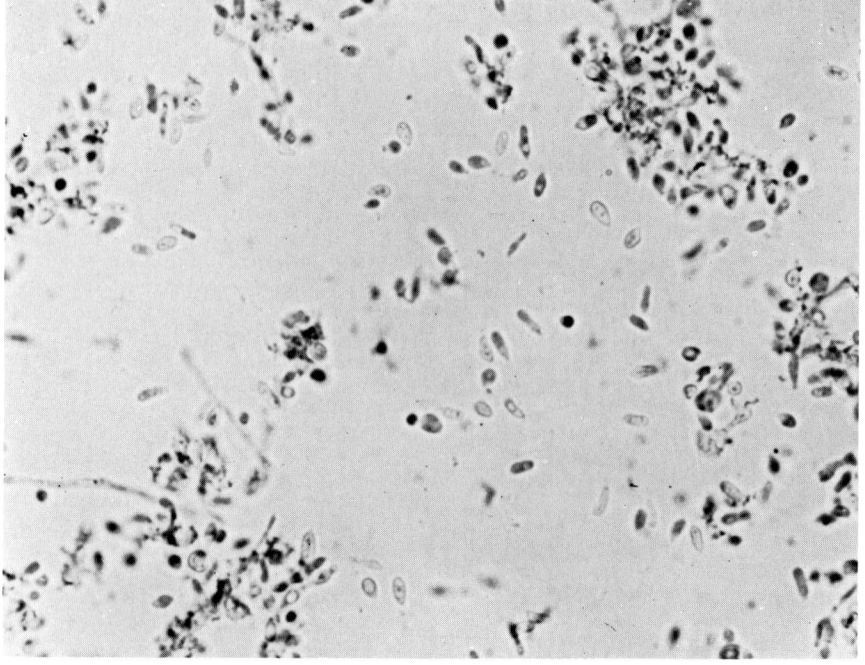

Fig. 104-13. Elongated budding cells of *Sporothrix schenkii* from culture at 37 C.

shaped) conidia develop laterally along the hyphae or terminally in rosette pattern (Fig. 104-12). The parasitic phase of *S. schenkii*, which is a yeastlike organism, can be obtained by culturing the organism at 37 C on brain-heart infusion agar or on blood agar enriched with 1% glucose and 0.1% cystine (Fig. 104-13).[30, 31] Microscopically these cells are about 3 μm in diameter; round, oval, or fusiform in shape; and they reproduce by bud formation. The yeastlike phase of this organism is sensitive to cyclo-heximide at 37 C. A moist agar surface and increased CO_2 tension facilitates the yeastlike conversion of the mold. Frequently several serial transfers must be made before this trans-formation is complete, and occasionally it may be necessary to rely on animal inoculations in order to obtain the yeast phase. In such a situation 0.2 ml dense suspension of mycelial elements, yeast cells, or pus is inoculated intratesticularly into several mice. These animals will develop an orchitis in a period of 2-3 weeks. The purulent fluid is aspirated and examined or is cultured at 37 C on enriched media.

Immunologic methods

Delayed hypersensitivity to extracts of S. schenkii has been demonstrated in naturally acquired and experimentally induced sporotri-chosis. Agglutinating, precipitating, and comple-ment-fixing antibodies have also been demon-strated in sera of patients and experimentally infected animals; however, these serologic methods are not routinely employed in the di-agnosis or prognosis of the disease. At present, skin tests and serologic tests have been limited to experimental investigations in the United States.[32]

Chromomycosis (chromoblastomycosis)

Most authors regard 5 dimorphic species of fungi as the etiologic agents of the subcutaneous fungus infection, chromomycosis. According to most taxonomic keys these organisms fall into the order Moniliales, family Dematiaceae, of the form class Fungi Imperfecti. They are slow-growing colonies, dark to dusky on the obverse side but jet black on the reverse side. Despite differences of opinion, species differentiation is based on the type and predominance of co-nidiophores that are produced. Three main types are formed: the *Phialophora*, the *Cladosporium*, and the *Acrotheca* (Table 104-5 and Fig. 104-14). Sporulation of any type of conidiophore is not mutually exclusive, since some of the strains may produce more than 1 type simultaneously.[33]

Fonsecaea pedrosoi, F. compacta, F. dermati-tidis, Phialophora verrucosa, and *Cladosporium carrioni*[34] are all recognized as causes of chromo-mycosis. The disease is a chronic, granulomatous infection of the skin and develops over a period of months to years. The route of infection is trau-matic implantation of the fungus into the skin or subcutaneous tissues.[35] The most frequent sites

Table 104-5. Types of sporulation found among agents of chromomycosis*

Type of sporulation	Description
Cladosporium	Conidia are borne consecutively on tips of conidiophore in moniliform appearance; most recently formed cell is distal; branched chains of conidia may be present; micro-scopic examination of conidia re-veals dark conspicuous site (**dis-junctor**) on spore wall, indicating point at which spore was attached
Phialophora	Conidia are borne within a flask-shaped structure (**phialide**) and extruded out through neck into re-ceptacle where conidia may ac-cumulate in a loosely bound mass; phialides attached laterally or terminally to hyphae and distinct in their morphology, consisting of enlarged spherical base, con-stricted neck, and receptacle
Acrotheca	Conidia are borne singly along lat-eral surfaces of conidiophore; when spores become detached from conidiophore, it has an irregu-lar appearance

*Based on data from Ajello, L., Georg, L. K., Kaplan, W., et al.: CDC Laboratory manual for medical mycology, PHS pub. no. 994, Washington, D.C., 1963, U.S. Government Printing Office.

of these localized infections are the legs, but cases have been described where lesions have appeared on other areas of the body. Advanced lesions have a warty, vegetative appearance; if the lymphatic channels are involved, stasis may develop and result in elephantiasis of the af-fected limb.

Laboratory methods

The most characteristic feature of histopatho-logic specimen is the presence of oval, brown, fungus cells seen in hematoxylin-eosin–stained sections (Fig. 104-15). These oval cells may occa-sionally be divided into halves or squares, indi-cating that their method of reproduction is most probably by fission. These organisms and other saprobic species in these genera grow well at room temperature on cycloheximide-containing agar. Animal inoculation and serologic methods are not performed in routine identification proce-dures.

The clinician can make a reliable diagnosis of the disease by the microscopic appearance of the oval, brown, fungus cells (sclerotic cells). De-finitive identification of the causative agent rests on the isolation of the organism by culture. Cul-tures may be made from biopsy material, crusts, or exudates. The agents of chromomycosis are not inhibited by cycloheximide or chloramphen-icol, and media containing these antibiotics may be used for the selective isolation of these fungi.

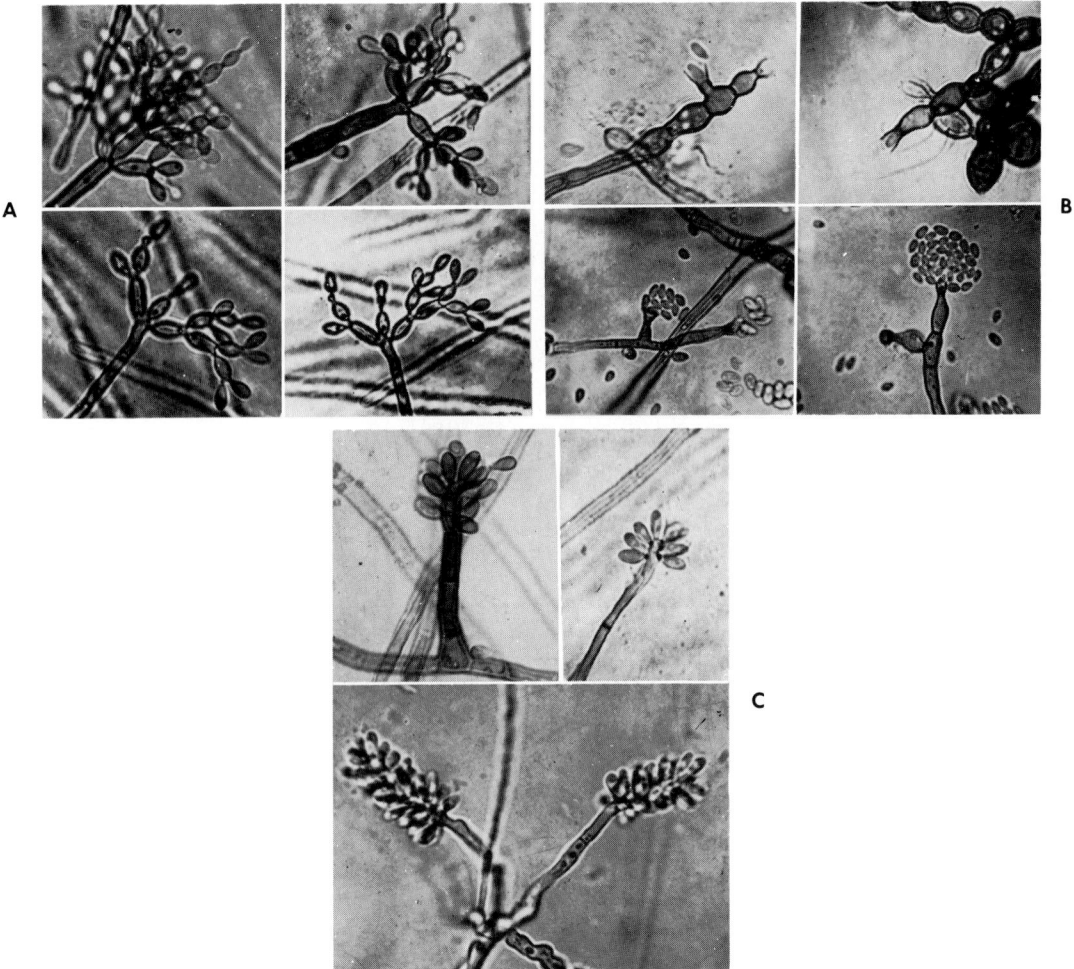

Fig. 104-14. A, *Cladosporium* type of sporulation. **B,** *Phialophora* type of sporulation. **C,** *Acrotheca* type of sporulation. (Courtesy Dr. A. L. Carrión.)

All cultures should be incubated at room temperature.

Immunologic methods

There are no useful immunologic methods available for the diagnosis of this disease.

Maduromycosis (maduromycotic mycetoma)

Several species of fungi have been identified as the etiologic agents of maduromycosis,[36-38] a localized disease characterized by deep-seated abscesses that rupture to form multiple draining sinuses.[39] As the disease progresses the skin, subcutaneous tissue, facia, and bone become involved. Examination of the serosanguineous fluid that drains from the sinuses reveals small pieces of fungus "granules." These granules may be white, yellow, brown, or black and can be well demonstrated on histopathologic sections of tissues by hematoxylin-eosin or periodic acid–Schiff stain. This disease is also called maduromycotic mycetoma and must be differentiated from actinomycotic mycetoma, a clinically similar infection. The etiologic agents of the latter are bacteria belonging to the family Actinomycetaceae.

Some of the causative fungi that have been identified are *Allescheria boydii, Phialophora jeanselmi,*[40] *Madurella mycetomi,*[41] *M. grisea* and *Cephalosporium falciforme.* The cultural characteristics are summarized in Table 104-6.

A. boydii is the ascogenous (ascus-bearing) state of the imperfect fungus *Monosporium apiospermum.*[42] Sexual reproduction can occur without the interaction of 2 different *thalli* (term denoting fungus bodies), i.e., the organism is self-fertile (homothallic). This fungus has been isolated from soil and is the most common cause of maduromycosis in the United States, whereas other species are predominant elsewhere. *A. boydii* has been implicated in diseases other than maduromycosis,[43-46] and because of its ubiquity,

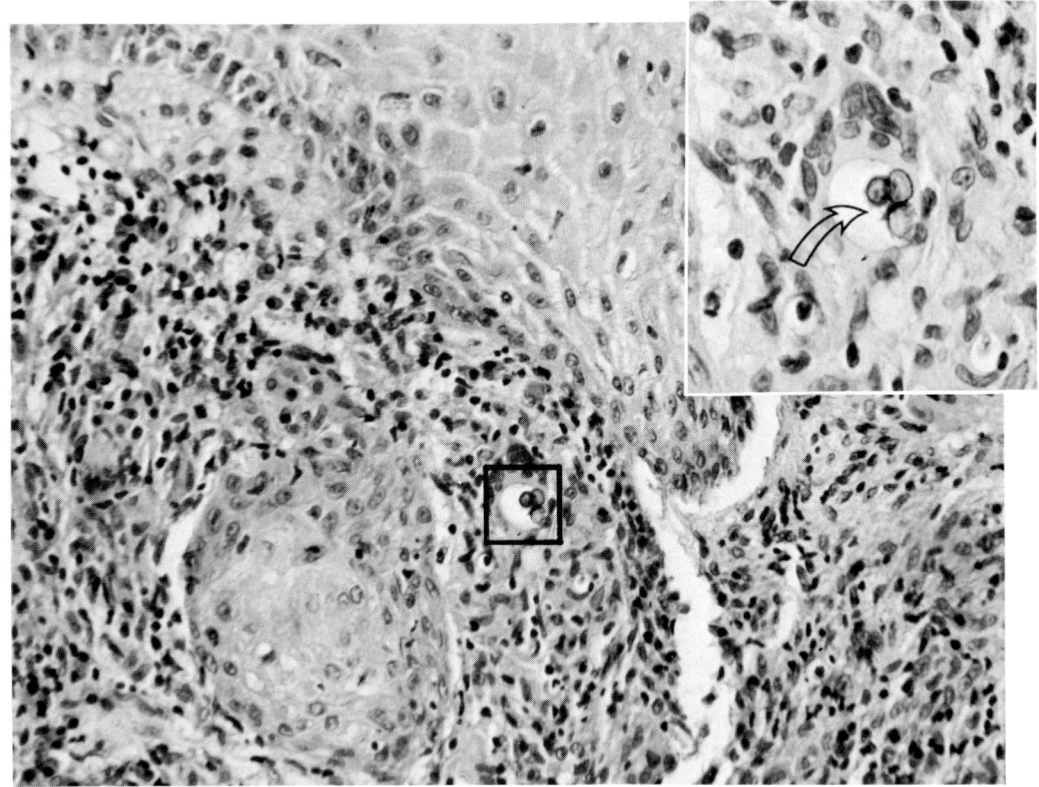

Fig. 104-15. Skin biopsy of chromomycosis illustrating pseudoepitheliomatous hyperplasia with marked chronic inflammation (×150). Insert shows high-powered view of giant cell (*arrow*) with intracytoplasmic sclerotic bodies of fungus (×500).

Table 104-6. Morphologic characteristics of the agents of maduromycosis*

Organisms	Macroscopic morphology	Microscopic morphology	Granules
Allescheria boydii (imperfect form, *Monosporium apiospermum*)	Rapid-growing, cottony colonies; white, turning gray to brown with age; cleistothecia (a closed ascocarp) may be produced in some strains	Hyphae, 1-3 μm in diameter; pear-shaped conidia borne singly brown in color, 4-9 μm × 6-10 μm	White or yellow
Cephalosporium falciforme	Slow-growing, cottony colony; pinkish to buff, reverse side currant red	Hyphae, 3-4 μm in diameter; sickle-shaped conidia borne singly at tips of conidiophores and successively pushed aside as they are formed, giving rise to clusters	White or yellow
Madurella grisea	Slow-growing colony; tan to gray, with velvety appearance	Hyphae, 1-3 μm in diameter, or dark thick chains of budding cells, 3-5 μm in diameter; no conidia	Black
M. mycetomi	Slow-growing colony; yellow to yellow-brown; may be membranous or fluffy in appearance	Hyphae variable, 1-6 μm in diameter; numerous chlamydospores; conidia may be produced from phialides	Black
Phialophora jeanselmi	Slow-growing, smooth colony; black, but develops velvety, gray aerial mycelium with age, reverse side black	Young culture contains many budding cells in chainlike arrangement; conidia borne in cylindrical phialides	Black

*Based on data from Ajello, L., Georg, L. K., Kaplan, W., et al.: CDC Laboratory manual for medical mycology, PHS pub. no. 994, Washington, D.C., 1963, U.S. Government Printing Office.

the organism must be repeatedly isolated from the lesion.

Laboratory methods

Clinical specimens, preferably granules or material aspirated from unopened lesions, should be cultured on Sabouraud dextrose agar containing **antibacterial** antibiotics such as chloramphenicol (0.05 mg/ml) or streptomycin (5000 U/ml). Granules taken from draining lesions are washed in sterile saline containing cloramphenicol or streptomycin prior to culture to reduce the potential bacterial flora that may be present. Media containing cycloheximide should not be used because some of these organisms are sensitive to this antibiotic. Cultures should be incubated at both 25 C and 37 C.

Sufficient clinical material must be cultured, preferably from widely separated areas of diseased tissue. Repeat cultures should be requested.

Immunologic methods

At present serologic and skin tests are unavailable.

YEASTLIKE FUNGI OF MEDICAL IMPORTANCE

Several genera of yeastlike fungi are of medical importance, and the technics used to identify these organisms are different from those employed in the identification of filamentous fungi. Medically, the most important of these genera are *Cryptococcus*,[47] *Candida*,[48] and *Trichosporon*.

In general the colonial and microscopic morphology of these organisms resembles those of the perfect yeasts. Since a sexual stage has not been observed in most of these yeastlike fungi, they are grouped in the form class Fungi Imperfecti, order Pseudosaccharomycetales, family Cryptococcaceae. The morphologic characteristics, laboratory methods for identification, and diseases produced by *Cryptococcus neoformans* and various species of *Candida* are discussed in the following sections. For the description of *T. cutaneum* see section on superficial mycoses.

Cryptococcosis
Cryptococcus neoformans[47]

The disease cryptococcosis, also known as torulosis or European blastomycosis, is of worldwide distribution. The etiologic agent is *C. neoformans*, the only medically important species of the genus *Cryptococcus*. The genus includes several species of yeastlike fungi that are nonfermentative and characteristically produce an extracellular polysaccharide capsule.

The disease can be manifest as a subclinical or clinical pulmonary infection or as a systemic infection with a predilection for the central nervous system. It occasionally involves the skin. A variety of laboratory media support the growth of *C. neoformans*, but it is inhibited by cycloheximide. On a chemically defined substrate this organism shows a growth requirement for thiamine. Specific patterns of nitrate and carbohydrate assimilation tests and pathogenicity for mice are important criteria for differentiating *C. neoformans* from other *Cryptococcus* species. The sexual stage of *C. neoformans* has been demonstrated and given the perfect name of *Filobasidiella neoformans*[49] (Fig. 104-16). The life cycle of this fungus and the morphology of the sexually produced fruiting structure (basidium) places the organism in the family Filoba-

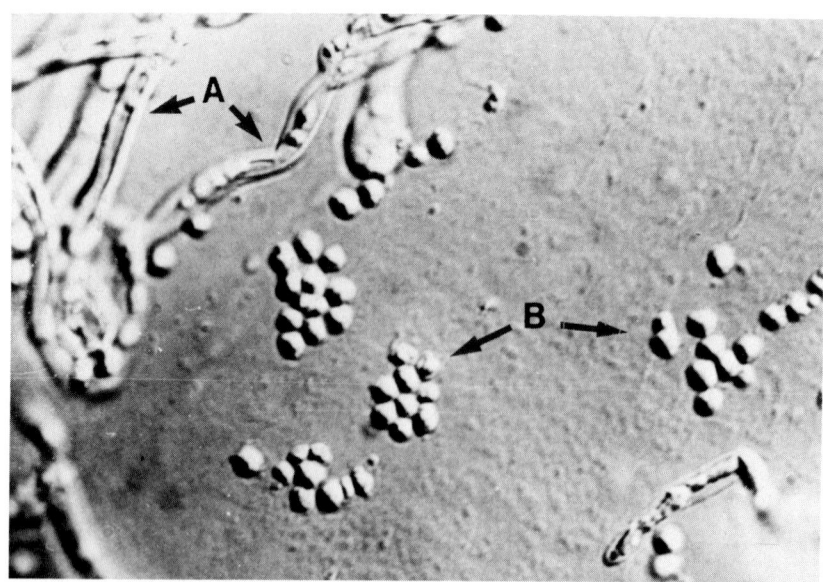

Fig. 104-16. *Filobasidiella neoformans,* the sexual stage of *Cryptococcus neoformans,* illustrating **A,** hyphae with clamp connections and terminal basidium, and **B,** basidiospores (×1200). (Courtesy Dr. J. K. Kwon-Chung.)

sidiaceae of the Ustilaginales. The asexual phase is typically yeastlike and the cells have varying degrees of capsular material; sexually mated strains produce hyphae with clamp connections and basidia.

Laboratory methods

Clinical materials should be examined for the presence of encapsulated, budding yeast cells. When body fluids, especially spinal fluid, are submitted for diagnostic studies, the material should be centrifuged and the resulting supernatant fluid discarded. A loopful of the sediment is placed on a slide, mixed with an equal amount of India ink, and covered with a cover slip. The cover slip is gently pressed with the aid of a rubber eraser to provide a thin film, which can be examined microscopically for the presence of encapsulated, yeastlike cells (Fig. 104-17). The colloidal carbon particles will highlight the transparent capsule by producing a dark background. The acidic polysaccharide capsular material may also be demonstrated histochemically by the mucicarmine stain.[49] This stain is most often employed to demonstrate mucin in tissue sections; the capsular material of *C. neoformans* will also stain an intense pink to red with mucicarmine.

C. neoformans does not utilize nitrate; it assimilates glucose, sucrose, and galactose but not melibiose. Urease is produced by the organism and can be demonstrated by culture on Christensen urea agar.[50-52] It grows both at room temperature and 37 C and is pathogenic for mice by intracerebral inoculation. A variant has been described that is almost indistinguishable from the pathogenic *C. neoformans*. This variant, however, does not grow at 37 C and is not patho-genic for laboratory animals. Other cryptococci grow at room temperature but usually not at 37 C.

Pathogenicity test for C. neoformans. Prepare saline suspension, using cells from 4-6 d old culture, usually in 1:100 dilution. Inoculate 4 mice intracerebrally with 0.03 ml suspension, using a ¼ in., 26-gauge needle. This results in death of the mice within 7-10 d. Perform necropsy on mice that die (or are sacrificed at end of 2 wk if death does not occur). Remove top of skull, mix brain tissue with drop of India ink, and examine for encapsulated, budding yeast cells.
NOTE: If pathogenicity test is satisfactory, assimilation tests may be omitted.

Serologic classification and identification by agglutination reactions[53] and fluorescent antibody technics[54] have been reported but are not in general use.

C. neoformans selective medium (for soil, etc.). *C. neoformans* has been isolated repeatedly from habitats contaminated by pigeon excreta.[55] A medium selective for the isolation of this organism from such samples has been devised and is prepared as follows[56]:

Dextrose	10 g
Creatinine	0.78 g
Extract of *Guizotia abyssinica* seed*	200 ml
Chloramphenicol	0.05 g
Agar	20 g
Distilled water	800 ml

Autoclave medium at 15 psi for 15 min and cool to about 56 C. Add 0.1 g diphenyl ($C_6H_5C_6H_5$) dissolved in

---

*Extract of *G. abyssinica* seeds ("niger seed," a constituent of canary feed) is prepared by pulverizing seeds in Waring blender. Seventy g pulverized powder is suspended in 350 ml distilled water and auto-claved at 10 psi for 10 min. Extract is clarified by filtration through gauze.

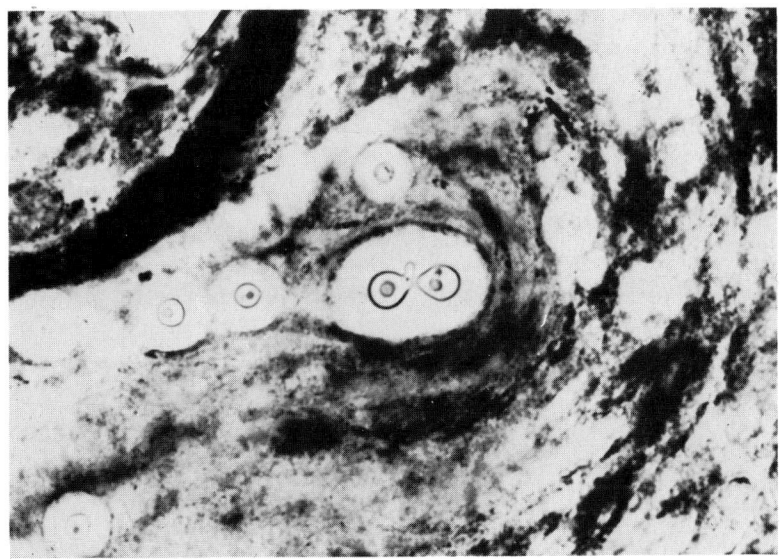

Fig. 104-17. Encapsulated, yeastlike cells of *Cryptococcus neoformans* in preparation of brain tissue from experimentally infected mouse. (×680.)

10 ml 95% ethanol to warm medium. Mix components thoroughly and then pour into Petri plates. Good growth of C. neoformans at 37 C is obtained on this medium, with the colonies developing a brown pigment. Growth of contaminating molds and bacteria is controlled by diphenyl and chloramphenicol, respectively.

Immunologic methods

At present only a few serologic tests are available for use in the study of cryptococcosis, and most of these are in the experimental stages of development.[53,54] As a rule serologic procedures are designed to detect antibodies in the sera of patients exposed to an antigen. In contrast, most serologic procedures employed in cryptococcosis detect the presence of antigen.[57] Sera from rabbits immunized with C. neoformans are employed in latex agglutination tests to detect the presence of cryptococcal antigen. This test is useful in cases of moderately severe cryptococcosis in that a good prognosis is indicated by a decrease in antigen titer concomitant with the detection of antibody.[58] Commercially prepared latex particles coated with cryptococcal antibody are available for the detection of antigen. In some cases of cryptococcosis, circulating antibodies[59] and skin test hypersensitivity[59] may be detected, but these tests have no established clinical significance.

Candidiasis[48]

Candidiasis (moniliasis, thrush) is most often seen as an acute or chronic infection of the skin, nails, or mucous membranes. It may also appear as a respiratory disease; under certain predisposing conditions, the fungus may disseminate to involve the central nervous system and viscera.[60]

Candidiasis is most frequently caused by the yeastlike fungus, Candida albicans, but other species of Candida have also been implicated. The genus is defined by Lodder as follows:

Budding cells and pseudomycelium; true mycelium may occur. Reproduction mainly by multilateral budding, besides fission may occur. Dissimilation either only oxidative or oxidative and fermentative.[61]

C. albicans may grow as a single budding yeast cell, or it may produce pseudohyphae and a true mycelium. This dimorphic characteristic may be found in culture or in infected tissues. The incidence of isolation of C. albicans from nonanimal habitats such as soil is low, whereas other members of the genus have been recovered from a variety of sources in nature such as plants, insects, soil, various processed foods, and occasionally from pathogenic processes. In healthy individuals C. albicans is rarely isolated from the skin but seems to be more common on the oral and vaginal mucous membranes and in feces.

Laboratory methods

Since Candida species are common in the normal oral cavity, sputum specimens that have been allowed to stand for any period of time are unsuitable for laboratory culture. These yeastlike organisms multiply rapidly in such an environment, and erroneous conclusions are obtained when large numbers of colonies are isolated.

All specimens should be examined microscopically for the presence of budding yeast cells or hyphae. Clinical materials should be cultured on Sabouraud dextrose agar with and without added antibiotics, since some species of Candida are sensitive to cycloheximide. Cultures should be incubated at room temperature. Occasionally more than 1 species of yeast may be present in the resulting growth. Only those colonies that are well isolated should be examined microscopically and subcultured to fresh medium. Nonencapsulated budding yeast cells must be identified by physiologic and morphologic criteria.

Only the yeastlike species C. albicans will produce chlamydospores with any regularity (Fig. 104-18), but certain isolates of C. stellatoideae and C. tropicalis may form these spores on rare occasions. Various media are available that enhance the **production of chlamydospores.** One such medium is prepared from cornmeal and is available commercially without added glucose. Petri plates of **cornmeal agar** are inoculated with the organism under study. The inoculum is taken from a well-isolated colony or a young (24 hour) broth culture with a stiff wire needle, and a single streak of about 4 cm is cut into the medium. The streak should penetrate to the bottom of the dish to ensure adequate growth under the surface of the agar. At least 4 specimens may be grown in 1 culture plate if care is taken to mark the plate off into quadrants, allowing sufficient area for growth of the individual test organisms. Each culture plate should be inoculated with a strain of C. albicans known to produce chlamydospores to serve as a control. Cultures are incubated at room temperature.

Germ tube formation. For a rapid, presumptive identification of C. albicans, the germ tube test is available.[62] A dilute suspension of the unknown yeast is inoculated into 0.5-1.0 ml serum. The suspension is incubated at 37 C for exactly 2 hours, after which time it is examined microscopically. C. albicans and occasionally C. stellatoideae produce short hyphal elements within this 2-hour period of incubation, whereas other species of Candida do not.

Carbohydrate fermentation and assimilation tests should be performed on all isolates that do not produce chlamydospores. Test organisms are inoculated into fermentation tubes containing 1% solutions of lactose, dextrose, maltose, or sucrose in beef extract broth (with 0.04% bromthymol blue indicator. (See Media for fungi, Chapter 72.) To ensure anaerobiosis, sterile petroleum jelly is melted and poured over the surface of each tube.

Assimilation studies are performed on a carbohydrate-free, nitrogen base, agar medium yeast nitrogen base, dehydrated [Difco]. A confluent lawn of the test organism is seeded onto

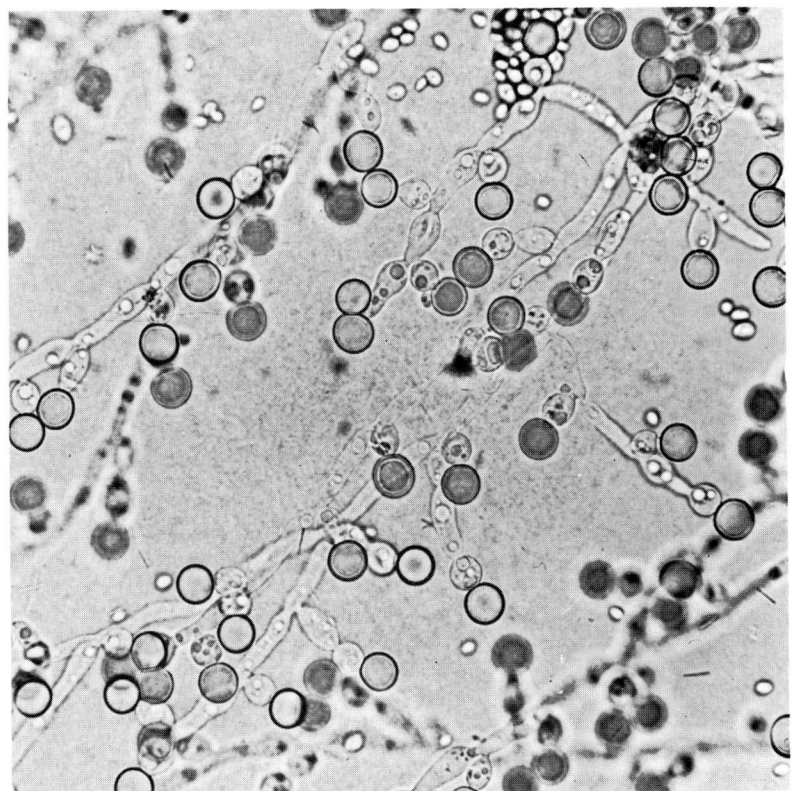

Fig. 104-18. Pseudohyphae, blastospores, and chlamydospores of *Candida albicans* from cultures on corn-meal agar at room temperature. (×680.)

Table 104-7. Morphologic and biochemical characteristics of *Candida* species

Species	Cornmeal agar (chlamydospore formation)	Sugar fermentation*				Sugar assimilation*						
		D	M	S	L	D	G	L	M	R	S	C
Candida albicans	+	a† g†	a g	a or −	−	+	+	−	+	−	+	−
Candida stellatoideae	+	a g	a g	a or −	−	+	+	−	+	−	−	−
Candida tropicalis	+	a g	a g	a g	−	+	+	−	+	−	+	+ or −
Candida guilliermondi	−	− or a‡ g‡	−	− or g‡ a‡	−	+	+	−	+	+	+	+
Candida krusei	−	a g	−	−	−	+	−	−	−	−	−	−
Candida parapsilosis	−	a g or a	− or a	− or a	−	+	+	−	+	−	+	−
Candida pseudotropicalis	−	a g	−	a g	a g	+	+	+	−	+	+	− or +

*D = dextrose; G = galactose; L = lactose; M = maltose; R = raffinose; S = sucrose; C = cellobiose.
†a = acid; g = gas.
‡Fermentation may be weak or delayed for 2-3 wk.

the agar, and filter paper disks (7 mm) saturated with test sugars (prepared carbohydrate disks available commercially [Difco, BBL]) are distributed on the surface. The sugars employed in assimilation studies are glucose, galactose, maltose, sucrose, lactose, raffinose, and cellobiose. The cultures are incubated at 27 C and examined for growth around the test sugar at 24 and 48 hours.

The most reliable results are obtained when suspensions of cells that have exhausted their endogenous metabolites are used. Several methods are available for obtaining such suspensions; however, a dense inoculum of cells placed in sterile saline and allowed to remain at room temperature overnight will suffice. A viability control of this inoculum should always accompany each test. Fermentation and assimilation patterns are presented in Table 104-7.

Animal studies are not routinely used in identification of the various species of *Candida*.

Immunologic methods

Routine serologic tests are not performed in the diagnostic laboratory to detect antibodies to antigenic preparation of *C. albicans*. Fluorescent antibody technics have been described to identify *C. albicans*, but these technics are not routinely used.[63]

Data from serologic studies with human sera reveal that a large number of the normal population possesses antibodies to antigens of *C. albicans*. Furthermore, skin test hypersensitivity may also be demonstrated in this group of people. It is felt that these immunologic tools are of little or no value in the diagnosis of the disease.

Culture isolates of *C. albicans* have been shown to fall into 1 of 2 antigenic groups, A and B.[64] Most of these studies have been performed with absorbed antisera; group A is identical with *C. tropicalis*, and group B with *C. stellatoideae*.

SYSTEMIC MYCOSES

The respiratory tract is the most common route of infection by the fungi responsible for systemic mycoses; however, there are a few documented cases in which cutaneous inoculation represented the primary focus. In general the disease is limited to the lungs as a mild subclinical or clinical infection. In a few cases the infection disseminates hematogenously or by direct extension to other organs and, under certain conditions, may be manifest in cutaneous lesions. The fungi most often responsible for systemic mycoses are dimorphic, with the exception of the yeastlike fungus, *Cryptococcus neoformans* (see Yeastlike fungi of medical importance). The dimorphic fungi exist in tissues in one phase, i.e., sporangia (*Coccidioides immitis*) or yeastlike cells (*Histoplasma capsulatum*, *Blastomyces dermatitidis*, *Paracoccidioides brasiliensis*), whereas in cultures at room temperature they will appear as filamentous molds.

All these fungi have been isolated from the soil where they exist saprobically. These infections are not contagious, i.e., no direct human-to-human transmission is known. Infection in man and animals follows the accidental inhalation or implantation of the organism from the saprobic environment. The spores produced in culture are easily airborne and may prove to be a laboratory hazard when these fungi are improperly handled.[65]

Coccidioidomycosis
Coccidioides immitis[66]

Coccidioides immitis, a dimorphic fungus, is found in the soil of certain geographically delimited areas of the southwestern United States, the northern states of Mexico, and a small endemic focus in South America and possibly in Central America. *C. immitis* is the etiologic agent of coccidioidomycosis (valley fever). In laboratory culture, the fungus grows rapidly in a filamentous form, producing a white, cottony mycelium, although considerable variation in appearance and color of colonies has been noted.[67] Older cultures may develop a powdery appearance and tend to darken to buff or brown, especially on the underside.

The route of infection in man and animals is almost entirely respiratory, but documented cases of primary cutaneous coccidioidomycosis are known. In infected tissues the organism is seen as a large thick-walled **spherule** (sporangium) measuring 10-100 μm in diameter, and occasionally larger variations are seen in the size of the spherule, depending on the stage of development of the fungus. Within these spherules are formed small, round to irregularly shaped **endospores** that may either line the inner walls or fill the entire structure. These are liberated apparently by rupture of the mature spherules.

Epidemiologic surveys in endemic areas reveal a high incidence of positive reactivity to **coccidioidin**, a culture filtrate of the organism.[68-70] Although the positive skin test is indicative of past or present exposure to the fungus, a majority of these individuals (60%) are asymptomatic and will give no history of infection. The remaining 40% will be symptomatic and present with a clinical picture ranging from an acute upper respiratory infection to a disseminated fatal disease.

Laboratory methods

Microscopic examination of sputum, bronchial washing, pus, pleural fluids, and gastric washings should be performed. Mature spherules containing endospores are distinguishable from tissue elements and other artifacts by their thick, highly refractile wall. However, it is difficult to demonstrate the presence of spherules with assurance in such specimens, since confusing artifacts are often present. It is sometimes helpful to seal the edges of the coverslip with petroleum jelly and incubate the slide at 37 C overnight. Several germ tubes may then be seen developing from single spherules (see section on *Blastomyces dermatitidis*).

A reliable diagnosis of the disease may be made by demonstrating the endosporulating spherule in histologic sections of biopsies. Spherules containing endospores are readily seen in hematoxylin-eosin–stained sections. These sections may also be stained by the periodic acid–Schiff stain or the Gomori methenamine–silver stain. Occasionally small spherules without endospores or enlarging endospores may be seen in the absence of mature spherules, at which time they may be confused with *B. dermatitidis*.

Clinical specimens should also be seeded onto culture media. *C. immitis* is not appreciably susceptible to cycloheximide and can therefore be grown on media containing this antibiotic. As a routine procedure, all clinical specimens should be cultured in duplicate in the presence and absence of antibiotic-containing media. **If there is a high index of suspicion that the clinical specimen harbors C. immitis, the material should be cultured in a screw-capped bottle or tube with Sabouraud antibiotic-containing selective agar, or the copper sulfate medium of Smith.**[71] The screw cap should be kept partially loosened to permit typical growth. The cultures are incu-

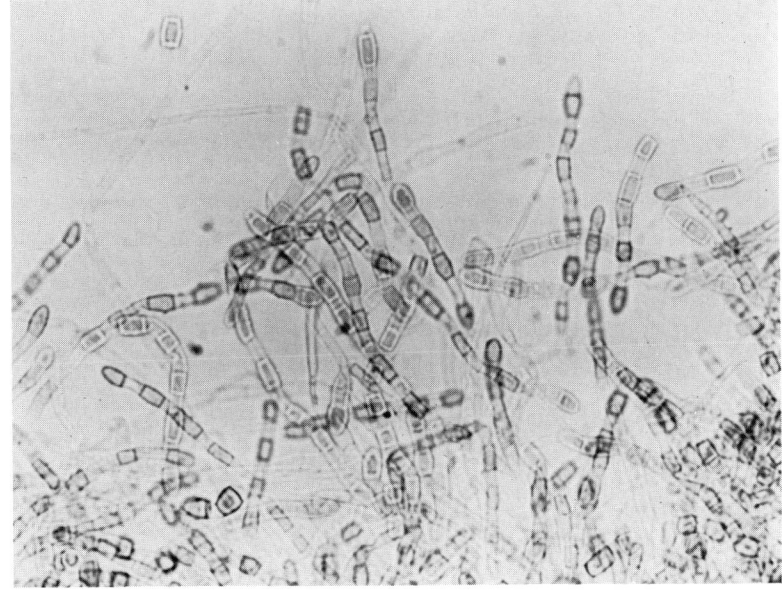

Fig. 104-19. Arthrospores of *Coccidioides immitis* from culture at room temperature. (×680.)

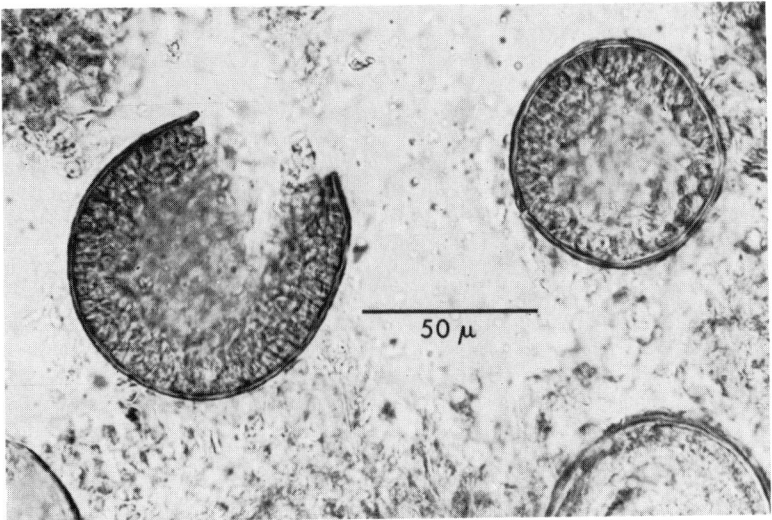

50 μ

Fig. 104-20. Spherules of *Coccidioides immitis* from lymph node of infected mouse.

bated at room temperature. Within 1-2 weeks small colonies appear, and these rapidly develop white, cottony aerial mycelia.[72] With age the colony may become tan to brown and develop a powdery appearance.

Microscopically, the cottony mycelium is made up of branching septate hyphae, which are segmented into arthrospores (Fig. 104-19). Pleomorphism may occur among some strains, and cultures should not be discarded if typical arthrospores are not seen. In general **any fungus that grossly resembles C. immitis must be handled with extreme care.** The organism is highly infectious, and the dry arthrospores are airborne very easily. Suspected cultures should be flooded with sterile saline and only the wetted material examined microscopically. Suspensions of the fungus may be injected intraperitoneally into mice. If the inoculated mice die, they should be examined for the presence of spherules in lesions. If they do not succumb within 2 weeks, some mice should be sacrificed and searched for spherules. Tiny fragments of tissue from lesions may be minced with iris scissors, placed in a drop of lactophenol–cotton blue, and examined between coverslip and slide.

In the infected animal the arthrospores become rounded, develop a thicker wall, and enlarge to form a spherule in 3-4 days. Within mature spherules are seen numerous endospores, which may either line the walls or completely fill the structure (Fig. 104-20). These endospores are formed by internal cleavage of the multinucleated cytoplasm. When released, each endospore is capable of maturation into a spherule within the animal tissues or if seeded onto suitable bacteriologic media, into a white filamentous mold.

Immunologic methods

Both skin tests and serologic tests are available for the study of coccidioidomycosis.[73] The skin test antigen used to detect delayed hypersensitivity is available commercially. This test is relatively specific, although some patients may react to other mycotic antigens (e.g., histoplasmin and blastomycin).[74-77]

Circulating antibodies in patients with coccidioidomycosis may be detected by precipitin tests or complement fixation (CF) tests. Precipitin antibodies are usually detected in the first to fourth week of illness, and they usually disappear in 1 or 2 months. In some cases these antibodies may be detected over a longer period of time. Complement fixing antibodies appear later, and their titer usually increases with increasing severity of the disease; thus the titer of the complement-fixing antibody is of prognostic value. Generally, when the titer reaches a certain critical level, extrapulmonary dissemination may be suspected. This critical level varies according to the serologic technic employed. In general these serologic studies are performed in laboratories where rigid controls and standards have been set (e.g., School of Medicine, University of California, Davis, Calif., and Communicable Disease Center, U.S.P.H.S., Atlanta, Ga., for description of CF test in coccidioidomycosis, see Smith, Saito, et al., 1950[78]).

The antigenic preparations employed in skin tests and the various serologic tests are prepared by growing static cultures of C. immitis in glucose-asparagine broth for several weeks. This medium is similar to that used in the commercial production of tuberculin. Cell-free filtrates prepared from this medium must be standardized before they are employed in these various immunologic tests. Other methods have been devised for the preparation of antigens from the mycelial[79] and spherule[80] phase of C. immitis.

Histoplasmosis
Histoplasma capsulatum[81]

The dimorphic fungus *Histoplasma capsulatum* has a worldwide distribution.[82,83] It is the etiologic agent of histoplasmosis, which is primarily a respiratory disease but which may rapidly spread to involve cells of the reticuloendothelial system as in the liver and spleen. This mycosis is usually an asymptomatic infection, but in a small number of cases it may be a chronic pulmonary disease or a widely disseminated and fatal one.

Within cells of the reticuloendothelial system the fungus grows in the form of small, budding yeast cells (about 2×4 μm) (Fig. 104-21). When cultured at room temperature on Sabouraud glucose agar, the fungus grows in a filamentous form. In young cultures the colonies are white, and as they age the colony tends to become buff to brown.

H. capsulatum has been isolated from the soil,[84] especially when it is contaminated with bat guano or chicken and starling droppings. Various animals, e.g., bats, dogs, and horses, have been proved to be naturally infected with this fungus. Although histoplasmosis occurs throughout the world, there are areas of high endemicity.[85] Such areas in the United States include the Ohio and Mississippi valleys.

The sexual phase of *H. capsulatum* has been observed. It is a heterothallic ascomycete whose perfect stage is *Emmonsiella capsulata* and it is placed in the family Gymnoascaceae.[49]

Laboratory methods

The unequivocal diagnosis of histoplasmosis requires isolation of the fungus in culture. Clinical specimens suspected of harboring the fungus include sputum, biopsies, blood, and bone marrow. These specimens should be cultured on brain-heart infusion blood agar or glucose cysteine blood agar with and without chloramphenicol. Cultures should also be prepared on antibiotic-containing Sabouraud (e.g., Mycosel) agar. It must be stressed that the yeast phase of *H. capsulatum* at 37 C is sensitive to cycloheximide. For this reason cultures should

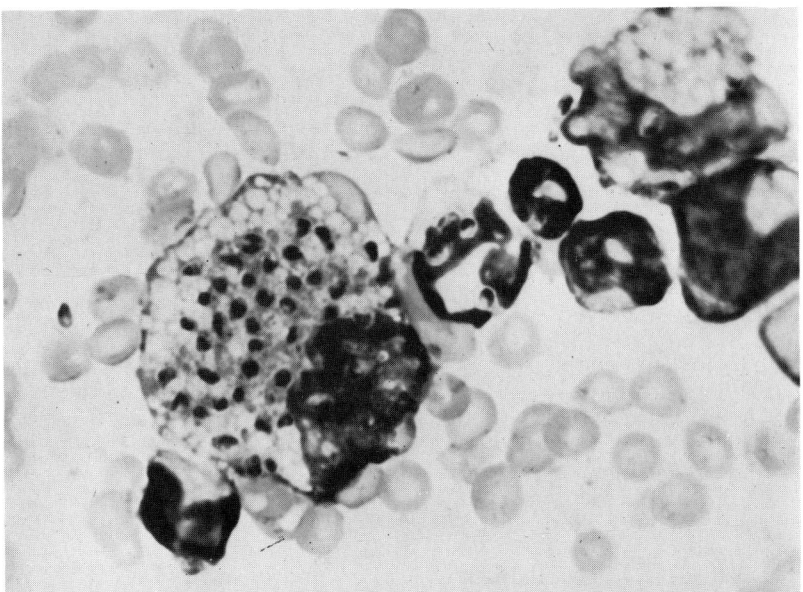

Fig. 104-21. Yeast cells of *Histoplasma capsulatum* within cytoplasm of mouse macrophage. (Wright's stain; ×1000.)

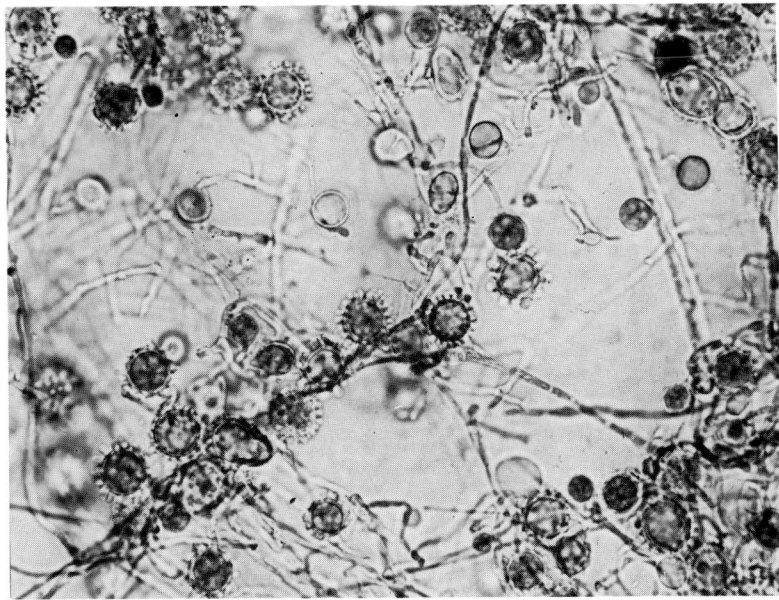

Fig. 104-22. Tuberculate chlamydospores of *Histoplasma capsulatum* in culture at room temperature. (×400.)

be seeded **in duplicate,** and 1 culture incubated at room temperature. The fungus will grow on antibiotic-containing Sabouraud agar at room temperature. Blood and bone marrow specimens should be cultured in a liquid medium (brain-heart infusion broth). All cultures should be held 4 weeks before they are discarded as negative. Clinical specimens should be processed and seeded onto an appropriate medium as soon as they are received. This consideration is impor-

tant, especially when sputum is to be cultured, since the organism appears to die rapidly in this fluid. *H. capsulatum* can be converted from the filamentous phase to the yeastlike phase by various methods.[86,87]

At room temperature the organism grows in a filamentous form, which consists of delicate, septate hyphae. Microconidia, round to pear-shaped, are borne laterally on these filaments. In older cultures large, round or pear-shaped macroconidia are formed.[88, 89] These large, thick-walled spores are covered with numerous tubercles (Fig. 104-22). In animal tissue the fungus reproduces as a small, budding, intracellular yeastlike organism. The unicellular phase of the fungus can be obtained in culture if incubated at 37 C.[90-92] Typical white to cream-colored, pasty colonies develop at this temperature.

Immunologic methods

Commercially prepared skin test antigens are available for the detection of delayed hypersensitivity in patients suffering from histoplasmosis. This immunologic tool should not be used recklessly, since it has been well established that skin testing with this material may result in a significant rise in antibody titer in individuals who are hypersensitive to the antigens of *H. calsulatum*.[93] For this reason the histoplasmin skin test has no place in the diagnostic work-up of patients and should not be used.

Several municipal and state health laboratories have services available for performing serologic studies for histoplasmosis. The precise tests vary, depending on the procedures employed. These tests may be qualitative or quantitative and include tube precipitin, agar gel diffusion, latex agglutination, and complement fixation.[94] In many instances these laboratories prepare their own antigenic materials.[95] For this reason it is necessary that serum samples be sent repeatedly to the same laboratory so that a comparison of serologic results will be meaningful.

Cross-reactions with other mycotic antigens have been demonstrated, e.g., blastomycin.[74, 96] However, increased reliability of serologic results is obtained when both histoplasmin (culture filtrate of mycelial phase) and whole, killed yeast cells are used as antigens. Several serum samples taken at varying intervals during the course of the disease should be submitted for serologic studies. A single serum sample provides little or no diagnostic value.

Another serologic test that may be of value in the rapid detection of the fungus in clinical specimens is the fluorescent antibody technic.[97, 98] At present this procedure is not routinely employed since special reagents and equipment are needed.

North American blastomycosis
Blastomyces dermatitidis

The etiologic agent of North American blastomycosis (Gilchrist's disease) is the dimorphic fungus, *Blastomyces dermatitidis*.[99, 100] The disease, which usually begins as a mild respiratory infection, may disseminate, usually involving osseous and cutaneous tissues.[101-103] Infection by this organism must be differentiated from other chronic granulomatous diseases, e.g., tuberculosis and other mycoses. The disease is almost entirely limited geographically to the North American continent, with areas of high endemicity restricted to the upper Mississippi valley, to the Ohio valley, and to a focus in the Middle Atlantic states. Cases have also been reported from Africa. The organism has been isolated from soil.

In culture at room temperature, the filamentous phase usually develops within 2 weeks. A white, downy to fluffy characteristic growth is soon apparent; with age, the colonies become tan to brown. Microscopic examination reveals characteristic conidia, 3-5 μm in size, borne along the side of hyphae or are terminal on short lateral filaments. They are short, knobby, round to piriform projections, which appear similar to chlamydospores in older cultures. In tissues or in

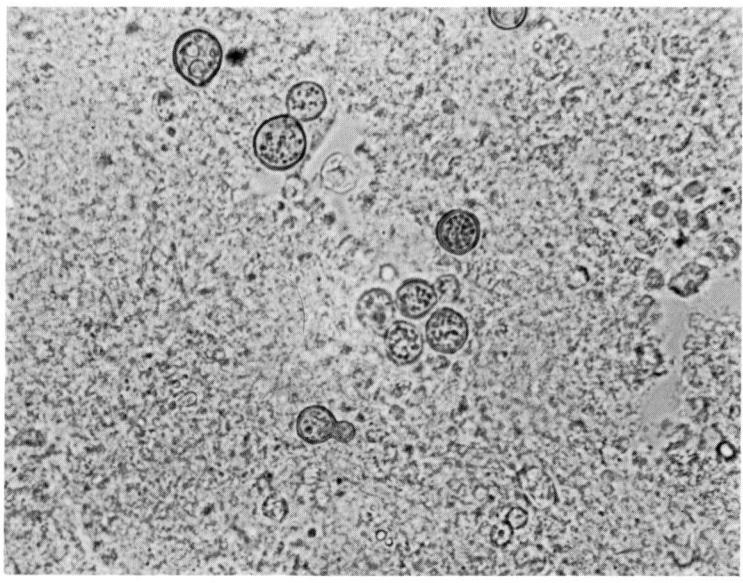

Fig. 104-23. Typical budding cells of *Blastomyces dermatitidis* grown on blood agar at 37 C. (×1000.)

culture at 37 C on enriched media the fungus appears as large, round to oval cells, which usually vary from 8-10 μm in diameter, but larger forms may also be seen. Small forms have also been described, varying from 2-4 μm in size. These cells characteristically bud by producing 1 daughter cell attached to the mother cell on a wide base. These daughter cells remain attached and rapidly attain the same size as the mother cell, the combination appearing much like the figure 8. The yeastlike cells are typically multinucleate.[104] The perfect stage of *B. dermatitidis* is *Ajellomyces dermatitidis*.[105] The sexual phase has been demonstrated to have the characteristics of the family Gymnoascaceae.

Laboratory methods

Direct microscopic examination of unstained clinical materials may reveal typical yeastlike cells with a single bud connected by a wide base (Fig. 104-23). These preparations must be carefully examined for the characteristic forms, since single fungus cells are difficult to differentiate from white blood cells. A modified slide culture technic may be employed to differentiate *B. dermatitidis* from lymphocytes. The cover slip is rimmed with petroleum jelly, and the slide incubated at 37 C for 4 hours. The yeastlike cells will produce single germ tubes. The fungus must be isolated in culture for definitive identification.

Clinical specimens are cultured in duplicate on media with added antibiotics (e.g., Mycosel agar) and without added antibiotics (e.g., brain-heart infusion blood agar or Kelley agar) and are incubated at room temperature and 37 C.[106] The yeastlike phase is sensitive to cycloheximide.

Animal inoculation is not a routine laboratory procedure but can be performed when difficulties are encountered with in vitro cultures.[107] A suspension of *B. dermatitidis* is inoculated intraperitoneally into mice. Penicillin, Streptomycin, or chloramphenicol may be added to clinical specimens such as sputum when bacterial contamination may produce death of animals. Animals that die are necropsied, and lesions are examined for characteristic yeastlike cells.

Immunologic methods

Serodiagnostic tools for the study of blastomycosis include skin tests with commercially available antigens and various serologic tests such as complement fixation, precipitation, and agglutination tests. It is important to remember that the serologic results from a single serum sample offer little if any diagnostic value. It is also important to remember that when sera are submitted for serologic studies, they should be sent to the same laboratory at which previous sera were analyzed. Differences in antigenic preparations may, and often do, yield different results. Serum antibodies from patients suffering from blastomycosis may cross react to a high degree with antigens prepared from other mycotic agents (e.g.,

histoplasmin).[74] The antigenic preparations of *B. dermatitidis* include culture filtrates and whole, killed yeast cells.[75] Sera should be tested with both types of antigenic preparations and additionally with coccidioidin and histoplasmin preparations.

Paracoccidioidal granuloma (paracoccidioidomycosis or South American blastomycosis)
Paracoccidioides brasiliensis

Paracoccidioides brasiliensis, a dimorphic fungus, is the etiologic agent of a chronic granulomatous infection of the oral mucous membranes, the lymph nodes, and the internal organs.[108,109] The disease is geographically limited to South America and has been known by several synonyms, e.g., Lutz-splendore-Almeida disease and Brazilian blastomycosis. Untreated, this disease may be fatal.

In culture at room temperature, the fungus develops slowly as a filamentous form with a short, white aerial mycelium that darkens with age. The mycelium is usually composed of undifferentiated, septate filaments, but intercalated and terminal chlamydospores may be found.

In tissue or in cultures at 37 C on enriched medium, the fungus grows as multipolar, budding yeast cells. The multiple daughter cells are attached to the mother cell by narrow connections. Occasionally a moniliform appearance results when several consecutive cells are connected together. One type of cell structure often observed is the "pilot's wheel," in which the daughter cells, usually very small, cover the entire surface of the mother cell. When these structures are focused on in a single plane, they have the appearance of a ship's steering wheel. Although multipolar bud formation is a characteristic of this fungus, cells with only 1 daughter are often seen. When the latter type of sporulation predominates, the organism may be mistaken for other yeastlike fungi that produce similar morphologic forms.

A cutaneous infection characterized clinically by the formation of keloids and histopathologically by the presence of numerous budding yeastlike cells has been called Lobo's disease. Some investigators consider it a variant form of South American blastomycosis, whereas others claim it to be an entirely different disease caused by another agent. Verified cultures have not been obtained from these lesions.

Laboratory methods

A direct examination of unstained clinical materials may reveal the characteristic multipolar budding cells (Fig. 104-24). All specimens should always be cultured in duplicate, on media with and without added antibiotics. One set of cultures should be incubated at room temperature, the other at 37 C. When incubated at 37 C, the yeast phase of the organism is sensitive to cycloheximide.

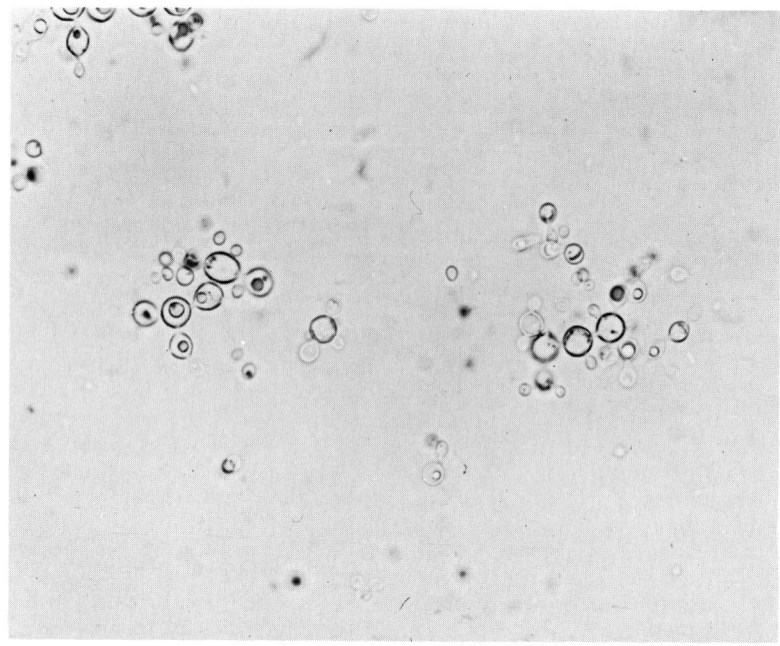

Fig. 104-24. Multipolar budding yeast cells of *Paracoccidioides brasiliensis* from culture at 37 C. (×680.)

Compact mold colonies develop slowly at room temperature, first appearing in about 10-14 days. They may be smooth and heaped at first, but as the colonies age, short, white aerial mycelia develop on the surface. Microscopically, the colonies are composed of nondescript, septate filaments, which readily dissociate. Swollen cells and chlamydospores may be found in large numbers. Since the filamentous phase is not distinctive in its morphology, conversion to the typical yeastlike form must be effective before any culture can be identified as *P. brasiliensis*.

The yeastlike phase is obtained by incubating cultures on enriched media such as blood agar or brain-heart infusion agar at 37 C. Cream to tan, soft, yeastlike colonies develop, which microscopically are composed of budding cells similar to those seen in tissue. The yeastlike phase may also be produced in experimental animals, i.e., intratesticular inoculation of guinea pigs; but animals are not routinely used for isolation or identification of the fungus.

Immunologic methods

Skin tests and serologic tests are available for the study of paracoccidioidal granuloma. Most of these tests are in various stages of experimental development.[110,111] Antigenic similarities common to *P. brasiliensis* and various species of *Emmonsia* have been shown to occur.[112] Sera from patients suffering from paracoccidioidal granuloma may cross react with mycotic antigens prepared from other fungi (e.g., histoplasmin, blastomycin).

OTHER MYCOSES*
Phycomycosis

Several genera of the class Phycomycetes have been implicated as etiologic agents in phycomycosis.[113,114] The clinical manifestations of this disease vary, depending on the route of infection, and include such entities as subcutaneous eosinophilic granulomas, respiratory infections, and involvement of facial and orbital tissues, the last condition leading eventually to cerebral invasion.

Definitive diagnosis of this disease rests on the isolation and identification of the organism in culture. The diagnosis of phycomycosis, however, is often presumptive and is made by histopathologic examination of postmortem specimens in which cultures of tissues are frequently neglected. In this situation one must rely on the ability of the pathologist to identify the characteristic broad, cenocytic hyphal elements in tissues. Discrepancies frequently arise in the interpretation of the fungal elements observed, and the agents with which they are most often confused are species of the genus *Aspergillus*.

Absidia, *Rhizopus*, *Mucor*, *Mortierella*, and *Basidiobolus* are the genera most often implicated in this disease. Species of fungi belonging to these genera are ubiquitous and are occasionally isolated as contaminants from clinical specimens. Careful evaluation and interpretation must be given to cultures that are isolated, especially from crusted lesions of the skin.

---

*Frequently opportunistic.

Laboratory methods

Tissues and exudates from suspected lesions must be examined microscopically and cultured on media that do not contain cycloheximide. These cultures are incubated at room temperature or at 37 C. The most striking morphologic features of this class of fungi are the absence of septa, the presence of relatively broad filaments (10-15 μm in width) branching at irregular intervals, and the production of spores within a sporangium.

Pathogenicity studies with animals are not performed as an aid to diagnosis. Experimentally, however, rabbits have been infected by intranasal instillation of *R. oryzae*, but this occurs only after the animals were made diabetic by treatment with alloxan. The resulting infection resembles that seen in nasal, pulmonary, and cerebral infections of man.

Aspergillosis

The medical importance of the genus *Aspergillus* has increased concomitantly with the increased use of antibiotic and steroid therapy.[61] Bird fanciers and poultry farmers have well appreciated the potential hazards of this group of fungi because many species of birds are highly susceptible to infection by these fungi. Recently a new area of interest has been created with the elucidation of the chemistry and pharmacologic properties of a group of toxins isolated from *Aspergillus flavus*. These toxins, **aflatoxins**, not only are toxic but also have been shown to be potent carcinogens.

Aspergillosis is an infection caused by any one of several species of *Aspergillus*. Depending on the focus of infection, the disease may be manifested as a cavitary pulmonary infection, otomycosis, sinusitis, mycetoma, or keratitis, *A. fumigatus* is most frequently isolated from lesions, but *A. flavus, A. niger, A. terreus*, and other species have also been implicated.[115]

Thermophilic forms of *Aspergillus* are known, and these are able to grow at temperatures up to 50 C. The genus contains ubiquitous fungi frequently found as contaminants in laboratory media. Histopathologic studies of clinical specimens reveal septate filaments (3-4 μm in diameter), which branch dichotomously. The hyphae are generally oriented in the same plane. These fungus elements may be confused with those produced by the class Phycomycetes.

Laboratory methods

Clinical specimens are examined microscopically for hyphae. Specimens consisting of purulent material from abscesses, bronchial washings, or of biopsy material can be cleared with 10% potassium hydroxide. This treatment has no visible deleterious effect on the fungus elements. Cultures are prepared on media that do not contain chloramphenicol and are incubated at room temperature or at 37 C. In the case of *A. fumigatus*, higher temperatures of incubation may be

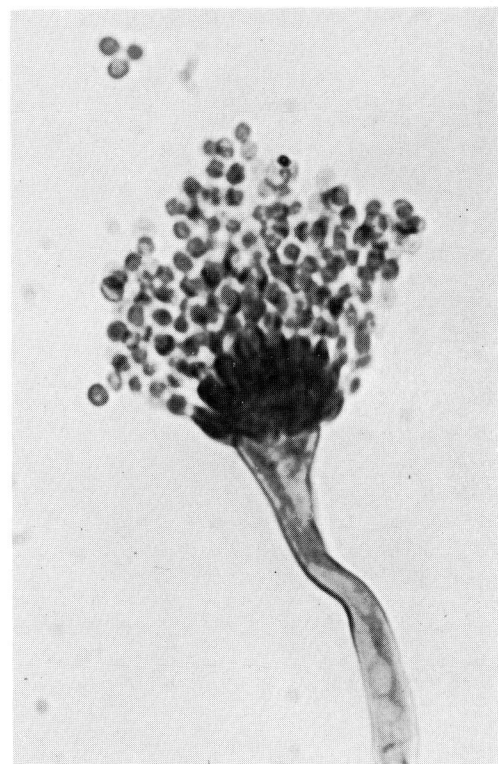

Fig. 104-25. Conidiophore and conidiospores of *Aspergillus* sp. (×680.)

employed. Sparsely isolated colonies from 1 clinical specimen do not indicate that the organism is the cause of the disease process. In such a situation, repeat cultures should be requested on fresh specimens.

Species identification rests on the mode of conidiospore formation (Fig. 104-25), the color of colony, and the morphology of the conidiospore. The sexual stages of some species of *Aspergillus* have been observed, and these species have been placed in the class Ascomycetes.

Geotrichosis
Geotrichum candidum

Geotrichum candidum is a common saprobic fungus often found on decaying fruits and vegetables and frequently isolated from the soil. *G. candidum* has been implicated in a variety of diseases such as bronchial, pulmonary, oral, and intestinal infections. Oral geotrichosis clinically simulates the infection caused by *Candida albicans*. Because of the ubiquitous nature of this organism, it is frequently difficult to assess the significance of its presence in clinical specimens in the absence of disease.

Laboratory methods

G. candidum grows readily on a variety of laboratory media. Clinical specimens may be seeded onto Sabouraud dextrose agar containing

Table 104-8. Source of specimens and media required for demonstration and isolation of fungi from specific types of fungus diseases*

Disease	Type of specimen	Isolation medium
Superficial mycoses		
Tinea versicolor	Skin scrapings	None available at present
Tinea nigra	Skin scrapings	Cycloheximide medium†
Piedra	Clipped hairs	Sabouraud dextrose agar
Cutaneous mycoses (dermatomycoses)		
Candidiasis	Skin scrapings	Cycloheximide medium
	Scrapings from mucocutaneous areas	Sabouraud dextrose agar (for *Candida*
	Vaginal scrapings	sp. inhibited by cycloheximide)
Onychomycosis	Nail scrapings	
Tinea capitis	Plucked hairs	Cycloheximide medium
Tinea corporis	Skin scrapings	
Tinea pedis	Skin scrapings	
Subcutaneous mycoses		
Sporotrichosis	Pus from ulcers	Cycloheximide medium
	Aspirated fluid from subcutaneous abscesses	
Chromoblastomycosis (Chromomycosis)	Crust and scrapings for warty outgrowths	Cycloheximide medium
	Exudate from lesions	
Mycetoma (maduromycosis)	Pus from draining sinuses	Sabouraud dextrose agar
	Aspirated fluids from unopened sinus tracts	BHI‡ agar
	Biopsy specimens	
Systemic mycoses		
Cryptococcosis	Spinal fluid	Sabouraud dextrose agar + chloramphenicol
	Sputum	
	Pus from abscesses	
	Pus from sinus tracts	
	Scrapings from skin lesions	
	Urine	
Candidiasis	Sputum	Cycloheximide medium
	Bronchial washings	Sabouraud dextrose agar (for *Candida*
	Spinal fluid	sp. inhibited by cycloheximide)
	Urine	
	Stools	
Coccidioidomycosis	Sputum	Cycloheximide medium
	Bronchial washings	Copper sulfate medium
	Spinal fluid	
	Urine	
	Scrapings from skin lesions	
	Pus from draining abscesses and sinuses	
Histoplasmosis	Blood	Cycloheximide medium
	Sternal marrow	BHI agar + C & S§
	Sputum	BHI (no antibiotics) for 37 C incubation
	Bronchial washings	
	Spinal fluid	
	Exudate from ulcers	
	Scrapings from skin lesions	
Blastomycosis, North American	Scrapings from edge of skin lesions	Cycloheximide medium
	Pus from open abscesses	BHI agar + C & S§
	Pus from sinus tracts	BHI (no antibiotics) for 37 C incubation
	Urine	
	Sputum	
	Bronchial washings	

*Modified from Ajello, L., Georg, L. K., Kaplan, W., et al.: CDC Laboratory manual for medical mycology, PHS pub. no. 994, Washington, D. C., 1963, U. S. Government Printing Office, pp. A-6 and A-7.
†Sabouraud dextrose agar + chloramphenicol and cycloheximide.
‡Brain-heart infusion.
§Chloramphenicol and cycloheximide.

Table 104-8. Source of specimens and media required for demonstration and isolation of fungi from specific types of fungus diseases—cont'd

Disease	Type of specimen	Isolation of medium
Paracoccidioidomycosis	Scrapings from edge of skin lesions Scrapings from mucous membranes Biopsied lymph nodes Sputum Bronchial washings	Same as for North American blasto-mycosis
Miscellaneous mycoses Mucormycosis (phycomycosis)	Sputum Bronchial washings Biopsy material	Sabouraud dextrose agar + chloramphenicol
Aspergillosis	Sputum Bronchial washings	Same as for mucormycosis
Geotrichosis	Sputum Bronchial washings Stools	Sabouraud dextrose agar + chloramphenicol

chloramphenicol. The fungus grows as a rapidly spreading, moist, wrinkled colony. Microscopically the colony is composed of septate, branching hyphae. Arthrospores fragment readily and appear as barrel-shaped or elliptical cells. Animal studies are usually not performed, unless *Coccidioides immitis* is suspected. In this case a suspension of the fungus should be inoculated into mice. *G. candidum* is not dimorphic, whereas in *C. immitis* inoculation spherules will be observed in diseased tissues.

Cladosporiosis
Cladosporium trichoides

Cladosporiosis is a rare mycotic disease caused by the dematiacious fungus *Cladosporium trichoides*. The term cladosporiosis is an unfortunate one because other species of the genus *Cladosporium* cause diseases unlike the clinical manifestations produced by *C. trichoides*. *C. wernecki* infect only the superficial layers of skin (see tinea nigra) and *C. carrioni* is one of the agents that causes a subcutaneous mycotic disease (see chromomycosis).

Infection with *C. trichoides* most frequently involves the brain, with no other apparent focus of disease. However, the fungus probably enters the body by way of the respiratory tract.

Laboratory methods

Dark hyphae, usually pale brown, are seen in smears and sections of the brain. *C. trichoides* grows well on a variety of laboratory media incubated at room temperature or 37 C. The fungus colony is characterized by a velvety surface and may be irregularly folded and olive gray to olive brown. Conidia and condiophores similar to those produced by *C. carrioni* are found on microscopic examination of the growth. *C. trichoides* is virulent for the mouse, and lesions in the brain are seen at necropsy.

SUMMARY

The increasing awareness of the role of fungi in disease processes and improved laboratory techniques for their diagnosis have made it imperative that the laboratory worker develop a degree of competence in this field. Fungi once thought to be passsing inhabitants of the laboratory environment cannot be discarded after only a cursory examination. Attemps must be made to identify all the fungi that are isolated, especially when they are repeatedly found in different specimens taken from the same patient. It is essential that all specimens be examined microscopically for the presence of fungus elements. The types of specimens received in the diagnostic laboratory and the isolation media to be used are summarized in Table 104-8.

REFERENCES

1. Keddie, F., and Shadomy, S.: Sabouraudia **3**:21, 1963.
2. Daly, J. F.: Arch. Dermatol. **75**:584, 1957.
3. Barlow, A. J. E., and Chattaway, F. W.: J. Invest. Dermatol. **24**:65, 1955.
4. Tate, P.: Parasitology **21**:31, 1929.
5. Vanbreuseghem, R.: Mycologia **44**:176, 1952.
6. Pipkin, J. L.: Arch. Dermatol. **66**:9, 1952.
7. Rothman, S., Smiljanic, A., Shapiro, et al.: J. Invest. Dermatol. **8**:81, 1947.
8. Emmons, C. W.: Arch. Dermatol. **30**:337, 1934.
9. Georg, L. K.: Mycologia **44**:470, 1952.
10. Georg, L. K., and Camp, L. B.: J. Bacteriol. **74**:113, 1957.
11. Dawson, C. O., and Gentles, J. C.: Nature **183**:1345, 1959.
12. Rebell, G., and Taplin, D.: Dermatophytes: their recognition and identification, rev. ed., Coral Gables, 1974, University of Miami Press.
13. Ajello, L.: Ann. N. Y. Acad. Sci. **89**:30, 1960.
14. English, M. P., and Gibson, M. S.: Br. Med. J. **1**:1442, 1959.
15. Georg, L. K., Hand, E. A., and Menges, R. A.: J. Invest. Dermatol. **27**:335, 1956.
16. Georg, L. K.: J. Invest. Dermatol. **23**:123, 1954.
17. Georg, L. K.: Trans. N. Y. Acad. Sci. **18**:639, 1956.
18. Kaplan, W., Georg, L. K., and Ajello, L.: Ann. N. Y. Acad. Sci. **70**:636, 1958.
19. Rook, A. J., and Frain-Bell, W.: Med. Illus. **8**:823, 1954.
20. Bentley, M. L.: J. Gen. Microbiol. **8**:365, 1953.

21. Robbins, W. J., and Ma, R.: Am. J. Bot. **32**:509, 1945.
22. Silva, M., and Benham, R. W.: J. Invest. Dermatol. **18**:453, 1952.
23. Chattaway, F. W., and Barlow, A. J. E.: J. Gen. Microbiol. **11**:506, 1954.
24. Chattaway, F. W., and Barlow, A. J. E.: Nature **181**:281, 1958.
25. Wolf, F. T.: Nature **180**:860, 1957.
26. Ajello, L., Georg, L. K., Kaplan, W., et al.: CDC Laboratory manual for medical mycology, PHS pub. no. 994, Washington, D. C., 1963, U. S. Government Printing Office.
27. Benham, R. W., and Kesten, B.: J. Infect. Dis. **50**:437, 1932.
28. Hansmann, G. H., and Schencken, J. R.: Am. J. Pathol. **10**:731, 1934.
29. Post, G. W., Jackson, A., Garber, P. E., et al.: Dis. Chest **34**:455, 1958.
30. Campbell, C. C.: J. Bacteriol. **50**:233, 1945.
31. Drouhet, E., and Mariat, F.: Ann. Inst. Pasteur **83**:506, 1952.
32. Kaplan, W., and Ivens, M. S.: J. Invest. Dermatol. **35**:151, 1960.
33. Silva, M.: Trans. N. Y. Acad. Sci. (ser. II) **21**:46, 1958.
34. Ridley, M. F.: Aust. J. Dermatol. **4**:23, 1957.
35. Borelli, D.: Arch. Dermatol. **76**:789, 1957.
36. Gammel, J. A.: Arch. Dermatol. **15**:241, 1927.
37. Mackinnon, J. E.: Trans. R. Soc. Trop. Med. Hyg. **48**:470, 1954.
38. Symmers, D., and Sporer, A.: Arch. Pathol. **37**:309, 1944.
39. Boyd, M. F., and Crutchfield, E. D.: Am. J. Trop. Med. **4**:215, 1921.
40. Emmons, C. W.: Arch. Pathol. **39**:364, 1945.
41. Hanan, E. B., and Zurett, S.: Arch. Dermatol. Syph. **37**:947, 1938.
42. Gordon, M. A.: J. Bacteriol. **73**:199, 1957.
43. Benham. R. W., and Georg, L. K.: J. Invest. Dermatol. **10**:99, 1948.
44. Pautler, E. E., Roberts, R. W., and Beamer, P. R.: Arch. Ophthalmol. **53**:385, 1955.
45. Scharyj, M., Levene, N., and Gordon, H.: J. Infect. Dis. **106**:141, 1960.
46. Tong, J. L., Valentine, E. H., Durrance, J. R., et al.: Am. Rev. Tuberc. **78**:604, 1958.
47. Littman, M. L., and Zimmerman, L. E.: Cryptococcosis-torulosis or European blastomycosis, New York, 1956, Grune & Stratton.
48. Winner, H. I., and Hurley, R.: Candida albicans, Boston, 1964, Little, Brown & Co.
49. Kwon-Chung, K. J.: Mycologia **67**:1197, 1975.
50. Mallory, F. B.: Pathological technique, Philadelphia, 1942, W. B. Saunders Co.
51. Littman, M. L.: J. Infect. Dis. **101**:51, 1957.
52. Seeliger, H. P. R.: J. Bacteriol. **72**:127, 1956.
53. Evans, E. E.: J. Immunol. **64**:423, 1950.
54. Kase, A., and Marshall, J. D.: Am. J. Clin. Pathol. **34**:52, 1960.
55. Emmons, C. W.: Am. J. Hyg. **62**:227, 1955.
56. Shields, A. B., and Ajello, L.: Science **151**:208, 1966.
57. Bennett, J., Hasenclever, H., and Tynes, B.: Trans, Assoc. Am. Physicians **77**:145, 1964.
58. Gordon, M. A.: Int. J. Dermatol. **9**:209, 1970.
59. Bennett, J., and Hasenclever, H.: Am. Rev. Resp. Dis. **91**:616, 1964.
60. Woods, J. W., Manning, I. H., and Patterson, C. N.: J.A.M.A. **145**:207, 1951.
61. Lodder, J., editor: The yeasts, Amsterdam, 1970, North-Holland Publishing Co.
62. Taschdjian, C. L., Burchall, J. J., and Kozinn, C. L.: A.M.A. J. Dis. Child. **99**:212, 1960.
63. Gordon, M. A.: Proc. Soc. Exp. Biol. Med. **97**:694, 1958.
64. Hasenclever, H. F., and Mitchell, W. O.: J. Bacteriol **82**:570, 1961.
65. Ibach, M. J., Larsh, H. W., and Furcolow, M. L.: Science **119**:71, 1954.
66. Fiese, M. J.: Coccidioidomycosis, Springfield, Ill., 1958, Charles C Thomas, Publisher.
67. Friedman, L., Pappagianis, D., Berman, R. J., et al.: J. Lab. Clin. Med. **42**:438, 1953.
68. Maddy, K. T., Crecelius, J. G., and Cornell, R. G.: Public Health Rep. **75**:955, 1960.
69. Smith, C. E., Pappagianis, D., and Saito, M. T.: In Proceedings of symposium on coccidioidomycosis, PHS pub. no. 575, Washington, D. C., 1957, U. S. Department of Health, Education and Welfare, pp. 3-9.
70. Smith, C. E., Beard, R. R., Rosenberger, H. C., et al.: J.A.M.A. **132**:833, 1946.
71. Smith, C. E.: Med. Clin. North Am. **27**:790, 1943.
72. Hampson, C. R.: J. Bacteriol. **67**:739, 1954.
73. Smith, C. E., Whiting, E. G., Baker, E. E., et al.: Am. Rev. Tuberc. **57**:330, 1948.
74. Campbell, C. C., and Binkley, G. E.: J. Lab. Clin. Med. **42**:896, 1953.
75. Knight, R. A., and Marcus, S.: Am. Rev. Tuberc. Pulmon. Dis. **77**:983, 1958.
76. Smith, C. E., Saito, M. T., Beard, R. R., et al.: Am. J. Public Health **39**:722, 1956.
77. Smith, C. E., Saito, M. T., and Simons, S. A.: J.A.M.A. **160**:546, 1956.
78. Smith, C. E., Saito, M. T., Beard, R. R., et. al.: Am. J. Hyg. **52**:1, 1950.
79. Pappagianis, D., Smith, C. E., Kobayashi, G. S., et al.: J. Infect. Dis. **108**:35, 1961.
80. Levine, H. B., Cobb, J. M., and Scalarone, G. M.: Sabouraudia **7**:20, 1969.
81. Sweany, H. C.: Histoplasmosis, Springfield, Ill., 1960, Charles C Thomas, Publisher.
82. Edwards, P. Q., and Klaer, J. H.: Am. J. Trop. Med. **5**:235, 1956.
83. Schwarz, J., and Drouhet, E.: Arch. Pathol. **64**:409, 1957.
84. Emmons, C. W.: Public Health Rep. **64**:892, 1949.
85. Christie, A., and Peterson, J. C.: J. Pediatr. **29**:417, 1946.
86. Larsh, H. W., Winton, A., and Silberg, S. L.: Proc. Soc. Exp. Biol. Med. **93**:612, 1956.
87. Rowley, D. A., and Huber, M.: J. Infect. Dis. **96**:174, 1955.
88. Dowding, E. S.: Can. J. Res. **26**:265, 1948.
89. Edwards, M. R., Hazen, E. L., and Edwards, G. A.: Can. J. Microbiol. **6**:65, 1960.
90. Scherr, G. H.: Exp. Cell. Res. **12**:92, 1957.
91. Campbell, C. C.: J. Bacteriol. **54**:263, 1947.
92. Pine, L., and Peacock, C. L.: J. Bacteriol. **75**:167, 1958.
93. Kaufman, L., Terry, R. J., Schubert, J. H., et al.: J. Bacteriol. **94**:798, 1967.
94. Hill, G. B., and Campbell, C. C.: J. Lab. Clin. Med. **48**:255, 1956.
95. Salvin, S. B., and Hottle, G. A.: J. Immunol. **60**:57, 1958.
96. Salvin, S. B.: Prog. Allergy. **7**:213, 1963.
97. Gordon, M. A.: J. Bacteriol. **77**:678, 1959.
98. Kaufman, L., and Kaplan, W.: J. Bacteriol. **82**:729, 1961.
99. Salvin, S. B.: Mycologia **61**:311, 1949.
100. Schwarz, J., and Baum, G. L.: Am. J. Clin. Pathol. **21**:999, 1959.

101. Martin, D. S., and Smith, D. T.: Am. Rev. Tuberc. **39**:275, 1939.
102. Watson, S. H., Moore, S., and Blank, F.: Can. Med. Assoc. J. **78**:35, 1958.
103. Wilson, J. W., Cawley, E. P., Weidman, F. D., et al.: Arch. Dermatol. **71**:39, 1955.
104. Bakerspigel, A.: Can. J. Microbiol. **3**:923, 1957.
105. McDonough, E. S., and Lewis, A. L.: Science **156**:528, 1967.
106. Halliday, W. J., and McCoy, E.: J. Bacteriol. **70**:464, 1955.
107. Baker, R. D.: Am. J. Trop. Med. **19**:547, 1939.
108. Mackinnon, J. E.: Trans. R. Soc. Trop. Med. Hyg. **53**:487, 1959.
109. Perry, H. O., Weed, L. A., and Kierland, R. R.: Arch. Dermatol. **70**:477, 1954.
110. Restrepo, A.: Infect. Immun. **2**:268, 1970.
111. Yarzabal, L. A., Biguet, J., Vaucelle, T., et al.: Sabouraudia **11**:80, 1973.
112. Josefiak, E. J., Foushee, J. H. S., and Smith, L. C.: Am. J. Clin. Pathol. **30**:547, 1958.
113. Lie Kian Joe, Njo-Injo Tjoei Eng, Sutoma Tjokronegoro, et al.: J. Trop. Med. Hyg. **9**:143, 1960.
114. Rabin, E. R., Lundberg, G. D., and Mitchell, E. T.: N. Engl. J. Med. **264**:1286, 1961.
115. Drake, C. H.: Mycopathologia **4**:103, 1948.

SEROLOGY OF
INFECTIOUS DISEASES

105

GENERAL CONSIDERATIONS

Alex C. Sonnenwirth

SOME BASIC PRINCIPLES

Immunology used to be defined as the study of resistance to disease-producing agents. Resistance is a complex state; it includes all the properties of the host that confer protection against infectious agents and is usually enhanced after recovery from a specific infection.

The terms immune and immunity (L., *immunis*, safe) were used for many decades to denote the fact that certain individuals who recovered from a particular disease would not again contract the same disease and that immunity could be actively induced by introducing the infectious agent, usually in altered form, into the host (Davis et al.[1]).

By the 15th century it was well known that those who recovered from an attack of smallpox would not become reinfected, i.e., they became immune, and therefore deliberate attempts were made to induce immunity by inoculating individuals with skin scrapings from smallpox lesions. Jenner (1790) finally showed that inoculation with pus from cowpox lesions (vaccination; L., *vacca*, cow) induced immunity to smallpox. His work and the subsequent findings of Pasteur, who used aged cultures to induce immunity, proved the realiability of immunization procedures and the main underlying principle: the need for using altered agents, i.e., agents the virulence of which has been attenuated by various means such as passage through unnatural hosts, aging, or killing by chemical or physical means.[1]

Toxins of both microbial and nonmicrobial origins were also shown to be usable for inducing immunity to these substances (diphtheria and tetanus toxins, snake venoms, etc.). Altered toxins (toxoids) are universally employed for immunization. Eventually it was found (1890) that the immune response to the introduction of infectious or toxic agents (**antigens**) was due to the appearance of certain substances (**antibodies**) in the serum of the host, which are specifically formed in response to the administration of antigen (Davis et al.[1]).

Soon thereafter it was also found that the **immune response,** instead of conferring resistance, may result in a state of **hypersensitivity** (due to cellular sensitization or antibody production or both), i.e., greater reactivity on subsequent exposure to the antigen, with sometimes untoward or dangerous consequences. It was finally realized that manifestations of the immune response and antibody formation are general phenomena: Many antibodies induced by infectious agents have no protective value and thus resistance is not an essential feature. In addition, specific antibodies and specific hypersensitivity may be brought about by an almost limitless number of nonliving, often harmless substances (pollen, foreign serum proteins, etc.).[2] Microbial antigens are only a minority of the antigenic substances. Thus exposure to antigen results in changed reactivity of the host, who is capable to "recognize and respond specifically to the foreignness of a wide range of biological substances that are not normally present in his own tissues" (Holborow[2]). This changed reactivity (the result of specific sensitization) in some cases manifests itself as immunity, in other cases as hypersensitivity; i.e., the results may be beneficial or harmful.

Starting in the 1950s, various aspects of the immune response have become of interest in areas different from the original concept, namely, resistance to infectious agents. For example, because of their high precision, immunologic and serologic* methods were applied in the analysis of complex macromolecules (e.g., antibody molecules are utilized as analytical reagents for the study of the structure of antigenic molecules, enzymes, etc.); antigen-antibody reactions serve as models for specific reactions such as those encountered in fertilization or in maternal-fetal interactions; antibody formation is studied as a model for protein synthesis and for cellular differentiation; and cellular responses such as the appearance of specifically altered lymphoid cells (lymphocytes, macrophages) are studied intensively.

*The 2 terms are often used interchangeably; serologic reaction refers to specific reactions of immune sera,[1] whereas immunologic methods encompass, in addition, other reactions also (cellular reactivity, etc.) See Part VI, Immunology.

Eventually it was recognized that many immunologic phenomena are involved in a variety of human diseases as well as in tumor development and in transplantation rejection. Thus, as stated by Rose,[3] "our understanding of the **immunological response** has broadened from its role in **protection against infection** to a **cause of several** (immunological) **diseases.** These may be allergic and immune complex diseases (due to extrinsic antigens) or autoimmune diseases (due to intrinsic antigens); malignant change or failure of the immunological response may also produce disease." The definition of immunology now encompasses the various aspects enumerated above. Gell et al.[4] consider immunology proper the study of "foreignness" and of the reaction against foreign substances, including all "immune" or "allergic" reactions. Autoimmunity, immune tolerance, and the immunologic competence of cells thus are all encompassed.

Chapters 60-67 (Part VI, Immunology) cover immunoglobulins and their assessment, complements, cell-mediated immunological responses, phagocytosis, autoantibodies, transplantation immunology, and tumor-associated antigens.

In this part (Chapters 105-108) only tests for serologic diagnosis of infectious diseases (mostly bacterial diseases) are discussed.

Serologic tests for the diagnosis of viral diseases are discussed in Chapter 93, those for rickettsial diseases in Chapter 95, those for parasitic diseases in Chapter 100, and those for fungal diseases in Chapters 104 and 107. Consult index for other serologic tests.

Serology deals with the specific reactions of antigens and antibodies and is a more restrictive term than immunology. It has been called the "handmaiden of immunology" and has been defined as the study of diagnostic and experimental procedures connected with immunology, involving serum reactions.

Serologic tests are employed both for (1) the **identification of microorganisms** (described in the sections on bacteriology, mycology, and viruses and rickettsiae) and for (2) the **demonstration of antibodies** in the serum of the host.

In certain diseases in which the causative agent cannot be isolated (such as syphilis), the finding of specific antibodies is important. The evidence furnished by serologic methods is indirect, and it should be kept in mind that prior vaccination may be responsible for the presence of antibodies. Serologic diagnosis is often of little aid in rapid or early diagnosis, since significant antibody response, with some exceptions, is not produced until the infection has persisted at least 7-10 days.

When an infectious agent invades the host, antibody formation is initiatied; it may continue for many months, and the presence of specific antibody therefore indicates only that infection has taken place sometime in the past. It is necessary to show a **change** in titer during the illness, i.e., an increase during the second and following weeks and a decrease afterwards. For this reason it is imperative to obtain a serum sample early in the disease (**acute phase**) and another one later (**convalescent phase**) and to test them preferably at the same time, using identical technics and reagents.

The **diagnostic uses of serology** now extend beyond the identification and measurement of antibodies in infectious disease. Using a variety of technics (see Antigen-antibody reactions), it is now possible to detect and measure antibodies in—among others—the autoimmune diseases (e.g., rhematoid factor, thyroid antibodies, etc.), to identify the offending agent in drug-induced thrombocytopenic purpura,[4] to perform immunoassay of hormones (e.g., immunoassay of human chorionic gonadotropin as a pregnancy test), and to diagnose various immunologic abnormalities (e.g., hypogammaglobulinemia, myeloma, macroglobulinemias, etc.). See Chapters 60-67.

Some important source material and references in immunology and serology are *Clinical Aspects of Immunology,*[5] *An ABC of Modern Immunology,*[6] *Manual of Clinical Immunology,*[3] *Clinical Immunology,*[7] *Principles of Immunology,*[8] *Methods in Immunodiagnosis,*[9] and *Research in Immunochemistry and Immunobiology.*[10]

RESISTANCE TO DISEASE

Natural resistance involves both passive and active factors. Some disease-producing agents infect only certain species of animals, whereas other species are unaffected: Hansen's disease (leprosy) and infectious hepatitis affect humans only, whereas lower animals possess passive resistance to the organisms that cause these infections.

Age and sex also influence natural resistance of the individual to disease. Males seem to have a higher incidence of infectious diseases than females. Similarly, older people are more susceptible to certain diseases than younger ones.

The **skin** is one of the most important natural passive defenses against infection. It forms an effective mechanical barrier, and it is dry and provides a temperature unfavorable for organisms that require a moist, warm environment. Perspiration and the excretion of other concentrated fluids onto the skin surface provide an unsuitable environment for growth of organisms.

A critical factor in the development of microorganisms is optimum oxygen tension. Oxygen tension within the body may be too high or too low for certain disease-producing agents. As a result, infection is greatly retarded or completely prevented.

Among the active factors of natural defense are the **mucous membranes,** which secrete specific bactericidal and virucidal agents. Minute cilia, present on these membranes, prevent the entrance of organisms by means of their constant waving and beating motion toward the outside. Bactericidal substances are also secreted by deeper tissues of the body.

Phagocytosis is an important defense mechanism. Certain white blood cells actually engulf and assimilate pathogenic organisms with which they come in contact. It is significant that an increased white cell count usually occurs during the course of an infection.

Fever is actually a very effective body defense. Many organisms that ordinarily could thrive at normal body temperature find it difficult to survive if the temperature of their environment is increased by a few degrees.

Response of the body to infection is manifested by the process of **inflammation,** consisting, among others, of an increase in the number of white blood cells, dilatation of blood vessels and increased permeability of capillaries and formation of fibrin, localizing bacteria and assisting the phagocytes. In addition, the lymph and blood flow increases, diluting and flushing away toxic substances.

Acquired resistance is associated with the state commonly termed **immunity.** When a disease-producing agent enters the human body, certain tissues respond (see **immunologic apparatus and lymphocytes,** Chapter 60) by producing **antibodies (immunoglobulins).** The antibodies act as distinct defensive mechanisms directed against the original infective agent. They represent an acquired defense against disease, since they occur only after a disease-producing agent has been introduced into the body.

Naturally acquired active immunity occurs through actual infection by a disease-producing agent. When the body is invaded by a microorganism, specific antibodies against this agent are produced and the body develops immunity to reinfection by these organisms. **Artificially acquired active immunity** occurs through the administration of the infective agent in an inactivated form. The protein of the organism is sufficient to stimulate the body to produce the specific antibody protectors.

Acquired passive immunity may be natural or artificial. The absorption of maternal antibodies by the fetus and the reception of these antibodies by infants from breast colostrum are examples of naturally acquired passive immunity. When immune serum, produced in other animals, is injected into an individual to provide preformed specific antibodies, this is referred to as **artificially acquired passive immunity.**

ANTIGENS

An antigen used to be defined as any substance that, when introduced into the body, will stimulate the animal's immune mechanism to produce a specific antibody that will react with this substance in some observable way. In more advanced terms, an **antigen** is "a macromolecule that will induce the formation of immunoglobulins or sensitized lymphocytes that will react specifically with the antigen" or, somewhat more specifically, "a substance that catalyzes B lymphocytes and T lymphocytes into specific adaptive responses to the antigen" (Barrett[11]). See also Chapter 60 for a more detailed discussion.

A chemical substance, to function as antigen, must be foreign ("not self," alien) to the animal body.

Practically all proteins are antigens, and it used to be said that most antigens are proteins. However, many lipoproteins, nucleoproteins, synthetic polypeptides, and polysaccharides are also antigenic. For example, the pneumococcus capsule, polysaccharide in nature, is an excellent antigen. A complete antigen is characterized by 2 indispensable properties: **antigenicity** (or **immunogenicity**), i.e., its capability to induce the formation of antibodies, and **specific reactivity,** its ability to react specifically with the antibodies it stimulates and with no other antibodies.[1]

Haptens are substances that are not antigenic (immunogenic) by themselves but do react selectively with antibodies of the appropriate specificity. For example (Davis et al.[1]), if a rabbit is injected with p-azobenzenearsenate-globulin, it will form antibodies that will react with the protein that was injected and with other proteins containing p-azobenzenearsenate substituents, but not with the proteins lacking the substituent. Benzenearsenate itself (the hapten), when injected, does **not** stimulate the formation of antibodies, but it will react with the antibodies formed when azobenzenearsenate proteins (the protein-hapten complex) are injected. Most haptens are small molecules with a molecular weight of 1000 or less. The specificity of antibody-antigen reactions depends on the **antigenic determinants,** i.e., portions of the antigen molecule. These are very small, probably of the order of magnitude of 4-5 amino acid residues. The number of specific reactive (determinant) sites on the antigen molecule varies. **Conjugated proteins** are proteins that have substituents linked to their amino acid chains; the substituents are termed **haptenic groups.** The haptenic group is part of an antigenic determinant, but it does not necessarily represent the complete antigenic determinant (Davis et al.[1]).

ANTIBODIES

Antibodies are substances, protein in nature, that are produced by the body in response to stimulation by antigens and that react specifically with the stimulating antigen. The capability of reacting with the antigen is used for actual detection and identification of the antibody.

Antibody activity was observed by Tiselius and Kabat (1939) to reside in the γ-globulins. These are relatively slow-moving fractions, on electrophoresis, of serum proteins. Since it was shown later, by immunoelectrophoresis, that other globulins beyond the γ range also possess antibody activity, all globulins with antibody activity are now called **immunoglobulins.**

According to the Committee on Nomenclature of Human Immunoglobulins (World Health Organization, WHO),[28] immunoglobulins are proteins of animal origin that possess antibody activity. Certain proteins related to them by chemical structure and thus antigenic specificity but with (as yet) no known antibody activity are also included, such as Bence Jones proteins and myeloma proteins.

Immunoglobulins may be found in the plasma and in other body fluids or tissues (urine, spinal fluid, lymph nodes, etc.).

IgG or γg (7Sγ, γ₂, microglobulin). IgG is the most abundant type, comprising about 75% of the immunoglobulin population. Electrophoretically, it is the slowest-moving γ-globulin; antibodies to many viruses, bacteria, and their toxic products (as well as the factor responsible for LE cells) belong in this class. γG antibody is characteristic of the **secondary response** in immunization or infection. γG molecules cross the placenta and furnish the newborn infant with a supply of maternal antibodies for the first few months of life. The molecular weight is about 150,000, and the sedimentation coefficient is 7S. Various subclasses have been identified. **IgG antibody is resistant to mercaptoethanol.**

IgG antibodies are highly effective **precipitins**, are strongly **complement fixing**, and **neutralize** viruses, exotoxins, and enzymes, but are relatively weak agglutinins and lysins.[12]

IgM or γM (19Sγ, β₂M, γ-macroglobulin). Cold agglutinins, blood group antibodies (isohemagglutinins), rheumatoid factors, and **anti-O antibodies formed against the O antigens of gram-negative** bacteria are usually, but not exclusively, found in the IgM class. **After antigenic stimulus, the IgM molecules are the first to appear;** this primary response, characterized by a low titer of IgM antibody (identifiable by its **destruction after treatment of serum with mercaptoethanol**) has been utilized to distinguish initial attacks of infections from recurrent attacks. Its detection in cord blood has also been suggested as a screening test for congenital prenatal infections,[13] since the normal, uninfected newborn has practically no IgM antibody (it does not cross the placenta).

IgM antibodies are most active in agglutination and lysis but poorly detectable by precipitation or complement fixation. They neutralize viruses but not toxins or enzymes.[12]

IgA or γA (β₂A, γ₁A). Thyroglobulin antibody in chronic thyroiditis, insulin antibody in diabetes mellitus, and some other antibodies have been found in this class (but also in γG and γM). A special form of γA antibody is present in the secretions of the parotid gland, in the saliva and colostrum. γA does **not** cross the placenta. The serologic activity of γA is limited; it is detectable mostly by direct or passive agglutination. It also neutralizes viruses.

IgD or γD. Discovered in 1965, this class represents about 0.2% of the total serum immunoglobulin.

IgE or γE. Described in 1966, γE is present in small quantities and is now known to be an atopic reagin antibody involved in skin sensitization. It was also found in serum from a patient with multiple myeloma and in normal serum. It has been detected by the radioimmunoassay technic and by the red cell–linked antigen-antiglobulin reaction. Its best-known actions are harmful; however, it is possibly beneficial in immunity to intestinal worms.

For further details, see Chapter 61.

ANTIGEN-ANTIBODY REACTIONS

The specificity of antigens was mentioned earlier. It is important, however, to point out that such specificity is not absolute. False-positive antigen-antibody reactions may occur due to **cross-reactivity.**

A single bacterium (fungus, rickettsia, etc.) contains a number of substances, many of which may be antigenic; thus a single organism may stimulate the production of several antibodies. When the serum containing the antibodies is tested, reactions may occur if an agent containing any of the original antigens is used. When the same antigen is possessed by several different infectious agents, **cross-reactivity** is a distinct possibility. All microorganisms containing the same antigen will stimulate the production of similar antibody, which will cross-react when tested with any substance possessing the original antigen.

Antibodies react more strongly with the **homologous antigen** (i.e., the antigen that stimulated their formation) than with a **heterologous antigen.**

False-negative reactions may occur in antigen-antibody testing because of **zonal reactions.** An optimum proportion of antigen and antibody exists for every serologic reaction. When the procedure is performed at this optimum, complete reactions occur. If, however, an excess of antigen or antibody is present, the resulting reactions may be weak or negative.

The antibody content may be so high in an undiluted serum that the antigen present may be insufficient in proportion to give a clear-cut reaction. Diluting the serum will result in a positive reaction. Such an occurrence is termed a **prozone** phenomenon or reaction. A **postzone** reaction is caused by a great excess of antigen. This can be corrected by diluting the antigen.

In many diseases the antibodies are distinctly protective and form a major part of the defense mechanism. In other conditions the relationship between antibody and protection has not been clearly established. In any case the antibodies appear as a response of the body to foreign substances.

The term **autoantibody** is applied to antibodies that react with antigens of the producer of the antibodies. Under certain conditions an individual is capable of producing antibodies against his own tissues. Such antibodies can be detected in vitro. The phenomenon is discussed more fully in Chapters 60-67.

Several types of **antigen-antibody reactions** are employed in serology.

Agglutination. This is a reaction in which the antigen (cellular or particulate) is in suspension. The antigen agglutinates (clumps) and settles out after it reacts with its specific antibody.

Precipitation. This reaction occurs when a soluble antigen (in solution) reacts with its antibody. It is manifested by precipitation and settling out of the antigen. **Flocculation** is a variety of precipitation; the reaction is manifested in the form of clumps instead of a precipitate.

Lysis. Lysis occurs when blood cells or bacterial cells are dissolved (lysed) after reacting with their antibodies.

Neutralization. In this reaction the effects of the antigen are stopped (neutralized) by its specific antibody. The term is also used for denoting the activity of antibodies that render the antigenic microorganism (usually viruses) noninfective.

These reactions—agglutination, precipitation (and flocculation), and lysis—are visible and can be directly observed. They are employed in a variety of procedures. Bacterial antibodies are identified most often with the aid of agglutination; toxin-antitoxin reactions employ precipitation, and lysis is employed in complement fixation and other tests.

Complement fixation. When an antigen combines with its appropriate antibody in the presence of complement (test system), the antigen-antibody complex binds and inactivates ("fixes") the complement. Binding (removal, "fixing") of free complement can be visualized by addition of a second antigen-antibody ("indicator") system such as red cells and appropriate red cell antibody (hemolysin) requiring complement for its completion (second stage of test). Failure of the red cells to lyse indicates that a specific antibody-antigen reaction has taken place in the first stage of the test. Conversely, if the red cells lyse, free complement is present, and this indicates that no antigen-antibody reaction occurred in the first stage of the test. The test is widely used for detection and measurement of unknown antibody using known antigen; it can also be employed to detect antigen using a known antiserum (Fig. 105-1).

Opsonization. This term refers to the combination of antibodies with surface components of cells, which makes them more readily phagocytosed.

Passive agglutination tests. Antigens can be attached to agglutinable particles ("coated particles") and antibodies to these attached antigens can be detected with greater sensitivity by the agglutination of the carrier cells. Polysaccharides extracted from bacterial cells attach to red blood cells (**bacterial hemagglutination,** Chapter 108). Protein antigens can be attached to red cells that are pretreated with tannic acid, or the proteins can be coupled to the red cell membrane with bis-diazotized benzidine (**hemagglutination with protein antigens,** Chapter 108). Many antigens, which apparently may be protein or polysaccharide,[5] can be adsorbed to other agglutinable particles such as bentonite or polystyrene latex, a spherical polymer (**latex tests,** Chapter 107).

Inhibition tests. In these tests mutual neutrali-

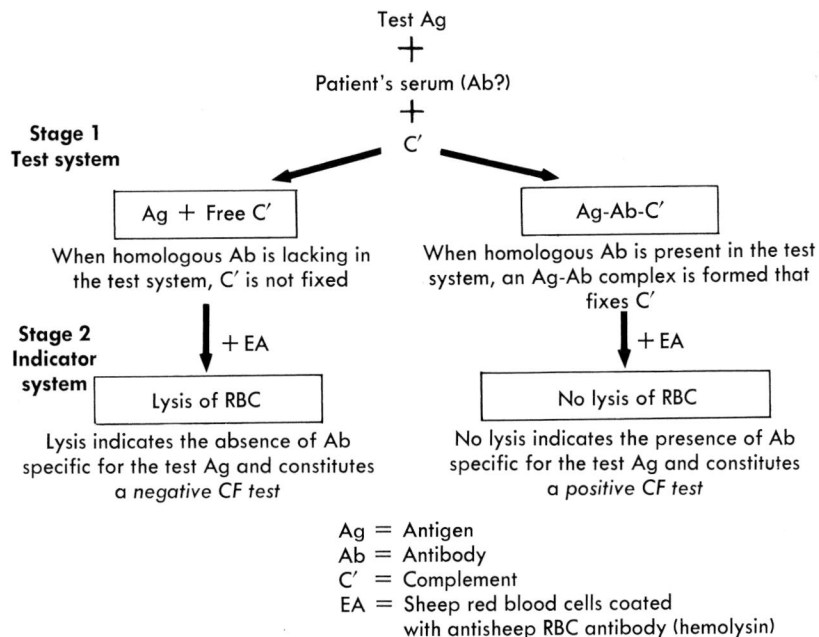

Fig. 105-1. Complement-fixation test. (From Palmer, D. F.: Fundamental nature of the antigen-antibody system, CDC Laboratory Update 78-30, Atlanta, 1978, Bureau of Laboratories, Center for Disease Control.)

zation of the antigen and antibody is detected by demonstration of the inhibition of characteristic reactions. Generally, any reaction between an antigen and its homologous antibody can be inhibited by 1 of 2 procedures: expose the antigen to the appropriate antibody or expose the antiserum to the appropriate antigen. When the neutralized antiserum is then added to its homologous antigen (or the neutralized antigen is mixed with its homologous antiserum), no reaction will take place. **Hemagglutination-inhibition and latex agglutination–inhibition**

tests are widely used because of their exquisite sensitivity (e.g., see immunologic pregnancy tests, Chapter 26, and serologic diagnosis of viral infections, Chapter 95).

Gel-diffusion (immunodiffusion) tests. These are modifications of the precipitin reaction and are immensely useful and sensitive. The precipitation takes place in a gel medium[14] (see Chapters 61, 74, 95, and also the index for the numerous gel-diffusion tests).

Immunoelectrophoresis. Described by Grabar and Williams,[15] this technic constitutes a com-

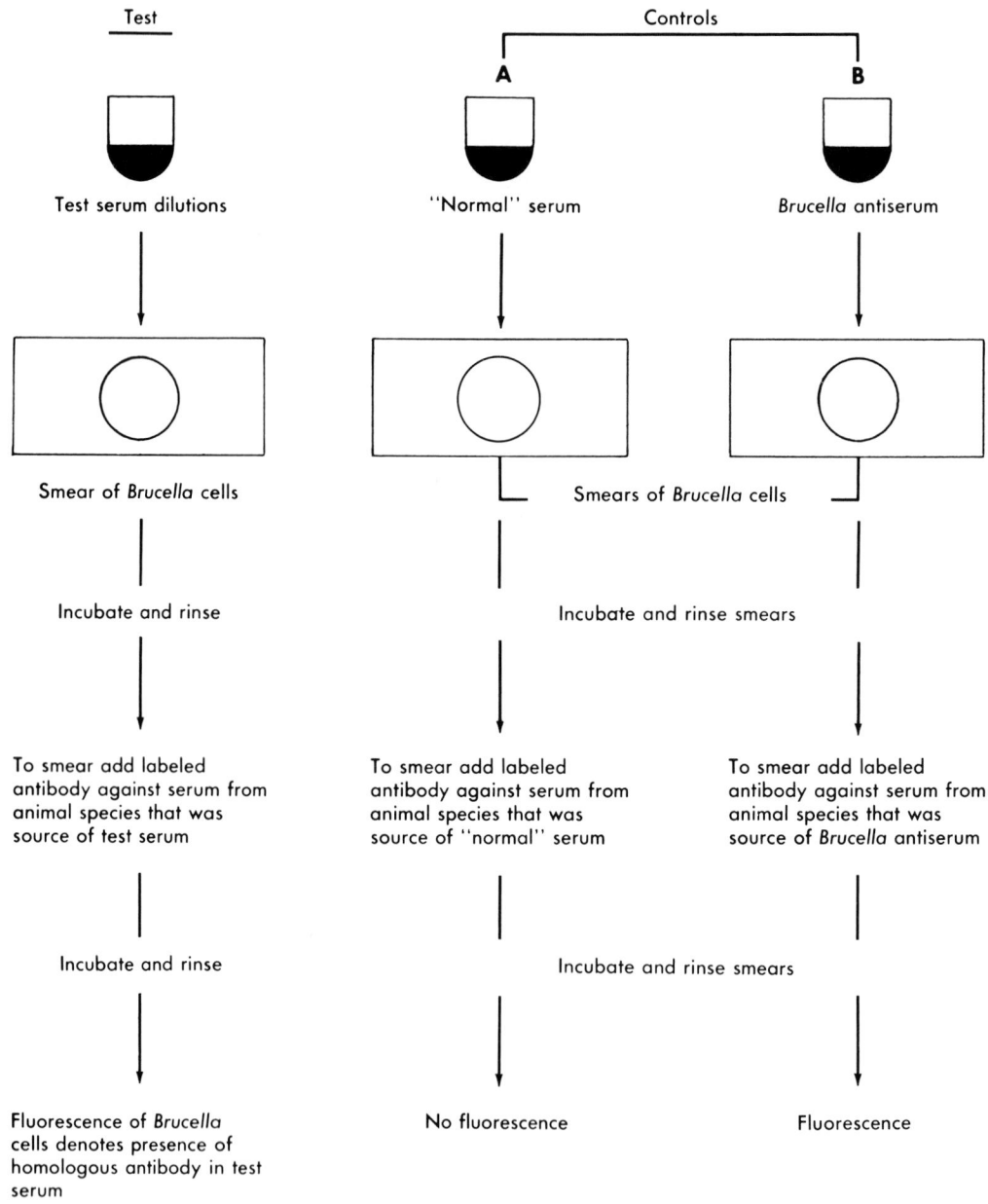

Fig. 105-2. Indirect fluorescent antibody (FA) test for detection of antibody in unknown serum. (From Cherry, W. B., Goldman, M., and Carski, T. R.: Fluorescent antibody techniques, Atlanta, 1960, Communicable Disease Center, Public Health Service Pub. no. 729.)

bination of physicochemical and immuno-chemical methods. The material to be examined (serum, etc.) is separated first by electrophoresis (on a translucent gel) and subsequently is subjected to the effect of a precipitating antiserum by placing the latter in a trough in the gel parallel to the electrophoretically separated proteins. The antigens and antibodies diffuse toward one another, forming sharply defined precipitin lines. The technic is used in protein chemistry, for determination of various serum protein fractions, and has become a powerful tool in clinical diagnosis. For details see Chapter 74, and the Immunology, Hematology, and Chemistry sections.

An important reference is Ouchterlony's *Handbook of Immunodiffusion and Immunoelectrophoresis.*[14]

Fluorescent antibody (FA) methods. The methods are discussed in detail in Chapter 70, particularly as used for detection of antigens (identification of bacteria, etc.). FA methods are also used to locate antibody in tissue and to detect and identify antibodies in serum. For detecting antibody in an unknown serum, the **indirect FA procedure** is used. Fig. 105-2 illustrates the principle and the steps involved in the indirect FA test for identifying unknown antibody (in this case, anti-*Brucella* antibody in the patient's serum). The test involves exposure of unlabeled antibody (presumed to be present in serum examined) to a known antigen, washing off the serum carefully, and addition of labeled anti-gamma globulin (antibody) directed against the globulin (serum) of animal species that was the source of the test serum. If the test serum was from a human being, labeled anti-human γ-globulin is used. Strict controls, including a known normal serum (free of the antibody looked for) an a known serum (containing the antibody) are employed.

Counterimmunoelectrophoresis (CIE). See Chapter 74 for a detailed discussion. Also, see index for various applications.

Enzyme-linked immunosorbent assay (EL-ISA). See Chapter 74 for detailed discussion. Consult index for various applications.

GLASSWARE

The various items of glassware must be properly selected for the procedure that is being carried out and must be scrupulously clean and free of any contaminants.

Glass tubes and slides

Glass tubes include Kahn tubes (12 × 75 mm), Wassermann tubes (13 × 100 mm), and graduated centrifuge tubes. Tests employing smaller final quantities of fluid are carried out in Kahn tubes; Wassermann tubes are utilized when final dilutions contain larger amounts of liquid. Graduated tubes are used for accurately preparing red cell suspensions of a specified percentage of cells in diluent. It is possible to prepare accurate suspensions by reading the packed cell volume from

the calibrations on the tube. Ungraduated tubes are used as containers for freshly drawn blood. After clotting, the cellular elements can be centrifuged out and the serum harvested with one transfer from the original tube.

All tubes must be clean and properly stored to protect against dust when not in use. Etched or scratched tubes should be discarded and replaced. Tubes should be examined for cracks and chips and damaged tubes should be discarded. Cracked and chipped centrifuge tubes may easily break while undergoing centrifugation.

Several types of glass slides are used in the serology laboratory. These include ordinary 25 × 75 mm slides, slides with ceramic rings fused into the glass, slides with paraffin rings, or single or double concavity slides. For each test described in the following section, the slides to be used are specified. All slides must be kept chemically clean and dust free. Etched or cloudy slides that interfere with proper viewing of a reaction should be discarded.

Safety pipetting devices[16]

Many pipetting outfits have been designed to protect the laboratorian from mouth contact with toxic or infectious materials. The laboratory worker should be familiar with these devices and adept in the use of at least one of them, as infectious or toxic materials must never be mouth-pipetted.

Pipetting devices
1. **Propipettes,** Safety Pipette Filler (commercially available, Fisher Scientific and others)
   a. Operation steps
      (1) Press on agate valve "A" and squeeze bulb to expel air and create vacuum.
      (2) Press on agate valve "S," which draws liquid to desired level.
      (3) Press on agate valve "E" to expel liquid. To deliver last drop, cover air inlet in front of "E," press "E," and squeeze small bulb on side.
2. **Caulfield pipettor** (commercially available, Fisher Scientific and others)
   a. Operation steps
      (1) Rub glycerine, with fingertip, on face of rubber bushing at bottom of Pipettor. Grip pipet well up at top and insert firmly into Pipettor.
      (2) Squeeze bulb between thumb and second and third fingers, holding index finger above and away from control button.
      (3) Press down with tip of index finger on valve control at top of bulb. Then, holding finger firmly down on top of bulb will automatically seal air vent. Place pipet into solution.
      (4) To draw up solution keep tip of index finger firmly over control valve, at same time allowing bulb to open gradually.
      (5) To release fluid accurately, rest tip of index finger on top and little to side of valve control button. Roll finger gently over onto control button to release liquid. Pipet may be emptied quickly by pressing finger firmly on valve control and squeezing bulb.
3. **Rubber bulbs** (commercially available, Scientific Products). This safety device is difficult to control

for accuracy, but is used to draw fluid into pipet. Bulb is then removed and fingertip is used in usual manner to deliver accurate volumes.

Other safety devices
1. **Fisher Safety Pipette Filler**
2. **Cornwall** Continuous Pipetting Outfit—Becton, Dickinson & Co.
3. **Fisher Pipet Adapter**
4. **Nalgene Pipetting aids**—Nalgene Labware Div.
5. **Eppendorf Automatic Pipets**—Arthur H. Thomas Co.

Pipets

The capacities most frequently utilized are 10, 5, 1, 0.2 and 0.1 ml, graduated to tip. Frequently a pipet is used to deliver a volume of fluid less than the total capacity. Most accurate results are obtained if the delivery is made point to point. That is, if 4 ml fluid are pipetted using a 5 ml pipet, is is better to pipet between the 0.4 ml graduation than from the 1 ml mark to the tip.

Pipetting technic
1. Check pipet to see if it is clean and dry. Inspect tips. Do not use chipped pipets.
2. Draw up fluid to be measured slightly above desired etched line.
3. Hold pipet in vertical position and wipe off outside of pipet tip with gauze.
4. Bring liquid down to mark, reading from bottom of meniscus while holding pipet vertically by releasing pressure of pipetting device just enough to allow fluid to flow slowly. Do not wipe tip. Make certain that no drops of fluid are hanging from pipet.
5. If level of liquid goes below desired mark, discharge contents of pipet into original container and repeat.
6. Introduce pipet into neck of container and allow to drain.

When using serologic pipets, use the smallest pipet that will hold the volume desired. The small amount of reagent adhering to the side could seriously affect the accuracy of the procedure; for this reason, wiping off the outside of the pipet is important.

Care of serologic glassware

The following procedure should be used for cleaning all glassware except pipets and the tubes used for the colloidal gold technic:

Collect dirty glassware in containers with detergent or germicidal solution (Roccal, etc.). It is important to keep glassware wet after use so that serum or blood clots do not dry. Dried proteinaceous material is difficult to remove.

Transport glassware to sink in laboratory and rinse with cold running tap water until all serum and blood clots are removed.

Soak all glassware in hot detergent solution overnight.

The following morning rinse tubes 6 times in cold running tap water and twice in distilled water.

Place tubes upside down in wire baskets and put in drying oven at 100-120 C for 3 h.*

---

*In conformity with the Systeme International (SI) and to conserve space, the following abbreviations will be used: s, second; h, hour; and d, day.

After removal from oven, let glassware cool before use.

Cleaning of pipets
1. Place used pipets in solution of detergent in large glass jar, the bottom of which is lined with cotton.
2. Wash pipets in pipet washer 1 h with cold running tap water.
3. Soak in concentrated chromic acid cleaning solution.
4. Transfer pipets to pipet washer and wash 2 h with cold running tap water.
5. Rinse in distilled water 3 times.
6. Place pipets in wire basket and dry in oven at 100-120 C for 2 h.

Routine glassware, in addition to pipets, should be soaked once every week in the sulfuric acid–potassium dichromate solution and thoroughly cleaned.

Plastic and disposable items

The use of disposable (single-use) test tubes, plastic beakers, etc. has gained wide popularity. For precautions in selecting the proper plastics and for a detailed discussion of the subject, see Chapter 70.

EQUIPMENT

Microscope. For use and care of microscope see Chapter 2.

Centrifuges. The centrifuge is an important piece of equipment in the serologic laboratory. In smaller laboratories tabletop instruments that accommodate 6 tubes are often used. The speed is controlled by means of a rheostat on the front panel. Top speeds of centrifuges vary; the top speed of a particular instrument should be known in order to use the speed control intelligently.

In larger laboratories, floor-mounted models are usually provided, and these can accommodate a large number of tubes at one time. The top speed of these instruments is higher than that of the table models. Because of the increased inertia of the larger models, they are equipped with a brake to facilitate stopping. In these units the tubes are placed in balanced receptacles that are in turn held by spokes emanating from the central hub.

A special type of high-speed centrifuge is required to spin capillary tubes. The microhematocrit employed in hematologic tests may be used. After the capillary tube is filled with blood, it is closed by heat-fusing at one end or by using a plastic cap on one end.

In all instances in which centrifugation is required, balancing the units is very important. Tubes must be placed exactly opposite from each other, they must be of identical weight, and they must contain the same amount of fluid.

If possible, centrifuges should be equipped with tachometers so that speed may be checked and controlled.

Constant temperature devices. A means of maintaining a constant temperature is required for serologic tests. Dry-air incubators or warm water baths are used. Such units are electrically operated and contain thermostats that hold the temperature within preset limits. These devices must be checked prior to use by installing a thermometer within the apparatus.

Refrigerators should be controlled in a similar manner.

Rotating machines. Rotating machines are required for proper performance of the various flocculation and agglutination tests. Such machines consist of a flat plate mounted over an electrically operated oscillating mechanism. The plate moves in a tight circle at a prescribed rate of speed. The number of oscillations/min is controlled by a knob located on the front of the machine. Rotation rate should be checked carefully at frequent intervals. This can be accomplished by counting the revolutions that take place during a timed interval of operation.

Equipment for sterilization. Certain items of equipment used in some serologic procedures require sterilization. Autoclaves, hot-air ovens, and hot-water sterilizers are used for this purpose. All items of glassware are sterilized in hot-air ovens. Test tubes, syringes, and pipets should be perfectly dry before hot-air sterilization to prevent breakage and reduce decomposition. Flasks should be plugged with cotton. Pipets and syringes may be wrapped in paper. Pipets may also be placed in special cans for sterilization.

The equipment to be sterilized is placed in a hot-air sterilizer and the temperature gradually raised to about 170 C. It is heated 2 h at this temperature. This is sufficient to turn white paper to a faint yellow color. See also Chapter 70.

Microtechnics
Microtitration (Microtiter, Microtitrator) technics

The original microtitration system was devised and introduced by Takatsy (1950).[17] In 1962 a number of refinements and modifications of the equipment were reported by Sever,[18] who established specific procedures that made the microtitration technic eminently suitable for the performance of complement fixation, hemagglutination, hemagglutination inhibition, and metabolic inhibition tests. The technic is also used in antibiotic susceptibility testing, blood group antibody titrations, phage titrations, etc.; it can be used in any procedure that requires serial dilutions. The system permits an 8-fold saving of reagents and rapid performance of microdilutions.

The essential components of the system[18] are as follows:

1. Plexiglas (or disposable plastic) plates (to be used in place of test tubes), each having 96 wells (8 rows of 12 wells), 6 mm in diameter, with a working capacity of 125 μl (0.125 ml). Plates are available with hemispherical bottom wells (U plates), designed for metabolic inhibition, complement fixation, and arbovirus hemagglutination-inhibition tests or with conical bottom wells (V plates), used for hemagglutination and hemagglutination-inhibition tests.
2. Pipet droppers, stainless steel, calibrated to deliver 0.025 ml/drop, and 0.05 ml.
3. Microdiluters (wire diluting loops), calibrated to pick up and deliver 25 μl (or 50 μl).
4. Go-no-go delivery testers, 0.025 and 0.05 ml.
5. Plate holders.

Dilutions are prepared by serial 2-fold transfers of fluid with a microtitration diluter that picks up and transfers a precise volume. Several serial dilutions may be performed simultaneously as the diluters are designed with a special taper to give the same diluter spacing as the wells contained in the plastic plate. The diluters may be rinsed and flamed to cleanse them for reuse.

A pipet dropper calibrated to deliver a precalibrated volume of fluid is used to deliver reagents such as buffers, antigens, and erythrocyte suspension. The pipet dropper is designed to be filled by mouth suction or with a safety-suction bulb. The drops are easily controlled by a bulb or with the fingertip. After the addition of all the reagents to a microtitration test the plates may be stacked or taped to prevent evaporation during incubation. The disposable plastic plates float on the surface of a water bath, thus providing an incubation comparable to standard macro methods.

Tests are read in the same manner as macro tests, and the plates may be centrifuged with the use of special carriers to read tests that are interpreted by the percent lysis of the indicator cell system.[16]

A brief description of the technic is as follows:

1. Place 1 drop (25 μl) appropriate diluent in each well, leaving first well empty, with pipet dropper.
2. Flame microdiluter, cool, and prewet in saline. Pick up solution (serum, etc.) to be diluted by immersing microdiluter loop into solution (fluid will be kept inside loop by surface tension). Several (up to 8) microdiluters can be handled simultaneously. Place microdiluters in wells of plates.
3. Rotate handle of microdiluter by fingertip control 4 times to obtain good mixing. Remove microdiluter and rotate in successive wells in same manner.
4. Depending on test, appropriate antigen, complement, etc. are added to each well with droppers.
5. Plate can be centrifuged by using special centrifuge carriers. Read results using concave mirror.

The great advantage of this technic is that it allows performance of dilutions with great ease and rapidity and that it uses 0.025 (or 0.05) ml volumes of serum, antigen, etc., instead of the customary 0.25 or 0.2 ml, thus resulting in considerable saving of reagents. The system has gained wide acceptance in the United States and has been adapted for use with a large variety of tests.

Detailed instructions are found in Sever's paper[18] and are available from several manufacturers, together with extensive bibliographies concerning use of the technic; Conrath's *Handbook of Microtiter Procedures*[19] is especially useful.

SPECIMENS FOR SEROLOGIC TESTS

Specimens include serum, cerebrospinal fluid, and plasma. **Serum** is the fluid portion of clotted blood, whereas **plasma** is the fluid portion of whole, unclotted blood. Plasma is obtained by treating fresh blood with an anticoagulant, centrifuging to remove cells, and separating of the supernatant fluid.

Venipuncture

All equipment (lancets, needles, syringes) used for collection of blood must be sterile. Sterilization should be accomplished by dry heat (2 h at 170 C) or autoclaving (15 min at 121 C, 15 psi). Boiling for 30 min can be employed if neither of these means for sterilization is available, but it is **not** recommended. Sterilization is necessary to prevent the transmission of serum hepatitis.

Disposable sterile equipment should be used wherever feasible, since it eliminates need for sterilization and excludes the possibility of serum hepatitis transmission.

Serum is obtained from clotted whole blood obtained by venipuncture. The procedure of venipuncture is described below. Another procedure, using the Vacutainer system,* can also be employed.

Equipment
1. Gauze squares, 2 × 2 in.
2. Tourniquet
3. Needle, 1½-2 in. 19-21 gauge (sterile)
4. Syringe (sterile)
5. Collecting tube

Procedure
1. Place label on collecting tube.
2. Wash hands with soap and water.
3. Assemble sterile syringe and sterile needle. Remove from wrapper and vial, using precaution not to contaminate needle or plunger. Keep needle covered with vial when not in use.
4. Place tourniquet on patient's arm above elbow. Tighten to check venous circulation. Take pulse at wrist to make certain that arterial circulation is not cut off. By opening and closing fist several times, patient increases circulation.
5. Locate vein by palpation. Cleanse skin with gauze soaked in 70% alcohol. Let skin dry before making puncture. Do not palpate area after cleaning! Have patient close his fist and straighten arm.
6. Inspect syringe and make certain that plunger is pushed to bottom of barrel, to prevent injection of air into vein. Place forefinger on hub of needle while holding syringe in right hand. With left hand grasp arm and hold skin taut with thumb. Insert needle at about 30° angle through skin next to vein to be punctured. Lower syringe and move needle parallel to vein for about 1.5 cm; direct it into vein. In "good" veins, blood will enter syringe immediately on puncture. In veins with low pressure, plunger may have to be withdrawn slightly to ascertain entry of needle in vein. Move needle into vein cautiously.
7. Steadying syringe with left hand, withdraw blood by pulling plunger back with right hand. Release tourniquet, place dry gauze square over puncture site, and withdraw needle. Let patient open hand and press gauze on puncture for 1-2 min.
8. Take needle off syringe and expel blood gently into tube.
9. Wash needle and syringe immediately afterward in cold tap water to prevent coagulation of blood in equipment. Separate needle, barrel, and plunger and place in cold water. If disposable, discard needle and syringe.

Capillary puncture

For certain serologic procedures blood is obtained by puncturing the lobe of an ear, the tip of the finger, or, in infants, the great toe or the heel.

_____
*Becton, Dickinson & Co., Rutherford, N.J.

Equipment
1. Gauze squares, 2 × 2 in.
2. Capillary tubes
3. Sterile lancet

Procedure
1. Rub site to be punctured with alcohol.
2. Puncture skin with blood lancet. In case of the ear, puncture edge of lobe, not side. Perform puncture with sharp instrument; if done with quick stab, it is practically painless.
3. Wipe off first drop of blood and collect second drop. Do not press site; allow blood to flow into capillary tube.
4. Fuse one end of capillary tube (or use plastic cap on one end) and centrifuge to separate cells.

Preparation and preservation of serum

1. Plug collecting tubes containing blood with sterile cork and set aside at room temperature.
2. Ream margin of blood clot free of tube by circling with applicator stick before centrifuging. This facilitates separation of cells and serum after coagulation has taken place. Care should be taken not to lyse any cells, since this might render serum unusable.
3. Centrifuge at 1500 rpm for 15 min.
4. After centrifugation carefully transfer serum to clean container using dry, sterile dropper.

For the majority of serologic tests the serum must be rendered free of **complement** by **inactivation.** Inactivation is important, since complement promotes lysis of erythrocytes and can contribute to false test results. To inactivate complement, place tubes of serum in 56 C water bath 30 min.

The following rules should be observed to assure clear specimens of serum:

1. Withdraw blood before meals. This will eliminate chyle, which appears in serum after fatty meal.
2. Use sterile needles and glassware.
3. Remove needle and run blood gently down side of tube to avoid rupture of cells.
4. Let specimen stand at room temperature 30 min to allow time for complete cloting.
5. Separate serum from cells as soon as possible.
6. Store serum specimens in refrigerator until test is performed.
7. Do not contaminate specimens with acid or alkali. Such substances will denature serum proteins and render specimens useless.
8. Do not contaminate specimens with heavy metals such as silver, mercury, etc.
9. Avoid heat and bacterial contamination. Excessive heat coagulates serum proteins. Bacterial growth causes alteration of protein molecules.

Serum that has been separated from the cells may be stored at ordinary refrigerator temperature for up to 72 h. When longer storage is required, the specimen may be preserved for an indefinite period of time by storage in a freezer. Seal and label the specimen container before storage.

Chemical preservatives can be added to serum to be stored. Suitable preservatives include Merthiolate powder (0.001 g/ml serum) and 5% solutions of either phenol or tricresol (0.1 ml/ml serum). Liquid serum can also be preserved by removal of the liquid portion by **lyophilization.** In this process the serum is completely dried from the frozen state, employing special equipment and vials that can be sealed. In powdered form proteins remain unchanged. The lyophilized serum can be satisfactorily reconstituted with sterile water. When this process is used, there is no detectable loss of potency even after several years of storage. Guinea pig serum, utilized in a number of serologic tests, is supplied by commercial sources in the dried state. Many other biologic products used in serologic tests are similarly processed.

Shipment of serologic specimens

Small laboratories often are limited in the diagnostic procedures that can be carried out and may have to ship serologic specimens to other laboratories for performance of diagnostic tests.

Serum, plasma, and cerebrospinal fluid should be handled as follows:
1. Collect and process specimens under sterile conditions.
2. Ship specimens by the fastest route, as soon after collection as possible.
3. Do not ship whole blood unless the test to be performed requires whole blood. Remove cells from plasma and clot from serum before shipment.
4. Do not inactivate serum or plasma before mailing. Heat destroys bactericidal properties.
5. Keep the specimen and packing container in the refrigerator until time of shipment.
6. If specimen is contaminated or shipment requires several days, preserve by refrigeration in transit. First, freeze specimen; then pack and ship in a well-insulated container with dry ice.

Unless contraindicated, chemical preservation can also be used, as described earlier. Merthiolate is the preservative of choice. Only fresh solutions prepared on the day to be utilized should be employed. Merthiolate may be added to the specimen in aqueous solution or may be introduced into specimen tubes and the fluid removed by desiccation. In either aqueous solution or crystalline form, Merthiolate does not interfere with the mechanism of the test and does not introduce a dilution factor.

To prepare shipping tubes for serologic specimens add (on day to be used) 1 g Merthiolate/100 ml distilled water. **Do not use commercially prepared tinctures or solutions.**

For serum and plasma use 12 × 75 mm tubes. Pipet 1% Merthiolate solution into each tube. Add solution at the rate of 0.1 ml for each 2-4 ml serum or plasma to be shipped.

CELL SUSPENSIONS AND SERIAL DILUTIONS

Information concerning the quantity of antibody present can be obtained by diluting the serum. By making the amount of dilution progressively greater in a series of tubes, a **serial dilution** is obtained. The dilution is performed by starting with a low dilution and proceeding through higher dilutions. The highest dilution of serum to give a positive reaction with the antigen is an index of antibody concentration. For example, if a serum reacts at 1:160 dilution with the appropriate antigen, it has a higher concentration of antibody than a serum that will react only at a concentration of 1-40 but not at a higher dilution. The reciprocal of the highest dilution is referred to as **titer** (in the case cited above, 160 and 40).

Red blood cells are used in many serologic reactions. In some the red blood cells contain the antigens involved and the antibodies looked for react with them directly (sheep red blood cells in

the heterophil agglutination test); in others red blood cells are used as part of an indicator system (complement-fixation tests).

Red blood cell suspensions

Equipment
1. Gauze sponges, 4 × 4 in.
2. Graduated centrifuge tubes
3. Aspirator (Richards pump or capillary pipet)

Reagents
1. Blood with anticoagulant (human, rabbit, or sheep)
2. Physiologic saline, 0.85%

Procedure
1. Filter blood through gauze into graduated centrifuge tube. Fill tube with physiologic saline. Centrifuge 5 min at speed sufficient to pack cells (1500-1800 rpm).
2. Remove supernatant fluid and thin upper layer of white cells by aspiration. Resuspend erythrocytes in 10 vol physiologic saline by gentle shaking (best mixing is obtained by corking tube and inverting several times) and centrifuge. Repeat this step 3 times.
3. Read and record packed cell volume before removing supernatant after last centrifugation. Remove as much of supernatant fluid as possible without disturbing packed cell volume. Supernatant fluid should be colorless after 3 washings. If color persists, cells are too fragile and cannot be used.

Calculation. The required volume of saline may be calculated for any desired concentration of cell suspension by using the following formula:

$$\text{Total volume} = \frac{\text{Packed cell volume} \times 100}{\text{Desired \% cell concentration}}$$

Assume that a 2% cell suspension is desired. After the last centrifugation the packed cell volume was 0.2 ml.

$$\text{Total volume} = \frac{0.2 \text{ ml} \times 100}{2}$$

$$= \frac{20 \text{ ml}}{2}$$

$$= 10 \text{ ml}$$

Total volume − Packed cell volume =
ml saline to be added
10 − 0.2 = 9.8 ml saline to be added

Comments

1. All glassware utilized in preparation of cell suspensions must be scrupulously clean. For cleaning glassware, potassium dichromate–sulfuric acid solution is recommended.

2. All reagents used must be pure and free from contaminating substances.

3. When not used, cell suspensions should be stored at 4-8 C.

4. Always mix suspension of cells well before using to ensure uniformity per unit volume.

5. Cell suspension should always be checked for hemolysis before using. Frequently an additional washing will suffice to render partially hemolyzed suspension usable. If hemolysis persists, fresh suspension must be prepared.

Standardization of erythrocyte suspensions by spectrophotometer*

The spectrophotometric method of standardizing erythrocyte suspensions is applicable and is recommended for **all** serologic tests employing red blood cells.

I. Calibration of spectrophotometer
A. *Mechanical operation of instrument*
1. Place instrument permanently away from direct light and in vibration-free location.
2. Keep optical parts of instrument as free from dirt and dust as possible. (Keep covered.)
3. Refer to manufacturer's manual for other important points concerning line voltage fluctuation, exciter lamp, and use of didymium standard for wavelength calibration.
4. Study instrument and attached diagram of instrument.
5. Locate all operating controls.

---

*From Palmer, D. F., Cavallaro, J. J., and Galt, R. H.: Laboratory diagnosis by serologic methods, Atlanta, 1975, Center for Disease Control.

B. *Zero transmittance adjustment*
1. Place line power ON-OFF switch in ON position. Allow instrument to warm up at least one-half hour.
2. Rotate COARSE control to approximately full-scale indication—position index spot near 100% T or near value to be used; fine control may be in any position, preferably midrange.
3. Raise and rotate cuvette adapter so that key of adapter is at right angles to cuvette well (5) keyway. Cover cuvette well with light shield.
4. Instrument should read exactly 0% transmittance (black scale).
5. If it is not exactly 0% transmittance, adjust with ZERO control lever (8, located under machine). This is coarse adjustment device and may not adjust to exactly 0% transmittance.
6. If necessary, adjust by sliding scale panel (3) (fine adjustment) left or right until zeros on each scale coincide exactly.

C. *Wavelength calibration with didymium standard*
NOTE: The procedures outlined below always must be followed after **installation** or **transportation** of instrument and on **disturbance** or **replacement** of exciter lamps.

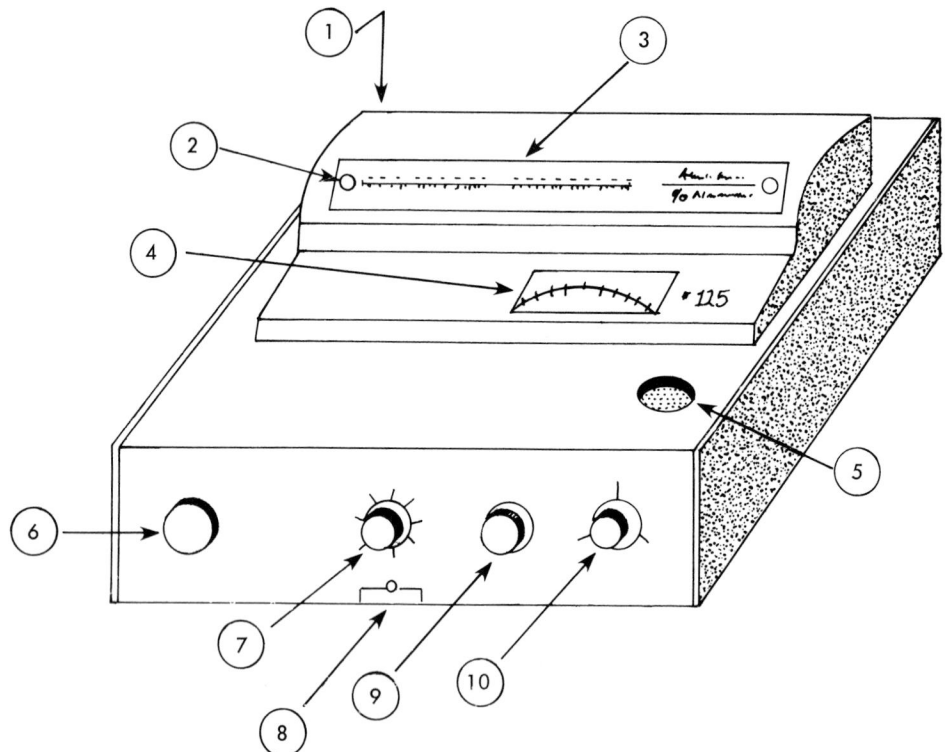

1. Line power on-off switch (rear instrument panel)
2. Friction spring
3. Scale panel
4. Wavelength dial
5. Cuvette well—covered by cylindrical light shield
6. Wavelength control
7. Coarse control
8. Zone lever control
9. Fine control
10. Filter selector

Fig. 105-3. Spectrophotometer. (From Palmer, D. F., Cavellaro, J. J., and Gaft, R. H.: Laboratory diagnosis by serologic methods, Atlanta, 1975, Center for Disease Control.)

1. Place line power ON-OFF switch in ON position and allow 30 min for warm-up of instrument.
2. Set wavelength scale to read exactly 540 nanometers (nm; formerly measured in millimicrons).
3. Adjust filter selector *(10)* to proper position for desired wavelength range according to list below:

Position	Wavelength range (nm)	Wavelength dial area color
UV	325-380	Blue
VIS	380-650	White
NIR	650-825	Red

Adjust to visible (VIS) range.
4. Check zero transmittance adjustment as above.
5. Remove cuvette adapter and cover cuvet well opening.
6. Adjust COARSE and FINE control knobs so meter needle points to 100% on transmittance (black) scale.
7. Clean surface of didymium calibrating standard thoroughly before using it by wiping with clean cleansing tissue, gently blowing off any lint.
8. Uncover cuvette well and place clean didymium calibrating standard in well so key enters cuvette well keyway. Make sure calibrating standard is fully seated in well.
9. Read and record % transmittance (black scale) of didymium calibrating standard.
10. Remove calibrating standard; insert opaque piece of white paper into cuvette well. Determine and record color of light entering well.
11. Wavelength calibration of instrument is correct within 1 nm and is satisfactory if:
    a. Indicated transmittance is within ±1.5 scale divisions of value of transmittance (T) marked on standard **and**
    b. Light entering cuvette well is orange.
12. If wavelength calibration is incorrect, see operating manual that comes with instrument for correction procedures.

*D. Calibrate series of tubes to obtain set of matched cuvettes**

1. Warm up spectrophotometer a minimum of 10 min and set wavelength at 540 nm.
2. Pipet 4 ml undiluted cyanmethemoglobin† standard into clean, unscratched cuvette. (Use plastic or neoprene-coated test tube rack to prevent scratching tubes.) Wipe outside of cuvette clean.
3. Place cuvette in sample well of instrument. Some cuvettes have etched line at lip that should be aligned with mark on sample well.
4. Adjust with COARSE and FINE adjustments until standard reads 50% T. If "zero adjust" control is present, use it to set pointer at 0% T when cuvette holder is empty and covered.
5. Pour standard solution into next cuvette to be calibrated.
6. Rotate this tube in cuvette holder until it reads as near to 50% T as possible. If it will not read within ± 0.5% T, discard tube.
7. If it falls within ± 0.5% T, etch a mark on tube at point where reading is nearest 50% T. Etching should line up with mark on sample well.

8. Continue this process until several cuvettes have been matched together.

II. Calculation of factor and target absorbance (A)*

A. Measure absorbance on standard and unknown solutions

1. Warm up instrument for at least 10 min.
2. Adjust wavelength control to 540 nm setting.
3. Carefully wipe lower third of calibrated 12 × 75 mm† cuvette containing at least 2.0 ml reference solution (cyanmethemoglobin reagent only). This solution is called "reagent blank." Properly position cuvette in cuvette well.
4. Adjust galvanometer COARSE and FINE controls until galvanometer index reads 100% on black transmittance scale (or zero on red absorbance scale). Many spectrophotometers employ additional control called "zero adjust," which is used to set needle on 0% T when cuvette well is empty and covered.
5. Remove reagent blank and replace it with matched cuvette containing sample solution. Again, wipe cuvette clean and properly position it as before.
6. Read absorbance of sample on absorbance scale.

B. Preparation of cyanmethemoglobin reagent (Hycel)

1. Dilute 1 vial of reagent in 2 L distilled water (instead of 1 L as indicated on label). This helps to overcome "resistant cell phenomenon."
2. Store this reagent in brown screw-capped polyethylene bottle or in dark, and at room temperature. (Do not use rubber or cork stoppers unless they are covered with parafilm, as there is a chemical reaction between cyanide and these materials, which results in contamination of reagent.
3. Discard reagent if it becomes cloudy or if precipitate forms after prolonged use.

C. Preparation of cyanmethemoglobin standard curve (Hycel) and calculation of target absorbances

1. The following concentrations of standard solutions should be used to calculate a factor: 80, 60, 40, 20, and 0 mg/dl cyanmethemoglobin.
2. Prepare these concentrations by diluting the 80.0 mg/dl‡ cyanmethemoglobin (undiluted) standard as follows:

Tube	Cyanmeth. conc (mg/dl)	Vol. 80 mg/dl standard (ml)	Vol. cyanmeth. reagent (ml)
1	80	4	0
2	60	3	1
3	40	2	2
4	20	1	3
5	0 (blank)	0	4

3. Wrap cork stoppers in parafilm and plug each tube. Standards will remain stable for several months provided they are kept refrigerated and free from contamination.
4. Read absorbance of standards at 540 nm. Be sure to use only matched and clean cuvettes.
5. Absorbance readings are used to calculate factor that will be used to convert absorbance of unknown samples to mg/dl cyanmethemoglobin.

---

*Cuvettes already calibrated to ±0.25% T may be purchased from several laboratory supply houses and from Hycel.

†The abbreviation "cmg" will be used for cyanmethemoglobin.

---

*In the original publication the term "optical density (O.D.) was used, but in this text the newer term "absorbance" (A) will be used.

†13 × 100 mm cuvettes (minimum volume 3.0 ml) are used in certain instruments.

‡Mg/dl is used in place of mg%.

Table 105-1. Target values for serologic tests employing standardized red blood cell suspensions

Desired % Susp		Target mg/dl cyanmeth. (all spectro-photometers)	Target A for your spectrophotometer	Test
Mammalian	3.0	37.537		
	2.8	35.035		All CFs (sheep)
	2.5	31.26		Toxoplasma IHA and *Mycoplasma* IHA (sheep)
	2.0	25.025		Paul-Bunnell heterophile aby test (sheep)
				Ox cell hemolysin test (cattle)
	0.4	5.005		Adenovirus HA-HI (monkey, rat)
				Measles virus HA-HI (monkey)
				Reovirus HA-HI (human)
				Enterovirus HA-HI (human)
				Myxovirus HA-HI (human, guinea pig, pig)
				Murine viruses HA-HI (human, guinea pig, sheep, mouse)
Goose	0.25	3.009		Arbovirus HA-HI
Chicken—baby chick	0.50	5.059		Poxvirus HA-HI (chicken)
				Myxovirus HA-HI (chicken)
	0.25	2.746		Rubella virus HA-HI (2-day chick)

This factor then enables calculation of target absorbance, which is needed to prepare standardized RBC suspensions. Calculate factor for converting absorbance to mg/dl cmg by dividing sum of concentrations of standards by sum of absorbance readings of standards. For example:

Conc of standards (mg/dl cyanmeth.)	A_{540} readings of standards
80.0	0.460
60.0	0.350
40.0	0.240
20.0	0.120
0.0	0.000
200.0	1.170

$$\text{Factor} = \frac{200.0 \text{ mg/dl cmg}}{1.170 \text{ A}} = 170.94 \text{ mg/dl cmg/A}$$

This factor may be used without change so long as same instrument is employed and has not been moved or repaired. Reliability of the instrument should be checked before each subsequent use by reading absorbance of 40 mg/dl cmg dilution and comparing it with previous 40 mg/dl cmg values.

6. Using factor computed for your spectrophotometer, fill in column 3 of Table 105-1; column 3 is target absorbance on your spectrophotometer for each cell suspension to be used.

Target absorbance (Table 105-1) =

$$\frac{\text{mg/dl cmg (Table 105-1)}}{\text{Factor}}$$

Examples (using factor of 170.94 computed previously):

2.8% Sheep cells: $\dfrac{35.035 \text{ mg/dl cmg}}{170.94 \text{ mg/dl cmg/A}} =$

0.205 Target A

0.4% Mammalian cells: $\dfrac{5.005 \text{ mg/dl cmg}}{170.94 \text{ mg/dl cmg/A}} =$

0.0293 Target A

0.25% Goose cells: $\dfrac{3.009 \text{ mg/dl cmg}}{170.94 \text{ mg/dl cmg/A}} =$

0.0176 Target A

0.50% Chicken cells: $\dfrac{5.059 \text{ mg/dl cmg}}{170.94 \text{ mg/dl cmg/A}} =$

0.0296 Target A

These target absorbances, as stated above, will be used for accurately diluting 4% suspensions to any lesser concentration.

III. **Preparation of standardized erythrocyte suspensions**

1. Obtain fresh cells (less than 4 days old for best HA results). Bleeding should be done using 1 vol blood to 4 vol modified Alsever solution.
2. Wash cells 3 times in PBS diluent in 12- or 15-ml conical centrifuge tube. One-half to full speed in any clinical centrifuge is satisfactory. Carefully remove buffy layer of white blood cells after each wash. Following last wash, read packed cell volume and dilute to approximately 4% suspension with PBS.
3. Mix well and carefully pipet (with long-tipped Mohr measuring pipet) 1.0 ml "4%" suspension into 25 ml volumetric flask.
4. QS to 25.0 ml with cyanmethemoglobin reagent. Mix well by inverting flask at least 10 times.
5. Allow to stand 20-60 min at room temperature.
6. Mix again. If avian cell solutions appear turbid, add a few milligrams (a "pinch") of saponin and mix. All avian cell solutions must be briefly centrifuged after lysis to remove cellular debris.
7. Warm up and check spectrophotometer by reading 40 mg/dl standard.
8. Pour enough of hemolyzed sample into calibrated, clean cuvette to nearly fill tube.
9. Read absorbance of sample against reagent blank at 540 nm, being careful to read red (logarithmic) scale. This is Test A.
10. Calculate dilution needed to obtain desired suspension:

(A of test susp.) ×

$$\frac{(\text{Original vol. of test susp.} - 1.0 \text{ ml})}{\text{Target A (Table 105-1, col. 3)}} =$$

Final vol. of desired suspension

Example:
  If 0.5% suspension of chicken erythrocytes is desired, and 20 ml of 4% suspension having test A of 0.358 is used:

$$\frac{(0.358 \times 19 \text{ ml})}{0.0296} =$$
  230 ml final vol. of desired 0.5% susp.

Volume calculated in this formula is total volume of 0.5% suspension, i.e., 19 ml of 4% suspension is diluted *to* final volume of 230 ml to give 230 ml of standardized 0.5% chicken RBC suspension. Be sure to mix test suspension thoroughly but gently before preparing diluted suspension. It is not necessary to check accuracy of dilutions spectrophotometrically.

Serial dilutions

As previously described, serial dilutions are prepared by progressively decreasing the volume of serum with the maintenance of a constant total volume of liquid.

Equipment
1. Test tubes
2. Test tube rack
3. Gauze sponges, 4 × 4 in.
4. Serologic pipets, 5 and 10 ml

Reagents
1. Physiologic saline, 0.85%
2. Serum
3. Red blood cell suspension, 2%

Procedure. An example of serial dilution is as follows:
1. With marking pencil, number test tubes 1-10 and place them in test tube rack.
2. Pipet 8 ml saline into tube 1. Into each of remaining tubes pipet 5 ml saline.
3. To tube 1 add 2 ml serum and mix.
4. Transfer 5 ml of contents from tube 1 to tube 2 and mix.
5. Transfer 5 ml of contents from tube 2 to tube 3 and mix. Continue this process from tube to tube through last tube in series. After mixing contents of tube 10, discard 5 ml from this tube.
6. Add 5 ml 2% red blood cell suspension to all tubes. This gives total volume of 10 ml in each tube.

Explanation of dilutions. Dilutions of serum are expressed as ratio of quantity of serum contained in total volume of fluid to total volume. In tube 1 above, before addition of cell suspension, 2 vol serum were contained in 10 vol **total** fluid. This is a dilution of 2:10 and can be expressed more simply as a 1:5 dilution. Even though 5 vol of contents of tube 1 were transferred to tube 2, serum dilution in tube 1 remains 1:5. Actual quantity of serum transferred to tube 2 above is 1 ml (i.e., 5 ml of a 1:5 dilution). After transfer to tube 2 there is 1 ml serum contained in 10 ml total fluid. Once again these values apply to tube **before** cell suspension has been added. Serum dilution in tube 2 therefore, is 1:10. If 5 ml of 1:10 serum dilution are transferred from tube 2 to tube 3, actual quantity of serum involved is 0.5 ml. After transfer to tube 3 there is 0.5 ml serum contained in 10 ml total fluid. Serum dilution in tube 3 (**before** addition of cell suspension) is 1:20. Amount of serum transferred to each succeeding tube in series is one-half amount present in previous tube. If quantity of serum is halved but total volume remains constant, then it follows that dilution is doubled.

In serial dilution that was performed, volume in each tube before addition of cell suspension was 5 ml. When 5 ml red cell suspension was added to each tube, total volume of fluid was doubled. Since serum content remained constant and total volume was doubled, serum dilution was therefore doubled. It is apparent, then, that although serial dilutions in first part of our example were 1:5, 1:10, 1:20, etc.; on doubling total volume, dilutions became 1:10, 1:20, 1:40, etc. Example given is representative, in principle, of **most** serial dilutions encountered in clinical serology.

When transferring from low dilution to higher dilution, using pipet, it is important that outside of pipet be wiped between tubes. Small quantity of diluted serum adhering to outside of pipet can in many cases drastically alter desired higher dilution.

Mixing of serum and saline can be conveniently performed by drawing up diluted serum into pipet and expelling it, repeating several times and avoiding bubble formation.

All tubes employed in preparing serial dilutions should be clearly labeled.

Serial dilution, along with being an effective means of quantitating antibody content, is also useful in discovering **zonal** reactions.

AUTOMATION IN SEROLOGY

The availability and widespread use of the AutoAnalyzer* system for clinical chemistry tests gave impetus to attempts for adapting the system to the performance of serologic tests. In 1965 Sturgeon et al.[20] described the AutoAnalyzer blood typing technic and Vargues et al.[21] devised a fully automatic technic, improved by Gaillon et al.[22] for performance of the complement-fixation test for syphilis.

An important development has been the successful **automation of a flocculation test for syphilis.** McGrew et al.[23,24] described the use of the AutoAnalyzer for the Automated Reagin test (ART), which employs Rapid Plasma Reagin (RPR) Card test antigen suspension.† According to their report, results obtained with the ART compare favorably (97-98% agreement) with the manual VDRL slide and RPR (circle) card test. The ART is a useful procedure in public health, blood bank, and hospital laboratories.

A **semiautomated system for the fluorescent treponemal antibody–absorption (FTA-ABS)** test has also been developed [25-27] that allows performance of 200 tests per day. The system automates the test (addition of unknown serum to antigen fixed on slide, incubation in moist chamber at 37 C for 30 min, rinsing, drying, addition of fluorescein-tagged conjugate, incubation, washing, drying, transfer to a special microscope stage), except for preparation of serum samples and reading of processed slides. However, the instrument is no longer manufactured or available (1977).

The successful automation of serologic tests for syphilis will undoubtedly also pave the way for improved diagnosis of other infectious diseases by serologic tests.

---

*Technicon Corp., Ardsley, N.Y.
†Hynson, Westcott & Dunning, Inc., Baltimore, Md.

The manual Microtiter system described earlier has also been automated by mounting 8 diluting loops on a motor-driven loop assembly drive and by adding a manifold for automatic addition of diluent and another for delivering test medium (red cells, etc.).

It is expected, in the light of these developments, that automated serologic tests may eventually replace certain manual serologic technics, especially in laboratories in which large numbers of tests are performed daily.

MATERIALS FOR SEROLOGIC TESTS

With regard to the performance of various serologic tests, it is important to remember that a large number and variety of reagents (antigens, control antisera, various red blood cell suspensions) are commercially available. Depending on the size of the laboratory, the equipment, and the manpower available, the decision whether the reagents should be prepared in the laboratory or should be purchased must be made by the individual responsible for the proper functioning of the laboratory. In many cases the decision will be a simple one. Certain antigens (such as those used in tests for the diagnosis of syphilis) are extremely laborious to prepare and difficult to standardize. For the average clinical laboratory, prepared antigens purchased commercially are the answer. In some other instances (e.g., certain antigens for fungal and parasitic diseases) the antigens are not readily available and may have to be prepared in the laboratory.

The procedures described in this section include, where feasible, both the preparation of antigens and also commercial sources. When commercially prepared antigens and other reagents are used, it is extremely important to note the instructions of the manufacturer carefully and to follow the details of the procedure as given in the accompanying descriptions. Preparations bearing the same name or designation made by different manufacturers are not always of the same sensitivity or specificity, and for this reason the instructions should be followed to the letter.

REFERENCES

1. Davis, B. D., Dulbecco, R., Eisen, H. N., et al.: Microbiology, ed. 2, New York, 1973, Harper & Row, publishers.
2. Holborow, E. J.: Lancet 1:833, 890, 942, 995, 1049, 1098, 1148, 1208, 1967.
3. Rose, N. R., and Friedmann, H., editors: Manual of clinical immunology, Washington, D.C., 1976, American Society for Microbiology, chap. 60.
4. Ackroyd, J. F., editor: Immunological methods, Philadelphia, 1964, F. A. Davis Co.
5. Gell, P. G. H., Coombs, R. R. A., and Lackman, P. J.: Clinical aspects of immunology, ed. 3, Oxford, 1975, Blackwell Scientific Publications.
6. Holborow, E. J.: An ABC of modern immunology, ed. 2, Boston, 1973, Little, Brown, & Co.
7. Freedman, S. O.: Clinical immunology, New York, 1971, Harper & Row, Publishers.
8. Rose, N. R., Milgrom, F., and van Oss, C. J., editors: Principles of immunology, New York, 1973, Macmillan Publishing Co.
9. Rose N. R., and Bigazzi, P., editors: Methods in immunodiagnosis, New York, 1973, John Wiley & Sons.
10. Kwapinski, J. E., editor: Research in immunochemistry and immunobiology, vols. 1 and 2, Baltimore, 1972, University Park Press.
11. Barrett, J. T.: Basic immunology and its medical application, St. Louis, 1976, The C. V. Mosby Co.
12. Pike, M.: Bacteriol. Rev. 31:157, 1967.
13. Janeway, C. A.: J. Pediatr. 72:885, 1968.
14. Ouchterlony, Ö.: Handbook of immunodiffusion and immunoelectrophoresis, Ann Arbor, Mich., 1968, Ann Arbor Science Publishers.
15. Grabar, P., and Williams, C. A.: Biochim. Biophys. Acta 10:193, 1953.
16. Palmer, D. F., Cavallaro, J. J., and Galt, H. R.: Laboratory diagnosis by serologic methods, Atlanta, 1975, Center for Disease Control.
17. Takatsy, G.: Kiserl. Orvostud. Bes. 2:393, 1950; Acta Microbiol. Acad. Sci. Hung. 3:191, 1955.
18. Sever, J. L.: J. Immunol. 88:320, 1962.
19. Conrath, T. B., editor: Handbook of microtiter procedures, Cambridge, Mass., 1972, Dynatech Corp.
20. Sturgeon, P., DuCros, M., McQuiston, D., and Smythe, W. In Automation in analytical chemistry, Technicon symposia 1965, White Plains, N.Y., 1966, Mediad.
21. Vargues, R., Studievic, C., and Ripault, J.: Ann. Biol. Clin. 23:623, 1965.
22. Gaillon, R., Ripault, J., Studievic, C., and Dausset, J.: Int. Arch. Allerg. 32:278, 1967.
23. McGrew, B. E., DuCros, M. J. F., Stout, G. W., and Falcone, V. H.: Am. J. Clin. Pathol. 50:52, 1968.
24. Stout, G. W., McGrew, B. E., and Falcone, V. H.: Public Health Lab. 26:7, 1968.
25. Roberts, M. E., Miller, J. N., and Brinnings, G. F.: J. Bacteriol. 96:1500, 1968.
26. Fisher Scientific Co.: The Laboratory 36:108, 1968.
27. Norins, L. In Automation in clinical chemistry, Technicon symposia 1967, vol. 1, White Plains, N.Y., 1968, Mediad.
28. Committee on nomenclature of human immunoglobulins: Bull. W. H. O. 30:447, 1964.

106

SEROLOGIC TESTS IN INFECTIOUS DISEASES— I. TESTS FOR SYPHILIS

Alex C. Sonnenwirth

COURSE OF SYPHILIS

Syphilis is a contagious venereal disease caused by a spirochete (*Treponema pallidum*) that leads to many structural and cutaneous lesions. The disease is transmitted through direct (usually sexual) contact with an infectious lesion. The organisms in most cases probably enter the body through a microscopic break in the epidermal layer (abraded skin) or through intact mucous membranes. Although some of the treponemes apparently remain at the site of infection immediately after entrance, others are carried away by the bloodstream and thus cause a systemic infection within a few hours after exposure.

A characteristic inflammatory response (primary lesion), known as the **chancre**, develops at the portal of entry about 3-4 weeks (range: 10-90 days) after the initial entrance of the treponeme into the host. This stage is known as **primary syphilis.** The chancre persists for 1-5 weeks and then heals spontaneously.

The chancre is found usually in the anogenital region; however, it may occur wherever the treponeme first entered the body (e.g., lip, tongue, tonsil). It is usually single but may be multiple. Although it is usually an eroded, hard papule, it may also be quite soft. Uncomplicated, it is almost always painless. Any anogenital lesion, however, must be suspected.

A common site for a chancre in women is the cervix of the uterus. The primary lesion, as mentioned above, will heal eventually without ther-

Much of the material in this chapter is based on *Syphilis, a synopsis,*[1] *Manual of tests for syphilis, 1969* (reprinted 1978),[2] and other publications and directives listed in the text, emanating from the Venereal Disease Program, and the Venereal Disease Research Laboratory, C.D.C., U.S.P.H.S.

apy, but the disease will continue its course. The only absolute criterion for the diagnosis of primary syphilis is a positive dark-field examination of the lesion and the detection of *T. pallidum.* (For demonstration of *T. pallidum* by **fluorescent antibody methods** in material from lesions see Chapter 80.) However, when there is a combination of healing lesion, lymphadenopathy, a rising antibody titer, and a history of exposure, a diagnosis of primary syphilis may be made for all practical purposes.

When the chancre first appears, serologic tests for syphilis are usually nonreactive (seronegative primary). The tests usually become reactive (seropositive primary) during the following 1-4 weeks.

A generalized or localized skin eruption usually appears about 6 weeks later (range: 2 weeks–6 months). *T. pallidum,* as a rule, can be demonstrated in these lesions. This stage of the disease is referred to as **secondary syphilis.** In some cases this stage may appear before the chancre is healed; in other cases it may be so minimal that it is missed. Enlarged lymph glands may occur along with papules, sore throat, patchy loss of hair, and headache. These secondary symptoms usually disappear within about 3 weeks and in untreated cases may reappear 1 or more times as relapses.

The diagnosis of secondary syphilis is dependent on the observation of the characteristic skin lesions, dark-field detection of *T. pallidum* in the lesions, and increasingly positive serologic tests for syphilis. The nontreponemal antigen tests are always reactive in this stage. Most of the treponemal tests will also be reactive.

Secondary syphilis usually develops into **latent syphilis,** which by definition is hidden syphilis. There are no clinical manifestations of syphilis. It is usually diagnosed by the presence of persistent reaction in the serologic tests for syphilis. A reactive (positive) serologic test must be considered diagnostic of latent syphilis until the reaction is proved to be caused by something else. The progress of latent syphilis depends largely on the physiology of the individual concerned. It may continue as such throughout the life of the individual, or it may result in the development of signs and symptoms of late syphilis.

The latent period is divided into early latent (duration under 4 years) and **late latent** (duration 4 years or more) syphilis. Early latent syphilis is infectious, especially when under 1 year's duration.

Late syphilis is not infectious (except for the fetus), and *T. pallidum* cannot be demonstrated from the lesion by dark-field examination. The lesions of late syphilis are chronic and destructive. Following adequate treatment of early syphilis, the serologic titer will become nonreactive in practically all cases. Following adequate treatment of late syphilis, the serologic titer will remain reactive indefinitely or will descend slowly over a period of years.

Influence of treatment on serologic reactions in syphilis

Treatment may change both the clinical course and the serologic pattern of the disease. If the patient is treated adequately before the appearance of a chancre, it is probable that none will appear and that his serologic test for syphilis will remain nonreactive. If he is treated at the seronegative primary stage, his serologic test will remain nonreactive. If he is treated in the seropositive primary stage, his serologic test (nontreponemal, reagin, standard test for syphilis [STS]) usually will become nonreactive within 12 months. And if he is treated during the secondary stage, usually his STS will become nonreactive in about 12-18 months. Effects of treatment after the secondary stage are variable, but, as a rule, the sooner the infected patient is treated, the more marked will be his serologic response.

On the other hand, if treatment is given 10 years after the onset of the disease, the posttreatment serologic titer could be expected to change little if any. The longer the patient goes untreated, the longer it will take his STS to reach negativity after adequate treatment, **if indeed it ever does.** Should he have clinical lesions, they will improve with therapy, although his serology remains unchanged.

Having received an optimum dosage of penicillin, it is extremely doubtful if any additional amount of antibiotics will alter the rate or nature of changes in serologic response; individuals infected 2 years or more before treatment may remain serologically reactive for life despite clinical cure and optimum doses of penicillin.

SEROLOGIC TESTS IN NONVENEREAL TREPONEMATOSES

Several infections with *Treponema* species are known in which the route of transmission is nonvenereal. **Yaws** is a disease found in most tropical areas of the world and is attributed to infection with *T. pertenue*. All nontreponemal and treponemal tests for syphilis are positive in this disease, and it cannot be differentiated from syphilis using these tests. **Pinta,** attributed to infection with *T. carateum,* is primarily a disease of the American tropics but is also found in other tropical and subtropical areas. The route of transmission is usually nonvenereal with rare occurrences of venereal and congenital transmission. Serologic tests for syphilis become positive more slowly in pinta than in syphilis; no differentiation between the 2 diseases is possible using serologic tests. **Bejel,** regarded as a nonvenereal form of syphilis most likely caused by *T. pallidum,* occurs mainly in the Near and Middle East, especially among Arabs. No chancres develop at the sites of inoculation; the results of serologic tests parallel those found in syphilis.

All the nonvenereal treponematoses respond to treatment with penicillin and other antisyphilitic compounds, and for this reason the serologic tests for syphilis are valuable in these conditions as guides in treatment. They are also valuable in the differential diagnosis of these diseases, especially in yaws that must be distinguished from cutaneous leishmaniasis, tuberculosis, and leprosy.

SEROLOGIC TESTS FOR SYPHILIS*

As a result of *T. pallidum* infection the host develops serum antibodies of various kinds. Serologic testing in syphilis aims at detecting one or another of these antibodies.

The tests are divided into 2 major groups based on the type of antigen used: (1) **nontreponemal** or **reagin** (lipoidal or cardiolipin) antigens and (2) **treponemal** antigens (treponemes or treponemal extracts).

Depending on the test system used, further classification of the 2 groups is possible (agglutination, complement fixation, immunofluorescence, etc.; see below).

The standardization and careful performance of these tests, with meticulous adherence to the details of the technics involved, is of extreme importance, since uniform interpretation would otherwise not be possible. Of the many syphilis tests described (probably over 200), only a few are now used. The physician needs to be familiar with only 2 or 3 tests; using these, he will be able to diagnose syphilis in practically any stage.

The **sensitivity** of a test refers to its ability to be reactive in the presence of syphilis, whereas the **specificity** of a test refers to its ability to be nonreactive in the absence of syphilis.

Some tests may be highly sensitive and may be particularly suited for screening, whereas others may be highly specific and more suited for use in making problem diagnoses. Such tests are a definite aid in the diagnosis of syphilis in any

---

*Based, in part, on *Syphilis, a synopsis,* 1968, Public Health Service Pub. no. 1660.[1]

stage, and they are used as almost the sole basis for the diagnosis of latent syphilis.

NOTE: Ongoing research has altered and continues to alter the usage and acceptance of various serologic tests and their interpretation by continual improvement of existing tests and search for tests that are both highly sensitive and specific.

Rapid changes have taken place in the last 10-15 years in terms of test usage patterns, and undoubtedly such changes will continue. Indications of such changes are the almost complete replacement of lipoidal antigens by cardiolipin antigens, the decline in the use of the nontreponemal complement fixation tests, and the rapidly expanding use of certain treponemal tests. In a span of a few years the popularity of the Reiter protein complement fixation test (RPCF or KRP) has declined sharply in the United States, as has the use of the treponemal immobilization test (TPI), albeit for entirely different reasons. Both have been superseded by the fluorescent treponemal antibody (FTA) test. The latter also has undergone significant changes; whereas in the early 1960s the FTA-200 technic was used, by around 1966 it was completely replaced by the FTA-ABS technic. More recently, *T. pallidum* hemagglutination tests have been introduced: a sheep-erythrocyte test (microhemagglutination assay for *T. pallidum;* **MHA-TP**) and a turkey-erythrocyte test (*T. pallidum* hemagglutination; **TPHA** and **HATTS**), both of which are gaining in popularity.

As more information is gained with each test by performance of tens of thousands of tests, it is inevitable that shortcomings are discovered and a more reliable, specific, and sensitive test is used instead.

Both the laboratorian and the clinician should keep in mind these changes and make every effort to keep familiar with newer and ongoing developments and improvements in the field of syphilis serology.

Nontreponemal antigen tests[1]

In response to invasion by *T. pallidum*, a substance called **Wassermann antibody** (or **reagin**), an antibody complex, appears in the serum of the syphilitic individual, on the average, 4-6 weeks after infection or 1-3 weeks after the appearance of the primary chancre. The presence of reagin in the patient's serum is measured by serologic tests for syphilis employing nontreponemal antigens (i.e., antigens prepared from beef heart rather than from *T. pallidum* or certain other treponemes).

The original **Wassermann test** was a complement fixation test that used as antigen a tissue extract of liver derived from congenital (stillborn) syphilitics. Wassermann and his coworkers believed that their antigen, which contained treponemes, was specific and detected antibody specifically directed against *T. pallidum*. This assumption was proved incorrect since soon afterward it was found that equally specific results could be obtained with the use of liver extracts from nonsyphilitic individuals and with tissue extracts in alcohol or ether derived from normal organs such as beef heart, human heart, and ox kidney. Although the Wassermann test as such is no longer performed, it is not uncommon to hear the term "Wassermann" applied to any nontreponemal serologic test for syphilis.

The antigens used in the nontreponemal tests are now prepared from beef heart lipids with cholesterol, cardiolipin (a phosphatide of beef heart muscle) reinforced by purified lecithin, a lecithinized and cholesterolized cardiolipin, or cardiolipin with synthetic or natural lecithins. Wassermann antibody (reagin) is thought to be a lipoprotein produced by the combination of certain microorganisms with proteins of the tissues. Although it is nonspecific, not being an antibody to treponemes, its detection by the nontreponemal antigens has been highly valuable in the diagnosis of syphilis.

Tests commonly used to detect and measure Wassermann antibody (reagin) are basically of 2 types: **flocculation** and **complement fixation.** Examples of **slide flocculation tests** are the VDRL slide test and the older Mazzini and Kline tests. Among the **card flocculation tests,** the RPR (circle) Card test is widely used (results are read macroscopically); the reagin screen test (RST) has recently been introduced. The **complement fixation** test (Kolmer test) is now rarely used.

Although these nontreponemal antigen tests are not absolutely specific or sensitive for syphilis, their performance is quite practical, they are widely available, and their findings are highly indicative.

Laboratory reports based on the slide flocculation tests are of 2 types—**qualitative** and **quantitative.** Qualitative reports will read simply as follows:

1. **Reactive,** or Positive, or 4+;
2. **Weakly Reactive,** or Weakly Positive, or 3+, 2+, or 1+; *or*
3. **Nonreactive,** or Negative.

Quantitative results are obtained by diluting or titrating the serum in geometric progression to an end point. The titer is usually reported as the highest dilution in which the test is fully reactive. A titer of 1:32 means that the serum was reactive in a dilution of 1 to 32. This may also be stated as "32 dils." RPR tests are reported only as Reactive or Nonreactive. **Prozone phenomena** due to antibody excess occasionally occur. In such cases the undiluted specimen will give a weakly reactive or nonreactive test result. Quantitative testing at higher dilutions will, however, result in reactive findings.

Quantitative serologic tests are helpful in treatment evaluation. In an early case the titer may be expected to decline with adequate treatment. On the other hand, if the titer rises persistently, one usually considers that the disease remains active and requires retreatment; it may also indicate reinfection in an adequately treated patient or relapse in an inadequately treated patient. Lastly, a rising titer may indicate a recent infection in the untreated patient or an acute false-positive reaction.

Reactive reagin tests are first obtained at about 4-6 weeks after infection or 1-3 weeks after the chancre appears. The tests should become nonreactive in 6-12 months after treatment for primary syphilis and in 12-18 months after treatment in secondary syphilis. The titer will decline slightly or not at all after treatment in late latent or late infection.

When using nontreponemal tests, it should be remembered that many cases of late latent or late syphilis give only weakly reactive results; **in 20-30% of such cases the STS may be nonreactive and could be missed if only reagin tests are used.**[4,5]

Ordinarily the titer is high in secondary syphilis, but there are exceptions to this. A high titer does not necessarily mean early syphilis or even syphilis, but it is strong evidence of the presence of syphilis. Some of the highest titers recorded have been in late benign visceral or cutaneous syphilis, (nonsyphilitic) infectious mononucleosis, hemolytic anemia, or systemic lupus erythematosus.

Various **rapid reagin tests** (for screening) have been developed. The RPR, RST, and the USR tests belong in this category. The RPR (circle) card test gained wide popularity in the late 1960s, and it may eventually replace the VDRL slide test.

In these rapid tests a modified VDRL antigen is used. Choline chloride is added to the antigen to inactivate or inhibit the substances in the unheated serum or plasma (used in the tests) that may interfere with the antibody-antigen reaction. EDTA (ethylenediaminotetraacetate) is added for preventing deterioration of the antigen. For the RPR (circle) card test, colloidal charcoal is added to the antigen, which makes macroscopic reading possible.

A recent (1976) survey of 10,604 laboratories in the United States showed that about 43% use the RPR card test and 50% use the VDRL test, with a definite trend toward adoption of the RPR card test.[3]

Treponemal antigen tests[1]

Because the antigens used in the nontreponemal antigen tests are not entirely specific for syphilis, antigens from treponemes were prepared to produce a **specific test.** Some treponemal antigen tests have been rather difficult and costly to perform, and some have lacked the sensitivity of the nontreponemal antigen tests. They have therefore been considered principally as **confirmatory tests** in cases of doubtful diagnoses and in diagnostic problem cases.

A partial list of tests employing T. pallidum or extracts of this treponeme as antigen is given below.

Complement fixation:
  Reiter protein complement fixation (RPCF)
  Kolmer with Reiter protein antigen (KRP)
  T. pallidum complement fixation (TPCF)
Immobilization:
  T. pallidum immobilization (TPI)
Agglutination:
  T. pallidum agglutination
Immunofluorescence:
  Fluorescent treponemal antibody (FTA-200)
  Fluorescent treponemal antibody-absorption (FTA-ABS)
Hemagglutination:
  Microhemagglutination assay for T. pallidum (MHA-TP)
  T. pallidum hemagglutination test (TPHA, HATTS)

In 1949 Nelson and Mayer published a report on the phenomenon of **Treponema pallidum immobilization (TPI).** This employs as the antigen T. pallidum obtained from rabbit syphilis orchitis. The treponemes are kept alive for a few hours in a special medium. When syphilitic serum and complement are added and incubated, the treponemes are immobilized; i.e., they stop moving. Present tests using this principle are considered to be specific because they employ the etiologic agent as the antigen; however, the TPI tests are less sensitive than the nontreponemal antigen tests and become reactive later in early syphilis than do nontreponemal antigen tests. Therefore it is possible to have a nonreactive TPI test in some cases of early syphilis.

The TPI test is technically difficult, time consuming, and very expensive to perform. Despite these drawbacks, it has become the final serologic arbiter and the standard by which all treponemal tests have been judged (see further comments below).

The **RPCF** or **KRP tests,** utilizing as antigen a protein fraction from the Reiter strain of treponeme (a nonpathogenic organism that can be cultivated), were widely employed in the mid 1960s. However, they were found not to be sufficiently specific. They also lack sensitivity, especially in late syphilis. The tests have been abandoned in the United States (see Nicholas and Beerman[6]).

The **FTA tests** are indirect fluorescent antibody technics, which detect specific treponemal antibody and allow its rapid recognition. The patient's serum is added to a suspension of dead T. pallidum (antigen) on a slide. If the patient's serum contains antibody against the organism, it will combine with the treponemes.

To visualize the reaction, i.e., the presence of antibody (human γ-globulin) on the treponemes, an antihuman globulin antibody "tagged" with a fluorescent dye (fluorescein isothiocyanate) is added to the carefully washed slide. The mixture is allowed to react, and the slide is again washed. When viewed through a microscope equipped with an appropriate light source (ultraviolet light) and filters, the treponemes that had reacted

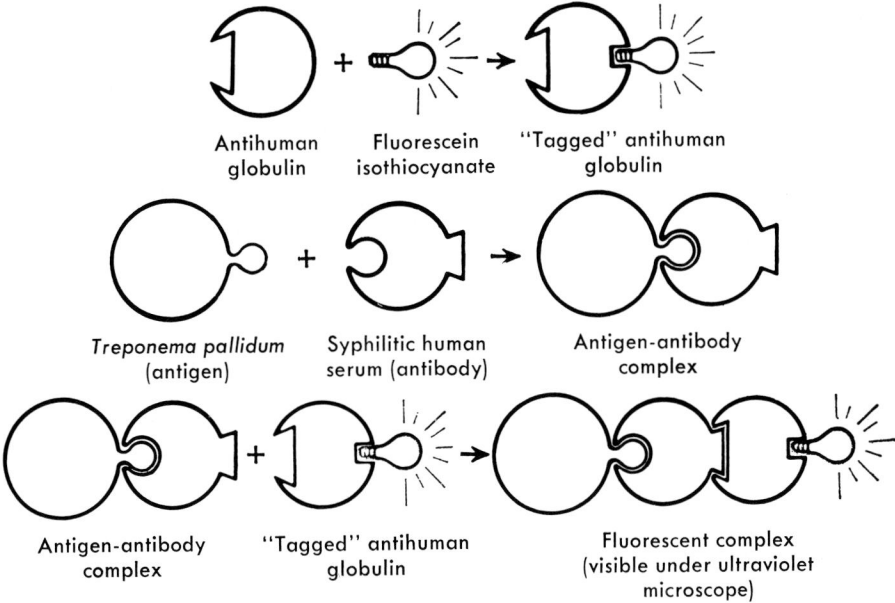

Antihuman   Fluorescein   "Tagged" antihuman
globulin   isothiocyanate   globulin

Treponema pallidum   Syphilitic human   Antigen-antibody
(antigen)   serum (antibody)   complex

Antigen-antibody   "Tagged" antihuman   Fluorescent complex
complex   globulin   (visible under ultraviolet
                              microscope)

Fig. 106-1. Principle of the indirect method of fluorescent antibody technic as used in the fluorescent treponemal antibody (FTA) test (schematic outline).

with the patient's antibody will fluoresce, since they are now coated, in addition, with the antihuman globulin–tagged antiserum. If the patient had no antibody against the treponemes, no globulin coating occurs, and the fluorescent antihuman serum will not combine with the treponemes; no fluorescence is observed. (A discussion of fluorescent antibody tests is found in Chapter 70.) Fig. 106-1 illustrates the principle involved.

The fluorescent treponemal antibody test has undergone several phases of development since its introduction in 1957.[7] Originally a 1:5 dilution of test serum was employed (**FTA test**); to prevent nonspecific reactions (with treponemes found in the normal human mouth, etc.), i.e., to improve specificity, the **FTA-200 test** was devised (1960),[8] in which a 1:200 dilution of the test serum was used. This eliminated the false-positive reactions but also greatly reduced the sensitivity of the test.

Eventually Hunter et al. (1964)[9] diluted the test serum 1:5 with a sonicated extract of non-pathogenic Reiter treponemes and thus absorbed out antibodies common to *T. pallidum* and normal flora treponemes ("group antibodies"). Antibodies "specific" for *T. pallidum* remain in the syphilitic serum (**fluorescent treponemal antibody–absorption [FTA-ABS] test**). For a recent evaluation of the FTA-ABS test, see Dans et al.[10]

As mentioned earlier, the TPI test has been the standard by which all treponemal antibody tests are judged, and it was recognized as the ultimate test in confirmation of problem cases. Some recent reports throw considerable doubt on this tenet. Tuffanelli et al.,[11] Atwood et al.,[4] and Harner et al.,[5] among others, have found that the fluorescent treponemal antibody absorption (FTA-ABS) test is more sensitive than the TPI test in latent and late syphilis (as well as in primary syphilis). It is also as specific as the TPI test and considerably simpler to perform. Thus they all, in essence, share the conclusion that the FTA-ABS test is the "confirmatory test of choice."

The *T. pallidum* **hemagglutination tests** (MHA-TP, TPHA, HATTS), employing blood cells coated with *T. pallidum* antigen, are easier to do than the FTA-ABS, require no expensive equipment, and, except for low sensitivity in primary syphilis, appear to be useful.[12-14]

NOTE: As of August 1978, the U.S. Center for Disease Control listed the status of serologic tests for syphilis as follows:

I. Standard tests (eligible to appear in the *Manual of Tests for Syphilis*)
   A. Nontreponemal
      Automated reagin test (ART), qualitative and quantitative
      Rapid plasma reagin (RPR; 18 mm circle) card test, qualitative and quantitative
      Unheated serum reagin (USR) test, qualitative
      Venereal Disease Research Laboratory (VDRL) slide test (serum), qualitative and quantitative
      Venereal Disease Research Laboratory (VDRL) slide test (spinal fluid), qualitative and quantitative
   B. Treponemal
      Fluorescent treponemal antibody-absorption (FTA-ABS) test (serum), qualitative

II. Provisional tests (warrant large-scale studies; suitable for reporting results to physicians)
   A. Nontreponemal
      Reagin screen test (RST), qualitative and quantitative (Fisher-Lederle)
   B. Treponemal
      Fluorescent antibody dark-field (FADF) test
      Microhemagglutination–*Treponema pallidum* (MHA-TP) test, qualitative (Ames)
III. Investigational tests (suitable for investigative studies in parallel with a standard test)
   A. Nontreponemal
      Rapid plasma reagin (RPR; 14 mm circle) card test (Hynson, Westcott & Dunning)
      Syphla-Chek Test (Hyland)
   B. Treponemal
      Hemagglutination treponemal tests for syphilis (HATTS) (Difco)
      Treponema pallidum hemagglutination (TPHA) test (Burroughs, Wellcome)

Spinal fluid examination[1]

The only means of diagnosing neurosyphilis accurately and evaluating its treatment is by spinal fluid examination. Examination of the cerebrospinal fluid should be part of the management in every case of syphilis. In early forms of the disease the examination is most meaningful 6 months to 1 year after treatment; in latent or late forms of the disease, examination should precede treatment. A diagnosis of latent syphilis cannot be made unless asymptomatic neurosyphilis is excluded by a negative cerebrospinal fluid.

Three tests of spinal fluid are essential for the diagnosis of neurosyphilis:

Cell count: Over 4 lymphocytes is abnormal.

Total protein: Protein is always elevated in active neurosyphilis. "Normal" values vary from laboratory to laboratory depending on the test used. Individuals vary considerably in their normal total protein values, but a total protein of more than 40 mg/100 ml is usually abnormal.

VDRL (or Kolmer) spinal fluid tests: A reactive spinal fluid VDRL (or Kolmer) is practically always an indication of central nervous system syphilis but not necessarily of its activity. False-positive reactions in the spinal fluid are **rare.**

The presence of reagin in the spinal fluid is the only finding that is pathognomonic of neurosyphilis, since any condition that causes meningeal irritation may result in an increase in the cell count and protein concentration of the spinal fluid. Consequently, reactive reagin in the spinal fluid is reliable evidence of past or present neurosyphilis. With the exception of late tabes dorsalis, the clinical syndrome is rarely so clear cut as to permit the diagnosis of neurosyphilis in the face of negative reagin serologic findings. Conversely, even in the absence of clinical signs or symptoms, a positive reagin test is indicative of asymptomatic neurosyphilis. After successful treatment and arrest of late neurosyphilis, it may take many years for the spinal fluid reagin test to become nonreactive.

The degree of activity of neurosyphilis is indicated by increased numbers of lymphocytes and increased protein in the spinal fluid. A cell count of more than $4/mm^3$ is usually abnormal and indicative of an active central nervous system infection.

Unless cell counts are made accurately and as soon as possible, there is little point in doing spinal fluid examinations for syphilis. **Spinal fluid that contains blood** or other contamination or has been kept in a warm place for hours will not provide an accurate cell count. Consequently, when spinal fluid is sent to a laboratory by mail or is left unexamined in a warm place for as much as a day, the cell count is unreliable. NOTE: A bloody tap, resulting in small quantities of **reactive** serum in spinal fluid, can produce a positive Kolmer or VDRL reaction, and red cells may be mistakenly interpreted as white cells.

Increased total protein in association with pleocytosis and reactive spinal fluid reagin is also indicative of active neurosyphilis. Following successful treatment, high total protein values decline slowly, and they may not become normal for a year or more. In general, the cell count may be expected to return first to normal followed by the protein and finally the serologic test.

Colloidal tests of spinal fluid such as the colloidal gold test, once widely utilized, are of no diagnostic significance and are not a reliable guide to the activity of neurosyphilis. These tests have no value in the management of neurosyphilis.[1]

NOTE: To date (1978) there is no standardized FTA (or TPI) technic for the detection of spinal fluid antibodies. It is known that FTA and TPI antibodies can be found in spinal fluid; however, neither test is recommended or generally performed on spinal fluid because (1) their specificity does not seem greater than the VDRL or Kolmer test, (2) the latter are considerably cheaper than the treponemal tests, and (3) the significance and interpretation of reactive tests are not yet clear.[15,16]

False-positive reactions[1,11,17-19]

For many years it has been suspected that sera of some individuals give false-positive reactions with reagin (STS) tests. This was verified when tests detecting treponemal antibodies became available, since treponemal tests are capable of distinguishing latent syphilis from false-positive reactions. If one of the less sensitive treponemal tests is reactive, syphilis may be diagnosed. Should this test be nonreactive, the diagnosis of syphilis may not be excluded until a nonreactive TPI or **preferably** FTA-ABS is obtained.

All normal sera may contain minute amounts of reagin. The sensitivity of nontreponemal tests is altered by varying the proportion of reagents, temperature, mixing time, etc. For these reasons about one-fourth of all false-positive reactions represent technical errors or day-to-day variability in testing. Such titers rarely exceed weakly reactive or reactive at 1 dil. These "technical" false-positive reactors may be excluded by repeating the same nontreponemal tests and obtaining nonreactive results.

The false-positive reactor is characterized by repeatedly reactive nontreponemal tests accompanied by nonreactive treponemal tests (FTA-ABS). The duration of reagin reactivity arbitrarily determines whether the false-positive reaction is acute (less than 6 months) or chronic (6 months or longer). Although false-positive reactions have been called "biologic," many such reactions are associated with specific diseases or follow vaccination or immunization; therefore this adjective is best discarded. The terms "acute false positive" or "chronic false positive" adequately describe what is observed.

Acute false-positive reactions are found in persons suffering from many viral and bacterial infections or who have had certain vaccinations and immunizations. Titers are generally less than 8 dils; the reaction lasts a few weeks to a few months. Often, no preexisting illness or specific cause may be recognized. (NOTE: A history of a prior infection or immunization in a patient with a low-titered STS in no way confirms a false-positive reaction. Syphilis is still the single most common cause of a reactive test for syphilis. Unless tests promptly become nonreactive or a nonreactive treponemal test result is obtained, syphilis cannot be reliably excluded.)

Chronic false-positive reactions are usually less frequent than "technical" false-positive or acute false-positive reactions. About half the chronic false-positive reactors reported in the literature were under 30 years of age, 70% were women, and about 10% had systemic lupus erythematosus; others had collagen diseases or autoimmune diseases.

Lepromatous leprosy, heroin addiction, and occasionally malaria are associated with chronic false-positive **nontreponemal tests** for syphilis. The nonvenereal treponematoses (yaws, pinta, bejel) characteristically give **reactive nontreponemal tests** as well as **reactive treponemal tests** and are not serologically distinguishable.

(NOTE: Often, if the patient has multisystem disease and a positive LE cell preparation, a reactive serologic test is considered automatically to be false. Syphilis and systemic lupus erythematosus or syphilis and leprosy can and do coexist. Each case must be determined individually by clinical appraisal and appropriate serologic tests.)

Passive reaginemia is defined as the placental transfer of maternal reagin to an uninfected newborn (congenital false-positive reactor). Antibodies crossing the placenta are predominantly of the type reacting in complement fixation tests; flocculation tests will give much lower titers in the neonate than in the maternal serum. Children born to women treated for syphilis during pregnancy are not always cured in utero (depending on drug, dosage, and duration of treatment). All children giving reactive tests at birth must be followed with serial serological tests. A falling titer represents loss of passively transferred reagin; rising titers indicate active infection requiring treatment. Immobilizing antibodies may also passively cross the placenta, and detectable levels may persist up to 6 months, occasionally giving reactive results for a longer period than the reagin tests.

False-positive and **borderline** results do occur in the FTA-ABS test.[17-20] Sera of some genital herpes patients,[11, 20] heroin addicts, and patients with autoimmune diseases, myeloma, and systemic lupus erythematosus, as well as sera of some pregnant women, sometimes give false-positive reactions with the FTA-ABS test. An atypical beading pattern in the FTA-ABS test with lupus erythematosus sera has also been reported.[21]

Use and interpretation of serologic tests in syphilis

All blood specimens submitted for syphilis testing should be tested with a standard test for syphilis using nontreponemal antigen (STS, e.g., the VDRL or RPR [circle] card test); the FTA-ABS test should **not** be used alone as a screening test. If the test is nonreactive, repeat it (quantitative VDRL), reexamine and requestion the patient, and check for results of STS reaction that may have been made previously. If the repeat VDRL test is again nonreactive, syphilis is unlikely. **However, note that in late latent and late syphilis the STS may be nonreactive in about 20-30% of cases.**[4,5] Therefore in problem cases a treponemal test (FTA-ABS, MHA-TP, or TPHA) should be performed, even if the VDRL tests repeatedly are nonreactive.

If the STS (VDRL slide test or other) is reactive or weakly reactive, the test should be repeated (quantitative). If the repeat test shows a significant rise in titer, it may mean syphilis or an acute false-positive reaction. The latter is transient and is easily evaluated clinically and with follow-up testing. In problem cases perform the FTA-ABS test.

If the VDRL test does not show a rise in titer, an FTA-ABS test should be done.

If the serum is reactive in the FTA-ABS (or the TPI, somewhat less sensitive than the former) test, the diagnosis of syphilis is indicated.

NOTE: In problem cases in which significant doubt exists, the serodiagnosis should **not** be made on the basis of a **single** treponemal test. Regardless of whether the reaction is reactive or nonreactive, a second specimen should be tested. **Reactive MHA-TP or TPHA tests** should be confirmed with the FTA-ABS.

It should be noted that **treponemal antibodies** (as detected by the FTA-ABS and, to a somewhat lesser extent, the TPI test) **persist for many** (20 or more) **years after presumably adequate treatment.** For this reason neither test can be used for evaluation of treatment.

It should also be kept in mind that because of the usual persistence of low-titered reactive reagin serologic tests and the persistence of treponemal antibodies, many cases are found that have some history of arsenical or bismuth therapy. If adequate therapy history cannot be obtained, as often is the case, the physician is justified in retreating these patients with fully adequate doses of penicillin.[1]

Also, in pregnancy, when any doubt exists about previous treatment or the presence of active infection, a course of treatment should be given to prevent congenital syphilis. NOTE: In 1972 the Center for Disease Control issued a Provisional Technique for performance of the **FTA-ABS IgM** test in congenital syphilis of the newborn. In 1975 the routine performance of the test was discontinued because of the need for further evaluation; the test is felt to be insufficiently sensitive for use as a screening test in infants at risk.[22,23]

GENERAL RULES FOR SYPHILIS TESTS*
Quality control of syphilis tests[2]

Syphilis serology standardization programs in the United States are at present conducted by the Center for Disease Control (Venereal Disease Control Division) and state public health laboratories. These programs had their inception in 1938 at the Assembly of Laboratory Directors and Serologists and have evolved to meet present needs. Standardization programs have promoted uniformity of tests for syphilis and have assisted laboratories to attain and maintain a high level of efficiency in serologic tests for syphilis. The achievement of these goals has ultimately depended on the individual laboratories' participation in these programs—their willingness and ability to incorporate recommended quality control measures and to take corrective action to eliminate deficiencies.

Quality control measures in syphilis serology are designed to ensure that reliable and reproducible test results are obtained within a laboratory and among different laboratories performing the same tests. Strict adherence to technic, recommendations, and use of standardized reagents will eliminate most technical errors. The behavior of control sera of predetermined reactivity patterns detects day-to-day variability in testing and indicates when corrective action is required but does not indicate the causative factors. Other quality control measures that are essential for reliable and reproducible test results are:

1. Clean, well-lighted, temperature-controlled laboratories, with adequate space for work and storage.

2. Equipment, instruments, and glassware that meet specifications and are of sufficient quantity for the types and volume of testing performed.

---

*Condensed from *Manual of tests for syphilis, 1969* (reprinted 1978).[2]

Dates of purchase, repair, and maintenance of equipment and instruments should be recorded.

3. Satisfactory glassware cleaning methods (see Glassware Specifications and Cleaning, below).

4. Test procedures selected on the basis of adaptability to the laboratory facilities and the qualifications of the personnel performing the tests.

5. Current published technics that are available for reference and are strictly followed without modification.

6. Careful and precise measurements of specimens and reagents to eliminate random errors.

7. Periodic **check readings** to maintain uniform reading levels among laboratory personnel.

8. Control of reagents.
   a. Adequate **check testing** of new lots of reagents for standard reactivity before being placed in routine use (see Reagent Control, below).
   b. Proper preparation, labeling, and storage of **reagents.** Shelf-life control should be exercised, and substandard, deteriorated, or outdated reagents should be discarded.
   c. Documenting steps in the preparation of new lots of reagents and control sera and recording the results of check testing of each lot.

9. **Control sera** with established reactivity patterns for each test performed. Include these each time serologic testing is performed to provide a stable baseline and day-to-day consistency. Control sera should be similar to the test specimens and should include at least a Reactive, an intermediate, and a Nonreactive control (duplicating the composition of patients' specimens at 2 clinically significant points of increased reactivity). The intermediate controls are the most important, since these reflect the difference in reactivity from 1 antigen suspension to another or from 1 test period to another (see Preparation of Control Sera, below).

10. Acceptable test **specimens.** Ensure acceptability by correct collection and identification, prompt transmission to the laboratory, and proper storage conditions and processing methods (see Collection, Submission, and Processing of Specimens, below).

11. **Daily work sheets.** Keep daily work sheets for recording the specimen numbers, results of all tests performed, control results, lot numbers of reagents, reagent titers, room temperature, and the worker's initials. As tests are read, record the actual results of all controls and specimens, not just the interpretation or final report.

12. Careful checking of all testing records and report forms for clerical errors. All records of testing should be identified with the laboratory accession number given the specimen.

13. **Periodic interlaboratory checks.** Continuous participation in a proficiency testing study in which the participating laboratory is provided

a means for periodic detection of problems by comparison of its test results with those of a reference laboratory; sending all specimens with any degree of reactivity to a reference laboratory for verification of reactivity; and the periodic sharing of split specimens of unknown reactivity with a peer laboratory for comparison of results.

14. Attendance of qualified laboratory personnel at basic and refresher training courses to obtain current information and instruction in new or modified test procedures.

Equipment maintenance and control[2]

Laboratories located in institutions with maintenance service should arrange for periodic inspections of all equipment for minor adjustments and replacement of worn parts. If this service is not available, a technical worker in the laboratory should be responsible for periodic checking and obtaining necessary maintenance. Records should be maintained that show dates of inspection, maintenance, and repairs. Laboratory workers should be instructed on the proper use and care of equipment and on routine checking procedures to determine that equipment is fulfilling test requirements.

Temperature. Check temperature of water bath each time it is used. If incubators, freezers, and refrigerators do not have recording thermometers, place thermometers in 1 or more areas; check temperature each day and at the time of use. Place a thermometer in the testing area so that room temperature can be observed and recorded when testing is performed.

Speed. Check speed of rotating machines before and during the time they are used and do not tolerate marked variations from prescribed speeds. Centrifuges should be equipped with tachometers so that speed may be checked and controlled. Clean the inside of centrifuges occasionally to prevent the accumulation of glass particles and dust that may be blown into specimens.

pH meter. Inspect the pH meter periodically to ensure that the reference electrode reservoir is filled with electrolyte. Keep glass electrode ready to use by storing with tip immersed in water. Before using, standardize the pH meter with 2 buffer solutions of different pH values.

Colorimeter or spectrophotometer. Check instruments periodically with a calibrating standard to verify instrument performance; include controls of known transmission values when test samples are analyzed.

Microscopes. Keep microscopes clean and protected from dust with appropriate covers when not in use. For fluorescence microscopy, check intensity of the mercury arc illumination periodically with a light meter.

Balances. Place balances in areas that are free of vibration and air currents and provide with covers for protection from dust. Store weights in a closed box and handle with forceps. Clean balances after each use.

Water still and demineralizer. Clean the still and replace the ion exchange cartridge in the demineralizer periodically to maintain the production of good quality distilled or demineralized water. The frequency will depend on the quality of local tap water and the number of hours per day that the still or demineralizer is in operation. Determine the quality of the effluent water with a purity meter daily and take corrective action when indicated.

Glassware specifications and cleaning[2]

Glassware for each serologic procedure should meet the recommended specifications, and sufficient quantities should be available for the volume of testing performed. Glassware that becomes etched or scratched to a degree that will interfere with observations should not be used. Clean glassware must be used to obtain reliable results. A qualified technical worker should supervise and be responsible for all glassware cleaning procedures. The methods to be used should be written in detail, step by step, posted in the working area for ready reference, and strictly followed.

Glassware cleaning methods will differ with the volume and variety of tests performed but all include certain basic steps: prerinsing, washing, rinsing with tap and distilled water, drying, and, finally, spot checking to determine whether cleaning agents have been adequately removed. The availability of excellent cleaning products and equipment makes routine use of acid cleaning unnecessary.

Suitable containers should be available at the laboratory bench for discarding glassware. Completely submerge items such as pipets and slides in water or a mild detergent solution to avoid drying of material on the glassware that makes cleaning more difficult.

Cleaning of glassware. Clean glassware by hand washing or by machine washing. Some laboratories are entirely dependent on hand washing for all glassware; others wash only special items by hand because of size, shape, or fragility. To wash items by hand, prerinse with tap water, soak in a glassware detergent solution, brush thoroughly with an appropriate size brush, rinse with tap water 6-8 times, and finally rinse with unused distilled or demineralized water.

Automatic machine washers. These machines should be of a type and size that will meet the specific washing requirements of the laboratory. The washer should be designed to withstand continuous use with minimum major maintenance, and it should be constructed so that glassware with restrictive openings can be thoroughly washed and rinsed. Make provisions for final rinsing of glassware with unused distilled or demineralized water. Follow directions of the manufacturer as to washing and rinsing. Manual preliminary rinsing may be necessary to remove gross foreign material before proceeding with machine washing.

Pipets. Soak pipets in detergent solution in an upright container or cylinder so that the solution will fill the inside of the pipet. Rinse with tap water for at least 30 min in a pipet rinser that operates on a siphon principle; such a rinser is inexpensive and efficient, provided there is sufficient water pressure for a turbulent fill-and-empty cycle. Give pipets a final rinse in unused distilled or demineralized water. Wash pipets in a glassware washing machine only if it is equipped with a specially built pipet header to permit the wash and rinse water to go through them under pressure; pipets cannot be adequately cleaned or rinsed by being placed loosely in a basket in a glassware washing machine.

Glass slides. Glass slides may be cleaned satisfactorily by several methods. In some laboratories, slides are placed in special racks for washing and rinsing in the glassware washing machines. Hand washing in detergent solution with adequate rinsing is also practiced. Slides should have grease-free surfaces, and sera should spread readily on the slides. If cleaned slides do not meet these criteria, scrub the slides with Bon Ami, dry, and polish with a clean lint-free cloth. To free slides of paraffin rings, soak in detergent solution to loosen. Discard glass slides with ceramic rings into water, wash with a mild detergent and soft hand brush, rinse, and dry; avoid prolonged soaking of these slides in detergent solution, since the ceramic rings will become brittle and will flake off.

Glass or polyethylene containers. Clean large containers periodically to prevent accumulation of debris and contaminants in stored distilled or demineralized water, phosphate-buffered saline, or other solutions. Dry glassware in a hot-air oven; arrange glassware so that it will drain. Spot check representative samples of glassware, after cleaning, with an appropriate color indicator solution to determine if rinsing has been adequate to remove cleaning agents.

Laboratory equipment and glassware should meet the specifications described in the technic for each test procedure. Establish and follow effective procedures for care and maintenance of equipment and cleaning of glassware. Keep equipment clean and in good working condition. Glassware should be scrupulously clean. Maintenance programs and cleaning methods should fit the needs of individual laboratories, but certain elements are common to all laboratories.

Preparation and calibration of needles for slide flocculation tests[2]

1. File a deep nick in needle just above bevel.
2. Break point off needle with pliers.
3. Using a 1 or 2 ml syringe containing material to be dispensed, check needle by counting number of drops in 1 ml reagent. Drops should be allowed to fall freely from tip of needle. Needle and syringe should be held **perpendicularly** to tabletop.
4. Adjust needles **not** meeting these specifications to deliver correct volumes before being used.
5. If too many drops/ml are delivered by needle, opening of tip is too small. Adjust by reaming out tip with sharp-pointed instrument such as sharpened end of triangular file.
6. If too few drops/ml are delivered by needle, opening of tip is too large. Adjust by pressing together slightly or by filing edges of needle inward.

7. Once calibrated, protect tips of needles against dropping on floor, sink, or to bottom of bottles.
8. Check needles **each day** before using and adjust if necessary.
9. Clean needles and syringes by rinsing with water, alcohol, and acetone. Remove needle from syringe after cleaning.

Reagent control[2]

It is **the responsibility of the laboratory** to ensure that reagents are of good quality and standard reactivity. Chemicals and distilled water should be of high quality, and solutions should be prepared according to directions specified in each technic. Each new lot of cardiolipin antigen or antigen suspension (nontreponemal tests), and antigen, sorbent, and conjugate for the FTA-ABS test should be check tested in parallel with a standard reagent to verify that it is of standard reactivity. Parallel testing should be performed on **more than 1 testing day** by using different specimens of graded reactivity for each test period. Tests should be performed in accordance with the technics described in this manual. Keep a permanent record of the results of all check testing.

NOTE: **Individual specimens of graded reactivity for check testing may be obtained by selecting specimens from daily test runs and storing them in the freezer.** Fresh specimens **from routine test runs** should be used for the **Nonreactive specimens.**

Chemicals. All chemicals should be of reagent quality and meet the specifications of the particular technic. Invalid results may be obtained when substandard chemicals are employed or when specific directions for preparation of reagents are not followed.

Distilled water. Distilled water of the highest quality should be used for the preparation of reagents. A purity meter, which is simple to operate, can be used daily to determine the relative purity of the water. A periodic check of pH will also indicate to some degree the quality of the distilled water. If stored, distilled water should be placed in Pyrex (or equivalent) or plastic containers that can be tightly stoppered, although freshly distilled water is preferred. Demineralized water of good quality may be used.

Saline. Sodium chloride for saline should be dried in the hot-air oven for 30 min at 160-180 C to remove absorbed moisture. Heating at higher temperatures should be avoided, since it may result in decomposition of the salt. The sodium chloride may be weighed and

Test	Reagents	Needle gauge	Size drop required (ml)	No. drops delivered/ml reagent
RPR (circle) Card	Antigen suspension	20	0.017 or 1/60	60 ± 2
USR	Antigen suspension	18	0.022 or 1/45	45 ± 1
VDRL (qualitative)	Antigen suspension	18	0.017 or 1/60	60 ± 2
VDRL (quantitative)	Antigen suspension	19	0.014 or 1/75	75 ± 2
VDRL	0.9% saline	23	0.010 or 1/100	100 ± 2
VDRL	Sensitized antigen suspension	21 or 22	0.010 or 1/100	100 ± 2

stored in corked test tubes to avoid daily weighing. Saline solutions should be prepared according to the specific directions given in each test technic. Dissolve salts in distilled or demineralized water and shake the solution thoroughly to ensure complete mixing. If stored, the solutions should be placed in Pyrex (or equivalent) or plastic containers that can be tightly stoppered. A pH determination should be made on each new lot of buffered saline prepared in the laboratory.

Check testing nontreponemal (cardiolipin) test antigens[2]
VDRL antigen

Criteria of acceptability
1. Reportable test results on individual specimens in qualitative and quantitative tests should be comparable with those obtained with the standard antigen.
2. The difference in the numbers of "rough" Nonreactive results obtained with the new antigen and with the standard antigen should not be greater than that obtained with duplicate suspensions of the standard antigen.

Procedure
1. Prepare 2 VDRL antigen suspensions from standard (S) VDRL antigen and buffered saline and 2 antigen suspensions from the new (X) VDRL antigen and buffered saline that produce the established reactivity pattern with control sera of graded reactivity.
2. Compare the 4 antigen suspensions (S1, S2, X1, and X2) by qualitative testing of individual sera of graded reactivity. Test at least 10 Reactive, 15 Weakly Reactive, and 25 Nonreactive sera.
3. Select 3 Reactive sera for **quantitative** testing. In test tubes, prepare serial dilutions of each serum in 0.9% saline (1.2, 1:4, 1:8, 1:16, 1:32, 1:64). Test each serum dilution with the 4 antigen suspensions in a qualitative test.
4. Prepare sensitized VDRL antigen suspension for spinal fluid testing from each of the 2 new antigen suspensions and the 2 standard antigen suspensions that produce established reactivity pattern on spinal fluid controls of graded reactivity.
5. Compare the 4 sensitized antigen suspensions by qualitative testing of at least 6 spinal fluid specimens of graded reactivity. (If necessary, simulated spinal fluid specimens may be prepared by diluting serum 1:80 or higher in 0.9% saline.)
6. For all testing, arrange specimens on slides so that reactivity of the 4 antigen suspensions can be examined side by side.
7. Record results of all testing.
8. Review test results and determine if new antigen meets criteria of acceptability.
When differences in reactivity between the new and standard antigen suspensions occur, check the pH of the VDRL buffered saline to determine if it is a contributing factor. VDRL buffered saline outside the range of pH 6.0 ± 0.1 is not satisfactory.

RPR card and USR antigen suspensions
Criteria of acceptability
1. When tested with the Nonreactive control serum, the antigen particles should be evenly dispersed and comparable with the standard antigen suspension in appearance.
2. Reportable test results on controls and indi-

vidual sera in qualitative tests should be comparable with those obtained with the standard antigen suspension.
3. The number of "rough" Nonreactive results obtained with the new antigen suspension should not be greater than that obtained with the standard antigen suspension.

Procedure
1. Test new lot of antigen suspension and standard antigen suspension with control sera of graded reactivity.
2. If established pattern of reactivity is obtained on control sera with both new and standard antigen suspensions, compare the 2 antigen suspensions by qualitative testing of individual sera of graded reactivity. Test at least 10 Reactive, 15 intermediate (Reactive "minimal" for RPR card, and Weakly Reactive for USR), and 25 Nonreactive sera.
3. For all testing, arrange specimens on slides or cards so that reactivity of the 2 antigen suspensions can be examined side by side.
4. Record results of all testing.
5. Review test results and determine if new antigen suspension meets criteria of acceptability.

Check testing FTA-ABS test reagents[2]
Treponema pallidum antigen

Criteria of acceptability
1. A sufficient number of organisms should remain on slides after staining so that tests may be read without difficulty.
2. The antigen should not contain background material that stains to the extent that it interferes with the reading of the test.
3. No significant change in the number or appearance of organisms should occur on antigen smears stored in the freezer at −20 C.
4. The antigen should not stain specifically with a standard conjugate at its working titer.
5. Reportable test results on controls and individual sera should be comparable with those obtained with the standard antigen.

Procedure
1. Reconstitute a sample of the new antigen according to the accompanying directions. Mix well to disperse treponemes evenly.
2. Observe gross appearance as to clarity and particulate matter.
3. Observe number and morphology of treponemes by dark-field microscopy. Note presence of spermatozoa, tissue particles, and other debris that may interfere with reading of tests.
4. Prepare required number of antigen smears with new antigen and with a standard antigen, and fix as for FTA-ABS test.
5. Reserve half of fixed slides for second testing to be performed 3 or more days later. Store at −20 C.
6. On both testing days, compare the 2 antigens by testing controls and individual sera of graded reactivity according to FTA-ABS technic. Test 5 Reactive (1+ − 4+) and 5 Nonreactive sera.
7. Read consecutively standard antigen slide and new antigen slide on each control and serum tested and compare results of both antigens. The Minimally Reactive (1+) control with standard antigen is used as reading control.

8. Record results of all testing.
9. Review test results and determine if new antigen meets criteria of acceptability.

FTA-ABS test sorbent

Criteria of acceptability
1. The new sorbent should remove nonspecific reactivity of the nonspecific control serum.
2. The new sorbent should not reduce the intensity of fluorescence of the Reactive (4+) control serum to less than 3+.
3. The Nonspecific staining control with new sorbent should be Nonreactive.
4. Reportable test results on controls and individual sera should be comparable with those obtained with standard sorbent.
5. The sorbent should be usable rehydrated to the indicated volume on the label or according to accompanying directions.

Procedure
1. Compare new sorbent with standard sorbent by testing controls and individual sera of graded reactivity. Select 3 Reactive (1+ − 4+), 3 Nonspecific (known to demonstrate at least 2+ Nonspecific reactivity when diluted 1:5 in phosphate-buffered saline [PBS; see FTA-ABS test]), and 4 Nonreactive sera.
2. Dilute Reactive (4+) and Nonspecific control sera 1:5 in new sorbent, standard sorbent, and PBS. Prepare Minimally Reactive (1+) control.
3. Prepare 1:5 dilutions of individual sera in new sorbent, standard sorbent, and PBS.
4. Test diluted controls and individual sera as described in Steps 6-20 of the FTA-ABS Test on Serum.
5. Read completed slides in following order: Reactive and Nonspecific control sera diluted in PBS, standard sorbent, and new sorbent; Nonspecific staining control; Minimally Reactive (1+) control; and each individual serum diluted in PBS, standard sorbent, and new sorbent.
6. Record results of all testing.
7. Review test results and determine if new sorbent meets criteria of acceptability.

Fluorescein-labeled antihuman globulin (conjugate)

Criteria of acceptability
1. A satisfactory conjugate should not stain a standard antigen nonspecifically at **3 doubling dilutions** below the working titer of the conjugate.
2. Reportable test results on controls and individual sera should be comparable with those obtained with the standard conjugate.

Most manufacturers designate on the label the working titer of the conjugate that was determined under the testing conditions and with the equipment in their laboratories. Since conditions and equipment vary from one laboratory to another, it is necessary to titer and check test a new lot of conjugate with the fluorescence microscope assembly available.

Titration
1. Prepare serial doubling dilutions of new con-

Table 106-1. Titration of new conjugate (fluorescein-labeled antihuman globulin)*

Conjugates	Controls Non-specific staining control (PBS)	Reactive (4+) control serum (1:5 in PBS)	Reactive (1+) control serum
Standard conjugate, titer 1:400	—	4+	1+
New conjugate dilution:			
1:12.5	< 1+	4+	
1:25	–	4+	
1:50	–	4+	
1:100	–	4+	
1:200	–	4+	
1:400	–	4+	
1:800	–	3+	

*From Manual of tests for syphilis, 1969.[2]

jugate in PBS containing 2% Tween 80 (see FTA-ABS test) to include titer indicated by manufacturer.

Examples:
(a) 1:2.5, 1:5, 1:10, 1:10, 1:20, 1:40, 1:80, 1:160
(b) 1:12.5, 1:25, 1:50, 1:100, 1:200, 1:400, 1:800

Prepare higher dilutions if necessary.
2. Test each conjugate dilution with the Reactive (4+) control serum diluted 1:5 in PBS in accordance with FTA-ABS technic.
3. Include a nonspecific staining control with each conjugate dilution (see FTA-ABS Test, Controls, Step 4a).
4. A standard conjugate, at its titer, is set up at the same time with a Reactive (4+) control serum, a Minimally Reactive (1+) control serum, and a nonspecific staining control with PBS for the purpose of controlling reagents and test conditions.
5. Read slides in following order:
   a. Examine the 3 control slides to ensure that reagents and testing conditions are satisfactory.
   b. Examine slides with new conjugate; start with lowest dilution of conjugate. Record readings in pluses.
6. The **end point** of the titration is the highest dilution giving maximum (4+) fluorescence. The **working titer** of the new conjugate is 1 doubling dilution below the end point. In Table 106-1 dilution selected for working titer is 1:200.
7. New conjugate should not stain nonspecifically at 3 doubling dilutions below working titer of conjugate. In Table 106-1 conjugate would meet this criterion, since there is no nonspecific staining with 1:25 dilution.
8. Dispense conjugate in not less than 0.3 ml quantities and store at −20 C or lower. (For practical purposes a conjugate with a working titer of 1:400 or higher may be diluted 1:10 with sterile PBS containing Merthiolate [Eli Lilly & Co., Indianapolis] in a concentration of 1:5000 before storage in freezer.)
9. Verify titer of conjugate after at least 3 d storage in freezer.

Check testing. If criterion of acceptability for nonspecific staining has been met and working titer has been determined, new conjugate should be check tested in parallel with standard conjugate before being placed in routine use.

1. Check test sample of new conjugate that has been stored in freezer for 3 or more d.*
2. Compare new conjugate and standard conjugate at their respective working titers by testing controls and individual sera of graded reactivity according to FTA-ABS technic. Test 5 Reactive (1+ − 4+) and 5 Nonreactive sera.
3. Read tests with standard conjugate and with new conjugate by comparing with Minimally Reactive (1+) reading controls tested with their respective conjugates.
4. Record results of all testing.
5. Review test results and determine if new conjugate meets criteria of acceptability.

Preparation of control sera[2]

Control sera of graded reactivity should be included each time serologic testing procedures are performed.

For the nontreponemal flocculation tests with serum and spinal fluid, the antigen suspension to be used each day is first examined with control sera. The results obtained with the controls should reproduce the established reactivity pattern. If the results are not acceptable, routine testing should be delayed until optimal reactivity has been established (by preparing another antigen suspension, correcting room temperature, adjusting equipment, etc.).

For the FTA-ABS test the control sera are included in the test run. If the pattern of reactivity is not acceptable, results of the tests on individual specimens are considered invalid and are **not** reported.

Control sera of graded reactivity for nontreponemal and treponemal test procedures are available from commercial sources or may be prepared from individual sera or sera pooled after testing. Reactive serum of high titer may be used to prepare spinal fluid controls. A pattern of reactivity should be established for each new lot of control serum prepared in the laboratory, or confirmed for each new lot of control serum obtained from a commercial source, by comparing the new control serum with standard control serum.

Control sera for nontreponemal antigen tests[2]

Collection and processing of serum

1. Collect clear sera giving Reactive (not Weakly Reactive) results from daily test runs or from individual donors. Store in Pyrex bottles (or equivalent) in freezer.
2. Collect and store Nonreactive sera in same manner.

Do not collect hemolyzed, contaminated, or chylous sera.

---

*In conformity with the Système International (SI) and to conserve space, the following abbreviations will be used: s, second; h, hour; and d, day.

Table 106-2. Example of results obtained with prepared serum dilutions

Dilution	Reactive serum (ml)	Nonreactive serum (ml)	RPR (circle) card test	USR test	VDRL slide test
1	1.0	1.0	R	R	R
2	0.5	1.5	R	R	R
3	0.25	1.75	R	R	R
4	0.20	1.80	R	R	R
5	0.15	1.85	R	R_m	R_m
6	0.12	1.88	R	W	W
7	0.09	1.91	R_m	W_m	W_m
8	0.06	1.94	N	N	N
9	0.03	1.97	N	N	N
10	0.00	2.00	N	N	N

R = Reactive   N = Nonreactive
W = Weakly Reactive   m = minimal

3. When control sera are to be prepared, thaw serum pools and mix each pool thoroughly.
4. Sterilize by filtration with suitable bacteriologic filter assembly. (To remove coarse, suspended particles that would rapidly clog sterilizing filter, clarifying filter or prefilter may be used in separate unit or superimposed on top of sterilizing filter in same filter holder, e.g., Seitz filters of 1.0 and 0.1 μm porosity.) Filter at refrigerator temperature (preferred) or at room temperature.
5. Measure volume of each filtered serum pool and add 1 mg Merthiolate powder for each ml serum.

Pretesting serum dilutions

1. Prepare preliminary dilutions of Reactive serum in Nonreactive serum (Table 106-2). Serial 2-fold dilutions may also be used. **Serum-in-serum dilutions do not mix as readily as serum-in-saline dilutions; therefore it is necessary to mix these dilutions thoroughly before testing.**

Based on the results indicated in Table 106-2, a set of serum dilutions suitable for the USR and VDRL Slide tests might be selected as follows:

> Control 1—Dilution 4
> Control 2—Dilution 6
> Control 3—Nonreactive pool

> *or*

For the RPR (circle) Card and the VDRL Slide tests:

> Control 1—Dilution 4
> Control 2—Dilution 6
> Control 3—Dilution 7
> Control 4—Nonreactive pool

2. Heat serum dilutions for 30 min at 56 C for VDRL slide test with serum. Do not heat dilutions for USR or RPR card tests.
3. Perform test(s) that are employed in the laboratory on these serum dilutions with antigen suspensions that reproduce reactivity patterns of standard control sera. Record test results.
4. Select 1 dilution that is a clear-cut Reactive and at least 1 dilution that shows intermediate reactivity for each test. If several tests are employed, 2 or more dilutions may be required to obtain intermediate reactivity in all tests.

Preparation of control sera

1. Calculate amount of each serum dilution to be prepared. This will be determined by quantity needed for each day's testing, period of time dur-

ing which controls will be used, and type of storage facility available. Control sera, properly stoppered, may be stored for 2-3 mo in freezer or 1 mo in freezing compartment of refrigerator.

2. Prepare calculated volumes of each serum dilution. Mix thoroughly by placing serum pool in Erlenmeyer flask or wide-diameter bottle having capacity 3-5 times volume of pool. Rotate flask on mechanical slide rotator for 30-60 min at approximately 100 rpm or mix with a magnetic stirrer. **Avoid foaming.**

3. Test a sample from each serum mixture in all of the tests in which it is to be used as a control. If necessary, adjust pools to higher or lower reactivity by addition of small quantity of Reactive or Nonreactive serum as required. Mix thoroughly and retest.

4. Dispense quantities of each dilution, **sufficient for 1 testing period,** into properly labeled tubes and stopper tightly with paraffin-coated corks. (Small Vacutainers [Becton, Dickinson & Co., Rutherford, N.J.] or equivalent may be used.)

5. Combine in sets and place in freezer.

6. Reset corks after 24 h and return sets to freezer.

Establishing pattern of reactivity

1. Remove a set of new control sera from freezer, thaw, and mix thoroughly.

2. Perform tests for which patterns are to be established on new control sera with antigen suspensions that reproduce reactivity patterns on standard control sera.

3. Repeat tests on 2 additional d with different set of new control sera on each testing day.

4. Compare results obtained in 3 testing runs.
   a. If identical results are obtained, no further testing is necessary.
   b. If discrepant results are obtained, perform additional testing as indicated to establish reactivity pattern.

Routine use of control serum

1. Each day tests are to be performed, remove 1 set of control sera from freezer, thaw, and mix thoroughly. Control sera must be at room temperature when tested.

2. Check reactivity of test antigen suspension with control sera as described in test technic

3. **Do not use** an antigen suspension that does **not** reproduce the established reactivity pattern of the control sera. If necessary, prepare a new antigen suspension that reproduces the reactivity pattern of control sera before performing routine tests on specimens.

Control sera for FTA-ABS test

Selection and preparation of reactive and nonspecific serum for controls

1. For Reactive control serum, select individual Reactice sera from FTA-ABS rest runs, or from individual syphilitic donors, that are Reactive 4+ when diluted in PBS and are no less than 3+ to 4+ when diluted in sorbent. Selected Reactive sera may be pooled and stored in freezer.

2. For Nonspecific control serum, collect individual tubes of Nonreactive sera from FTA-ABS test runs or from individual nonsyphilitic donors. Pretest for Nonspecific reactivity by testing each serum diluted 1:5 in both PBS and sorbent. Select sera that are Reactive 2+ or greater when diluted in PBS and Nonreactive (complete absence of fluorescence) when diluted in sorbent. Selected Nonspecific sera may be pooled and stored in freezer.

Do not collect hemolyzed, contaminated, or chylous sera.

3. When control sera are to be prepared, process sera as given in Control Sera for Nontreponemal Antigen Tests, Collection and Processing of Serum, Steps 3-5, in quantities sufficient for 2-3 mo.

4. Confirm reactivity of processed Reactive and Nonspecific sera diluted 1:5 in both PBS and sorbent.

5. Dispense quantities of Reactive serum and Nonspecific serum sufficient for 1 testing period (0.3-0.4 ml) into properly labeled tubes and stopper tightly with paraffin-coated corks (small Vacutainers or equivalent may be used).

6. Combine in sets and store in freezer.

Pretesting for minimally reactive (1+) control

1. Heat standard control sera and new Reactive serum at 56 C for 30 min.

2. To determine range of reactivity of new Reactive serum, prepare serial 2-fold dilutions of serum from 1:100 to 1:3200 in PBS.

3. Add 0.03 ml serum dilution to correspondingly labeled antigen slides and complete tests, as described in Steps 6-20 of the FTA-ABS Test on Serum.

4. Set up standard controls for FTA-ABS test.

5. Read and compare reactivity of each dilution against Minimally Reactive (1+) control.

6. Select dilutions of new Reactive serum that approximate degree of fluorescence of **standard** Minimally Reactive (1+) control serum.

7. Prepare and test additional intermediate dilutions in indicated range to obtain one with identical reactivity to standard Minimally Reactive (1+) control serum.

Establishing pattern of reactivity

1. Remove a set of new control sera and a set of standard control sera from freezer; thaw, mix thoroughly, and heat at 56 C for 30 min.

2. Reactive control serum
   a. Dilute new Reactive serum 1:5 in both PBS and sorbent.
   b. Prepare 3 dilutions of Reactive serum in PBS; one should be that dilution selected in pretesting that corresponds to standard Minimally Reactive (1+) control serum; other 2 should be a dilution slightly above and a dilution slightly below the selected dilution.

3. Dilute Nonspecific control serum 1:5 in both PBS and sorbent.

4. Perform tests on new control sera and standard control sera according to directions for testing controls in FTA-ABS technic.

5. Verify reactivity by repeat testing on at least 2 additional d; use a different set of new control sera on each testing day.

6. Compare results obtained in the 3 test runs.
   a. If identical results are obtained, no further testing is necessary.
   b. If discrepant results are obtained, perform additional testing as indicated to establish reactivity pattern.

Control sera for serologic tests on spinal fluid specimens

1. Select an individual serum or serum pool that is Reactive in spinal fluid test when diluted 1:80 or higher in 0.9% saline.

2. Dispense small quantities of Reactive serum, sufficient for 1 testing period, into labeled tubes and stopper tightly with paraffin-coated corks

(small Vacutainers of equivalent may be used). Store in freezer.

3. After 3 or more d storage, thaw 1 tube of Reactive serum and mix thoroughly.
4. Prepare serial dilutions of serum in 0.9% saline; start at 1:80.
5. Test serum dilutions in parallel with standard controls by using spinal fluid technic.
6. Select 3 serum dilutions that produce Reactive, Minimally Reactive, and Nonreactive test results. respectively.
7. Confirm reactivity pattern of these 3 dilutions by testing in parallel with standard controls on at least 3 testing days. Use a different tube of new control serum each test day.

Proficiency testing study samples[2]

Syphilis serology proficiency testing study samples may be prepared similarly to control serums of graded reactivity. It is recommended that these be distributed monthly or bimonthly to participating laboratories and that a set of standard control sera of graded reactivity be included with the first set of proficiency testing samples and periodically thereafter, if possible. These proficiency testing samples should be of graded reactivity for each test in the study, and all or part of the samples should be submitted in duplicate. The recommended range of reactivity in each year's study is this: Reactive, not more than 40%; intermediate or Weakly Reactive, 20-30%; and Nonreactive, 30-40%.

Source
1. Reactive and Nonreactive sera may be collected from daily test runs and stored in freezer.
2. Blood may be obtained from individual donors and processed to separate serum. (Plasma from blood banks has been satisfactory when treated as follows: add 4-5 g kaolin to 30 ml of plasma and shake well to form chalky white suspension. Refrigerate at 2-10 C for 48 h and shake occasionally. Recover plasma by centrifugation.) Store in freezer.

Processing and distribution of prepared serum samples
1. When proficiency testing samples are to be prepared, process sera as for Control Serums for Nontreponemal Antigen Tests, Collection and Processing of Serum, Steps 3-5.

Observe sterile precautions with pools of Reactive and Nonreactive serums.
2. Prepare preliminary dilutions of Reactive serum in Nonreactive serum and perform all tests included in study on each dilution.
3. Select appropriate dilutions of graded reactivity. Choose dilutions that are clear-cut in reactivity and on which reproducible results can be obtained.
4. Calculate amount of each serum dilution needed for study. This will depend on number of participating laboratories and use of single or duplicate samples.
5. Prepare serum pools of calculated volumes needed for use in study by diluting Reactive in Nonreactive serum and mixing thoroughly. Nonreactive pool may be used for some specimens. These pools should be sterile.
6. Test duplicate samples of each serum pool with each of tests to be included in study. If necessary,

adjust pool to higher or lower reactivity and test new samples.
7. Observe sterile precautions in dispensing samples of prepared serum to tubes with prenumbered, gummed labels (Professional Tape Co., Riverside, Ill.). Vacutainers (or equivalent) or tubes with paraffin-coated corks or screw caps may be used.
   NOTE: At the Venereal Disease Research Laboratory, serum pools are dispensed through a closed system from an aspirator bottle (fitted with rubber tubing attached to a 20-gauge, 1 in. needle) into 2 ml Vacutainers.
8. Check samples for sterility before distribution (tubed samples may be placed in 35 C incubator for 24 h and examined for contaminating growth).
9. Test a tubed sample of each serum pool to determine if changes in reactivity have occurred.
10. Package samples in careful, orderly manner with checks to prevent errors. Include instructions for heating, suggested date for testing, required date for return of test results, and report forms.
11. Ship samples so that they will not arrive at their destination on a weekend or holiday.

Collection, submission, and processing of specimens[2]
Collection and submission of specimens

Blood specimens for RPR (circle) Card, USR, VDRL Slide, and FTA-ABS tests
1. Syringes, needles, and collection tubes should be clean, dry, and sterile to prevent contamination and hemolysis of specimen. Vacutainers (or equivalent) or tubes with corks may be used and should have labels attached securely for patient identification.
2. Draw at least 5-8 ml blood, place in tube, and allow to clot at room temperature. Blood should not be taken for 1 h after a meal to avoid chylous serum. Identify specimen with name of patient immediately after collection to avoid error.
3. Store specimens in refrigerator until sent to laboratory and do not place them in the mail over long weekends or holidays when delivery may be delayed. Stopper specimen tube tightly; wrap carefully in cotton or some other suitable material to prevent breakage and absorb any leaking fluid and include request slip identifying patient and specific test(s) desired. Ship specimens in mailing cartons approved by postal service.
4. If **serum** is sent to laboratory, submit information as to whether or not it has been heated (time and temperature) and if preservatives have been added.

Spinal fluid specimens for VDRL Slide test and total protein determination
1. Collection tubes should be clean, dry, and sterile (Merthiolated tubes may be prepared for collection of specimens; see below).
2. Aseptically collect approximately 5 ml spinal fluid. Identify specimen tube with name of patient.
3. If specimen is to be centrifuged before sending to laboratory, note on request slip the original condition or appearance of specimen.
4. Package specimen tube and request slip and ship as for blood specimen.

Use of Merthiolate as a bacteriostatic agent

Grossly contaminated serum or spinal fluid specimens are unsatisfactory for testing in serologic tests for syphilis because of the unpredictable effect of contamination on test reactivity. Although specimens are usually drawn with reasonable attention to sterility, many specimens mailed to central testing laboratories, especially during the warmer months, show evidence of gross bacterial contamination on arrival. Removal of bacteria from contaminated specimens by centrifuging or filtration is ineffective, since products of bacterial metabolism remaining in the supernatant fluid may alter reactivity.

Harris and Mahoney[24] reported on the use of dry Merthiolate as a bacteriostatic agent for spinal fluid preservation. The compound (sodium ethylmercurithiosalicylate) curtails bacterial growth without interfering with the mechanisms of the usual serologic tests for syphilis either through chemical action or the introduction of a dilution factor. Furthermore, its presence does not affect the results obtained with the turbidimetric methods for determining total proteins in spinal fluids. Collection tubes containing Merthiolate are prepared as follows:

1. Prepare necessary amount of Merthiolate solution on the day it is to be used by adding 1.0 g Merthiolate powder to each 100 ml distilled water. Do not use commercially prepared tinctures or solutions.
2. Pipet 0.1 ml 1% aqueous Merthiolate solution to bottom of sterile 13 × 100 mm tubes. Place tubes in vacuum dessicator over calcium chloride at room temperature and protect from light. Dehydration will be complete in 24-48 h or less if adequate vacuum is established.
3. Prepare paraffin-coated corks by submerging corks in hot, but not smoking, paraffin for 1 min and removing excess paraffin by rolling corks on heavy paper or cloth while hot.
4. Remove tubes from dessicator and stopper tightly with paraffin-coated corks.
5. Store tubes in dark. They will remain usable for several months.

The concentration of Merthiolate obtained when 2.0-8.0 ml spinal fluid or serum is added to these tubes is sufficient to inhibit most bacterial growth.

Preparation of specimens for testing

Number specimen tubes with prenumbered self-adhesive labels (Flex material, K1 adhesive, Avery Label Co., Monrovia, Calif.) that can be transferred from tube to tube with the specimen as it is being processed. Do not use wax pencil numbers, names, etc., for identification, since these can be smudged or wiped off, resulting in a possible error in identification.

Processing
1. Centrifuge specimens and decant clear serum or spinal fluid to clean tube; transfer numbered label with specimens.
2. Specimens to be heated at 56 C before testing should be at room temperature (23-29 C) when placed in water bath.
3. Thaw frozen specimens and mix thoroughly before heating or testing.
4. Allow specimens to return to room temperature before testing (10-30 min after thawing or heating).
5. Examine all specimens and recentrifuge those found to contain particulate debris.

Criteria of acceptability
1. Serum specimens that are excessively hemolyzed, grossly contaminated with bacteria, or extremely turbid are unsatisfactory for testing. An acceptable specimen should not contain particulate matter that would interfere with reading test results. A specimen is too hemolyzed for testing when printed matter cannot be read through it.
   NOTE: **Hemolysis may be caused by wet or dirty syringes, needles, or tubes; chemicals; freezing or extreme heat.**
2. Spinal fluids that are grossly contaminated with blood or bacteria are unsatisfactory for testing.
3. Do not test specimens that are not acceptable for testing but report as **Unsatisfactory.** Note condition of specimen on report form.

Nontreponemal antigen tests

FLOCCULATION TESTS

The VDRL (Venereal Disease Research Laboratory) test detects the presence of syphilitic reagin by means of a reaction between reagin and a standard antigen. The antigen used in this test is composed of cardiolipin and lecithin that have been extracted from beef heart and purified. Cholesterol is added to the alcoholic mixture of the cardiolipin and lecithin for the purpose of increasing the antigen's effective reacting surface.

Syphilitic reagin is capable of producing changes in the dispersion of the cardiolipin-lecithin antigen that result in visible **flocculation.** The tests, as described below, have been carefully standardized, and it is mandatory that the technics be adhered to as outlined.

VDRL slide tests[2]

Before performing these tests consult the section on General Rules for Syphilis Tests.

Equipment and glassware
1. Rotating machine, adjustable to 180 rpm, circumscribing a circle ¾ inch in diameter on a horizontal plane
2. Ringmaker, to make paraffin rings approximately 14 mm in diameter
3. Slide holder, for 2 × 3 inch microscope slides
4. Hypodermic needles, without bevels
   a. For serum test: 18-, 19-, and 23-gauge
   b. For spinal fluid test: 21- or 22-gauge
5. Slides, 2 × 3 inch, with 12 paraffin or ceramic rings,* approximately 14 mm in diameter, for serum test
6. Slides,† agglutination, approximately 2 × 3 inch, with concavities measuring 16 mm in diameter and 1.75 mm in depth, for spinal fluid test
7. Syringe, Luer-type, 1 or 2 ml
8. Bottles‡: 30 ml, round, glass stoppered, narrow

---

*Glass slides with ceramic rings may also be used with the following precautions. Rings must be high enough to prevent spillage when slides are rotated at prescribed speed. Slides must be cleaned so that serum will spread to inner surfaces of ceramic rings. This type of slide should be discarded if or when ceramic rings begin to flake off.
†Clay-Adams, New York (catalog no. A-1474 or A-1474/X).
‡Corning Glass Works, Corning, New York (catalog no. LG-1, MW-90530).

mouth, approximately 35 mm in diameter, with flat interbottom surfaces (NOTE: Some of the bottles now available are unsatisfactory for preparing antigen suspension because of the convex interbottom surface that causes saline to be distributed only at periphery.)

Reagents

1. VDRL antigen*
   a. The antigen is a colorless, alcoholic solution containing 0.03% cardiolipin, 0.9% cholesterol, and sufficient purified lecithin to produce standard reactivity. During recent years, this amount of lecithin has been 0.21% ± 0.01%. Each lot of antigen must be serologically standardized by proper comparison with an antigen of known reactivity.
   b. Antigen is dispensed in screw-capped (Vinylite liners) bottles or hermetically sealed glass ampules and should be stored in the dark at either refrigerator (6-10 C) or room temperature. Components of this antigen remain in solution at these temperatures, so that any precipitate noted will indicate changes resulting from factors such as evaporation or additive materials contributed by pipets. Antigen that contains precipitate should be discarded.
   c. A new lot of antigen should be compared with an antigen of standard reactivity before being placed in routine use (see Check Testing Nontreponemal [cardiolipin] Test Antigens, above).
2. VDRL buffered saline containing 1% sodium chloride, pH 6.0 ± 0.1

Formaldehyde, neutral (A.C.S.)	0.5 ml
Secondary sodium phosphate, anhydrous (A.C.S.), (Na$_2$HPO$_4$)	0.037 g
Primary potassium phosphate, (A.C.S.) (KH$_2$PO$_4$)	0.170 g
Sodium chloride (A.C.S.)	10 g
Distilled water	1000 ml

   a. Check pH of solution and store in screw-capped or glass-stoppered bottles. (NOTE: When an unexplained change in test reactivity occurs, check pH of VDRL buffered saline to determine if this is a contributing factor. Saline outside range of pH 6.0 ± 0.1 should be discarded.)
3. Saline, 0.9%
   a. Add 900 mg dry sodium chloride (ACS) to each 100 ml distilled water.
4. Saline, 10%
   a. Add 10 g dry sodium chloride (ACS) to each 100 ml distilled water.

VDRL slide tests with serum

Antigen suspension

Temperature of buffered saline and antigen should be in the range of 73-85 F (23-29 C) at time antigen suspension is prepared.

1. Pipet 0.4 ml buffered saline to bottom of a 30 ml, round, glass-stoppered bottle.
2. Add 0.5 ml antigen (from lower half of 1.0 ml pipet graduated to tip) directly onto saline while continuously but gently rotating bottle on flat surface.

NOTE: Antigen is added drop by drop, but rapidly, so that approximately 6 s are allowed for each 0.5 ml antigen. Pipet tip should remain in upper third of bottle, and rotation should not be vigorous enough to splash saline onto pipet. Proper speed of rotation is obtained when center of bottle circumscribes a 2 in. diameter circle approximately 3 times/s.

3. Blow last drop of antigen from pipet without touching pipet to saline.
4. Continue rotation of bottle for 10 s.
5. Add 4.1 ml buffered saline from 5 ml pipet.
6. Place top on bottle and shake from bottom to top and back approximately 30 times in 10 s.
7. Antigen suspension is ready for use and may be used during 1 d.
8. Double volume of antigen suspension may be prepared at 1 time by using doubled quantities of antigen and saline. A 10 ml pipet should be used for delivering the 8.2 ml vol saline. If larger quantities are required, more than 1 antigen suspension should be prepared. Test these suspensions with control sera and pool the ones with satisfactory reactivity.
9. Mix antigen suspension gently each time it is used. Do not mix suspension by forcing back and forth through syringe and needle, since this may cause breakdown of particles and loss of reactivity.

Testing accuracy of delivery needles

1. Needles used each day should be checked. Practice will allow rapid delivery of antigen suspension and saline, but care should be exercised to obtain drops of uniform size.
2. For slide qualitative test on serum, dispense antigen suspension from syringe fitted with 18-gauge needle without bevel that will deliver 60 drops ± 2 drops antigen suspension/ml when syringe and needle are held vertically.
3. For slide quantitative test on serum, dispense antigen suspensions from syringe fitted with 19-gauge needle without bevel that will deliver 75 drops ± 2 drops of antigen suspension/ml when syringe and needle are held vertically. (Saline may be delivered from 19-gauge needle [0.02 ml/drop] and 15-gauge needle [0.03 ml/drop].)
4. For slide quantitative test on serum, dispense 0.9% saline from syringe fitted with 23-gauge needle (with or without bevel) that will deliver 100 drops ± 2 drops saline/ml when syringe and needle are held vertically.
5. Adjust needles not meeting these specifications to deliver correct volumes before being used (see Preparation and Calibration of Needles for Slide Flocculation Tests, above).

Preliminary testing of antigen suspension

1. Test control sera* of graded reactivity as described under VDRL Slide Qualitative Test on Serum. Whole serum controls may be prepared as described under Control Sera for Nontreponemal Antigen Tests.
2. Reactions with control sera should reproduce established reactivity pattern. Nonreactive serum should show complete dispersion of antigen particles.
3. Do not use an unsatisfactory antigen suspension or pool of antigen suspensions.

---

*Antigen can be obtained from the following manufacturers: BBL, Division of BioQuest, Cockeysville, Md.; Difco Laboratories, Detroit; Hyland Division, Travenol Laboratories, Costa Mesa, Calif.; Lederle Laboratories, Pearl River, N.Y.; The Sylvana Co., Millburn, N.J.; Texas Biological Laboratories, Fort Worth, Tex.

---

*BBL, Division of BioQuest, Cockeysville, Md.; Dade Reagents, Miami; Difco Laboratories, Detroit; and Hyland Division, Travenol Laboratories, Los Angeles.

NOTE: Control sera of graded reactivity (Reactive, Weakly Reactive, and Nonreactive) are always included during testing period to ensure proper reactivity of antigen suspension at time tests are performed.

Preparation of serum

1. Heat clear serum, obtained from centrifuged, clotted blood, in 56 C water bath for 30 min before testing.
2. Examine all sera when removed from water bath and recentrifuge those found to contain particulate debris.
3. Reheat at 56 C for 10 min those sera to be tested more than 4 h after original heating period.
4. When tested, sera must be at room temperature.

VDRL slide qualitative test with serum

Slide flocculation tests for syphilis are affected by room temperature. For reliable and reproducible results, tests should be performed within temperature range of 73-85 F (23-29 C). At lower temperatures, test reactivity is decreased; at higher temperatures, test reactivity is increased.

Procedure

1. Pipet 0.05 ml heated serum into 1 ring of paraffin-ringed or ceramic-ringed slide.
Glass slides with concavities, wells, or glass rings are not recommended for this test.
2. Add 1 drop (1/60 ml) antigen suspension onto each serum with 18-gauge needle and syringe.
3. Rotate slides for 4 min. (Mechanical rotators that circumscribe a ¾ in. diameter circle should be set at 180 rpm.)
When tests are performed in a dry climate, slides may be covered with box lid containing moistened blotter during rotation to prevent excessive evaporation.
4. Read tests microscopically with 10× ocular and 10× objective, immediately after rotation.
5. Report results as follows:

Reading	*Report*	
Medium and large clumps	Reactive	(R)
Small clumps	Weakly Reactive	(W)
No clumping or very slight roughness	Nonreactive	(N)

6. **A prozone reaction** is encountered occasionally. This type of reaction is demonstrated when complete or partial inhibition of reactivity occurs with undiluted serum and maximum reactivity is obtained only with diluted serum. This prozone phenomenon may be so pronounced that only a Weakly Reactive or "rough" Nonreactive result is produced in the qualitative test by a serum that will be strongly Reactive when diluted.
It is recommended **that all sera producing Weakly Reactive or "rough" Nonreactive results in qualitative test be retested by using quantitative procedure before a report of the VDRL slide test is submitted.** When a Reactive result is obtained on some dilution of a serum that produced only a Weakly Reactive or "rough" Nonreactive result before dilution, report test as Reactive and include quantitative titer (see examples, Step 12, VDRL Slide Quantitative Test on Serum).

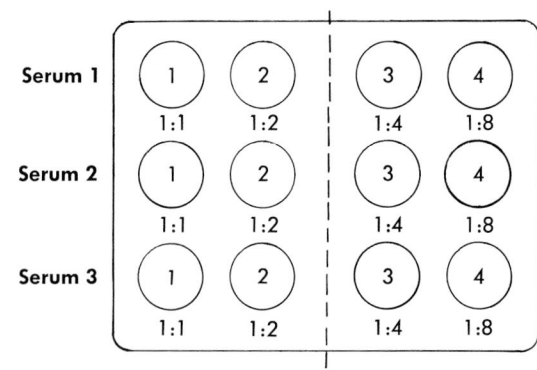

Fig. 106-2. Diagram of slide for quantitative VDRL Slide test. (From 1975 Identical memorandum, Atlanta, 1975, Bureau of Laboratories, Center for Disease Control.)

VDRL slide quantitative test on serum (safety pipetor method)[25]

Test quantitatively, **to an end-point titer,** all sera that produce Reactive, Weakly Reactive, or "rough" Nonreactive results in the **qualitative VDRL slide test.** The dilutions of the serum to be tested are undiluted (1:1), 1:2, 1:4, etc. Three serum quantitative tests through 1:8 dilution (Fig. 106-2) or 2 serum quantitative tests through 1:32 dilution (Fig. 106-3) may be performed on 1 slide.

Procedure

1. Select tubes of serum for quantitation and place in rack.
2. Measure 0.05 ml of 0.9% saline onto second, third, and fourth paraffin rings in row on slide. Do not spread saline. Saline may be delivered from 18-gauge needle without point (0.025 ml/drop; use 2 drops), or use large needle or calibrated dropper that delivers 0.05 ml in a single drop; these should be checked daily for accuracy of delivery.
3. Using safety pipetor device with disposable tip (should deliver 0.05 ml or 50 μl), measure 0.05 ml of serum to first and second rings. Avoid contamination of instrument with serum.
4. Use same pipetor and tip to prepare serial 2-fold dilutions by drawing serum/saline mixture up and down in tip 5 or 6 times. Avoid excess bubbles. (Use clean plastic tip for each serum tested.)
5. Mix serum and saline in ring 2 (1:2 dil); transfer 0.05 ml of 1:2 dilution to ring 3 and mix (1:4 dil); transfer 0.05 ml of 1:4 dilution to ring 4, mix (1:8 dil), and discard 0.05 ml. Additional serial dilutions may be set up for strongly reactive sera. (If the 0.05 ml of serum dilution has not spread within entire area of paraffin ring, spread this with pipetor tip before proceeding to next ring.)
6. Add 1 drop (1/60 ml) of VDRL antigen suspension to each ring with 18-gauge needle and syringe (used for antigen suspension in qualitative test).
7. Rotate slides for 4 min (mechanical rotators that circumscribe a ¾ in. diameter circle should be set at 180 rpm).
NOTE: When tests are performed in a dry climate, slides may be covered with moisture chamber during rotation to prevent excessive evaporation.

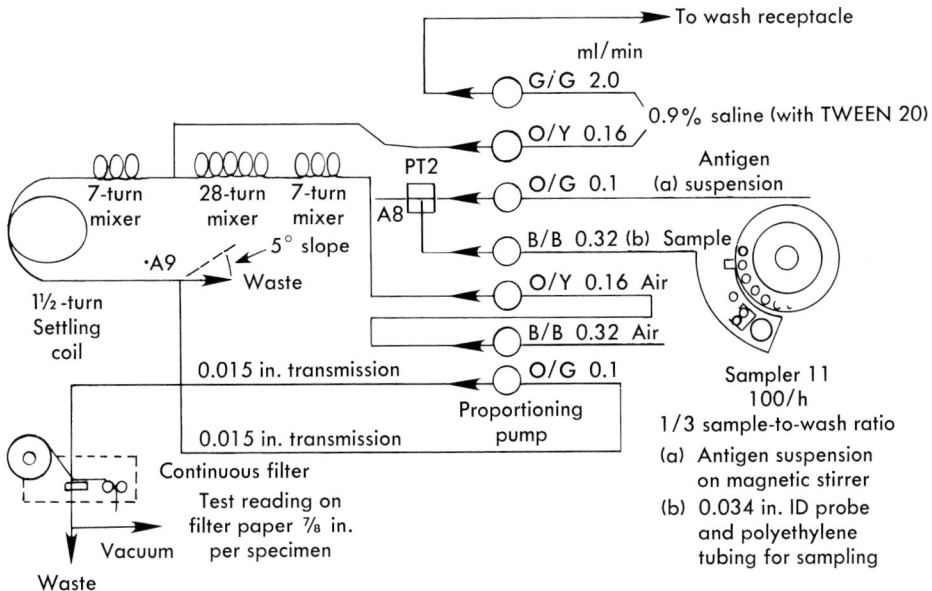

Fig. 106-3. Flow diagram: automated reagin test (ART) for syphilis. (Courtesy Technicon Corp., Tarrytown, N.Y.)

8. Read tests microscopically with 10× ocular and 10× objective immediately after rotation. Record reading for each dilution tested.

9. Report titer in terms of greatest serum dilution that produces a Reactive (not Weakly Reactive) result, in accordance with the examples shown at the bottom of the page.

VDRL slide tests with spinal fluid

Preparation of "sensitized antigen suspension"

1. Prepare antigen suspension as described for VDRL Slide tests (see Antigen Suspension).

2. Add 1 part 10% saline to 1 part VDRL slide test suspension.

3. Mix by gently rotating bottle or inverting tube and allow to stand at least 5 min but not more than 2 h before use.

Testing of delivery needles

1. It is of primary importance that the proper amount of reagent be used, and for this reason needles used each day should be checked. Practice will allow rapid delivery of antigen suspension, but care should be exercised to obtain drops of uniform size.

2. For slide qualitative and quantitative tests on spinal fluid, dispense sensitized antigen suspension from syringe fitted with a 21- or 22-gauge needle that will deliver 100 drops ± 2 drops sensitized antigen suspension/ml when syringe and needle are held vertically.

3. Adjust needles not meeting these specifications to deliver correct volume before being used (see Preparation and Calibration of Needles for Slide Flocculation Tests).

Preliminary testing of sensitized antigen suspension

1. Satisfactory control sera* for spinal fluid test are conveniently prepared by diluting serum in 0.9% saline (see Control Sera for Serologic Tests on Spinal Fluid Specimens).

2. For daily use, remove 1 tube of Reactive control serum from freezer, thaw, and mix thoroughly. Prepare designated serum dilutions in 0.9% saline. Controls are tested without preliminary heating in slide test.

3. Test control serum dilutions as described under VDRL Slide Qualitative Test on Spinal Fluid.

4. Reactions on control serum dilutions should reproduce established reactivity pattern, and Nonreactive dilution should show complete dispersion of antigen particles.

5. Do not use an unsatisfactory sensitized antigen suspension.

NOTE: Control serum dilutions of graded reactivity (Reactive, Minimally Reactive, and Nonreactive) are always included during testing period to ensure proper reactivity of sensitized antigen suspension at time tests are performed.

*BBL, Division of Bio-Quest, Cockeysville, Md.

Undiluted Serum (1:1)	Serum dilutions					Report
	1:2	1:4	1:8	1:16	1:32	
R	W	N	N	N	N	Reactive, undiluted only, or 1 dil
R	R	W	N	N	N	Reactive, 1:2 dilution, or 2 dils
R	R	R	W	N	N	Reactive, 1:4 dilution, or 4 dils
W	W	R	R	W	N	Reactive, 1:8 dilution, or 8 dils
N (rough)	W	R	R	R	N	Reactive, 1:16 dilution, or 16 dils
W	N	N	N	N	N	Weakly Reactive, undiluted only, or 0 dils

Preparation of spinal fluid. Centrifuge and decant each spinal fluid. The spinal fluid is tested without preliminary heating. Spinal fluids that are visibly contaminated or contain gross blood are unsatisfactory for testing.

VDRL slide qualitative test on spinal fluid

Slide flocculation tests for syphilis are affected by room temperature. For reliable and reproducible results, tests should be performed within temperature range of 73-85 F (23-29 C). At lower temperatures, test reactivity is decreased; at higher temperatures, test reactivity is increased.

1. Pipet 0.05 ml spinal fluid into 1 concavity of agglutination slide.
2. Add 1 drop (0.01 ml) sensitized antigen suspension to each spinal fluid with 21- or 22-gauge needle.
3. Rotate slides for 8 min on mechanical rotator at 180 rpm.

When tests are performed in a dry climate, slides may be covered with box lid containing moistened blotter during rotation to prevent evaporation.

4. Read tests microscopically with a 10× ocular and a 10× objective immediately after rotation.
5. Report results as follows:

Reading	Report	
Definite clumping	Reactive	(R)
No clumping or very slight roughness	Nonreactive	(N)

VDRL slide quantitative test on spinal fluid

Quantitative tests are performed on all spinal fluids found to be Reactive in the qualitative test.

1. Prepare spinal fluid dilutions as follows:
   a. Pipet 0.2 ml 0.9% saline into each of 5 or more tubes.
   b. Add 0.2 ml unheated spinal fluid to tube 1, mix well, and transfer 0.2 ml to tube 2.
   c. Continue mixing and transferring 0.2 ml from 1 tube to the next until last tube is reached. The respective dilutions are 1:2, 1:4, 1:8, 1:16, 1:32, etc.
2. Test each spinal fluid dilution and undiluted spinal fluid as described under VDRL Slide Qualitative Test on Spinal Fluid.
3. Report results in terms of the greatest spinal fluid dilution (dils) that produces a Reactive result.

Rapid reagin tests[26]

The rapid reagin tests are performed on unheated serum or plasma, simplifying the processing of specimens.

The antigen used is a modified VDRL antigen suspension with choline chloride and EDTA added; the RPR card test antigen also contains charcoal for making macroscopic reading possible.

Rapid plasma reagin (RPR) test.[27] The original test used unmeasured amounts of plasma and was used as a field procedure for screening large numbers of persons. The test proved to be about 10% more reactive than the VDRL slide test.

Unheated serum reagin (USR) test.[28] The USR is a modification of the RPR test. It has a somewhat lower level of reactivity than the VDRL slide test. The test is performed on measured volumes of unheated serum.

RPR (circle) Card test.[29] Testing is performed on unheated serum (less often on plasma) and is performed in the laboratory instead of the field. The card used for the test is rotated on a mechanical rotator, and the tests are read macroscopically (the antigen contains charcoal).

The test is about as specific and sensitive as the VDRL Slide test. In fact, there are indications that the test may be more sensitive than the VDRL Slide test, as shown by testing specimens that were VDRL nonreactive and RPR (circle) Card test reactive, with the FTA-ABS test; thus the RPR (circle) Card test may detect more cases of syphilis than the VDRL test.[30]

Automated reagin test (ART). See below.

Unheated serum reagin (USR) test on serum[2,27,28]

Before performing this test, consult section on general rules for syphilis tests.

Equipment and glassware
1. Centrifuge, angle-head: Sorvall SS-1, type XL (Ivan Sorvall, Norwalk, Conn.), or equivalent, and tachometer
2. Tubes (Ivan Sorvall, Norwalk, Conn.), stainless-steel, 50 ml capacity, without flange
3. Cotton gauze
4. Rotating machine, adjustable to 180 rpm, circumscribing a circle ¾ in. in diameter on a horizontal plane
5. Ringmaker, to make paraffin rings approximately 14 mm in diameter
6. Slide holder, for 2 × 3 inch microscope slides
7. Hypodermic needle, 18-gauge, without bevel
8. Slides,* 2 × 3 inch, with paraffin rings approximately 14 mm in diameter
9. Syringe, Luer-type, 1 or 2 ml
10. Bottles, 30 ml, round, glass stoppered, narrow mouth, approximately 35 mm in diameter, with flat innerbottom surface

Some of the bottles now available are unsatisfactory for preparing antigen suspension because of the convex innerbottom surface that causes the saline to be distributed only at the periphery.

Reagents
1. VDRL antigen
2. VDRL buffered saline
3. Phosphate (0.02M), Merthiolate (0.2%) solution
   a. Dissolve 1.42 g Na_2HPO_4, 1.36 g KH_2PO_4, and 1.00 g Merthiolate in distilled water to final volume of 500 ml. The pH of this solution should be 6.9. Store in dark at room temperature. May be used for a period of 3 mo.
4. Choline chloride solution (40%)
   a. Because of its hygroscopic nature, entire contents of previously unopened bottle may be used in preparing solution. Example: dissolve

---

*Glass slides with ceramic rings may also be used with the following precautions. Rings must be high enough to prevent spillage when slides are rotated at prescribed speed. Slides must be cleaned so that serum will spread to inner surfaces of ceramic rings. This type of slide should be discarded if or when ceramic rings begin to flake off.

entire contents of 250 g bottle of choline chloride in distilled water to final volume of 625 ml.

    b. Filter and store at room temperature. May be used for 1 y. Refilter if visible particles form.

5. EDTA (0.1M)

    a. Dissolve 3.72 g EDTA ([ethylenedinitrol] tetraacetic acid, disodium salt) to volume of 100 ml in distilled water. May be used for 1 y.

6. Resuspending solution

To prepare 10 ml resuspending solution, combine the following:

0.1M EDTA	1.25 ml
Choline chloride (40%)	2.5 ml
Phosphate (0.02M), Merthiolate (0.2%)	5.0 ml
Distilled water	1.25 ml

    a. **Prepare this solution each time antigen suspensions are made.**

Preparation of antigen suspension*

1. Prepare antigen suspension as for VDRL Slide tests.

Bulk batches of 100 ml VDRL antigen suspension may be prepared for USR antigen suspension in a 250 ml glass-stoppered Pyrex bottle (or equivalent) by using appropriate amounts of antigen and buffered saline. Add antigen rapidly with 10 ml pipet directly onto buffered saline while continuously rotating bottle. Time and speeds of rotation and shaking after addition of antigen are same as for VDRL antigen suspension preparation.

2. Centrifuge measured amounts of antigen suspension in stainless-steel tubes in angle centrifuge at room temperature at relative centrifugal force of approximately $2000 \times g$ for 15 min. Start timing when centrifuge reaches desired speed. Centrifuge from 5-30 ml in single centrifuge tube.

3. Locate sediment and decant supernatant fluid by inverting tube away from side containing sediment. While holding tube in an inverted position, wipe inside with cotton gauze without disturbing sediment.

4. Resuspend with a volume of **resuspending solution** equal to that of original volume of antigen suspension that was centrifuged.

5. If more than 1 centrifuge tube is used, combine all suspensions in bottle, stopper tightly, and shake gently a few seconds to obtain an even suspension. This is the completed antigen suspension.

6. A new lot of antigen suspension should be compared with an antigen suspension of known reactivity before being placed in routine use (see Check Testing Nontreponemal [Cardiolipin] Test Antigens).

7. Store antigen suspension at 3-10 C. Antigen suspension stored in this manner has been found to give satisfactory results for at least 6 mo. However, do not use antigen suspension if, at any time, expected results are not obtained with control sera of graded reactivity.

Testing accuracy of delivery needles

1. It is of primary importance that proper amounts of reagents be used, and for this reason, needles used should be checked each day. Practice will allow rapid delivery of antigen suspension, but care should be exercised to obtain drops of uniform size.

2. For USR test, dispense antigen suspension from syringe fitted with 18-gauge needle without bevel that will deliver 45 drops ± 1 drop antigen suspension/ml when checked with 1 or 2 ml syringe held vertically.

3. Adjust needles not meeting these specifications to deliver correct volume before using (see Preparation and Calibration of Needles for Slide Flocculation Tests).

Preliminary testing of antigen suspension

1. For daily use, withdraw sufficient antigen suspension from stock bottle for 2 d testing and return stock bottle to refrigerator. Keep antigen suspension at room temperature for not less than 30 min before it is used.

2. Test control sera* of graded reactivity each day as described under Unheated Serum Reagin (USR) Test on Serum. Whole serum controls may be prepared as described under Control Sera For Nontreponemal Antigen Tests.

3. Reactions with control sera should reproduce established reactivity pattern. Nonreactive serum should show complete dispersion of antigen particles.

4. Do not use an unsatisfactory antigen suspension.

Preparation of sera

1. Centrifuge blood specimens at room temperature at a force sufficient to separate serum from cellular elements. Generally, a force of 1500-2000 rpm for 5 min is adequate.

2. Sera may be retained in original collection tube. NOTE: Sera are tested without heating and should be at 73-85 F (23-29 C) at time of testing.

USR test on serum

Slide flocculation tests for syphilis are affected by room temperature. For reliable, reproducible results, control sera, USR antigen suspension, and test specimens should be at room temperature, 73-85 F (23-29 C), when tests are performed.

1. Pipet 0.05 ml unheated serum from original collecting tube into 1 ring of paraffin-ringed glass slide.

2. Add 1 drop ($1/45$ ml) antigen suspension onto each serum.

3. Rotate slide on rotating machine for 4 min at 180 rpm.

4. Read tests microscopically with 10× ocular and 10× objective immediately after rotation.

5. Report results as follows:

Reading	*Report*	
Medium and large clumps	Reactive	(R)
Small clumps	Weakly Reactive	(W)
No clumping, or very slight roughness	Nonreactive	(N)

NOTE: Specimens giving any degree of clumping should be subjected to further serologic study, including quantitation.

Rapid Plasma Reagin (RPR) (circle) Card test on serum[29, 31, 32]†

Before performing this test, consult section on general rules for syphilis.

---

*BBL, Division of BioQuest, Cockeysville, Md.; Difco Laboratories, Detroit; Sylvana Co., Milburn, N.J.

*BBL, Division of BioQuest, Cockeysville, Md.; Dade Reagents, Miami; Difco Laboratories, Detroit.

†From *Manual of tests for syphilis*, 1969 (reprinted 1978).[2]

Equipment, glassware, and reagents. All equipment and supplies necessary to perform the RPR 18 mm (circle) card test are contained in a kit (Hynson, Westcott & Dunning, Baltimore), with the exception of controls, rotating machine, and cover.

1. The kit contains:
   a. RPR card test antigen
      This antigen suspension is similar to that prepared for the USR test. It also contains a suspension of specially prepared charcoal particles.* Store antigen suspension in ampules or in plastic dispensing bottle at 2-8 C. An unopened ampule has a shelf life of at least 12 mo from date of manufacture; antigen suspension in plastic dispensing bottle (refrigerated) usually remains satisfactory for approximately 3 mo. Do not use antigen suspension beyond expiration date on ampule. A new lot of antigen suspension should be compared with an antigen suspension of known reactivity before being placed in routine use (see Check Testing Nontreponemal [Cardiolipin] Test Antigen).
   b. 20-gauge needle without bevel
   c. Plastic dispensing bottle
   d. Plastic-coated cards, each with ten **18 mm circle** spots
   e. Dispenstirs, 0.05 ml/drop
   f. Capillary pipets, 0.05 ml capacity
   g. Rubber bulbs
   h. Stirrers
2. Rotating machine—fixed speed or adjustable to 100 rpm, circumscribing a ¾ in. diameter circle on a horizontal plane
3. Humidifier cover—any convenient cover containing a moistened blotter may be used to cover cards during rotation
4. Pipets (optional)—any of the following may be used instead of Dispenstirs or capillary pipets:
   0.2 ml, graduated in 0.01 ml subdivisions
   0.5 ml, graduated in 0.01 ml subdivisions
   1.0 ml, graduated in 0.01 ml subdivisions

Testing of delivery needles
1. It is of primary importance that proper amounts of reagents be used, and for this reason, needles used should be checked each day.
2. For RPR Card test, dispense antigen suspension from plastic dispensing bottle with 20-gauge disposable needle without level. These needles should deliver 60 drops ± 2 drops antigen suspension/ml when held in vertical position. Practice will allow rapid delivery of antigen suspension, but care should be exercised to obtain drops of uniform size.
3. To check accuracy of needle, place needle on 2 ml syringe or on 1 ml pipet. Fill syringe or pipet with antigen suspension and, holding in verticle position, count number of drops delivered in 0.5 ml. Needle is considered to be satisfactory if 30 drops ± 1 drop are obtained in 0.5 ml.

Editor's note: This is a 0.25% suspension of specially prepared charcoal (available only from Hynson, Westcott & Dunning, Baltimore) in distilled water. It is added to the "resuspending solution" (see USR test) as follows:[33]

0.25M EDTA	0.5 ml
Choline chloride, 40%	2.5 ml
Phosphate (0.02M), Merthiolate, 0.2%	5.0 ml
Distilled water	1.0 ml
Charcoal suspension, 0.25%	1.0 ml

4. A needle not meeting this specification should be replaced with another needle that does meet this specification (see Preparation and Calibration of Needles for Slide Flocculation Tests).

Preliminary testing of antigen suspension
1. Attach needle hub to tapered fitting on plastic dispending bottle. Shake antigen ampule to resuspend antigen particles, snap ampule neck at break line, and withdraw all the RPR card antigen suspension into dispensing bottle by suction, collapsing bottle and using it as a bulb. Shake dispenser gently before each series of antigen drops is delivered.
2. Test control sera (Hynson, Westcott & Dunning, Baltimore) of graded reactivity each day as described under Rapid Plasma Reagin (RPR [circle] Card Test and Serum). Whole serum controls may be prepared as described under Control Sera for Nontreponemal Antigen Tests.
3. Use only those suspensions that have given designated reactions with controls.

Preparation of sera
1. Centrifuge blood specimens at room temperature at a force that is sufficient to separate serum from cells. Generally, 1500-2000 rpm for 5 min is sufficient.
2. Specimens may be retained in original collection tube.
NOTE: Sera are tested without heating and should be at 73-85 F (23-29 C) at time of testing.

RPR (circle) Card test on serum

Slide flocculation tests for syphilis are affected by room temperature. For reliable and reproducible results, controls, RPR card antigen suspension, and test specimens should be at room temperature, 73-85 F (23-29 C), when tests are performed.

1. Place 0.05 ml unheated serum onto a **18 mm circle** of test card, using a Dispenstir, a 0.05 ml capillary pipet with attached rubber bulb, or serologic pipet.
2. Spread serum with inverted Dispenstir (closed end) or stirrer (broad end) to fill entire circle (specimen may be spread with serologic pipet if tip is smooth and will not scratch card surface).
3. Add exactly 1 drop ($^1/_{60}$ ml) RPR card test antigen suspension to each test area containing serum. Do not stir.
4. Place card on rotator and cover with humidifier cover.
5. Rotate 8 min at 100 rpm on mechanical rotating machine.
6. Read tests without magnification immediately after rotation. A **brief** rotating and tilting of card by hand should be used to aid in differentiating Nonreactive from Minimally Reactive results.
7. Report results as follows:

Reading	*Report*	
Small to large clumps	Reactive	(R)
No clumping or very slight roughness	Nonreactive	(N)

Specimens giving any degree of clumping should be subjected to further serologic study, including quantitation.

8. Upon completion of daily tests, remove needle, rinse in water, and air-dry. (Avoid wiping needle, since this removes silicone coating.) Recap dispensing bottle and store in refrigerator.

Rapid Plasma Reagin (RPR) (circle) Card test with serum, quantitative

Quantitative testing with this method was described by Portnoy.[29,31] The quantitative test was not included in the *Manual of Tests for Syphilis, 1969*,[2] but it is now an accepted standard test.

Procedure[29]

1. For each specimen to be tested, place 0.05 ml 0.9% saline solution into rings numbered 2 to 5. Serologic pipet, 1 ml or less, or an 18-gauge needle without point may be used; latter should deliver 0.025 ml/drop. **Do not spread saline solution.**
2. Using capillary pipet graduated at 0.05 ml (to tip) and rubber bulb, place 0.05 ml unheated serum or plasma in ring 1. NOTE: Serum should not be drawn into rubber bulb, since this may cause incorrect results on subsequent tests.
3. Refill capillary and, holding in vertical position, prepare serial 2-fold dilutions by drawing mixture up and down capillary 5-6 times, transferring 0.05 ml from ring 2 to ring 3 to ring 4 to ring 5. Discard 0.05 ml after mixing contents in ring 5.
4. Place 1 drop ($1/60$ ml) RPR card antigen suspension onto each ring.
5. Using broad end of clean stirrer for each specimen, start at highest dilution of serum (ring 5) and mix RPR card antigen suspension and serum, filling entire surface of ring. Proceed to rings 4, 3, 2, and 1 and do similar stirring.
6. Rotate for 8 min at 100 rpm on mechanical rotator.
7. Read tests and report in terms of highest dilution yielding reactive result.
8. If highest dilution tested (1:16) is reactive, proceed as follows:
   a. Prepare 1:50 dilution of nonreactive serum in 0.9% saline solution. (This is to be used for making 1:32 and higher dilutions of specimens to be quantitated.)
   b. Prepare 1:16 dilution of test specimen by adding 0.1 ml serum or plasma to 1.5 ml 0.9% saline solution. Mix throughly.
   c. Place 0.05 ml of 1:50 nonreactive serum in rings 2, 3, 4, and 5.
   d. Using capillary pipet, place 0.05 ml of 1:16 dilution of test specimen in ring 1.
   e. Refill capillary, make serial 2-fold dilutions, and complete tests as described in steps 3 to 7.
9. Highest dilutions are prepared if necessary in 1:50 nonreactive serum.

Automated reagin test (ART)*

Equipment

1. AutoAnalyzer Equipment† (see Fig. 106-3)
   a. Sampler II without mixing unit. Use cam with sampling rate of 100/h and 1:3 sample-to-wash ratio.
   b. Proportioning pump with single-speed or 2-speed motor.
   c. Automated Reagin Test (ART) manifold.
   d. Continuous-filter modified by removing mixing assembly and using microprobe, 0.02 in. ID, to dispense tests on filter paper. With set-speed filter unit, filter paper speed should be

approximately ⅞ in./36 s; variable speed unit should be adjusted to this speed.
2. Roll of special filter paper, no. 402, 1 in. width (no substitutes).
3. Magnetic stirrer, small, equipped to maintain room temperature. Insulating material such as Styrofoam may be placed on stirrer to prevent transfer of heat to antigen bottle.
4. Micro stirring bar, length ½ in., and diameter ⅛ in., **or** length ¼ in., and diameter ⅛ in.
5. Vacuum pump, suitable for continuous operation at a vacuum of 15-20 in. (380-510 mm) Hg. Central vacuum source may be used if negative pressure is relatively constant and does not fall below 15 in. (380 mm) Hg.
6. Wooden blocks or racks to hold sample cups in rows of 10.

Glassware

1. Bottles, 30 ml, round, screw capped or glass stoppered, narrow mouth, with flat bottom; 25 ml Erlenmeyer flasks may be used if inner surface of bottom is flat.
2. Dropping bottles with droppers.
3. Sample cups, disposable, polystyrene. Cups must be free from dust and lint. Routinely check for holes in bottom of cups.
   a. For qualitative tests: 0.5 ml size
   b. For quantitative tests: 2.0 ml size

Reagents

1. Rapid Plasma Reagin (RPR) Card test antigen suspension (Hynson, Westcott & Dunning, Baltimore) with charcoal particles, 10 ml ampule size. Store antigen suspension in refrigerator at 3-10 C. Remove sufficient antigen suspension for 1 d testing and keep at room temperature.
2. 0.9% Saline. Dissolve 9 g dry sodium chloride in each 1000 ml distilled water.
3. Tween 20 (Technicon Corp., Tarrytown, N.Y.). Add to saline as wetting agent.
4. Saline and Tween 20. Add 0.05 ml Tween 20 from dropping bottle to each liter of 0.9% saline. Mix well. Prepare solution each testing day for use in wash receptacle and as diluent in manifold. During testing period, maintain saline and Tween 20 at 24-29 C.
5. Dye solution. Use food color (McCormick and Co., Baltimore), which is a vegetable dye, as marker on filter-paper strip. Make 1:5 dilution of dye in distilled water and store in dropping bottle with dropper. (If diluted dye solution becomes contaminated or changes viscosity, it should be discarded.) For use in the test, add 1 or 2 drops to sample cup and fill with saline solution. Final concentration of dye should be **minimal** amount that can be easily observed on filter paper.
6. Cleaning solution, 2.5% urea in 0.05N sodium hydroxide. Add 2.5 g urea to 100 ml 0.05N sodium hydroxide in distilled water. Food color may be added so that cleaning solution can be monitored in system.

Collection and preparation of specimens

1. Test may be run on serum or plasma. To perform the ART on plasma, collect blood in tubes containing an anticoagulant (EDTA, [Na2]* or potassium oxalate and sodium fluoride†). Other anticoagu-

---

*From National Communicable Disease Center: Technique for the Automated Reagin Test (ART), U.S. Department of Health, Education and Welfare, Public Health Service, Atlanta, 1970.
†Technicon Corp., Tarrytown, N.Y.

---

*B-D Vacutainer tube no. 3204Q, Becton, Dickinson & Co., Rutherford, N.J.
†B-D Vacutainer tube no. 3204PS, Becton, Dickinson & Co., Rutherford, N.J.

lants should not be used until evaluated for this technic.

2. Specimens must be clear and free from particulate material. If serum or plasma has been stored in refrigerator, examine and recentrifuge if it is not clear.

3. Test specimens **unheated.** If specimens have been refrigerated, keep at room temperature for at least 30 min before testing.

Control serums*

1. Control serums for the ART may be prepared from individual or pooled serums. Selected dilutions of reactive serum in nonreactive serum may be prepared, dispensed in quantities sufficient for 1 testing period, and stored in freezer (see *Manual of Tests for Syphilis, 1969*). A reactive serum or pool on which a quantitative pattern has been established may be used. A pattern of reactivity must be established for each new lot of control serum prepared in the laboratory, or confirmed for each new lot of control serum obtained from a commercial source, by comparing new control serum with standard control serum.

2. Use control serums of graded reactivity at beginning of each test run. When tests are run continuously, include a set of control serums with every 150 specimens. Results obtained should reproduce an established pattern of reactivity.

3. In addition to prepared serums, test 2-4 individual nonreactive specimens to give a more complete picture of test patterns as an aid in reading.

4. A test run not producing predetermined reactivity in control serums under conditions of technic should be considered invalid.

Automated reagin qualitative test

NOTE: The automated reagin test for syphilis is affected by room temperature. For reliable and reproducible test results, tests should be performed within a room temperature range of 24-29 C.

Procedure

1. Bring reagents and specimens to room temperature (24-29 C) before use.

2. Pump saline and Tween 20 mixture into all tubing lines. **Check bubble pattern after all lines are filled.** Follow diagram for further steps (Fig. 106-3).

3. Fill 0.5 ml cups with specimens. Tap cup on tabletop to release air bubble if present. Do not test a specimen of less than 0.1 ml quantity.

4. Place control sera, test sera, and dye markers in proper sequence in sampler tray. Place dye marker at beginning and end of test specimens in tray, after control sera, and between every 10 specimens.

5. Place 10 ml antigen suspension in 30 ml bottle or flask with flat bottom. Add stirring bar and place on magnetic stirrer. Adjust to slow, even rotation and begin pumping antigen. Replenish antigen supply when stirring bar is seen at surface of liquid.

6. Start sampler when antigen suspension is seen in mixing coil. Adjust specimen probe if necessary.

7. Start continuous-filter unit after antigen suspension is decanted at A9 fitting. **Adjust dispensing probe** to give a 0.3-0.5 cm wide stream on filter paper before tests are deposited. Smooth deposition of antigen suspension on filter paper strip is essential for satisfactory reading of test run.

8. Periodically check for charcoal deposit in system to help prevent clogging of tubing. In particular, check antigen feed system, A9 decant fitting, and subsequent feed system between this fitting and filter paper. Segments drawn off A9 fitting **must** be discrete and unbroken to assure easy and accurate reading of tests.

9. Rinse system between every 2 sample trays by pumping saline and Tween 20 through all tubing lines for 1-2 min.

10. At end of testing day, pump urea cleaning solution into antigen suspension, sample, and diluent lines for 5 min. (**Do not pump cleaning solution into wash receptacle.**) Pump distilled water into all lines for 20-30 min.

If a 2-speed pump is used, pump cleaning solution into system as above, using rapid-wash cycle. Pump distilled water into **all** lines for 10 min at slow speed, and complete distilled water rinse with rapid-wash cycle.

In addition, clean sample and dispensing probes and metal connections; these may be cleaned by flushing with distilled water using specially adapted syringe. (Connect 6 in. length of .030 Tygon tubing to 2 in. length of .0625 Tygon tubing with cyclohexanone; attach free end of .0625 tubing to tip of a 10 ml syringe with cyclohexanone.) An appropriate-size stylet (from a 22- or 23-gauge needle) may be used to clean excessively clogged connections.

Reading of results

1. Number filter-paper strips at first and last position of each 10 specimens with appropriate specimen number. Space taken by each specimen should be approximately ⅞ in. and can be marked off at side of strip.

2. Tests can be read at the convenience of the serologist and can be kept as a permanent record if desired.

3. Read and report results as follows:

Reactive	Granularity and increased density of charcoal deposit
Nonreactive	Even distribution of charcoal particles; compare with nonreactive controls if slight increase in density is seen

4. Retest specimen showing any reactivity that follows a strongly reactive specimen to avoid giving a false-reactive report caused by carry-over of reagin.

Automated reagin quantitative test

All specimens reactive in Automated Reagin qualitative test should be quantitatively retested to end point titer. Undiluted specimen should be included in quantitative test to serve as check on original testing.

1. Prepare serial 2-fold dilutions of reactive specimens in following manner:

a. Pipet 0.2 ml of 0.9% saline (without Tween 20) into each of 4 or more 2 ml conical plastic sample cups.

b. Using a 0.2 ml pipet or an automatic diluter, add 0.2 ml of serum or plasma to first cup and mix 4 or more times (1:2 dilution; a Micro-Pipette [Alfred Bicknell Associates, Cambridge, Mass.] has been used interchangeably with a 0.2 ml pipet in this laboratory with satisfactory results).

c. Transfer 0.2 ml of 1:2 dilution to second cup and mix. Continue transferring and mixing until all dilutions are made.

---

*Hynson, Westcott & Dunning, Baltimore.

2. Place cups in sampler tray in following order: undiluted, 1:2, 1:4, 1:8, etc.
3. Place dye marker between each series of dilutions, as well as at beginning and end of tests in sampler tray.
4. Test undiluted specimen and each dilution as described in ART qualitative procedure.
5. Read test reactions in same manner as in ART qualitative procedure.
6. Report results in terms of greatest dilution giving a reactive result, as in following examples:

Undi-luted	Dilutions				Report
	1:2	**1:4**	**1:8**	**1:16**	
R	N	N	N	N	Reactive, undiluted only, or 1 dil
R	R	N	N	N	Reactive, 1:2 dilution, or 2 dils
R	R	R	R	N	Reactive, 1:8 dilution, or 8 dils

7. If greatest dilution tested gives a reactive result, prepare additional dilutions for testing.

A prozone reaction caused by excess antibody, occasionally seen in flocculation tests for syphilis, has not been observed in the ART system.

Kahn tests

A detailed description of Kahn tests was included in the *1959 Manual, Serologic Tests for Syphilis* (U.S. Public Health Service)[34] but was removed from its 1964 edition,[35] in which it was listed as a test "which will serve adequately as an aid in diagnosis." In the 1969 edition,[2] the Kahn tests are described as "tests of historical interest." For details of the procedure, the reader is referred to the seventh edition of this text[36] and Kahn.[37-42]

Hinton tests

The Hinton reagin tests are of historical interest.

For details of the procedure the interested reader is referred to Stuart et al.,[43] Hinton et al.,[44] and the *1964 Manual, Serologic Tests for Syphilis*.[35]

Mazzini tests

For details of the Mazzini tests, which are now used rarely, see Mazzini and the *1964 Manual, Serologic Tests for Syphilis*.[35]

Kline tests

For details of the Kline tests see Kline[46] and the *1964 Manual, Serologic Tests for Syphilis*.[35]

• • •

For a discussion of **Kolmer complement fixation tests,** see Complement Fixation Tests.

Treponemal antigen tests

FLUORESCENT TREPONEMAL ANTIBODY-ABSORPTION (FTA-ABS) TEST

A general discussion of fluorescent antibody tests is found in Chapter 70. The FTA-ABS test and its rationale and place in the serodiagnosis of syphilis is discussed earlier in this chapter. Automation of the FTA-ABS test is discussed in Chapter 105.

Fluorescent treponemal antibody–absorption (FTA-ABS) test on serum[9,47,48*]

Before performing this test, consult the section on general rules for syphilis tests.

Equipment, supplies, and glassware
1. Incubator, adjustable to 35-37 C
2. Dark-field fluorescence microscope assembly
3. Bibulous paper
4. Diamond-point pencil (optional)
5. Template, used as guide for cutting circles 1.0 cm ID on glass slides (optional)
6. Slide board or holder
7. Moist chamber—place moistened paper inside convenient cover fitting slide board
8. Loop, bacteriologic, standard 2 mm, 26-gauge, platinum
9. Oil, immersion, low fluorescence, nondrying
10. Microscope slides, 1 × 3 in., frosted end, approximately 1 mm thick†
11. Coverslips, no. 1, 22 mm square
12. Dish, staining, glass or plastic, with removable slide carriers
13. Glass rods, approximately 100 × 4 mm, both ends fire-polished

Reagents. See "Check Testing FTA-ABS Test Reagents."
1. *Treponema pallidum* antigen‡§
   a. Antigen for FTA-ABS test is a suspension of *T. pallidum* (Nichols strain) extracted from rabbit testicular tissue. Extract should contain a minimum of 30 organisms/high-dry field. Antigen may be stored at 6-10 C or processed by lyophilization.
   b. Store lyophilized antigen at 6-10 C and hydrate for use according to accompanying directions.
   c. Discard antigen suspension if it becomes bacterially contaminated or does not demonstrate proper reactivity with control sera.
2. FTA-ABS test sorbent‡
   a. Sorbent is a standardized product prepared from cultures of Reiter treponemes. This may be purchased in lyophilized or liquid state.
   b. Store sorbent, and rehydrate if lyophilized, according to accompanying directions.
3. Fluorescein-labeled antihuman globulin‖ (conjugate)
   a. Conjugate should be of proved quality for FTA-ABS test. Test each new lot of conjugate to determine its working titer and to verify that it

---

*From *Manual of tests for syphilis*, 1969 (reprinted 1978).[2]

†Glass slides with 2 etched circles, 1 cm ID, catalog no. A-1447/10, Clay-Adams, New York.

‡BBL, Division of BioQuest, Cockeysville, Md.; Difco Laboratories, Detroit; Fisher Scientific Co., Pittsburgh; The Sylvana Co., Millburn, N.J.

§Beckman Instruments, Diagnostic Operations, Fullerton, Calif.

‖BBL, Division of BioQuest, Cockeysville, Md.; Difco Laboratories, Detroit; Fisher Scientific Co., Pittsburgh; The Sylvana Co., Millburn, N.J.; Lederle Laboratories, Pearl River, N.Y.; Hyland Division, Travenol Laboratories, Los Angeles.

meets criteria concerning nonspecific staining and standard reactivity.

b. Store lyophilized conjugate at 6-10 C. Dispense rehydrated conjugate in not less than 0.3 ml quantities and store at −20 C or lower. For practical purposes a conjugate with a working titer of 1:400 or higher may be diluted 1:10 with sterile phosphate-buffered saline (containing Merthiolate in a concentration of 1:5000) before storage.

c. When conjugate is thawed for use, do not refreeze but store at 6-10 C. It may be used as long as satisfactory reactivity is obtained with test controls.

d. If a change in FTA-ABS test reactivity is noted in routine laboratory testing, conjugate should be retitered to determine if it is the contributing factor.

4. Phosphate-buffered saline (PBS), pH 7.2 ± 0.1 Formula per liter:

NaCl	7.65 g
Na_2HPO_4	0.724 g
KH_2PO_4	0.21 g

Several liters may be prepared and stored in a large Pyrex (or equivalent) or polyethylene bottle. Determine pH of each lot of PBS prepared for FTA-ABS test. PBS outside the range of pH 7.2 ± 0.1 should be discarded.

5. *Tween 80**

a. To prepare PBS containing 2% Tween 80, heat the 2 reagents in 56 C water bath. To 98 ml PBS, add 2 ml Tween 80 by measuring from bottom of pipet, and rinse out pipet. The 2% Tween 80 solution should be pH 7.0-7.2. Check pH periodically since solution may become acid. This solution keeps well at refrigerator temperature; discard if precipitate develops or if pH changes.

6. Mounting medium, which consists of 1 part PBS, pH 7.2, plus 9 parts glycerin (reagent quality)

7. Acetone (ACS)

Preparation of T. pallidum antigen smears

1. Mix antigen suspension well with disposable pipet and rubber bulb by drawing suspension into and expelling it from pipet at least 10 times to break treponemal clumps and ensure even distribution of treponemes. Determine by dark-field examination that treponemes are adequately dispersed before making slides for FTA test. Additional mixing may be required.

2. On clean slides cut 2 circles 1 cm ID with diamond-point pencil. Wipe slides with clean gauze to remove loose glass particles. Slide with preetched circles may be used.

3. Smear 1 loopful of *T. pallidum* antigen evenly within each circle by using standard 2 mm, 26-gauge, platinum wire loop. Experience with individual lots of antigen may indicate that a smaller or larger quantity should be spread in each circle. Allow to air-dry at least 15 min.

4. Fix smear† in acetone for 10 min and allow to

air-dry thoroughly. (Not more than 60 slides should be fixed with 200 ml acetone.) Store acetone-fixed smears at −20 C or below. Fixed, frozen smears are usable indefinitely, provided that satisfactory results are obtained with controls. Do not thaw and refreeze antigen smears.

Preparation of sera. Bacterial contamination or excessive hemolysis may render specimens unsatisfactory for testing.

1. Heat test and control sera at 56 C for 30 min before testing.

2. Reheat previously heated test sera for 10 min at 56 C on day of testing.

Controls. Store and use control sera from commercial sources* according to accompanying directions. Whole serum controls may be prepared as described under Control Sera for the FTA-ABS Test. Include the following controls in each test run:

1. Reactive (4+) control Reactive serum or a dilution of Reactive serum demonstrating strong (4+) fluorescence when diluted 1:5 in PBS and only slightly reduced fluorescence† when diluted 1:5 in sorbent.

a. Using a 0.2 ml pipet and measuring from bottom, add 0.05 ml Reactive control serum into tube containing 0.2 ml PBS. Mix well, at least 8 times.

b. Using 0.2 ml pipet and measuring from bottom, add 0.05 ml Reactive control serum into tube containing 0.2 ml sorbent. Mix well, at least 8 times.

2. Minimally Reactive (1+) control Dilution of Reactive serum demonstrating **minimal degree of fluorescence reported as "Reactive" for use as a reading standard.** The Reactive (4+) control serum may be used for this control when diluted in PBS according to directions.

3. Nonspecific serum controls A nonsyphilitic serum known to demonstrate at least 2+ nonspecific reactivity in FTA test at dilution in PBS of 1:5 or higher.

a. Using 0.2 ml pipet and measuring from bottom, add 0.05 ml Nonspecific control serum into tube containing 0.2 ml PBS. Mix well, at least 8 times.

b. Using another 0.2 ml pipet and measuring from bottom, add 0.05 ml Nonspecific control serum into tube containing 0.2 ml sorbent. Mix well, at least 8 times.

4. Nonspecific staining controls
a. Antigen smear treated with 0.03 ml PBS.
b. Antigen smear treated with 0.03 ml sorbent.

Controls 1, 3, and 4 are included for purpose of controlling reagents and test conditions. Control 2 (Minimally Reactive [1+] control serum) is included as reading standard. If a gradual decrease of fluorescence in Reactive controls is observed over a period of time, this may indicate deterioration of control sera, reagents, or light source.

---

*Hill Top Laboratories, Cincinnati.

†Smears may be fixed for 20 s in a solution of 10% methyl alcohol in distilled water. (Not more than 20 slides should be fixed with 200 ml 10% methyl alcohol; this solution should be prepared on day of use.) Antigen smears to be fixed by this method should be prepared on day of test.

---

*BBL, Division of BioQuest, Cockeysville, Md.; Difco Laboratories, Detroit; Fisher Scientific Co., Pittsburgh; The Sylvana Co., Milburn, N.J.

†A reduction of no more than 1+ fluorescence, i.e., 4+ changing to 3+.

Control pattern illustration	Reaction
Reactive control	
a. 1:5 PBS dilution	R4+
b. 1:5 sorbent dilution	R (4+ to 3+)
Minimally reactive (1+) control	R1+
Nonspecific serum controls	
a. 1:5 PBS dilution	R (2+ to 4+)
b. 1:5 sorbent dilution	N
Nonspecific staining controls	
a. Antigen, PBS, and conjugate	N
b. Antigen, sorbent, and conjugate	N

Test runs in which these control results are not obtained are considered unsatisfactory and should not be reported.

FTA-ABS test on serum

1. Identify previously prepared slides by numbering frosted end with a lead pencil (see Preparation of *Treponema pallidum* Antigen Smears, above).
2. Number tubes to correspond to sera and control sera being tested and place in racks.
3. Prepare Reactive (4+), Minimally Reactive (1+), and Nonspecific control serum dilutions in sorbent and/or PBS according to directions (see Controls).
4. Pipet 0.2 ml sorbent into test tube for each test serum.
5. Using 0.2 ml pipet and measuring from bottom, add 0.05 ml heated test serum into appropriate tube and mix 8 times.
6. Cover appropriate antigen smears with 0.03 ml Reactive (4+), Minimally Reactive (1+), and Nonspecific control serum dilutions.
7. Cover appropriate antigen smears with 0.03 ml PBS and 0.03 ml sorbent for "Nonspecific staining controls *a* and *b*," respectively.
8. Cover appropriate antigen smears with 0.03 ml test serum dilutions.
9. Prevent evaporation by placing slides within moist chamber.
10. Place slides in incubator at 35-37 C for 30 min.
11. Rinsing procedure
    a. Place slides in slide carriers and rinse slides with running PBS for approximately 5 s.
    b. Place slides in staining dish containing PBS for 5 min.
    c. Agitate slides by dipping them in and out of PBS at least 10 times.
    d. Using fresh PBS, repeat Steps *b* and *c*.
    e. Rinse slides in running distilled water for approximately 5 s.
12. Gently blot slides with bibulous paper to remove all water drops.
13. Dilute conjugate to its working titer in PBS containing 2% Tween 80.
14. Place approximately 0.03 ml diluted conjugate on each smear. Spread uniformly with glass rod to cover entire smear.
15. Repeat Steps 9-12.
16. Mount slides immediately by placing small drop of mounting medium on each smear and applying coverslip.
17. Examine slides as soon as possible. If a delay in reading is necessary, place slides in a darkened room and read within 4 h.
18. Study smears microscopically using mercury arc illumination and high-power dry objective. Combination of BG 12 exciting filter, not greater

than 3 mm in thickness, and OG 1 barrier filter (or their equivalents*) has been found to be satisfactory for routine use.
19. Check Nonreactive smears by using illumination from a tungsten light source to verify presence of treponemes.
20. Using Minimally Reactive (1+) control slide as reading standard, record intensity of fluorescence of treponemes according to chart below.

Reading	Intensity of fluorescence	Report	
2+ to 4+	Moderate to strong	Reactive	(R)
1+	Equivalent to Minimally Reactive (1+) control	Reactive	(R)†
<1+	Weak but definite, less than Minimally Reactive (1+) control	Borderline	(B)†
−	None or vaguely visible	Nonreactive	(N)

Reporting scheme. The FTA-ABS reporting scheme is illustrated below.

Test reading	Repeat	Report
4+		R
3+	—	R
2+		R
1+	1+ or greater	R
	<1+ or −	B
<1+	1+, <1+, or −	B
−		N

Suggested attachment to reports of Borderline test results. The Borderline report of the FTA-ABS test performed in our laboratory on the specimen obtained from *(patient's name)* means that the results cannot be interpreted as either Reactive or Nonreactive.

If this is the first specimen you have submitted for FTA-ABS testing on this patient, another specimen should be submitted for FTA-ABS testing.

If this is a second specimen from this patient on which an FTA-ABS test has been made and the report is again Borderline, it is impossible to state definitely that the patient does or does not have serologic evidence of syphilitic infection. A careful review of the patient's history and physical findings is suggested, and diagnosis will necessarily rest upon the clinical evidence in view of the Borderline serologic findings.

TREPONEMA PALLIDUM HEMAGGLUTINATION TESTS[12-14]

As discussed earlier in this chapter (Treponemal Antigen Tests), as of August 1978 the

---

*Filter equivalents:
   Exciting filters—BG 12 =o= AO 702
   Barrier filters—OG 1 =o= AO 724 or 1124
   =o= B&L Y-8 =o= Zeiss 50/- (II/0).

†Retest all specimens with intensity of fluorescence of 1+ or less. When a specimen initially read as 1+ is retested and is subsequently read as 1+ or greater, test is reported as "Reactive." All other results on retest are reported as "Borderline." It is not necessary to retest nonfluorescent (Nonreactive) specimens.

Center for Disease Control classified the *T. pallidum* hemagglutination tests either in the Provisional Test status (MHA-TP) or in the Investigational Test status.

Microhemagglutination assay for Treponema pallidum antibodies (MHA-TP test)[49-54]*

Before performing this test, the technologist should become familiar with the introductory chapter and the chapter on equipment and glassware in the *Manual of Tests for Syphilis, 1969*[2] and with the *Microtiter Instruction Manual.*[55]

Equipment and supplies
1. Microdiluters (0.025 ml)†
2. Pipet droppers calibrated to deliver 0.025 ml†
3. Go-no-go delivery testers for 0.025 ml (blotters)†
4. Tray viewer‡
5. Disposable, clear plastic trays with 8 rows of 15 cups each‡; round-bottom (U-shaped) cups should be smooth and free from dust and lint
6. 12 × 75 mm test tubes
7. 1.0 ml serologic pipets graduated in 1/100 ml
8. 0.1 ml or 0.2 ml serologic pipets graduated in 1/100 ml

To avoid mouth pipetting of serum, use push-button automatic pipets with disposable tips calibrated to deliver 0.025 ml (25 μl) and 0.020 ml (20 μl).

Reagents. Rehydrate the lyophilized reagents with sterile distilled water according to the manufacturer's instructions. Store lyophilized and rehydrated reagents at 2-8 C. These reagents should be discarded if they become contaminated or do not demonstrate the proper reactivity with control sera.

1. Absorbing diluent (liquid).§ This consists of sonicated cell membranes from sheep and ox erythrocytes, normal rabbit testicular extract, sonicated Reiter treponemes, normal rabbit serum, and Tween 80 and acacia powder in phosphate buffered saline (PBS), pH 7.2. This reagent is used to preabsorb and dilute sera and to prepare working dilutions of sensitized and unsensitized cell suspensions.
2. Antigen. *Treponema pallidum* sensitized sheep cells (lyophilized).§
   a. Rehydrated antigen is a 2.5% suspension of formalinized, tanned sheep erythrocytes that have been sensitized with sonicated *T. pallidum* (Nichols strain). Reconstituted reagents should be used within 5 d.
   b. Prepare working dilution of antigen **for 1 test day** by adding 1 part rehydrated suspension to 5.5 parts absorbing diluent (1:6.5 dilution). Quantity of working dilution needed is 0.075 ml for each serum dilution tested plus a slight excess.

3. Unsensitized sheep cells (lyophilized).*
   a. When rehydrated, this is a 2.5% suspension of formalized, tanned sheep erythrocytes (**not** sensitized with *T. pallidum* antigen). Reconstituted reagents should be used within 5 d.
   b. Prepare working dilution (1:6.5) for 1 test day, allowing 0.075 ml for each serum tested plus a slight excess.
4. Sterile distilled water.
5. 0.85% Saline.

Controls
1. Lyophilized control sera.* Store lyophilized control sera at 2-8 C. When rehydrated, control sera may be stored at −20 C. These sera are supplied unabsorbed.
   a. Reactive control serum should not vary more than ±1 doubling dilution from the end-point titer established for that serum (dilutions are expressed in terms of **final serum dilution** obtained after addition of all reagents).
   b. Nonreactive control serum should be nonreactive at 1:80 serum dilution.
2. Unsensitized-erythrocyte serum control. Each test and control serum tested with sensitized sheep erythrocytes (antigen) is also tested at its lowest dilution with unsensitized erythrocytes. This serum control should be nonreactive.
3. Reagent controls. Both sensitized erythrocytes (antigen) and unsensitized erythrocytes mixed with absorbing diluent should give nonreactive test results.

Preparation of sera for testing
1. Add 0.02 ml unheated test and control sera to 0.38 ml absorbing diluent in test tubes (1:20 dilutions).
2. Mix at least 8 times and incubate at room temperature (25 C ± 5 C) for 30 min.
3. Absorbed test and control sera (1:20 dilutions) are now ready to be tested. Residual of absorbed sera may be stored at 2-8 C and can be retested on same day. Absorbed sera should be at room temperature when tested.

Preparation of microdiluting equipment[53]
1. Microdiluter preparation
   a. Rotate microdiluters in distilled water to clean.
   b. Flame microdiluters to incandescence over Bunsen burner, quench in distilled water to cool, and blot to expel liquid.
2. Go-no-go delivery test (delivery test and prewetting are accomplished in same operation).
   a. Fill each microdiluter by touching it to surface of 0.85% saline. Do not wet canopy (top) of loop.
   b. Touch microdiluter to marked center of one of circles on go-no-go delivery tester (blotter) and observe dampened area within circle.
   c. Properly prepared microdiluter will deliver all contained fluid, which will be sufficient to **immediately** dampen area within circle. Solution from an improperly prepared microdiluter will not be sufficient to dampen entire area within circle.
3. Calibrated pipet dropper must be clean. To assure proper delivery of fluid, gently blot excess solution from outside of pipet dropper with cleansing tissue after filling. Hold dropper in vertical position when adding fluid to tray cups.

---

*From Bureau of Laboratories: Micro-Hemagglutination Assay for *Treponema pallidum* antibodies (MHA-TP). Provisional technique, (revised Jan. 1977), Atlanta, U.S. Department of Health, Education and Welfare, Public Health Service, Center for Disease Control.
†Cooke Engineering Co., Alexandria, Va.
‡Ames Co., Division of Miles Laboratories, Elkhart, Ind.
§Prepared by Fuji Zoki Pharmaceutical Co., Tokyo; distributed by Ames Co., Division of Miles Laboratories, Elkhart, Ind.

---

*Prepared by Fuji Zoki Pharmaceutical Co., Tokyo; distributed by Ames Co., Division of Miles Laboratories, Elkhart, Ind.

Table 106-3. Outline of MHA-TP Qualitative Test

					Diluted (1:6.5) unsensitized cells (ml)	Diluted (1:6.5) sensitized cells (ml)	Final serum dilution
Absorbed test serums (1:20)				ml			
Serum test	(Rows A, C, E, G)			0.025	—	0.075	1:80
Serum control	(Rows B, D, F, H)			0.025	0.075	—	1:80
	Absorbed control serums (1:20)						
Cup no.	Reactive control serum (ml)	+	Absorbing diluent (ml)	Control serum dilution			
1	0.025 (1:20)		—	1:20	—	0.075	1:80
2	0.025 (1:20)		0.025	1:40	—	0.075	1:160
3	0.025 (1:40)		0.025	1:80	—	0.075	1:320
4	0.025 (1:80)		0.025	1:160	—	0.075	1:640
5	0.025 (1:160)		0.025	1:320	—	0.075	1:1,280
6	0.025 (1:320)		0.025	1:640	—	0.075	1:2,560
7	0.025 (1:640)		0.025	1:1,280	—	0.075	1:5,120
8	0.025 (1:1,280)		0.025	1:2,560	—	0.075	1:10,240
9	0.025 (1:2,560)		0.025	1:5,120	—	0.075	1:20,480
10	0.025 (1:5,120		0.025	1:10,240	—	0.075	1:40,960
11	0.025 (1:20)		—	1:20 C*	0.075	—	1:80
	Nonreactive control serum (ml)						
1	0.025 (1:20)		—	1:20	—	0.075	1:80
2	0.025 (1:20)		—	1:20 C*	0.075	—	1:80
Reagent controls							
1	—		0.025	—	—	0.075	—
2	—		0.025	—	0.075	—	—

*Control.

MHA-TP qualitative assay on serum

Refer to Table 106-3.
1. Record control and serum numbers on daily work sheets to correspond to their respective tray and cup numbers.
2. Place 0.025 ml of each absorbed test serum (1:20 dilution) into 2 adjacent cups in tray; e.g., cup no. 1 in rows A and B; cup no. 2 in rows A and B; etc.
3. Using pipet dropper calibrated to deliver 0.025 ml, add 0.075 ml (3 drops) of working dilution of sensitized cells (antigen) to each cup in rows A, C, E, and G (absorbed test serum).
4. Add 0.075 ml (3 drops) of working dilution of unsensitized cells to each cup in rows B, D, F, and H (absorbed control serum).
5. **Final serum dilution** in each test and control cup is 1:80.
6. Set up Reactive and Nonreactive control sera (Table 106-3).
   a. Prepare 2-fold dilutions of absorbed Reactive control serum (1:20 dilution) in absorbing diluent to exceed end-point titer (final serum dilution) established for this serum; e.g., 1:80, 1:160, 1:320, 1:640, etc. (dilutions may be prepared in 0.025 ml quantities in tray cups with microtiter equipment; or these may be prepared in test tubes and 0.025 ml transferred to cups). Measure 0.025 ml of absorbed Reactive control serum (1:20 dilution) into another cup for unsensitized-erythrocyte serum control.
   b. Measure 0.025 ml of absorbed Nonreactive control serum (1:20 dilution) into each of 2 adjacent cups (test and serum control.)
   c. Add 0.075 ml of unsensitized cells to each cup for Reactive and Nonreactive unsensitized-erythrocyte serum controls.
   d. Add 0.075 ml sensitized cells to all other cups containing Reactive control serum dilutions and Nonreactive control serum dilution.
7. Set up reagent controls.
   a. Add 0.075 ml sensitized erythrocytes to 0.025 ml absorbing diluent in 1 cup.
   b. Add 0.075 ml unsensitized erythrocytes to 0.025 ml absorbing diluent in another cup.
   NOTE: Other methods of adding 0.075 ml quantities of sensitized cells and unsensitized cells may be used if delivery is checked for accuracy.
8. Shake trays gently, stack, and cover with empty tray.
9. Incubate trays at room temperature (25 C ± 5 C) for at least 4 h. Incubation period may be extended to overnight.
10. Read settling patterns of red blood cells using angled mirror (tray viewer) to visualize patterns from below.
11. Readings are scored on a scale of − to 4+, and degree of hemagglutination is judged according to following criteria:

Degree of hemagglutination	*Reading*	*Interpretation*
Smooth mat of cells covering entire bottom of cup, edges sometimes folded	4+	Reactive
Smooth mat of cells covering smaller area of cup	3+	Reactive
Smooth mat of cells surrounded by red circles	2+	Reactive
Smooth mat of cells surrounded by smaller red circle with agglutination outside circle	1+	Reactive
Button of cells having small "hole" in center	±	Nonreactive
Definite compact button in center of cup or may have very small "hole" in center	–	Nonreactive

12. Results of the controls included for each test day should conform to criteria outline under Controls.
13. Reporting scheme for qualitative test.
    a. Report as Reactive a serum showing hemagglutination of 1+ or higher with sensitized cells (antigen), provided there is no hemagglutination with unsensitized cells.
    b. Report as Nonreactive a serum showing no hemagglutination (– or ±) with sensitized cells and unsensitized cells.
14. If nonspecific hemagglutination occurs with unsensitized cells (serum control), retest serum and report results as described under Quantitative Assay on Serum, (Step 10, below).

MHA-TP quantitative assay on serum

Presently available data suggest that no additional valuable diagnostic information is obtained with the quantitative test. The following technic is included, however, because it is needed for control purposes in the qualitative test.

Procedure

1. Place 0.025 ml absorbing diluent in each cup required for dilutions, leaving cups in first and last rows empty.
2. Add 0.050 ml absorbed test and control serums (1:20 dilution) to appropriate cups in first row; add 0.025 ml of each to last row of cups (serum controls).
3. Prepare serial dilutions of serum with microdiluters. Place 0.025 ml microdiluters in cups containing 0.050 ml absorbed serum. Rotate 4 s to fill microdiluter. Remove microdiluters, place in next cups of same row, and rotate. Prepare further dilutions of serum by transferring 0.025 ml from 1 cup to the next, discarding excess from last cup by checking delivery on blotter.
4. After completing dilutions in each tray, clean microdiluters by rotating in distilled water, blotting, dipping in 0.85% saline, and blotting to check delivery.
5. Add 0.075 ml unsensitized cells to cups in last row (serum controls).
6. Add 0.075 ml sensitized cells (antigen) to all other cups containing absorbed serum dilutions.
7. Set up reagent controls (see Qualitative Assay on Serum, Step 7).
8. Complete tests and read in manner described for qualitative microhemagglutination assay (see Qualitative Assay on Serum, Steps 8-12).
9. Quantitative tests showing nonreactive results in control cup are reported in terms of highest dilution giving a Reactive result (1+, 2+, 3+, or 4+) as illustrated below.

Final serum dilution

1:80	1:160	1:320	1:640	1:1280	1:2560	Report
4+	4+	3+	1+	±	—	R 1:640
3+	2+	1+	—	—	—	R 1:320
1+	—	—	—	—	—	R 1:80
±	—	—	—	—	—	N
—	—	—	—	—	—	N
2+	4+	4+	4+	2+	±	R 1:1280

10. If nonspecific hemagglutination occurs with unsensitized erythrocytes (serum control), retest serum in following manner:
    a. Prepare dilutions of absorbed serum in 2 rows of cups.
    b. Add 0.075 ml sensitized cells to each cup in 1 row.
    c. Add 0.075 ml unsensitized cells to other row.
    d. Report as Reactive, without reference to titer, if:
       (1) Hemagglutination with sensitized cells is at least 2 doubling dilutions greater than with unsensitized cells;

    and

       (2) First dilution showing no hemagglutination with unsensitized cells has a 3+ or 4+ reaction with sensitized cells.
    e. Report as Inconclusive, nonspecific hemagglutination in serum control if:
       (1) Hemagglutination with sensitized cells is

	Serum	Final serum dilution					Report
		1:80	1:160	1:320	1:640	1:1280	
1	Sensitized cells	4+	4+	4+	3+	1+	Reactive
	Unsensitized cells	4+	4+	2+	—	—	
2	Sensitized cells	4+	3+	2+	—	—	Inconclusive, nonspecific hemagglutination in serum control
	Unsensitized cells	4+	2+	—	—	—	
3	Sensitized cells	4+	—	—	—	—	
	Unsensitized cells	4+	—	—	—	—	

only 1 doubling dilution greater than with unsensitized cells;

or

(2) Hemagglutination with sensitized cells is at same dilution as with unsensitized cells.

Examples are shown at the bottom of the facing page.

TPHA (Treponema pallidum hemagglutination) test[12-14]*

In the TPHA test, turkey erythrocytes are used; it does not require an absorbing diluent. Studies for its evaluation are in progress.

• • •

For discussion of the treponemal complement fixation (Reiter) test, see Complement Fixation Tests.

TREPONEMA PALLIDUM IMMOBILIZATION TEST

The *Treponema pallidum* immobilization test (TPI) has proved to be a valuable aid in diagnosing and excluding the diagnosis of syphilis. The procedure is performed by placing the serum, which contains the specific mobilizing antibody, in a test tube with the live treponemes and complement. After incubation in an oxygen-free atmosphere, a syphilitic patient's serum will immobilize the spirochetes, whereas a normal patient's serum will not. The resulting living and/or dead spirochetes are then examined by the dark-field method to determine the percent of motility. The immobilizing antibody develops only in response to the treponematoses: syphilis, yaws, pinta, and bejel. This test is highly specific for the treponematoses.

The antibody measured by the test is distinct from syphilitic reagin and is a specific antitreponemal antibody. The test is difficult to perform, it is expensive, and it is presently performed only by a few reference laboratories well equipped for the test.

Specimens should not be drawn from patients for at least 1 wk after the last dose of an oral antibiotic or 1 mo after the last dose of an injected antibiotic. Traces of antibiotics in the serum may render the TPI test inconclusive.

The FTA-ABS test has replaced the TPI test as the best confirmatory test in the serodiagnosis of syphilis.

For details of the technic see Nelson and Mayer,[56] Harris et al.,[57] the *1964 Manual, Serologic Tests of Syphilis*,[35] or the sixth edition (1963) of this text.

COMPLEMENT FIXATION TESTS

The complement fixation technic had its beginning with the discovery by Pfeiffer in 1894 of what has been termed the Pfeiffer phenomenon or bacteriolysis.

Pfeiffer showed that, with the development of immunity by an animal to bacteria, its body fluids develop the property of dissolving these bacteria. He immunized guinea pigs to cholera organisms. After immunizing these animals he injected the same cholera vibrios into their peritoneal cavities and found, when he punctured the abdominal cavity with sterile glass capillary tubes and withdrew peritoneal fluid, that this fluid dissolved the cholera vibrios. Nonimmunized pigs did not show this phenomenon. This was an example of bacteriolysis.

Mechnikoff further proved that this same phenomenon could be detected in the test tube; i.e., by mixing cholera vibrios in a test tube containing the peritoneal fluid of an immunized guinea pig, the same bacteriolysis could be observed. Bordet showed that on heating the cholera-immunized serum to 56 C and adding fresh, unheated blood serum plus cholera organisms, bacteriolysis occurred; on heating the immune serum, not adding blood or serum, and adding cholera organisms, there followed no bacteriolysis. Thus he demonstrated that there were 2 substances concerned with the bacteriolytic test—a specific thermostable antibody that could withstand heating at 56 C and another that could not withstand such heating, the latter substance, which is thermolabile, could be replaced by fresh normal blood or blood serum. He first showed that the thermolabile substance is present at all times in normal blood and is not a product of the immunization injections, but the substance that is thermostable is a product to immunization injections and is not normally found in blood or blood serum. This phenomenon of bacteriolysis was found similar to that of hemolysis that was first noted by Bordet and Gengou.[31] They showed that hemolysis could be developed by the interaction between a substance, e.g., sheep cells, and a corresponding "substance sensibilatrice" produced by injecting a rabbit with repeated quantities of sheep cells in the presence of a third substance called **complement**. In other words, an antibody formed by the organism in response to the injection of the sheep cells, the "substance sensibilatrice," now called generally **hemolysin** (or amboceptor), would hemolyze the sheep cells in the presence of a sufficient amount of **complement** found in various quantities in practically all animals. It was further shown that the heating of the serum containing hemolysin at 56 C for $\frac{1}{2}$ hour destroyed the complement but did not affect the antiserum or hemolysin in any way. It was upon this so-called hemolytic system, which was only mildly interesting to research workers for a number of years, that Wassermann, Neisser, and Bruck based the famous test named after the first of these investigators, which is commonly considered the classic serologic test for the diagnosis of syphilis.

Wassermann, Neisser, and Bruck believed that in the blood of all syphilitic patients there was a

---

*Burroughs, Wellcome & Co., Research Triangle Park, N.C.

substance, or antibody, which in the presence of specific extract of the *Treponema pallidum* was sufficient **to so bind or fix complement that the later addition of the hemolysin and the homologous cell (sheep cell) was followed by no hemolysis or lack of hemolysis;** furthermore, that if the blood serum came from a patient who was not syphilitic, the antigenic extract supposedly derived from a suspension of *T. pallidum* would not bind complement, which would be free later to hemolyze the specific hemolysin and cellular mixture (sheep cells). This was a valuable application of the well-known Bordet-Gengou phenomenon and has served exceedingly well for many years to assist in the diagnosis of syphilis.

As discussed earlier, the theory on which the Wassermann test was based (the need for treponemal extract) was not correct, since extracts of normal tissues yield excellent antigenic extracts for performance of the test.

Despite the use of a nonspecific antigen, the Wassermann test and its later modifications served exceedingly well in the diagnosis of syphilis.

It should also be kept in mind that complement fixation tests **employing specific antigens** but based on the same principles as encountered in the complement fixation test for syphilis are used in the diagnosis of many diseases, including amebiasis, glanders, typhus, echinococcosis, malaria, filariasis, Rocky Mountain spotted fever, and trypanosomiasis, as well as various viral diseases. Variations exist, of course, in the antigen employed and the antibody detected.

Complement and complement fixation

Complement is a complex system of proteins. At least 11 discrete serum proteins have been identified as components of the complement system. These are not antibodies; immunization does not increase their concentration. The components of complement are designated by the symbols C1, C2, etc. The numbers following the symbol C refer to the sequence of discovery. See Chapter 62 for details.

Complement occurs in the blood of various species of animals, and the complement in the serum of **guinea pigs** is widely used in the laboratory. Of the various components of complement, the best proportions of each seem to be present in the guinea pig serum. It has been determined that lysis of cells (some bacterial red cells, tissue cells) after combination with a specific lysin will not occur unless complement is present. The lysin antibody combines with the cells, but the reaction will not go to completion unless complement becomes a part of the combination. The lytic activity of complement, in conjunction with specific antibody, is dependent on the presence of certain ions, namely, magnesium and calcium.

Complement becomes bound or fixed in antigen-antibody reactions. This process, leading to the removal of free complement from the system, is referred to as **complement fixation**

(stage 1). It provides a sensitive means of detecting antigen-antibody reactions. To determine whether complement has been removed from a system, sensitized sheep erythrocytes (sheep cells plus suitable hemolysins, which are used as an **indicator,** are added to the system (stage 2). If hemolysis occurs, free complement is present, and the unknown serum contains no antibody. If hemolysis does not develop, complement has been bound by the antigen-reagin complex, and the unknown serum is considered to be reactive (positive). For a schematic diagram of the CF test, see Fig. 75-1.

In the complement fixation test for syphilis, the serum to be tested is heated (**inactivated**) to destroy its complement. Therefore the only source of complement is the guinea pig serum. This source of complement must be carefully titrated so that a 4+ syphilitic serum will utilize all of the complement. A weakly positive serum will use only part of the complement, leaving some available to produce partial hemolysis of the sheep cells.

For a discussion of complement and the complement fixation reaction see Davis et al.[58] and Yachnin,[59] as well as Chapter 62.

Preparation and preservation of complement

Pooled, dried complement sera are widely employed and are commercially available. They are usually quite satisfactory, although occasionally unsatisfactory lots of complement are encountered. If preparation of complement in the laboratory is preferred, proceed as described below.

Preparation.* Select 3 or more large, healthy male guinea pigs. With a needle and syringe remove 5 ml blood from the heart and place in individual tubes identified by number.

After the blood has clotted at room temperature, ring with applicator stick and refrigerate for at least 1 h. Centrifuge and remove clear serum from the clot. Pool sera from all tubes, recentrifuge, and preserve. Or—

If animals are to be exsanguinated, stun to anesthetize, cut the external jugular veins, and collect blood in Petri dishes or 50 ml centrifuge tubes.

Allow clotting to take place for 1 h at room temperature. Loosen clot from wall of container and refrigerate for 1-2 h. Decant and filter serum through gauze, centrifuge, pool clear serum, and preserve.

Preservation

Method 1. Dehydrate complement serum from the frozen state, in vacuo, by the lyophile or Cryochem method.

Method 2. Add an equal part of the following solution to the complement serum:

Sodium acetate	12 g
Boric acid	4 g
Sterile distilled water	100 ml

For use, dilute 1 ml preserved complement serum with 14 ml saline solution to prepare a 1:30 dilution. Store in refrigerator.

---

*From *1959 Manual, Serologic methods for syphilis,* Public Health Service Pub. no. 411 (revised), U.S. Government Printing Office.

Method 3. Add 1 g sodium chloride for every 10 ml guinea pig serum. Store in refrigerator.

Method 4. Freeze complement serum and retain in the frozen state until used; 2 g/100 ml sodium acetate is added before dehydration or storage to complement serum at the Venereal Disease Research Laboratory.

Technic of bleeding guinea pig
1. Assemble the following materials.
   a. Guinea pig and animal board
   b. 5 ml Luer syringe with 1½ inch 21-gauge needle, sterilized in dry-heat oven at 170 C for 2 h
   c. Test tube for collecting blood
   d. Sterile sponges
   e. Alcohol or iodine
   f. Ether anesthetic
   g. Sterile saline in test tubes for emergency injection or for opening needle if it becomes plugged
2. Place animal on animal board.
3. Shave skin over area of heart.
4. Locate heartbeat (left ventricle) by palpation.
5. Give animal a light anesthetic.
6. Disinfect skin with alcohol or iodine.
7. Plunge needle attached to syringe into heart, taking care that needle is in left ventricle.
8. Slowly withdraw 5 or 10 ml blood from heart.
9. Eject contents of syringe into sterile test tube.
10. Inject 5 ml saline into abdominal wall of guinea pig and release it from board.

Procedure
1. Allow blood to clot.
2. Loosen clot from side of tube with sterile wooden applicator.
3. Centrifuge at high speed to separate serum from clot.
4. Remove clear supernatant serum from clot by means of sterile dropper, placing it in sterile test tube.
5. If there are any blood cells in serum, recentrifuge it, and decant cell-free serum.

Collection and preservation of sheep blood[60,61]

Sheep cells may be too resistant or too susceptible to the hemolytic action of complement and hemolysin. Since the reactivity level of a complement fixation test is influenced by the quality of sheep cells employed, particular attention should be given to the sheep cells. Only aseptically collected sheep blood in sterile containers is recommended for use in complement fixation testing.

Red cells from an occasional sheep will be found to be exceptionally resistant to the hemolytic action of complement and hemolysin. Whenever blood from an untested sheep is drawn, comparative complement and hemolysin titrations should be made, employing other sheep cells of acceptable quality. Sheep cells are too fragile for use when a saline suspension of washed cells, prepared as prescribed by a test technic, shows any degree of hemolysis when stored overnight at 6-10 C.

Discard unsatisfactory cells and obtain another supply of sheep blood.

Equipment and glassware
1. Bleeding flask, Erlenmeyer, 2 L capacity, fitted with a no. 10 2-hole rubber stopper, filter funnel (2.5 cm in diameter, 6.4 cm stem), rubber and glass tubing, and 13-gauge hypodermic needle
2. Dispensing assembly consisting of rubber tubing, clamp, and filling mantle, plus air filter tube

Reagent
1. 3.8% Sodium citrate solution
   a. Dissolve 3.8 g sodium citrate (ACS) in each 100 ml distilled water.
   b. Sixty ml of this solution is required for each 50 ml sheep blood collected.

Assembly of bleeding flask
1. Draw a line on the 2 L flask with a wax pencil, marking off 880 ml vol. This will provide for collection of 400 ml blood in 480 ml citrate solution.
2. Pour 480 ml 3.8% sodium citrate solution into flask. Cut a small piece of wire screening and place in funnel. Tie a piece of gauze over mouth of funnel.
3. Assemble bleeding flask by inserting stopper of bleeding apparatus into flask and securing it with string ties. Sterilize entire unit at 15 psi for 20 min.

Collection of blood
1. Immobilize sheep in standing position. Raise head until nose and center of neck form straight line. Turn head slightly and clip wool from puncture area.
2. Apply digital pressure above collarbone to cause dilation of external jugular vein. Sterilize area directly over located vein with weak iodine solution or 70% alcohol.
3. Apply digital pressure just below point to be punctured and insert sterile needle into skin and then into vein. Rotate flask continuously during collection of blood and for 5 min afterward to prevent clotting. Allow blood to cool to room temperature (23-29 C).
4. Replace glass suction mouthpiece with previously sterilized filling mantle. Replace hypodermic needle with section of sterile glass tubing containing loosely packed sterile cotton. Invert and suspend flask. Dispense blood aseptically into sterile rubber-stoppered vaccine bottles and store in refrigerator. Remove blood mixtures from these bottles, as required, with sterile syringe and needle.

Sheep blood of good quality, collected and stored in manner described, has been found satisfactory for use over a 3 mo period.

In many laboratories where animal facilities are unsatisfactory or inadequate, it will be advisable to procure sheep cell suspensions widely available from biologic supply houses.

Hemolysis and hemolysin

Hemolysis is the digestion or dissolution of blood cells by various agents. Hemolysis may be caused by chemical or bacteriologic factors. For instance, blood cells are hemolyzed by the addition of distilled water and mineral acids. A specific blood cell, e.g., the sheep cell, would be hemolyzed or digested in the presence of the specific antisheep hemolysin and sufficient complement. Excessive or prolonged heat, toxins of certain bacteria, undue agitation, age, and other factors cause hemolysis of blood cells.

Hemolysin is a substance, either present normally or artificially produced in the blood serum of animals, that is capable of dissolving the blood cells against which it has a specific action. This reaction does not take place unless complement is used. Hemolysin is artificially produced by the injection of blood cells of 1 species of animal into the bloodstream of another animal at definite intervals. The blood serum of the animal injected contains the hemolysin that is specific in dissolving the blood cells of the species of animal whose cells were used for injection.

For example, if sheep cells are injected into the bloodstream of a rabbit, the rabbit blood serum develops antisheep hemolysin. This hemolysin is capable of dissolving sheep cells (if complement is present in the reaction). Any other type of hemolysin is produced in a similar fashion.

Preparation of hemolysin. The following method[62] gives consistently satisfactory results. Whole sheep blood is injected intracutaneously into rabbits, followed by intravenous inoculation of washed sheep cells. Blood from several sheep is used during the course of injections.

Select 6 or 8 medium-sized young rabbits weighing about 2 kg each. Defibrinate a small amount of sheep blood with glass beads. Give each rabbit a series of 5 intracutaneous injections of whole sheep blood every other day, beginning with a dosage of 0.5 ml and increasing this each time by 0.5 ml (Table 106-4).

Prepare a 20% suspension of sheep cells by washing red cells thoroughly with a 0.85% saline solution to which 0.01% magnesium sulfate has been added (see Reagents, saline solution, **Kolmer tests**).

Two intravenous injections of 1 ml 20% sheep cell suspension are given at 3 d intervals after the last injection of whole sheep blood (Table 106-4). Test bleedings are made, beginning 3 d after the second intravenous injection, by piercing the marginal ear vein with a stylet and collecting approximately 1 ml blood in a small tube. Serum is separated from these blood samples by centrifuging after clotting is completed.

Each rabbit serum is titrated for hemolysin content by the method described in the Kolmer complement fixation technic.

Exsanguinate those rabbits having a hemolysin titration unit of 1:5000 dilution or higher. Separate sera from blood clots, pool, and preserve by the addition of an equal amount of glycerin.

Keep in refrigerator, where activity is maintained over long periods of time or preserve by lyophilization. Aliquots of 4 ml are dehydrated, sealed in an atmosphere of nitrogen, and stored in the refrigerator. For use, an ampule is opened, and the dried hemolysin is dissolved in 4 ml distilled water. The restored material

is further diluted with an equal volume of glycerin and stored in the refrigerator.

Repeat the intravenous injections of 20% washed cells in the rabbits with a low hemolysin titer.

Stock glycerinated (50%) sheep red cell hemolysin can be stored at refrigerator temperature for long periods of time with little loss of reactivity. When a marked drop in titer is found or if precipitate is seen in the diluted hemolysin, the reagent should be discarded and reprepared from stock hemolysin.

Method of bleeding rabbit from carotid artery

1. Prepare the following sterile instruments.
   a. 1 pair sharp-pointed small scissors
   b. 1 pair sharp-pointed long scissors
   c. 2 seraphine clamps
   d. 2 fine-pointed hemostats
   e. 1 pair tissue forceps
   f. Several pieces of linen thread about 20 cm long
   g. 3 or 4 Rockefeller centrifuge tubes with corks
   h. Gauze sponges
   i. 2 groove directors or probes
2. Also assemble material for anesthetic, iodine, shaving material, and rabbit board.
3. Place animal on rabbit board and give rabbit a light anesthetic. Ether is preferable to chloroform.
4. Shave hair over entire front area of neck.
5. Pour on a generous quantity of iodine. If too small a quantity of iodine is used, the blood may become contaminated from bacteria on rabbit's skin. Make a long incision through skin over neck. The incision should be at least 10 cm in length and extend in a lateral line in center of neck.
6. Grasp probes at center and probe down into muscles until carotid artery is visible. It will be easily recognized by arterial beat and vagus nerve that is adjacent to it. Do not mistake jugular vein for carotid artery.
7. Lift artery on probes, placing probes sidewise under artery to lift it.
8. Separate artery from nerve.
9. Tie off upper end of artery with linen thread that has been previously dipped in iodine. Do not tie too tightly or arterial wall may be broken. Tie tightly enough so that artery does not retract through suture.
10. Clamp other end of artery about 3.8 cm below thread with seraphine clamp.
11. Cut thread so that about 0.6 cm remains protruding from double knot.
12. Pick up 1 wall of artery between thread and clamp with hemostat. Be sure not to close entire artery during this process.
13. Cut artery in about center of space between thread and clamp.
14. Place a small amount of iodine on end of cut artery nearer clamp. This procedure must not consume too much time.
15. Direct end of artery into a sterile Rockefeller tube, and loosen seraphine clamp.
16. Blood spurts through artery into tube. Be sure to keep animal under a light anesthetic during this process. Do not give too heavy an anesthetic.
17. Allow blood to run from artery, filling as many tubes as necessary, until animal is dying; then give a heavy anesthetic, sacrificing rabbit.
18. Bottle is stoppered with a sterile cork immediately after blood is obtained.

Shipley[64] has devised a board for studies requiring repeated injections into the ear veins of rabbits. It has the advantage of effectively holding rabbits and

Table 106-4. Schedule of injections[63]

Day	Dosage (ml)	Route of inoculation	Material injected
1	0.5	Intracutaneous	Whole blood
3	1.0	Intracutaneous	Whole blood
5	1.5	Intracutaneous	Whole blood
7	2.0	Intracutaneous	Whole blood
9	2.5	Intracutaneous	Whole blood
12	1.0	Intravenous	20% washed cells
15	1.0	Intravenous	20% washed cells
18	Test bleeding		

immobilizing their ears for bleeding or injection procedures.

The significant feature of the apparatus is a mask, shaped to accommodate the anterior three-fourths of the rabbit's head. An inverted U-shaped collar holds the head firmly in the mask so that the position of the ears is correspondingly stabilized. The head holder is made by molding a liquid thermo-setting plastic (plaster of Paris may also be used) around a plaster of Paris model that has been shaped to conform to the head of a rabbit weighing about 2.5 kg. Provisions are made for leaving a hole from the nose to the outside. Within the 2 horizontal, tubular supports that are included in the plastic casting run two 0.5 cm ball chains 30 cm long. The anterior three-fourths of the rabbit's head is held in the cast by a horse collar–shaped neckpiece to which are attached the ball chains. Once the rabbit's head is placed in the cast, the operator exerts traction on the chains, and under moderate tension the latter are secured by fitting them into 2 narrow vertical slots on the ends of the horizontal support tubes.

The body of the rabbit is confined in a 13 × 13 × 30 cm metal box with a hinged lid and clasp. Two flanges fastened to the front of the box prevent the rabbit's legs from reaching the area about the ears. All parts are mounted on a piece of 30 × 69 × 1.9 cm plywood, the top and edges of which are covered with sheet metal 0.013 mm thick. For maximum rigidity, durability, and ease in cleaning, stainless steel, chrome-plated brass, and plastic were used. In using this box, by transilluminating the rabbit's ear from below, locating and visualizing particularly the smaller veins are greatly facilitated. It is rarely necessary to clip or shave the hair over the vein in preparation for injection. A flexible arm with a small socket and bulb attached may be brought into any desired position beneath either ear.

Laboratory Branch complement fixation (LBCF) method[65]

A standardized complement fixation (CF) procedure, useful with **all** diagnostic CF antigens **(bacterial, fungal, rickettsial, and viral)**, has been developed by a task force in the Laboratory Branch of the Center for Disease Control, U.S. Public Health Service.

The method uses the 50% end-point hemolytic complement technics and serves well as a practical day-to-day working tool with all antigens tested. It is, however, **not generally used in serologic testing for syphilis**. Readers interested in the details of the technic, as well as its adaptation to a microtechnic, are referred to the original publication[65]; see also Chapter 93.

REITER PROTEIN COMPLEMENT FIXATION TEST[66-69]*
One-fifth volume Kolmer tests [70, 71]†

This small-volume Kolmer test may be used with Reiter protein (treponemal) antigen (KRP) as well as with cardiolipin (nontreponemal) antigen.

---

*Referred to as the RPCF or KRP test.
†From *1964 Manual, Serologic tests for syphilis*.[35] The test was removed from the 1969 manual,[2] but it is retained here since it is still used in laboratories outside the United States.

Equipment and glassware
1. Racks, test tube, galvanized wire, for 72 tubes
2. Test tubes, Pyrex, 12 × 75 mm
3. Test tubes, Pyrex, 15 × 85 mm or 13 × 100 mm
4. Tubes, centrifuge, graduated, 15 ml capacity, Pyrex
5. Tubes, centrifuge, round bottom, 50 ml capacity

Reagents
1. Reiter protein antigen
   This antigen is prepared from a culture of Reiter treponemes by cryolysis and ammonium sulfate precipitation.[68,69]
2. Kolmer saline
   Dissolve 8.5 g dried sodium chloride (ACS) and 0.1 g magnesium sulfate or chloride in 1 L freshly distilled water. Freshly prepared saline should be used for each test run. Place in refrigerator a portion of saline sufficient for diluting complement to be used in tests.
3. Sheep red cells
   See Collection and Preservation of Sheep Blood. Freshly collected sheep blood should be refrigerated 48 h before being used. To determine if a new lot of cells is satisfactory, comparative hemolysin and complement titrations should be performed with other sheep cells of acceptable quality. Sheep cells are too fragile for use when a 2% suspension of washed cells shows hemolysis when stored overnight at 6-10 C.
4. Antisheep red cell hemolysin (immune rabbit serum)
   Stock glycerinated (50%) antisheep red cell hemolysin can be stored at refrigerator temperature for long periods of time with little loss of reactivity. See Preparation of Hemolysin.
5. Complement*
   See Preparation and preservation of Complement.

• • •

Cell-free guinea pig serum can be obtained by centrifuging the tubes of blood and decanting serum from the clots when the laboratory practice is to bleed guinea pigs the day before the complement fixation tests are performed. The serum from 3 or more guinea pigs should be pooled and returned to the refrigerator.

Dehydrated complement serum should be restored to **original serum volume** by dissolving in the proper amount of buffered diluent or distilled water and storing in the refrigerator.

Complement serum stored in the frozen state should be returned to the liquid state by being left at room temperature or at 37 C only long enough to melt. As protein content of these sera will tend to collect at the bottom of the tube during thawing, these tubes of serum should be adequately mixed by inversion and returned to the refrigerator (6-10 C).

Complement stored in the frozen state should be divided into quantities sufficient for 1 day's use to avoid complement destruction due to repeated thawing and refreezing.

Antigen dilution. The **Reiter protein antigen** dilution should be prepared just prior to its use in the test. The test dose is 0.1 ml antigen diluted to titer.
1. Place required amount of saline in flask or tube.
2. Draw up 0.05 ml or more of Reiter protein antigen in bottom half of a 0.1 or 0.2 ml pipet, graduated to tip, and add to saline.
3. Mix well by filling and emptying pipet a few times in diluted antigen.

---

*Available from biologic supply houses.

Preparation of 2% sheep red cell suspension. For each day's testing, prepare a fresh 2% sheep red cell suspension.

Filter an adequate quantity of preserved sheep blood through gauze into a 50 ml, round-bottom centrifuge tube. Add 2 or 3 vol saline to the tube. Centrifuge tubes at a force sufficient to sediment cells in 5 min (I.E.C. centrifuge size 1 at 2000 rpm or I.E.C. centrifuge size 2 at 1700 rpm). Remove supernatant fluid by suction, taking off upper white cell layer.

Fill tube with saline and resuspend cells by inverting and gently shaking tube. Recentrifuge tube and repeat the process for a total of 3 washings. If supernatant fluid is not colorless on third washing, cells are too fragile and should not be used. After supernatant fluid is removed from third washing, cells are poured or washed into a 15 ml graduated centrifuge tube. Fill tube with saline and resuspend cells by inverting. Centrifuge at previously used speed for 10 min to pack cells firmly and evenly.

Read the volume of packed cells in the centrifuge tube and carefully remove supernatant fluid.

Prepare a 2% suspension of sheep cells by washing the cells into a flask with 49 vol saline. Shake flask to ensure even suspension of cells. Example:

2.1 ml (packed cells) × 49 =
  102.9 ml (saline solution required)

Pipet 15 ml 2% cell suspension into a graduated centrifuge tube and centrifuge at previously used speed for 10 min. A 15 ml aliquot of a properly prepared cell suspension will produce 0.3 ml ± 0.01 ml packed cells.

CAUTION: Use only centrifuge tubes that have been tested for proper calibration in 15 ml and cell-pack volume zones.

When the packed cell volume is beyond the tolerable limits stated above, the cell suspension concentration should be adjusted. The quantity of saline solution that must be removed or added to the cell suspension to accomplish adjustment is determined according to the following formula:

$$\frac{\text{Actual reading of centrifuge tube}}{\text{Correct reading of centrifuge tube}} \times$$
$$\text{Volume of cell suspension} =$$
$$\text{Corrected volume of cell suspension}$$

Example 1:
  Volume of cell suspension   100 ml
  Centrifuge tube (15 ml) reading   0.27 ml

$$\frac{0.27 \text{ ml}}{0.3 \text{ ml}} \times 100 \text{ ml} = 90 \text{ ml}$$

Therefore 10 ml saline solution should be removed from each 100 ml cell suspension. Saline solution may be removed by centrifuging an aliquot of the cell suspension and pipetting off the desired volume of saline solution for discard.

Example 2:
  Volume of cell suspension   100 ml
  Centrifuge tube (15 ml) reading   0.33 ml

$$\frac{0.33 \text{ ml}}{0.3 \text{ ml}} \times 100 \text{ ml} = 110 \text{ ml}$$

Therefore 10 ml saline solution should be added to each 100 ml cell suspension. An adjusted cell suspension should be rechecked by centrifuging a 15 ml portion.

Place flask of cell suspension in refrigerator when not in use. Always shake before using to secure an even suspension since the corpuscles settle to the bottom of the flask when allowed to stand.

Preparation of stock hemolysin dilution. Prepare 1:100 stock hemolysin dilution as follows:

Kolmer saline	94 ml
Phenol solution (5% in Kolmer saline)	2 ml
Glycerinized hemolysin (50%)	2 ml

Mix phenol solution well with the saline before glycerinized hemolysin is added. This stock dilution keeps well at refrigerator temperature but should be discarded if it is found to contain precipitate or if a marked drop in titer occurs. Each new lot of stock hemolysin dilution (1:100) should be checked by parallel titration with the previous stock hemolysin dilution before it is placed into routine use.

Dilutions of hemolysin of 1:1000 or greater are prepared by further diluting the 1:100 dilution.

Preparation of sera. All specimens are lined up and properly labeled.

The sera are removed from the clots with capillary pipets to test tubes properly labeled. Great care is required to prevent errors in labeling and confusion of sera. Each serum should be free of corpuscles; otherwise, it is necessary to break up the clots with wooden applicators (1 for each serum) and centrifuging for clear serum. Slight tinging with hemoglobin does no harm. Sera containing large amounts of hemoglobin are likely to be anticomplementary.

Heat serum at 56 C for 30 min. Previously heated sera should be reheated for 10 min at 56 C on day of testing.

Hemolysin and complement titrations

1. Place 10 tubes (numbered 1 to 10) in rack.
2. Prepare 1:1000 dilution of hemolysin by placing 4.5 ml saline in test tube and adding 0.5 ml 1:100 stock hemolysin dilution. Mix well. Add 0.5 ml 1:1000 hemolysin dilution in tubes 2 through 5.
3. Add saline to tubes 2 through 10 and prepare dilutions as follows:

Tube	Saline (ml)	Process	Final hemolysin dilution
1	—	None	1:1,000
2	0.5	Mix	1:2,000
3	1.0	Mix; transfer 0.5 ml to tube 6	1:3,000
4	1.5	Mix; transfer 0.5 ml to tube 7	1:4,000
5	2.0	Mix; transfer 0.5 ml to tube 8	1:5,000
6	0.5	Mix; transfer 0.5 ml to tube 9	1:6,000
7	0.5	Mix; transfer 0.5 ml to tube 10	1:8,000
8	0.5	Mix	1:10,000
9	0.5	Mix	1:12,000
10	0.5	Mix	1:16,000

4. Perform hemolysin and complement titrations simultaneously in same rack.
5. Use 12 × 75 mm tubes. Place 10 tubes (numbered 1 to 10) in 1 side of rack for hemolysin titration and 6 tubes (numbered 1 to 6) in other side for complement titration. Add 1 tube to rack for cell control. Pipet 0.1 ml of each of hemolysin dilutions (1:1,000 to 1:16,000) into each of corresponding 10 tubes of hemolysin titration.

Table 106-5. Hemolysin titration*

Tube	Hemoly-sin (0.1 ml)	Comple-ment 1:50 (ml)	2% sheep red cell suspension (ml)	Saline (ml)
1	1:1000	0.1	0.1	0.4
2	1:2000	0.1	0.1	0.4
3	1:3000	0.1	0.1	0.4
4	1:4000	0.1	0.1	0.4
5	1:5000	0.1	0.1	0.4
6	1:6000	0.1	0.1	0.4
7	1:8000	0.1	0.1	0.4
8	1:10,000	0.1	0.1	0.4
9	1:12,000	0.1	0.1	0.4
10	1:16,000	0.1	0.1	0.4

*From Serologic tests for syphilis, 1964 manual.

Table 106-6. Preparation of diluted hemolysin*

Dilution containing 1 unit/ 0.1 ml	Dilution containing 2 units/0.1 ml	To prepare 2-unit hemolysin dilution, mix	
		1:100 Hemolysin solution (ml)	Saline solution (ml)
1:4000	1:2000	0.1	1.9
1:5000	1:2500	0.1	2.4
1:6000	1:3000	0.1	2.9
1:8000	1:4000	0.1	3.9
1:10,000	1:5000	0.1	4.9
1:12,000	1:6000	0.1	5.9
1:16,000	1:8000	0.1	7.9

*From Serologic tests for syphilis, 1964 manual.[35]

Table 106-7. Complement titration*

Tube	Complement 1:50 (ml)	Saline (ml)	1 h in 37 C water bath	Hemolysin 2 units (ml)	2% sheep red cell suspension (ml)	½ h secondary incubation in 37 C water bath
1	0.25	0.25		0.1	0.1	
2	0.20	0.30		0.1	0.1	
3	0.15	0.35		0.1	0.1	
4	0.13	0.37		0.1	0.1	
5	0.12	0.38		0.1	0.1	
6	0.10	0.40		0.1	0.1	

*From Serologic tests for syphilis, 1964 manual.[35]

6. Prepare a 1:50 dilution of complement by adding 0.1 ml complement to 4.9 ml saline. Mix thoroughly. Pipet 0.1 ml 1:50 complement into each of the 10 tubes of hemolysin titration.

7. Add the following amounts of 1:50 complement and saline to complement titration tubes in this order, being sure to wash down all complement adhering to wall of tube:

Tube	1	2	3	4	5	6
Complement 1:50 (ml)*	0.25	0.20	0.15	0.13	0.12	0.10
Saline (ml)	0.25	0.30	0.35	0.37	0.38	0.40

*The quantity of 1:50 complement in the first 2 tubes may be measured with a 0.5 ml or a 0.25 ml pipet and in the last 4 tubes with a 0.2 ml pipet.

8. Add 0.1 ml 2% sheep red cell suspension to each tube of hemolysin titration and to cell control tube and 0.4 ml saline to hemolysin titration tubes and 0.6 ml saline to cell control tube. Shake each tube of hemolysin titration to ensure even distribution of cells and place rack containing the 2 titrations in 37 C water bath for 1 h. Shake rack after 30 min. Completed hemolysin titration is shown in Table 106-5.

9. Remove rack from water bath and read hemolysin titration. **The unit of hemolysin is the highest dilution that gives complete hemolysis.** Hemolysin for the complement titration and the test is diluted so that 2 units are contained in 0.1 ml, and dilution should be at least 1:2000.

10. Prepare diluted hemolysin, containing 2 units/ 0.1 ml, sufficient for complement titration as shown in Table 106-6.

11. Add 0.1 ml diluted hemolysin (containing 2 units of hemolysin) to each of the 6 tubes of the complement titration.

12. Add 0.1 ml 2% sheep red cell suspension to each tube of the complement titration. The addition of hemolysin and cells to the complement titration should be completed without delay, preferably **within 5 min** after rack is removed from the water bath.

13. Shake each tube of the complement titration to ensure even distribution of the cells and return the rack to the 37 C water bath for 30 min. The complete complement titration is shown in Table 106-7.

14. Remove rack from water bath and read complement titration. **The smallest amount of 1:50 complement giving complete hemolysis is the exact unit.** For use in the test, complement is diluted so that 2 exact units are contained in 0.2 ml.

Example:

Exact unit	0.15 ml
Two exact units (dose)	0.30 ml
Complement dilution used in titration	1:50

Table 106-8. Limits of usable complement dilutions and preparation*

1:50 complement dilution (ml)		Dilution containing 2 exact units in 0.2 ml	Preparation	
Exact unit	2 exact units		Undiluted complement (ml)	Saline (ml)
0.25	0.5	1:20	1.0	19.0
0.20	0.4	1:25	1.0	24.0
0.15	0.3	1:33	1.0	32.0
0.13	0.26	1:38	1.0	37.0
0.12	0.24	1:42	1.0	41.0
0.10	0.2	1:50	1.0	49.0

*From Serologic tests for syphilis, 1964 manual.[35]

15. Calculate dilution of complement to be employed in test proper by dividing 50 (reciprocal of complement dilution) by dose, and multiplying by volume in which dilution is to be contained, i.e., $\frac{50}{0.3} \times 0.2 = 33$ or a 1:33 dilution of guinea pig serum. The limits of usable complement dilutions and preparation are given in Table 106-8.

16. **Tubes of the complement or hemolysin titrations showing complete hemolysis may be removed and placed in refrigerator for later use as hemoglobin solutions for the reading standards.**

Qualitative tests with serum (one-fifth volume Kolmer; RPCF or KRP)[35]

1. Arrange 12 × 75 mm test tubes in wire racks so that there are 2 tubes for each serum and for control sera of graded reactivity. Number first row of tubes to correspond to sera and control sera being tested. Three additional tubes are included for reagent controls (antigen, hemolytic system, and cell control).

2. Prepare a **1:5 dilution of each test serum** by adding 0.2 ml serum to 0.8 ml Kolmer saline. Mix well. Pipet 0.2 ml of each of **diluted control sera** into appropriate tubes in first (test) and second (control) rows. Add 0.2 ml **1:5 dilution of each serum to be tested** to appropriate tubes in first and second rows; then add 0.1 ml **Kolmer saline** to each tube of second row (individual serum controls).

3. Pipet saline into the 3 reagent control tubes as follows:

Antigen control	0.2 ml
Hemolytic system control	0.3 ml
Cell control	0.6 ml

4. Add 0.1 ml antigen dilution to each tube of first row (individual serum tests) and to antigen control tube.

5. Allow test racks to stand for 10-15 min at room temperature.

6. During this interval, prepare **diluted complement** to titer with **cold** Kolmer saline. Amount of complement dilution is calculated by determining number of tubes in test run and allowing 0.2 ml for each tube plus a slight excess.

7. Using 2 ml pipet add 0.2 ml diluted complement (containing 2 exact units) to all tubes of test run except cell control tube as follows: add diluted complement to 1 rack of tubes. Mix by shaking rack and place in refrigerator. Repeat same for each rack of tubes.

8. Refrigerate test **(primary incubation)** at 6-10 C for at least 15 h but not longer than 18 h.

9. The following morning, prepare reading standards by heating hemoglobin solution saved from previous day's titration in 56 C water bath for 5 min. Then make a 1:7 dilution of 2% cell suspension by adding 0.5 ml 2% cell suspension to 3.0 ml saline. Prepare reading standards by mixing hemoglobin and 1:7 cell suspension in proportions given in Table 106-9.

10. Prepare diluted hemolysin to titer with saline. Amount of hemolysin dilution is calculated by determining number of tubes in test run and allowing 0.1 ml for each tube plus a slight excess.

11. Remove racks of tubes from refrigerator at regular 5 or 10 min intervals and place immediately in 37 C water bath for 10 min.

12. Remove each rack from water bath and add 0.1 ml diluted hemolysin to all tubes of test except cell control tube. Shake rack.

13. Add 0.1 ml 2% sheep red cell suspension (prepared the previous day) to all tubes. The 2% cell suspension should be agitated occasionally to ensure

Table 106-9. Preparation of reading standards*

1:7 cell suspension (ml)	Hemoglobin solution (ml)	Complement fixed (%)	Reading
0.7	None	100	4+
0.35	0.35	50	3+
0.35†	1.05†	25	2+
0.07	0.63	10	1+
0.07†	1.33†	5	±
None	0.7	0	–

*From Serologic tests for syphilis, 1964 manual.[35]
†Double quantities are pipetted and 0.7 ml removed from each tube after adequate mixing.

even suspension of cells during the period when this reagent is being added to the CF tests.

14. Mix contents of tubes thoroughly by shaking each rack before returning it to 37 C water bath for **secondary incubation.**

15. Examine antigen and hemolytic system controls at **5 min intervals** to determine "clearing time"; i.e., length of time necessary to produce complete hemolysis. At no time should hemolysis occur in cell control.

16. Examine control serums of graded reactivity at **5 min intervals** to determine "reading time." Reading time is length of time necessary to reproduce predetermined reactivity pattern of control sera. **Reading time should be at least 10 min more than clearing time but should not exceed a total of 60 min.**

17. Remove each rack of tubes from water bath at reading time and read results by comparing with reading standards. If reading falls between 2 tubes of reading standards, it is recorded as lower value.

18. For any specimen with incomplete hemolysis in control tube, return both tubes to 37 C water bath for not more than 60 min incubation. Read control tubes at 5 min intervals and record test results when complete hemolysis is observed in control tube.

19. Report results of qualitative tests as shown in Table 106-10. For an outline of the one-fifth volume Kolmer test with serum see Table 106-11.

Quantitative tests with serum (Kolmer one-fifth volume; RPCF or KRP)[35]

1. Place 12 × 75 mm test tubes in racks, allowing 8 tubes for each serum to be tested. Include reagent controls (antigen, hemolytic system, and cell control) and control sera of graded reactivity.

2. Pipet indicated amount of saline into each of the following reagent control tubes:

Antigen control	0.2 ml
Hemolytic system control	0.3 ml
Cell control	0.6 ml

3. For each serum, pipet 0.2 ml saline into tubes 2 through 7 and 0.1 ml into tube 8. Pipet 0.2 ml serum (**diluted 1:5**) into tubes 1, 2, and 8. Mix contents of tube 2, transfer 0.2 ml to tube 3, and so on to tube 7. Mix contents of tube 7 and discard 0.2 ml.

4. Add 0.1 ml diluted antigen to first 7 tubes of each serum test, to **test** tubes of control sera, and to antigen control tube. Shake rack to mix thoroughly.

5. Allow racks to stand at room temperature for 10-15 min.

6. During this interval, prepare diluted complement with **cold** Kolmer saline (calculate amount of complement dilution by determining number of tubes in test run and allowing 0.2 ml for each tube plus a slight excess).

Table 106-10. Kolmer qualitative test reporting*

Test tube reading	Control tube reading	Report	Test tube reading	Control tube reading	Report
4+	−	Reactive	3+	3+	Anticomplementary
3+	−	Reactive	3+	2+	Anticomplementary
2+	−	Reactive	3+	1+	Weakly Reactive
1+	−	Reactive	3+	±	Reactive
±	−	Weakly Reactive	2+	2+	Nonreactive
−	−	Nonreactive	2+	1+	Nonreactive
4+	4+	Anticomplementary	2+	±	Weakly Reactive
4+	3+	Anticomplementary	1+	1±	Nonreactive
4+	2+	Weakly Reactive	±	±	Nonreactive
4+	1+	Reactive			

*From Serologic tests for syphilis, 1964 manual.[35]

Table 106-11. Outline of one-fifth volume Kolmer test with serum*

Tube		Saline (ml)	Diluted antigen (ml)	Shake rack well. Allow to stand at room temperature for 10-15 min.	Complement 2 exact units (ml)	Incubate 15-18 h at 6-10 C followed by 10 min in 37 C water bath.	Hemolysin 2 units (ml)	Sheep cell suspension (2%) (ml)	Shake rack well. Secondary incubation in 37 C water bath.
Serum (1:5), ml)									
Test	0.2	None	0.1		0.2		0.1	0.1	
Control	0.2	0.1	None		0.2		0.1	0.1	
Reagent controls									
Antigen		0.2	0.1		0.2		0.1	0.1	
Hemolytic system		0.3	None		0.2		0.1	0.1	
Cell		0.6	None		None		None	0.1	

*From Serologic test for syphilis, 1964 manual.[35]

7. Add 0.2 ml diluted complement (containing 2 exact units) to all tubes except cell control.

8. Shake racks to mix thoroughly and place in refrigerator at 6-10 C for 15-18 h (**primary incubation**).

9. **Complete tests the following morning as indicated for qualitative tests.**

Quantitative tests showing complete hemolysis in the control tube are reported in terms of the highest dilution giving a Reactive result (1+, 2+, 3+, or 4+). The first tube is considered to be undiluted, or 1 dil. Additional dilutions may be prepared and tested if no end point is obtained.

For any specimen with incomplete hemolysis in the control tube, return all tubes to the 37 C water bath for a total of not more than 60 min incubation. Read control tubes at 5 min intervals and record test results when complete hemolysis is observed in the control tube.

Retesting of anticomplementary sera. Anticomplementary sera may be retested by preparing doubling dilutions in saline. Each dilution of serum is tested in 2 tubes, as test and control, as described for the qualitative test. Results of these tests may be interpreted as Reactive, without reference to titer, if the first serum dilution showing complete hemolysis in the control tube has a 3+ or 4+ reaction in the tube containing antigen. All other reactions would be reported as Anticomplementary.

REFERENCES

1. Syphilis, a synopsis, 1968, Venereal Disease Program, Natioanl Communicable Disease Center, Public Health Service Pub. no. 1660, Washington, D.C., 1968, U.S. Government Printing Office.

2. Manual of tests for syphilis, 1969, Public Health Service Pub. no. 411, reprinted 1978, HEW Pub. no. CDC 78-8347, Atlanta, Center for Disease Control.

3. Bauer, H.: Survey on current usage of tests for syphilis, 1976, Association of State and Territorial Public Health Laboratory Directors.

4. Atwood, W. G., Miller, J. L., Stout, G. W., and Norins, L. C.: J.A.M.A. **203**:549, 1968.

5. Harner, R. E., Smith, J. L., and Israel, C. W.: J.A.M.A. **203**:545, 1968.

6. Nicholas, L., and Beerman, H.: Am. J. Med. Sci. **249**:466, 1965.

7. Deacon, W. E., Falcone, V. H., and Harris, A.: Proc. Soc. Exp. Biol. Med. **96**:477, 1957.

8. Deacon, W. E., Freeman, E. M., and Harrris, A.: Proc. Soc. Exp. Biol. Med. **103**:827, 1960.

9. Hunter, E. F., Deacon, W. E., and Meyer, P. E.: Public Health Rep. **79**:410, 1964.

10. Dans, P. E., Judson, F. N., Larsen, S. A., and Lantz, M. A.: South. Med. J. **70**:312, 1977.

11. Tuffanelli, D. L., Wuepper, K. D., Bradford, L. L., and Wood, R. M.: N. Engl. J. Med. **276**:258, 1967.

12. Jaffe, H. W., Larsen, S. A., Jones, O. G., and Dans, P. E.: Am. J. Clin. Pathol. **70**:230, 1978.

13. Rathlev, T.: WHO/VDT/RES 77. **65**:1, 1965.

14. Sequiera, P. J. L., and Eldridge, A. E.: Br. J. Vener. Dis. **49**:242, 1973.

15. Falcone, V. H.: Public Health Lab. **26**:39, 1968.

16. Fiumara, N. J.: J.A.M.A. **192**:1111, 1965.

17. Burns, R. E.: J.A.M.A. **234**:617, 1975.

18. Soldman, J. N., and Lantz, M. A.: J.A.M.A. **217**:53, 1971.

19. Drew, F. L., and Sarandria, J. L.: J. Am. Vener. Dis. Assoc. **1**:165, 1975.
20. Peter, R., Thompson, M. A., and Wilson, D. L.: J. Clin. Microbiol. **9**:369, 1979.
21. Kraus, S. J., Haserick, J. R., and Lantz, M. A.: N. Engl. J. Med. **282**:1287, 1970.
22. Kaufman, B.: J. Am. Vener. Dis. Assoc. **1**:79, 1974.
23. Reimer, N.: Ann. N.Y. Acad. Sci. **251**:77, 1975.
24. Harris, A., and Mahoney, J. F.: J. Vener. Dis. Inform. **25**:46, 1944.
25. Identical memorandum. Director, Bureau of Laboratories, Center for Disease Control, Atlanta, Jan. 2, 1975.
26. Wallace, A. L.: Am. J. Clin. Pathol. **44**:712, 1965.
27. Portnoy, J., Garson, W., and Smith, C. A.: Public Health Rep. **72**:761, 1957.
28. Portnoy, J., Bossak, H. N., Falcone, V. H., and Harris, A.: Public Health Rep. **76**:933, 1961.
29. Portnoy, J.: Am. J. Clin. Pathol. **40**:473, 1963.
30. Portnoy, J., and Garson, W.: Public Health Rep. **75**:985, 1960.
31. Portnoy, J.: Public Health Lab. **23**:43, 1965.
32. Falcone, V. H., Stout, G. W., and Moore, M. B., Jr.: Public Health Rep. **79**:491, 1964.
33. Portnoy, J., Brewer, J. H., and Harris, A.: Public Health Rep. **77**:645, 1962.
34. Serologic tests for syphilis, 1959 Manual, Public Health Service Pub. no. 411, Washington, D.C., 1959, United States Government Printing Office.
35. Serologic tests for syphilis, 1964 Manual, Public Health Service Pub. no. 411 (rev. 1964), Washington, D.C., 1964, U.S. Government Printing Office.
36. Frankel, S., Reitman, S., and Sonnenwirth, A. C.: Gradwohl's clinical laboratory methods and diagnosis, ed. 7, St. Louis, 1970, The C. V. Mosby Co.
37. Kahn, R. L.: Proc. Soc. Exp. Biol. Med. **20**:325, 1923.
38. Kahn, R. L.: Proc. Soc. Exp. Biol. Med. **21**:76, 1923.
39. Kendrick, P. L., and Kahn, R. L.: J. Vener. Dis. Inform. **31**:104, 1950. McDermott, E. B., et al.: Br. J. Vener. Dis. **33**:182, 1957.
40. Kahn, R. L., and McDermott, E. B.: Am. J. Clin. Pathol. **18**:364, 1948.
41. Kahn, R. L., and McDermott, E. B.: J. Lab. Clin. Med. **33**:1220, 1948.
42. Kahn, R. L.: Serology with lipid antigens, Baltimore, 1950, The Williams & Wilkins Co.
43. Stuart, G. O., Grant, J. F., and Hinton, W. A.: J. Vener. Dis. Inform. **29**:27, 1948.
44. Hinton, W. A., Stuart, G. O., and Grant, J. F.: Am. J. Syph., Gonor. Vener. Dis. **33**:587, 1949.
45. Mazzini, L. Y.: J. Immunol. **66**:261, 1951.

46. Kline, B. S.: Am. J. Clin. Pathol. **16**:68, 1946.
47. Deacon, W., Lucus, J. B., and Price, E. V.: J.A.M.A. **198**:624, 1966.
48. Stout, G. W., Kellogg, D. S., Jr., Falcone, V. H., et al.: Health Lab. Sci. **4**:5, 1967.
49. Tomizawa, T., and Kasamatsu, S.: Jpn. J. Med. Sci. Biol. **19**:305-308, 1966.
50. Cox, P. M., Logan, L. C., and Norins, L. C.: Appl. Microbiol. **18**:485, 1969 (also WHO document, WHO/VDT/RES/69.174).
51. Tomizawa, T., Kasamatsu, S., and Yamaya, S.: Jpn. J. Med. Sci. Biol. **22**:341-350, 1969.
52. Logan, L. C., and Cox, P. M.: Am. J. Clin. Pathol. **53**:163-166, 1970. (Also WHO document, WHO/VDT/RES/69.175.)
53. West, B. S., and Pagano, A. D.: HSMHA Health Reports **87**(1):93-96, 1972.
54. Coffey, E. M., Bradford, L. L., Naritomi, L. S., and Wood, R. M.: Appl. Microbiol. **24**:26-30, 1972.
55. Microtiter instruction manual, ed. 3, Alexandria, Va., Oct. 1965, Cooke Engineering Co.
56. Nelson, R. A., Jr., and Mayer, M. M.: J. Exp. Med. **89**:369, 1949.
57. Harris, A., Bossak, H. N., and Olansky, S.: Public Health Lab. **13**:63, 1955.
58. Davis, B. D., Dulbecco, R., Eisen, H. N., et al.: Microbiology, New York, 1967, Harper & Row, Publishers.
59. Yachnin, S.: N. Engl. J. Med. **274**:140, 1966.
60. Portnoy, J., Bossak, H. N., and Harris, A.: J. Vener. Dis. Inform. **28**:137, 1947.
61. Bossak, H. N.: Am. J. Clin. Pathol. **19**:496, 1949.
62. Darter, L. A.: J. Lab. Clin. Med. **41**:653, 1953.
63. Serologic tests for syphilis, 1959 Manual, Public Health Service Pub. no. 411 (rev. 1959), U.S. Government Printing Office, Washington, D.C.
64. Shipley, J.: Proc. Soc. Exp. Biol. Med. **63**:75, 1946.
65. Standardized diagnostic complement fixation method and adaptation to micro test, Public Health Service (rev. 1974), Atlanta, Center for Disease Control.
66. Cannefax, G. R., and Garson, W.: Public Health Rep. **72**:335, 1957.
67. Bossak, H. N., Falcone, V. H., Duncan, W. P., and Harris, A.: Public Health Lab. **16**:39, 1958.
68. D'Alessandro, G., and Dardanoni, L.: Am. J. Syph., Gonor. Vener. Dis. **37**:137, 1953.
69. Wallace, A. L., and Harris, A.: Public Health Lab. **16**:27, 1958.
70. Kolmer, J. A., and Lynch, E. R.: J. Vener. Dis. Inform. **29**:166, 1948.
71. Kolmer, J. A.: Am. J. Clin. Pathol. **12**:109, 1942.

107

SEROLOGIC TESTS IN INFECTIOUS DISEASES—II

Alex C. Sonnenwirth

In this chapter a number of antigen-antibody reactions are described that are useful in the diagnosis of a variety of bacterial and fungal diseases. Tests for syphilis are discussed in Chapter 106, those for viral diseases in Chapter 94, and for parasitic diseases in Chapter 100.

The human (and animal) body responds to infection by the formation of specific antibodies. The most significant and direct evidence of infection is that obtained by the isolation and identification of the causative agent. However, this is not always successful or feasible. By demonstrating the presence of a specific antibody in the patient's serum, serologic tests using **known antigens** supply indirect evidence of the disease-producing agent or antigen that stimulated the formation of the (unknown) **antibody.** By exposing the patient's serum to various known antigens and using a variety of procedures, the presence or absence of antibody to the antigens can be determined (**serologic diagnosis by antibody determination).**

Another use of **serologic** technics is in the **identification of microorganisms;** in addition to morphologic and biochemical tests, known antisera are employed for aiding in determining the identity of the microorganism. Known serum antibodies, usually prepared in animals, bring about the agglutination of the unknown organism, and serologic identification is thus achieved.

Agglutination tests are commonly employed in the identification or determination of specific serotypes of *Salmonella, Shigella,* enteropathogenic *Escherichia coli, Brucella, Bordetella pertussis, Francisella tularensis,* and others. **Precipitin tests** are employed for the grouping of streptococci, whereas **quellung** tests are used for the identification of pneumococci, *Klebsiella,* and *Haemophilus influenzae.* **Fluorescent antibody tests** are used increasingly for the identification and detection of various organisms (Chapter 70). Antisera for the use of these procedures are commercially available. Details of the procedures are described in the section on bacteriology under the respective organisms.

The test for presence or absence of antibody is usually most successful some time after the onset of the disease since antibodies develop gradually. **Agglutination reactions** are sometimes helpful in infections due to gram-negative enteric organisms. **Complement fixation** tests are most useful in the diagnosis of rickettsial and viral diseases as well as in certain parasitic and fungal infections. **Flocculation** tests are extremely useful in the diagnosis of syphilis, as is the indirect **fluorescent antibody** test. The success and applicability of many of the tests depend on the availability and quality of the antigens needed. Fortunately, many antigens are now commercially available. Some others, especially for various fungal and parasitic infections, are not available and have to be prepared whenever needed in the laboratory.

AGGLUTINATION TESTS FOR INFECTIOUS DISEASES "FEBRILE AGGLUTINATION" TESTS

Agglutination tests have been widely used for the detection of antibodies in the patient's serum against various disease-producing microorganisms. The early example of such procedures was the **Widal test,** devised for the diagnosis of typhoid fever. It employed as antigen a suspension of killed *Salmonella typhi* organisms.

Essentially the same technic is used in many other diseases; the antigen used is a suspension of the bacteria causing the suspected disease. The tests, commonly referred to as **"febrile agglutination" tests,*** are employed in the indirect diagnosis of various enteric fevers (typhoid and paratyphoid), brucellosis, tularemia, pertussis, glanders, leptospirosis, and various rickettsial diseases such as Rocky Mountain spotted fever, typhus fever, and tsutsugamushi fever (for bacterial hemagglutination tests see Chapter 108).

The *Proteus* antigens listed below have been widely used in a procedure known as the **Weil-Felix** reaction for the diagnosis of diseases caused by rickettsiae. *Proteus* organisms possess antigens in common with the rickettsiae and thus have been used to detect rickettsial antibodies (*Proteus* antigens are easier to prepare than are the rickettsial antigens).

The choice of antigens to be used in febrile diseases depends on the disease suspected and also on the geographic area in which the laboratory is situated. Certain diseases or types of organisms are more frequent in one locale than in another. The use of paratyphoid A (*Salmonella* A) antigen in the northern part of the United States is somewhat superfluous, since this disease is practically nonexistent in that area. On the other hand, in this era of rapid transportation and the large-scale movement of military and business personnel from one continent to another, the frequent occurrence of diseases in distant places should be kept in mind, since the patient may have recently returned from a distant area.

Certain rules are essential in performance and evaluation of "febrile agglutination" tests:

1. A single agglutination test is of little value. **At least 2 and preferably more tests should be performed every 3-5 days after the onset of the disease to demonstrate a change in antibody titer.** Many individuals possess agglutinins in their sera to several of the antigens commonly used. These agglutinins are usually of low titer (with *Salmonella* antigens, usually 20-80 or occasionally 160). Others have agglutinins due to immunization. A definite change, usually a significant rise, occurs in the first 8-15 days of the illness. **A progressive increase in titer is the prime evidence of infection.** If the tests are performed late

in the disease, a gradual decline in the titer will be noted over a period of time.

2. Antibodies are occasionally produced through stimulation by a new and unrelated infection (**anamnestic reaction** due to group bacterial antigens).

3. The tests have usually been performed as a battery. Such a battery includes titrations with a number of antigens. **Slide agglutination tests** are used as screening procedures. **Any positive or doubtful reaction should be repeated** with the macroscopic **tube agglutination test.** In recent years the battery usually includes the following antigens:

Salmonella group A	Paratyphoid A (a)
Salmonella group B	Paratyphoid B (b,1,2)
Salmonella group C	Paratyphoid C (c,1,5)
(C_1 and C_2)	Typhoid H (d)
Salmonella group D	*Brucella abortus*
(typhoid)	*Francisella tularensis*
Salmonella group E	

The *Salmonella* group antigens are **somatic (O)** antigens; the paratyphoid and typhoid (d) antigens are **flagellar (H)** antigens; both should be used. Some laboratories use only *Salmonella* A, B, and D antigens, **both** O and H, and the last 2 antigens in each column.

Value of and discrepancies in salmonella and other "febrile agglutination" tests

The value of the salmonella agglutination tests has declined as (1) the incidence of typhoid fever has decreased, at least in the developed world, (2) the general use of vaccines has increased, and (3) ever increasing numbers of antigenically related serotypes of *Salmonella* have been recognized. The sensitivity of the salmonella agglutination test is poor, and the titers of antibody against O and H antigens at times have been misleading and lacking correlation with (cultural) diagnosis.

Considerable documentation is available underlining the poor sensitivity and specificity of the salmonella agglutination tests.[2-5]

The value of the Weil-Felix (*Proteus*) test for diagnosis of Rocky Mountain spotted fever has recently been challenged by Hechemy et al.,[6] who found very extensive differences in results obtained by the classic Weil-Felix procedure and by the recently described specific microimmunofluorescence test employing rickettsial antigens.[7] The Weil-Felix agglutinin and rickettsial complement fixation tests are rarely positive until 10-14 days after onset of illness; despite questions about their specificity and sensitivity, they remain the only **widely** available laboratory methods for confirming suspected cases.[8]

On the other hand, there is little doubt about the value of agglutination tests in suspected cases of **brucellosis, tularemia,** or **leptospirosis.** Antibodies to these organisms can usually be demonstrated with considerably higher speci-

---

*Although widely used, the term "febrile agglutination" is semantically incorrect. Hamburger[1] suggests that agglutination tests should be ordered for the specific disease(s) indicated.

ficity and sensitivity than those against *Salmonella*.

It is recommended that febrile agglutinins should **not** be used as a routine battery but should be used only in select cases in which there is evidence of specific disease (tularemia, brucellosis, leptospirosis; the laboratory confirmation of typhoid or other salmonelloses depends essentially on bacterial culture).

Preparation of antigens

The antigens listed are available from several biological houses.* For laboratories that prefer to prepare their own antigens, a number of technics are outlined below.

Living antigens. Satisfactory antigens can be prepared by growing an organism in broth and using it without alteration. They can also be prepared by growing organisms on agar, washing them off with sterile saline, and using the suspension without further treatment. The use of living antigens is not recommended because there is definite danger involved in handling them.

Phenol-killed antigen. The organism can be grown on suitable solid medium or liquid broth. With the use of 0.5% phenol-containing saline, the growth from the agar surface is washed off, or, in the case of liquid medium, phenolized saline is added to the centrifuged sediment of the culture. It is important that the resulting suspension be clump free and that no particles of medium be present. Clumps can be broken up by shaking with sterile glass beads. The suspension is diluted to correspond to the density of tube 10 of the barium sulfate nephelometer (McFarland) and incubated for 24 h at 37 C. A test for sterility is made by inoculating a tube of fluid thioglycollate medium. Sterilization usually occurs if no spores are present. For use, dilute 1:3 with phenolized saline; the turbidity should approximate that of tube 3 of the McFarland nephelometer.

Formalin-killed antigen. Usually 0.3% **final** concentration of formalin (formaldehyde, USP) is sufficient to kill the bacteria; more may be necessary if a whole broth culture is used. In the case of motile bacteria, the formalin-killed preparation yields the flagellar or H antigen. It has been found that a formalinized broth suspension yields a more stable H preparation than one prepared from cells grown on agar.

Heat-killed antigen. The bacterial suspension is prepared with sterile saline and is heated in a water bath at 70-80 C for 30-60 min.

To prevent drying of the bacteria on the sides of the tube above the suspension, it is recommended that a stopper be inserted above the cotton plug, thus keeping the atmosphere in the tube saturated during the heating process.

Special antigens. Some antigens are best prepared in a manner that enhances their value as diagnostic agents. Motile bacteria, notably species of *Salmonella*, yield additional information if the flagellar (H) antigens and the somatic (O) antigens are studied separately. The flagella contain 1 set of antigens, and the body of the cell contains a different set. Flagellar antigens withstand formalin but are destroyed by heat, phenol, or alcohol. Somatic antigens are not affected by any of these. Hence it is possible to prepare an antigen that retains the flagellar components by killing an actively

motile culture with 0.3% formalin. This antigen will also have somatic factors present. On the other hand, an antigen containing only somatic factors may be prepared either from a nonmotile strain or from a motile strain, provided the latter is subjected to treatment that will destroy the flagellar components.

*Flagellar (H) antigens.** Select a smooth, typical, actively motile strain. If necessary, transfer it daily for several days to enhance its motility. It should then be grown on a suitable moist agar medium or in broth for 18 h. If on agar, the growth is washed off with a minimum amount of physiologic saline and may, if necessary, be filtered through cotton or coarse filter paper to remove the coarse particles. If a broth culture is used, it may be killed without further treatment, or the cells may be packed by centrifugation and resuspended in saline solution. The bacteria may be killed either before or after centrifugation. In either instance, 0.3% (final concentration) formalin (formaldehyde, USP) is added to the concentrated suspension, which is then left at room temperature or at 37 C for 24 h. Sterility tests should be made, especially if the preparation is to be kept as a stock antigen. Concentrated stock antigens, so prepared, may be kept refrigerated for months. If necessary, as much as 2% formalin may be used as a killing agent, but the antigen must be so diluted that the concentration of formalin is reduced to 0.3% or less at the time of use. At the time of use, the turbidity of the antigen should correspond to that of tube 3 of the McFarland barium sulfate nephelometer scale (Chapter 70).

Somatic (O) antigens. A nonmotile strain of the organism should be used. The bacteria are grown for 18-24 h on a suitable solid medium, preferably one that is not moist. The growth is washed off in a small amount of physiologic saline and an equal volume of absolute ethyl alcohol added. It should be mixed well and allowed to stand at room temperature overnight. The next day physiologic saline equivalent to half the volume of the alcohol-antigen mixture is added, thus reducing the alcohol concentration to 33%. For preservation 0.5% phenol (final concentration) is added. The concentrated antigen may be kept for months, but for use must be diluted with saline until the alcohol concentration is not more than 12% and the turbidity corresponds to that of tube 3 of the McFarland nephelometer.

Antigens for special organisms. Brucella antigens are prepared by growing the organisms on a suitable solid medium. They are killed by heat (80 C for 1 h) and preserved with 0.5% phenol.

Francisella tularensis antigen is prepared by growing the organism on blood dextrose cystine agar and killing it in suspension with 0.3% formalin or 0.5% phenol. (Strain no. 456, National Institutes of Health, is recommended.)

Proteus OX-19, OX-2, and OX-K antigens are prepared from nonmotile strains by killing with heat (80 C for 1 h) and preserving with phenol or by the method described above for the preparation of somatic (O) antigens.

For additional information, see ref. 9.

---

*Various antigens are available from many biological houses (Lederle, Difco, Markham, Lee, B. B. L.).

---

*For preparation of *Salmonella* H antigens, a motile smooth strain should be selected. Monophasic variants of diphasic types, such as *Salmonella paratyphi* B and *S. paratyphi* C, are available from the Center for Disease Control, Atlanta, and the International Salmonella Center, Copenhagen. The recommendations of these centers with regard to the particular strain to be used should be followed.

Slide agglutination test

A number of investigators have claimed that a simple, quantitative slide agglutination test for the detection or exclusion of serum agglutinins developed during certain febrile infections is as informative as the tube agglutination procedure. The rapid slide agglutination test is used as a **screening** procedure. (Some commercial tularemia antigens are to be used only for tube agglutination tests.) The technic described is based on the use of commercial antigens; the technic for the use of antigens of various manufacturers is, with minor variations, generally the same.

Procedure*

1. Use antigens in stock form purchased. Most commercial antigen bottles contain droppers standardized to deliver approximately 0.03 ml antigen.
2. Conduct tests on a large sheet of plate glass (30 × 41 cm) that has been ruled into 3.8 cm squares with a diamond-point or wax pencil.
3. Using a 0.2 ml pipet, deliver 0.08, 0.04, 0.02, 0.01, 0.005, and 0.002 ml quantities of serum to squares or rings of 1 row, from left to right. Do this with serum to be tested for as many rows as there are antigens to be used. **Use clear, unheated serum.**
4. Mix antigen vials by shaking. With dropper of antigen vial place 1 drop antigen on each quantity of serum on each row, from left to right.

When the antigen (1 drop) is mixed with quantities of serum indicated, the test will approximate the results of the conventional tube dilution test, in the following dilutions: 1:20, 1:40, 1:80, 1:160, and 1:320. Further dilutions may be prepared by using a 1:10 dilution of serum in physiologic saline and the volumes described above.

5. Proceeding from right to left, mix contents of each square of 1 horizontal row with wooden applicator stick or glass rod. Use new applicator or wipe glass rod clean before mixing contents of squares of another horizontal row.
6. Hold glass plate near an adequate light source. Slowly rock and tilt and observe for a period **not to exceed 3 min.**
7. Record all observed degrees of agglutination as follows:

100% (complete) agglutination	4 plus (++++)
Approximately 75% agglutination	3 plus (+++)
Approximately 50% agglutination	2 plus (++)
Approximately 25% agglutination	1 plus (+)
No agglutination	Negative (−)

NOTE: If the source of light used to provide satisfactory visibility furnishes a considerable quantity of heat, care should be taken to avoid drying at the edges of the serum-antigen film; such drying may be mistaken for partial agglutination.

The smallest quantity of serum that exhibits a 2 plus (++) or 50% agglutination is considered the "end point" of serum reactivity or serum titer.

*Condensed from Clinical laboratory aids manual, Pearl River, N.Y., 1968, Lederle Laboratories (now out of print).

Table 107-1. Agglutination pattern of a serum against 3 different antigens

Serum (ml)	Equivalent dilution	Antigen X	Antigen Y	Antigen Z
0.08	1:20	4+	4+	3+
0.04	1:40	4+	3+	2+
0.02	1:80	4+	2+	2+
0.01	1:160	2+	1+	—
0.005	1:320	—	—	—
0.002	1:640	—	—	—

Therefore if a serum specimen showed the pattern given in Table 107-1, it would be reported as the following serum titers:

Antigen X	1:160
Antigen Y	1:80
Antigen Z	1:80

For interpretation see Tube Agglutination Test.

Tube agglutination test

The macroscopic tube agglutination test represents more work than the rapid slide agglutination test. However, it is the **definitive** procedure in confirming or ruling out results of the slide test. False-positive slide tests are usually ruled out by the tube test. It is useful in clarifying erratic or equivocal agglutination or prozone reactions obtained in the slide test and in the accurate determination of the variations in serum antibody titers that occur during the various stages of infection.

Procedure. The **commercial** antigens described under the slide test can be used in the tube test also. If preferred, phenol-killed, heat-killed, or formalinized antigens can be prepared as described earlier. For H antigens of motile organisms, the formalin method should be used. For O antigens, use the ethyl alcohol method. The procedure with one of the commercial antigens (Lederle Laboratories, Pearl River, N.Y.) follows:

1. Dilute stock antigens 1:100 with physiologic saline. Prepare only a sufficient quantity for the day's work.
2. Prepare serum dilutions.
   a. Place 0.9 ml saline in the first tube of a series of 10 tubes (13 × 100 mm) and place 0.5 ml saline in each of the 9 remaining tubes.
   b. With a 1 ml pipet (graduated to tip), place 0.1 ml of clear, **unheated** serum in tube 1. Mix by aspiration. Remove 0.5 ml of mixture and transfer it to tube 2.
   c. Mix and transfer 0.5 ml of tube 3. Continue this procedure until contents of tube 10 have been mixed.
   d. Discard 0.5 ml of contents of tube 10.

The series of 10 tubes now contain 0.5 ml each of serum dilutions ranging as follows: 1:10, 1:20, 1:40, 1:80, 1:160, 1:320, 1:640, 1:1280, 1:2560, and 1:5120.

As an antigen control, use 1 or 2 tubes containing 0.5 ml saline only (no serum). If possible, include a positive serum control (consisting of the serial dilutions noted above), using a serum specimen of known reactivity.

3. Add 0.5 ml diluted antigen to each tube. Final serum dilutions now range as follows: 1:20, 1:40,

1:80, 1:160, 1:320, 1:640, 1:1280, 1:2560, 1:5120, 1:10,240.

4. Shake rack of tubes to mix antigen and serum thoroughly and incubate them in water bath. Incubation temperatures and length of time are as follows: Tubes with somatic (O) *Salmonella* antigens and *Proteus* OX-19 antigens should be incubated 18-24 h at 48-50 C. Tubes with flagellar (H) *Salmonella* antigens (paratyphoid and Group D flagellar) should be incubated 2 h at the same temperature. Those with somatic *Brucella abortus* antigen should be incubated at 37 C for 48 h. *P. tularensis* (tularemia) antigen test tubes should be incubated at 37 C for 2 h and then placed in refrigerator for 18 h (overnight).

5. Remove racks of tubes and allow them to stand at room temperature while results are being read. Read results of all control tubes first. Remove 2 or 3 tubes at a time from racks, hold them in front of a suitable source of light, and estimate degree of agglutination as follows:

   4 plus (++++): complete agglutination and sedimentation; supernatant fluid clear

   3 plus (+++): nearly complete agglutination and sedimentation; supernatant fluid about 75% clear

   2 plus (++): marked sedimentation; supernatant fluid about 50% clear

   1 plus (+): distinct sedimentation; supernatant fluid about 25% clear

   Trace (±): slight sedimentation on tube wall; supernatant fluid practically as dense as antigen control

   Negative (−): no evidence of agglutination; supernatant fluid same density as antigen control

The end-point titer of the serum is designated as the highest dilution of serum (the smallest quantity of undiluted serum) that exhibits a 50% degree of agglutination (2 plus, or ++).

Upon gentle shaking of the tubes, large flaky aggregates will be noted with the H agglutinins, which are easily broken up. The O agglutinins produce granular or small flaking agglutination.

Interpretation. It is important that there be close communication between the physician and the laboratory. Results should always be interpreted with reference to clinical data.

A single test result is not diagnostically significant unless the titer is unusually high. In the unvaccinated patient a serologic diagnosis is usually made if either there is a **4-fold rise in O antigen** titer or the titer for O antigen is higher than 1:50 or 1:100 on a single specimen taken in the first 2-3 weeks of infection. Antibiotic treatment in typhoid fever often prevents a rise in titer, or it may inhibit the development of detectable antibody.

Negative results. Negative results may be due to the absence of the agglutinin sought (patient does not have infection for which test was made) or because the blood was taken too early in the disease (before the appearance of sufficient agglutinin in the serum). It should be remembered that a positive result following a negative one after several days (rise in titer) is usually significant. Negative results do not necessarily rule out infection, and such results are best used as baselines for subsequent comparative titrations.

Positive results. Past history of immunization or infection is important in the correct interpretation of positive results.

In **brucellosis** a titer of 1:160 is **suggestive** of recent infection. Persistently low titers are significant if previous tests were negative. Individuals who had brucellosis may be nonspecifically restimulated by subsequent nonbrucellar infections, with their *Brucella* titer rising rapidly (1:160) and then dropping precipitously in 10-15 days.

In suspected **acute** brucellosis, the following should be noted[10]:

1. Little or no titer may develop during the first 10 days of illness.
2. Acute and convalescent phase serum specimens, taken 2-4 weeks apart and tested in the same test run, are essential for demonstration of active infection. **A 4-fold rise in titer is significant.**
3. The titer may decline after the sixth week or may persist as high as 1:160 for years after apparent clinical recovery. Therefore a titer of 1:160 or above is indicative of *Brucella* infection at some time but not necessarily of current or recent infection.

In chronic brucellosis there is no definite criterion whereby the significance of an agglutination test titer may be judged. No diagnostic question is likely to be raised about persons yielding high titers (titers higher than 1:160) and clinical findings that are compatible with modern knowledge of brucellosis while showing no symptoms of tularemia. Even though a titer of 1:20 is obtained, infection with *Brucella* cannot be ruled out on the basis of agglutination tests alone. In fact, some individuals, although infected, do not develop agglutinins.

Persons who have recovered from brucellosis may have *Brucella* antibodies restimulated nonspecifically by any subsequent febrile illness. In such instances agglutination titers may rise to 1:160 or sometimes higher in a few days and drop to negative or 1:20 within 10 days. Such reactions confuse test interpretation.

In **tularemia,** serum agglutinin titers of 1:80 or 1:160 usually appear in the second week of the disease and increase considerably during the fourth to seventh week (1:640-1:10,240) with gradual dropping in titer at the end of 1 year. Uninfected individuals may have titers of 1:40. If a single specimen only is available, a titer of **1:160 or above** is indicative of a *Francisella* infection at some time but not necessarily of current or recent infection. Agglutinins decline slowly but may be detectable for life.

Cross-reactions often occur and must be considered. Vaccination with typhus (rickettsial) antigen will evoke the formation of *Proteus* OX-19 antibodies. Cholera vaccine may produce *B. abortus* antibodies. Tularemia agglutinins may agglutinate *B. abortus*, whereas *Brucella* agglutinins may react with *P. tularensis*.

Agglutination tests in **acute shigellosis (dys-**

Table 107-2. Significance of serum titers*

Disease	Febrile antigen	Serum agglutinins		
		Appear	Maximum	Titer and significance
Typhoid fever	Salmonella group D (typhoid O)	7-10 d	3-5 wk	1:80† (in early stages) = suspicious 1:160† and rising = definitely indicative
	Typhoid H (flagellar d)	Later	Later	1:40‡ = suspicious 1:80‡ = definitely indicative
Paratyphoid fever and other Salmonella infections	Salmonella groups A, B, C, and E (somatic); paratyphoid A, B, and C (flagellar)	Those characterized by prolonged fever and typhoidlike symptoms present antibodies of titers similar to above; lower titers may be more significant, depending on prevalence of particular Salmonella species. Similar titers are also encountered in gastrointestinal infections, but significance is somewhat different since patient may be well by the time antibodies are fully developed.		
Typhus fevers	Proteus OX-19	7-10 d	By 14th d	1:40-1:80 (early) = suspicious 1:160 = definitely indicative
Rocky Mountain spotted fever	Proteus OX-19	7-10 d	By 14th d	Peak titers usually not above 1:160-1:320
Brucellosis	B. abortus	2-3 wk	3-5 wk	1:80-1:60 = indicative 1:320 or more in single specimen = conclusive

*From Clinical laboratory aids manual, Pearl River, N.Y., 1968, Lederle Laboratories.
†May be higher in vaccinated individuals.
‡Much higher in vaccinated individuals.

entery) are not useful. The antibodies develop irregularly, and the multiplicity of species and types capable of causing the disease would necessitate agglutination tests against a large number of shigellae suspensions. **Bacterial hemagglutination tests** have shown positive reactions with 4- to 16-fold increases of agglutinin within 10 days after the onset of illness in about 75% of children who had Shigella sonnei dysentery (Chapter 108).

Comments

1. Titers of sera from the same patient, when obtained with **commercial antigens of different manufacturers,** may not be comparable. DeVillier et al.[11] found 2- to 4-fold differences in titer of the same serum when using 4 different commercially prepared antigens. This makes interpretation of test results difficult. It is good practice to keep a record of the antigen preparation used and its manufacturer so that on inquiry from another laboratory or physician the proper identification of the antigen can be furnished.

2. **High slide test titers** often **cannot** be confirmed by the tube test. If such is the case, dilute problem serum in 30% bovine albumin (1:10 or 1:20) and repeat slide test.

Vi agglutination

Many known carriers of typhoid bacilli possess antibody against the Vi (virulence) antigen of S. typhi. This is a surface antigen, easily lost during cultivation. Vi titers seem to correlate better with the carrier state than do O or H titers. For this reason, Felix et al.[11a] suggested the use of Vi agglutination for detection of carriers. A false-positive reaction rate of 6-8% and the fact that up to 30% of known carriers have a negative Vi test[12] have led Schroeder[4] to minimize the usefulness of the test as a screening device for detection of carriers in the community. An elevated Vi titer may be indicative of the typhoid carrier state; the titer usually disappears within a few weeks after the termination of the carrier state.

Unfortunately, no 2 authors have performed this test alike. Brower divided the methods for the detection of the Vi antibodies in the serum into the following groups:

1. **Absorption technic,** used by Felix, in which serum is first absorbed with an **S. typhi** strain rich in O and H antigens, and then Vi titer is determined by agglutination with a Vi strain.
2. **Direct titration of antibodies** with a strain that contains only Vi antigens; e. g., Bhatnagar strain of S. typhi.
3. **Direct titration** with a strain from which O antigens have been eliminated by growing in broth containing O serum and H antigens separated by repeated centrifugation and washing, according to method of Detre.
4. **Precipitation tests,** using antigenic extracts from Vi strains.

Because of technical difficulties involved in the other methods, the third method was found to be the most satisfactory. However, it requires considerable work. The cultures must be tested and transferred frequently, and their V-W variation cannot be prevented easily.

The technic of the Vi agglutination test is that of tube agglutination tests. The dilutions of the sera, however, are lower: 1:5, 1:10, 1:20, and 1:40. A suspension of the Bhatnagar Vi strain in 0.85% sodium chloride is used. The antigen is adjusted to tube 3 of the McFarland nephelometric standard. The tubes are incubated for 2 h at 37 C and then left in the refrigerator overnight. A hand lens is used to facilitate the reading.

Vi hemagglutination tests[13-15] have also been investigated for the detection of typhoid carriers. They seem to be more reliable and more sensitive than the agglutination test (Chapter 108).

Vi agglutinations are not routinely performed, and when the test is needed, sera should be submitted to central or reference laboratories.

SEROLOGIC DIAGNOSIS IN BRUCELLOSIS

In the absence of positive cultures the most reliable indicator of *Brucella* infection is the agglutination test. This is particularly true in cases of acute brucellosis in which a high serum agglutinin titer will be found in most cases. The agglutinins appear as early as the fifth day of illness and have a tendency to increase on subsequent tests, but it must be kept in mind that in some cases agglutinins fail to appear even when brucellae have been isolated. As a rule, agglutinins are also detected in relatively high titers during the subacute stage or during recurrences. The titers become lower with time except in certain chronic cases in which the symptomatology depends on the presence of active foci of infection. On the other hand, it has been observed that in some patients the agglutinin titer may remain high even if recovery has been apparent for months or even years.

Whatever the interpretation that might be given to the agglutination test, we must take into consideration the fact that a relatively high incidence of *Brucella* agglutinins can exist in a healthy population or in persons suffering from an unrelated illness. In such circumstances, even if the titers are generally below 1:100, this may cause confusion. It is therefore required to have titers above 1:100 to attribute some value to an agglutination test. In this respect it may be helpful to know that according to the experience acquired at the clinics of the University of Minnesota and the Brucellosis Center of Mexico City, a titer of 1:320 has been found in the majority of bacteriologically proved cases.

During the evolution of the disease one may find considerable variations in titers of agglutinins from 1 week to the next. Titers may drop to less than 1:100 and even be entirely negative and then rise again to significant levels. There has been considerable controversy in the interpretation of the agglutination test during the so-called hyperergic sequences of brucellosis. Titers are generally under 1:100, which, as previously indicated, have no diagnostic value. The disturbing facts concerning the low titers and even complete lack of agglutination in some cases proved by isolation of *Brucella* have to be considered in the light of findings concerning **incomplete and blocking antibodies.** The **prozone phenomenon** (which may extend to 1:400 dilution) may occur in certain cases and may cause confusion if the test is performed with an insufficient number of tubes. This can be avoided by using a sufficient number of dilutions. To reduce the frequency of prozone the use of a 5% sodium chloride solution has been recommended.

For a comprehensive review and detailed procedures pertaining to serologic technics in brucellosis, see *Laboratory Techniques in Brucellosis,*[16] Kerr et al.,[17] and Farrell et al.[18]

Selection and standardization of antigens

Most of the conflicting reports concerning the **agglutination test** depend on the lack of uniformity in the selection and standardization of the antigens. Due to exhaustive investigation it has been agreed that antigens have to be prepared with smooth cultures. The Bureau of Animal Industry, United States Department of Agriculture, has obtained good results with antigens prepared with *B. abortus* strain 1119, although smooth strains of any of the 3 species may be used. The medium recommended is potato infusion, but liver infusion agar is quite satisfactory. Cultures are incubated in Roux bottles for 48 h at 37 C, and the growth is washed with saline, filtered through cotton, and heated for 1 h at 60 C. Phenol is added to a final concentration of 0.5%, and after tests for sterility the suspension is centrifuged, the supernatant fluid discarded, and the sediment resuspended in a small volume of saline containing 0.5% phenol. This stock suspension is usually kept several days before standardization.

It is desirable that the antigen should be diluted to give a titer of 1:1000 with the International Standard Serum supplied by Weybridge Veterinary Laboratory, but this is not necessary. Any dilution selected may be properly tested with the standard serum. A suspension corresponding to tube 2 of the McFarland scale is about the best concentration of brucellae in the antigen.

The selected suspension is tested with serial dilutions of the standard serum, and the 50% agglutination end point is used for calculation of the factor by which any 50% end-point titration of unknown sera should be multiplied to obtain the equivalent of the titer in international units. If, for instance, the end point of the new antigen is 1:500, the factor will be

$$\frac{1000}{500} = 2$$

If the end point of the new antigen is 1500, the factor will be 0.66. Therefore an unknown serum giving a titer of 640 with the 1:500 antigen will be designated as having a titer of 1280, adjusted to international units. If, on the other hand, the antigen with the 1500 end point is used in the test, the titer in international units will be only 422.

The degree of agglutination expressed in international units not only helps to reduce error to a minimum but serves to compare results with those obtained in other laboratories or other countries.

Because of the usefulness of the agglutination test, there has been considerable interest in various attempts to simplify the technic and reduce the time needed to observe results. The test developed by Huddleson has enjoyed great favor, but according to observations at the University of Minnesota, this method be used only as a screening test because false-positive reactions were often found.

Agglutination methods

Rapid screening procedure. Use slide agglutination method above.

Preliminary testing. Many workers recommend the **tube test** for preliminary screening. Stokes[19] recommends the use of 4 serum dilutions (1:20, 1:200, 1:400, and 1:800).

Standard tube method. The test recommended by FAO/WHO[20] is the tube dilution method with a properly standardized antigen. Used venous blood obtained under aseptic conditions; take care to avoid hemolysis.

1. Place a series of 10 tubes (13 × 100 mm) in a rack and add 0.9 ml isotonic saline to the first and 0.5 ml to the remaining tubes.
2. Add 0.1 ml serum to tube 1, mix thoroughly, and transfer 0.5 ml to tube 2 and so on. Discard the last 0.5 ml removed from tube 10.
3. Add 0.5 ml standardized antigen to each of the 10 tubes. Mix contents of each tube and place rack in water bath at 37 C for 48 h. Final serum dilutions are from 1:20 (first tube) to 1:10,240 (last tube).
4. For antigen control, prepare a tube with equal amounts of antigen and saline. Use also a known positive serum and a known negative serum (make serial dilutions of latter 2 sera) in manner described for test serum.
5. Read results at room temperature.

The end point (titer) is designated as the (2+) tube containing the highest dilution of serum, showing 50% or more agglutination (i.e., 50% clearing of supernatant). The degree of agglutination is determined by reading the degree of clearing without shaking the tubes. Complete agglutination and clear supernatant is recorded as 4+; 75% clearing and almost complete agglutination, as 3+; 50% clearing and marked agglutination, as 2+; 25% with some sediment, as 1+. No clearing is recorded as negative. A **control tube** to simulate 50% clearing can be set up by mixing 0.25 ml antigen in a tube with 0.75 ml saline.[16]

Comments

1. According to Hall and Manion,[21] the action of **blocking antibodies** can be overcome if the tests are incubated in the usual manner and the tubes then are centrifuged at 4000 rpm for 15 minutes.

2. Schubert and Colvin[22] reported that both blocking and prozone can be eliminated if the tubes are centrifuged at 850 × g (2000 rpm) for 15 minutes, after 24 hours' incubation at 37 C. Thus centrifugation may overcome the need for 48 hours' incubation.

3. When looking for blocking antibodies, set up a duplicate row, using **inactivated** serum (56 C, 15 minutes).[23]

Spot test

Rapid tests should be considered as screening tests; a further simplification in the preparation of the antigen and the performance of the test has been used with satisfactory results at the Brucellosis Center of Mexico City and the laboratories of the University of Minnesota. The antigen prepared by Castañeda[24-26] is a suspension of brucellae that has been fixed with formalin and stained with methylene blue. The antigen is standardized in concentration and color. It is a rather thick emulsion of brucellae, and the color is a deep blue; the aim is that a mixture of antigen and blood made on a slide with a loopful of each should take on a greenish color. The mixture is rotated by moving the slide, and the results can be detected within 1-2 min. In a negative reaction the red cells have a tendency to accumulate at the periphery of the mixture, forming a reddish ring surrounding the greenish mixture. In positive reactions the antigen is agglutinated and forms a blue ring at the periphery surrounding a red or reddish mixture at the center. The test has been standardized to produce visible agglutination only when agglutinins are present in titer higher than 1:100, which eliminates weak or false-positive reactions. A negative reaction in patients suffering from an acute illness is an indication of an infection not related to brucellosis. A positive reaction is a good indication of active brucellosis. Details of the preparation and standardization of the antigen can be found elsewhere.[26]

Surface fixation

Another alternate method for the serologic diagnosis of human brucellosis is the so-called "**surface fixation**" or **Castañeda strip test**.[27] This serologic method has been extensively used at the Brucellosis Center of Mexico with satisfactory results. It has been successfully used as a screening test in febrile diseases, and often it has been the first indication of brucellosis. Briefly, this test is performed on a strip of filter paper on which the *Brucella* antigen has been printed as a black spot. When normal serum is applied to this antigen and the paper is placed over a layer of isotonic saline, the fluid

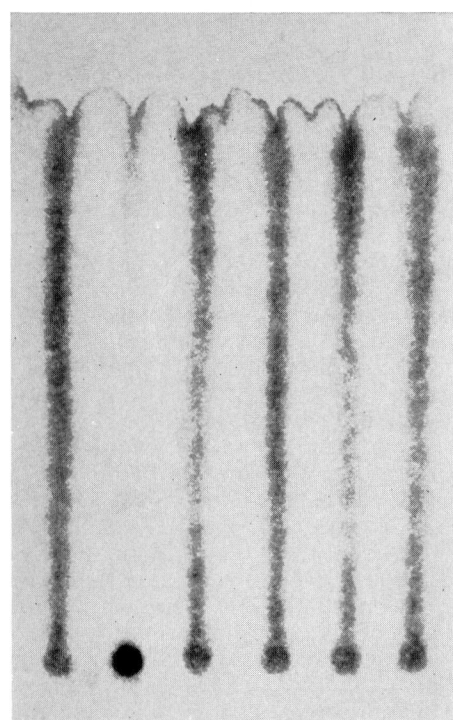

Fig. 107-1. Surface fixation or Castañeda strip test. (Courtesy Dr. M. R. Castañeda.)

washes up the antigen, leaving a trace that looks like a comet. If a strong, positive serum is used, the spot remains fixed. Intermediate strengths of fixation may be gauged according to the length of the trace of the displaced antigen (Fig. 107-1). A strong positive reaction may be seen among several negative reactions.

Antihuman globulin (Coombs) test for Brucella antibodies

Several workers recommend performance of the indirect Coombs (AHG) test,[28] especially in chronic brucellosis in which the agglutination test may be negative.

In the test, serial dilutions of the unknown serum are incubated (37 C, 30-60 minutes) with a suitably diluted suspension (1:20 or 1:50) of standard *B. abortus* antigen to allow adherence of the antibodies to the surface of the antigen. Kerr et al.[29] recommend the use of 2 × ½ inch or 2 × ⅜ inch round-bottomed tubes. The tubes are centrifuged lightly; the sedimented cells are washed and resuspended 3 times in physiologic saline to remove all traces of the serum proteins. Resuspension is accomplished by drawing the suspension up and down in a Pasteur pipet 10 times.[29] One drop of the washed cell suspensions from each tube is mixed with 1 drop of optimal dilution of a Coombs antihuman globulin serum. The mixture is incubated at 37 C (30-60 minutes) and then centrifuged and examined for agglutination. For control, drops of a diluted normal serum are added to drops of cell suspension. The dilution of the Coombs serum is determined by a checkerboard titration of antigen and serum of known antibody titer.

In the Kerr et al. series[29] the standard agglutination test was of little value in chronic brucellosis, whereas the AHG test detected antibodies that were incapable of agglutinating in the standard agglutination test. Out of 14 cases in which the agglutination titer was 1:80 or less (in 9, it was less than 1:20), the AHG titers ranged from 1:320 to 1:5120. Coghlan and Weir[29a] reported that in acute brucellosis IgG, IgA, and IgM type immunoglobulins are involved, whereas in the chronic cases the serum reactivity is confined mostly to IgG (and IgA), low-molecular-weight immunoglobulins. The AHG test does measure IgG agglutinins in sera that do not agglutinate in the standard agglutination test. Thus by using the Coombs (AHG) and complement fixation test (see below), it may be possible to detect cases of chronic brucellosis.

Complement fixation (CF) test for brucellosis

The CF test is a good indicator of the IgG immunoglobulin class. Thus its use is recommended in conjunction with the standard tube and AHG test for detection of chronic brucellosis.

Both the AHG and the CF tests are time consuming; however, there seems to be justification for their use in problem cases.

SEROLOGIC TESTS IN LEPTOSPIROSIS

The reader is advised to study the section on *Leptospira* (Chapter 80) before proceeding to undertake serologic tests for leptospirosis.

Two comprehensive sources on details of serologic tests in leptospirosis are Babudieri's[30]

review and the monographs of Galton et al.[31] and Sulzer and Jones.[32]

Since cultivation of leptospirae and animal inoculation are time-consuming procedures and useful only during the acute phase of the disease, it is often necessary to demonstrate antibodies in the patient's serum. Antibodies in leptospirosis generally appear from the sixth to the twelfth day of disease and increase rapidly, reaching maximum titers by the third or fourth week. After infection, low agglutinin titers may persist for months or years. For this reason it is frequently impossible to determine whether current leptospiral infection exists or antibodies are due to past experience with the disease unless at least 2 blood samples are examined, one during the early stages of illness and another 10 days to 2 weeks later to detect a rise in titer. Serodiagnostic tests will not provide an early diagnosis, but, when carefully evaluated, together with clinical and epidemiologic data, they are helpful in confirming active or past leptospiral infections.[31] Antibiotic treatment seems to have a marked effect on the appearance and persistence of antibodies.

Procedures for leptospiral antibodies

Among a variety of tests available the one most widely used and regarded as the choice technic is the **microscopic agglutination (MA) test with live antigen** (previously known as the **agglutination-"lysis"** test; however, it is now known that true lysis does not occur[33]). The test has some practical disadvantages; it is time consuming and hazardous, and the antigens used are frequently unstable. The **microscopic agglutination test with formalin-killed antigens** is less hazardous, the antigens are more stable, and the results of the 2 tests compare favorably.[31]

The **macroscopic agglutination** test of Galton et al.[31,33] is performed easily and rapidly and is valuable for screening. A modified semi-micro method[34] and a microtechnic[35] for the MA test are being used in many laboratories; these will save time and materials. A modification of the microtechnic[36] has proved to be beneficial in that the serologic test can be carried out in a tissue culture plate with 96 flat-bottom wells and can be read easily on the stage of the dark-field microscope by using an AU.22UM-long-working-distance objective.[32]

In the original microtechnic, U-bottom plastic plates (Linbro Chemical Co., New Haven, Conn.) were employed. In this technic 0.05 ml serum was added to wells in the first row, and 0.025 ml saline was added to the remainder of the wells. With the 0.025 microdiluters, serial dilutions of the serum were made through 1:12,800 through the eleventh well, leaving the twelfth well for a saline control for each antigen used. The test was read in these plates by using a 3.5× objective and 10× oculars. A **latex-agglutination test**[37,38] and an **indirect fluorescent antibody (IF)** test have also been reported. Other tests such as the sonic-vibrated leptospiral **complement fixation test**[39] and the **hemolytic test**[40] are difficult to perform and are not generally used in the clinical laboratory.

Complement fixation (CF) test

The CF test is not used extensively. Killed antigens or chemical extracts are employed. The test is usually inferior to the agglutination test; however, since agglutinins persist for longer periods than CF antibodies, th CF test is more reliable as a diagnostic indicator of current infection.[33]

Hemolytic (HL) test [40]

In the hemolytic test chemical extracts of loptospirae are used to sensitize sheep red blood cells that agglutinate in the presence of leptospiral agglutinins.

Macroscopic agglutination test [32]*

A rapid macroscopic slide agglutination test[31,39] can be used to screen human and animal serum samples. If this test is positive, the titer is determined by the microscopic agglutination test with live or formalinized antigens. The 12 leptospiral strains used to prepare antigens for both tests are representatives of each serogroup in which there is cultural or serologic evidence to indicate the presence of some member of the group in the United States. They include the following serotypes: *ballum*, S-102; *canicola*, Ruebush; *icterohaemorrhagiae*, Wijnberg; *bataviae*, Van Tienen; *grippotyphosa*, Andaman; *pyrogenes*, Salinem; *autumnalis*, Akiyami A; *pomona*, Johnson; *wolffi*, 3705; *australis*, Ballico; *tarassovi*, Perepelicin; and *georgia*, LT117. Serotypes representative of other serogroups are added to the battery as needed.

Cross-agglutination studies with 17 slide test antigens and antisera against 68 leptospiral serotypes or subserotypes indicate that with most of the antisera some degree of cross-reactivity occurred with one or more of the 12 antigens. *L. cynopteri* and *celledoni* antisera failed to cross with any of the 12 antigens, but serum from 2 of 3 patients infected with *celledoni* were positive with *canicola* and *javanica* antigens. Thus in certain areas of the world it may be desirable to include tests for *cynopteri*, *celledoni*, *javanica*, and *butembo* serotypes. The only other exceptions were *semeranga* and *andamana;* there is ample evidence, however, indicating that these 2 serotypes are more closely related to the saprophytic leptospires than to the pathogenic types.

Microscopic agglutination (MA) test [32]

Preparation of antigens. The 12 serotypes referred to above are used routinely. However, if paired serum samples appear positive by the slide test and negative by the microscopic test with these 12 antigens, a second

---

*A commercial kit containing 4 pools of 3 antigens each is available from Difco Laboratories, Detroit.

battery of antigens should also be used. These include *javanica, cynopteri, sentot, djasiman, alexi, borincana*, and *celledoni* serotypes.

Leptospiral strains used for antigen production are maintained in EMJH (or Stuart's) medium and transferred every 7 d. A 4-d-old culture appears to lose the "breeding nests." Such actively growing seed cultures are used in approximately a 1:10 ratio to inoculate the desired amount of Tween 80 medium[41,42] in 170.1 g screw-capped prescription bottles. The inoculated bottles are incubated 4-6 d at 28-30 C in a slanted position and then examined by dark-field microscopy for density, smoothness, and purity. If the antigens appear too dense, they may be diluted with Ellinghausen medium or buffered 0.85% saline solution. Very dense antigens will be undersensitive, but, if very light, they tend to be too sensitive, and titers will be higher. A desirable antigen should contain 100-200 organisms per high-power field or as measured against a no. 20 Roessler standard[43] on a nephelometer. A ½ MacFarland standard can be used to check the density of antigens for serology. Some cultures develop small clumps of leptospires; frequent, successive transfer, however, tends to eliminate development of these aggregates. Contaminated cultures should not be used.

The sensitivity of each lot of antigen should be checked against the homologous antiserum before use, preferably at the beginning of each week. A satisfactory antigen should react within a 2-fold dilution above or below the known titer of the antiserum. If a 4-fold or greater difference in titer exists, the antigen should not be used. If live antigens are to be used, they may be added to the diluted serum after standardizing and should never be used after 8 d. If killed antigens are to be used, formalin is added to the cultures in a final concentration of 0.25% formaldehyde, and they are allowed to stand 1-2 h, then centrifuged for 10 min at 1500 × g to remove extraneous materials, and then tested for sensitivity against homologous antisera. These formalinized antigens usually remain stable for 1-2 wk. They should be checked with positive and negative control sera before use and watched closely for spontaneous agglutination. Although comparable, titers obtained with the formalinized antigens usually appear somewhat lower than titers obtained with live antigens. In addition, more cross-reactions with heterologous serotypes occur with the killed antigens.

Agglutination test procedure with live antigens. Serial 2-fold dilutions of serum are prepared with buffered 0.85% saline to provide dilutions of 1:25 through 1:3200 (higher, if necessary, to reach the end point). To 0.2 ml of each serum dilution, 0.2 ml antigen is added. The tubes are shaken, incubated at room temperature for 2 h, and examined. A drop from each tube is examined by dark-field microscopy with a low-power objective and 10× or 15× oculars without a coverslip. The degree of agglutination is read as negative 1+, 2+, 3+, 4+. A reaction is recorded as 4+ when 75-100% of the leptospires appear clumped, 3+ when approximately 75% of the organisms are agglutinated, 2+ with about 50% agglutinated, and 1+ with at least 25% agglutinated. The titer is the last dilution showing a 2+ reaction.

Agglutination test procedure with formalinized antigens. Serial 2-fold dilutions of serum are prepared in buffered 0.85% saline, starting with 1:25 through 1:3200 (higher, if necessary) to a final volume of 0.2 ml. To each serum dilution, 0.2 ml antigen is added. The tubes are shaken, incubated in a water bath at 52 C for 2 h, and then refrigerated for 1 h. Drops of the respective dilutions are placed on a slide, and agglutination is read as described above. With formalin-killed antigens, agglutination appears different from that with live antigens. The clumps tend to be larger and less tightly packed, giving a lacy appearance. A new modified MA test (see below) can be used that saves time, effort, and materials.

Modified semimicro test for the MA test[32]

Everything is done as in the MA test in standardizing the antigen and reading the semimicro test. The difference is in the test procedure.

Procedure
1. Serial 2-fold or 4-fold dilutions (depending on type of results needed) are made in tubes with buffered 0.85% saline by using Cornwall syringe of proper size equipped with a 7.62 cm cannula. Size of syringe depends on amount of serum needed. Amount of serum needed depends on number of antigens (serotypes against which serum is being tested).
2. Next, 0.05 ml of each serial dilution is added to U-shaped depressions in a plastic plate containing 96 wells. (Linbro Chemical Co., New Haven, Conn.) This amount is added with a plastic 0.5 ml Mohr type pipet (Falcon Plastics, Los Angeles) held in vertical position. One pipet can be used if you begin at highest serum dilution. Number of rows of wells used depends on number of antigens to be used.
3. With a similar plastic pipet, add an equal volume of antigen (0.05 ml). Shake plates gently to mix serum and antigen and cover with sheets of paper or plastic; then let them incubate on tabletop at room temperature for 2 h. Test is read as above.

Comments
1. The test is especially desirable for those laboratories that find it expensive to grow large amounts of antigen.
2. If the plates and pipets are to be used again at the end of the tests, they can be placed in 10% Clorox solution for 2 hours to kill organisms. Then pour off the liquid contents in a discard pan and rinse the materials thoroughly with tap water several times, twice with distilled water, and dry.

Microtiter method for the MA test

A modification of the original microtiter technic test[36] has proved to be useful. A tissue culture plate that has 96 wells with flat bottoms is used for serology. The tests are easily read with the dark-field microscope by using an AU.22UM-long-working-distance objective. In the original microtiter technic. U-bottom plastic plates (Linbro Chemical Co., New Haven, Conn.) were used; 0.05 ml serum was added to well on the first row, and 0.025 ml saline was added to the remaining wells. With the 0.025 ml diluters, serial dilutions of the serum were made through 1:12,800 (eleventh well), leaving the twelfth well for a saline control for each antigen used. The test is read in these plates by using a 3.5× objective and a 10× ocular.

Hemagglutination (HA) test[32, 34a–34c]

1. **Preparation of antigen**
   a. Prepare serotype *andamana* by seeding a 10%

inoculum of each into 2-liter flat-bottom flasks containing 1-liter amounts of medium. Let stand in a 30 C incubator for 6 to 8 d; then check for contamination.
b. Kill the organisms by immersing each flask in a 56 C water bath for 30 min; then centrifuge the contents of each flask at 5,000 × g to pack the organisms.
c. Discard the supernatant; reconstitute the packed organisms to 1/30th of the original volume with 0.15M NaCl and add absolute alcohol to bring alcohol content to 50% alcohol. Let stand in a 56 C water bath for 1-2 h.
d. Let stand in 4 C refrigerator overnight; centrifuge the next day as above and save the supernatant. Discard packed particulate.
e. Add cold absolute alcohol to the supernatant to bring the alcohol content up to 90% and let stand in 4 C refrigerator for 6-9 d or until a fine, white grayish precipitate forms.
f. At the end of this period centrifuge as before and save the precipitate, which is the HA or HL antigen.
g. Decide whether you wish to store immediately or use. If the antigen is to be stored, reconstitute to 1/30th the original volume with distilled water; then add 2% human albumin. Dispense into 1.0 ml amounts to be lyophilized. Be careful not to leave the antigen at extended lyophilization (18 h). The antigen can be tested before lyophilization to determine the antigen unitage to be used to sensitize human red blood cells (RBC); then lyophilize.
h. Check RBC for hemolysis and prepare them for the test. Sheep RBC as well as human O-negative RBC can be used with success.
i. Sensitize with the correct dilution of antigen for 1 h in 37 C water bath or 20 min in 56 C water bath. Bulk amounts of the antigen can be handled this way by predetermining the optimal dilution of the antigen that is needed to agglutinate the RBC you wish to use. The RBC are used at a 10% concentration. A block titration of serum and antigen is needed to determine optimal antigen unitage for use in the HA test.
j. After sensitization do a check test in test tubes by reacting the homologous antisera (preabsorbed with these cells to get rid of heterophile) with the sensitized cells. If titer is sufficiently high, wash the sensitized cells 3 times with 0.15M saline and fix with 40% pyruvic aldehyde; if HRBC are used, let sit in a 4 C refrigerator for 48 h, concentrate to 10 times, then store in Kent buffer at 4 C refrigeration; fix with gluteraldehyde if SRBC are used at a 0.5% final concentration, let stand at room temperature for 2-3 h. This eliminates the necessity for fresh cells in daily work. Add a 1:10,000 final concentration of merthiolate of sodium azide as a preservative during storage. Nonsensitized cells are prepared in a similar manner for controls and can also be sensitized with antigen after fixation. The test is easily done by the microtiter system. The antigen is diluted to 1:10 for use in test. This dilution has been found by repeated testing to be comparable to that of the tube test, which is done with a 1:10 dilution.

2. **Comparison of the microdilution plates and tube method for the HA test.**

a. Dilute each serum to 1:10 and then inactivate in a 56 C water bath for 1 h. Next absorb with 1.0 ml of a 1% suspension of RBC for every 0.1 ml of serum used, finish diluting to 1:25 with 0.5 ml of Kent buffer, and place in a 37 C water bath for 20 min. The serum dilution is centrifuged and drawn off the RBC and is now ready for either the **tube** or **microtiter** test.

b. The antigen is resuspended and diluted as above.

c. 0.1 ml serum is added to each well in the first row in the plate; 0.4 ml of serum is added in each of the first and second tubes.

d. 0.05 ml Kent buffer with bovine serum albumin (BSA) or any good buffered saline is added to rest of plate for serial dilution; 0.4 ml of buffer is added to all other tubes.

e. Leave eleventh place for initial serum dilutions and nonsensitized antigen for heterophile control (0.05 ml of 1:25 serum dilution for microtiter and 0.4 ml of 1:25 serum [initial] to tube 11).

f. Other controls are (1) sensitized cells with saline in well 12 or tube 12, (2) nonsensitized cells with saline, and (3) a titrated row each of known positive and known negative serum controls.

g. 0.1 ml of 1:10 antigen dilution (sensitized cells) was added to each tube, and 0.025 ml of 1:10 antigen dilution is used in each well in the microtiter system. Nonsensitized cells were added to the eleventh row of wells or tubes containing the initial 1:25 serum dilution.

h. Duplicate each test serum as well as known test sera.

i. A 1:25 dilution is considered positive if heterophile is negative.

j. The test is read as early as 3 h.

k. To save time and materials a screening test can be done on each serum by testing only a serum at 1:25 dilution with its heterophile test and a saline control; then if positive, the serum can be titrated later as described above.

l. The test is positive (+) if it has good agglutination and negative (−) if a smooth mat (button) is formed on bottom of well or tube. The titer is the highest dilution with a 2+ agglutination.

Indirect fluorescent antibody (IF) test

Torten et al.[44] reported the development of an IF screening test for human leptospirosis, which employs a genus-specific antigen, *L. patoc* I. This is a saprophytic strain, easily cultivable and presenting no hazard to laboratory personnel. Torten et al. found that slides with fixed antigen could be kept up to 3 months at 4 C without deterioration. Some limitations and the need for further evaluation of the IF method were pointed out by Hirschberg et al.[45]

Interpretation of serologic findings[32]

In leptospirosis, antibodies generally appear from the sixth to the twelfth day of disease, as detected by the MA test, and increase rapidly, reaching maximum titers by the third or fourth week; however, with the HA test, antibodies are detected as early as the fourth day after the onset of illness. After infection, low agglutinin titers may persist for months or years, as measured by the MA test but not with the HA test. For this reason, determining whether current leptospiral infection exists or whether antibodies are due to past experience with the disease is frequently impossible unless at least 2 blood samples are examined, one taken during the early stages of illness and another 2 weeks to 19 days later. Serodiagnostic tests will not provide an early diagnosis, but, when carefully evaluated together with clinical and epidemiologic data, they are helpful in differentiating active from past leptospiral infections. The HA test seems to detect antibodies early in the course of illness but does not detect antibodies late in convalescence. These antibodies have been shown by 2-mercaptoethanol treatment and column fractionation of the serum to be in the IgM fraction of the immunoglobulins.

One should never depend entirely on the serologic reactions of the patient's serum to determine the infecting serotype. For example, during the acute phase of *icterohaemorrhagiae* infections, paradoxical reactions may occur with serotypes, such as some strains of *sejroe*, and *andamana*. Such reactions have been observed even with *biflexa*. Therefore the infecting serotype can obviously be determined with certainty only by isolating and serologically identifying the leptospires. A negative reaction, even on serial samples, does not rule out the possibility of infection, since the patient may be infected with a serotype not included in the battery of testing antigens. Neither does failure to demonstrate a rise in titer eliminate the possibility of current infection. Some evidence indicates that early antibiotic treatment may suppress the development of leptospiral antibodies to such an extent that they appear late and show no increase or fail to appear at all.[30]

• • •

Leptospirosis may be much more prevalent than formerly realized. The classic symptoms of Weil's disease apparently are not always present; it has been estimated that as many as 30% of *L. icterohaemorrhagiae* infections do not cause Weil's disease. Apparently a not insignificant number of cases go undiagnosed, and the opinion has been expressed that in the United States 5-10% of aseptic meningitis cases may be due to *Leptospira*. It is thus important to test for agglutinins for leptospirae or to submit sera for testing to laboratories equipped to do one or more of the test described, in addition to the use of bacteriologic methods for the isolation of leptospirae from the patient.

WEIL-FELIX AGGLUTINATION TEST

One of the earliest tests to be devised for the serologic diagnosis of rickettsial infections is the Weil-Felix test. The antigen employed is **nonspecific** and represents the O variant of nonmotile strains of *Proteus vulgaris* designated as

Table 107-3. Interpretation of Weil Felix reaction

Rickettsial infection	Proteus antigen		
	OX-19	OX-2	OX-K
Rocky Mountain spotted fever	++++ or +	+ or ++++	–
Epidemic typhus	++++	+	–
Murine typhus	++++	+	–
Brill-Zinsser disease*	–	–	–
Scrub typhus	–	–	++++
Rickettsialpox	–	–	–
Q fever	–	–	–

*= A positive OX-19 reaction is occasionally observed.

++++ = Fourfold or greater rise in titer; − = no reaction.

OX-19, OX-2, and OX-K. These antigens are thought to be agglutinated by antibody developing in blood of patients infected with typhus fever and certain other rickettsial diseases.

Epidemic and endemic typhus show marked agglutination of OX-19 and OX-2 but do not agglutinate OX-K. Rocky Mountain spotted fever induces a variety of responses to OX-19 and OX-2 but not to OX-K. Q fever and rickettsialpox fail to induce agglutinins to the *Proteus* antigens. These reactions are summarized in Table 107-3.

The Weil-Felix test is of no value in separating murine typhus, epidemic typhus, and Rocky Mountain spotted fever; it only indicates the presence of a rickettsial infection.

Presumptive evidence is obtained earlier as *Proteus* agglutinins appear 4-5 days after onset and rise rapidly by the tenth to twelfth day. Antibody declines to a nondiagnostic level 1-4 months later.

Preparation of antigen

1. Streak *P. Vulgaris* on dry agar containing 0.5% phenol to develop and maintain nonmotile variants.
2. Suspend growth from an 18-24 h culture in 0.85% saline and adjust turbidity to tube 3 of McFarland nephelometer scale.
3. Use as live antigen or kill by adding 0.5% formalin.
4. Store under refrigeration. On prolonged storage, antigen becomes hyperagglutinable.

Procedure

1. Prepare serial 2-fold serum dilution ranging from 1:20-1;640.
2. Mix 0.5 ml of each dilution with 0.5 ml *Proteus* OX-19 antigen.
3. Repeat setup using *Proteus* OX-2 and OX-K antigens.
4. To permit correct reading of reactions, prepare turbidity controls as shown below:

Antigen	0.5 ml	0.25 ml	0.125 ml
Saline	0.5 ml	0.75 ml	0.975 ml
Agglutination	0	2+	3+

5. Incubate test and control tubes at 50 C in water bath for 18-24 h with tubes submerged to a depth of one-third the column of liquid so as to create circulation of serum-antigen mixture by temperature differential.

6. After incubation allow tubes to cool to room temperature and read degree of agglutination as 0, 1+, 2+, 3+, or 4+ by comparing supernatant fluid with that of control tubes.

Interpretation. The titer is determined as the reciprocal of the highest serum dilution at which a 2+ or greater reaction is obtained.

A 4-fold or greater rise in antibody titer between acute and convalescent phase serum specimens is essential for a presumptive diagnosis. The titer of a single serum specimen has no significance unless the titer is 1:160 or greater.

A low static titer usually indicates a past *Proteus* infection.

For recent criticism and challenge of the validity of Weil-Felix (Proteus) tests, see "Value of Febrile Agglutinin Tests," above.

TESTS FOR ANTIBODIES IN GLANDERS AND MELIOIDOSIS

Glanders (caused by *Pseudomonas mallei*) is a disease of horses, but it is occasionally transmitted to other domestic animals and man. Melioidosis resembles glanders and was first described in man with chief features of septicemia, pyemia, and granulomatous nodules in all parts of the body. It occurs in guinea pigs and rabbits in certain laboratories as well as among wild rats. Melioidosis is caused by *Pseudomonas pseudomallei* (formerly *Malleomyces pseudomallei*).

The demonstration of elevated or rising titers in both diseases is an important diagnostic aid. The method of Cravitz and Miller[50a] is useful for both agglutination and complement fixation tests.

Preparation of antigens

Agglutinating antigen from P. mallei. Heavily seeded beef extract glycerol agar plates (or glycerin-potato-veal agar) are incubated at 37 C for 24 h. The growth is harvested in 0.5% phenolized saline, shaken with glass beads until homogeneous, and then incubated at 37 C for 2-4 d. When sterile, it is filtered through coarse filter paper. For use in the test the antigen is diluted to equal the turbidity of tube 3 of the McFarland nephelometer (approximately 1 billion organisms/ml).

Agglutinating antigen from P. pseudomallei. The antigen is prepared as the A. mallei antigen and is suspended in formalinized (0.1%) saline instead of phenolized saline to preserve the flagellar antigens.

Complement-fixing antigen. The 24 h growth of heavily seeded plates is suspended in saline containing 0.5% concentration of formalin and is kept at 37 C for 4 d (or until sterile). After high-speed centrifugation the supernatant fluid is preserved with Merthiolate (1:5000 final concentration) and used as complement-fixing antigen.

Agglutination test

Serial 2-fold dilutions of serum are made, beginning with 1:5 and ending with 1:1280. Both antigen and serum are used in 0.5 ml quantities/tube. Final dilutions of the serum are 1:10 through 1:2560. Shake tubes and incubate for 24 h at 37 C. Reading is performed by means of reflected light, using a microscope lamp and mirror.

Complement fixation technic

The technic is standard and conforms to that described under complement fixation tests, Chapter 106. The antigen, hemolysin, and complement are titrated. The test is performed by setting up 15 tubes. Serum dilutions are used in the first 9 tubes, the tenth and eleventh are used for anticomplementary controls of the serum and the antigen, and the remaining 4 tubes are used as controls of the hemolytic system.

Known positive and negative sera should be included in the tests. Results of the complement fixation test are read after overnight incubation.

Results in glanders. Normal individuals have agglutinins that can range up to 1:320 against *P. mallei*. the complement fixation test is apparently less sensitive, since normal sera are negative at 1:10 dilution. In individuals who show titers higher than 1:320 in the agglutination test or a rise from a lower titer, the findings are considered diagnostic. Titers of 1:1280 and 1:2560 have been observed in acute cases. The complement fixation test, usually negative in normal sera, becomes positive slower than does the agglutination test (3-6 wk in complement fixation, 1-3 wk in agglutination tests) and many reach titers of 1:320 or 1:640.

Results in melioidosis. Normal sera have agglutinins against *P. pseudomallei* to about the same extent as against *A. mallei*. Complement-fixing antibodies to *P. pseudomallei* are not found in normal sera with the technic described. There is considerable cross-reaction between the antigens prepared from the 2 organisms, especially in the complement fixation test. In the agglutination tests there is usually a higher titer for the homologous antigen (in the case of melioidosis, the titer is higher with *P. pseudomallei* antigen than with *P. mallei* antigen). This seems to hold true for the complement fixation test also.

• • •

Indirect hemagglutination test for melioidosis: See Alexander et al.[46] or Jones and Hambie (in reference 9).

TEST FOR DIAGNOSIS OF PERTUSSIS

Powell and Jamieson[47] reported their results with a simple agglutination test for the diagnosis of pertussis. This test was suggested by the typhus bedside test of Castañeda et al.[48] The test can be carried out with a drop of blood from the patient's finger or ear or with a drop of serum if the blood is drawn and sent to a central laboratory.

Antigen. The antigen consists of a homogeneous suspension in sodium citrate solution of pertussis bacilli standardized against strongly positive, weakly positive, and negative agglutinating sera and usually adjusted to a turbidity of about 100 billion bacilli/ml, colored to a desired intensity with methylene blue, and preserved with 1:10,000 Merthiolate. This antigen may be kept in capillary tubes similar to those used to dispense smallpox vaccine, or it may be dispensed in small dropper bottles. A capillary tube of antigen (approximately 1/40 ml) is sufficient for 1-drop test, and multiple tests may be done, each with a single drop from a bulk dropper bottle. With proper care and cleanliness, the antigen in dropper bottles will not readily become contaminated in the presence of the Merthiolate preservative.

Agglutinating antibody. This may be tested for in a single small drop of blood from the finger or ear as obtained with a Bard-Parker blade for blood count or a similar drop of serum or citrated blood if the blood is sent to a central laboratory.

Procedure

1. Place a small drop (approx. 1/40 ml) of the blue pertussis antigen on a microscope slide. With match stick, toothpick, or probe quickly spread the drop of antigen to form a circle about 1.25 cm in diameter.
2. Add a similar drop of blood or serum to the drop of antigen, stir mixture a few seconds, and then rock or tilt slide, holding drops, back and forth for 1 min.

The sodium citrate in the antigen-suspension prevents coagulation of the blood.

Reactions. A **positive** result is readily observed as granulation or clumping of the blue antigen. If blood is used, read against a reddish background; if serum is used, read against a white background. Overly long agitation of test-drop mixture giving a positive reaction may cause the clumped antigen to form a blue ring at the margin of the drop. A **negative** reaction shows a diffuse blue color modified with red if blood is used.

After agitation and observation of the antigen-blood mixture for about 1 min, set aside the drop mixture and allow to dry without disturbing. After partial drying has taken place, additional agitation may produce artifacts in the negative reactions.

The entire test may be conducted and read in 2 or 3 min, since only 1 min agitation suffices for the incubation period. The test card or paper holding the drop mixture, after drying, comprises a permanent record that may be glued to the patient's record, or the original test may be done directly on a blank area of the record, if this is not quickly wetted through.

Further details regarding the demonstration of pertussis antibodies in patient's sera can be found in the publication of Lautrop and Lacey[49] and Manclark's chapter.[9]

LEGIONNAIRES' DISEASE—INDIRECT FLUORESCENT ANTIBODY TEST*

The indirect fluorescent antibody (IFA) test was first applied to Legionnaires' disease studies by McDade et al.[50] The demonstration of titers in the sera of patients with Legionnaires' disease established the newly isolated bacterium as the causative agent of the disease.

The IFA test for detection of antibodies in human serum to the Legionnaires' disease bacterium (LDB) appears to be specific; however, if possible, all positive results should be accompanied by isolation[50] or direct demonstration of the LDB.[51,52] Until recently LDB isolates were serologically similar, and only 1 representative antigen was needed for competent IFA screening. The discovery of distinct serogroups (4 at the time of writing) means that several antigens are now required for IFA screening and that even more may be required later when more serogroups are defined.

The IFA test for the LDB is already a primary diagnostic tool although basic research is incomplete. Modifications in technic will continue to

_____
*From Jones, J. L., and Hebert, G. A., editors: "Legionnaires'"—the disease, the bacterium and the methodology, Atlanta, May 1978 (revised Oct. 1978), Center for Disease Control.

appear as research progresses. However, the following procedures and technics have proven reliable and can be used diagnostically.

Antigens. All manipulations with live bacteria must be done in a biological safety cabinet. Cultures of the Philadelphia 1 strain of the initial LDB group and the Togus 1 strain are plated on F-G agar[53] and incubated 72 h at 35-37 C in a candle jar.

The growth is harvested as follows:

1. Scrape growth off each plate with bent glass rod using 2-3 ml phosphate-buffered saline (PBS), pH 7.2, per plate.
2. Kill cells by adding equal volume of ethyl ether. Shake mixture vigorously by hand for 10 min. Allow to settle for 30 min and then remove aqueous layer with pipet and excess ether by vacuum.
3. Wash 3 times and resuspend with PBS.
4. Plate on blood agar and F-G agar. No growth after 10 d indicates a sterile suspension of LDB.
5. Dilute LDB suspension with normal yolk sac (NYS) and sodium azide for a final concentration of 1% NYS and 0.05 NaN$_3$. At dilution, suspension should contain approximately 40 bacteria per oil immersion field (1000×).

   NOTE: A batch of antigen prepared from 16 agar plates (13 × 100 mm) will yield approximately 4 L final antigen by this procedure.
6. Dispense in small amounts and store at −20 C.

Control sera. Two positive human sera are required, one of each serogroup. To conserve reagent, high-titered sera may be diluted with normal human serum to give an IFA titer of 1:512. The negative control may be any human serum that gives less than 1+ fluorescence at dilutions ≥ 1:32.

Reagents

1. Fluorescent antibody reagent (antihuman conjugate). Reagent used in our laboratories is the globulin fraction of a rabbit antihuman globulin, labeled with fluorescein isothiocyanate (FITC) and preserved with 0.01% thimerosal. Many antihuman conjugates for other IFA tests are available from commercial sources. Some of these may prove reliable in the IFA test for LDB antibody. An LDB-positive human serum of known titer obtained with standard antigen and conjugate should be used to titer the antihuman conjugate to determine its routine test dilution. The conjugate should also be screened for nonspecific staining of the antigen suspension by performing the test without a human serum.
2. Normal yolk sac (NYS). Homogenize normal chicken egg yolk sacs in PBS, pH 7.2, to give a 10% (wt/vol) suspension. Higher dilutions may prove to be as satisfactory. Add sodium azide to a final concentration of 0.05% and store at 4 C.

Preparation of antigen slides

1. Prepare smears on multiwell slides (acetone resistant).
2. Air-dry.
3. Fix smears by placing slides in acetone for 15 min.
4. Air-dry.

Dilution of control sera

1. Negative control sera
   a. Prepare 1:16 dilution in 10% NYS.
   b. Make further 2-fold dilutions of 1:32 and 1:64 in PBS.
2. Positive control sera
   a. Prepare a 1:16 dilution in 10% NYS.
   b. Make further 2-fold dilutions of 1:32 to 1:1024 in PBS.

Filtration of patients' sera

1. Prepare a 1:16 dilution of each serum specimen in 10% NYS. Make additional 2-fold dilutions of 1:32 to 1:1024 in PBS. To save time and reagents you can screen sera by examining only the 1:64 and 1:128 dilutions.
2. Number antigen slides and add each patient's serum dilution to its well on slides. Mark control slides and add 1:32 and 1:64 dilutions of negative control serum and 1:32 through 1:1024 dilutions of positive control sera to their designated antigen wells.
3. Incubate slides in moist chamber at 35-37 C for 30 min.
4. Rinse slides briefly with PBS and place them in fresh PBS for 10 min. Rinse slides with distilled water. Allow slides to air-dry.
5. Prepare antihuman conjugate by following manufacturer's instructions and, if necessary, adjust to predetermined use dilution. Add conjugate to each well of slides.
6. Incubate slides in moist chamber at 35-37 C for 30 min.
7. Rinse slides briefly with PBS and place them in fresh PBS for 10 min. Rinse slides with distilled water. Allow slides to air-dry.
8. Add buffered glycerol to each slide and mount a no. 1 coverslip (24 × 60 mm) to cover all wells.
9. Examine slides with appropriately equipped fluorescence microscope.

Examination of slides. The stained bacteria are small rods and filamentous forms. Record the predominant staining intensity seen in each antigen well. Grade the fluorescence as follows:

4+ = Maximum or brilliant yellow-green
3+ = Bright yellow-green
2+ = Definite but dim staining
1+ = Barely visible staining
0 = No staining

The serum titer or end point is the highest dilution giving a 1+ fluorescence of at least half the LDB per 40× oil immersion field. The intensity of fluorescence observed may vary depending on the fluorescent microscope assembly used. With reference antigen and a standard conjugate the positive control serum should have the expected titer within one 2-fold dilution, and the negative control serum should read no more than ± at 1:64.

Interpretation. A 4-fold or greater increase in titer to ≥1:128 from acute phase serum to convalescent phase serum is considered indicative of recent infection with LDB. A titer of ≥1:256 for a single serum specimen is considered presumptive evidence of infection at some undetermined time.

NOTE: At the time of this writing (1978), direct and indirect fluorescent antibody reagents for Legionnaires' disease were available from the Center for Disease Control (Attn: Biological Products Division, Bureau of Laboratories), Atlanta, Ga. 30333.

LATEX AGGLUTINATION TEST FOR CRYPTOCOCCUS NEOFORMANS ANTIGEN[54–58]

Cryptococcosis is a systemic infection caused by the pathogenic fungus *Cryptococcus neofor-*

mans (Chapter 104). The organism gains entrance to the body by causing a brief, inflammatory lung infection. From there it rapidly disseminates and shows a preference for the central nervous system. *C. neoformans* is usually a secondary invader, which coexists with tuberculosis, hematologic malignant diseases, and diabetes. Therapy with corticosteroids, other immunosuppressive agents, or broad-spectrum antibiotics may also reduce a patient's resistance to this disease. Thus the symptoms of cryptococcosis may be masked by those of the primary affliction.

Until recently, the sole method of diagnosis of cryptococcosis was the culturing of *C. neoformans* from blood or cerebrospinal fluid (CSF). Cryptococcosis, however, is one of the diseases in which **antigens** of the infective agent circulate within the host, and the latex agglutination (LA) test for *Cryptococcus** detects these antigens.

The LA test provides a technic for detecting the polysaccharide antigen of *C. neoformans* in serum or CSF. This techic gives more rapid results than isolation of *C. neoformans* from serum or CSF, and antigen is occasionally detected in patients from whom no organism can be isolated. Rheumatoid factor in the patient's serum may interfere with the test.

The test is an indirect agglutination procedure that uses latex particles sensitized with either normal or anticryptococcal rabbit globulin. When the **anticryptococcal globulin–sensitized latex** comes in contact with the polysaccharide antigen of *C. neoformans* in the specimen, the globulin-polysaccharide complex reacts, causing the sensitized latex to agglutinate. Latex sensitized with **normal** rabbit globulin should **not** be agglutinated by the polysaccharide antigen. Serum or CSF specimens that show agglutination with both the anticryptococcal globulin–sensitized latex and the normal globulin–sensitized latex are usually showing interference due to rheumatoid factor (RF) in the sample. Any samples that show agglutination with **both** the sensitized latex reagents should be titrated with both reagents through a series of 2-fold dilutions. If the titer of the serum when tested with anticryptococcal globulin–sensitized latex is at least 4-fold higher than when tested with normal globulin–sensitized latex, cryptococcosis is suspected, although a positive diagnosis cannot be made due to the interference. Nearly equal titers with the 2 reagents give an equivocal test, and subsequent samples should be tested for a rising titer with the anticryptococcal globulin–sensitized latex.

An important feature of the test is the consistency of titers obtained using different lots of reagents to test the same serum or CSF specimen. This is due to the fact that the latex particles

*Crypto LA Kit, International Biological Laboratories, Cranbury, N.J.

in each lot of reagents are sensitized with an optimal dilution of globulin, and thus all have the same degree of reactivity. This consistency is further reinforced by the inclusion of a standard for checking the reactivity of the sensitized latex before titering serum or CSF specimens. Thus if for any reason the reactivity of the sensitized latex has been altered, incorrect results are avoided.

A description of the test,* including preparation of reagents, is included here for illustration of the principles involved. At the same time it should be noted that **a commercial kit** (Crypto LA Kit, International Biological Laboratories, Cranbury, N.J.) **is available and is widely used.** Only those laboratories with expertise should undertake preparation of the reagents; otherwise, the commerical kit should be used, with meticulous attention to directions.

Reagents
1. Glycine buffered saline (GBS), pH 8.4
2. GBS, pH 8.4, containing 0.1% bovine serum albumin
3. Polystyrene latex particle suspension ($0.81\mu m$, Difco Laboratories, Detroit)
4. Rabbit anti-*C. neoformans* globulin adjusted to 4 g/100 ml protein and demonstrating a tube agglutination titer of 1:1024 or greater
5. Rabbit normal globulin adjusted to 4 g/100 ml protein
6. Specimens and controls
   a. Positive specimen for positive control
   b. Normal serum for negative control
   c. Serum positive for rheumatoid factor
   d. Unknown serum, cerebrospinal fluid, and/or urine
7. 1N NaOH

Equipment
1. Test tubes (13 × 100 mm)
2. Test tube racks
3. Glass slides (2 × 3 in.)
4. Wax, glass-marking pencil
5. Serologic pipets
   a. 0.5 ml graduated in hundredths
   b. 1.0 ml graduated in hundredths
   c. 5.0 ml graduated in tenths
6. Water bath (56 C)
7. Toothpicks or applicator sticks
8. Graduates (glass stoppered), 10 ml
9. Spectrophotometer (Coleman, Jr., Coleman Systems, Irvine, Calif.) with round cuvettes (12 × 75 mm)
10. Rotary shaker with platform
11. pH meter

Preparation of reagents
1. Glycine buffered saline (GBS), pH 8.4
   a. Mix 9.0 g NaCl and 7.5 g glycine.
   b. Add distilled water to 1000 ml.
   c. Adjust to pH 8.4 with 1N NaOH.
2. GBS, pH 8.4, with 0.1% bovine serum albumin (GBS/BSA)
   a. Add 1 g BSA (fraction V)/liter of GBS.
   b. Mix thoroughly.

*From Kaufman, L., and Blumer, S. O. In Palmer, D. F., Cavallaro, J. J., and Galt, R. H., editors: Laboratory diagnosis by serologic methods, Atlanta, 1975, Center for Disease Control.

3. Standardized polystyrene latex suspension
   a. To determine whether latex suspension is of correct concentration, thoroughly mix commercial latex particle suspension and dilute 1:100 with GBS (0.1 ml latex suspension + 9.9 ml GBS) using glass-stoppered 10 ml graduate.
   b. Measure absorbance of 1:100 dilution of latex in 12 × 75 mm cuvettes using a Coleman, Jr., spectrophotometer at a wavelength of 650 nm. If absorbance is 0.3 ± 0.02, undiluted latex suspension is properly standardized.
   c. If absorbance reading is not 0.3 ± 0.02, calculate dilution of commerical latex suspension needed to obtain desired standardized suspension.

Final volume of standardized suspension =

$$\frac{\text{Actual absorbance of 1:100 dilution} \times \text{Volume of commercial latex}}{\text{Desired absorbance}}$$

Example:
   Absorbance of 1:100 dilution reads 0.50, and there is 5.0 ml of commercial latex suspension:

$$\frac{0.50 \times 5.0}{0.30} = 8.3 \text{ ml final volume of standardized suspension}$$

   Therefore 8.3 ml of standardized suspension would be obtained by adding 3.3 ml GBS to 5.0 ml commercial latex suspension. Repeat Steps 3, 3a, and 3 to verify that correct concentration of latex particles has been attained.

4. Sensitized latex
   a. Dilutions of rabbit anti-*C. neoformans* globulin are made in GBS as follows:
      0.1 ml antiglobulin + 9.9 ml GBS = 1:100
      1 ml, 1:100 dilution + 1 ml GBS = 1:200
      1 ml, 1:100 dilution + 2 ml GBS = 1:300
      1 ml, 1:100 dilution + 3 ml GBS = 1:400
   One ml of each dilution of antiglobulin is mixed thoroughly with 1.0 ml standardized latex suspension and allowed to stand at room temperature for 15 min.
   b. Using GBS/BSA, make serial 2-fold dilutions of known positive specimen.
      (1) Set up row of 8 tubes (13 × 100) and add 0.5 ml GBS/BSA to each.
      (2) Add 0.5 ml positive control specimen to first tube, mix, and transfer 0.5 ml to second tube.
      (3) Continue mixing and transferring 0.5 ml through tube.
      (4) Discard 0.5 ml from tube 8.
   c. Determine optimally reactive dilution of rabbit anti-*C. neoformans* globulin needed for sensitization.
      (1) Test each dilution of known positive specimen against each latex preparation sensitized with various dilutions of antiglobulin.
         (a) On 2 × 3 in. slides, mark off six 1 in. squares with wax pencil. In a 1 in. square mix 0.04 ml 1:2 dilution of positive specimen with 0.02 ml latex sensitized with 1:100 dilution of antiglobulin.
         (b) In other squares mix 0.04 ml of each of remaining dilutions of specimen with 0.02 ml of same reagent. Place slides on

rotary shaker platform and rotate at 125 ± 25 rpm for 5 min. Record as positive all dilutions of specimen showing agglutination equal to or greater than 2+ (i.e., small but definite clumps against a slightly cloudy background). Repeat this same procedure with latex sensitized with 1:200, 1:300, and 1:400 dilutions of antiglobulin.
      (2) Optimally sensitized latex preparation is that which shows 2+ agglutination with highest dilution of positive specimen. This dilution of positive specimen will serve as 2+ positive control for screening and titering unknown specimens.

5. Control latex (LC)
   a. Control latex (LC) reagent is prepared by mixing equal volumes of normal rabbit globulin, **prepared at same dilution as antiglobulin,** and standardized latex suspension. In general a total volume of 2.0 ml LC will be sufficient for test.
   Example:
      (1) Optimal dilution of antiglobulin = 1:200, so normal rabbit globulin is likewise diluted 1:200.
      (2) Mix 1.0 ml normal rabbit globulin (1:200) and 1.0 ml standardized 1% latex suspension.

Performance of test
1. Inactivate all **serum** and **cerebrospinal fluid** specimens at 56 C in a water bath for 30 min. **Urine** specimens should be inactivated by boiling for 10 min.
2. Mark off a 2 × 3 inch slide into 6 one inch sections using wax pencil.
3. In a single 1 inch square mix 0.04 ml unknown undiluted specimen with 0.02 ml latex reagent.
4. On same slide, on other squares, mix additional unknown specimens, plus positive control (2+) specimen and negative control (normal serum), as above. Place slide on rotary shaker platform and rotate at 100-150 rpm for 5 min.
5. Record as positive only those specimens that show agglutination equal to or greater than 2+ positive control.
6. In same manner (Steps 2-5) test all positive serum specimens with LC reagent to rule out false-positive reactions due to rheumatoid factor. Use positive rheumatoid factor serum as positive control for LC reagent.
7. Positive undiluted cerebrospinal fluid and urine specimens and all sera positive with latex reagent and negative with LC should be titered.
   a. Set up a row of 4 tubes (13 × 100 mm) for each specimen to be titered. Label tubes.
   b. To tubes of each row, add 0.5 ml GBS/BSA as diluent.
   c. Add 0.5 ml of each specimen to be tested to first tubes, mix, and transfer 0.5 ml to second tubes. Continue mixing and transferring 0.5 ml through tube 4. **Do not** discard 0.5 ml from fourth tube.
   d. On marked slide mix 0.04 ml of each dilution of each specimen with 0.02 ml latex reagent and rotate as above. One slide will be sufficient to test 4 dilutions of each positive specimen plus positive and negative controls.
   e. Titer of a positive specimen is highest dilution that shows an agglutination equivalent to 2+ positive control. If reaction of 1:16 dilution

(tube 4) is stronger than 2+, continue diluting specimen through 4 more tubes (1:32-1:256) and repeat testing procedure until a titer is determined.

Precautions and suggestions
1. The LA test should always be performed under carefully standardized conditions. Maintain constancy of latex concentration, volume of reactants, reaction time, rotating speed, and degree of agglutination of 2+ positive control.
2. Both latex and LC reagents are stable at 4 C for 12 mo. or more. Freezing, however, will destroy these reagents. It is always necessary to include a negative control in each run to verify stability of latex reagents. If negative control fails to show a homogeneous, milky suspension with no agglutination when reacted with LC and latex reagents, then test is not valid.
3. Likewise, test is invalid if positive control shows agglutination greater or less than established 2+ degree or latex reagent fails to yield a given titer with a known positive specimen previously tested.
4. It is advisable to centrifuge or filter all specimens that contain any visible amount of particulate matter. All specimens not to be cultured should also be preserved with merthiolate (1:10,000).

Interpretation
1. The LA test for cryptococcal antigen appears to have diagnostic as well as prognostic value in that increasing titers reflect progressive disease, while declining titers indicate response to chemotherapy and progressive recovery. Cryptococcal antigen in body fluids of the untreated patient indicates active disease; however, in some instances LA titers remain positive at a low level for an indefinite period of time during which the fungus is no longer viable in the treated patient.
2. LA tests in which serum specimens react with both latex and LC reagents should be considered equivocal. However, since it is possible that cryptococcosis and arthritic conditions can occur concomitantly, titers with both latex reagent and LC should be determined.

    If a 4-fold or greater titer occurs with the latex reagent, this may suggest that cryptococcosis is a real possibility, and additional specimens should be examined for titer change.

    Reactions of less than 2+ in undiluted spinal fluids should be regarded as highly suggestive of cryptococcosis, and additional specimens should be examined for evidence of increasing titer.
3. The properly controlled LA test appears to be 100% specific. Hundreds of serum and cerebrospinal fluid specimens from patients with a variety of bacterial, viral, and fungal infections other than cryptococcosis have been found to be nonreactive. The LA test has generally been shown to be a reliable and valuable adjunct to the diagnosis of cryptococcosis.

4. A negative reaction should not exclude a diagnosis of cryptococcosis, particularly if only a single specimen has been tested and the patient shows symptoms consistent with those of cryptococcosis.

AGAR-GEL IMMUNODIFFUSION TEST FOR HISTOPLASMOSIS[59-67]*

Histoplasmosis is caused by a yeastlike fungus, *Histoplasma capsulatum* (Chapter 104). Due to the varying clinical manifestations of histoplasmosis, laboratory procedures are essential to diagnosis. **Dermal sensitivity** to histoplasmin persists for years after recovery and may be of little use in an endemic area due to the high incidence of positive but otherwise healthy reactors. The skin test is also complicated by frequent cross-reactions with other mycoses, such as blastomycosis, and coccidioidomycosis. **Culturing** of *H. capsulatum* is probably the most conclusive laboratory procedure, but it is not always easy to accomplish. The **agar-gel precipitin test** in conjunction with other serologic procedures, e.g., the complement fixation test, is of considerable value in the diagnosis and prognosis of histoplasmosis. It can be performed with relative ease and in most cases will distinguish hypersensitivity and chronic infection from an active case of histoplasmosis. It is especially useful when the complement fixation test is negative or the patient's serum is anticomplementary.

Principles
1. Homologous antigen and antibody, diffusing toward each other through a semisolid medium, will mix at some point in optimal or near optimal proportions to form a visible band of precipitate.
2. *Histoplasma* antibodies in a patient's serum will precipitate one or more antigens present in a histoplasmin preparation.
3. *Histoplasma* antibodies in a patient's serum can be identified by allowing the patient's serum and the known histoplasmin antigen to diffuse toward each other through a semisolid medium and then comparing the resulting bands of precipitation with those of a reference antiserum.

Reagents
1. Agar medium
2. Histoplasmin antigen (prepared from mycelial phase of *H. capsulatum*)
3. Sera
    a. Positive (containing H and M precipitins)
    b. Negative
    c. Patient's

Equipment
1. 2 × 3 in. glass slides, precleaned
2. Pipets, Pasteur
3. Serologic pipets, 10 ml
4. Applicators, cotton tipped
5. Pattern for cutting wells in agar medium

---

*Condensed from Palmer, D. F., Cavallaro, J. J., and Galt, R. H., editors: Laboratory diagnosis by serologic methods, Atlanta, 1975, Center for Disease Control.

6. Die (3 mm) for cutting wells in agar medium
7. Reading box containing fluorescent light source*

Preparation of reagents and materials

1. 1% Agar medium
   a. 0.9 g Sodium chloride
   b. 1.0 g Purified agar (Noble's Special Agar or equivalent)
   c. 0.4 g Sodium citrate ($Na_3C_6H_5O_7 \cdot 2H_2O$)
   d. 0.25 ml Phenol (88%)
   e. 7.5 g Glycine
   f. Distilled water to 100 ml (heat to dissolve)
      Before use, autoclave at 15 psi for 10 min. Final pH = 6.7-6.8.
2. 0.2% Agar dilution
   Add 2 ml melted 1% agar to 8 ml distilled water (heated to 70-80 C).

Performance of test

1. Swab hot 0.2% agar onto 2 clean 2 × 3 in. slides and place in 37 C incubator for 30 min to dry.
2. Pipet 7 ml 1% agar onto each precoated slide (temperature of agar should be 60-65 C).
3. Allow agar to harden.
4. Cut 2 patterns in agar on each slide as shown in drawing:

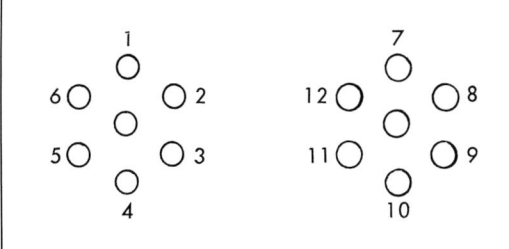

The 6 outer wells should be 4 mm from each other and 4 mm from center well. Each well is 3 mm in diameter.

To remove agar from wells, use Pasteur pipets connected to light suction.

5. Using Pasteur pipets, fill wells with reagents as follows:

Slide 1

Well	Reagents
Center	Histoplasmin
1 and 4	Known positive serum
7 and 10	Known positive serum
2 and 8	Known negative serum
3 and 9	Known negative serum
5 and 11	Unknown serum 1
6 and 12	Unknown serum 2

Slide 2

Well	Reagents
Center	Histoplasmin
1 and 4	Known positive serum
7 and 10	Known positive serum
2 and 8	Known negative serum
3 and 9	Unknown serum 3
5 and 11	Unknown serum 4
6 and 12	Unknown serum 5

---

*A 22 W 20.3 cm circular fluorescent tube mounted 5 cm below top of reading box. Background beneath light source should be a flat black finish.

6. Incubate at room temperature (25 C) in a moist chamber.
7. Read slides at 24 and 48 h.
8. Look for lines of precipitation. To facilitate reading reactions, view box containing fluoresecent bulb above black background may be used.

Precautions and suggestions

1. Be sure that temperature of agar medium is 60-65 C.
2. Top of each slide should be marked so that wells can be identified. Scratch glass slide or label in some manner that will not be affected by moisture. Label slide, not Petri dish containing slide.
3. When removing agar from wells, use light vacuum. Do not touch bottom of well with pipet when removing agar.
4. Completely fill wells with reagents, but **do not** overfill.
5. Agar medium may be added to slides and slides stored for later use, provided they are kept in moist chamber at 4 C. (This is conveniently accomplished by placing slides in Petri Dishes, which are placed in can containing wet paper towel or equivalent.) Prepared slides should be kept at 4 C and used within 2 wk.
6. Agar medium may be prepared, autoclaved, and stored at 4 C for later use. However, once the agar medium has been remelted it must be used or discarded. Storing agar in small amounts eliminates unnecessary waste of media.

Interpretation. Appearance of one or more thin opaque lines or bands of precipitation between the antigen and serum wells is a positive reaction. The M band generally occurs nearer the antigen well and usually indicates hypersensitivity or chronic infection. The H band generally occurs nearer the antiserum (patient's serum) well and is usually due to active histoplasmosis. An H band rarely occurs in the absence of an M band.

The precipitin reactions will usually occur in 16-18 hours and should be read within 2 days.

A pattern of typical reactions of (1) active histoplasmosis and (2) a positive but otherwise healthy reactor (dermal sensitivity or chronic infection) is shown below.

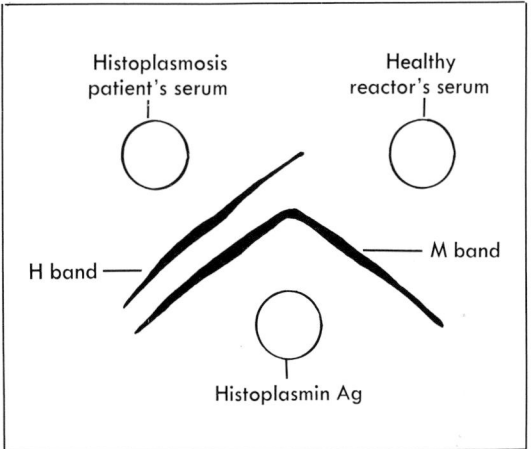

DIRECT IMMUNOFLUORESCENT IDENTIFICATION OF TREPONEMA PALLIDUM IN BODY FLUIDS AND TISSUE SECTIONS[68,69]*
Provisional technic

Equipment
1. Dark-field fluorescence microscope assembly
2. Cryostat (IEC) for tissue sections
3. Diamond-point pencil
4. Slide board or holder
5. Moist chamber
6. Bibulous paper
7. Rubber bulbs, approximately 2 ml capacity
8. Loop, bacteriologic, standard 2 mm, 26-gauge, platinum

Glassware
1. Microscope slides, 1 × 3 inch, frosted end, approximately 1 mm thick
2. Coverslips, no. 1, 22 mm square
3. Dish, staining, with removable slide carriers
4. Glass rods, both ends fire-polished
5. Disposable capillary pipets, 5¾ in. in length

Reagents
1. Sterile distilled water
2. Phosphate-buffered saline, pH 7.2 (Bacto Hemagglutination Buffer no. 0512, Difco Laboratories, Detroit)
3. Phosphate-buffered saline pH 7.2, with 2% Tween 80
4. Acetone, reagent grade
5. Mounting media consisting of 1 part buffered saline plus 9 parts glycerine (reagent quality), pH 7.2-9
6. Fluorescein-labeled anti-T. pallidum globulin (rabbit origin; lyophilized) of proven quality, which has been absorbed with nonpathogenic Reiter treponeme
7. Lyophilized conjugate should be rehydrated with distilled water and diluted with PBS with 2% Tween 80 according to accompanying directions

Preparation of specimens
1. Body fluids, lesion exudates, suspensions of macerated tissue or other materials to be used for preparing smears should be well mixed with a disposable pipet and rubber bulb to ensure even distribution of material. If quantity allows and if it appears advantageous, organisms in spinal fluids and aqueous humor fluids should be concentrated by centrifugation.
2. Fresh-frozen (unfixed) tissues are cut on a cryostat at 2-5 μm thickness for preparing specimens for tissue stain.

Controls
NOTE: **Appropriate controls must be included in each test run and should be performed in duplicate.**
1. Positive control
   a. Smear controls consist of suspensions of T. pallidum prepared by reconstituting lyophilized FTA-ABS test antigen or testicular aspirations made from T. pallidumen infected rabbits. Extracts of rabbit testicular syphilomas prepared for the T. pallidum immobilization (TPI) test may also be used.
   b. If tissue sections are being studied, a known infected tissue section must be included. The

Venereal Disease Research Laboratory, Center for Disease Control, uses fresh-frozen (unfixed), infected rabbit testicle sections cut on a cryostat at 2-5 μm thickness.
2. Negative control
   a. Smears made from nonpathogenic Reiter treponeme cultures or freshly obtained human mouth treponemes may be used.
   b. A normal tissue section is included when tissues are to be studied.

Direct immunofluorescent identification of T. pallidum in fluids
Procedure
1. On a grease-free slide, cut 2 circles approximately 1 cm in diameter with a diamond-point pencil.
2. With capillary pipet or loop, smear approximately 0.01 ml test material within each circle and allow to air-dry. Four smears should be prepared for each specimen.
3. Immerse slides in acetone for 10 min, remove, and air-dry. (If slides are not to be stained and read immediately, they should be stored at −20 C. When testing is to be performed, they should be allowed to thaw and dry thoroughly at room temperature [24-29 C] before staining.)
4. Cover each circle with approximately 0.03 ml diluted conjugate or enough to sufficiently cover antigen.
5. Prevent evaporation and contact with direct light by covering slides with moist chamber.
6. Allow slides to remain at room temperature for 30 min.
7. Rinse slides gently with buffered saline, soak in 2 changes of buffered saline for a total of 10 min, and follow with a final rinse in distilled water.
8. Blot slides gently with bibulous paper.
9. Place a very small drop of mounting medium on each circle and apply coverslip.

Direct immunofluorescent identification of Treponema pallidum in tissues
Procedure
1. On a grease-free slide, gently pick up 1 tissue section per slide from frozen microtome blade. Each specimen to be studied should have at least 4 sections stained.
2. With a diamond-point pencil, cut a circle that encompasses entire section.
3. Allow tissue sections to thoroughly dry.
4. Continue as for Direct Immunofluorescent Identification of T. Pallidum in Fluids, steps 3-9.

Reading test results
1. A microscope equipped with ultraviolet and tungsten light sources is used for observations. When using UV light, the Venereal Disease Research Laboratory, Center for Disease Control, uses a BG-12 exciter filter (2 mm thickness is preferred) in combination with a Euphos barrier filter (eye cap)* for tissue sections, and an OG-1 barrier filter (eye cap) for smear slides.
2. A 10× objective is used for scanning the area and a 45× or 54× high dry objective for verification. Oil immersion is used only in rare cases (mainly in

---

*From Venereal Disease Research Laboratory, Center for Disease Control: Provisional Technique, Atlanta, Jan. 1971.

---

*Optional; some investigators prefer the OG-1 for tissue sections.

tissues) where higher magnification is needed for absolute identification.

NOTE: With control and unknown specimens that do not demonstrate fluorescent treponemes, slide must be observed with tungsten light in order to ascertain if spiral organisms are, in fact, present. See Reporting Test Results, steps 3 and 4.

Reporting test results

1. Strongly fluorescent spiral organisms: slides containing spiral organisms equally fluorescent as positive controls.
2. Weakly fluorescent spiral organisms: spiral organisms showing degrees of fluorescence that are definitely below control reading.
   NOTE: In doubtful or questionable cases, test should always be repeated using freshly prepared slides of known and unknown materials. Any uncertainty is usually resolved by looking at either 4 smear or 4 tissue preparations.
3. Nonfluorescent spiral organisms: materials in which spiral organisms can readily be seen and identified with tungsten light but in which organisms do not fluoresce when observed with UV light.
4. Negative for spiral organisms: no organisms that can be identified as treponemes or spirochetes are observed in material tested using either tungsten or UV light.
   NOTE: Depending on material examined and its source, some slides may demonstrate weak or slightly fluorescent artifacts or debris substances. These materials can for the most part be clearly seen by tungsten light not to have morphologic characteristics of treponemes.

STREPTOCOCCAL ANTIBODY TESTS
Tests for serologic detection of infection by group A β-hemolytic streptococci*

At present, the 2 most suitable serologic tests for the detection of infection by group A β-hemolytic streptococci are the **antistreptolysin O (ASO)** test and the **antideoxyribonuclease B (ADN-B)** test.

The ASO test is the most suitable for several reasons. It has good reproducibility and is well known, and the antigen concerned in the test is produced by most strains of group A streptococci. In addition, the antigen reagent employed is available commercially and has been standardized.

The ADN-B test is suitable because it has good reproducibility and is the test of choice for streptococcal pyoderma and its complications. In addition, the antigen concerned in the test is produced by most strains of group A streptococci, and the antigen reagent employed is commercially available.[70]

The ADN-B test appears to be the best single test for the serologic detection of streptococcal infection,[71] but it is not as well known, has not been as widely used, and is not as well standardized as the ASO test. Until these deficiences are corrected, a safe approach to the serologic detection of group A streptococcal infection is to use the ASO test and another test (ADN-B, antibody to other streptococcal enzymes, or a multienzyme).

The **Streptozyme*** test is a well-known, commercially available **multienzyme test** in which erythrocytes are coated with a mixture of unpurified, streptococcal, extracellular antigens, including streptolysin, deoxyribonucleases, nicotinamide adenine dinucleotidase, hyaluronidase, streptokinase, and probably others. The Streptozyme test is a valuable screening test when used as an adjunct to the ASO test (or, in the future, the ADN-B test). It can detect multiple antibodies and requires only a few minutes to complete. It is therefore particularly useful for laboratories that perform only the ASO test. These laboratories can use it to screen specimens with low ASO titers (≤ 170) for antibodies to other streptococcal products.[72] This test could be recommended as a single presumptive test for use in lieu of either the ASO or ADN-B test, or both, after it has been shown that it is as sensitive as the ASO and ADN-B tests, that quantitation is accurate, that performance of the test by technologists who use it is good, and that the test has been standardized.

However the Center for Disease Control now recommends that laboratories use the ASO test and an additional test. Later it may be possible to recommend either the ADN-B or Streptozyme test as a single test for serologic detection of infection by group A β-hemolytic streptococci.

Antistreptolysin O (ASO) titer determination

Most strains of serologic group A streptococci produce 2 hemolytic factors, streptolysin O and S. Both are capable of disrupting (hemolyzing) red blood cells. When an individual has a group A streptococcal infection, streptolysin O will stimulate the development of a specific antibody, antistreptolysin O, whereas streptolysin S does not stimulate the formation of antibody. The serum titers of antistreptolysin O may be of diagnostic value in patients having, or having had in the recent past, a streptococcal group A infection. This assumes some importance when it is remembered that the sequels of such infections include **rheumatic fever, glomerulonephritis,** and **erythema nodosum.**

Antistreptolysin O antibody is present in most individuals in low titers since streptococcal infections are common. When a patient has signs suggesting rheumatic fever, it is important to determine whether or not he has had a recent streptococcal infection. Elevated titers or increasing titers (with a maximum level at 4-6 weeks after infection) indicate recent infection.

---

*From Bureau of Laboratories, Current item no. 258, Atlanta, Dec. 27, 1977, Center for Disease Control.

*Use of trade names is for identification only and does not constitute endorsement by the Public Health Service or by the U.S. Department of Health, Education and Welfare.

Table 107-4. Serum dilutions

	1:10		1:100					1:500				
Diluted serum (ml)	0.8	0.2	1.0	0.8	0.6	0.4	0.3	1.0	0.8	0.6	0.4	0.2
Isotonic buffer (ml)	0.2	0.8	0.0	0.2	0.4	0.6	0.7	0.0	0.2	0.4	0.6	0.8
Reduced lysin (ml)	0.5	0.5	0.5	0.5	0.5	0.5	0.5	0.5	0.5	0.5	0.5	0.5
Unit/tube	12	50	100	125	166	250	333	500	625	833	1250	2500

The test is considered a valuable aid in the differential diagnosis of early rheumatic fever and rheumatoid arthritis (in which it is not elevated and usually no increase occurs) when the clinical picture is not decisive. Serial determinations at biweekly intervals yield more valuable information than a single determination. The test can be used in the differential diagnosis of acute glomerulonephritis and infectious asthma, both of which show elevated titers, and other diseases presenting similar clinical pictures, without elevated titers.

When streptolysin O in its reduced form is added to red blood cells, hemolysis occurs. If a patient's serum containing antistreptolysin O antibody is added to the streptolysin, an antigen-antibody reaction will occur, the antibody neutralizing the streptolysin O, in part or completely, depending on the level of antibody present. A constant quantity of streptolysin (antigen) is added to progressively decreasing amounts of serum, and if the antibody present is sufficient to neutralize the antigen, no hemolysis will occur when red blood cells are subsequently added. When the antigen exceeds the antibody, the excess streptolysin will cause hemolysis. The ASO antibody titer is the reciprocal of the highest serum dilution that prevents hemolysis of the cells. The ASO titer is measured in **Todd units** (originally defined as the amount of serum just neutralizing 2½ minimum hemolytic doses of a standardized streptolysin).

It is difficult, if not impossible, to state the normal ASO values in man. The level of healthy individuals is generally considered to be 0-125 Todd units (TU), but higher titers have been found in individuals without rheumatic fever or other disease. A titer of 400 U or higher is considered definitely elevated. Single determinations, as pointed out earlier, have little if any value. If an individual shows a rise from 50-250 TU in a relatively short time, it is of diagnostic significance. Persistently low Todd units (50 or less) are helpful in excluding rheumatic fever. Three technics are described below.

ASO macrotechnic of Rantz and Randall [73]

The ASO macrotechnic of Rantz and Randall is widely used.

Preparation of lysin. Grow Richards strain, or any other strain of known good hemolysin-producing streptococci belonging to group A, in meat infusion broth containing 0.2% dextrose and 2% proteose-peptone, and buffered by the addition, after autoclaving, of 0.2% sodium bicarbonate in sterile solution.

Centrifuge after 24 h. To each 100 ml supernatant fluid add 42.9 g ammonium sulfate and let stand at 20 C. Centrifuge and dissolve the sediment in phosphate buffer, pH 7.0, and make up to $^1/_{25}$ of the original volume of the culture with the buffer solution. Dialyze in cellophane sacks for 18 h against running tap water. Add 9 g sodium chloride to each liter of the dialyzed material and sterilize by passing through Seitz filter.

Phosphate buffer, pH 7.0, is made by dissolving 14.2 g disodium phosphate · $12H_2O$ and 3.63 g monopotassium phosphate in 1 L distilled water.

Determination of combining unit. Dissolve 1.6 g sodium hydroxide in 1000 ml isotonic buffer of pH 6.5.

Buffer, pH 6.5, is made by dissolving 4.2 g sodium chloride, 3.17 g monopotassium phosphate, and 3.58 g disodium phosphate · $12H_2O/L$ solution.

Make a fresh solution of 0.15 g cysteine hydrochloride in 25 ml of this solvent.

Set up mixtures of the lysin and the buffered cysteine:

Lysin (ml)   0.35 0.30 0.25 0.20 0.15 0.10
Cysteine (ml) 0.15 0.20 0.25 0.30 0.35 0.40

After 10 min add to each tube 1 ml standard antistreptolysin containing 1 U/ml. Incubate for 15 min in the water bath at 37 C. Add to each tube 0.5 ml 5% suspension of rabbit blood cells in the pH 6.5 buffer without sodium hydroxide. Incubate for 45 min. Centrifuge. That amount of lysin that just failed to produce hemolysis is the combining unit.

Determination of antistreptolysin titer. Dilute the concentrated lysin above to the degree determined in the previous test with isotonic buffer. A further dilution is carried out in the buffered cysteine solution at the time of use, so that the combining unit will be present in a final volume of 0.5 ml. The lysin is ready for use after 10 min exposure to the reducing agent (alkaline cysteine) and does not deteriorate within 60 min.

Set up the reaction as shown in Table 107-4.

Incubate in the water bath at 37 C for 15 min. **Add to each tube 0.5 ml buffered rabbit red blood cells.** Incubate for an additional 45 min.

The last tube in which hemolysis has **not** occurred indicates the antistreptolysin titer of the serum (usually expressed as Todd units).

A control serum of known titer should be included as a check.

Streptolysin O reagent is available from a number of biological houses. Buffer and control serum are usually supplied with the reagent, together with detailed instructions. Essentially the performance of the test remains unchanged. The addition of a thirteenth tube for red cell control, containing buffer and red cells only, is advocated to assure that no hemolysis occurs due to some technical error in the absence of streptolysin. A fourteenth tube, containing buffer, streptolysin O, and red cells, is also used, to show complete hemolysis. A standard control serum is always included in the titration and is handled exactly like the patient's serum.

Capillary ASO microtechnic

A **microtechnic for ASO determination** has been described by Jablon et al.[74] It obviates the necessity of drawing venous blood.

Procedure

1. Use thin-walled 1.25 mm ID capillaries, 90 mm long.
2. Obtain blood by puncture of earlobe or finger and let it run into duplicate capillaries. Use sterile disposable lancet. Run column of blood into center of capillary.
3. Seal one end by pushing capillary into softened modeling clay or heat-seal in Bunsen flame.
4. Place capillaries inside standard Wassermann tube; label with patient's name.
5. Allow blood to clot (about 8-10 min).
6. Centrifuge Wassermann tube, containing capillaries, for 10 min at 1000 rpm.
7. Remove one of capillaries, holding duplicate one in reserve. Nick capillary with file at junction of serum and clot. Break off capillary.
8. Allow serum to run from capillary into standard 0.1 ml pipet graduated in 0.001 ml increments, to 0.03 mark. Hold end of capillary opposite bore of pipet and tilt capillary and pipet slightly to permit serum to run from capillary into pipet.
9. Expel 0.03 ml serum into standard Kahn tube, 10 × 75 mm. Add 0.27 ml streptolysin O buffer (Difco Laboratories, Detroit). This is **solution A** (1:10 dilution).
10. To 0.5 ml serum dilution A add 0.45 ml buffer. This is **solution B** (1:100 dilution).
11. To 0.09 ml solution B add 0.36 ml buffer. This is **solution C** (1:500 dilution).
12. Add to each of above tubes 0.05 ml Bacto streptolysin O reagent (Difco Laboratories, Detroit).
13. Shake tubes gently and place in water bath at 37 C for 15 min.
14. Add to each tube 0.05 ml 5% suspension of saline-washed human red blood cells, group O, previously prepared in streptolysin O buffer.
15. Shake tubes gently and return to water bath for 15 min.
16. Again shake tubes and return to water bath for additional 30 min.
17. Centrifuge at 1500 rpm for 1 min.
18. Read as in the standard Rantz and Randall macrotechnic.

ASO microtitration technic

A micro ASO test, using the Microtiter equipment, was reported by Klein et al.[75] Advantages of the test are savings in reagents and time; about twice as many microtests as macrotests can be carried out in a given period of time.

The technic is performed at the Center for Disease Control as follows.*[76-80]

Reagents

1. Gelatin-barbital buffer
2. Cold distilled water
3. Ice

*From Palmer, D. F., Cavallaro, J. J., and Galt, R. H., editors: Laboratory diagnosis by serologic methods, Atlanta, 1975, Center for Disease Control.

4. Streptolysin O
5. 2.5% suspension of sheep or rabbit red blood cells
6. Standard antiserum
7. Test sera

Equipment

1. Microtitration equipment
   a. Calibrated pipet droppers: one 0.05 ml and two 0.025 ml droppers
   b. Calibrated microdiluters: six 0.05 ml diluters
   c. U plates (disposable or Lucite): 1 plate per 6 specimens, 1 cover plate
   d. Microdiluter testers (go-no-go), 0.05 ml
   e. Cotton swabs
   f. Centrifuge carriers
   g. Test-reading mirror
   h. Stand for microdiluters and pipets
   i. Vibratory mixer
2. Incubator (37 C)
3. Centrifuge: International size 2 with no. 976 head
4. Serologic pipets: 0.2 ml, 1.0 ml, and 2.0 ml
5. Test tubes: 15 × 85 mm or 13 × 100 mm
6. Test tube supports
7. Interval timer
8. Burner
9. Beakers
10. Cleansing tissues
11. Fine tip felt marking pen
12. Pink fluorescent lamps, Fadex

Preparation of reagents and materials

1. Preparation of gelatin-barbital buffer (GB)
   a. Stock barbital buffer solution

Barbital (diethylbarbituric acid)	3.3 g
Sodium barbital (sodium diethylbarbiturate)	1.4 g
Sodium chloride	42.5 g
Distilled water, qs to	1000 ml

   Add barbital and sodium barbital to approximately 500 ml distilled water. Heat to just below boiling with constant stirring until barbital dissolves. Add sodium chloride; mix thoroughly until sodium chloride dissolves. Remove from heat and add approximately 400 ml distilled water. Cool solution to room temperature. Transfer to 1000 ml volumetric flask and bring to volume with distilled water. Determine pH. It should be 7.2 ± 0.05. Store at 4 C. Discard at first sign of contamination.
   b. Stock gelatin solution

Gelatin	1.25 g
Distilled water, qs to	1000 ml

   Add gelatin to approximately 200 ml distilled water. Heat to boiling with constant stirring to prevent scorching gelatin. Remove from heat and add approximately 300 ml distilled water. Cool to room temperature. Transfer to 1000 ml volumetric flask and bring to volume with distilled water. Store at 4 C. Prepare **only** enough gelatin water to last 7-10 d, as it is easily contaminated. **Discard** at first sign of bacterial or mold growth.
   c. Working solution of GB
   Prepare working solution as needed by adding 1 part stock barbital solution to 4 parts gelatin solution, e.g., 20 ml buffer solution to 80 ml of gelatin solution. Store in refrigerator. Discard at first sign of contamination.
2. Preparation of 2.5% red blood cell suspension
   a. Pipet 3-4 ml citrated rabbit or sheep blood through 2 layers of clean gauze into 15 ml graduated centrifuge tube. Add 2 or 3 vol GB

to each volume of blood. Centrifuge at 600 × g **for 5 min.**

b. Remove supernatant and layer of white blood cells. Fill centrifuge tube with GB. Resuspend cells by mixing gently with pipet. Centrifuge at 600 × g for 5 min. **Repeat washing process twice.** If supernatant is not colorless after 2 washings, cells are too fragile and should not be used.

c. After second washing, add GB to packed cells up to 10 ml graduated mark. Resuspend cells with pipet. Centrifuge at 600 × g for 10 min. Record column of packed cells and remove supernate. Prepare 2.5% suspension by adding 3.9 ml buffered diluent to each 0.1 ml packed cells.

d. Store cell suspension at 4 C. Discard at first sign of hemolysis or contamination.

3. Preparation of initial serum dilutions
a. The **initial** serum dilutions of 1:10, 1:60, and 1:85 are prepared in **test tubes.** Subsequent dilutions are carried out in ∪ **plates.** Both serum and GB should be at room temperature when preparing dilutions. Include standard serum of known titer in each day's run to serve as positive control.

b. Prepare dilutions as shown below. Mix thoroughly.

Tube no.	Initial dilution	GB	Undiluted serum	1:10 serum
1	1:10	0.9 ml	0.1 ml	—
2	1:60	1.0 ml	—	0.2 ml
3	1:85	1.5 ml	—	0.2 ml

Procedure

1. Label microtiter ∪ plate as indicated in plate pattern (Fig. 107-2) so that each specimen is assigned 2 rows (1:60 row and a 1:85 row), with 6 wells per row.
   Label 6 wells on bottom row of each plate as specimen hemolysin controls. Also label well for streptolysin control and well for RBC control on 1 plate in each run (**not for each plate**).

2. Add GB, at room temperature, as follows:
   a. 0.05 ml (0.05 ml dropper) to wells 2-6 of each row assigned to specimens and to streptolysin 0 control well
   b. 0.025 ml (0.025 ml dropper) to each serum hemolysin control well
   c. 0.075 ml (0.025 ml dropper) to RBC control well

3. Pipet (0.2 ml pipet) 0.1 ml of each 1:60 serum dilution into labeled test well.

4. Pipet 0.1 ml of each 1:85 serum dilution into labeled test well and 0.05 ml into serum hemolysin control wells.

5. Test 0.05 ml microdiluter for accuracy.

6. Transfer 0.05 ml from first well to second well.

7. Prepare serial 2-fold dilutions through sixth well. Serum dilutions for each serum are **first row—** 1:60, 1:120, 1:240, 1:480, 1:960, 1:1920; **second row—**1:85, 1:170, 1:340, 1:680, 1:1360, 1:2720.

8. Check microdiluters for accuracy and place in distilled water for rinsing.

9. Repeat any dilution series that gives an inaccurate diluter check.

10. Reconstitute streptolysin O reagent according to package directions with **cold** distilled water. Mix gently to avoid aeration. Keep reconstituted reagent in ice water.

11. Add 0.025 ml cold streptolysin O reagent to all wells **except** RBC and serum hemolysin controls.

12. Turn on vibrator.

13. Place plate on vibrator for 20 s. Remove plate **before** stopping vibrator. CAUTION: extended agitation may cause oxidation and inactivation of streptolysin O.

14. Cover plate with empty plate. If there is more than one test plate, 3 plates may be stacked and cover placed on top.

15. Place covered plate in 37 C incubator for 15 min.

16. Remove plate from incubator and add 0.025 ml (0.025 ml dropper) of cold 2.5% red blood cells to **all** wells. Do not add RBC to more than 6 plates at a time before mixing on vibrator because RBC will settle out and be more difficult to resuspend.

17. Mix on vibrator for 15-20 s or until all cells are in suspension.

18. Restack and cover plates.

19. Incubate at 37 C for 15 min.

20. Remove plates from incubator.

21. Mix on vibrator for 15-20 s or until all cells are in suspension.

22. Restack and/or cover plates.

23. Reincubate at 37 C for 30 min.

24. Centrifuge plates for 2 min at 250 × g to pack RBC (1200 rpm in size 2 international centrifuge with no. 976 head).

25. Read for presence or absence of hemolysis, using reading mirror and fluorescent lamp.

Reading of test

1. Examine streptolysin control for **presence of complete hemolysis.**

2. Examine **cell control for absence of hemolysis.**

3. Examine **serum control for absence of hemolysis.**

4. Validity: the test must be repeated on all sera in the run if:
   a. Titer of reference serum is not as stated by manufacturer.
   b. Streptolysin O control does not show complete hemolysis of RBC.
   c. RBC control shows any **hemolysis.**

5. If there is hemolysis in serum hemolysin control, test on that specimen is not valid unless there is at least one well above 1:85 dilution in test (for that particular serum) that has no hemolysis. Hemolysis in serum hemolysin control well indicates presence of natural hemolysin for RBC in patient's serum. This hemolysin is usually diluted out at dilutions above 1:85 and does not interfere with determination of end point.

Reporting results. The titer may be expressed in Todd units (TU) if the potency of the streptolysin O used in the test had been adjusted against the Todd standard **or** in international units (IU) if the potency of the streptolysin O used in the test had been adjusted against the WHO international standard. For practical purposes, these 2 units are equivalent.

Precautions and suggestions
Streptolysin

1. Avoid shaking or aeration of streptolysin solution. Mix **gently** when reconstituting. Oxidation reduces hemolytic activity.

2. Leftover streptolysin solution must be discarded. It is not reusable.

Red blood cell suspension

1. Do **not** use same pipet dropper for red blood cells that was used for streptolysin solution. Trace of streptolysin in dropper can cause some lysis of cells.

2. Do **not** add cells to more than 6 plates at a time

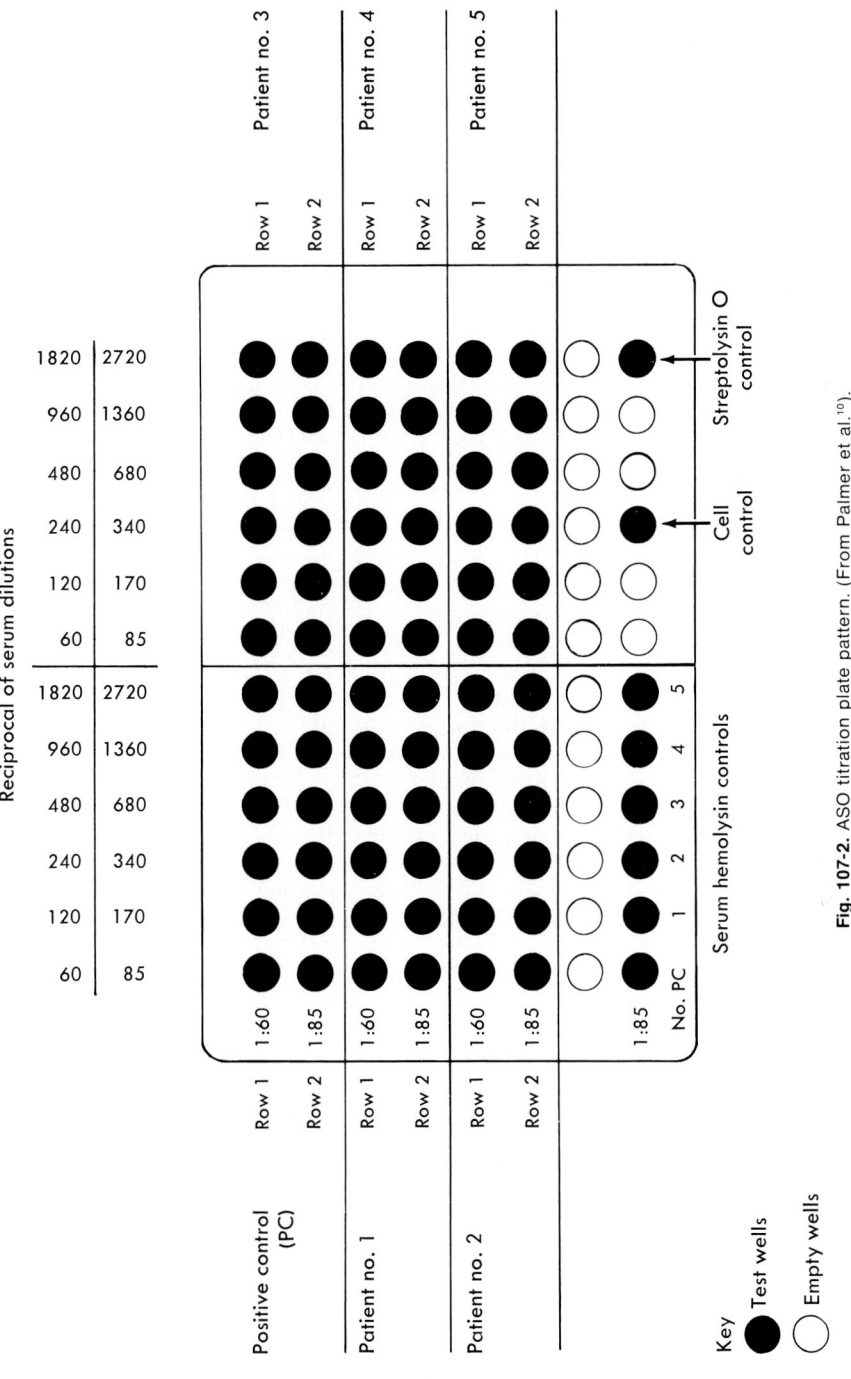

Fig. 107-2. ASO titration plate pattern. (From Palmer et al.[10]).

before mixing plates; cells settle out and are difficult to resuspend.

Incubation

1. To ensure proper incubation temperature for all plates, do not put more than 3 plates (plus cover) in a stack.
2. Keep a pan of water in incubator to provide a moist atmosphere to prevent evaporation from plates.

Vibrator

1. Syntron paper jogger (or equivalent) or Thomas Shaking apparatus is satisfactory.

Interpretation. The most convincing serologic evidence suggestive of a recent group A streptococcal infection is a rise in titer of 2 dil steps or more between acute and convalescent phase sera. A rise in titer occurs about 1 week after infection and peaks 2-4 weeks later. In the absence of complications or reinfection, the ASO titer will usually fall to preinfection levels within 6-12 months.

If only a single specimen is available, or in the absence of a 2 dil rise (or fall) in titer, then the upper "limit of normal" titer is a useful guide for determining the significance of the ASO titer.

The upper "limit of normal" value represents the highest ASO titer obtained in 85% of a "normal" population with no apparent recent streptococcal infection. Thus an ASO titer above the upper limit has an 85% chance of being due to a recent streptococcal infection.

It should be recognized that an ASO titer of a single specimen below the upper limit of normal cannot definitely rule out a streptococcal infection since a significant increase in titer (2-fold or more dilutions) may occur even though the titers do not exceed the "normal" range.

The upper "limit of normal" for ASO titers varies with age and may also vary with geographic location.

The upper limit of normal ASO titers in young adults is in the range of 200. Approximately 80% of this population will have titers below the 200 level. Youngsters from 6-14 years of age may have somewhat higher titers; the upper limit of normal for this age group is approximately 250. Normally, as age increases above 17 years, the ASO titer falls eventually to a level below 100.

Over 80% of patients with acute rheumatic fever and over 95% of patients with acute glomerulonephritis have elevated ASO titers. These titers have been reported to range between 159-1585 or higher.

False-positive ASO titers can be caused by increased levels of β-lipoproteins in serum due to liver disease, by contamination of the sera by *B. cereus* or with several species of *Pseudomonas*, and by oxidation of the streptolysin O.

ASO latex agglutination test*

A commercial kit (Calbiochem-Behring Corp., La Jolla, Calif.) is now available for the latex ASO test.

---

*From Calbiochem-Behring Corp. product description, 1976.

Principle. The principle of the test is an immunologic reaction between ASO as an antibody and the corresponding antigen (streptolysin O) coated on the surface of biologically inert latex particles.

Since only sera with ASO titers greater than 200 IU/ml are of interest for adult testing, sufficient streptolysin O is added to the test specimen to neutralize approximately 200 IU/ml of ASO prior to the addition of the ASO latex reagent.

Reagents

1. ASO latex reagent: a suspension of polystyrene latex particles in glycine buffer, pH 8.2. Latex particles are coated with streptolysin O (β-hemolytic streptococci, group C).
2. Streptolysin O (β-hemolytic streptococci, group C), lyophilized. Reconstitute with normal saline as indicated on label.
3. ASO positive control: a stabilized human serum protein preparation containing ASO at a concentration above 200 IU/ml.
4. ASO negative control: a stabilized, diluted human serum containing ASO at a concentration below 100 IU/ml.

Procedure

Qualitative determinations

1. Bring all reagents and serum samples to room temperature.
2. Add normal saline as indicated on label to a vial of lyophilized streptolysin O. Shake gently to dissolve.
3. Pipet 0.3 ml of solution into 3 small test tubes.
4. Add 0.1 ml patient's serum to first tube; 0.1 ml ASO positive control to second tube; and 0.1 ml ASO negative control to third tube.
5. Mix by shaking. Let tubes stand for 15 min at room temperature.
6. Place 1 drop (~0.05* ml) of each mixture on 3 separate fields on test slide.
7. Shake ASO latex reagent to obtain uniform suspension. Expel contents of dropper, refill, and add 1 drop to each field containing sample to be tested. Mix well with stirring rod, spreading mixture over most of field. Tilt slide through several planes for 5 min. Rotary shaker may also be used.
8. Examine for agglutination **immediately** using direct light (e.g., high-intensity lamp) at distance of approximately 10-15 cm from surface of slide. Suitable equipment for analysis of agglutination tests may also be used. Reaction of test serum is compared to ASO positive and negative control sera.

Quantitative determinations (latex kit titration)

1. Number 6 tubes I, II, III, IV, V, and VI. Dispense 0.5 ml normal saline into tubes I, III, IV, V, and VI, and 1.0 ml saline into tube II.
2. Dispense 0.5 ml patient's serum into tubes I and II, and pipet as follows (mix well at each step):
   a. From tube I : 0.5 ml into tube III, then 0.5 ml from tube III into tube V; discard 0.5 ml from tube V.
   b. From tube II: 0.5 ml into tube IV, then 0.5 ml from tube IV into tube VI; discard 0.5 ml from tube VI.

---

*If a Pasteur pipet is used to dispense serum/streptolysin O mixture, 2 drops may have to be used to obtain required volume (0.05 ml).

3. Number 6 tubes 1, 2, 3, 4, 5, and 6. Pipet 0.1 ml patient's serum dilution from tube I into tube 1, 0.1 ml from tube II into tube 2, continuing through tube 6.
4. Reconstitute streptolysin O with normal saline as indicated on label, mix well, and dispense 0.3 ml into tubes 1-6.
5. Mix tubes well and allow to stand at room temperature for 15 min.
6. Place a drop (~0.05 ml) of diluted serum/streptolysin O mixture from tubes 1-6 on their respective fields on test slide.
7. Shake ASO latex reagent to obtain uniform suspension and add 1 drop to each field containing mixture.
8. In each field, mix 2 drops evenly over 2 cm² area using clean stirring rod.
9. Tilt slide through several planes for 5 min. Read **immediately** as indicated in Qualitative Determinations, step 8.

Quality control. ASO positive and negative controls should be included in each test series. Satisfactory performance is indicated by agglutination with the ASO positive control and a lack of agglutination with the ASO negative control.

Results

Qualitative determinations. An agglutination of the latex particle suspension is a positive result indicating that ASO is present in the specimen in a concentration of or greater than 200 IU/ml (±15%). Lack of agglutination indicates an ASO concentration below 200 IU/ml (±15%). In the concentration range of 170-230 IU/ml, positive or negative results may appear.

Quantitative determinations. The antistreptolysin O content of the patient's serum is based on the highest dilution showing distinct agglutination and can be taken from the following:

Reaction square no.	Serum dilution	ASO titer IU/ml (±15%)
1	1:2	≥ 400
2	1:3	≥ 600
3	1:4	≥ 800
4	1:6	≥ 1200
5	1:8	≥ 1600
6	1:12	≥ 2400

Limitations of procedure. Reaction times longer than 5 min may produce false-positive reactions. Markedly lipemic or contaminated sera may also cause false-positive reactions. Care should be taken to keep the ASO latex reagent dropper vial tightly closed to prevent flocculation due to evaporation of the suspension.

Strength of agglutination reaction is not indicative of the ASO concentration.

In the qualitative test, weak reactions may occur with slightly or markedly elevated concentrations. In some cases of greatly increased ASO titer (more than 2000 IU/ml), agglutination may be inhibited due to antibody excess (prozone). When this is suspected, it is advisable to dilute the patient's serum 1:4 with normal saline and repeat the procedure.

Expected values. An ASO titer of 200 IU/ml is usually regarded as the upper limit of normal since less than 20% of healthy subjects yield titers of greater than 200 IU/ml. In newborns, the titer is usually higher than in the mother but falls sharply during the first few weeks of life as the IgG acquired from the maternal circulation is eliminated. The normal adult ASO level is gradually attained by age 5 or 6, but a considerable drop in titer is seen in the elderly.

A rise in ASO titer generally takes place 1-4 weeks after the onset of infection with β-hemolytic streptococci, group A. When the disease has subsided the titer gradually declines, returning to normal levels within 6 months. If the titer does not decrease, a recurrence of the infection may be indicated.

Increased ASO titers may be associated with ankylosing spondylitis. (Bechterew's disease), glomerulonephritis, scarlet fever, and tonsilitis. An extremely low ASO titer is observed in the nephrotic syndrome and in antibody deficiency syndromes. Elevated ASO levels are not generally found in rheumatoid arthritis except during acute attacks.

Specific performance characteristics. Bach et al.[81] compared the Rapi/tex-ASO Kit (qualitative method) with the tube dilution hemolysis method of Rantz and Randall[73] in measurement of ASO antibody levels. Although the latex procedure is standardized on the basis of international units,[82] the results they presented with their study were expressed in Todd units (TU). All sera with 250 TU or above were positive with the ASO latex reagent.[81] At ASO titers of 166 TU, a frequently used upper limit of normal,[83] 10% of the sera tested were negative by latex agglutination. Specimens with titers in the range of 100-125 TU showed variable agglutination patterns. All of the sera with an ASO titer below 100 TU were negative.[81]

Multienzyme test (Streptozyme) for detection of antibodies to streptococcal extracellular antigens*

The Streptozyme test described below is a qualitative test, but it can also be used for determining a quantitative Streptozyme antibody titer.

Streptozyme (STZ) offers a simple, rapid screen or titration method for detection of antibodies to the extracellular antigens of streptococcus A, such as may develop in streptococcal pharyngitis, rheumatic fever, pyoderma, glomerulonephritis, and other related conditions.

The antistreptolysin O (ASO) test is the most widely used serologic test for the detection of streptococcus A sequelae. Since streptolysin is only one of several streptococcus A exoenzymes, the ASO test will not detect the other antibodies to exoenzymes of streptococcus A.

Examinations of over 1000 sera[84-88] have shown that approximately 80% of the sera positive by Streptozyme at a 1:100 dilution (100 STZ U) have an antistreptolysin O titer of 166 TU or above, while an additional 10% showed an antistreptokinase (ASK) and/or antihyaluronidase (AH) titer also above 166. Positive agglutination in the case of the other 10% is speculated to be caused by the

---

*From product description, Wampole Laboratories, Division of Carter-Wallace, Cranbury, N.J.

presence of antibodies to other streptococcal extracellular antigens[84,86] or to the combined effect of several antibodies, which individually would fall below the 166 titer. Practically no sera with an elevated ASO titer can be missed by the Streptozyme slide test. Thus the accuracy of detection of antibodies to extracellular antigens of streptococcus A is superior for streptozyme as compared to the conventional ASO test used alone.[88,89]

Streptozyme detects more positive specimens than any single test for streptococcal exoenzyme antibodies.[85,88] It is recognized that a single determination of antibodies to streptococcal A extracellular antigens is not as significant as serial titrations performed at weekly or biweekly intervals for up to 6 weeks following the streptococcal infection. Positive sera should be further diluted in order to determine the titer. Sequential determinations can give the trend of the patient's antibody production to allow clinical conclusions with regard to the progress of the disease and treatment.

Cholesterol and β-lipoproteins that may cause false-positive titers with the classic antistreptolysin test do not interfere with the streptozyme test.[85]

Principle. The Streptozyme reagent consists of a standardized suspension of aldehyde-fixed sheep cells sensitized with streptococcus A extracellular antigens including some of the classic exoenzymes, such as streptolysin, streptokinase, hyaluronidase, DNase, and NADase that will react with antibodies to these antigens to give a positive agglutination reaction.

Reagents
1. Streptozyme reagent (standardized sheep cells sensitized with streptococcus A extracellular antigens). Cell concentration = 3-5%; contains buffer and preservative.
2. Positive control serum (human). Contains preservative; reconstitute to 1.0 ml.

Precautions
1. Before use, read instructions carefully.
2. For indications of deterioration, read instructions.

Specimen collection and preparation
1. Fresh or inactivated serum or plasma as well as peripheral blood from fingertip or earlobe may be used.
2. If serum is to be tested, fresh serum should be used. If serum cannot be tested within 24 h after collection, it should be stored frozen. If sample to be tested is to be mailed, a preservative such as sodium azide 0.1% or thimerosal 1:10,000 should be added. In frozen state, serum may be kept for extended periods.
3. When performing test with blood, a heparinized capillary or the plain capillary supplied in the kit may be used.

Materials
1. Reagent
2. Positive control serum
3. Calibrated capillary tubes and bulbs
4. Mirrored glass slide
5. Isotonic saline (0.85% sodium chloride)
6. Stirrers
7. Pipets or syringes with large hypodermic needles
8. Conventional test tubes

Testing of samples. In order to obtain accurate and reproducible results, the test procedure must be carefully followed.

Procedure for serum or plasma
1. Dilute serum sample 1:100 with isotonic saline.
2. Fill capillary to mark (0.05 ml) with diluted serum and expel into section of slide.
3. Add 1 drop of reagent.
4. Using disposable stirrer, thoroughly mix fluids. Use clean stirrer for each mixture.
5. Rock mirror slide back and forth gently and evenly for 2 min at rate of 8-10 times/min., then stop rocking, and gently place slide on flat surface and observe for agglutination within 10 s.
NOTE: Direct light source above slide facilitates reading.

Procedure for blood (peripheral)
1. Draw blood from fingertip, earlobe, or other suitable area.
2. Allow capillary supplied to fill to line (0.05 ml).
3. Without allowing blood to clot and using bulb supplied, expel sample into tube containing 2.5 ml isotonic saline. On a basis of a 50% hematocrit, this 1:50 blood dilution is equivalent to a 1:100 serum dilution.
4. Proceed as with Steps 2-5 under procedure for Serum or Plasma.
Positive results with Streptozyme, compared with positive results for ASO, ADNase-B, and AH individually tested, agreed in over 96% of the cases; overall agreement was approximately 93% for both positive (elevated) and negative (nonelevated) titers.[84]
The accuracy of Streptozyme in a group of 76 patients with streptococcal disease, including acute rheumatic fever, acute glomerulonephritis, pharyngitis, and pyoderma, was found to be 95%.[85]

Titration procedure*
Serum or plasma. To obtain the level of Streptozyme antibody (STZ titer) prepare the dilutions illustrated below, using conventional test tubes and a pipet or syringe with a large-gauge hypodermic needle.

Preparation of dilutions for STZ titer		Resulting dilution
0.1 ml Serum or plasma (primary dilution)	+ 9.9 ml Saline =	1:100
1.0 ml Primary dilution	+ 1.0 ml Saline =	1:200
0.5 ml Primary dilution	+ 1.5 ml Saline =	1:400
0.5 ml Primary dilution	+ 2.5 ml Saline =	1:600
0.5 ml Primary dilution	+ 3.5 ml Saline =	1:800

Test each dilution as described under Procedure for Serum or Plasma.

The last dilution to show positive agglutination on the slide is taken as the STZ titer.

Blood (peripheral). To test blood collected from fingertip or earlobe, follow the dilution procedure described for serum without allowing blood to clot if no anticoagulant is used. On the basis of a 50% hematocrit, the final blood dilution represents half the serum dilution shown above, i.e., the 1:100 dilution of blood represents a 1:200 serum dilution. Test each dilution as described under Procedure for Blood (peripheral). The

---

*This should be reported in STZ units. An STZ unit is equivalent to reciprocal of last dilution showing agglutination. For example, if 1:100 dilution of serum is positive while higher dilutions are negative, sample contains 100 STZ U.

last dilution to show positive agglutination on the slide is taken as the STZ titer.

Results. Positive sera show readily visible agglutination, and negative sera are uniformly turbid or slightly granular.

Limitations of procedure. The value of a single determination is limited in that sequential determinations can give the trend of the patient's antibody production to better allow clinical conclusions with regard to the progress of the disease and thus treatment.

Expected values. ASO titer is commonly expressed in Todd units (TU), which refer to the reciprocal value of the highest serum dilution that shows no hemolysis in the test originally described by Todd.[90]

Todd units specifically refer to ASO and only ASO. Streptozyme detects antibodies to multiple streptococcal extracellular antigens (only one of these antigens is streptolysin O). **It is technically incorrect to express the Streptozyme dilution in Todd units.**

Since ASO only measures 1 antibody while Streptozyme detects antibodies to multiple antigens, it is possible for a patient to have a significant STZ titer while showing a negative ASO response. As a rule an elevated STZ titer (100 units or higher) can be expected to occur in 20% of patients showing a negative ASO titer (less than 166 TU). Titers considered within normal limits for STZ and ASO may vary according to geographic location, season of the year, and age group of patients.[85]

• • •

For a comparative study of ASO, antideoxyribonuclease B, and multienzyme (Streptozyme) tests, see Golubjatnikov et al.[91]

Antihyaluronidase (AHT) test

Most group A streptococci produce the enzyme hyaluronidase. Many individuals, after a group A streptococcal infection, develop an increasing titer of antihyaluronidase, an antibody that inhibits the activity of the enzyme.

The AHT procedure is based on measurement of the specific inhibition of hyaluronidase by antihyaluronidase in the patient's serum and is regarded as a valuable adjunctive test to the ASO procedure in the detection of antecedent group A streptococcal infections.

A mucin clot prevention test, slightly modified form that of Quinn and Liao,[93] consists of (1) combination of a constant volume of standardized hyaluronidase with serial dilutions of the patient's serum; (2) incubation of the mixture at 37 C for 15 minutes, followed by refrigeration for 10 minutes; (3) addition of AHT substrate (potassium hyaluronate solution); (4) incubation at 37 C for 20 minutes followed by refrigeration for 30 minutes; (5) addition of 0.1 ml 2N acetic acid and vigorous shaking; (6) observation of the tubes for presence or absence of clot formation and clarity.

The AHT titer is the reciprocal of the highest serum dilution showing a clot, i.e., the highest dilution of the serum (containing antihyaluronidase) that will inhibit the hyaluronidase and thereby prevent it from dissolving the clot formed in each tube in which there is no free hyaluronidase.

Healthy individuals may exhibit titers up to 250. A titer of 1024 or higher is significant in rheumatic fever.[92] It is advisable to perform more than 1 determination to demonstrate changes in the titer. The ASO test will detect about 80% of group A streptococcal infections; if the AHT test is added, the detection rate can be increased to 90%.

Standardized reagents for the test, together with detailed instructions for performance of the procedure, are now commercially available (Difco Laboratories, Detroit).

Streptococcal antideoxyribonuclease B determination

Deoxyribonuclease B (DNase B) is produced by group A streptococci; the titer of antibodies to the enzyme increases in the serum of many individuals after infection with group A streptococci. The DNase B test was shown to be a valuable adjunct to other streptococcal antibody tests in establishing the occurrence of a prior streptococcal infection.

For details of the test see Ayoub and Wannamaker[93] and for a microtechnic, see Nelson et al.[94]

The test is now commercially available (ADB Test System, Beckman Instruments, Fullerton, Calif.).

SEROLOGIC TESTS FOR DIAGNOSIS OF MYCOPLASMIC INFECTIONS
(George E. Kenny)

Serologic procedures for detection of antibody in *M. pneumoniae* infections will be emphasized because of the importance of this agent and because considerable information is available on the antigens of this organism.[95] Much less information is available concerning serologic methods for measuring human serum antibody to *M. hominis* and *Ureaplasma urealyticum*. Three methods are available for use in serology with the Mycoplasmatales: complement fixation, metabolic inhibition, and fluorescent antibody. Other more complex procedures have been developed, which are of less immediate use in serodiagnosis.[95] Serodiagnosis of *M. pneumoniae* infections is carried out by 2 methods: complement fixation with lipid or whole organism antigen and metabolic inhibition testing. Both tests appear to measure antibody to the same determinant, the lipid antigen, and results of the two tests correlate well.[96]

Complement fixation test for M. pneumoniae

Antibody testing is carried out on paired sera using a standard microtiter complement fixation (CF) test. Whole organism antigens are commercially available, although lipid extracts of whole organisms have proven to give a more sensitive test.[97] Details for preparing lipid antigens are presented elsewhere[97]; the procedure is simple and readily reproduced. For the CF test 4 units of antigen are employed with 2 full units of complement with overnight fixation at 4 C. Fourfold antibody rises in paired sera correlate well with infection with the organism: 58% of pneumonia patients with *M. pneumoniae* isolates showed 4-fold antibody rises.[98] Since antibody levels decline slowly after infection, presence of antibody cannot be used as an index of recent infection; however, titers of 1:256 or greater are suggestive of recent infection. Paired sera should be collected as close to onset as possible and again 3 weeks later. The specificity of the complement fixation test is excellent for diagnosis of pneumonia.[98] However, certain startling cross-reactions of *M. pneumoniae* lipids have been observed that suggest a note of caution in serodiagnosis of other infections. Lipids from *M. neurolyticum,* a rodent organism unrelated to *M. pneumoniae,* cross react strongly with *M. pneumoniae* lipids.[99] Additionally, glyceroglycolipids obtained from spinach cross-react with *M. pneumoniae* lipid, and the spinach lipids can be used for serodiagnosis of *M. pneumoniae* infections.[100]

Metabolic inhibition testing

The metabolic inhibition test measures the ability of antibody to stop growth of the organism. The end point of the test is measured by observing the failure of the organism to produce a normal metabolic product (ammonia from arginine or urea, acid from glucose, or the failure to reduce tetrazolium); this failure is conveniently indicated by a color change in a pH or redox indicator in the medium. Specific details of tests are described elsewhere for glycolytic organisms,[101] arginine-utilizing organisms,[102] and *U. urealyticum.*[103] The general principle of the tests is that a small amount of live organisms (with a specific titer in terms of color-changing units) is mixed with dilutions of antibody. That dilution of antibody which prevents the color change associated with the normal production of a metabolite is the end point of the reaction. It is imperative that paired sera be run in the same test and that the amount of organisms be carefully controlled because the end point of the test changes with incubation time. The role of accessory factors such as complement has been difficult to establish, but addition of fresh guinea pig serum may stabilize titers. The presence of antibiotics in the serum will give a false positive-reaction, but this problem can be circumvented by use of antibiotic-resistant variants in the case of *M. pneumoniae.*[104] Although metabolic inhibition tests measure antibody well in hyperimmune animal antisera prepared against either *M. hominis* or *U. urealyticum,* the tests are less successful in measuring antibody to these organisms in human sera. A portion of this problem is due to

the antigenic heterogeneity of *M. hominis* [105] and the large number of serotypes of *U. urealyticum.*[106] Additionally, infections with these organisms may be more superficial than infections with *M. pneumoniae.* Thus serologic testing for *M. hominis* and *U. urealyticum* infections is still in the developmental stage.

Cold agglutinin test

The cold agglutinin test has long been used for diagnosis of *M. pneumoniae* infections because an increase in antibodies is found in 34-68% of *M. pneumoniae* infections.[98] The test is not specific for *M. pneumoniae,* however, a variety of other diseases will also produce a 4-fold rise.

Procedure. The cold agglutinin test of Schmidt et al.[107] is recommended.
1. Blood to be tested for cold agglutinins should be stored at room temperature before separation of the clot. Storage at 4 C will result in absorption of antibodies onto red cells, but warming to 37 C will release cold agglutinins.[107]
2. Twofold serial dilutions of serum are prepared in saline and dispensed in 0.1 ml volumes into test tubes.
3. A 0.1 ml volume of 1.0% human O erythrocytes is added to each tube.
4. Tubes are incubated at 4 C for 1 h.
5. Tests are read immediately upon removal from cold. Positive test will result in a shield pattern on bottom of tube that is difficult to disrupt by gentle shaking. Reversibility of agglutination is tested by incubation at 37 C for 15-30 min.
6. Highest dilution of antibody that agglutinates red cells and that is reversible at 37 C is termed the "end point" of the test.

Interpretation. A 4-fold or greater rise in cold agglutinins is suggestive of a recent *M. pneumoniae* infection. High titers (greater than 1:32) may indicate infection with *M. pneumoniae* but are frequently present in the absence of such infection.

C-REACTIVE PROTEIN

C-reactive protein (CRP) is an abnormal protein that appears in blood in the **acute stages of various inflammatory disorders but is undetectable in the blood of healthy persons.** The name of the protein is derived from the fact that it forms a precipitate with the non-type-specific somatic C polysaccharide of the pneumococcus. It is probably an α-globulin, consisting of at least 2 components, and its production is stimulated by bacterial infections, various pyrogenic agents (typhoid vaccine), or the products of injured tissue (as in myocardial infarction).

The C-reactive protein was isolated and purified by MacLeod and Avery in 1941.[108] By injecting the purified protein into rabbits, an antiserum is obtained (C-reactive protein antiserum, CRPA). This antiserum is used for the demonstration of C-reactive protein in human serum by the employment of a simple precipitation test.[109]

C-reactive protein is invariably present in the sera of patients with frank rheumatic activity as well as in the sera of patients with low-grade rheumatic activity. The presence of CRP in the serum of a rheumatic patient is an "extremely reliable and sensitive indicator of rheumatic activity." The test is not specific since CRP appears in blood as a response to other inflammatory conditions; however, in the case of questionable rheumatic fever with minimal or no clinical signs, the presence of CRP may be of diagnostic value. The absence of CRP rules out rheumatic activity.

In following the course of treatment in rheumatic fever, the disappearance of CRP from the patient's serum is a true reflection of lack of inflammatory activity as a result of therapy or spontaneous remission.

The advantages of the CRP test over the erythrocyte sedimentation rate are (1) the sedimentation rate may be elevated without inflammation, as in anemia, pregnancy, convalescent stage of infectious disease, nephrotic syndrome, and hyperglobulinemia, and (2) it may be normal in cases with frank rheumatic activity in the presence of congestive heart failure. In such cases, CRP, which is present **only** in inflammatory conditions, is a valuable adjunct or substitute for the sedimentation test.

In rheumatic patients treated with ACTH and cortisone, C-reactive protein reappears when the treatment is discontinued. This is due in most cases to the so-called "rebound phenomenon," which disappears within days. When CRP is present in such cases for a period longer than 2 weeks, treatment is renewed, since the persistence of CRP is considered evidence of the persistence of rheumatic activity.

In Sydenham's chorea the CRP test is negative, a positive test being indicative of associated carditis. In cases of coronary insufficiency **without myocardial necrosis,** the CRP test is negative. In cases of myocardial infarction the test is positive.

CRP is present in widespread malignancies and usually but not always (70-80%) in active rheumatoid arthritis, gout, various virus infections (especially infectious hepatitis), pneumococcal pneumonia, active tuberculosis, and the acute stage of cirrhosis of the liver. It was found in a large percentage of patients with the active lepromatous form of Hansen's disease and in a smaller percentage of patients with the clinically inactive lepromatous form of Hansen's disease. In the common contagious diseases the test if most often positive in acute tonsillitis, scarlet fever, varicella, and mumps.

At the present time the CRP test is accepted as a valuable aid in the diagnosis of low-grade, questionable rheumatic fever, in observation of the course of this disease during treatment, and in the differential diagnosis of coronary insufficiency, particularly as to the presence or absence of myocardial infarction and cessation of inflammation.

Excellent discussions and reviews of C-reactive protein were published by Hedlund[110] and Fischel.[111]

A number of technics have been devised for the detection of C-reactive protein in the serum. Of these, the most widely used are the capillary serum technic and the latex fixation slide test.

NOTE: Nakamura et al.[112] found that CRPA from different animal sources gave varying reactivity with the same acute phase serum samples. Also, different lots of CRPA from the same manufacturer and lots of serum from various manufacturers had wide variations in antibody content. They pointed out the need for standardization of CRP antisera.

Capillary tube serum technic[109]

Draw up the CRPA* to one-third of a 90 mm long, 0.4 mm ID capillary tube length. Place the finger over the tube. Wipe the tube clean.

Draw an equal amount of the patient's serum into capillary.

Invert the tube several times, slowly, to ensure proper mixture of CRPA and serum. Do not let an air pocket form between CRPA and serum.

Insert the capillary tube (upright) in the capllary tube rack, making sure that the bottom meniscus of the fluid column in the capillary tube is 5-10 mm above the clay. Wipe the capillary tube clean to facilitate subsequent reading.

Place the rack in an incubator at 37 C for 2 h. At the end of this time preliminary reading can be made to determine whether the reaction is positive or negative; presence of precipitate indicates a positive reaction.

Remove the rack from the incubator and place in a refrigerator at 4 C overnight. At the end of this time a final reading may be made as to the relative quantitative aspect of the reaction. It must be borne in mind that packing may not have occurred. In such cases when the precipitate is dispersed throughout the fluid column, the reading may be obtained from the summation of the total dispersal precipitate. Semiquantitative as well as definite equalitative readings are best made against a dark background, using oblique illumination.

The readings may be evaluated as follows:

No visible reaction	0
Definite but slight reaction (1 mm column of precipitate)	1+
Moderately strong (2 mm)	2+
Strong reaction (3 mm)	3+
Very strong reaction (4 mm)	4+

Fingertip technic[113]

A modification of this method, known as the fingertip method, has been worked out by Goldin and Kaplan; it can be used for children and debilitated adults.

Draw the blood into capillary tubes larger than those used for the CRP test, preferably blood-collecting tubes. Seal the tip of the tube with paraffin or in a flame. After the blood has clotted it may be centrifuged or allowed to stand overnight at room temperature. The inside diameter of these special tubes should be large enough to allow transfer of the serum directly to the capillaries in which the CRP test is being made. The

---

*C-reactive protein antiserum available from BBL, Division of BioQuest, Cockeysville, Md.; Difco Laboratories, Detroit; Hyland Laboratories, Los Angeles.

evaluation of the test is as in the technic described above.

Latex fixation technic

Singer et al.[114] reported results of a study with a latex fixation test for C-reactive protein and a comparison with the capillary precipitin tube method. The study was performed to develop a simple quantitative method for measuring C-reactive protein that would eliminate error often noted when visually reading the capillary tube test. Their first objective was to avoid such complicated serologic methods as complement fixation tests and gel diffusion methods. The authors were successful in coating or sensitizing polystyrene latex with antibody to C-reactive protein. They then studied the reaction of the sensitized latex particles and test sera in electrolytes of various ionic strengths with varying levels of pH. By these procedures they were able to demonstrate a sensitive and quantitative technic for detection of C-reactive protein.

In their studies it was noted that a prozone sometimes occurred in patients with excessive amounts of antigen. The 2 methods yielded well-correlated results.

The test, in a modified rapid slide test form, has gained wide acceptance, particularly with the availability of commercially prepared kits (Hyland Laboratories, Los Angeles) containing sensitized latex particles and the required glycine-saline diluent. The **original procedure of Singer et al.** follows.[114]

Polystyrene latex particles of uniform size (0.81 μm).* Add 20 ml distilled water to 2 ml suspension of latex and filter through Whatman no. 40 filter paper. When 0.1 ml is added to 10 ml 0.85% solution of sodium chloride, the diluted suspension should match a light transmittance of 5% in a spectrophotometer at 650 nm.

Procedure
1. Dilute test serum (2-fold dilutions with saline) 1:10 to 1:5120. Each tube should contain 0.5 ml diluted serum.
2. Mix 10 ml physiologic saline, 0.05-0.1 ml C-reactive protein antiserum, and 0.1 ml latex stock suspension.
3. Add 0.5 ml of mixture just described to each of the tubes of diluted serum and to control tube (0.5 ml saline).
4. Shake tubes thoroughly and incubate for 90 min at 56 C.
5. If the larger amount of antiserum was used (0.1 ml or more), centrifuge tubes at 2300 rpm for 3 min. Observe macroscopically the agglutination of the latex particles (grade from 0 to 4 plus). Agglutination in 1:20 or higher dilution is considered a positive test.
6. If less than 0.1 ml antiserum was used, refrigerate tubes for 18 h after incubation, centrifuge, and observe as above.

Rapid slide latex test

The use of a commercially available kit (CR test, Hyland Laboratories, Los Angeles) is recom-

mended for this test. The test is much more rapid and convenient than the tube test or the capillary test. It can be employed either as a screening test to detect the presence of C-reactive protein or as a quantitative test to determine its level in the patient's serum.

Accuracy with this method depends in part **on inactivation of the test serum for 30 minutes at 56 C.** Uninactivated sera frequently exhibit false-positive reactions.

Procedure
Qualitative procedure
1. Inactivate test serum at 56 C for 30 min.
2. Prepare a 1:5 dilution of serum under test by adding 0.1 ml serum to 0.4 ml glycine-saline buffer diluent.
3. Using one of the capillary pipets supplied, place a drop of **diluted** serum in 1 section of divided slide. Using same pipet, place a drop of **undiluted** serum in another section of slide. Same capillary pipet may be used for transferring both samples, provided it is used for diluted one first and then emptied as completely as possible before it is used for undiluted.
4. Add 1 drop of latex–anti-C-reactive protein reagent* to each section. With a wooden applicator or toothpick, mix each reaction mixture (diluted sample first) and spread over area approximately 20 × 25 mm.
5. Tilt slide slowly from side to side for 1-2 min and observe for macroscopic clumping.

INTERPRETATION. The test is an antigen-antibody reaction, which is most marked when the reactants are in optimal concentrations. Prozones may be encountered, in which case flocculation will be seen with diluted serum and a weak or negative reaction with undiluted serum. Visible flocculation in either or both sections indicates the presence of C-reactive protein. Serum devoid of this abnormal protein will give a smooth suspension with no visible flocculation in either section. Interpretation of results may be made as shown in Table 107-5.

Quantitative procedure
1. Prepare dilutions of serum in glycine-saline buffer diluent. Serum specimens are tested at dilutions of 1:2, 1:4, 1:8, 1:16, 1:32, 1:64. Occasionally, greater dilutions may be necessary.
2. Using a capillary pipet, transfer 1 drop of each serum dilution to successive sections of divided slide. Same capillary pipet may be used for a series of dilutions if transfer is started with highest dilution and continued toward lowest dilution.
3. Add 1 drop of latex–anti-C-reactive protein reagent to each drop of serum dilution. Using

---

*Latex particles precoated with anti-CRPA (serum hyperimmune to C-reactive protein).

---

*Dow Chemical Co., Midland, Mich.

Table 107-5*

Undiluted serum	Diluted serum	
0 to 2+	2+ to 4+	Strongly positive
3+ to 4+	0 to 2+	Positive
1+ to 2+	Negative	Weakly positive
Negative	Negative	Negative

*From CR Test, Hyland Laboratories, Los Angeles.

wooden applicator or toothpick and starting with highest serum dilution, mix each reaction mixture and spread it over an area approximately 20 × 25 mm.

4. Tilt slide slowly from side to side for 1-2 min and observe for macroscopic agglutination.

INTERPRETATION. The highest serum dilution showing visible flocculation is taken as the C-reactive protein titer of the specimen.

• • •

NOTE: The latex slide tests for CRP are more sensitive than the capillary precipitin tests.

REFERENCES

1. Hamburger, M.: Arch. Intern. Med. **124:**114, 1969.
2. Bokkenheuser, V., Suit, P., and Richardson, N.: Am. J. Public Health **54:**1507-1513, 1964.
3. Freter, R.: Agglutinin titration (Widal) for the diagnosis of enteric fever and other enterobacterial infections. In Rose, N. R., and Friedman, H., editors: Manual of clinical immunology, Washington, D.C., 1976, American Society for Microbiology; pp. 285-288.
4. Schroeder, S. A.: J.A.M.A. **206:**839-840, 1968.
5. Vogel, H., Cherubin, C. E., and Millian, S. J.: Am. J. Clin. Pathol. **53:**932-935, 1970.
6. Hechemy, K. E., Stevens, R. W., Sasowski, S., et al.: J. Clin. Microbiol. **9:**292, 1979.
7. Philip, R. N., Casper, E. A., Ormsbee, R. A., et al.: J. Clin. Microbiol. **3:**51-61, 1976.
8. Center for Disease Control: Morbidity and Mortality Weekly Report **28:**182, April 27, 1979.
9. Rose, N., and Friedman, M.: Manual of Clinical Immunology, Washington, D. C., 1976, American Society for Microbiology.
10. Palmer, D. F., Cavallaro, J. J., and Galt, R. H., editors: Laboratory diagnosis by serologic methods, Atlanta, 1975, Center for Disease Control.
11. Devillier, A. B., Deupree, R. H., Dickinson, C., and Beeler, M. F.: Am. J. Clin. Pathol. **44:**410, 1965.
11a. Felix, A., Krikorian, K. S., and Reitler, R.: J. Hyg. **35:**421, 1935.
12. Bokkenheuser, V., Smith, P., and Richardson, N.: Am. J. Public Health **54:**1507, 1964.
13. Staach, H. H., and Spaun, J.: Acta Pathol. Microbiol. Scand. **32:**420, 1953.
14. Landy, M., and Lamb, E.: Proc. Soc. Exp. Biol. Med. **82:**593, 1953.
15. Schubert, J. H., Edwards, P. R., and Ramsey, C. H.: J. Bacteriol. **77:**648, 1949.
16. Alton, G. G., and Jones, L. M.: Laboratory techniques in brucellosis, Geneva, 1967, World Health Organization, Monograph Series no. 55.
17. Kerr, W. R., McCaughey, W. J., Coghlan, J. D., et al.: J. Med. Microbiol. **1:**181, 1968.
18. Farrell, I. D., Robertson, L., and Hinchcliffe, P. M.: J. Hyg. (Camb.) **74:**23, 1975.
19. Stokes, E. J.: Clinical bacteriology, ed. 3, Baltimore, 1968, The Williams & Wilkins Co.
20. Joint FAP/WHO Expert Panel on Brucellosis, First, second, and third reports, FAO Agricultural Studies no. 14, 1951, no. 67, 1953, and no. 148, 1958.
21. Hall, W. H., and Manion, R. E.: J. Clin. Invest. **32:**96, 1953.
22. Schubert, J. H., and Calvin, J. F.: Health Lab. Sci. **1:**309, 1964.

23. Spink, W. W.: The nature of brucellosis, Minneapolis, 1956, University of Minnesota Press.
24. Castañeda, M. R.: Brucellosis, Mexico, D. F., 1954, La Prensa, Medica Mexicana.
25. Castañeda, M. R.: Bull. W.H.O. **24:**73, 1961.
26. Castañeda, M. R.: Bull. W.H.O. **9:**399, 1953.
27. Castañeda, M. R.: Proc. Soc. Exp. Biol. Med. **83:**36, 1953.
28. Wilson, M. M., and Merrifield, E. V. O.: Lancet **2:**913, 1951.
29. Kerr, W. R., Coghlan, J. D., Payne, D. J. H., and Robertson, L.: Lancet **2:**1181, 1966.
29a. Coghlan, J. D., and Weir, D. M.: Br. Med. J. **2:**269, 1967.
30. Babudieri, B.: Bull. W.H.O. **24:**45, 1961.
31. Galton, M. M., Menges, R. W., Shotts, E. B., et al.: Leptospirosis, P.H.S. Pub. no. 951, Atlanta, 1962, Center for Disease Control.
32. Sulzer, C. R., and Jones, W. L.: Leptospirosis. Methods in laboratory diagnosis (HEW Pub. no. CDC 79-8275), Atlanta, 1978, Center for Disease Control.
33. Joint FAO/WHO Expert Committee on Zoonoses: W.H.O. Tech. Rep. Ser. **378:**57, 1967.
34. Sulzer, C. R., and Jones, W. L.: Health Lab. Sci. **10:**13-17, 1973.
34a. Baker, L. A., and Cox, C. D.: Appl. Microbiol. **25:**697, 1973.
34b. Sulzer, C. R., and Jones, W. L.: Appl. Microbiol. **26:**655, 1973.
34c. Sulzer, C. R., Glosser, J. W., Rogers, F., et al.: J. Clin. Microbiol. **2:**218, 1975.
35. Galton, M. M., Sulzer, C. R., Santa Rosa, C. A., and Fields, M. J.: Appl. Microbiol. **13:**81-85, 1965.
36. Cole, J. K., Jr., Sulzer, C. R., and Pursell, A. R.: Appl. Microbiol. **25:**976-980, 1973.
37. Muraschi, T. F.: Proc. Soc. Exp. Biol. Med. **99:**235, 1968.
38. Klein, A. E., and Labzoffsky, N. A.: Can. J. Microbiol. **6:**463, 1960.
39. Galton, M. M., Powers, D. K., Hall, A. D., and Cornell, R. G.: Am. J. Vet. Res. **19:**505, 1958.
40. Cox, C. D.: Proc. Soc. Exp. Biol. Med. **90:**610, 1955.
41. Ellinghausen, H. C., Jr., and McCullough, W. G.: Am. J. Vet. Res. **26:**45-51, 1965.
42. Johnson, R., and Harris, V. G.: J. Bacteriol. **94:**27-31, 1967.
43. Roessler, W. G., and Brewer, C. R.: Appl. Microbiol. **15:**1114-1121, 1967.
44. Torten, M., Shenberg, E., and Van der Hoeden, J.: J. Infect. Dis. **116:**537, 1966.
45. Hirschberg, N., Galton, M. M., and Sulzer, C. R.: Health Lab. Sci. **5:**89, 1968.
46. Alexander, A. D., Huxsoll, D. D., Warner, A. R., et al.: Appl. Microbiol. **20:**825, 1970.
46a. Cravitz, L., and Miller, W. R.: J. Infect. Dis. **86:**46, 52, 1950.
47. Powell, H. M., and Jamieson, W. A.: J. Immunol. **43:**13, 1942.
48. Castañeda, M. R., Silva, R., and Monnier, A.: Rev. Med. Hosp. Gen. **2:**382, 1940.
49. Lautrop, H., and Lacey, B. W.: Bull. W.H.O. **23:**15, 1960.
50. McDade, J. E., Shepard, C. C., Fraser, D. W., et al.: N. Engl. J. Med. **297:**1189-1197, 1977.
51. Chandler, F. W., Hicklin, M. D., and Blackmon, J. A.: N. Engl. J. Med. **297:**1218-1220, 1977.
52. Cherry, W. B., Pittman, B., Harris, P. P., et al.: J. Clin. Microbiol. **8:**329, 1978.
53. Feeley, J. C., Gorman, G. W., Weaver, R. E., et al.: J. Clin. Microbiol. **8:**320-325, 1978.

54. Bennett, J. E., and Bailey, J. W.: Am. J. Clin. Pathol. **56:**360-365, 1971.
55. Bloomfield, N., Gordon, M. A., and Elmendorf, D. F.: Proc. Soc. Exp. Biol. Med. **114:**64-67, 1963.
56. Goodman, J. S., Kaufman, L., and Koenig, M. G.: N. Engl. J. Med. **285:**434-436, 1971.
57. Gordon, M. A., and Vedder, D. K.: J.A.M.A. **197:**961-967, 1966.
58. Kaufman, L., and Blumer, S.: Appl. Microbiol. **16:**1907-1912, 1968.
59. Bennett, D. E.: South. Med. J. **59:**922-926, 1966.
60. Busey, J. F., and Hinton, P. F.: Am. Rev. Respir. Dis. **92:**637-639, 1965.
61. Burnett, G. W., and Scherp, H. W.: Oral microbiology and infectious disease, Baltimore, 1962, The Williams & Wilkins Co.
62. Heiner, D. C.: Pediatrics **22:** 616-627, 1958.
63. Kaufman, L.: Public Health Rep. **81:**177-185, 1966.
64. Kaufman, L., Brandt, B., and McLaughlin, D.: Am. J. Hyg. **79:**181-185, 1964.
65. Schubert, J. H., Lynch, H. J., Jr., and Ajello, L.: Am. Rev. Respir. Dis. **84:**845-849, 1961.
66. Wiggins, G. L., and Schubert, J. H.: J. Bacteriol. **89:**589-596, 1965.
67. Pan American Health Organization: Manual of standardized serodiagnostic procedures for systemic mycosis. Part I. Agar immunodiffusion tests, 1972.
68. Mothershed, S. M., and Bullard, J. C.: Br. J. Vener. Dis. **44:**201-207, 1968.
69. Yobs, A. R., Brown, L., and Hunter, E. F.: Arch. Pathol. **77:**220-225, 1964.
70. Klein, G. C.: Immune response to streptococcal infection. In Rose, N. R., and Friedman, H., editors: Manual of clinical immunology, Washington, D.C., 1976, American Society for Microbiology, pp. 264-273.
71. Kaplan, E. J., Anthony, B. F., Chapman, S. S., et al.: J. Clin. Invest. **49:**1405-1414, 1970.
72. Klein, G. C., and Jones, W. L.: Appl. Microbiol. **21:**257-259, 1971.
73. Rantz, L. A., and Randall, E.: Proc. Soc. Exp. Biol. Med. **59:**22, 1945.
74. Jablon, J. M., Saul, M., and Saslaw, M. S.: Am. J. Clin. Pathol. **30:**83, 1958.
75. Klein, G. C., Moody, M. M., Baker, C. N., and Addison, B. V.: Appl. Microbiol. **16:**184, 1968.
76. Hallen, J.: Acta Pathol. Microbiol. Scand. **57:**301-306, 1963.
77. Klein, G. C., Baker, C. N., and Jones, W. L.: Appl. Microbiol. **21:**999-1001, 1971.
78. Lofgren, S.: Acta Pathol. Microbiol. Scand. **21:**768-774, 1944.
79. Spaun, J., Bentzon, M. W., Larsen, S. O., and Hewitt, L. F.: Bull. W.H.O. **24:**271-279, 1961.
80. Todd, E. W.: J. Exp. Med. **55:**267-280, 1932.
81. Bach, G. L., et al.: Am. J. Clin. Pathol. **39:**126-128, 1969.
82. Spaun, J. M., et al.: Bull. W.H.O./O.M.S. **24:**271-279, 1961.
83. Davidsohn, I., and Wells, B. B., editors: Todd-Sanford clinical diagnosis by laboratory methods, Philadelphia, 1966, W. B. Saunders Co., p. 896.

84. Klein, G. C., and Jones, W. L.: Appl. Microbiol. **21:**257, 1971.
85. Bisno, A. L., and Ofek, I.: Am. J. Dis. Child. **127:**676, 1974.
86. Janeff, J., Janeff, D., Taranta, A., and Cohen, H.: Lab. Med. **2:**32, 1971.
87. Collins, O. D., III: Am. J. Clin. Pathol. **57:**598, 1972.
88. Dodge, W. F., Spargo, B. H., Travis, L. B., et al.: N. Engl. J. Med. **286:**273, 1972.
89. Ofek, I., Kaplan, O., Bergner-Rabinowitz, S., et al.: Clin. Pediatr. (Phila.) **12:**341, 1973.
90. Todd, E. W.: J. Exp. Med. **55:**267, 1932.
91. Golubjatnikov, R., Koehler, R., and Buccowich, J.: Health Lab. Sci. **14:**284, 1977.
92. Quinn, R., and Liao, S.: J. Clin. Invest. **29:** 1156, 1950.
93. Ayoub, E. M., and Wannamaker, L. W.: Pediatrics **29:**527, 1952.
94. Nelson, J., Ayoub, E. M., and Wannamaker, L. W.: J. Lab. Clin. Med. **71:**867, 1968.
95. Kenny, G. E. In Sela, M., editor: The antigens, vol. 3, New York, 1975, Academic Press.
96. Senterfit, L. B., Pollack, J. D., and Somerson, N. L.: Proc. Soc. Exp. Biol. Med. **140:**1294, 1972.
97. Kenny, G. E., and Grayston, J. T.: J. Immunol. **95:**19, 1965.
98. Grayston, J. T., Foy, H. M., and Kenny, G. E. In Hayflick, L., editor: The mycoplasmatales and L-phase of bacteria, New York, 1969, Appleton-Century-Crofts.
99. Kenny, G. E.: Infect. Immun. **4:**149, 1971.
100. Kenny, G. E., and Newton, R. M.: Ann. N.Y. Acad. Sci. **225:**54, 1973.
101. Taylor-Robinson, D., Purcell, R. H., Wong, D. C., and Chanock, R. M.: J. Hyg. (Camb.) **64:**91, 1966.
102. Purcell, R. H., Taylor-Robinson, D., Wong, D. C., and Chanock, R. M.: Am. J. Epidemiol. **84:**51, 1966.
103. Purcell, R. H., Taylor-Robinson, D., Wong, D. C., and Chanock, R. M.: J. Bacteriol. **92:**6, 1966.
104. Niitu, Y., Hasegawa, S., and Kubota, H.: Antimicrob. Agents Chemother. **5:**111, 1974.
105. Hollingdale, M. R., and Lemcke, R. M.: J. Hyg. **68:**469, 1970.
106. Shepard, M. C., Lunceford, C. D., Ford, D. K., et al.: Int. J. Sys. Bacteriol. **24:**160, 1974.
107. Schmidt, N. J., Lenette, E. H., Dennis, J., and Gee, P. S.: J. Immunol. **97:**95, 1966.
108. MacLeod, C. M., and Avery, O. T.: J. Exp. Med. **73:**183, 1941.
109. Anderson, H. C., and McCarty, M.: Am. J. Med. **8:**45, 1950.
110. Hedlund, P.: Acta Med. Scand. **169**(suppl. 361):1, 1961.
111. Fischel, E. E. In Cohen, A. S., editor: Laboratory diagnostic procedures in the rheumatic diseases, Boston, 1967, Little, Brown & Co.
112. Nakamura, R. M., Magsaysay, R., Ford, J., and Kunitake, G. M.: Am. J. Clin. Pathol. **44:**290, 1965.
113. Goldin, M., and Kaplan, M. A.: Am. J. Clin. Pathol. **25:**1432, 1965.
114. Singer, J. M., Plotz, C. M., Pader, E., and Elster, S. K.: Am. J. Clin. Pathol. **28:**611, 1957.

108

BACTERIAL HEMAGGLUTINATION TESTS

Erwin Neter

A variety of microorganisms, including bacteria, viruses, rickettsiae, and fungi, cause agglutination of red blood cells. Two principal different types of hemagglutination reactions have been observed. In the first type, bacteria or viruses agglutinate erythrocytes in the absence of antibodies or other biologic factors. This type of reaction has been referred to as **direct** microbial hemagglutination. Best known is the agglutination of erythrocytes by certain groups of viruses, but the reaction is not restricted to this group of microorganisms and occurs with bacteria as well. The second type of microbial hemagglutination is based on a different mechanism. In the first phase of this reaction, microbial antigens become attached to red blood cells, either naturally or artificially, and thus bring about the acquisition of new serologic specificities of the erythrocytes. On the addition of homologous microbial antibodies, hemagglutination ensues, and with certain erythrocytes hemolysis takes place in the presence of hemolytic complement. This type of microbial hemagglutination reaction has been referred to as **indirect, conditioned,** and **passive** hemagglutination. Antigens that do not become attached spontaneously to red blood cells may be combined with erythrocytes experimentally by means of tannic acid, chemical linkages, or nonagglutinating antibodies. It is noteworthy that direct viral hemagglutination has been studied much more intensively than direct bacterial hemagglutination, whereas the reverse is true with regard to indirect microbial hemagglutination reactions. The subject of bacterial hemagglutination and hemolysis has been extensively reviewed.[1,2] Only the more important bacterial hemagglutination tests are described in this chapter. These procedures presently are useful in research and, in certain cases, in the clinical laboratory.

DIRECT BACTERIAL HEMAGGLUTINATION

It has been known for many years that certain bacteria cause agglutination of red blood cells.

Since antibodies are not involved in the reaction, the term "direct bacterial hemagglutination" has been suggested for this reaction. It has been demonstrated that special structures on the surface of bacteria, referred to as fimbriae, are responsible for this reaction. Fimbriae are distinctly different from flagella and may be present even in nonmotile strains. However, it remains to be determined whether all hemagglutinating bacteria possess fimbriae. Hemagglutination has been demonstrated with a variety of bacterial species, notably staphylococci, certain Enterobacteriaceae, and *Haemophilus aegyptius*. Bacteria may be grown in fluid or on solid culture media to obtain material for this reaction. Obviously a suitable medium for the particular species to be tested has to be employed. Attention should be called to the fact that various strains and species of bacteria do not agglutinate red blood cells from all animal species or even individuals. The direct bacterial hemagglutination test may be carried out in test tubes as well as on slides. The slide test and test tube methods have yielded satisfactory results.

Slide test[3]

Procedure. Red blood cells are separated by centrifugation from citrated blood (from guinea pig or other suitable animals), washed twice in 0.85% NaCl solution, and made up to a 3% suspension in saline.

Tests are made in depressions on a white porcelain tile. A drop of red blood cell suspension is mixed with a drop of broth culture, centrifuged broth culture deposit, or surface growth from agar, and tile rocked to and fro at room temperature for at least 5 min.

Results. Hemagglutination reaction is designated ++++ when coarse clumping commences within a few seconds, +++ when moderate clumping commences within 1-2 min, ++ when fine clumping appears only after 1 min, and + when very fine granules appear after 3-5 min. Full fimbriation is indicated when a drop of uniformly mixed, uncentrifuged broth culture gives a ++ or +++ reaction. Nonfimbriate cultures give no reaction, even when a large loopful of solid growth material from agar is mixed with red blood cells.

Test tube method[4]

Procedure. Red blood cell suspension is prepare from citrated whole blood by washing cells 3 times and suspending them in physiological saline solution. Cells may be stored as a 10% suspension at 4 C for short periods.

Test is performed by adding equal quantities (0.2 or 0.5 ml) of an 0.5% suspension of red blood cells to a broth culture or saline suspension of organisms in a 12 × 75 mm test tube.

Tubes are shaken vigorously by hand for a few minutes and allowed to stand at room temperature.

Results. Usually gross clumping occurs immediately and can be readily observed in an oblique light beam. If reaction is less marked, agglutination is detected after standing, by pattern of red blood cells on bottom of tube. Agglutinated cells form a thin uniform blanket covering entire bottom, whereas unagglutinated cells form a small compact disk.

At the present time the direct bacterial hemagglutination test remains largely a tool for research. The test appears to be useful for the differentiation of *H. aegyptius* from related species, notably *H. influenzae*. The role of fimbriae in pathogenicity has not yet been elucidated. It is noteworthy that direct bacterial hemagglutination may be inhibited by specific bacterial antibodies.

INDIRECT, CONDITIONED, OR PASSIVE BACTERIAL HEMAGGLUTINATION

Numerous bacterial antigens, polysaccharide in nature, become readily attached to red blood cells. The erythrocytes thus acquire new serologic specificities. As a result, these modified (sensitized) erythrocytes are agglutinated on the addition of homologous bacterial antibodies. This hemagglutination reaction takes place with red blood cells from a variety of warm-blooded animal species. Modified sheep red blood cells are lysed in the presence of homologous bacterial antibodies and guinea pig complement. It is noteworthy that several antigens may be fixed simultaneously to the surface of erythrocytes. This indirect, conditioned, or passive hemagglutination test has been used for the determination and titration of either bacterial antibodies or bacterial antigens.

It should be emphasized that 19S (IgM) antibodies agglutinate these antigenically modified erythrocytes significantly better than 7S (IgG) antibodies.

Sera to be tested by these procedures must not agglutinate or lyse nonmodified erythrocytes; if heterologous red blood cells are used, the erythrocyte antibodies must be removed by preceding absorption unless the dilutions of the serum are sufficiently high to avoid their interference with the test. Best known among bacterial hemagglutination tests is the application of this procedure for the detection of tuberculopolysaccharide antibodies, the so-called Middlebrook-Dubos test.[5] For a listing of microorganisms used in such tests see Neter.[1] More recently the method has been utilized for the detection of *Pasteurella pseudotuberculosis*, leptospiral, and certain teichoic acid antibodies.[6-8]

With certain bacteria such as Enterobacteriaceae the test may be carried out as follows:[9]

Bacteria are grown on nutrient agar, in infusion broth, or in other suitable media, depending on the nutritional requirements of the species. For enteric microorganisms brain veal agar in Kolle flasks has been employed. The resulting growth is suspended in 25 ml physiological saline solution or Difco hemagglutination buffer (pH 7.3). To effect release of antigen the bacterial suspension is heated in boiling water for 1 hour. The supernatant fluid obtained after centrifugation (preferably high-speed centrifugation) is used for modification of red blood cells. A suitable dilution of this antigen has to be determined. For the supernate of enteric bacteria a dilution of 1:10 has been found satisfactory. Purified antigens such as the lipopolysaccharides of certain gram-negative bacilli have also been used; approximately 10 µg/ml for a 2.5% erythrocytes suspension has yielded satisfactory results. Certain enterobacterial lipopolysaccharides are available commercially (Difco Laboratories, Detroit).

When red blood cells homologous to the serum to be tested are used, interference from "normal" erythrocyte antibodies is usually not encountered, and absorption of such antibodies is not necessary. Blood from group O, Rh-negative donors is suitable in tests with human sera. When heterologous erythrocytes are employed, serum and complement in the dilutions used must be free of red blood cell antibodies. With high-titered sera it is usually not necessary to carry out absorption of these antibodies prior to the test, since the antiserum has a markedly higher titer of bacerial than of eythrocyte antibodies. Alternately, it is necessary to absorb serum with nonmodified red blood cells prior to performing the bacterial hemagglutination and hemolysis tests. Appropriate controls with nonmodified red blood cells and known antisera must always be included in the tests.

Formalin-treated erythrocytes, which can be stored, are also suitable as carriers of certain bacterial antigens for the hemagglutination test.[10] Recently titration of bacterial antibodies by means of hemagglutinating Autoanalyzer was described.[11]

Bacterial hemagglutination test[10]

Procedure. Whole blood (from humans or various warm-blooded animals) in a dilution of 1:20 (equal to a 2.5% erythrocyte suspension) is washed 3 times to remove plasma, which may interfere with antigen modification. To sediment of this suspension is added antigen in a volume sufficient to make again a 2.5% red blood cell suspension.

Mixture is then incubated at 37 C for 30 min and washed 3 times with either of above-mentioned diluents to remove excess antigen. This modified (sensitized) red blood cell suspension is then ready for use.

Serial dilutions of serum to be studied (vol 0.2 ml) are mixed with an equal amount of modified erythrocytes.

Mixtures are incubated in a water bath at 37 C for 30 min. Agglutination may be read at this stage, but centrifugation is recommended at 1000 rpm for 1-2 min because it markedly enhances agglutination reaction. Agglutination is observed grossly. Marked agglutination results in formation of 1 single clump of red blood cells or a few large clumps. Control suspensions are not agglutinated. Grades of agglutination may be gauged from 0 to 4+. For example:

1. Wash 0.5 ml whole blood with 19.5 ml saline solution or buffer.
2. Repeat washing twice.
3. To sediment add 20 ml 1:10 diluted antigen.
4. Incubate in water bath at 37 C for 30 min.
5. Wash 3 times with 20 ml diluent as above.
6. Prepare serial dilutions of test serum (0.2 ml) from 1:10 to 1:2560; use 0.2 ml diluent in an additional test tube for control purposes.
7. Add modified erythrocytes (0.2 ml) to all test tubes.
8. For control purposes add nonmodified, washed red blood cells from identical source to serum in serial diultions as above.
9. Incubate in water bath at 37 C for 30 min.
10. Centrifuge all test tubes at 1000 rpm for 1-2 min.
11. Read and record resulting agglutination.

Bacterial microtiter hemagglutination test[12]

This technic has been employed by several investigators for the titration of antibodies against certain Enterobacteriaceae. The method has the advantages of economy and simplicity. (For a general discussion of the microtitration technic and equipment see Chapter 105.)

Procedure. Plastic disposable plates containing 96 wells with conical bottoms are used. (Cooke Engineering Co., Alexandria, Va.; Linbro Manufacturing Co., New Haven, Conn.) An antigen control of sensitized red cells and known positive serum, a serum control of serum and unsensitized cells, and a cell control of sensitized cells and phosphate-buffered saline (PBS) should be included in each test.

With a calibrated pipet, 0.025 ml PBS is delivered to each well. Same pipet is used to perform all tests to minimize errors introduced by differences in drop size.

Calibrated loop is used to deliver 0.025 ml serum specimen to first well and to make serial 2-fold dilutions.

Calibrated pipet is used to add 0.025 ml sensitized red cell suspension to each well.

Plates are sealed tightly with tape and agitated gently to ensure thorough mixing. Rapid performance of entire procedure is necessary because evaporation will seriously affect results.

Plates are left undisturbed at room temperature for 16 h before hemagglutination patterns in bottoms of wells are read with aid of a reflecting mirror and an overhead high-intensity light.

Degrees of hemagglutination are recorded as follows:

4+ = A homogeneous scatter of clumped red cells without a central button of cells. Occasionally a 4+ reaction is formed as a tight, irregular button that can be distinguished from a negative reaction by tilting the plate. A 4+ button slides as an intact unit, whereas a negative button runs like a teardrop.

3+ = A small button in midst of a homogeneous scatter of clumped cells.

2+ = A more well-developed button than 3+ with less peripheral scattering of clumped cells.

1+ = A button with minimal circumferential scatter.

0 = No hemagglutination. A smooth button surrounded by a clear supernatant.

Endpoint is highest dilution showing definite hemagglutination, i.e., 2+ or greater.

Various authors utilized effectively the Microtiter test with some modifications.[13-17]

Hemolytic modification of bacterial hemagglutination test

This test is carried out as described under Bacterial Hemagglutination Test, with the following 3 exceptions:

Procedure. Add guinea pig complement (0.1 ml) in a suitable dilution to all test tubes immediately after or before addition of serum under study and modified red blood cells. A dilution of 1:20 of freshly prepared guinea pig serum or lyophilized complement has proved to be satisfactory.

Incubate in water bath at 37 C for 1 h.

Read hemolysis after incubation for 30 min and 1 h. Suitable controls, including nonmodified erythrocytes and a known antiserum, must be used.

Recently this procedure has been used for the titration of gonococcal antibodies in human sera.[18]

Polyvalent bacterial hemagglutination test

It is possible to prepare a polyvalent red blood cell suspension by treating red blood cells with a mixture of different bacterial antigens, each in a suitable dilution. Such an erythrocyte suspension is agglutinated by antibodies against any one of the corresponding antigens. This test may be useful for screening sera for antibodies against one or another bacterial antigen.

Enzyme bacterial hemagglutination test

It has been shown that treatment of red blood cells with certain proteoltic enzymes, either before or after antigen modification, may increase the sensitivity of the test. As a result, the titers of serum and particularly of human γ-globulin are higher than those obtained with the hemagglutination test itself.[19] The following enzymes were found to be effect when used in amounts of approximately 500-1000 μg/ml: trypsin, chymotrypsin, pancreatic protease, and, to a lesser degree, ficin and papain. It is conceivable that the method may detect "incomplete" Rh antibodies in a way similar to the detection of "incomplete" Rh antibodies with enzyme-treated Rh-positive erythrocytes.

Procedure. Red blood cells are washed and treated with bacterial antigen as described in discussion on Bacterial hemagglutination test. Cells are then washed 3 times, and to sediment is added 1 of above enzymes (500-1000 μg/ml) in amounts sufficient to make again a 2.5% erythrocyte suspension.

Cells are incubated in a water bath at 37 C for 30 min, washed 3 times, and then added to serum or γ-globulin in serial dilutions as previously described under bacterial hemagglutination test.

Resulting agglutination is read after centrifugation at 1000 rpm for 1-2 min.

Coombs' bacterial hemagglutination test

Human erythrocytes modified by bacterial antigen as previously described under bacterial hemagglutination test and tested with certain human sera, notably cord serum, and with human γ-globulin may be agglutinated upon the addition of human γ-globulin antiserum (Coombs' serum),[20] when the hemagglutination test itself yields negative results. The procedure is the same as that described for the bacterial hemagglutination test.

After completion of the test the mixtures of modified red blood cells and cord serum are washed 3 times, and 0.1 ml suspension is mixed with an equal amount of commercial Coombs' serum. Agglutination may occur after short incubation with or without centrifugation, depending on the particular Coombs' serum used.

This procedure has made possible the demonstration of bacterial antibodies in cord serum and human γ-globulin titers exceeding those obtained by means of hemagglutination and conventional agglutination tests.

Tuberculopolysaccharide hemagglutination and hemolysis tests

The hemagglutination test first described by Middlebrook and Dubos[5] has been employed for the detection and titration of antibodies to a polysaccharide fraction of the tubercle bacillus.

In brief, red blood cells are modified with old tuberculin or a purified fraction thereof and then tested with serum in serial dilutions. The resulting hemagglutination is read and recorded. A hemolytic modification of the test using tuberculopolysaccharide has been described by Middlebrook.[21]* These tests may be carried out as described in the following discussions.

Tuberculopolysaccharide hemagglutination test with homologous erythrocytes. Red blood cells are washed 3 times with several volumes of phosphate-buffered saline (PBS) solution (0.01M dibasic sodium phosphate solution containing 0.8% sodium chloride and adjusted to pH 7.0 with 1N HCl). One aliquot of 0.05 ml of these Packed, washed red cells is added to 2.4 ml 1:12 dilution of a special "tuberculin" Lederle Laboratories, Pearl River, N.Y.) preparation in PBS. This mixture is incubated at 37 C for 2 h and agitated every 15 min. It is then centrifuged; supernatant fluid is discarded, and sedimented red cells are washed 3 times by resuspending in several volumes of PBS and centrifuging. Finally, washed, sensitized red blood cells are resuspended in 10 ml PBS; this constitutes 0.5% suspension of modified red cells.

Twofold serial dilutions of serum to be tested are prepared in above-mentioned diluent. For control purposes diluent alone is used in an additional test tube. To each tube is added an aqual volume of 0.5% suspension of modified red blood cells.

All tubes are incubated at 37 C for 2 h; after complete settling of red blood cells occurs, rack of tubes is shaken vigorously and allowed to stand undisturbed at room temperature overnight.

The results are read and recorded in terms of hemagglutination.

Tuberculopolysaccharide hemagglutination test with sheep red blood cells. Sheep blood is collected aseptically in 1.2 vol sterile, modified Alsever solution:

Glucose	2.05 g
Sodium citrate	0.8 g
Sodium chloride	0.42 g
Distilled water	100 ml

The pH is adjusted to 6.1 with 10% citric acid solution. It is autoclaved at 10 psi for 15 min.

Alsever–sheep's blood mixture is stored at 4 C; it is not used until at least 3 d after collection. If kept sterile, the mixture remains suitable as a source of sheep red blood cells for at least 3 mo.

An appropriate amount of this mixture is washed 3 times with at least 5 vol PBS.

A special tuberculin (Lederle Laboratories) preparation is diluted with 11 vol PBS. To 48 vol of this diluted antigen, 1 vol packed, washed sheep red cells is added. The mixture is incubated at 37 C and agitated every 15 min for 2 h to ensure uniform modification of cells. This mixture is centrifuged; sedimented red blood cells are washed 3 times in large volumes of PBS. Finally, washed, modified (sensitized) cells are resuspended in 200 vol PBS. This 0.5% erythrocyte suspension is ready for use or may be stored at 4 C for up to 3 d unless hemolysis occurs.

To 4 ml 1:4 dilution of inactivated serum to be tested is added 0.2 ml packed, washed, untreated sheep cells. After thorough agitation suspension is kept at room temperature for 10 min and then centrifuged at high speed (2000-2500 rpm) for 10 min; without removal of supernatant fluid another 0.2 ml packed, washed, untreated sheep cells is added and mixed with supernatant fluid with as little disturbance of first 0.2 ml packed red cells as possible. This suspension is allowed to stand at room temperature for 10 min and centrifuged at high speed as before. Supernatant fluid is removed and represents a 1:4 dilution of absorbed test serum.

Twofold serial dilutions (vol 0.5 ml) of absorbed test serum are made in PBS, from 1:4-1:128 or higher. Added to each tube is an equal volume of 0.5% suspension of modified sheep cells. Two control tubes are included in test: (1) 0.5 ml 1:4 dilution absorbed test serum and 0.5 ml unmodified sheep erythrocyte control suspension and (2) 0.5 ml PBS and 0.5 ml modified sheep red blood cells. A known positive serum in serial dilution and should be included as a positive control.

All tubes are incubated at 37 C for 2 h; after complete settling of red blood cells has occurred, rack of tubes is shaken vigorously and allowed to stand undisturbed overnight at room temperature.

Results are recorded in terms of agglutination.

Hemolytic modification of the tuberculopolysaccharide hemagglutination test. This test is carried out with sheep erythrocytes as previously described, except that to each tube is added an excess of absorbed complement prepared as follows.

One vol packed, washed, unsensitized sheep cells (from same batch as used in hemagglutination test is mixed with 15 vol 1:3 dilution pooled, fresh guinea pig serum in PBS. Mixture is allowed to stand at about 4 C for 10 min; it is then centrifuged at high speed (2000-3000 rpm) for 10 min. Without removal of supernatant fluid another equal volume of packed, washed, unsensitized sheep cells is added and suspended in

---

*Editor's note:** The tuberculopolysaccharide test and its modifications were used in attempts to develop a diagnostic test for tuberculosis. However, the tests are not considered sufficiently reliable or valid for that purpose.

supernatant fluid with as little disturbance as possible of sedimented first aliquot of packed sheep cells. This suspension is allowed to stand another 10 min at 4 C and then centrifuged at high speed. Supernatant fluid thus obtained is used as absorbed complement. Little or no hemolysis should occur during absorption. Absorbed complement should be used immediately after it is prepared or stored at refrigerator temperature and used within 3-4 h.

To each tube of serum (0.5 ml), modified sheep erythrocytes (0.5 ml), and appropriate controls a 1/20 vol (0.05 ml) absorbed complement is added.

Tubes are incubated at 37 C for 1 h; each rack is shaken vigorously at 15-20 min intervals. Test is read for hemolysis after allowing red blood cells to settle at room temperature onto bottom of tubes.

Presence of hemolysis indicates that antibody is present in test serum for component(s) of tubercle bacillus that has been absorbed onto red blood cells, provided that appropriate controls are negative. As in other tests, an antibody containing serum should be included as a positive control.

Applications

The indirect bacterial hemagglutination test has been applied to the study of antibodies against various bacteria and also to the antigenic analysis of certain microorganisms. Comparative studies of conventional agglutination and indirect hemagglutination methods have revealed that generally speaking, the latter procedure is somewhat more sensitive than the former for the titration of antibodies against enteric pathogens such as enteropathogenic *Escherichia coli*, shigellae, and salmonellae as well as against other bacteria such as *Pseudomonas aeruginosa*, *Pasteurella tularensis*, and other microorganisms, including opportunistic pathogens.[10,22-33] Furthermore, in some instances antibodies and the increase in the titers of antibodies during early stages of infection are demonstrated only by the hemagglutination method. Another advantage of the hemagglutination procedure is the fact that red blood cells can be modified with several antigens (see discussion on Polyvalent Hemagglutination Test), making multiple monovalent agglutination tests unnecessary. This procedure appears to be applicable particularly to the screening of serum specimens.[34] It appears, then, that with standardized antigens and methods the hemagglutination tests may find practical applications in the future. Irrespective of the procedure chosen, the detection of the antibody response of patients with certain infections can be of value to the clinician. For example, when 2 or more pathogens are isolated from the feces of a patient with diarrheal disease, determination of the antibody response may supply information as to the presence of single or dual infection. This approach also aids in the recognition of mild and subclinical infection.[26-29] The study of the immune response of patients with urinary tract and opportunistic infections has been utilized also for clarification of etiologic and pathogenetic problems.[35-37]

The hemagglutination procedure, with the use of known antisera, also lends itself to the study of antigens in various bacteria. For example, a widely distributed hetrerogenetic bacterial antigen has been detected by means of this method.[38] It may be mentioned, too, that this method may be useful for antigenic analysis of autoagglutinated bacteria, which are unsuitable for agglutination reactions.

TANNIC ACID HEMAGGLUTINATION TESTS

Protein antigens, which do not spontaneously modify untreated erythrocytes, become attached to tannic acid–treated red blood cells. Homologous protein antibodies will then cause hemagglutination. This test, first introduced by Boyden,[39] has been used extensively for the determination and titration of antibodies against **bacterial and nonbacterial proteins.** Recently, Chen and Meyer[40] utilized the procedure for the confirmation of plague infections.

In principle, suitable red blood cells are treated first with tannic acid and then with the antigen under investigation. These protein-modified erythrocytes are then added to serum in serial dilutions, and the resulting hemagglutination is read after standing according to the pattern of sedimentation of the red blood cells.

The procedure has been adapted as a micromethod, for example, by Sanborn and Vedros.[41] The tanned cell hemagglutination test has been used successfully for the demonstration of chlamydial antibodies, among others.[42]

NOTE: Antigens may be attached to the surface of erythrocytes also by **coupling with bisdiazotized benzidine (BDB)**[43,44] or **chromium chloride.**[45-49] These procedures have been used for the titration of antibodies against flagellar antigens from *Salmonella*, acidic capsular polysaccharides from *Klebsiella*, teichoic acid from *Staphylococcus*, polysaccharides from *Streptococcus pneumoniae*, and *Mycoplasma* antigens, among others. Conversely, antigens may be quantitated by hemagglutination-inhibition. See following discussion for procedure in Tannic Acid Hemmagglutination Test.[50]

Tannic acid hemagglutination test

Blood cells. Either sterile, defibrinated sheep blood or sheep blood diluted with Alsever solution is employed. Blood in Alsever solution often can be used satisfactorily for 3-6 wk if collected aseptically and kept at 5 C. Human, rabbit, and rat red blood cells have been used successfully and advantageously, since their use may eliminate necessity to absorbe "normal" erythrocyte antibodies of sera under study.

Standardization of erythrocytes. Because concentration of erythrocytes affects endpoint of hemagglutination titration, standardization of cell concentration is necessary. Cells are washed 3 times with saline. If hemolysis occurs, cells should be discarded, since they usually are too fragile for later treatment. One ml packed cells (or some multiple thereof) is then diluted with about 40 ml (or some multiple thereof) buffered saline of pH 7.2, so that 1 ml of this diluted cell suspension plus 5 ml distilled water give a scale reading of 400 in Klett-Summerson colorimeter. These cells can often be kept at 5 C for 2-3 d without extensive hemolysis but are usually used within 18-24 h. Erythrocytes may also be standardized in Beckman spectrophotometer.

Tannic acid. Merck or Mallinkrodt reagent grade tannic acid is recommended. A 1:100 dilution in saline is kept at 5 C as a stock solution, from which 1-20,000 dilution is made daily.

Buffered saline solutions, pH 6.4 and 7.2. These solutions are made by mixing 100 ml of respective 0.15M buffer.

Preparation of tannic acid–treated erythrocytes. One ml standardized cells plus 1 ml 1:20,000 tannic acid are incubated in a water bath at 3 C for 10 min. Cells are then centrifuged gently and washed with 1 ml buffered saline, pH 7.2, and resuspended gently in 1 ml saline. These tannic acid cells can be kept at 5 C for up to 18 h before use. Concentration of tannic acid required to alter cell surface for protein modification (sensitization) apparently varies with different antigens. Thus various authors employ 1:20,000, 1:30,000, or 1:40,000 tannic acid for various purposes. It is therefore advisable when employing this method for first time with a particular antigen to test various concentrations of tannic acid for their ability to yield stable, nonhemolyzed, and optimally modified suspensions for agglutination by specific antisera.

Sensitization of tannic acid–treated cells with protein. Four ml buffered saline, pH 6.4, plus 1 ml protein under study in suitable dilution in saline plus 1 ml tannic acid–treated cells are mixed in that order and kept at room temperature for 10 min. The cells are then centrifuged, washed once with 2 ml 1:100 normal rabbit serum, and resuspended gently in 1 ml 1:100 normal rabbit serum.

Diluents. Sera usually are diluted in 1:100 normal rabbit serum, as recommended by Boyden. It is found, however, that 0.2% solutions in saline of gelatin, bovine γ-globulin, bovine serum albumin, and rabbit γ-globulin often can be employed for stabilization. If serum or γ-globulin is employed, these materials are inactivated at 56 C for 30 min. They are then absorbed for 10 min at room temperature with an equal volume of washed, packed, untreated sheep erythrocytes to remove "normal" red cell antibodies. This absorption can be omitted if preliminary tests reveal that 1:100 serum or diluted globulin solutions do not agglutinate protein-conjugated erythrocytes.

Performance of test. Serial dilutions of serum under investigation (e.g., 1:10-1:2560 or higher) in vol 0.5 ml are prepared in 10 × 100 or 18 × 100 mm test tubes. Tannic acid–treated, protein-conjugated erythrocytes (vol 0.05 ml) are added to each tube. Tubes are carefully shaken so as to disperse cells homogeneously. Suitable controls, including serum diluent and unmodified erythrocytes, are also used.

Reading of test. Usually hemagglutination reaction is read after tubes have stood at room temperature for 3-12 h. However, reaction can be accelerated by centrifugation in 8 place head of an International no. 2 centrifuge at 400 rpm for 2 min.

With experience it is found that reaction is most sensitive and can be read and graded best according to pattern formed by agglutinated cells on bottom of tubes. Various grades are as follows:

++++ Compact, granular agglutinate
+++ Smooth mat on bottom of tube with folded edges
++ Smooth mat, edges somewhat ragged
+ Narrow ring of red around edge of smooth mat

± or − Smaller area of tube covered than +, heavier ring around edge, to discrete button in center of tube

This method has been used as a satisfactory, sensitive, and specific procedure for the titration of diphtheria and tetanus antitoxins and antibodies against a variety of bacterial proteins. For a list of bacterial antigens see Neter.[1] The procedure has also proved particularly useful for studies of antibodies against many protein antigens of nonbacterial origin, e.g., for the detection and titration of thyroid autoantibodies.[51]

Tannic acid hemagglutination test with formalin-preserved erythrocytes

It has been shown by Fulthorpe[52] and others that protein-modified tannic acid–treated red blood cells can be preserved for several months by formalin treatment.

Procedure. Sheep red blood cells are treated with tannic acid and modified by protein antigen as described above. After final washing, sensitized cells are resuspended in a minimum vol 0.85% saline and poured into a solution of isotonic 0.05M sodium borate–succinic acid buffer saline, pH 7.5, containing 1% normal horse serum and 20% formalin. This mixture is left in contact with cells for 3 d, with frequent shaking to break up cell clumps. Supernatant fluid is withdrawn and replaced with 1% normal horse serum saline every 2 d for 1 wk; thereafter concentration of free formalin is negligible. Such cells remain apparently unchanged and with a constant sensitivity for up to 4 mo.

This procedure has been used recently with antigen from pathogenic *T. pallidum* (Nichols strain) for the serodiagnosis of syphilis.[53-56]

The method has been modified by the use of erythrocytes stabilized with pyruvic aldehyde, treated with tannic acid, and fixed with glutaraldehyde for the demonstration of antibodies to *Plasmodium* antigen.[57]

Finally, attention is called to the fact that certain bacterial antigens, notably the protein A antigen from *Staphylococcus aureus*, interact with immunoglobulins by a nonspecific mechanism, namely, by combining with the Fc fragment. As a result, erythrocytes sensitized with antibodies are agglutinated by this antigen.[58] More recently it has been shown that certain streptococci, including those of groups A, B, and C, also agglutinate antibody-sensitized erythrocytes.[59]

REFERENCES

1. Neter, E.: Bacteriol. Rev. **20**-166, 1956.
2. Neter, E.: Pathol. Microbiol. **28**:859, 1965.
3. Gillies, R. R., and Duguid, J. P.: J. Hyg. **56**:20, 1958.
4. Davis, D. J., Pittman, M., and Griffitts, J. J.: J. Bacteriol. **59**:427, 1950.
5. Middlebrook, G., and Dubos, R. J.: J. Exp. Med. **88**:521, 1948.
6. Currie, J. A., Marshall, J. D., and Crozier, D.: J. Infect. Dis. **116**:117, 1966.
7. Chorpenning, F. W., and Stamper, H. B.: Immunochemistry **10**:15, 1973.

8. Sulzer, C. R., and Jones, W. L.: Appl. Microbiol. **26**:655, 1973.
9. Neter, E., Westphal, O., Lüderitz, O., et al.: Ann. N.Y. Acad. Sci. **66**:141, 1956.
10. Young, V. M., Gillem, H. C., Massey, E. D., et al.: Am. J. Public Health **50**:1866, 1960.
11. Douglas, R., Miller, T., and Scott, L.: J. Infect. Dis. **130**:651, 1974.
12. Haltalin, K. C., Matteck, B. M., and Nelson, J. D.: J. Immunol. **97**:517, 1966.
13. Kunin, C. M., and Beard, M. V.: J. Bacteriol. **85**-541, 1963.
14. Sever, J. L.: J. Immunol. **88**:320, 1962.
15. Rauss, K., and Ketyi, I.: Schweiz. Z. Allg. Pathol. Bakteriol. **22**:20, 1959.
16. Lee, M. R., Ikari, N. S., Branche, W. C., and Young, V. M.: J. Bacteriol. **91**:463, 1966.
17. Bellanti, J. A., Buescher, E. L., Brandt, W. E., et al.: J. Immunol. **98**:171, 1967.
18. Maeland, J. A.: Acta Pathol. Microbiol. Scand. **67**:102, 1966.
19. Neter, E., Drislane, A. M., Harris, A. H., et al.: Am. J. Public Health **49**:1050, 1959.
20. Neter, E.: Proc. Soc. Exp. Biol. Med. **96**:488, 1957.
21. Middlebrook, G.: J. Clin. Invest. **29**:1480, 1950.
22. Neter, E., Drislane, A. M., Harris, A. H., et al.: N. Engl. J. Med. **261**:1162, 1959.
23. Gaines, S., and Landy, M.: J. Bacteriol. **69**:628, 1955.
24. Havlik, J., Kott, B., and Potuznik, V.: J. Clin. Pathol. **12**:440, 1959.
25. Saslaw, S., and Carlisle, H. N.: Am. J. Med. Sci. **242**:166, 1961.
26. Sieburth, J. McN.: J. Immunol. **78**:380, 1957.
27. Torlone, V.: Sperimentale **108**:315, 1958.
28. Wentworth, F. H., Brock, D. W., Stulberg, C. S., et al.: Proc. Soc. Exp. Biol. Med. **91**:586, 1956.
29. Yamada, C.: Jpn. J. Med. Sci. Biol. **13**:77, 1960.
30. Belikova-Aldakova, V. D., Blumel, N. F., Zherikova, A. D., et al.: J. Hyg. Epidemiol. Microbiol. Immunol. **16**:404, 1972.
31. Schipper, I. A., Kelling, C., Ebeltoft, H., et al.: Appl. Microbiol. **25**:458, 1973.
32. Caceres, A., and Mata, L. J.: J. Infect. Dis. **129**:439, 1974.
33. Surgalla, M. J., Neter, E., and Fitzpatrick, J. E.: J. Clin. Microbiol. **1**:298-301, 1975.
34. Neter, E., Harris, A. H., and Drislane, A. M.: Am. J. Public Health **55**:1164, 1965.
35. Neter, E., Oberkircher, O. R., Rubin, M. I., et al.: Pediatr. Res. **4**:500, 1970.
36. Neter, E.: Yale J. Biol. Med. **44**:241, 1971.
37. Neter, E.: In Prier, J. E., and Friedman, H., editors: Opportunistic pathogens, Baltimore, 1974, University Park Press.
38. Neter, E.:, Anzai, H., and Gorzynski, E. A.: Proc. Soc. Exp. Biol. Med. **105**:131, 1960.
39. Boyden, S. V.: J. Exp. Med. **93**:107, 1951.
40. Chen, T. H., and Meyer, K. F.: Bull. W.H.O. **34**:911, 1966.
41. Sanborn, W. R., and Vedros, N. A.: Health Lab. Sci. **3**:111, 1966.
42. Belden, E. L., and McKercher, D. G.: Infect. Immun. **7**:141, 1973.
43. Johnson, H. M., Brenner, K., Angelotti, R., et al.: J. Bacteriol. **91**:967, 1966.
44. Lam. G. T., and Morton, H. E.: Appl. Microbiol. **27**:356, 1974.
45. Brock, J. H., and Reiter, B.: Immunochemistry **8**:933, 1971.
46. Langman, R. E.: J. Immunol. Methods **2**:59, 1972.
47. Eriksen, J.: Acta Pathol Microbiol. Scand. **81**:309, 1973.
48. Baker, P. J., Stadhak, P. W., and Prescott, B.: Appl. Microbiol. **17**:422, 1969.
49. Poole, G. M., Counter, F. T., and Baker, R. S.: Appl. Microbiol. **25**:159, 1973.
50. Stavitsky, A. B., and Arquilla, E. R.: Int. Arch. Allergy Appl. Immunol. **13**:1, 1958.
51. Witebsky, E., Rose, N. R., Terplan, K., et al.: J.A.M.A. **164**:1439, 1957.
52. Fulthorpe, A. J.: J. Hyg. **55**:382, 1957.
53. LeClair, R. A.: J. Infect. Dis. **123**:668, 1971.
54. Blum, G., Ellner, P. D., McCarthy, L. R., et al.: J. Infect. Dis. **127**:321, 1973.
55. Cox, P. M., Logan, L. C., and Stout, G. W.: Public Health Lab. **29**:43, 1971.
56. Coffey, E. M., Bradford, L. L., Naritomi, L. S., et al.: Appl. Microbiol. **24**:26, 1972.
57. Farshy, D. C., and Kagan, I. G.: Am. J. Trop. Med. Hyg. **21**:868, 1972.
58. Winblad, S., and Ericson, C.: Acta Pathol. Microbiol. Scand. **81**:150, 1973.
59. Christensen, P., and Kronvall, G.: Acta Pathol. Microbiol. Scand. **82**:19, 1974.

INDEX

Page numbers in *italics* indicate illustrations.

Page numbers followed by *n* indicate footnotes.

Page numbers followed by *t* indicate tables.

1